诊断免疫组织化学
Diagnostic Immunohistochemistry

注 意

由于医药科学的持续进步，新的科研成果和临床经验不断加深着我们对疾病的认识，因此有必要及时地对治疗方案和临床用药加以改进。除了要遵循常规的用药安全注意事项外，建议读者要查对药品制造商所提供的每种药物的最新说明，核实所使用药物的剂量、方法、疗程及用药禁忌。医务工作者的责任是依据对患者病情的了解和治疗经验来决定每一位患者的用药剂量和最佳治疗方案。本书出版者及作者对患者由于阅读本书后可能产生的人身伤害和造成的经济损失概不负责。

诊断免疫组织化学
Diagnostic Immunohistochemistry

第二版

主　编　David J. Dabbs

主　译　周庚寅

　　　　翟启辉

　　　　张庆慧

北京大学医学出版社

图书在版编目（CIP）数据

诊断免疫组织化学：第2版/（美）戴博斯（Dabbs, D. J.）主编；
周庚寅，翟启辉，张庆慧主译.—北京：北京大学医学出版社，2008.7
书名原文：Diagnostic Immunohistochemistry
ISBN 978-7-81071-750-2
Ⅰ.诊… Ⅱ.①戴…②周…③翟…④张… Ⅲ.免疫学－组织化学－免疫诊断
Ⅳ. R446.8 R392.11
中国版本图书馆 CIP 数据核字（2008）第 065681 号

北京市版权局著作权合同登记号：图字：01-2006-5593

Diagnostic Immunohistochemistry, 2nd edition
David J.Dabbs
ISBN-13: 978-0-443-06652-8
ISBN-10: 0-443-06652-3
Copyright © 2006 by Elsevier Limited. All rights reserved.

Authorized Simplified Chinese translation from English language edition published by the Proprietor.
978-981-259-745-8
981-259-745- X

Elsevier (Singapore) Pte Ltd.
3 Killiney Road, #08-01 Winsland House I, Singapore 239519
Tel: (65) 6349-0200, Fax: (65) 6733-1817
First Published 2008
2008 年初版

Simplified Chinese translation Copyright © 2008 by Elsevier (Singapore) Pte Ltd. and Peking University Medical Press. All rights reserved.

Published in China by Peking University Medical Press under special agreement with Elsevier (Singapore) Pte Ltd. This edition is authorized for sale in China only, excluding Hong Kong SAR and Taiwan. Unauthorized export of this edition is a violation of the Copyright Act. Violation of this Law is subject to Civil and Criminal Penalties.

本书简体中文版由北京大学医学出版社与 Elsevier (Singapore) Pte Ltd.在中国境内（不包括香港特别行政区及台湾）协议出版。本版仅限在中国境内(不包括香港特别行政区及台湾)出版及标价销售。未经许可之出口，是为违反著作权法，将受法律之制裁。

诊断免疫组织化学

主　　译：	周庚寅　翟启辉　张庆慧
出版发行：	北京大学医学出版社（电话：010-82802230）
地　　址：	(100191) 北京市海淀区学院路 38 号　北京大学医学部院内
网　　址：	http://www.pumpress.com.cn
E-mail：	booksale@bjmu.edu.cn
印　　刷：	北京圣彩虹制版印刷技术有限公司
经　　销：	新华书店
责任编辑：	药　蓉　　责任校对：金彤文　　责任印制：张京生
开　　本：	889 mm × 1194 mm　1/16　印张：54.5　字数：1699 千字
版　　次：	2008 年 9 月第 1 版　2008 年 9 月第 1 次印刷
书　　号：	ISBN 978-7-81071-750-2
定　　价：	580.00 元

版权所有，违者必究

（凡属质量问题请与本社发行部联系退换）

译者名单（以姓氏笔画为序）

刘志艳	孙妍琳	牟　坤	吴晓娟	吴澄宇	张　询	张庆慧
张廷国	张建平	张翠娟	李　丽	李劲松	杨　斌	杨熙明
连瑞虹	陈方杰	周庚寅	孟　斌	郝春燕	夏成青	郭成浩
高　鹏	黄教悌	甄军晖	翟启辉			

编写秘书： 吴晓娟　　张翠娟

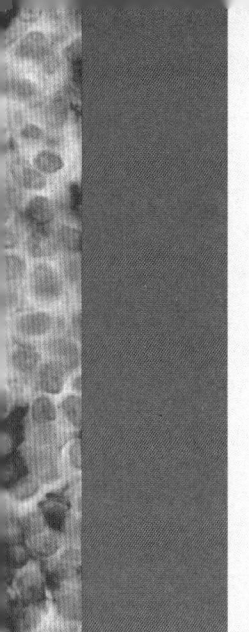

原著者名单

Leon Barnes MD
Professor of Pathology and Otolaryngology
University of Pittsburgh School of Medicine
Professor and Chairman
Department of Medicine and Pathology
University of Pittsburgh School of Dental Medicine
Chief, Division of Head and Neck Pathology
University of Pittsburgh Medical Center
Pittsburgh, PA, USA

Nancy J Barr MD
Assistant Professor of Clinical Pathology
Department of Pathology
Keck School of Medicine
University of Southern California Medical Center
Los Angeles, CA, USA

Deborah Belchis MD
Pathologist
Pathology Department
Northwest Hospital Center
Randallstown, MD, USA

Parul Bhargava MD
Instructor in Pathology
Harvard Medical School
Beth Israel Deaconess Medical Center
Boston, MA, USA

David S Bosler MD
Pathologist
Department of Anatomic Pathology
William Beaumont Hospital
Royal Oak, MI, USA

David G Bostwick MD MBA
Medical Director
Bostwick Laboratories
Richmond, VA, USA

Lisa A Cerilli MD
Pathologist
Health Partners Regional Laboratory
Richmond, VA, USA

Cheryl Coffin MD
Professor of Pathology and Division Head of Pediatrics
Pathology Department
Primary Children's Medical Center
Salt Lake City, UT, USA

David J Dabbs MD
Professor and Chief of Pathology
Department of Pathology
Magee-Women's Hospital
Pittsburgh, PA, USA

Ronald A DeLellis MD
Professor of Pathology and Laboratory Medicine
Pathologist in Chief
Department of Pathology
Rhode Island Hospital
Providence, RI, USA

Eduardo J Eyzaguirre MD
Assistant Professor
Department of Pathology
University of Texas Medical Branch
Galveston, TX, USA

Christopher Gocke MD
Associate Professor
Department of Pathology
Johns Hopkins Medical Institutes
Baltimore, MD, USA

Neal S Goldstein MD
Staff Anatomic Pathologist
Department of Anatomic Pathology
William Beaumont Hospital
Royal Oak, MI, USA

vii

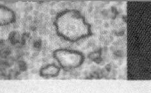

原著者名单

Samuel P Hammar MD
Pathologist and Director
Diagnostic Specialties Laboratory
Bremerton, WA, USA

Jennifer L Hunt MD
Assistant Professor of Pathology and Otolaryngology
Department of Pathology
UPMC Presbyterian Hospital
Pittsburgh, PA, USA

Christina Isacson MD
Pathologist, Virginia Mason Medical Center
Department of Pathology
Seattle, WA, USA

Deborah Josefson MD
Associate Medical Director
Bostwick Laboratories
Glen Allen, VA, USA

Marshall E Kadin MD
Associate Professor of Pathology
Harvard Medical School
Boston, MA, USA

Lina Liu MD
Staff Pathologist
Bostwick Laboratories
Glen Allen, VA, USA

Jun Ma MD
Staff Pathologist
Bostwick Laboratories
Glen Allen, VA, USA

Paul E McKeever MD
Professor of Pathology
Chief Section of Neuropathology
Department of Pathology
University of Michigan Medical Center
Ann Arbor, MI, USA

James W Patterson MD
Professor and Director of Dermatopathology
University of Virginia Medical Center
Charlottesville, VA, USA

Junqi Qian MD
Director of Molecular Diagnostics
Bostwick Laboratories
Glen Allen, VA, USA

Shan-Rong Shi MD
Associate Professor of Clinical Pathology
Department of Pathology
Keck School of Medicine
University of Southern California
Los Angeles, CA, USA

Sandra J Shin MD
Assistant Professor of Pathology and Laboratory Medicine
Department of Pathology and Laboratory Medicine
Weill Medical College of Cornell University
New York, NY, USA

Robert A Soslow MD
Associate Attending Pathologist
Department of Pathology
Memorial Sloane Kettering Cancer Center
New York, NY, USA

Paul E Swanson MD
Professor and Director of Anatomic Pathology
University of Washington Medical Center
Seattle, WA, USA

Clive R Taylor MD PhD
Professor and Chairman of Pathology
Senior Associate Dean for Educational Affairs
Keck School of Medicine
University of Southern California
Los Angeles, CA, USA

David Walker MD
Professor and Chairman
Department of Pathology
University of Texas Medical Branch
Galveston, TX, USA

Mark R Wick MD
Professor & Associate Director of Surgical Pathology
Director of Diagnostic Immunohistochemistry
Division of Surgical Pathology
University of Virginia Medical Center
Charlottesville, VA, USA

Nancy Wu MD
Assistant Professor of Clinical Pathology
Department of Pathology
Kenneth Norris Jr Hospital
Los Angeles, CA, USA

Sherif R Zaki MD
Chief, Infectious Disease Pathology Activity
National Center for Infectious Diseases
Centers for Disease Control and Prevention
Atlanta, GA, USA

Charles F Zaloudek MD
Professor of Pathology
Department of Pathology
University of California, San Francisco
San Francisco, CA, USA

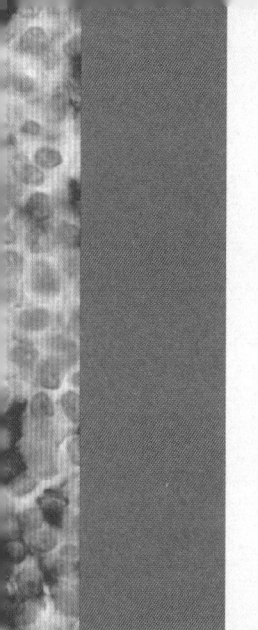

译者序言

20世纪60年代初免疫荧光技术问世，实现了人们用已知抗体检测未知抗原的梦想。由于标记荧光的自然淬灭，染色切片不能长期存留；此外，因无法显示背景组织或细胞，而不能进行精确定位，限制了其广泛应用。相隔十年后，免疫酶标化学出现，由于其不可替代的优越性，很快风靡了全球病理界。随着检测方法的不断改进，其特异性和敏感性不断提高。现今，没有免疫组织化学的辅助，对许多肿瘤几乎不能作出精确的诊断和分类。同时，免疫组化在临床病理诊断中的广泛应用也推动了免疫组化技术自身的快速发展。

随着抗体的商品化，几乎每一天都有新的抗体出现，使病理学家们应接不暇，需要解决的问题接踵而至：用一种抗体不可能作出病理诊断，更没有单一抗体可鉴别肿瘤的良恶性，区分一线和二线抗体、恰当地进行抗体组合已不再是纯技术问题和技巧问题；设立严格的阳性和阴性对照的重要性不言而喻，但并没有在各级医院严格实施；如何识别假阳性和假阴性结果，怎样把握一种标志物跨组织甚至跨胚层的交叉免疫反应，如何对免疫组化的结果进行分析和描述需要进一步提高和规范；抗原修复增加了免疫组化技术的敏感性，但又可使某些抗原出现假阳性结果，CD117就是其中的范例。

《诊断免疫组织化学》一书从临床病理学的角度，对上述问题作出了全面科学的回答。本书介绍了免疫组化技术的进展、原理和误区，分系统介绍了每一抗体的应用范围、抗体组合、每一肿瘤的免疫组化诊断要点。图随文排，清晰地显示免疫组化的细胞定位，便于医生一边诊断一边翻阅，是一部兼具权威性和实用性的免疫组化技术和诊断用书。

本书由我教研室和美国的华裔病理学者合作完成，由于免疫学知识的欠缺，个别段落和词句的译文反复斟酌仍感词不达意，虽经多次审校，力求译意准确，但错误之处在所难免，望广大读者和同道指正。

周庚寅

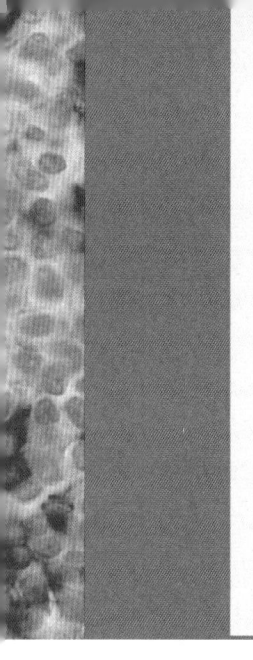

原著序言

在过去很多年里，病理学家们在传统的福尔马林固定、石蜡包埋和HE染色的基础上，应用许多特殊技术，对上述方法得出的结果进行确认、补充和完善。这些技术在兴起时，往往被赋予过高的热情，随之而来的则是失望，最终发展为冷静而客观的评价。许多技术对病理诊断产生了永久的影响，尽管它们并不像当初想象的那样深刻和广泛。这些技术包括特殊染色、组织培养、电镜、免疫组化和分子生物学技术。我们对前三项技术期望很多，对后者更是寄予厚望。公平来讲，迄今为止，没有哪一项特殊技术像免疫组化技术那样对病理诊断产生如此深刻的影响。我想，说它是一种革命，特别是在肿瘤病理学领域的革命，是毫不夸张的。那些亲身经历过免疫组化时代的病理学家们一定会有同样的感受。现在新一代病理学家们能够如此方便地使用HMB-45或CD31染色，以鉴别黑色素细胞和内皮细胞，他们很难体会在此之前病理学家们为了鉴别这两种细胞所需要付出的努力。这项技术有许多明显的优点，对于常规方法处理的人体组织标本来说，是一种接近理想的生物技术。这些优点包括：这项技术可以与标准的固定和包埋相匹配，可以对保存多年的标本进行回顾性研究，由此得来的结果灵敏而特异。实际上，这项技术可以应用于任何免疫原性分子，并且在病理学家们所熟悉的形态学基础上对标记结果进行评价。

与医学上许多其他突破性进展相似，免疫组织化学的兴起也来源于卓越而简单的想法：将抗体与特异性抗原结合，并通过与荧光物结合抗体在镜下显现。之后，对其技术方法不断进行调整，比如非荧光染料的使用、反应的放大和抗原的修复，都仅仅代表技术的改进，尽管每一种改进的意义都是不可忽视的。正是由于这些技术进步，才使得免疫组化这项技术从科研领域推广到了病理临床应用，其应用范围也遍布全球。当然，这项技术也存在着缺陷。曾经认为在某种细胞中特异表达的抗原，后来被发现在其他组织中也有表达；无关的抗原间可能发生交叉反应；抗体出现时非特异性着色亦伴随发生；位于肿瘤组织中的非肿瘤细胞与特异性标记物反应可能会被误认为是肿瘤的一部分。最不可靠的是，抗原可能会超出正常细胞的范围而进入邻近的肿瘤细胞中。以上任何一种错误都可能导致对实验结果的误判，并导致误诊；更糟糕的是，它可能导致在最初苏木精-伊红染色得出正确诊断的基础上最终出现错误诊断。防止出现这些危险的一个好方法是熟悉这些抗体的局限性，并懂得如何避免这些问题的出现。更重要的预防方法是，掌握扎实的基础解剖病理学知识。这将使观察者对任何意外的免疫组化结果的正确性提出质疑，无论其结果为阳性或是阴性。没有任何情况比一个病理学新手只根据免疫组化结果，而忽略病变部位的细胞形态就作出诊断更危险的事情了。同样，任何其他应用于人体组织诊断的特殊技术也存在同样问题，分子生物学技术就是最新和最明显的例证。然而，当审慎选择使用时，免疫组化技术是非常有力的辅助诊断工具，另外还会在经济上获益。事实上，病理学家的工作已经很依赖于免疫组化了，原因之一是如果由于忽略了某个关键性免疫组化染色而造成误诊，可能会成为一种医疗渎职行为。

在列举免疫组化的优点时如果不包括这一方法给人带来的视觉享受，那么将是不全面的。给予这个评论，我是认真的。毫无疑问，组织学技术拥有美学成分，这正如技术大师 Pio del Rio Hortega 和 Pierre

Masson曾经说过的那样。遗憾的是，这些卓越的形态学"艺术家"们没有机会感叹完美的免疫组化技术所带来的美学震撼就先行离去了。作为他们的幸运的后继者，让我们来享受这本由一流的免疫组化专家主编、一批优秀的病理学家参与编写的精彩论著吧。本书以清晰、流畅的思路对这一领域的知识进行了概括性描述，内容涵盖技术介绍和应用两个方面。

本书的第一版出版于2002年，并迅速成为该领域的权威著作之一。第二版以更加标准化的形式，涵盖更多的器官系统和最新标记物的介绍。本书具有大量实用的表格，将各种不同的抗体进行了归纳，并对所有主要疾病的鉴别诊断和诊断要点进行了系统阐述。值得注意的是，本书对前瞻性生物标记物（如Her-2/neu在乳腺癌中的意义以及CD117在胃肠间质肿瘤诊断中的意义）也进行了详细的描述，它们在协助病理医生进行肿瘤诊断与评价中起到越来越重要的作用。总之，作者们成功地编写了一本权威的、全面的和反映最新进展的著作，病理医生们将发现，它不仅在阐述技术理论方面，同时在协助日常诊断工作方面都将是必不可少的。

Juan Rosai

连瑞虹　译
翟启辉，周庚寅　审校

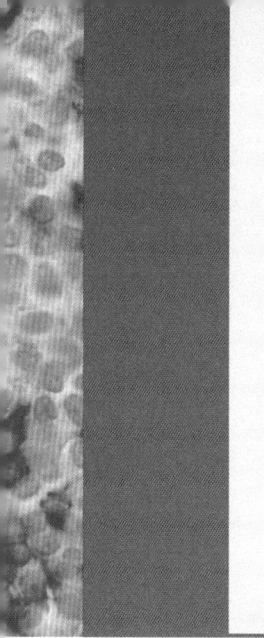

第二版前言

重新编写《诊断免疫组织化学》的挑战性在于继续将大量对诊断病理学家有价值的免疫组化知识编纂于本书中。世界各地的诊断病理学家对本书的编写形式非常认可。病理学家们普遍反映：这本书确实具有实用价值，能够帮助他们解决日常诊断工作中遇到的问题。

实际上，世界各地的病理学家们应该感谢他们自己积累了大量资料，用于本书内容。

与第一版相同，这项工作的挑战在于本书出版后的很长时间里，每一章节中的基本知识都仍然是恰当和富有生命力的。本书的作者都是其各自领域的专家，因为他们的贡献才使这种可能成为现实。本书每章都包含经过时间检验的基本知识和专家们的最新经验总结。

本书的目的仍然是为那些从事外科病理和细胞病理诊断的解剖病理和外科病理医生们提供一本参考书籍。

除了少数例子外，每一章的编纂自成一体。这种结构使得每章的内容具有可重复性并且丰富。这将帮助医生及受训人员不必寻遍全书就可获得想要的信息。每章的内容都从诊断的角度对全面的知识进行理解。本书按照器官系统的结构顺序对肿瘤病理学进行介绍。每章都有章节目录、引言和对该器官系统疾病诊断的系统性阐述。每一专题介绍之后都会插入"诊断要点"进行归纳，这既是对这部分内容的总结，同时也为快速寻找重要的诊断信息提供参考。

我衷心感谢世界各地所有通过电话、写信或以 e-mail 方式对本书提出建议的病理工作者们。

我也衷心感谢那些为本书辛勤工作的编者和著者，他们付出了时间和才智来帮助诊断病理学的同仁们。

David J. Dabbs

陈方杰　　译

翟启辉　　审校

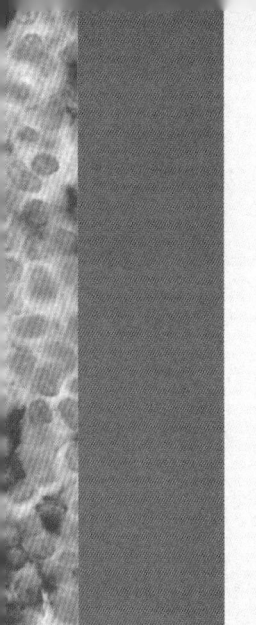

第一版前言

编写《诊断免疫组织化学》这本书的一个挑战是如何将过去十年间所发表的大量免疫组化知识进行系统的、有条理的介绍。由于免疫组化技术对患者诊断和治疗的巨大贡献，使得诊断病理学产生了重大变化。在现实工作中，我们所有的病理工作者都在不断推动着这一知识体系的发展，这也是本书出版的第二个挑战。

我们意识到，《诊断免疫组织化学》一个潜在的危险在于能否确认每一章节中的基本知识在本书出版之后仍有生命力。专家们以其在各自领域的贡献才使这种希望成为现实。本书每章都包含经过时间检验的基本知识和作者的最新经验总结。

本书的目的在于为那些外科病理和细胞病理诊断医生提供一本参考书籍。每章的内容都力争从诊断的角度进行全面阐述；但我们并不试图对免疫组化知识进行百科全书式的笼统介绍，而是按照器官系统的结构顺序对肿瘤病理学进行撰写，每章自成体系，以方便检索，让使用者不必查遍全书便可找到有价值的诊断信息。采用这种体系，使得内容非常丰富，这不仅可以提高使用效率，还能够帮助使用者加深概念，尤其是对于那些初学者。

David J. Dabbs

连瑞虹　译
翟启辉，周庚寅　审校

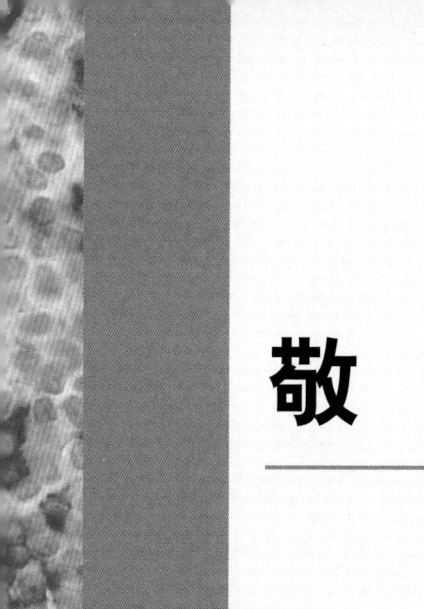

敬 献

题献

谨将此书献给借助于本书而使患者受益的同仁们。

特别献给

Annette 和 Kirstie，本书的合作者们。

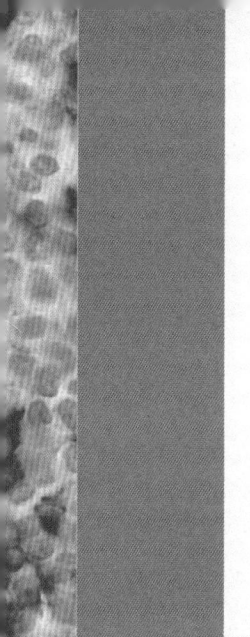

如何使用本书

第一章详细介绍了免疫组织化学技术及其发展历史。第二章概要论述免疫组织化学技术在感染性疾病的解剖病理学研究中的应用。其余的章节按照器官、系统主要介绍与肿瘤病理相关的诊断免疫组织化学。

每章的排列顺序为：章节目录、引言、抗原和抗体生物学以及与其相关的文献回顾。在每一章中，用"免疫组织分析谱"来描述肿瘤的免疫染色类型，并附以大量的表格以便于参考。在相关的部分使用了诊断规则。在许多部分插入了"诊断要点"。诊断易犯错误也在相关部分予以阐述。

为使各章节所使用的名词一致，在文章和表格中使用了下列缩写和符号：

+，结果几乎总是弥漫强阳性；

S，有时为阳性；

R，很少阳性，如果为阳性，少数细胞呈阳性；

N 或（-），阴性。

我衷心希望本书为不断提高外科病理医生的知识和诊断质量提供帮助。

David J.Dabbs

连瑞虹　译

翟启辉，周庚寅　审校

目 录

1 免疫组织化学技术：原理、局限性和标准化 1
2 感染性疾病的免疫组织化学 38
3 软组织和骨肿瘤的免疫组织化学 62
4 霍奇金淋巴瘤的免疫组织化学 119
5 非霍奇金淋巴瘤的免疫组织化学 136
6 黑色素细胞肿瘤的免疫组织化学 164
7 不明来源转移癌的免疫组织化学 183
8 头颈部肿瘤的免疫组织化学 233
9 内分泌肿瘤的免疫组织化学 266
10 纵隔的免疫组织化学 306
11 肺和胸膜肿瘤的免疫组织化学 334
12 皮肤肿瘤的免疫组织化学 406
13 胃肠道、胰腺、胆管、胆囊和肝的免疫组织化学 446
14 前列腺、膀胱、睾丸和肾的免疫组织化学 515
15 小儿肿瘤的免疫组织化学 628
16 女性生殖系统的免疫组织化学 655
17 乳腺组织的免疫组织化学 716
18 神经系统的免疫组织化学 767

索 引 837

1 免疫组织化学技术：原理、局限性和标准化

原作者：Clive R. Taylor, Shan-Rong Shi, Nancy J. Barr and Nancy Wu

译　者：吴澄宇，黄教悌，夏成青

审校者：张建平，孙妍琳

目　录

引言	1
免疫组织化学的基本原理	2
抗体——特异性染色试剂	2
封闭非特异性背景染色	3
检测系统	5
质量控制	13
组织固定、处理程序和抗原修复	15
免疫组织化学染色的技术	17
结语	30
附录A：简化程序	31
附录B：双重染色	31

引　言

免疫组织化学（IHC）或免疫细胞化学是基于抗原-抗体相互识别，在光学显微镜的水平上利用抗体特异性结合，对组织或细胞内的特异性抗原进行定位的一种方法。免疫组织化学应用的历史悠久，自1940年Coons建立免疫荧光技术检测冰冻切片的相应抗原，至今已有半个多世纪的历史[1]。然而，直到20世纪90年代初，该方法才广泛应用于病理诊断[2-4]。同时免疫组织化学的一系列技术进步为病理诊断提供了敏感的检测系统。如Avrameas等[5,6]建立的酶标技术（辣根过氧化物酶标记），是在适当的发光底物存在的情况下，使得标记的抗体能在传统光学显微镜下观察。这一系列发展的新方法都具有较高的敏感性，从最简单的直接连接的一步法到多步检测方法，如过氧化物酶-抗过氧化物酶（PAP）法、抗生物素蛋白-生物素连接（ABC）法和生物素-链卵白素（B-SA）法，以及信号放大方法（如酪胺）和高敏感的"基于聚合体"的标记系统等[4,7-19]。

杂交瘤技术[20]的出现为免疫组织化学技术的发展及高特异性单克隆抗体的大量生产提供了可能。特异性抗体最初应用于组织染色，开始在冰冻切片应用的抗体最终均扩展应用到常规石蜡、火棉胶或其他材料包埋的组织切片。当免疫组织化学技术应用于常规福尔马林固定、石蜡包埋组织切片的诊断时，引发了一场"棕色技术革新"[21]。1974年Taylor等[22]发现有些抗原可通过免疫组织化学染色在常规处理的组织中被检测到，并阐述了免疫组织化学染色应用于常规石蜡切片的重要意义。世界各地的病理学家基于这些研究，对在福尔马林固定、石蜡包埋组织切片上进行免疫组织化学染色方法进行了广泛而深入的研究[22-27]。其中很重要的研究是寻找能较好保持抗原性而不使组织形态学受到影响的固定剂代替福尔马林，但到目前为止仍没有发现理想的固定剂。关于这一点，Larsson指出"适合于所有抗原的免疫细胞化学固定剂可能永远都找不到"[28]。主要是由于新的固定剂在形态学的保存方面不能和福尔马林相媲美。

Huang及他的同事[29]引进了酶消化法作为免疫组织化学染色的预处理，以暴露某些因福尔马林固定而隐蔽的抗原。然而，虽然酶消化法被广泛应用，Leong等[30]发现，该方法并不能改善大部分免疫组织化学染色的效果，而且单个的组织切片当染色不同抗原时酶消化的最佳条件难以控制。因此需要建立一种新的、比酶消化效率更高、适用范围更广泛、使用更方便的并能将其标准化的技术。另外，新的方法还要能使常

规福尔马林固定、石蜡包埋组织切片的免疫组织化学染色具有可重复性和稳定性，以改进抗原隐蔽现象。

Shi和他的合作者于1991年[34]在Fraenkel-Conrat等[31-33]生物化学研究的基础之上创建了抗原修复（AR）技术。与酶消化法不同，抗原修复是一种在免疫组织化学染色前常规处理的石蜡切片进行高温加热的方法（如微波炉加热），而火棉胶包埋的组织不用加热的方法进行抗原修复[35-37]。已有一百多篇报道认为，抗原修复使得免疫组织化学染色信号明显增强[38-42]。抗原修复有很多的改良方法，但大部分方法都是用不同的缓冲液作为抗原修复液以代替具有某些毒性的金属盐溶液[38, 39, 42-53]。AR-IHC在世界范围的应用证实了AR-IHC的可能性，并使其在分子形态学方面应用更广泛，但同时有些基本问题和操作方法需要得到进一步解决[2, 3, 38, 39, 54-60]。

本章将重点介绍免疫组织化学染色在福尔马林固定、石蜡包埋组织切片病理诊断中的应用。同时也对免疫组织化学染色的原理和实际应用技术、应用的局限性及缺点进行讨论，以便为免疫组织化学的进一步发展，特别是标准化及定量免疫组织化学的发展提供借鉴。

免疫组织化学的基本原理

病理学家们早已意识到目前传统病理诊断技术的局限性[2, 3, 24, 25]，因此一直在寻找更好的形态学诊断方法。大量"特殊染色"的发明为细胞的正确识别及诊断提供必要的方法。早期染色方法，大多是建立在冰冻切片的细胞和组织中的成分发生化学反应的基础上（组织化学）。这些组织化学染色对特定细胞的识别具有重要价值；大多数情况下组织化学染色是被用来显示细胞或组织的结构以支持特定的诊断而不是用来识别真正的细胞组织的成分。随着免疫组织化学染色新领域的出现，将会越来越广泛地应用多种特异性的特殊染色，对细胞组织的特异性成分进行识别。

免疫组织化学染色是建立在组织化学染色基础上的，作为组织化学染色的重要补充方法，其大大增加了检测细胞组织切片中特异性成分的种类。正如在功能形态学领域中的先驱者们强调的那样，"所有染色的目的都是在微量化学水平上辨认那些在常量化学水平已知的物质的存在和分布"[61]。和其他特殊染色方法一样，免疫组织化学染色的最重要的原则是在满意的信-噪比基础上，在细胞和组织中清楚地定位靶成分。放大信号的同时消减非特异性染色背景（噪）是获得满意的和实际有用的结果的主要策略。经过二十多年的发展，免疫组织化学染色技术已成为病理实验室的"常规"染色技术（见附录A）。

抗体 —— 特异性染色试剂

抗体是一个分子，具有和抗原分子特异性结合的性质，并且动物抗体的产生是由外在抗原的刺激而引起的，这是免疫反应的基础。抗原-抗体的识别是建立在蛋白质（抗原）的三维结构上，这对理解免疫组织化学染色的有效性（特别是福尔马林引起的蛋白质构象的改变，即"遮蔽"）和抗原修复的原理非常重要。

抗体是一种免疫球蛋白分子，由两部分组成：一对轻链（κ或λ）和一对重链（γ、α、μ、δ和ε）。抗原也是一种具有复杂结构的分子，能保持其相对的三维刚性结构，对宿主而言是外源异物。结构复杂并具有特定三维结构的蛋白质和碳水化合物具有较好的抗原性，可拥有一个以上能诱导抗体形成的独特的三维结构（图1.1）。抗原分子中这些特定的部位称作抗原决定簇（或表位），具有不同的氨基酸残基[61]，是与抗体相应对位结合的精确部位[62]。一个表位是一个功能单位，并非蛋白质的一个固定的结构，并且不能单独与其对应的抗体识别[62]。抗原决定簇（或表位）可以分为连续性和间断性两种。前者由多肽链上连续的氨基酸残基组成，而后者由多肽链中不同部位的氨基酸残基通过蛋白质构象折叠结合到一起构成[63]。这可能反映在福尔马林固定对不同蛋白质的抗原性产生不同的影响上。

抗体分子的任何刚性结构均可作为抗原决定簇诱导抗体的产生。免疫球蛋白分子既可以作为抗体，与组织抗原特异性结合，同时也可作为抗原，提供抗原决定簇，与新的抗体结合。免疫组织化学染色正是利用免疫球蛋白的这一特性来进行的（图1.2）。

抗体能否应用于免疫组织化学染色基于免疫组织化学染色时抗原-抗体反应的敏感性及特异性。杂交瘤技术的发展和应用[20]提供了大量生产高特异性抗体的可能。尽管不同的抗原具有相似或交叉反应的表位，单克隆抗体也不能保证对相应抗原反应的特异性，但大多数单克隆抗体对免疫组织化学染色反应的特异性均较好。"多克隆抗体"实际上是一种抗血清，包括不同亲和力的或针对免疫动物的不同抗原决定簇

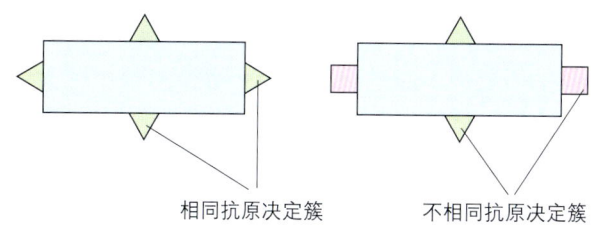

图1.1 抗原和抗原决定簇。1个抗原分子由1个免疫"惰性"载体和1个或多个相同的(左)或不同的(右)抗原决定簇组成(引自Taylor CR, Cote RJ. Immunomicroscopy: A Diagnostic Tool for the Surgical Pathologist, 3rd ed. Philadelphia: WB Saunders, 2005:6)

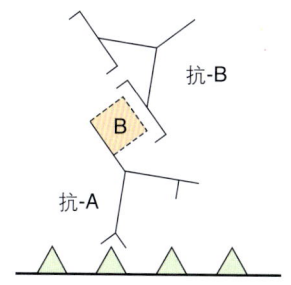

图1.2 作为抗原的抗体。抗-A抗体和组织切片中的A抗原特异性结合。抗原B(B)是抗-A分子中的第二个抗原决定簇,是抗-A分子的一部分;第二种动物产生的抗-B抗体将与之结合。因此抗-B(所谓的第二抗体,二抗)可用于定位组织切片中抗-A(第一抗体,一抗)结合的位点(引自Taylor CR, Cote RJ. Immunomicroscopy: A Diagnostic Tool for the Surgical Pathologist, 3rd ed. Philadelphia: WB Saunders, 2005:9)

的不同特异性的多种分子类型的抗体,也可能包含数量不等的针对所有抗原的抗体。因此,多克隆抗体非特异性染色背景比单克隆抗体的染色更深。同理,在固定组织中某些"难以标记"的抗原如果用单克隆抗体经抗原修复以后仍不能获得满意结果时,用多种抗体混合的多克隆抗体有时比单克隆抗体效果要好。因此,用高度纯化的抗原生产高亲和性的传统的多克隆抗体(抗血清)然后通过多步骤回收,以获得尽可能高特异性的抗体,有时非常有用。对这种抗血清的评估,用免疫扩散法检测其特异性可能难以检测到微量抗体的特异性,只有当抗血清应用于含多种不同抗原的组织时其特异性才能显现出来。可用冰冻切片和石蜡切片作免疫组织化学染色,或Western blotting技术来评估这类抗体的敏感性及特异性。

比较而言,多克隆抗体比单克隆抗体具有更高的敏感性,但特异性较低。原因是多克隆抗体(实际上是由多种抗体组成的)能识别单一蛋白质(抗原)上的数个不同的结合位点(表位),而单克隆抗体只能识别一种表位。信号放大技术及抗原修复技术的应用将会大大提高单克隆抗体检测的敏感性。

尽管单克隆抗体可能和非靶分子发生交叉反应[63],但绝大多数商业化用于免疫组织化学染色的抗体还是非常可靠的。可设立严格的对照来观察切片的染色是否为预期的结果,从而检测单克隆抗体的特异性。Johnson[64]推荐了一种简单的检测抗体特异性的方法,就是将染色结果与已报道的抗原的分布进行比较,并与已知的和同一抗原不同表位结合的第二种抗体的染色进行比较。

封闭非特异性背景染色

封闭组织背景染色有两个目的:减少非特异性抗体结合和内源性酶的影响。由于有多种不需要的抗体可能存在于抗血清中,非特异性抗体结合对多克隆性抗体来说更常见。抗体的稀释度增高,背景则相应减弱。如有必要,可在和第一抗体孵育之前先将组织切片用同种动物的正常血清孵育,这样可封闭"不需要的"结合位点。另一种非特异性结合的形式是,由于抗体为带电荷的分子,与组织中带异种电荷的成分(如胶原)非特异性结合,这种非特异性结合可导致一抗或标记部分(连接物、PAP,以及其他方法)与胶原等成分结合,引起胶原和其他组织成分产生假阳性染色,从而掩盖了特异性染色(图1.3A)。预先用动物正常血清孵育也可减弱这种非特异性结合。理论上,正常血清中的蛋白覆盖了组织切片中的带电位点,去除(至少是减弱)一抗和相继加入的抗体的非特异性黏附。工作中常用同种动物的正常血清作为桥接抗体(PAP法)或第二抗体(共轭和ABC法)是因为这种血清既不干扰也不参与免疫组织化学染色过程中的免疫反应。

内源性酶的存在对非特异性背景的产生也有重要影响。酶在固定过程中变性和失活的程度不同,如过氧化物酶,在冰冻切片和石蜡切片中均能保存活性;而碱性磷酸酶通过常规固定和石蜡包埋时则完全失活。当用同种或相似的酶作标记时,为了消除假阳性反应,免疫组织化学染色时要先将这些内源性酶的残留活性消除。过氧化物酶活性存在于很多正常细胞和肿瘤细胞中,包括红细胞、中性粒细胞、嗜酸性粒细胞和肝细胞。当对富含红细胞的组织(如骨髓)进行免疫组织化学染色时,应将过氧化物酶封闭与空白对照(仅用过氧化氢和显色剂的混合物处理切片以显示内源性过氧化物酶的活性）同时应用。或者用其他方法，如免疫金或葡萄糖氧化酶法，以与内源性酶活性产生的背景相区别。

在加入酶标记的抗体或 PAP 复合物以前封闭内源性酶的活性很重要，否则封闭时会将标记酶也灭活，导致假阴性结果。有很多方法可抑制过氧化物酶的活性。Streefkerk[65]建议在染色前用甲醇和过氧化氢的混合物孵育切片；Burns[66]用梯度 H_2O_2（浓度最高到10%）来漂白正铁血红素；Weir 等[67]则在染色前于室温下用乙醇配制的 0.075% 的盐酸孵育切片 15 分钟，这些方法都能有效消除内源性过氧化物酶的活性，并能很好地保存免疫球蛋白的抗原性。

一般常用一定比例的甲醇和 H_2O_2 混合物孵育 15 分钟可获得满意效果。

一些研究者[68-70]认为甲醇-H_2O_2 法太强烈，可能会引起一些抗原变性。Strauss[69, 70]提议用苯肼来代替，可能保存大多数分子的抗原性，但缺点是不能完全抑制嗜酸性粒细胞的内源性过氧化物酶。联合应用苯肼、由葡萄糖氧化酶-葡萄糖混合物产生的新鲜 H_2O_2 和叠氮钠可抑制内源性过氧化物酶活性而对淋巴细胞表面抗原基本无损伤[71]。用 0.1% 叠氮钠配制 H_2O_2（0.3%）也是一种简单、有效的方法[72]。最近的研究表明单氢环丙烷能抑制内源性过氧化物酶，并且对抗原性不产生影响[73]。Robinson 和 Dawson[74]在胃泌素的研究中，通过先用 4-氯-1-萘酚（显示蓝灰色）处理内源性过氧化物酶来避免抗原变性，然后进行免疫组织染色，用双氨对二氨基联苯（产生棕色反应产物）建立过氧化物酶标记。也有人用 α-萘酚派诺宁处理内源性过氧化物酶（粉色），再将双氨对二氨基联苯（棕色）用于辣根过氧化物酶标记[22, 23]，可以显示石蜡切片的 Ig 抗原。

Heyderman 和 Neville[75, 76]介绍了一种方法，首先用蒸馏水配制的 7.5% H_2O_2 孵育切片以抑制酸性正铁血红素，再用蒸馏水配制的 2.28% 高碘酸溶液封闭内源性过氧化物酶。由于在高碘酸处理过程中可形成醛类物质，而导致非特异性染色现象。在加抗体之前用 0.02% 的硼氢化钠[77]溶液孵育切片。这一方法在癌胚抗原（CEA）、上皮细胞膜抗原的染色上取得了良好效果，但可能使碳水化合物的抗原决定簇（如血型抗原）变性。另有研究表明，用低浓度（0.28%）高碘酸短时间（45秒）孵育病人小肠活检标本的冰冻切片能有效抑制内源性过氧化物酶活性，而不会使淋巴细胞表面标志抗原丢失[78]。比较用于冰冻和石蜡切片的多种抑制内源性过氧化物酶活性的方法，Hittmair 和 Schmid[79]报道，甲醛-H_2O_2 对细胞组织中的某些较敏感的抗原如中间丝蛋白抗原有破坏作用。

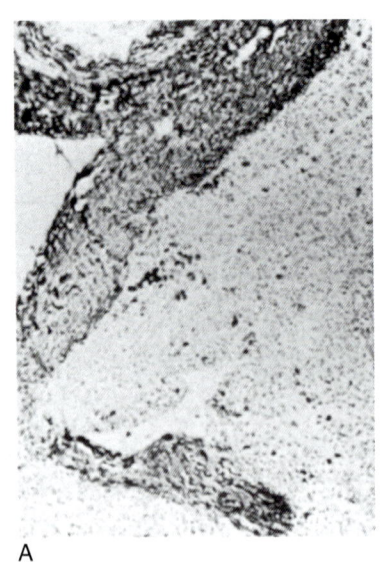 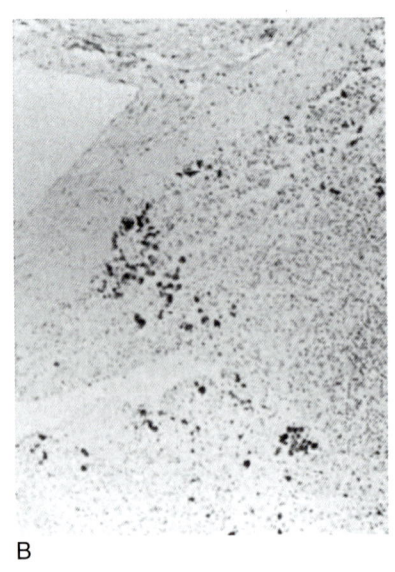

A B

图1.3 封闭第一和第二抗体非特异性结合效果举例。(A) 脾切片 PAP 法染 IgG，可见散在浆细胞阳性（封闭），但胶原束着色深。(B) 相邻的切片除了在加一抗前用同种动物正常血清封闭外其他处理方法相同（本例用正常猪血清与猪抗兔 Ig 连接抗体搭配使用）。这种情况下因为胶原束的非特异性染色明显减弱，使得浆细胞的染色更清楚。石蜡切片，DAB 显色，苏木精复染（×60）（引自 Taylor CR, Cote RJ. Immunomicroscopy: A Diagnostic Tool for the Surgical Pathologist, 2nd ed. Philadelphia: WB Saunders, 1994: 68）

检测系统

抗体分子在没有标记的情况下不能在光学显微镜甚至电镜下观察到。检测系统是对一抗或二抗进行标记，将其靶抗原-抗体结合的位点显示出来。人们已经用过很多标记物，包括与底物反应时能产生有色产物特性的荧光复合物和活性酶标记，然后在显微镜下观察。如果通过适当的处理可产生电子致密物，也可适用于电镜观察；也可采用能直接用于电镜观察的标记物，如金、铁蛋白、病毒颗粒等。

另外，通过信号放大可提高检测系统的敏感性，下面将进一步阐述。

直接连接-标记抗体法

通过化学方法使标记物与抗体结合，然后直接将标记抗体用于检测组织切片的方法（图1.4），已广泛应用于免疫组织学诊断。在准备标记抗体时，目标是使每个抗体分子带上黏附的标记分子数得到最大化。理想的状态是100%的抗体分子都被标记，并且标记过程中不会使任何一个分子失去免疫活性。同时，标记过程中也不能使标记物失去活性（如损坏辣根过氧化物酶的活性位点）。最终的标记产物不应含有游离的标记物，以避免与组织切片发生非特异性结合。同样也不应有没被标记的抗体或标记物失活的抗体分子。

这些要求在常规病理实验室很难做到。然而，自20世纪80年代早期以来，这种连接反应的方法有了很大改进，高质量的连接物，如过氧化物酶、葡萄糖氧化酶、碱性磷酸酶都有商业化产品。

直接连接法（直接法）具有快速和容易操作等优点。对于这种方法，抗体或抗血清（多克隆抗体）的纯度（专一的特异性）非常重要。如前述，抗血清除了需要的特异性抗体外还含有多种具有不同特异性的其他抗体分子。这些抗体在标记过程中都会被标记，并且有可能产生假阳性反应。直接标记更适合于单克隆抗体标记。对于通过腹水（与体外培养相比）制备的单克隆抗体应注意，其中可能含有未知特异性的鼠免疫球蛋白（抗体）。

直接标记抗体在实际应用中的缺点是检测不同抗原时必须分别对一抗进行标记。与间接标记和不标记抗体方法相比，直接标记需要较高浓度的抗体。

间接法或三明治法

间接标记法（间接法）或三明治法（图1.5）是对直接标记法的改良，具有以下优点：

1. 功能增强，因为标记的抗体可和不同的一抗联合使用。
2. 只标记第二抗体。
3. 一抗常常可用稀释度高的工作液（与直接标记相比）。
4. 由同种动物产生的第二抗体对第一抗体具有较高的特异性和亲和性，目前商业化标记的第二抗体种类丰富。
5. 该方法能用自身特异性对照，可省去一抗，或用另一种抗体代替一抗，可为各种染色模式提供有效性评估。

所有间接标记法的原理均非常相似；过氧化物酶和荧光间接标记方法分别如图1.5A和B所示。抗靶抗原的特异性抗体（如兔抗-A）加在切片上，然后洗去多余的抗体。加上标记的第二抗体（如猪抗兔免疫

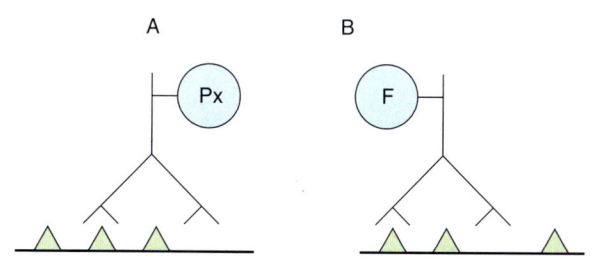

图1.4 (A,B)直接连接法。标记物直接与能特异性结合靶抗原的抗体连接。Px，过氧化物酶；F，荧光素（引自Taylor CR, Cote RJ. Immunomicroscopy: A Diagnostic Tool for the Surgical Pathologist, 3rd ed. Philadelphia: WB Saunders, 2005: 19）

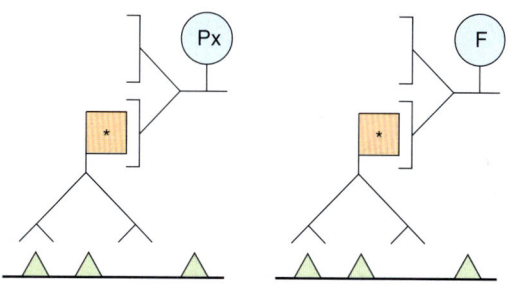

图1.5 (A,B)间接（三明治）法。一抗不标记，该方法用标记的第二抗体，第二抗体特异性抗第一抗体。方框内为一抗的抗原决定簇。Px，过氧化物酶标记；F，荧光标记（引自Taylor CR, Cote RJ. Immunomicroscopy: A Diagnostic Tool for the Surgical Pathologist, 3rd ed. Philadelphia: WB Saunders, 2005: 20）

球蛋白），其能特异性结合兔抗体的抗原决定簇，标记的二抗与一抗特异结合，而一抗则和抗原结合。

不标记抗体法

酶桥接技术

化学结合的缺点可通过将标记的部分只与抗原通过免疫结合而连接的方法予以避免。为达到这一目的，Mason和他的同事们[80]建立了称作酶桥接法的技术。但这一方法目前已很少应用（原理见图1.6）。

过氧化物酶 - 抗过氧化物酶法

PAP法（图1.7）是第二种不标记抗体的方法，也可避免化学连接的内在问题。PAP系统首先由Sternberger及其同事用来检测抗螺旋体抗体[81]，据报道该方法比相应的连接法的敏感性高100～1000倍。其原理与酶桥接法相似（图1.6）。PAP是过氧化物酶-抗过氧化物酶（peroxidase antiperoxidase）的缩写，代表这一染色方法的第三步。

PAP试剂包括以稳定的小的免疫复合物形式存在的抗辣根过氧化物酶抗体和辣根过氧化物酶抗原。典型的复合物结构包含2个抗体分子和3个辣根过氧化物酶分子，如图1.7所示。PAP和一抗必须来自同一种动物（或者具有共同抗原决定簇的密切相关的动物物种），而桥接抗体（桥抗）来自第二种动物，并特异性抗第一抗体（如兔抗体），同时免疫球蛋白整合到PAP复合物中（如兔抗过氧化物酶）。如图1.7A：第一抗体由兔产生，桥接抗体由猪产生（即猪抗兔IgG抗体），而PAP系统为兔抗辣根过氧化物酶（兔抗过氧化物酶）和辣根过氧化物酶抗原的复合物。桥接抗体扮演"特种胶"的角色，将PAP的标记部分与第一抗体连接，而第一抗体则和靶抗原连接。这种方法具有较高敏感性和特异性，也有较好的稳定性，目前已广泛应用于常规石蜡切片。

PAP法的缺点之一是结合到PAP的抗体和第一抗体必须来自同种动物。在使用不同的试剂来源时会造成不必要的浪费，如一个试剂盒里的兔PAP不能连接另外一个试剂盒里的山羊一抗，即使使用所谓的广谱桥接抗体（2种或2种以上桥接抗体的混合物液）也一样。为了能将鼠或山羊抗体和兔PAP一起使用，必须采用四步法（图1.7B），如鼠一抗与兔抗鼠免疫球蛋白连接，接着是桥接抗体，然后是兔PAP。

用山羊、小鼠、大鼠、黑猩猩（与人免疫球蛋

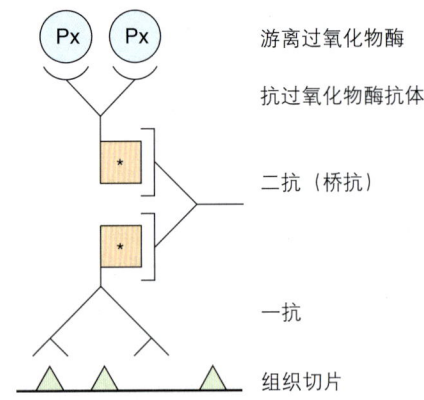

图1.6 酶桥接法。二抗用于连接一抗和抗过氧化物酶抗体，后者和游离的过氧化物酶结合。方框内的 * 代表一抗和二抗的抗原决定簇。Px，过氧化物酶标记（引自 Taylor CR, Cote RJ. Immunomicroscopy: A Diagnostic Tool for the Surgical Pathologist, 2nd ed. Philadelphia: WB Saunders, 1994:12）

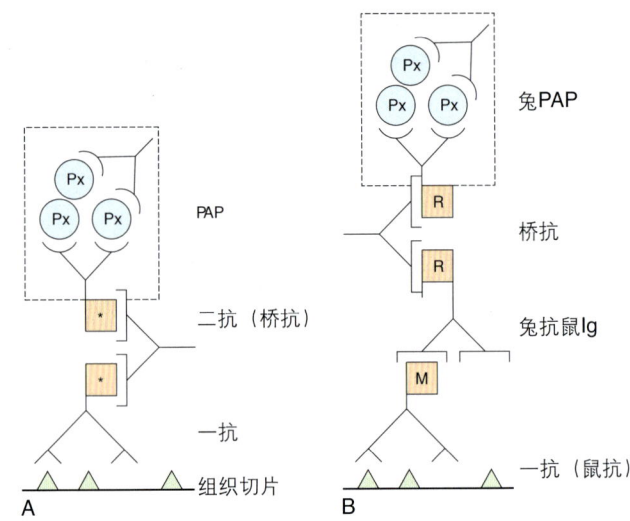

图1.7 （A）过氧化物酶-抗过氧化物酶（PAP）法（三步）。PAP试剂（虚线）是1个稳定的免疫复合物；它通过桥抗与一抗连接。（B）PAP法（四步）。PAP试剂（虚线）是1个稳定的免疫复合物。本例一抗来源于鼠（鼠Ig为单克隆抗体[M]）；该抗体后接兔抗鼠Ig（R），1个桥抗（如猪抗兔Ig）和兔PAP。Px，过氧化物酶标记（引自 Taylor CR, Cote RJ. Immunomicroscopy: A Diagnostic Tool for the Surgical Pathologist, 2nd ed. Philadelphia: WB Saunders, 1994:12）

有交叉反应）生产的PAP目前都可分别用于山羊、小鼠、大鼠、人的第一抗体。

生物素 - 抗生物素蛋白法

生物素-抗生物素蛋白法（图1.8）利用了生物素与抗生物素蛋白之间的高亲和性。生物素可通过化学方法连接到一抗上（图1.8A），产生生物素化复合物，

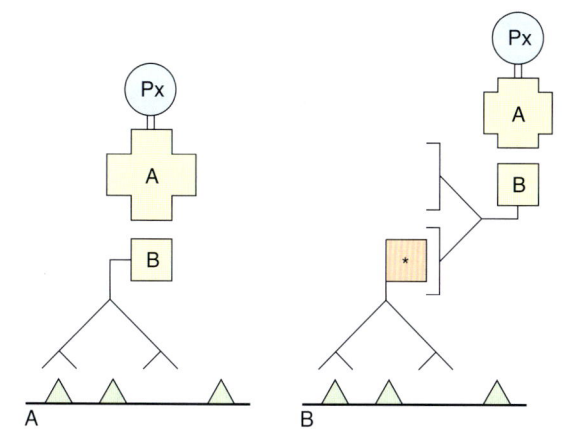

图1.8 （A）直接生物素-抗生物素蛋白法。一抗和生物素连接（B），然后加上抗生物素-过氧化物酶复合物（A-Px）。（B）间接生物素-抗生物素蛋白法。用于单克隆抗体的一抗不标记，用生物素标记的二抗来定位。方框内 * 表示一抗的抗原决定簇。Px，过氧化物酶标记；A，抗生物素蛋白；B，生物素（引自 Taylor CR, Cote RJ. Immunomicroscopy: A Diagnostic Tool for the Surgical Pathologist, 3rd ed. Philadelphia: WB Saunders, 2005:21）

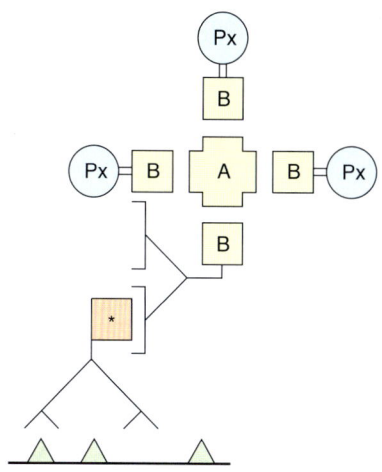

图1.9 抗生物素蛋白-生物素连接（ABC）法。生物素标记二抗将一抗连接到一个大的抗生物素蛋白-生物素-过氧化物酶复合物上。方框内 * 表示一抗的抗原决定簇。A，抗生物素蛋白；B，生物素；Px，过氧化物酶标记（引自Taylor CR, Cote RJ. Immunomicroscopy: A Diagnostic Tool for the Surgical Pathologist, 3rd ed. Philadelphia: WB Saunders, 2005:22）

当加到组织切片上时，可定位组织切片内的抗原位点。接着加上与辣根过氧化物酶标记的抗生物素蛋白；抗生物素蛋白与生物素化的抗体紧密结合，可显示组织切片上与抗原结合的过氧化物酶。这一方法快捷，特别适用于间接标记法（图1.8B）。

该方法存在两个缺点：第一，不同批次的生物素和不同批次的抗生物素蛋白间的亲和性不同，造成不同实验室间该方法的敏感性和稳定性差异很大；第二，有些组织含有较多的内源性生物素，将直接和抗生物素蛋白-过氧化物酶结合，产生非特异性染色（假阳性）。为避免这两个缺点，可通过封闭技术来解决。

抗生物素蛋白-生物素连接（ABC）法

Hsu 和同事[13, 14]改良了生物素-抗生物素蛋白系统，大大提高了敏感性。该方法既可用于直接标记法，也可用于间接标记法。在间接标记法中（图1.9），先加入第一抗体，再加入生物素标记的第二抗体，接着加入预先形成的抗生物素蛋白和生物素辣根过氧化物酶复合物。这一复合物可对存在于抗原部位的辣根过氧化物酶分子进行定位。ABC法染色时间较 PAP 法短，但与内源性生物素结合的问题仍未解决。

生物素-链卵白素系统

生物素-链卵白素（B-SA）法通过用链卵白素代替抗生物素蛋白，将链卵白素直接与酶分子结合等方法克服了ABC法存在的一些问题。链卵白素是从链霉菌中提取的分子质量为60kD的四聚体，是抗生物素蛋白的类似物，能以非常高的亲和力和生物素结合。理论上，它们之间的亲和力是多数抗原-抗体之间亲和力的10倍以上，并能提供非常特异的检测手段及放大抗原-抗体间结合的信号。用链卵白素代替抗生物素蛋白出于以下几个理由：

1. 链卵白素不含能和肾、肝、脑和肥大细胞中的植物血凝素非特异性结合的碳水化合物。

2. 链卵白素的等电点接近中性，而在生理情况下抗生物素蛋白的等电点为10；因此链卵白素结合不存在生理条件下抗生物素蛋白结合具有的静电非特异性结合。

3. 在B-SA方法中，因为酶是直接与链卵白素结合的，试剂的稳定性较高，可稀释成即用型试剂并能长期保存。

在 B-SA 方法中，可对二抗及标记试剂进行修饰，以使生物素和酶标的数量大大增加，提高检测的敏感性。同时也节省昂贵的一抗用量。过氧化物酶和碱性磷酸酶都可用做酶标。目前已有多家公司生产该系统的成套试剂如 BioGenex、Shandon-Lipshaw、Immunon 和 DAKO 等公司。

多价系统

目前很多供应商提供多价检测系统（BioGenex,

Shandon-Lipshaw, Immunon, DAKO)。这些系统提供由抗不同种动物免疫球蛋白组成的混合型二抗。这样使得一种二抗既可用于单克隆抗体也可用于多克隆抗体。

碱性磷酸酶 – 抗碱性磷酸酶法

碱性磷酸酶-抗碱性磷酸酶（APAAP）法除了用APAAP代替PAP外，其原理和PAP法相同（图1.10）。该方法首先由Cordell等建立[82]，采用的是猪抗小牛碱性磷酸酶特异性抗体。APAAP法有三个主要用途：①用于含高水平内源性过氧化物酶的组织的染色，②与过氧化物酶联合使用进行双重染色，③用于那些适合于碱性磷酸酶鲜红色底物的特殊细胞的染色[4]。

碱性磷酸酶标记适用于富含内源性过氧化物酶的组织，如骨髓、髓系细胞浸润的淋巴组织，尤其适用于冰冻切片，因为完全封闭血及骨髓涂片中髓样白细胞的内源性过氧化物酶非常困难，同时封闭可引起一些抗原决定簇变性。APAAP法对骨髓染色有用。如Erber和McLachlan[83]采用APAAP法成功对常规处理、脱钙、石蜡包埋的72例骨髓标本进行14种单克隆抗体染色获得满意的结果。

对于双重标记，联合应用APAAP法和免疫过氧化物酶染色方法较为简单（见附录B）。用碱性磷酸酶作为第二标记可以避免使用两种过氧化物酶引起的交叉反应。另外，进行同步双重染色也可应用不同种类抗体，如多克隆和单克隆抗体作为一抗（图1.10）。用固红和固蓝进行APAAP法双重染色[84]，应注意避免混合颜色染色（即红色变成紫色）；为此，染色较弱的一抗应先染色，第二抗体的孵育时间应较短（10～15分钟，显微镜下观察控制）。

碱性磷酸酶底物产生的鲜红色（固红或新品红）比传统的过氧化物酶染色更清晰。APAAP法也可应用于细胞核的染色或只有少数细胞阳性染色的细胞涂片。Wong等[85]对48例人乳腺癌组织雌激素受体（ER）进行了研究，结果显示APAAP法明显改善了显色结果，因为与传统的DAB棕色反应产物相比，APAAP法的碱性磷酸酶染色剂的红色更清晰。这种免疫组织化学染色结果与以细胞质为基础的右旋糖酐包被的木炭法（DCC）具有相似的结果。另外Vaediman等[86]用单克隆抗体Leu-M5（CD11c）对毛细胞性白血病患者的外周血及骨髓涂片进行染色，能检测到极少数的肿瘤细胞。

APAAP法的这种显色优点，可用于碱性磷酸酶结合抗生物素蛋白或链卵白素而改良的ABC或B-SA法。前述的PAP的技术也可应用于APAAP法。和PAP复合物一样，应考虑APAAP法的特异性并测定合适的浓度。PAP的复合物是3个抗原分子（过氧化物酶）结合2个抗体分子，而APAAP法复合物由2个分子的抗原（碱性磷酸酶）结合1个分子抗体。这一构象和二价抗体的结合反应相似。APAAP复合物性质稳定，可长时间保存。

有两种方法可增加APAAP标记法的免疫染色强度。第一种方法是"双桥联"技术，也可用于PAP法，即简单地重复免疫染色过程的第二和第三步［加第二（桥联）抗体和标记复合物][87,88]。APAAP法增加敏感性并非是形成双桥联所致，而是由于结合了剩余的未被结合的一抗。第二种增加敏感性的方法是由Davidoff等人[89]建立的，联合应用APAAP技术和抗生物素蛋白-生物素-碱性磷酸酶复合物（ABAP）技术。这种放大过程是在一抗孵育后，相继加入生物素化抗鼠IgG（Vector)和鼠APAAP（DAKO），然后加入ABAP复合物（Vector）标记，Davidoff应用该方法对人睾丸冰冻切片进行desmin和vimentin免疫标记，发现联合应用APAAP和ABAP法与单独应用APAAP或ABAP法相比，能显示更少量的固有层肌纤维母细胞中的靶抗原。

蛋白A法

从葡萄球菌中获得的蛋白A能和多种免疫球蛋白分子保守区（Fc）紧密结合。唯一的条件是一抗与蛋白A结合，绝大多数IgG分子都结合蛋白A，只是

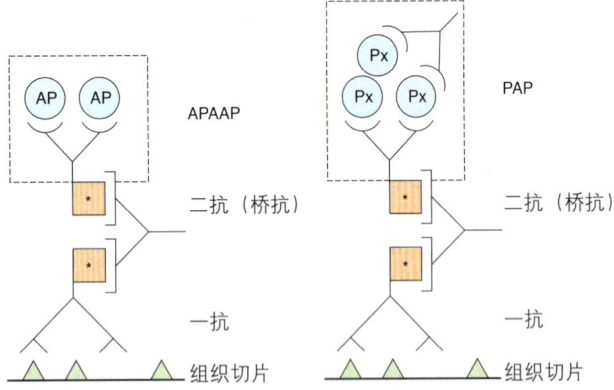

图1.10 APAAP法和PAP法显示用不同一抗和二抗进行双标记的可行性，如鼠抗vimentin，马抗鼠IgG，鼠APAAP（左）；兔抗keratin（多克隆山羊抗兔IgG），兔PAP（右）。AP，碱性磷酸酶；Px，过氧化物酶（引自Taylor CR, Cote RJ. Immunomicroscopy: A Diagnostic Tool for the Surgical Pathologist, 3rd ed. Philadelphia: WB Saunders, 2005:20）

不同动物不同的IgG亚型与蛋白A的亲和力不同（图1.11和1.12）。蛋白A-过氧化物酶或蛋白A-PAP法并没有PAP、ABC或链卵白素的方法敏感，但在某些特殊情况下仍具有其优点。

酶标记抗原法

酶标记抗原法是免疫过氧化物酶法中最具特异性的方法。它的应用原理如图1.13示。只用一种抗体，该方法利用抗体分子具有两个化合价，一个在研究条件下可和靶抗原结合，另一个则可和后加抗原结合，它就是和辣根过氧化物酶连接的抗原。因而此法是抗原标记过程。

此法所需第一抗原的工作浓度相对较高，一抗的用量较大，因此用于抗原和抗体来源丰富的抗原检测。该法的一个主要优点是一抗纯度要求不高，用这种方法，与组织结合的非特异性的抗体不会被检测出来；由于缺乏对A抗原特异性，也不会和A抗原-过氧化物酶复合物结合，因而不能检测出来。

该方法适用于用2个标记抗体（如κ-过氧化物酶和λ-碱性磷酸酶）同时检测同一切片上的2种抗原的双标技术（图1.14）。

多聚体标记二步法

对于免疫组织化学染色方法，人们一直在不断寻求新的、更敏感可靠、更简单的方法，试图在不影响敏感性的情况下简化传统多步骤检测系统，缩短染色时间。在实际工作中，实验步骤减少时，敏感性也会降低。新的方法，如催化沉淀法或酪氨酸信号放大（TSA）[7, 8]、免疫多聚酶链反应（Immuno-PCR）[90]和终产物放大[91]等方法虽提高了检测的敏感性，但同时

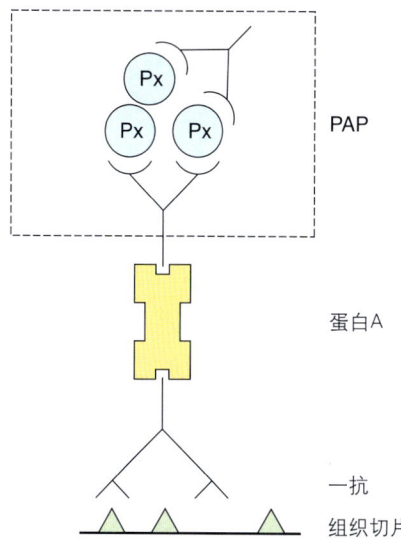

图1.12 蛋白A-PAP法。蛋白A用于连接一抗（Fc）和PAP复合物内的抗体（Fc）。Px，过氧化物酶标记（引自Taylor CR, Cote RJ. Immunomicroscopy: A Diagnostic Tool for the Surgical Pathologist, 2nd ed. Philadelphia: WB Saunders, 1994: 14）

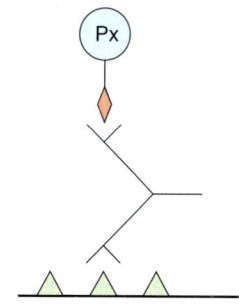

图1.13 标记抗原法。加入过量的抗体，抗体的一个化合价与组织切片中的抗原结合，另一个化合价与随后加入的标记抗原结合。Px，过氧化物酶标记（引自 Taylor CR, Cote RJ. Immunomicroscopy: A Diagnostic Tool for the Surgical Pathologist, 2nd ed. Philadelphia: WB Saunders, 1994: 14）

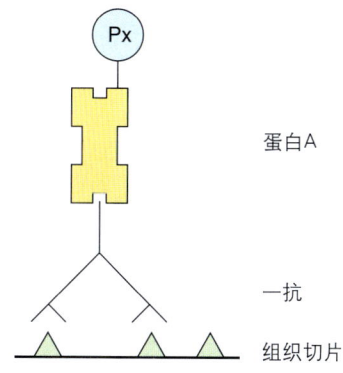

图1.11 蛋白A结合法。蛋白A，用过氧化物酶标记，和一抗Fc片段结合。Px，过氧化物酶（引自 Taylor CR, Cote RJ. Immunomicroscopy: A Diagnostic Tool for the Surgical Pathologist, 2nd ed. Philadelphia: WB Saunders, 1994: 14）

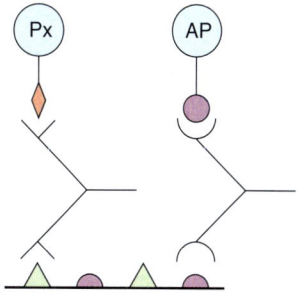

图1.14 标记抗原双重染色。2个不同的抗体分别识别组织切片中各自的抗原，然后只和相应的标记抗原结合［用过氧化物酶（Px）或碱性磷酸酶（AP）标记］（引自 Taylor CR, Cote RJ. Immunomicroscopy: A Diagnostic Tool for the Surgical Pathologist, 2nd ed. Philadelphia: WB Saunders, 1994: 15）

增加了检测过程的复杂程度，并常常产生过高的非特异性染色。也有人尝试利用天然或合成多聚体载体增加和改变连接抗体配对的酶或配体的数量的方法优化检测方法。

伴信号放大的一步或两步法检测的发展反映了提倡信号放大的趋势，这将有利于 IHC 的标准化，简单的技术比复杂的技术要好。

新的多聚体标记二步法是一种高度信号放大、相对简单的免疫组织化学染色方法。最初于 1995 年建立了一种强化的多聚体二步法免疫组织化学染色检测系统（EnVision, DAKO, Carpinteria, CA）[12, 16, 19]。然而，由于连接酶和连接抗体的右旋糖酐载体分子质量过大，会形成空间障碍，使得显色效果较差。1999年，出现了一种新的称之为 PowerVision 的多聚体标记系统（ImmunoVision Technologies, Daly City, CA）应用该检测系统和现有的多步骤检测系统进行比较研究[91]，发现 PowerVision 的检测效率较高，如在稀释度为 1∶320 条件下用 PowerVision 可获得中等强度的染色结果，而其他方法显示弱阳性或阴性结果。另外，联合应用 AR 和这一新的二步检测法检测长期保存的石蜡切片的 p53（Pab-1801）、p27^{Kip1}、p21^{WAF1}，其染色结果与新鲜石蜡切片的染色结果相似。

PowerVision 系统的基础是紧密结合的酶-抗体连接复合物，每个连接抗体都结合了大量的酶分子。用某些特殊方法可连接抗体和酶聚合成紧密压缩状态使其空间体积尽可能减小，以增加结果的可靠性（图 1.15）[92]。二步检测系统的优点是方法简单和敏感性高。

应用任何所谓的"超敏感"检测系统均应注意尽可能稀释一抗的有效工作浓度，以避免非特异性染色[93, 94]。

酪氨酸信号放大系统

根据 20 世纪 80 年代采用的酶免疫测定法中的酶放大法原理，Bobrow 等[8, 93]建立了催化报告沉淀技术（CARD）在固相免疫测定系统和膜免疫测定系统中获得信号放大。1992 年 CARD 技术被应用于免疫组织化学染色[7]。

CARD 中的信号放大是通过形成自由基而产生的生物素化酪氨酸沉积，该过程由辣根过氧化物酶氧化作用催化。活化的生物素化酪氨酸与某些富含电荷的成分如酪氨酸、苯丙氨酸、色氨酸等共价结合，由此再引起另外的生物素化分子在抗原-抗体反应部位沉

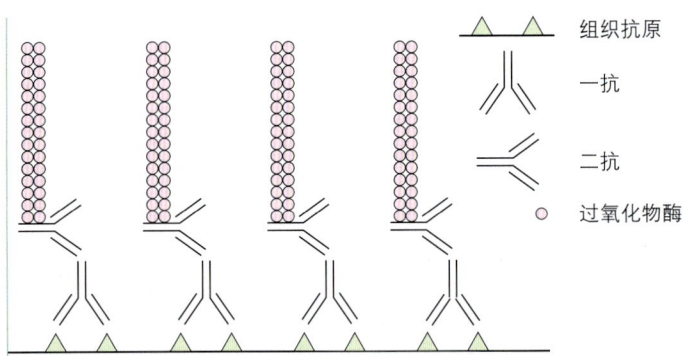

图 1.15　PowerVision 检测系统模式图。酶连接抗体比其他多聚体复合物的分子结构紧密，因此允许多种复合物紧密结合在一起。丰富的结合在一起的酶分子沉积在每个抗原位置，就像一个大城市的轮廓（引自 Shi S-R, et al. Appl Immunohistochem Mol Morphol,1999, 7:201-208）

积，称为信号放大（图 1.16）[95-98]。

酪氨酸信号放大（TSA）已开始在免疫组织化学染色中应用，能使一些长期保存的石蜡切片中难以检测的抗原获得阳性染色结果[95]。TSA 试剂已商品化（NEN Life Science Products, Boston, MA; CSA system, DAKO, Carpinteria,CA）。这些 TSA 检测过程类似于辣根过氧化物酶结合的检测系统，即将切片与生物素标记的酪氨酸孵育后，彻底洗净，再和辣根过氧化物酶结合的链卵白素孵育，最后由显色剂（DAB、AEC 等）对组织切片中放大的信号进行显色。

虽然，TSA 法增加免疫组织化学染色和原位杂交的敏感性，但由于某些原因[94]，还没有广泛应用于诊断病理学领域。其原因包括以下几个方面：

1. 步骤增加，延长了实验时间。
2. 在信号增强的同时，也增加非特异性背景染色。
3. 现有技术结合适当的抗原修复可获得同样的结果。

另外还有 ImmunoMax 技术，可联合应用抗原修复和 TSA 系统来检测某些难测的抗原，也可能减少昂贵的一抗的用量[95-98]。

一抗的滴度和检测系统

免疫组织化学染色时抗体的最佳稀释度是指能获得特异性染色与非特异性背景染色间的最大对比度的抗体稀释度。稀释度的选择具有一定的主观性，不是简单获得最强信号，而是根据最大对比度来决定。对于只用一种抗体的直接标记法，滴度相对简单（表 1.1）。像间接标记和 PAP 法等应用 2 种和 3 种抗体的方法，每一个试剂都必须用其最佳稀释度。另外，就整个染色过程获得的对比度来说，第一

抗体和第二抗体的稀释度是相互依存的，应该比较几种稀释度的标记试剂（二抗）和不同稀释度的一抗搭配使用的染色结果；比较是通过棋盘滴定法等方法获得的（表1.2和1.3）。

非连接方法：所谓的不标记抗体法

所有多步骤法的原理都相似，这里以三步法的PAP法为例作一说明。

<u>过氧化物酶-抗过氧化物酶试剂的滴度</u>　由于PAP试剂广泛的商业来源，有必要对选择的试剂预先进行滴度测定以确定用于某个检测系统中获得理想染色的试剂的稀释度，在这一系统中其他试剂已最优化（表1.3）。理想情况下，所有的滴度应以活性试剂的微克数计；实际工作中这一设想很难做到。当然一个实验室成套试剂中的某种试剂的稀释度，并不能自动地用于另一个实验室，除非所有的试剂都是相同的。

一旦确定了理想的稀释度，浓缩试剂应分装成适量的包装储存，以备使用前稀释成工作液。另外，若没有加入蛋白或其他稳定剂来保持活性，最好不要将试剂以高浓度的形式保存，因为活性将随保存时间而减弱。商品化的免疫染色试剂盒包含预先稀释的试剂，这些试剂的有效期为一年或更长，也证明了高度稀释的试剂是稳定的。

应用准备的分装新鲜制备的试剂的一个主要原因

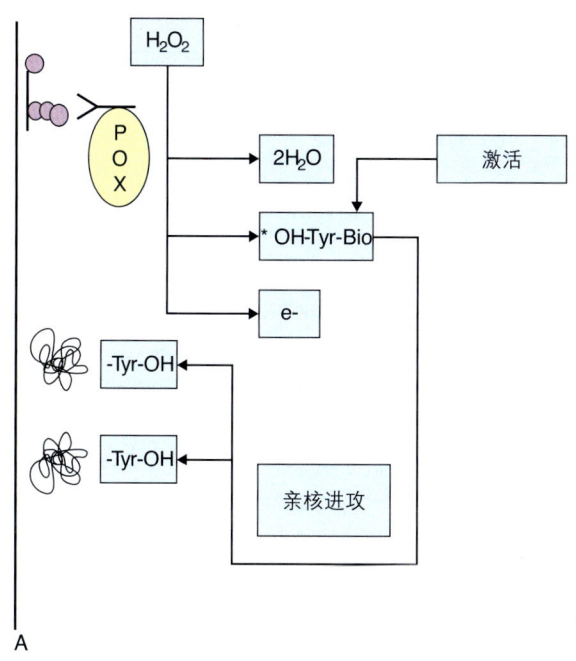

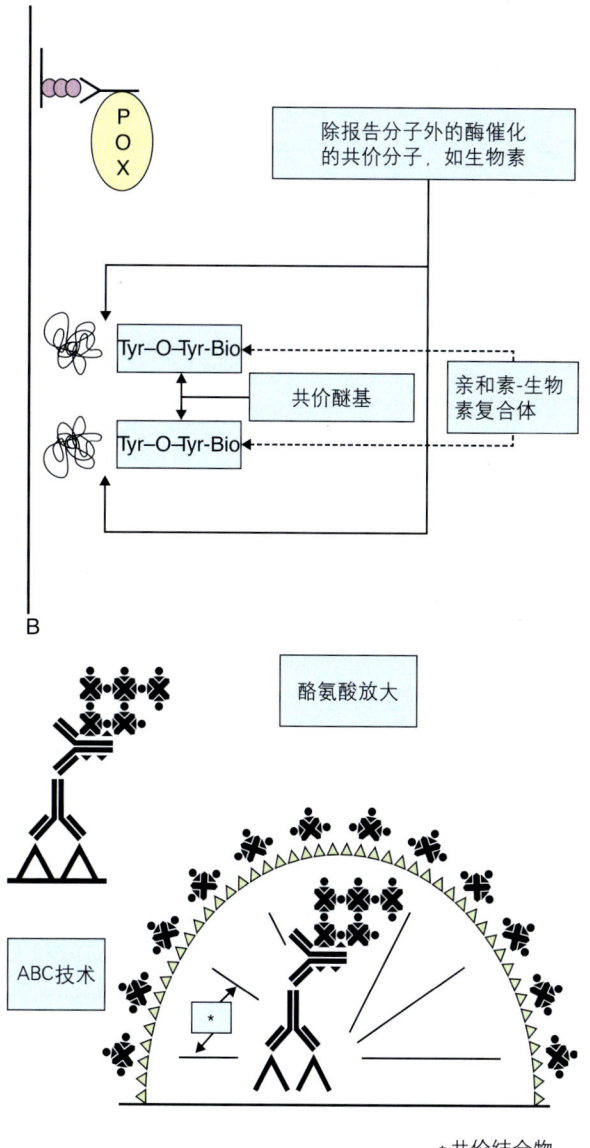

图1.16　(A)酪氨酸放大的激进模式。(B)酪氨酸-报告物沉积。(C)和ABC法比较（引自 Merz H, et al. Chapter 14. In: Shi S-R, Giu J, Taylor CR, eds. Antigen Retrieval Techniques: Immunohistochemistry and Molecular Morphology. Natick, MA: Eaton; 2000: 228-229）

是避免用巴斯德吸管从一个试剂管（瓶）中重复取样。此方法无一例外地造成细菌污染和试剂失活（不可预测的和令人烦恼的）。"真正的"科学家能从他的教训中吸取经验，采用密封的稀释试剂，这样试剂可以直接从滴瓶中滴出来，从而在很大程度上克服了污染问题。我们毫不犹豫地在实验室借鉴了此技术，当我们制备用于一段时间或几天的新的稀释度的试剂时，应用这些小的塑料滴瓶。

表1.1　确定用于直接连接法抗体理想浓度的稀释度

染色强度[*]	一抗的系列稀释度					
	1/5	1/20	1/80	1/320	1/1280	1/2560
不需要的背景染色[a]	++	+	±	±	±	±
特异性抗原[b]	+++	++++	++++	+++	++	+

[*] 染色强度采用半定量，级别由0到++++；±表示意义不明的弱阳性
[a] 不需要的背景染色可能由几种不同的机制造成（见正文）
[b] 特异性抗原染色强度（如用一定稀释度的抗κ抗体，特异性染色应存在于浆细胞）
（引自Taylor CR, Cote RJ.Immunomicroscopy: A Diagnosis Tool for the Surgical Pathologist, 2nd ed. Philadelphia: WB Saunders, 1994:23）

表1.2　间接免疫过氧化物酶法理想抗体浓度的确定——棋盘滴定法

二抗稀释度（连接）↓		一抗的系列稀释度					
		1/5	1/20	1/80	1/320	1/1280	阴性对照[*]
	1/10	切片1	切片2	切片3	切片4	切片5	切片16
		+++[a]	++++	+++	++	+	±
		(++)	(++)	(++)	(++)	(++)	(++)
	1/40	切片6	切片7	切片8	切片9	切片10	切片17
		+++	+++	++++	++++	++	-
		(+)	(+)	(+)	(±)	(±)	(±)
	1/160	切片11	切片12	切片13	切片14	切片15	切片18
		++	++	+	±	±	-
		(+)	(±)	(±)	(-)	(-)	(-)

18个切片滴度举例
[*] 阴性对照（不用一抗，用免疫前血清，或特异性不相关血清代替；见文中阴性对照）
[a] 特异性染色强度用0到++++等级别表示，非特异性背景染色强度用括号内相同的级别表示0到++++；例如+++/(+)表示强特异性染色（+++）伴中等背景染色（+）
注：该例切片9的滴度为理想滴度
（引自Taylor CR, Cote RJ.Immunomicroscopy: A Diagnostic Tool for the Surgical Pathologist, 2nd ed. Philadelphia: WB Saunders, 1994:29）

表1.3　过氧化物酶-抗过氧化物酶法棋盘滴定法[*]

一抗稀释度（例：兔抗胰岛素）	二抗稀释度（例：猪抗兔IgG）	PAP稀释度（兔PAP）		
		1/20	1/80	1/160
		（切片号）		
1/80	1/10	1	2	3
	1/40	4	5	6
	1/160	7	8	9
1/320	1/10	10	11	12
	1/40	13	14	15
	1/160	16	17	18
1/1280	1/10	19	20	21
	1/40	22	23	24
	1/160	25	26	27
对照（省去一抗）	1/10	28	29	30
	1/40	31	32	33
	1/160	34	35	36

[*] 显示36个切片方格图案；根据切片显示最佳对比度选择理想的试剂稀释度。根据经验，可简化这样复杂的抗体滴定，根据经验（也就是以前用过的来源相同的类似试剂）省去不太可能成为理想稀释度的一些稀释度
（引自Taylor CR, Cote RJ.Immunomicroscopy: A Diagnostic Tool for the Surgical Pathologist, 2nd ed. Philadelphia: WB Saunders, 1994:29）

免疫组织化学技术：原理、局限性和标准化

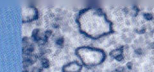

质量控制

美国病理学家学会定义，质量控制是"发现、减少并纠正分析过程中缺陷的方法和技术的结合"[99]。这是针对实验的过程和方法质量保证体系的一部分。对于免疫组织化学染色，质量控制涉及整个实验过程中的每个步骤，包括组织的获取、固定、脱水、切片、染色和最后染色结果的解释与报告。实验的所有步骤都应分别描述，确立并监测每一实验步骤的参数，以保证实验结果的稳定性和可重复性。应每天记录质量控制结果，发现错误时应立即采取纠正措施，并记入档案。本节将讨论有关抗体确认及对照应用等方面的质量控制。

在临床实验室已很好地建立了试剂的质量控制参考标准。例如，血清检验结果可用标准血清来验证，如美国病理学家学会建立的"样本检查"程序。最近，人们已经考虑建立免疫组织化学质量控制参考标准。然而，实行起来并不简单。和血清标本不同，不可建立病理组织库，并且组织标本的量是有限的。另外，形态学相似的肿瘤，其抗原性不一定相同，多组织包埋块所包含的组织也很有限，不能完全解决问题。为克服这一难题，有人提出建立由人工肿瘤或人类肿瘤细胞系组成的能无限供应的标准参考对照[100]。

每一个实验和实验室用的抗体（包括每一个新抗体）均必须经过验证研究（经过验证的即用型试剂不需要验证，如试剂盒中的部分试剂）。这样的研究是必需的，因为试剂的来源、组成、浓度和/或特异性可能都不清楚[101]。实验的性能参数包括敏感性、特异性、精确性、稳定性。建议应用包括已知阳性和阴性的正常和肿瘤组织的多组织对照块进行研究，利用其结果检验受试抗体的特异性和准确性。抗体染色的特异性可通过多组织对照块中某些细胞、组织和肿瘤等出现预期阴性着色来显示。相反，精确性则验证整个染色过程的有效性，通过同一张切片对照中同时存在预期的阳性或阴性成分。敏感性测试是检测少量抗原，通过已知弱阳性染色组织的阳性结果来确定。精确性通过非特异性背景染色来评价，可用阴性对照代替一抗来检测精确性。如果不同实验获得相同的结果，说明实验是稳定的。

生物染色委员会（BSC）及食品和药品管理局（FDA）联合发表了试剂包装内说明书指南，包括对生产厂家在试剂的检测、销售以及阳性和阴性对照的用途等方面的指导意见（表 1.4）[102]。BSC 认为，因为组织固定、脱水过程、包埋等内在影响因素的变化，不可能建立一个通用的免疫组织化学染色程序。因此，必须将对照片与实验切片同时染色和解

表 1.4　免疫组织化学日常质量控制的类型和目的

质控类型	抗原（分析目标）	抗体（试剂）	目的
阳性	含待检测及定量的抗原的非病人组织或细胞	抗体试剂（试剂盒中的）的组成和用于病人标本的一样	对所有步骤进行控制
	预期结果已知		对使用者进行阳性反应的表现进行培训和比较半定量
	和病人样本用同样的处理程序		验证分析的所有步骤，包括固定和脱水
	用对靶抗原起保护作用的程序处理样本		验证除各实验室用的固定和脱水以外的所有步骤
阴性（特异性）	组织或细胞抗体（试剂盒中的）染色预期阴性	抗体试剂（试剂盒中的）的组成和用于病人标本的一样	检测不需要抗体与细胞或细胞成分的交叉反应
	和病人标本用同样的方法处理		
	可能是病人标本的一部分		
阴性（非特异性）	病人标本中含有要研究的组织同样的成分	稀释液（和抗体稀释液一样）中无抗体	检测不需要的背景染色
	病人标本用同样的方法处理	不与靶抗原特异性结合的抗体，稀释度和试剂盒中的抗体一样	

（引自 Taylor CR, Cote RJ.Immunomicroscopy: A Diagnostic Tool for the Surgical Pathologist, 2nd ed. Philadelphia: WB Saunders, 1994:27）

释。对照可保证所用染色技术适当和所用染色方法的特异性，因此对免疫组织化学染色结果的正确解释非常重要。

应同时进行阳性和阴性对照实验，阳性对照是指已经含有待检测抗原的组织。这些对照组织的固定和处理过程应和待检测组织的固定及处理过程相似，可防止对实验标本的假阴性结果。例如，实验组织过度固定，导致抗原性减弱或消失，而对照组织固定适当，可导致假阴性结果。为此，生产商提供的阳性对照片不能代替实验室自己的阳性对照片，因为它们的处理过程不一定和实验组织相同，只能证实试剂的有效性，不能证明组织固定及处理程序是否合适。

一般来说，最好的阳性对照应该由实验室自己制备。使用和常规外科手术标本一起固定和处理的组织作对照是较好的选择。通常用肿瘤组织作对照，因为正常组织可能比其相应的肿瘤组织含更多的抗原。因此用正常组织作对照可能造成待测的肿瘤组织假阴性结果。另外，理想的阳性对照不应该表现为强度一致的阳性染色，其染色强度应该是不均匀的，在很多区域是弱阳性。这些弱的染色区域可用来比较观察一抗敏感性的细微改变，这也有助于减少假阴性结果的发生。

很多类型的组织都能用做阳性对照。总体来说外科切除标本比尸体解剖标本好，因为后者可能包含组织自溶区域，影响染色结果。对于体液和细针穿刺标本的免疫细胞学检测来说，未固定的细胞离心涂片或细胞块经固定、包埋后可用做细胞对照材料。选择合适的对照组织最重要的条件是对照组织含有待检测的抗原，并且其固定和处理过程和实验样本一样。

阴性对照是在不含一抗的情况下对实验组织进行染色，对确定使用方法的特异性和评价非特异性染色背景的存在有重要意义。可通过不同的方法进行阴性对照实验。吸收对照是用高纯度的用于产生一抗的蛋白质或肽类抗原来吸收一抗的阴性对照。该方法的目的是消除抗体和组织中蛋白的结合。然而研究发现吸收对照不能确定结合于组织中的蛋白和用于吸附的蛋白是否同一蛋白。单克隆抗体可能结合表位相似的无关蛋白，特别是组织固定以后。因此吸收对照不能保证组织蛋白抗体的特异性[103-105]。

其他的阴性对照包括用稀释的抗体（缓冲液加牛血清白蛋白载体蛋白）代替一抗，或者从同种动物获取的同种稀释度的非免疫性免疫球蛋白代替一抗。用无关的抗体替代一抗也可作为阴性对照。另外，有些研究者认为在同一组织上应用一系列不同抗体时，不同一抗的染色结果可相互作为阴性对照（只要抗体是同型免疫球蛋白，来自同种动物，并且稀释度相当）。最后，对于阴性对照，如果同一次免疫染色采用微波抗原修复、胰蛋白酶消化等不同处理方法时，应根据不同的方法分别进行阴性对照切片的染色。

另一个有效的对照方法是用多组织对照切片。每一个多组织对照切片含有按棋盘或香肠方式排列的样本。棋盘对照切片包括指定组织类型和它们特定的位置。香肠对照切片伴有显示不同组织类型分布，组织通常呈束状排列。如前述，多组织对照切片对验证新试剂特别有用，也可用于日常质量控制。但该方法费用较高，对标本如何固定和处理无法控制[106,107]。

通过"微组织阵列"制备的改进，以上的缺点已被发现，尤其是商品化的仪器有利于提供包含有多个精细组织芯的微阵列组织块（如 Beecham Instruments, Hackensack, NJ, USA）。内处理组织中200～300个芯通过该方法合并为"微组织阵列块"，这可用于许多抗体的对照。因为每个芯体积小（一般直径0.6～1.5mm），一个原始的活检组织块可作为多芯样本的来源，而且也能为档案资料提供许多原始组织块。这项技术的优缺点在 Skacel 等[108]发表的《Applied Immunohistochemistry and Molecular Morphology》进一步讨论。在最新一版的《Applied Immunohistochemistry and Molecular Morphology》中对组织微阵列的制备、商业化用途和此方法的优缺点进行了精彩的综述[108,109]。

当含有待测抗原的实验组织与正常组织相邻时，应作内对照。内对照的细胞阳性染色反映免疫反应是否合适。对于广泛存在的抗原，如波形蛋白（vimentin），阳性内对照染色可用做这一抗体的阳性对照。因为其广泛存在，波形蛋白染色也可作为报告分子，以评估组织的固定和处理是否合适[110]。如前讨论的那样，过度固定或固定不充分均可造成染色结果不同。波形蛋白表位多种多样，对过度固定特别敏感，可改变或破坏抗原表位。波形蛋白的一个单克隆抗体 V9 可识别这一敏感的表位。因此 V9 染色的强度可用来评估福尔马林固定的程度，也可用于检测福尔马林过度固定后抗原修复方法对抗原的修复情况。波形蛋白内对照染色的强度可用于确定组织切片固定程度不同对实验结果的不同影响。

从上述讨论来看，理解并应用适当的阳性和阴性对照是免疫组织化学染色过程中最重要的方面。对照的恰当应用是正确解释免疫组织化学染色结果的基础。

组织固定、处理程序和抗原修复

组织处理包括固定、脱水、石蜡包埋（为切片提供介质）。为了使组织保存最佳化，组织在包埋于石蜡之前应"固定"，这是一个对形态和免疫组织学结果影响深远的程序。理想的固定剂不仅应供应便利，还应能最大范围地适用于各种免疫组织化学染色标本。固定剂应该能保持抗原的完整性，并限制在以后的处理过程中抗原聚集、弥散或异位，还应该使抗原在包埋于支持介质（如石蜡）以后能保持形态结构的完整。

常用的组织病理固定剂分为两类：凝固性固定剂（如乙醇）和交联固定剂（如甲醛）。两类固定剂都能改变蛋白质的空间构象，可掩盖抗原位点（表位），对抗体结合产生不利影响。目前已知交联固定剂改变很多抗原的免疫组织化学染色结果，而乙醇这样的凝固性固定剂则影响则较少[34, 111-113]。大多数外科病理的固定剂是10%中性福尔马林（NBF）（交联固定剂），随后用100%乙醇固定一段时间，因此组织被福尔马林和乙醇"双重固定"。对于福尔马林固定的组织，很多抗原在免疫组织化学染色时，其信号的强度与固定时间有关[111, 113, 114]。福尔马林作为固定剂的历史悠久，具有以下优点：

1. 即使在长时间固定后，对很多组织的形态保存仍很好，需要说明的是，"很好"的含义在某种程度上带有一定的主观性，包括各种各样的人工假象造成的病理学家乐于见到的形态学特征，因为病理学家已经习惯了这种固定程序。

2. 福尔马林是廉价的化学品，比其他固定剂便宜。

3. 福尔马林固定对组织标本的消毒作用比其他固定剂可靠，特别是对病毒。

4. 对碳水化合物类的抗原保存更好[115]。

5. 使蛋白质在原位交联，能防止蛋白质在水或酒精中渗出和弥散，保存其抗原性。很多低分子量的抗原（肽）被非交联固定剂如乙醇或甲醇固定而改变性状，但可被福尔马林以交联衍生物形式很好地保存下来[28]。一般认为，为保持一些大分子的免疫反应性，如中间丝和免疫球蛋白，非交联沉淀固定剂比醛类固定剂更好。

对于形态学和免疫组织化学染色来说，福尔马林均被认为是令人满意的固定剂，并且通过简单有效的抗原修复技术就能恢复被减弱或修饰的抗原。

抗原修复

一种简单的热诱导的抗原修复技术（在水中将组织切片加热）目前被广泛应用[38, 39, 55, 58]。在病理诊断中，已将抗原修复成功应用于福尔马林固定组织的免疫组织化学染色，从而不再急于寻找替代福尔马林的固定剂。1997年，Prento和Lyon[116]比较了6种作为福尔马林替代品的商品化固定剂。结论是，最好的免疫组织化学染色是联合应用福尔马林固定和抗原修复，并且6种福尔马林替代品没有一个满足组织病理诊断方面的要求（主要是使形态学发生变化）。

Williams等人[117]用经不同方法保存和固定、处理的扁桃体组织切片，详细研究了组织处理方法对免疫组织化学染色的影响。发现微波抗原修复技术缓解了因固定、脱水和切片制作的变化引起的不良影响。他们报道10%的中性缓冲福尔马林、10%的锌福尔马林和10%福尔马林盐溶液固定显示总体效果较好，并有非常好的抗原保护作用。相反，10%乙酸福尔马林、B5、Bouin固定液则对抗原保护欠佳，即使经过抗原修复也一样。其他研究也显示用其他固定剂将减弱抗原修复的效果[114-116]。

虽然Williams等人没有研究组织切片的保存[117]，但有研究认为组织切片经长期保存后，会减弱某些抗原的染色强度[121-126]。笔者认为此情况不常见，并且多数可通过抗原修复加以恢复。例如，即使长时间保存的切片，联合应用抗原修复和敏感的多聚体标记二步法检测系统仍能获得满意的p53（Pab-1801）、$p21^{WAF1}$（Ab-1，癌基因）和$p27^{Kip1}$（DCS-72.F6，NeoMarker）等的染色结果。

抗原修复能提高保存样本的免疫组织化学染色强度，可用于常规免疫组织化学染色的标准化操作过程[17, 38, 39, 92]。免疫组织化学染色中的标准化处理和抗原修复的恰当应用是影响抗原修复效果的重要因素。

影响抗原修复 - 免疫组织化学染色效果的主要因素有加热的温度和时间（加热条件 T × t）以及修复液的 pH 值。在某些情况下，修复液的组成成分和摩尔浓度也是影响抗原修复 - 免疫组织化学染色效果的因素。

加热条件

如前述，加热抗原修复-免疫组织化学染色是建立在 Fraenkel-Conrat 等的生物化学研究的基础上的，他们证实发生在蛋白质和福尔马林之间的化学反应至少部分可通过加热或强碱水解逆转[31-33]。用传统的加热到100℃的方法可获得与微波加热同样的效果。蒸馏水也可用做修复液，但效果稍差[34]。随后有报道，用传统加热方法得到了相似的结果[39,125,126]。Malmstrom 等人[122]在常规处理的膀胱癌组织石蜡切片上用蒸馏水作修复液进行增殖细胞核抗原（PCNA）（PC10和19F4）的免疫组织化学染色获得了较好的结果。

福尔马林在固定过程中发生的化学反应还不清楚。Mason和O'Leary[124]证明在交联过程中用量热法和红外光谱分析并没有观察到可见的蛋白质二级结构的改变。他们还注意到没有固定的蛋白质样品在70~90℃范围内发生了明显的变性，而同样的温度对福尔马林固定标本无任何不良影响（即福尔马林固定蛋白质具有热稳定性）。抗原修复方法利用这一特性，当标本进行高温加热时，由福尔马林固定的蛋白质的一级和二级结构能免受加热引起的变性，同时使蛋白质分子表面交联受到一定程度的减弱，从而恢复其免疫原性。虽然抗原修复的原理不清楚，但不完全是 Cattoretti 等人[43]提出的"蛋白质变性是唯一的机制"。

因此，加热条件可能是影响抗原修复效果的最重要的因素[37-41,54-56,125-130]。其现象表明：

1. 在蒸馏水中高温加热常规处理、石蜡包埋的组织切片可明显增加免疫组织化学染色的强度[34,125,131-133]。

2. 在一定范围内，随温度的增高，能产生更好的染色结果[38,39,55-57,125,128]。理想的抗原修复效果与加热的温度（T）和持续的时间（t）有关（T × t）[110,129]。

3. 用不同的缓冲液作修复液，如果 pH 值相同，可获得同样的免疫组织化学染色强度，表明化学成分不一定是影响结果的关键因素[47-49]。

4. 即使延长石蜡切片在枸橼酸缓冲液（或任何缓冲液）中存放的时间，但不加热，对抗原修复的效果亦无明显影响[52,54,134]。

修复液的 pH 值和化学成分

对一些抗原来说，修复液的 pH 值亦很关键[49,50]。根据1995年的一项对比研究及修复液pH值对抗原的不同影响，可分为三种情况：

1. 大多数抗原，修复液的 pH 值在 1.0~10.0 的范围内对修复效果无明显影响。

2. 某些抗原，特别是细胞核内抗原（如 MIB-1、ER），在pH为中等范围时抗原修复-免疫组织化学染色的强度大幅度减弱，低 pH 值时效果则较理想。

3. 少数抗原（MT-1、HMB-45）在低 pH 值（1.0~2.0）条件下显示阴性或仅呈灶状弱阳性染色，而在高pH值条件下可获得非常好的染色效果（图 1.17、1.18）。

Evers和Uylings也发现抗原修复免疫组织化学染色效果依赖 pH 和温度的变化。他们测试了两种抗体，MAP-2 和 SMI-32，显示 MAP-2 的最佳 pH 值是 4.5，而 SMI-32 的最佳 pH 值是 2.5，并且只要 pH 适当，修复液的种类并不重要。

总之，影响抗原修复的主要因素是加热的温度和时间（T × t），以及修复液的 pH 值。在某些情况下修复液的成分和摩尔浓度可能影响抗原修复-免疫组织化学染色效果，当用常规修复液不能得到满意结果时，应考虑修复液的成分和浓度的影响。

抗原修复的试验组合法

试验组合法是抗原修复技术的初步试验，检验两种主要因素：加热条件（T × t）和 pH 值，为待测抗原建立最佳的修复方案。

通常，应用低、中、高三种加热条件和 pH 值为待测抗原筛选最佳的抗原修复-免疫组织化学染色方案，如表 1.5 所示。试验组合也可用连续的二步法进行：①如前文所列出的那样，用一标准温度（100℃ 10分钟）对同一修复液的不同pH值进行试验，以便为修复液找到最佳的 pH 值；②在确立 pH 基础上对加热条件进行试验。

微波、微波高压锅、蒸汽和高压消毒锅加热法等[38,39]不同的加热方法亦可通过类似的方式进行评估，通过改善条件，产生满意的抗原修复-免疫组织化学染色结果。

试验组合法可作为待测抗原确定理想的抗原修复方案的快速筛选方法。目的是在福尔马林固定时间不清楚的情况下使被福尔马林处理后隐藏的抗原获得最大程度的修复，使结果更令人满意[47-50]。另外，试验组合法也可鉴定抗原修复-免疫组织化学染色的假阴性或假阳性结果。

免疫组织化学技术：原理、局限性和标准化

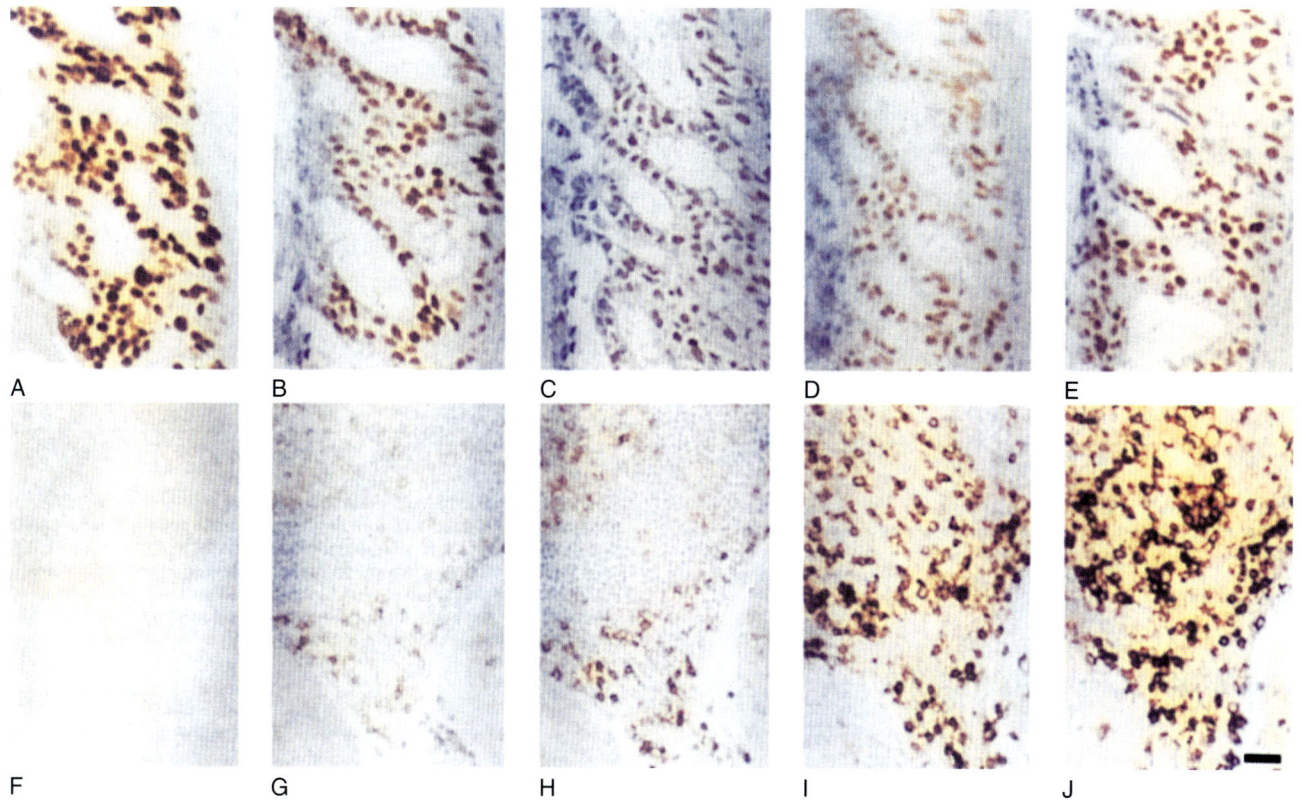

图 1.17　用抗 ER 单克隆抗体（MAb）对常规福尔马林固定石蜡包埋乳腺组织切片（A～E）和用 MT-1 单克隆抗体对淋巴结（F～J）进行抗原修复 - 免疫组织化学染色的染色强度比较。两种抗体均用盐酸巴比妥钠作抗原修复液。抗原修复液的 pH 值是 2、3、4、6 和 8，对于 ER 来说，对应的染色强度分别是 ++++、+++、+、++、+++，为 B 型模式（A～E）。F～J 显示 C 型模式，抗原修复液的 pH 值是 2、3、4、6 和 8，MT-1 对应的染色强度分别是 -、+、++、+++、++++。一些细胞核显示很弱的假阳性染色（F）。DAB 为染色剂，苏木精复染（原始放大倍数 ×100，bar=20μm，授权自 Shi, S-R, Imam SA, Young L, et al. Antigen retrieval immunohistochemistry under the influence of pH using monoclonal antibodies. Journal of Histochemistry &Cytochemistry 1995; 43:193-201）

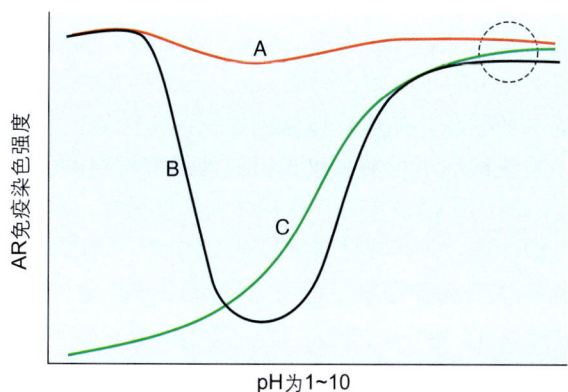

图 1.18　pH 值影响抗原修复免疫染色三种模式示意图。线 A（A 模式）显示在 pH 为 3 到 6 之间染色模式稳定，染色强度仅轻微减弱。线 B（B 模式）显示在 pH 为 3 到 6 之间染色强度显著减弱。线 C（C 模式）显示随着修复液 pH 值的增加，抗原修复免疫染色的强度相应增强。圆圈（右）显示用高 pH 值抗原修复液的优势（授权自 Shi S-R, Imam SA, Yong L, et al. Antigen retrieval immunohistochemistry under the influence of pH using monoclonal antibodies. Journal of Histochemistry & Cytochemistry 1995;43:193-201）

表 1.5　建议用于筛选理想的抗原修复程序的试验组合法

TRIS-HCl 缓冲液	pH 1～2	pH 7～8	pH 10～11
超高温，120℃*	切片 1	切片 4	切片 7
高温，100℃，10 分钟	切片 2	切片 5	切片 8
中高温，90℃，10 分钟†	切片 3	切片 6	切片 9

* 超高温 120℃可用高压锅或延长微波炉加热时间达到
† 中高温 90℃可通过水浴或用温度计监测微波炉加热达到
注：可用 1 张以上的切片作不经抗原修复的对照。可用 pH6.0 枸橼酸缓冲液代替 pH7～8 的 TRIS-HCl 缓冲液，因为结果一样
（引自 Shi S-R, Cote RJ, Taylor CR. Antigen retrieval immunohistochemistry: Past, present, and future. J Histochem Cytochem 1997; 45:327-343）

免疫组织化学染色的技术

以下的论述主要是针对长期保存的石蜡包埋组织切片的免疫组织化学染色技术。新鲜冰冻切片除了不需要抗原修复和脱蜡外，其基本原理与程序和石蜡切片一样，抗体的滴度（稀释度）也可能有所不同。

成功的免疫组织化学染色取决于正确应用组织学和免疫学技术，建议在进行免疫组织化学实验前，应熟悉相关受试抗原的基本背景知识。以下信息特别重要：

1. 抗原在细胞内的定位。
2. 一抗的特异性。
3. 以前的免疫组织化学染色结果（从文献，特别是有经验的实验室获得）中关于组织固定对抗原的不良影响，以及预处理的价值，如热诱导的抗原修复的效果等信息。

另外，应该知晓实验试剂的详细信息，特别是一抗和显色系统的厂商、单克隆抗体的克隆号、推荐使用浓度等信息。

抗原修复方法

微波加热法（Shi 等，1991）[34, 94]

1. 脱蜡后的切片放在装有修复液的塑料缸内；建议每次用同样数量的切片，必要时可用"空白"片以保证加热条件不变。
2. 染缸用松的旋钮盖盖好，在微波炉内加热10分钟。每5分钟为一循环，中间间隔1分钟以检查缸内的液体水平。必要时在5分钟后再加入一些修复液以免切片变干。建议从液体沸腾时开始计时以使加热时间标准化，这样可避免不同实验室用不同的微波炉引起的差异。
3. 加热时间结束后，将染缸从微波炉内移出，自然冷却15分钟。
4. 切片用蒸馏水洗2次，置PBS内5分钟，然后可进行免疫组织化学染色。

包括传统的水浴加热、高压锅加热、蒸汽锅和高压消毒锅加热等在内的多种加热方法均可以采用，并能获得相似的免疫组织化学染色结果。研究证明，只要将加热条件调整适当，不同的加热方法可获得相似的免疫组织化学染色结果[38, 39]。

封闭非特异性结合

脱蜡后立即用甲醇-过氧化氢灭活内源性过氧化物酶。可在加入生物素结合连接物之前用抗生物素蛋白-生物素或脱脂牛奶对内源性生物素进行封闭（孵育10分钟）[119]。

也可用来自于二抗（连接抗体）同源的正常血清对非特异性结合位点进行封闭。

洗涤步骤

清洗步骤至关重要，每步均应彻底清洗。常用pH7.4的0.01mol/L的PBS清洗。在盛有PBS的缸内清洗切片2次，每次5分钟（共10分钟）。也可在切片上滴加PBS在湿盒内放置10分钟，中间换一次PBS。自动免疫组织化学染色，清洗程序也是自动的，采用多步清洗。

一抗孵育

孵育的时间由抗体的敏感性和浓度以及组织切片的质量决定。第一抗体的浓度根据前面描述的滴定试验，并参考供应商的说明书来决定。总体来说，冰冻切片孵育的时间比库存石蜡切片短。常用的孵育时间是室温下30分钟。多步骤方法，如PAP法连续孵育和清洗导致总的时间较长。在37℃的湿盒内孵育可缩短孵育时间，每步孵育的时间可缩短到10分钟或更短。湿盒可放在37℃烤箱内，但比热盘的效率低，因为需要较长的时间使温度达到37℃。一些自动染色仪用37℃或42℃来加速染色。微波加速免疫组织化学染色过程被称为快速免疫组织化学染色[140-143]，但是一般情况下并不便利。

在37℃孵育切片的关键是将切片放在湿盒里，一般在室温下孵育。如果切片不能保持湿润，会引起过强的非特异性背景染色。应注意液体的蒸发将导致抗体浓度相对增加，也会产生非特异性背景染色。含水平切片架的湿盒可以购买，也可用玻璃棒和树胶玻璃或玻璃板用防水胶黏合而成。抗体孵育时染色架必须保持水平状态，以防抗体流到组织以外区域。

某些情况下可孵育过夜（或延长孵育时间），保持盒内湿润显得很重要。将抗体高滴度稀释，孵育过夜，常可减轻非特异性背景染色（例如一个抗体孵育30分钟达到满意结果，可将之稀释10倍甚至100倍，然后孵育12至24小时）。这一方法可节约昂贵的抗体，同时降低了抗体的非特异性结合而使背景染色减弱（抗体浓度低时有利于高亲和性的免疫反应性结合）。这种方法只需要延长一抗的孵育时间，其他步骤正常。一抗孵育过夜对于很多商业实验室来说是个很好的选择，具有工作安排上的方便，同时由于使用高稀释度一抗，降低了成本。

检测试剂的孵育

如前所述，试剂须按照一定浓度，遵守供应商提供的每种试剂的浓度和操作程序。孵育应小心，通常是室温条件下每步（连接和标记）孵育30分钟。将试剂滴到切片上，并要完全覆盖组织。必须仔细确认整个组织包括边缘都浸在试剂中，并且没有气泡，自动染色时应特别予以注意（例如毛细管自动染色机）。

底物和染色剂

有几种不同的染色剂可供使用（表1.6）。对于辣根过氧化物酶来说，推荐用DAB，因为这种棕色产物不溶于乙醇，因而适用于多数复染剂和封片剂。AEC，染色显示红色，也已经广泛应用，虽然溶于乙醇，但比DAB致癌危险性低，因而受到免疫组织化学供应商的推崇。

一般情况下，我们常规用DAB或AEC染色。AEC产生鲜红色，与用苏木精复染可形成鲜明的对比[注意应用不含乙醇的苏木精（如Mayer，而不用Harris）以避免将溶于乙醇的AEC有色反应产物溶解]。当抗原-抗体-酶浓度高时，AEC可能产生棕黄色产物（AEC有两个反应位点，当其中一个被转变时，变成红色；当两个都和过氧化物酶反应时，产生棕绿色产物）。pH值为4.8的乙酸缓冲液能减轻这一反应。切片应用水性介质（如80%甘油）封片。水性封片剂含有少量有机溶剂，可使染色慢慢溶解或消失。注意不能用乙醇脱水。甘油封片可用指甲油将盖玻片边缘密封以长期保存。

DAB可用于特殊目的；因其不溶于乙醇，可进行染色、脱水和封片。另外因为其电子密度高，可用于电子显微镜观察。一些研究者建议将DAB反应产物锇酸化，以产生更强的颜色。但也有人认为用光镜观察并不需要这样处理；事实上，这样处理也有缺点，因为背景染色也被加强，其对比度反而减弱。类似的效果还可以通过用硫酸镍或氯化钴进行后处理，以产生更好的对比度[144, 145]。

如果用DAB，液体配制应在通风橱内进行，操作者应戴口罩和手套。多余溶液应在稀释后丢弃。一般认为工作液危害较小；但粉剂危害较大。有些供应商提供定量的用密封管分装的DAB，但价格较贵。目前市场上可买到即用型DAB溶液，具有方便、安全、环境污染少等优点。

其他染色剂还有α-萘酚派若宁（粉色）、4-氯-1-萘酚（蓝色）和Hanker-Yates以及大量"广谱"染色剂（表1.6）。反应底物也适用于碱性磷酸酶。有些底物在酶位点上持续反应，产生颗粒状有色物质，从而使碱性磷酸酶系统反应更敏感。但如果反应过度，这些颗粒可能使组织形态模糊。

复染和封片

复染和封片是最后的步骤。多数免疫组织化学染色用苏木精进行核复染。在对核抗原进行免疫定位时应避免复染过度（苏木精浅染对辨认核内染色信号很关键）。苏木精的复染时间要依据苏木精配制的时间（新配制的苏木精复染的时间比久置的苏木精复染时间短得多）。必要时在显微镜下对染色过程进行监控以确定理想的复染时间。对于溶于乙醇的染色剂（如AEC或固红）应用水性封片剂。封片剂在加热板上加热使之溶化。有两种封片方法：一种是在切片的组织上滴一滴封片剂，再将盖玻片慢慢地盖在切片上；另一种是将盖玻片放在纸巾上，在其中央滴一滴封片剂，再将切片有组织的面朝下慢慢放在盖玻片上。使用这两种方法时都应小心，避免在组织和盖玻片间出现气泡。对于不溶于乙醇的染色（如DAB、新品红），可用永久性封片剂。组织切片先用梯度乙醇脱水：

表1.6　免疫组织化学染色：常用"染色剂"或底物*

程序	颜色	溶于乙醇
过氧化物酶		
二氨基联苯胺（DAB）	棕色	不溶
DAB加增强剂	黑色	不溶
3-氨基-9-乙基咔唑（AEC）	红色†	溶
4-氯-1-萘酚（4-CN）	蓝-黑	溶
Hanker-Yates试剂	蓝色	不溶
α-萘酚派若宁	红色	溶
3,3′,5,5′-四甲基联苯胺（TMB）	蓝色	不溶
碱性磷酸酶		
固蓝BB	蓝色	溶
固红TR	红色	溶
新品红	红色	不溶
BCIP-NBT	蓝色	不溶
葡萄糖氧化酶		
四唑	蓝色	不溶
TNBT	黑色	不溶
免疫金		
用银增强	黑色	不溶

*还有其他"染色剂"，但是这里所列的均经过充分论证。从几个公司的目录上可找到多种商业化产品
†AEC有2个反应位点：在过量酶存在的情况下2个都起反应，颜色由红变成棕绿
（引自 Taylor CR, Cote RJ. Immunomicroscopy: A Diagnostic Tool for the Surgical Pathologist, 2nd ed. Philadelphia: WB Saunders, 1994: 67）

90%、100%乙醇各2次；然后在二甲苯中清洗2次，每次3分钟。按前述水性封片剂封片方法封片。注意应在通风橱内操作。

免疫组织化学染色的具体操作步骤见本章附录A。

双重免疫酶标技术

检测石蜡组织切片中第二种抗原常常通过对连续切片中的相邻两个切片进行过氧化物酶染色（图1.19）。虽然这种方法可满足普通用途，但有时，特别是研究的细胞体积小，或者散在分布于其他细胞之间时，要确定相邻切片中特定细胞群的染色模式可能显得困难（图1.20）。

双重免疫酶标技术可在同一张切片上显示两种抗原，并由结合抗体法和不标记抗体法两种方法修改而成。例如，首先采用DAB作反应底物对第一抗原进行染色（呈棕色），第二种抗原的染色可用不同的过氧化物酶底物，如4-氯-1-萘酚（呈蓝色反应产物）。

滴加第二个抗体系列前，是否需洗净第一个抗体（和DAB反应以后）还存在争议。如果必要，清洗可用酸性溶液（通常用pH2.2的氨基乙酸-盐酸缓冲液或1 mol/L 盐酸孵育1小时）或氧化剂溶液（0.15mol $KMnO_4$，0.005mol/L H_2SO_4溶于140V蒸馏水中，pH为1.8）孵育切片，再用1%的Na_2SO_4孵育1分钟。然而

Sternberger 和 Joseph[18]在没有清洗第一套试剂的情况下成功地同时检测了两种抗原。第二个一抗和第一个一抗来自同种动物，检测两种抗原用的是同样的PAP标记试剂。其原理可能是因为DAB多聚体氧化产物（用于第一个抗原-PAP方法）封闭了第一个PAP复合物的催化位点，同时也削弱了第一套抗体的抗原性，因而阻止了和第二套抗体及第二套显色系统的反应。

Lan和同事[142]通过在两个免疫组织化学染色之间增加微波加热程序（10分钟）开发了一个简单、可靠、敏感的多重免疫组织化学染色方法（用于消除前一个免疫组织化学染色试剂），这一方法确保彻底阻止抗体的交叉反应。

为防止第二套抗体和第一套抗体间的交叉反应，可使用不同动物产生的两种特异性一抗，并分别使用种特异性的二抗和相应的不同的酶（如过氧化物酶和葡萄糖氧化酶，或过氧化物酶和碱性磷酸酶）。这种方法的优点是方便，有些试剂（如第一抗体）可以同时滴加以节省时间[147]。

双标记抗原可以同时进行两种抗原染色[148]。Behringer等[149]开发了半抗原-抗半抗原桥联（HAB）方法并用ABC法来进行双重免疫染色。但是，如果要达到同样的免疫染色强度，需要更高的一抗浓度。

当使用双免疫酶标染色时，有时很难辨认同一细胞的两种染色，因为一种染色的反应产物可能覆盖另

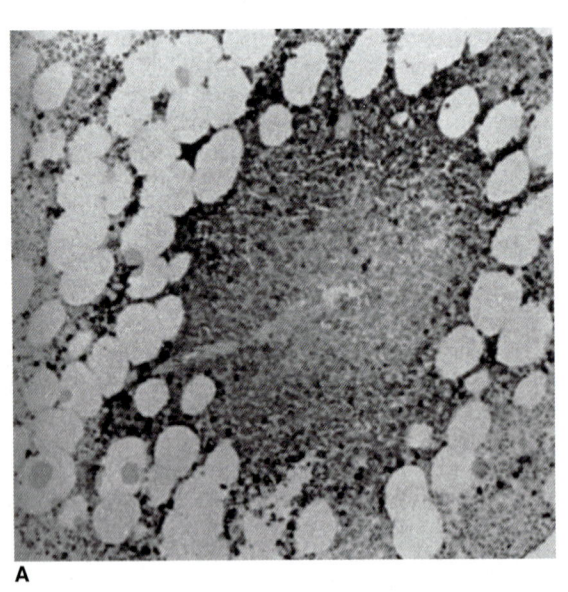 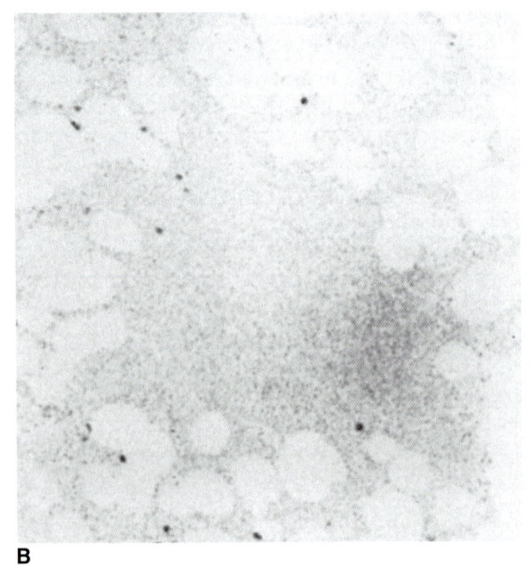

图1.19 （A,B)B5固定骨髓穿刺切片，显示小的孤立结节，由淋巴细胞和少量淋巴浆样淋巴细胞组成，周围有散在浆细胞。很多淋巴和淋巴浆样细胞与抗λ抗体强反应（A）。抗κ抗体只和结节周围的散在浆细胞反应（B，小黑点）。该病人最终显示有小肠孤立性淋巴浆细胞性淋巴瘤（也是λ型）。石蜡切片DAB显色，苏木精复染（×125）；当时未检测到血清副蛋白；可能是因为肿瘤细胞少，不足以产生可检测到的副蛋白；然而疾病的后期出现了"单克隆"IgM（引自Taylor CR, Cote RJ. Immunomicroscopy: A Diagnostic Tool for the Surgical Pathologist, 2nd ed. Philadelphia: WB Saunders, 1994:59）

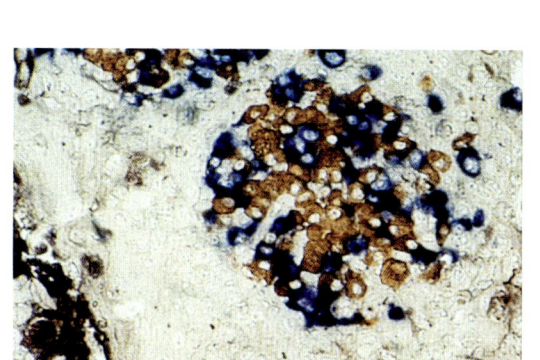

图 1.20　用辣根过氧化物酶和碱性磷酸酶法对淋巴结反应性增生石蜡切片进行 κ（棕色）和 λ（蓝色）双重染色

一染色。在这种情况下可用一个简单的方法加以区别，即在显微镜下观察第一抗原的染色并照相，然后再将第二种抗原染色，对切片重新观察，在相同视野进行照相并进行对比。

也可改进或灵活应用这些染色方法。例如在同一切片中可对 6 种不同的抗原进行染色[150]。联合应用免疫金-银染色（黑色）和免疫过氧化物酶-AEC（红-棕色）或免疫碱性磷酸酶-固红或固蓝进行双重或三重染色[151]。联合应用免疫过氧化物酶-AEC（红色）和免疫碱性磷酸酶-固蓝（蓝色）染色对比度可能更好。在显微镜下仔细观察并控制第二种（和第三种颜色）显色反应，选择应用较敏感的检测系统可在同一张切片上获得最佳对比度的多重染色。在实际工作中，如果应用双重标记方法进行免疫病理诊断时，最好有计算机辅助图像分析系统，能对双重染色的染色强度进行精确测定，对染色信号进行精确定位。在图像分析方面，"光谱图像分析"功能强大，使双重染色更具有可操作性和实用性[152]。

单克隆抗体双重染色的适用方法见附录 B。

自动化

不同实验室间标本固定及处理的方法差异较大，目前还不可能建立一个通用的免疫组织化学染色标准方法。只能在实验室内部建立一个标准的方法。如前述，选择恰当的对照及严格遵照实验各方面的要求，包括试剂的准备和应用、孵育时间的控制等。这些实验室内部的标准可保证实验的准确性和可重复性。这些标准需要进行反复多次而且是快速、准确的试验，因而对自动化仪器有所需求。

自动免疫染色设备出现在 20 世纪 80 年代早期，这一曾经仅小范围应用于科研实验室的设备得到了广泛的应用。为满足日益增长的诊断的需要，有必要使用自动染色设备。随着软件设计的改进、硬件的不断完善，美国大多数免疫组织化学实验室已经应用自动设备，也出现自动细胞图像系统和自动抗原修复系统等设备。

就染色过程而言，人工染色方法的大多数步骤依赖技术人员的熟练程度，为保证染色结果的质量，每一步骤都要求技术人员按规程仔细操作，包括切片的准备、试剂和抗体的应用、孵育时间的控制、切片的清洗和擦拭等，这些步骤大多是缓慢和重复的，如果忽略某一步骤，或操作的顺序错误，或在染色过程中没有保持切片湿度，孵育时间过长或过短，抗体稀释度太高或太低，底物反应不足或过度等，都会大大增加出现错误的可能性。除了这些技术上的影响因素外，还有试剂的影响，如不同的染色剂、缓冲液、酶以及抗体的不同活性等。随着自动化设备的出现，这些步骤大都可进行标准化操作。

自动染色仪的设计模仿人工染色方法。适合自动化流程的步骤包括添加试剂、组织孵育、切片清洗。这一程序可在一天内完成[153]。切片可以垂直排放，试剂由上加入通过重力作用和由顶端到底部的毛细管的作用向下，代替了切片和盖玻片之间的液体。相反，试剂可从下面的槽中通过底部到顶端的毛细管的作用，在相邻的垂直夹在一起的两个切片之间向上攀升。用第二种方法时，液体由切片的底端吸干。第三种方法是切片水平放在平台上，试剂和缓冲液用一个探头、一次性吸管，或者试剂测试包加在切片的上面，再通过一个水平的吸管吸走。

毛细管染色仪的效率与毛细管的充盈和排空能力有关，在一定程度上依赖于所用试剂的张力。如水溶性溶液表面张力较大，比乙醇溶液难以充盈毛细管，这可能会造成试剂上升不足，影响染色结果。因此，使用从下面抽吸试剂的毛细管染色仪时，应注意这一问题。由于此原因，建议使用双层切片，将对照切片放在上层。这样可监控试剂上升的高度。利用重力的毛细管设备不存在这一问题。用这种仪器，对照切片最好放在底层，以便对试剂用量是否充分进行监测。这两种毛细管方法的缺点是不能用在厚的、疏松的或组织有皱褶的切片，这些都可能影响毛细管的空间，导致染色不好或气泡的存在。有些毛细管染色仪要求使用特制载玻片，这种载玻片夹在一起时具有一定的空隙，用来解决这类问题。

根据不同实验室的需要，可选择不同用途的自动染色仪[154]。总体来说，操作标准应满足所有实验室。首先，在自动免疫染色仪使用前，应进行平行研究，自动染色的结果应该相当于或好于人工染色结果，用同一抗体对同一组织（如阳性对照）的自动染色结果在实验室内应具有重复性；染色仪应能适用于多种抗体和检测系统，并适用于各种各样的抗原和染色方法；软件应具备灵活的程序，使用方便；理想的染色仪使用简单，染色过程中不需技术人员花费过多的时间；应能精确添加试剂，并完全覆盖组织；试剂的蒸发丢失和加样时带走的试剂量的损失应保持最少状态。如果染色过程发生错误，染色仪还应具有错误追溯程序并能报告问题。很多厂商供应专用的试剂、酶、染色剂和复染剂，与染色仪配合使用。专用试剂的染色方案不能随意改变，通常这些试剂较贵。有些即用型试剂印有条码，利于计算机跟踪和控制试剂的体积、编号和有效期，有助于质量控制。相反，开放的自动染色系统更灵活，允许使用其他试剂和染色方法。这些方案可以客户化，并能储存以便随时使用。

免疫染色自动化有几个优点：自动化的价值在于提供了标准的微环境，使得实验室内不同染色间具有一致性，避免重复操作；精确加入昂贵的试剂，更为经济；不需要守候机器，不仅节约时间，也节省人力；自动染色仪可通过软件界面指导操作过程，节省技术培训的费用和时间；从安全角度来说，使用稳定、密封的自动化工作站能减少污染，并协助处理有害的化学物质，增加生物安全性。其他优点还包括增加每次染色的切片数量，通过加热和混匀加快了反应速度，节约实验时间。最后，大多数系统还对染色过程中的每一步骤提供计算机检测的说明和报告[155,156]。

抗原修复的自动化最近已开始应用。抗原修复方法始见于20世纪90年代。由于该技术自身多种不确定性，标准化一直比较困难。这些不确定因素包括微波炉的体积和功率、修复液的温度、修复的时间和冷却的速度等；也包括微波炉内切片和容器的数量以及这些容器的体积和材料。控制这些不确定因素才能获得稳定可靠的结果。

目前也出现了自动定量免疫组织化学染色等技术。这些技术对诊断、预后判断和治疗有较大价值。自动细胞图像系统可用于检测分子标志物、激素受体，或肿瘤的微转移[157,158]。这种自动化系统使用标准的免疫细胞化学染色方法，并应用自动显微镜技术，即通过对靶细胞的一百多种形态学参数进行评估，进行标准化打分和定量报告染色结果。细胞的图像和分析结果可以储存，以便必要时进行复查、确认。

尽管出现了这些新的自动化技术，但仍然存在一些问题。如实验组织选择的不恰当、组织固定错误，或脱水或切片过程中的问题，这些都会影响抗原的检测结果。这些自动化技术并不能代替病理医师选择适当的实验方法进行正确判断，因而，也并非是提高实验室质量控制标准的必要手段，只是在高水平的实验室更能发挥自动染色仪的效用。然而，自动化技术能够提供可重复的、标准的结果，以此为基础，将能发展和完善定量免疫组织化学染色和计算机图像分析，使组织形态学和化学方法能综合应用于疾病的诊断、预后和治疗。

技术问题

免疫组织化学是多步骤的实验诊断程序，包括适当的选材、固定、脱水和染色等，但仍然需要有经验的病理医师作最后的诊断。在确认结果时，应根据细胞内特异性抗原 - 抗体反应的有色产物的存在与否、分布的模式和强度进行正确判断。染色结果可能是局限的或弥漫的，可以是细胞核着色、胞浆着色或膜着色。如因技术问题没有获得预期的染色结果，必须系统地寻找问题，这一过程中的每一个不确定因素都应该逐步地分别检查（表1.7）。

表1.7 各种问题的发现与解决措施

组 织	预处理	检测系统
病人组织	二甲苯	连接和标记
固定	乙醇	兼容性
组织处理	水	失效期
对照组织	抗原修复	染色剂
固定		准备
组织处理		孵育时间
		失效期
固 定	**封 闭**	**实验结果**
固定适当	过氧化物酶封闭	阳性染色
固定过度	生物素封闭	阴性染色
固定不足	背景封闭	灶状或弱阳性
延迟固定		背景染色
		人工假象染色
组织处理	**抗 体**	**结果对照**
脱水	预先稀释浓度	阳性染色
包埋	失效期	阴性染色
切片	储存	背景染色
封片	污染	人工假象染色
组织切片	孵育	

技术问题一般可分为两类，分别发生在染色前和染色时。未及时固定、固定过度、固定不充分及固定不均匀等都可影响结果，这在前面已经讨论。目前，大多数实验室固定后的脱水过程由仪器自动完成，但组织脱水过程对结果的影响可能没有得到足够认识。如石蜡包埋之前组织脱水不充分可严重影响结果，定期配制新的乙醇溶液可减少或防止脱水不充分。其他一些在处理过程中出现的问题包括使用不适当的载玻片导致脱片，切片不仔细造成的组织皱褶或折叠可导致染色不均匀。组织脱水后和染色前对切片进行的一系列处理过程中（如酶消化和/或抗原修复）也有较多的不稳定因素，技术问题同样不可避免。由个人操作或仪器故障引起的错误对免疫组织化学染色结果的影响还没有得到充分的研究。

根据实验切片和阳性对照片染色结果的模式，错误的染色结果大致可分下列五种情况[151]，我们将逐一讨论：

1. 实验组织和阳性对照都不着色。
2. 实验组织不染色，阳性对照阳性染色适当。
3. 实验组织染色过浅，阳性对照阳性染色适当。
4. 实验组织和/或阳性对照有背景染色。
5. 实验组织和/或阳性对照存在人为染色（假性染色）。

样本和对照均不着色

当样本和对照都不着色时，必须检查是否遵循正确的染色程序，即检查所有的染色步骤次序是否正确，孵育时间是否充分，是否遗漏任何试剂；查看抗体特别是第一抗体的稀释度；也应检查抗体的失效期和储存条件，过期的抗体可能引起假阴性结果；另外，储存在自动除霜的冰箱内的抗体经反复冻融，可导致抗体失效；检查各种缓冲液及pH值是否适当，如用于过氧化物酶的缓冲液不应含叠氮钠；应尽量避免实验过程中样本干燥；试剂用量是否正确、有无应用湿盒等。另外，还有染色剂问题，必须确定染色剂溶液配制是否适当，可通过向少量的配制好的染色剂溶液中加入标记试剂，观察有无颜色变化来检测染色剂，注意染色剂溶液有效期很短。最后，不染色的原因可能因免疫组织化学染色前不当的预处理、复染或封片引起。例如AEC不能和含乙醇、二甲苯或甲苯的复染剂和封片剂一起使用，因为这些化学物质可溶解AEC和底物反应产生的可溶性有色沉淀物。

实验组织不着色，阳性对照阳性染色适当

如果只是阳性对照显示阳性染色结果，可假定染色程序操作正确，并且试剂有效。在这种情况下，问题发生在染色前而不是在染色过程中。因此，可能是组织固定不当、脱水过程不当或预处理不当，或者上述几种原因综合造成的。

福尔马林固定的问题包括固定不及时、固定过度、固定不充分和固定不均匀[155]。有些靶抗原易发生自溶现象，由于这一原因，标本应尽快固定，最好在离体30分钟以内，固定不及时会使抗原、抗体不能进行有效反应和染色。过度固定也可导致不染色，可能由于抗原交联和固定剂的污染。因此福尔马林固定时间不应超过48小时。在固定不充分时，只有标本边缘的组织有时间吸收固定剂，而组织的中央区域仍未固定。在这些中央区域标本会在组织脱水时被乙醇进行凝固性固定，这将造成染色不均，有时使用不同抗体或不当应用抗原修复技术也能造成中央染色过强或边缘区染色过强。

不着色也可能是组织处理过程造成的，可能是没有因固定出现的问题重要，所以对这个问题的研究较少。组织处理过程存在的问题主要是用久置的乙醇引起脱水不完全。另外，热敏感的表位可能因包埋时蜡温过高而丢失。因此包埋时蜡温不应超过56℃（表1.8）。

实验组织染色过浅，阳性对照阳性染色适当

实验组织固定和/或脱水不当可造成标本染色过浅，而对照染色正常。上述所分析的引起不着色的原因都适用于染色过弱这一情况。需要强调的是对照切片和实验组织的固定与脱水方法必须一样。另一个造成实验组织染色过浅的原因是实验组织抗原含量过少。如果发现是由于固定不当导致实验组织的抗原浓度低，可提高抗体的浓度，延长孵育的时间，或提高反应的温度。这些措施都可提高染色的强度。另外，如果在加抗体前切片仍遗留过多的缓冲液可导致抗体稀释而使实验组织染色过浅（表1.8）。

背景染色

任何不是特异性抗原-抗体反应结果的染色都是非特异性背景染色。这种染色结果可用阴性对照染色来确认。有很多情况可引起背景染色，最常见的原因是抗体与组织中的结缔组织(如胶原)的带电成分间的非特异性结合。这种情况，可用与二抗来源相同的非

免疫性动物的血清封闭以减少非特异性染色；提高缓冲液中的盐浓度也可能有帮助。另一个常见的背景染色的原因是实验组织中存在过氧化物酶，如红细胞（假过氧化物酶）和白细胞（内源性过氧化物酶）的过氧化物酶没有清除，可能增加背景染色[160]。某些组织中富含内源性生物素（如肝和肾），常可引起假阳性信号，这种情况可通过更换另一种不含抗生物素蛋白-生物素的检测系统或者用抗生物素蛋白预处理组织来减少背景信号的产生。切片过厚、固定不好的组织或坏死组织背景染色都比较高；抗体溶液本身因素也可能引起染色背景的增高，如溶液里存在抗体微粒（由于抗体反复冻融造成）或抗体浓度过高。其他少见的背景染色过高的原因和组织脱水过程有关，如石蜡去除不完全，可通过组织以外的弥漫的背景阳性染色来识别。背景染色还可由实验步骤间切片清洗不彻底或缓冲液被污染而造成。另一个引起非特异性染色的原因是染色剂未完全溶解或浓度过高引起染色剂-底物过度反应，可通过过滤染色剂溶液或降低其浓度来解决（表1.9）。

假性染色

组织细胞中某些特殊物质可能导致非特异性假性染色。如有未溶解的色素沉淀，可以通过过滤去除；有时，B5固定的组织可能由于脱锌不完全出现弥漫性黑色沉淀，可在染色前通过除汞来解决这一问题。有时内源性色素，如含铁血黄素或黑色素的信号和免疫组织化学的染色信号难以区别，但是这种染色在阴性对照片中也可见到。如果没有阴性对照比较，可用与色素颜色不同的显色剂（如染成红色的AEC）加以区别。有时，某些微生物如细菌或真菌污染也可导致假性染色（表1.10）。

因为免疫组织化学染色的多步骤特点，会出现多

表1.8 技术问题和解决措施：不着色或着色浅

问　题	解决措施
固定不当	避免固定延迟（>30分钟）或固定过度（>40小时）
脱水不完全	检查脱水程序，按常规换试剂（如乙醇）
石蜡过热	监测石蜡温度（<56℃）
加热时间太长	调整抗原修复时间
未遵守染色步骤	查看实验操作程序
试剂无效	查看失效期，查看储存条件，查看和其他试剂是否配套，检查pH值
抗体过度稀释	检查抗体的滴度，增加抗体浓度，延长孵育时间，升高反应温度，检查切片上残留缓冲液的量
染色中组织干燥	遵照操作手册，保持标本湿润；用湿盒以防水分蒸发
孵育时间不足	延长孵育时间直至获得预期染色强度，加热，提高抗体浓度
染色剂无效	向标记物溶液中加染色剂，监测颜色变化

表1.9 技术问题和解决措施：背景染色

问　题	解决措施
非特异性蛋白结合	用同种动物非免疫血清作二抗，向缓冲液中加盐
石蜡去除不完全	只用完全脱蜡的切片
固定不佳或组织坏死	确认组织固定适当，避开组织坏死区
抗体浓度不当	检查抗体滴度，降低抗体浓度，缩短孵育时间，降低反应温度
内源性生物素	用抗生物素蛋白封闭
切片清洗不彻底	根据实验程序适当清洗切片
染色剂染色太深	检查染色剂-底物反应时间，过滤染色剂，降低染色剂浓度

表1.10 技术问题和解决措施：人工假染色

问　题	解决措施
存在染色剂或复染液沉淀	过滤染色剂或复染液沉淀
B5固定组织黑色沉淀	染色之前去除汞
内源性色素与特异性阳性染色混淆	在阴性对照中寻找这些色素，用对比度好的染色剂
微生物污染	经常更换试剂，用新鲜试剂，检查失效期

免疫组织化学技术：原理、局限性和标准化

种技术问题。严格遵守质量控制规程，并避免大部分问题的发生，同时应认真判断染色结果，作出正确诊断（图1.21～1.36）。

免疫组织化学染色定量及标准化

免疫组织化学染色标准化主要是将其定量或半定量，应将其标准化，这也越来越受到基础和临床研究的重视。免疫组织化学染色的转化型研究依赖于回顾性研究，可利用现存的样本及对以前公布的临床数据和长期有效随访的系列数据进行研究。对世界各地保存的各种大量病理切片标本进行回顾性调查和转化型研究，可大大促进免疫组织化学技术对各种预后因素的研究。

在这一研究中，"标准化"是一个巨大的挑战，很难作到完善，因为从标本固定和脱水程序、抗原修复、免疫组织化学染色试剂和方法的选择直到最后的

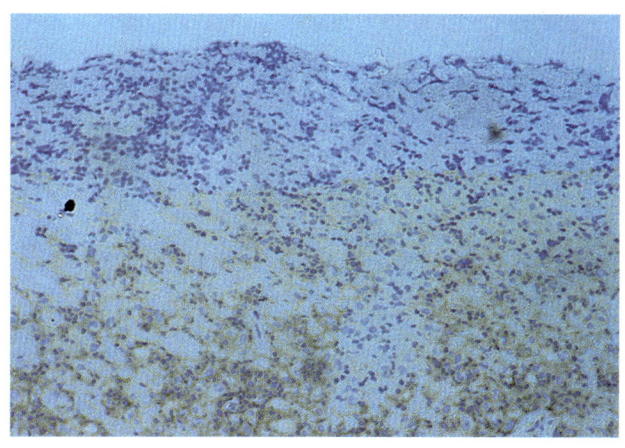

图1.21 用采用毛细吸管原理的自动染色仪染的切片，显示试剂上升不足

"评分"及意义评估等均受很多因素的影响。免疫组织化学染色标准化的方法之一是南加州一个实验室推行的一种称之为"总体实验"的方法[2]。其要点是要求

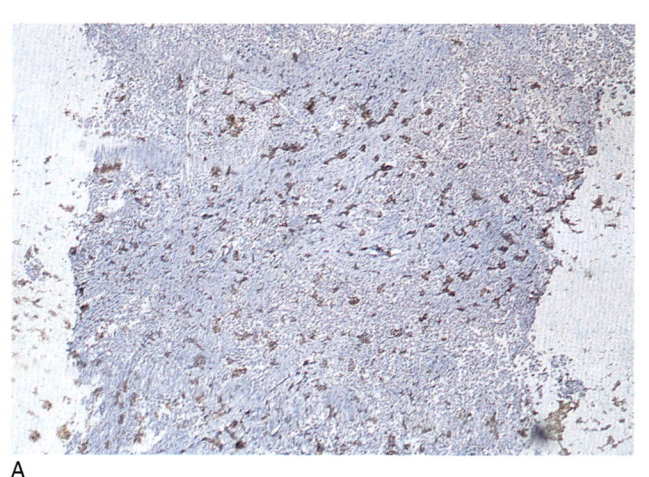

A

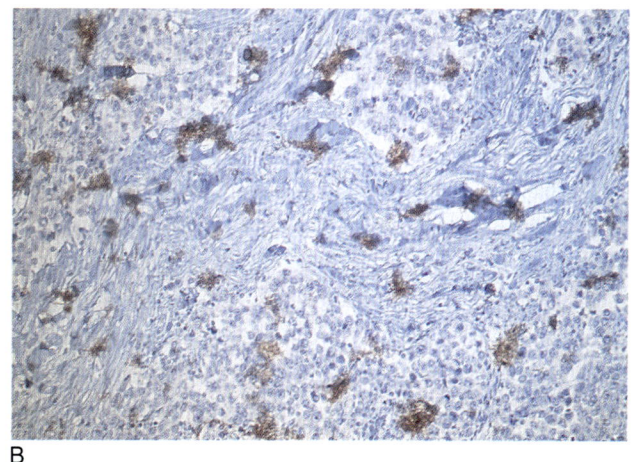

B

图1.22 (A,B)"染料斑点"，由染料沉淀未被完全溶解造成的人工假象

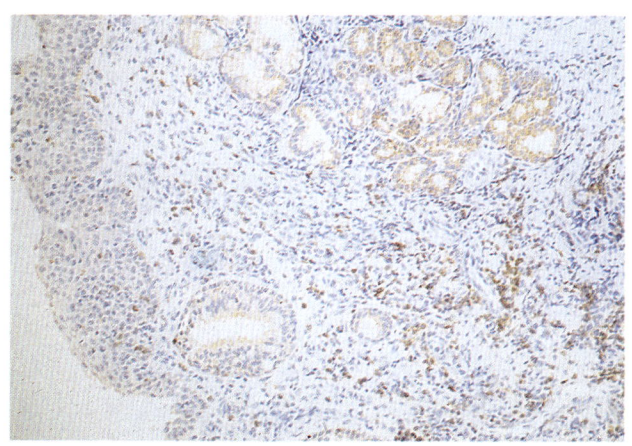

图1.23 腮腺组织切片CD3染色显示散在T淋巴细胞和腺上皮非特异性胞浆颗粒样着色

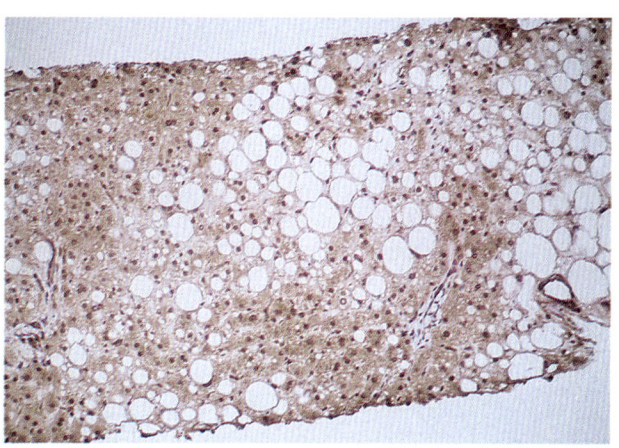

图1.24 肝组织切片，显示内源性过氧化物酶引起的非特异性背景染色

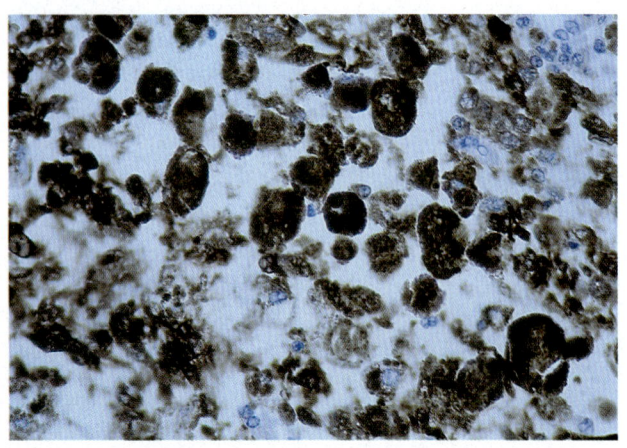

图 1.25 含色素的嗜色素细胞，不要和染色剂混淆

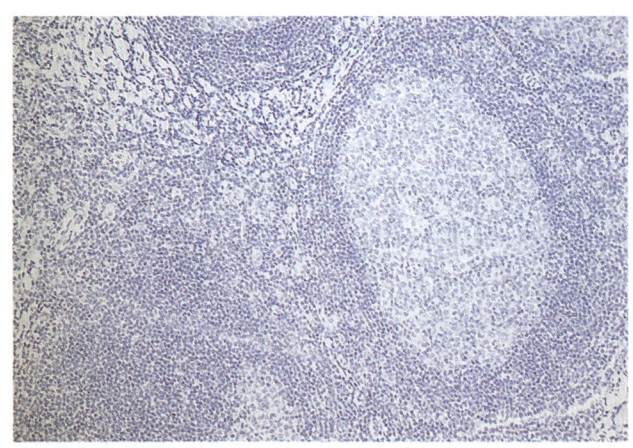

图 1.26 未使用一抗的淋巴结切片

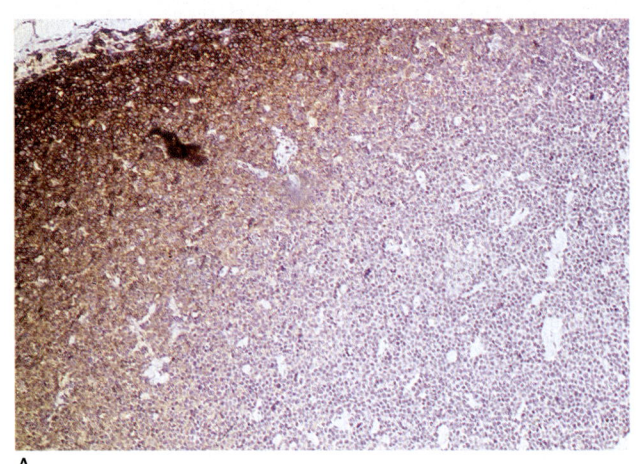

A

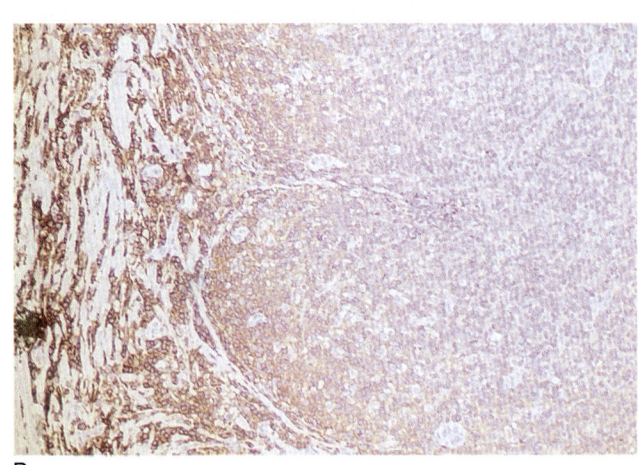

B

图 1.27 淋巴结切片 CD45 染色（A 和 B）显示固定引起的假象。包膜下区显示清楚的胞膜染色（A）和组织固定不充分的切片边缘区（B）

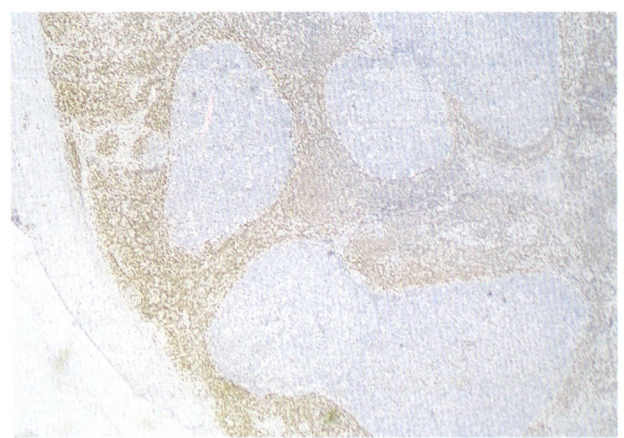

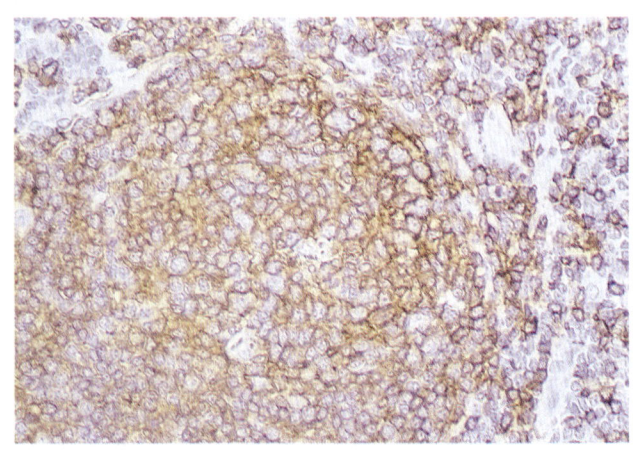

图 1.28 另 1 个淋巴结切片 bcl-2 染色显示类似的固定引起的假象，（由边缘）向淋巴结中央逐渐丢失可见的染色信号

图 1.29 淋巴结切片 CD20 染色，显示生发中心区 B 细胞胞膜强着色

免疫组织化学技术：原理、局限性和标准化

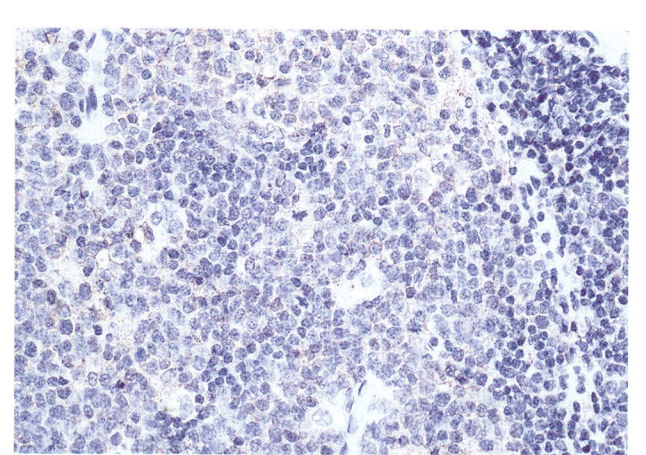

图 1.30 相似的淋巴结切片 CD20 染色，显示生发中心区 B 淋巴细胞染色不理想，生发中心可通过散在的吞噬细胞可染体的存在来识别

病理医师必须注意标本的取材、固定的方法和时间、抗原修复的方法、试剂的选择和实验的具体操作、对照的应用、染色结果的解释和确认等每一环节和每一个步骤（表 1.11）。

从实际操作看，库存标本的免疫组织化学染色标准化最难之处是福尔马林对组织标本的影响和抗原修复对这一影响的修复程度。用试验组合法对抗原修复程序的优化已讨论过。标准的抗原修复程序对整个免疫组织化学染色的标准化尤为关键。

免疫组织化学染色标准化的另一关键因素是要从无数商品化的检测和放大系统中选择一种并合理应用。我们将放大和加强系统分成三类（表 1.12），分别称为检测前放大（一抗孵育前）、检测放大（从一

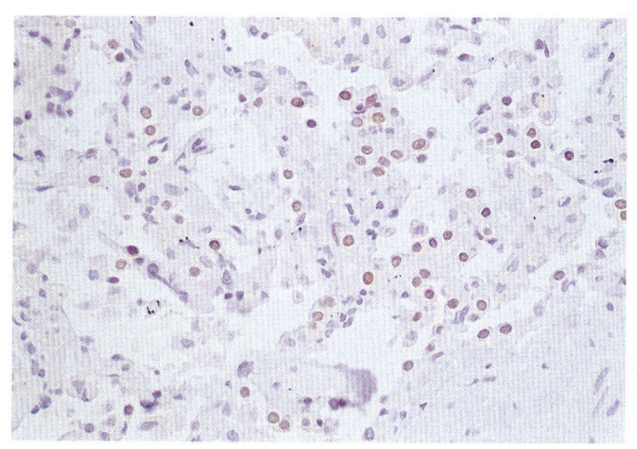

图 1.31 正常肺组织的 TTF-1 染色，显示肺泡表面细胞（肺泡细胞）特异性核染色

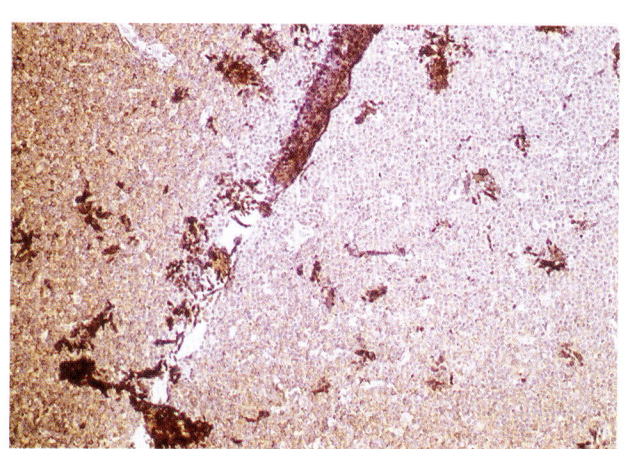

图 1.32 淋巴结切片 CD43 染色，显示脱水问题造成的组织裂痕和折叠，引起染色不均和染料沉淀。所有这些假象都影响对结果的解释

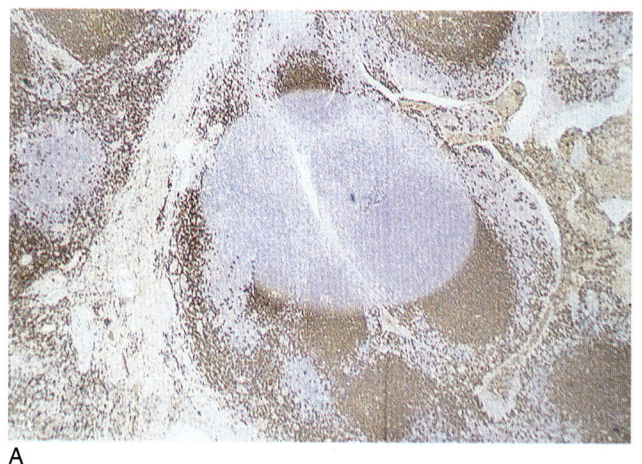

A

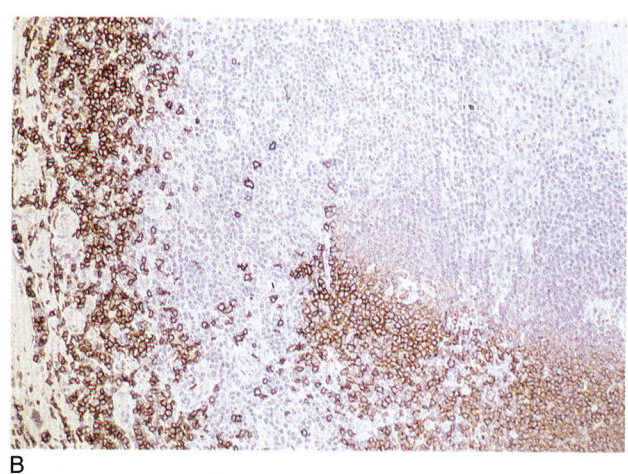

B

图 1.33 (A,B) 淋巴结切片 CD20 染色，显示低倍和高倍镜下"气泡假象"，是染色过程中形成的非亲水性气泡

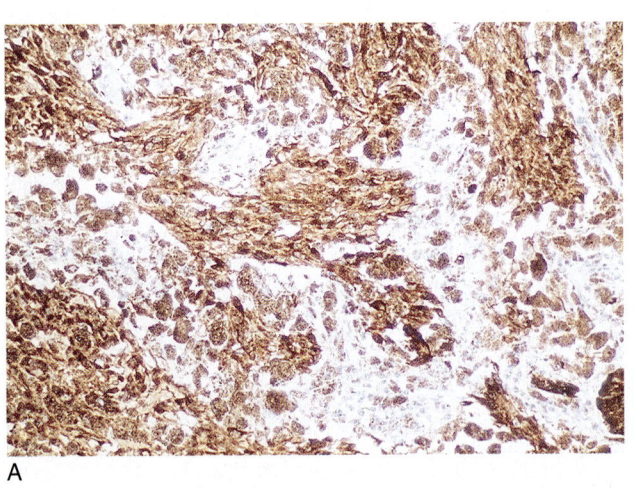
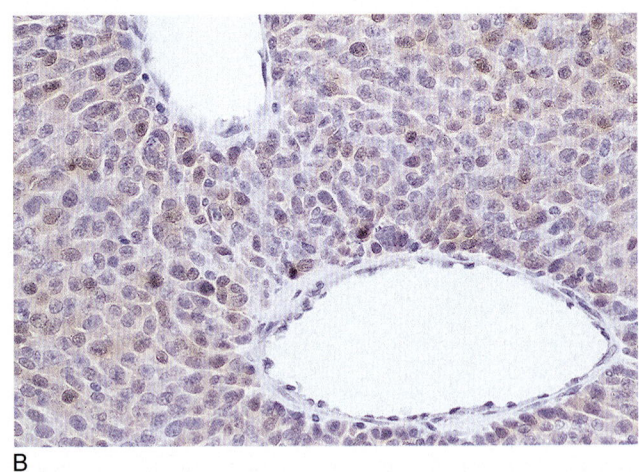

图1.34 (A,B) 恶性黑色素瘤S-100染色。左图的梭形肿瘤细胞染色过度,以至于很难辨认是否是核染色,同样右图血管周围的梭形肿瘤细胞显示逐渐增强的染色,很容易判断为核阳性染色

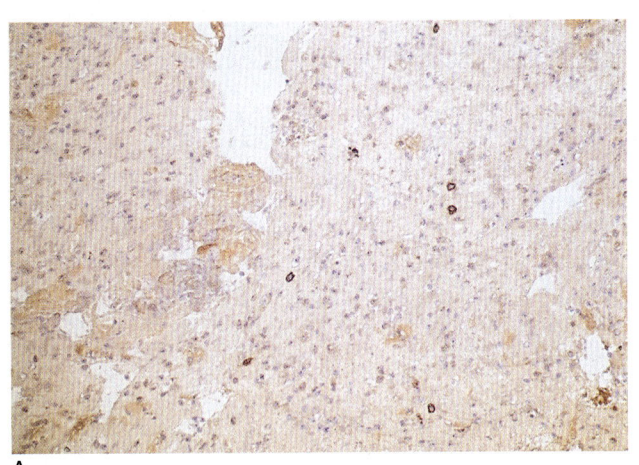
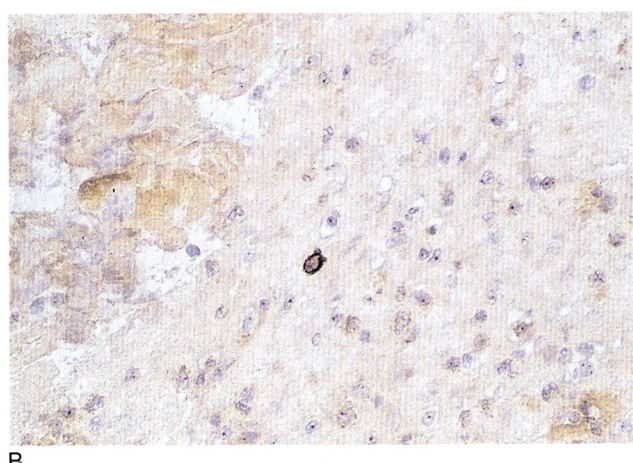

图1.35 (A,B) 细胞块切片CD20染色。可见均质的蛋白质样物质背景染色。B图中高倍镜突出显示阳性B淋巴细胞和CD20本应阴性着色的散在T淋巴细胞呈核异常阳性

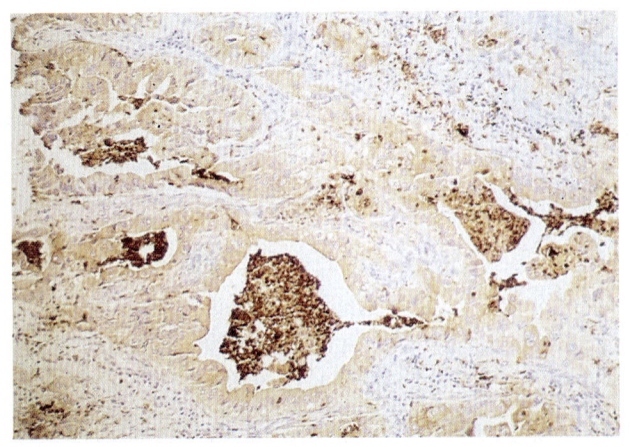

图1.36 腺癌切片CEA染色,显示阳性染色的多形核中性粒细胞表现为强内源性过氧化物酶染色,间质内也有散在分布

抗孵育到标记物孵育)和检测后放大(标记后)[91]。

检测前放大

抗原修复是有效、简单的检测前放大[38, 39, 54-57, 92]。抗原修复产生的信号放大是福尔马林处理影响的某些抗原表位的恢复而使抗原性增加[59, 60]。在某种意义上,抗原修复是恢复自然的抗原-抗体反应,更有利于特异性结合,但并不增加非特异性结合,因而可提高信-噪比。

检测期放大

如前所述,随着染色方法的快速发展,也逐渐反映

免疫组织化学技术：原理、局限性和标准化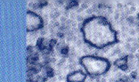

表 1.11 免疫组织化学"总体实验"的内容

实验程序	质量保证	责任者
临床问题，实验选择	免疫组织化学必要性，选择染色	外科病理医师，有时为临床医师
标本的获取及处理	标本收集、固定、脱水、切片	病理医师／病理技术员
问题分析	称职的医师与技术员，实验室内和实验室间实验程序的熟练测试	病理医师／病理技术员
结果的校准和报告	根据对照确定阳性／阴性的标准，报告的内容及形式，出报告的时间	病理医师／病理技术员
解释，意义	有经验的合格的病理医师，熟练解释；诊断、预后意义，适当的相关性	外科病理医师和／或临床医师

（引自 Taylor CR. Biotech Histochem 1992: 67:110-117）

表 1.12 免疫组织化学三种基本信号放大方法分类

分 类	基本原理和作用模式	优点和问题
检测前放大：		
抗原修复	修复福尔马林引起的蛋白质结构改变，在减轻背景染色的同时显著放大信号	是所有放大方法中最简单、最经济的方法（加热），对有些抗体／抗原无效
检测期放大：	增加标记信号的积累（酶或其他）	多重标记技术系统和多聚体基础上的多步骤检测系统更简单，作为非生物素检测，避免了内源性生物素反应问题
其他多步骤检测系统；PAP、ABC、APAAP、B-SA	PAP，增强 2～50 倍；ABC，2～100 倍	
逐步放大	重复检测循环	
多聚体和多标记放大系统	目前有 EnVision、PowerVision、EPOS 试剂盒；平均一抗稀释度提高 2～5 倍，我们实验 PCNA 稀释度提高 1：160	
检测后放大		程序复杂，涉及重复反应周期，逐步放大的缺点是消耗劳动力及经费，随信号的放大增强背景染色增加
用金属、咪唑等增加 DAB 显色反应和 CARD	增强显色反应	
	HRP 催化生物素化酪氨酸在 HRP 部位的沉积	
抗终产物（EP）	抗 EP ＋生物素化连接物＋ HRP 标记，信号增强 16 倍	
金／银增强法	增强银染色	

PAP，过氧化物酶-抗过氧化物酶；ABC，抗生物素蛋白-生物素复合物；APAAP，碱性磷酸酶-抗碱性磷酸酶；B-SA，生物素-链卵白素；PCNA，增殖细胞核抗原；EPOS，增强的多聚体一步染色（DAKO）；CARD，催化报告沉淀；HRP，辣根过氧化物酶
（引自 Shi S-R, Guo J, Cote RJ, et al.Sensitivity and detection efficiency of a novel two-step detection system (PowerVision) for immunohistochemistry. Appl Immunohistochem Mol Morphology 1999; 7: 201-208）

出目前使用的三步检测系统的一些不足，如复杂耗时的染色程序，难以定量，一些难检抗体的检测效率低下，以及内源性生物素和酶活性对检测系统的影响等。另外，如前述一些计算机辅助自动染色系统的出现部分解决了稳定性、实验室工作劳动强度和费用等问题，并使实验的可重复性有大幅度改进。然而，有时这些反而给结果总体的可重复性带来不利影响。因为，目前"任何实验室"都可在缺乏必要背景知识的情况下开展免疫染色实验，完全依赖自动染色程序和质量控制方法，而对免疫染色过程和影响因素没有足够的认识。如果在科学术语中出现这种现状就难以令人满意，必须指出，著名的大型生产商将继续对试剂的质量进行改进。另外，说明书也更加全面并且在染色和分析结果时更具实用价值。或许，最大的问题是技术人员和病理医生常常忽视阅读说明书，或者忽略了其中的内容。就作者的经验，由于忽略了阅读说明书详

细内容而最常造成滥用的是由DAKO公司生产的HER-2试剂盒。

检测后放大

检测后放大的方法试图增加染色剂反应。其主要缺点是增加免疫组织化学实验的复杂程度（增加了较难控制的染色步骤）和增加非特异性染色背景，信－噪比降低，使判断更加困难。一般不建议常规使用这种方法。

"参考标准"的建立和组织切片抗原含量评估曲线

如前所述，目前仅是实验室内质量控制，如果应用得当，可提高实验室的质量控制水平，但由于实验方法和实验产品的局限性，不能保证不同实验室间的重复性。理论上，可能生产蛋白纯品（抗原），进行稀释后为Western blotting和免疫组织化学染色提供一系列已知参考标准。"矩阵模型"[161]技术可为待测蛋白（抗原）建立有效的人工对照（见下文）。通过这一方法，用"标准曲线"得出一转化公式来计算包括抗原修复在内的各种染色条件下福尔马林固定、石蜡包埋组织切片中待测抗原的精确含量。这种方法也可用做"预实验"来建立免疫组织化学染色的标准程序，也可用做质量控制的参考标准。主要的生产商在测试试剂盒时开始包括监控原材料，特别是分级说明（量化）的地方。这对判断阳性程度是有价值的。计算机图像分析技术也有了改进，在量化方面它明显优于人的眼睛，前提条件是必须设定内对照。

"人工组织"（图1.37）是一种在离心培养条件下生长的人造组织块，为整个实验过程对照提供了一种新的方式。"人工组织"由两到三种或者更多种细胞系构成，在标准条件下共培养，产生一种人造组织块（如可包括纤维母细胞、乳腺癌细胞和内皮细胞），作为一种标准参照物，可大量供应，为多种常用抗体提供对照，包括组织固定和操作步骤的对照。

抗原矩阵模型：人工阳性组织对照

为了对在不同时间、不同实验室、不同技术人员所做的免疫组织化学染色进行质量控制，需要有一个"通用"的阳性对照或"参考标准"，现已用纯品蛋白质的矩阵模型系统生产的"人工组织"建立参考标准，该"人工组织"可用福尔马林固定、石蜡包埋，并可用与待检实验标本相同的免疫组织化学染色步骤来处理。以这些阳性对照组织切片（抗原含量已知）的免

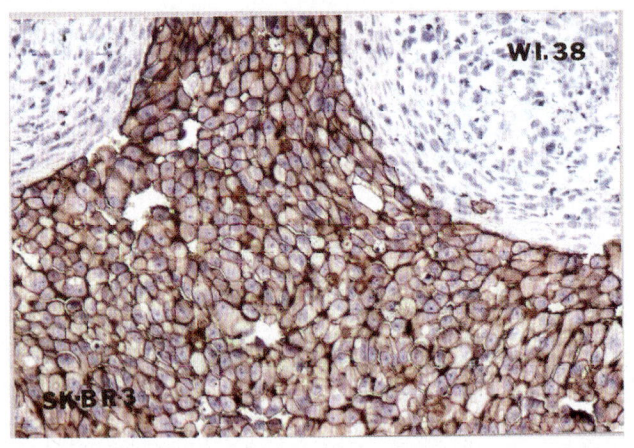

图1.37 人造类乳腺组织HER-2染色，乳腺上皮成分（MCF-7细胞系）呈阳性染色，但纤维母细胞呈阴性（合作项目，Dr. Ingram M, Dr. Imam A, Dr. Taylor C, 2002, 美国国家肿瘤研究所IMAT项目资助）

疫组织化学染色强度来计算检测标本的抗原含量。

Battifora等人创建了"Quicgel"方法，是用乳腺癌细胞系制作人工组织对照块，该组织块和临床待检标本放在同一组织盒内，同时进行预处理和免疫组织化学染色[162]。与"Quicgel"法相比较，矩阵模型有以下几个优点：

1. "Quicgel"法必须有适当的表达待测抗原的细胞系，该细胞系在细胞培养和储存过程中生物学性质应保持不变。

2. 纯蛋白矩阵模型建立在不同稀释度的精确蛋白质含量的基础上，有蛋白质含量恒定的优点。

矩阵模型组织和"Quicgel"法一样，可用和常规石蜡包埋组织一样的方法脱水和储存。两种方法都有其实际应用价值，但目前还未广泛应用。

结　语

目前，免疫组织化学染色方法使得外科诊断病理更加科学，但仍不完善。其主要缺点是缺少对靶抗原的定量评估，特别是在临床和实验病理研究中，对定量免疫组织化学染色方法对影响疾病的预后和转归的标志物进行研究时显得尤为重要。值得注意的是，有关免疫组织化学标准化的方法同样适用于原位杂交技术。目前，应建立标准化检测体系，结合反应产物计算机辅助分析，对待测抗原进行精确定量，也为分子形态学（显微镜下定位蛋白质、DNA和RNA）的研究提供可靠的实验方法。

免疫组织化学技术：原理、局限性和标准化

附录 A：简化程序

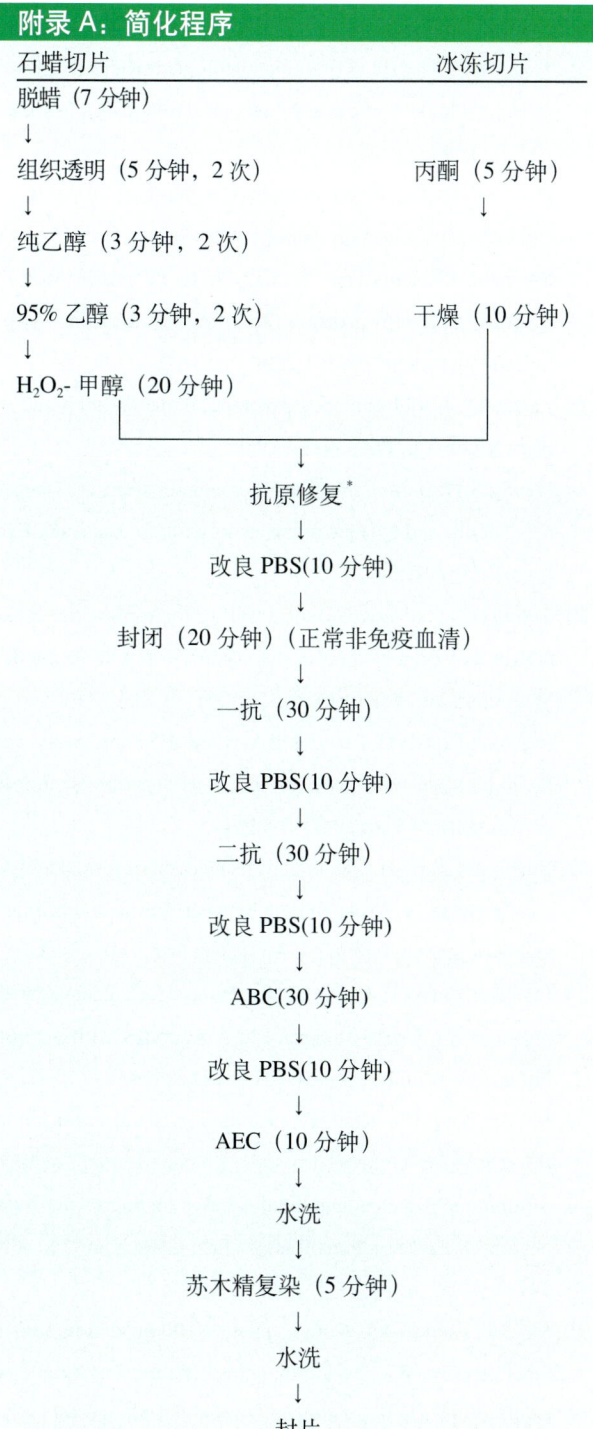

石蜡切片	冰冻切片
脱蜡（7分钟）	
↓	
组织透明（5分钟，2次）	丙酮（5分钟）
↓	↓
纯乙醇（3分钟，2次)	
↓	
95% 乙醇（3分钟，2次)	干燥（10分钟）
↓	
H_2O_2-甲醇（20分钟）	

↓
抗原修复*
↓
改良 PBS(10 分钟)
↓
封闭（20 分钟）（正常非免疫血清）
↓
一抗（30 分钟）
↓
改良 PBS(10 分钟)
↓
二抗（30 分钟）
↓
改良 PBS(10 分钟)
↓
ABC(30 分钟)
↓
改良 PBS(10 分钟)
↓
AEC（10 分钟）
↓
水洗
↓
苏木精复染（5 分钟）
↓
水洗
↓
封片

* 多种方法
PBS，磷酸盐缓冲液；ABC，抗生物素蛋白-生物素复合物；AEC，3-氨基-9-乙基咔唑
（引自 Taylor CR, Cote RJ. Immunomicroscopy: A Diagnostic Tool for the Surgical Pathologist, 2nd ed. Philadelphia: WB Saunders, 1994:422)

附录 B：双重染色

有一段时间用鼠单克隆抗体作双重标记在我们实验室已成为常规。该方法可用于冰冻切片，也可用于细胞离心涂片。

简单地说，染色程序相继应用两种不同的染色系统，一抗均采用鼠单克隆抗体。第一种标记是间接ABC过氧化物方法，用生物素化马抗鼠IgG连接ABC过氧化物酶，AEC为底物。第二种标记是间接共轭法，用山羊抗鼠 IgG 连接碱性磷酸酶，固蓝作为底物。对照显示未能检测到第二标记系统（山羊抗鼠 Ig-碱性磷酸酶）和第一抗体结合；这种情况可能归功于原子的空间干扰。由于使用可溶于乙醇的 AEC，封片剂用缓冲甘油胶。

ABC，抗生物素蛋白-生物素复合物；AEC，3-氨基-9-乙基咔唑
（引自 Taylor CR, Cote RJ. Immunomicroscopy: A Diagnostic Tool for the Surgical Pathologist, 2nd ed. Philadelphia: WB Saunders, 1994:424)

参考文献

1. Coons AH, Creech HJ, Jones RN. Immunological properties of an antibody containing a fluorescent group. Proc Soc Exp Biol Med 1941; 47:200.
2. Taylor CR. The current role of immunohistochemistry in diagnostic pathology. Adv Pathol Lab Med 1994; 7:59.
3. Taylor CR. An exaltation of experts: Concerted efforts in the standardization of immunohistochemistry. Hum Pathol 1994; 25:2.
4. Taylor CR, Cote RJ, eds. Immunomicroscopy: a diagnostic tool for the surgical pathologist, 2nd edn. Philadelphia: WB Saunders; 1994.
5. Avrameas S. Enzyme markers: Their linkage with proteins and use in immunohistochemistry. Histochem J 1972; 4:321.
6. Nakane PK, Pierce GBJ. Enzyme-labeled antibodies for the light and electron microscopic localization of tissue antigens. J Cell Biol 1967; 33:307.
7. Adams JC. Biotin amplification of biotin and horseradish peroxidase signals in histochemical stains. J Histochem Cytochem 1992; 40:1457.
8. Bobrow MN, Harris TD, Shaughnessy KJ, et al. Catalyzed reporter deposition: A novel method of signal amplification: Application to immunoassays. J Immunol Methods 1989; 125:279.
9. Colvin RB, Bhan AK, McCluskey RT, eds. Diagnostic immunopathology, 2nd edn. New York: Raven Press; 1995.
10. DeLellis RA, Sternberger LA, Mann RB, et al. Immunoperoxidase techniques in diagnostic pathology:

Report of a workshop sponsored by the National Cancer Institute. Am J Clin Pathol 1979; 71:483.
11. Elias JM, ed. Immunohistopathology: a practical approach to diagnosis. Chicago: American Society of Clinical Pathologist Press; 1990.
12. Heras A, Roach CM, Key ME. Enhanced polymer detection system for immunohistochemistry. Mod Pathol 1995; 8:165A.
13. Hsu SM, Raine L, Fanger H. A comparative study of the peroxidase-antiperoxidase method and an avidin-biotin complex method for studying polypeptide hormones with radioimmunoassay antibodies. Am J Clin Pathol 1981; 75:734.
14. Hsu S-M, Raine L, Fanger H. Use of avidin-biotin-peroxidase complex (ABC) in immunoperoxidase techniques: A comparison between ABC and unlabeled antibody (PAP) procedures. J Histochem Cytochem 1981; 29:577.
15. Polak JM, van Noorden S, eds. Immunocytochemistry: modern methods and applications, 2nd edn, Bristol: Wright; 1986.
16. Sabattini E, Bisgaard K, Ascani S, et al. The EnVision system: A new immunohistochemical method for diagnostics and research: Critical comparison with the APAAP, ChemMate, CSA, LABC, and SABC techniques. J Clin Pathol 1998; 51: 506.
17. Shi S-R, Cote RJ, Taylor CR. Standardization and further development of antigen retrieval immunohistochemistry: Strategies and future goals. J Histotechnol 1999; 22:177.
18. Sternberger LA, Joseph SA. The unlabeled antibody method: Contrasting color staining of paired pituitary hormones without antibody removal. J Histochem Cytochem 1979; 27:1424.
19. Vyberg M, Nielsen S. Dextran polymer conjugate two-step visualization system for immunohistochemistry. Appl Immunohistochem 1998; 6:3.
20. Kohler G, Milstein C. Continuous cultures of fused cells secreting antibody of predefined specificity. Nature 1975; 256:495.
21. Leong AS-Y. Commentary: Diagnostic immunohistochemistry – problems and solutions. Pathology 1992; 24:1.
22. Taylor CR, Burns J. The demonstration of plasma cells and other immunoglobulin containing cells in formalin-fixed, paraffin-embedded tissues using peroxidase labeled antibody. J Clin Pathol 1974; 27:14.
23. Taylor CR. The nature of Reed-Sternberg cells and other malignant 'reticulum' cells. Lancet 1974; 2:802.
24. Taylor CR. A history of the Reed-Sternberg cell. Biomedicine 1978; 28:196.
25. Taylor CR, Kledzik G. Immunohistologic techniques in surgical pathology: A spectrum of new special stains. Hum Pathol 1981;1 2:590.
26. Pinkus GS. Diagnostic immunocytochemistry of paraffin-embedded tissues. Hum Pathol 1982; 13:411.
27. Swanson PE. Editorial: Methodologic standardization in immunohistochemistry: A doorway opens. Appl Immunohistochem 1993; 1:229.
28. Larsson L-I, ed. Immunocytochemistry: theory and practice. Boca Raton, FL: CRC Press; 1988.
29. Huang S-N. Immunohistochemical demonstration of hepatitis B core and surface antigens in paraffin sections. Lab Invest 1975; 33:88.
30. Leong AS-Y, Milios J, Duncis CG. Antigen preservation in microwave-irradiated tissues: A comparison with formaldehyde fixation. J Pathol 1988; 156:275.
31. Fraenkel-Conrat H, Brandon BA, Olcott HS. The reaction of formaldehyde with proteins. IV: Participation of indole groups. J Biol Chem 1947; 168:99.
32. Fraenkel-Conrat H, Olcott HS. The reaction of formaldehyde with proteins. V: Cross-linking between amino and primary amide or guanidyl groups. J Am Chem Soc 1948; 70:2673.
33. Fraenkel-Conrat H, Olcott HS. Reaction of formaldehyde with proteins. VI: Cross-linking of amino groups with phenol, imidazole, or indole groups. J Biol Chem 1948; 174:827.
34. Shi SR, Key ME, Kalra KL. Antigen retrieval in formalin-fixed, paraffin-embedded tissues: An enhancement method for immunohistochemical staining based on microwave oven heating of tissue sections. J Histochem Cytochem 1991; 39: 741.
35. Shi SR, Tandon AK, Cote C, et al. S-100 protein in human inner ear: Use of a novel immunohistochemical technique on routinely processed, celloidin-embedded human temporal bone sections. Laryngoscope 1992; 102:734.
36. Shi SR, Tandon AK, Haussmann RR, et al. Immunohistochemical study of intermediate filament proteins on routinely processed, celloidin-embedded human temporal bone sections by using a new technique for antigen retrieval. Acta Otolaryngol (Stockh) 1993; 113:48.
37. Shi SR, Cote C, Kalra KL, et al. A technique for retrieving antigens in formalin-fixed, routinely acid-decalcified, celloidin-embedded human temporal bone sections for

immunohistochemistry. J Histochem Cytochem 1992; 40:787.

38. Taylor CR, Shi SR, Chen C, et al. Comparative study of antigen retrieval heating methods: Microwave, microwave and pressure cooker, autoclave, and steamer. Biotech Histochem 1996; 71:263.
39. Taylor CR, Shi S-R, Cote RJ. Antigen retrieval for immunohistochemistry: Status and need for greater standardization. Appl Immunohistochem 1996; 4:144.
40. Boon ME, Kok LP. Breakthrough in pathology due to antigen retrieval. Mal J Med Lab Sci 1995; 12:1.
41. Evers P, Uylings HB, Suurmeijer AJ. Antigen retrieval in formaldehyde-fixed human brain tissue. Methods 1998; 15:133.
42. Gown AM, de Wever N, Battifora H. Microwave-based antigenic unmasking: A revolutionary new technique for routine immunohistochemistry. Appl Immunohistochem 1993; 1:256.
43. Cattoretti G, Pileri S, Parravicini C, et al. Antigen unmasking on formalin-fixed, paraffin-embedded tissue sections. J Pathol 1993; 171:83.
44. Leong AS-Y, Milios J. An assessment of the efficacy of the microwave antigen-retrieval procedure on a range of tissue antigens. Appl Immunohistochem 1993; 1:267.
45. Merz H, Rickers O, Schrimel S, et al. Constant detection of surface and cytoplasmic immunoglobulin heavy and light chain expression in formalin-fixed and paraffin-embedded material. J Pathol 1993; 170:257.
46. Shi SR, Chaiwun B, Young L, et al. Antigen retrieval using pH 3.5 glycine-HCl buffer or urea solution for immunohistochemical localization of Ki-67. Biotech Histochem 1994; 69:213.
47. Shi S-R, Cote RJ, Yang C, et al. Development of an optimal protocol for antigen retrieval: A 'test battery' approach exemplified with reference to the staining of retinoblastoma protein (pRB) in formalin-fixed paraffin sections. J Pathol 1996; 179:347.
48. Shi SR, Cote RJ, Young L, et al. Use of pH 9.5 TRIS-HCl buffer containing 5% urea for antigen retrieval immunohistochemistry. Biotech Histochem 1996; 71:190.
49. Shi SR, Imam SA, Young L, et al. Antigen retrieval immunohistochemistry under the influence of pH using monoclonal antibodies. J Histochem Cytochem 1995; 43:193.
50. Shi S-R, Gu J, Kalra KL, et al. Antigen retrieval technique: A novel approach to immunohistochemistry on routinely processed tissue sections. Cell Vision 1995; 2:6.
51. Suurmeijer AJ, Boon ME. Notes on the application of microwaves for antigen retrieval in paraffin and plastic tissue sections. Eur J Morphol 1993; 31:144.
52. Taylor CR, Shi S-R, Chaiwun B, et al. Strategies for improving the immunohistochemical staining of various intra-nuclear prognostic markers in formalin-paraffin sections: Androgen receptor, estrogen receptor, progesterone receptor, p53 protein, proliferating cell nuclear antigen, and Ki-67 antigen revealed by antigen retrieval techniques. [see comments] Hum Pathol 1994; 25:263.
53. von Wasielewski R, Werner M, Nolte M, et al. Effects of antigen retrieval by microwave heating in formalin-fixed tissue sections on a broad panel of antibodies. Histochemistry 1994; 102:165.
54. Shi SR, Cote RJ, Taylor CR. Antigen retrieval immunohistochemistry: Past, present, and future. J Histochem Cytochem 1997; 45:327.
55. Shi S-R, Cote RJ, Young LL, et al. Antigen retrieval immunohistochemistry and molecular morphology in the year 2001. Appl Immunohistochem Mol Morphol 2001; 9:107.
56. Shi S-R, Cote RJ, Taylor CR. Antigen retrieval techniques: current perspectives. J Histochem Cytochem 2001; 49:931.
57. Shi S-R, Gu J, Kalra KL, et al. Antigen retrieval technique: A novel approach to immunohistochemistry on routinely processed tissue sections. In: Gu J, ed. Analytical morphology: theory, applications & protocols. Natick, MA: Eaton; 1997: 1-40.
58. Shi Y, Li G-D, Liu W-P. Recent advances of the antigen retrieval technique. Linchuang yu Shiyan Binglixue Zazhi (J Clin Exp Pathol) 1997; 13:265.
59. Shi S-R, Gu J, Taylor CR, eds. Antigen retrieval techniques: immunohistochemistry and molecular morphology. Natick, MA: Eaton; 2000.
60. Shi S-R, Gu J, Turrens F, et al. Development of the antigen retrieval technique: philosophy and theoretical base. In: Shi S-R, Gu J, Taylor CR, eds. Antigen retrieval techniques: immunohistochemistry and molecular morphology. Natick, MA: Eaton; 2000:17-39.
61. Mann G, ed. Physiologic histology. Oxford: Oxford University Press; 1902.
62. van Regenmortel MHV. The recognition of proteins and peptides by antibodies. In: van Oss CJ, van Regenmortel MHV,

eds. Immunochemistry. New York: Marcel Dekker; 1994:277-300.
63. Barlow DJ, Edwards MS, Thornton JM. Continuous and discontinuous protein antigenic determinants. Nature 1986; 322: 747.
64. Johnson CW. Issues in immunohistochemistry. Toxicol Pathol 1999; 27:246.
65. Streefkerk JG. Inhibition of erythrocyte pseudoperoxidase activity by treatment with hydrogen peroxide following methanol. J Histochem Cytochem 1972; 29:829.
66. Burns J. Background staining and sensitivity of the unlabeled antibody-enzyme (PAP) method: Comparison with the peroxidase-labeled antibody sandwich method using formalin-fixed paraffin embedded material. Histochemistry 1975; 43: 291.
67. Weir EE, Pretlow TG, Pitts A. Destruction of endogenous peroxidase activity in order to locate cellular antigens by peroxidase-labeled antibodies. J Histochem Cytochem 1974; 22: 51.
68. McMillan EM, Martin D, Wasik R, et al. Demonstration in situ of 'T' cells and 'T' cell subsets in lichen planus using monoclonal antibodies. J Cutan Pathol 1981; 8:228.
69. Straus W. Phenylhydrazine as inhibitor of horseradish peroxidase for use in immunoperoxidase procedures. J Histochem Cytochem 1972; 20:949.
70. Straus W. Use of peroxidase inhibitors for immunoperoxidase procedures. In: Feldman R, ed. First international symposium on immunoenzymatic techniques. Amsterdam, Holland; 1976: 117.
71. Andrew SM, Jasani B. An improved method for the inhibition of endogenous peroxidase non-deleterious to lymphocyte surface markers: Application to immunoperoxidase studies on eosinophil-rich tissue preparations. Histochem J 1987; 35:426.
72. Li C-Y, Zeismer SC, Lacano-Villareal O. Use of azide and hydrogen peroxide as an inhibitor for endogenous peroxidase method. J Histochem Cytochem 1987; 35:1457.
73. Schmid KW, Hittmair A, Schmidhammer H, et al. Non-deleterious inhibition of endogenous peroxidase activity (EPA) by cyclopropanone hydrate: A definitive approach. J Histochem Cytochem 1989; 37:473.
74. Robinson G, Dawson I. Immunochemical studies of the endocrine cells of the gastrointestinal tract. I: The use and value of peroxidase-conjugated antibody techniques for the localization of gastrin-containing cells in human pyloric antrum. Histochem J 1975; 7:321.
75. Heyderman E. Immunoperoxidase technique in histopathology: Applications, methods, and controls. J Clin Pathol 1979; 32:971.
76. Heyderman E, Neville MA. A shorter immunoperoxidase technique for the demonstration of carcinoembryonic antigen and other cell products. J Clin Pathol 1977; 30:138.
77. Lillie RD, Pizzolato P. Histochemical use of borohydride as aldehyde blocking reagent. Stain Technol 1976; 13:16.
78. Kelly J, Whelan CA, Weir DG, et al. Removal of endogenous peroxidase visualization of monoclonal antibodies. J Immunol Methods 1987; 96:127.
79. Hittmair A, Schmid KW. Inhibition of endogenous peroxidase for the immunocytochemical demonstration of intermediate filament proteins (IFP). J Immunol Methods 1989; 116: 199.
80. Mason TE, Phifer RF, Spicer SS, et al. An immunoglobulin enzyme bridge method for localizing tissue antigens. J Histochem Cytochem 1969; 17:573.
81. Sternberger LA, ed. Immunocytochemistry. Englewood Cliffs, NJ: Prentice-Hall; 1974.
82. Cordell JL, Falini B, Erber WN, et al. Immunoenzymatic label of monoclonal antibodies using immune complexes of alkaline phosphatase and monoclonal anti-alkaline phosphatase (APAAP) complexes. J Histochem Cytochem 1984; 32:219.
83. Erber WN, McLachlan J. Use of APAAP technique on paraffin wax embedded bone marrow trephines. J Clin Pathol 1989; 42:1201.
84. Wagner L, Worman CP. Color-contrast staining of two different lymphocyte subpopulations: A two-color modification of alkaline phosphatase monoclonal anti-alkaline phosphatase complex technique. Stain Technol 1988; 63:129.
85. Wong SY, Carrol EDS, Ah-See SY, et al. Detection of estrogen receptor proteins in breast tumors using an improved APAAP immunohistochemical technique. Cancer 1988; 62: 2171.
86. Vardiman JW, Gilewski TA, Ratain MJ, et al. Evaluation of Leu-M5 (CDIIc) in hairy cell leukemia by the alkaline phosphatase anti-phosphatase technique. Am J Clin Pathol 1988; 90:250.

87. Ordronneau P, Lindstrom D, Petrusz P. Four unlabeled antibody bridge techniques: A comparison. J Histochem Cytochem 1984; 32:172.
88. Vacca LL, Hewett D, Woodson G. A comparison of methods using diaminobenzidine (DAB) to localize peroxidases in erythrocytes, neutrophils, and peroxidase-anti-peroxidase complex. Stain Technol 1978; 53:331.
89. Davidoff MS, Schulze W, Holstein AF. Combination of alkaline phosphatase anti-alkaline phosphatase (APAAP) and avidin-biotin-alkaline phosphatase complex (ABAP)-techniques for amplification of immunocytochemical staining of human testicular tissue. Andrologia 1991; 23:353.
90. Sano T, Smith CL, Cantor CR. Immuno-PCR: Very sensitive antigen detection by means of specific antibody-DNA conjugates. Science 1992; 258:120.
91. Chen B-X, Szabolcs MJ, Matsushima AY, et al. A strategy for immunohistochemical signal enhancement by end-product amplification. J Histochem Cytochem 1996; 44:819.
92. Shi S-R, Guo J, Cote RJ, et al. Sensitivity and detection efficiency of a novel two-step detection system (PowerVision) for immunohistochemistry. Appl Immunohistochem Mol Morphol 1999; 7:201.
93. Bobrow MN, Shaughnessy KJ, Litt GJ. Catalyzed reporter deposition, a novel method of signal amplification. II: Application to membrane immunoassays. J Immunol Methods 1991; 137:103.
94. Shi S-R, Gu J, Cote RJ, et al. Standardization of routine immunohistochemistry: where to begin? In: Shi S-R, Gu J, Taylor CR, eds. Antigen retrieval technique: immunohistochemistry and molecular morphology. Natick, MA: Eaton; 2000:255–272.
95. Toda Y, Kono K, Abiru H, et al. Application of tyramide signal amplification system to immunohistochemistry: A potent method to localize antigens that are not detectable by ordinary method. Pathol Int 1999; 49:479.
96. Mengel M, Werner M, von Wasielewski R. Concentration dependent and adverse effects in immunohistochemistry using the tyramine amplification technique. Histochem J 1999; 31:195.
97. Kawai K, Osamura RY. Antigen retrieval versus amplification techniques in diagnostic immunohistochemistry. In: Shi S-R, Gu J, Taylor CR, eds. Antigen retrieval techniques: immunohistochemistry and molecular morphology. Natick, MA: Eaton; 2000:249–253.
98. Merz H, Ottesen K, Meyer W, et al. Combination of antigen retrieval techniques and signal amplification of immunohistochemistry in situ hybridization and FISH techniques. In: Shi S-R, Gu J, Taylor CR, eds. Antigen retrieval techniques: immunohistochemistry and molecular morphology. Natick, MA: Eaton; 2000:219–248.
99. College of American Pathologists: Standard for laboratory accreditation. Skokie, IL: 1987.
100. Taylor CR. The total test approach to standardization of immunohistochemistry. [editorial] Arch Pathol Lab Med 2000; 124:945.
101. Cote RJ, Taylor CR. Immunohistochemistry and related marking techniques. In: Damjanov I, Linder J, eds. Anderson's pathology, 10th edn. St. Louis: CV Mosby; 1996:136–175.
102. Taylor CR. Report of the Immunohistochemistry Steering Committee of the Biological Stain Commission. 'Proposed format: Package insert for immunohistochemistry products.' Biotech Histochem 1992; 67:323.
103. Burry RW. Specificity controls for immunocytochemical methods. J Histochem Cytochem 2000; 48:163.
104. Swaab DF, Pool CW, VanLeenwen FW. Can specificity ever be proven in immunocytochemical staining? J Histochem Cytochem 1977; 25:388.
105. Willingham MC. Conditional epitopes: Is your antibody always specific? J Histochem Cytochem 1999; 47:1233.
106. Battifora H. The multitumor (sausage tissue block): Novel method for immunohistochemical antibody testing. Lab Invest 1986; 55:244.
107. Battifora H, Mehta P. The checkerboard tissue block: An improved multitissue control block. Lab Invest 1990; 63:722.
108. Skacel M, Skilton B, Peltay JD, et al. Tissue microarrays: A powerful tool for high-throughput analysis of clinical specimens: A review of the method with validation data. AIMM 2002; 10:1.
109. Mengel M, Kreipel M, von Wasielewski R. Rapid and large-scale transition of new tumor biomarker to clinical biopsy material by innovative tissue microarray systems. AIMM 2003; 11:261.
110. Battifora H. Assessment of antigen damage in immunohistochemistry: The vimentin internal control. Am J Clin Pathol 1991; 96:669.
111. Battifora H, Kopinski M. The influence of protease digestion

and duration of fixation on the immunostaining of keratins: A comparison of formalin and ethanol fixation. J Histochem Cytochem 1986; 34:1095.

112. Cuevas EC, Bateman AC, Wilkins BS, et al. Microwave antigen retrieval in immunocytochemistry: A study of 80 antibodies. J Clin Pathol 1994; 47:448.

113. Leong AS-Y, Gilham PN. The effects of progressive formaldehyde fixation on the preservation of tissue antigens. Pathology 1989; 21:266.

114. Shi S-R, Cote RJ, Chaiwun B, et al. Standardization of immunohistochemistry based on antigen retrieval technique for routine formalin-fixed tissue sections. Appl Immunohistochem 1998; 6:89.

115. Yokoo H, Nakazato Y. A monoclonal antibody that recognizes a carbohydrate epitope of human protoplasmic astrocytes. Acta Neuropathol 1996; 91:30.

116. Prento P, Lyon H. Commercial formalin substitutes for histopathology. Biotech Histochem 1997; 72:273.

117. Williams JH, Mepham BL, Wright DH. Tissue preparation for immunocytochemistry. J Clin Pathol 1997; 50:801.

118. Allison RT, Best T. p53, PCNA and Ki-67 expression in oral squamous-cell carcinomas – the vagaries of fixation and microwave enhancement of immunocytochemistry. J Oral Pathol Med 1998; 27:434.

119. Miller RT, Kubier P, Reynolds B, et al. Blocking of endogenous avidin-binding activity in immunohistochemistry. Appl Immunohistochem Mol Morphol 1999; 7:63.

120. Zhang PJ, Wang H, Wrona EL, et al. Effects of tissue fixatives on antigen preservation for immunohistochemistry: A comparative study of microwave antigen retrieval on Lillie fixative and neutral buffered formalin. J Histotechnol 1998; 21:101.

121. Cote RJ, Shi Y, Groshen S, et al. Association of p27^{kip1} levels with recurrence and survival in patients with stage C prostate carcinoma. J Natl Cancer Inst 1998; 90:916.

122. Grabau KA, Nielsen O, Hansen S. Influence of storage temperature and high-temperature antigen retrieval buffers on results of immunohistochemical staining in sections stored for long periods. Appl Immunohistochem 1998; 6:209.

123. Jacobs TW, Prioleau JE, Stillman IE, et al. Loss of tumor marker-immunostaining intensity on stored paraffin slides of breast cancer. J Natl Cancer Inst 1996; 88:1054.

124. Kato J, Sakamaki S, Niitsu Y. More on p53 antigen loss in stored paraffin slides. N Engl J Med 1995; 333:1507.

125. Prioleau J, Schnitt SI. p53 antigen loss in stored paraffin slides. N Engl J Med 1995; 332:1521.

126. Malmstrom PU, Wester K, Vasko J, et al. Expression of proliferative cell nuclear antigen (PCNA) in urinary bladder carcinoma: Evaluation of antigen retrieval methods. APMIS 1992; 100:988.

127. Wester K, Wahlund E, Sundstrom C, et al. Paraffin section storage and immunohistochemistry. Appl Immunohistochem Mol Morphol 2000; 8:61.

128. Mason JT, O'Leary TJ. Effects of formaldehyde fixation on protein secondary structure: A calorimetric and infrared spectroscopic investigation. J Histochem Cytochem 1991; 39:225.

129. Igarashi H, Sugimura H, Maruyama K. Alteration of immunoreactivity by hydrated autoclaving, microwave treatment, and simple heating of paraffin-embedded tissue sections. APMIS 1994; 102:295.

130. Kawai K, Serizawa A, Hamana T, et al. Heat-induced antigen retrieval of proliferating cell nuclear antigen and p53 protein in formalin-fixed, paraffin-embedded sections. Pathol Int 1994; 44:759.

131. Evers P, Uylings HB. Microwave-stimulated antigen retrieval is pH and temperature dependent. J Histochem Cytochem 1994; 42:1555.

132. Lucassen PJ, Ravid R, Gonatas NK, et al. Activation of the human supraoptic and paraventricular nucleus neurons with aging and in Alzheimer's disease as judged from increasing size of the Golgi apparatus. Brain Res 1993; 632:105.

133. Shi SR, Cote RJ, Taylor CR. Antigen retrieval immunohistochemistry used for routinely processed celloidin-embedded human temporal bone sections: Standardization and development. Auris Nasus Larynx 1998; 25:425.

134. Werner M, Von Wasielewski R, Komminoth P. Antigen retrieval, signal amplification and intensification in immunohistochemistry. Histochem Cell Biol 1996; 105:253.

135. Katoh A, Breier S. Nonspecific antigen retrieval solutions. J Histotechnol 1994; 17:378.

136. O'Reilly PE, Raab SS, Niemann TH, et al. p53, proliferating cell nuclear antigen, and Ki-67 expression in extrauterine leiomyosarcomas. Mod Pathol 1997; 10:91.

137. Shin R-W, Iwaki T, Kitamoto T, et al. Hydrated autoclave pretreatment enhances TAU immunoreactivity in formalin-fixed normal and Alzheimer's disease brain tissues. Lab

Invest 1991; 64:693.

138. Biddolph SC, Jones M. Low-temperature, heat-mediated antigen retrieval (LTHMAR) on archival lymphoid sections. Appl Immunohistochem Mol Morphol 1999; 7:289.

139. Miller RT, Swanson PE, Wick MR. Fixation and epitope retrieval in diagnostic immunohistochemistry: A concise review with practical considerations. Appl Immunohistochem Mol Morphol 2000; 8:228.

140. Boon ME, Kok LP, Moorlag HE, et al. Accelerated immunogold-silver and immunoperoxidase staining of paraffin sections with the use of microwave irradiation: Factors influencing results. Am J Clin Pathol 1989; 91:137.

141. Chiu KY. Use of microwaves for rapid immunoperoxidase staining of paraffin sections. Med Lab Sci 1987; 44:3.

142. Choi T-S, Whittlesey MM, Slap SE, et al. Advances in temperature control of microwave immunohistochemistry. Cell Vision 1995; 2:151.

143. Leong AS-Y, Milios J. Rapid immunoperoxidase staining of lymphocyte antigens using microwave irradiation. J Pathol 1986; 148:183.

144. Adams JC. Heavy metal intensification of DAB-based HRP reaction product. J Histochem Cytochem 1981; 29:775.

145. Hsu SM, Soban E. Color modification of diaminobenzidine (DAB) precipitation by metallic ions and its application for double immunohistochemistry. J Histochem Cytochem 1982; 30:1079.

146. Lan HY, Mu W, Nikolic-Paterson DJ, et al. A novel, simple, reliable, and sensitive method for multiple immunoenzyme staining: Use of microwave oven heating to block antibody crossreactivity and retrieve antigens. J Histochem Cytochem 1995; 43:97.

147. Mason DY, Sammons R. Alkaline phosphatase and peroxidase for double immunoenzymatic labeling of cellular constituents. J Clin Pathol 1978; 31:454.

148. Falini B, De Solas I, Halverson C. Double-labeled antigen method for demonstration of intracellular antigens in paraffin-embedded tissues. J Histochem Cytochem 1982; 30:21.

149. Behringer DM, Meyer KH, Veh RW. Antibodies against neuroactive amino acids and neuropeptides. II: Simultaneous immunoenzymatic double staining with labeled primary antibodies of the same species and a combination of the ABC methods and the hapten-anti-hapten bridge (HAB) technique. J Histochem Cytochem 1991; 39:761.

150. Van Rooijen N. Six methods for separate detection of two different antigens in the same tissue section. J Histochem Cytochem 1980; 28:716.

151. Krenacs T, Laszik Z, Dobo E. Application of immunogold-silver staining and immunoenzymatic methods in multiple labeling of human pancreatic Langerhans islet cells. Acta Histochem 1989; 85:79.

152. Lehr HA, van der Loos CM, Teeling P, et al. Complete chromogen separation and analysis in double immunohistochemical stains using Photoshop-based image analysis. J Histochem Cytochem 1999; 47:119.

153. Herman GE, Elfont EA, Floyd AD. Overview of automated immunostainers. Methods Mol Biol 1994; 34:383.

154. Le Neel T, Moreau A, Laboisse C, et al. Comparative evaluation of automated systems in immunohistochemistry. Clin Chim Acta 1998; 278:185.

155. Fetsch PA, Abati A. Overview of the clinical immunohistochemistry laboratory: Regulations and troubleshooting guidelines. Methods Mol Biol 1999; 115:405.

156. Moreau A, Le Neel T, Joubert M, et al. Approach to automation in immunohistochemistry. Clin Chim Acta 1998; 278: 177.

157. Bauer KD, Hawes D, de la Torre-Bueno J, et al. Analysis of occult bone marrow metastases using automated cellular imaging. Mod Pathol 2000; 13:220A.

158. Makarewicz K, McDuffe L, Shi S-R, et al. Immunohistochemical detection of occult metastases using an automated intelligent microscopy system. Presented at the 88th annual meeting of the American Association of Cancer Research, San Diego, CA, 1997:269.

159. Martin W, Chon A, Fabiono A, et al. Effect of formalin tissue fixation and processing on immunohistochemistry. Am J Surg Pathol 2000; 24:1016.

160. Rickers RR, Malinisk RM. Intralaboratory quality assurance of immunohistochemical procedures: Recommended practices for daily application. Arch Pathol Lab Med 1989; 113:673.

161. van der Ploeg M, Duijndam WAL. Matrix models: Essential tools for microscopic cytochemical research. Histochemistry 1986; 84:283.

162. Riera J, Simpson JF, Tamayo R, et al. Use of cultured cells as a control for quantitative immunocytochemical analysis of estrogen receptor in breast cancer: The Quicgel method. Am J Clin Pathol 1999; 111:329.

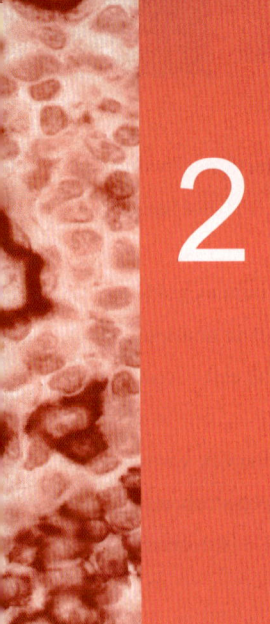

2 感染性疾病的免疫组织化学

原作者：Eduardo J. Eyzaguirre, David H. Walker and Sherif R. Zaki

译　者：陈方杰，翟启辉

审校者：陈方杰，周庚寅

目　录

引言	38
病毒性感染	39
细菌性感染	43
真菌感染	45
原虫感染	46
新型感染性疾病	46
病理学家、免疫组化和生物恐怖	48

引　言

自20世纪80年代起，病理学家们已经处理了大量的来源于一种或多种病原感染的病理标本[1]。在本章节中，病理学家们业已成为认识感染病原的重要角色。在很多的病例中，无新鲜组织可用做培养，病理学家们可提供及时的形态学诊断，以便于对病人诊治[2]。并且，病理学家们在分辨新出现和再出现的感染病原和描述病理致病过程，如汉坦病毒肺综合征及其他的病毒性出血热、钩端螺旋体病、立克次体以及于2001年所发生的炭疽热生物恐怖袭击的诊断中已成为中心角色[3-7]。

传统上，感染性疾病的微生物鉴别基本采用血清学分析和培养技术。但是，血清学结果在免疫抑制或单个样本存在的情况下可能会难以解释。另外，新鲜组织也并非总是可用于培养，难以培养的病原体可能几星期甚至几个月才产生结果。此外，培养不能区别是否来源于组织的浸润。有些微生物拥有特有的形态，可在福尔马林固定组织中，由常规和特殊染色加以鉴别。然而，在一些特例中传统的形态学方法难以甚至根本无法判定感染原。

免疫组化在外科手术病理中是最有效的技术之一。越来越多的特异性抗体用于探测和鉴别传染性疾病中的致病原，如病毒、细菌、真菌及寄生虫的抗体。Coons等[8]第一次使用特异性抗体在组织中检测出微生物抗原——肺炎双球菌。相对于传统染色，免疫组化拥有很多优势（表2.1），并体现在感染性疾病的诊断上（表2.2）。需要重点指出的是无论单克隆或多克隆抗体都须检验可能的交叉性反应。现已获得了广泛发生于细菌和致病真菌的抗原[1,9]。最后非常重要的是要理解免疫组化有多个步骤，每一步都可影响最后的结果。但总之，免疫组化的局限性来源于可利用的特异性抗体及抗原决定簇的保持情况[1,10]。众所周知，对于较大的微生物如原虫、真菌和一些细菌，福尔马林固定的蜡块组织不需要预处理。与此相反，对于较小的感染原，如微生物中的病毒和衣原体，必须用蛋白水解酶或热抗原修复以增强免疫反应。表2.3列举了目前外科手术病理中可用于诊断的抗体。

表2.1　免疫组化在感染性疾病中的诊断优势
结果迅速
可在福尔马林固定、石蜡包埋的组织上操作，降低暴露于严重感染性疾病的危险
高敏感性：甚至在形态改变之前，即可鉴定出感染原
可用于单个病人的回顾性诊断和对疾病的深入性研究
特异性：单克隆或某些多克隆抗体可用于感染原的特异性诊断

表2.2　免疫组化在感染性疾病诊断中的作用
可用于新型人类病原体的辨别
微生物/形态学的相互关系可确立感染原的致病作用
提供快速的形态诊断可用于严重感染性疾病的早期治疗
提供对于感染性疾病的发病机制的认识
当无新鲜组织或组织培养时可提供诊断

感染性疾病的免疫组织化学

表2.3 可用于感染性疾病免疫组化诊断的抗体

微生物	抗体/克隆	稀释度	预处理	来源
腺病毒	Mab/20/11 和 2/6	1:2000	蛋白激酶 K	Chemicon
曲霉菌	Mab/WF-AF-1	1:200	HIAR*	Dako
亨氏巴尔通体	Mab	1:100	HIAR	Biocare Medical
BK 病毒	Mab/BK T.1	1:8000	Trypsin	Chemicon
白色念珠菌	Mab/1B12	1:400	HIAR	Chemicon
肺炎衣原体	Mab/RR402	1:200	HIAR	Accurate
隐孢子虫	Mab/Mabc1	1:100	HIAR	Novocastra
巨细胞病毒	Mab/DDG9/CCH2	1:50	HIAR	Novocastra
肠贾第虫	Mab/9D5.3.1	1:50	HIAR	Novocastra
乙型肝炎 B 核心抗原	Rabbit polyclonal	1:2000	HIAR	Dako
乙型肝炎 B 表面抗原	Mab/3E7	1:100	HIAR	Dako
单纯疱疹病毒 1 和 2	Rabbit polyclonal	1:3200	HIAR	Dako
幽门螺杆菌	Rabbit polyclonal	1:40	Protase I	Dako
HHV8	Mab/LNA-1	1:500	HIAR	Novocastra
产单核细胞李斯特菌	Rabbit polyclonal	1:5000	蛋白激酶 K	Difco
细小病毒 B19	Mab/R92F6	1:500	HIAR	Novocastra
肺孢子虫	Mab/3F6	1:20	HIAR	Novocastra
呼吸道合胞病毒	Mab/5H5N	1:200	HIAR	Novocastra
弓形虫	Rabbit polyclonal	1:320	HIAR	Biogenex
西尼罗病毒	Mab/5H10	1:400	蛋白激酶 K	Bioreliance

* 热抗原修复

病毒性感染

免疫组化在诊断许多病毒感染性疾病和研究其发病机制及流行病学中均起到重要作用。传统上，病毒感染的诊断依赖于日常组织病理学中的细胞变化。几种病毒感染原产生特异性的细胞内包涵体，病理学家可据此作出病毒感染的推断性诊断。但是，一些病毒感染的特征性细胞学变化常常不明显，必须进行仔细的搜寻[11]。并且只有50%的已知病毒性疾病与特异性细胞内包涵体有关[12]。另外，福尔马林，这种在组织病理中最常用的固定剂，难以保留病毒包涵体的形态及颜色特征。当病毒包涵体无法在苏木精-伊红染色组织切片中发现时，或当呈现的病毒包涵体无法区别于其他病毒感染性疾病时，免疫组化技术便成为可供选择的方法。

乙型肝炎病毒

乙型肝炎病毒（乙型病毒，HBV）感染是慢性肝炎的重要诱发因素。在许多病例中，由乙肝病毒诱发的肝细胞形态学改变不足以成为乙肝病毒感染的假定性诊断依据。另外一些病例中，可能只有很少量的乙肝病毒表面抗原（HBsAg），所以不能由地衣红染色技术显示。在这些情况下，免疫组化技术相较于其他组织化学技术探测HBsAg更加敏感，对于作出诊断更加有帮助[13]。HBsAg已用于诊断乙肝及对病毒携带者的研究[14, 15]。80％或更多的HBsAg血清学阳性的病例，使用免疫组化可显示细胞质内HBsAg（图2.1）[16]。免疫过氧化物酶定位，乙肝病毒核心抗原（HBcAg）可被显示于肝细胞核或胞浆中，或两者兼之（图2.2）。胞浆显示明显的核心抗原与严重的活动性肝炎有关[17]。

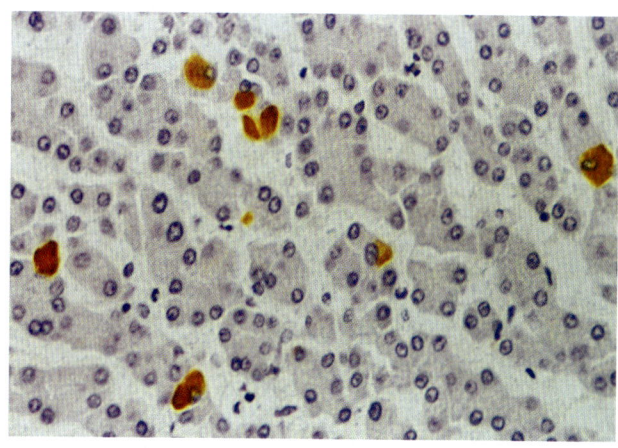

图2.1 肝活检组织来源于慢性乙肝病人，使用抗HBsAg单抗，分散的肝细胞显示胞浆内反应 [二氨基联苯胺（DAB）过氧化物酶染色和苏木精复染，×400]

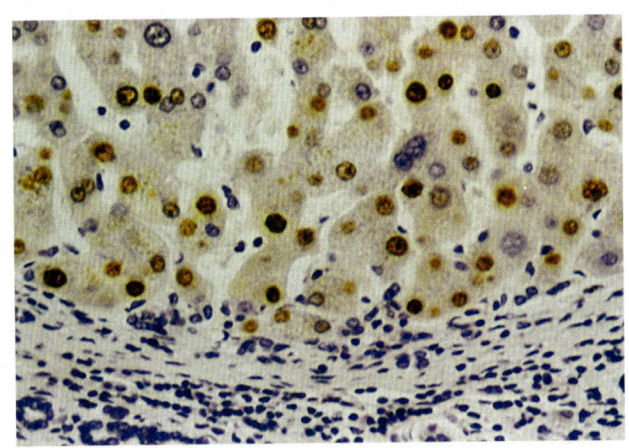

图2.2 慢性活动性乙肝，多克隆抗体抗乙肝核心抗原（HBcAg）显示大量的肝细胞胞核阳性（二氨基联苯胺过氧化物酶染色和苏木精复染，×400）

丙型肝炎病毒

临床诊断丙型肝炎病毒（HCV）感染基于血清学抗HCV抗体的显示及在血清中探测到HCV RNA。但是，抗HCV抗体在免疫抑制的病人中可能探测不到[18]。几种多克隆和单克隆抗体抗HCV非结构蛋白已被生产应用于免疫组化。然而，与RT-PCR探测HCV RNA相比较，大多数抗体敏感性低而不能在临床上使用[18-21]。而且，与非HCV抗原决定簇的交叉反应已被发现于单克隆抗体TORDJI-22[21-22]。弥漫或粗颗粒细胞浆染色多见于慢性丙型肝炎病人中数目不等的肝细胞内[19, 23, 24]，很少见于胆管上皮细胞、淋巴细胞和窦内皮细胞中。

最近一种单克隆抗体抗HCV E2衣糖蛋白已被证实具高敏感性，可用于临床诊断及随访慢性丙型肝炎病人，如与EnVision技术联合使用，准确率达95%[25]。这种抗体可用于早期探测HCV相关肝硬化后肝移植的再感染，与移植排斥反应的再感染进行鉴别。

疱疹病毒

单纯疱疹病毒（HSV）感染，可查见多核巨细胞内包含特征性毛玻璃样核及Cowdry A型核内包涵体。当大量的病毒包涵体位于感染细胞内时，比较容易作出诊断。但是当特异性核内包涵体、多核细胞，或两者缺少时，或当活检组织较小时，HSV的诊断却非常困难[26]。在这些病例中，应用免疫组化技术来探测HSV抗原具有明显优势。

应用多克隆或单克隆抗HSV抗体的免疫组织化学技术诊断HSV感染，已被证实是一种敏感而特异的技术方法（图2.3）[29, 30]。尽管多克隆抗体对主要的HSV糖蛋白抗原是敏感的，但它并不能区分HSV-1和HSV-2，因为这两种病毒抗原性相似[31]。另外，HSV感染的组织特征并无特异性，也可发生于水痘-带状疱疹（VZV）感染的病人中。单克隆抗体抗VZV衣糖蛋白gp1敏感性和特异性很高，可用于鉴别HSV和VZV感染[27, 32, 33]。

免疫组化技术可以证明人类疱疹病毒8（HHV8）与Kaposi肉瘤、原发性渗出性淋巴瘤、多中心性Castleman病相关[34-38]。Kaposi肉瘤组织形态表现多样，相似于其他的良性及恶性血管肿瘤，诊断有一定困难。Kaposi肉瘤相关核抗原-1（LANA-1）有助于确立诊断，尤其是在诊断困难的早期病变或当肿瘤位于不常见的部位时，可用来区分Kaposi肉瘤与几种形态相似的血管增生性病变（见第12章）[39, 40]，免疫染色限定于梭形细胞和裂隙血管内皮细胞的细胞核。免疫组化亦可显示HHV-8 LANA-1表达于HIV相关性复发性胸膜渗出病变的间皮细胞[41]和原发性肺高压丛状病变的细胞中[42]。

巨细胞病毒（CMV）在免疫抑制病人中是非常重要的机会性病原体。固定组织中的CMV组织学诊断通常取决于辨认特异性细胞病变，包括细胞核及细胞质包涵体，或两者兼而有之。但是，组织学检查缺乏敏感性，在某些病例中不典型细胞病变特征可与反应性或退行性病变相混淆[43]。在这些病例中，免疫组化使用单克隆抗体抗早期或晚期CMV抗原可探测到CMV抗原位于被感染的细胞核或细胞浆内（图2.4），另外，当细胞在早期未显示病变时，免疫组化亦可探测到CMV抗原[44-49]。例如，CMV早期核抗原表达于

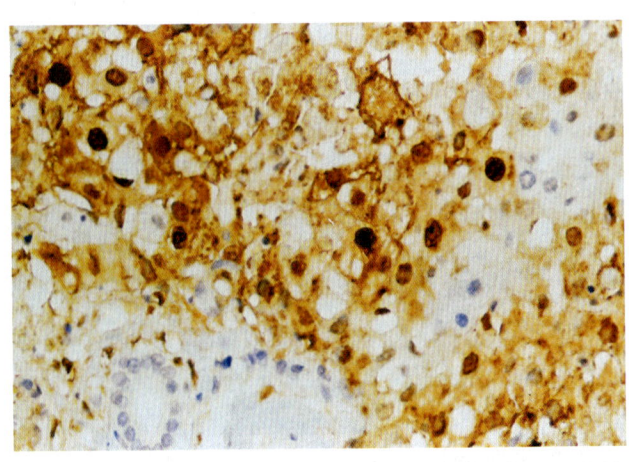

图2.3 单纯疱疹性肝炎。许多肝细胞和库普弗细胞的细胞核和细胞浆中呈现单纯疱疹抗原强免疫染色（二氨基联苯胺过氧化物酶染色和苏木精复染，×400）

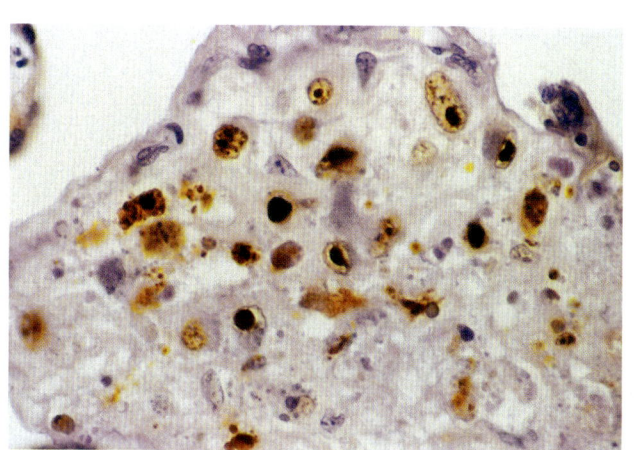

图2.4 先天性巨细胞病毒感染中的绒毛炎。间质细胞和霍夫包尔（Hofbauer）细胞胞核和胞质中的CMV抗原阳性（二氨基联苯胺过氧化物酶染色和苏木精复染，×400）

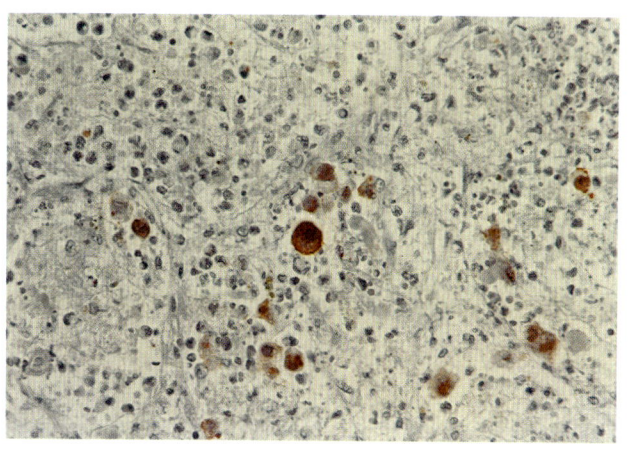

图2.5 腺病毒肺炎。被感染细胞位于坏死渗出中，显示腺病毒细胞核阳性（AEC过氧化物酶染色和苏木精复染，×400）

细胞感染后9～96小时并显示早期活动性病毒复制。对于检测类固醇难治性溃疡性结肠炎CMV的感染、肝移植病人发生神经性并发症、中枢神经系统潜伏CMV感染，免疫组化技术都非常有帮助[50, 51]。也可用于证明前3个月流产组织中高频度的CMV抗原[52]。免疫组化的敏感性高于光镜下鉴定病毒包涵体，也不亚于组织培养与原位杂交[44, 46, 47, 49, 53]。另外，免疫组化分析快于贝壳试管（shell vial）技术，与免疫荧光或培养技术协同可迅速得到结果，这对于早期抗CMV治疗非常重要。

腺病毒

在移植导致的免疫抑制和先天性免疫缺陷病人中，腺病毒感染导致发病甚至死亡越来越受到重视[54, 55]。文献中腺病毒感染在HIV感染病人中很少得到描述[56-58]。特征性腺病毒包涵体呈双染性，位于核内，呈均一和玻璃状。但是在一些病例中，特征性细胞病变仅限于极少的细胞中[57]。另外，其他的病毒包涵体，包括CMV、人类乳头瘤病毒、HSV和VZV也可被误诊为腺病毒包涵体，反之亦然。况且免疫抑制病人合并其他病毒感染几率很高。在这些情况下，免疫组化分析对于确定诊断是必要的手段。一种可与全部41种腺病毒血清型反应的单克隆抗体已用于证明免疫抑制病人核内腺病毒抗原（图2.5）[57-61]。组织学诊断腺病毒性肠炎非常困难，通常不能作出诊断。免疫组化染色在鉴别腺病毒肠炎和CMV肠炎方面具有重要价值[57, 62]。另外一些使用免疫组化技术进行诊断的疱疹病毒感染包括Epstein-Barr病毒感染和人类疱疹病毒-6感染[64]。

细小病毒B19

细小病毒B19与非症状性感染、传染性红斑、急性关节病、再生障碍性贫血危机、胎儿水肿、慢性贫血和红细胞再生障碍性贫血有关。诊断细小病毒感染可根据鉴别骨髓样本的特异性发现，包括前体红细胞、巨原红细胞、红细胞样的细胞内嗜酸或嗜碱性核内包涵体的降低或缺失[65, 66]。由于静脉内注射免疫球蛋白治疗非常有效，因此获得一种快速而准确的诊断手段极为重要。单克隆抗体抗VP1和VP2壳蛋白免疫组化已被作为一种快速而敏感的方法使用，可在福尔马林固定蜡块组织上诊断细小病毒B19的感染[67-70]。免疫组化在包涵体稀疏的病例尤为有帮助，如常规组织切片染色不能确诊的病例，或胎儿水肿晚期细胞溶解的病例（图2.6）[67, 71, 72]。几项研究已发现形态学、免疫组化、原位杂交和PCR之间的相关性[66, 67, 70, 72]。

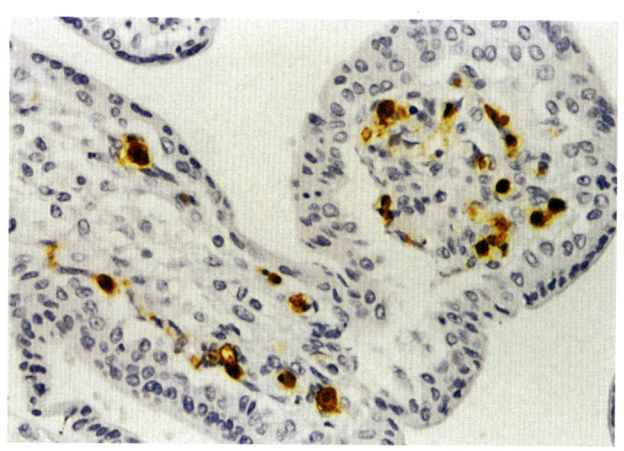

图2.6 细小病毒感染所致胎儿水肿。绒毛血管中幼红细胞细胞核阳性（二氨基联苯胺过氧化物酶染色和苏木精复染，×600）

病毒性出血热

自20世纪80年代以来，大量新出现或再出现的病毒性出血热物质已引起病理学家的重视[3-5]。这些研究人员在鉴定这些物质方面扮演重要角色，有利于新的病毒性出血热物质的流行病学、临床和发病机制的研究[4, 5, 7]。病毒性出血热往往是致命的，在缺乏出血或器官征象的情况下，这些疾病临床上很难诊断并且经常需要处理和测试潜在危险的生物学标本。另外，组织病理特征为非特征性，它们可相似于其他病毒、立克次体和细菌（如钩端螺旋体病）的感染。免疫组化是必要的手段，并已成功和安全地应用于诊断和研究这些疾病的发病机制。

几项研究已经应用免疫组化作为一种敏感、安全和快捷的方法诊断病毒性出血热，如黄热病（图2.7）[73-75]、登革出血热[75, 76]、Crimean-Congo 出血热、阿根廷出血热[77]、委内瑞拉出血热[79]和马尔堡病[80]。另外，一种敏感、特异和安全的免疫染色方法可在福尔马林固定的皮肤活检组织中诊断埃博拉出血热（图2.8）[81]。免疫组化证实拉沙热病毒靶细胞主要为内皮细胞、单核炎性细胞和肝细胞（图2.9）[81-83]。

乳头瘤病毒

免疫组化在福尔马林固定组织上检测人类乳头瘤病毒（HPV）已被更加敏感的诊断分子技术如原位杂交所替代[84-87]。另外，与分子技术相比，免疫组化敏感度较低，仅能探测大量而非潜伏性的感染，而且不能判断病毒类型（图2.10）。

BK病毒感染多发于幼儿期，在有免疫能力的个体中病毒潜伏于肾、中枢神经系统和B淋巴细胞。在

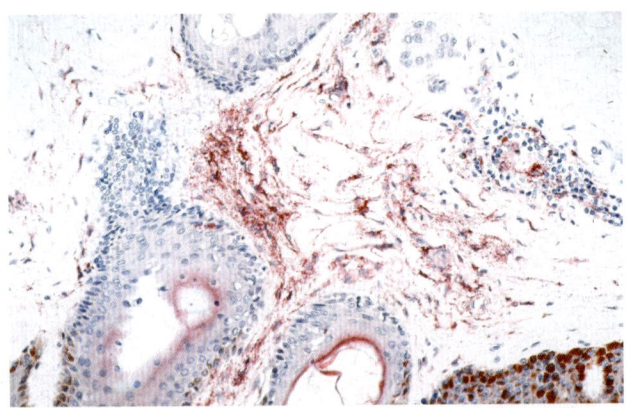

图2.8 埃博拉病毒。广泛的埃博拉病毒抗原主要见于真皮成纤维细胞，皮肤标本来源于致命的埃博拉出血热病例（免疫碱性磷酸酶染色、萘酚快红底物和苏木精复染，×20）

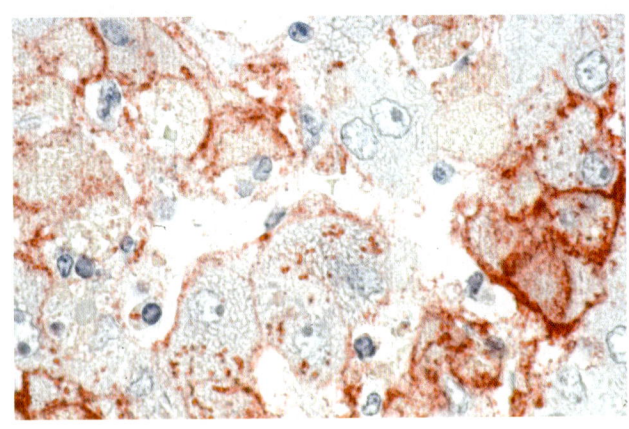

图2.9 拉沙热。拉沙热病人的肝脏中，散在的肝细胞和网状内皮细胞呈现单克隆抗体抗拉沙热病毒阳性（萘酚快红底物和苏木精复染，×100）

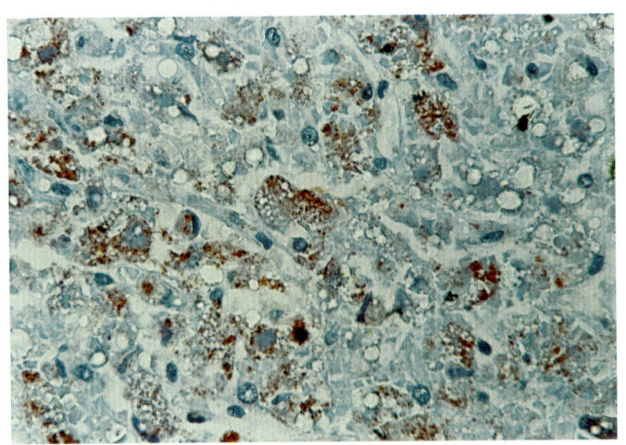

图2.7 黄热病。大量黄热病病毒抗原见于肝细胞和库普弗细胞（AEC过氧化物酶染色和苏木精复染，×400）

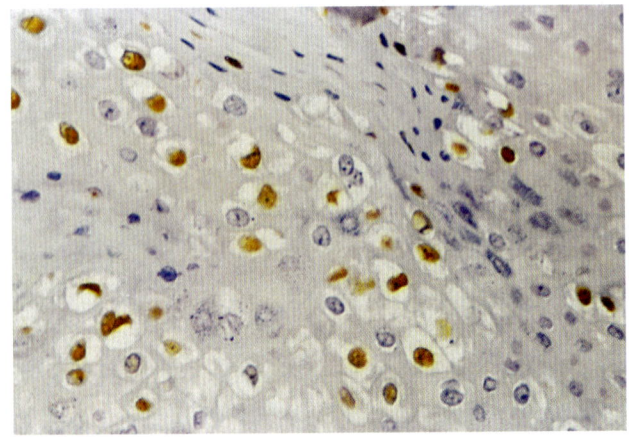

图2.10 人类乳头瘤病毒。HPV抗原位于轻度异型增生的鳞状上皮凹空细胞的核内（DAB与苏木精复染，×600）

免疫抑制的病人中，感染活性增高并扩散到其他器官。在肾脏，感染与单核间质炎性浸润和肾小管萎缩有关，很难与急性移植排斥鉴别。此外，BK病毒感染观察到的细胞病变不是诊断性的，也可在其他病毒感染中发现。在这种情况下，免疫组化可有效证明BK病毒感染[88-91]。

人类多瘤病毒JC病毒是一种双链DNA病毒，可引起多灶性进行性脑白质病（PML）。这种致命的脱髓鞘疾病以少突胶质细胞和奇异性巨星形胶质细胞的病变为特征。免疫组化采用多克隆兔抗血清抗VP1蛋白证实PML诊断，是一种特异、敏感和快捷的手段[92-95]。JC病毒抗原常见于少突胶质细胞，偶见于星形胶质细胞，并且抗原携带细胞更多见于早期病灶。

其他病毒

当没有培养的情况下，免疫组化技术亦用于确认呼吸病毒性疾病如流感A病毒和呼吸道合胞病毒感染[96-99]。狂犬病的确诊很大程度上依赖于组织病理发现特异性细胞质包涵体（尼克小体）。在相当比例的病例中，尼克小体可能不醒目并极其稀少，用于确诊狂犬病极为困难。况且，在一些非发病区狂犬病的诊断往往被临床上所忽略，或病人呈现上行型麻痹。在这种情况下，免疫组化染色是一种非常敏感、安全而特异的狂犬病诊断工具（图2.11）[100-104]。另外一些可利用免疫组化方法诊断的病毒物质包括肠道病毒[105-108]、东部马脑脊髓炎[109-111]和轮状病毒[112-114]。

细菌性感染

在细菌性感染中，大量的免疫组化研究应用于研究幽门螺杆菌。几项研究已评估了免疫组化在其他细菌、分枝杆菌、立克次体和螺旋体感染的应用。

应用免疫组化在固定的组织上检验细菌通常不要求抗原修复。由于一些抗体可与其他细菌产生交叉反应，使结果的解释变得困难。另外，抗体可能仅与细菌和螺旋体的某些成分发生反应，即便这些病原体不成活，仍可以对其残留部分标记。

幽门螺杆菌

胃幽门螺杆菌感染可导致慢性活动性胃炎，并与淋巴组织增生、胃淋巴瘤和胃腺癌密切相关。大量细菌所引起的严重感染在日常的HE染色的组织上很容易检测到；但检测率仅为66%，而且伴有许多假阳性和假阴性结果。传统组织化学方法如银染色较HE染色在检测幽门螺杆菌方面更加敏感。对于检测少量的细菌，免疫组化技术已被证明更加特异和敏感，综合考虑该方法更便宜，比传统的组织化学方法更有优越性（图2.12）[116,117]。治疗慢性活动性胃炎

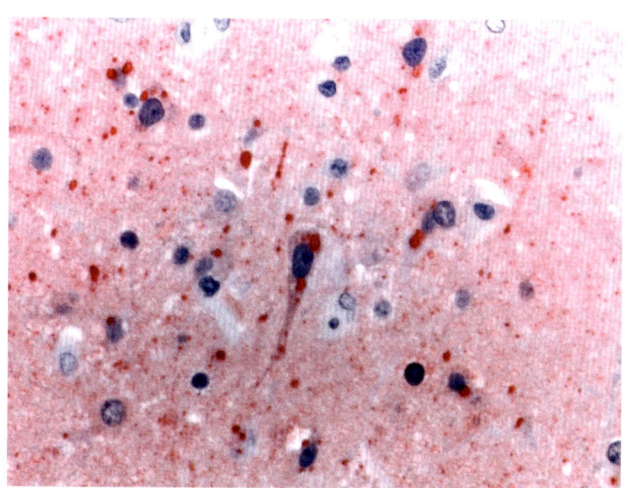

图2.11 狂犬病。兔多克隆抗体免疫染色显示，狂犬病病毒位于中枢神经系统的神经元细胞中，红色沉淀与尼克包涵体在苏木精-伊红染色中一致（免疫碱性磷酸酶染色、萘酚快红底物和苏木精复染，×40）

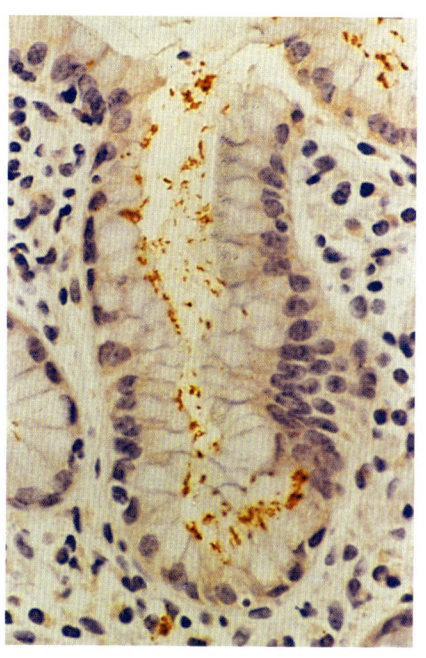

图2.12 免疫过氧化物酶染色可清楚显示，大量弯曲的幽门螺杆菌位于慢性活动性胃炎表面黏液中（DAB与苏木精复染，×600）

和幽门螺杆菌感染可使细菌形态发生改变，使其与细胞外碎屑或黏液小球区别非常困难。在这些病例中，即使组织检查或细菌培养呈现假阴性，免疫组化技术也可提高细菌的检出率[118-121]。

Whipple 病

Whipple 病主要累及小肠和肠系膜淋巴结，一般较少累及其他器官，如心脏和中枢神经系统。大量泡沫状巨噬细胞为这种疾病的特征性改变，诊断通常依据细胞浆内查见 PAS 阳性的细菌。然而，PAS 阳性巨噬细胞的出现是非特异性的；它们也可见于其他的疾病，如鸟分枝杆菌复合感染、组织胞浆菌病、马红球菌感染及巨球蛋白血症。使用兔多克隆抗体免疫组化染色可提供一种敏感和特异的方法，用于快速诊断小肠和小肠外的 Whipple 病，并可对治疗反应进行随访。

落基山斑疹热

确诊落基山斑疹热（Rocky Mountain spotted fever，RMSF）通常依靠血清学方法检测抗斑疹热（SFG）立克次体抗体，但是相当部分患有 RMSF 的病人在疾病的第一周缺乏诊断滴度。用免疫组化技术已在福尔马林固定的组织切片上成功检出 SFG 立克次体（图 2.13）[125, 126]。在使用皮肤活检诊断可疑 RMSF 病例，或确诊血清阴性的致命性 RMSF 病例方面，几项研究已证实了免疫组化具有应用价值。

巴尔通体属感染

巴尔通体属是一种生长缓慢、较难培养的革兰阴性、Warthin-Starry 着色细菌，与杆菌性血管瘤病、肝紫癜、猫抓病及血培养阴性心内膜炎有关。用免疫组化技术成功地在血培养阴性心内膜炎的心瓣膜上检出了亨森巴尔通体和五日热巴尔通体（图 2.14）[129, 130]。这种多克隆兔抗体虽不能用于鉴别亨森巴尔通体和五日热巴尔通体，但可用于探测猫抓病、杆菌性血管瘤病和肝紫癜中的致病菌。一种特异性巴尔通体属的单克隆抗体已用于检测由这种病菌所导致的脾破裂[133]。

其他细菌感染

用免疫组化技术在福尔马林固定的组织上可检出的其他细菌感染性疾病，包括钩端螺旋体病。该病为一种动物传染性疾病，通常表现为急性热病症状，但偶尔可有不同寻常的表现如肺出血伴发呼吸衰竭或腹部疼痛[134-136]。在非典型临床表现的病人胆囊和肺组织中，免疫组化采用兔多克隆抗体可检测钩端螺旋体抗原（图 2.15）[134-137]。

莱姆病具有变化无常的临床表现，伯氏疏螺旋菌在组织和体液中非常难培养。另外，在潜伏期前 2~4 周培养极少阳性。采用多克隆或单克隆抗体免疫染色可在组织上辨别伯氏疏螺旋菌。尽管免疫组化较银染

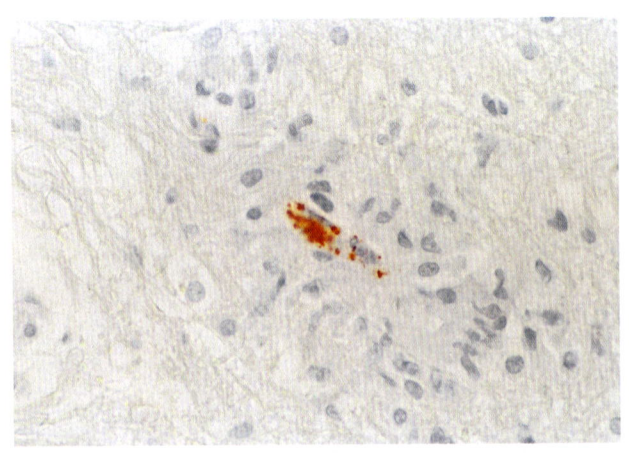

图 2.13　病人患致命性落基山斑疹热的脑干。免疫组化显示立克次体位于内皮细胞，被小胶质细胞结节环绕（AEC 过氧化物酶染色和苏木精复染，×600）

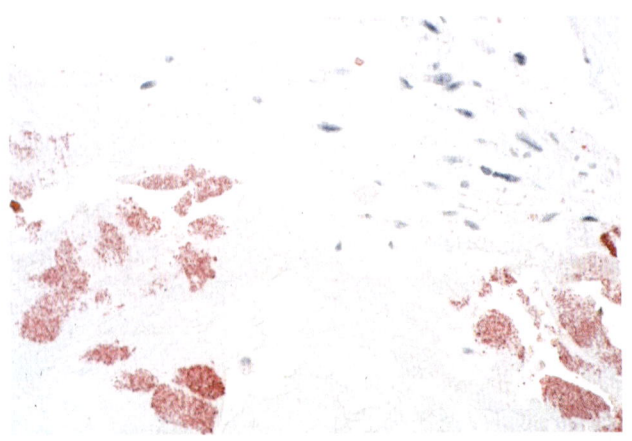

图 2.14　巴尔通体属。病人患组织培养阴性的心内膜炎，免疫组化显示小鼠单抗亨森巴尔通体属位于心瓣膜上（萘酚快红底物和苏木精复染，×40）

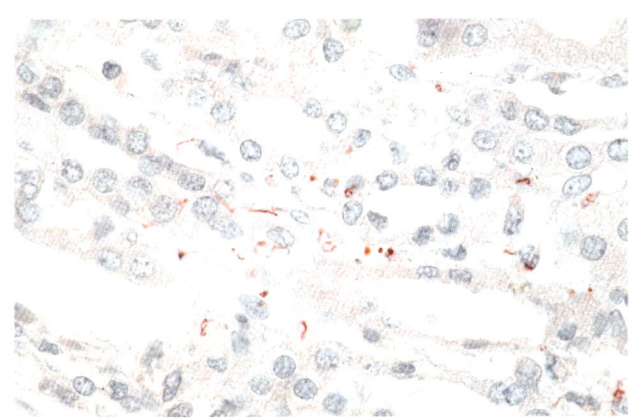

图2.15 钩端螺旋体。免疫染色显示完整的钩端螺旋体和颗粒状的钩端螺旋体抗原位于肾中，病人死于肺出血（兔多克隆抗血清免疫碱性磷酸酶染色、萘酚快红底物和苏木精复染，×63）

色更加特异，但其敏感性不佳，细菌因其在组织切片上的低数量而难以探测[138, 139]。免疫组化在鉴定流感杆菌[140-142]、衣原体属[143-145]、嗜肺军团菌和杜氏军团菌[146-148]、李斯特菌[149-151]、沙门菌属[152, 153]、分枝杆菌属[154-159]、立克次体等感染方面比非落基山斑疹热如南欧斑疹热、斑疹伤寒热[160]、立克次体[161, 162]、南非蜱咬热[125]、恙虫病[163]及梅毒病人的螺旋体更具有应用价值[164-166]。

真菌感染

大多数真菌可较容易地由HE染色或组织化学染色［PAS和银染（GMS）］确定。但是，这些染色不能鉴别形态相似但对抗真菌药物治疗敏感性不同的真菌。另外，真菌在组织切片中因几种因素而形态特点不够典型、包括排列的方向性、真菌感染部位时间的长短、抗真菌化学疗效、感染组织的类型和宿主免疫反应[167]的不同。目前，真菌感染的最后诊断依赖于培养技术，但是，培养可持续几天甚至更长才能确定结果，并且病理学家经常不能获得新鲜组织。

在过去的几年中，免疫组化技术已被用于在福尔马林固定、石蜡包埋的组织上鉴别各类真菌[168-170]，免疫组化方法具有提供快速的特异鉴别几种真菌的优势，并可使病理学家能够鉴别特殊的菌丝和真菌感染，并准确地与人工产物相鉴别[169, 172]。另外，免疫组化可使病理学家把真菌感染的微生物学和组织学发现与非损害性菌落相区分。免疫组化在多种真菌出现的情况下亦有帮助；在这些病例中，双重免疫染色技术可鉴别组织中不同的真菌类型[173]。众所周知免疫组化在鉴别真菌中有其自身的局限性，广泛出现的致病真菌共同抗原经常与多抗，甚至有些单抗产生交叉免疫反应[169, 171-174]。因此，使用一组抗真菌抗体检验交叉反应是评价免疫组化方法的一个非常重要的步骤[169, 170]。

念珠菌属在HE染色组织切片中经常着色较弱，有时其形态较难与荚膜组织胞浆菌、新型隐球菌，甚至卡氏肺囊虫鉴别。抗念珠菌属抗原的单抗和多抗敏感且反应强烈并且与其他真菌无交叉反应[169, 170, 175, 176]。特别是两种抗白色念珠菌甘露糖蛋白的单克隆抗体显示出很高的敏感性和特异性。单抗3H8主要识别白色念珠菌的菌丝，而单抗1B12显示菌体[176, 177]。

当新型隐球菌产生黏液卡红阳性荚膜时，对其鉴别并不困难。但是，荚膜阴性菌种感染却难以诊断，并且易与组织胞浆菌病、芽生菌病、丝状菌病相混淆。而且，在长时间的感染中，真菌经常碎裂或呈现不典型的形态结构。抗新型隐球菌多抗非常敏感和特异[169, 170]。目前，已生产的单抗可在福尔马林固定组织上用来诊断和鉴别不同种类的新型隐球菌。抗体具有非常高的敏感性（97%）和特异性（100%），可区分新型隐球菌的新生变种[178, 179]。

申克孢子丝菌在组织切片上可能易与皮炎芽生菌和皮肤丝状菌相混淆。另外，申克孢子丝菌可能在组织上很稀疏。特异性抗申克孢子丝菌体抗体虽然敏感但与念珠菌属呈现交叉反应。然而，经过与白色念珠菌孢子抗体的特异性吸附，交叉反应性可被去除[169, 170]。

浸润性曲霉病是一种经常发生的真菌感染，在免疫抑制的病人中具有很高的致病率和死亡率。诊断通常很困难，很大程度上依赖于组织学鉴别和组织培养查见具有分隔的菌丝。然而，几种丝状真菌如镰刀菌属、*Pseudallescheria boydii*和足放线菌属在HE染色的组织上与曲霉菌具有相似的形态。另外，组织学培养能够证实的病例数较低，阳性率从30%到50%不等[180, 181]。几种抗曲霉菌抗原的多抗和单抗已在福尔马林固定组织上验证具有不同的敏感性，大多数与其他真菌属具有交叉反应[174, 182, 183]。目前，单克隆（WF-AF-1、164G和611F）抗曲霉菌半乳甘露聚糖鉴别烟曲霉菌、黄曲霉菌和黑曲霉菌，在福尔马林固定组织上显示很高的敏感性和特异性，与其他丝状真菌无交叉反应性[181, 184]。

使用单克隆抗体可在支气管肺泡灌洗标本中检测肺孢子虫囊肿和滋养体，在检测肺孢子虫囊肿上，结果敏感于六亚甲基四胺银（GMS）、姬姆萨（Giemsa）染色或巴帕尼科拉乌（Papanicolaou）染色（图2.16）

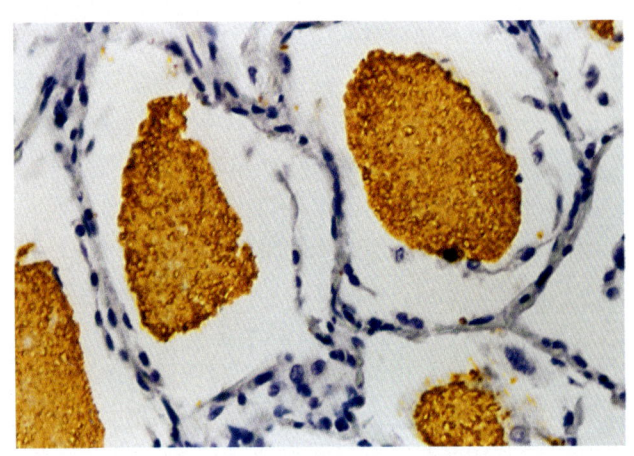

图 2.16 HIV 感染免疫缺陷患者并发肺孢子虫肺炎。单抗抗肺孢子虫免疫过氧化物酶显示孢子虫和滋养体在肺泡内聚集（DAB 与苏木精复染，×400）

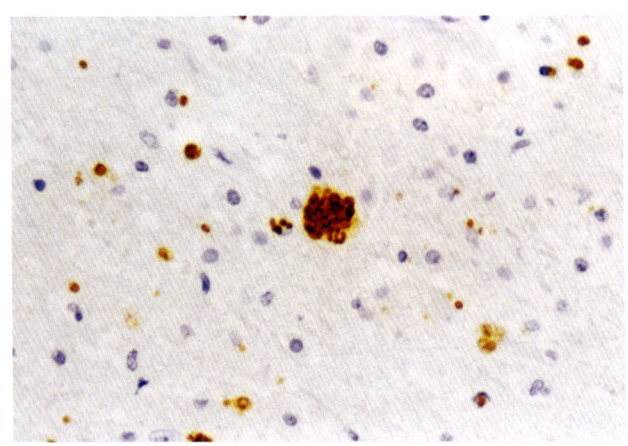

图 2.17 HIV 感染患者并发弓形虫脑炎。免疫过氧化物酶显示假囊和散在的速殖体（DAB 与苏木精复染，×400）

[170, 185, 186]。当非典型性病理特征如肉芽肿性肺孢子虫肺炎，或出现玻璃状膜或肺外肺孢子虫病时，抗体对于诊断肺孢子虫肺炎非常有帮助。

马尔尼菲青霉菌在免疫抑制病人中经常引起播散性感染，临床上与组织胞浆菌病或利什曼病相似[171, 187]。形态学上，它必须与荚膜组织胞浆菌、新型隐球菌、白色念珠菌相区分。单抗 EBA-1 抗曲霉菌半乳甘露聚糖在组织切片上与马尔尼菲青霉菌有交叉反应[182, 188]。免疫组化亦用来检测芽生菌病、球孢子菌病和组织胞浆菌病[169, 170, 189]。但是，抗体与其他几种真菌有很强的交叉反应性。

原虫感染

原虫通常可在 HE 染色或 Giemsa 染色的组织切片上鉴定，但是，因其体积小和不易明显辨别的特征，经常难以作出明确的诊断。免疫组化检测原虫感染局限于因组织坏死或自溶致使原虫形态结构扭曲的病例中。另外，在一些免疫抑制的病人中，弓形虫病可有非同寻常的扩散型表现，只存在大量的速殖体而无缓殖体（图 2.17）[190, 191]。免疫组化也可应用在一些表现特殊的病例中[192]。

在日常工作中利什曼病的诊断并不困难，但是在某些情况下，如慢性肉芽肿性利什曼病原虫数目很少，微生物不出现于通常的位置，或在由于坏死而扭曲疾病的形态学表现的病例中，病理诊断可能较为困难[193]。在这些病例中，免疫组化染色成为非常有价值的诊断工具[193-196]。高敏感性和特异性的单抗 p19-11 可

识别不同种类的利什曼原虫并可区分与之形态相似的微生物（弓形虫、克式锥虫和马尔尼菲青霉菌）[193]。

免疫组化在福尔马林固定、石蜡包埋的组织上也应用于鉴别隐孢子虫属[197]、溶组织内阿米巴[198]、克式锥虫[199-201]、巴贝虫属[202]和兰式贾第鞭毛虫[203]。

新型感染性疾病

1992 年，医疗机构定义新型感染性疾病（EID）为由新型的、从未认知的微生物引起的疾病或那些发病率在过去的 20 年有所增加或不久的将来有可能增加的疾病[204]。1973 以来，新确认的致病菌不断增加。认识新型感染性疾病是一项挑战，因为很多致病原在新型感染性疾病成为公共健康问题之前多年未被认识[205]。EID 成为全球现象，应要求全球作出反应。疾病控制中心已建立战略性措施来预防和监测 EID[205]。病理解剖实验室承担最初和快速探测 EID 的关键角色[206, 207]。免疫组化除帮助鉴别新型感染物质之外，对于认识 EID 的致病机制和流行病学亦作出贡献。

汉坦病毒肺综合征

1993 年，在美国的西南部出现了几例以前健康的个体死于快速渐进性肺水肿、呼吸困难和休克的病例[208, 209]。免疫组化成为鉴定以前未知的汉坦病毒抗原的中心角色。免疫组化分析对于鉴别 1993 年前未知的汉坦病毒肺综合征病例，并且显示病毒抗原

分布于微循环尤其是肺部微循环的内皮细胞，起到重要作用（图 2.18）[210, 212]。

西尼罗病毒性脑炎

西尼罗病毒（WNV）最初于 1937 年鉴定于非洲，第一例 WNV 脑炎在美国被描述于 1999 年。临床征象各异且不典型，症状从亚临床到弛缓瘫痪型和脑炎。形态表现为血管周围单核细胞炎性浸润，神经元坏死，水肿和小胶质细胞结节，尤多见于脑干、小脑和脊髓[213-217]。诊断 WNV 通常依据在脑脊液或血清中发现特异性 IgM，并显示病毒 RNA 存在于血清、脑脊液或其他组织中[218]。免疫染色使用单抗或多抗已成功应用于免疫抑制病人，在缺乏适当的抗体反应的情况下，可诊断 WNV 感染（图 2.19）[214]。

肠病毒 71 脑脊髓炎

肠病毒 71（EV71）与口蹄疫、疱疹性咽峡炎、无菌性脑膜炎和脊髓灰质炎样弛缓性麻痹密切相关。最近发现 EV71 与一些特殊病例的暴发性脑炎、肺水肿出血，以及心力衰竭有关[219, 220]。严重的、广泛的脑皮质、脑干和脊髓的脑脊髓炎已被描述。单抗抗 EV71 免疫染色在联系 EV71 感染和暴发性脑炎中起到关键性作用（图 2.20）。病毒抗原见于神经元、神经细胞树突和单核炎性细胞内[221-223]。

尼派病毒感染

尼派病毒为最近所描述的副黏病毒，可引发急性发热性脑炎综合征，具有很高的死亡率[224, 226]。病理在鉴别致病因素方面起到关键性作用。组织病理发现包括含有血栓的脉管炎、微梗塞、合体巨细胞和病毒包涵体。合体巨内皮细胞为特征性改变，尽管只见于 25% 的病例[224]，病毒包涵体也可见于其他副黏病毒感染。免疫染色对疾病作出明确诊断提供了有力的帮助，可显示病毒抗原位于神经元细胞和大多数器官的内皮细胞内（图 2.21）[5, 224]。

埃利希病

埃利希和微粒孢子虫属细菌分别可引起人类单核细胞性埃利希病和人类粒细胞性微粒孢子虫病。急性发热性疾病通常表现为血细胞减少、肌痛和轻到中度的肝炎[227-230]。

诊断埃利希病依赖于发现典型单核细胞和粒细胞内

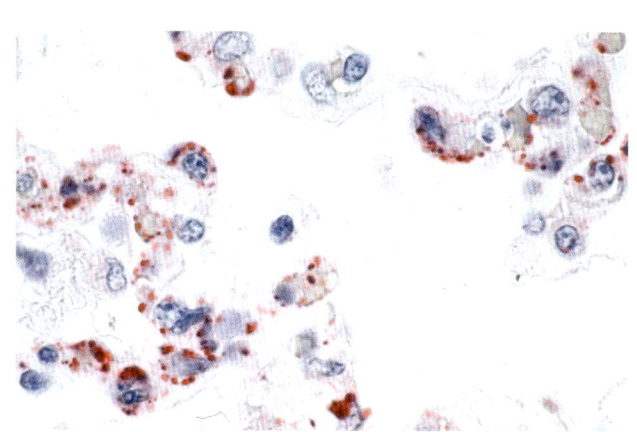

图 2.18 鼠单抗免疫组化显示汉坦病毒位于肺微循环血管内皮细胞内（免疫碱性磷酸酶与萘酚快红底物和苏木精染色，×100）

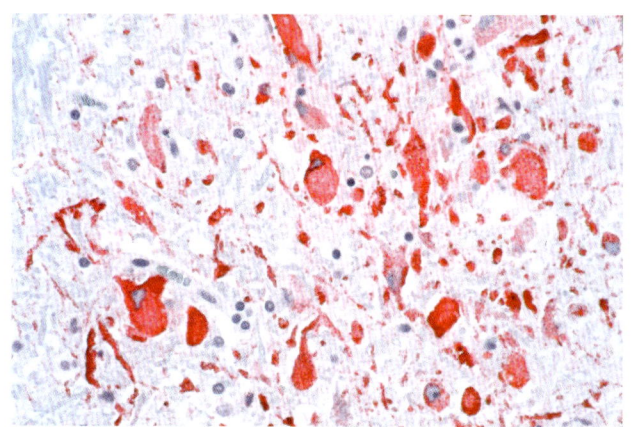

图 2.19 西尼罗病毒。免疫染色黄病毒抗原位于中枢神经组织的神经元和神经突起中，来自西尼罗病毒脑炎的免疫抑制患者（黄病毒超免疫小鼠腹水，萘酚快红底物和苏木精复染，×40）

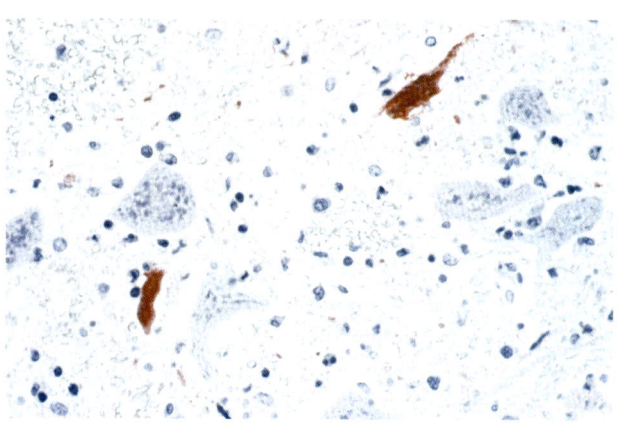

图 2.20 肠病毒 71。肠病毒脑炎致死病例，EV71 阳性染色位于神经元和神经细胞树突中（免疫碱性磷酸酶与萘酚快红底物和苏木精复染，×40）

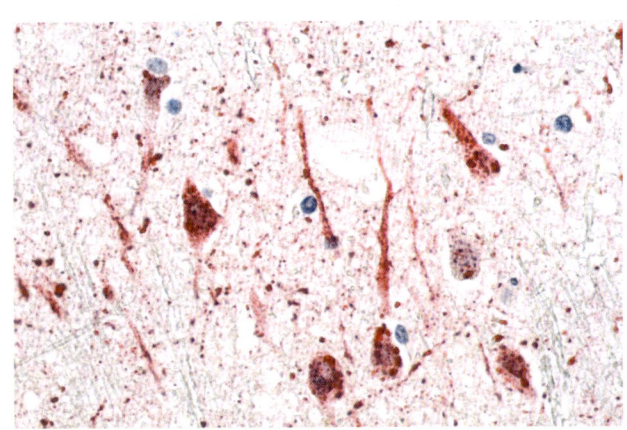

图2.21 尼派病毒。尼派病毒脑炎致死病例,免疫染色尼派病毒抗原位于中枢神经组织的神经元和神经细胞树突中(萘酚快红底物和苏木精复染,×63)

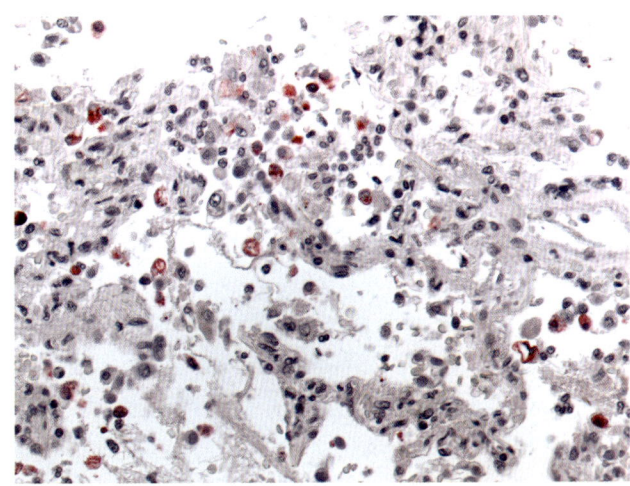

图2.22 SARS。冠状病毒抗原阳性肺细胞和巨噬细胞位于SARS患者的肺组织中(免疫碱性磷酸酶与萘酚快红底物和苏木精复染,×63)

包涵体(桑葚体),PCR分析可检出血液中的特异性抗体。但是,桑葚体非常稀少而且经常被忽略。HE染色经常不能显示该病菌,即使免疫组化呈现大量的埃利希抗原,抗体滴度经过几个星期才可上升到诊断水平[227]。另外,免疫抑制病人死亡之前可能不产生抗埃利希抗体[227,229]。在这种病例中,埃利希病和微粒孢子虫病的免疫染色已表明其是一种敏感和特异的诊断方法[227,229-231]。

免疫组化已被证实为一种非常有价值的鉴别和研究手段,用于许多的新型感染性疾病,如埃博拉出血热[81-83,227]、亨德拉病毒性脑炎[5,232,233]、钩端螺旋体病[135-137]和最近鉴定的与严重急性呼吸性综合征(SARS)相关的一种新型冠状病毒[224,235]。SARS首次被发现于全球暴发的严重肺炎中,首例发生于2002年末中国广州,随后暴发于2003年2月,先后发现于亚洲、欧洲、北美和南美洲二十余个国家。发病初始的临床、病理和实验室研究主要集中于已知的呼吸系统疾病的病因,相继,从SARS患者的鼻咽部分离出病毒,经超微结构证实为冠状病毒。多个报告描述了弥漫性肺泡损伤为其主要的组织病理改变。应用免疫组化(图2.22)和原位杂交(ISH)在人和实验动物的组织上可检出与SARS相关的冠状病毒(SARS-CoV)[236-245]。

病理学家、免疫组化和生物恐怖

当前,人们越来越关注使用感染性物质作为可能的生物武器。生物战剂从稀有的外来病毒到普通的细菌物质。故意使用生物因子引起的疾病,可相似于自然状态的疾病暴发,或可能拥有非同寻常的特征[246]。美国CDC已颁布对于生物袭击的一套完整的公共健康应对措施。非常重要的两部分应对方案包括迅速诊断和确定生物因子特征。病理学家使用最新的诊断技术如免疫组化、原位杂交和PCR对于快速探测和控制新出现的感染性疾病产生重要影响,无论这些疾病出于自然状态或人为所致。无论是在调查或追溯生物恐怖,还是加速实施有效的公共健康反应措施方面,免疫组化提供了一种简便、安全、敏感和特异的快速探测方法。

炭疽

免疫组化单抗抗细胞壁和荚膜抗原标记炭疽杆菌,已成功应用于鉴定与生物恐怖有关的炭疽病例,成为在早期诊断和治疗此类疾病非常重要的一个环节[5,250-254]。革兰染色和细菌培养分离炭疽杆菌是诊断炭疽的通常方法;然而,先期抗生素治疗会影响细菌培养和革兰染色结果[252]。免疫组化已被证实为高敏感和特异的方法,用于皮肤活检、胸腔活检、经支气管活检和胸腔积液中探测炭疽杆菌(图2.23)[251-253]。

另外,免疫染色亦可有效地检测细菌的感染途径和鉴别疾病的扩散方式[252,255]。

兔热病

免疫组化染色可在福尔马林固定的组织切片上快速检测野兔热弗朗希斯菌。兔热病可拥有不同类型的临床和病理表现,与其他感染性疾病如炭疽、鼠疫、猫抓病或性病性淋巴肉芽肿相似。而且,这些微生物即使使用革兰染色或银染色方法仍难以在切片上显示。

感染性疾病的免疫组织化学 **2**

一种小鼠单抗抗野兔热弗朗希斯菌脂多糖已被用于显示肺、脾、淋巴结和肝中完整的细菌或颗粒状细菌抗原，并具有极高的敏感性和特异性（图2.24）[256, 257]。

鼠疫

一种小鼠单抗抗鼠疫耶尔森菌片段-1抗原已被应用于探测位于血管、肺、淋巴结、脾和肝细胞内或细胞外的细菌（图2.25）[258-262]。这种技术在福尔马林固定的皮肤活检组织上快速诊断鼠疫具有潜在应用价值，另外，根据鉴定耶尔森菌位于肺部不同区域（如肺泡或间质）免疫组化可鉴别初发和再发肺部鼠疫[258]。

免疫组化方法使用多抗和单抗已被应用于鉴别几种其他可能性生物恐怖因子，包括布鲁菌病[5]、Q热[5, 125, 263, 264]、病毒性脑炎（东部马脑炎）（图2.26）[5, 109-111]、立克次体病（伤寒和落基山斑疹热）[125-128, 160]和病毒性出血热（埃博拉病、马尔堡病）[5, 77-83]。

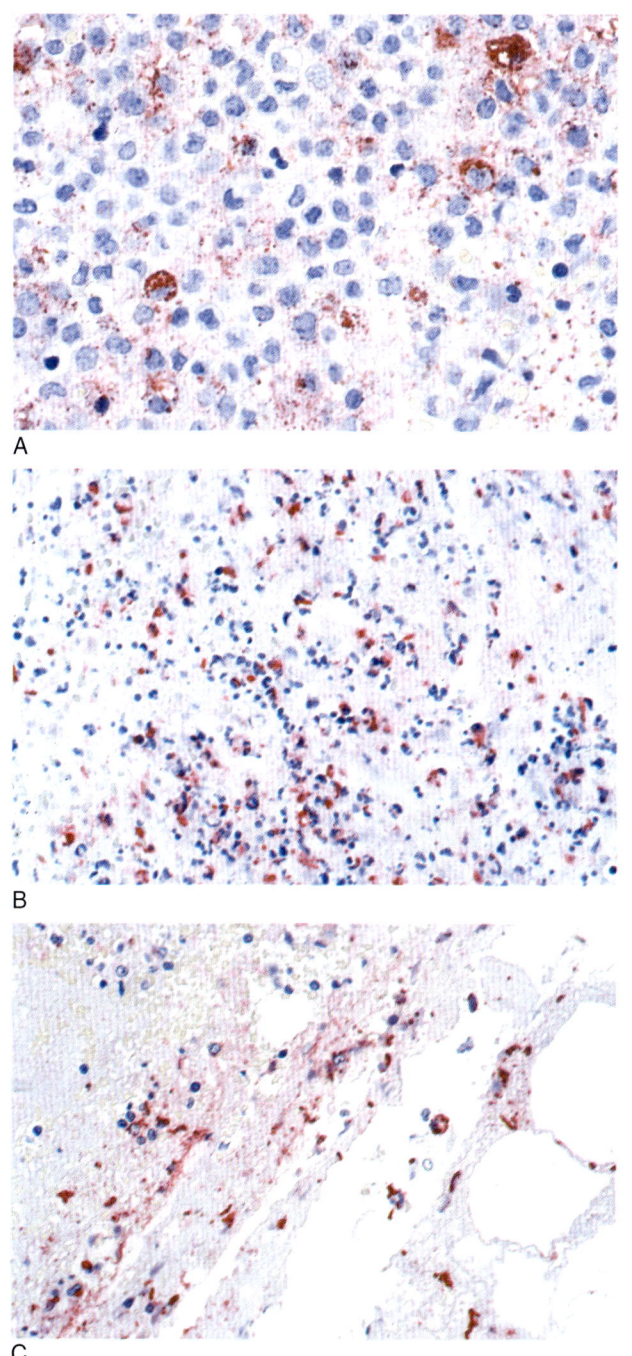

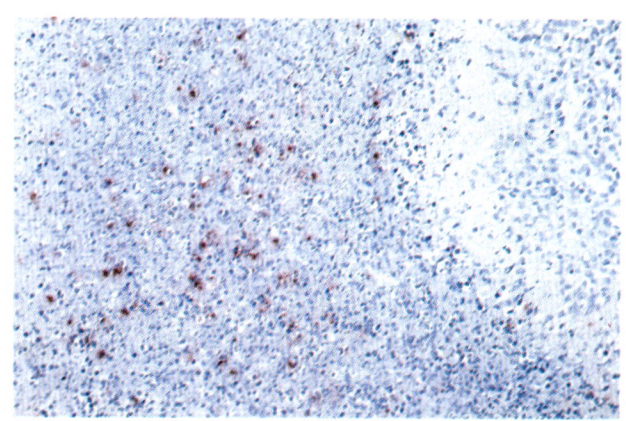

图2.24 兔热病。淋巴结免疫染色显示星状脓肿，小鼠单抗抗野兔热弗朗希斯菌脂多糖显示，含有野兔弗朗希斯菌抗原的巨噬细胞位于中心坏死区（免疫碱性磷酸酶与萘酚快红底物和苏木精复染，×10）

图2.23 炭疽。（A）胸膜渗漏细胞显示抗炭疽杆菌荚膜抗原染色的杆菌片段和颗粒（免疫碱性磷酸酶与萘酚快红底物和苏木精复染，×63）；（B）抗炭疽杆菌细胞壁抗体显示皮肤炭疽活检大量颗粒抗原染色和杆菌片段（免疫碱性磷酸酶与萘酚快红底物和苏木精复染，×40）；（C）抗炭疽杆菌细胞壁抗体显示纵隔淋巴结大量颗粒抗原和杆菌片段（免疫碱性磷酸酶与萘酚快红底物和苏木精复染，×63）

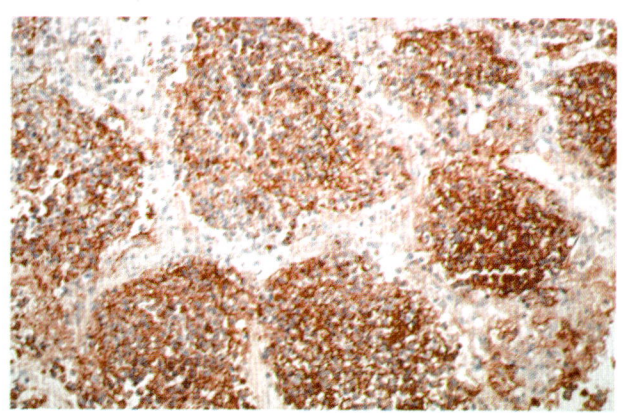

图2.25 鼠疫。小鼠单抗抗鼠疫耶尔森菌片段-1肺部免疫染色显示，大量细菌和颗粒抗原位于肺泡中（免疫碱性磷酸酶与萘酚快红底物和苏木精复染，×20）

49

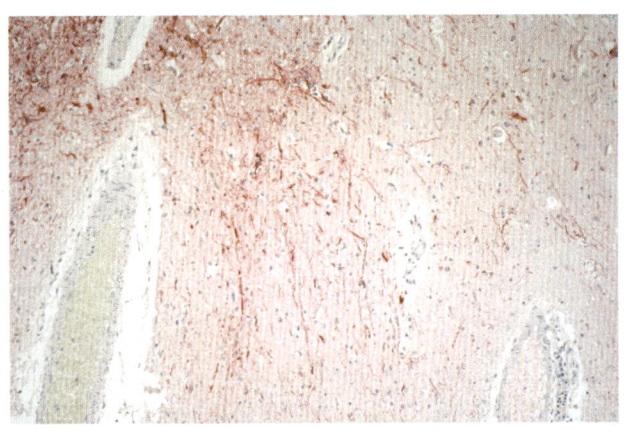

图2.26 小鼠抗东部马脑炎菌抗体显示，病毒抗原位于中枢神经组织的神经元和神经细胞树突中（免疫碱性磷酸酶与萘酚快红底物和苏木精复染，×10）

参考文献

1. Cartun RW. Use of immunohistochemistry in the surgical pathology laboratory for the diagnosis of infectious diseases. Pathol Case Rev 1999; 4:260–265.
2. Watts JC. Surgical pathology in the diagnosis of infectious diseases (Editorial). Am J Clin Pathol 1994; 102:711–712.
3. Schwartz DA, Bryan RT. Infectious disease pathology and emerging infections: Are we prepared? Arch Pathol Lab Med 1996; 120:117–124.
4. Schwartz DA. Emerging and reemerging infections: Progress and challenges in the subspecialty of infectious disease pathology. Arch Pathol Lab Med 1997; 121:776–784.
5. Zaki SR, Paddock CD. The emerging role of pathology in infectious diseases. In: Scheld WM, Armstrong D, Hughes JM, eds. Emerging infections 3. Washington, DC: ASM Press; 1999:181–200.
6. Medical Examiners, Coroners, and Biologic Terrorism: A Guidebook for Surveillance and Case Management. MMWR Morbidity and Mortality Weekly Report 2004; 53(RR-8):1–53.
7. Zaki SR, Peters CJ. Viral hemorrhagic fevers. In: Connor DH, Chandler FW, Schwartz DA, et al., eds. Pathology of infectious diseases. Stamford, CT: Appleton and Lange; 1997:347–364.
8. Coons AH, Creech HJ, Jones RN, et al. The demonstration of pneumococcal antigen in tissues by use of fluorescent antibodies. J Immunol 1942; 45:159–170.
9. Jeavons L, Hunt L, Hamilton A. Immunochemical studies of heat-shock protein 80 of *Histoplasma capsulatum*. J Med Vet Mycol 1994; 32:47–57.
10. Werner M, Chott A, Fabiano A, et al. Effect of formalin tissue fixation and processing on immunohistochemistry. Am J Surg Pathol 2000; 24:1016–1019.
11. Woods GL, Walker DH. Detection of infection or infectious agents by use of cytologic and histologic stains. Clin Microbiol Rev 1996; 9:382–404.
12. Chandler FW. Invasive microorganisms. In: Spicer SS, ed. Histochemistry in pathology diagnosis. New York, NY: Marcel Dekker; 1987:77–101.
13. Clausen PP, Thomsen P. Demonstration of hepatitis B surface antigen in liver biopsies. A comparative investigation of immunoperoxidase and orcein staining on identical sections on formalin-fixed, paraffin-embedded tissue. Acta Pathol Microbiol Scand [A] 1978; 86A:383.
14. Thomsen P, Clausen PP. Occurrence of hepatitis B-surface antigen in consecutive material of 1539 liver biopsies. Acta Pathol Microbiol Immunol Scand. [A] 1983; 91:71.
15. Al Adnani MS, Ali SM. Patterns of chronic liver disease in Kuwait with special reference to localization of hepatitis B surface antigen. J Clin Pathol 1984; 37:549.
16. Taylor C. Lung, pancreas, colon and rectum, stomach, liver. In: Taylor CR, Cote RJ, eds. Immunomicroscopy: a diagnostic tool for the surgical pathologist. 2nd edn. Philadelphia, PA: WB Saunders; 1994:292–317.
17. Park YN, Han KH, Kim KS, et al. Cytoplasmic expression of hepatitis B core antigen in chronic hepatitis B virus infection: role of precore stop mutants. Liver 1999; 19:199–205.
18. Dries V, von Both I, Müller M, et al. Detection of hepatitis C virus in paraffin-embedded liver biopsies of patients negative for viral RNA in serum. Hepatology 1999; 29:223–229.
19. Brody RI, Eng S, Melamed J, et al. Immunohistochemical detection of hepatitis C antigen by monoclonal antibody TORDJI-22 compared with PCR viral detection. Am J Clin Pathol 1998; 110:32–37.
20. Nuovo GJ, Holly A, Wakely P, et al. Correlation of histology, viral load, and in situ viral detection in hepatic biopsies from patients with liver transplants secondary to hepatitis C infection. Hum Pathol 2002; 33:277–284.
21. Komminoth P, Adams V, Long AA, et al. Evaluation of methods for hepatitis C virus detection in archival liver biopsies.

Comparison of histology, immunohistochemistry, in-situ hybridization, reverse transcriptase polymerase chain reaction (RT-PCR) and in-situ RT-PCR. Pathol Res Pract 1994; 190:1017–1025.
22. Doughty AL, Painter DM, McCaughan GW. Nonspecificity of monoclonal antibody TORDJI-22 for the detection of hepatitis C virus in liver transplant recipients with cholestatic hepatitis. Liver Transpl Surg 1999; 5:40–45.
23. Sansonno D, Iacobelli AR, Cornacchiulo V, et al. Immunohistochemical detection of hepatitis C virus-related proteins in liver tissue. Clin Exp Rheumatol 1995; 13 (Suppl 13):S29–S32.
24. Blight K, Rowland R, Hall PD, et al. Immunohistochemical detection of the NS4 antigen of hepatitis C virus and its relation to histopathology. Am J Pathol 1993; 143:1568–1573.
25. Verslype C, Nevens F, Sinelli N, et al. Hepatic immunohistochemical staining with a monoclonal antibody against HCV-E2 to evaluate antiviral therapy and reinfection of liver grafts in hepatitis C viral infection. J Hepatol 2003; 38:208–214.
26. Feiden W, Borchard F, Burrig KF, et al. Herpes esophagitis: I. Light microscopical immunohistochemical investigations. Virchows Arch [A] 1984; 404:167–176.
27. Nikkels AF, Delvenne P, Sadzot-Delvaux C, et al. Distribution of varicella zoster virus and herpes simplex virus in disseminated fatal infections. J Clin Pathol 1996; 49:243–248.
28. Greenson JK, Beschorner WE, Boitnott JK, et al. Prominent mononuclear cell infiltrate is characteristic of herpes esophagitis. Hum Pathol 1991; 22:541–549.
29. Wang JY, Montone KT. A rapid simple in situ hybridization method for herpes simplex virus employing a synthetic biotin-labeled oligonucleotide probe: a comparison with immunohistochemical methods for HSV detection. J Clin Lab Anal 1994; 8:105–115.
30. Kobayashi TK, Ueda M, Nishino T, et al. Brush cytology of herpes simplex virus infection in oral mucosa: use of the ThinPrep processor. Diag Cytopath 1998; 18:71–75.
31. Nicoll JAR, Love S, Burton PA, et al. Autopsy findings in two cases of neonatal herpes simplex virus infection: detection of virus by immunohistochemistry, in situ hybridization and the polymerase chain reaction. Histopathology 1994; 24: 257–264.
32. Nikkels AF, Debrus S, Sadzot-Delvaux C, et al. Comparative immunohistochemical study of herpes simplex and varicella-zoster infections. Virchows Archiv A Pathol Anat 1993; 422:121–126.
33. Cohen PR. Tests for detecting herpes simplex virus and varicella-zoster virus infections. Dermat Clin 1994; 12:51–68.
34. Katano H, Sato Y, Kurata T, et al. Expression and localization of human herpesvirus 8-encoded proteins in primary effusion lymphoma, Kaposi's sarcoma, and multicentric Castleman's disease. Virology 2000; 269:335–344.
35. Katano H, Suda T, Morishita Y, et al. Human herpesvirus 8-associated solid lymphomas that occur in AIDS patients takes anaplastic large cell morphology. Mod Pathol 2000; 13: 77–85.
36. Ely SA, Powers J, Lewis D, et al. Kaposi's sarcoma-associated herpesvirus-positive primary effusion lymphoma arising in the subarachnoid space. Hum Pathol 1999; 30:981–984.
37. Katano H, Sato Y, Kurata T, et al. High expression of HHV-8-encoded ORF73 protein in spindle-shape cells of Kaposi's sarcoma. Am J Pathol 1999; 155:47–52.
38. Said JW, Shintaku IP, Asou H, et al. Herpesvirus 8 inclusions in primary effusion lymphoma: report of a unique case with T-cell phenotype. Archiv Pathol Lab Med 1999; 123: 257–260.
39. Cheuk W, Wong KOY, Wong CSC, et al. Immunostaining for human herpesvirus 8 latent nuclear antigen-1 helps distinguishing Kaposi sarcoma from its mimickers. Am J Clin Pathol 2004; 121:335–342.
40. Robin YM, Guillou L, Michels JJ, et al. Human herpesvirus 8 immunostaining. A sensitive and specific method for diagnosing Kaposi sarcoma in paraffin-embedded sections. Am J Clin Pathol 2004; 121:330–334.
41. Bryant-Greenwood P, Sorbara L, Filie AC, et al. Infection of mesothelial cells with human herpesvirus 8 in human immunodeficiency virus-infected patients with Kaposi sarcoma, Castleman disease, and recurrent pleural effusions. Mod Pathol 2003; 16:145–153.
42. Cool CD, Pradeep RR, Yeager ME, et al. Expression of human herpesvirus 8 in primary pulmonary hypertension. N Engl J Med 2003; 349:1113–1122.
43. Anwar F, Erice A, Jessurun J. Are there cytopathic features associated with cytomegalovirus infection predictive of resistance to antiviral therapy? Ann Diag Pathol 1999; 3:19–22.

44. Sheehan MM, Coker R, Coleman DV. Detection of cytomegalovirus (CMV) in HIV+ patients: comparison of cytomorphology, immunohistochemistry and in situ hybridization. Cytopathology 1998; 9:29–37.

45. Kutza AS, Muhl E, Hackstein H, et al. High incidence of active cytomegalovirus infection among septic patients. Clin Infect Dis 1998; 26:1076–1082.

46. Saetta A, Agapitos E, Davaris PS. Determination of CMV placentitis: Diagnostic application of the polymerase chain reaction. Virchows Arch 1998; 432:159–162.

47. Solans EP, Yong S, Husain AN, et al. Bronchioloalveolar lavage in the diagnosis of CMV pneumonitis in lung transplant recipients: an immunocytochemical study. Diagn Cytopath 1997; 16:350–352.

48. Nebuloni M, Pellegrinelli A, Ferri A, et al. Etiology of microglial nodules in brains of patients with acquired immunodeficiency syndrome. J Neurovirol 2000; 6:46–50.

49. Rimsza LM, Vela EE, Frutiger YM, et al. Rapid automated combined in situ hybridization and immunohistochemistry for sensitive detection of cytomegalovirus in paraffin-embedded tissue biopsies. Am J Clin Pathol 1996; 106:544–548.

50. Kambhan N, Vij R, Cartwright CA, et al. Cytomegalovirus infection in steroid-refractory ulcerative colitis. A case-control study. Am J Surg Pathol 2004; 28:365–373.

51. Ribalta T, Martinez AJ, Jares P, et al. Presence of occult cytomegalovirus infection in the brain after orthotopic liver transplantation. An autopsy study of 83 cases. Virchows Arch 2002; 440:166–171.

52. Cruz-Spano L, Lima-Pereira FE, Gomes da Silva-Basso N, et al. Human cytomegalovirus infection and abortion: an immunohistochemical study. Med Sci Monit 2002; 8:BR230–235.

53. Colina F, Juca NT, Moreno E, et al. Histological diagnosis of cytomegalovirus hepatitis in liver allografts. J Clin Pathol 1995; 48:351–357.

54. Flomenberg P, Babbitt J, Drobyski WR, et al. Increasing incidence of adenovirus disease in bone marrow transplant recipients. J Infect Dis 1994; 169:775–781.

55. Strickler JG, Singleton TP, Copenhaver GM, et al. Adenovirus in the gastrointestinal tracts of immunosuppressed patients. Am J Clin Pathol 1992; 97:555–558.

56. Yi ES, Powell HC. Adenovirus infection of the duodenum in an AIDS patient: an ultrastructural study. Ultrastruct Pathol 1994; 18:549–551.

57. Yan Z, Nguyen S, Poles M, et al. Adenovirus colitis in human immunodeficiency virus infection: an under-diagnosed entity. Am J Surg Pathol 1998; 22:1101–1106.

58. Dombrowski F, Eis-Hubinger AM, Ackermann T, et al. Adenovirus-induced liver necrosis in a case of AIDS. Virchows Archiv 1997; 431:469–472.

59. Simsir A, Greenebaum E, Nuovo G, et al. Late fatal adenovirus pneumonitis in a lung transplant recipient. Transplantation 1998; 65:592–594.

60. Saad RS, Demetris AJ, Lee RG, et al. Adenovirus hepatitis in the adult allograft liver. Transplantation 1997; 64:1483–1485.

61. Ohori NP, Michaels MG, Jaffe R, et al. Adenovirus pneumonia in lung transplant recipients. Hum Pathol 1995; 26:1073–1079.

62. Wang WH, Wang HL. Fulminant adenovirus hepatitis following bone marrow transplantation. A case report and brief review of the literature. Arch Pathol Lab Med 2003; 127:e246–e248.

63. Lones MA, Shintaku IP, Weiss LM, et al. Posttransplant lymphoproliferative disorder in liver allograft biopsies: a comparison of three methods for the demonstration of Epstein-Barr virus. Hum Pathol 1997; 28:533–539.

64. Challoner PB, Smith KT, Parker JD, et al. Plaque-associated expression of human herpesvirus 6 in multiple sclerosis. Proc Natl Acad Sci USA 1995; 92:7440–7444.

65. Brown KE, Young NS. Parvovirus B19 infection and hematopoiesis. Blood Rev 1995; 9:176–182.

66. Jordan JA, Penchansky L. Diagnosis of human parvovirus B19-induced anemia: correlation of bone marrow morphology with molecular diagnosis using PCR and immunohistochemistry. Cell Vision 1995; 2:279–282.

67. Morey AL, O'Neil HJ, Coyle PV, et al. Immunohistological detection of human parvovirus B19 in formalinfixed, paraffin-embedded tissues. J Pathol 1992; 166:105–108.

68. Puvion-Dutilleul F, Puvion E. Human parvovirus B19 as a causative agent for rheumatoid arthritis. Proc Natl Acad Sci USA 1998; 95:8227–8232.

69. Yufu Y, Matsumoto M, Miyamura T, et al. Parvovirus B19-associated haemophagocytic syndrome with lymphadenopathy resembling histiocytic necrotizing lymphadenitis (Kikuchi's diease). Br J Haematol 1997; 96:868–871.

70. Vadlamudi G, Rezuke N, Ross JW, et al. The use of mono-

clonal antibody R92F6 and polymerase chain reaction to confirm the presence of parvovirus B19 in bone marrow specimens of patients with acquired immunodeficiency syndrome. Arch Pathol Lab Med 1999; 123:768–773.

71. Wright C, Hinchliffe SA, Taylor C. Fetal pathology in intrauterine death due to parvovirus B19 infection. Br J Obstet Gynaecol 1996; 103:133–136.

72. Essary LR, Vnencak-Jones CL, Manning SS, et al. Frequency of parvovirus B19 infection in nonimmune hydrops fetalis and utility of three diagnostic methods. Hum Pathol 1998; 29:696–701.

73. Monath TP, Ballinger ME, Miller BR, et al. Detection of yellow fever viral RNA by nucleic acid hybridization and viral antigen by immunohistochemistry in fixed human liver. Am J Trop Med Hyg 1989; 40:663–668.

74. De Brito T, Siqueira SA, Santos RT, et al. Human fatal yellow fever. Immunohistochemical detection of viral antigens in the liver, kidney, and heart. Pathol Res Practice 1992; 188:177–181.

75. Hall WC, Crowell TP, Watts DM, et al. Demonstration of yellow fever and dengue antigens in formalin-fixed paraffin-embedded human liver by immunohistochemical analysis. Am J Trop Med Hyg 1991; 45:408–417.

76. Ramos C, Sanchez G, Pando RH, et al. Dengue virus in the brain of a fatal case of hemorrhagic dengue fever. J Neurovirol 1998; 4:465–468.

77. Burt FJ, Swanepoel R, Shieh W-J, et al. Immunohistochemical and in situ localization of Crimean-Congo hemorrhagic fever (CCHF) virus in human tissues and implications for CCHF pathogenesis. Arch Pathol Lab Med 1997; 121:839–846.

78. Maiztegui JI, Laguens RP, Cossio PM, et al. Ultrastructural and immunohistochemical studies in five cases of Argentine hemorrhagic fever. J Infect Dis 1975; 132:35–53.

79. Hall WC, Geisbert TW, Huggins JW, et al. Experimental infection of guinea pigs with Venezuelan hemorrhagic fever virus (Guanarito): a model of human disease. Am J Trop Med Hyg 1996; 55:81–88.

80. Geisbert TW, Jaax NK. Marburg hemorrhagic fever: report of a case studied by immunohistochemistry and electron microscopy. Ultrastruct Pathol 1998; 22:3–17.

81. Zaki SR, Shieh W-J, Greer PW, et al. A novel immunohistochemical assay for the detection of Ebola virus in skin: implications for diagnosis, spread, and surveillance of Ebola hemorrhagic fever. J Infect Dis 1999; 179(Suppl 1):S36–S37.

82. Ksiazek TG, Rollin PE, Williams AJ, et al. Clinical virology of Ebola hemorrhagic fever (EHF): virus, virus antigen, and IgG and IgM antibody findings among EHF patients in Kikwit, Democratic Republic of Congo. J Infect Dis 1999; 179:S177–S187.

83. Wyers M, Formenty P, Cherel Y, et al. Histopathological and immunohistochemical studies of lesions associated with Ebola virus in a naturally infected chimpanzee. J Infect Dis 1999; 179(Suppl 1):S54–S59.

84. Delvenne P, Fontaine M-A, Delvenne C, et al. Detection of human papillomaviruses in paraffin-embedded biopsies of cervical intraepithelial lesions: analysis by immunohistochemistry, in situ hybridization, and the polymerase chain reaction. Mod Pathol 1994; 7:113–119.

85. Lopez-Beltran A, Escudero AL, Carrasco-Aznar JC, et al. Human papillomavirus infection and transitional cell carcinoma of the bladder. Immunohistochemistry and in situ hybridization. Pathol Res Pract 1996; 192:154–159.

86. Meyer MP, Markiw CA, Matuscak RR, et al. Detection of human papillomavirus DNA in genital lesions by using a modified commercially available in situ hybridization assay. J Clin Microbiol 1991; 29:1308.

87. Wilbur DC, Reichman RC, Stoler MH. Detection of infection by human papillomavirus in genital condyloma. A comparison study using immunohistochemistry and in situ nucleic acid hybridization. Am J Clin Pathol 1988; 89:505.

88. Pappo O, Demetris AI, Raikow RB, et al. Human polyomavirus infection of renal allografts: histopathologic diagnosis, clinical significance and literature review. Mod Pathol 1996; 9:105–109.

89. Nebuloni M, Tosoni A, Boldorini R, et al. BK virus renal infection in a patient with the acquired immunodeficiency syndrome. Arch Pathol Lab Med 1999; 123:807–811.

90. Elli A, Banfi G, Battista-Fogazzi G, et al. BK polyomavirus interstitial nephritis in a renal transplant patient with no previous acute rejection episodes. J Nephrol 2002; 15:313–316.

91. Boldorini R, Omodeo-Zorini E, Sunno A, et al. Molecular characterization and sequence analysis of polyomavirus strains isolated from needle biopsy specimens of kidney allograft recipients. Am J Clin Pathol 2001; 116:489–494.

92. Jochum W, Weber T, Frye S, et al. Detection of JC virus by

92. anti-VP1 immunohistochemistry in brains with progressive multifocal leukoencephalopathy. Acta Neuropathol 1997; 94: 226–231.
93. Chima SC, Agostini HT, Ryschlkeewitsch CF, et al. Progressive multifocal leukoencephalopathy and JC virus genotypes in West African patients with acquired immunodeficiency syndrome. A pathologic and DNA sequence analysis of 4 cases. Arch Pathol Lab Med 1999; 123:395–403.
94. Aoki N, Mori M, Kato K, et al. Antibody against synthetic multiple antigen peptides (MAP) of JC virus capsid protein (VP1) without cross reaction to BK virus: a diagnostic tool for progressive multifocal leukoencephalopathy. Neurosci Letts 1996; 205:111–114.
95. Silver SA, Arthur RR, Rozan YS, et al. Diagnosis of progressive multifocal leukoencephalopathy by stereotactic brain biopsy utilizing immunohistochemistry and the polymerase chain reaction. Acta Cytolog 1995; 39:35–44.
96. Guarner J, Shieh W-J, Dawson J, et al. Immunohistochemical and in situ hybridization studies of influenza A virus infection in human lungs. Am J Clin Pathol 2000; 114:227–233.
97. Cartun RW, Tahhan HR, Knibbs DR, et al. Immunocytochemical identification of respiratory syncytial virus (RVS) in formalin-fixed, paraffin-embedded tissue from immunocompromised hosts. Mod Pathol 1989; 2:15.
98. Nielson KA, Yunis EJ. Demonstration of respiratory syncytial virus in an autopsy series. Pediatr Pathol 1990; 10:491–502.
99. Wright C, Oliver KC, Fenwick FI, et al. A monoclonal antibody pool for routine immunohistochemical detection of human respiratory syncytial virus antigens in formalin-fixed, paraffin-embedded tissue. J Pathol 1997; 182:238–244.
100. Jogai S, Radotra BD, Banerjee AK. Immunohistochemical study of human rabies. Neuropathology 2000; 20:197–203.
101. Jogai S, Radotra BD, Banerjee AK. Rabies viral antigen in extracranial organs: a postmortem study. Neuropathol Appl Neurobiol 2002; 28:334.
102. Warner CK, Zaki SR, Shieh WJ, et al. Laboratory investigation of humans from vampire bat rabies in Peru. Am J Trop Med Hyg 1999; 60:502–507.
103. Sinchaisri TA, Nagata T, Yoshikawa Y, et al. Immunohistochemical and histopathological study of experimental rabies infection in mice. J Vet Med Sc 1992; 54:409–416.
104. Jackson AC, Ye H, Phelan CC, et al. Extraneural organ involvement in human rabies. Lab Invest 1999; 79:945–951.
105. Yousef GE, Mann GF, Brown IN, et al. Clinical and research application of an enterovirus group-reactive monoclonal antibody. Intervirol 1987; 28:199–205.
106. Hohenadl C, Klingel K, Rieger P, et al. Investigation of the coxsackievirus B3 nonstructural proteins 2B, 2C, and 3AB: generation of specific polyclonal antisera and detection of replicating virus in infected tissue. J Virol Methods 1994; 47:279–295.
107. Zhang H, Li Y, Peng T, et al. Localization of enteroviral antigen in myocardium and other tissues from patients with heart muscle disease by an improved immunohistochemical technique. J Histochem Cytochem 2000; 48:579–584.
108. Li Y, Bourlet T, Andreoletti L, et al. Enteroviral capsid protein VP1 is present in myocardial tissues from some patients with myocarditis or dilated cardiomyopathy. Circulation 2000; 101:231–234.
109. Del Piero F, Wilkins PA, Dubovi EJ, et al. Clinical, pathologic, immunohistochemical, and virologic findings of Eastern equine encephalitis in two horses. Vet Pathol 2001; 38:451-456.
110. Patterson JS, Maes RK, Mullaney TP, et al. Immunohistochemical diagnosis of Eastern equine encephalomyelitis. J Vet Diag Invest 1996; 8:156–160.
111. Garen PD, Tsai TF, Powers JM. Human Eastern equine encephalitis: immunohistochemistry and ultrastructure. Mod Pathol 1999; 12:646–652.
112. Tatti KM, Gentsch J, Shieh WJ, et al. Molecular and immunological methods to detect rotavirus in formalin-fixed tissue. J Virol 2002; 105:305–319.
113. Morrison C, Gilson T, Nuovo GJ, et al. Histologic distribution of fatal rotaviral infection: an immunohistochemical and reverse transcriptase in situ polymerase chain reaction analysis. Hum Pathol 2001; 32:216–221.
114. Cioc AM, Nuovo GJ. Histologic and in situ viral findings in the myocardium in cases of sudden, unexpected death. Mod Pathol 2001; 15:914–922.
115. El-Zimaity HMT, Graham DY, Al-Assis MT, et al. Interobserver variation in the histopathological assessment of *Helicobacter pylori* gastritis. Hum Pathol 1996; 27:35–41.
116. Barbosa AJ, Queiros DMM, Mendes EN, et al. Immunocytochemical identification of *Campylobacter pylori* in gastri-

tis and correlation with culture. Arch Pathol Lab Med 1988; 11:288–291.
117. Toulaymant M, Marconi S, Garb J, et al. Endoscopic biopsy pathology of *Helicobacter pylori* gastritis. Arch Pathol Lab Med 1999; 123:778–781.
118. Marcio L, Angelucci D, Grossi L, et al. Anti-*Helicobacter pylori* specific antibody immunohistochemistry improves the diagnostic accuracy of *Helicobacter pylori* in biopsy specimen from patients treated with triple therapy. Am J Gastroenterol 1998; 93:223–226.
119. Tokunaga Y, Shirahase H, Yamamoto E, et al. Semiquantitative evaluation for diagnosis of *Helicobacter pylori* infection in relation to histological changes. Am J Gastroenterol 1998; 93:26–29.
120. Chan WY, Hui PK, Leung KM, et al. Coccoid forms of *Helicobacter pylori* in the human stomach. Am J Clin Pathol 1994; 102:503–507.
121. Goldstein NS. Chronic inactive gastritis and coccoid *Helicobacter pylori* in patients treated for gastroesophageal reflux disease or with H. pylori eradication therapy. Am J Clin Pathol 2002; 118:719–726.
122. Baisden BL, Lepidi H, Raoult D, et al. Diagnosis of Whipple disease by immunohistochemical analysis. A sensitive and specific method for the detection of *Tropheryma whipplei* (the Whipple bacillus) in paraffin-embedded tissue. Am J Clin Pathol 2002; 118:742–748.
123. Lepidi H, Fenollar F, Gerolami R, et al. Whipple disease: immunospecific and quantitative immunohistochemical study of intestinal biopsy specimens. Hum Pathol 2003; 34:589–596.
124. Lepidi H, Costedoat N, Piette JC, et al. Immunohistological detection of *Tropheryma whipplei* (Whipple bacillus) in lymph nodes. Am J Med 2002; 113:334–336.
125. Dumler JS, Walker DH. Diagnostic tests for Rocky Mountain spotted fever and other rickettsial diseases. Dermat Clin 1994; 12:25–36.
126. White WL, Patrick JD, Miller LR, et al. Evaluation of immunoperoxidase techniques to detect *Rickettsia rickettsii* in fixed tissue sections. Am J Clin Pathol 1994; 101:747–752.
127. Procop GW, Burchette JL Jr, Howell DN, et al. Immunoperoxidase and immunofluorescent staining of *Rickettsia rickettsii* in skin biopsies. Arch Pathol Lab Med 1997; 121:894–899.
128. Paddock CD, Greer PW, Ferebee TL, et al. Hidden mortality attributable to Rocky Mountain spotted fever: immunohistochemical detection of fatal, serologically unconfirmed disease. J Infect Dis 1999; 179:1469–1476.
129. Lepidi H, Fornier PE, Raoult D. Quantitative analysis of valvular lesions during *Bartonella* endocarditis. Am J Clin Pathol 2000; 114:880–889.
130. Baorto L, Payne RM, Slater LN, et al. Culture-negative endocarditis caused by *Bartonella henselae*. J Pediatr 1998; 132:1051–1054.
131. Reed JA, Brigati DJ, Flynn SD, et al. Immunohistochemical identification of *Rochalimaea henselae* in bacillary (epithelioid) angiomatosis, parenchymal bacillary peliosis, and persistent fever with bacteremia. Am J Surg Pathol 1992; 16:650–657.
132. Min KW, Reed JA, Welch DF, et al. Morphologically variable bacilli of cat scratch disease are identified by immunohistochemical labeling with antibodies to *Rochalimaea henselae*. Am J Clin Pathol 1994; 101:607–610.
133. Daybell D, Paddock CD, Zaki SR, et al. Disseminated infection with *Bartonella henselae* as a cause of spontaneous splenic rupture. Clin Infect Dis 2004; 39:21–24.
134. Zaki SR, Shieh W-J, and the Epidemic Working Group. Leptospirosis associated with an outbreak of acute febrile illness and pulmonary hemorrhage, Nicaragua 1995. Lancet 1996; 347:535–536.
135. Trevejo RT, Rigau-Perez JG, Ashford DA, et al. Epidemic leptospirosis associated with pulmonary hemorrhage – Nicaragua, 1995. J Infect Dis 1998; 178:1457–1463.
136. Guarner J, Shieh WJ, Morgan J, et al. Leptospirosis mimicking acute cholecystitis among athletes participating in a triathlon. Hum Pathol 2001; 32:750–752.
137. Nicodemo AC, Duarte MI, Alves VA, et al. Lung lesions in human leptospirosis: microscopic, immunohistochemical, and ultrastructural features related to thrombocytopenia. Am J Trop Med Hyg 1997; 56:181–187.
138. Lebech AM, Clemmensen O, Hansen K. Comparison of in vitro, immunohistochemical staining, and PCR for detection of *Borrelia burgdorferi* in tissue from experimentally infected animals. J Clin Microbiol 1995; 33:2328–2333.
139. Aberer E, Kersten A, Klade H, et al. Heterogeneity of *Borrelia burgdorferi* in the skin. Am J Dermpath 1996; 18:571–

579.

140. Terpstra WJ, Groeneveld K, Eijk PP, et al. Comparison of two nonculture techniques for detection of *Haemophilus influenzae* in sputum: In situ hybridization and immunoperoxidase staining with monoclonal antibodies. Chest 1988; 94:126S.

141. Groeneveld K, van Alphen L, van Ketel RJ, et al. Non-culture detection of *Haemophilus influenzae* in sputum with monoclonal antibodies specific for outer membrane lipoprotein P6. J Clin Microbiol 1989; 27:2263.

142. Forsgren J, Samuelson A, Borrelli S, et al. Persistence of nontypeable *Haemophilus influenzae* in adenoid macrophages: a putative colonization mechanism. Act Oto-Laryngol 1996; 116:766–773.

143. Shurbaji MS, Dumler JS, Gage WR, et al. Immunohistochemical detection of chlamydial antigens in association with cystitis. Am J Pathol 1990; 93:363.

144. Paukku M, Puolakkainen M, Paavonen T, et al. Plasma cell endometritis is associated with *Chlamydia trachomatis* infection. Am J Clin Pathol 1999; 112:211–215.

145. Naas J, Gnarpe JA. Demonstration of *Chlamydia pneumoniae* in tissue by immunohistochemistry. APMIS 1999; 107:882–886.

146. Suffin SC, Kaufmann AF, Whitaker B, et al. *Legionella pneumophila*. Identification in tissue sections by a new immunoenzymatic procedure. Arch Pathol Lab Med 1980; 104:283–286.

147. Maruta K, Miyamoto H, Hamada T, et al. Entry and intracellular growth of *Legionella dumoffii* in alveolar epithelial cells. Am J Respir Crit Care Med 1998; 157:1967–1974.

148. Fiore AE, Nuorti JP, Levine OS, et al. Epidemic legionaire's disease two decades later: Old sources, new diagnostic methods. Clin Infect Dis 1998; 26:426–433.

149. Parkash V, Morotti RA, Joshi V, et al. Immunohistochemical detection of *Listeria* antigens in the placenta in perinatal listeriosis. Int J Gynecol Pathol 1998; 17:343–350.

150. Chiba M, Fukushima T, Koganei K, et al. *Listeria monocytogenes* in the colon in a case of fulminant ulcerative colitis. Scan J Gastroenterol 1998; 33:778–782.

151. Weinstock D, Horton SB, Rowland PH. Rapid diagnosis of *Listeria monocytogenes* by immunohistochemistry in formalin-fixed brain tissue. Vet Pathol 1995; 32:193–195.

152. Pospischil A, Wood RL, Anderson TD. Peroxidase-antiperoxidase and immunogold labeling of *Salmonella typhimurium* and *Salmonella cholerasuis* var *kunzendorf* in tissues of experimentally infected swine. Am J Vet Res 1990; 51:619–624.

153. Thygesen P, Martinsen C, Hougen HP, et al. Histologic, cytologic, and bacteriologic examination of experimentally induced *Salmonella typhimurium* infection in Lewis rats. Comp Med 2000; 50:124–132.

154. Carabias E, Palenque R, Serrano JM, et al. Evaluation of an immunohistochemical test with polyclonal antibodies raised against mycobacteria used in formalin-fixed tissue compared with mycobacterial specific culture. APMIS 1998; 106:385–388.

155. Kim KM, Lee A, Choi KY, et al. Intestinal tuberculosis: clinicopathologic analysis and diagnosis by endoscopic biopsy. Am J Gastroenterol 1998; 93:606–609.

156. Osaki M, Adachi H, Gomyo Y, et al. Detection of mycobacterial DNA in formalin-fixed, paraffin-embedded tissue specimens by duplex polymerase chain reaction: application to histopathologic diagnosis. Mod Pathol 1997; 10:78–83.

157. Barbolini G, Bisetti A, Colizzi V, et al. Immunohistologic analysis of mycobacterial antigens by monoclonal antibodies in tuberculosis and mycobacteriosis. Hum Pathol 1989; 20:1078–1083.

158. Lockwood DN, Colston MJ, and Khanolkar-Young SR. The detection of *Mycobacterium leprae* protein and carbohydrate antigens in skin and nerve from leprosy patients with type 1 (reversal) reactions. Am J Trop Med Hyg 2002; 66:409–415.

159. Verhagen C, Faber W, Klatser P, et al. Immunohistological analysis of in situ expression of mycobacterial antigens in skin lesions of leprosy patients across the histopathological spectrum. Association of mycobacterial lipoarabinomannan (LAM) and *Mycobacterium leprae* phenolic glycolipid-I (PGL-I) with leprosy reactions. Am J Pathol 1999; 154:1793–1804.

160. Walker DH, Feng HM, Ladner S, et al. Immunohistochemical diagnosis of typhus rickettsioses using an anti-lipopolysaccharide monoclonal antibody. Mod Pathol 1997; 10:1038–1042.

161. Koss T, Carter EL, Grossman ME, et al. Increased detection of rickettsialpox in a New York city hospital following the anthrax outbreak of 2001: use of immunohistochemistry for the rapid confirmation of cases in an era of bioterrorism. Arch

Dermatol 2003; 139:1545–1552.

162. Walker DH, Hudnall SD, Szaniawski WK, et al. Monoclonal antibody-based immunohistochemical diagnosis of rickettsialpox: the macrophage is the principal target. Mod Pathol 1999; 12:529–533.

163. Moron CG, Popov VL, Feng-HM, et al. Identification of the target cells of *Orientia tsutsugamushi* in human cases of scrub typhus. Mod Pathol 2001; 14:752–759.

164. Guarner J, Southwick K, Greer P, et al. Testing umbilical cords for funisitis due to *Treponema pallidum* infection, Bolivia. Emerg Infect Dis 2000; 6:487–492.

165. Chung KY, Lee MG, Chon CY, et al. Syphilitic gastritis: demonstration of *Treponema pallidum* with the use of fluorescent treponemal antibody absorption complement and immuno-peroxidase stains. J Am Acad Derm 1989; 21:183–185.

166. Guarner J, Greer PW, Bartlett J, et al. Congenital syphilis in a newborn: an immunopathologic study. Mod Pathol 1999; 12:82–87.

167. Schwarz J. The diagnosis of deep mycoses by morphological methods. Hum Pathol 1982; 13:519–533.

168. Marques MEA, Coelho KIR, Bacchi CE. Comparison between histochemical and immunohistochemical methods for the diagnosis of sporotrichosis. J Clin Pathol 1992; 45:1089–1093.

169. Reed JA, Hemaan BA, Alexander JL, et al. Immunomycology: rapid and specific immunocytochemical identification of fungi in formalin-fixed, paraffin-embedded material. J Histochem Cytochem 1993; 41:1217–1221.

170. Jensen HE, Schonheyder H, Hotchi M, et al. Diagnosis of systemic mycosis by specific immunohistochemical tests. APMIS 1996; 104:241–258.

171. Cooper CR, McGinnis MR. Pathology of *Penicillium marneffei*: an emerging acquired immunodeficiency syndrome-related pathogen. Arch Lab Pathol Med 1997; 121:798–804.

172. Fukuzawa M, Inaba H, Hayama M, et al. Improved detection of medically important fungi by immunoperoxidase staining with polyclonal antibodies. Virchows Arch 1995; 427:407–414.

173. Kauffman L. Immunohistologic diagnosis of systemic mycosis: an update. Eur J Epidemiol 1992; 8:377–382.

174. Verweij PE, Smedts F, Poot T. Immunoperoxidase staining for identification of *Aspergillus* species in routinely processed tissue sections. J Clin Pathol 1996; 49:798–801.

175. Breier F, Oesterreicher C, Brugger S, et al. Immunohistochemistry with monoclonal antibody against *Candida albicans* mannan antigen demonstrates cutaneous *Candida granulomas* as evidence of *Candida* sepsis in an immunosuppressed host. Dermatology 1997; 194:293–296.

176. Marcilla A, Monteagudo C, Mormeneo S, et al. Monoclonal antibody 3H8: a useful tool in the diagnosis of candidiasis. Microbiol 1999; 145:695–701.

177. Monteagudo C, Marcilla A, Mormeneo S, et al. Specific immunohistochemical identification of *Candida albicans* in paraffin-embedded tissue with a new monoclonal antibody (1B12). Am J Clin Pathol 1995; 103:130–135.

178. Kockenberger MB, Canfield PJ, Kozel TR, et al. An immunohistochemical method that differentiates *Cryptococcus neoformans* varieties and serotypes in formalinfixed paraffin-embedded tissues. Med Mycol 2001; 39:523–533.

179. Tsunemi T, Kamata T, Fumimura Y, et al. Immunohistochemical diagnosis of *Cryptococcus neoformans* var. *gatti* infection in chronic meningoencephailitis: the first case in Japan. Intern Med 2001; 40:1241–1244.

180. Tarrand JJ, Lichterfeld M, Warraich I, et al. Diagnosis of invasive septate mold infections. A correlation of microbiological culture and histologic or cytologic examination. Am J Clin Pathol 2003; 119:854–858.

181. Choi JK, Mauger J, McGowan KL. Immunohistochemical detection of Aspergillus species in pediatric tissue samples. Am J Clin Pathol 2004; 121:18–25.

182. Pierard GE, Arrese-Estrada J, Pierard-Franchimont C, et al. Immunohistochemical expression of galactomannan in the cytoplasm of phagocytic cells during invasive aspergillosis. Am J Clin Pathol 1991; 96:373–376.

183. Phillips P, Weiner MH. Invasive aspergillosis diagnosed by monoclonal and polyclonal reagents. Hum Pathol 1987; 18:1015–1024.

184. Fenelon LE, Hamilton AJ, Figueroa JI, et al. Production of specific monoclonal antibodies to *Aspergillus* species and their use in immunohistochemical identification of aspergillosis. J Clin Microbiol 1999; 37:1221–1223.

185. Wazir JE, Brown I, Martin-Bates E, et al. EB9, a new antibody for the detection of trophozoites of *Pneumocystis carinii* in bronchoalveolar lavage specimens in AIDS. J Clin Pathol

1994; 47:1108–1111.

186. Wazir JE, Macrorie SG, Coleman DV. Evaluation of the sensitivity, specificity, and predictive value of monoclonal antibody 3F6 for the detection of *Pneumocystis carinii* pneumonia in bronchoalveolar lavage specimens and induced sputum. Cytopathol 1994; 5:82–89.

187. Chaiwun B, Khunamornpong S, Sirivanichai C, et al. Lymphadenopathy due to *Penicillium marnerffei* infection: Diagnosis by fine needle aspiration cytology. Mod Pathol 2002; 15:939–943.

188. Arrese EJ, Stynen D, Pierard-Franchimont C, et al. Immunohistochemical identification of *Penicillium marneffei* by monoclonal antibodies. Int J Dermatol 1992; 31:410–412.

189. Burke DG, Emancipator SN, Smith MC, et al. Histoplasmosis and kidney disease in patients with AIDS. Clin Infect Dis 1997; 25:281–284.

190. Arnold SJ, Kinney MC, McCormick MS, et al. Disseminated toxoplasmosis: unusual presentations in the immunocompromised host. Arch Pathol Lab Med 1997; 121:869–873.

191. Warnke C, Tuazon CU, Kovacs A, et al. Toxoplasma encephalitis in patients with acquired immunodeficiency syndrome: diagnosis and response to therapy. Am J Trop Med Hyg 1987; 36:509.

192. Ganji M, Tan A, Maitar ML, et al. Gastric toxoplasmosis in a patient with acquired immunodeficiency syndrome. A case report and review of the literature. Arch Pathol Lab Med 2003; 127:732–734.

193. Hofman V, Brousset P, Mougneau E, et al. Immunostaining of visceral leishmaniasis caused by *Leishmania infantum* using monoclonal antibody (19-11) to the leishmania homologue of receptors for activated c-kinase. Am J Clin Pathol 2003; 120:567–574.

194. Azadeh B, Sells PG, Ejeckman GC, et al. Localized *Leishmania lymphadenitis* immunohistochemical studies. Am J Clin Pathol 1994; 102:11–15.

195. Kenner JR, Aronson NE, Bratthauer GL, et al. Immunohistochemistry to identify *Leishmania parasites* in fixed tissues. J Cutan Pathol 1999; 26:130–136.

196. Amato VS, Duarte MIS, Nicodemo AC, et al. An evaluation of clinical, serologic, anatomopathologic and immunohistochemical findings for fifteen patients with mucosal leishmaniasis before and after treatment. Rev Inst Med Trop S Paulo 1998; 40:23–30.

197. Bonnin A, Petrella T, Dubremetz JF, et al Histopathologic methods for diagnosis of cryptosporidiosis using monoclonal antibodies. Eur J Clin Microbiol Infect Dis 1990; 9:664–665.

198. Perez de Suarez E, Perez-Schael I, Perozo-Ruggeri G, et al. Immunocytochemical detection of *Entamoeba histolytica*. Trans R Soc Trop Med Hyg 1987; 81:624–626.

199. Guarner J, Bartlett J, Zaki SR, et al. Mouse model for Chagas disease: immunohistochemical distribution of different stages of *Trypanosoma cruzi* in tissues throughout infection. Am J Trop Med Hyg 2001; 65:152–158.

200. Anez N, Carrasco H, Parada H, et al. Myocardial parasite persistence in chronic chagasic patients. Am J Trop Med Hyg 1999; 60:726–732.

201. Reis MM, Higuchi M de L, Benvenuti LA, et al. An in situ quantitative immunohistochemical study of cytokines and IL-2R+ in chronic human chagasic myocarditis: correlation with the presence of myocardial *Trypanosoma cruzi* antigens. Clin Immun Immunopathol 1997; 83:165–172.

202. Torres-Velez FJ, Nace EK, Won KY, et al. Development of an immunohistochemical assay for the detection of babesiosis in formalin-fixed, paraffin-embedded tissue samples. Am J Clin Pathol 2003; 120:833–838.

203. Sanad MM, Darwish RA, Nasr ME, et al. Giardia lamblia and chronic gastritis. J Egypt Soc Parasitol 1996; 26:481–495.

204. Institute of Medicine. Emerging infections: microbial threats to health in the United States. Washington, DC: National Academy Press; 1992.

205. CDC. Preventing emerging infectious diseases: a strategy for the 21st century. MMWR 1998; 47 No. RR-15.

206. Perkins BA, Flood JM, Danila R, et al. Unexplained deaths due to possibly infectious causes in the United States: defining the problem and designing surveillance and laboratory approaches. Emerg Infect Dis 1998; 2:47–53.

207. Houpikina P, Raoult D. Traditional and molecular techniques for the study of emerging bacterial diseases: one laboratory's perspective. Emerg Infect Dis 2002; 8:122–131.

208. Khan AS, Khabbaz RF, Armstrong RC, et al. Hantavirus pulmonary syndrome: the first 100 US cases. J Infect Dis 1996; 173:1297–1303.

209. Moolenaar RL, Dalton C, Lipman HB, et al. Clinical features that differentiate hantavirus pulmonary syndrome from three other acute respiratory illnesses. Clin Infect Dis 1995;

21:643–649.

210. Nolte KB, Feddersen RM, Foucar K, et al. Hantavirus pulmonary syndrome in the United States: a pathological description of a disease caused by a new agent. Hum Pathol 1995; 26:110–120.

211. Zaki SR, Greer PW, Coffield LM, et al. Hantavirus pulmonary syndrome. Pathogenesis of an emerging infectious disease. Am J Pathol 1995; 146:552–579.

212. Zaki SR, Khan AS, Goodman RA, et al. Retrospective diagnosis of hantavirus pulmonary syndrome, 1978–1993. Implications for emerging infectious diseases. Arch Pathol Lab Med 1996; 120:134–139.

213. Shieh WJ, Guarner J, Layton M, et al. The role of pathology in an investigation of an outbreak of West Nile encephalitis in New York, 1999. Emerg Infect Dis 2000; 6:370–372.

214. Cushing MM, Brat DJ, Mosunjac MI, et al. Fatal West Nile virus encephalitis in an renal transplant recipient. Am J Clin Pathol 2004; 121:26–31.

215. Petersen RL, Roehrig JT, Hughes JM. West Nile virus encephalitis. N Engl J Med 2002; 347:1225–1226.

216. Sampson BA, Ambrosi C, Charlot A, et al. The pathology of human West Nile virus infection. Hum Pathol 2000; 31:527–532.

217. Guarner J, Shieh WJ, Hunter S, et al. Clinicopathologic study and laboratory diagnosis of 23 cases with West Nile virus encephalomyelitis. Hum Pathol 2004; 35:983–990.

218. Lanciotti RS, Kerst AJ, Nasci RS, et al. Rapid detection of West Nile virus from human clinical specimens, field-collected mosquitoes, and avian samples by a TaqMan reverse transcriptase PCR assay. J Clin Microbiol 2000; 38:4066–4071.

219. Ho M, Chen ER, Hsu KH, et al. An epidemic of enterovirus 71 infection in Taiwan. Taiwan enterovirus epidemic working group. N Engl J Med 1999; 341:929–935.

220. Chan LG, Parashar UD, Lye MS. Deaths of children during an outbreak of hand, foot, and mouth disease in Sarawak, Malaysia: clinical and pathological characteristics of the disease. Clin Infect Dis 2000; 31:678–683.

221. Wong KT, Chua KB, Lam SK. Immunohistochemical detection of infected neurons as a rapid diagnosis of enterovirus 71 encephalomyelitis. Ann Neurol 1999; 45:271–272.

222. Yan JJ, Wang JR, Liu CC, et al. An outbreak of enterovirus 71 infection in Taiwan 1998: a comprehensive pathological, virological, and molecular study on a case of fulminant encephalitis. J Clin Virol 2000; 17:13–22.

223. Shieh WJ, Jung SM, Hsueh C, et al. Pathologic studies of fatal causes in outbreak of hand, foot, and mouth disease, Taiwan. Emerg Infect Dis 2001; 7:146–148.

224. Wong KT, Shieh WJ, Kumar S, et al. Nipah virus infection. Pathology and pathogenesis of an emerging paramyxoviral zoonosis. Am J Pathol 2002; 161:2153–2167.

225. Goh KJ, Tan CT, Chew NK, et al. Clinical features of Nipah virus encephalitis among pig farmers in Malaysia. N Engl J Med 2000; 342:1229–1235.

226. Chua KB, Bellini WJ, Rota PA, et al. Nipah virus: a recently emergent deadly paramyxovirus. Science 2000; 288:1432–1435.

227. Dawson JE, Paddock CD, Warner CK, et al. Tissue diagnosis of Ehrlichia chaffeensis in patients with fatal ehrlichiosis by use of immunohistochemistry, in situ hybridization, and polymerase chain reaction. Am J Trop Med Hyg 2001; 65:603–609.

228. Walker DH, Dumler JS. Human monocytic and granulocytic ehrlichiosis. Discovery and diagnosis of emerging tick-borne infections and the critical role of the pathologist. Arch Pathol Lab Med 1997; 121:785–791.

229. Paddock CD, Suchard DP, Grumbach KL, et al. Fatal seronegative ehrlichiosis in a patient with HIV infection. N Engl J Med 1993; 329:1164–1167.

230. Lepidi H, Bunnell JE, Martin ME, et al. Comparative pathology and immunohistology associated with clinical illness after *Ehrlichia phagocytophila*-group infections. Am J Trop Med Hyg 2000: 62:29–37.

231. Sehdev AE, Dumler JS. Hepatic pathology in human monocytic ehrlichiosis. *Ehrlichia chaffeensis* infection. Am J Clin Pathol 2003; 119:859–865.

232. Hooper PT, Russell GM, Selleck PW, et al. Immunohistochemistry in the identification of a number of new diseases in Australia. Vet Microbiol 1999; 68:89–93.

233. Williamson MM, Hooper PT, Selleck PW, et al. Experimental hendra virus infection in pregnant guinea-pigs and fruit bats (*Pteropus poliocephalus*). J Comp Pathol 2000; 122:201–207.

234. Ksiazek TG, Erdman D, Goldsmith CS, et al. A novel coronavirus associated with severe acute respiratory syndrome. N Engl J Med 2003; 348:1953–1966.

235. Peiris JS, Lai ST, Poon LL, et al. Coronavirus as a possible cause of severe acute respiratory syndrome. Lancet 2003; 361: 1319–1325.

236. Nakajima N, Asahi-Ozaki Y, Nagata N, et al. SARS coronavirus-infected cells in lung detected by new in situ hybridization technique. Jpn J Infect Dis 2003; 56:139–141.

237. Kuiken T, Fouchier RA, Schutten M, et al. Newly discovered coronavirus as the primary cause of severe acute respiratory syndrome. Lancet 2003; 362:263–270.

238. Chong PY, Chui P, Ling AE, et al. Analysis of deaths during the severe acute respiratory syndrome (SARS) epidemic in Singapore: challenges in determining a SARS diagnosis. Arch Pathol Lab Med 2004; 128:195–204.

239. McAuliffe J, Vogel L, Roberts A, et al. Replication of SARS coronavirus administered into the respiratory tract of African green, rhesus and cynomolgus monkeys. Virology 2004; 330: 8–15.

240. Roberts A, Vogel L, Guarner J, et al. SARS coronavirus infection of golden Syrian hamsters. J Virol 2005; 79:503–511.

241. Chen PC, Hsiao CH, et al. Tissue and cellular tropism of the coronavirus associated with severe acute respiratory syndrome: an in-situ hybridization study of fatal cases. J Pathol 2004; 203:729–730; author reply 730–721.

242. To KF, Tong JH, Chan PK, et al. Tissue and cellular tropism of the coronavirus associated with severe acute respiratory syndrome: an in-situ hybridization study of fatal cases. J Pathol 2004; 202:157–163.

243. Chow KC, Hsiao CH, Lin TY, et al. Detection of severe acute respiratory syndrome-associated coronavirus in pneumocytes of the lung. Am J Clin Pathol 2004; 121:574–580.

244. Ding Y, He L, Zhang Q, et al. Organ distribution of severe acute respiratory syndrome (SARS) associated coronavirus (SARS-CoV) in SARS patients: implications for patho-genesis and virus transmission pathways. J Pathol 2004; 203: 622–630.

245. Sheih W-J, Cheng-Hsiang H, Paddock CD, et al. Immunohistochemical, in situ hybridization, and ultrastructural localization of SARS-associated coronavirus in lung of a fatal case of severe acute respiratory syndrome in Taiwan. Hum Pathol 2005; 36:303–309.

246. Ashford DA, Kaiser RB, Bales ME, et al. Planning against biological terrorism: lessons from outbreak investigations. Emerg Infect Dis 2003; 9:515–519.

247. Inglesby TV, O'Toole T, Henderson DA. Preventing the use of biological weapons: improving response should prevention fail. Clin Infect Dis 2000; 30:926–929.

248. Lillibridge SR, Bell AJ, Roman RS. Thoughts for the new millennium: Bioterrorism. Centers for Disease Control and prevention, bioterrorism preparedness and response. Am J Infect Control 1999; 27:463–464.

249. Franz DR, Zajtchuk R. Biological terrorism: understanding the threat, preparation, and medical response. Dis Month 2000; 46:125–190.

250. Ezzell JW, Abshire TG, Little SF, et al. Identification of *Bacillus anthracis* by using monoclonal antibodies to cell wall galactose-N-acetylglucosamine polysaccharide. J Clin Microbiol 1990; 28:223–231.

251. Shieh WJ, Guarner J, Paddock C, et al. The critical role of pathology in the investigation of bioterrorism-related cutaneous anthrax. Am J Pathol 2003; 163:1901–1910.

252. Guarner J, Jernigan JA, Shieh WJ, et al. Pathology and pathogenesis of bioterrorism-related inhalational anthrax. Am J Pathol 2003; 163:701–709.

253. Jernigan JA, Stephens DS, Ashford DA, et al. Bioter-rorism-related inhalational anthrax: the first 10 cases reported in the United States. Emerg Infect Dis 2001; 7:933–944.

254. Jernigan DB, Raghunathan PL, Bell BP, et al. Investigation of bioterrorism-related anthrax, United States, 2001: epidemiologic findings. Emerg Infect Dis 2002; 8:1019–1028.

255. Grinberg LM, Abramova FA, Yampolskaya OV, et al. Quantitative pathology of inhalational anthrax I: quantitative microscopic findings. Mod Pathol 2001; 14:482–495.

256. Guarner J, Greer PW, Bartlett J, et al. Immunohistochemical detection of *Francisella tularensis* in formalin-fixed paraffin-embedded tissue. Appl Immun Mol Morphol 1999; 7:122–126.

257. DeBey BM, Andrews GA, Chard-Bergstrom C, et al. Immunohistochemical demonstration of *Francisella tularensis* in lesions of cats with tularaemia. J Vet Diagn Invest 2002; 14: 162–164.

258. Guarner J, Shieh WJ, Greer PW, et al. Immunohisto-chemical detection of *Yersinia pestis* in formalin-fixed paraffin-embedded tissue. Am J Clin Pathol 2002; 117:205–209.

259. Davis KJ, Vogel P, Fritz DL, et al. Bacterial filamentation of *Yersinia pestis* by b-lactam antibiotics in experimentally infected mice. Arch Pathol Lab Med 1997; 121:865–868.

260. Davis KJ, Fritz DL, Pitt ML, et al. Pathology of experimental pneumonic plague produced by fraction 1-positive and fraction 1-negative *Yersinia pestis* in African green monkeys (*Cercopithecus aethiops*). Arch Pathol Lab Med 1996; 120: 156–163.

261. Williams ES, Mills K, Kwiatkowski DR, et al. Plague in black-footed ferret (*Mustela nigripes*) J Wild Dis 1994; 30:581–585.

262. Gabastou JM, Proaño J, Vimos A, et al. An outbreak of plague including cases with probable pneumonic infection, Ecuador, 1998. Trans R Soc Trop Med Hyg 2000; 94:387–391.

263. van Moll P, Baumgartner W, Eskens U, et al. Immunocytochemical demonstration of *Coxiella burnetii* antigen in the fetal placenta of naturally infected sheep and cattle. J Comp Pathol 1993; 109:295–301.

264. Brouqui P, Dumler JS, Raoult D. Immunohistologic demonstration of Coxiella burnetii in the valves of patients with Q fever endocarditis. Am J Med 1994; 97:451–458.

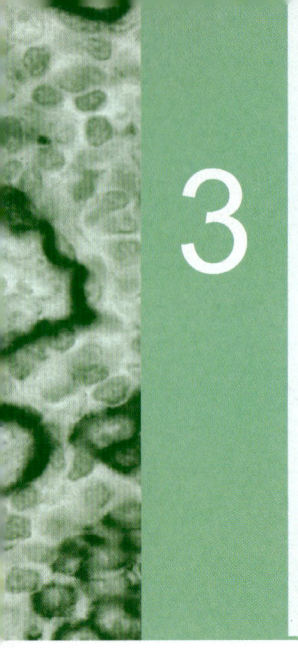

3 软组织和骨肿瘤的免疫组织化学

原作者：Lisa A. Cerilli and Mark R. Wick

译　者：李劲松

审校者：张建平，孟　斌

目　录

引言	62
抗原/抗体生物学	62
软组织特殊肿瘤	74

引　言

　　软组织和骨肿瘤种类繁多，变化多样，随着知识的积累，其分类也精细到肿瘤的分化模式，分类的复杂性也不断增加，因此对其生化基本特征也需有所了解。本章正是对该主题的实用总结，但内容并非广博或全面。皮肤和皮下常见肿瘤主要在第12章讨论。形态特征明显、诊断不需免疫组化的病变不在讨论之列。需要强调的是免疫组化仅是间叶肿瘤组织学诊断的辅助，而不是替代。

抗原/抗体生物学

中间丝蛋白

　　中间丝蛋白（intermediate filament proteins，IFPs）与微丝、微管均为人类所有细胞的结构成分[1, 2]，直径7～10nm，在胞质内常排列成束状，在富含高分子量角蛋白的上皮细胞中常可观察到平行排列的IFPs，形成电镜下张力细丝或张力原纤维[3]。此外，各种IFPs在超微结构水平上不能区分。在生化和功能上IFPs至少有6种不同组分——角蛋白、波形蛋白、结蛋白、神经丝蛋白（NFPs）、胶质纤维酸性蛋白（GFAP）和层蛋白（核封装蛋白）[4]，前5种IFPs在病理诊断中已有很好应用，在此予以讨论。

　　所有IFPs在结构上同源[5]，但特性及功能显著不同。各种IFPs的分子量介于40～200kD之间，其等电pH值也不同。应特别注意的是各种IFPs在非肿瘤细胞和人类肿瘤细胞中具有的特征性分布形式[2]。在IFPs家族中，角蛋白和NFPs是由两种或多种蛋白形成的异聚体，而其他IFPs则是一种蛋白单体的同聚物[6]。IFPs由位于不同染色体的多个基因编码（如染色体12q和17q编码角蛋白、染色体2q编码结蛋白、10p编码波形蛋白、17q编码GFAP）[7-10]，对IFPs共同的生化特性来说，这种情况有些出乎意外。

　　起初，人们认为IFPs在肌细胞中作为"细胞骨架"，仅具结构功能，并假设它们能维系胞浆蛋白之间的正常关系，以及将胞浆内的收缩结构固定在胞膜上。然而，随着细胞生物学的进展，人们已对此提出严重质疑[11]。现已知中间丝具有核酸结合功能，而且易受钙激活蛋白酶作用，并作为环腺苷酸依赖性蛋白激酶的底物，故提出所有IFPs都可调节细胞外钙离子进入细胞（继而激活蛋白酶）并在转录或翻译水平上调节核功能[12]。在形态学上，IFPs与胞膜和核周胞浆的关系支持这一理论并使"细胞骨架"的作用降至次要地位。现在的观点倾向于认为，IFPs的原纤维并非作为细胞的"骨架"，而是伴随细胞周期活性有效发挥其核酸结合功能。一些中间丝插入细胞间的含有结蛋白的桥粒斑中（桥粒负责保持组织的完整性），并非一定执行结构生物学功能，而是因为细胞间连接点是细胞内外环境"生化信息交流"的部位[13]。

角蛋白

作为上皮细胞和上皮性肿瘤中基本的IFPs，角蛋白（keratin）对于恶性肿瘤中癌的诊断具有高度特异性和敏感性。细胞角蛋白（cytokeratin，CK）在各种类型上皮细胞中均为典型的成对表达，一个为酸性（Ⅰ型），另一个为碱性（Ⅱ型）[14]。角蛋白分子量从 40～60kD 不等，由 Moll 及其同事给予其序号名称。这样在每一种类型组中它们都是按分子量由低到高顺序编号[15]。酸性等电点的Ⅰ型角蛋白有12个，碱性的Ⅱ型角蛋白有8个。正如 Miettinen 所描述的，细胞角蛋白在细胞生长过程中可自行配对，由一个Ⅰ型角蛋白与一个比其大 7～9kD 的Ⅱ型角蛋白相结合[14]。

从待测组织或肿瘤中可以检测到特殊的角蛋白亚型，结合可预测的、已知的基因表达类型，就可以部分确定含有这些成分的细胞（表3.1）。需特别强调的是，非上皮细胞在生理状态下确实能检测到部分细胞角蛋白（如CK8和CK18，偶尔CK19），但通常需要用特殊技术来保存或检测这些含量极低的IFPs（如丙酮固定、冰冻切片免疫组化或扩增性免疫检测方法）。部分间叶肿瘤同样也可表达角蛋白，且表达谱较宽，例如CK1、CK7、CK8、CK13、CK14、CK18和CK19，均可见于滑膜肉瘤[14, 16]。其他常表达细胞角蛋白的软组织肿瘤或骨肿瘤包括上皮样肉瘤（CK8、CK18和CK19）、脊索瘤（CK8、CK18、CK19、CK4、CK5可阳性也可阴性）、副脊索瘤（CK8），以及骨内造釉细胞瘤（CK19）[14-19]。上述肿瘤与滑膜肉瘤构成的这一组病变，有些作者建议将其称为软组织和骨原发性"癌肉瘤"。

自20世纪90年代以来，发现还有其他一些"典型"缺乏角蛋白表达的间叶肿瘤在某些情况下可用反常的方式合成这类IFPs（表3.2）。据报道，的确实际上所有肉瘤形态的肿瘤都显示了合成此类IFPs的潜能。然而，应当强调的是，在常规诊断情况下仅有少部分恶性间叶肿瘤有"异常"角蛋白活性，主要有平滑肌肉瘤（LMS）、恶性外周神经鞘瘤（MPNST）、上皮样血管肉瘤，甚至Ewing肉瘤/原始神经外胚层肿瘤（ES/PNET）[20]。据以前的文献所述，此类肿瘤最常出现的是CK8、CK18和CK19。需要强调的是，异常的IFPs表达并不常见。许多有关报道实际上为免疫组化技术中使用的角蛋白抗体浓度过高或方法过于敏感而导致的假阳性。由于IFPs在结构上相互关联[21]，一些抗角蛋白抗体与波形蛋白、结蛋白、NFPs或GFAP发生交叉反应也就不足为奇了。根据有关中间丝种系间相互关系及共性方面的资料，Geisler和Weber[22]对其单克隆抗体的不同类型概括如下：

1. 组织特异（中间丝特异）但种系非特异；
2. 组织和种系均特异；
3. 组织非特异而种系特异；
4. 组织和种系均非特异。

从比较生物学的角度出发，以上抗体均有应用价值，但仅有前两类能用于外科病理诊断。

已有大量有关人类肿瘤IFPs表达的临床数据报

表3.1　各种非肿瘤细胞细胞角蛋白亚型表达

Ⅱ型（碱性）细胞角蛋白*		分布	Ⅰ型（酸性）细胞角蛋白*	
（Moll分类号）	（分子量）		（Moll分类号）	（分子量）
—	—	手掌和足底表皮	CK9	64kD
CK1	67kD	表皮和所有其他部位的角化鳞状上皮	CK10	56.5kD
CK2	65kD		CK11	56kD
CK3	63kD	角膜	CK12	55kD
CK4	59kD	内脏非角化上皮	CK13	51kD
CK5	58kD	鳞状上皮和腺上皮的基底细胞、肌上皮细胞和间皮	CK14	50kD
CK6	56kD	鳞状上皮	CK16	48kD
CK7	54kD	单层上皮	—	—
—	—	腺上皮基底细胞和肌上皮细胞	CK17	46kD
CK8	52kD	单层上皮	CK18	45kD
		单层上皮、大多数腺上皮和某些鳞状上皮细胞	CK19	40kD
		胃肠道单层上皮细胞、皮肤Merkel细胞	CK20	46kD

*在同一行中显示了在同一细胞类型中成对表达的特征性角蛋白

表3.2 间质细胞和肿瘤中"异常"表达的细胞角蛋白亚型

细胞角蛋白 Moll 分类号	识别的单克隆抗体	可能的分布部位
8	CAM5.2(Becton-Dickinson) AE3(PROGEN) KL1(Serotec) F12~19 (Biogenesis) RCK102(Biogenesis) DC10 (BioGenex) MAK-6 (Medac) 5D3 (Biogenesis) NCL-5D3 (Medac) 6D7/3F3 (Medac) 2A4 (Biohit) M20 (Accurate) KS8.7 (Paesel) NCL-CK8(Novocastra) UCD/AB6.01 (ATCC) C22 (Biogenesis) 4.1.18 (BioGenex) H1 (Bioprobe) C51 (Neomarkers) 34βH11 (Enzo) Lu5 (Sera-Lab) C11 (Neomarkers)	胎儿纤维细胞，浆膜下成纤维细胞，子宫肌层，血管平滑肌，胎儿心肌，血管内皮细胞，部分淋巴器官网状细胞，肿瘤性浆细胞和CD30+的淋巴样细胞（很罕见），部分平滑肌肉瘤，上皮样血管内皮瘤，上皮样血管肉瘤，原始神经外胚层肿瘤和Ewing肉瘤；恶性外周神经鞘瘤，透明细胞肉瘤
18	MFN116(Axcel) PKK1 (LabSystems) CK18(Novocastra) KS18.4(Paesel) KS18.8 (Biotest) DC10(BioGenex) K918.04(Cymbus) KS-B17.2(Sigma) 4B11(Biohit) DA7 (Bioprobe) KS18.18(Camon) 34βH11 (DiagBiosys) F12~19 (Biogenesis) C11(Neomarkers) LP34(Medac)	胎儿成纤维细胞，子宫肌层，血管平滑肌，胎儿心肌，血管内皮细胞，部分淋巴器官网状细胞，部分CD30+的淋巴样细胞（罕见），部分平滑肌肉瘤，上皮样血管内皮瘤，上皮样血管肉瘤，原始神经外胚层肿瘤和Ewing肉瘤，恶性外周神经鞘瘤和透明细胞肉瘤
19	AE1(BM; ICN) PKK1 (LabSystems) CK19(Novocastra) RCK108(BioGenex) BA17(DAKO) KS19.1(Serotec) F12~19(Biogenesis) MAK-6(Medac)	子宫肌层，胎儿心肌，部分肿瘤性髓样细胞，部分平滑肌肉瘤，极少数原始神经外胚层肿瘤和Ewing肉瘤

表3.3 作者在研究软组织肿瘤中应用的抗体试剂

试剂	来源	稀释度	抗原修复	主要的诊断应用原则
抗角蛋白（M）				
AE1/AE3	Boehringer-Mannheim	1:150	MWER	识别上皮样肉瘤、滑膜肉瘤和部分其他软组织肉瘤中散在的上皮样分化
CAM5.2	Becton-Dickinson	1:200	MWER	
MAK-6	Medac	1:75	MWER	
DC10	BioGenex	1:50	MWER	
CK18	Novocastra	1:50	MWER	
CK19	Novocastra	1:50	MWER	
CK7	BioGenex	1:75	MWER	
抗结蛋白（M）	BioGenex	1:2000	MWER	识别平滑肌和横纹肌肿瘤
抗波形蛋白（M）	BioGenex	1:2000	MWER	在软组织肿瘤中普遍存在的中间丝蛋白，作为阳性标本对照
抗上皮细胞膜抗原（M）	DAKO	1:400	NT	识别上皮样肉瘤、滑膜肉瘤和部分外周神经鞘肿瘤
抗肌特异性肌动蛋白（HHF-35 克隆）（M）	Enzo	1:8000	MWER	识别平滑肌和横纹肌肿瘤以及肌纤维母细胞分化
抗α-单体肌动蛋白（1A4 克隆）（M）	DAKO	1:200	MWER	识别平滑肌肿瘤和肌纤维母细胞分化
抗肌红蛋白（P）	DAKO	1:800	MWER	识别横纹肌肿瘤
抗Myo-D1（M）	DAKO	1:10	MWER	识别横纹肌肿瘤
抗肌细胞生成素（M）	Novocastra	1:30	MWER	识别横纹肌肿瘤
抗h-钙调素结合蛋白（M）	DAKO	1:200	MWER	识别平滑肌肿瘤
抗S-100 蛋白（P）	DAKO	1:1000	NT	识别黑色素细胞、施万细胞和软骨肿瘤
抗CD57（M）	Becton-Dickinson	1:20	MWER	识别施万细胞肿瘤
抗Ⅳ型胶原（M）	BioGenex	1:40	MWER	识别滑膜、肌源性、外周神经鞘和内皮肿瘤
抗层粘连蛋白（M）	Sigma	1:20	MWER	识别滑膜、肌源性、外周神经鞘和内皮肿瘤
抗Ⅷ因子相关抗原（M）	DAKO	1:20	MWER	识别内皮肿瘤
抗CD34（M）	DAKO	1:800	MWER	识别内皮肿瘤、皮肤隆突性纤维肉瘤、孤立性纤维性肿瘤、部分外周神经鞘肿瘤和上皮样肉瘤
抗CD31（M）	DAKO	1:40	MWER	识别内皮肿瘤
抗血栓调节素1（M）	DAKO	1:200	MWER	识别内皮肿瘤和间皮瘤
抗荆豆凝集素1（P）	DAKO	1:4000	NT	识别与荆豆凝集素相关的内皮肿瘤
荆豆凝集素1	DAKO	1:1000	NT	识别内皮肿瘤
抗CD68	DAKO	1:800	MWER	纤维组织细胞肿瘤的可能标志（见正文）
抗骨连接素（M）	BioDesign	1:100	MWER	成骨细胞可能分化的敏感标志物
抗骨钙素（M）	Biogenesis	1:100	MWER	成骨细胞分化的特异标志物
抗突触素（M）	BioGenex	1:40	MWER	检测神经外胚层分化
抗CD99（M）	DAKO	1:20	MWER	识别几乎全部的神经外胚层肿瘤和Ewing 肉瘤，标记约50%的滑膜肉瘤和恶性外周神经鞘肿瘤，也存在于软组织中的淋巴母细胞性淋巴/白血病

M，单克隆；P，多克隆（杂抗血清）；MWER，微波抗原修复；NT，未预处理的组织切片

道。从重要的哲学方法论的角度考虑，如果将此数据应用于病理诊断，就必须保持获得以上数据的技术方法。因此，在实际工作中使用新技术时，不考虑对最终诊断的作用和影响是不可取的。简而言之，病理诊断的目的不是判断肿瘤中IFPs的多寡，而是建立一个免疫组化诊断标准，使交叉反应最小、诊断价值最大。如能掌握其质控标准，那么在常规包埋的临床标本中间叶肿瘤异常角蛋白的表达就会降低。

结蛋白

结蛋白（desmin）是一种胞浆 IFP，特征性表达于肌细胞及相关肿瘤[23-25]。在平滑肌细胞中结蛋白见于胞浆致密体和膜下致密斑中，在横纹肌中结蛋白细丝连接于肌小节 Z 盘上。

Small 和 Sobieszek 于 1977 年首次发现结蛋白，认为结蛋白是一种独特的生化成分[26]。在体外去除肌动蛋白和肌球蛋白的肌细胞中，他们发现结蛋白是一种残留的丝状蛋白，并暂时命名为"骨架蛋白"，其等电点大约为 4，对热稳定，并难溶于富盐溶液中。氨基酸分析发现其含有高浓度的谷氨酸和天冬氨酸，并且与胶质纤维和 NFPs 有明显的化学同源性。此研究的一个重要发现是去除骨架蛋白（结蛋白）后的肌细胞仍然可以在三磷腺苷和钙离子的作用下反应性收缩。此发现使其作者认为该蛋白并无收缩作用，而是将肌动蛋白和肌球蛋白丝保持和固定在质膜上。

此发现被其他研究者证实并加以拓展[27-29]。现已知结蛋白分子量为 53kD，形成以 36～37kD/nm 为单位的团块。它由一个 N- 末端"头片段"和 C- 末端"尾片段"组成，均为非螺旋构型，两者构成呈α-螺旋的中间域的支架，中间域由大约 300 个氨基酸残基组成。头部生化组成在不同物种间差异很大，而螺旋部分则高度"保守"，提示此部分在物种间有着惊人的同源性。鸡和猪的结蛋白生化差异不到 9%。事实上，种内不同 IFPs 之间也表现出类似的同源性；然而，所有 5 种 IFPs 的氨基酸序列的同源性大约为 30%[29]。

同其他中间丝一样，结蛋白也表现出 20～22nm 的轴向周期性。Ip 和 Heuser 提出结蛋白是以纤维交联四聚体的方式聚合成异聚体[30]。结蛋白呈并行排列，有半个单位的滑动余地，其中头部与相邻的中间域相连。结蛋白的螺旋部分形成螺线管样的三级分子结构，其实，这种构象也可由生化模型预测出来。疏水性的氨基酸残基被暴露在外侧，因而解释了结蛋白具有与非亲水性的核膜与胞膜相连的能力。

结蛋白出现于横纹肌生长过程中的肌管形成阶段，肌母细胞在这一阶段相互融合[31]。它取代了大部分波形蛋白，因为波形蛋白是一种几乎所有胚胎间质细胞中首先表达的中间丝。结蛋白丝最初呈纵向排列，随着肌细胞的成熟转而集中于 Z 盘周围[32]。Fischman 和 Danto[33]应用单克隆抗体（D3 和 D76）对胚胎和成人的肌细胞中的结蛋白免疫反应活性进行了分析。D3 可以识别出胚胎细胞中的结蛋白，而对成人细胞无反应。D76 的结果恰好与之相反。这些数据提示或者是结蛋白在细胞成熟过程中发生了生化改变，或者是胚胎和成人细胞中的抗原决定簇不同。

虽然结蛋白最常表达于肌源性细胞中，但体外培养的鸡胚细胞和仓鼠肾成纤维细胞中也有结蛋白的表达[34]。这些细胞所具有的肌成纤维细胞特性可很好地解释此现象。然而有报道，在完整的肌成纤维细胞组织中，用免疫荧光检测却未发现结蛋白活性。因此，并不是所有的肌细胞都含有结蛋白。例如，Schmid 及其同事报道哺乳动物的血管（大动脉）平滑肌中有 3 种独立的细胞类型：只表达波形蛋白的细胞、同时表达波形蛋白和结蛋白的细胞及只表达结蛋白的第 3 种细胞[35]。免疫电镜研究证明适当的特异性抗结蛋白抗体可以与肌细胞及其肿瘤中的中间丝结合[36]。这些试剂应当与相关的收缩蛋白如肌动蛋白和肌球蛋白之间无交叉反应性；这一点非常重要，因为这 3 种蛋白共享一部分抗原决定簇。

结蛋白 3 种最具有特征性的单克隆抗体分别为 D33、DER-11 和 DEB-5。通过 Western blot 技术，显示其可识别结蛋白 324～415 残基间的抗原决定簇，并与其他 IFPs 无交叉反应，这些抗体具有组织特异性但无种间特异性。

通常认为结蛋白是软组织肿瘤中肌源性分化的一种特异性标记物。因而它可见于大多数的横纹肌瘤、平滑肌瘤、横纹肌肉瘤以及平滑肌肉瘤（LMSs）[23-25,37-39]。由于在超微结构上肌纤维瘤病也有部分肌源性的特性，所以像硬纤维瘤和肌纤维瘤之类的病变中可能会有结蛋白表达[40]。然而，肌上皮细胞却典型地缺乏结蛋白表达。结蛋白也可异源性共表达于其他肿瘤，例如原始神经外胚层肿瘤（PNETs）、促纤维增生性小圆细胞肿瘤（PNETs 的亚型）、上皮样肉瘤、恶性外周神经鞘瘤（MPNSTs）和一些恶性"横纹肌样"瘤[41-45]。

波形蛋白

波形蛋白（vimentin）是一个 50kD 的蛋白质，最初由鼠成纤维细胞培养分离而来[2,46]。它的名字来源于拉丁语 vimentum，用来描述一排有弹性的杆子。该蛋白被认为是中间丝家族"最原始的"成员，因为它见于大多数（即使不是全部）胚胎发育早期的细胞中。除此之外，当在细胞系或肿瘤中同时表达两种或更多的 IFPs 时，波形蛋白总是其中之一[47]。因此，波形蛋白被认为无细胞类型特异性。从间叶肿瘤病理学的角度看，波形蛋白的意义在于它与结蛋白、

NFPs 和 GFAP 之间的氨基酸同源性要比与角蛋白之间的大很多[22, 46]。

波形蛋白在软组织中的普遍存在限制了它在肿瘤病理诊断中的应用。然而波形蛋白可作为实用的"对照标记物"以判断组织保存和处理是否良好[48]。如果在常规制片组织中波形蛋白应为阳性的非肿瘤性内皮细胞、成纤维细胞以及其他间质成分中不能很容易地检测到波形蛋白，则不能正确判断其相伴随的肿瘤细胞是阳性还是阴性。偶尔波形蛋白的表达形式也可以很独特，例如，在软组织恶性"横纹肌样"瘤中，波形蛋白通常在胞浆内形成致密的球形结构，并压迫肿瘤细胞核[45]。表 3.3 ~ 3.7 列出了波形蛋白的系列商业化抗体，其中应用最广泛的是 V9 和 3B4 克隆[47, 49-54]。

神经丝蛋白

神经丝蛋白（nerofilament proteins，NFPs）是由分子量分别为 68kD、150kD 和 200kD 的 3 个碱性亚基构成的[55, 56]，所以，明显大于其他 IFPs。3 个 NFPs 的每个亚基都是单独基因编码，而不是另外两个的衍生物[57]。在 IFPs 中，NFPs 家族的表达与胚胎期神经"母"细胞或肿瘤细胞向神经元分化有关[58, 59]。NFPs 的另一个特征是 3 个亚基中的每一个在生

表 3.4　软组织和骨的恶性小圆细胞肿瘤相关免疫标记物的阳性率*

抗原/肿瘤	KER	EMA	VIM	DES	MSA	MYOGN	SYN	CD57	S-100P	CD45	CD99	OCN
RMS	<10[a]	<1[a]	93	94	96	92	0	17	7	0	19	0
ES/PNET	7	0	75	<1[b]	<1[b]	<1[b]	65	30	<10[a]	0	91	0
PSRCT	50[a]	30[a]	75[a]	50[a]	50[a]	50[a]	75[a]	30[a]	<10[a]	0	90[c]	0
MCS	<5[a]	0	98	0	0	0	0	58	97[d]	0	13	0
SCOS	<1[a]	0	100	<1	<5[a]	0	0	50[a]	33	0	35	73
ML/LEUK	0	0	75[a]	0	0	0	0	<5[a]	0	98	50[a]	0
SCSS	75[e]	75	100	0	0	0	0	90	30[a]	0	0	0

* 除了特别标注外，该表中所有数据显示各种肿瘤免疫标记物的阳性率；这些数据均来自于名为"Immunoquery"的网站（Frisman D；http://www.immunoquery.com）
[a] 数据来自于作者的经验
[b] 许多作者将表达 DES/MSA，或 MYOGN 的周围神经外胚层肿瘤归类为多表型小圆细胞肿瘤
[c] 多表型小圆细胞肿瘤的促结缔组织增生性小圆细胞肿瘤通常为 CD99 阴性
[d] S-100 蛋白只见于间叶性软骨肉瘤中的软骨岛
[e] 角蛋白 7、13 和 19 见于 45%~50% 的小细胞滑膜肉瘤病例中，但鉴别诊断应用少于 10%。KER，角蛋白，可用抗体 CAM5.2、MAK-6 和 AE1/AE3 混合检测；EMA，上皮细胞膜抗原；VIM，波形蛋白；DES，结蛋白；MSA，肌特异性肌动蛋白；MYOGN，肌细胞生成素；SYN，突触素；S-100P，S-100 蛋白；OCN，骨钙素；RMS，胚胎性和腺泡状横纹肌肉瘤；ES/PNET，Ewing 肉瘤/原始神经外胚层肿瘤；PSRCT，多表型小圆细胞肿瘤；MCS，间叶性软骨肉瘤；SCOS，小细胞骨肉瘤；ML/LEUK，恶性淋巴瘤/白血病；SCSS，小细胞低分化滑膜肉瘤

表 3.5　软组织和骨的恶性梭形细胞肿瘤相关免疫标记物的阳性率*

抗原/肿瘤	KER	EMA	VIM	DES	MSA	SMA	CALD	S-100P	CD57	Collagen type IV	LM	CD34	CD31	UL	CD99	OCN
SCRMS	<10[a]	<1[a]	95	95	96	25	<1	7	17	98[a]	100	0	0	0	20	0
FS	0	0	100	0	0	<5[a]	0	2	0	0	0	0	0	0	0	0
LMS	<10[a]	0	91	75[a]	90	88	85	8	50	75	63	16	<1[a]	0	20	0
MPNST	<10[a]	25	100	11	18	<1	<1	63	43	83	80	9	0	0	50[a]	0
MSS	76	75	100	0	0	12	<1[a]	30[a]	90	100	95	0	0	0	50[a]	0
SCAS	<5[a]	0	100	0	<10[a]	<10[a]	<5[a]	1[a]	0	10	55	80	80	70	0	0
KS	0	0	100	0	0	100	<5[a]	0	0	50[a]	50[a]	86	53	10	0	0
FOS	<1[a]	0[a]	100	<1[a]	<1[a]	<1[a]	<1[a]	10[a]	50[a]	0	0	0	0	0	0	80[a]

* 该表中的所有数据显示了每种肿瘤中免疫标记物的阳性率，除了特殊标注外，这些数据均来自于名为"Immunoquery"的网站（Frisman D；htth://www.immunoquery.com）
[a] 数据来自于作者的经验
KER，角蛋白，用抗体 CAM5.2、MAK-6 和 AE1/AE3 混合检测；EMA，上皮细胞膜抗原；VIM，波形蛋白；DES，结蛋白；MSA，肌特异性肌动蛋白；SMA，平滑肌（α单体）肌动蛋白；CALD，h-钙调素结合蛋白；S-100P，S-100 蛋白；OCN，骨钙素；LM，层粘连蛋白；UL，荆豆凝集素；FS，纤维肉瘤；SCRMS，梭形细胞横纹肌肉瘤；LMS，平滑肌肉瘤；MPNST，恶性外周神经鞘瘤；MSS，单相梭形细胞滑膜肉瘤；SCAS，梭形细胞血管肉瘤；KS，Kaposi 肉瘤；FOS，成纤维细胞性骨肉瘤

表3.6 软组织和骨的恶性上皮样肿瘤相关免疫标记物的阳性率*

抗原/肿瘤	KER	EMA	VIM	DES	MSA	SMA	CALD	S-100P	CD57	HMB-45	TY	M1	CD31	CD34	Collagen type IV	OCN
EPS	100	96	100	10	39	33	25[a]	<5[a]	0	0	0	0	<1[a]	52	50[a]	0
EPSS	95[a]	99[a]	100	0	0	0	0	10[a]	50[a]	0	0	0	0	0	100	0
EAS	10[a]	0	100	0	0	0	0	<1[a]	0	0	0	0	80	80	65[a]	0
EMPNST	<10[a]	20	100	11	18	<1	<1	63	43	<1[a]	<1[a]	<1[a]	0	9	83	0
CCS	<1[a]	0	100	0	30	0	0	90[a]	17	85	90[a]	70[a]	0	4	0	0
SEFS	<1[a]	0[a]	100	0[a]	0[a]	0[a]	0[a]	0[a]	0[a]	0[a]	0[a]	0[a]	0[a]	0[a]	0[a]	0[a]
ELMS	<10[a]	0	90	75	90	85	75	8	50[a]	0	0	0	0[a]	16	75	0
ASPS	0	0	50[a]	20	<10[a]	0[a]	0	30	0	0	0	0	0	0	0	0
HMFH	<1[a]	0	100	<10[a]	17	18	<5[a]	<1[a]	0	0	0	0	0	0	0	0
EOS	<1[a]	0[a]	100	<1[a]	<1[a]	<1[a]	0	<5[a]	50[a]	0	0	0	0	0	0	82

* 该表中的所有数据显示了每种肿瘤中免疫标记物的阳性率。这些数据均来自于名为"Immunoquery"的网站(Frisman D; http://www.immunoquery.com)
[a] 数据来自于作者的经验

KER,角蛋白,用抗体CAM5.2、MAK-6和AE1/AE3混合检测;EMA,上皮细胞膜抗原;VIM,波形蛋白;DES,结蛋白;MSA,肌特异性肌动蛋白;SMA,平滑肌(α单体)肌动蛋白;CALD,h-钙调素结合蛋白;S-100P,S-100蛋白;OCN,骨钙素;TY,酪氨酸激酶;MI,MART-1(黑色素-A);EPS,上皮样肉瘤;EPSS,上皮样滑膜肉瘤;EAS,上皮样血管肉瘤;EMPNST,上皮样恶性外周神经鞘瘤;CCS,透明细胞肉瘤;SEFS,硬化性上皮样纤维肉瘤;ELMS,上皮样平滑肌肉瘤;ASPS,腺泡状软组织肉瘤;HMFH,组织细胞性恶性纤维组织细胞瘤;EOS,上皮样骨肉瘤

表3.7 软组织和骨的恶性多形性肿瘤相关免疫标记物的阳性率*

抗原/肿瘤	KER	EMA	VIM	DES	MSA	SMA	CALD	S-100P	CD57	Collagen type IV	LM	CD34	CD31	UL	CD99	OCN
PRMS	<10[a]	<1[a]	100	95	96	25	<1	7	17	98[a]	100	0	0	0	20	0[a]
PLPS/DLPS	0	0	100	0	<1[a]	<1[a]	<1[a]	70[b]	0	20[a]	10[a]	0	0	0	0	0[a]
PLMS/DLMS	<10[a]	0	91	75[a]	90	88	75	8	50	75	63	16	<1	0	20	0[a]
MPNST	<10[a]	20	100	11	18	<1	<1	63	43	83	80	9	0	0	10[a]	0[a]
MFH	76[b]	75[b]	100	0	0	12	<1[a]	30[a]	90[b]	100[b]	95[b]	0	0	0	50[b]	0[a]
DCHOR	<1[a]	0	100	<10[a]	17	18	<5[a]	<1[a]	0[a]	0	0	0	0	0	0[a]	0[a]
DCHS	100[b]	94[b]	100	3	0	0	0	88[b]	32[b]	13	10	0	0	10[ab]	0[a]	0[a]
POGS	<1[a]	0[a]	100	0	0	0	0	97[b]	58[b]	10[ab]	5[ab]	0	0	0	0[a]	0[a]
	<1[a]	<1[a]	100	11	0	0	50	0	32[b]	50[b]	0	0	0	0	35	82

* 该表中的全部数据显示了每种肿瘤中免疫标记物的阳性率。除了特殊标记外,这些数据均来自于名为"Immuoquery"的网站(Frisman D; http://www.immunoquery.com)
[a] 数据来源于作者的经验
[b] 对特定抗原决定簇仅局灶阳性

KER,角蛋白,用抗体CAM5.2、MAK-6和AE1/AE3混合检测;EMA,上皮细胞膜抗原;VIM,波形蛋白;DES,结蛋白;MSA,肌特异性肌动蛋白;SMA,平滑肌(α单体)肌动蛋白;CALD,h-钙调素结合蛋白;S-100P,S-100蛋白;LM,层粘连蛋白;UL,荆豆凝集素;OCN,骨钙素;PRMS,多形性横纹肌肉瘤;PLPS/DLPS,多形性和去分化脂肪肉瘤;PLMS/DLMS,多形性和去分化平滑肌肉瘤;MPNST,多形性恶性外周神经鞘瘤;DMSS,去分化单相梭形细胞滑膜肉瘤;MFH,恶性纤维组织细胞瘤;DCHOR,去分化脊索瘤;DCHS,去分化软骨肉瘤;POGS,多形性骨肉瘤

物体内都可由磷酸化或者非磷酸化两种形成[60],而其他中间丝(除GFAP外)不具备该特征。相应地,NFPs的抗体也可特异性地仅针对其中的一种[61,62]。

实际上,NFPs在福尔马林固定石蜡包埋的组织中,即使用现代的免疫组化技术和商业化抗体也不易检测。据我们的经验,"SMI"系列的单克隆抗体[63]对常规处理的外科病理标本阳性反应最稳定。现已知,在软组织肿瘤中只有神经母细胞瘤的各种亚型、神经节瘤、副神经节瘤和转移性神经内分泌癌NFPs呈阳性[64-67]。

胶质纤维酸性蛋白

胶质纤维酸性蛋白(glial fibrillary acidic protein, GFAP),在软组织肿瘤诊断中意义不大。该蛋白有51kD大小,为星形细胞、室管膜细胞和视网膜Müller细胞的主要成分,在成熟的少突胶质细胞中一般不表达[67-69]。非胶质组织中若出现GFAP假阳性则为施万细胞、库普弗细胞和一些软骨细胞[69]。因此,在部分包括上述成分的肿瘤(外周神经鞘瘤和软

骨样肿瘤)[70-75]中偶尔可出现GFAP阳性。虽然此种情况很少发生，但我们还是认为GFAP不宜作为软组织病理诊断常规抗体。

上皮相关标记物

上皮细胞膜抗原

上皮细胞膜抗原（epithelial membrane antigen, EMA）是从乳腺上皮中分离得到的，为几种人乳脂肪球蛋白（HMFGPs）中的一种。HMFGPs分子量差别很大（由51kD到>1000kD不等），它们大多为糖蛋白[76]，并构成上皮细胞紧密连接处的部分胞膜[77]。除此之外，由于HMFGPs在高尔基复合体中被包装，免疫组化可见其特征性球形结构[77]。包括EMA在内的HMFGPs的功能仍未完全明了，据认为可能在分泌过程中起作用，或者对细胞行使保护功能[76]。

大部分（并非全部）人非肿瘤性上皮细胞中至少表达一种HMFGPs，但胃肠表面上皮、宫颈管上皮、前列腺腺泡上皮、附睾、生殖细胞、肝细胞、肾上腺皮质细胞、睾丸网、表皮的鳞状上皮细胞及甲状腺滤泡上皮除外[78]。

EMA（应用最广泛的一种HMFGPs）最具特征性的单抗为E29。它标记一种大小约为450kD的糖蛋白。特异性方面，在非肿瘤性成分的软组织中，只有脊索、神经周的成纤维细胞和浆细胞可能为EMA阳性[79-81]。然而有更多的肿瘤组织EMA阳性。滑膜肉瘤、上皮样肉瘤、部分外周神经鞘肿瘤（"神经束膜瘤"和一些神经鞘黏液瘤）、脊索瘤、副脊索瘤和部分浆细胞瘤均为阳性[82]。需要强调的是，"真正的" EMA阳性（一般等同于上皮分化）必须是细胞膜阳性，单纯胞浆阳性而胞膜阴性应为假阳性，不能作为诊断的依据[83]。

其他的上皮标记物

如果"标准的"上皮性标记物（如CK和EMA）染色结果不确定，则需其他上皮标记物染色，尤其是当形态学特征提示上皮分化明显或怀疑有假阳性时。对其他上皮标记物了解最多的是桥粒斑蛋白（desmoplakin）、桥粒芯糖蛋白（desmoglein）和E-钙黏素。前两者是"桥粒芯胶蛋白（desmocollins）"或者桥粒复合体中的成分，代表了特化的细胞间连接结构[84,85]。钙黏素则是钙依赖性的细胞间跨膜黏附分子，分为3个亚类：E-、P-和N-钙黏素，具有各自

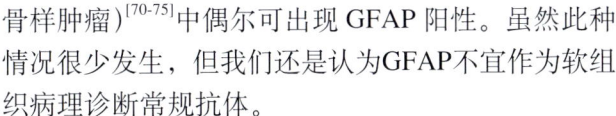

的免疫学特征和组织分布[86,87]。这些分子在细胞连接中具有各自的亚型特征并和细胞选择性黏附有关。E-钙黏素是一种典型的与上皮分化相关的亚型。由编码钙黏素的cDNA核苷酸序列对其氨基酸序列进行分析，已证实它们有共同的序列，因此将它们视为一个具有不同特性的黏附分子家族。除个别情况外，桥粒斑蛋白或桥粒芯糖蛋白和E-钙黏素一般只在上皮性肿瘤和具有上皮特征的间叶肿瘤中表达。

其他的肌源性标记物

肌动蛋白

除结蛋白外，另一个对于确定肌源性分化最有用的胞浆标记物为肌动蛋白（actin）家族[25,88]。这些微丝收缩多肽有6个主要异构体，分别命名为：骨骼肌α、平滑肌α、平滑肌γ、心肌α、非肌源性β和非肌源性γ肌动蛋白[88,89]。α和γ异构体见于"纯"肌源性分化的组织中，但它们也可表达于具有肌纤维母细胞或肌上皮特性的细胞中[90-93]，其分子量约为45kD，它们也可被识别保守性氨基酸序列的抗体或异构体选择性识别抗体所标记[88-90]。显然，诊断需要的是异构体抗体。然而，由于在对异聚蛋白的免疫组化检测中会出现一些不可避免的问题，甚至一些抗肌动蛋白抗体也并非"纯粹"肌源性分化所特异的。例如常用的商业性试剂克隆1A4就是如此，该抗体作为抗（α-）平滑肌肌动蛋白抗体广为人知[91]，实际上，它还能与一些非平滑肌细胞反应，包括肌纤维母细胞、肌上皮细胞和其他细胞。另外一个抗体命名为HHF-35，或称为抗肌特异性肌动蛋白抗体，在常规处理的标本中显示更为严格的肌特异性[25,90]。

其他的肌小节收缩蛋白

骨骼肌的收缩机制由一个蛋白复合物来完成，该复合物包括肌球蛋白II（分子量为460kD）、肌动蛋白、原肌球蛋白（分子量为70kD）和肌钙蛋白。肌钙蛋白分子有3个亚单位，分别为肌钙蛋白I、肌钙蛋白T和肌钙蛋白C，分子量在18~35kD之间[94]。肌球蛋白是一个肌动蛋白结合蛋白，有两个球形的头和一个延长的尾，尤其是肌球蛋白II由两条重链和4条轻链（两条磷酸化的和两条碱性的）组成。肌球蛋白重链的N-末端部分形成球形的头，每一个头部都有一个肌动蛋白结合位点和一个酸性位点，以水解ATP。肌球蛋白分子的头与肌动蛋白形成交叉的桥状结构[95]。在肌小节中央两侧

肌球蛋白分子形成对称结构。肌小节细丝是两条肌动蛋白链以双螺旋形式形成的多聚体。原肌球蛋白分子位于两条肌动蛋白链的间槽内。肌钙蛋白沿着原肌球蛋白分散排布[96]。肌钙蛋白T与肌球蛋白结合其他的肌钙蛋白成分，肌钙蛋白I抑制肌球蛋白和肌动蛋白的相互作用，肌钙蛋白C含有能启动肌肉收缩的钙粒子结合位点。辅肌动蛋白有190kD大小，可连接肌动蛋白到肌小节的Z线。另一蛋白为连接素（tinin），连接Z线到M线并提供粗丝形成的基质[97]。由于这些标记物敏感性相对较差，所以一般不用于诊断目的[98-103]。

肌红蛋白

肌红蛋白（myoglobin）是一个分子量为17.8kD的蛋白质，仅发现于骨骼肌中，并与铁分子形成复合物[104]。这种分子的浓度在具有持续性收缩特点的肌肉中最高。由于肌红蛋白在横纹肌成熟过程中出现相对较晚，所以在显示朝向肌源性分化的胚胎性肿瘤中免疫组化常显示为阴性。而多形性"成人型"横纹肌肉瘤和横纹肌瘤肌红蛋白常为阳性[98, 99, 101, 106-111]。

Myo-D1 和成肌素（myogenin）

转录因子是一个"超家族"，可调节特异性细胞系增生。横纹肌中的转录因子称为Myo-D家族[112-114]。它们由位于染色体1、11和12上的基因编码，并且是碱性螺旋-环-螺旋（BHLH）模序多肽复合物的一部分，它们都是由220~320个氨基酸组成的小蛋白。自20世纪90年代后，此类核内蛋白的两个成员Myo-D1和myogenin就被用于人类肿瘤中横纹肌分化的特异性标记物[112-115]。它们激活自身转录及其他BHLH蛋白的转录，与视网膜母细胞瘤基因相配合，控制细胞离开细胞周期以及启动向横纹肌方向分化。

由于抗Myo-D1和myogenin的抗体必须进入核浆，因此在常规外科标本中应用困难。然而，抗原修复液的修饰以及热介导的抗原决定簇增强作用，使这些抗体可应用于诊断[114]。需要强调的是，就像激素受体蛋白一样，Myo-D1和myogenin严格定位于细胞核内，因此，在胞浆的阳性标记（这是抗体应用中经常性的问题，尤其是抗Myo-D1抗体）必须视为假阳性染色而不予考虑。

钙调素结合蛋白

钙调素结合蛋白（caldesmon）是一种胞浆蛋白，包括两个异构体，其中之一主要见于平滑肌细胞以及其他具有部分肌源性分化的细胞中。高分子量异构体大小在89~93kD之间，能与肌动蛋白、原肌球蛋白、钙调蛋白、肌球蛋白和磷脂结合，其功能为阻碍肌动蛋白-原肌球蛋白-活化肌球蛋白-ATP酶的作用，因此是钙依赖性平滑肌收缩的抑制调节子[116]。

针对钙调素结合蛋白的商业性抗体现已应用于外科病理诊断中。它们对于平滑肌、肌纤维母细胞和肌上皮分化细胞均具有特异性，因而是结蛋白和肌动蛋白免疫组化染色的辅助标记物[116, 117]。

施万细胞分化标记物

S-100 蛋白

S-100 蛋白的命名来源于它可溶于饱和（100%）的硫酸铵溶液中。最初是从中枢神经系统中分离而来，现在已知其在人体组织中分布广泛，包括神经节、神经元、软骨细胞、施万细胞、黑色素细胞、固有吞噬或抗原提呈单核细胞、朗格汉斯组织细胞、肌上皮细胞、脊索和各种上皮（尤其是乳腺、唾液腺、汗腺和女性生殖系统）[118]。S-100蛋白具有二聚体特性，有α和β两个亚单位。因此它有3种异构体——S-100ao（α-二聚体）、S-100a（α-β异构体）和S-100b（β-二聚体）。该蛋白两个亚单位的分子量均为约10.5kD，S-100蛋白的基本功能是对钙流入的调节[119]。

S-100 蛋白的单克隆抗体和异种抗血清都可用于诊断，有些单克隆抗体是分别针对α或者β亚单位的特异性抗体，因此与多克隆抗血清相比它们表现出相对窄谱的反应性。例如，β亚单位特异性抗体主要标记神经节细胞和施万细胞[120]。所以在临床病理诊断应用并不广泛。临床实践中最常应用的是S-100蛋白的异种抗血清。一般情况下，S-100可作为判断肿瘤来源分化的抗体组合之一，是识别软组织和骨肿瘤中施万细胞、黑色素细胞或软骨细胞确有价值的指标[121-125]。

CD57（Leu7，HNK-1）

CD57是一种膜抗原，见于约20%的外周血中具有"自然杀伤"活性的单核白细胞中，其分子量为95kD。该组抗体的原型称为HNK-1（后命名为Leu7）[126]，该抗体也可以与一些分子量为19~72kD不等的神经分子反应[127-130]。其中一部分与5'-核苷酸酶活性相关[129]，其他的则为髓磷脂相关糖蛋白（myelin-associated glycoproteins，MAGs）[127-130]。最大的MAGs（MAG-72）在结构上与免疫球蛋白超家族基因产物以及神经黏附分子和具有自身磷酸化位点的表皮生长因子受体相关。MAGs是整合的细胞膜蛋白，正常见于少突胶质细胞。其功能是参与介导髓鞘形成过程中轴突间或轴突-神经胶质间的相互作用，因此，与施万细胞和神经肿瘤相关联也就不足为奇了。然而，在神经周的（非施万细胞）外周神经鞘病变中也有HNK-1阳性的报道[131]。一般情况下，CD57不仅可以作为外周神经鞘肿瘤的潜在标记物，也可见于Ewing肉瘤和PNETs中，因为神经内分泌颗粒和突触小泡的基质蛋白中含有HNK-1的一种靶蛋白[71, 73, 132-140]。

需要强调的是，CD57并不仅限于软组织肿瘤中的神经鞘细胞或神经外胚层成分，而是最常见于这些细胞类型。其他如滑膜肉瘤、平滑肌肉瘤和一些转移性癌也可以被HNK-1标记[132]。因此，可将CD57抗体用于检测肌源性、上皮性和神经性分化的配套抗体中。CD57最常用于鉴别纤维肉瘤和MPNST、恶性纤维组织细胞瘤（MFH）和MPNST以及黏液性神经鞘肿瘤（良性和恶性）和非神经性的黏液性肿瘤。

IV型胶原纤维和层粘连蛋白

从含量上看，无论在哪种细胞中，IV型胶原都是基底膜的主要成分。其分子量为550kD，有3个螺旋，末端呈球形，并有两个非胶原结构域，其中之一定位于分子羧基末端330nm处，在该处有一个"弯曲点"使该部分形成"曲棍球杆"样[141]。IV型胶原与其他类型胶原不同之处在于它不形成原纤维，其螺旋结构是间断性的，并且有一个不同的氨基酸区域，编码该分子螺旋链的基因定位于染色体13q[142]。

层粘连蛋白（laminin）是基底膜的另一种重要成分，其分子量为1000kD，有3个短臂和1个长臂，都具有球形末端。层粘连蛋白与氨基葡萄糖相连，作为连接基底膜IV型胶原与周围基质的桥梁[143]。层粘连蛋白在基底膜中的确切位置还有争议，有些研究者认为它是致密层的成分，另一些则认为其位于透明层，还有一些人认为它同时分布于两部分中[144]。除了简单的"分界"和锚定功能，层粘连蛋白可能还影响细胞之间的相互作用及细胞形态的改变[145]。

软组织中的内皮细胞、平滑肌细胞和施万细胞周围具有完整的基底膜[146, 147]。因此，抗IV型胶原和层粘连蛋白抗体是检测这些细胞系的成套抗体的有效成员。尤其是在难以鉴别的纤维肉瘤和MFH与MPNSTs的诊断上，由于并不是所有的MPNSTs对S-100蛋白或CD57都有反应，所以在鉴别诊断中，IV型胶原或层粘连蛋白阳性将支持外周神经鞘肿瘤的诊断。在此特殊情况下我们最常使用这两种标记物，因此IV型胶原和层粘连蛋白属于辅助性"神经"标记物。

内皮标记物

内皮细胞几个相关标记物已用于软组织中血管肿瘤的鉴别诊断。其敏感性和特异性程度各异，讨论如下。

VIII因子相关抗原（vWF）

VIII因子相关抗原或vWF是一个大的多聚蛋白，仅由内皮细胞和巨核细胞合成。它包括3个多聚亚单位，分子量大于10 000kD。生理情况下，它们通过蛋白水解在血浆中形成小片段[148]。vWF具有双重功能。首先，它与抗血友病因子形成循环复合物，又称为VIII因子促凝蛋白。抗血友病因子是肝细胞合成的分子量为265kD的蛋白质，影响内源性凝血途径中X因子的激活。其次，vWF在血小板凝聚中起重要作用，因此该蛋白水平降低或功能不全的病人，临床上表现为出血体质，称之为von Willebrand综合征[149]。

在软组织病理学中，vWF主要用于血管肿瘤和与其形态相似肿瘤的鉴别[150-152]。因为vWF主要在内皮细胞中的Weibel-Palade小体（WPBs）中包装，所以从逻辑上说该因子的免疫组化阳性程度应与该细胞器的超微结构相平行。事实也的确如此。由于WPBs在低分化的血管肿瘤中很少，这也解释了为什么vWF在高级别血管肉瘤病变中有如此低的敏感性（约为10%~15%）[151, 152]。因而，该标记物用于鉴别良性和交界性内皮肿瘤时更加实用，如血管瘤亚型和"血管内皮瘤家族"的鉴别诊断[153]。

CD34

CD34或人类造血干细胞抗原，可被包括My10、QBEND-10和BI-3C5在内的几种单克隆抗体所识别[154-157]。它是一个110kD的蛋白质，如其名称所示，是由造血系统未成熟细胞[155, 158]，包括淋巴样和髓性成分以及内皮细胞所表达。在相应的软组织肿瘤中，CD34也是血管分化的潜在标记物。不论肿瘤级别如何，CD34对内皮分化都具有高度敏感性，能识别出85%以上的血管肉瘤和Kaposi肉瘤（KS）[153-155, 157]。然而CD34并非十分特异，据报道在一些LMSs、外周神经鞘肿瘤和上皮样肉瘤中可呈阳性[155, 158, 159]，这些肿瘤在某种程度上可能与血管肉瘤或血管内皮瘤类似。除此之外，CD34在隆突型皮肤纤维肉瘤（及其变型）、梭形细胞脂肪瘤和孤立性纤维瘤中也很常见，可常规地作为这些肿瘤诊断的辅助标记物[160-162]。因此，作为内皮标记物，CD34抗体在用于鉴别诊断时最好与其他抗体配套使用。

CD31

血小板内皮细胞黏附分子-1（PECAM-1），也称CD31[163]，是一个130kD的跨膜糖蛋白，可见于血管内皮细胞、巨核细胞、血小板和其他部分造血成分中，可被单克隆抗体JC/70A识别[164]。在所有软组织肿瘤中，CD31对内皮性肿瘤高度特异，而且其敏感性也很高[165]。就我们所知，无论级别或亚型如何，血管肉瘤实际上100%为CD31阳性，血管瘤和血管内皮瘤的各亚型也是如此[166,167]。然而，必须承认，CD34对Kaposi肉瘤（KS）的标记一致性比CD31高[167]，其原因未知。

血栓调节素

血栓调节素（TMN）是一个75kD的糖蛋白，分布于内皮细胞、间皮细胞、成骨细胞、单核巨噬细胞和部分上皮细胞[168-173]。其生理作用是将血栓素从促凝蛋白转变为抗凝蛋白[170]。由于在一些转移性癌和大多数间皮瘤中TMN都可能存在[172,173]，而这两者都可能与上皮样血管肉瘤相混淆，故不能作为血管肿瘤的单一标记物。然而，已证明TMN是内皮分化，尤其是分化差的血管恶性肿瘤的一个敏感指标[171,174]。KS对TMN具有同样的免疫反应性[175]，因此，在配套抗体中TMN具有一定的应用价值。

荆豆凝集素

荆豆凝集素（UEAI）不是抗体，而是由荆豆所产生的植物凝集素。它能识别岩藻寡糖化的Fuc-α-1-2-Gal链，该寡糖是各种糖蛋白的组成部分[176]。尤其是H血型抗原和癌胚抗原，与内皮细胞表达的岩藻糖化蛋白一样能与UEAI常规结合[152,171,176]。生物素化的Ulex可作为组化试剂用于外科病理检测，或者也可用未标记的植物凝集素先与组织结合，再通过生物素化的抗-Ulex和卵白素-生物素-过氧化物酶复合物检测。如前所述，由于UEAI对内皮分化并非特异，故只能作为组化/免疫组化配套检测的组分之一。例如除血管肿瘤外，上皮样肉瘤和各种转移性癌也可与Ulex结合[177,178]。然而，由于UEAI的高度敏感性使其仍可作为内皮标记物而继续使用。

"纤维组织细胞"标记物

自1985年以来，各种单克隆抗体和异种抗血清不断取得进展，石蜡切片中"组织细胞"或"纤维组织细胞"的标记物也一样，被用于识别良性或恶性纤维组织细胞瘤、非典型纤维黄瘤和皮肤及软组织的"组织细胞瘤"等病变。这些抗体的靶点包括α-1-抗胰蛋白酶、溶菌酶、α-1-抗糜蛋白酶、组织蛋白酶B、CD68、CD163、XIIIa因子和HAM56抗原等成分[179-189]。

虽然大多数纤维组织细胞肿瘤确实能被这些特定的标记物标记，但其特异性均较差。除CD163外[189]，癌、黑素瘤和其他肉瘤形态的肿瘤对这些标记物也可有比较高的表达率[190,191]。鉴于多种肿瘤与纤维组织细胞肿瘤形态极其相似，现行诊断方式还是采用排除法。因此，对于免疫染色或电镜观察波形蛋白阳性的肿瘤只有在排除了上皮性、肌源性、神经和内皮分化后，才可以诊断为纤维组织细胞性病变。在此情况下，再应用针对"组织细胞"标记物的其他抗体是多余的，而且可能有误导作用。因此，我们并不提倡应用。

成骨分化标记物

在骨和软组织肿瘤病理中，最大的困难就是在恶性病变中确定骨基质的形成，因为出现真正的类骨质就等同于骨肉瘤的诊断，因此至关重要。自20世纪90年代后期，在相关文献中可看到许多被认为是特异性成骨标记物的研究报道，包括骨形成蛋白、Ⅰ型胶原、COL-I-C肽、核心蛋白多糖、骨钙素（OCN）、骨连接素（ONN）、骨桥蛋白、蛋白多糖Ⅰ和Ⅱ、骨涎蛋白和骨糖蛋白75[192]。但其中只有ONN和OCN能较好地用于石蜡切片，从而应用于免疫组化诊断。

骨钙素（OCN）

骨钙素（OCN）是最普遍的非胶原性骨内蛋白之一，主要位于成骨细胞中。其分子量为9kD，是富含γ-羧基谷氨酸残基的胞浆蛋白。在成骨性分化和类骨质形成的最后步骤中，螺旋-环-螺旋形转录因子下调其表达，而维生素D的类似物，如1,25-(OH)$_2$-Vit D$_2$和24-epi-1,25-(OH)$_2$-Vit D$_2$则上调其表达[192-198]。OCN的各种异种抗血清和单克隆抗体均已用于免疫组化分析[193,196,193-202]，结果显示在某些解剖部位的成纤维细胞能表达与OCN多克隆抗体起交叉反应的抗原决定簇，因此，那些选择性识别多肽片段的单克隆抗体更适合用于诊断工作[199]。一般情况下

OCN对成骨性分化有比较好的敏感性（大约70%），从实用角度看，它对骨形成细胞和肿瘤实际上是完全特异的[201, 202]。因此，可作为此类肿瘤的单独标记物。

骨连接素（ONN）

骨连接素（ONN）是一种与调节成骨细胞和骨板与细胞外基质黏附以及早期基质钙化有关的蛋白质。在骨细胞和巨核细胞，ONN在翻译后进行不同的修饰，形成具有不同寡糖亚结构的分子；而两种细胞的ONN相关基因组DNA序列、核内RNA序列和mRNA序列则是完全相同的[192, 201-207]。其他一些细胞也可以合成ONN相关抗原。一项研究发现，成纤维细胞、血管外膜细胞、内皮细胞、软骨细胞、部分上皮细胞和神经均可呈ONN阳性反应[202]。总之，据报道ONN对成骨性肿瘤诊断的敏感性为90%，特异性为54%[201, 202]。另外，由于ONN抗血清存在交叉反应的可能[202, 208-210]，因此在诊断中应使用其单克隆抗体。即使这样，由于没有证实ONN有与OCN相关的选择性表达，所以它仅能作为几个分化相关蛋白抗体的配套成员。

软组织和骨肿瘤的其他标记物

用于软组织和骨肿瘤病理鉴别诊断的其他常用标记物如下：黑色素细胞相关标记物如melan-A（MART-1）、酪氨酸酶和HMB-45[211-216]，神经内分泌和神经外胚层的产物如突触素、神经元特异性（γ-二聚）烯醇化酶、蛋白基因产物9.5和NB84[217-223]，造血系统标记物如CD1a、CD45、CD138、HLA-DR和免疫球蛋白轻链[224-231]。其内容详见本书皮肤、内分泌器官和造血系统有关章节。在此着重讨论另一个淋巴网状内皮标记物——CD99，又称为p30/32糖蛋白或MIC2蛋白[232-234]。它是由位于X和Y染色体上的基因编码的一种细胞表面蛋白[235, 236]。CD99表达于胞膜上，大部分Ewing肉瘤和PNETs都可表达CD99，但在淋巴母细胞性淋巴瘤、孤立性纤维瘤和滑膜肉瘤以及其他的间质肿瘤和部分上皮性病变中可有特殊类型的表达[229, 232, 233, 237-244]。CD99商业性单抗有12E7、O13和HBA-71（表3.3）。

另一个标记物来源于血液病理学领域，即间变性淋巴瘤激酶-1（ALK-1），是一种蛋白酪氨酸激酶，又称为"p80"，是异常的ALK-NPM融合基因的产物，由系统性间变性大细胞（"Ki-1"）淋巴瘤中t（2;5）（p23;q35）染色体易位产生[245]。出乎意料的是，ALK-1并不局限于造血系统病变，尤其是在许多"炎性肌纤维母细胞肿瘤"（IMTs，以前称为"炎性假瘤"）中也发现了ALK-1，可能是因为IMTs在染色体2p23位点上常出现异常所致[246, 247]。尽管开始人们期望p80是所有梭形细胞增生性病变的一种特异性标记物，但现在发现ALK-1也可见于平滑肌肉瘤、横纹肌肉瘤和恶性纤维组织细胞瘤中[248]。因此，该标记物在鉴别诊断中的应用价值有限。但ALK-1阳性在IMTs的鉴别诊断中可排除如下病变：结节性筋膜炎、硬纤维瘤、婴儿肌纤维瘤病和婴儿型纤维肉瘤（所有这些病变p80呈阴性）[246]。

诊断要点：软组织抗原/抗体

1. 结蛋白是软组织肿瘤中肌源性分化的特异性标记物，见于几乎所有的横纹肌肉瘤/平滑肌肉瘤、横纹肌瘤/平滑肌瘤。
2. 结蛋白可见于肌纤维瘤病和多表型肿瘤。
3. 波形蛋白在软组织肿瘤中广泛存在，并作为最原始的胞浆原纤维出现于低分化的肉瘤中。
4. GFAP可见于施万细胞和软骨细胞。
5. 角蛋白常见于滑膜肉瘤、脊索瘤、副脊索瘤、上皮样肉瘤和造釉细胞瘤，而平滑肌肉瘤、恶性外周神经鞘瘤、上皮样血管肉瘤和多表型肿瘤如PNET中通常少见。
6. EMA常规表达于滑膜肉瘤、上皮样肉瘤、神经束膜瘤、神经鞘黏液瘤、脊索瘤/副脊索瘤和浆细胞瘤。
7. （α-）平滑肌肌动蛋白（SMA）肌源性分化特异性低于h-钙调素结合蛋白或HHF-35及肌特异性肌动蛋白（MSA）。
8. Myo-D1和成肌素是核转录因子，对横纹肌分化高度特异。
9. Ⅷ因子相关抗原仅见于内皮细胞和巨核细胞。
10. CD31高度局限于内皮肿瘤中，并有很好的敏感性。
11. 血栓调节素可见于间皮细胞和癌，因此不是血管分化的特异性标记物。
12. 虽然CD34对内皮分化检测敏感，但是由于可与各种间叶细胞反应而缺乏特异性。
13. ALK-1可见于平滑肌肉瘤、横纹肌肉瘤和恶性纤维组织细胞瘤中，但是在结节性筋膜炎、硬纤维瘤、婴儿肌纤维瘤病和婴儿纤维肉瘤中阴性。

软组织特殊肿瘤

软组织良性肿瘤

增生性纤维母细胞病变

纤维瘤病以细长的纤维母细胞平行排列成束，并有多少不等的胶原将其分隔为特征。现已知纤维瘤病有几种形式，包括先天性肌纤维瘤病和几种成人的变型，其区别仅在于位置不同：腹部、阴茎、足底和手掌。其他少见形式包括玻璃样变、牙龈和指端纤维瘤病。该类病变与血管外皮细胞瘤、平滑肌瘤、纤维瘤和外周神经鞘肿瘤相似。由于这些病变无独特的免疫表型，其鉴别诊断很大程度上仍要靠组织病理和临床表现。如期望的那样，这些病变波形蛋白均为强阳性，但部分病变结蛋白（图3.1）和肌选择性肌动蛋白可阳性。外周神经鞘肿瘤（神经纤维瘤和施万细胞瘤）为S-100蛋白阳性，可用于与纤维母细胞性病变的鉴别诊断。

腱鞘纤维瘤和胶原性纤维瘤（促纤维增生性纤维母细胞瘤）通常从临床上就足以与纤维瘤病鉴别。这些肿瘤的肌特异性肌动蛋白[249]和平滑肌肌动蛋白[250]常呈弥漫性或局灶阳性，S-100也可呈弱阳性[251]。但结蛋白为阴性[249, 251]。腱鞘纤维瘤和胶原性纤维瘤除了有共同的免疫表型外，还有相同的染色体11q12的异常[252]。

外周神经鞘肿瘤

在儿童和成人中最常见的外周神经鞘肿瘤就是神经纤维瘤和施万细胞瘤，但二者鉴别诊断略有不同：神经纤维瘤一般易于和黏液瘤、非色素性梭形细胞或"神经化的"黑色素细胞痣、富于细胞性和器官样瘢痕组织相混淆，而施万细胞瘤更易与平滑肌瘤相混淆。

在这种情况下，S-100蛋白非常有用，在施万细胞中S-100呈强阳性，在神经纤维瘤中则强弱不一。大多数外周神经鞘肿瘤CD57也为阳性。因黑色素细胞痣和平滑肌瘤S-100蛋白和CD57也可阳性，需要与外周神经鞘肿瘤鉴别。外周神经鞘肿瘤HMB-45、酪氨酸酶和肌源性标记物包括结蛋白、肌相关肌动蛋白均为阴性，可分别用于区分黑色素细胞痣和平滑肌瘤。应用HMB-45的一个例外是砂粒体型色素性施万细胞瘤，此肿瘤好发于肠道、软组织和骨组织，由充满黑色素颗粒的细胞组成，但却是典型的外周神经鞘细胞。Carney报道的31例病例中HMB-45几乎全部为阳性[253]。在神经纤维瘤和黑色素细胞痣鉴别有困难的病例中，应用ⅩⅢa因子则易于诊断，因为ⅩⅢa因子仅见于神经纤维瘤。Fine等还发现钙结合蛋白（calretinin）在施万细胞瘤中呈典型的弥漫阳性，而神经纤维瘤为阴性或仅为弱阳性[254]。

神经纤维瘤的神经束膜细胞含有EMA，在这些肿瘤的小部分细胞中可用免疫组化方法检测到。因为在神经鞘黏液瘤肿瘤细胞团周围有神经束膜成分，因此EMA对于"经典的"神经鞘黏液瘤诊断也有一定价值。偶尔，神经鞘肿瘤GFAP阳性，而其他良性软组织肿瘤阴性。尽管文献尚存在一定分歧，髓磷脂碱性蛋白在神经鞘肿瘤的诊断中也有一定的价值，但我们并不推荐将GFAP和髓磷脂碱性蛋白用于良性软组织肿瘤常规免疫表型分析。

> **诊断要点**：神经鞘肿瘤
> 1. 神经性黑色素细胞痣与神经纤维瘤的鉴别：ⅩⅢa因子神经纤维瘤阳性，黑色素细胞痣阴性。
> 2. 神经鞘肿瘤可偶尔有GFAP和EMA阳性细胞。

梭形细胞脂肪瘤

尽管梭形细胞脂肪瘤的诊断通常是明确的，但也有部分病例类似于其他梭形细胞增生。梭形细胞脂肪瘤为CD34强阳性[255, 256]，但一些在形态上类似梭形细胞脂肪瘤的其他肿瘤也可为CD34阳性，包括孤立性纤维瘤、神经纤维瘤、隆突型皮肤纤维肉瘤、巨细胞

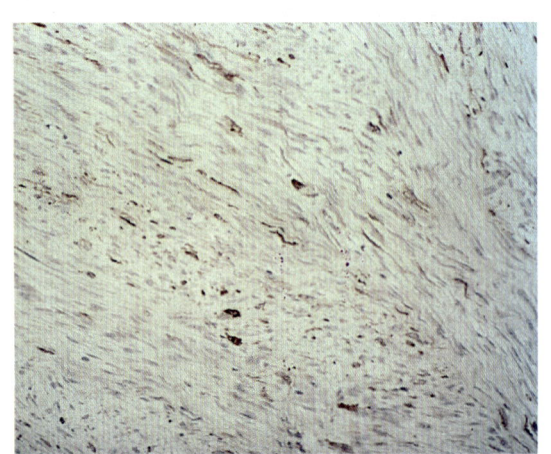

图3.1 硬纤维瘤结蛋白多灶性阳性

纤维母细胞瘤、巨细胞血管纤维瘤和血管脂肪瘤。梭形细胞中S-100蛋白阴性，可与神经纤维瘤鉴别。另外，梭形细胞脂肪瘤bcl-2强阳性，但许多孤立性纤维瘤也可为阳性。应用一组免疫组化染色及细致的组织学观察，通常可对梭形细胞脂肪瘤作出正确诊断。

平滑肌瘤

除了结蛋白、钙调素结合蛋白和肌相关肌动蛋白（MSA）之外，也有一些对肌源性分化特异的标记物可用于平滑肌瘤的诊断，但一般不作为常规免疫病理诊断方法，有些人推荐使用平滑肌肌球蛋白和Z线蛋白，尤其是当病变的组织学类型特殊（如黏液样或玻璃样病变）或其他染色无法确定是否为肌源性病变时。

颗粒细胞瘤

颗粒细胞瘤是一种良性肿瘤，在临床病理中少有恶性，对其已有大量免疫组化研究。颗粒细胞瘤除了易与组织细胞病变混淆外，还与平滑肌瘤[257]和某些癌如肾细胞癌的颗粒细胞亚型相似。成人型颗粒细胞瘤 S-100 蛋白（核和胞浆）、NSE、波形蛋白、α-抑制素、calretinin 和 CD68 均为一致性弥漫阳性[258-262]，大部分 CD57 和/或髓磷脂碱性蛋白也阳性[258]。

有一种病变在组织学上与成人型颗粒细胞瘤相同，沿牙槽嵴分布，几乎全部发生于女性新生儿或婴幼儿，特称为先天性颗粒细胞瘤。其与成人病变的不同之处在于S-100蛋白和NSE完全为阴性。成人型和先天性病变均为α-1-抗胰蛋白酶、CD68和波形蛋白阳性。虽然通常认为CD68为"组织细胞"标记物，其阳性与吞噬溶酶体的富集有关，但在颗粒细胞瘤呈明显特征性阳性。因此，单独应用CD68不能鉴别真性颗粒细胞瘤和反应性组织细胞性颗粒细胞增生。

血管瘤

对细胞结构致密，无明显管腔的良性血管病变诊断有一定困难。幼年性毛细血管瘤和上皮样血管瘤都可能与低级别的血管肉瘤、上皮样肉瘤或血管外皮细胞瘤相混淆。因为上皮样肉瘤 UEAI 凝集素常为阳性，因此当考虑该诊断时需用几个内皮标记物进行鉴别，Ⅷ因子相关抗原和CD31阴性有助于诊断。上皮样肉瘤的上皮性标记物呈特征性阳性，而良性血管增生阴性。血管外皮肿瘤由于部分内皮标记物阴性而易于诊断。

葡萄糖转运蛋白1（GLUT1）作为幼年性血管瘤

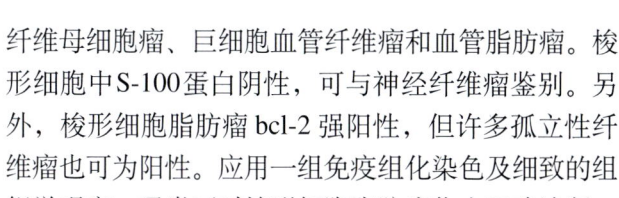

软组织和骨肿瘤的免疫组织化学 3

的标记物令人关注，但并不特异，各种人类实体肿瘤中均有GLUT1表达的报道[263-266]。一项研究发现97%（139/143）的幼年性血管瘤内皮细胞GLUT1强阳性，而66例血管畸形为阴性[256]。迄今为止，还没有实用的免疫组化方法能将血管瘤和与其组织学上相似（"轻微异型"）的血管肉瘤区别开。

FLI-1是近期报道的内皮标记物，较为独特的是其细胞核定位。FLI-1是DNA结合转录因子中"ETS"家族的一个成员，涉及不同的生理功能，包括细胞生长和分化以及器官发育。几项研究显示 FLI-1 在各种良性、居间型/中间性和恶性血管肿瘤中均为阳性[267-270]。

> **诊断要点**：血管肿瘤
>
> 1. CD31 对内皮高度特异而且非常敏感。
> 2. FLI-1是核转录因子，在良性、居间型/中间性和恶性血管肿瘤中呈一致性阳性。在Ewing肉瘤/PNET和淋巴母细胞性淋巴瘤中也呈一致性表达。

横纹肌瘤

横纹肌瘤是具有横纹肌分化的良性肿瘤，镜下分为"成人"、"幼年"或"胎儿"3型。成人型横纹肌瘤细胞有丰富的嗜酸性胞浆；而胎儿型则含有未分化的小细胞，并与形似胎儿肌肉的其他细胞相混合；幼年型在组织学上是这些类型的混合，可能是一个过渡性病变。其鉴别诊断有时包括颗粒细胞瘤、冬眠瘤、副神经节瘤和横纹肌肉瘤。

根据我们的经验，各型横纹肌瘤波形蛋白、结蛋白、肌特异性肌动蛋白、Myo-D1、成肌素均为阳性，以及不同程度的肌红蛋白阳性。尽管有报道少数细胞SMA阳性，但平滑肌肌动蛋白、波形蛋白、GFAP、CD57、CD68、细胞角蛋白和EMA一般均为阴性[271-273]。CD56可呈灶性阳性[274]。虽然部分横纹肌瘤病例S-100蛋白阳性，但仅为少量小灶性阳性[271]，因此与副神经节瘤和颗粒细胞瘤S-100阳性不易混淆。肌源性标记物阳性及CD68阴性也有助于横纹肌瘤的诊断。如同血管肿瘤，免疫组化不能区分骨骼肌良恶性肿瘤，大部分病例依据临床病理学标准足以作出明确诊断。

血管肌纤维母细胞瘤

血管肌纤维母细胞瘤（angiomyofibroblastoma，

AMF）是好发于外阴浅表软组织的独特病变，波形蛋白、结蛋白（图3.2）、肌动蛋白（图3.3）和雌激素受体蛋白均显示为阳性[275, 276]。部分研究[277-279]也显示CD34和黄体酮受体阳性[277, 278]。XⅢa因子、角蛋白、S-100蛋白、CD57、GFAP或CD68阴性[277]。其免疫组化特征与平滑肌瘤相同，但与大多数的其他黏液样肿瘤包括黏液样脂肪肉瘤、黏液样MFH、黏液样神经纤维瘤和黏液样MPNST不同。

尽管血管肌纤维母细胞瘤与侵袭性血管黏液瘤临床特征部分重叠，但通常根据其形态表现足以鉴别。血管肌纤维母细胞瘤体积较小，界限清楚，而侵袭性血管黏液瘤却有明显的浸润并向深处侵袭。血管周围间质细胞聚集是血管肌纤维母细胞瘤的典型病变，而侵袭性血管黏液瘤中无此现象。与血管肌纤维母细胞瘤结蛋白阳性相反，侵袭性血管黏液瘤一般为阴性。因此，免疫组化还是有一定帮助的，但鉴别诊断最终要靠常规的形态学表现。侵袭性血管黏液瘤有较强的复发潜能，而血管肌纤维母细胞瘤则不复发，因此二者鉴别尤为重要。

> **诊断要点**：血管肌纤维母细胞瘤
>
> 依据形态学观察通常可以区别血管肌纤维母细胞瘤（AMF）和侵袭性血管黏液瘤（AAM），但是在AMF的血管周围细胞中结蛋白常为阳性，而AAM为阴性。

软组织交界性肿瘤

血管外皮细胞瘤

血管外皮细胞瘤少见，以致密钝圆的梭形细胞增生伴丰富的血管间质为特征，营养血管常呈"鹿角状"结构。血管外皮细胞瘤中的卵圆形瘤细胞无明显形态特征，易与其他软组织肿瘤细胞相混淆（图3.4）。其免疫学表型既无特异性也无特征性。一般来说，血管外皮细胞瘤的诊断是通过免疫组化排除其他可能的病变后的一个形态学诊断。

尽管瘤与瘤之间染色强度会有所差异，但血管外皮瘤的瘤细胞波形蛋白呈一致性阳性[280]。正常的外皮细胞表达XⅢa因子和HLA-DR，大约50%的血管外皮细胞瘤也呈阳性[281-283]。XⅢa因子也可见于一些纤维组织细胞增生，但脑膜瘤和血管球瘤为阴性，而这些病变均需与血管外皮细胞瘤鉴别。已证实少数血管外皮细胞瘤的肌相关肌动蛋白呈灶性阳性[284]，CD34和

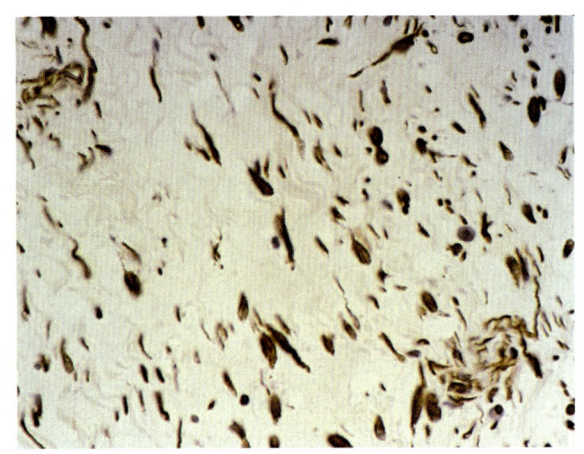

图3.2　血管肌纤维母细胞瘤的梭形细胞为结蛋白阳性

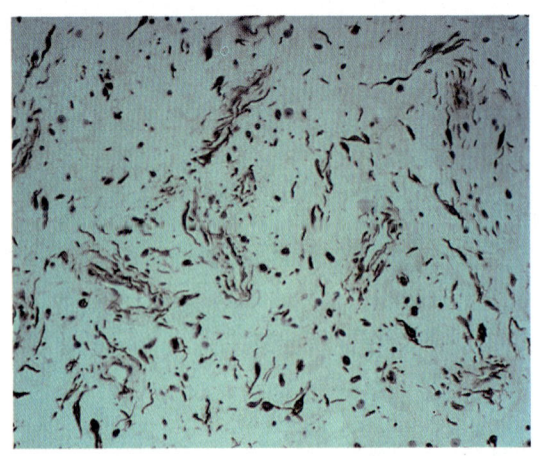

图3.3　在血管肌纤维母细胞瘤梭形细胞和血管中α异构体（"平滑肌"）肌动蛋白阳性

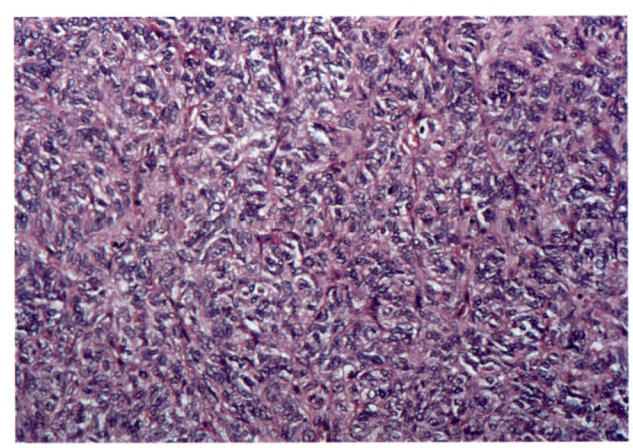

图3.4　血管外皮瘤由卵圆形细胞构成，与不同类型多种肿瘤组织学图像相似

CD57约50%的病例阳性，但结蛋白、CD31、细胞角蛋白和S-100蛋白均为阴性[281, 283]。

血管外皮细胞瘤中可有胰岛素样生长因子-Ⅱ（IGF-Ⅱ）过表达，并认为在该肿瘤相关的低血糖中起重要作用。此类病例免疫组化可检测到IGF-Ⅱ多肽。

孤立性纤维瘤

虽然该病变于1931年作为一种间叶性胸膜病变首次描述[285]，但在20世纪90年代，越来越多的肺外孤立性纤维瘤被认识。有些先前报道的胸外"血管外皮细胞瘤"可能为孤立性纤维瘤，而以往这种胸外的病变没有被认识。其他需要在组织学上作鉴别诊断的病变包括滑膜肉瘤、富于细胞性血管纤维瘤、神经纤维瘤和梭形细胞脂肪瘤。孤立性纤维瘤中的瘤细胞CD34（图3.5）和波形蛋白呈强阳性，bcl-2也常为阳性。细胞角蛋白、CD31和肌动蛋白均为阴性[162, 286-288]。CD99可显示为弥漫强阳性[289]。

为排除与孤立性纤维瘤组织学形态相似的其他梭形细胞增生性病变，需要一组抗体染色。神经纤维瘤bcl-2和CD34可能阳性，但与孤立性纤维瘤不同的是其特征性的S-100蛋白和/或CD57阳性。滑膜肉瘤bcl-2也常为阳性[287]，但CD34为阴性且上皮标记物常为阳性，至少为灶性阳性[162]。梭形细胞脂肪瘤是另一种CD34阳性的肿瘤，一般从组织学上就能将其与孤立性纤维瘤区分，但是偶尔其形态也可能与后者十分相似。但是，梭形细胞脂肪瘤中的脂肪细胞成分S-100蛋白阳性，甚至在该肿瘤的"富细胞"型中也是如此。

孤立性纤维瘤的黏液型可能与其他黏液样病变相混淆，如低级别纤维黏液样肉瘤、黏液样脂肪肉瘤和黏液样MPNST。黏液样脂肪肉瘤和纤维黏液样肉瘤CD34阴性。S-100蛋白、CD56或CD57阳性有助于黏液样MPNST的诊断，然而，约25%的病例可为阴性，并不排除MPNST的诊断。

软组织骨化性纤维黏液瘤

软组织骨化性纤维黏液瘤（OFMT）是一种生长缓慢的间叶病变，好发于四肢深部的皮下组织或骨骼肌。镜下，呈致密的小叶状排列，形态温和的圆细胞分布于多少不等的黏液样或致密玻璃样的间质中。通常以形成不完整的板层骨壳为特征，但部分病例可缺乏此结构。

大部分病例的OFMT瘤细胞S-100蛋白和波形蛋白呈弥漫强阳性[290-296]。此外也可见CD57、NSE[290, 294]、突触素[290]和GFAP阳性[294, 293]。某些病例可有肌源性分化，表现为结蛋白和α-平滑肌肌动蛋白阳性[290, 291, 296, 297]。OFMT中细胞角蛋白、EMA[292, 293, 296]和HMB-45[293]均阴性。

上皮样血管内皮瘤

在血管肿瘤中，上皮样血管内皮瘤（EHE）被分类为具有"居间型/中间性"生物学行为的肿瘤，介于上皮样血管瘤和上皮样血管肉瘤之间。EHE是一种血管中心性肿瘤，表现出原始的血管分化。按发生频率排列其好发部位为：肝、肺、骨和浅表软组织（图3.6）。显然，明确的内皮分化证据是诊断EHE的基本标准。有许多血管标记物如vWF、CD31、CD34、UEAI和FLI-1可用于诊断，而且大部分EHEs显示vWF和UEAI两者均为阳性[298, 299]。

由于EHE中细胞内原始血管空泡与腺癌内所见的黏液空泡相似，所以可与癌相混淆。有上皮样表现

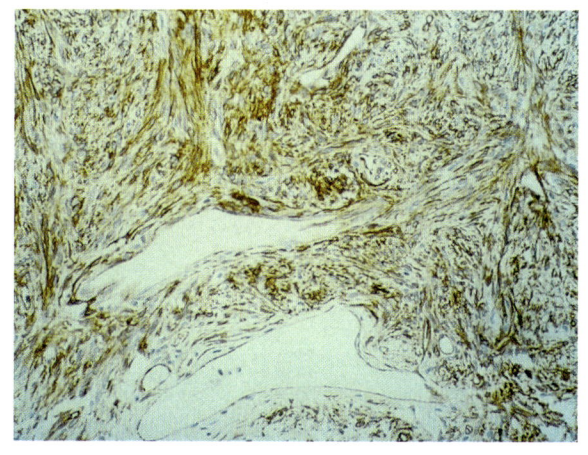

图3.5 孤立性纤维瘤显示一致性CD34阳性

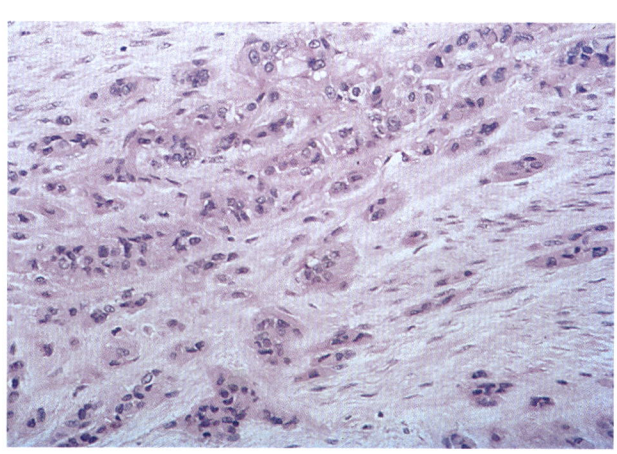

图3.6 上皮样血管内皮瘤由肥胖的多边形细胞构成，细胞特征温和并有胞浆内管腔形成

的其他肉瘤也需鉴别，而最难鉴别的类似病变为上皮样肉瘤。该肿瘤同 EHE 一样均呈结节样生长，胖圆的嗜酸性细胞排列成索状或巢状。EHE 角蛋白阳性（与上皮样肉瘤所见一样）是争论的焦点。确实有关于 EHE 共表达内皮和上皮性标记物的报道[300,301]。Gray 及其同事研究发现大多数 EHEs 角蛋白染色阳性[300]。另一项皮肤和软组织 30 例标本的研究发现 26% 的病例角蛋白阳性[302]。这些发现均表明对疑为 EHEs 的免疫组化诊断，除了几个内皮标记物外还需上皮标记物。缺乏 EMA、E-钙黏素和桥粒斑蛋白表达也是有用的指标，尤其是同时伴 CD31 和/或 CD34 阳性时。

上皮样肉瘤样的血管内皮瘤

Billings 等描述了一种特殊的血管肿瘤，常规镜下形态更加类似上皮样肉瘤[303]。因此称为"上皮样肉瘤样血管内皮瘤"（ESLH）。确实该病变与真正的上皮样肉瘤（EPS）一样角蛋白和波形蛋白阳性，但 ESLH 反常性的 CD34 阴性（CD34 见于 EPS 和大多数其他血管内皮瘤中）。此外，CD31 和 FLI-1 阳性（见第 12 章）。

卡波西型血管内皮瘤

最初认为卡波西型（kaposiform）血管内皮瘤（KHE）全部发生于儿童和婴幼儿[304]，但近来发现也是累及成人的少见肿瘤[305]。许多病例都与淋巴血管瘤病以及贺卡-梅综合征（Kasabach-Merritt syndrome，一种消耗性凝血综合征）有关，实际上，后者是引发很多 KHE 患者死亡的原因[306]。肿瘤由梭形细胞呈小结节状生长，如同卡波西肉瘤（Kaposi's sarcoma, KS）和梭形细胞血管瘤，但含有散在巢状具有嗜酸性空泡状胞浆的上皮样大细胞，也可见含铁血黄素和玻璃样小滴。

KHE 瘤细胞有部分内皮标记物表达。一般 CD34 和 FLI-1 阳性，但Ⅷ因子相关抗原和 UEAI 通常阴性[304]。在 KHE 中未检测到 KS 相关的与疱疹病毒[KSHV（HHV8）]有关的核酸或蛋白质[306]。如同其他内皮性增生，KHE 也表达血管内皮生长因子受体-3[307]。

侵袭性血管黏液瘤

侵袭性血管黏液瘤（AAM）是一种好发于女性盆腔和会阴软组织的特殊肿瘤。由嵌于黏液样基质中排列疏松、形态温和的星状细胞组成，基质中有许多明显的小静脉和毛细血管大小的血管，使人联想起黏液性脂肪肉瘤（图 3.7）。AAM 缺乏在一些明显的恶性黏液瘤中所见到的分枝状血管。AAM 的一些形态学和免疫学表型特征也可见于部分肌内黏液瘤[308,309]。

AAM 的免疫组化显示肌动蛋白阳性而 S-100 蛋白阴性，提示其为肌源性或肌纤维母细胞性分化[310]。但结蛋白一般为阴性。AAM 的超微结构研究[308]也支持为纤维母细胞性或肌纤维母细胞性分化。

软组织的恶性肿瘤

基于肉瘤最初的组织学生长方式可将其分为 4 组，包括：小圆细胞肿瘤、上皮样多边形细胞肿瘤、梭形细胞肿瘤和多形性肿瘤。通过免疫组化可对每一种肿瘤在组织学基础上作出判断。

小圆细胞肿瘤

软组织的小圆形细胞肿瘤（图 3.8，表 3.4）是一组不同来源的肿瘤，瘤细胞形态特征相似，主要发生于儿童和青少年。横纹肌肉瘤、PNET/ES 和淋巴瘤/白血病是该组病变的典型成员。另一病变是 PNET 的变型，称为腹腔内促纤维增生性小圆细胞肿瘤。

横纹肌肉瘤

胚胎性横纹肌肉瘤（E-RMS）占全部横纹肌肉瘤的一半以上，是诊断的最大难题之一。基于其不同的分化程度、细胞构成和生长方式，E-RMS 的形态学图像差别很大。灶性的条带状细胞、大的嗜酸性肌母细胞和黏液样基质可见于 E-RMS，但在与其形态学相似的其他肿瘤中不出现。许多 E-RMS 病例仅由密集

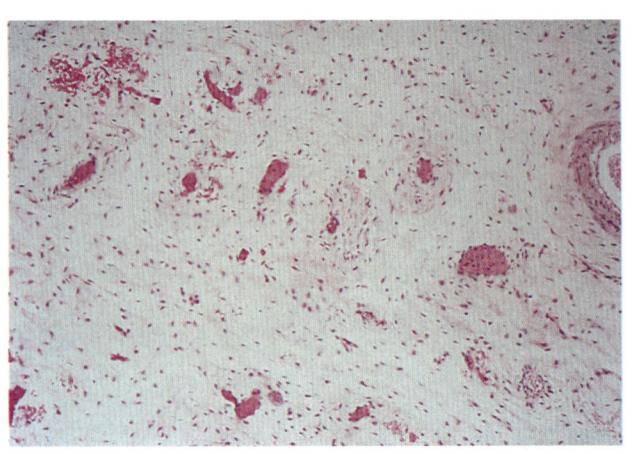

图 3.7　盆腔软组织侵袭性血管黏液瘤——需鉴别诊断的病变包括血管肌纤维母细胞瘤、黏液样平滑肌肿瘤、外周神经鞘肿瘤和黏液样脂肪肉瘤。免疫组化仅对排除单纯肌源性和神经源性病变有帮助

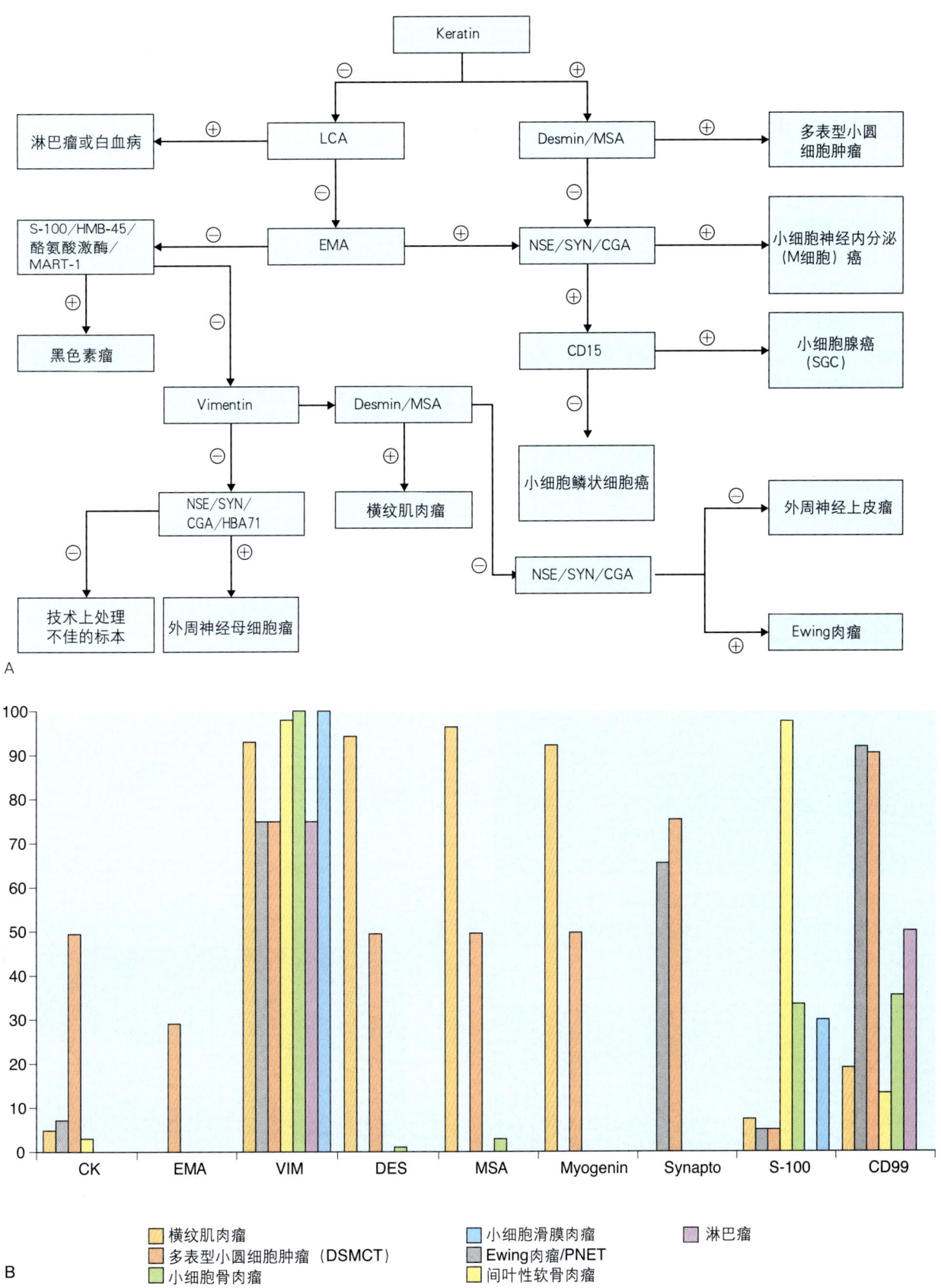

图3.8 （A）恶性小圆细胞肿瘤免疫组化诊断略图。（B）小圆细胞肿瘤常用标记物的免疫组化阳性率图示。CK，细胞角蛋白；EMA，上皮细胞膜抗原；VIM，波形蛋白；DES，结蛋白；MSA，肌特异性肌动蛋白；Synapto，突触素

排列的未分化小细胞组成（图3.9），需与多种肿瘤鉴别，包括神经母细胞瘤、ES、滑膜肉瘤、黑色素瘤、婴儿黑色素性神经外胚瘤、粒细胞肉瘤和恶性淋巴瘤。此外，E-RMS也可能与腺泡状横纹肌肉瘤的实性变型相混淆（图3.10），但二者预后不同。成人病例还需要与小细胞癌和分化差的小细胞血管肉瘤鉴别。

对于分化差的E-RMS，免疫组化尤为重要。横纹肌肉瘤以顺序渐增的方式表达横纹肌标记物（波形蛋白、myogenin/Myo-D1、结蛋白、快速肌球蛋白和肌红蛋白），重现正常肌发生模式。虽然波形蛋白诊断意义不大，但是恒定阳性。在肌源性标记物中，myogenin和结蛋白在石蜡切片中检测最恒定，实际上所有的E-RMS以及腺泡状和多形性横纹肌肉瘤均显示明显可见的染色（图3.11）[24]。这些标记物除了腹腔内促纤维增生性小圆形细胞肿瘤阳性外，其他小圆形细胞肿瘤均为阴性。

Myo-D1为横纹肌肉瘤高度特异性和敏感性的标记物，在82%~100%的病例中细胞核阳性[115, 311-313]。Myo-D1是DNA结合核调节蛋白，在间叶干细胞中启动肌源性分化。在E-RMS细胞中Myo-D1的染色形

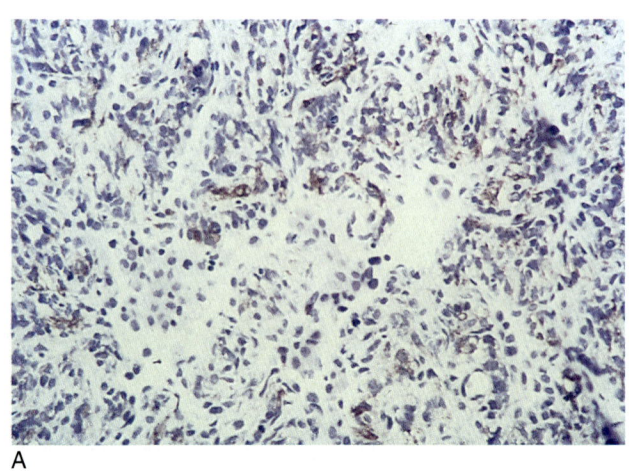

A

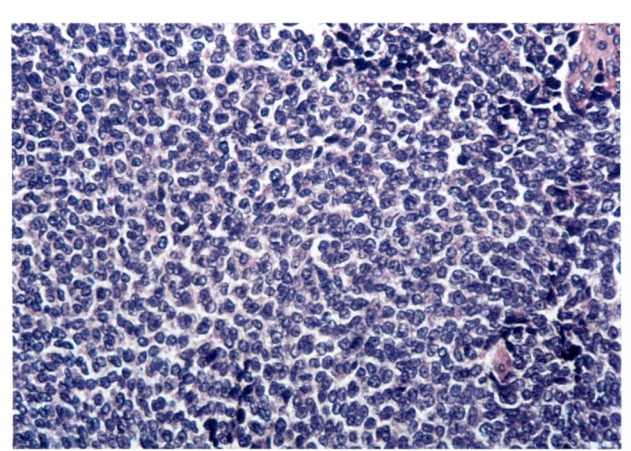

图3.9　原始的胚胎性或腺泡性横纹肌肉瘤的"实性"形式为小圆细胞恶性肿瘤原型的代表，需要其他辅助诊断

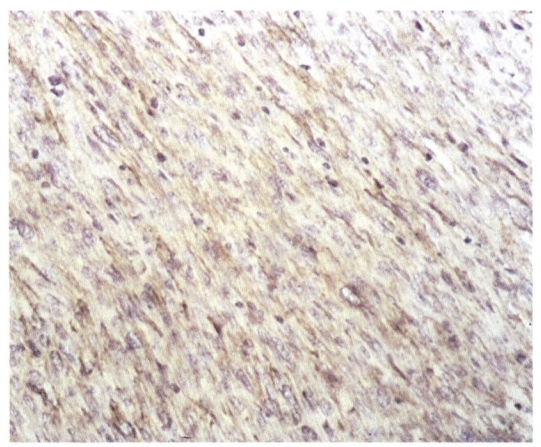

B

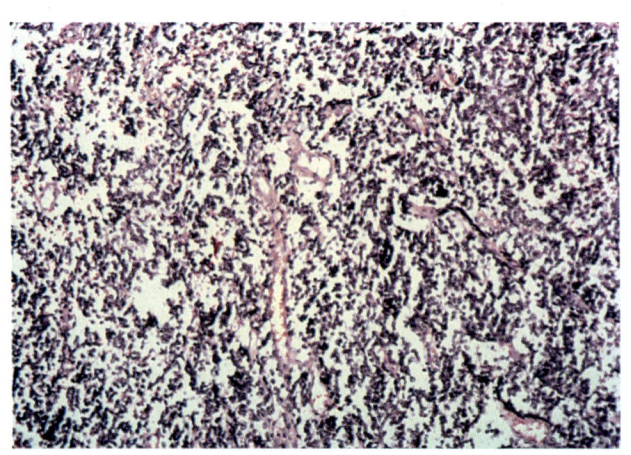

图3.10　腺泡状横纹肌肉瘤的典型图像

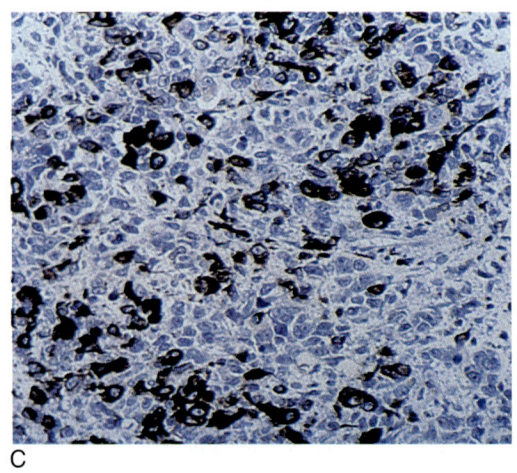

C

图3.11　横纹肌肉瘤所有亚型结蛋白一致性阳性，包括胚胎性（A）、腺泡性（B）和多形性（C）

式是不同的[312]，在小而原始的肿瘤细胞中核染色最致密，而在有更明显骨骼肌分化的大细胞中一般无反应[115]。有时，Myo-D1 可与一些小圆细胞肿瘤中的未知胞浆抗原发生交叉反应，在神经母细胞瘤和 ES/PNET 的细胞浆中呈丝状染色[114]。除此之外需要记住的是，部分PNET病例确实可以同时表达肌源性和神经外胚层的标记物[313]。

在其他肌源性标记物中，myogenin（MYG）在E-RMS 中可能敏感性最强。MYG 核阳性比 Myo-D1 更强[115]。据我们的经验，在横纹肌肉瘤中，MYG 的敏感性比得上结蛋白和肌相关肌动蛋白。ES/PNET 典型的呈 MYG 阴性[115]，如果 MYG 阳性则可以排除 ES/PNET 的诊断。尽管实际上在其他儿童肿瘤中应用 PCR 的技术已发现 MYG 相关的 mRNA，但并不影响免疫组化的判断[314]。

微丝相关蛋白纽带蛋白（vinculin）是肌肉组织的一个主要成分，在肌小节的肌纤维排列中起作用。在横纹肌肉瘤的不同组织学亚型中，纽带蛋白主要表达于分化的肿瘤中，而在 E-RMS 中仅为灶性阳性[315]。在平滑肌肉瘤纽带蛋白也可阳性。肌营养不良蛋白是杜氏肌营养不良基因位点的蛋白产物，是骨骼肌细胞主要的细胞骨架蛋白。对于该标记物在横纹肌肉瘤诊断中的应用仅有有限的研究[316]。肌营养不良蛋白在大部分横纹肌肉瘤的冰冻切片中呈阳性，在其他小细胞肿瘤包括淋巴瘤、PNET 和 Wilms 瘤中为阴性[316, 317]。

"未分化"横纹肌肉瘤为结蛋白阴性的小细胞肿瘤，但Myo-D1或MYG阳性，目前也可以用其他不同抗体标记。巢蛋白是一种表达于未成熟骨骼肌细胞、内皮和一些与肿瘤毗邻的间质细胞中的丝状蛋白[318]。部分研究提示，巢蛋白也见于未分化横纹肌肉瘤[318]，与胰岛素样生长因子-Ⅱ（IGF-Ⅱ）相似，原位杂交显示IGF-Ⅱ的表达与横纹肌肉瘤的细胞分化程度相反[319]。胎儿型乙酰胆碱受体也可能有助于低分化横纹肌肉瘤与其他小细胞肿瘤的鉴别[320]。在成熟的横纹肌中胎儿型乙酰胆碱受体为阴性。最后，在横纹肌肉瘤的冰冻切片和部分石蜡切片中，已发现CD56、CD57和神经原纤维异构体的存在，但不影响诊断[321]。

治疗常常会导致各种不同肿瘤的细胞分化，并且可减少各型横纹肌肉瘤的有丝分裂活性。确实在E-RMS病例中，免疫组化Ki-67检测其治疗后的增殖活性未变化或有所增加代表该肿瘤具有侵袭性生物学潜能。在治疗后未发现肿瘤肌源性标记物表达有所改变[322]，但根据我们经验，"异向"分化更为常见，尤其是神经外胚层的标记物如CD56、CD57和突触素在治疗后的横纹肌肉瘤中并非少见。

此现象使人想到，值得注意的 E-RMS 诊断陷阱，即伴有部分肌源性分化的"多表型"小圆细胞肿瘤。这些病变可同时表达不同细胞系的多种标记物，将于本节后面详述（图 3.12）。

> **诊断要点**：横纹肌肉瘤
>
> 横纹肌分化标记物以顺序方式表达：波形蛋白、myogenin/Myo-D1、结蛋白、快速肌球蛋白和肌红蛋白。

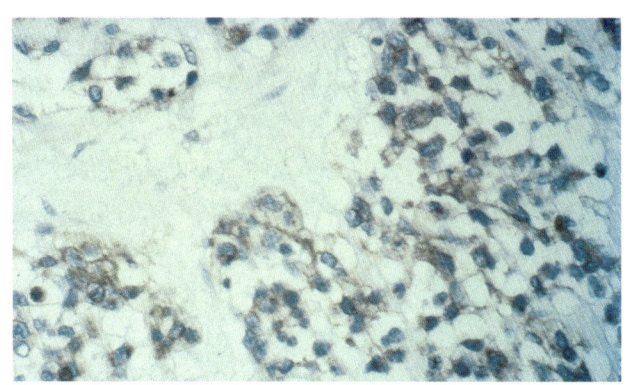

图 3.12　小细胞横纹肌肉瘤 CD57 阳性并不多见

Ewing 肉瘤和原始神经外胚层肿瘤（PNET）

Ewing 家族肿瘤包括骨和软组织的小圆细胞肿瘤，部分病例是由一种特殊的染色体异常[t（11;22）]及其变异而定义的。经过15年的研究，现已明确 ES 和外周PNET为同一谱系肿瘤[221, 323, 324]。除了上述核型特征外，二者在组织培养上表现出相同的神经外胚层特征，原癌基因的表达也相似。按照经典的定义，ES 与 PNET 的区别在于 ES 缺乏假菊形团样结构，电镜或免疫组化无神经外胚层特征，但目前认为此鉴别要点已过时并被弃用。

在 ES/PNET，EWS 和 FLI-1 基因位于染色体易位断裂点的两侧。用RT-PCR的方法可检测到由此融合基因转录的 mRNA，大约存在于 75% 的病例中[325, 326]，在其他小细胞肿瘤并未发现此转录体。部分 ES/PNET 病例有 EWS-FLI-1 和 PAX3-FKHR 两种基因转录体的双表达,二者分别是Ewing肉瘤家族和腺泡状横纹肌肉瘤特有的表型[327,328],同时这些病变也在免疫组化水平上表现出异常的肌源性分化。

Ewing肉瘤家族更明显的特征是MIC2/CD99高表达,此糖蛋白可用多种单克隆抗体检测,包括HBA71、12E7、RFB-1[329]和013(表3.3)。MIC2/CD99为细胞膜弥漫阳性,几乎见于所有的ES/PNET中(>95%)[329-331]。尽管最初认为CD99是ES/PNET的特异性标记物,但目前发现许多肿瘤也表达CD99。除ES/PNET外,儿童小细胞肿瘤、淋巴母细胞性淋巴瘤和部分腺泡状横纹肌肉瘤CD99均为阳性。显然MIC2必须结合其他标记物染色才能作出最后诊断。

典型的ES/PNET对嗜铬素、细胞角蛋白、胶质纤维酸蛋白(GFAP)、结蛋白、肌特异性肌动蛋白、myogenin、CD31和CD45呈阴性反应[332,333]。然而,在一项50例肿瘤的研究中发现在分子水平上有t(11;22)的易位,免疫组化显示20%的ES/PNET病例细胞角蛋白阳性[334],以我们的经验,在这些肿瘤中若有角蛋白出现也仅为灶性阳性。

整合素是一组大的、异源性细胞膜糖蛋白家族,表达形式复杂多样。整合素亚单位在不同的儿童小细胞肿瘤中表达各异。ES/PNET显示为β1+、α1−、α3−、α5+和α6−表达类型[335]。此表达形式与横纹肌肉瘤有部分重叠,但与神经母细胞瘤β1+、α1+、α3+、α5−和α6−明显不同。ILK(β1-整合素连接激酶)是一种与β1-整合素胞浆结构域相互作用的蛋白,一项研究发现ILK在所有的ES/PNET及三分之一的神经母细胞瘤中表达[336]。与此相反,其他儿童小细胞肿瘤不表达这种标记物。Trk受体属于三聚体蛋白家族,在ES/PNET和神经母细胞瘤中呈不同表达,ES/PNET免疫组化倾向于TrkA(A+/B-/C+),而神经母细胞瘤则表现为(A-/B-/C+)表型。

间叶性软骨肉瘤

间叶性软骨肉瘤(MCS)是一种侵袭性软骨肿瘤,常见于青年人,通常发生于骨外。瘤组织以大量小细胞成分为特征,实际上难以与经典的ES区别,除非有明显的原始软骨岛形成,这些软骨岛似乎是以模仿胚胎软骨发生的方式由小细胞生成。MCS的另一突出特征是出现血管外皮细胞瘤样的脉管结构,通过染色体核型和分子学研究,目前将其归类为"Ewing肉瘤家族"的另一成员。

与其他软骨肉瘤不同,MCS的S-100并不呈弥漫阳性,阳性部位仅局限在软骨母细胞岛,而小细胞成分阴性[337,338]。肿瘤所有成分CD57可能阳性,大多数病例NSE阳性[337]。ⅩⅢα因子也呈阳性,但为非特异性[338]。有人认为发生在中枢神经系统的MCS有25%的病例显示细胞角蛋白和神经纤维酸蛋白阳性[339],但根据我们的经验,对此结论表示置疑。

典型的MCS不表达结蛋白、肌动蛋白、细胞角蛋白或者EMA[337]。与ES/PNET不同,MCS突触素[337]阴性,但二者CD99均为阳性[340,341]。

> **诊断要点**:PNET/Ewing肉瘤
> 1. FLI-1、CD99、NSE、突触素呈典型阳性。
> 2. 20%的病例角蛋白灶性阳性。
> 3. 鉴别诊断抗体组包括肌源性标记(阴性)。

"多表型小圆细胞肿瘤"

有确切的证据表明,成人和儿童小圆细胞肿瘤的一部分有多向分化能力。我们遇到大约25例多表型肿瘤,其表型与经典的ES/PNET不易区别,但都同时伴有上皮性、肌源性和神经外胚层标记物的表达。此组病例均为侵袭性肿瘤,甚至比一般的ES/PNET侵袭性更强。其他研究者也有类似病理变异的描述,既有少见的多向分化的组织学证据(包括PNET中的腺样结构),也有某些特殊解剖部位特有的形态学特征[342-344]。"多表型小圆细胞肿瘤"这一术语对描述此类肿瘤的一般特性似乎是最合适的。

"促纤维增生性小圆细胞肿瘤"(DSRCT)被认为是这组肿瘤的典型代表,该肿瘤以EWS/WT-1融合基因转录体为特点,并具有独特的形态学特征,即在分散的肿瘤细胞巢周围围绕着反应性的纤维组织(图3.13)。DSRCT的免疫表型相当复杂,不同标记物的阳性率分别为:角蛋白(86%),EMA(93%),NSE(81%),波形蛋白(97%),结蛋白(90%)[345]。有趣的是,仅有少部分病例CD99为阳性[41,345,346]。除少数病例外,肌动蛋白、成肌素和嗜铬素在DSRCT通常为阴性。

我们观察了肿瘤复发的连续过程,其中一例肿瘤从PNET的表型特点转变到DSRCT的图像。而且,我们研究的另一例DSRCT显示经过化疗后其形态学特征和免疫学表型都发生了显著改变。在这些特殊肿

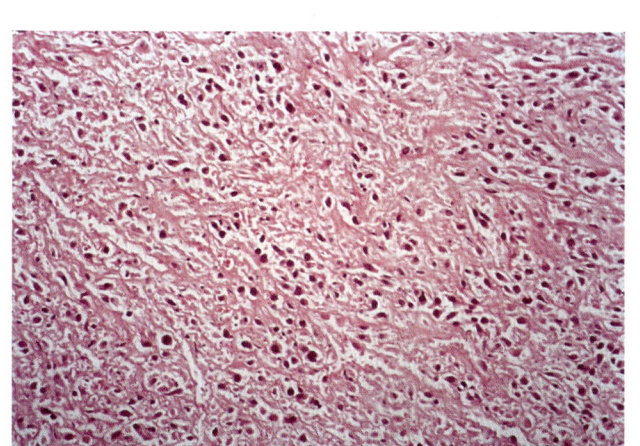

图 3.13 促纤维增生性小圆细胞肿瘤是一个独特的小圆细胞恶性肿瘤，表现为致密的纤维性间质

瘤中，与结蛋白、突触素、calretinin 和 HBME-1 共表达的标记物通常与腺上皮相关（角蛋白7、MOC31抗原、BerEP4抗原、CD15和CA72-4）。这些发现支持DSRCT具有多潜能分化的概念，并受多种细胞毒性剂作用的调节。

诊断要点：DSRCT

1. 特征性WT-1、角蛋白8/18、EMA、NSE、波形蛋白/结蛋白阳性。
2. 偶尔 CD99 或成肌素阳性。

低分化小细胞滑膜肉瘤

分化差的滑膜肉瘤（PDSS）的小细胞亚型常与其他小圆细胞肿瘤混淆，如 ES/PNET 及高级别恶性外周神经鞘瘤（MPNST）。更复杂的问题是，有些报道在神经肿瘤中也有独特的t（x;18）染色体易位，而该易位通常与滑膜肉瘤相关[347, 348]。如果不了解CD99常表达于 PDSS，那么 CD99 阳性也会使诊断更加困难[349]。此时多种细胞角蛋白染色可能有助于鉴别诊断，例如，据报道 CK7 在近 50% 的 PDSS 中阳性，而 PNET 阴性[350]。

淋巴造血系统恶性肿瘤

造血系统肿瘤很少表现为软组织肿块，在儿科病人尤其少见，而最常见的是其他小圆细胞肿瘤。由于CD45 在造血细胞中普遍存在，且有极高的特异性，因此是非常有价值的标记物。并不是所有的CD45抗体都能够识别出常规组织处理的抗原，但"鸡尾酒"式的单克隆抗体 PD7/26; 2B11（表 3.3）在石蜡切片中的染色效果确实较好。

实际工作中CD45 可作为诊断造血细胞系分化的标记物，相反，淋巴瘤和白血病细胞一般不表达其他的系标记物。如前所述，需要注意淋巴母细胞性淋巴瘤通常为CD99阳性（与ES/PNET相同），因此可能形成诊断陷阱[351, 352]，但淋巴母细胞性淋巴瘤末端脱氧核糖核酸转移酶也呈阳性，而其他小圆细胞肿瘤一般为阴性（但不是全部）[353]，因此可以鉴别。淋巴瘤可表现为各种意外的形态学图像，可与上述肉瘤相似，也可具有印戒细胞特征[354]，可伴有黏液样基质[355]，或纤维样基质[356]。

梭形细胞样肉瘤

深部软组织的梭形细胞肉瘤（图3.14）包括纤维肉瘤、平滑肌肉瘤（LMS）、MPNST、单相性梭形细胞滑膜肉瘤、恶性纤维组织细胞瘤（MFH）以及梭形细胞血管肉瘤。尽管免疫组化在不断发展，但这些肿瘤类型间的鉴别诊断仍面临困难。

纤维肉瘤　在 20 世纪 60 年代后期，纤维肉瘤也许是"最常见"的软组织恶性肿瘤。然而随着时间的推移，其诊断标准已有显著进展。目前已将纤维肉瘤列为最少见的肉瘤。先前诊断的纤维肉瘤中，有很大一部分是 MFH、纤维瘤病和结节性筋膜炎等。纤维肉瘤最常表现为中年人的缓慢增生性肿块，发生部位广泛。该病变也可作为先天性肿瘤而见于婴儿，但被认为是一独立类型。

"经典的"纤维肉瘤其形态学诊断是基于梭形细胞交叉排列形成"鱼骨"样外观和不同程度的胶原间质，不伴有其他特异分化迹象。在此定义下，病变仅波形蛋白阳性，其他任何系标记物均为阴性。相反，肠系膜及腹膜后的"炎症型纤维肉瘤"显示有肌纤维母细胞分化，肌动蛋白为阳性[357]，因此，应认为其是一种"肌纤维肉瘤"[358]。纤维肉瘤的另一种变异是所谓的"硬化性上皮样"亚型，将在本章后面讨论。

平滑肌肉瘤　平滑肌肉瘤最常见于成人腹膜后，在四肢的深部软组织不常发生，但可见于更表浅的部位，特别是在真皮和皮下。LMS的鉴别诊断传统的包括由梭形细胞交叉排列构成的其他肉瘤，包括纤维肉瘤、MPNST、滑膜肉瘤和梭形细胞横纹肌肉瘤。此外如炎性假瘤、神经纤维瘤和血管外皮瘤（图3.4）也应考虑在内。

当前是根据结蛋白（图3.14）、α-平滑肌肌动蛋白和h-钙调素结合蛋白免疫组化阳性来证实平滑肌肉瘤的平滑肌分化的。一些研究显示肌动蛋白和钙调素结合蛋白在检测平滑肌肿瘤的肌源性分化方面可能比结蛋白更敏感。然而，依我们的经验，绝大部分LMS病例确实被结蛋白标记。结蛋白阳性的梭形细胞横纹肌肉瘤（一种罕见的肿瘤）应从LMS中鉴别出来，可以依据其钙调素结合蛋白和SMA阴性，而

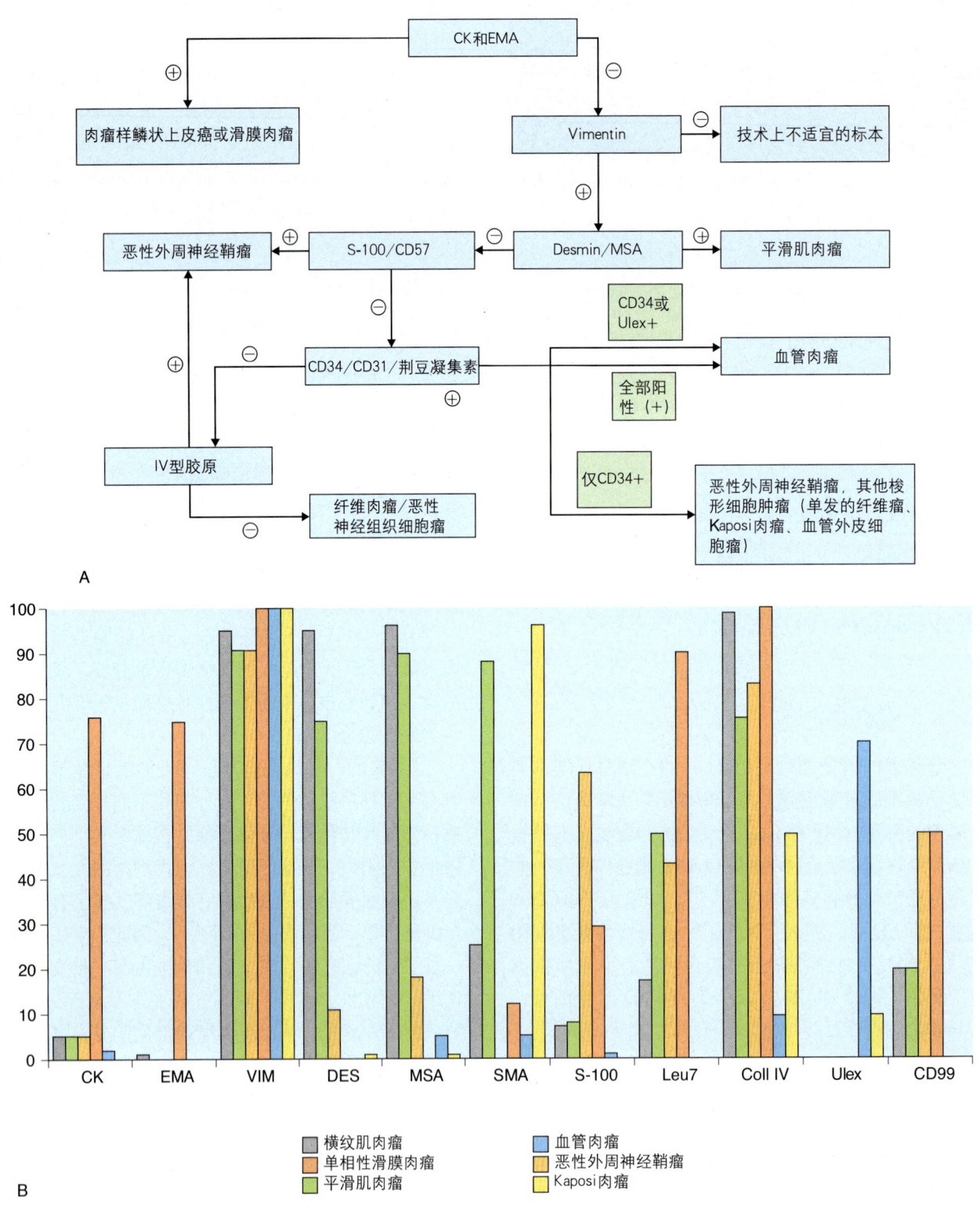

图3.14 （A，B）具有梭形细胞形态的肉瘤

肌红蛋白、Myo-D1 和成肌素阳性相鉴别。

LMS 与许多其他软组织肿瘤的部分免疫学表型相似是很常见的，例如在浅表性平滑肌肿瘤中 S-100 和 CD57 可呈阳性，而 MPNST 也为阳性。偶尔 LMS 可能会表达所谓的"组织细胞"标记物如 CD68，有些可能标记 CD30 和 CD34[359]。据我们的经验，LMS 中可能出现的角蛋白和 EMA 似乎与解剖部位的影响有关。来源于骨盆软组织和盆腔内脏的 LMS 有 40%～50% 的病例显示异常的"上皮性"免疫表型，而其他部位的病变则很少见，但并未见其他学者有类似报道。

Calponin 是另一平滑肌特异性蛋白，进展性地表达至 4 种异构体，以钙依赖的方式与肌动蛋白强力结合[360]。在肿瘤实质细胞和血管平滑肌细胞中表达，也见于肌纤维母细胞[361]。滑膜肉瘤也可显示 calponin 阳性，但其他标记物可将该肿瘤与 LMS 鉴别。

LMS 偶尔可呈 CD99 强阳性，但为点状胞浆着色[362,363]。此外，平滑肌肉瘤雌激素和孕激素受体均可阳性，不论其发生在内脏还是肢体软组织[363,364]。

GLUT-1 的高表达在很多人类恶性肿瘤中已有报道，包括非小细胞肺癌[365]、结直肠癌[366]、血管肉瘤[367]和甲状腺癌[368]，并且 GLUT-1 过表达与预后较差相关[365]。部分软组织 LMS 也呈现 GLUT-1 阳性，而平滑肌瘤均为阴性[364]。尽管此类报道较少，但提示 GLUT-1 标记与 LMS 远处转移危险因素相关[364]。

良、恶性平滑肌肿瘤可能更常见于人类免疫缺陷病毒（HIV）感染患者，且常发生于不常见的部位，并显示有 EB 病毒潜在感染[369]。几种 EBV 抗原在 HIV 相关性 LMS 中有表达，包括潜伏抗原 EBNA-1、即刻早期抗原 BZFL1 和早期抗原 EA-D，同时也表达病毒衣壳抗原 p160、gp125 和膜抗原 gp350[370]。这些发现显示 EB 病毒能够选择性溶解感染间叶细胞，并在一定条件下在平滑肌肉瘤发生中起作用。值得注意的是，在 HIV 患者的 Kaposi 肉瘤病变中未见瘤细胞与 EBV 整合[369]。

恶性外周神经鞘瘤 恶性外周神经鞘瘤（也被称为神经纤维肉瘤、恶性神经鞘瘤或神经源性肉瘤，MPNST）是一种具有高度多样组织学图像的肿瘤。恶性外周神经鞘瘤可能与纤维肉瘤或 MFH 很难区别，常显示出腺样结构及非神经鞘间叶成分的不同分化。然而，许多 MPNST 确实单独从形态学上就可诊断，尤其是与大神经相关联时。

与非肿瘤性施万细胞和良性神经鞘肿瘤相关的标记物在 MPNST 中也常被检测到。50%～70% 的病例 S-100 蛋白阳性，但通常仅为少部分肿瘤细胞阳性[44]。同样在 50% 的 MPNST 中 CD56 和 CD57 也呈阳性（图 3.15）[73]，髓基质蛋白（myelin basic protein）阳性不常见。应该记住：仅用神经鞘相关标记物并不能确定 MPNST 的诊断，只有当波形蛋白也阳性时，其诊断才较可靠。大约三分之二的 MPNST 可被包括 S-100 蛋白、CD56、CD57 或髓磷脂基质蛋白在内的一组抗体标记[44]。然而，至少两种抗体均阳性者不足 35%。因此，多数情况下免疫组化不能提供强有力的诊断依据。而且，如前所述，神经鞘恶性肿瘤有潜在的多向分化趋势，也可被上皮和肌源性标记物标记。需要重申的是，LMS 也可能呈 S-100 蛋白和 CD57 阳性，因此鉴别诊断特别重要[371,372]。

另一个与 MPNST 有共同免疫表型特征的梭形细胞肿瘤是单相性滑膜肉瘤（MSS）。大约 40% 的 MSS 病例 S-100 蛋白阳性，约 30% 的病例 CD57 阳性[373]。多种细胞角蛋白亚型检测对疑难病例可有帮助，因为多数滑膜肉瘤 CK17 和/或 CK19 阳性[373]。相反，MPNST 典型的呈阴性。

伴有血管肉瘤样图像的 MPNST 也有报道[374]，免疫组化证实有内皮分化。

MPNST 与梭形细胞（肉瘤样）恶性黑色素瘤的鉴别诊断特别困难，无论是皮肤还是转移部位[375]。外周神经鞘细胞和黑色素细胞之间有某些胚胎学联系，其肿瘤学表现为：色素性神经纤维瘤和黑色素性神经鞘瘤、嗜神经性黑色素瘤、黑色素瘤样的上皮样 MPNST 以及在 Carney 综合征中联合发生的上皮样蓝痣和砂粒体样黑色素性神经鞘瘤。在实际工作中，组

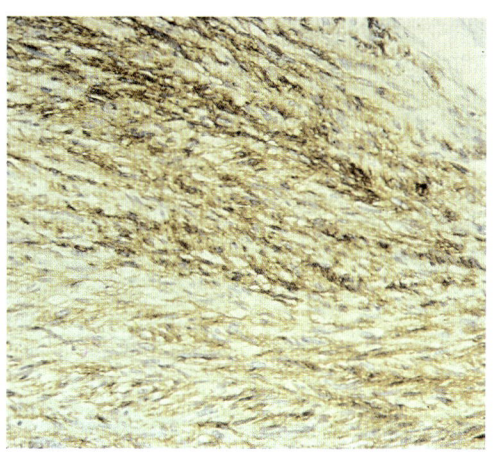

图 3.15 恶性外周神经鞘瘤（MPNST）CD57 阳性。S-100 蛋白、CD57、髓基质蛋白和 Ⅳ 型胶原在 MPNST 中的阳性率大于 85%

织学上与MPNST相似，S-100蛋白弥漫强阳性的肿瘤一般应考虑为黑色素瘤，尤其是伴有HMB-45、HMB-50、酪氨酸酶或MART-1阳性，因为后面4个标记物与神经鞘肿瘤极少相关。尽管神经鞘细胞能产生Ⅳ型胶原，但此标记物对神经鞘肿瘤的诊断价值有限，因为伴有平滑肌、内皮和肌纤维母细胞分化的细胞均能合成Ⅳ型胶原。

> **诊断要点：恶性外周神经鞘瘤（MPNST）**
>
> 1. 三分之二的病例 S-100 蛋白和 CD56/CD57 阳性，常呈局灶性。
> 2. S-100蛋白在黑色素瘤中也阳性，其他黑色素瘤特异标记物是关键的诊断抗体。
> 3. MPNST 的 CK7 表达阴性（滑膜肉瘤阳性）。

单相性梭形细胞滑膜肉瘤（MSS） 单相性梭形细胞（所谓的"纤维样"）滑膜肉瘤代表了这种肿瘤的形态学谱系的一端。典型的双相性滑膜肉瘤诊断不成问题，而 MSS 的图像与其他的几种软组织肿瘤有相似之处，包括纤维肉瘤、MPNST、血管外皮瘤和LMS。

EMA 在 MSS 中典型表达（图 3.16）。与双相滑膜肉瘤不同，梭形细胞滑膜肉瘤的CK仅呈灶性散在阳性，尤其是对 CK7、CK8、CK18 和 CK19 也可呈阳性[349, 376]。尽管偶尔在双相性滑膜肉瘤的上皮成分中癌胚抗原可呈阳性，但所有梭形细胞病例均为阴性[377]。然而，Ⅳ型胶原和 E-钙黏素可在 MSS 中弥漫阳性[379]。

CD99在MSS中常为阳性[264, 378, 379]，但在许多其他梭形细胞肿瘤中也有表达。如上所述，少部分MSS病例CD57和S-100蛋白也可阳性[36]。bcl-2蛋白的强阳性也引起了人们的注意[380, 381]，一项荧光原位杂交（FISH）分析也证实其存在t（X；18）易位。79%的MSS病例bcl-2阳性，而20例LMS、4例MPNST和4例纤维肉瘤阴性[381]。尽管如此，在许多其他软组织肿瘤中也确实观察到bcl-2阳性，例如梭形细胞脂肪瘤、Kaposi肉瘤、孤立性纤维瘤和胃肠间质瘤[380]。有趣的是，所有这些病变也典型表达CD34，而MSS总是阴性，因此可成为一个实用的鉴别诊断依据。

梭形细胞血管肉瘤 梭形细胞血管肉瘤是血管肉瘤的少见组织学类型[382]。大多数病例 UEAI 标记阳性，但是不到10%的病例vWF阳性。实际上，所有病例均可见到 CD31、CD34 和血栓调节素相互间的联合表达（见第 12 章）。

Kaposi 肉瘤 Kaposi 肉瘤（KS）临床有 4 种类型："经典型"（地中海型）、淋巴结病型、移植相关型和获得性免疫缺陷综合征（AIDS）相关型，其镜下特点相同。KS 晚期很容易与梭形细胞血管肉瘤、Kaposi样血管内皮瘤相混淆。这些肿瘤一般CD34均为阳性，但只有KS表现为疱疹病毒8型潜伏核抗原-1 核阳性[383, 384]（见第 12 章）。

具有上皮样形态的肉瘤

许多软组织肉瘤（图 3.17，表 3.6）由多边形大细胞组成，形态与癌相似。这些病变包括上皮样肉瘤、上皮样单相性滑膜肉瘤、透明细胞肉瘤、腺泡状软组织肉瘤、上皮样LMS、上皮样血管肉瘤、上皮样

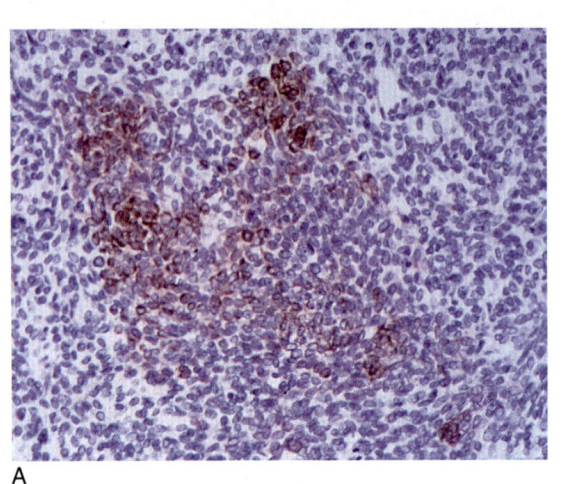

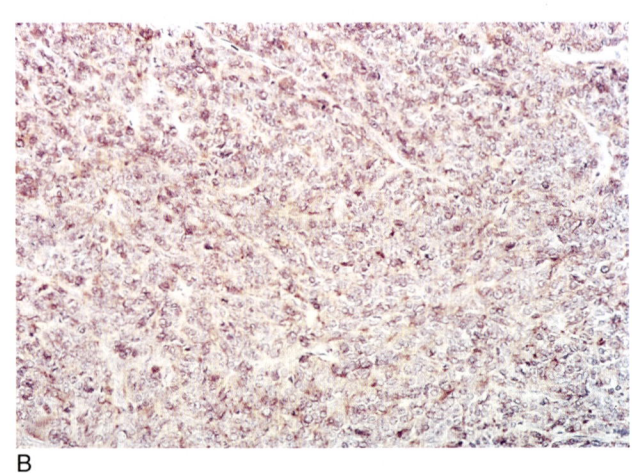

图 3.16 （A）滑膜肉瘤角蛋白阳性（B）上皮细胞膜抗原（EMA）阳性

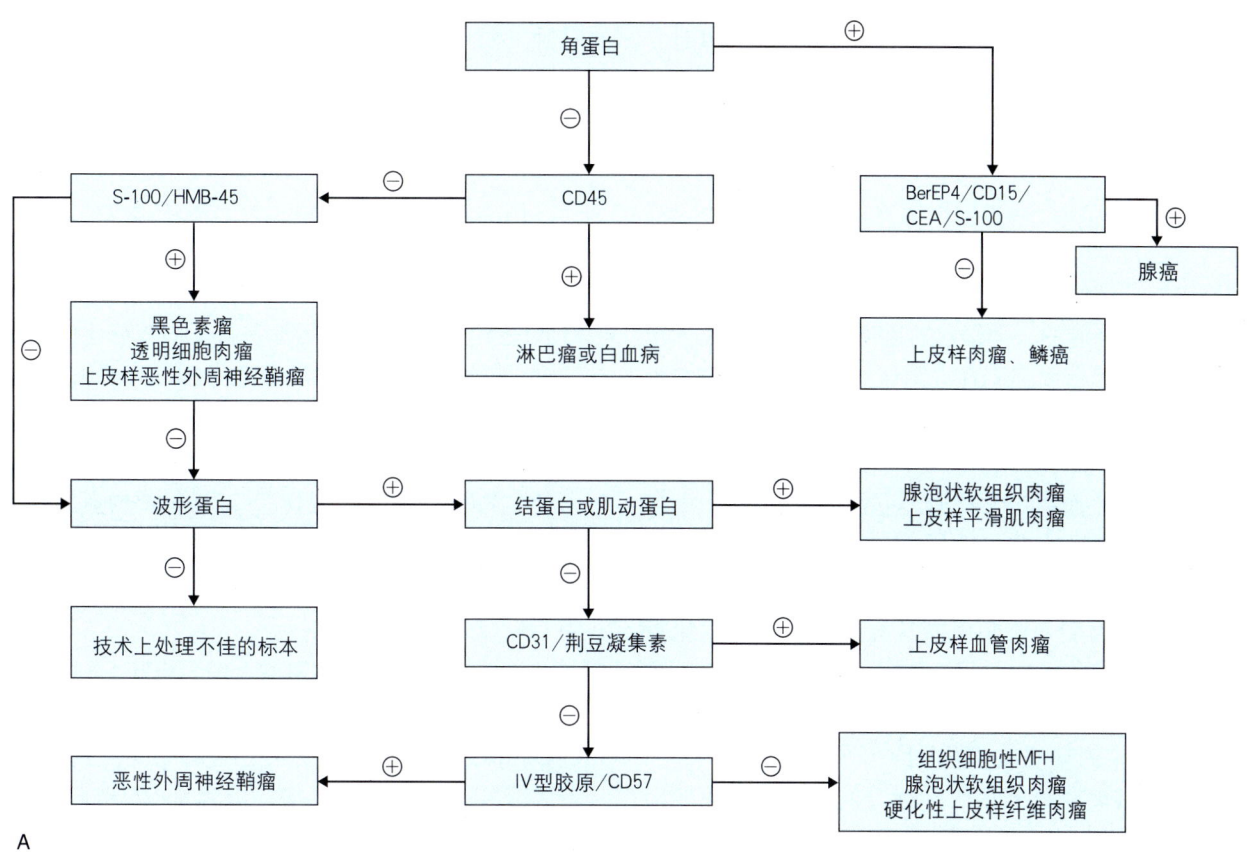

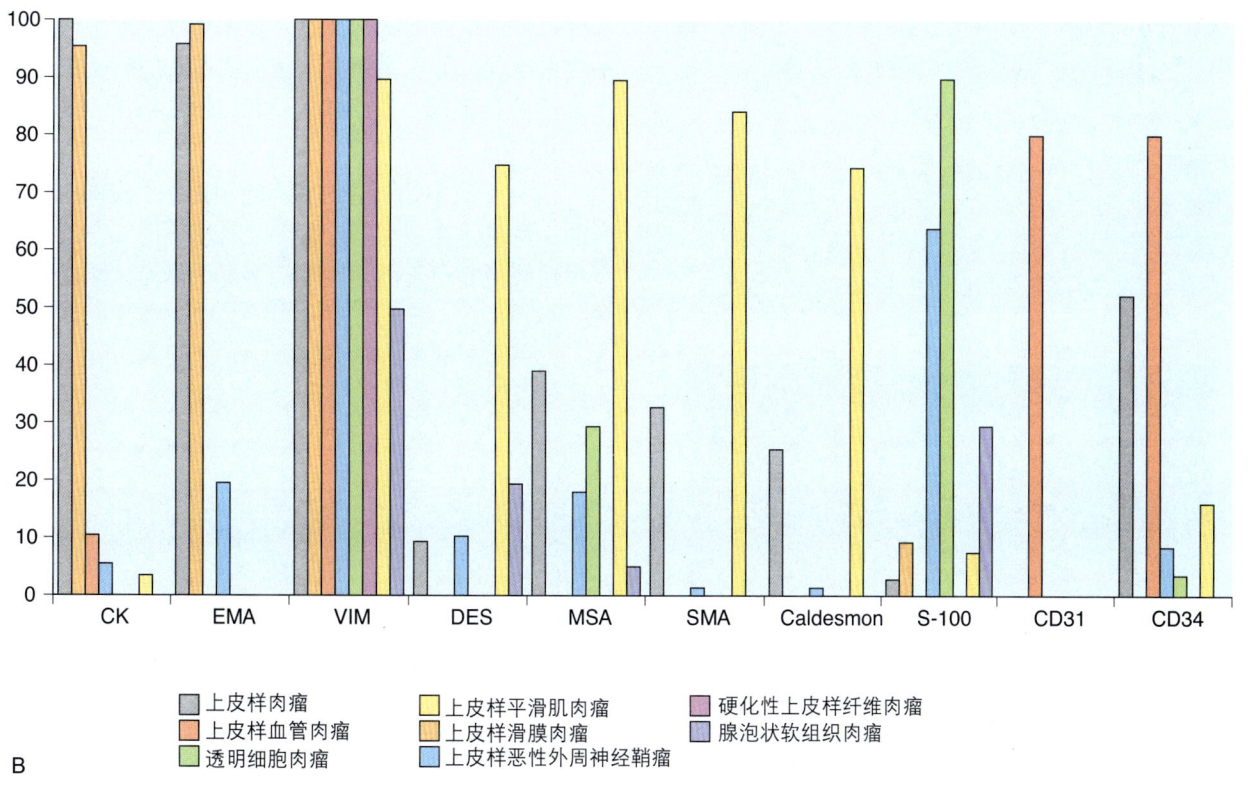

图 3.17 （A）恶性上皮样细胞肿瘤的免疫组化诊断方略图；（B）恶性梭形细胞肿瘤常见免疫组化结果直方图

MPNST、恶性颗粒细胞瘤和"组织细胞型"MFH。

上皮样肉瘤　上皮样肉瘤（EPS）组织学上以中心坏死的融合结节为特征。其图像与渐进性坏死性肉芽肿、黑色素瘤或转移性癌有些相似。偶尔肿瘤胞浆出现空泡会误诊为血管内皮瘤或血管肉瘤[385]。少数病例可出现罕见的组织学改变，例如软骨样基质[386]或横纹肌样的细胞[387]。

上皮样肉瘤的一个恒定的免疫表型特点是波形蛋白和角蛋白呈核周强阳性（图3.18），超微结构水平可见核周中间丝蛋白聚集。每例肿瘤细胞角蛋白的标记范围有所不同（图3.19），p63、CK5和CK6在EPS中倾向阴性，而组织学相似的癌常为阳性[388]。大多数EPS中CD34表达阳性[159,389]，也有神经丝蛋白阳性的个例报道[390,391]。

上皮样肉瘤与滑膜肉瘤具有共同的免疫组化特征，二者细胞角蛋白和EMA均呈阳性。另外，二者均偶尔癌胚抗原和S-100蛋白阳性[392]。大多数EPS和滑膜肉瘤E-钙黏素也呈强阳性[393,394]。

免疫组化有助于EPS和孤立的渐进性坏死性肉芽肿（如"深部"环形肉芽肿和细胞性风湿小结）的鉴别诊断。肉芽肿CD45和CD163阳性，而EPS的肿瘤细胞阴性，反之，渐进性坏死性肉芽肿EMA、细胞角蛋白[395]和CD34均为阴性[396]。

由于上皮样血管肿瘤可异常表达角蛋白，因而可与上皮样肉瘤相混淆。确如前述，上皮样血管瘤为与EPS形态相似的血管内皮瘤的一个特殊变型[303]。与FLI-1蛋白一样，CD31阳性是真正内皮分化的强有力证据。然而，由于EPS常表现为CD34阳性，与血管肿瘤相似，所以CD34不能用于这两组肿瘤的鉴别。

由Kato等人在91%的上皮样肉瘤中意外发现了一种名为CA-125的标记物[396]。该标记物典型的与苗勒上皮肿瘤相关，尤其是在卵巢中，而在间质肿瘤中的表达让人费解。所有其他所提及的多边形细胞肿瘤中CA-125均为阴性[396]。

上皮样单相性滑膜肉瘤　由于EPS（尤其是近端型）[397]与单纯上皮样滑膜肉瘤之间在临床病理上有许多相似之处[398]，所以，很难通过免疫表型分析将二者区分。二者鉴别的实用标记物是CD34，EPS为CD34阳性而上皮样滑膜肉瘤为阴性。另如上述，Kato等发现在几乎所有的EPS病例中CA-125均为阳性[396]，而滑膜肉瘤则为阴性。

上皮样血管肉瘤　血管肉瘤的上皮样变型与上皮样血管内皮瘤的区别在于其临床病理学的不同，它们均可累及深部软组织。其他需要鉴别的病变包括无色素性黑色素瘤、低分化癌和其他的多边形细胞肉瘤（图3.20）。

与"典型的"的血管肉瘤相比，上皮样血管肉瘤的免疫组化类型在一定程度上有所不同。尤其是上皮样血管肉瘤角蛋白阳性更为多见。然而，如其他的内

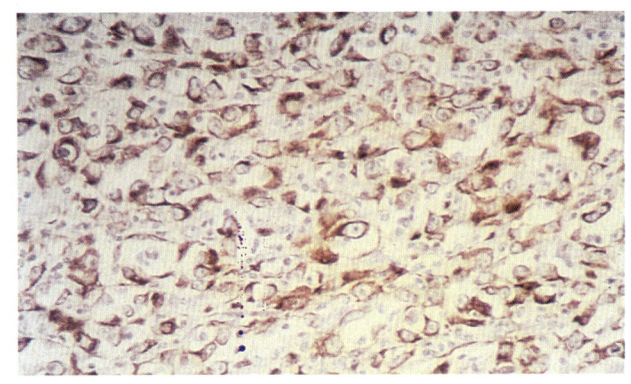

图3.18　上皮样肉瘤波形蛋白阳性并呈核周染色增强

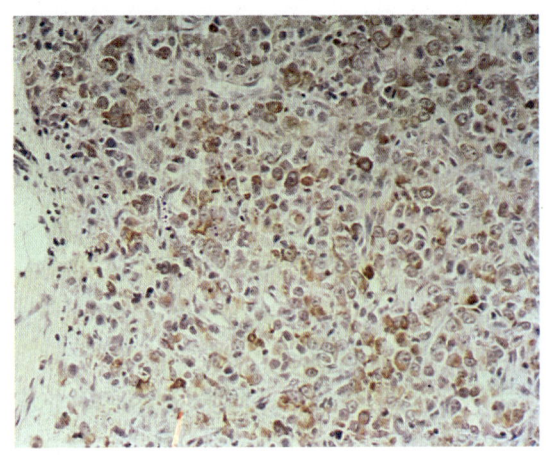

图3.19　上皮样肉瘤角蛋白阳性

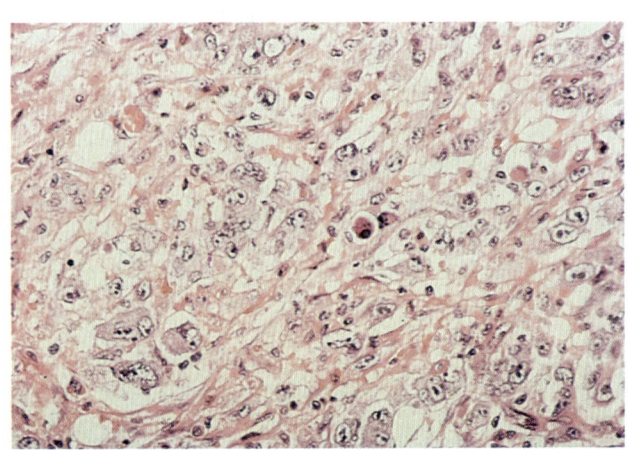

图3.20　上皮样血管肉瘤诊断上易与软组织中转移的恶性黑色素瘤或低分化癌相混淆

皮增生一样，CD31 和 FLI-1 是上皮样血管肉瘤敏感而特异的标记物（图3.21）[165, 399, 400]。

CD34 在各种多边形软组织肿瘤中都可能出现，包括上皮样LMS、上皮样MPNST、透明细胞肉瘤和上皮样肉瘤，这就降低了其作为内皮分化指标的可用性[399]。我们也观察到上皮样血管肉瘤可表达腺上皮相关蛋白CA72-4，单克隆抗体B72.3可识别此蛋白[401]。此现象的生物学意义还不清楚，但可能是一诊断陷阱。

上皮样恶性外周神经鞘肿瘤（MPNST） 上皮样MPNST是一种极为少见的肿瘤类型，在组织学上类似于黑色素瘤及转移癌、CCS和肾外横纹肌样瘤（图3.24）。因此，上皮样MPNST是难以识别的诊断类型。

上皮样 MPNST 的 S-100 蛋白阳性率至少为70%，高于MPNST肿瘤的其他类型[405]。NSE和蛋白基因产物 9.5 在大部分上皮样 MPNST 中也呈阳性[405, 406]，但CD56和CD57（图3.25）阳性少见。尽管细胞呈现多边形形态，但上皮样MPNST中细胞角蛋白和癌胚抗原阴性，而部分病例 EMA 阳性。由于MPNST结蛋白、肌动蛋白、UEAI、FLI-1和CD31均呈阴性，所以可排除上皮样平滑肌肉瘤和血管肉瘤。少数上皮样MPNST即使缺乏黑色素，其酪氨酸酶和HMB-45 也可呈阳性[407]。然而如果肿瘤同时表达CD56 或 CD57 就不支持 CCS 或黑色素瘤的诊断。

硬化性上皮样纤维肉瘤（SEF） SEF是见于深部软组织的一种特殊肿瘤，发生部位与筋膜板、滑膜或骨骼肌紧密相关[408-410]。它由呈小索状和巢状的均

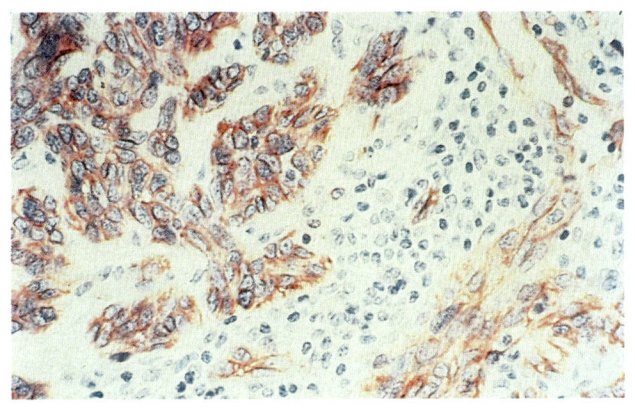

图 3.21 上皮样血管肉瘤中 UEAI 阳性

> **诊断要点**：上皮样肉瘤/滑膜肉瘤/血管肉瘤
>
> 1. 3 种肿瘤角蛋白均可阳性。
> 2. 血管肉瘤CD31+/FLI-1阳性；上皮样肉瘤CD34阳性；滑膜肉瘤 CD31/CD34/FLI-1 均为阴性。

透明细胞肉瘤 以前认为透明细胞肉瘤（clear cell sarcoma, CCS）是软组织原发的与皮肤恶性黑色素瘤相对应的肿瘤。然而，目前已知CCS具有特征性的t（12;22）染色体易位，而皮肤的黑色素瘤无此改变。CCS以上皮样细胞成分为特征，胞浆透明或淡嗜酸性伴有纤细的纤维血管间质，有或无黑色素沉着。

CCS 的免疫组化特性与恶性黑色素瘤完全相同，包括波形蛋白、S-100蛋白（图3.22）、酪氨酸酶、MART-1、HMB-45、HMB-50和小眼转录因子均呈阳性（图3.23），而EMA及肌源性、神经和内皮标记物均阴性。尽管有一项研究报道29%的病例角蛋白阳性[402]，但一般来说，CCS 中角蛋白阴性[402]。

如上所述，t（12;22）（q13;q12）易位（形成EWS/ATF-1 杂合基因）是CCS的特征[403, 404]。通过原位杂交及PCR方法可检测此杂合基因，为免疫组化提供了实用的辅助诊断。

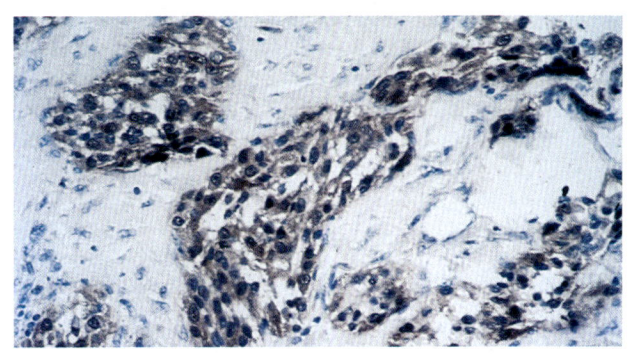

图 3.22 透明细胞肉瘤 S-100 阳性，见证了其为软组织恶性黑色素瘤的观点

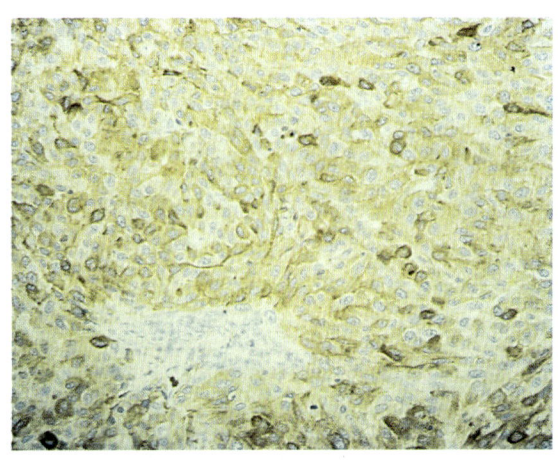

图 3.23 透明细胞肉瘤 HMB-45 阳性

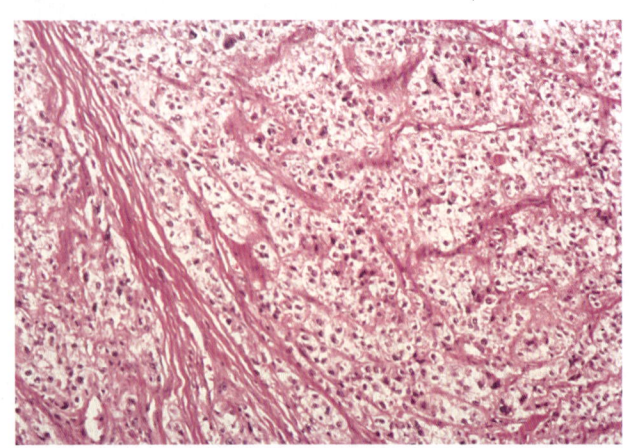

图3.24 上皮样MPNST缺乏明显的组织学特征，正确诊断需其他辅助依据

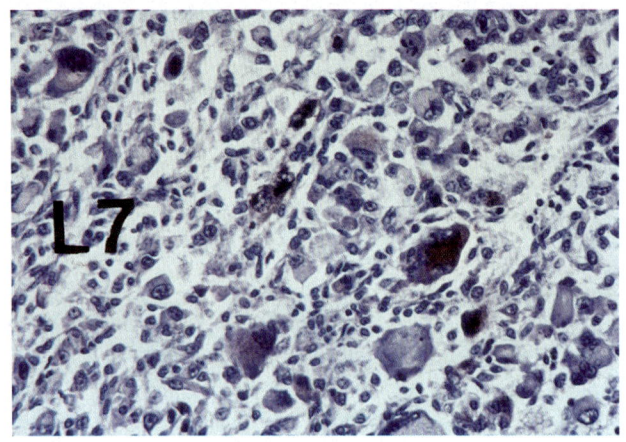

图3.25 上皮样MPNST中CD57阳性

一的小多边形细胞组成，胞浆透明，位于致密的胶原化和玻璃样变的间质中，可以呈骨样构型。SEF也可含有一般纤维肉瘤形态特征的区域，并且有些也可显示车辐状结构或黏液区。其鉴别诊断包括结节性筋膜炎、骨化性肌炎、硬纤维瘤、玻璃样变的平滑肌瘤、硬化性淋巴瘤、转移性乳腺小叶癌、骨化性纤维黏液瘤、单相性滑膜肉瘤、透明细胞肉瘤、骨外骨肉瘤和骨外黏液样软骨肉瘤。

SEF的免疫组化资料有限[408, 411]，大约50%的病例呈散在的瘤细胞EMA局灶弱阳性，29%的病例S-100蛋白也呈局灶弱阳性。细胞角蛋白、NSE、CD45、HMB-45、CD68和结蛋白阴性[408]。我们认为SEF免疫组化诊断问题尚未解决。

上皮样平滑肌肉瘤 平滑肌肿瘤中通常可见上皮样改变，一般为局灶性，偶尔为主要成分。此类肿瘤曾被命名为平滑肌母细胞瘤，但当前的信息提示即使形态相对温和，肿瘤也有转移的潜能。因此，如果瘤细胞有任何程度的核分裂及细胞异型性均应诊断为上皮样LMS。

我们诊断的10例上皮样LMS中肌特异性肌动蛋白或结蛋白阳性，但二者均阳性者仅有3例，与其他研究结果相同[412]，可能与超微结构中许多肿瘤细胞仅有幼稚肌丝结构有关。上皮样LMS对非肌源性标记物呈一致性阴性，如对S-100蛋白、细胞角蛋白、EMA、UEAI植物凝集素、vWF、CD 31或癌胚抗原均没有显示任何阳性[412, 413]。此外，我们的病例中还观察到钙调素结合蛋白和α-平滑肌肌动蛋白阳性。

腺泡状软组织肉瘤（ASPS） 自1952年对ASPS的诊断描述后，其细胞分化来源一直有争议。尽管长期以来试图证明该肿瘤的神经外胚层或内分泌性质，但是大部分近期研究支持其肌源性分化表型。

ASPS中有多种肌相关蛋白表达，如结蛋白、肌动蛋白、肌球蛋白、Z线蛋白和肌酸激酶的MM同工酶阳性，为肌源性分化提供了有力证据。然而，对于其是否为横纹肌肉瘤的一种类型仍未被证实[25, 105, 414-416]。有关该病变中α-肌小节肌动蛋白和α-平滑肌肌动蛋白的研究均有报道[417-419]。

ASPS的另外一些研究探讨了Myo-D1和成肌素的表达[418, 420, 421]。大多数研究发现Myo-D1的核染色完全阴性[422, 423]。在大部分ASPS中发现Myo-D1的抗体"58A"有颗粒性的胞浆阳性，但被认为是一种非特异性人工假象。

我们的8例ASPS病例中均无NSE、CD57、CK、嗜铬素、S-100蛋白、EMA、vWF、CD31、UEAI或癌胚抗原的标记，也无黑色素细胞特异性的标记物[415]。

"组织细胞性"恶性纤维组织细胞瘤 MFH偶尔可完全由多边形细胞组成并呈片状生长（图3.26），称为"组织细胞性"变型。我们研究的病例中没有一例组织细胞性MFH表现出特异性标记物，且仅有波形蛋白阳性。如本章前述，几种蛋白水解酶和所谓的"组织细胞选择性"标记物（CD68；HAM56）也可见于MFH，但并非特异及诊断必需，只要排除了上皮、肌源性和神经来源即可。

软组织多形性肿瘤

可出现多形性组织学形态的软组织肉瘤（图3.27，表3.7）包括：MFH、多形性横纹肌肉瘤、

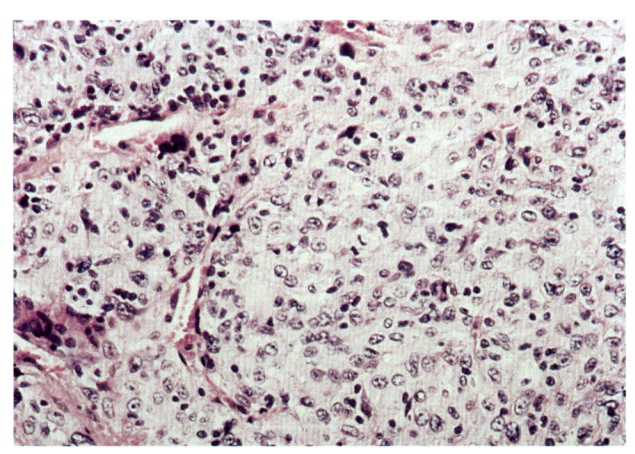

图3.26 "组织细胞性"恶性纤维组织细胞瘤（MFH）由片状相对单一的上皮样细胞组成，需要与多种病变相鉴别

多形性或去分化脂肪肉瘤、去分化LMS和多形性MPNST。

恶性纤维组织细胞瘤（MFH） 在常规染色组织形态下，MSF是成人最常见的软组织肉瘤。根据最初的描述，对多种蛋白酶（图3.28）和铁蛋白的反应与MFH"纤维组织细胞性"分化的结论相关。但是现在的研究认为该论点有严重问题。Roholl及其同事认为MFH的免疫表型最接近于肌纤维母细胞[424]。这一观点得到了其他研究的支持，这些研究在MFH中确定了具有肌特异性肌动蛋白和结蛋白反应的细胞亚群[425]同时超微结构显示肿瘤细胞具有肌纤维母细胞样特征[426]。

然而，从实际应用上，MFH最好限定于仅波形蛋白阳性而缺乏其他系特异性标记物的肿瘤，这样也解决了关于"MFH"是否是一组均一性肿瘤的问题。现在已经清楚，其他典型肿瘤如神经源性、肌源性或脂肪母细胞性肿瘤都可能出现MFH样区域。这些观察使人相信有些MFH反映了其他类型软组织肉瘤分化的最终共同途径（曾被错误地称为"去分化"）[427]。细胞培养以及肿瘤裸鼠移植的研究都从另一角度支持此假说，肿瘤形态一致的MFH移植后出现了其他的免疫表型，有些出现了肌源性分化，而另一些则出现了神经甚至上皮特征[428]。

多形性横纹肌肉瘤（PRMS） 在横纹肌肉瘤中，多形性横纹肌肉瘤最少见，几乎仅见于成人（图3.29）。该肿瘤免疫组化诊断相对容易，因其一致性表达结蛋白、肌特异性或肌小节肌动蛋白、肌球蛋白或肌红蛋白（图3.30）[429]，在PRMS的特征性大"条带状"细胞及梭形细胞或上皮样病灶中均为阳性。由于

MFH偶尔也可表达结蛋白和肌特异性肌动蛋白，因此在诊断PRMS时阳性范围也很重要。MFH为明显灶性阳性，而多形性横纹肌肉瘤为广泛弥漫阳性。PRMS缺乏S-100蛋白、CD56、CD57和髓磷脂碱性蛋白，此4种标记物中若有任何一种阳性则应考虑MPNST的可能。

多形性和"去分化"脂肪肉瘤 除了散在的肿瘤性脂肪母细胞外，多形性脂肪肉瘤与MFH相似，脂肪母细胞可呈"桑葚状"或"印戒样"。另一方面，"去分化"脂肪肉瘤则具有混合性组织学形态，多形性MFH样的病灶和分化良好的脂肪肉瘤相邻。"去分化"形态最常见于复发肿瘤，说明是由原始间叶细胞的继发性肿瘤克隆的过度增生而成。多形性和去分化脂肪肉瘤也可出现类似于MFH的免疫反应模式，然而，与MFH不同，脂肪肉瘤的脂肪母细胞呈灶性S-100阳性[430]，而上皮、施万细胞及肌源性相关的标记物全部阴性。

多形性恶性外周神经鞘瘤 MPNST同样也可表现出多形性形态。大多数病例与分化较好的（梭形细胞）MPNST一样，S-100蛋白、CD56、CD57和髓磷脂碱性蛋白呈阳性[431]。

软组织的其他原发肿瘤

有些软组织原发肿瘤不能清楚地归入前面的类型，这些肿瘤包括恶性肾外横纹肌样瘤、脊索瘤、骨外黏液样软骨肉瘤（"脊索样"肉瘤）、骨外骨肉瘤以及部分脂肪肉瘤和血管肉瘤的变型。

颗粒细胞血管肉瘤

血管肉瘤的颗粒细胞变型极为少见（图3.31）[432]。免疫组化发现此病变UEAI、CD31、FLI-1和CD34阳性，证实了该肿瘤的内皮特性。CD68也可阳性，说明肿瘤细胞的胞浆颗粒有溶酶体性质。未见有关角蛋白在颗粒细胞血管肉瘤的报道。

肾外横纹肌样肿瘤（ERT）

发生于儿童肾脏、组织学上确定为"恶性横纹肌样瘤"的肿瘤也可发生在成人肾外各部位，包括软组织[433]。其特征为核周胞浆玻璃样嗜酸性包涵体，核圆形，偏位，染色质空泡状，核仁明显（图3.32），免疫表型复杂。

ERT常显示上皮分化，有些肿瘤与"近端"上皮样肉瘤难以鉴别[434]。大多数波形蛋白、EMA（图3.33）

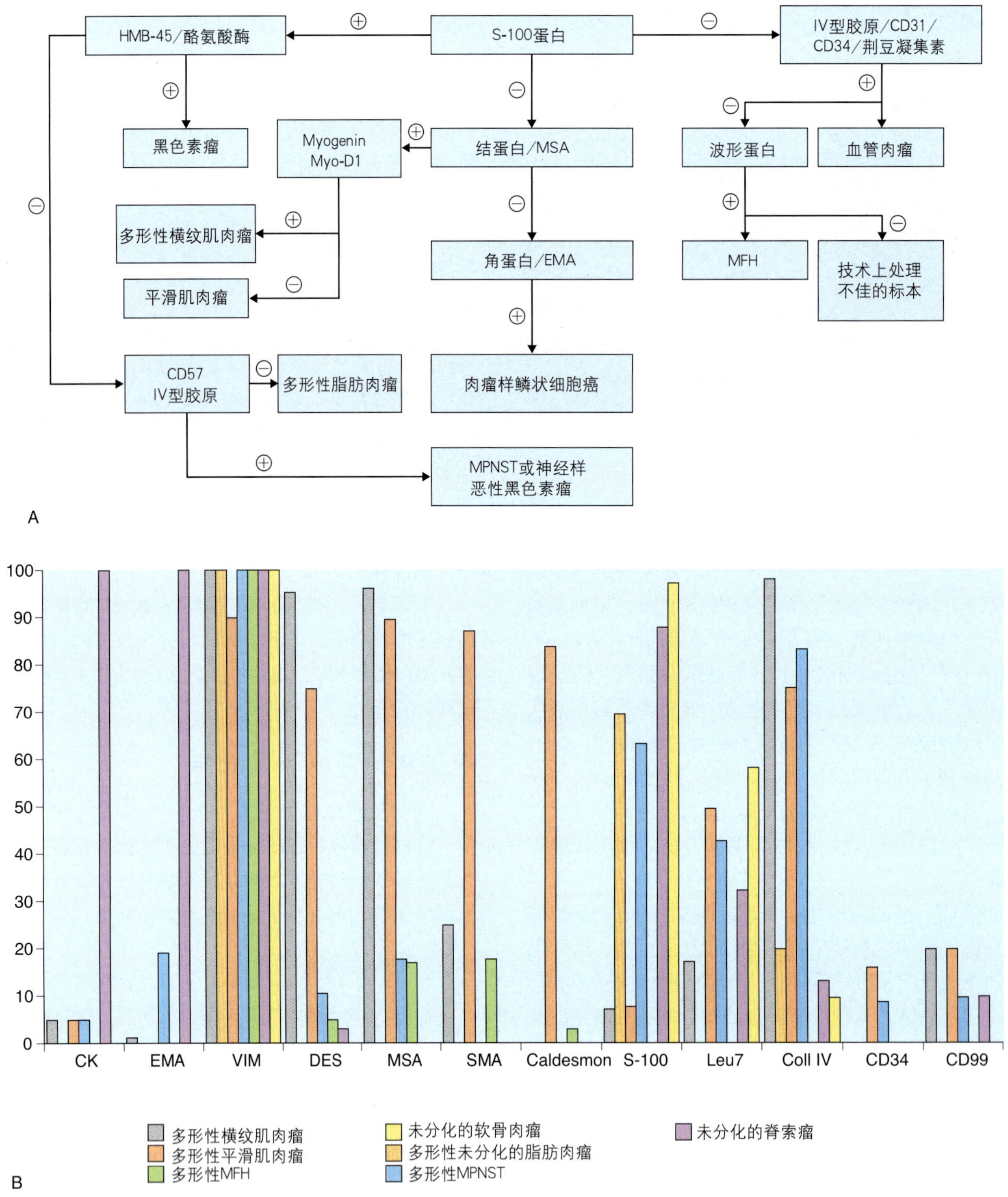

图 3.27 （A）恶性多形性肿瘤免疫组化诊断方略图；（B）多形性肿瘤常见免疫组化结果直方图

和角蛋白（图3.34）阳性[435,436]，并且核周染色增强。部分病例肌特异性肌动蛋白、癌胚抗原、α-平滑肌肌动蛋白、CD99、突触素、CD57、NSE和S-100蛋白也呈阳性。HMB-45、嗜铬素、肌红蛋白和CD34阴性。虽然ERT免疫表型与其他肉瘤和低分化癌重叠，但肿瘤的形态学表现一般足以作出鉴别诊断。

脂肪肉瘤变型

大多数病理学者均可通过典型脂肪分化诊断脂肪肉瘤。然而，当黏液样和圆形细胞变型脂肪母细胞较

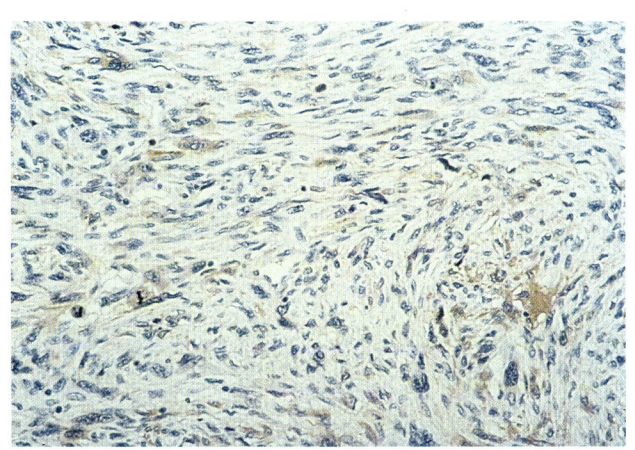

图 3.28 MFH 可被几种与单核巨噬细胞相关的标记物标记，如图示的 α-1-抗胰凝乳蛋白酶阳性。然而这些标记物完全没有特异性，重要的是诊断MFH时应首先排除其他系标记物阳性的病变

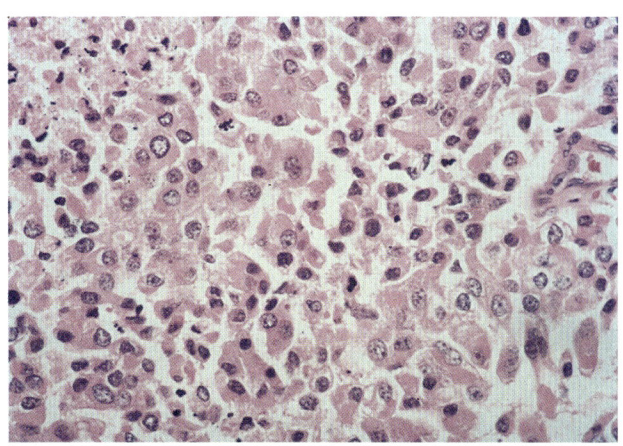

图 3.31 颗粒细胞血管肉瘤罕见，鉴别诊断包括颗粒细胞瘤、转移的黑色素瘤和上皮样平滑肌肉瘤

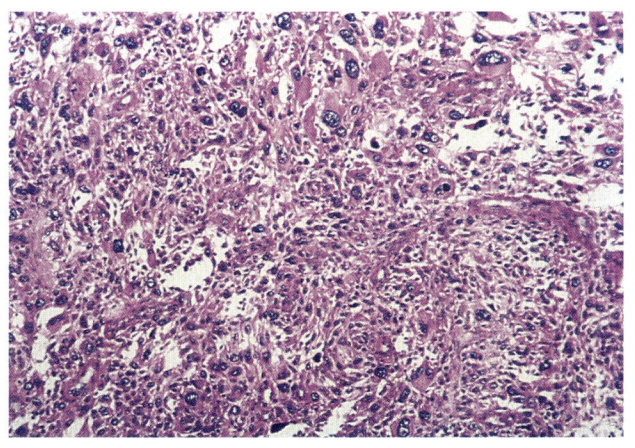

图 3.29 多形性横纹肌肉瘤，常规形态易与 MFH 混淆

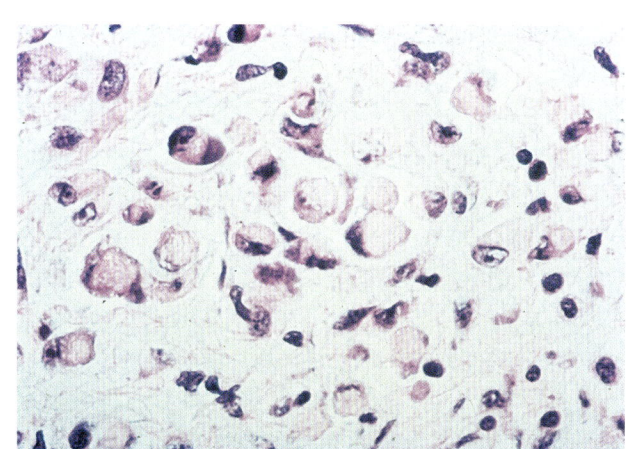

图 3.32 肾外横纹肌样瘤组织学图像，显示特征性的大细胞，胞浆嗜酸性，核空泡状偏位，核仁明显

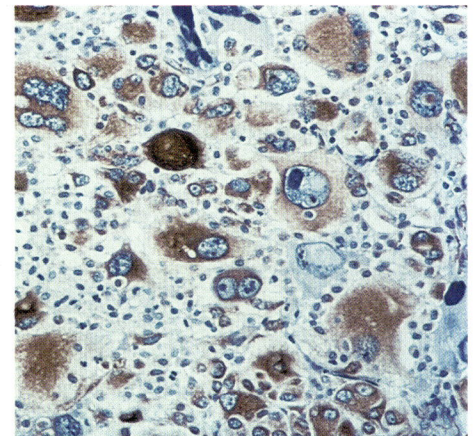

图 3.30 多形性横纹肌肉瘤，肌红蛋白阳性

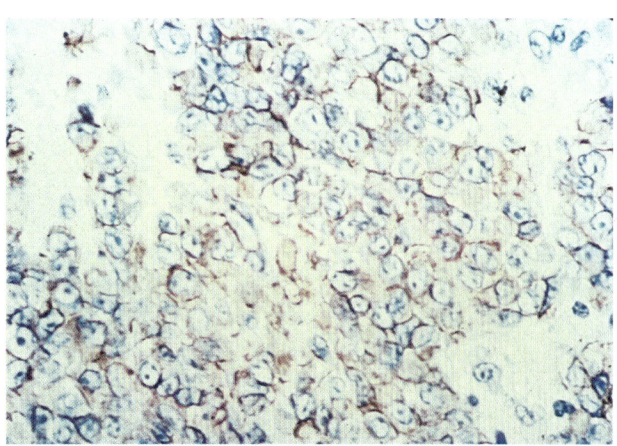

图 3.33 肾外横纹肌样瘤EMA可阳性，可能与上皮样肉瘤变型和转移癌相混淆

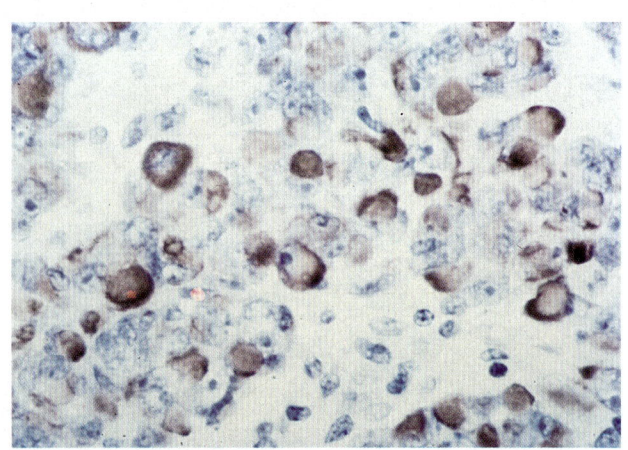

图3.34 横纹肌样瘤角蛋白阳性，易与其他软组织肉瘤或转移癌混淆

骨及软组织的软骨样肿瘤（图3.35）

脊索瘤 脊索瘤是具有脊索样分化的恶性肿瘤，主要发生于中轴骨，周围病变少见[438,439]。其鉴别诊断包括转移性腺癌（尤其是肾细胞癌）、软骨肉瘤、黏液乳头状室管膜瘤和血管内皮细胞瘤[440]。

脊索瘤角蛋白恒定阳性显示其上皮性质，该肿瘤可能阳性的角蛋白亚型包括CK1、CK5、CK8、CK10、CK14～16、CK18和CK19，尤以CK5突出（图3.36）[441]。脊索瘤也特征性地表达EMA（图3.37）[441,442]，以及HBME-1（另一种胞膜糖蛋白抗原），HBME-1在转移性肾细胞癌中阴性[19]。软骨肉瘤对上皮标记物阴性，但S-100蛋白阳性。此外，脊索瘤几乎总是表达N-钙黏素，而软骨肉瘤极少表达[86]。血管内皮瘤可以合成角蛋白，但其CD31和FLI-1阳性并缺乏S-100蛋白。室管膜瘤GFAP阳性[440]，与需鉴别的其他肿瘤均不相同。

在1973年，Heffelfinger及其同事描述了一种特殊的脊索瘤变型，具有软骨性区域，外观类似于软骨肉瘤[444,445]，他们将此病变命名为软骨样脊索瘤并认为比传统的脊索瘤预后较好。尽管形态学特点不同，但软骨样脊索瘤的免疫组化染色模式基本上与传统脊索瘤一致[443,445-447]。

"去分化"脊索瘤（图3.38）出现了与MFH免疫表型相同的间变成分，但此肿瘤新克隆细胞仍偶尔会有S-100蛋白阳性，而去分化区的细胞少见细胞角蛋白阳性（图3.39）。

少或不清楚时，可能难以诊断。

黏液样脂肪肉瘤（MLPS）波形蛋白和S-100蛋白阳性，后者仅限于脂肪母细胞阳性。此外，具有特征性的t（12;16）的MLPS也可灶性表达结蛋白、肌特异性肌动蛋白（MSA）和α-平滑肌肌动蛋白[437]。MLPS显示CD34和CD56阴性，但我们的部分病例CD57阳性。

圆形细胞脂肪肉瘤是一种异源性肿瘤，可类似于骨外软骨肉瘤或富细胞性外周神经鞘瘤。3种肿瘤S-100蛋白和波形蛋白均为阳性，但是CD57只见于软骨肉瘤中。镜下MPNST与圆形细胞脂肪肉瘤相似，但是与脂肪细胞病变不同的是MPNST可表达CD56或髓磷脂碱性蛋白。

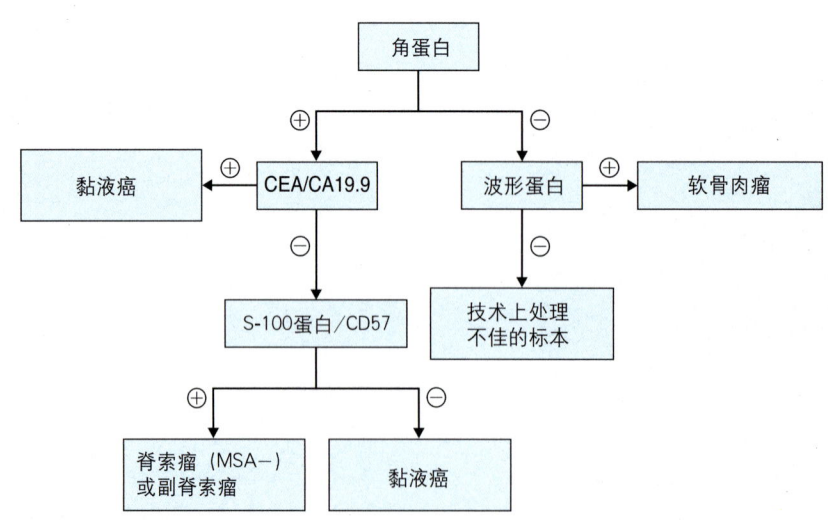

图3.35 软组织的脊索样及黏液样肿瘤的免疫组化诊断方略图

软组织和骨肿瘤的免疫组织化学 3

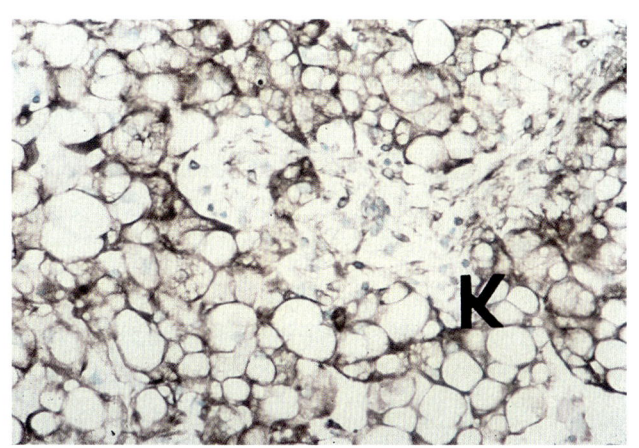

图 3.36 脊索瘤角蛋白阳性

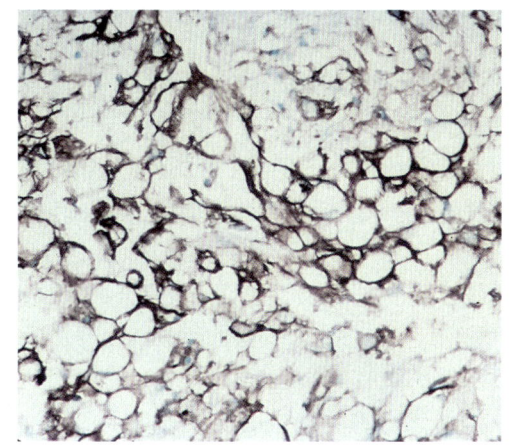

图 3.37 脊索瘤 EMA 阳性

副脊索瘤 副脊索瘤罕见，发生在肢体深部软组织中，生长缓慢。其鉴别诊断主要包括骨外黏液样软骨肉瘤和外周脊索瘤。然而，软骨样脂肪瘤、骨化纤维黏液瘤、肌上皮瘤和皮下黏液乳头状室管膜瘤有时

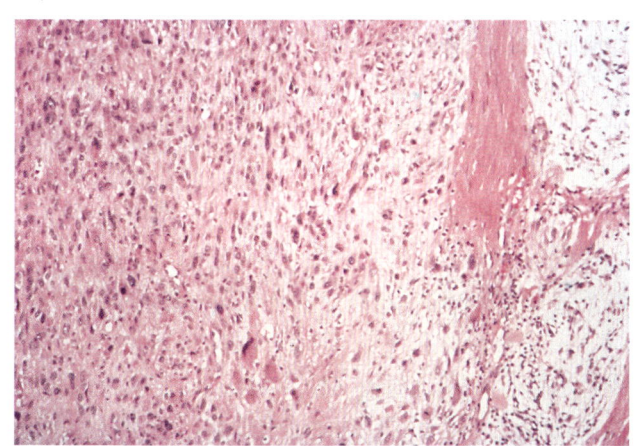

图 3.38 个别脊索瘤发生间变性转化（"去分化"），并获得了与 MFH 非常相似的免疫表型

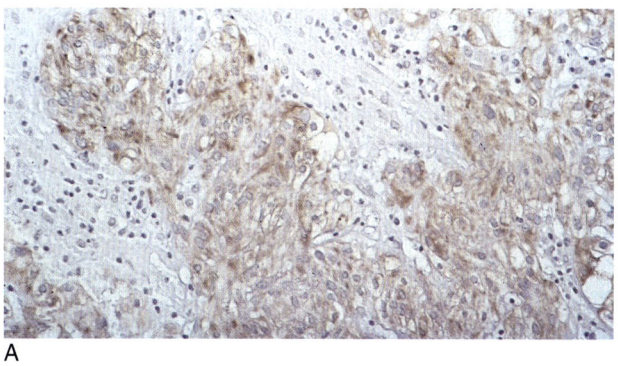

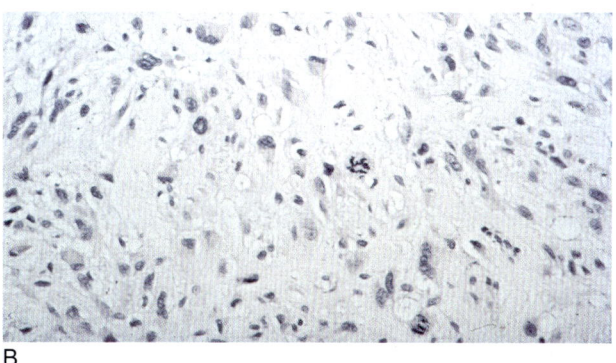

图 3.39 （A）去分化脊索瘤分化好的区域角蛋白阳性，（B）而间变灶同一标记物阴性

> **诊断要点：脊索瘤**
>
> 1. 脊索瘤典型的呈 CK+、S-100+、HMBE+。
> 2. 鉴别诊断包括转移性肾细胞瘤（HBME-1-）、软骨肉瘤（CK-）、黏液乳头状室管膜瘤（GFAP+）和血管内皮瘤（CD31+/FLI-1+）

也需考虑。副脊索瘤具有与骨外黏液样软骨肉瘤不同的独特免疫表型。副脊索瘤 CK8、CK18、EMA、S-100 蛋白、Ⅳ型胶原和波形蛋白典型阳性[17, 18, 450-453]。相反，骨外黏液样软骨肉瘤角蛋白阴性[17]，偶有Ⅳ型胶原阳性。

另一方面，副脊索瘤和外周脊索瘤免疫表型大多重叠，包括角蛋白亚型、EMA、波形蛋白、S-100蛋白和Ⅳ型胶原。事实上，Scolyer等推断两种肿瘤不能用免疫组化区分[454]。

软骨母细胞瘤 软骨母细胞瘤在软组织中少见[455]。可与巨细胞修复性肉芽肿和巨细胞肿瘤相混淆。软骨母细胞瘤波形蛋白、NSE 和 S-100 蛋白强阳性，如后面两个标记物阴性时则应考虑其他诊断[456-458]。尤其是软骨母细胞瘤中增生的间质细胞显示

95

S-100蛋白强阳性，使其与骨巨细胞瘤和修复性肉芽肿更易鉴别[458,459]。

异常CK的表达是软骨母细胞瘤的一个潜在特征[458,460]。单核的软骨母细胞性瘤细胞CD68阴性[457,461]。据说部分软骨母细胞瘤胞浆显示肌特异性肌动蛋白阳性[162]。

骨外软骨肉瘤，普通型 软组织的普通型软骨肉瘤的鉴别诊断包括伴有软骨样特征的反应性和良性增生，例如软骨瘤、软骨母细胞型骨肉瘤、上皮样血管内皮瘤（EHE）和外周脊索瘤，部分鉴别诊断前面已述。除了骨化生性病灶之外，普通型软骨肉瘤骨粘连蛋白（ONN）阴性，此特征与软骨母细胞性骨肉瘤不同[212]。免疫组化并不能将普通型软骨肉瘤与其他软骨病变区分，但可与EHE和脊索瘤区分。EHE表达内皮标记物而脊索瘤上皮标记物阳性。

骨外黏液样软骨肉瘤（"脊索样肉瘤"） 虽然骨的和骨外黏液样软骨肉瘤具有相同的形态学特征，但在超微结构和分子水平有根本区别，提示为两种类型肿瘤。骨外黏液样软骨肉瘤（EMC）证实有t(9;22)染色体交互易位，从而导致EWS和CHN基因的融合[463-465]，免疫组化S-100蛋白和CD57常仅呈灶性阳性；而骨黏液性软骨肉瘤S-100蛋白和CD57呈弥漫阳性。两种软骨肉瘤变型均显示角蛋白、E-钙黏素和N-钙黏素阴性[86]。EMC的免疫组化特征倾向于"奇异的"神经内分泌分化，突触素或嗜铬素阳性[466-468]。此表现原因未知，但若为阳性则对鉴别诊断有重要意义。

透明细胞软骨肉瘤 透明细胞软骨肉瘤（CCC）是一种少见亚型——尤其是在软组织中——具有特殊的临床病理特征并且预后相对较好[469]。该肿瘤的组织学特征为透明多边形细胞呈小叶状排列，伴明显化生性成骨区和散在类似软骨母细胞瘤的区域。CCC瘤细胞显示S-100蛋白、波形蛋白、CD57和溶菌酶阳性[464]。与普通型软骨肉瘤和间叶性软骨肉瘤不同，部分病例ONN强阳性[470,471]。

其他骨或软组织肿瘤

骨肉瘤 骨外骨肉瘤非常罕见，与骨内骨肉瘤一样也具有各种组织学类型，包括纤维母细胞性、软骨母细胞性、小细胞性和血管扩张性骨肉瘤。

这些肿瘤的免疫组化显示无明显病理诊断及鉴别诊断特征。骨外骨肉瘤波形蛋白阳性，且肿瘤实质成分常常CD57阳性。α-平滑肌肌动蛋白可灶性阳性，部分结蛋白同时阳性[472]，或许与肿瘤肌纤维母细胞性分化有关。S-100蛋白仅在明显软骨区域阳性[472]。个别病例上皮性标记物阳性[472-474]。GFAP和神经丝蛋白阴性。

以往常用碱性磷酸酶的骨同工酶标记来鉴别骨外骨肉瘤与其他多形性肉瘤[470]。其主要缺点是仅适用冰冻切片或印片，而不适于石蜡切片。

骨基质蛋白ONN和骨钙素已经引起人们很大兴趣，但是它们在识别骨肉瘤中的作用还需要进一步证实。已观察到骨肉瘤和骨母细胞瘤的肿瘤性成分ONN阳性，但在骨巨细胞瘤和软骨母细胞瘤中的单核瘤细胞也为阳性[475]。部分多形性和纤维肉瘤性骨肉瘤ONN也呈灶性阳性[476]。后者说明ONN的产生是骨母细胞分化的早期事件。总之，在诊断成骨性肿瘤时，ONN和OCN的特异性阳性分别约为40%和95%[203,204]。这两种标记物可能在确认骨外骨肉瘤诊断的抗体组合中较为实用。

骨和软组织的巨细胞瘤 骨的巨细胞瘤为局部潜在浸润性肿瘤，以累及长管状骨的骨骺或邻近的干骺端为特征。原发于深部软组织形态类似的巨细胞瘤少见，而较常见的是发生于浅部腱鞘的巨细胞瘤。软组织巨细胞瘤、恶性软组织巨细胞瘤和巨细胞型MFH均为深部软组织的骨外巨细胞肿瘤，与腱鞘巨细胞瘤不同，但是它们的免疫组化表现类似。

免疫组化研究主要集中于基质单核细胞和多核巨细胞成分。破骨细胞样的巨细胞通常CD68强阳性[477-481]，但单核细胞成分阳性强度大为减弱。基质细胞显示α-平滑肌肌动蛋白可为阳性，但CD45、S-100蛋白、结蛋白和溶菌酶均为阴性[477,479]。部分巨细胞瘤出现血管浸润引起了对其合成基质金属蛋白酶（MMPs）和金属蛋白酶组织抑制物（TIMP）的关注，二者均与肿瘤细胞浸润性有关。巨细胞瘤的多核细胞为MMP-9（明胶酶B）阳性，但在其单核细胞成分中仅为灶性阳性[477,482,483]。部分研究显示在复发和转移的巨细胞瘤中TIMP的阳性表达比MMP的阳性表达增多[477,484]。

造釉细胞瘤 长骨造釉细胞瘤为一类罕见肿瘤，主要发生于青年人胫骨中段。典型结构为"骨纤维结构不良"（Campanacci病）中连续病变谱的一部分[485,486]。在富细胞性的间质中可见不规则排列的上皮样或鳞状细胞样致密细胞巢（图3.40）。过去认为该肿瘤为内皮性增生或上皮性病变，但现在已清楚其为上皮增生病变。所有造釉细胞瘤CK均为阳性，以CK14和CK19为主（图3.41）[487-491]。另外，内皮标记物完全阴性。因为其形态学上倾向于上皮样和梭形细胞双相分化，以及上皮的免疫表型，所以有人推测造釉细胞瘤是否为骨内的滑膜肉瘤。然而，二者具有完全不同的细胞遗传学改变[490, 491]，是完全不同的两种具有上皮分化的间叶肿瘤。

从病理学的角度，活检标本可能会有疑问，即造釉细胞瘤是否是转移癌而非骨原发性肿瘤。迄今为止，对两组病变尚未作过系统的免疫组化比较。然而，对该问题最直接的解决方法就是对照影像学研究，造釉细胞瘤具有独特的影像学表现[486]，与转移癌明显不同。当造釉细胞瘤出现明显硬化时（为"骨纤维结构不良"的极端病变），需用免疫组化鉴别，因为此时单独常规染色难以发现浸润的上皮。

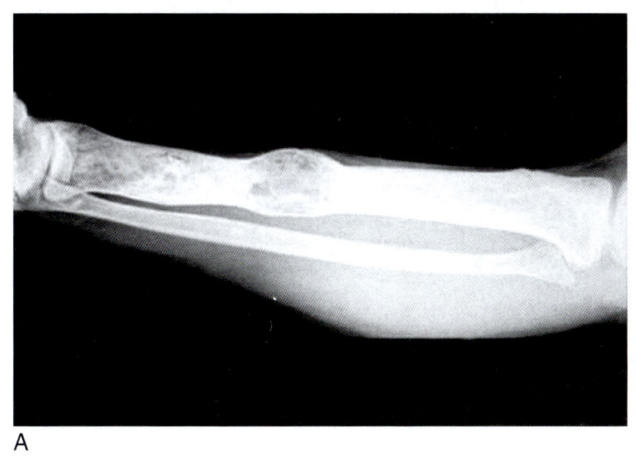

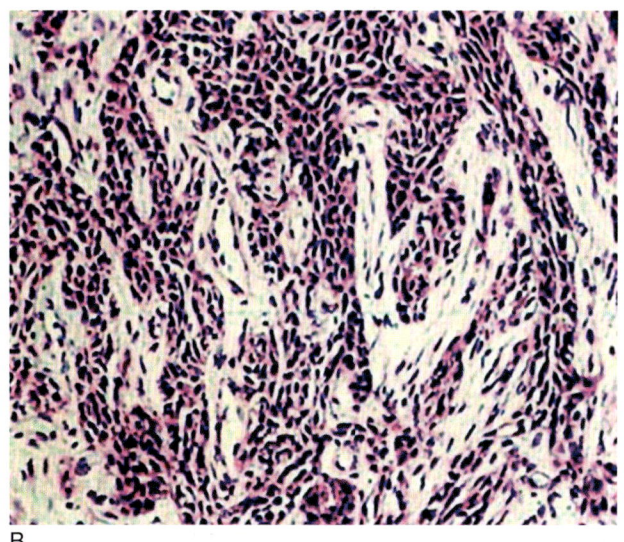

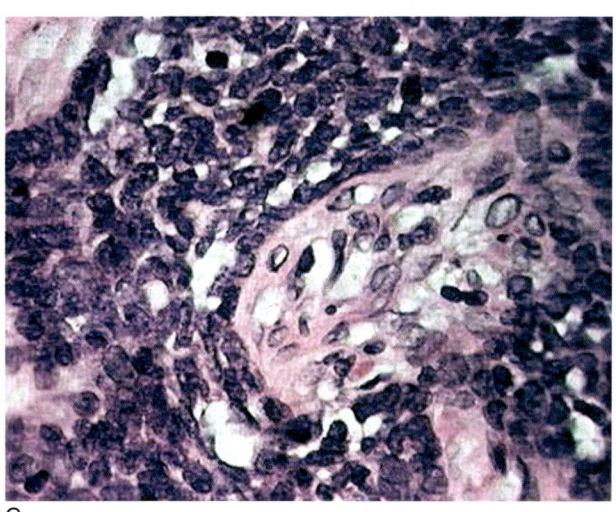

图 3.40 （A）长骨造釉细胞瘤的 X 线照片和（B,C）组织学图像

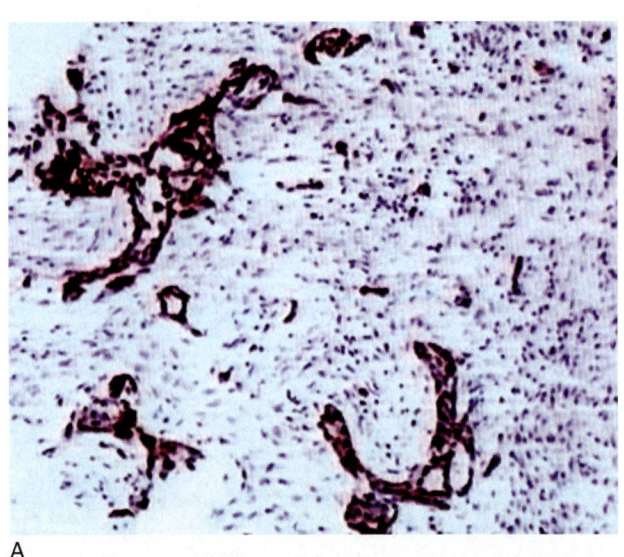 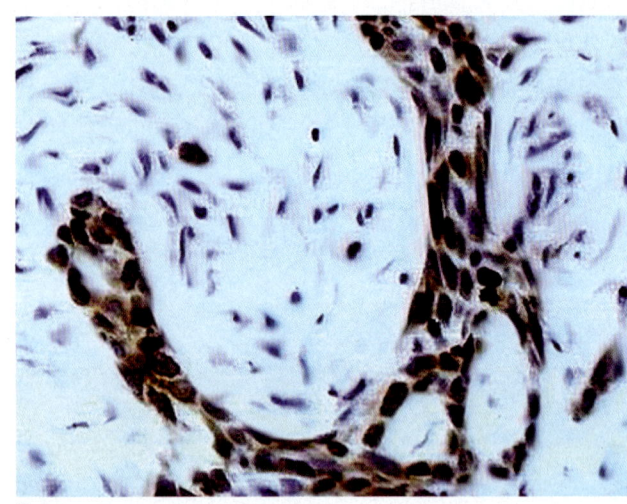

图 3.41 （A）长骨造釉细胞瘤 CK14 阳性和（B）CK19 阳性

参考文献

1. Denk H, Krepler R, Artlieb U, et al. Proteins of intermediate filaments: An immunohistochemical and biochemical approach to the classification of soft tissue tumors. Am J Pathol 1983; 110:193–208.

2. Lazarides E. Intermediate filaments: A chemically heterogeneous, developmentally regulated class of proteins. Annu Rev Biochem 1982; 51:219–250.

3. Erlandson RA. Diagnostic transmission electron micro-scopy of tumors. New York: Raven; 1994:165.

4. Osborn M, Weber K. Biology of disease: Tumor diagnosis by intermediate filament typing: A novel tool for surgical pathology. Lab Invest 1983; 48:372–394.

5. Anderton BH. Intermediate filaments: A family of homologous structures. J Muscle Res Cell Motil 1981; 2:141–166.

6. Hermann H, Aebi U. Intermediate filaments and their associates: Multitalented structural elements specifying cytoarchitecture and cytodynamics. Curr Opin Cell Biol 2000; 12:79–90.

7. Mischke D. The complexity of gene families involved in epithelial differentiation: Keratin genes and the epidermal differentiation complex. Subcell Biochem 1998; 31:71–104.

8. Saavedra-Matiz CA, Chapman NH, Wijsman EM, et al. Linkage of hereditary distal myopathy with desmin accumulation to 2q. Hum Hered 2000; 50:166–170.

9. Ferrari S, Cannizzaro LA, Battini R, et al. The gene encoding human vimentin is located on the short arm of chromosome 10. Am J Hum Genet 1987; 41:616–626.

10. Yoshime T, Maruno M, Kumura E, et al. Stochastic determination of the chromosomal region responsible for expression of human glial fibrillary acidic protein in astrocytic tumors. Neurosci Lett 1998; 247:29–32.

11. Goldman R, Goldman AE, Green K, et al. Intermediate filaments: Possible functions as cytoskeletal connecting links between the nucleus and the cell surface. Ann NY Acad Sci 1985; 455:1–17.

12. Osborn M. Summary: Intermediate filaments 1984. Ann NY Acad Sci 1985; 455:669–681.

13. Vandenburgh HH. Cell shape and growth regulation in skeletal muscle: Exogenous versus endogenous factors. J Cell Physiol 1983; 116:363–371.

14. Miettinen M. Keratin immunohistochemistry: Update of applications and pitfalls. Pathol Annu 1993; 28(Pt. 2):113–143.

15. Moll R, Franke WW, Schiller DL, et al. The catalogue of human cytokeratins: Patterns of expression in normal epithelia, tumors, and cultured cells. Cell 1982; 31:11–24.

16. Miettinen M, Limon J, Niezabitowski A, et al. Patterns of keratin polypeptides in 110 biphasic, monophasic, and poorly-differentiated synovial sarcomas. Virchows Arch 2000; 437: 275–283.

17. Folpe AL, Agoff SN, Willis J, et al. Parachordoma is

immunohistochemically and cytogenetically distinct from axial chordoma and extraskeletal myxoid chondrosarcoma. Am J Surg Pathol 1999; 23:1059–1067.

18. Fisher C, Miettinen M. Parachordoma: A clinicopathologic and immunohistochemical study of four cases of an unusual soft tissue neoplasm. Ann Diagn Pathol 1997; 1:3–10.

19. O'Hara BJ, Paetau A, Miettinen M. Keratin subsets and monoclonal antibodies HBME-1 in chordoma: Immunohistochemical differential diagnosis between tumors simulating chordoma. Hum Pathol 1998; 29:119–126.

20. Swanson PE, Dehner LP, Sirgi KE, et al. Cytokeratin immunoreactivity in malignant tumors of bone and soft tissue. Appl Immunohistochem 1994; 2:103–112.

21. Pruss RM, Mirsky R, Raff MC, et al. All classes of intermediate filaments share a common antigenic determinant defined by a monoclonal antibody. Cell 1981; 27:419–428.

22. Geisler N, Weber K. Comparison of the proteins of two immunologically distinct intermediate-sized filaments by amino acid sequence analysis: desmin and vimentin. Proc Natl Acad Sci USA 1981; 78:4120–4123.

23. Wick MR. Antibodies to desmin in diagnostic pathology. In: Wick MR, Siegal GP, eds. Monoclonal antibodies in diagnostic immunohistochemistry. New York: Marcel Dekker; 1988:93–114.

24. Truong LD, Rangdaeng S, Cagle P, et al. The diagnostic utility of desmin: A study of 584 cases and review of the literature. Am J Clin Pathol 1990; 93:305–314.

25. Rangdaeng S, Truong LD. Comparative immunohistochemical staining for desmin and muscle specific actin: A study of 576 cases. Am J Clin Pathol 1991; 96:32–45.

26. Small JV, Sobieszek A. Studies on the function and composition of the 10-nm (100 A) filaments of vertebrate smooth muscle. J Cell Sci 1977; 23:243–268.

27. Geisler N, Weber K. Purification of smooth muscle desmin and a protein-chemical comparison of desmins from chicken gizzard and hog stomach. Eur J Biochem 1980; 111:425–433.

28. Lazarides E, Balzer DR Jr. Specificity of desmin to avian and mammalian muscle cells. Cell 1978; 14:429–438.

29. Geisler N, Weber K. The amino acid sequence of chicken muscle desmin provides a common structural model for intermediate filament proteins. EMBO J 1982; 1:1649–1656.

30. Ip W, Heuser JE. Subunit structure of desmin and vimentin protofilaments and how they assemble into intermediate filaments. Ann NY Acad Sci 1985; 455:185–199.

31. Ngai J, Capetanaki YG, Lazarides E. Expression of the genes encoding for the intermediate filament proteins vimentin and desmin. Ann NY Acad Sci 1985; 455:144–155.

32. Tokuyasu KT, Maher PA, Dutton AH, et al. Intermediate filaments in skeletal and cardiac muscle tissue in embryonic and adult chicken. Ann NY Acad Sci 1985; 455:200–212.

33. Fischman DA, Danto SI. Monoclonal antibodies to desmin: Evidence for stage-dependent intermediate filament immunoreactivity during cardiac and skeletal muscle development. Ann NY Acad Sci 1985; 455:167–184.

34. Tuszynski GP, Frank ED, Damsky CD, et al. The detection of smooth muscle desmin-like protein in BHK21/C13 fibroblasts. J Biol Chem 1979; 254:6138–6143.

35. Schmid E, Osborn M, Rungger-Brandle E, et al. Distribution of vimentin and desmin filaments in smooth muscle tissue of mammalian and avian aorta. Exp Cell Res 1982; 137:329–340.

36. Richardson FL, Stromer MH, Huiatt TW, et al. Immunoelectron and immunofluorescence localization of desmin in mature avian muscles. Eur J Cell Biol 1981; 26:91–101.

37. Daste G, Gioanni J, Lauque D, et al. GC12, marker of cells of mesodermal origin: Value and application to cytodiagnosis of serous effusions. Arch Anat Cytol Pathol 1997; 45:185–191.

38. Pollock L, Rampling D, Greenwald SE, et al. Desmin expression in forms: Influence of the desmin clone and immunohistochemical method. J Clin Pathol 1995; 48:535–538.

39. Chang TK, Li CY, Smithson WA. Immunocytochemical study of small round cell tumors in routinely processed specimens. Arch Pathol Lab Med 1989; 113:1343–1348.

40. Granter SR, Badizadegan K, Fletcher CDM. Myofibromatosis in adults, glomangiopericytoma, and myopericytoma: A spectrum of tumors showing perivascular myoid differentiation. Am J Surg Pathol 1998; 22:513–525.

41. Ordi J, de Alava E, Torne A, et al. Intraabdominal desmoplastic small round-cell tumor with EWS/ERG fusion transcripts. Am J Surg Pathol 1998; 22:1026–1032.

42. Parham DM, Dias P, Kelly DR, et al. Desmin positivity in primitive neuroectodermal tumors of childhood. Am J Surg Pathol 1992; 16:483–492.

43. Manivel JC, Wick MR, Dehner LP, et al. Epithelioid sarcoma:

An immunohistochemical study. Am J Clin Pathol 1987; 87: 319–326.

44. Wick MR, Swanson PE, Scheithauer BW, et al. Malignant peripheral nerve sheath tumor: An immunohistochemical study of 62 cases. Am J Clin Pathol 1987; 87:425–433.

45. Fanberg-Smith JC, Hengge M, Hengge UR, et al. Extrarenal rhabdoid tumors of soft tissue: A clinicopathologic and immunohistochemical study of 18 cases. Ann Diagn Pathol 1998; 2:351–362.

46. Geisler N, Plessmann U, Weber K. Amino acid sequence characterization of mammalian vimentin, the mesenchymal intermediate filament protein. FEBS Lett 1983; 163: 22–24.

47. Gereben B, Leuheiber K, Rausch WD, et al. Inverse hierarchy of vimentin epitope expression in primary cultures of chicken and rat astrocytes: A double immunofluorescence study. Neurobiology 1998; 6:141–150.

48. Battifora H. Assessment of antigen damage in immunohistochemistry: The vimentin internal control. Am J Clin Pathol 1991; 96:669–671.

49. Gereben B, Gerics B, Galfi P, et al. Species specificity of glial vimentin, as revealed by immunocytochemical studies with the VIM3B4 and V9 monoclonal antibodies. Neurobiology 1995; 3:151–164.

50. Olah I, Glick B. Anti-vimentin monoclonal antibodies differentiate two resident cell populations in chicken spleen. Dev Comp Immunol 1994; 18:67–73.

51. Heatley M, Whiteside C, Maxwell P, et al. Vimentin expression in benign and malignant breast epithelium. J Clin Pathol 1993; 46:441–445.

52. Bohn W, Wiegers W, Beuttenmuller M, et al. Species-specific recognition patterns of monoclonal antibodies directed against vimentin. Exp Cell Res 1992; 201:1–7.

53. Carbone A, Gloghini A, Volpe R, et al. Anti-vimentin antibody reactivity with Reed-Sternberg cells of Hodgkin's disease. Virchows Arch A 1990; 417:43–48.

54. Meyer SA, Ingraham CA, McCarthy KD. Expression of vimentin by cultured astroglia and oligodendroglia. J Neurosci Res 1989; 24:251–259.

55. Dahl D. Immunohistochemical differences between neurofilaments in perikarya, dendrites, and axons: Immunofluorescence study with antisera raised to neurofilament polypeptides (200 kD, 150 kD, and 70 kD) isolated by anion exchange chromatography. Exp Cell Res 1983; 149:397–408.

56. Hickey WF, Lee V, Trojanowski JQ, et al. Immunohistochemical application of monoclonal antibodies against myelin basic protein and neurofilament triplet protein subunits: Advantage over antisera and technical limitations. J Histochem Cytochem 1983; 31:1126–1135.

57. Shaw G. Neurofilaments: Abundant but mysterious neuronal structures. Bioessays 1986; 4:161–166.

58. Tapscott SJ, Bennett GS, Toyama Y, et al. Intermediate filament proteins in the developing chick spinal cord. Dev Biol 1981; 86:40–54.

59. Tremblay GF, Lee VMY, Trojanowski JQ. Expression of vimentin, glial filament, and neurofilament proteins in primitive childhood brain tumors: A comparative immunoblot and immunoperoxidase study. Acta Neuro-pathol 1985; 68:239–244.

60. Lee VMY, Carden MJ, Trojanowski JQ. Novel monoclonal antibodies provide evidence for the in-situ existence of a non-phosphorylated form of the large neurofilament subunit. J Neurosci 1986; 6:850–858.

61. Brown A. Contiguous phosphorylated and non-phosphorylated domains along axonal neurofilaments. J Cell Sci 1998; 111:455–467.

62. Sternberger LA, Sternberger NH. Monoclonal antibodies distinguish phosphorylated and non-phosphorylated forms of neurofilaments in situ. Proc Natl Acad Sci USA 1983; 80: 6126–6130.

63. Ulfig N, Nickel J, Bohl J. Monoclonal antibodies SMI311 and SMI312 as tools to investigate the maturation of nerve cells and axonal patterns in human fetal brain. Cell Tissue Res 1998; 291:433–443.

64. Trojanowski JQ, Lee VMY. Anti-neurofilament monoclonal antibodies: Reagents for the evaluation of human neoplasms. Acta Neuropathol 1983; 59:155–158.

65. Trojanowski JQ, Lee VMY, Schlaepfer WW. An immunohistochemical study of central and peripheral nervous system tumors with monoclonal antibodies against neurofilaments and glial filaments. Hum Pathol 1984; 15:248–257.

66. Trojanowski JQ, Lee VMY. Expression of neurofilament antigens by normal and neoplastic human adrenal chromaffin cells. N Engl J Med 1985; 313:101–104.

67. Osborn M, Altmannsberger M, Shaw G, et al. Various sympathetic derived human tumors differ in neurofilament

expression: Use in diagnosis of neuroblastoma, ganglioneuroblastoma, and pheochromocytoma. Virchows Arch B Cell Pathol 1982; 40:141–156.
68. Shaw G, Weber K. The intermediate filament complement of the brain: A comparison between different mammalian species. Eur J Cell Biol 1984; 33:95–104.
69. Trojanowski JQ. Neurofilament and glial filament proteins. In: Wick MR, Siegal GP, eds. Monoclonal antibodies in diagnostic immunohistochemistry. New York: Marcel Dekker; 1988:115–146.
70. Dolman CL. Glial fibrillary acidic protein and cartilage. Acta Neuropathol 1989; 79:101–103.
71. Yasuda T, Sobue G, Ito T, et al. Human peripheral nerve sheath neoplasms: Expression of Schwann cell-related markers and their relation to malignant transformation. Muscle Nerve 1991; 14:812–819.
72. Lodding P, Kindblom LG, Angervall L, et al. A clinicopathologic study of 29 cases. Virchows Arch A 1990; 416:237–248.
73. Giangaspero F, Fratamico FC, Ceccarelli C, et al. Malignant peripheral nerve sheath tumors and spindle cell sarcomas: An immunohistochemical analysis of multiple markers. Appl Pathol 1989; 7:134–144.
74. Kawahara E, Oda Y, Ooi A, et al. Expression of glial fibrillary acidic protein (GFAP) in peripheral nerve sheath tumors: A comparative study of immunoreactivity of GFAP, vimentin, S100 protein, and neurofilament in 38 schwannomas and 18 neurofibromas. Am J Surg Pathol 1988; 12:115–120.
75. Memoli VA, Brown EF, Gould VE. Glial fibrillary acidic protein (GFAP) immunoreactivity in peripheral nerve sheath tumors. Ultrastruct Pathol 1984; 7:269–275.
76. Swanson PE. Monoclonal antibodies to human milk fat globule proteins. In: Wick MR, Siegal GP, eds. Monoclonal antibodies in diagnostic immunohistochemistry. New York: Marcel Dekker; 1988:227–283.
77. Petersen OW, VanDeuers B. Characterization of epithelial membrane antigen expression in human mammary epithelium by ultrastructural immuno peroxidase cytochemistry. J Histochem Cytochem 1986; 34:801–809.
78. Sloane JP, Ormerod MG. Distribution of epithelial membrane antigen in normal and neoplastic tissues and its value in diagnostic tumor pathology. Cancer 1981; 47:1786–1795.
79. Ormerod MG, Steele K, Westwood JH, et al. Epithelial membrane antigen: Partial purification, assay, and properties. Br J Cancer 1983; 48:533–541.
80. Heyderman E, Strudley I, Powell G, et al. A new monoclonal antibody to epithelial membrane antigen (EMA)-E29: A comparison of its immunocytochemical reactivity with polyclonal anti-EMA antibodies and another monoclonal antibody, HMFG-2. Br J Cancer 1985; 52:355–361.
81. Cordell J, Richardson TC, Pulford KAF, et al. Production of monoclonal antibodies against human epithelial membrane antigen for use in diagnostic immunocytochemistry. Br J Cancer 1985; 52:347–354.
82. Wick MR, Swanson PE, Manivel JC. Immunohistochemical analysis of soft tissue sarcomas: Comparisons with electron microscopy. Appl Pathol 1988; 6:169–196.
83. Swanson PE, Manivel JC, Scheithauer BW, et al. Epithelial membrane antigen in human sarcomas: An immunohistochemical study. Surg Pathol 1989; 2:313–322.
84. Franke WW, Moll R, Mueller H, et al. Immunocytochemical identification of epithelium-derived human tumors with antibodies to desmosomal plaque proteins. Proc Natl Acad Sci USA 1983; 80:543–547.
85. Arnemann J, Spurr NK, Magee AI, et al. The human gene (DSG2) coding for HDGC, a second member of the desmoglein subfamily of the desmosomal cadherins, is, like DSG1 coding for desmoglein DG1, assigned to chromosome 18. Genomics 1992; 13:484–486.
86. Laskin WB, Miettinen M. Epithelial-type and neural-type cadherin expression in malignant noncarcinomatous neoplasms with epithelioid features that involve the soft tissues. Arch Pathol Lab Med 2002; 126:425–431.
87. Sata H, Hasegawa T, Abe Y, et al. Expression of E-cadherin in bone and soft tissue sarcomas: a possible role in epithelial differentiation. Hum Pathol 1999; 30:1344–1349.
88. Miettinen M. Antibody specificity to muscle actins in the diagnosis and classification of soft tissue tumors. Am J Pathol 1988; 130:205–215.
89. Schurch W, Skalli O, Seemayer TA, et al. Intermediate filament proteins and actin isoforms as markers for soft tissue tumor differentiation and origin. I. Smooth muscle tumors. Am J Pathol 1987; 128:91–103.
90. Tsukada T, McNutt MA, Ross R, et al. HHF35, a muscle actin-specific monoclonal antibody. II. Reactivity in normal, reactive, and neoplastic human tissue. Am J Pathol 1987; 127:

389–402.

91. Jones H, Steart PV, DuBoulay CE, et al. Alpha-smooth muscle actin as a marker for soft tissue tumors: A comparison with desmin. J Pathol 1990; 162:29–33.

92. Cintorino M, Vindigni C, DelVecchio MT, et al. Expression of actin isoforms and intermediate filament proteins in childhood orbital rhabdom- yosarcomas. J Submicrosc Cytol Pathol 1989; 21:409–419.

93. Bussolati G, Papotti M, Foschini MP, et al. The interest of actin immunocytochemistry in diagnostic histopathology. Basic Appl Histochem 1987; 31:165–176.

94. Ogut O, Granzier H, Jin JP. Acidic and basic troponin-T isoforms in mature fast-twitch skeletal muscle and effect on contractility. Am J Physiol 1999; 276:C1162–C1170.

95. Lutz GJ, Lieber RL. Skeletal muscle myosin-II structure and function. Exerc Sport Sci Rev 1999; 27:63–77.

96. Lefevre G. Troponins: Biological and clinical aspects. Ann Biol Clin 2000; 58:39–48.

97. Atkinson RA, Joseph C, Dal Piaz F, et al. Binding of alpha-actinin to titin: Implications for Z-disk assembly. Biochemistry 2000; 39:5255–5264.

98. Dodd S, Malone M, McCulloch W. Rhabdomyosarcoma in children: A histological and immunohistochemical study of 59 cases. J Pathol 1989; 158:13–18.

99. Lai R, Tian Y, An J, et al. A comparative study on morphology and immunohistochemistry of rhabdomyosarcoma and embryonal skeletal muscles. Chin Med J 1997; 110:392–396.

100. Gruchala A, Niezabitowski A, Wasilewska A, et al. Rhabdomyosarcoma: Morphologic, immunohistochemical, and DNA study. Gen Diagn Pathol 1997; 142:175–184.

101. Carter RL, Jameson CF, Philp ER, et al. Comparative phenotypes in rhabdomyosarcoma and developing skeletal muscle. Histopathology 1990; 17:301–309.

102. Saku T, Tsuda N, Anami M, et al. Smooth and skeletal muscle myosins in spindle cell tumors of soft tissue: An immunohistochemical study. Acta Pathol Jpn 1985; 35:125–136.

103. Osborn M, Hill C, Altmannsberger M, et al. Monoclonal antibodies to titin in conjunction with antibodies to desmin separate rhabdomyosarcomas from other tumor types. Lab Invest 1986; 55:101–108.

104. Moczygemba C, Guidry J, Wittung-Stafshede P. Heme orientation affects holo-myoglobin folding and unfolding kinetics. FEBS Lett 2000; 470:203–206.

105. Parham DM, Webber B, Holt H, et al. Immunohistochemical study of childhood rhabdomyosarcomas and related neoplasms: Results of an Intergroup Rhabdomyosarcoma Study project. Cancer 1991; 67:3072–3080.

106. Carter RL, McCarthy KP, Machin LG, et al. Expression of desmin and myoglobin in rhabdomyosarcomas and in developing skeletal muscle. Histopathology 1989; 15:585–595.

107. Coindre JM, deMascarel A, Trojani M, et al. Immunohistochemical study of rhabdomyosarcoma: Unexpected staining with S100 protein and cytokeratin. J Pathol 1988; 155:127–132.

108. Seidal T, Kindblom LG, Angervall L. Myoglobin, desmin, and vimentin in ultrastructurally proven rhabdomyomas and rhabdomyosarcomas: An immunohistochemical study utilizing a series of monoclonal and polyclonal antibodies. Appl Pathol 1987; 5:201–219.

109. Brooks JJ. Immunohistochemistry of soft tissue tumors: Myoglobin as a tumor marker for rhabdomyosarcoma. Cancer 1982; 50:1757–1763.

110. Tsokos M, Howard R, Costa J. Immunohistochemical study of alveolar and embryonal rhabdomyosarcoma. Lab Invest 1983; 48:148–155.

111. Kraevsky NA. Use of immunohistochemical methods in the diagnosis of myogenous tumors. Acta Histochem Suppl 1984; 30:79–80.

112. Hosoi H, Sugimoto T, Hayashi Y, et al. Differential expression of myogenic regulatory genes, Myo-D1 and myogenin, in human rhabdomyosarcoma sublines. Int J Cancer 1992; 50:977–983.

113. Newsholme SJ, Zimmerman DM. Immunohistochemical evaluation of chemically induced rhabdomyosarcomas in rats: Diagnostic utility of Myo-D1. Toxicol Pathol 1997; 25:470–474.

114. Wang NP, Marx J, McNutt MA, et al. Expression of myogenic regulatory proteins (myogenin and Myo-D1) in small blue round cell tumors of childhood. Am J Pathol 1995; 147:1799–1810.

115. Cui S, Hano H, Harada T, et al. Evaluation of new monoclonal anti-Myo-D1 and anti-myogenin antibodies for the diagnosis of rhabdomyosarcoma. Pathol Int 1999; 49:62–68.

116. Dias P, Chen B, Dilday B, et al. Strong immunostaining for myogenin in rhabdomyosarcoma is significantly associated with tumors of the alveolar subclass. Am J Pathol 2000; 156:

399–408.

117. Watanabe K, Kusakabe T, Hoshi N, et al. h-Caldesmon in leiomyosarcoma and tumors with smooth muscle-like differentiation: Its specific expression in the smooth muscle cell tumors. Hum Pathol 1999; 30:392–396.

118. Huber PA. Caldesmon. Int J Biochem Cell Biol 1997; 29:1047–1051.

119. Shiro B, Siegal GP. The use of monoclonal antibodies to S100 protein in diagnostic immunohistochemistry. In: Wick MR, Siegal GP, eds., Monoclonal antibodies in diagnostic immunohistochemistry, New York: Marcel Dekker; 1988:455–503.

120. Fujii T, Machino K, Andoh H, et al. Calcium-dependent control of caldesmon-actin interaction by S100 protein. J Biochem 1990; 107:133–137.

121. Loeffel SC, Gillespie GY, Mirmiran SA, et al. Cellular immunolocalization of S100 protein within fixed tissue sections by monoclonal antibodies. Arch Pathol Lab Med 1985; 109:117–122.

122. Masui F, Ushigome S, Fujii K. Clear cell chondrosarcoma: A pathological and immunohistochemical study. Histo-pathology 1999; 34:447–452.

123. Abramovici LC, Steiner GC, Bonar F. Myxoid chondrosarcoma of soft tissue and bone: A retrospective study of 11 cases. Hum Pathol 1995; 26:1215–1220.

124. Swanson PE, Wick MR. Clear cell sarcoma: An immunohistochemical analysis of six cases and comparison with other epithelioid neoplasms of soft tissue. Arch Pathol Lab Med 1989; 113:55–60.

125. Kahn HJ, Marks A, Thom H, et al. Role of antibody to S100 protein in diagnostic pathology. Am J Clin Pathol 1983; 79:341–347.

126. Van den Berg LH, Sadiq SA, Thomas FP, et al. Characterization of HNK-1 bearing glycoproteins in human peripheral nerve myelin. J Neurosci Res 1990; 25:295–299.

127. Weiss SW, Langloss JM, Enzinger FM. Value of S100 protein in the diagnosis of soft tissue tumors, with particular reference to benign and malignant Schwann cell tumors. Lab Invest 1983; 49:299–308.

128. Hammer JA, O'Shannessy DJ, DeLeon M, et al. Immunoreactivity of PMP22, P0, and other 19 to 28 kD glycoproteins in peripheral nerve myelin of mammals and fish with HNK-1 and related antibodies. J Neurosci Res 1993; 35:546–558.

129. Merkouri E, Matsas R. Monoclonal antibody BM89 recognizes a novel cell surface glycoprotein of the L2/HNK-1 family in the developing mammalian nervous system. Neuroscience 1992; 50:53–68.

130. Vogel M, Kowalewski HJ, Zimmermann H, et al. Association of the HNK-1 epitope with 5-nucleotidase from Tomarmorata (electric ray) electric organ. Biochem J 1991; 278:199–202.

131. Abo T, Balch CM. A differentiation antigen of human NK and killer cells, identified by a monoclonal antibody (HNK-1). J Immunol 1981; 127:1024–1029.

132. Hirose T, Scheithauer BW, Sano T. Perineurial malignant peripheral nerve sheath tumor (MPNST): A clinicopathologic, immunohistochemical, and ultrastructural study of seven cases. Am J Surg Pathol 1998; 22:1368–1378.

133. Swanson PE, Manivel JC, Wick MR. Immunoreactivity for Leu7 in neurofibrosarcoma and other spindle cell sarcomas of soft tissue. Am J Pathol 1987; 126:546–560.

134. Michels S, Swanson PE, Robb JA, et al. Leu7 in small cell neoplasms: An immunohistochemical study. Cancer 1987; 60:2958–2964.

135. Amann G, Zoubek A, Salzer-Kuntschik M, et al. Relation of neural marker expression and EWS gene fusion types in MIC2/CD99-positive tumors of the Ewing family. Hum Pathol 30: 1058–1064.

136. Abe S, Imamura T, Park P, et al. Small round cell type of malignant peripheral nerve sheath tumor. Mod Pathol 1998; 11:747–753.

137. Gardner LJ, Polski JM, Fallon R, et al. Identification of CD56 and CD57 by flow cytometry in Ewing's sarcoma or primitive neuroectodermal tumor. Virchows Arch A 1998; 433:35–40.

138. Sangueza OP, Requena L. Neoplasms with neural differentiation: A review. Part II: Malignant neoplasms. Am J Dermatopathol 1998; 20:89–102.

139. Devaney K, Vinh TN, Sweet DE. Small cell osteosarcoma of bone: An immunohistochemical study with differential diagnostic considerations. Hum Pathol 1993; 24:1211–1225.

140. Pettinato G, Manivel JC, d'Amore ESG, et al. Melanotic neuroectodermal tumor of infancy: A reexamination of a histogenetic problem based on immunohistochemical, flow cytometric, and ultrastructural study of 10 cases. Am J Surg Pathol 1991; 15:233–245.

141. Salzer JL, Holmes WP, Colman DR. The amino acid sequences of the myelin-associated glycoproteins: Homology to the immunoglobulin gene superfamily. J Cell Biol 1987; 104:959–965.

142. Dixit SN, Mainardi CL, Beachey EH, et al. 7S domain constitutes the amino-terminal end of type IV collagen: An immunohistochemical study. Coll Rel Res 1983; 3:263–273.

143. Griffin CA, Emanuel BS, Hansen JR, et al. Human collagen genes encoding basement membrane alpha-1 (IV) and alpha-2 (IV) chains map to the distal long arm of chromosome 13. Proc Natl Acad Sci USA 1987; 84:512–516.

144. Terranova VP, Rohrbach DH, Martin GR. Role of laminin in the attachment of PAM212 (epithelial) cells to basement membrane collagen. Cell 1980; 22:719–726.

145. Foidart JM, Bere EW, Yaar M Jr, et al. Distribution and immunoelectron microscopic localization of laminin, a noncollagenous basement membrane glycoprotein. Lab Invest 1980; 42:336–342.

146. McGarvey ML, Baron-Van Evercooren BV, Kleinman KH, et al. Synthesis and effects of basement membrane components in cultured rat Schwann cells. Dev Biol 1984; 105:18–28.

147. Nigar E, Dervan PA. Quantitative assessment of basement membranes in soft tissue tumors: Computerized image analysis of laminin and type IV collagen. J Pathol 1998; 185:184–187.

148. Ogawa K, Oguchi M, Yamabe H, et al. Distribution of collagen type IV in soft tissue tumors: An immunohistochemical study. Cancer 1986; 58:269–277.

149. d'Ardenne AJ, Kirkpatrick P, Sykes BC. Distribution of laminin, fibronectin, and interstitial collagen type III in soft tissue tumors. J Clin Pathol 1984; 37:895–904.

150. Fischer BE, Thomas KB, Schlokat U, et al. Triplet structure of human von Willebrand factor. Biochem J 1998; 331:483–488.

151. Kaufman RJ, Pipe SW. Regulation of factor VIII expression and activity by von Willebrand factor. Thromb Haemost 1999; 82:201–208.

152. Mukai K, Rosai J. Factor VIII-related antigen: An endothelial marker. In: DeLellis RA, ed. Diagnostic immunohistochemistry. New York: Masson; 1984:243–261.

153. Sehested M, Hou-Jensen K. Factor VIII-related antigen as an endothelial cell marker in benign and malignant diseases. Virchows Arch A 1981; 391:217–225.

154. Ordonez NG, Batsakis JG. Comparison of *Ulex europaeus* I lectin and factor VIII-related antigen in vascular lesions. Arch Pathol Lab Med 1984; 108:129–132.

155. Swanson PE, Wick MR. Immunohistochemical evaluation of vascular neoplasms. Clin Dermatol 1991; 9:243–253.

156. Ramani P, Bradley NJ, Fletcher CDM. QBEND10, a new monoclonal antibody to endothelium: Assessment of its diagnostic utility in paraffin sections. Histopathology 1990; 17:237–242.

157. Traweek ST, Kandalaft PL, Mehta P, et al. The human hematopoietic progenitor cell antigen (CD34) in vascular neoplasms. Am J Clin Pathol 1991; 96:25–31.

158. Sirgi KE, Wick MR, Swanson PE. B72.3 and CD34 immunoreactivity in malignant epithelioid soft tissue tumors: Adjuncts in the recognition of endothelial neoplasms. Am J Surg Pathol 1993; 17:179–185.

159. Miettinen M, Lindenmayer AE, Chanbal A. Endothelial cell markers CD31, CD34, and BNH9 antibody to H- and Y-antigens: Evaluation of their specificity and sensitivity in the diagnosis of vascular tumors and comparison with von Willebrand factor. Mod Pathol 1994; 7:82–90.

160. Natkunam Y, Rouse RV, Zhu S, et al. Immunoblot analysis of CD34 expression in histologically diverse neoplasms. Am J Pathol 2000; 156:21–27.

161. Arber DA, Kandalaft PL, Mehta P, et al. Vimentin-negative epithelioid sarcoma: The value of an immunohistochemical panel that includes CD34. Am J Surg Pathol 1993; 17:302–317.

162. Harvell JD, Kilpatrick SE, White WL. Histologic relations between giant cell fibroblastoma and dermatofibrosarcoma protuberans: CD34 staining showing the spectrum and a simulator. Am J Dermato- pathol 1998; 20:339–345.

163. Templeton SF, Solomon AR Jr. Spindle cell lipoma is strongly CD34-positive: An immunohistochemical study. J Cutan Pathol 1996; 23:546–550.

164. Hasegawa T, Matsuno Y, Shimoda T, et al. Extrathoracic solitary fibrous tumors: Their histological variability and potentially aggressive behavior. Hum Pathol 1999; 30:1464–1473.

165. Metzelaar MJ, Korteweg J, Sizma JJ, et al. Biochemical characterization of PECAM-1 (CD31 antigen) on human platelets. Thromb Haemost 1991; 66:700–707.

166. Parums DV, Cordell JL, Michlein K, et al. JC70: A new monoclonal antibody that detects vascular endothelium associated antigen on routinely processed tissue sections. J Clin Pathol 1990; 43:752–757.

167. Ohsawa M, Naka N, Tomita Y, et al. Use of immunohistochemical procedures in diagnosing angiosarcomas: Evaluation of 98 cases. Cancer 1995; 75:2867–2874.

168. DeYoung BR, Wick MR, Fitzgibbon JF, et al. CD31: An immunospecific marker for endothelial differentiation in human neoplasms. Appl Immunohistochem 1993; 1:97–100.

169. DeYoung BR, Swanson PE, Argenyi ZB, et al. CD31 immunoreactivity in mesenchymal neoplasms of the skin and subcutis. J Cutan Pathol 1995; 22:215–222.

170. Takahashi Y, Hosaka Y, Niina H, et al. Soluble thrombomodulin purified from human urine exhibits a potent anticoagulant effect in vitro and in vivo. Thromb Haemost 1995; 73:805–811.

171. Kurosawa S, Galvin JB, Esmon NC, et al. Proteolytic formation and properties of functional domains of thrombomodulin. J Biol Chem 1987; 262:2206–2212.

172. Karmochkine M, Boffa MC. Thrombomodulin: Physiology and clinical applications. Rev Med Interne 1997; 18:119–125.

173. Yonezawa S, Maruyama I, Sakae K, et al. Thrombomodulin as a marker for vascular tumors: Comparative study with factor VIII and *Ulex europaeus* I lectin. Am J Clin Pathol 1987; 88:405–411.

174. Kim SJ, Shiba E, Ishii H, et al. Thrombomodulin is a new biological and prognostic marker for breast cancer: An immunohistochemical study. Anticancer Res 1997; 17:2319–2323.

175. Ordonez NG. Value of thrombomodulin immunostaining in the diagnosis of mesothelioma. Histopathology 1997; 31:25–30.

176. Appleton MA, Attanoos RL, Jasani B. Thrombomodulin as a marker of vascular and lymphatic tumors. Histopathology 1996; 29:153–157.

177. Zhang YM, Bachmann S, Hemmer C, et al. Vascular origin of Kaposi's sarcoma: Expression of leukocytic adhesion molecule-1, thrombomodulin, and tissue factor. Am J Pathol 1994; 144:51–59.

178. Holthofer H, Virtanen I, Kariniemi AL, et al. Ulex europaeus I lectin as a marker for vascular endothelium in human tissues. Lab Invest 1982; 47:60–66.

179. Leader M, Collins M, Patel J, et al. Staining for factor VIII-related antigen and *Ulex europaeus* I (UEA-I) in 230 tumors: An assessment of their specificity for angiosarcoma and Kaposi's sarcoma. Histopathology 1986; 10:1153–1162.

180. Wick MR, Manivel JC. Epithelioid sarcoma and epithelioid hemangioendothelioma: An immunohistochemical and lectin-histochemical comparison. Virchows Arch A 1987; 410:309–316.

181. DuBoulay CEH. Demonstration of alpha-1-antitrypsin and alpha-1-antichymotrypsin in fibrous histiocytomas using the immunoperoxidase technique. Am J Surg Pathol 1982; 6:559–564.

182. Kindblom LG, Jacobsen GK, Jacobsen M. Immunohistochemical investigations of tumors of supposed fibroblastic-histiocytic origin. Hum Pathol 1982; 13:834–840.

183. Meister P, Nathrath W. Immunohistochemical characterization of histiocytic tumors. Diagn Histopathol 1981; 4:79–87.

184. Pulford KAF, Rigney EM, Micklem KJ, et al. KP1: A new monoclonal antibody that detects a monocyte/macrophage-associated antigen in routinely processed tissue sections. J Clin Pathol 1989; 42:414–421.

185. Gloghini A, Volpe R, Carbone A. Ki-M6 immunos-taining in routinely processed sections of reactive and neoplastic human lymphoid tissue. Am J Clin Pathol 1990; 94:734–741.

186. Gown AM, Tsukada T, Ross R. Human atherosclerosis. II: Immunocytochemical analysis of the cellular composition of human atherosclerotic lesions. Am J Pathol 1986; 125:191–207.

187. Takeya M, Yamashiro S, Yoshimura T, et al. Immunophenotypic and immunoelectron microscopic characterization of major constituent cells in malignant fibrous histiocytoma using human cell lines and their transplanted tumors in immunodeficient mice. Lab Invest 1995; 72:679–688.

188. Nemes Z, Thomazy V. Factor XIIIa and the classic histiocytic markers in malignant fibrous histiocytoma: A comparative immunohistochemical study. Hum Pathol 1988; 19:822–829.

189. Lau SK, Chu PG, Weiss LM. CD163: a specific marker of macrophages in paraffin-embedded tissue samples. Am J Clin Pathol 2004; 122:794–801.

190. Reid MB, Gray C, Fear JD, et al. Immunohistologic demonstration of factors XIIIa and XIIIs in reactive and neoplastic

fibroblastic and fibrohistiocytic lesions. Histopathology 1986; 10:1171–1178.
191. Thewes M, Engst R, Boeck K, et al. Expression of cathepsins in dermal fibrous tumors: An immunohistochemical study. Eur J Dermatol 1998; 8:86–89.
192. Gloghini A, Rizzo A, Zanette I, et al. KP1/CD68 expression in malignant neoplasms including lymphomas, sarcomas, and carcinomas. Am J Clin Pathol 1995; 103:425–431.
193. Doussis IA, Gatter KC, Mason DY. CD68 reactivity of non-macrophage-derived tumors in cytological specimens. J Clin Pathol 1993; 46:334–336.
194. Schulz A, Loreth B, Battmann A, et al. Bone matrix production in osteosarcoma. Verh Dtsch Ges Pathol 1998; 82:144–153.
195. Park YK, Yang MH, Kim YW, et al. Osteocalcin expression in primary bone tumors: In situ hybridization and immunohistochemical study. J Korean Med Sci 1995; 10:263–268.
196. Lian JB, Stein GS. Development of the osteoblast phenotype: Molecular mechanisms mediating osteoblast growth and development. Iowa Orthop J 1995; 15:118–140.
197. Tamura T, Noda M. Identification of a DNA sequence involved in osteoblast-specific gene expression via interaction with helix-loop-helix (HLH)-type transcription factors. J Cell Biol 1994; 126:773–782.
198. Garnero P, Grimaux M, Seguin P, et al. Characterization of immunoreactive forms of human osteocalcin generated in vivo and in vitro. J Bone Miner Res 1994; 9:255–264.
199. Mahonen A, Jaaskelainen T, Maenpaa PH. A novel vitamin D analog with two double bonds in its side chain: A potent inducer of osteoblastic cell differentiation. Biochem Pharmacol 1996; 51:887–892.
200. Arbour NC, Darwish HM, DeLuca HF. Transcriptional control of the osteocalcin gene by 1/25 dihydroxyvitamin D-2 and its 24-epimer in rat osteosarcoma cells. Biochim Biophys Acta 1995; 1263:147–153.
201. Bradbeer JN, Virdi AS, Serre CM, et al. A number of osteocalcin antisera recognize epitopes on proteins other than osteocalcin in cultured skin fibroblasts: Implications for the identification of cells of the osteoblastic lineage in vitro. J Bone Miner Res 1994; 9:1221–1228.
202. Takada J, Ishii S, Ohta T, et al. Usefulness of a novel monoclonal antibody against human osteocalcin in immunohistochemical diagnosis. Virchows Arch A 1992; 420:507–511.
203. Fanburg JC, Rosenberg AE, Weaver DL, et al. Osteocalcin and osteonectin immunoreactivity in the diagnosis of osteosarcoma. Am J Clin Pathol 1997; 108:464–473.
204. Fanburg-Smith JC, Bratthauer GL, Miettinen M. Osteo-calcin and osteonectin immunoreactivity in extraskeletal osteosarcoma: A study of 28 cases. Hum Pathol 1999; 30:32–38.
205. Naylor SL, Helin-Davies D, Charoenworawat P, et al. The human osteonectin gene (OSN) has Taq I and Msp I polymorphisms. Nucleic Acids Res 1989; 17:6753.
206. Rodan GA, Noda M. Gene expression in osteoblastic cells. Crit Rev Eukaryot Gene Expr 1991; 1:85–98.
207. Villarreal XC, Grant BW, Long GL. Demonstration of osteonectin mRNA in megakaryocytes: The use of the polymerase chain reaction. Blood 1991; 78:1216–1222.
208. Kelm RJ Jr, Hair GA, Mann KG, et al. Characterization of human osteoblast and megakaryocyte-derived osteonectin (SPARC). Blood 1992; 80:3112–3119.
209. Kamihagi K, Katayama M, Ouchi R, et al. Osteonectin/SPARC regulates cellular secretion rates of fibronectin and laminin extracellular matrix proteins. Biochem Biophys Res Commun 1994; 200:423–428.
210. Serra M, Morini MC, Scotlandi K, et al. Evaluation of osteonectin as a diagnostic marker of osteogenic bone tumors. Hum Pathol 1992; 23:1326–1331.
211. Wuisman P, Roessner A, Bosse A, et al. Osteonectin in osteosarcomas: A marker for differential diagnosis and/or prognosis? Ann Oncol 1992; 3(Suppl 2):S33–S35.
212. Bosse A, Vollmer E, Bocker W, et al. The impact of osteonectin for differential diagnosis of bone tumors: An immunohistochemical approach. Pathol Res Pract 1990; 186: 651–657.
213. Fetsch PA, Marincola FM, Filie A, et al. Melanoma-associated antigen recognized by T-cells (MART-1): The advent of a preferred immunocytochemical antibody for the diagnosis of metastatic malignant melanoma with fine needle aspiration. Cancer 1999; 87:37–42.
214. Kaufmann O, Koch S, Burghardt J, et al. Tyrosinase, melan-A, and KBA62 as markers for the immunohistochemical identification of metastatic amelanotic melanomas in paraffin sections. Mod Pathol 1998; 11:740–746.
215. Zelger BG, Steiner H, Wambacher B, et al. Malignant melanomas simulating various types of soft tissue tumors.

Dermatol Surg 1997; 23:1047–1054.
216. Fetsch JF, Michal M, Miettinen M. Pigmented (melanotic) neurofibroma: A clinicopathologic and immunohistochemical analysis of 19 lesions from 17 patients. Am J Surg Pathol 2000; 24:331–343.
217. Cangul IT, van Garderen E, Van der Poel HJ, et al. Tyrosinase gene expression in clear cell sarcoma indicates a melanocytic origin: Insight from the first reported canine case. APMIS 1999; 107:982–988.
218. Papas-Corden P, Zarbo RJ, Gown AM, et al. Immunohistochemical characterization of synovial, epithelioid, and clear cell sarcomas. Surg Pathol 1989; 2:43–58.
219. Gould VE, Wiedenmann B, Lee I, et al. Synaptophysin expression in neuroendocrine neoplasms as determined by immunocytochemistry. Am J Pathol 1987; 126:243–257.
220. Ladanyi M, Heinemann FS, Huvos AG, et al. Neural differentiation in small round cell tumors of bone and soft tissue with the translocation t(11;22)(q24]2): An immunohistochemical study of 11 cases. Hum Pathol 1990; 21:1245–1251.
221. Parham DM, Hijazi Y, Steinberg SM, et al. Neuroectodermal differentiation in Ewing's sarcoma family of tumors does not predict tumor behavior. Hum Pathol 1999; 30:911–918.
222. Roessner A, Jurgens H. Round cell tumors of bone. Pathol Res Pract 1993; 189:111–136.
223. Dierick AM, Roels H, Langlois M. The immunophenotype of Ewing's sarcoma: An immunohistochemical analysis. Pathol Res Pract 1993; 189:26-32.
224. Wang AR, May D, Bourne P, et al. PGP9.5: A marker for cellular neurothekeoma. Am J Surg Pathol 1999; 23:1401–1407.
225. Miettinen M, Chatten J, Paetau A, et al. Monoclonal antibody NB84 in the differential diagnosis of neuroblastoma and other small round cell tumors. Am J Surg Pathol 1998; 22: 327–332.
226. Gerbig AW, Zala L, Hunziker T. Tumor-like eosinophilic granuloma of the skin. Am J Dermatopathol 2000; 22:75–78.
227. Stefanato CM, Andersen WK, Calonje E, et al. Langerhans cell histiocytosis in the elderly: A report of three cases. J Am Acad Dermatol 1998; 39:375–378.
228. Knowles DM II. Lymphoid cell markers: Their distribution and usefulness in the immunopathologic analysis of lymphoid neoplasms. Am J Surg Pathol 1985; 9(Suppl):85–108.
229. Weiss LM, Bindl JM, Picozzi VJ, et al. Lymphoblastic lymphoma: An immunophenotypic study of 26 cases with comparison to T-cell acute lymphoblastic leukemia. Blood 1986; 67:474–478.
230. Picker LJ, Weiss LM, Medeiros LJ, et al. Immunophenotypic criteria for the diagnosis of non-Hodgkin's lymphoma. Am J Pathol 1987; 128:181–201.
231. Orosz Z, Kopper L. Syndecan-1 expression in different soft tissue tumors. Anticancer Res 2001; 21:733–737.
232. Ozdemirli M, Fanburg-Smith JC, Hartmann DP, et al. Precursor B-lymphoblastic lymphoma presenting as a solitary bone tumor and mimicking Ewing's sarcoma: A report of four cases and review of the literature. Am J Surg Pathol 1998; 22:795–804.
233. Petruch UR, Horny HP, Kaiserling E. Frequent expression of hematopoietic and non-hematopoietic antigens by neoplastic plasma cells: An immunohistochemical study using formalin-fixed, paraffin-embedded tissue. Histopathology 1992; 20:35–40.
234. Robertson PB, Neiman RS, Worapongpaiboon S, et al. O13 (CD99) positivity in hematologic proliferations correlates with TdT positivity. Mod Pathol 1997; 10:277–282.
235. Soslow RA, Bhargava V, Warnke RA. MIC2, TdT, bcl-2, and CD34 expression in paraffin-embedded high-grade lymphoma/acute lymphoblastic leukemia distinguishes between distinct clinicopathologic entities. Hum Pathol 1997; 28:1158–1165.
236. Hibshoosh H, Lattes R. Immunohistochemical and molecular genetic approaches to soft tissue tumor diagnosis: A primer. Semin Oncol 1997; 24:515–525.
237. Smith MJ, Goodfellow PN. MIC2R: A transcribed MIC2-related sequence associated with a CpG island in the human pseudoautosomal region. Hum Mol Genet 1994; 3:1575–1582.
238. Smith MJ, Goodfellow PJ, Goodfellow PN. The genomic organization of the human pseudoautosomal gene MIC2 and the detection of a related locus. Hum Mol Genet 1993; 2: 417–422.
239. Fellinger EJ, Garin-Chesa P, Su SL, et al. Biochemical and genetic characterization of the HBA-71 Ewing's sarcoma cell surface antigen. Cancer Res 1991; 51:336–340.
240. Amann G, Zoubek A, Salzer-Kuntschik M, et al. Relation of neurological marker expression and EWS gene fusion types

in MIC2/CD99-positive tumors of the Ewing family. Hum Pathol 1999; 30:1058–1064.
241. Renshaw AA. O13 (CD99) in spindle cell tumors: Reactivity with hemangiopericytoma, solitary fibrous tumor, synovial sarcoma, and meningioma, but rarely with sarcomatoid mesothelioma. Appl Immunohistochem 1995; 3:250–256.
242. Soslow RA, Wallace M, Goris J, et al. MIC2 gene expression in cutaneous neuroendocrine carcinoma (Merkel cell carcinoma). Appl Immunohistochem 1996; 4:235–240.
243. Lumadue JA, Askin FB, Perlman EJ. MIC2 analysis of small cell carcinoma. Am J Clin Pathol 1994; 102:692–694.
244. Nicholson SA, McDermott MB, Swanson PE, et al. CD99 and cytokeratin-20 in small-cell and basaloid tumors of the skin. Appl Immunohistochem Mol Morphol 2000; 8:37–41.
245. Shiota M, Fujimoto J, Semba T, et al. Hyperphosphorylation of a novel 80 kDa protein-tyrosine kinase similar to Ltk in a human Ki-lymphoma cell line, AMS3. Oncogene 1994; 9: 1567–1574.
246. Cessna MH, Zhou H, Sanger WG, et al. Expression of ALK-1 and p80 in inflammatory myofibroblastic tumor and its mesenchymal mimics: a study of 135 cases. Mod Pathol 2002; 15:931–938.
247. Sigel JE, Smith TA, Reith JD, et al. Immunohistochemical analysis of anaplastic lymphoma kinase expression in deep soft tissue calcifying fibrous pseudotumor: evidence of a late sclerosing stage of inflammatory myofibroblastic tumor? Ann Diagn Pathol 2001; 5:10–14.
248. Li XQ, Hisaoka M, Shi DR, et al. Expression of anaplastic lymphoma kinase in soft tissue tumors: an immunohistochemical and molecular study of 249 cases. Hum Pathol 2004; 35:711–721.
249. Eckert F, Schaich B. Tendon sheath fibroma: A case report with immunohistochemical studies. Hautarzt 1992; 43:92–96.
250. Ide F, Shimoyama T, Horie N, et al. Collagenous fibroma (desmoplastic fibroblastoma) presenting as a parotid mass. J Oral Pathol Med 1999; 28:465–468.
251. Neilsen GP, O'Connell JX, Dickersin GR, et al. Collagenous fibroma (desmoplastic fibroblastoma): A report of seven cases. Mod Pathol 1996; 9:781–785.
252. Sciot R, Samson I, van der Berghe H, et al. Collagenous fibroma (desmoplastic fibroblastoma): Genetic link with fibroma of tendon sheath? Mod Pathol 1999; 12:565–568.
253. Carney JA. Psammomatous melanotic schwannoma: A distinctive, heritable tumor with special associations, including cardiac myxoma and the Cushing syndrome. Am J Surg Pathol 1990; 14:206–222.
254. Fine SW, McClain SA, Li M. Immunohistochemical staining for calretinin is useful for differentiating schwannomas from neurofibromas. Am J Clin Pathol 2004; 122:552–559.
255. Templeton SF, Solomon AR Jr. Spindle cell lipoma is strongly CD34 positive: An immunohistochemical study. J Cutan Pathol 1996; 23:546–550.
256. Suster S, Fisher C. Immunoreactivity for the human hematopoietic progenitor cell antigen (CD34) in lipomatous tumors. Am J Surg Pathol 1997; 21:195–200.
257. Shimokama T, Watanabe T. Leiomyoma exhibiting a marked granular change: Granular cell leiomyoma versus granular cell schwannoma. Hum Pathol 1992; 23:327–331.
258. Mazur MT, Shultz JJ, Myers JL. Granular cell tumor: Immunohistochemical analysis of 21 benign tumors and one malignant tumor. Arch Pathol Lab Med 1990; 114:692–696.
259. Cavaliere A, Sidoni A, Ferri I, et al. Granular cell tumor: An immunohistochemical study. Tumori 1994; 80:224–228.
260. Kurtin PJ, Bonin DM. Immunohistochemical demonstration of the lysosome-associated glycoprotein CD68 (KP-1) in granular cell tumors and schwannomas. Hum Pathol 1994; 25:1172–1178.
261. Filie AC, Lage JM, Azumi N. Immunoreactivity of S100 protein, alpha-1-antitrypsin, and CD68 in adult and congenital granular cell tumors. Mod Pathol 1996; 9:888–892.
262. Fine SW, Li M. Expression of calretinin and the alpha-subunit of inhibin in granular cell tumors. Am J Clin Pathol 2003; 119:259–264.
263. Younes M, Lechago LV, Lechago J. Overexpression of the human erythrocyte glucose transporter occurs as a late event in human colorectal carcinogenesis and is associated with an increased incidence of lymph node metastases. Clin Cancer Res 1996; 2:1151–1154.
264. Haber RS, Weiser KR, Pritsker A, et al. GLUT1 glucose transporter expression in benign and malignant thyroid nodules. Thyroid 1997; 7:363–367.
265. North PE, Waner M, Mizeracki A, et al. GLUT1: A newly discovered immunohistochemical marker for juvenile hemangiomas. Hum Pathol 2000; 31:11–22.
266. Younes M, Brown RW, Stephenson M, et al. Overexpression

of Glut1 and Glut3 in stage I nonsmall cell lung cancer is associated with poor survival. Cancer 1997; 80:1046–1051.
267. Sato Y. Role of ETS family transcription factors in vascular development and angiogenesis. Cell Struc Funct 2001; 26:19–24.
268. Folpe AL, Chand EM, Goldblum JR, et al. Expression of FLI-1, a nuclear transcription factor, distinguishes vascular neoplasms from potential mimics. Am J Surg Pathol 2001; 25:1061–1066.
269. Rossi S, Orvieto E, Furlanetto A, et al. Utility of the immunohistochemical detection of FLI-1 expression in round cell and vascular neoplasms using a monoclonal antibody. Mod Pathol 2004; 17:547–552.
270. Lelievre E, Lionneton F, Mattot V, et al. Ets-1 regulates FLI-1 expression in endothelial cells: identification of ETS binding sites in the FLI-1 gene promoter. J Biol Chem 2002; 277:25143–25151.
271. Kapadia SB, Meis JM, Frisman DM, et al. Fetal rhabdomyoma of the head and neck: A clinicopathological and immunophenotypic study of 24 cases. Hum Pathol 1993; 24:754–765.
272. Tanda F, Rocca PC, Bosincu L, et al. Rhabdomyomas of the tunica vaginalis of the testis: A histologic, immunohistochemical, and ultrastructural study. Mod Pathol 1997;10:608–611.
273. Bastian BC, Brocker EB. Adult rhabdomyoma of the lip. Am J Dermatopathol 1998; 20:61–64.
274. Gibas Z, Miettinen M. Recurrent parapharyngeal rhabdomyoma: Evidence of neoplastic nature of the tumor from cytogenetic study. Am J Surg Pathol 1192; 16:721–728.
275. Ockner DM, Sayadi H, Swanson SE, et al. Genital angiomyofibroblastoma: Comparison with aggressive angiomyxoma and other myxoid neoplasms of skin and soft tissue. Am J Clin Pathol 1997; 107:36–44.
276. Fletcher CDM, Tsang WTW, Fisher C, et al. Angiomyofibroblastoma of the vulva: A benign neoplasm distinct from aggressive angiomyxoma. Am J Surg Pathol 1992; 16:373–382.
277. Neilsen GP, Rosenberg AE, Young RH, et al. Angiomyofibroblastoma of the vulva and vagina. Mod Pathol 1996; 9:284–291.
278. Granter SR, Nucci MR, Fletcher CD. Aggressive angiomyxoma: Reappraisal of its relationship to angiomyofibroblastoma in a series of 16 cases. Histopathology 1997; 30:3–10.
279. Laskin WB, Fetsch JF, Tavassoli FA. Angiomyofibroblastoma of the female genital tract: Analysis of 17 cases including a lipomatous variant. Hum Pathol 1997; 28:1046–1055.
280. Enzinger FM, Weiss SW. Fibrous tumors of infancy and childhood. In: Enzinger FM, Weiss SW, eds. Soft tissue tumors, 2nd edn. St Louis: Mosby-Yearbook; 1995:722.
281. Nemes Z. Differentiation markers in hemangiopericytoma. Cancer 1992; 69:133–140.
282. Molnar P, Nemes Z. Hemangiopericytoma of the cerebellopontine angle: Diagnostic pitfalls and the diagnostic value of the subunit A of factor XIII as a tumor marker. Clin Neuropathol 1995; 14:19–24.
283. Catalano PJ, Brandwein M, Shah DK, et al. Sinonasal hemangiopericytomas: A clinicopathologic and immunohistochemical study of seven cases. Head Neck 1996; 18: 42–53.
284. Middleton LP, Duray PH, Merino MJ. The histological spectrum of hemangiopericytoma: Application of immunohistochemical analysis including proliferative markers to facilitate diagnosis and predict prognosis. Hum Pathol 1998; 29:636–640.
285. Klempreer P, Rabin CB. Primary neoplasms of the pleura: A report of five cases. Arch Pathol 1931;1 1:385–412.
286. Hanau CA, Miettinen M. Solitary fibrous tumor: Histological and immunohistochemical spectrum of benign and malignant variants presenting at different sites. Hum Pathol 1995; 26:440–449.
287. Hasegawa T, Matsuno Y, Shimoda T, et al. Frequent expression of bcl-2 protein in solitary fibrous tumors. Jpn J Clin Oncol 1998; 28:86–91.
288. Brunnemann RB, Ro JY, Ordonez NG, et al. Extrapleural solitary fibrous tumor: A clinicopathologic study of 24 cases. Mod Pathol 1999; 12:1034–1042.
289. de Saint Aubain Somerhausen N, Rubin BP, Fletcher CD. Myxoid solitary fibrous tumor: A study of seven cases with emphasis on differential diagnosis. Mod Pathol 1999; 12:463–471.
290. Matsumoto K, Yamamoto T, Min W, et al. Ossifying fibromyxoid tumor of soft parts: Clinicopathologic, immunohistochemical and ultrastructural study of four cases. Pathol Int 1999; 49:742–746.

291. Ekfors TO, Kulju T, Aaltonen M, et al. Ossifying fibromyxoid tumour of soft parts: Report of four cases including one mediastinal and one infanile. APMIS 1998; 106:1124–1130.

292. Yang P, Hirose T, Hasegawa T, et al. Ossifying fibromyxoid tumor of soft parts: A morphological and immunohistochemical study. Pathol Int 1994; 44:448–453.

293. Miettinen M. Ossifying fibromyxoid tumor of soft parts: Additional observations of a distinctive soft tissue tumor. Am J Clin Pathol 1991; 95:142–149.

294. Fukunaga M, Ushigome S, Ishikawa E. Ossifying subcutaneous tumor with myofibroblastic differentiation: A variant of ossifying fibromyxoid tumor of soft parts? Pathol Int 1994; 44:727–734.

295. Schofield JB, Krausz T, Stamp GW, et al. Ossifying fibromyxoid tumour of soft parts: Immunohistochemical and ultrastructural analysis. Histopathology 1999; 22:101–112.

296. Williams SB, Ellis GL, Meis JM, et al. Ossifying fibromyxoid tumour (of soft parts) of the head and neck: A clinicopathological and immunohistochemical study of nine cases. J Laryngol Otol 1993; 107:75–80.

297. Folpe AL, Weiss SW. Ossifying fibromyxoid tumor of soft parts: a clinicopathologic study of 70 cases with emphasis on atypical and malignant variants. Am J Surg Pathol 2003; 27:421–431.

298. Hamakawa H, Omori T, Sumida T, et al. Intraosseous epithelioid hemangioendothelioma of the mandible: A case report with an immunohistochemical study. J Oral Pathol Med 1999; 28:233–237.

299. Siddiqui MT, Evans HL, Ro JY, et al. Epithelioid haemangioendothelioma of the thyroid gland: A case report and review of literature. Histopathology 1998; 32:473–476.

300. Gray MH, Rosenberg AE, Dickerson GR, et al. Cytokeratin expression in epithelioid vascular neoplasms. Hum Pathol 1990; 21:212–217.

301. Van Haelst UJ, Pruszczynski M, ten Cate LN, et al. Ultrastructural and immunohistochemical study of epithelioid hemangioendothelioma of bone: Coexpression of epithelial and endothelial markers. Ultrastruct Pathol 1990; 14:141–149.

302. Mentzel T, Beham A, Calonje E, et al. Epithelioid hemangioendothelioma of skin and soft tissues: Clinicopathologic and immunohistochemical study of 30 cases. Am J Surg Pathol 1997; 21:363–374.

303. Billings SD, Folpe AL, Weiss SW. Epithelioid sarcoma-like hemangioendothelioma. Am J Surg Pathol 2003; 27:48–57.

304. Zukerberg LR, Nickoloff BJ, Weisee SW. Kaposiform hemangioendothelioma of infancy and childhood: An aggressive neoplasm associated with Kasaback-Merritt syndrome and lymphangiomatosis. Am J Surg Pathol 1993; 17:321–328.

305. Mentzel T, Mazzoleni G, Dei Tos AP, et al. Kaposiform hemangioendothelioma in adults. Clinicopathologic and immunohistochemical analysis of three cases. Am J Clin Pathol 1997; 108:450–455.

306. Lyons LL, North PE, MacMoune-Lai F, et al. Kaposiform hemangioendothelioma: a study of 33 cases emphasizing its pathologic, immunophenotypic, and biologic uniqueness from juvenile hemangioma. Am J Surg Pathol 2004; 28:559–568.

307. Folpe AL, Veikkola T, Valtola R, et al. Vascular endothelial growth factor receptor-3 (VEGFR-3): a marker of vascular tumors with presumed lymphatic differentiation, including Kaposi's sarcoma, kaposiform and Dabska-type hemangioendotheliomas, and a subset of angiosarcomas. Mod Pathol 2000; 13:180–185.

308. Begin LR, Clement PB, Kirk ME, et al. Aggressive angiomyxoma of pelvic soft parts: A clinicopathologic study of nine cases. Hum Pathol 1985; 16:621–628.

309. Sementa AR, Gambini C, Borgiani L, et al. Aggressive angiomyxoma of the pelvis and perineum: Report of a case with immunohistochemical and electron microscopic study. Pathologica 1989; 81:463–469.

310. Ockner DM, Sayadi H, Swanson PE, et al. Genital angiomyofibroblastoma. Comparison with aggressive angiomyxoma and other myxoid neoplasms of skin and soft tissue. Am J Clin Pathol 1997; 107:36–44.

311. Tsang WY, Chan JK, Lee KC, et al. Aggressive angiomyxoma: A report of four cases occurring in men. Am J Surg Pathol 1992; 16:1059–1065.

312. Tallini G, Parham DM, Dias P, et al. Myogenic regulatory protein expression in adult soft tissue sarcomas: A sensitive and specific marker of skeletal muscle differentiation. Am J Pathol 1994; 144:693–701.

313. Dias P, Parham DM, Shapiro DN, et al. Myogenic regulatory protein (MyoD1) expression in childhood solid tumors: Diagnostic utility in rhabdomyosarcoma. Am J Pathol 1990; 13:1283–1291.

314. Sorensen PH, Shimada H, Liu XF, et al. Biphenotypic sarcomas with myogenic and neural differentiation express the

Ewing's sarcoma EWS/FLI1 fusion gene. Cancer Res 1995; 15:1385–1392.

315. Gattenlohner S, Muller-Hernelink HK, Marx A. Polymerase chain reaction-based diagnosis of rhabdomyosarcomas: Comparison of fetal type acetylcholine receptor subunits and myogenin. Diagn Mol Pathol 1998; 7:129–134.

316. Meyer T, Brinck U. Immunohistochemical detection of vinculin in human rhabdomyosarcomas. Gen Diagn Pathol 1997; 142:191–198.

317. Pinto A, Paslawski D, Sarnat HB, et al. Immunohistochemical evaluation of dystrophin expression in small round cell tumors of childhood. Mod Pathol 1993; 6:679–683.

318. Bowman F, Champigneulle J, Schmitt C, et al. Clear cell rhabdomyosarcoma. Pediatr Pathol Lab Med 1996; 16:951–959.

319. Kobayshi M, Sjoberg G, Soderhall S, et al. Pediatric rhabdomyosarcomas express the intermediate filament nestin. Pediatr Res 1998; 43:86–92.

320. Yun K. A new marker for rhabdomyosarcoma: Insulin-like growth factor II. Lab Invest 1992; 67:653–664.

321. Gattenlohner S, Vincent A, Leuschner I, et al. The fetal form of the acetylcholine receptor distinguished rhabdomyosarcomas from other childhood tumors. Am J Pathol 1998; 152:437–444.

322. Molenaar WM, Muntinghe FL. Expression of neural adhesion molecules and neurofilament protein isoforms in skeletal muscle tumors. Hum Pathol 1998; 29:1290–1293.

323. Coffin CM, Rulon J, Smith L, et al. Pathologic features of rhabdomyosarcoma before and after treatment: A clinicopathologic and immunohistochemical analysis. Mod Pathol 1997; 10:1175–1187.

324. Navarro S, Cavazzana AO, Llombart-Bosch A, et al. Comparison of Ewing's sarcoma of bone and peripheral neuroepithelioma: An immunocytochemical and ultrastructural analysis of two primitive neuroectodermal neoplasms. Arch Pathol Lab Med 1994; 118:608–615.

325. Lizard-Nacol S, Justrabo E, Mugneret F, et al. Immuno-cytologic study of light cell lines established in vitro from Ewing's sarcoma: Identification of neural markers. C R Seances Soc Biol Fil 1988; 182:118–125.

326. Lee CS, Southey MC, Waters K, et al. EWS/FLI-1 fusion transcript detection and MIC2 immunohistochemical staining in the detection of Ewing's sarcoma. Pediatr Pathol Lab Med 1996; 16:379–392.

327. Scotlandi K, Serra M, Manara MC, et al. Immunostaining of the p30/32MIC2 antigen and molecular detection of EWS rearrangements for the diagnosis of Ewing's sarcoma and peripheral neuroectodermal tumor. Hum Pathol 1996; 27:408–416.

328. de Alava E, Lozano MD, Sola I, et al. Molecular features in a biphenotypic small cell sarcoma with neuroectodermal and muscle differentiation. Hum Pathol 1998; 29:181–184.

329. Knezevich SR, Hendson G, Methers JA, et al. Absence of detectable EWS/FLI1 expression after therapy-induced neural differentiation in Ewing sarcoma. Hum Pathol 1997; 29:289–294.

330. Ambros IM, Ambros PF, Strehl S, et al. MIC2 is a specific marker for Ewing's sarcoma and peripheral primitive neuroectodermal tumors: Evidence for a common histogenesis of Ewing's sarcoma and peripheral primitive neuroectodermal tumors from MIC2 expression and specific chromosome aberration. Cancer 1991; 67:1886–1893.

331. Fellinger EJ, Garin-Chesa P, Triche TJ, et al. Immunohistochemical analysis of Ewing's sarcoma cell surface antigen p30/32MIC2. Am J Pathol 1991; 139:317–325.

332. Halliday BE, Slagel DD, Elsheikh TE, et al. Diagnostic utility of MIC-2 immunocytochemical staining in the differential diagnosis of small blue cell tumors. Diagn Cytopathol 1998; 19:410–416.

333. Miettinen M, Lehto VP, Virtanen J. Histogenesis of Ewing's sarcoma: An evaluation of intermediate filaments and endothelial cell markers. Virchows Arch Cell Pathol 1988; 41:277.

334. Navas-Palacios JJ, Aparicio-Duque R, Valdes MD. On the histogenesis of Ewing's sarcoma: An ultrastructural, immunohistochemical, and cytochemical study. Cancer 1984; 53:1882.

335. Gu M, Antonescu CR, Guiter G, et al. Cytokeratin immunoreactivity in Ewing's sarcoma: Prevalence in 50 cases confirmed by molecular diagnostic studies. Am J Surg Pathol 1999; 24;410–416.

336. Barth T, Moller P, Mechtersheimer G. Differential expression of beta 1, beta 3, beta 4 integrins in sarcomas of the small round blue cell category. Virchows Arch 1995; 426:19–25.

337. Chung DH, Lee JI, Kook MC, et al. ILK (beta 1 integrin-linked protein kinase): A novel immunohistochemical marker

338. Swanson PE, Lillemoe TJ, Manivel JC, et al. Mesenchymal chondrosarcoma: An immunohistochemical study. Arch Pathol Lab Med 1990; 114:943–948.
339. Kurotaki H, Tateoka H, Takeuchi M, et al. Primary mesenchymal chondrosarcoma of the lung: A case report with immunohistochemical and ultrastructural features. Acta Pathol Jpn 1992; 42:364–371.
340. Rushing EJ, Armonda RA, Ansari Q, et al. Mesenchymal chondrosarcoma: A clinicopathologic and flow cytometric study of 13 cases presenting in the central nervous system. Cancer 1996; 77:1884–1891.
341. Brown RE, Boyle JL. Mesenchymal chondrosarcoma: molecular characterization by a proteomic approach, with morphogenic and therapeutic implications. Ann Clin Lab Sci 2003; 33:131–141.
342. Granter SR, Renshaw AA, Fletcher CD, et al. CD99 reactivity in mesenchymal chondrosarcoma. Hum Pathol 1996; 27:1273–1276.
343. Lyon DB, Dortzbach RK, Gilbert-Barness E. Polyphenotypic small-cell orbitocranial tumor. Arch Ophthalmol 1991; 111:1402–1408.
344. Pearson JM, Harris M, Eyden BP, et al. Divergent differentiation in small round-cell tumours of the soft tissues with neural features – an analysis of 10 cases. Histopathology 1993; 23:1–9.
345. Frydman CP, Klein MJ, Abdelwahab IF, et al. Primitive multipotential primary sarcoma of bone: A case report and immunohistochemical study. Mod Pathol 1991; 4:768–772.
346. Gerald WL, Ladanyi M, de Alava E, et al. Clinical, pathologic, and molecular spectrum of tumors associated with t(11;22)(p13]2): Desmoplastic small round-cell tumor and its variants. J Clin Oncol 1998; 16:3028–3036.
347. Katz RL, Quezado M, Senderowicz AM, et al. An intra-abdominal small round cell neoplasm with features of primitive neuroectodermal and desmoplastic round cell tumor and a EWS/FLI-1 fusion transcript. Hum Pathol 1997; 28:502–509.
348. Noguera R, Navarro S, Cremades A, et al. Translocation (X:18) in a biphasic synovial sarcoma with morphologic features of neural differentiation. Diagn Mol Pathol 1998; 7:16–23.
349. Pelmus M, Guillou L, Hostein I, et al. Monophasic fibrous and poorly differentiated synovial sarcoma: immunohistochemical reassessment of 60 t(X;18)(SYT-SSX)-positive cases. Am J Surg Pathol 2002; 26:1434–1440.
350. Masui F, Matsuno Y, Yokoyama R, et al. Synovial sarcoma, histologically mimicking primitive neuroectodermal tumor/Ewing's sarcoma at distant sites. Jpn J Clin Oncol 1999; 29:438–441.
351. Ozdemirli M, Fanburg-Smith JC, Hartmann DP, et al. Differentiating lymphoblastic lymphoma and Ewing's sarcoma: lymphocyte markers and gene rearrangement. Mod Pathol 2001; 14:1175–1182.
352. Lucas DR, Bentley G, Dan ME, et al. Ewing sarcoma vs. lymphoblastic lymphoma: a comparative immunohistochemical study. Am J Clin Pathol 2001; 115:11–17.
353. Mathewson RC, Kjeldsberg CR, Perkins SL. Detection of terminal deoxynucleotidyl transferase (TdT) in nonhematopoietic small round cell tumors of children. Pediatr Pathol Lab Med 1997; 17:835–844.
354. Machen SK, Fisher C, Gautam RS, et al. Utility of cytokeratin subsets for distinguishing poorly differentiated synovial sarcoma from peripheral primitive neuroectodermal tumour. Histopathology 1998; 33:501–507.
355. Ramnani D, Lindberg G, Gokaslan ST, et al. Signet-ring cell variant of small lymphocytic lymphoma with a prominent sinusoidal pattern. Ann Diagn Pathol 1999; 3:220–226.
356. Tse CC, Chan JK, Yuen RW, et al. Malignant lymphoma with myxoid stroma: A new pattern in need of recognition. Histopathology 1991; 18:31–35.
357. Tsang WY, Chan JK, Tang SK, et al. Large cell lymphoma with a fibrillary matrix. Histopathology 1992; 29:80–82.
358. Fisher C. Myofibroblastic malignancies. Adv Anat Pathol 2004; 11:190–201.
359. Meis JM, Enzinger FM. Inflammatory fibrosarcoma of the mesentery and retroperitoneum: A tumor closely simulating inflammatory pseudotumor. Am J Surg Pathol 1991; 15:1146–1156.
360. Mechtersheimer G, Moller P. Expression of Ki-1 antigen (CD30) in mesenchymal tumors. Cancer 1990; 66:1732–1737.
361. Winder SJ, Walsh MP. Calponin: Thin filament-linked regulation of smooth muscle contraction. Cell Signal 1993; 5:677–686.
362. Miettinen MM, Sarloma-Rikala M, Kovatich AJ, et al. Calponin and h-caldesmon in soft tissue tumors: Consistent

h-caldesmon immunoreactivity in gastrointestinal stromal tumors indicates traits of smooth muscle differentiation. Mod Pathol 1999; 12:756–762.

363. Kaddu S, Baham A, Cerroni L, et al. Cutaneous leiomyosarcoma. Am J Surg Pathol 1997; 21:970–987.

364. Oliai BR, Tazelaar HD, Lloyd RV, et al. Leiomyosarcoma of the pulmonary veins. Am J Surg Pathol 1999; 23:1082–1088.

365. Rao UN, Finkelstein SD, Jones MW. Comparative immunohistochemical and molecular analysis of uterine and extrauterine leiomyosarcomas. Mod Pathol 1999;1 2:1001–1009.

366. Younes M, Brown RW, Stephenson M, et al. Overexpression of Glut1 and Glut2 in stage I nonsmall cell lung carcinoma is associated with poor survival. Cancer 1997; 80:1046–1051.

367. Younes M, Lechago LV, Lechago J. Overexpression of the human erythrocyte glucose transporter occurs as a late event in human colorectal carcinogenesis and is associated with an increased incidence of lymph node metastases. Clin Cancer Res 1996; 2:1151–1154.

368. North PE, Waner M, Mizeracki A, et al. GLUT1: A newly discovered immunohistochemical marker for juvenile hemangiomas. Hum Pathol 2000; 31:11–22.

369. Haber RS, Weiser KR, Pritsker A, et al. GLUT1 glucose transported expression in benign and malignant thyroid nodules. Thyroid 1997; 7:363–367.

370. Bowman F, Gultekin H, Dickman PS. Latent Epstein-Barr virus infection demonstrated in low-grade leiomyosarcomas of adults with acquired immunodeficiency syndrome, but not in adjacent Kaposi's lesion or smooth muscle tumors in immunocompetent patients. Arch Pathol Lab Med 1997; 121: 834–838.

371. Jenson HB, Montalvo EA, McClain KL, et al. Characterization of natural Epstein-Barr virus infection and replication in smooth muscle cells from a leiomyosarcoma. J Med Virol 1999; 57:36–46.

372. Swanson PE, Wick MR, Dehner LP. Leiomyosarcoma of somatic soft tissues in childhood: An immunohistochemical analysis of six cases with ultrastructural correlation. Hum Pathol 1991; 22:569–577.

373. Swanson PE, Stanley MW, Scheihauer BW, et al. Primary cutaneous leiomyosarcoma: A histological and immunohistochemical study of 9 cases, with ultrastructural correlation. J Cutan Pathol 1988; 15:129–141.

374. Smith TA, Machen SK, Fisher C, et al. Usefulness of cytokeratin subsets for distinguishing monophasic synovial sarcoma from malignant peripheral nerve sheath tumor. Am J Clin Pathol 1999; 112:641–648.

375. Morphopoulos GD, Banerjee SS, Ali HH, et al. Malignant peripheral nerve sheath tumour with vascular differentiation: A report of four cases. Histopathology 1996; 28:401–410.

376. King R, Busam K, Rosai J. Metastatic malignant melanoma resembling malignant peripheral nerve sheath tumor: Report of 16 cases. Am J Surg Pathol 1999; 23:1499–1505.

377. Lopes JM, Bjerkehagen B, Holm R, et al. Immunohistochemical profile of synovial sarcoma with emphasis on the epithelial-type differentiation: A study of 49 primary tumours, recurrences, and metastases. Pathol Res Pract 1994; 190:168–177.

378. Machen SK, Fisher C, Gautam RS, et al. Utility of cytokeratin subsets for distinguishing poorly differentiated synovial sarcoma from peripheral primitive neuroectodermal tumour. Histopathology 1998; 33:501–507.

379. Ordonez NG, Mahfouz SM, MacKay B. Synovial sarcoma: An immunohistochemical and ultrastructural study. Hum Pathol 1990; 21:733–749.

380. Nicholson AG, Goldstraw P, Fisher C. Synovial sarcoma of the pleura and its differentiation from other primary pleural tumours: A clinicopathological and immunohistochemical review of three cases. Histopathology 1998; 33:508–513.

381. Suster S, Fisher C, Moran CA. Expression of bcl-2 oncoprotein in benign and malignant spindle cell tumors of soft tissue, skin, serosal surfaces, and gastrointestinal tract. Am J Surg Pathol 1998; 22:863–872.

382. Morgan MB, Swann M, Somach S, et al. Cutaneous angiosarcoma: a case series with prognostic correlation. J Am Acad Dermatol 2004; 50:867–874.

383. Robin YM, Guillou L, Michels JJ, et al. Human herpesvirus 8 immunostaining: a sensitive and specific method for diagnosing Kaposi sarcoma in paraffin-embedded sections. Am J Clin Pathol 2004; 121:330–334.

384. Cheuk W, Wong KO, Wong CS, et al. Immunostaining for human herpesvirus 8 latent nuclear antigen-1 helps distinguish Kaposi sarcoma from its mimickers. Am J Clin Pathol 2004; 121:335–342.

385. Hirakawa N, Naka T, Yamamoto I, et al. Overexpression of bcl-2 protein in synovial sarcoma: A comparative study of other soft tissue spindle cell sarcomas and an additional analy-

sis by fluorescence in situ hybridization. Hum Pathol 1996; 27:1060–1065.

386. Von Hochstetter AR, Meyer VE, Grant JW, et al. Epithelioid sarcoma mimicking angiosarcoma: The value of immunohistochemistry in the differential diagnosis. Virchows Arch A Pathol Anat Histopathol 1991; 418:271–278.

387. Chetty R, Slavin JL. Epithelioid sarcoma with extensive chondroid differentiation. Histopathology 1994; 24:400–401.

388. Laskin WB, Miettinen M. Epithelioid sarcoma: new insights based on an extended immunohistochemical analysis. Arch Pathol Lab Med 2003; 127:1161–1168.

389. Guillou L, Wadden C, Coindre JM, et al. 'Proximal type' epithelioid sarcoma: A distinctive aggressive neoplasm showing rhabdoid feature: Clinico- pathologic, immunohistochemical, and ultrastructural study of a series. Am J Surg Pathol 1997; 21:130–146.

390. Gerharz CD, Moll R, Meister P, et al. Cytoskeletal heterogeneity of an epithelioid sarcoma with expression of vimentin, cytokeratins, and neurofilaments. Am J Surg Pathol 1990; 14:274–283.

391. Domagala W, Weber K, Osborn M. Diagnostic significance of coexpression of intermediate filaments in fine needle aspiration. Acta Cytol 1988; 32:49–59.

392. Judkins AR, Montone KT, LiVolsi VA, et al. Sensitivity and specificity of antibodies on necrotic tumor tissue. Am J Clin Pathol 1997; 110:641–646.

393. Smith ME, Brown JI, Fisher C. Epithelioid sarcoma: Presence of vascular-endothelial cadherin and lack of epithelial cadherin. Histopathology 1998; 33:425–431.

394. Saito T, Oda Y, Itakura E, et al. Expression of intercellular adhesion molecules in epithelioid sarcoma and malignant rhabdoid tumor. Pathol Int 2001; 51:532–542.

395. Wick MR, Manivel JC. Epithelioid sarcoma and isolated necrobiotic granuloma: a comparative immunocytochemical study. J Cutan Pathol 1986; 13:253–260.

396. Kato H, Hatori M, Kokubun S, et al. CA125 expression in epithelioid sarcoma. Jpn J Clin Oncol 2004; 34:149–154.

397. Lee MW, Jee KJ, Ro JY, et al. Proximal-type epithelioid sarcoma: case report and results of comparative genomic hybridization. J Cutan Pathol 2004; 31:67–71.

398. Weidner N, Goldman R, Johnston J. Epithelioid monophasic synovial sarcoma. Ultrastruct Pathol 1993; 17:287–294.

399. Cerilli LA, Huffman HT, Anand A. Primary renal angiosarcoma: A case report with immunohistochemical, ultrastructural, and cytogenetic features and review of the literature. Arch Pathol Lab Med 1998; 122:929–935.

400. Poblet E, Gonzalez-Palacios F, Jimenez FJ. Different immunoreactivity of endothelial markers in well and poorly differentiated areas of angiosarcomas. Virchows Arch 1996; 428: 217–221.

401. Sirgi KE, Wick MR, Swanson PE. B72.3 and CD34 immunoreactivity in malignant epithelioid soft tissue tumors: adjuncts in the recognition of endothelial neoplasms. Am J Surg Pathol 1993; 17:179–185.

402. Mooi WJ, Deenik W, Peterse JL, et al. Keratin immuno-reactivity in melanoma of soft parts (clear cell sarcoma). Histopathology 1995; 27:61–65.

403. Hiraga H, Nojima T, Abe S, et al. Establishment of a new continuous clear cell sarcoma cell line: Morphological and cytogenetic characterization and detection of chimaeric EWS/ATF-1 transcripts. Virchows Arch 1997; 431:45–51.

404. Stenman G, Kindblom LG, Angervall L. Reciprocal translocation t(12;22)(q13]3) in clear-cell sarcoma of tendons and aponeuroses. Genes Chromosomes Cancer 1992; 4:122–127.

405. Laskin WB, Weiss SW, Bratthauer GL. Epithelioid variant of malignant peripheral nerve sheath tumor (malignant epithelioid schwannoma). Am J Surg Pathol 1991; 15:1136–1145.

406. Hoang MP, Sinkre P, Albores-Saavedra J. Expression of protein gene product 9.5 in epithelioid and conventional malignant peripheral nerve sheath tumors. Arch Pathol Lab Med 2001; 125:1321–1325.

407. Boyle JL, Haupt HM, Stern JB, et al. Tyrosinase expression in malignant melanoma, desmoplastic melanoma, and peripheral nerve sheath tumors. Arch Pathol Lab Med 2002; 126:816–822.

408. Meis-Kindblom JM, Kindblom LG, Enzinger FM. Sclerosing epithelioid fibrosarcoma: A variant of fibrosarcoma simulating carcinoma. Am J Surg Pathol 1995; 19:979–993.

409. Hindermann W, Katenkamp D. Sclerosing epithelioid fibrosarcoma. Pathologe 2003; 24:103–108.

410. Antonescu CR, Rosenblum MK, Pereira P, et al. Sclerosing epithelioid fibrosarcoma: a study of 16 cases and confirmation of a clinicopathologically distinct tumor. Am J Surg Pathol 2001; 25:699–709.

411. Eyden BP, Manson C, Banerjee SS, et al. Sclerosing epithelioid fibrosarcoma: A study of five cases emphasizing diag-

nostic criteria. Histopathology 1998; 33:354–360.
412. Suster S. Epithelioid leiomyosarcoma of the skin and subcutaneous tissue: Clinicopathologic, immunohistochemical, and ultrastructural study of five cases. Am J Surg Pathol 1994; 18:232–240.
413. Lopez-Barea F, Rodriguez-Peralto JL, Sanchez-Herrera S, et al. Primary epithelioid leiomyosarcoma of bone: Case report and literature review. Virchows Arch 1999; 434:367–371.
414. Mukai M, Torikata C, Iri H, et al. Histogenesis of alveolar soft-part sarcoma: An immunohistochemical and biochemical study. Am J Surg Pathol 1986; 10:212–218.
415. Miettinen M, Ekfors T. Alveolar soft part sarcoma: Immunohistochemical evidence for muscle cell differentiation. Am J Clin Pathol 1990; 93:32–38.
416. Hurlimann J. Desmin and neural marker expression in mesothelial cells and mesotheliomas. Hum Pathol 1994; 25:753–757.
417. Foschini MP, Ceccarelli C, Eusebi V, et al. Alveolar soft-part sarcoma: Immunological evidence of rhabdomyoblastic differentiation. Histopathology 1988; 13:101–108.
418. Foschini MP, Eusein V. Alveolar soft part sarcoma: A new type of rhabdomyosarcoma? Semin Diagn Pathol 1994; 4:58–68.
419. Hirose T, Kudo E, Hasaegawa T, et al. Cytoskeletal properties of alveolar soft part sarcoma. Hum Pathol 1990; 21:204–211.
420. Menesce LP, Eyden BP, Edmondson D, et al. Immuno-phenotype and ultrastructure of alveolar soft part sarcoma. J Submicrosc Cytol Pathol 1993; 2593:377–387.
421. Rosai J, Dias P, Parham DM, et al. MyoD1 protein expression in alveolar soft part sarcoma as confirmatory evidence of its skeletal muscle nature. Am J Surg Pathol 1991; 15:974–981.
422. Nakano H, Tateishi A, Imamura T, et al. RT-PCR suggests human skeletal muscle origin of alveolar soft part sarcoma. Oncology 2000; 58:319–323.
423. Ordonez NG, Mackay B. Alveolar soft-part sarcoma: A review of the pathology and histogenesis. Ultrastruct Pathol 1998; 22:275–292.
424. Roholl PJ, Prinsen I, Rademakers LP, et al. Two cell lines with epithelial cell-like characteristics established from malignant fibrous histiocytomas. Cancer 1991; 68:1963–1972.
425. Hasegawa T, Hasegawa F, Hirose T, et al. Expression of smooth muscle markers in so-called malignant fibrous histiocytomas. J Clin Pathol 2003; 56:666–671.
426. Nakanishi I, Katsuda S, Ooi A, et al. Diagnostic aspects of spindle-cell sarcomas by electron microscopy. Acta Pathol Jpn 1983; 33:425–437.
427. Brooks JJ. The significance of double phenotypic patterns and markers in human sarcomas: a new model of mesenchymal differentiation. Am J Pathol 1986; 125:113–123.
428. Schneider P, Busch U, Meister H, et al. Malignant fibrous histiocytoma (MFH): a comparison of MFH in man and animals. A critical review. Histol Histopathol 1999; 14:845–860.
429. Gaffney EF, Dervan PA, Fletcher CD. Pleomorphic rhabdomyosarcoma in adulthood: Analysis of 11 cases with definition of diagnostic criteria. Am J Surg Pathol 1993; 17:601–609.
430. Gloghini A, Rizzo A, Zanette I, et al. KP1/CD68 expression in malignant neoplasms including lymphomas, sarcomas, and carcinomas. Am J Clin Pathol 1995; 103:425–431.
431. Fisher C, Carter RL, Ramachandra S, et al. Peripheral nerve sheath differentiation in malignant soft tissue tumours: An ultrastructural and immunohistochemical study. Histopathology 1992; 20:115–125.
432. Hitchcock MG, Hurt MA, Santa Cruz DJ. Cutaneous granular cell angiosarcoma. J Cutan Pathol 1994; 21:256–262.
433. Kodet R, Newton WA Jr, Sachs N, et al. Rhabdoid tumors of soft tissues: A clinicopathologic study of 26 cases enrolled on the Intergroup Rhabdomyosarcoma Study. Hum Pathol 1991; 22:674–684.
434. Shiratsuchi H, Oshiro Y, Saito T, et al. Cytokeratin subunits of inclusion bodies in rhabdoid cells: immunohistochemical and clinicopathological study of malignant rhabdoid tumor and epithelioid sarcoma. Int J Surg Pathol 2001; 9:37–48.
435. Fanburg-Smith JC, Hengge M, Hengge UR, et al. Extrarenal rhabdoid tumors of soft tissue: A clinicopathologic and immunohistochemical study of 18 cases. Ann Diagn Pathol 1998; 2:351–362.
436. Perrone T, Swanson PE, Twiggs L, et al. Malignant rhabdoid tumor of the vulva: Is distinction from epithelioid sarcoma possible? A pathologic and immunohistochemical study. Am J Surg Pathol 1989; 13:848–858.
437. Gibas Z, Miettinen M, Limon J, et al. Cytogenetic and immunohistochemical profile of myxoid liposarcoma. Am J Clin

Pathol 1995; 103:20–26.

438. Miettinen M, Gannon FH, Lackman R. Chordoma- like soft tissue sarcoma in the leg: A light and electron microscopic and immunohistochemical study. Ultrastruct Pathol 1992; 16: 577–586.

439. Tong G, Perle MA, Desai P, et al. Parachordoma or chordoma periphericum? Diagn Cytopathol 2003; 29:18–23.

440. Coffin CM, Swanson PE, Wick MR, et al. An immuno-histochemical comparison of chordoma with renal cell carcinoma, colorectal adenocarcinoma, and myxopapillary ependymoma: a potential diagnostic dilemma in the diminutive biopsy. Mod Pathol 1993; 6:531–538.

441. Naka T, Iwamoto Y, Shinohara N, et al. Cytokeratin subtyping in chordomas and the fetal notochord: An immunohistochemical analysis of aberrant expression. Mod Pathol 1997; 10: 545–551.

442. Hu Y, Gao Y, Zhang X. A clinicopathological and immunohistochemical study of 34 cases of chordoma. Chung Hua Ping li Hsueh Tsa Chih 1996; 25:142–144.

443. Mi C. An immunohistochemical and ultrastructural study of 20 chordomas. Chung Hua Ping li Hsueh Tsa Chih 1992; 21: 106–108.

444. Heffelfinger MJ, Dahlin DC, MacCarty CS, et al. Chordomas and cartilaginous tumors at the skull base. Cancer 1973; 32:410–420.

445. Rosenberg AE, Brown GA, Bhan AK, et al. Chondroid chordoma – a variant of chordoma: A morphologic and immunohistochemical study. Am J Clin Pathol 1994; 101:36–41.

446. Wojno KJ, Hruban RH, Garin-Chesa P, et al. Chondroid chordomas and low-grade chondrosarcomas of the craniospinal axis: An immunohistochemical analysis of 17 cases. Am J Surg Pathol 1992; 16:1144–1152.

447. Ishida T, Dorfman HD. Chondroid chordoma versus low-grade chondrosarcoma of the base of the skull: Can immunohistochemistry resolve the controversy? J Neuro-oncol 1994; 18:199–206.

448. Meis JM, Raymond AK, Evans HL, et al. 'Dedifferentiated' chordoma: a clinicopathologic and immunohistochemical study of three cases. Am J Surg Pathol 1987; 11:516–525.

449. Crapanzano JP, Ali SZ, Ginsberg MS, et al. Chordoma: a cytologic study with histologic and radiologic correlation. Cancer 2001; 93:40–51.

450. Niezabitowski A, Limon J, Wasilewska A, et al. Parachordoma – a clinicopathologic, immunohistochemical, electron microscopic, flow cytometric, and cytogenetic study. Gen Diagn Pathol 1995; 141:49–55.

451. Wiebe BM, Jensen K, Laursen H. Parachordoma of the sacrococcygeal region – a neuroepithelial tumor. Clin Neuropathol 1995; 14:343–346.

452. Karabela-Bouropoulou V, Skourtas C, Liapi-Avgeri G, et al. Parachordoma: A case report of a very rare soft tissue tumor. Pathol Res Pract 1996; 192:972–978.

453. Ishida T, Oda H, Oka T, et al. Parachordoma: An ultrastructural and immunohistochemical study. Virchows Arch A Pathol Anat Histopathol 1993; 422:239–245.

454. Scolyer RA, Bonar SF, Palmer AA, et al. Parachor- doma is not distinguishable from axial chordoma using immunohistochemistry. Pathol Int 2004; 54:364–370.

455. Granados R, Martin-Hita A, Rodriguez-Barbero JM, et al. Fine-needle aspiration cytology of chondroblastoma of soft parts. Diagn Cytopathol 2003; 28:76–81.

456. Nakamura Y, Becker LE, Marks A. S-100 protein in tumors of cartilage and bone: An immunohistochemical study. Cancer 1983; 52:1820–1824.

457. Posl M, Amling M, Ritzel H, et al. Morphologic characteristics of chondroblastoma: A retrospective study of 56 cases of the Hamburg bone tumor register. Pathologe 1996; 17:26–34.

458. Semmelink HJ, Pruszczynski M, Wiersma-van Tilburg A, et al. Cytokeratin expression in chondro- blastomas. Histopathology 1990; 16:257–263.

459. Monda L, Wick MR. S-100 protein immunostaining in the differential diagnosis of chondroblastoma. Hum Pathol 1985; 16:287–293.

460. Edel G, Ueda Y, Nakanishi J, et al. Chondroblastoma of bone: A clinical, radiological, light and immunohistochemical study. Virchows Arch A Pathol Anat Histopathol 1992; 421:355–366.

461. Brecher ME, Simon MA. Chondroblastoma: An immunohistochemical study. Hum Pathol 1988; 19:1043–1047.

462. Povysil C, Tomanova R, Matejovsky Z. Muscle-specific actin expression in chondroblastoma. Hum Pathol 1997; 28:316–320.

463. Kilpatrick SE, Inwards CY, Fletcher CD, et al. Myxoid chondrosarcoma (chordoid sarcoma) of bone: A report of two cases and review of the literature. Cancer 1997; 79:1903–1910.

464. Antonescu CR, Argani P, Erlandson RA, et al. Skeletal and extraskeletal myxoid chondrosarcoma: A comparative clinicopathologic, ultrastructural, and molecular study. Cancer 1998; 83:1504–1521.

465. Orndal C, Carlen B, Akerman M, et al. Chromosomal abnormality t(9;22)(q22]2) in an extraskeletal myxoid chondrosarcoma characterized by fine needle aspiration cytology, electron microscopy, immunohistochemistry and DNA flow cytometry. Cytopathology 1991; 2:261–270.

466. Domanski HA, Carlen B, Mertens F, et al. Extraskeletal myxoid chondrosarcoma with neuroendocrine differentiation: a case report with fine-needle aspiration biopsy, histopathology, electron microscopy, and cytogenetics. Ultrastruct Pathol 2003; 27:363–368.

467. Goh YW, Spagnolo DV, Platten M, et al. Extraskeletal myxoid chondrosarcoma: a light microscopic, immuno-histochemical, ultrastructural, and immunoultrastructural study indicating neuroendocrine differentiation. Histo-pathology 2001; 39: 514–524.

468. Algros MP, Collonge-Rame MA, Bedgejian I, et al. Neuro-ectodermal differentiation of extraskeletal myxoid chondrosarcoma: a classical feature? Ann Pathol 2003; 23: 244–248.

469. Swanson PE. Clear cell tumors of bone. Semin Diagn Pathol 1997; 14:281–291.

470. Wang LT, Liu TC. Clear cell chondrosarcoma of bone: A report of three cases with immunohistochemical and affinity histochemical observations. Pathol Res Pract 1993; 189:411–415.

471. Bosse A, Ueda Y, Wuisman P, et al. Histogenesis of clear cell chondrosarcoma: An immunohistochemical study with osteonectin, a non-collagenous structure protein. J Cancer Res Clin Oncol 1991; 117:43–49.

472. Lidang Jensen LM, Schumacher B, Jensen MO, et al. Extraskeletal osteosarcomas: A clinicopathologic study of 25 cases. Am J Surg Pathol 1998; 22:588–594.

473. Dardick I, Schatz JE, Colgan TJ. Osteogenic sarcoma with epithelial differentiation. Ultrastruct Pathol 1992; 16:463–474.

474. Hasegawa T, Hirose T, Hizawa K, et al. Immuno- phenotypic heterogeneity in osteosarcomas. Hum Pathol 1991; 22: 583–590.

475. Serra M, Morini MC, Scotlandi K, et al. Evaluation of osteonectin as a diagnostic marker of osteogenic bone tumors. Hum Pathol 1992; 23:1326-1331.

476. Schulz Z, Jundt G, Berghauser KH, et al. Immunohistochemical study of osteonectin in various types of osteo-sarcoma. Am J Pathol 1988; 132:233–238.

477. Masui F, Ushigome S, Fujii K. Giant cell tumor of bone: An immunohistochemical comparative study. Pathol Int 1998; 48:355–361.

478. Fornasier VL, Protzner K, Zhang I, et al. The prognostic significance of histomorphometry and immunohistochemistry in giant cell tumors of bone. Hum Pathol 1996;2 7:754–760.

479. Watanabe K, Tajino T, Kusakabe T, et al. Giant cell tumor of bone: Frequent actin immunoreactivity in stromal tumor cells. Pathol Int 1997; 47:680–684.

480. Paulino AF, Spiro RH, O'Malley B, et al. Giant cell tumour of the retropharynx. Histopathology 1998; 33:344–348.

481. Folpe AL, Weiss SW, Fletcher CD, et al. Tenosynovial giant cell tumors: Evidence for a desmin-positive dendritic cell subpopulation. Mod Pathol 1998; 11:939–944.

482. Ueda Y, Imai K, Tsuchiya H, et al. Matrix metallo- proteinase 9 (gelatinase B) is expressed in multinucleated giant cells of human giant cell tumor of bone and is associated with vascular invasion. Am J Pathol 1996; 148:611–622.

483. Rao VH, Singh RK, Delimont DC, et al. Transcriptional regulation of MMP-9 expression in stromal cells of human giant cell tumor of bone by tumor necrosis factor-alpha. Int J Oncol 1999; 14:291–300.

484. Schoedel DE, Greco MA, Stetler-Stevenson WG, et al. Expression of metalloproteinases and tissue inhibitors of metalloproteinases in giant cell tumor of bone: An immunohistochemical study with clinical correlation. Hum Pathol 1996; 27:1144–1148.

485. Kahn LB. Adamantinoma, osteofibrous dysplasia, and differentiated adamantinoma. Skeletal Radiol 2003; 32:245–258.

486. Hazelbag HM, Hogendoorn PC. Adamantinoma of the long bones: an anatomicoclinical review of its relationship to osteofibrous dysplasia. Ann Pathol 2001; 21:499–511.

487. Kuruvilla G, Steiner GC. Osteofibrous dysplasia-like adamantinoma of bone: a report of five cases with immunohistochemical and ultrastructural studies. Hum Pathol 1998; 29: 809–814.

488. Jundt G, Remberger K, Roessner A, et al. Adamantinoma of long bones: a histopathological and immunohistochemi-cal study of 23 cases. Pathol Res Pract 1995; 191:112–120.

489. Benassi MS, Campanacci L, Gamberi G, et al. Cytokeratin expression and distribution in adamantinoma of the long bones and osteofibrous dysplasia of tibia and fibula: an immunohistochemical study correlated to histogenesis. Histopathology 1994; 25:71–76.
490. Ishida T, Iijima T, Kikuchi F, et al. A clinicopathological and immunohistochemical study of osteofibrous dysplasia, differentiated adamantinoma, and adamantinoma of long bones. Skeletal Radiol 1992; 21:493–502.
491. Knapp RH, Wick MR, Scheithauer BW, et al. Adamantinoma of bone: an electron microscopic and immuno-histochemical study. Virchows Arch A 1982; 398:75–86.

4 霍奇金淋巴瘤的免疫组织化学

原作者：Parul Bhargava and Marshall E. Kadin

译　者：郝春燕

审校者：周庚寅，张翠娟

目　录

引言	119
H/RSCs 新的生物学标记物	124
总结	130

引　言

霍奇金淋巴瘤（HL）大多数是 B 淋巴细胞的恶性克隆性增殖，少数是 T 淋巴细胞的恶性克隆性增殖，围绕着多少不等的炎细胞和纤维性背景。因此，被分为 2 种主要的组织学类型：①经典型 HL（CHL）和②结节性淋巴细胞为主型 HL（NLPHL）。其中，经典型 HL 又分为 4 种亚型：a. 结节硬化型，b. 混合细胞型，c. 富于淋巴细胞型（LRCHL）和 d. 淋巴细胞消减型（图 4.1、4.2）[1-3]。

结节性淋巴细胞为主型霍奇金淋巴瘤是一种 B 细胞肿瘤，由生发中心 B 细胞经过持续的免疫球蛋白基因体细胞突变发展形成[3-5]。富于淋巴细胞型霍奇金淋巴瘤属于生发中心/生发中心后 B 细胞淋巴瘤，该组肿瘤还包括结节硬化型、混合细胞型和淋巴细胞消减型霍奇金淋巴瘤，霍奇金/R-S 细胞（H/RSCs）发生了广泛的免疫球蛋白基因体细胞突变[6]。结节性淋巴细胞为主型霍奇金淋巴瘤中的 H/RSCs（因其特殊的形态又称作爆米花样细胞）表达 bcl-6，一种生发中心 B 细胞转录因子，但不表达生发中心后 B 细胞相关多糖蛋白 CD138/syndecan-1[7]。相反，经典型霍奇金淋巴瘤中的 H/RSCs 则不同，同时表达 bcl-6 和 CD138，提示它们是生发中心或生发中心后细胞混合起源。

在所有的结节性淋巴细胞为主型霍奇金淋巴瘤病例和少数经典型霍奇金淋巴瘤病例中，都存在 H/RSCs 的 B 细胞抗原（CD20、CD79a）表达（图 4.3）[8-11]。另外，结节性淋巴细胞为主型霍奇金淋巴瘤中 H/RSCs 周围经常围绕着一些活化的辅助性记忆 T 细胞（CD4+、CD57+、CD45R+、CD45-），通常局限于次级滤泡生发中心的明区（图 4.4）[4]。

少部分（10%~20%）经典型霍奇金淋巴瘤病例中，H/RSCs 有 T 细胞亚型的特点，表达多种 T 细胞抗原（CD2、CD3、CD4、CD8）和细胞毒性分子相关抗原（粒酶B、穿孔素和TIA-1）（图 4.5）[12-18]。通过单一 H/RSCs 的多聚酶链反应扩增 T 细胞受体基因证明，约 1%~2% 的 CHL 病例 H/RSCs 是 T 细胞来源的[19-21]。然而，在一些经典型霍奇金淋巴瘤病例通过免疫球蛋白基因重排也可检测到异常的 B 细胞抗原，推测可能是 B 细胞来源的。

所有的经典型霍奇金淋巴瘤病例中肿瘤细胞都表达 CD30，是肿瘤坏死因子超家族成员之一（图 4.6）[22-24]。通过天然 CD30L 或者 EB 病毒潜伏膜蛋白 1（EBV-LMP-1）激活 CD30 可以导致 NFκB 转录因子的激活，NFκB 转录因子对 H/RSCs 有抗凋亡、促进细胞增殖和细胞因子表达上调的作用[25, 26]。H/RSCs 也表达 CD40[27]，CD40 是一种 B 细胞抗原，具有生发中心后 B 细胞的特点，被激活后可以抑制凋亡（图 4.7，4.17F）[28]。经证实 H/RSCs 不同程度地表达 CD25（Tac，p55），CD25 是白细胞介素2（IL-2）受体的 α 单位[29, 30]。最后，通过 LeuM1 抗体在 60%~85%，平均 68% 的 CHL 中检测到 H/RSCs 表达 CD15（图 4.8）[31-34]。LeuM1 的抗原决定簇是一种三糖：3-岩藻糖-N-乙酰乳糖胺，是由 2 型血型组中的 1-3 岩

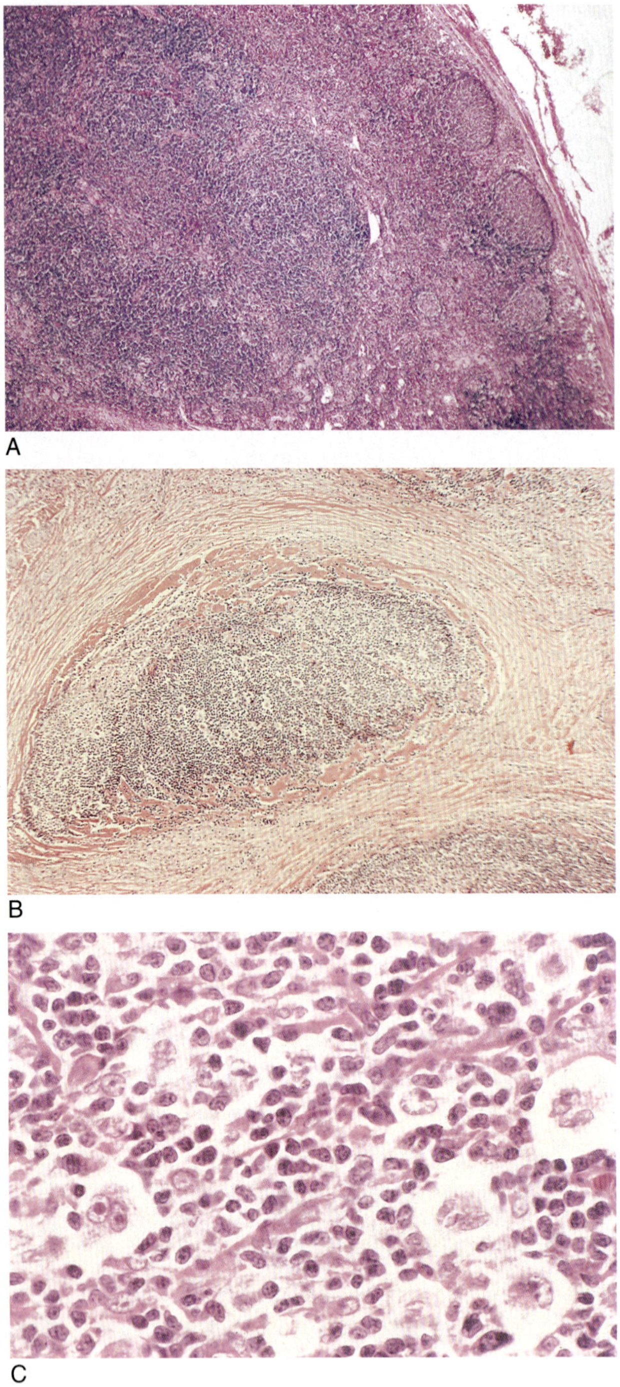

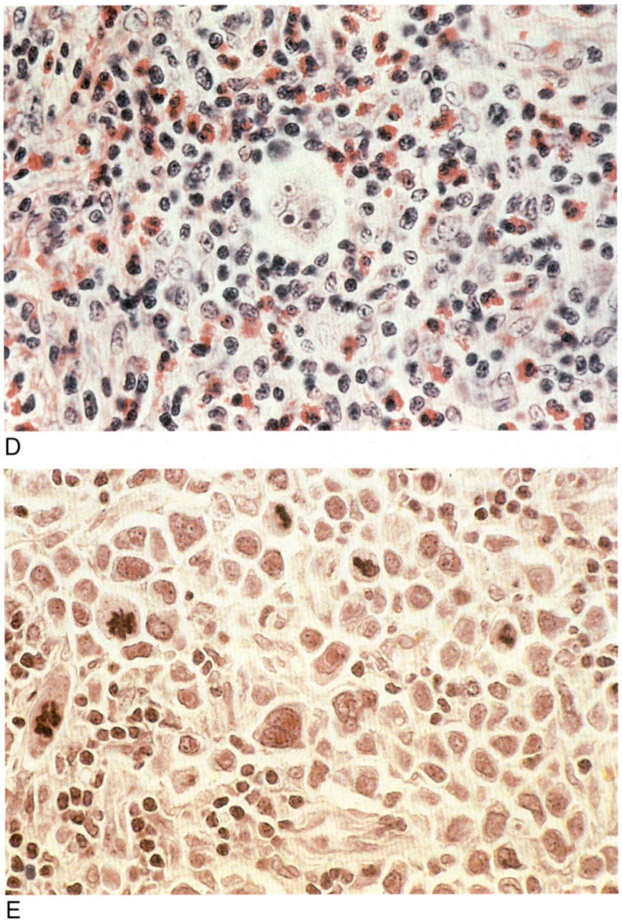

图4.1 经典型霍奇金淋巴瘤（HL）。（A）富于淋巴细胞型；（B）结节硬化型；（C）结节硬化型中的陷窝细胞；（D）混合细胞型；（E）淋巴细胞消减型

藻糖形成的；其糖链等同于Lewis X的糖链，又称作X-半抗原[35]。Ree和其合作者比较性研究发现：抗Lewis X（Bg7）（Signet实验室；Dedham，MA）H/RSCs着色效果要比LeuM1好，阳性率为87%，而LeuM1只有68.5%的H/RSCs着色（图4.9）[36]。

fascin是用来标记经典型霍奇金淋巴瘤中H/RSCs的一种新的敏感标记物[37]，它是一种55kD的肌动蛋白绑定蛋白，主要位于非肿瘤组织中的树突状细胞中。fascin染色阳性显示，霍奇金淋巴瘤（主要是结节硬化型HL）的肿瘤细胞可能是树突状细胞尤其是指状突树突状细胞来源的（图4.10）。但是，既然fascin的表达可由B细胞EBV感染介导，那么由病毒介导的fascin在淋巴样细胞或其他类型细胞中表达的可能性也要考虑到[37]。

EBV被认为与霍奇金淋巴瘤的发病和EBV-LMP-1有关，EBV的小RNAs又称为EBERs。在约50%的经典型霍奇金淋巴瘤病例中可以检测到EBERs（图4.11）[38]。H/RSCs通常表达EBV基因产

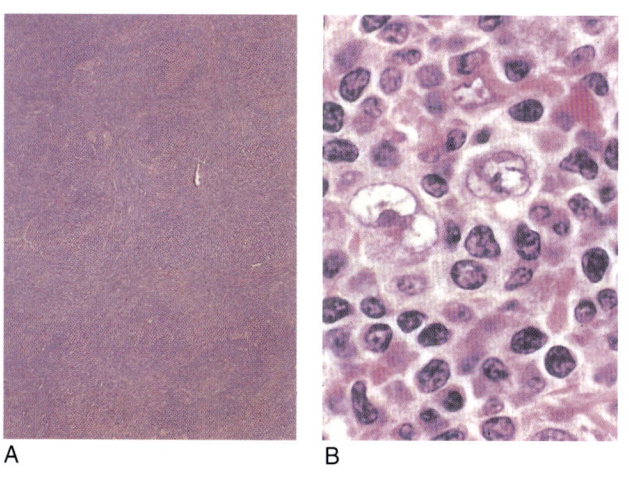

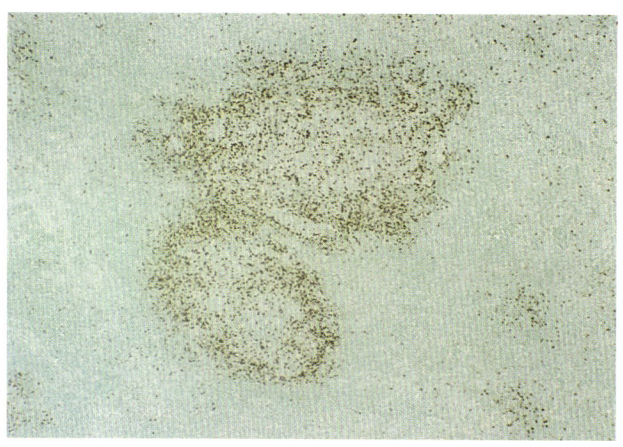

图4.2 结节性淋巴细胞为主型霍奇金淋巴瘤。(A) 低倍镜下显示结节样分布;(B) 爆米花样霍奇金/R-S 细胞

图4.4 在结节性淋巴细胞为主型 HL 中 Leu7+(CD57+)的 T 淋巴细胞围绕着 H/RSCs

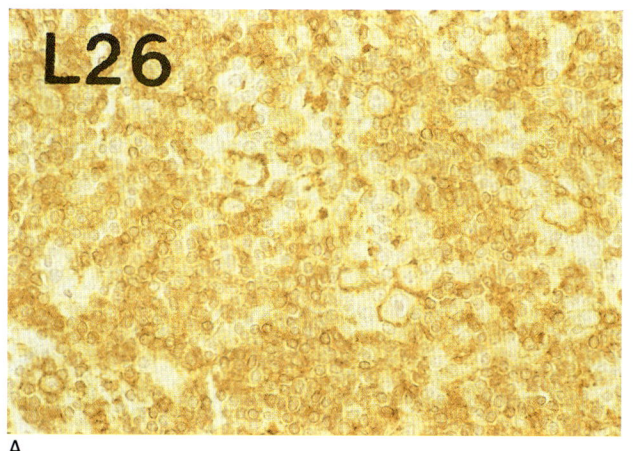

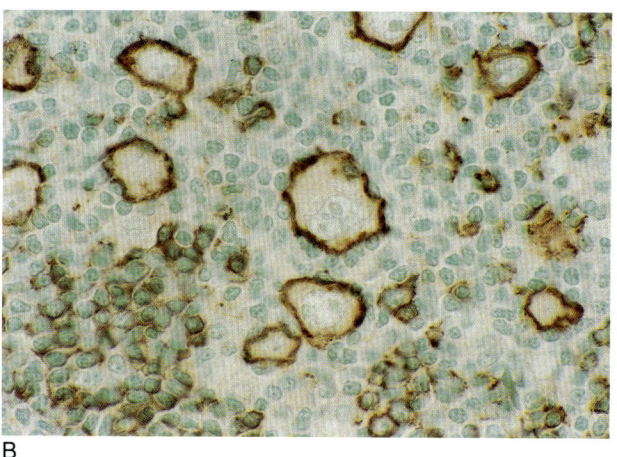

图4.3 淋巴细胞为主型HL中B细胞抗原表达。(A) L26+(CD20+)的小B淋巴细胞围绕着大的H/RSCs;(B) 淋巴细胞为主型HL中 H/RSCs CD20 阳性

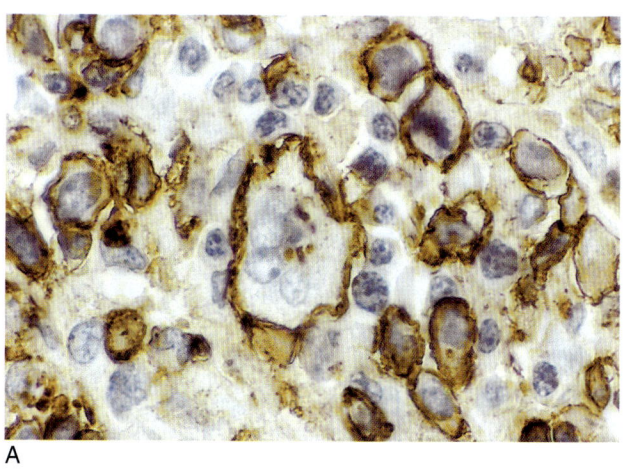

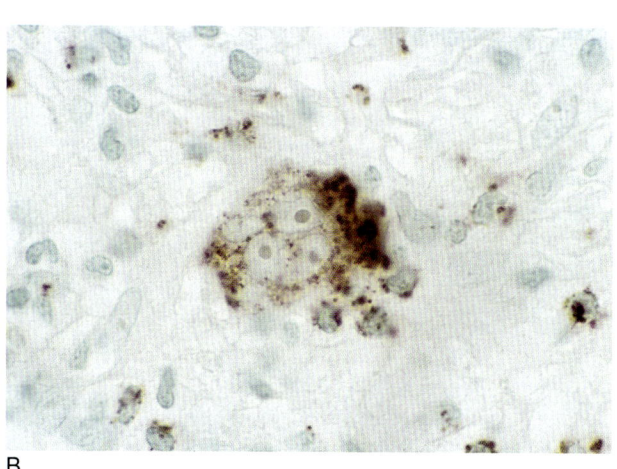

图4.5 具有T细胞表型的HL。(A) H/RSCs 的 UCHL1(CD45RO)染色阳性;(B) H/RSCs 及其周围小淋巴细胞中的细胞毒分子 TIA-1 的表达

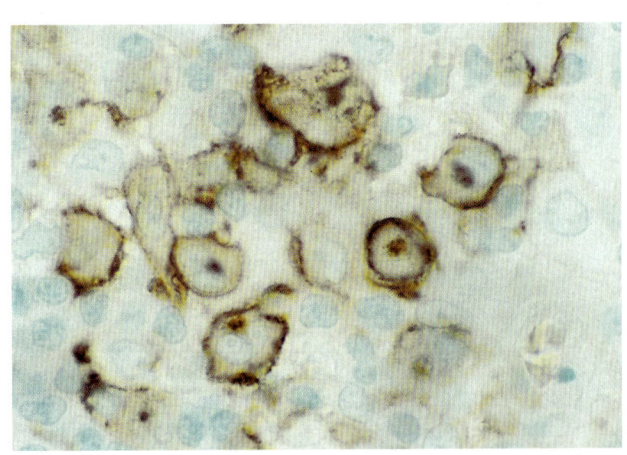

图 4.6 经典型 HL 中用 Ber-H2 标记 H/RSCs 的 CD30 表达

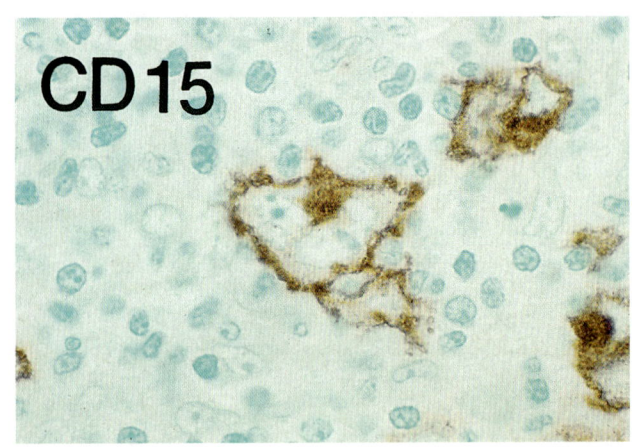

图 4.8 经典型 HL 中用 LeuM1 标记 H/RSCs 的 CD15 表达

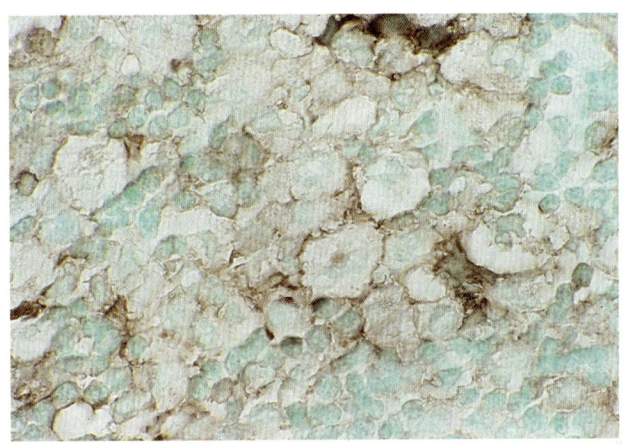

图 4.7 H/RSCs 的 CD40 表达

物潜伏膜蛋白 1（LMP-1），LMP-1 是一种使 H/RSCs 具有生长优势的转化蛋白[39, 40]。EBV 在混合细胞型和淋巴细胞消减型 HL 中的检出率明显高于结节硬化型 HL[40-42]。免疫状态低下的经典型霍奇金淋巴瘤患者较易检测到 EBV，例如感染了人类免疫缺陷病毒（HIV）的患者和移植后发生免疫增生性疾病的患者[43]。EBV 在发展中国家的霍奇金淋巴瘤患者中也有很高的检出率[41, 42]。

与经典型霍奇金淋巴瘤相反，结节性淋巴细胞为主型霍奇金淋巴瘤的爆米花样细胞不表达 CD15、CD25 或 CD30，而白细胞共同抗原（LCA）或 CD45，以及上皮细胞膜抗原（EMA）通常表达阳性（图 4.12）。经典型霍奇金淋巴瘤中 H/RSCs 通常不表达 LCA 和 EMA（图 4.13）[44, 45]。德国的霍奇金研究小组发现免疫组织化学技术在正确诊断淋巴细胞为主型霍奇金

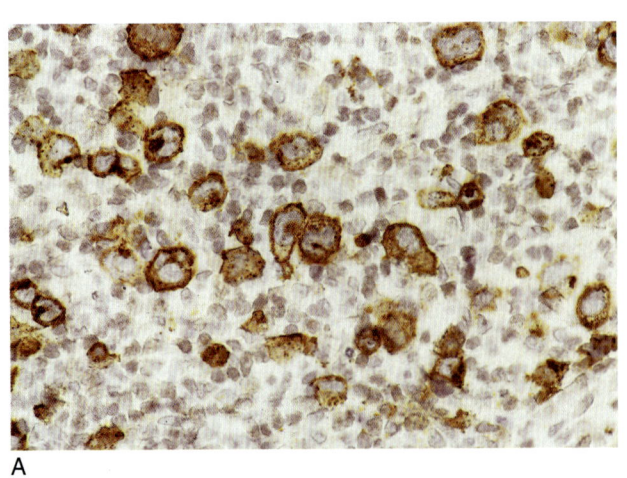

A

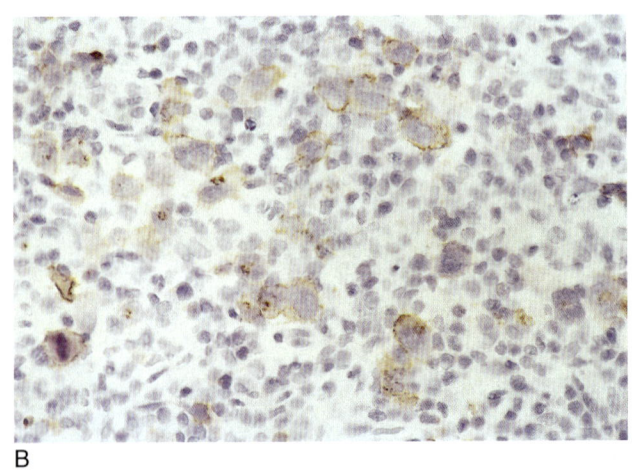

B

图 4.9 在一例淋巴细胞消减型霍奇金淋巴瘤中，分别用（A）抗 Lewis X 和（B）抗 LeuM1 抗体检测 H/RSCs 的 CD15 表达，结果显示抗 Lewis X 抗体具有更高的敏感性

霍奇金淋巴瘤的免疫组织化学 4

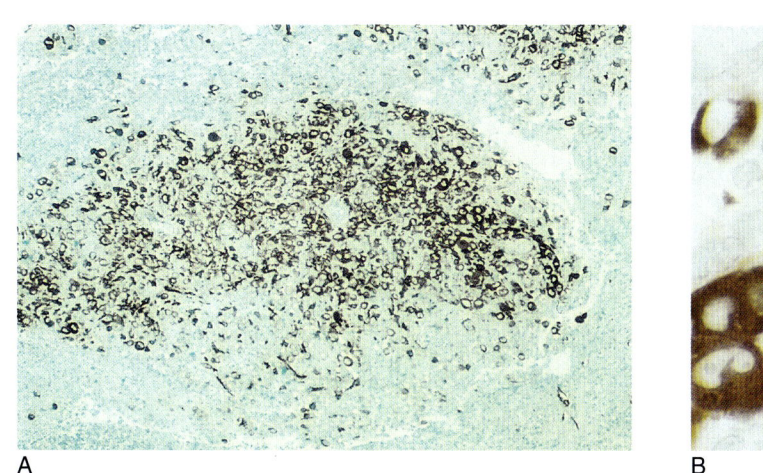
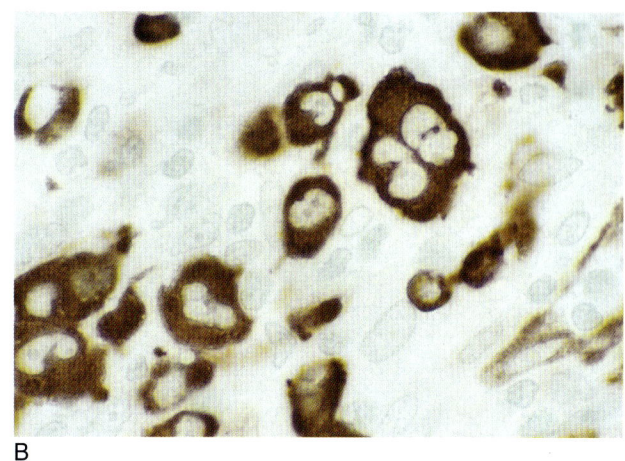

图 4.10　fascin 在结节硬化型霍奇金淋巴瘤中的表达。(A) 低倍镜下的硬化结节；(B) 高倍镜下显示 H/RSCs 细胞阳性

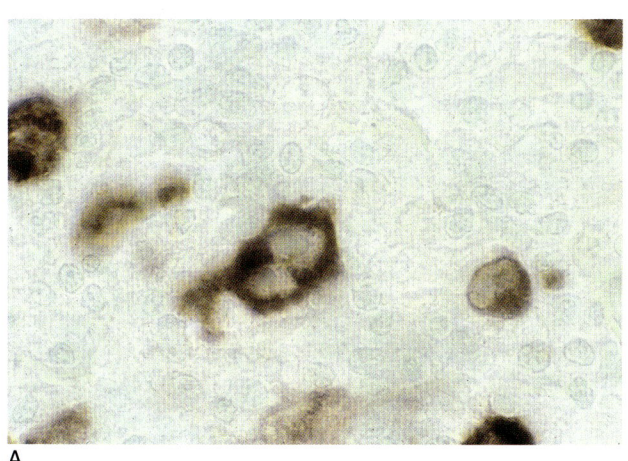
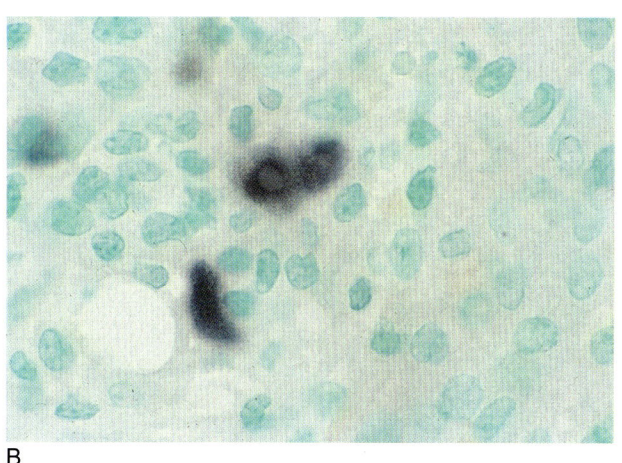

图 4.11　HL 的 EB 病毒检测。(A) 潜伏膜蛋白 1 (LMP-1) 的表达；(B) EBV 的小 RNAs(EBERs) 的表达

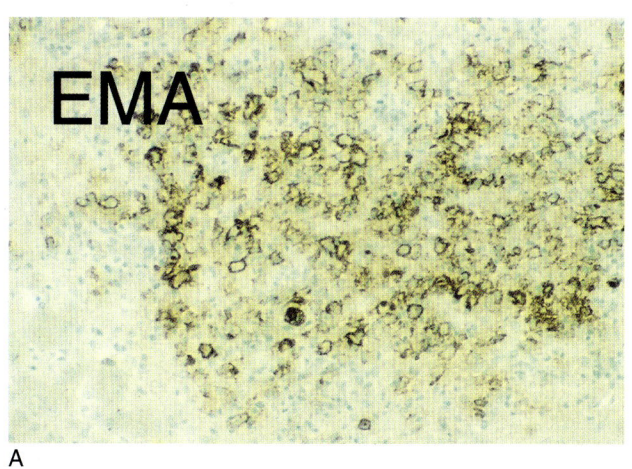
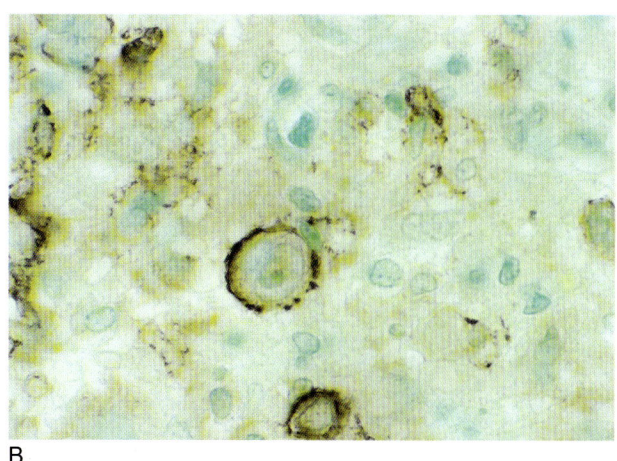

图 4.12　结节性淋巴细胞为主型 HL 中上皮细胞膜抗原 (EMA) 的表达。(A) 低倍镜显示结节；(B) 高倍镜显示 H/RSCs 阳性

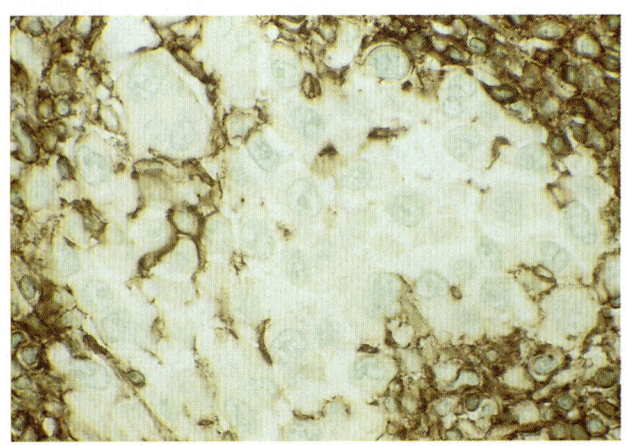

图 4.13 经典型 HL 中 H/RSCs 缺乏 LCA（白细胞共同抗原）的表达

病中起着十分重要的作用。由专家小组通过传统形态学方法诊断的104例淋巴细胞为主型霍奇金病中，其中25例应用免疫组化技术否定了形态学诊断结果，而13例最初没有诊断为淋巴细胞为主型霍奇金病的患者表达明显的淋巴细胞为主型霍奇金病样免疫表型，并且其生存率明显高于经典型霍奇金淋巴瘤[46]。

> 诊断要点：CHL 和 NLPHL
>
> 1. NLPHL：B细胞肿瘤，来源于突变的生发中心细胞。
> 2. 典型的 NLPHL bcl-6、CD20、CD79a、CD45（LCA）和 EMA 表达阳性，CD15（LeuM1）、CD25、CD138 和 CD30 表达阴性。
> 3. CHL 的 RSC 不同程度地表达 CD138、bcl-6，很少表达 CD20、CD79a。
> 4. CHL 的 RSC 很少表达与 T 细胞亚型有关的 CD 分子如 CD2、CD3、CD4、CD8。
> 5. 典型的 CHL 的 RSC 表达 CD15、CD30、CD40+，有时表达 CD25+。
> 6. CHL 的 RSC 表达 Bg7 抗体优于 LeuM1

H/RSCs 新的生物学标记物

转录因子：Oct-2、BOB.1、BSAP、NFκB、JunB

Oct-2是一种转录因子，与它的共激活因子BOB.1/OBF.1 一起，位于免疫球蛋白基因的 octomer 位点上，编码免疫球蛋白合成[47]。生发中心B细胞高表达Oct-2和BOB.1。结节性淋巴细胞为主型霍奇金淋巴瘤中的L&H细胞，因为起源于生发中心B细胞，因此也相应地表达这两个标记物[48]。相反，经典型霍奇金淋巴瘤中的 H/RSCs（80%）都不表达或者仅少量（20%）表达其中一种免疫球蛋白[49, 50]，基因缺失突变被认为是H/RSCs不表达的原因，转录激活因子如Oct-2/BOB.1的缺失可能是产生免疫球蛋白异常调节的一种新机制[49]。尽管绝大多数T细胞淋巴瘤Oct-2阴性，但在一些外周T淋巴瘤、NOS 以及部分（≈50%）ALK 阳性的间变性大细胞淋巴瘤中都存在不同程度的表达[51]。

B 细胞特异激活蛋白（BSAP）是 B 细胞及 B 细胞起源淋巴瘤的另一个转录子，它是由PAX-5基因编码的，具有影响 B 细胞抗原表达、免疫球蛋白表达及类别转换的功能，它在大多数经典型霍奇金淋巴瘤中的 H/RSCs[52]及结节性淋巴细胞为主型霍奇金淋巴瘤中的 L&H 细胞都表达[48]，进一步证实了它们来源于 B 细胞。相反，BSAP在正常的或恶性的T细胞中均不表达，因此在T/裸细胞间变性大细胞淋巴瘤中（ALCL）也不表达[52]。

增强 κ 轻链核因子（NFκB）正常存在于多种细胞中，在应激反应、免疫低下及感染的刺激下可以短暂性活化。现已发现NFκB在培养的 H/RSCs 细胞中活化[25]，主要是由于它的天然抑制物IκB的基因发生了突变或者大量的逆转[53]。NFκB导致抗凋亡基因过表达，使得H/RSCs细胞尽管丧失了合成免疫球蛋白的能力，也能逃脱凋亡。

JunB和c-Jun是转录因子激活蛋白-1（AP-1）家族的成员。AP-1 蛋白被大量激活生长因子通路的细胞外信号或者是应激信号（例如紫外线）快速短暂激活，促进有丝分裂诱导的细胞周期进程并调节细胞凋亡。近来人们发现经典型霍奇金淋巴瘤中的 H/RSCs 过表达含有 c-Jun 和 JunB 的 AP-1 蛋白（图4.14），相反，结节性淋巴细胞为主型霍奇金淋巴瘤中的恶性细胞既不表达c-Jun 也不表达 JunB[54]。然而，我们手中的资料表明（尚未公开发表），JunB在少量结节性淋巴细胞为主型霍奇金淋巴瘤病例中有表达。另外JunB 在散在的淋巴细胞特别是在进行性转化的生发中心细胞中也有染色，JunB 或者c-Jun除了在t（2；5）阳性的ALCL强表达外，在大部分其他的B或者T淋巴细胞的 NHL 中不表达或者仅微弱表达[54]。

化学活化因子受体CCR7是在B、T及活化的树

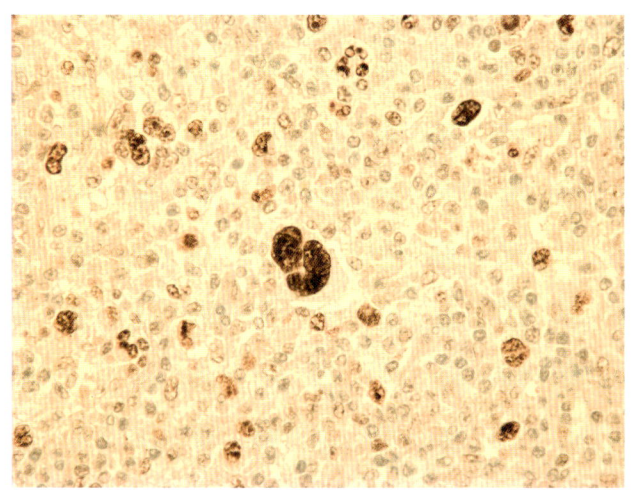

图 4.14 JunB 在 HL 中的表达

表 4.1 H/RSCs 的新生物学标记

抗原	经典型 HL	NLPHL	TCRLBCL	ALCL
NFκB	+	UK	UK*	N
JunB/c-Jun	+	S	UK	+
CCR7	+	N	UK	UK
Oct-2/BOB.1	S**	+	+	N
J chain	N	S	S	N
BSAP	S	+	+	N

+，几乎所有病例都阳性；S，有时阳性；N，没有病例阳性；NK，不知其表达
* 在 DLBCL 中为±，在 TCRLBCL 中没有直接的研究
** 两者均阴性（80%），只有一个阳性（20%）

突细胞中均有表达的淋巴细胞归巢受体，并对淋巴细胞迁移到第二淋巴器官有调节作用。CCR7的启动子绑定在 AP-1 和 NFκB 上。同 c-Jun/JunB 在经典型霍奇金淋巴瘤中过表达一致，CCR7在大部分CHL中的H/RSCs过表达（图4.15）[55]。

J链是一个分子量15kD的酸性蛋白，是由分泌多聚免疫球蛋白的 B 细胞和浆细胞合成的。J 链蛋白在绝大多数结节性淋巴细胞为主型霍奇金淋巴瘤中的 RSCs 表达，但由于免疫球蛋白基因失调，在经典型霍奇金淋巴瘤中的 H/RSCs 中不表达[49, 56, 57]。

新的生物学标记物在HL和其他病变中的表达特征在HL鉴别诊断中的应用，归纳如表4.1。

诊断要点：新标记物

1. NLPHL 中的 L&H 细胞 Oct-2 和 BOB.1 恒定阳性，经典型HL中的RSCs绝大部分都阴性或仅表达一种。
2. BSAP 在 NLPHL 和 CHL 中都阳性，而在 T 细胞间变性淋巴瘤中阴性。
3. CHL 通常表达 JunB 和 CCR7，但是 NLPHL 很少表达。
4. J 链蛋白在大多数 NLPHL 中表达。

抗体和方法学总结

诊断 HL 通常使用的抗体有 Ber-H2、LeuM1、LCA、fascin、L26、LN1、LN2、UCHL1、CD3、ALK-1和EBV-LMP-1。EMA和CD57在识别结节性淋巴细胞为主型霍奇金淋巴瘤时很有效。单克隆抗体LN1可以与大约1/3的HL的H/RSCs起反应，在结节性淋巴细胞为主型霍奇金淋巴瘤中表达率较高（超过75%）[10]，单克隆抗体LN2可以识别MHC II 型抗原的恒定链，可以与将近2/3的HL中的H/RSCs起反应[10]。所有先前提到的抗体都可用于福尔马林固定、石蜡包埋的组织，另外抗体BNH.9[58]和CBF.78[59]一般用于疑难病例的诊断（图4.16，表4.2）。

对于抗原修复，我们已用蒸汽锅加热玻片到95～98℃取代了微波修复，玻片被浸在广口瓶中的枸橼酸盐缓冲液中（pH6，0.01mol/L），在蒸汽中加热20分钟，然后，在室温下放置30分钟，双蒸水冲洗2遍，再放到磷酸盐缓冲液中（pH7.4）。

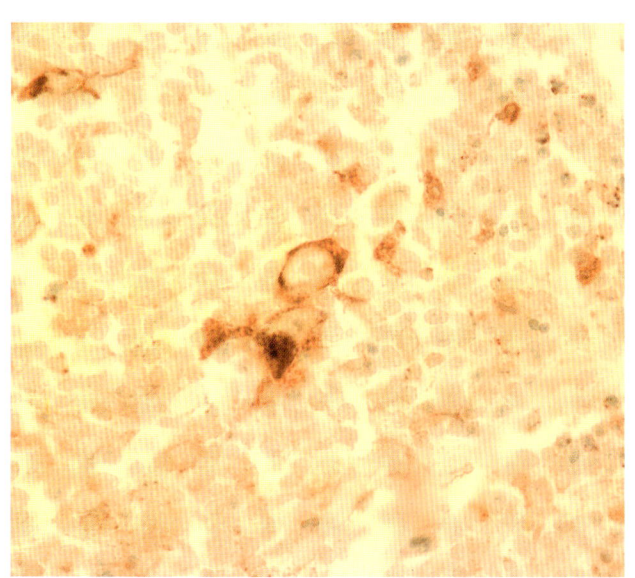

图 4.15 H/RSCs 表达 CCR7

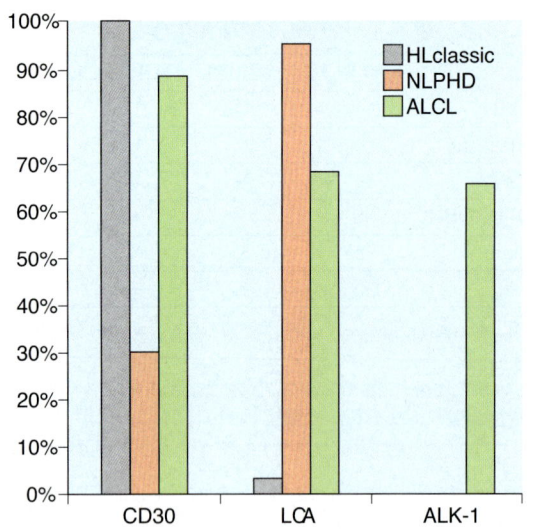

图 4.16 抗原在经典型 HL、NLPHD 及 ALCL 中的阳性率

免疫组化的诊断缺陷

免疫表型的不稳定性

H/RSCs 免疫表型的不稳定性在同时活检和连续性活检的相同病人的石蜡切片标本中已有报道，Chu 与合作者发现，在同时活检的 39 例标本中有 11 例（28%）H/RSCs 免疫表型相同，在连续活检的 21 例标本中只有 4 例（19%）是稳定的。差异主要与细胞的种系特异性抗原有关，而 CD15 和 CD74 抗原的差异较小。

CD15 抗原

依赖 CD15 的表达去诊断一个 HL 是很困难的，因为高达 30% 的经典型霍奇金淋巴瘤不表达 CD15 但却能被 LeuM1 检测到，我们和其他人已发现检测 Lewis X 抗原更敏感[36]。辨别 CD15 阳性的细胞同样是非常重要的。因为粒细胞 CD15 阳性率很高[31]，而且可以在许多肿瘤包括 HL 中存在。

白介素-2 受体

白介素-2 受体（CD25）是 HL 免疫治疗的靶点之一。这种治疗方案的缺陷是，尽管 H/RSCs 细胞表达的 CD25 是治疗的直接靶点，但检测 CD25 的表达有时很困难。事实上，在 HL 中活化的肿瘤浸润性淋巴细胞（TILs）呈 CD25 阳性，因此把它们与 H/RSCs 区分开是非常重要的，我们发现使用生物素化的酪氨酸增强步骤[62]，大部分福尔马林固定、石蜡包埋[30]的组织可以解决这个问题[30]。

表 4.2　霍奇金淋巴瘤相关抗原的抗体检测

抗体	克隆	制造商	稀释度	抗原修复方法
CD30	Ber-H2	DAKO	1:20	蒸汽/枸橼酸盐缓冲液 pH6，20 分钟，95~98℃
CD15	LeuM1	Becton-Dickinson	1:25	同 CD30
CD45（LCA）	2B11	DAKO	1:200	同 CD30
CD20	L26	DAKO	1:100	同 CD30
CD45RO	UCHL1	DAKO	1:200	胃蛋白酶消化 10 分钟，37℃
CD3	UCHT1	DAKO	1:30	蒸汽/枸橼酸盐缓冲液 pH6，20 分钟，95~98℃
CD40	MAB89	Immunotech	1:40	同 CD3
ALK-1	ALK-1	DAKO	1:25	同 CD3
Fascin	55K-2	DAKO	1:75	同 CD3
Lewis X type2 chain（Bg7）	P12	Signet	1:40	蒸汽/枸橼酸盐缓冲液 pH8，20 分钟，95~98℃
EBV-LMP-1	CS1-4	DAKO	1:50	蒸汽/枸橼酸盐缓冲液 pH6，20 分钟，95~98℃
bcl-6	PG-B6p	DAKO	1:10	同 EBV-LMP-1
CD57	Leu7	DAKO	1:10	同 EBV-LMP-1
EMA	E29	DAKO	1:50	胃蛋白酶消化 12 分钟，37℃
CDw75	LN1	ICN Biomedicals	未稀释	蒸汽/枸橼酸盐缓冲液 pH6，20 分钟，95~98℃
CD74	LN2	ICN Biomedicals	未稀释	同 CDw75
NFκB	P65C	Zymed Lab	1:200	同 CDw75
CCR7	CCR7.6B3	eBioscience, SanDiego, CA	1:200	在 1mmol/L EDTA pH8.0 中蒸汽 30 分钟（参考 Blood 2003；2473）
Jun B	SC8051	from Dako Santa Cruz,CA	1:75	HIER（蒸汽/靶修复液 30 分钟）

霍奇金淋巴瘤的免疫组织化学

CD30 抗原

用抗原修复的方法使用单克隆抗体Ber-H2，可以提高检测福尔马林固定、石蜡包埋的组织中CD30的敏感性。然而，有些血液病理学家更推崇使用B5固定组织，B5是一种含汞的氯化物，在免疫染色前需要脱汞，通常用Lugol方法然后再用硫代硫酸盐。Facchetti及其合作者研究发现，省略Lugol步骤检测CD30可取得满意的结果，甚至不需要微波加热修复或者蛋白酶水解消化切片[63]。

免疫组化的鉴别诊断

非淋巴组织肿瘤

CD30，最稳定的H/RSCs标记物，很容易在福尔马林固定、石蜡包埋的组织中检测，然而，在一些非淋巴组织恶性肿瘤如胚胎性癌、恶性黑色素瘤及胰腺癌中也可以表达CD30[64, 65]。由于CD30阳性的间变性大细胞淋巴瘤有浸润淋巴窦的特征，因此有可能与少量表达CD30的转移癌混淆[22]。另外，因为恶性黑色素瘤可以表达CD30，有时可能把低分化的恶性黑色素瘤，误认为原发的CD30阳性的间变性大细胞淋巴瘤[65]。

CD15在H/RSCs中的阳性表达也和多种癌有关系[66]，幸运的是，很少会碰到被误诊为HL的癌，相反的，结节硬化型HL合体细胞变型的黏附性瘤细胞，偶尔会被误诊为CD15阳性的转移癌。

非霍奇金淋巴瘤

间变性大细胞淋巴瘤

CD30在间变性大细胞淋巴瘤（ALCL）的瘤细胞中显色，间变性大细胞淋巴瘤是一种非霍奇金淋巴瘤，与霍奇金淋巴瘤具有不同的生物学特征[22, 67-70]。尽管间变性大细胞淋巴瘤具有黏附性的生长方式和浸润淋巴窦的显著组织学特征，但经验表明，仍有少数病例易于与富于细胞型霍奇金淋巴瘤，尤其是那些被英国国家研究所分类为结节硬化Ⅱ型[71]或合体细胞变型[72]及一些淋巴细胞消减型HL的病例相混淆（图4.17）[73]。这些病例，可以用抗体组合进行鉴别（表4.1和4.3），或许最有用的是多克隆抗体p80NPM/ALK，或者是单克隆抗体ALK-1，一种抗由t (2;5)(p23;q35) 染色体或其他更少见染色体易位产生的融合蛋白NPM/ALK的抗体（图4.18）[74, 75]。这种融合蛋白即便是在HL的恶性细胞中，表达也非常少见。

外周T细胞淋巴瘤的淋巴上皮样细胞变型（Lennert淋巴瘤）是另外一种T细胞淋巴瘤，由于存在H/RS样细胞、嗜酸性粒细胞及浆细胞而与经典型霍奇金淋巴瘤相似。小簇的上皮样组织细胞形成肉芽肿样结构是它的显著特征，Lennert淋巴瘤中H/RS样细胞表达CD4+的T细胞表型[76]。

原发纵隔的B细胞大细胞淋巴瘤

原发纵隔的B细胞淋巴瘤（PMBCL）可以和HL混淆，因为它也是好发于年轻人前纵隔的实体包块，在富含胶原的硬化性背景上含有H/RS样细胞（图4.19）[77]。在一项研究中发现51例中有35例H/RS样细胞表达CD30（69%）[78]。但是原发纵隔的B细胞淋巴瘤是可以和HL鉴别开的，因为它弥漫地强表达CD20，不表达CD15，没有EBV（EBERs和LMP-1），缺乏炎性背景，特别是HL中特征性的嗜酸性粒细胞。

富于T细胞的B细胞淋巴瘤

富于T细胞的B细胞淋巴瘤（TCRBCL）是一种非霍奇金淋巴瘤，多发生在50岁以上临床晚期（Ⅲ或Ⅳ期）的老年病人。富于T细胞的B细胞淋巴瘤对治疗HL的化疗方案反应很差，因此，把它与HL特别是结节性淋巴细胞为主型霍奇金淋巴瘤或者富于淋巴细胞型霍奇金淋巴瘤（图4.20）[78,79]区分开是十分重要的。富于T细胞的B细胞淋巴瘤中的瘤细胞不表达CD30和CD15以及波形蛋白，但在经典型HL中的H/RSCs都有表达。另外，在富于淋巴细胞型霍奇金淋巴瘤和经典型HL中富于TIA-1+的淋巴细胞浸润，在结节性淋巴细胞为主型霍奇金淋巴瘤中却很少见到，而且结节性淋巴细胞为主型霍奇金淋巴瘤中的特征性的CD57+淋巴细胞在富于T细胞的B细胞淋巴瘤中也不多见[80]。

具有H/RS样细胞的移植后霍奇金样淋巴组织增生紊乱（HL-PTLD）（图4.21），在异体移植病人，使用甲氨蝶呤化疗[81]及HIV病人中已有报道，在这些情况下均可发生经典型HL，不同在于形态学和免疫表型特征[82]。经典型HL中H/RSCs表达CD30和CD15，HL-PTLD中的细胞常表达活化的B细胞表型，比如CD20和CD30阳性，但CD15阴性，事实上在所有HL-PTLD中EBV阳性。

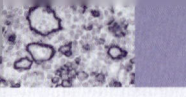

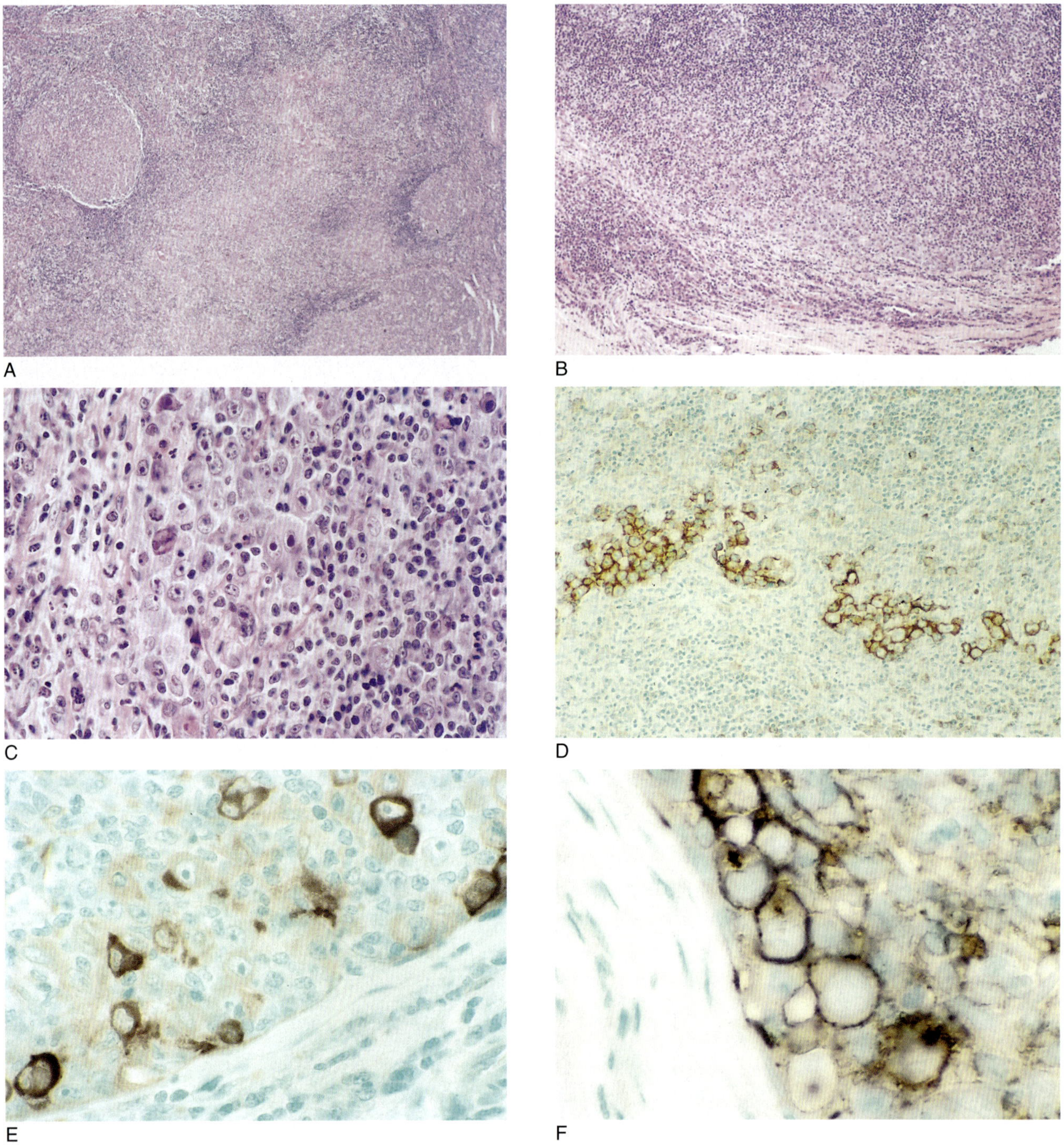

图4.17 富于细胞型HL，滤泡间及窦内分布的瘤细胞。(A) 低倍镜下滤泡间浸润；(B) 低倍镜下淋巴窦内的浸润；(C) 高倍镜下淋巴窦内的H/RSCs；(D) 淋巴窦内H/RSCs CD30的表达；(E) H/RSCs fascin的表达；(F) 淋巴窦内H/RSCs CD40的表达

假瘤性增生的免疫组化鉴别诊断

传染性单核细胞增多症

传染性单核细胞增多症中的H/RS样细胞在组织形态上，在EBERs、EBV-LMP-1和CD30的表达及LCA的低表达[83]上与HL相似，然而，传染性单核细胞增多症中的H/RS样细胞CD15阴性，并且缺乏HL中环绕H/RSCs的特征性的玫瑰花环T淋巴细胞[84]。

巨细胞病毒感染性淋巴结炎

巨细胞病毒感染的淋巴结由于病毒包涵体的原因含有H/RS样细胞，这些细胞免疫组化染色CD15和CD30都是阴性的，易于与HL区别（图4.22）。

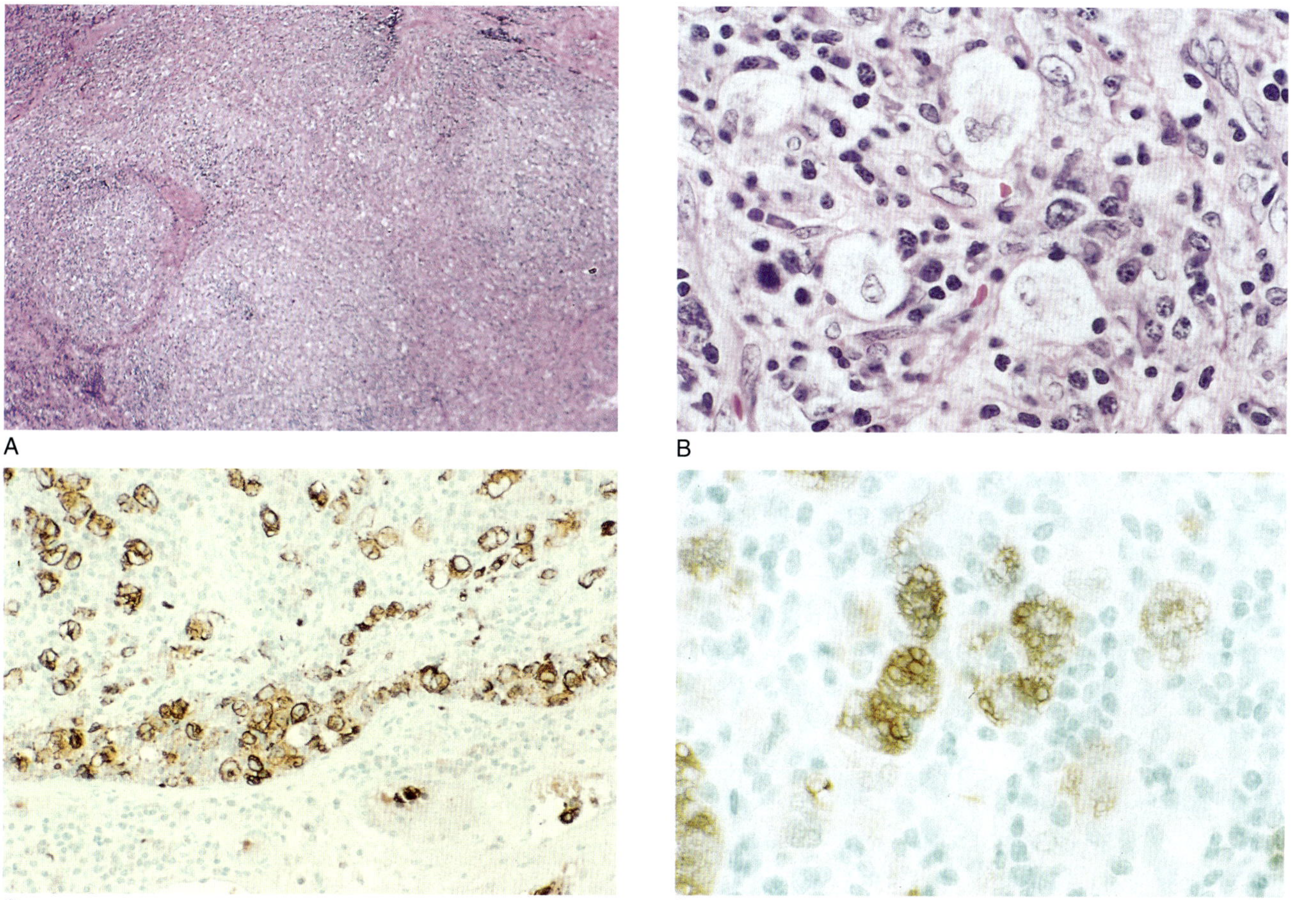

霍奇金淋巴瘤的免疫组织化学 4

图4.18 霍奇金样间变性大细胞淋巴瘤。(A) 结节样分布;(B) 陷窝细胞;(C) 淋巴窦内瘤细胞的CD30染色;(D) 陷窝中瘤细胞 p80NPM/ALK 的表达

滤泡间淋巴结炎

形似霍奇金病的淋巴结炎被看做一种良性的淋巴结病,形似滤泡间HL[85,86]。颈部淋巴结经常被累及,一般不会进展为淋巴瘤,淋巴结滤泡增生,滤泡间可见上皮样组织细胞、淋巴细胞、嗜酸性粒细胞及免疫母细胞。某些免疫母细胞像H/RSCs一样有较明显的核仁,但是,它们的核仁比较小而且是嗜碱性的,和H/RS样细胞的嗜酸性核仁形成对照。免疫组化可以把这种病变与HL区别开,因为其中的H/RS样细胞表达B

表4.3 霍奇金淋巴瘤鉴别诊断抗体一览表

	HL	ALCL	MLCBCL	TCRBCL
CD30	+	+	S	N
CD15	+	R	N	N
CD20	S	N	+	+
CD3	R	+	N	N
CD40	+	N	+	+
CD45 (LCA)	N	S	+	+
EBV-LMP-1	S	N	N	N
ALK	N	+	N	N
Fascin	+	S	N	N

+,几乎所有病例都阳性; S,有时阳性; R,很少阳性(<5%); N,阴性
HL,霍奇金淋巴瘤;ALCL,间变性大细胞淋巴瘤;MLCBCL,纵隔大细胞 B 细胞淋巴瘤;TCRBCL,富于 T 细胞的 B 细胞淋巴瘤

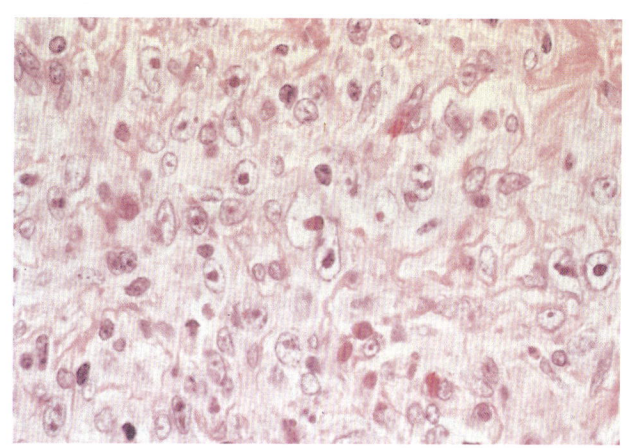

图 4.19 原发于纵隔的 B 细胞大细胞淋巴瘤中的 H/RS 样细胞

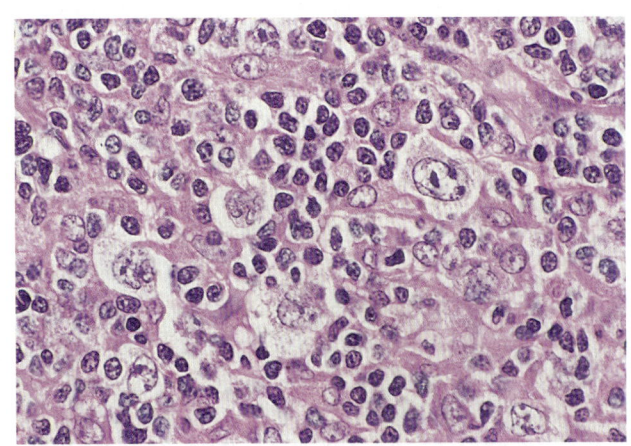

图4.20　富于T细胞的B细胞淋巴瘤中的H/RS样细胞

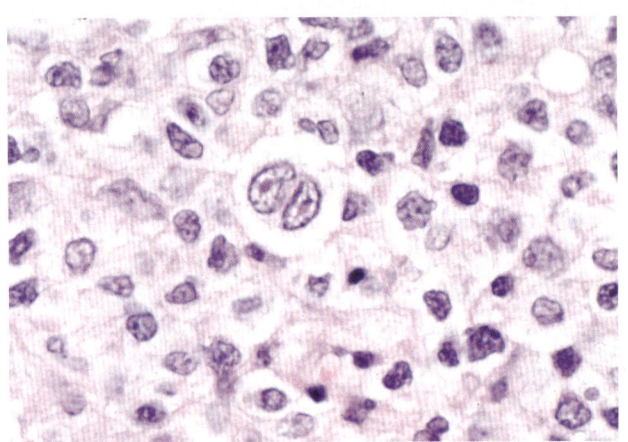

图4.21　移植后霍奇金样淋巴组织增生紊乱

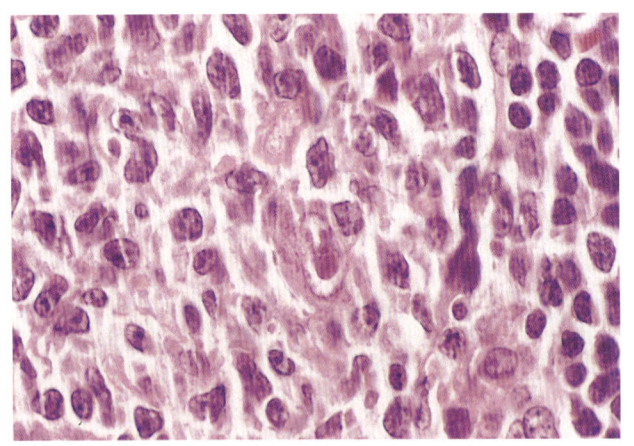

图4.22　巨细胞病毒感染的淋巴结内H/RS样细胞

或者T细胞抗原，并且缺乏CD15的表达[86, 87]。

肉芽肿性淋巴结炎

在非造血性及造血性恶性肿瘤包括HL中，非干酪样坏死性肉芽肿是非常常见的组织学特征（图4.23）。在HL中接近15%的病人有肉芽肿，可以出现

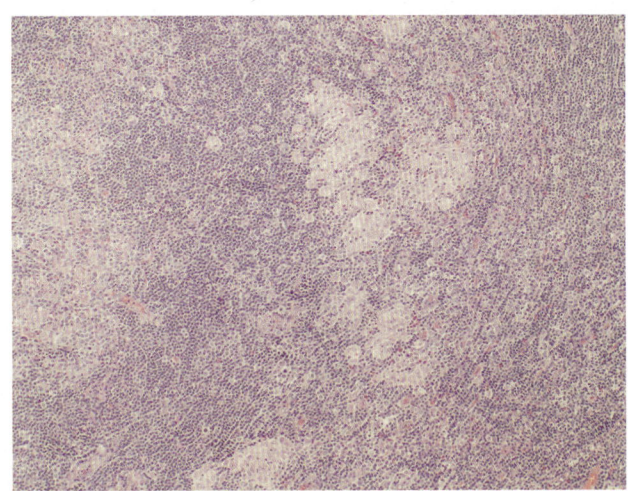

图4.23　HL淋巴结中的肉芽肿

在淋巴结和未被HL累及的结外部位[88]。缺乏诊断性的H/RSCs，仅出现肉芽肿，不能被看做诊断HL的依据。然而，在HL累及的部位可以出现肉芽肿反应，而且有时会很明显，这就需要全面复习形态学图像，从中找到小的HL病灶，这些区域的H/RSCs具有典型的免疫表型（CD30+、CD15+、LCA-、CD20-）与免疫母细胞截然不同（LCA+、CD20+、CD30+、CD15-）。

总　结

高质量的HE切片是诊断HL类型的前提，同时要避免免疫组化的陷阱。本章提出的HL和假瘤性淋巴组织增生性病变的诊断流程提供了应用免疫组化进行诊断的思路和方法（图4.24、4.25）。

参考文献

1. Lukes RJ, Butler JJ. The pathology and nomenclature of Hodgkin's disease. Cancer Res 1966; 26:1063–1083.
2. Harris NL, Jaffe ES, Stein H, et al. A revised European-American classification of lymphoid neoplasms: a proposal from the International Lymphoma Study Group. Blood 1994; 84: 1361–1392.
3. Mason DY, Banks PM, Chan J, et al. Nodular lymphocyte predominance Hodgkin's disease. A distinct clinicopathological entity. Am J Surg Pathol 1994; 18:526–530.
4. Poppema S. The nature of the lymphocytes surrounding Reed-Sternberg cells in nodular lymphocyte predominance and in other types of Hodgkin's disease. Am J Pathol 1989; 135:

霍奇金淋巴瘤的免疫组织化学 4

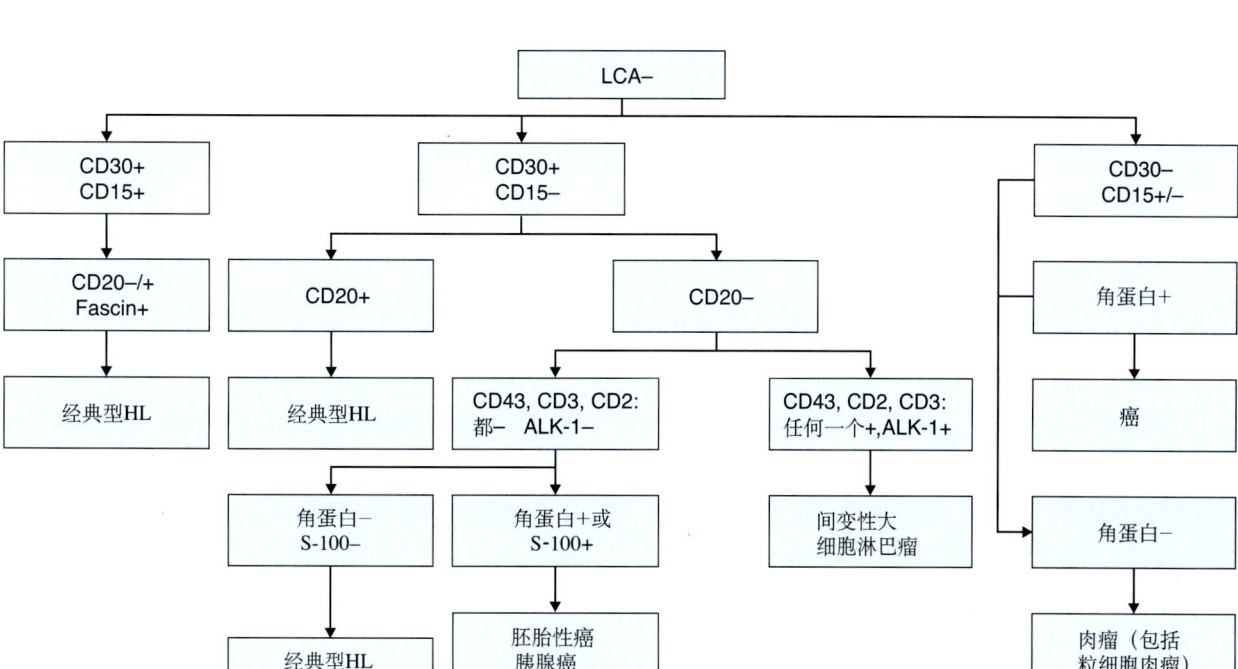

图 4.24　诊断流程：经典型霍奇金淋巴瘤

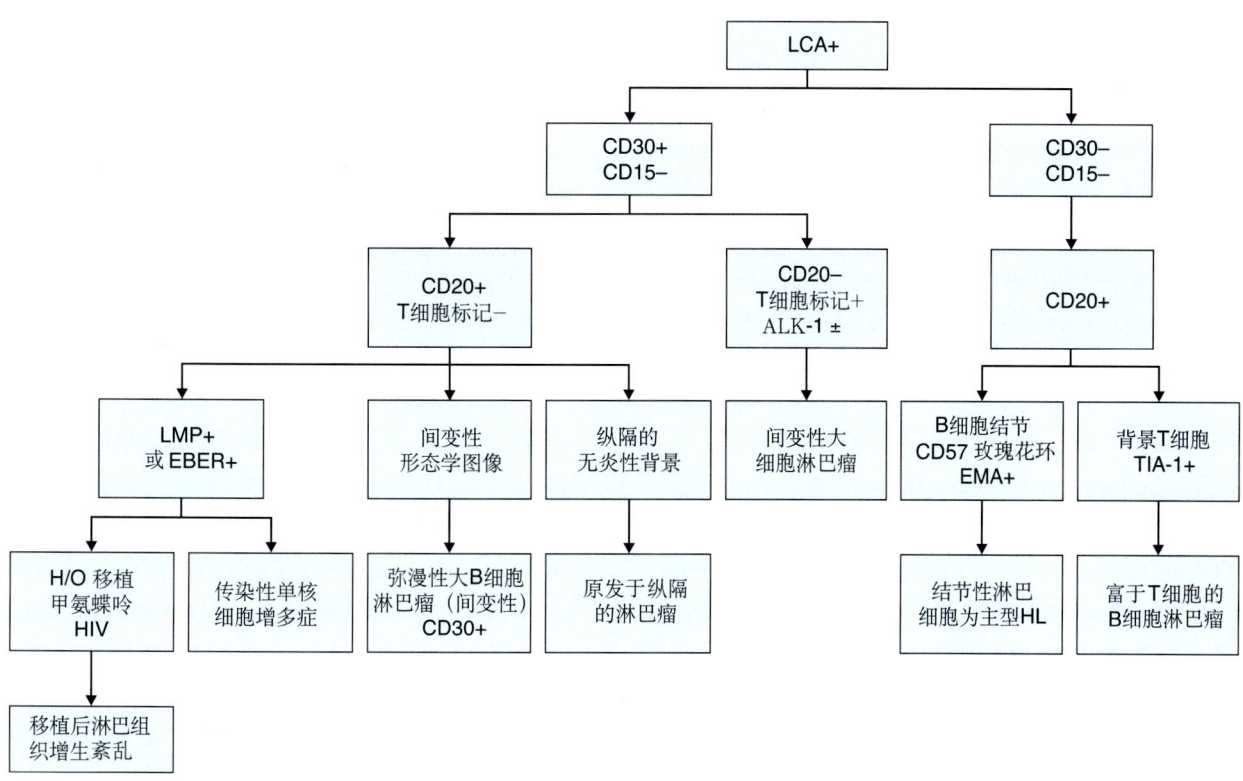

图 4.25　诊断流程：B 细胞淋巴瘤、结节性淋巴细胞为主型霍奇金淋巴瘤、假瘤性淋巴组织反应性增生性疾病

351–357.

5. Marafioti T, Hummel M, Anagnostopoulos I, et al. Origin of nodular lymphocyte-predominant Hodgkin's disease from a clonal expansion of highly mutated germinal-center B cells. N Engl J Med 1997; 337:453–458.

6. Kanzler H, Kuppers R, Hansmann ML, et al. Hodgkin and Reed-Sternberg cells in Hodgkin's disease represent the outgrowth of a dominant tumor clone derived from (crippled) germinal center B cells. J Exp Med 1996; 184:1495–1505.

7. Carbone A, Gloghini A, Gaidano G, et al. Expression status of BCL-6 and syndecan-1 identifies distinct histogenetic subtypes of Hodgkin's disease. Blood 1998; 92:2220–2228.

8. Pinkus GS, Said JW. Hodgkin's disease, lymphocyte predominance type, nodular – further evidence for a B cell derivation. L & H variants of Reed-Sternberg cells express L26, a pan B cell marker. Am J Pathol 1988; 133:211–217.

9. Epstein AL, Marder RJ, Winter JN, et al. Two new monoclonal antibodies (LN-1, LN-2) reactive in B5 formalin-fixed, paraffin-embedded tissues with follicular center and mantle zone human B lymphocytes and derived tumors. J Immunol 1984; 133:1028–1036.

10. Marder RJ, Variakojis D, Silver J, et al. Immunohistochemical analysis of human lymphomas with monoclonal antibodies to B cell and Ia antigens reactive in paraffin sections. Lab Invest 1985; 52:497–504.

11. Korkolopoulou P, Cordell J, Jones M, et al. The expression of the B-cell marker mb-1 (CD79a) in Hodgkin's disease. Histopathology 1994; 24:511–515.

12. Kadin ME, Muramoto L, Said J. Expression of T-cell antigens on Reed-Sternberg cells in a subset of patients with nodular sclerosing and mixed cellularity Hodgkin's disease. Am J Pathol 1988; 130:345–353.

13. Casey TT, Olson SJ, Cousar JB, et al. Immunophenotypes of Reed-Sternberg cells: a study of 19 cases of Hodgkin's disease in plastic-embedded sections. Blood 1989; 74:2624–2628.

14. Dallenbach FE, Stein H. Expression of T-cell-receptor beta chain in Reed-Sternberg cells. Lancet 1989; 2:828–830.

15. Oka K, Mori N, Kojima M. Anti-Leu-3a antibody reactivity with Reed-Sternberg cells of Hodgkin's disease. Arch Pathol Lab Med 1988; 112:139–142.

16. Oudejans JJ, Kummer JA, Jiwa M, et al. Granzyme B expression in Reed-Sternberg cells of Hodgkin's disease. Am J Pathol 1996; 148:233–240.

17. Krenacs L, Wellmann A, Sorbara L, et al. Cytotoxic cell antigen expression in anaplastic large cell lymphomas of T- and null-cell type and Hodgkin's disease: evidence for distinct cellular origin. Blood 1997; 89:980–989.

18. Felgar RE, Macon WR, Kinney MC, et al. TIA-1 expression in lymphoid neoplasms. Identification of subsets with cytotoxic T lymphocyte or natural killer cell differentiation. Am J Pathol 1997; 150:1893–1900.

19. Muschen M, Rajewsky K, Brauninger A, et al. Rare occurrence of classical Hodgkin's disease as a T cell lymphoma. J Exp Med 2000; 191:387–394.

20. Seitz V, Hummel M, Marafioti T, et al. Detection of clonal T-cell receptor gamma-chain gene rearrangements in Reed-Sternberg cells of classic Hodgkin disease. Blood 2000; 95: 3020–3024.

21. Willenbrock K, Ichinohasama R, Kadin ME, et al. T-cell variant of classical Hodgkin's lymphoma with nodal and cutaneous manifestations demonstrated by single-cell polymerase chain reaction. Lab Invest 2002; 82:1103–1109.

22. Stein H, Mason DY, Gerdes J, et al. The expression of the Hodgkin's disease associated antigen Ki-1 in reactive and neoplastic lymphoid tissue: evidence that Reed-Sternberg cells and histiocytic malignancies are derived from activated lymphoid cells. Blood 1985; 66:848–858.

23. Durkop H, Latza U, Hummel M, et al. Molecular cloning and expression of a new member of the nerve growth factor receptor family that is characteristic for Hodgkin's disease. Cell 1992; 68:421–427.

24. Smith CA, Gruss HJ, Davis T, et al. CD30 antigen, a marker for Hodgkin's lymphoma, is a receptor whose ligand defines an emerging family of cytokines with homology to TNF. Cell 1993; 73:1349–1360.

25. Bargou RC, Leng C, Krappmann D, et al. High-level nuclear NF-kappa B and Oct-2 is a common feature of cultured Hodgkin/Reed-Sternberg cells. Blood 1996; 87:4340–4347.

26. Bargou RC, Emmerich F, Krappmann D, et al. Constitutive nuclear factor-kappa B-RelA activation is required for proliferation and survival of Hodgkin's disease tumor cells. J Clin Invest 1997; 100:2961–2969.

27. Carbone A, Gloghini A, Gattei V, et al. Expression of functional CD40 antigen on Reed-Sternberg cells and Hodgkin's disease cell lines. Blood 1995; 85:780–789.

28. Banchereau J, Bazan F, Blanchard D, et al. The CD40 antigen and its ligand. Annu Rev Immunol 1994; 12:881–922.
29. Hsu SM, Tseng CK, Hsu PL. Expression of p55 (Tac) interleukin-2 receptor (IL-2R), but not p75 IL-2R, in cultured H-RS cells and H-RS cells in tissues. Am J Pathol 1990; 136: 735–744.
30. Levi E, Butmarc J, Kourea HP, et al. Detection of interleukin-2 receptors on tumor cells in formalin-fixed, paraffin-embedded tissues. Appl Immunohistochem 1997; 5:234.
31. Stein H, Uchanska-Ziegler B, Gerdes J, et al. Hodgkin and Sternberg-Reed cells contain antigens specific to late cells of granulopoiesis. Int J Cancer 1982; 29:283–290.
32. Hsu SM, Jaffe ES. Leu M1 and peanut agglutinin stain the neoplastic cells of Hodgkin's disease. Am J Clin Pathol 1984; 82:29–32.
33. Pinkus GS, Thomas P, Said JW. Leu-M1 – a marker for Reed-Sternberg cells in Hodgkin's disease. An immunoperoxidase study of paraffin-embedded tissues. Am J Pathol 1985; 119: 244–252.
34. von Wasielewski R, Mengel M, Fischer R, et al. Classical Hodgkin's disease. Clinical impact of the immunophenotype. Am J Pathol 1997; 151:1123–1130.
35. Gooi HC, Feizi T, Kapadia A, et al. Stage-specific embryonic antigen involving alpha 1 goes to 3 fucosylated type 2 blood group chains. Nature 1981; 292:156–158.
36. Ree HJ, Teplitz C, Khan A. The Lewis X antigen. A new paraffin section marker for Reed-Sternberg cells. Cancer 1991; 67:1338–1346.
37. Pinkus GS, Pinkus JL, Langhoff E, et al. Fascin, a sensitive new marker for Reed-Sternberg cells of Hodgkin's disease. Evidence for a dendritic or B cell derivation? Am J Pathol 1997; 150:543–562.
38. Weiss LM, Movahed LA, Warnke RA, et al. Detection of Epstein-Barr viral genomes in Reed-Sternberg cells of Hodgkin's disease. N Engl J Med 1989; 320:502–506.
39. Wang D, Liebowitz D, Kieff E. An EBV membrane protein expressed in immortalized lymphocytes transforms established rodent cells. Cell 1985; 43:831–840.
40. Pallesen G, Hamilton-Dutoit SJ, Rowe M, et al. Expression of Epstein-Barr virus latent gene products in tumour cells of Hodgkin's disease. Lancet 1991; 337:320–322.
41. Ambinder RF, Browning PJ, Lorenzana I, et al. Epstein-Barr virus and childhood Hodgkin's disease in Honduras and the United States. Blood 1993; 81:462–467.
42. Gulley ML, Eagan PA, Quintanilla-Martinez L, et al. Epstein-Barr virus DNA is abundant and monoclonal in the Reed-Sternberg cells of Hodgkin's disease: association with mixed cellularity subtype and Hispanic American ethnicity. Blood 1994; 83:1595–1602.
43. Herndier BG, Sanchez HC, Chang KL, et al. High prevalence of Epstein-Barr virus in the Reed-Sternberg cells of HIV-associated Hodgkin's disease. Am J Pathol 1993; 142:1073–1079.
44. Dorfman RF, Gatter KC, Pulford KA, et al. An evaluation of the utility of anti-granulocyte and anti-leukocyte monoclonal antibodies in the diagnosis of Hodgkin's disease. Am J Pathol 1986; 123:508–519.
45. Chittal SM, Caveriviere P, Schwarting R, et al. Monoclonal antibodies in the diagnosis of Hodgkin's disease. The search for a rational panel. Am J Surg Pathol 1988; 12:9–21.
46. von Wasielewski R, Werner M, Fischer R, et al. Lymphocyte-predominant Hodgkin's disease. An immunohistochemical analysis of 208 reviewed Hodgkin's disease cases from the German Hodgkin Study Group. Am J Pathol 1997; 150: 793–803.
47. Laumen H, Nielsen PJ, Wirth T. The BOB.1/OBF.1 co-activator is essential for octamer-dependent transcription in B cells. Eur J Immunol 2000; 30:458–469.
48. Steimle-Grauer SA, Tinguely M, Seada L, et al. Expression patterns of transcription factors in progressively transformed germinal centers and Hodgkin lymphoma. Virchows Arch 2003; 442:284–293.
49. Stein H, Marafioti T, Foss HD, et al. Down-regulation of BOB.1/OBF.1 and Oct2 in classical Hodgkin disease but not in lymphocyte predominant Hodgkin disease correlates with immunoglobulin transcription. Blood 2001; 97:496–501.
50. Hertel CB, Zhou XG, Hamilton-Dutoit SJ, et al. Loss of B cell identity correlates with loss of B cell-specific transcription factors in Hodgkin/Reed-Sternberg cells of classical Hodgkin lymphoma. Oncogene 2002; 21:4908–4920.
51. Marafioti T, Ascani S, Pulford K, et al. Expression of B-lymphocyte-associated transcription factors in human T-cell neoplasms. Am J Pathol 2003; 162:861–871.
52. Foss HD, Reusch R, Demel G, et al. Frequent expression of the B-cell-specific activator protein in Reed-Sternberg cells of classical Hodgkin's disease provides further evidence for

its B-cell origin. Blood 1999; 94:3108–3113.
53. Skinnider BF, Mak TW. The role of cytokines in classical Hodgkin lymphoma. Blood 2002; 99:4283–4297.
54. Mathas S, Hinz M, Anagnostopoulos I, et al. Aberrantly expressed c-Jun and JunB are a hallmark of Hodgkin lymphoma cells, stimulate proliferation and synergize with NF-kappa B. Embo J 2002; 21:4104–4113.
55. Hopken UE, Foss HD, Meyer D, et al. Up-regulation of the chemokine receptor CCR7 in classical but not in lymphocyte-predominant Hodgkin disease correlates with distinct dissemination of neoplastic cells in lymphoid organs. Blood 2002; 99:1109–1116.
56. Poppema S. The diversity of the immunohistological staining pattern of Sternberg-Reed cells. J Histochem Cytochem 1980; 28:788–791.
57. Stein H, Hansmann ML, Lennert K, et al. Reed-Sternberg and Hodgkin cells in lymphocyte-predominant Hodgkin's disease of nodular subtype contain J chain. Am J Clin Pathol 1986; 86:292–297.
58. Delsol G, Blancher A, al Saati T, et al. Antibody BNH9 detects red blood cell-related antigens on anaplastic large cell (CD30+) lymphomas. Br J Cancer 1991; 64:321–326.
59. al Saati T, Tkaczuk J, Krissansen G, et al. A novel antigen detected by the CBF.78 antibody further distinguishes anaplastic large cell lymphoma from Hodgkin's disease. Blood 1995; 86:2741–2746.
60. Chu WS, Abbondanzo SL, Frizzera G. Inconsistency of the immunophenotype of Reed-Sternberg cells in simultaneous and consecutive specimens from the same patients. A paraffin section evaluation in 56 patients. Am J Pathol 1992; 141:11–17.
61. Tepler I, Schwartz G, Parker K, et al. Phase I trial of an interleukin-2 fusion toxin (DAB486IL-2) in hematologic malignancies: complete response in a patient with Hodgkin's disease refractory to chemotherapy. Cancer 1994; 73:1276–1285.
62. Merz H, Malisius R, Mannweiler S, et al. ImmunoMax. A maximized immunohistochemical method for the retrieval and enhancement of hidden antigens. Lab Invest 1995; 73:149–156.
63. Facchetti F, Alebardi O, Vermi W. Omit iodine and CD30 will shine: a simple technical procedure to demonstrate the CD30 antigen on B5-fixed material. Am J Surg Pathol 2000; 24:320–322.
64. Schwarting R, Gerdes J, Durkop H, et al. BER-H2: a new anti-Ki-1 (CD30) monoclonal antibody directed at a formol-resistant epitope. Blood 1989; 74:1678–1689.
65. Polski JM, Janney CG. Ber-H2 (CD30) immunohistochemical staining in malignant melanoma. Mod Pathol 1999; 12:903–906.
66. Sheibani K, Battifora H, Burke JS, et al. Leu-M1 antigen in human neoplasms. An immunohistologic study of 400 cases. Am J Surg Pathol 1986; 10:227–236.
67. Kadin ME, Sako D, Berliner N, et al. Childhood Ki-1 lymphoma presenting with skin lesions and peripheral lymphadenopathy. Blood 1986; 68:1042–1049.
68. Nakamura S, Takagi N, Kojima M, et al. Clinicopathologic study of large cell anaplastic lymphoma (Ki-1-positive large cell lymphoma) among the Japanese. Cancer 1991; 68:118–129.
69. Gascoyne RD, Aoun P, Wu D, et al. Prognostic significance of anaplastic lymphoma kinase (ALK) protein expression in adults with anaplastic large cell lymphoma. Blood 1999; 93:3913–3921.
70. Falini B, Pileri S, Zinzani PL, et al. ALK+ lymphoma: clinico-pathological findings and outcome. Blood 1999; 93:2697–2706.
71. Haybittle JL, Hayhoe FG, Easterling MJ, et al. Review of British National Lymphoma Investigation studies of Hodgkin's disease and development of prognostic index. Lancet 1985; 1:967–972.
72. Strickler JG, Michie SA, Warnke RA, et al. The 'syncytial variant' of nodular sclerosing Hodgkin's disease. Am J Surg Pathol 1986; 10:470–477.
73. Rudiger T, Jaffe ES, Delsol G, et al. Workshop report on Hodgkin's disease and related diseases ('grey zone' lymphoma). Ann Oncol 1998; 9(Suppl 5):S31–S38.
74. Shiota M, Fujimoto J, Takenaga M, et al. Diagnosis of t(2;5)(p23;q35)-associated Ki-1 lymphoma with immunohistochemistry. Blood 1994; 84:3648–3652.
75. Pulford K, Lamant L, Morris SW, et al. Detection of anaplastic lymphoma kinase (ALK) and nucleolar protein nucleophosmin (NPM)-ALK proteins in normal and neoplastic cells with the monoclonal antibody ALK1. Blood 1997; 89:1394–1404.
76. Suchi T, Lennert K, Tu LY, et al. Histopathology and immu-

77. nohistochemistry of peripheral T cell lymphomas: a proposal for their classification. J Clin Pathol 1987; 40:995–1015.
77. Paulli M, Strater J, Gianelli U, et al. Mediastinal B-cell lymphoma: a study of its histomorphologic spectrum based on 109 cases. Hum Pathol 1999; 30:178–187.
78. Higgins JP, Warnke RA. CD30 expression is common in mediastinal large B-cell lymphoma. Am J Clin Pathol 1999; 112:241–247.
79. Chittal SM, Brousset P, Voigt JJ, et al. Large B-cell lymphoma rich in T-cells and simulating Hodgkin's disease. Histopathology 1991; 19:211–220.
80. Rudiger T, Ott G, Ott MM, et al. Differential diagnosis between classic Hodgkin's lymphoma, T-cell-rich B-cell lymphoma, and paragranuloma by paraffin immunohistochemistry. Am J Surg Pathol 1998; 22:1184–1191.
81. Chevrel G, Berger F, Miossec P, et al. Hodgkin's disease and B cell lymphoproliferation in rheumatoid arthritis patients treated with methotrexate: a kinetic study of lymph node changes. Arthritis Rheum 1999; 42:1773–1776.
82. Kamel OW, Weiss LM, van de Rijn M, et al. Hodgkin's disease and lymphoproliferations resembling Hodgkin's disease in patients receiving long-term low-dose methotrexate therapy. Am J Surg Pathol 1996; 20:1279–1287.
83. Strickler JG, Fedeli F, Horwitz CA, et al. Infectious mononucleosis in lymphoid tissue. Histopathology, in situ hybridization, and differential diagnosis. Arch Pathol Lab Med 1993; 117:269–278.
84. Reynolds DJ, Banks PM, Gulley ML. New characterization of infectious mononucleosis and a phenotypic comparison with Hodgkin's disease. Am J Pathol 1995; 146:379–388.
85. Fellbaum C, Hansmann ML, Lennert K. Lymphadenitis mimicking Hodgkin's disease. Histopathology 1988; 12:253–262.
86. Doggett RS, Colby TV, Dorfman RF. Interfollicular Hodgkin's disease. Am J Surg Pathol 1983; 7:145–149.
87. Chan JKC, Tsang WYW. Reactive lymphadenopathies. In: Weiss LM, ed. Pathology of lymph nodes. Contemporary issues in surgical pathology. Philadelphia: Churchill Livingstone; 1996.
88. Kadin ME, Donaldson SS, Dorfman RF. Isolated granulomas in Hodgkin's disease. N Engl J Med 1970; 283:859–861.

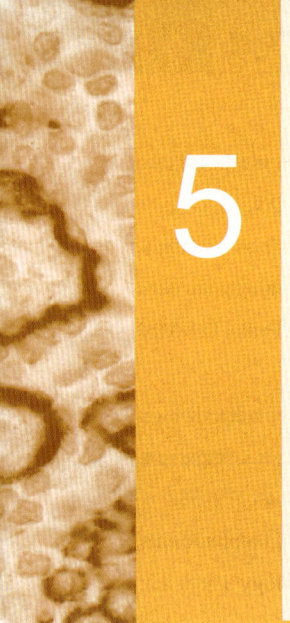

5 非霍奇金淋巴瘤的免疫组织化学

原作者：Christopher D.Gocke

译　者：周庚寅

审校者：郝春燕，孙妍琳

目　录

引言	136
非霍奇金淋巴瘤诊断中的抗原/抗体生物学	137
非霍奇金淋巴瘤和其他恶性肿瘤	143

引　言

作为一种诊断指标，免疫组织化学的发展从一开始就与人们对非霍奇金淋巴瘤的认识联系在一起。一方面，淋巴细胞可以产生免疫研究的试剂，另一方面从人类和动物体内获得淋巴细胞作为研究对象是可行的。这是一个相互促进的过程：淋巴细胞转化和淋巴瘤分类的研究要求有更多的诊断性试剂的出现，同时诊断试剂的快速发展促进了非霍奇金淋巴瘤更好的分类。

在过去的十年中，对非霍奇金淋巴瘤的诊断方案发生了一些变化。Kiel和Lukes-Collins分类法、事实分类法和工作分类，已经被1994年修订的欧美淋巴瘤（REAL）分类法所取代[1]。国际血液病理专家组根据淋巴瘤形态学、免疫表型、遗传学特征和临床表现，经过归纳和整理提出了新的淋巴瘤分类。形态学表现、免疫表型和遗传学特点都可以用于特定类型淋巴疾病的诊断，许多淋巴疾病仅依靠其形态学表现就可以作出诊断，而其他的一些淋巴疾病的确诊就需要分子生物学或免疫学方面的信息。尽管对REAL分类仍有不同意见[2-4]，但REAL分类却由于它在临床方面的实用性而得到了认可[5,6]。

在欧洲血液病理协会和北美血液病理协会的协作下，2001年世界卫生组织发表了修订的REAL分类法[7]。相比较REAL分类法，该造血和淋巴组织肿瘤的WHO分类法作了一些小的变动，它列出了所有已被认识的血液系统的恶性肿瘤[8,9]。由于WHO分类法已被广泛接受，该分类体系明确地（部分地）以免疫表型作为分类的基础，因此本章所涉及的非霍奇金淋巴瘤的免疫表型将会以WHO分类为指导。当大家所公认的变型与主要疾病显著不同时，这些变型将会被提到。

在免疫组织化学中，抗体组合的应用得到了广泛的认可。特别在造血和淋巴系统疾病的诊断中更是如此。细胞学/组织学的特点结合单一抗体的应用不足以区分良恶性或淋巴瘤类型[10,11]。没有一个单一的抗体组合可以满足所有的情况，但是一系列不同的适量的抗体组合却可以给我们提供有用的信息。如同病理学的其他领域一样，免疫组织化学常常在淋巴瘤的诊断中发挥着辅助形态学诊断的作用。此外，血液病理学家可采用分子生物学、流式细胞术和细胞基因的检测辅助诊断。需要强调的是，患者的病史与实验室检查的联系具有极其重要的价值。

淋巴瘤免疫学表型的术语与很多其他类型的肿瘤略有不同。白细胞的细胞表面抗原被命名为白细胞分化抗原群（CD），其中的每一种都可以结合不同数目的诊断抗体[12]。令病理学家们普遍感到烦恼的是，CD这一术语还没有和细胞或组织类型相对应。因此，一些相互分离的数字可能与相似的细胞类型相关，例如，B细胞限制性抗原决定簇CD20和CDw75。除了根据相应的CD分化抗原靶点命名外，抗体还可以根据任意克隆命名（例如，4C7）或根据起源地点命名（例如，Ki-1源于Kiel，德国）。

以往由于抗体不能够识别被固定剂交联遮蔽的抗

原决定簇，许多血液病理学诊断需要冰冻组织或丙酮固定的冰冻组织。由于在制备和解释冰冻切片免疫组织化学方面水平的限制，很少有常规病理实验室可以提供这种服务。然而，现在已经有了许多可以用于甲醛或汞固定组织的商品化的抗体。本章将主要介绍可用于石蜡包埋固定组织的有效抗体开展的免疫组织化学。对于大多数病理学实验室来说，该技术非常容易掌握。然而，良好的细胞形态的免疫组织化学分析结果在冰冻切片中不易获得。酶对蛋白的部分消化为一些抗体提供了更好的免疫标记效果[13]。一些抗原暴露或抗原修复也可有助于固定组织的免疫组织化学分析[14, 15]。当然如果必要，快速冰冻组织可被保留起来，送到相关的实验室进行进一步研究。

对于淋巴细胞分化、成熟和迁移的理解为淋巴瘤的免疫学表型提供了依据，因为淋巴细胞成熟的阶段，部分是根据它们产生的大分子所决定的。其细节[18-21]可参照经典的病理学著作[16,17]。恶性淋巴细胞可表达与某一分化阶段淋巴细胞表达相似的抗原成分。事实上，Lukes&Collins和Kiel淋巴瘤分类明确地把正常淋巴细胞分化的阶段作为分类的参考和原则[22-24]。一般来说，淋巴瘤是由阻滞在某个分化阶段的细胞组成[25]。这是一个有用的概念，尽管许多专家认为这样的表述不够完善，不能够代表所有淋巴瘤分型的真实状况。

非霍奇金淋巴瘤诊断中的抗原/抗体生物学

B 细胞

CD19

CD19 是 B 分化谱系中最早应用的免疫化学标记。抗体不能用于石蜡切片。

CD20

CD20抗原表位出现在B细胞成熟过程的前B细胞后期阶段，而且在B细胞分化的大多数阶段保留在细胞上，但是在浆细胞阶段这种抗原表位消失了。由于可以被抗体L26所识别，CD20在以下情况为强阳性：约半数的淋巴母细胞淋巴瘤/白血病，几乎所有的成熟 B 细胞淋巴瘤（浆细胞型除外），大约 1/4 的

经典霍奇金淋巴瘤的 Reed-Sternberg 细胞，大多数非 T 细胞淋巴瘤（图 5.1）。

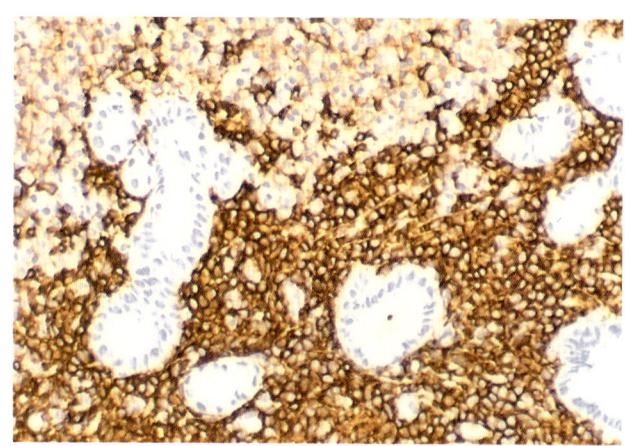

图5.1　黏膜相关性淋巴组织边缘区B细胞淋巴瘤的CD20免疫标记。细胞浆阳性的 B 细胞在胃腺间浸润。注意朝向腔面的浆细胞成分染色较浅或缺失（见顶部）

CD21

CD21抗体识别补体成分C3d的受体，此受体介导对补体包被颗粒的吞噬作用。滤泡树突细胞和一些B淋巴细胞CD21阳性。CD21对于在FL中识别滤泡树突细胞网是非常有用的，同时可以帮助识别血管免疫母细胞性 T 细胞淋巴瘤中增生的树突状细胞岛。

CD22

CD22是一种跨膜分子，可以抑制B细胞受体介导的信号转导，发挥分子开关的作用，使受到刺激的B细胞从增生状态变为凋亡状态[26]。它和CD19的表达大致一致，在毛细胞白血病表达为强阳性。

CD23

CD23是一种膜蛋白，可以和IgE低亲和力结合，同时调节单核细胞释放细胞因子。它在B细胞CLL/SLL和其他病变的鉴别诊断中是非常有用的，在CLL/SLL向大细胞转化的过程中仍表达。

CD79a

最近发现，CD79a的抗体在石蜡切片上可很好地检测出B细胞（图5.2A）[27]。其抗原与免疫球蛋白分子相关，表达于B淋巴细胞发生的早期。几乎所有前驱B淋巴母细胞淋巴瘤/白血病都为CD79a阳性，T细胞阴性。成熟B细胞淋巴瘤也为阳性。

DBA.44

DBA.44是一种B细胞亚群抗体，大多数毛细胞白血病（HCL）的胞浆表现为强阳性。然而这对于毛细胞白血病并不是特异的，因为在一些边缘区淋巴瘤和大细胞淋巴瘤中同样可以阳性。

免疫球蛋白轻链

抗κ和λ型免疫球蛋白轻链的抗体是最早用于免疫学诊断的试剂之一，同时也被过度地应用。

成熟 B 细胞产生免疫球蛋白，并将免疫球蛋白运送到细胞表面作为抗原的受体。这种由一条轻链和一条重链组成异源二聚体的免疫球蛋白分子在每一个细胞都是独特的。产生免疫球蛋白分子的基因重排过程可以导致产生κ的基因，或产生λ的基因。经重排机制产生的κ型免疫球蛋白细胞的数量是产生λ型免疫球蛋白细胞数量的两倍左右[28]。在正常或反应性B细胞群中，这个比例是保持不变的，但恶性 B 细胞淋巴瘤则不然。尽管正常轻链比例的范围已经被流式细胞术确定[29, 30]，但是定量分析却很难用于组织切片。在异常的多数细胞上仅出现一种轻链时，即轻链的限制性或者单型性。虽然与单克隆性含义不同，但通常认为单型性是恶性增殖的证据。实际上，当B细胞或浆细胞群的比例超过正常的 2：1 的 4 倍时（即超过大约85%的细胞κ阳性，或者超过65%的细胞λ阳性），就可以准确地作出单型性的诊断。这是一种大家认可的主观判断。

尽管大多数成熟B细胞和恶性B细胞表达两种轻链的一种，石蜡切片的免疫组化方法通常在检测淋巴细胞表面的轻链时仍不够敏感。然而，浆细胞因其免疫球蛋白位于细胞内和相对丰富而更容易分析。轻链免疫组织化学因背景染色的增加，使其分析判断较为复杂，这要归因于各种各样的细胞非特异性的摄取免疫球蛋白、细胞外血清的染色或间质的免疫球蛋白分子。免疫球蛋白轻链抗体应该理解为是一对抗体。一个抗体的缺失或缺乏与另一抗体的过度表达几乎同样重要。以下两种情况是相同的：这一对抗体对大多数细胞都染色或者没有抗体对任何细胞染色。上述两种情况下的任何一种都无法提供合理的解释。

免疫球蛋白轻链的免疫组织化学的低信号和较强的背景染色对病理学家提出了挑战。应该像对轻链抗体染色结果的分析一样，精心选择订购轻链抗体。因为免疫球蛋白轻链 mRNA 的原位杂交技术没有细胞外背景，这为病理学家提供了一个选择[31-34]。

T 细胞

CD2

CD2，E玫瑰花环受体，是一种T细胞广泛表达的细胞标记。它的抗体可以免疫标记绝大多数 T 细胞和NK细胞的恶性肿瘤，但是用于石蜡切片需要免疫学方法进行信号的放大（图 5.2B）[35]。一些胸腺B细胞也表现为 CD2 阳性。

CD3

在细胞膜上，T细胞抗原受体与CD3蛋白复合物相结合。一种商品化的抗CD3的多克隆抗体，可以与固定组织的多数 T 细胞淋巴瘤相互作用，但一些间变性大细胞淋巴瘤和 NK 细胞白血病／淋巴瘤例外。

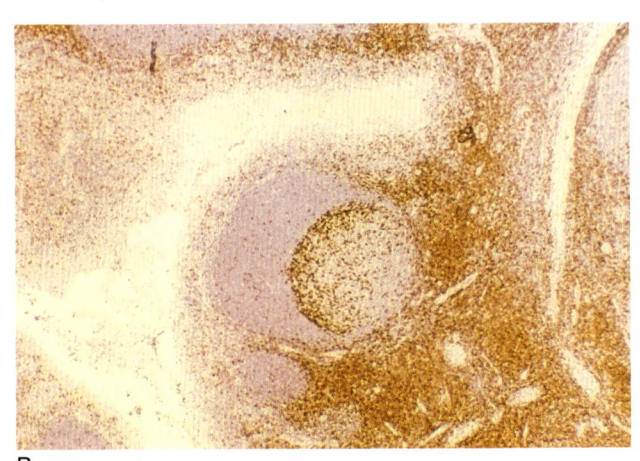

图 5.2 （A）正常淋巴结CD79a 表达。套淋巴细胞、多数生发中心细胞和散在的滤泡间 B 淋巴细胞表达早期 B 细胞抗原；（B）正常淋巴结内 CD2 表达。大多数滤泡间淋巴细胞和生发中心亮区的散在的 T 细胞表达早期 T 细胞抗原

CD3是T细胞非常特异的标记物。

CD4

在抗原的识别过程中，CD4分子与HLA II分子相互作用，标记辅助性T细胞亚群。CD4同样可以在一系列单核细胞系细胞，如朗格汉斯细胞和其他树突状细胞中表达。CD4抗原在不成熟的胸腺细胞中不表达，它表达于T细胞的分化过程中。虽然前驱T淋巴母细胞淋巴瘤CD4的表达不一，但是大多数成熟T细胞淋巴瘤CD4阳性，除外侵袭性NK细胞白血病、结外NK细胞淋巴瘤、λδ-T细胞淋巴瘤、皮下脂膜炎样T细胞淋巴瘤和肠病型T细胞淋巴瘤。该抗体可用于石蜡切片，但不如用于流式细胞术或冰冻切片敏感[36]。由于分别应用了抗体CD134/CD69[37]和CD30/CD184[38]，从而发现了T_H1和T_H2亚群。

CD5

CD5是一种信号转导分子，它存在于大多数胸腺细胞和不成熟的外周T细胞的表面。在循环的B细胞小的亚群中，CD5也可以是阳性。CD5最初用于B细胞CLL/SLL和套细胞淋巴瘤免疫组织化学诊断。需要进行抗原修复。

CD7

CD7可检测恶性肿瘤经常丢失的T细胞亚群标记物，尤其是蕈样霉菌病[39]。非T细胞恶性淋巴瘤包括NK细胞淋巴瘤和急性髓性白血病同样可表达CD7。CD7可以用于石蜡切片，但是有一定的困难。

CD8

CD8抗原界定抑制性/细胞毒T细胞亚群。它与CD4一同表达于胸腺细胞，但是这种情况只在一小部分的外周细胞中得以维持。CD4：CD8的比例与B细胞恶性淋巴瘤中免疫球蛋白轻链的比例并不相似；感染和炎症背景可以显著地改变2:1的比例。在固定组织中检测到的CD8的β链与流式细胞术检测的结果具有相似的敏感性。

其他抗体在非霍奇金淋巴瘤诊断中的应用

ALK

ALK是间变性淋巴瘤激酶基因的蛋白产物，最初是作为间变性大细胞淋巴瘤（ALCL）的t（2;5）染色体异位的伴随特征被人们所认识的。正常情况下，不应该在中枢神经系统以外的组织中发现这种蛋白。在间变性大细胞淋巴瘤（ALCL）中，ALK的表达因NPM基因与ALK基因的融合而上调，结果产生了这种血液病理学中少有的肿瘤特异性标记。ALK在淋巴瘤中的表达局限于间变性大细胞淋巴瘤（ALCL）和少数弥漫性大B细胞淋巴瘤[40]。该抗体可用于固定的组织，肿瘤细胞的胞浆和胞核均呈阳性[41]。几乎所有ALK阳性的淋巴瘤同时也表现为CD30和EMA阳性，CD15阴性（图5.3）。

cyclin D1

cyclin D1蛋白，又被称为bcl-1和PRAD1，是一种细胞周期调节蛋白，通过套细胞淋巴瘤中t（11;14）染色体异位确认。cyclin D1是一种可以在石蜡切片上检测的核蛋白，在大多数套细胞淋巴瘤中均表达（图5.4）。毛细胞白血病和浆细胞瘤也可弱表达cyclin

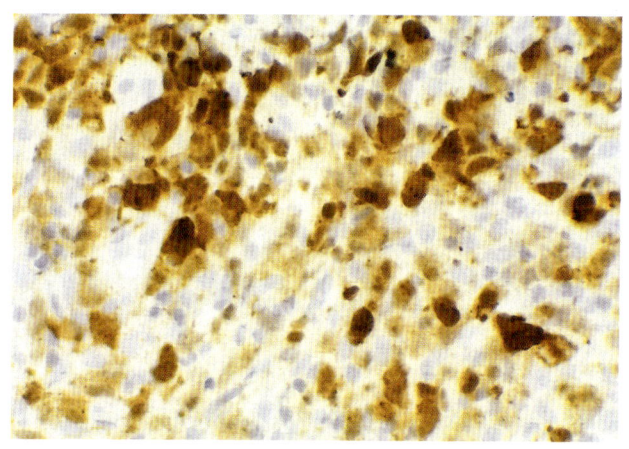

图5.3 ALK抗体显示，间变性大细胞淋巴瘤淋巴组织细胞变型（T细胞，原发性系统性）的瘤细胞胞浆和胞核均阳性。其间的小淋巴细胞和组织细胞为阴性

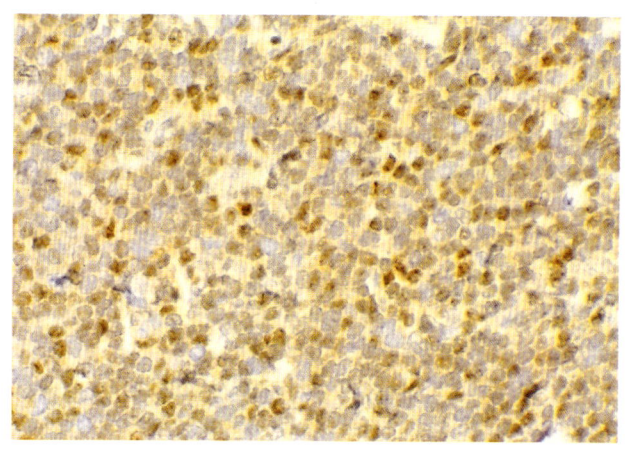

图5.4 套细胞淋巴瘤中cyclin D1的表达，请注意胞核为阳性

D1。许多B细胞淋巴瘤出现非特异性细胞浆染色,这与mRNA表达无相关性。

bcl-2

在淋巴瘤中,bcl-2是人们认识的第一个易位相关蛋白。大约3/4的滤泡性淋巴瘤(FL)发生了t(14;18)染色体易位,使bcl-2基因和免疫球蛋白重链基因并列,导致了bcl-2的过度表达(图5.5)。bcl-2为一种异源二聚体的一部分,该二聚体通过与一些配偶体的结合被调节,发挥机制尚未完全明了的抗凋亡作用。bcl-2通常表达于滤泡套层B淋巴细胞的胞浆,偶见于生发中心细胞和许多T淋巴细胞。bcl-2在多数小淋巴细胞淋巴瘤和80%的滤泡性淋巴瘤有较强的表达。bcl-2在其他淋巴瘤的表达归因于基因表达上调而非t(14;18)染色体易位。

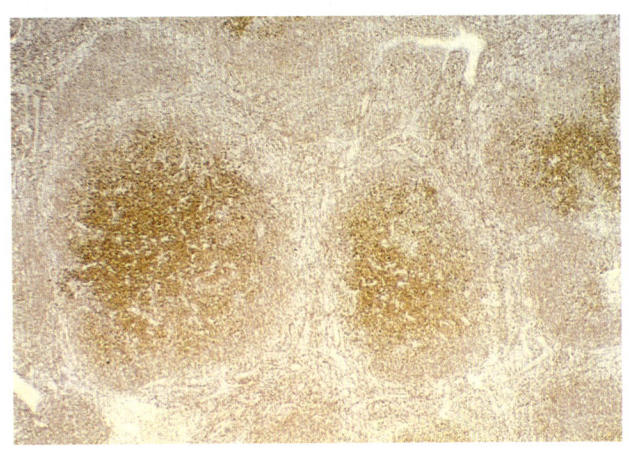

图5.5 bcl-2在滤泡性淋巴瘤中的表达。瘤性滤泡bcl-2阳性,但其周围的多数淋巴细胞为阴性。而在滤泡增生的淋巴结,情况恰好相反

bcl-6

bcl-6蛋白一般表达于生发中心淋巴细胞[42],发挥转录调节蛋白的作用。在正常淋巴结,bcl-6的分布方式与bcl-2相反。在一系列B细胞淋巴瘤,它表达于肿瘤细胞的细胞核,并在滤泡性淋巴瘤演进过程中丢失。bcl-6也可表达于结节性淋巴细胞为主型霍奇金病的L&H变型中。

CD1a

CD1a是一种跨膜抗原,一般表达于胸腺皮质细胞和朗格汉斯细胞。CD1a与β2巨球蛋白相关,可能在胸腺细胞的发育过程中发挥作用。可在前驱T淋巴母细胞淋巴瘤/白血病的亚群中发现CD1a。

CD10(CALLA)

CD10是急性淋巴母细胞白血病的共同抗原,是表达于早期淋巴祖细胞和正常生发中心细胞的一种锌金属肽酶。CD10常见于前驱B淋巴母细胞淋巴瘤和Burkitt淋巴瘤细胞的表面,较少见于前驱T淋巴母细胞白血病/淋巴瘤中。许多滤泡性淋巴瘤、一些弥漫性大B细胞淋巴瘤和多发性骨髓瘤均呈阳性。CD10和bcl-6通常作为生发中心起源的标记物。

CD15

CD15,X半抗原或Lewis X抗原,可以被LeuM1抗体识别。CD15最初作为单核/髓样细胞标记,同时也是经典霍奇金淋巴瘤R-S细胞的标记。除了一些皮肤原发性间变性大细胞淋巴瘤和其他外周T细胞淋巴瘤,CD15在大多数非霍奇金淋巴瘤中为阴性。着色的方式为典型的胞膜着色,同时核旁高尔基体点状阳性。外科病理学家将会注意到这种抗体也可用于腺癌染色。

CD25

白介素-2的受体被命名为CD25。最初是从T淋巴细胞中分离出来的。现在已知,CD25表达于毛细胞白血病和成人T淋巴细胞白血病/淋巴瘤。该抗体不能用于石蜡切片。

CD30

CD30抗原是肿瘤坏死因子受体超家族的成员之一,并对携带它的细胞有基因多效性作用。在一系列疾病中发现了越来越多的可溶性CD30。在外科病理实验室,CD30在冰冻组织中可由Ki-1抗体所识别或在石蜡切片上由抗体Ber-H2所识别。可接受的染色形式为胞膜着色或核周点状着色;胞浆着色应该看做结果可疑(图5.6)。在正常淋巴结和扁桃体特别是在生发中心的边缘,分散的大和小的活化的淋巴细胞CD30阳性。CD30表达于间变性大细胞淋巴瘤(ALCL)和淋巴瘤样丘疹病,同时表达于95%的经典型霍奇金淋巴瘤的一些R-S细胞(如同CD15,不是全部细胞阳性)。CD30也可以标记散在的非间变性淋巴瘤细胞。CD30还可以出现在一些胚细胞肿瘤和一些黑色素瘤中,因而它既不是肿瘤特异性标记物也不是淋巴瘤特异性标记物。CD30一直被认为是T_H2型细胞亚群的标记物或调节者。

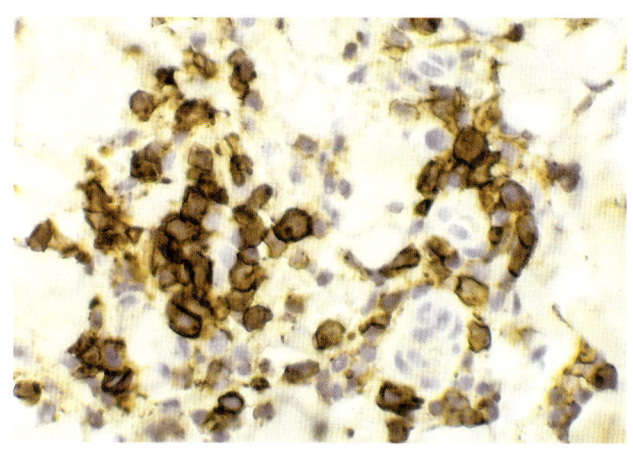

图5.6 在一例原发性皮肤T细胞间变性大细胞淋巴瘤（ALCL）中，抗体 Ber-H2 标记 CD30。一些细胞除胞膜强阳性外，还表现为核旁高尔基体着色

CD43

CD43可以作为一种抗黏附分子，介导白细胞之间的相互排斥。CD43又被称作白涎素，这种修饰的蛋白表达于除一些静止B细胞之外的所有白细胞的表面。CD43在淋巴瘤中的表达与CD5密切相关。因此，大多数T细胞恶性淋巴瘤、一组小淋巴细胞B细胞恶性淋巴瘤（CLL/SLL）、套细胞淋巴瘤（MCL）和前淋巴细胞白血病经常表现为阳性。而滤泡性淋巴瘤很少阳性（图5.7）。CD43在大多数白细胞中的广泛表达使它作为分类标记的作用变小。但CD43是异常B细胞群非常敏感的指示物。

CD45

CD45是一种具有酪氨酸磷酸酶活性的膜蛋白，在所有白细胞中均可发现。由于 mRNA 剪接方式的不同，从而形成了 RA、RB 和 RC，以及没有任何剪接的外显子 RO 4 种形式。CD45RB 在白细胞中广泛存在，因此它的抗体属全白细胞抗体。CD45RA 主要表达于B淋巴细胞，而CD45RO定位于髓细胞和T细胞。被称为抗-LCA的抗体复合物 2B11/PD7，在鉴别除大约 30% 的间变性大细胞淋巴瘤（ALCL）和大多数霍奇金病外的大多数淋巴瘤方面是有用的。抗 CD45RA 的抗体 4KB5 对于 B 细胞淋巴瘤不像 CD20 那样敏感，它可以标记大约 5% 的 T 细胞淋巴瘤。抗 CD45RO 的抗体 OPD4 和 UCHL1，其特异性与 4KB5 相比，大致上是相反的。

CD56

神经细胞黏附分子被命名为CD56。CD56是自然杀伤细胞（NK细胞）的理想标记物，但是也可以在CD4和CD8阳性的T细胞亚群中发现CD56。许多结外的外周 T 细胞和 NK 细胞白血病/淋巴瘤表达CD56，与其活化状态无关。一些良性和恶性浆细胞同样也是 CD56 阳性。

CD57

CD57抗体也可以识别正常NK细胞和T细胞亚群。因此，CD57阳性的恶性淋巴瘤包括：一小部分 T 淋巴母细胞白血病/淋巴瘤、大约3/4 的惰性 T 细胞大颗粒淋巴细胞性白血病和一小部分 NK 细胞淋巴瘤[43]。因而，一个 NK 细胞的典型表型为CD3-、CD5-、CD56+ 和 CD57-[44]。

CD99

CD99 是 MIC2 基因的产物，发挥调节细胞间黏

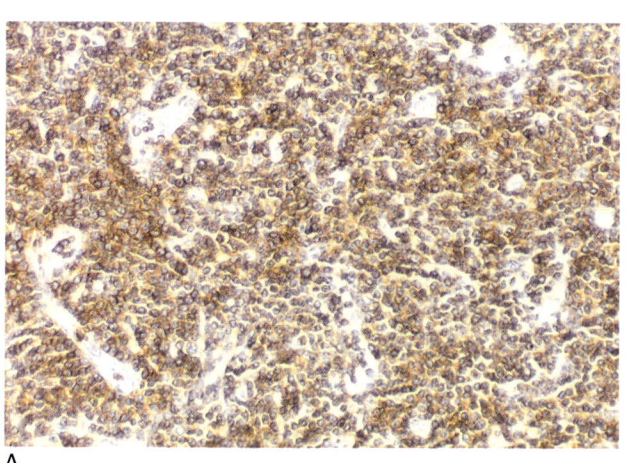
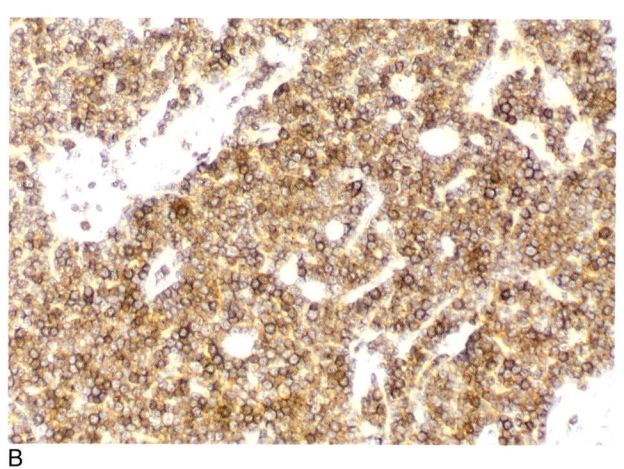

A　　　　　　　　　　　　　　　　　　B

图 5.7 在小淋巴细胞性淋巴瘤中 CD43（A）和 CD20（B）的联合表达

附分子相互作用的功能。CD99可在许多淋巴母细胞白血病/淋巴瘤、急性髓性白血病、一些低级别B细胞淋巴瘤和一些实体肿瘤中表达。

EB病毒潜伏膜蛋白1

EB病毒潜伏膜蛋白1（LMP-1）是一种病毒性蛋白，通过上调bcl-2来保护感染的细胞逃避凋亡。通常，LMP-1是作为EB病毒感染的标记。有报道说，对许多疾病采用免疫组织化学法检测LMP-1和用原位杂交的方法检测EB病毒RNA，二者结果密切相关，但是对NK/T细胞淋巴瘤，二者相关性很差。这可能与病毒的潜伏状态有关。

T细胞限制性细胞内抗原（TIA-1）

TIA-1表达于NK细胞和细胞毒T细胞，是一种细胞毒颗粒相关蛋白。它的表达与细胞的活化状态无关。B细胞恶性淋巴瘤均为TIA-1阴性，而NK细胞和一些T细胞淋巴瘤表现为胞浆颗粒样阳性。

穿孔素/粒酶B

这对颗粒相关蛋白同样定位于细胞毒T细胞和NK细胞。它们对于凋亡和通过使细胞膜发生穿孔诱导靶细胞死亡来说都是非常重要的。然而穿孔素/粒酶B的表达被认为是细胞活化状态的证据。它们标记皮下脂膜炎样T细胞淋巴瘤、侵袭性NK细胞白血病和结外NK/T细胞淋巴瘤（鼻型）。

Ki-67

Ki-67抗体识别一种参与细胞增殖周期的核蛋白。Ki-67抗体可以用来通过阳性细胞数量与总细胞数量比值来测定生长指数。这个指数大致与肿瘤的分级相关，对一些肿瘤（如Burkitt淋巴瘤）的鉴别诊断是重要的。Ki-67指数和结果之间相关已经用于MALT淋巴瘤和弥漫性大细胞淋巴瘤。

末端脱氧核苷酸转移酶（TdT）

末端脱氧核苷酸转移酶在前驱B细胞或T细胞早期的免疫球蛋白形成和T细胞受体基因重排的过程中具有DNA多聚酶活性。一般来说，只有早期B和T淋巴母细胞标记TdT。着色方式为细胞核着色。TdT是淋巴母细胞淋巴瘤/白血病的敏感性和特异性抗体，因为只有一小部分髓细胞性白血病为TdT阳性（图5.8）。

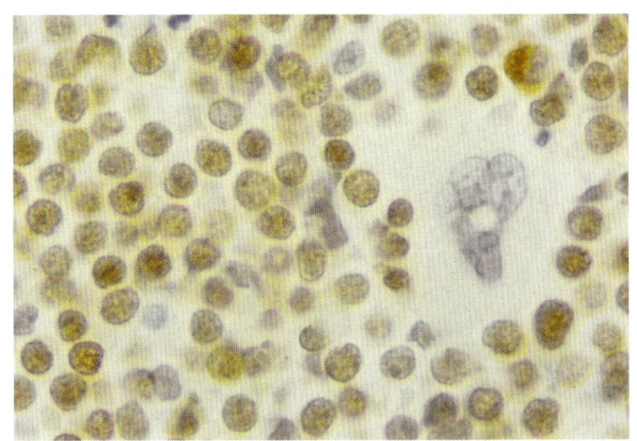

图5.8 TdT抗体标记前驱B淋巴母细胞白血病，细胞核阳性

一般问题

非霍奇金淋巴瘤和反应性病变

可以肯定地说，在血液病理学中，没有其他领域像不典型反应性淋巴病变和淋巴瘤之间的区分那样令病理学家担忧和寝食不安[45]。这其中最大的困难之一就是鉴别明显的淋巴结内的结节状病变，是滤泡性淋巴瘤还是显著的滤泡性增生。当通常的形态学无法解决这个问题时，可以用一组抗体来进行有效的辅助诊断。bcl-2特征性地表达于滤泡性淋巴瘤的瘤细胞胞浆（根据一项大规模研究，依其级别高低不同，74%~97%的病例为阳性[46]），在增生性滤泡的中心细胞和中心母细胞bcl-2表达缺失[47]。值得注意的是，正常套淋巴细胞和很多T细胞也表达bcl-2（尽管一般来说染色不像滤泡性淋巴瘤细胞那样强），因此在反应性滤泡中发现散在阳性细胞不应被过度诊断。反之，在一部分滤泡性淋巴瘤中，大转化细胞可能不标记bcl-2，这种情况不应该否定诊断。CD10和bcl-6在大多数滤泡性淋巴瘤的副皮质区和滤泡为阳性，但在增生性滤泡不会出现这种情况[48]。免疫球蛋白轻链限制是恶性淋巴瘤有用的提示物[49]，但令人遗憾的是，在用石蜡切片免疫组化研究的滤泡性淋巴瘤中却相对不常用。CD45RA抗体和bcl-2抗体有着相似的分布方式，可用来区分滤泡性淋巴瘤和滤泡性增生[50]。

滤泡间反应性病变常常需要和霍奇金淋巴瘤鉴别，但其中一部分与非霍奇金淋巴瘤相似。单核样细胞聚集或朗格汉斯组织细胞增生症偶尔需与边缘区淋巴瘤累及部分淋巴结鉴别。另外bcl-2阳性是一项重要的提示，因为79%的边缘区淋巴瘤bcl-2阳性，而增生则不然[46]。恶性朗格汉斯细胞表现为典型的 S-100 阳性和 CD1a 阳性[51]。显著的副皮质免疫母细胞增生，如传染性单核细胞增生症，需要和非霍奇金淋巴瘤和霍奇金淋巴瘤鉴别。尤其当成片的 B 细胞出现时，用全 B 或全 T 标记物进行染色可能是非常有帮助的[111]。反应性病变典型地表现为 B 和 T 细胞混合或以 T 免疫母细胞为主。弥漫性大 B 细胞淋巴瘤的变型之一，富于 T 细胞的 B 细胞淋巴瘤可能被误诊为良性病变，但是在应用一组全 B 细胞标记和免疫球蛋白轻链抗体之后，可以被适时地诊断出来[52]。

> **诊断要点**：滤泡性淋巴瘤与反应性增生
>
> 1. 在淋巴瘤中，可见增大的淋巴滤泡中 bcl-2 为阳性；而反应性增生的典型表现为滤泡周 bcl-2 阳性。
> 2. 对于区分滤泡性病变，免疫球蛋白轻链染色通常帮助不大。
> 3. 注意良性的、小的初级滤泡和滤泡内 T 细胞 bcl-2 可阳性。

非霍奇金淋巴瘤和其他恶性肿瘤

低分化大细胞恶性肿瘤与非霍奇金淋巴瘤常常需要鉴别诊断。通过应用抗 CD45RB（白细胞共同抗原）抗体、S-100 蛋白和细胞角蛋白（如 AE1/AE3 或 CAM5.2），多数淋巴瘤可以被诊断或排除。间变性大细胞淋巴瘤（ALCL）是特别需要注意的诊断陷阱，当瘤细胞在窦内分布，瘤细胞黏附成巢（尤其细胞呈单型性时），和上皮性恶性肿瘤很相似。白细胞共同抗原经常缺失[53, 54]，许多病例为裸细胞（既不表达 T 细胞抗原也不表达 B 细胞抗原）[54]，有大约 80% 的病例表达上皮细胞膜抗原（尽管是局灶性的）[55]。如果病理学家拟诊断 ALCL 时，那么 CD30 的应用将会很好地解决这一问题。波形蛋白在许多组织中都呈阳性，它可以作为抗原保存的对照指标[56]，但对淋巴瘤的诊断作用很小。

非霍奇金淋巴瘤的分类

WHO 分类最初将淋巴瘤分为 B 细胞型、T 细胞型和霍奇金型（见第 4 章）。这种区分基于免疫学分析，不需要免疫组织化学或流式细胞术检查。例如滤泡性淋巴瘤均为 B 细胞恶性肿瘤，一般来说不需要免疫表型进行诊断。这对于节省时间和资金来说是重要的，因为在美国相当比例的淋巴瘤为滤泡性淋巴瘤[57]。其他淋巴瘤也主要依据常规形态学研究进行初步诊断，然后进行免疫检查确认。很少有病例需要经过分析淋巴细胞本质的免疫组织化学和鉴定细胞遗传分类来进行最终的亚分类。

B 细胞肿瘤

B 细胞和 T 细胞肿瘤被分为前驱性病变（淋巴母细胞白血病和淋巴瘤）；以及成熟型或外周型恶性淋巴瘤。前者在最原始的骨髓和胸腺有其类似成分，后者其肿瘤细胞与正常胸腺外细胞、淋巴结细胞、脾细胞或循环淋巴细胞相似。本文着重讨论的是要用免疫组织化学进行诊断的恶性肿瘤，即"实体"瘤。

前驱 B 细胞肿瘤

前驱 B 淋巴母细胞白血病/淋巴瘤 典型表型：CD19+、CD79a+、CD20 − /+、CD22+/ −、CD10+、TdT+、免疫球蛋白 −

淋巴母细胞淋巴瘤和急性淋巴母细胞白血病在形态学和免疫表型上是同一种疾病，可根据其临床背景进行区分[58]。尽管大多数淋巴母细胞白血病属于 B 系，但仅有大约 20% 的淋巴母细胞淋巴瘤表达可被免疫组化检测的 B 细胞标记[59, 60]。实际上，所有的淋巴母细胞白血病/淋巴瘤在基因重排的过程中产生一种酶，即末端脱氧核苷酸转移酶（TdT）[61-65]。TdT 标记淋巴母细胞的胞核。CD19 在几乎所有的淋巴母细胞淋巴瘤中均表达，但是在石蜡切片上却检测不出。CD20+ 和 CD45RB 阳性对诊断来说不可靠[62-64, 66, 67]。CD74（LN2）[68]和 CD79a[63]抗体是 B 细胞或前驱 B 细胞淋巴母细胞淋巴瘤有用的标记。抗 CD43 的抗体被认为是一种 T 细胞的标记，但是其特异性不高。大多数前驱 B 细胞淋巴母细胞淋巴瘤/白血病表达 CD43，但 CD3 为阴性[63]。MIC2 基因的产物 CD99 在淋巴母细胞淋巴瘤中与 TdT 的表达是相同的[69, 70]，但其表达方式为胞膜阳性而非胞核阳性。当然，其他小圆细胞肿瘤，特别是在儿童也表现为 CD99 阳性。大多数前驱 B 细胞肿瘤为 CD10（CALLA）阳性，但是一些前驱 T 细胞肿瘤也同样表达 CD10[71]。其他有时在前驱 B 细胞淋巴瘤中发现的抗原包括：CD34[65]、细胞角蛋白[62]、NK 细胞抗原、CD56[72]和 Fas 配体[73]。bcl-2 通常表达于瘤细胞的胞浆，可以辅助前体 B 细胞肿瘤与 Burkitt 淋巴瘤/白血病的鉴别诊断[74]；然而，其他"淋巴母细胞"肿瘤，如套细胞淋巴瘤的母细胞变型 bcl-2 也可以阳性。

> **诊断要点**：淋巴母细胞淋巴瘤/白血病
>
> 1. 在前驱 B 细胞淋巴母细胞白血病/淋巴瘤中 CD20 和 LCA 可能为阴性。
> 2. TdT 几乎总是表达于淋巴母细胞淋巴瘤细胞的细胞核（尽管在双表型和一些髓性白血病中也可以发现 TdT）。
> 3. 通常表达 CD10 和 CD99。

成熟 B 细胞肿瘤

B 细胞慢性淋巴细胞白血病/小淋巴细胞淋巴瘤

典型表型：CD20+、CD23+、CD79a+、CD5+、CD43+

如同淋巴母细胞白血病/淋巴瘤，B 细胞 CLL 和 SLL 的免疫表型确实难以鉴别。这些成熟小 B 细胞恶性肿瘤一般为惰性病程。该肿瘤全 B 细胞标记阳性，尽管与其他 B 细胞淋巴瘤相比，CD20 胞浆阳性强度要弱一些。早期研究发现，只有 39% 的成熟小 B 细胞恶性肿瘤表达 Leu22（CD43）[49]，但是新近报告在 79%~100% 的病例中发现了 CD43 的表达[75-77]。随着用于固定组织的 CD5 抗体的出现（特别是用于抗原修复方法的 4C7），大多数 SLL 可以表现为阳性，尽管一些病例仅表现为细胞的弱阳性或不完全阳性[78, 79]。流式细胞术检测出的 CD5 阴性，经常是引起对 B 细胞 CLL/SLL 诊断重新复查的原因[80]，然而石蜡切片的免疫组化的结果一般是可信的。CD23（BU38）阳性可与套细胞淋巴瘤鉴别[75, 77, 81-84]，但是同时应该想到滤泡性树突状细胞和滤泡性淋巴瘤也表达 CD23。在发生了大细胞转化的 SLL 仍然表达 CD23[85]，bcl-2 为阳性[83]，CD10[75, 86]、cyclin D1[83, 87-90] 和 bcl-6[91] 阴性。尽管不经常见到，但癌蛋白 p53 水平的提高与临床预后不良有关[92]。近来报道，趋化因子受体 CXCR3 表达于 39 例 CLL/SLL 中的 37 例，在套细胞、滤泡性和小无裂细胞淋巴瘤中表达缺失[93]。非受体酪氨酸激酶 ZAP-70 表达于 B 细胞 CLL 的一种亚型的正常的和恶性 T 细胞，少见于其他 B 细胞恶性淋巴瘤。免疫组化的结果为胞核和胞浆阳性[94, 95]。ZAP-70 在 CLL 中的表达与病程缩短和预后不良有关[96, 97]。无论是与免疫球蛋白重链基因突变[96-99]还是与 CD38[97]的表达相比，ZAP-70 蛋白对估计病人预后来说都是更好的标记物。

> **诊断要点**：成熟 B 细胞淋巴瘤
>
> 1. CD20 和 bcl-2 标记 B 细胞 CLL/SLL、套细胞、滤泡和一些边缘区淋巴瘤。
> 2. B 细胞 CLL/SLL 中 CD23+ 和 cyclin D1-，与套细胞淋巴瘤加以区分。
> 3. B 细胞 CLL/SLL 中 CD5/CD43+ 和 CD10-，与滤泡性淋巴瘤加以区分。
> 4. ZAP-70 提示 B 细胞 CLL 的预后不良。

B 细胞前淋巴细胞白血病
典型表型：与 B 细胞 CLL/SLL 相同，但可能 CD5-、CD22+

在淋巴结中，B 细胞前淋巴细胞白血病的诊断很少出现困难，尽管脾的累及可能会增加脾淋巴瘤诊断的可能性，但是根据白细胞数的增高和典型的细胞学涂片可以排除这种可能。B 细胞前淋巴细胞白血病可表现为 CD5 和 CD23 阴性，同时 CD22 的阳性率可能高于 B 细胞慢性淋巴细胞白血病/小淋巴细胞淋巴瘤[100]。不难理解，有丝分裂指数如 Ki-67[101]，B 细胞前淋巴细胞白血病要高于 B 细胞慢性淋巴细胞白血病/小淋巴细胞淋巴瘤。

淋巴浆细胞性淋巴瘤
典型表型：通常局灶性 IgM+、CD20+、CD22+、CD79a+、CD5-、CD10-、CD43+/-

这种小淋巴细胞和浆细胞样淋巴细胞的肿瘤是与临床综合征 Waldenstrom 巨球蛋白血症相关的病理类型。正如人们所预期的，浆细胞样淋巴细胞的胞浆中表达的免疫球蛋白重链是典型的 IgM 型[102]。特别是在分化较好的细胞，总是可以呈现免疫球蛋白轻链限制性反应[103, 104]。CD20 阳性，但是相比 B 细胞慢性淋巴细胞白血病/小淋巴细胞淋巴瘤（B 细胞 CLL/SLL）CD23 和 CD43 更易缺失（仅表达于 20%~40% 的病例）[76, 77, 86, 105]。正常情况下，CD5、CD10 为阴性，但也有例外[103]。有趣的是，CD138（多配体蛋白聚糖，正常浆细胞和恶性浆细胞的标记物）在所有检测的 17 例 B 细胞前淋巴细胞白血病病例中均缺失。Fas 配体在淋巴浆细胞性淋巴瘤弱表达[73]，但是 Fas 本身（CD95，一种跨膜受体，肿瘤坏死因子受体超家族的成员之一）经常表达[107]。而 bcl-2 在 80% 的病例中为阳性[11]。

脾边缘区 B 细胞淋巴瘤
典型表型：免疫球蛋白-/+、B 细胞抗原+、CD5-、CD10-、CD23-、CD43-/+、CD11c+/-

脾边缘区 B 细胞淋巴瘤（SMZL）是原发性脾淋巴瘤的一种，外周血可能含有"绒毛状淋巴细胞"成分[108]。这些绒毛状淋巴细胞的胞浆突起可能导致与毛细胞白血病的混淆，但是两者的免疫表型是不同的。脾边缘区 B 细胞淋巴瘤（SMZL）中，成熟 B 细胞抗原典型地表达（CD20和CD79a），但DBA.44（CD72）（一种表达于许多低级别 B 细胞淋巴瘤的 B 细胞标记，大多与毛细胞白血病密切相关），只表达于30%的 SMZL 病例的细胞胞浆[109]。CD43 少有表达[46]。大约半数的 SMZL 病人有 CD11 c 阳性[110-113]，而毛细胞白血病几乎为全部阳性，但是抗体只对流式细胞术或冰冻切片有效。Ki-67呈现典型的低表达[114, 115]。bcl-2在多数 SMZL 中呈现阳性[109, 116, 117]，而 cyclin D1 在全部 SMZL 中均为阴性[89, 115, 118]。在固定组织中检测抗酒石酸磷酸酶的抗体已经有了进展，据报道说对毛细胞白血病非常敏感[119, 120]，但是少数呈现弱表达的 SMZL 病例已见于文献报道[121]。

毛细胞白血病　典型表型：B细胞抗原+、CD5-、CD10-、CD23-、CD11c+（强阳性）、CD25+、FMC7+、CD103+

白血病患者由于没有累及脾白髓，故不容易与原发性脾淋巴瘤相混淆，但是经常会广泛累及骨髓；细针穿刺难以获得病变组织，骨髓环钻活检的标本可以区分毛细胞白血病和其他低级别B细胞恶性肿瘤。毛细胞白血病表达大多数全B细胞抗原和白细胞共同抗原[122]，T 细胞标记和 CD43 为阴性[123,124]。CD20 标记可用于检测骨髓微小残留病变[125]。如上所述，DBA.44 在毛细胞白血病中常为阳性（50%~100%）[121, 126, 127]。TRAP 阳性在毛细胞白血病中比在 SMZL 和 MALT 型淋巴瘤中更强，也更常见（尽管有文献报告发现一个病例不是所有的毛细胞都着色）[121]，TRAP 和 DBA.44 共同阳性对毛细胞白血病是特异的[121, 128]。cyclin D1在许多毛细胞白血病病例中过度表达，尽管比在套细胞淋巴瘤中的表达程度低[129, 130]。一些报道认为毛细胞白血病检测不到cyclin D1[89, 90]，而另有人报道多数或全部的毛细胞白血病可表现出对 cyclin D1 呈弱阳性标记[130]。

浆细胞骨髓瘤 / 浆细胞瘤　典型表型：胞浆免疫球蛋白+（强阳性）、CD19-、CD20-、CD22-、CD79 a+/-、CD45RB-/+、EMA-/+、CD43-/+、CD56+/-、CD30+

多数浆细胞骨髓瘤/浆细胞瘤不存在诊断上的困难。浆细胞骨髓瘤/浆细胞瘤中含有丰富的细胞内免疫球蛋白。单一型轻链抗体可将它们与反应性或感染性病变区分开来，而且轻链强阳性，CD20 和（通常是）白细胞共同抗原表达缺失可将浆细胞骨髓瘤/浆细胞瘤与大B细胞淋巴瘤区分开来（图 5.9）。CD138 可以辅助诊断，因为它对浆细胞样分化非常敏感和特异[106, 131]。CD38在大多数浆细胞中呈现阳性[132]。bcl-2 常为阳性[133]。

诊断要点：B 细胞和浆细胞

1. 与成熟 B 淋巴细胞有关的抗原如 CD45 RB 和 CD20 在许多浆细胞中表达缺失。
2. 在不成熟或间变性骨髓瘤中，不要被上皮细胞膜抗原阳性所误导。
3. CD30 阳性（典型的胞浆阳性而不是胞膜或核旁）不应作出 ALCL 的诊断。

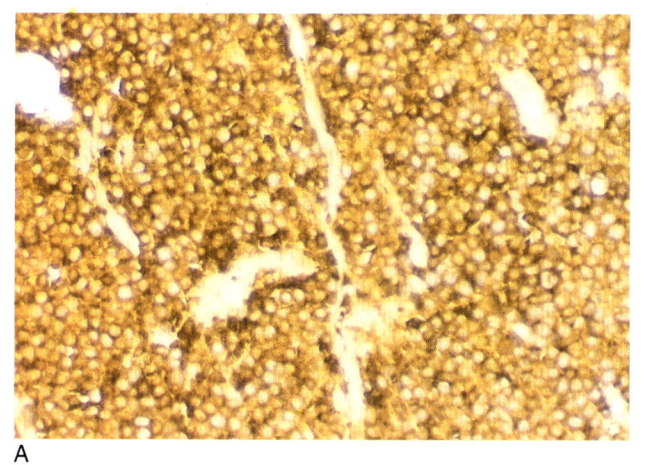

A

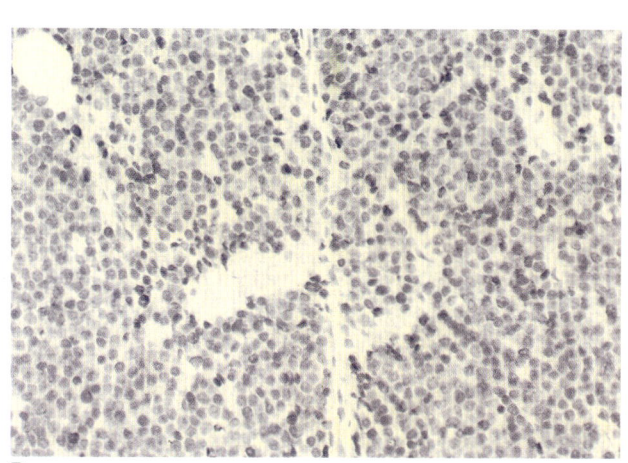

B

图 5.9　在该多发性骨髓瘤中，λ（A）和 κ（B）免疫球蛋白轻链抗体明确显示浆细胞的单型性

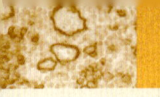

黏膜相关淋巴组织结外边缘区 B 细胞淋巴瘤 (MALT) 典型表型：免疫球蛋白+（40%，可能是淋巴细胞或浆细胞成分，或两者都有）、CD20+、CD79a+、CD5-、CD10-、CD23-、CD43-/+、CD11c+/-

结外边缘区 B 细胞淋巴瘤亦被称为 MALT 型淋巴瘤，在成人表现为局灶性病变，通常位于胃肠道，在其他有黏膜的部位，如泪腺、肺和乳腺出现的可能性较胃肠道小，另外偶见于非黏膜性部位如皮肤和甲状腺。MALT 型结外边缘区 B 细胞淋巴瘤呈现出异质性的细胞图像，其中有丰富的小边缘区（"中心细胞样"）细胞，有较丰富胞浆和肾形核的单核样 B 细胞，以及浆细胞。中心细胞样细胞常浸润腺上皮，形成淋巴上皮病变，细胞角蛋白抗体染色可以清晰地显示这一病变。免疫球蛋白轻链染色可以用于辅助鉴别反应性胃炎或相似的情况，这是小的内镜活检经常遇到的问题。40% 或更多的病例为单型性免疫球蛋白轻链[1, 134]；同时，皮肤结外边缘区淋巴瘤有 70% 的病例呈单型性[135]。应检测小细胞成分和浆细胞成分的单型性；淋巴细胞的染色可能会弱一些，因此对两种抗体应仔细比较，着重观察细胞浆而不是周围间质染色。浆细胞通常位于上皮下。在约 40% 的病例中，浆细胞呈单型性，通常比小细胞成分更易诊断[1]。浆细胞中可出现 Dutcher 小体。而在其他病变中，浆细胞为反应性增生且不呈单型性。

除极少数病例外，结外边缘区淋巴瘤不表达 CD5 也不表达 CD43[136, 137]；CD5 和 CD43 确实可能显示的是更具有侵袭性的疾病[138]。与滤泡性淋巴瘤不同，结外边缘区淋巴瘤为 CD10 阴性[137]。像其他小细胞淋巴瘤一样，结外 MZL 为 bcl-2 阳性[139-143]；然而，高级别或有大细胞转化的 MZL，bcl-2 阳性率会低很多[142]。相反的，与低级别 MALT 型淋巴瘤相比，高级别 MALT 型淋巴瘤的 p53 常过表达，同时增殖相关抗原如 Ki-67 阳性细胞明显增多[142, 144, 145]。淋巴细胞分化的癌蛋白调节因子 bcl-6，在大细胞淋巴瘤的一个亚型中过表达，同时在一些高级别 MALT 型淋巴瘤的大的转化的淋巴细胞中也发现它的表达[144]。MALT 型淋巴瘤中常见生发中心，在进行 CD21 染色后，生发中心会变得更明显，特别是在有大量滤泡的病例中。趋化因子受体 CXCR3 可以表达于结外 MZL 的单核样细胞和浆细胞中[93]。

免疫增生性小肠病（IPSID），是与结外 MALT 型淋巴瘤相关的一种疾病，它流行于居住在地中海沿岸的人群中。尽管黏膜浆细胞表达 IgA 缺乏轻链单型性，但是在不同的阶段，IPSID 有与非地中海 MALT 型淋巴瘤相似的边缘区淋巴细胞和大转化细胞[146]。

淋巴结边缘区 B 细胞淋巴瘤 典型表型：免疫球蛋白+、CD20+、CD79a+、CD5-、CD10-、CD23-、CD43-/+、CD11c+/-

淋巴结 MZL 的细胞学和免疫表型构成与其结外 MZL 基本相同，尽管一部分病例可能富有中等大小单核样细胞并相对缺少小的结节边缘区细胞。和胃肠道一样，免疫球蛋白轻链分析经常有效，大约有 30% 的病例表现单型性[49, 147, 148]。单型性特征有助于鉴别淋巴结 MZL 与具有单核细胞样 B 细胞的反应性滤泡增生。除去 B 细胞 CLL/SLL 和滤泡性淋巴瘤外，CD5、CD10 和 CD23 很少为阳性[79, 86, 149-152]。同样，CD43 也在 20%~40% 的淋巴结 MZL 中表达[76]。cyclin D1 表达缺失可以排除套细胞淋巴瘤。如 MALT 型淋巴瘤一样，大多数淋巴结 MZL 过表达 bcl-2（一项大型研究发现 79% 的病例阳性[46]），尽管该病与滤泡性淋巴瘤相比着色会弱一些，淋巴结 MZL 和滤泡性淋巴瘤可同时存在[153]。同结外 MZL 一样，肿瘤的一小部分可表达 p53（虽然基因未发生点突变，提示存在其他上调机制[154]）。这与经常发生 p53 突变的脾边缘区淋巴瘤是相反的[110, 155]。淋巴结 MZL 的表型类似于毛细胞白血病，但多数病例不表达 DBA.44[127]。

滤泡性淋巴瘤 典型表型：B 细胞抗原+、CD10+/-、CD5-、CD23-/+、CD43-、CD11c-

在北美，滤泡性淋巴瘤是非霍奇金淋巴瘤中最常见的类型[57]。幸运的是，大多数情况下根据其特征性的形态学表现，可以将其与反应性增生以及其他淋巴瘤直接区分开来。当标本组织过小或其他限制使诊断变得困难时，其特征性的免疫学表型可以解决这个问题。全 B 细胞抗原如 CD20 和 CD79a 总是阳性，并且有 90%~95% 的由甲醛固定的组织的病例表达 CD10（CALLA）[75, 156]。后者可与套细胞和小淋巴细胞性淋巴瘤相鉴别；并且，滤泡性淋巴瘤 CD43 和 CD5 不常为阳性（＜5% 的病例）也有助于诊断[49, 75, 76, 79, 80, 149, 157]。在 28% 的病例中可见轻链单型性，无助于和其他淋巴瘤鉴别[49]。

bcl-2 蛋白首先在滤泡性淋巴瘤中被分离出来，并且在我们对非霍奇金淋巴瘤的认识过程中起了非常重要的作用。现在，bcl-2 已作为一种诊断疾病的工具应用于日常工作中。bcl-2 与一系列包括 bcl-X 在内的相关蛋白组成异源二聚体；bcl-2 基因位于 18 号染色体，并且参与了滤泡性淋巴瘤特征性的14和18号染色体基因易位。多数滤泡性淋巴瘤由于发生了基因易位而过度表达bcl-2蛋白，包括97%的Ⅰ级FL，83%的Ⅱ级FL和74%的Ⅲ级FL[46, 158-161]。有趣的是，尽管发生的几率很低[162]，但是没有基因易位而出现bcl-2过表达的现象提示可能存在其他的上调机制。并不是所有小细胞都着色[163]，小裂细胞着色更强。甚至滤泡性淋巴瘤的变型都可被抗bcl-2的抗体所标记[164]。尽管bcl-2表达情况随肿瘤分级不同而改变，但是它并不能提示临床预后[165]。像正常滤泡中心细胞一样[91]，大多数FL也表达基因转录调节因子bcl-6[162, 166]。多数其他低级别B细胞淋巴瘤不表达bcl-6[91]。滤泡性淋巴瘤向弥漫性大B细胞淋巴瘤转化的过程中伴有bcl-6表达的降低[167]。

cyclin D1是套细胞淋巴瘤的标记，在滤泡性淋巴瘤中不表达[88, 89]。肿瘤抑制基因产物如p53[159, 161]、RB（视网膜母细胞瘤蛋白）[161]以及p53结合蛋白MDM2[168]在高级别FL中比低级别FL中有更多的表达。其他有助于诊断的要点包括：CD57阳性T细胞在滤泡性淋巴瘤中很少见（与结节性淋巴细胞为主型霍奇金病相比[169]），抗CD21的抗体显示FL中滤泡树突状细胞形成的完整网状结构[170]，CXCR3表达缺失[93]，以及CD30阳性细胞的出现，尤其是在滤泡外围[171, 172]。最后，当着色较强且一致时，bcl-2可用来作为滤泡性淋巴瘤骨髓中微小残留灶的指示物[173]。

> **诊断要点：** 滤泡性淋巴瘤
>
> 1. 对于滤泡性淋巴瘤，bcl-2表达是敏感的但不是特异的。
> 2. CD43或CD5、cyclin D1、bcl-6以及CD10应用的增加，可以有效地区分小淋巴细胞淋巴瘤

套细胞淋巴瘤　典型表型：表面IgM/D+、B细胞抗原+、CD5+、CD10-/+、CD23-、CD43+、CD11c-

正常套细胞被认为起源于滤泡的套淋巴细胞的内层，所以通常的成熟B细胞标记（CD20，CD79a）在套细胞淋巴瘤中强阳性表达就不足为奇了（尽管DBA.44可能只表达于少部分病例[121]）。免疫球蛋白轻链在40%的石蜡切片的病例中阳性[49]。CD23表达于活化B淋巴细胞的一个亚群和滤泡树突状细胞，在套细胞淋巴瘤中特征性地表现为阴性，尽管大约5%~10%的该肿瘤还可表现为阳性[75, 77, 82-84, 149, 174-176]。

CD10常不表达[149, 174, 177]。在石蜡切片免疫组化中，最有用的发现是cyclin D1在核内的表达（76%~100%的病例）和CD5在胞浆中的表达（73%~100%，但其中有一些较弱）[75, 79, 83, 87, 89, 90, 149, 174, 176, 178]。像在其他小淋巴细胞淋巴瘤中一样，CD43常与CD5共同表达[49, 75-77, 83]。不常见的套细胞淋巴瘤包括母细胞变型（特征性的核染色质分散的大细胞）和定位于黏膜的肿瘤[175, 177, 179]，它们与典型的套细胞淋巴瘤表达相同的抗原类型，可与前驱B细胞淋巴母细胞淋巴瘤[65, 180]和转化的SLL[85]相鉴别。此外，TdT和CD99在母细胞变型套细胞淋巴瘤中不表达，但在淋巴母细胞淋巴瘤/白血病中表达[66]。大约90%的套细胞淋巴瘤表达bcl-2，因此需要病理学家对可能与FL或SLL发生的混淆提高警惕[83, 175]。p53基因的突变会导致p53蛋白的过度表达[181]，这与更有侵袭性的病程相关[182-184]。Ki-67指数变化较大，可从5%至40%[185]。

> **诊断要点：** 套细胞淋巴瘤
>
> 1. 除了套细胞淋巴瘤，其他淋巴瘤几乎不表达cyclin D1。
> 2. 套细胞淋巴瘤cyclin D1的阳性不像甲状旁腺或乳腺对照组织那样强。

弥漫性大B细胞淋巴瘤　典型表型：B细胞抗原+、CD45RB+（除了一些间变性和纵隔淋巴瘤）、CD5-/+、CD10-/+

弥漫性大B细胞淋巴瘤有若干种形态学类型，免疫表型也随之改变[186, 187]。以下是对大范围的不同大细胞淋巴瘤的观察：尽管有例外，CD5通常为阴性[79]，形态上不像套细胞淋巴瘤或SLL[188]；bcl-2（24%~74%）、BAX、CD44[193]和caspase[194]的表达与预后不良有关[162, 188-192]；CD43表达于15%~30%[49, 76]的典型B细胞抗原阳性的病例，DBA.44[121]和CD99也可在一些病例中表达[70]。Ki-67指数比小淋巴细胞淋巴瘤高[195]。bcl-6是与滤泡中心细胞的生长和FL转化相关的蛋白[91, 166]，可在70%~80%的弥漫性大B细胞淋巴瘤中表达[48, 162]。50%的肿瘤表达CD10[48]。细胞角蛋白在大细胞淋巴瘤中很少阳性[196]。CD30阳性大B细胞淋巴瘤，间变性或其他类型在WHO分类中目前还没有从其他DLBCL中区分出来，因为其预后的意义尚未得到证实[197]。

富于T细胞的B细胞淋巴瘤除了上皮细胞膜抗原可阳性外，与其他DLBCL没有免疫表型的差别

[198]。DLBCL 亚型的免疫表型介绍如下：

纵隔大 B 细胞淋巴瘤[199]：这种独特的病变位于纵隔，被认为来自胸腺髓质 B 细胞。该淋巴瘤 CD20 和 CD22 阳性，但 CD21 阴性[200-202]。无 CD43 共表达[200]。典型者 CD20 的免疫标记非常强。CD30 在半数以上的病例中表达[203]，着色方式为弥漫性胞浆着色而非点状着色。

原发性渗出性淋巴瘤[204]：由人类疱疹病毒 8（Kaposi 肉瘤相关疱疹病毒）引起，肿瘤局限于病毒感染的免疫抑制病人的腹膜、胸膜和心包。大多数病例既不表达 B 细胞也不表达 T 细胞标记，CD30 常为阳性[205, 206]。

血管内大 B 细胞淋巴瘤[207, 208]：尽管也有 T 细胞表达的报道，大多数血管内大 B 细胞淋巴瘤病例表达 B 细胞标记[209]。在细胞表面发现许多淋巴细胞归巢受体，这使人们可以假定一种使淋巴细胞限定于血管内空间的机制[208, 210]。

> **诊断要点：弥漫性大 B 细胞淋巴瘤**
>
> 1. CD45RB、CD20 或 CD79a、S-100、细胞角蛋白、CD3 和 CD30，组成对大细胞淋巴瘤诊断的有效组合。
> 2. 在大 B 细胞淋巴瘤中，CD30 阳性通常只出现于少部分 B 细胞，阳性可能与浆细胞分化有关[211]，没有预后意义。
> 3. 在反应性背景中，片状大 B 细胞不常见，应提高对其是否是淋巴瘤的注意[39]。

伯基特淋巴瘤/白血病　典型表型：B 细胞抗原+、CD10+/−、CD5−

尽管伯基特（Burkitt）和伯基特样淋巴瘤的自然病史可能有一定的特征性，但仅依靠形态学表现进行区分的重复性很差，所以在 WHO 分类中被分为同一类型[7]。CD19、CD20 和 CD79a 都表达，CD5、CD23 通常表达缺失。与淋巴母细胞淋巴瘤/白血病相比，一个重要的区别在于伯基特细胞的胞核中未发现 TdT[212]。伯基特淋巴瘤 Ki-67（可给出生长分数）高表达，Ki-67 指数接近 100%[7]。bcl-2 和 CD10 在伯基特淋巴瘤/白血病的两种变型中有截然相反的关系：CD10 在伯基特淋巴瘤中阳性率高，在伯基特样淋巴瘤中阳性率低，bcl-2 在伯基特样淋巴瘤中阳性率高而在伯基特淋巴瘤中阳性率低[46]。CD43 也可以用来区分两种免疫表型：CD43 常在伯基特淋巴瘤中表达而在伯基

特样淋巴瘤中的表达率不到 50%[76]。

淋巴瘤样肉芽肿病　典型表型：B 细胞抗原+、CD30+/−、CD15−、LMP+

淋巴瘤样肉芽肿病是一种发生于结外部位的淋巴增生性病变，特别是在肺；患者为获得性或遗传性免疫缺陷。现在认为，EB 病毒转化的 B 细胞激发了活跃的 T 细胞反应[213]。这导致了血管中心性梗死、多形性淋巴组织浸润和一系列从炎症到明显大细胞淋巴瘤的表现。石蜡切片免疫组化对于识别这种在 T 细胞背景中大的、不典型的 B 细胞（CD20+ 和 LMP+）是非常重要的。尽管这些大细胞在细胞学上不典型而且可能为 CD30+，但是没有发现真正的 R-S 细胞。

T 和 NK 细胞肿瘤

前驱 T 细胞肿瘤

前驱 T 淋巴母细胞白血病/淋巴瘤　典型表型：CD1a+/−、CD2+/−、CD3+（CD3+ 总是表现为胞浆着色）、CD4/CD8 双阳性或双阴性、CD5+/−、CD7+、CD10−/+、TdT+、CD16−/+、CD57−/+、B 抗原−

这种疾病的淋巴母细胞与前驱 B 淋巴母细胞淋巴瘤/白血病的淋巴母细胞在形态学上不能区分，需要免疫学分析辅助鉴别。TdT 呈一致性地表达。除了通常的 B 和 T 系特异性抗体外，TAL-1（SCL）蛋白和 c-kit 受体可以用来鉴别恶性肿瘤的性质。上述每一种蛋白的抗体在大约 40%~50% 的 T 淋巴母细胞肿瘤中阳性，而 B 淋巴母细胞瘤阴性[214, 215]。与其他母细胞性恶性肿瘤的鉴别诊断通常比较容易：母细胞变型套细胞淋巴瘤 TdT 阴性，并且表达成熟 B 细胞肿瘤的标记；粒细胞肉瘤 TdT 阴性，而且髓过氧化物酶或溶菌酶常为阳性。需要注意的是 CD43 分子，除了可以标记 T 细胞恶性肿瘤外，也是许多髓内病变的标记[214]。CD99 的表达在前驱 T 细胞 ALL 中非常普遍[70]；在对小儿小细胞肿瘤进行鉴别诊断时必须想到这一现象。

成熟 T 细胞肿瘤

免疫组织化学分析非常有助于外周（或成熟）T 细胞肿瘤的诊断和分类。尽管没有与免疫球蛋白轻链相似的 T 细胞克隆免疫标记，但也会出现抗原的异常表达，而这种抗原异常表达方式在正常成熟 T 细胞中极少出现[39, 216]。通常 CD4 和 CD8 双阳性（二者皆表达）或双阴性（二者皆不表达）的细胞在胸腺外的数

量很少。相似的是，单个或者更多全T细胞抗原的丢失，譬如CD2、CD3、CD5、TCRαβ或者更常见的CD7，都支持T细胞淋巴瘤的诊断。当然也有规则之外的良性病例存在。大多数这样的分析只有在新鲜或冰冻组织中才能应用，而且其应用在一般的病理实验室中受到了限制。因此，应用流式细胞术或咨询标准实验室是必要的。

一些成熟T细胞白血病在外科病理标本中非常少见，因此只能得到它们的一般表型。

T细胞前淋巴细胞白血病　典型表型：CD2+、CD3+、CD4+（65%）、CD5+、CD7+、CD8+（21%）、CD25−

T细胞大颗粒淋巴细胞白血病　典型表型：CD2+、CD3+、CD4−、CD5−、CD7−、CD8+、TCRαβ+、CD16+、CD56−、CD57+/−、CD25−

侵袭性NK细胞白血病　典型表型：CD2+、CD3−、CD4−、CD8+/−、TCRαβ−、CD16+、CD56+/−、CD57+/−

这种白血病可以表达细胞毒性颗粒相关蛋白TIA-1。TIA-1蛋白正常表达于自然杀伤细胞和细胞毒T淋巴细胞，但与这些细胞的活化状态无关[217]。肿瘤细胞通常有EB病毒感染[218]。

成人T细胞淋巴瘤/白血病　典型表型：CD2+、CD3+、CD4+（大多数病例）、CD5+、CD7−、CD25+

另外一种病毒诱发的白血病/淋巴瘤（归因于HTLV1病毒感染），ATLL常有血白细胞计数的升高，也可形成单纯的淋巴瘤。在两者的任何一种情况下，通过分子生物学方法对肿瘤细胞中克隆性病毒DNA的证实可以作出有说服力的诊断。组织学上的异质性使得这种肿瘤与缺少特异性临床表现的非特异性外周T细胞淋巴瘤在实际操作中不易区分[219]。CD25的表达为典型的强阳性。大约20%的成人T细胞淋巴瘤/白血病CD30阳性，常表现为结外生长并且缺乏白血病的表现，但是与CD30阴性的病例具有相似的生存率[220]。

结外NK/T细胞淋巴瘤（鼻型）　典型表型：CD2+、CD3−、CD4−/+、CD8−/+、CD5−/+、CD7−/+、CD56+、CD43+、TCRαβ−、EBV-LMP-1+/−

像大多数T细胞淋巴瘤一样，特殊的临床表现（在亚洲常见，侵袭性结外病变，多在面部中线，伴有坏死）对该疾病的诊断非常重要[218]。这种淋巴瘤以前称为血管中心性淋巴瘤或淋巴瘤样肉芽肿病。血管中心性和侵入血管（导致梗死性坏死）是常见的特征，但不具有特异性。该类肿瘤与EB病毒感染密切相关（在分子学上已被证实），而且经石蜡切片的免疫组织化学证实[221-223]，某些病例的肿瘤细胞中携带有EBV-LMP-1。细胞毒性颗粒抗原（也可通过免疫组织化学检测）的表达，例如TIA-1、粒酶B和穿孔素，提示这种淋巴瘤来源于活化的自然杀伤细胞或者不太常见的细胞毒T细胞前体[217, 224-226]。与肺有关的病例更多地倾向于B细胞大细胞淋巴瘤[213]。

肠病型T细胞淋巴瘤　典型表型：CD3+、CD4−、CD7+、CD8+/−、CD56−/+、CD103+

肠道T细胞淋巴瘤多发生于有谷麸质过敏性肠病的病人，在空肠表现为顽固的穿孔性溃疡。肿块可明显或不明显。组织学表现为异质性，尽管部分病例包含单形性中等大小的细胞。上皮组织分化的标记阳性。大部分肠道淋巴细胞表现为细胞毒T细胞表型（TIA-1和粒酶B阳性）而CD56的表达相对较少[217, 227, 228]。通过免疫组织化学或者原位杂交的方法很少能检测到EB病毒的感染[229]。累及胃肠道的ALCL（间变性大细胞淋巴瘤）已被报道过[230]，但是这些肿瘤是否归属于肠病型T细胞淋巴瘤还不明确。p53几乎普遍过表达[231]。CD103作为一条完整的α链，出现于90%以上的正常肠道上皮内淋巴细胞，可能起到使淋巴细胞"归巢"上皮的作用，在所有的肠病型T细胞淋巴瘤中均有表达。能够识别这种抗原的B-ly-7抗体在固定的组织中无效。

肝脾T细胞淋巴瘤　典型表型：CD2+、CD3+、CD4−、CD5−、CD7+、CD8+/−、CD56+/−、TCRγδ+（部分TCRαβ+）、EBV-LMP-1−

这种少见的原发性肝淋巴瘤是由CD56+的T细胞构成的，可以检测到TIA-1阳性，而缺乏穿孔素和粒酶B的表达，这些细胞大部分处于非激活状态[224, 225, 232]。这种淋巴瘤一个不寻常的特征就是γδ型T细胞受体的表达，而不是更常见的αβ异源二聚体[233]。利用令人满意的抗体（βF1和TCRγδ），上述受体的表达可以在固定的石蜡包埋的组织中得以证实。

皮下脂膜炎样T细胞淋巴瘤　典型表型：CD3+、CD4−、CD8+/−、CD30−/+、CD43+、CD45RO+、CD56−/+、TIA-1+、穿孔素+、粒酶B+、TCRαβ+

顾名思义，皮下脂膜炎样T细胞淋巴瘤，有特殊的累及部位和形态学结构。表皮通常不被累及，肿瘤细胞围绕在真皮脂肪细胞周围但不破坏它们，同时有淋巴细胞侵犯血管但不形成梗死。大部分病例为CD8型并且通常不表达CD56[234, 235]。所有病例都有活化的细胞毒T细胞外观，但有趣的是，仅有少数病例表达CD30[235]。与其他类型可累及脂肪的T细胞淋巴瘤例如鼻型NK/T细胞淋巴瘤的免疫学区别，部分是依据CD56的缺失（尽管某些皮肤血管中心性淋巴瘤的CD56阴性，且与EB病毒无关[236]），部分是依据表皮成分的缺失或血管破坏。原发性皮肤间变性大细胞淋巴瘤可以扩展至皮下组织并且很像SPTCL（皮下脂膜炎样T细胞淋巴瘤），但是对CD30染色的正确分析判断可以帮助我们加以区分。

蕈样霉菌病/Sézary综合征　　典型表型：CD2+、CD3+、CD4+、CD5+、CD7-/+、CD8-、CD25-、TCRαβ+

蕈样霉菌病（MF）以及与它相似的白血病类型——Sézary综合征从免疫表型方面几乎不能将二者区分开来，而且在美国二者皆可同时查见T细胞淋巴瘤。蕈样霉菌病诊断的主要困难在于将早期病变与假性淋巴瘤或其他病因所致的反应性病变相区分。除了常规的形态依据和T细胞基因重排的分子检测外，免疫组织化学方法也可以提供一些指导性帮助。与正常的T细胞相比，蕈样霉菌病细胞常表现出一种或更多种表型上的异常：CD7常常缺失[237]，近2/3的病例存在其他抗原的缺失（CD2、CD3和/或CD5）[238]，βF1和CD3（正常联合表达）的不一致[239]。反应性病变中B细胞和CD8阳性淋巴细胞同时存在比蕈样霉菌病更为常见[238]。更具特征的是，S-100和CD1a+的朗格汉斯细胞和指状突网状细胞在真皮和Pautrier微脓肿中伴随蕈样霉菌病细胞出现[240]。蕈样霉菌病的大细胞转化可能与免疫组化中检测到的p53的表达有关[241]。

> **诊断要点：蕈样霉菌病**
> 1. 应用冰冻切片免疫组织化学方法，许多蕈样霉菌病病例可查见全T细胞抗原的丢失。
> 2. 大量的B细胞和CD8+的T细胞不支持蕈样霉菌病的诊断。

原发性皮肤CD30+的T细胞淋巴组织增生性疾病　　典型表型：CD3+、CD4+、CD8-、CD15-、CD30+、EMA-、ALK-

CD30分子的表达有助于识别原发性皮肤间变性大细胞淋巴瘤、CD30+相关性淋巴组织增生疾病和淋巴瘤样丘疹病[242,243]。这种区别对病人的治疗非常重要，因为应用保守疗法治疗增生病变效果非常显著。间变性细胞可能是单形性的或多形性的，而且数量变化范围从很少（在A型淋巴瘤样丘疹病中）到很多甚至呈片样分布（在C型淋巴瘤样丘疹病和原发性皮肤间变性大细胞淋巴瘤中）。尽管表现为CD4阳性和CD8阴性，但淋巴细胞因为有TIA-1和粒酶B的表达而呈现活化的细胞毒细胞的表型[244,245]。EMA和ALK[间变性淋巴瘤激酶；该基因与大约40%~80%的间变性大细胞淋巴瘤的t（2;5）染色体易位有关]可见于皮肤CD30+间变性大细胞淋巴瘤，但是这些并不是典型的原发性皮肤淋巴瘤的类型，而且预后较差[55,246,247]。CD30阴性大细胞淋巴瘤因其预后较差也不属于原发性皮肤间变性大细胞淋巴瘤的范畴[248,249]。经LMP-1证实，EB病毒感染在这种疾病中不起作用[250]。HECA-452抗体在多数正常的皮肤淋巴细胞中检测到一种抗原，这种抗原见于差不多半数的原发性皮肤间变性大细胞淋巴瘤，但未在淋巴结间变性大细胞淋巴瘤中查见[55]。

血管免疫母细胞性T细胞淋巴瘤　　典型表型：CD2+、CD3+、CD4+、CD8-/+、CD21和CD23+（在增生的滤泡树突细胞中）

主要临床特征（显著的全身性症状、中度全身淋巴结肿大、多克隆丙种球蛋白病和自身抗体与感染引发的并发症）可将其与其他类型的外周T细胞淋巴瘤区分开来。典型形态学可见显著的高内皮血管呈树枝状增生，淋巴细胞一般减少，增生的树突细胞岛伴有成片的中等大小胞浆透明的淋巴细胞。后者CD4+的T细胞的标记阳性，没有细胞毒T细胞分化的证据[217,225]。增生的滤泡树突细胞岛是该淋巴瘤特征之一，并且可被CD21和CD23的抗体所标记[251]。可见散在的大B细胞，不要由此误诊为是富于T细胞的B细胞淋巴瘤。近2/3的病例显示LMP-1阳性，B细胞和T细胞均可被感染[252]。有资料显示EB病毒的感染并不是疾病的原因，而是与免疫抑制有关；由EB病毒的感染引发的B细胞克隆性增生可以解释在这些病例中所形成的偶见的B免疫母细胞淋巴瘤[253]。

外周T细胞淋巴瘤（非特异性）　　典型表型：类型不一的T细胞抗原，CD4+>CD8+（可能双阴性），少见的B细胞抗原+

外周T细胞淋巴瘤作为胸腺后T细胞淋巴瘤的一个"废纸篓"种类[219]，是指所有非特异性外周T淋巴瘤。T细胞大小不一，呈现广谱性改变，有时混有组织细胞或嗜酸性粒细胞。应用免疫组化区分外周T细胞淋巴瘤和反应性病变可能是困难的，除非冰冻组织可检测出抗原缺失或T细胞淋巴瘤标记的不适当表达[39, 239, 254, 255]。TIA-1 在少数病例特别是结外部位可以表达[217]，LMP-1 较少表达[256]。

间变性大细胞淋巴瘤 典型表型：CD45RB+/-、CD3-/+、类型不一的T细胞抗原、CD15-/+、CD21-、CD25+/-、CD30+、CD43-/+、CD45RO-/+、EMA+/-、CD68-、溶菌酶-、ALK+/-

系统性间变性大细胞淋巴瘤（ALCL）是非霍奇金淋巴瘤中较为常见的一个类型，但是由于其早期在淋巴结内局限于窦内，且细胞构成呈多形性，因而它可能完全不被考虑为淋巴瘤。间变性淋巴瘤细胞较大，核仁明显，可见折叠状R-S样的胞核，细胞之间相互黏附。这些特征很容易辨认，但也容易忽视造成诊断困难[53, 257]。LCA（CD45RB）在大多数病例中表达，一个回顾性分析报道，阳性比例占70%～80%，但是石蜡包埋的组织阳性比例可能会低一些[258]。就细胞来源而言，T细胞比"裸"细胞（缺少B细胞和T细胞标记）更常见。70%的ALCL病例为T细胞家系，B细胞家系占15%（这些被看做是弥漫性大B细胞淋巴瘤），B和T细胞家系占5%，"裸"细胞占10%[257]。CD30为诊断该瘤的必需条件，CD15通常阴性[54, 259]。CD30细胞膜着色，同时以核旁点状方式标记高尔基体区域；弥漫性的胞浆阳性可能代表非特异性背景着色或良性大转化细胞的着色。在许多病例中，EMA 局灶性表达，极少数病例显示细胞角蛋白抗体在核周区域染色[259]。如前所述，表皮淋巴细胞抗体HECA-452只在少于20%的原发性系统性间变性大细胞淋巴瘤中表达[55]。EB病毒潜伏膜蛋白的检测结果不一[54, 260]。小细胞变型和淋巴组织细胞性变型都比经典的病例含更少的大细胞，但是恶性细胞保持了预期的表型[261-263]。ALK蛋白在43%～75%的间变性大细胞淋巴瘤中过表达；ALK表达与EMA表达相关，可延长病人的生存时间[264-267]。像很多其他成熟T细胞淋巴瘤一样，由于表达TIA-1和粒酶素B，原发性系统性ALCL常呈现细胞毒T细胞表型[217, 268-270]。p53在胞浆中明显（>60%的病例），但是尚未分离出该基因的突变[271, 272]。CD30和EMA的表达被用作该肿瘤骨髓微小病变的免疫组织化学标记[273]。

在系统性ALCL的诊断中，霍奇金病是最需要鉴别的。如果免疫组化呈现典型的LCA+/CD15-/T细胞标记+/EMA+/ALK+，则免疫表型是极有价值的。然而，还是有一些交界性病例即使进行分子学分析也很难进行鉴别。通过细胞角蛋白（在淋巴瘤中少见）的表达和常见特异性淋巴细胞抗原的缺失，可以将癌和ALCL鉴别开来。据报道CD30可在生殖细胞肿瘤和黑色素瘤中表达。当然黑色素瘤可以通过S-100和HMB-45的表达与ALCL相鉴别。

> **诊断要点：间变性大细胞淋巴瘤**
>
> 1. 多数系统性ALCL为：LCA+、CD3+、CD43+ 和 CD30+。
> 2. 寻找 CD30 在高尔基体和细胞膜的染色形式。
> 3. EMA、ALK 和 T 细胞标记阳性可以帮助区分 ALCL 和霍奇金病；fascin 在 ALCL 中通常为阴性。

参考文献

1. Harris NL, Jaffe ES, Stein H, et al. A revised European-American classification of lymphoid neoplasms: a proposal from the International Lymphoma Study Group. Blood 1994; 84(5):1361–1392.
2. Poppema S. Lymphoma classification proposal. Blood 1996; 87(1):412–413.
3. Meijer CJ, van der Valk P, de Bruin PC, et al. The revised European-American lymphoma (REAL) classification of non-Hodgkin's lymphoma: a missed opportunity? Blood 1995; 85(7):1971–1972.
4. Rosenberg SA. Classification of lymphoid neoplasms. Blood 1994; 84(5):1359–1360.
5. Pittaluga S, Bijnens L, Teodorovic I, et al. Clinical analysis of 670 cases in two trials of the European Organization for the Research and Treatment of Cancer Lymphoma Cooperative Group subtyped according to the Revised European-American Classification of Lymphoid Neoplasms: a comparison with the Working Formulation. Blood 1996; 87(10):4358–4367.
6. [No authors listed]. A clinical evaluation of the Inter-national Lymphoma Study Group classification of non-Hodgkin's lymphoma. The Non-Hodgkin's Lymphoma Classification Project. Blood 1997; 89(11):3909–3918.
7. Jaffe ES, Harris NL, Stein H, et al. editors. Pathology and genetics of tumours of haematopoietic and lymphoid tissues. Lyon: IARC Press; 2001.
8. Jaffe ES, Harris NL, Diebold J, et al. World Health Organization Classification of lymphomas: a work in progress. Ann Oncol 1998; 9(Suppl 5):S25–S30.
9. Harris NL, Jaffe ES, Diebold J, et al. The World Health Or-

ganization classification of hematological malignancies report of the Clinical Advisory Committee Meeting, Airlie House, Virginia, November 1997 World Health Organization classification of neoplastic diseases of the hematopoietic and lymphoid tissues. A progress report. Mod Pathol 2000; 13(2):193–207.

10. Abbondanzo SL. Paraffin immunohistochemistry as an adjunct to hematopathology. Ann Diagn Pathol 1999; 3(5):318–327.

11. Chu PG, Chang KL, Arber DA, et al. Practical applications of immunohistochemistry in hematolymphoid neoplasms. Ann Diagn Pathol 1999; 3(2):104–133.

12. Leucocyte Typing VI: White Cell Differentiation Antigens. In: Kishimoto T, Goyert S, Kikutani H, et al. eds. Sixth International Workshop and Conference; 1997; Kobe, Japan: Garland Publishers Inc; 1997.

13. Pileri SA, Roncador G, Ceccarelli C, et al. Antigen retrieval techniques in immunohistochemistry: comparison of different methods. J Pathol 1997;1 83(1):116–123.

14. Shi SR, Cote RJ, Taylor CR. Antigen retrieval immunohistochemistry: past, present, and future. J Histochem Cytochem 1997; 45(3):327–343.

15. Shi SR, Key ME, Kalra KL. Antigen retrieval in formalin-fixed, paraffin-embedded tissues: an enhancement method for immunohistochemical staining based on microwave oven heating of tissue sections. J Histochem Cytochem 1991; 39(6):741–748.

16. Johnson K, Chensue S, Ward P. Immunopathology. In: Rubin E, Farber J, eds. Pathology. 3rd edn. Philadelphia: Lippincott-Raven; 1999:104–153.

17. Inghirami G, Knowles D. The immune system: structure and function. In: Knowles D, ed. Neoplastic hematopathology. Baltimore: Williams & Wilkins; 1992:27–72.

18. Benoist C, Mathis D. T lymphocyte differentiation and biology. In: Paul W, ed. Fundamental immunology. 4th edn. Philadelphia: Lippincott-Raven Publishers; 1999:367–410.

19. DeFranco A. B lymphocyte activation. In: Paul W, ed. Fundamental Immunology. 4th edn. Philadelphia: Lippincott-Raven Publishers; 1999:225–261.

20. Melchers F, Rolink A. B-lymphocyte development and biology. In: Paul W, ed. Fundamental immunology. 4th edn. Philadelphia: Lippincott-Raven Publishers; 1999:183–224.

21. Rudin CM, Thompson CB. B-cell development and maturation. Semin Oncol 1998; 25(4):435–446.

22. Lennert K, Feller A. Histopathology of non-Hodgkin's lymphomas. 2nd edn. Berlin: Springer-Verlag; 1992.

23. Lukes R, Collins R. A functional approach to the classification of malignant lymphoma. Recent Results Cancer Res 1974; 46:18–30.

24. Lukes RJ, Collins RD. Immunologic characterization of human malignant lymphomas. Cancer 1974; 34(4 Suppl):1488–1503.

25. Stetler-Stevenson M, Medieros L, Jaffe E. Immunophenotypic methods and findings in the diagnosis of lymphoproliferative diseases. In: Jaffe E, ed. Surgical pathology of the lymph nodes and related organs. 2nd edn. Philadelphia: WB Saunders; 1995:22–57.

26. Nitschke L, Tsubata T. Molecular interactions regulate BCR signal inhibition by CD22 and CD72. Trends Immunol 2004; 25(10):543–550.

27. Mason DY, Cordell JL, Brown MH, et al. CD79a: a novel marker for B-cell neoplasms in routinely processed tissue samples. Blood 1995; 86(4):1453–1459.

28. Dorshkind K. Chapter 8 – B-Cell Development. In: Hoffman R, ed. Hematology: basic principles and practice. 3rd edn. New York: Churchill Livingstone; 2000:xxxi, 2584 p., [2524] p. of plates.

29. Chizuka A, Kanda Y, Nannya Y, et al. The diagnostic value of kappa/lambda ratios determined by flow cytometric analysis of biopsy specimens in B-cell lymphoma. Clin Lab Haematol 2002; 24(1):33–36.

30. Samoszuk MK, Krailo M, Yan QH, et al. Limitations of numerical ratios for defining monoclonality of immunoglobulin light chains in B-cell lymphomas. Diagn Immunol 1985; 3(3):133–138.

31. Aguilera NS, Kapadia SB, Nalesnik MA, et al. Extramedullary plasmacytoma of the head and neck: use of paraffin sections to assess clonality with in situ hybridization, growth fraction, and the presence of Epstein-Barr virus. Mod Pathol 1995; 8(5):503–508.

32. Beck RC, Tubbs RR, Hussein M, et al. Automated colorimetric in situ hybridization (CISH) detection of immunoglobulin (Ig) light chain mRNA expression in plasma cell (PC) dyscrasias and non-Hodgkin lymphoma. Diagn Mol Pathol 2003; 12(1):14–20.

33. Lee LH, Cioc A, Nuovo GJ. Determination of light chain

restriction in fine-needle aspiration-type preparations of B-cell lymphomas by mRNA in situ hybridization. Appl Immunohistochem Mol Morphol 2004; 12(3):252–258.

34. Pringle JH, Ruprai AK, Primrose L, et al. In situ hybridization of immunoglobulin light chain mRNA in paraffin sections using biotinylated or hapten-labelled oligonucleotide probes. J Pathol 1990; 162(3):197–207.

35. Malisius R, Merz H, Heinz B, et al. Constant detection of CD2, CD3, CD4, and CD5 in fixed and paraffin-embedded tissue using the peroxidase-mediated deposition of biotin-tyramide. J Histochem Cytochem 1997; 45(12):1665–1672.

36. Macon WR, Salhany KE. T-cell subset analysis of peripheral T-cell lymphomas by paraffin section immunohistology and correlation of CD4/CD8 results with flow cytometry. Am J Clin Pathol 1998; 109(5):610–617.

37. Dorfman DM, Shahsafaei A. CD69 expression correlates with expression of other markers of Th1 T cell differentiation in peripheral T cell lymphomas. Hum Pathol 2002; 33(3):330–334.

38. Weng AP, Shahsafaei A, Dorfman DM. CXCR4/CD184 immunoreactivity in T-cell non-Hodgkin lymphomas with an overall Th1- Th2+ immunophenotype. Am J Clin Pathol 2003; 119(3):424–430.

39. Picker LJ, Weiss LM, Medeiros LJ, et al. Immunophenotypic criteria for the diagnosis of non-Hodgkin's lymphoma. Am J Pathol 1987; 128(1):181–201.

40. Delsol G, Lamant L, Mariame B, et al. A new subtype of large B-cell lymphoma expressing the ALK kinase and lacking the 2;5 translocation. Blood 1997; 89(5):1483–1490.

41. Falini B, Bigerna B, Fizzotti M, et al. ALK expression defines a distinct group of T/null lymphomas ('ALK lymphomas') with a wide morphological spectrum. Am J Pathol 1998; 153(3):875–886.

42. Falini B, Fizzotti M, Pileri S, et al. Bcl-6 protein expression in normal and neoplastic lymphoid tissues. Ann Oncol 1997; 8(Suppl 2):101–104.

43. Arber D, Weiss L. CD57: a review. Appl Immunohistochem 1995; 3:137–152.

44. Frizzera G, Wu CD, Inghirami G. The usefulness of immunophenotypic and genotypic studies in the diagnosis and classification of hematopoietic and lymphoid neoplasms. An update. Am J Clin Pathol 1999; 111(1 Suppl 1):S13–S39.

45. Troxel DB, Sabella JD. Problem areas in pathology practice. Uncovered by a review of malpractice claims. Am J Surg Pathol 1994; 18(8):821–831.

46. Lai R, Arber DA, Chang KL, et al. Frequency of bcl-2 expression in non-Hodgkin's lymphoma: a study of 778 cases with comparison of marginal zone lymphoma and monocytoid B-cell hyperplasia. Mod Pathol 1998;1 1(9):864–869.

47. Wang T, Lasota J, Hanau CA, et al. Bcl-2 oncoprotein is widespread in lymphoid tissue and lymphomas but its differential expression in benign versus malignant follicles and monocytoid B-cell proliferations is of diagnostic value. APMIS 1995; 103(9):655–662.

48. Dogan A, Bagdi E, Munson P, et al. CD10 and BCL-6 expression in paraffin sections of normal lymphoid tissue and B-cell lymphomas. Am J Surg Pathol 2000; 24(6):846–852.

49. Gelb AB, Rouse RV, Dorfman RF, et al. Detection of immunophenotypic abnormalities in paraffin-embedded B-lineage non-Hodgkin's lymphomas. Am J Clin Pathol 1994; 102(6):825–834.

50. Browne G, Tobin B, Carney DN, et al. Aberrant MT2 positivity distinguishes follicular lymphoma from reactive follicular hyperplasia in B5- and formalin-fixed paraffin sections. Am J Clin Pathol 1991; 96(1):90–94.

51. Emile JF, Wechsler J, Brousse N, et al. Langerhans' cell histiocytosis. Definitive diagnosis with the use of monoclonal antibody O10 on routinely paraffin-embedded samples. Am J Surg Pathol 1995; 19(6):636–641.

52. Ng CS, Chan JK, Hui PK, et al. Large B-cell lymphomas with a high content of reactive T cells. Hum Pathol 1989; 20 (12):1145–1154.

53. Falini B, Pileri S, Stein H, et al. Variable expression of leucocyte-common (CD45) antigen in CD30 (Ki1)-positive anaplastic large-cell lymphoma: implications for the differential diagnosis between lymphoid and nonlymphoid malignancies. Hum Pathol 1990; 21(6):624–629.

54. Clavio M, Rossi E, Truini M, et al. Anaplastic large cell lymphoma: a clinicopathologic study of 53 patients. Leuk Lymphoma 1996; 22(3–4):319–327.

55. de Bruin PC, Beljaards RC, van Heerde P, et al. Differences in clinical behaviour and immunophenotype between primary cutaneous and primary nodal anaplastic large cell lymphoma of T-cell or null cell phenotype. Histopathology 1993; 23(2): 127–135.

56. Battifora H. Assessment of antigen damage in immuno-

histochemistry. The vimentin internal control. Am J Clin Pathol 1991; 96(5):669–671.
57. Anderson JR, Armitage JO, Weisenburger DD. Epidemiology of the non-Hodgkin's lymphomas: distributions of the major subtypes differ by geographic locations. Non-Hodgkin's Lymphoma Classification Project. Ann Oncol 1998; 9(7):717–720.
58. Medeiros LJ. Intermediate and high-grade diffuse non-Hodgkin's lymphomas in the Working Formulation. In: Jaffe E, ed. Surgical pathology of the lymph nodes and related organs. 2nd edn. Philadelphia: WB Saunders; 1995:283–343.
59. Weiss LM, Bindl JM, Picozzi VJ, et al. Lymphoblastic lymphoma: an immunophenotype study of 26 cases with comparison to T cell acute lymphoblastic leukemia. Blood 1986; 67(2):474–478.
60. Cossman J, Chused TM, Fisher RI, et al. Diversity of immunological phenotypes of lymphoblastic lymphoma. Cancer Res 1983; 43(9):4486-4490.
61. Braziel RM, Keneklis T, Donlon JA, et al. Terminal deoxynucleotidyl transferase in non-Hodgkin's lymphoma. Am J Clin Pathol 1983; 80(5):655–659.
62. Ozdemirli M, Fanburg-Smith JC, Hartmann DP, et al. Precursor B-lymphoblastic lymphoma presenting as a solitary bone tumor and mimicking Ewing's sarcoma: a report of four cases and review of the literature. Am J Surg Pathol 1998; 22(7):795–804.
63. Iravani S, Singleton TP, Ross CW, et al. Precursor B lymphoblastic lymphoma presenting as lytic bone lesions. Am J Clin Pathol 1999; 112(6):836–843.
64. Chimenti S, Fink-Puches R, Peris K, et al. Cutaneous involvement in lymphoblastic lymphoma. J Cutan Pathol 1999; 26(8):379–385.
65. Soslow RA, Zukerberg LR, Harris NL, et al. BCL-1 (PRAD-1/cyclin D-1) overexpression distinguishes the blastoid variant of mantle cell lymphoma from B-lineage lympho-blastic lymphoma. Mod Pathol 1997; 10(8):810–817.
66. Soslow RA, Baergen RN, Warnke RA. B-lineage lymphoblastic lymphoma is a clinicopathologic entity distinct from other histologically similar aggressive lymphomas with blastic morphology. Cancer 1999; 85(12):2648–2654.
67. Van Eyken P, De Wolf-Peeters C, Van den Oord J, et al. Expression of leukocyte common antigen in lymphoblastic lymphoma and small noncleaved undifferentiated non-Burkitt's lymphoma: an immunohistochemical study. J Pathol 1987; 151(4):257–261.
68. Taubenberger JK, Cole DE, Raffeld M, et al. Immuno-phenotypic analysis of acute lymphoblastic leukemia using routinely processed bone marrow specimens. Arch Pathol Lab Med 1991; 115(4):338–342.
69. Robertson PB, Neiman RS, Worapongpaiboon S, et al. 013 (CD99) positivity in hematologic proliferations correlates with TdT positivity. Mod Pathol 1997; 10(4):277–282.
70. Riopel M, Dickman PS, Link MP, et al. MIC2 analysis in pediatric lymphomas and leukemias. Hum Pathol 1994; 25(4):396-399.
71. Sheibani K, Nathwani BN, Winberg CD, et al. Antigenically defined subgroups of lymphoblastic lymphoma. Relationship to clinical presentation and biologic behavior. Cancer 1987; 60(2):183–190.
72. Tsang WY, Chan JK, Ng CS, et al. Utility of a paraffin section-reactive CD56 antibody (123C3) for characterization and diagnosis of lymphomas. Am J Surg Pathol 1996; 20(2):202–210.
73. Mullauer L, Mosberger I, Chott A. Fas ligand expression in nodal non-Hodgkin's lymphoma. Mod Pathol 1998; 11(4):369–375.
74. Soslow RA, Bhargava V, Warnke RA. MIC2, TdT, bcl-2, and CD34 expression in paraffin-embedded high-grade lymphoma/acute lymphoblastic leukemia distinguishes between distinct clinicopathologic entities. Hum Pathol 1997; 28(10):1158–1165.
75. de Leon ED, Alkan S, Huang JC, et al. Usefulness of an immunohistochemical panel in paraffin-embedded tissues for the differentiation of B-cell non-Hodgkin's lymphomas of small lymphocytes. Mod Pathol 1998; 11(11):1046–1051.
76. Lai R, Weiss LM, Chang KL, et al. Frequency of CD43 expression in non-Hodgkin lymphoma. A survey of 742 cases and further characterization of rare CD43+ follicular lymphomas. Am J Clin Pathol 1999; 111(4):488–494.
77. Kumar S, Green GA, Teruya-Feldstein J, et al. Use of CD23 (BU38) on paraffin sections in the diagnosis of small lymphocytic lymphoma and mantle cell lymphoma. Mod Pathol 1996; 9(9):925–929.
78. Kaufmann O, Flath B, Spath-Schwalbe E, et al. Immunohistochemical detection of CD5 with monoclonal antibody 4C7 on paraffin sections. Am J Clin Pathol 1997; 108(6):669–673.

79. Dorfman DM, Shahsafaei A. Usefulness of a new CD5 antibody for the diagnosis of T-cell and B-cell lymphoproliferative disorders in paraffin sections. Mod Pathol 1997; 10(9):859–863.
80. Huang JC, Finn WG, Goolsby CL, et al. CD5- small B-cell leukemias are rarely classifiable as chronic lymphocytic leukemia. Am J Clin Pathol 1999; 111(1):123–130.
81. Orazi A, Cattoretti G, Polli N, et al. Distinct morphophenotypic features of chronic B-cell leukaemias identified with CD1c and CD23 antibodies. Eur J Haematol 1991; 47(1):28–35.
82. Singh N, Wright DH. The value of immunohistochemistry on paraffin wax embedded tissue sections in the differentiation of small lymphocytic and mantle cell lymphomas. J Clin Pathol 1997; 50(1):16–21.
83. Aguilera NS, Chu WS, Andriko JA, et al. Expression of CD44 (HCAM) in small lymphocytic and mantle cell lymphoma. Hum Pathol 1998; 29(10):1134–1139.
84. Dorfman DM, Pinkus GS. Distinction between small lymphocytic and mantle cell lymphoma by immunoreactivity for CD23. Mod Pathol 1994; 7(3):326–331.
85. Dunphy CH, Wheaton SE, Perkins SL. CD23 expression in transformed small lymphocytic lymphomas/chronic lymphocytic leukemias and blastic transformations of mantle cell lymphoma. Mod Pathol 1997; 10(8):818–822.
86. Watson P, Wood KM, Lodge A, et al. Monoclonal antibodies recognizing CD5, CD10 and CD23 in formalin-fixed, paraffin-embedded tissue: production and assessment of their value in the diagnosis of small B-cell lymphoma. Histopathology 2000; 36(2):145–150.
87. Swerdlow SH, Yang WI, Zukerberg LR, et al. Expression of cyclin D1 protein in centrocytic/mantle cell lymphomas with and without rearrangement of the BCL1/cyclin D1 gene. Hum Pathol 1995; 26(9):999–1004.
88. Yang WI, Zukerberg LR, Motokura T, et al. Cyclin D1 (Bcl-1, PRAD1) protein expression in low-grade B-cell lymphomas and reactive hyperplasia. Am J Pathol 1994; 145(1):86–96.
89. Vasef MA, Medeiros LJ, Koo C, et al. Cyclin D1 immunohistochemical staining is useful in distinguishing mantle cell lymphoma from other low-grade B-cell neoplasms in bone marrow. Am J Clin Pathol 1997; 108(3):302–307.
90. Zukerberg LR, Yang WI, Arnold A, et al. Cyclin D1 expression in non-Hodgkin's lymphomas. Detection by immunohistochemistry. Am J Clin Pathol 1995; 103(6):756–760.
91. Raible MD, Hsi ED, Alkan S. Bcl-6 protein expression by follicle center lymphomas. A marker for differentiating follicle center lymphomas from other low-grade lymphoproliferative disorders. Am J Clin Pathol 1999; 112(1):101–107.
92. Aguilar-Santelises M, Magnusson KP, Wiman KG, et al. Progressive B-cell chronic lymphocytic leukaemia frequently exhibits aberrant p53 expression. Int J Cancer 1994; 58(4):474–479.
93. Jones D, Benjamin RJ, Shahsafaei A, et al. The chemokine receptor CXCR3 is expressed in a subset of B-cell lymphomas and is a marker of B-cell chronic lymphocytic leukemia. Blood 2000; 95(2):627–632.
94. Admirand JH, Rassidakis GZ, Abruzzo LV, et al. Immunohistochemical detection of ZAP-70 in 341 cases of non-Hodgkin and Hodgkin lymphoma. Mod Pathol 2004; 17(8):954–961.
95. Sup SJ, Domiati-Saad R, Kelley TW, et al. ZAP-70 expression in B-cell hematologic malignancy is not limited to CLL/SLL. Am J Clin Pathol 2004; 122(4):582–587.
96. Crespo M, Bosch F, Villamor N, et al. ZAP-70 expression as a surrogate for immunoglobulin-variable-region mutations in chronic lymphocytic leukemia. N Engl J Med 2003; 348(18):1764–1775.
97. Wiestner A, Rosenwald A, Barry TS, et al. ZAP-70 expression identifies a chronic lymphocytic leukemia subtype with unmutated immunoglobulin genes, inferior clinical outcome, and distinct gene expression profile. Blood 2003; 101(12):4944–4951.
98. Rassenti LZ, Huynh L, Toy TL, et al. ZAP-70 compared with immunoglobulin heavy-chain gene mutation status as a predictor of disease progression in chronic lymphocytic leukemia. N Engl J Med 2004; 351(9):893–901.
99. Carreras J, Villamor N, Colomo L, et al. Immunohistochemical analysis of ZAP-70 expression in B-cell lymphoid neoplasms. J Pathol 2005; 205(4):507–513.
100. Bennett JM, Catovsky D, Daniel MT, et al. Proposals for the classification of chronic (mature) B and T lymphoid leukaemias. French-American-British (FAB) Cooperative Group. J Clin Pathol 1989; 42(6):567–584.

101. de Melo N, Matutes E, Cordone I, et al. Expression of Ki-67 nuclear antigen in B and T cell lymphoproliferative disorders. J Clin Pathol 1992; 45(8):660–663.

102. Harris NL, Bhan AK. B-cell neoplasms of the lymphocytic, lymphoplasmacytoid, and plasma cell types: immunohistologic analysis and clinical correlation. Hum Pathol 1985; 16(8):829–837.

103. Hall PA, D'Ardenne AJ, Richards MA, et al. Lympho-plasmacytoid lymphoma: an immunohistological study. J Pathol 1987; 153(3):213–223.

104. Zukerberg LR, Medeiros LJ, Ferry JA, et al. Diffuse low-grade B-cell lymphomas. Four clinically distinct subtypes defined by a combination of morphologic and immunophenotypic features. Am J Clin Pathol 1993; 100(4):373–385.

105. Tworek JA, Singleton TP, Schnitzer B, et al. Flow cytometric and immunohistochemical analysis of small lymphocytic lymphoma, mantle cell lymphoma, and plasmacytoid small lymphocytic lymphoma. Am J Clin Pathol 1998; 110(5):582–589.

106. Chilosi M, Adami F, Lestani M, et al. CD138/syndecan-1: a useful immunohistochemical marker of normal and neoplastic plasma cells on routine trephine bone marrow biopsies. Mod Pathol 1999; 12(12):1101–1106.

107. Nguyen PL, Harris NL, Ritz J, et al. Expression of CD95 antigen and Bcl-2 protein in non-Hodgkin's lymphomas and Hodgkin's disease. Am J Pathol 1996; 148(3):847–853.

108. Catovsky D, Matutes E. Splenic lymphoma with circulating villous lymphocytes/splenic marginal-zone lymphoma. Semin Hematol 1999; 36(2):148–154.

109. Hammer RD, Glick AD, Greer JP, et al. Splenic marginal zone lymphoma. A distinct B-cell neoplasm. Am J Surg Pathol 1996; 20(5):613–626.

110. Baldini L, Fracchiolla NS, Cro LM, et al. Frequent p53 gene involvement in splenic B-cell leukemia/lymphomas of possible marginal zone origin. Blood 1994; 84(1):270–278.

111. Matutes E, Morilla R, Owusu-Ankomah K, et al. The immunophenotype of hairy cell leukemia (HCL). Proposal for a scoring system to distinguish HCL from B-cell disorders with hairy or villous lymphocytes. Leuk Lymphoma 1994; 14(Suppl 1):57–61.

112. Matutes E, Morilla R, Owusu-Ankomah K, et al. The immunophenotype of splenic lymphoma with villous lymphocytes and its relevance to the differential diagnosis with other B-cell disorders. Blood 1994; 83(6):1558–1562.

113. Rosso R, Neiman RS, Paulli M, et al. Splenic marginal zone cell lymphoma: report of an indolent variant without massive splenomegaly presumably representing an early phase of the disease. Hum Pathol 1995; 26(1):39–46.

114. Piris MA, Mollejo M, Campo E, et al. A marginal zone pattern may be found in different varieties of non-Hodgkin's lymphoma: the morphology and immunohistology of splenic involvement by B-cell lymphomas simulating splenic marginal zone lymphoma. Histopathology 1998; 33(3):230–239.

115. Mollejo M, Lloret E, Menarguez J, et al. Lymph node involvement by splenic marginal zone lymphoma: morphological and immunohistochemical features. Am J Surg Pathol 1997; 21(7):772–780.

116. Wu CD, Jackson CL, Medeiros LJ. Splenic marginal zone cell lymphoma. An immunophenotypic and molecular study of five cases. Am J Clin Pathol 1996; 105(3):277–285.

117. Pawade J, Wilkins BS, Wright DH. Low-grade B-cell lymphomas of the splenic marginal zone: a clinicopathological and immunohistochemical study of 14 cases. Histopathology 1995; 27(2):129–137.

118. Savilo E, Campo E, Mollejo M, et al. Absence of cyclin D1 protein expression in splenic marginal zone lymphoma. Mod Pathol 1998; 11(7):601–606.

119. Janckila AJ, Cardwell EM, Yam LT, et al. Hairy cell identification by immunohistochemistry of tartrate-resistant acid phosphatase. Blood 1995; 85(10):2839–2844.

120. Janckila AJ, Lear SC, Martin AW, et al. Epitope enhancement for immunohistochemical demonstration of tartrate-resistant acid phosphatase. J Histochem Cytochem 1996; 44(3):235–244.

121. Hoyer JD, Li CY, Yam LT, et al. Immunohistochemical demonstration of acid phosphatase isoenzyme 5 (tartrate-resistant) in paraffin sections of hairy cell leukemia and other hematologic disorders. Am J Clin Pathol 1997; 108(3):308–315.

122. Stroup R, Sheibani K. Antigenic phenotypes of hairy cell leukemia and monocytoid B-cell lymphoma: an immunohistochemical evaluation of 66 cases. Hum Pathol 1992; 23(2):172–177.

123. Kreft A, Busche G, Bernhards J, et al. Immunophenotype of hairy-cell leukaemia after cold polymerization of methyl-methacrylate embeddings from 50 diagnostic bone marrow

biopsies. Histopathology 1997; 30(2):145–151.

124. Segal GH, Stoler MH, Fishleder AJ, et al. Reliable and cost-effective paraffin section immunohistology of lymphoproliferative disorders. Am J Surg Pathol 1991; 15(11):1034–1041.

125. Hakimian D, Tallman MS, Kiley C, et al. Detection of minimal residual disease by immunostaining of bone marrow biopsies after 2-chlorodeoxyadenosine for hairy cell leukemia. Blood 1993; 82(6):1798–1802.

126. Hounieu H, Chittal SM, al Saati T, et al. Hairy cell leukemia. Diagnosis of bone marrow involvement in paraffin-embedded sections with monoclonal antibody DBA.44. Am J Clin Pathol 1992; 98(1):26–33.

127. Ohsawa M, Kanno H, Machii T, et al. Immunoreactivity of neoplastic and non-neoplastic monocytoid B lymphocytes for DBA.44 and other antibodies. J Clin Pathol 1994; 47(10):928–932.

128. Yaziji H, Janckila AJ, Lear SC, et al. Immunohistochemical detection of tartrate-resistant acid phosphatase in non-hematopoietic human tissues. Am J Clin Pathol 1995; 104(4):397–402.

129. Bosch F, Campo E, Jares P, et al. Increased expression of the PRAD-1/CCND1 gene in hairy cell leukaemia. Br J Haematol 1995; 91(4):1025–1030.

130. de Boer CJ, Kluin-Nelemans JC, Dreef E, et al. Involvement of the CCND1 gene in hairy cell leukemia. Ann Oncol 1996; 7(3):251–256.

131. Costes V, Magen V, Legouffe E, et al. The Mi15 mono-clonal antibody (anti-syndecan-1) is a reliable marker for quantifying plasma cells in paraffin-embedded bone marrow biopsy specimens. Hum Pathol 1999; 30(12):1405–1411.

132. Vallario A, Chilosi M, Adami F, et al. Human myeloma cells express the CD38 ligand CD31. Br J Haematol 1999; 105(2):441–444.

133. Hamilton MS, Barker HF, Ball J, et al. Normal and neoplastic human plasma cells express bcl-2 antigen. Leukemia 1991; 5(9):768–771.

134. Diss TC, Wotherspoon AC, Speight P, et al. B-cell monoclonality, Epstein-Barr virus, and t(14;18) in myoepithelial sialadenitis and low-grade B-cell MALT lymphoma of the parotid gland. Am J Surg Pathol 1995; 19(5):531–536.

135. Baldassano MF, Bailey EM, Ferry JA, et al. Cutaneous lymphoid hyperplasia and cutaneous marginal zone lymphoma: comparison of morphologic and immunophenotypic features. Am J Surg Pathol 1999; 23(1):88–96.

136. Berger F, Felman P, Thieblemont C, et al. Non-MALT marginal zone B-cell lymphomas: a description of clinical presentation and outcome in 124 patients. Blood 2000; 95(6):1950–1956.

137. Arends JE, Bot FJ, Gisbertz IA, et al. Expression of CD10, CD75 and CD43 in MALT lymphoma and their usefulness in discriminating MALT lymphoma from follicular lymphoma and chronic gastritis. Histopathology 1999; 35(3):209–215.

138. Ferry JA, Yang WI, Zukerberg LR, et al. CD5+ extranodal marginal zone B-cell (MALT) lymphoma. A low grade neoplasm with a propensity for bone marrow involvement and relapse. Am J Clin Pathol 1996; 105(1):31–37.

139. Ashton-Key M, Biddolph SC, Stein H, et al. Heterogeneity of bcl-2 expression in MALT lymphoma. Histopathology 1995; 26(1):75–78.

140. Cerroni L, Signoretti S, Hofler G, et al. Primary cutaneous marginal zone B-cell lymphoma: a recently described entity of low-grade malignant cutaneous B-cell lymphoma. Am J Surg Pathol 1997; 21(11):1307–1315.

141. Chetty R, O'Leary JJ, Biddolph SC, et al. Immunohistochemical detection of p53 and Bcl-2 proteins in Hashimoto's thyroiditis and primary thyroid lymphomas. J Clin Pathol 1995; 48(3):239–241.

142. Nakamura S, Akazawa K, Kinukawa N, et al. Inverse correlation between the expression of bcl-2 and p53 proteins in primary gastric lymphoma. Hum Pathol 1996; 27(3):225–233.

143. Navratil E, Gaulard P, Kanavaros P, et al. Expression of the bcl-2 protein in B cell lymphomas arising from mucosa associated lymphoid tissue. J Clin Pathol 1995; 48(1):18–21.

144. Omonishi K, Yoshino T, Sakuma I, et al. bcl-6 protein is identified in high-grade but not low-grade mucosa-associated lymphoid tissue lymphomas of the stomach. Mod Pathol 1998; 11(2):181–185.

145. Nakamura S, Akazawa K, Yao T, et al. A clinicopathologic study of 233 cases with special reference to evaluation with the MIB-1 index. Cancer 1995; 76(8):1313–1324.

146. Isaacson PG. Gastrointestinal lymphomas of T- and B-cell types. Mod Pathol 1999; 12(2):151–158.

147. Davis GG, York JC, Glick AD, et al. Plasmacytic differentiation in parafollicular (monocytoid) B-cell lymphoma. A study of 12 cases. Am J Surg Pathol 1992; 16(11):1066–1074.

148. Nizze H, Cogliatti SB, von Schilling C, et al. Monocytoid B-cell lymphoma: morphological variants and relationship to low-grade B-cell lymphoma of the mucosa-associated lymphoid tissue. Histopathology 1991; 18(5):403–414.

149. Kurtin PJ, Hobday KS, Ziesmer S, et al. Demonstration of distinct antigenic profiles of small B-cell lymphomas by paraffin section immunohistochemistry. Am J Clin Pathol 1999; 112(3):319–329.

150. Ballesteros E, Osborne BM, Matsushima AY. CD5+ low-grade marginal zone B-cell lymphomas with localized presentation. Am J Surg Pathol 1998; 22(2):201–207.

151. Dierlamm J, Pittaluga S, Wlodarska I, et al. Marginal zone B-cell lymphomas of different sites share similar cytogenetic and morphologic features. Blood 1996; 87(1):299–307.

152. Campo E, Miquel R, Krenacs L, et al. Primary nodal marginal zone lymphomas of splenic and MALT type. Am J Surg Pathol 1999; 23(1):59–68.

153. Hernandez AM, Nathwani BN, Nguyen D, et al. Nodal benign and malignant monocytoid B cells with and without follicular lymphomas: a comparative study of follicular colonization, light chain restriction, bcl-2, and t(14;18) in 39 cases. Hum Pathol 1995; 26(6):625–632.

154. Levy V, Miller C, Koeffler HP, et al. p53 in lymphomas of mucosal-associated lymphoid tissues. Mod Pathol 1996; 9(3):245–248.

155. Baldini L, Guffanti A, Cro L, et al. Poor prognosis in non-villous splenic marginal zone cell lymphoma is associated with p53 mutations. Br J Haematol 1997; 99(2):375–378.

156. McIntosh GG, Lodge AJ, Watson P, et al. NCL-CD10-270: a new monoclonal antibody recognizing CD10 in paraffin-embedded tissue. Am J Pathol 1999; 154(1):77–82.

157. Contos MJ, Kornstein MJ, Innes DJ, et al. The utility of CD20 and CD43 in subclassification of low-grade B-cell lymphoma on paraffin sections. Mod Pathol 1992; 5(6):631–633.

158. Ashton-Key M, Diss TC, Isaacson PG, et al. A comparative study of the value of immunohistochemistry and the polymerase chain reaction in the diagnosis of follicular lymphoma. Histopathology 1995; 27(6):501–508.

159. Cooper K, Haffajee Z. bcl-2 and p53 protein expression in follicular lymphoma. J Pathol 1997; 182(3):307–310.

160. Gaulard P, d'Agay MF, Peuchmaur M, et al. Expression of the bcl-2 gene product in follicular lymphoma. Am J Pathol 1992; 140(5):1089–1095.

161. Nguyen PL, Zukerberg LR, Benedict WF, et al. Immunohistochemical detection of p53, bcl-2, and retinoblastoma proteins in follicular lymphoma. Am J Clin Pathol 1996; 105(5):538–543.

162. Skinnider BF, Horsman DE, Dupuis B, et al. Bcl-6 and Bcl-2 protein expression in diffuse large B-cell lymphoma and follicular lymphoma: correlation with 3q27 and 18q21 chromosomal abnormalities. Hum Pathol 1999; 30(7):803–808.

163. Logsdon MD, Meyn RE Jr, Besa PC, et al. Apoptosis and the Bcl-2 gene family – patterns of expression and prognostic value in stage I and II follicular center lymphoma. Int J Radiat Oncol Biol Phys 1999; 44(1):19–29.

164. Goates JJ, Kamel OW, LeBrun DP, et al. Floral variant of follicular lymphoma. Immunological and molecular studies support a neoplastic process. Am J Surg Pathol 1994; 18(1):37–47.

165. Pezzella F, Jones M, Ralfkiaer E, et al. Evaluation of bcl-2 protein expression and 14;18 translocation as prognostic markers in follicular lymphoma. Br J Cancer 1992; 65(1):87–89.

166. Cattoretti G, Chang CC, Cechova K, et al. BCL-6 protein is expressed in germinal-center B cells. Blood 1995; 86(1):45–53.

167. Szereday Z, Csernus B, Nagy M, et al. Somatic mutation of the 5' noncoding region of the BCL-6 gene is associated with intraclonal diversity and clonal selection in histological transformation of follicular lymphoma. Am J Pathol 2000; 156(3):1017–1024.

168. Moller MB, Nielsen O, Pedersen NT. Oncoprotein MDM2 overexpression is associated with poor prognosis in distinct non-Hodgkin's lymphoma entities. Mod Pathol 1999; 12(11):1010-1016.

169. Kamel OW, Gelb AB, Shibuya RB, et al. Leu 7 (CD57) reactivity distinguishes nodular lymphocyte predomi-nance Hodgkin's disease from nodular sclerosing Hodgkin's disease, T-cell-rich B-cell lymphoma and fol-licular lymphoma. Am J Pathol 1993; 142(2):541–546.

170. Scoazec JY, Berger F, Magaud JP, et al. The dendritic reticulum cell pattern in B cell lymphomas of the small cleaved, mixed, and large cell types: an immunohistochemical study of 48 cases. Hum Pathol 1989; 20(2):124–131.

171. Miettinen M. CD30 distribution. Immunohistochemical study on formaldehyde-fixed, paraffin-embedded Hodgkin's and

172. Piris M, Gatter KC, Mason DY. CD30 expression in follicular lymphoma. Histopathology 1991; 18(1):25–29.
173. Chetty R, Echezarreta G, Comley M, et al. Immunohistochemistry in apparently normal bone marrow trephine specimens from patients with nodal follicular lymphoma. J Clin Pathol 1995; 48(11):1035–1038.
174. Kurtin PJ. Mantle cell lymphoma. Adv Anat Pathol 1998; 5(6):376–398.
175. Lavergne A, Brouland JP, Launay E, et al. Multiple lymphomatous polyposis of the gastrointestinal tract. An extensive histopathologic and immunohistochemical study of 12 cases. Cancer 1994; 74(11):3042–3050.
176. Pittaluga S, Wlodarska I, Stul MS, et al. Mantle cell lymphoma: a clinicopathological study of 55 cases. Histopathology 1995; 26(1):17–24.
177. Fraga M, Lloret E, Sanchez-Verde L, et al. Mucosal mantle cell (centrocytic) lymphomas. Histopathology 1995; 26(5):413–422.
178. Yatabe Y, Suzuki R, Tobinai K, et al. Significance of cyclin D1 overexpression for the diagnosis of mantle cell lymphoma: a clinicopathologic comparison of cyclin D1-positive MCL and cyclin D1-negative MCL-like B-cell lymphoma. Blood 2000; 95(7):2253–2261.
179. Kumar S, Krenacs L, Otsuki T, et al. bcl-1 rearrangement and cyclin D1 protein expression in multiple lymphomatous polyposis. Am J Clin Pathol 1996; 105(6):737–743.
180. Singleton TP, Anderson MM, Ross CW, et al. Leukemic phase of mantle cell lymphoma, blastoid variant. Am J Clin Pathol 1999; 111(4):495–500.
181. Gronbaek K, Nedergaard T, Andersen MK, et al. Concurrent disruption of cell cycle associated genes in mantle cell lymphoma: a genotypic and phenotypic study of cyclin D1, p16, p15, p53 and pRb. Leukemia 1998; 12(8):1266–1271.
182. Chang CC, Liu YC, Cleveland RP, et al. Expression of c-Myc and p53 correlates with clinical outcome in diffuse large B-cell lymphomas. Am J Clin Pathol 2000; 113(4):512–518.
183. Louie DC, Offit K, Jaslow R, et al. p53 overexpression as a marker of poor prognosis in mantle cell lymphomas with t(11;14)(q13;q32). Blood 1995; 86(8):2892–2899.
184. Hernandez L, Fest T, Cazorla M, et al. p53 gene mutations and protein overexpression are associated with aggressive variants of mantle cell lymphomas. Blood 1996; 87(8):3351–3359.
185. Fiel-Gan MD, Almeida LM, Rose DC, et al. Proliferative fraction, bcl-1 gene translocation, and p53 mutation status as markers in mantle cell lymphoma. Int J Mol Med 1999; 3(4):373–379.
186. Stein H, Lennert K, Feller AC, et al. Immunohistological analysis of human lymphoma: correlation of histological and immunological categories. Adv Cancer Res 1984; 42:67–147.
187. Doggett RS, Wood GS, Horning S, et al. The immunologic characterization of 95 nodal and extranodal diffuse large cell lymphomas in 89 patients. Am J Pathol 1984; 115(2):245–252.
188. Taniguchi M, Oka K, Hiasa A, et al. De novo CD5+ diffuse large B-cell lymphomas express VH genes with somatic mutation. Blood 1998; 91(4):1145–1151.
189. Fang JM, Finn WG, Hussong JW, et al. CD10 antigen expression correlates with the t(14;18)(q32;q21) major breakpoint region in diffuse large B-cell lymphoma. Mod Pathol 1999; 12(3):295–300.
190. Martinka M, Comeau T, Foyle A, et al. Prognostic significance of t(14;18) and bcl-2 gene expression in follicular small cleaved cell lymphoma and diffuse large cell lymphoma. Clin Invest Med 1997; 20(6):364–370.
191. Gascoyne RD, Adomat SA, Krajewski S, et al. Prognostic significance of Bcl-2 protein expression and Bcl-2 gene rearrangement in diffuse aggressive non-Hodgkin's lymphoma. Blood 1997; 90(1):244–251.
192. Gascoyne RD, Krajewska M, Krajewski S, et al. Prognostic significance of Bax protein expression in diffuse aggressive non-Hodgkin's lymphoma. Blood 1997; 90(8):3173–3178.
193. Drillenburg P, Wielenga VJ, Kramer MH, et al. CD44 expression predicts disease outcome in localized large B cell lymphoma. Leukemia 1999; 13(9):1448–1455.
194. Donoghue S, Baden HS, Lauder I, et al. Immunohistochemical localization of caspase-3 correlates with clinical outcome in B-cell diffuse large-cell lymphoma. Cancer Res 1999; 59(20):5386–5391.
195. Weiss LM, Strickler JG, Medeiros LJ, et al. Proliferative rates of non-Hodgkin's lymphomas as assessed by Ki-67 antibody. Hum Pathol 1987; 18(11):1155–1159.
196. Frierson HFJ, Bellafiore FJ, Gaffey MJ, et al. Cytokeratin in anaplastic large cell lymphoma. Mod Pathol 1994; 7(3):317–

321.

197. de Bruin PC, Gruss HJ, van der Valk P, et al. CD30 expression in normal and neoplastic lymphoid tissue: biological aspects and clinical implications. Leukemia 1995; 9(10):1620–1627.

198. Krishnan J, Wallberg K, Frizzera G. T-cell-rich large B-cell lymphoma. A study of 30 cases, supporting its histologic heterogeneity and lack of clinical distinctiveness. Am J Surg Pathol 1994; 18(5):455-465.

199. Suster S. Primary large-cell lymphomas of the mediastinum. Semin Diagn Pathol 1999; 16(1):51–64.

200. Davis RE, Dorfman RF, Warnke RA. Primary large-cell lymphoma of the thymus: a diffuse B-cell neoplasm presenting as primary mediastinal lymphoma. Hum Pathol 1990; 21(12):1262–1268.

201. Rodriguez J, Pugh WC, Romaguera JE, et al. Primary mediastinal large cell lymphoma. Hematol Oncol 1994; 12(4):175–184.

202. Rodriguez J, Pugh WC, Romaguera JE, et al. Primary mediastinal large cell lymphoma is characterized by an inverted pattern of large tumoral mass and low beta 2 microglobulin levels in serum and frequently elevated levels of serum lactate dehydrogenase. Ann Oncol 1994; 5(9):847–849.

203. Higgins JP, Warnke RA. CD30 expression is common in mediastinal large B-cell lymphoma. Am J Clin Pathol 1999; 112(2):241–247.

204. Knowles DM. Immunodeficiency-associated lymphoproliferative disorders. Mod Pathol 1999; 12(2):200–217.

205. Green I, Espiritu E, Ladanyi M, et al. Primary lym-phomatous effusions in AIDS: a morphological, immunophenotypic, and molecular study. Mod Pathol 1995; 8(1):39–45.

206. Nador RG, Cesarman E, Chadburn A, et al. Primary effusion lymphoma: a distinct clinicopathologic entity associated with the Kaposi's sarcoma-associated herpes virus. Blood 1996; 88(2):645–656.

207. DiGiuseppe JA, Nelson WG, Seifter EJ, et al. Intravascular lymphomatosis: a clinicopathologic study of 10 cases and assessment of response to chemotherapy. J Clin Oncol 1994; 12(12):2573–2579.

208. Ferry JA, Harris NL, Picker LJ, et al. Intravascular lymphomatosis (malignant angioendotheliomatosis). A B-cell neoplasm expressing surface homing receptors. Mod Pathol 1988; 1(6):444–452.

209. Domizio P, Hall PA, Cotter F, et al. Angiotropic large cell lymphoma (ALCL): morphological, immunohistochemical and genotypic studies with analysis of previous reports. Hematol Oncol 1989; 7(3):195–206.

210. Kanda M, Suzumiya J, Ohshima K, et al. Intravascular large cell lymphoma: clinicopathological, immuno-histochemical and molecular genetic studies. Leuk Lymphoma 1999; 34(5-6):569–580.

211. Rudinger T, Ott G, Ott M, et al. Reply to: B-cell anaplastic large cell lymphoma – the forgotten entity. Am J Surg Pathol 2000; 24:159–160.

212. Suzumiya J, Ohshima K, Kikuchi M, et al. Terminal deoxynucleotidyl transferase staining of malignant lymphomas in paraffin sections: a useful method for the diagnosis of lymphoblastic lymphoma. J Pathol 1997; 182(1):86–91.

213. Guinee D Jr, Jaffe E, Kingma D, et al. Pulmonary lymphomatoid granulomatosis. Evidence for a proliferation of Epstein-Barr virus infected B-lymphocytes with a prominent T-cell component and vasculitis. Am J Surg Pathol 1994; 18(8):753–764.

214. Chetty R, Pulford K, Jones M, et al. An immunohistochemical study of TAL-1 protein expression in leukaemias and lymphomas with a novel monoclonal antibody, 2TL 242. J Pathol 1996; 178(3):311–315.

215. Sykora KW, Tomeczkowski J, Reiter A. C-kit receptors in childhood malignant lymphoblastic cells. Leuk Lymphoma 1997; 25(3-4):201–216.

216. Chan J, Tsang W. Reactive lymphadenopathies. In: Weiss L, ed. Pathology of lymph nodes. New York: Churchill Livingstone; 1996:81–167.

217. Chan AC, Ho JW, Chiang AK, et al. Phenotypic and cytotoxic characteristics of peripheral T-cell and NK-cell lymphomas in relation to Epstein-Barr virus association. Histopathology 1999; 34(1):16–24.

218. Chan JK, Sin VC, Wong KF, et al. Nonnasal lymphoma expressing the natural killer cell marker CD56: a clinicopathologic study of 49 cases of an uncommon aggressive neoplasm. Blood 1997; 89(12):4501–4513.

219. Chan JK. Peripheral T-cell and NK-cell neoplasms: an integrated approach to diagnosis. Mod Pathol 1999; 12(2):177–199.

220. Takeshita M, Akamatsu M, Ohshima K, et al. CD30 (Ki-1)

expression in adult T-cell leukaemia/lymphoma is associated with distinctive immunohistological and clinical characteristics. Histopathology 1995; 26(6):539–546.

221. Tao Q, Ho FC, Loke SL, et al. Epstein-Barr virus is localized in the tumour cells of nasal lymphomas of NK, T or B cell type. Int J Cancer 1995; 60(3):315–320.

222. de Bruin PC, Jiwa M, Oudejans JJ, et al. Presence of Epstein-Barr virus in extranodal T-cell lymphomas: differences in relation to site. Blood 1994; 83(6):1612–1618.

223. Sabourin JC, Kanavaros P, Briere J, et al. Epstein-Barr virus (EBV) genomes and EBV-encoded latent membrane protein (LMP) in pulmonary lymphomas occurring in non-immunocompromised patients. Am J Surg Pathol 1993; 17(10):995–1002.

224. Kanavaros P, Vlychou M, Stefanaki K, et al. Cytotoxic protein expression in non-Hodgkin's lymphomas and Hodgkin's disease. Anticancer Res 1999; 19(2A):1209–1216.

225. Boulland ML, Kanavaros P, Wechsler J, et al. Cytotoxic protein expression in natural killer cell lymphomas and in alpha beta and gamma delta peripheral T-cell lymphomas. J Pathol 1997; 183(4):432–439.

226. Macon WR, Williams ME, Greer JP, et al. Natural killer-like T-cell lymphomas: aggressive lymphomas of T-large granular lymphocytes. Blood 1996; 87(4):1474–1483.

227. Chott A, Vesely M, Simonitsch I, et al. Classification of intestinal T-cell neoplasms and their differential diagnosis. Am J Clin Pathol 1999; 111(1 Suppl 1):S68–S74.

228. de Bruin PC, Connolly CE, Oudejans JJ, et al. Enteropathy-associated T-cell lymphomas have a cytotoxic T-cell phenotype. Histopathology 1997; 31(4):313–317.

229. Ilyas M, Niedobitek G, Agathanggelou A, et al. Non-Hodgkin's lymphoma, coeliac disease, and Epstein-Barr virus: a study of 13 cases of enteropathy-associated T- and B-cell lymphoma. J Pathol 1995; 177(2):115–122.

230. Carey MJ, Medeiros LJ, Roepke JE, et al. Primary anaplastic large cell lymphoma of the small intestine. Am J Clin Pathol 1999; 112(5):696–701.

231. Murray A, Cuevas EC, Jones DB, et al. Study of the immunohistochemistry and T cell clonality of enteropathy-associated T cell lymphoma. Am J Pathol 1995; 146(2):509–519.

232. Wu H, Wasik MA, Przybylski G, et al. Hepatosplenic gamma-delta T-cell lymphoma as a late-onset posttransplant lymphoproliferative disorder in renal transplant recipients. Am J Clin Pathol 2000; 113(4):487–496.

233. Cooke CB, Krenacs L, Stetler-Stevenson M, et al. Hepatosplenic T-cell lymphoma: a distinct clinicopathologic entity of cytotoxic gamma delta T-cell origin. Blood 1996; 88(11):4265–4274.

234. Salhany KE, Macon WR, Choi JK, et al. Subcutaneous panniculitis-like T-cell lymphoma: clinicopathologic, immunophenotypic, and genotypic analysis of alpha/beta and gamma/delta subtypes. Am J Surg Pathol 1998; 22(7):881–893.

235. Kumar S, Krenacs L, Medeiros J, et al. Subcutaneous panniculitic T-cell lymphoma is a tumor of cytotoxic T lymphocytes. Hum Pathol 1998; 29(4):397–403.

236. Kinney MC. The role of morphologic features, phenotype, genotype, and anatomic site in defining extranodal T-cell or NK-cell neoplasms. Am J Clin Pathol 1999; 111(1 Suppl 1):S104–S118.

237. Chang K, Weiss L. CD7: a review. Appl Immunohistochem 1994; 2:146–156.

238. Bakels V, van Oostveen JW, van der Putte SC, et al. Immunophenotyping and gene rearrangement analysis provide additional criteria to differentiate between cutaneous T-cell lymphomas and pseudo-T-cell lymphomas. Am J Pathol 1997; 150(6):1941–1949.

239. Picker LJ, Brenner MB, Weiss LM, et al. Discordant expression of CD3 and T-cell receptor beta-chain antigens in T-lineage lymphomas. Am J Pathol 1987; 129(3):434–440.

240. Bani D, Giannotti B. Differentiation of interdigitating reticulum cells and Langerhans cells in the human skin with T-lymphoid infiltrate. An immunocytochemical and ultrastructural study. Arch Histol Cytol 1989; 52(4):361–372.

241. Li G, Chooback L, Wolfe JT, et al. Overexpression of p53 protein in cutaneous T cell lymphoma: relationship to large cell transformation and disease progression. J Invest Dermatol 1998; 110(5):767–770.

242. Kempf W, Dummer R, Burg G. Approach to lymphoproliferative infiltrates of the skin. The difficult lesions. Am J Clin Pathol 1999; 111(1 Suppl 1):S84–S93.

243. Krishnan J, Tomaszewski MM, Kao GF. Primary cutaneous CD30-positive anaplastic large cell lymphoma. Report of 27 cases. J Cutan Pathol 1993; 20(3):193–202.

244. Kummer JA, Vermeer MH, Dukers D, et al. Most primary cutaneous CD30-positive lymphoproliferative disorders have

a CD4-positive cytotoxic T-cell phenotype. J Invest Dermatol 1997; 109(5):636–640.

245. Boulland ML, Wechsler J, Bagot M, et al. Primary CD30-positive cutaneous T-cell lymphomas and lymphomatoid papulosis frequently express cytotoxic proteins. Histopathology 2000; 36(2):136–144.

246. Vergier B, Beylot-Barry M, Pulford K, et al. Statistical evaluation of diagnostic and prognostic features of CD30+ cutaneous lymphoproliferative disorders: a clinicopathologic study of 65 cases. Am J Surg Pathol 1998; 22(10):1192–1202.

247. Herbst H, Sander C, Tronnier M, et al. Absence of anaplastic lymphoma kinase (ALK) and Epstein-Barr virus gene products in primary cutaneous anaplastic large cell lymphoma and lymphomatoid papulosis. Br J Dermatol 1997; 137(5):680–686.

248. Beljaards RC, Kaudewitz P, Berti E, et al. Primary cutaneous CD30-positive large cell lymphoma: definition of a new type of cutaneous lymphoma with a favorable prognosis. A European Multicenter Study of 47 patients. Cancer 1993; 71(6):2097–2104.

249. Brice P, Cazals D, Mounier N, et al. Primary cutaneous large-cell lymphoma: analysis of 49 patients included in the LNH87 prospective trial of polychemotherapy for high-grade lymphomas. Groupe d'Etude des Lymphomes de l'Adulte. Leukemia 1998; 12(2):213–219.

250. Anagnostopoulos I, Hummel M, Kaudewitz P, et al. Low incidence of Epstein-Barr virus presence in primary cutaneous T-cell lymphoproliferations. Br J Dermatol 1996; 134(2):276–281.

251. Leung CY, Ho FC, Srivastava G, et al. Usefulness of follicular dendritic cell pattern in classification of peripheral T-cell lymphomas. Histopathology 1993; 23(5):433–437.

252. Anagnostopoulos I, Hummel M, Finn T, et al. Heterogeneous Epstein-Barr virus infection patterns in peripheral T-cell lymphoma of angioimmunoblastic lymphadenopathy type. Blood 1992; 80(7):1804–1812.

253. Nathwani B, Jaffe E. Angioimmunoblastic lymphadenopathy (AILD) and AILD-like T-cell lymphomas. In: Jaffe E, ed. Surgical pathology of the lymph nodes and related organs. 2nd edn. Philadelphia: WB Saunders; 1995:390–412.

254. Borowitz MJ, Newby S, Brynes RK, et al. Multiinstitution study of non-Hodgkin's lymphomas using frozen section immunoperoxidase: the Southeastern Cancer Study Group experience. Blood 1984; 63(5):1147–1152.

255. Strickler JG, Weiss LM, Copenhaver CM, et al. Monoclonal antibodies reactive in routinely processed tissue sections of malignant lymphoma, with emphasis on T-cell lymphomas. Hum Pathol 1987; 18(8):808–814.

256. Hamilton-Dutoit SJ, Pallesen G. A survey of Epstein-Barr virus gene expression in sporadic non-Hodgkin's lymphomas. Detection of Epstein-Barr virus in a subset of peripheral T-cell lymphomas. Am J Pathol 1992; 140(6):1315–1325.

257. Kadin ME. Primary Ki-1-positive anaplastic large-cell lymphoma: a distinct clinicopathologic entity. Ann Oncol 1994; 5(Suppl 1):25–30.

258. Perkins PL, Ross CW, Schnitzer B. CD30-positive, anaplastic large-cell lymphomas that express CD15 but lack CD45. A possible diagnostic pitfall. Arch Pathol Lab Med 1992; 116(11):1192–1196.

259. Biernat W. Ki-1-positive anaplastic large cell lymphoma: a morphologic and immunologic study of 14 cases. Patol Pol 1994; 45(1):39–44.

260. Brousset P, Rochaix P, Chittal S, et al. High incidence of Epstein-Barr virus detection in Hodgkin's disease and absence of detection in anaplastic large-cell lymphoma in children. Histopathology 1993; 23(2):189–191.

261. Bayle C, Charpentier A, Duchayne E, et al. Leukaemic presentation of small cell variant anaplastic large cell lymphoma: report of four cases. Br J Haematol 1999; 104(4):680–688.

262. Kinney MC, Collins RD, Greer JP, et al. A small-cell-predominant variant of primary Ki-1 (CD30)+ T-cell lymphoma. Am J Surg Pathol 1993; 17(9):859–868.

263. Piris M, Brown DC, Gatter KC, et al. CD30 expression in non-Hodgkin's lymphoma. Histopathology 1990; 17(3):211–218.

264. Gascoyne RD, Aoun P, Wu D, et al. Prognostic significance of anaplastic lymphoma kinase (ALK) protein expression in adults with anaplastic large cell lymphoma. Blood 1999; 93(11):3913–3921.

265. Hodges KB, Collins RD, Greer JP, et al. Transformation of the small cell variant Ki-1+ lymphoma to anaplastic large cell lymphoma: pathologic and clinical features. Am J Surg Pathol 1999; 23(1):49–58.

266. Nakagawa A, Nakamura S, Ito M, et al. CD30-positive anaplastic large cell lymphoma in childhood: expression of p80npm/alk and absence of Epstein-Barr virus. Mod Pathol

267. Nakamura S, Shiota M, Nakagawa A, et al. Anaplastic large cell lymphoma: a distinct molecular pathologic entity: a reappraisal with special reference to p80(NPM/ALK) expression. Am J Surg Pathol 1997; 21(12):1420–1432.
268. Foss HD, Anagnostopoulos I, Araujo I, et al. Anaplastic large-cell lymphomas of T-cell and null-cell phenotype express cytotoxic molecules. Blood 1996; 88(10):4005–4011.
269. Foss HD, Demel G, Anagnostopoulos I, et al. Uniform expression of cytotoxic molecules in anaplastic large cell lymphoma of null/T cell phenotype and in cell lines derived from anaplastic large cell lymphoma. Pathobiology 1997; 65(2): 83–90.
270. Krenacs L, Wellmann A, Sorbara L, et al. Cytotoxic cell antigen expression in anaplastic large cell lymphomas of T- and null-cell type and Hodgkin's disease: evidence for distinct cellular origin. Blood 1997; 89(3):980–989.
271. Cesarman E, Inghirami G, Chadburn A, et al. High levels of p53 protein expression do not correlate with p53 gene mutations in anaplastic large cell lymphoma. Am J Pathol 1993; 143(3):845–856.
272. Inghirami G, Macri L, Cesarman E, et al. Molecular characterization of CD30+ anaplastic large-cell lymphoma: high frequency of c-myc proto-oncogene activation. Blood 1994; 83(12):3581–3590.
273. Fraga M, Brousset P, Schlaifer D, et al. Bone marrow involvement in anaplastic large cell lymphoma. Immunohistochemical detection of minimal disease and its prognostic significance. Am J Clin Pathol 1995; 103(1):82–89.

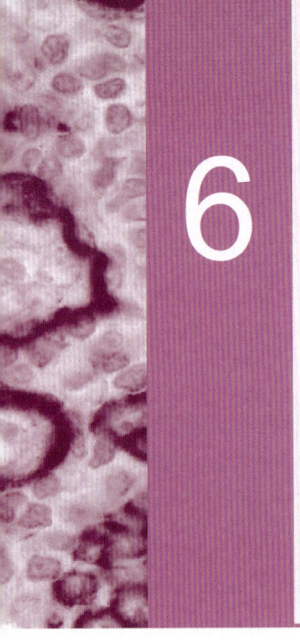

6 黑色素细胞肿瘤的免疫组织化学

原作者：Mark R. Wick
译　者：张廷国
审校者：甄军晖，刘志艳

目　录

引言	164
抗原/抗体生物学	164
黑色素细胞病变中的神经内分泌标记物	170
转移性黑色素瘤的"前哨"淋巴结活检	171
判断黑色素瘤预后的标记物	171

引　言

恶性黑色素瘤（MM）一直是外科病理诊断中最大的难点之一。无论是皮肤的原发性病变还是其他部位的转移性病灶，此类肿瘤均可以表现出多种不同的大体及组织学形态。原发性恶性黑色素瘤的组织学类型包括表浅扩散型、结节型、雀斑型、气球样（透明）细胞型、多形性肉瘤样型、梭形细胞/促纤维组织增生性/神经样型、小细胞（神经内分泌样）型、血管外皮细胞样型、印戒细胞型、黏液样型、腺样假乳头状型、化生型、横纹肌样，以及痣样型（图6.1、6.2、6.3）[1-3]。因为上述所有类型可能并无色素，所以这类病例的鉴别诊断比较困难。因此，电子显微镜、免疫组化和细胞遗传学的分析对于黑色素瘤的正确诊断相当重要。本章重点讨论免疫组化特征，一般而言在黑色素细胞肿瘤的诊断中，免疫组化是指导性的和主要的检测手段。同时，也简要地讨论关于恶性黑色素瘤的"预后"指标。

抗原/抗体生物学

黑色素细胞肿瘤中的丝状蛋白

近二十年来，中间丝蛋白（IFP）分析是免疫组织化学检测的重要里程碑。一般来说，keratin、vimentin、desmin、NF以及GFAP的免疫染色呈不同谱系的表达，利用不同的谱系可以鉴别组织学特征类似的肿瘤[4, 5]。

对黑色素细胞肿瘤来说，特别需要注意的是，痣和恶性黑色素瘤只有波形蛋白表达，缺乏其他四项中间丝状蛋白的表达（图 6.4、6.5）[5-7]。另外，在黑色素肿瘤中波形蛋白的密度高，大部分病例对这种标记呈强阳性免疫反应。事实上，许多学者都发现使用冰冻组织或特别固定（非福尔马林）的标本，恶性黑色素瘤中可检测到不同数量的包括角蛋白在内的其他中间丝[2, 8, 9]。然而，在一项本文作者参加的多研究所的合作研究中发现，使用石蜡切片和现代免疫组织化学方法，小于3%的黑色素瘤角蛋白阳性（图6.6），且这些病变表达IFP一般呈局灶阳性。同样，有报道认为极少数（<1%）的恶性黑色素瘤表达GFAP和结蛋白[2]，这些肿瘤通常表现出"化生性"肉瘤样显微镜下特征，或相反地表现出促纤维组织增生性和神经样的特性。出于实际应用的目的和根据应用石蜡切片对IFP染色研究的专门资料显示，即使应用先进的技术例如热抗原修复，波形蛋白仍然是95%以上的黑色素细胞肿瘤唯一的中间丝蛋白标记物。

因为 SMA（可被单克隆抗体 HHF-35 识别）和 α-异构重整（平滑肌）actin（可被 1A4 抗体识别），

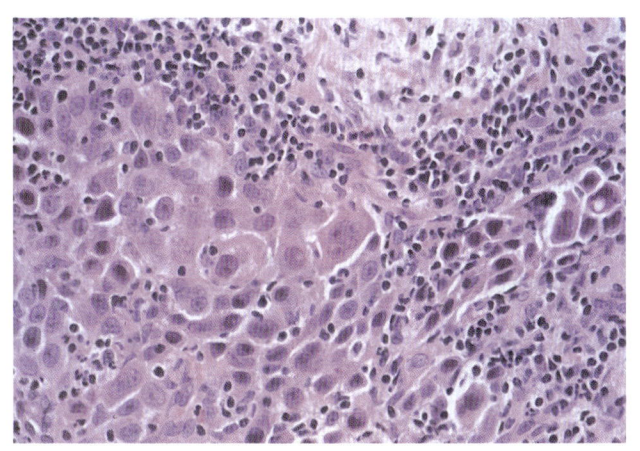

图6.1 大细胞上皮样无色素性恶性黑色素瘤，最常见的组织学类型

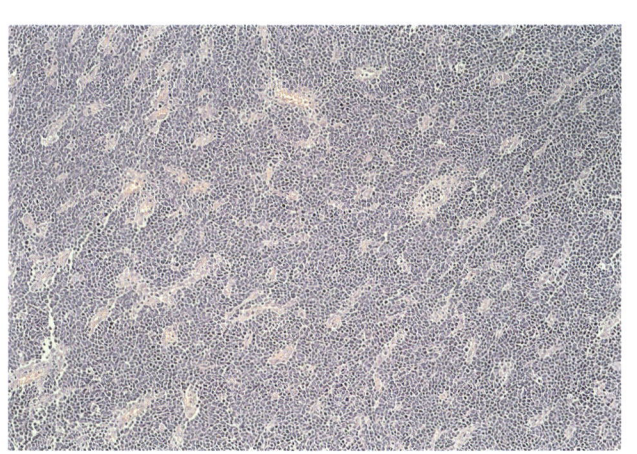

图6.2 小细胞无色素性黑色素瘤，形似神经内分泌癌

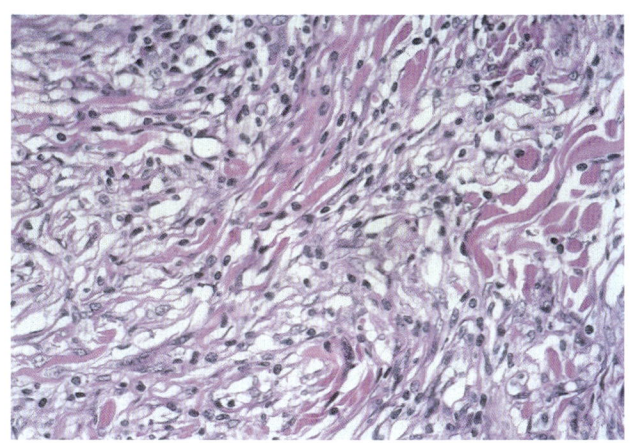

图6.3 肉瘤样/促纤维组织增生型无色素性黑色素瘤，形似肉瘤

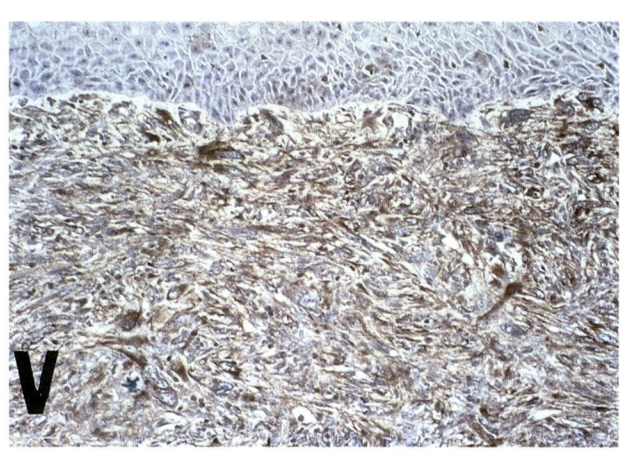

图6.4 如图所示，几乎所有的恶性黑色素瘤波形蛋白（V）均呈强阳性

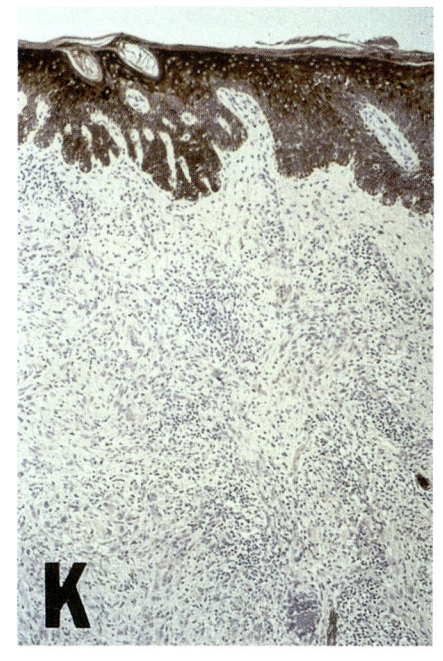

图6.5 在石蜡切片中，97%以上的黑色素瘤不表达角蛋白（K）

以及 caldesmon 主要在非上皮性、非黑色素细胞性、非神经胶质组织常见，所以在黑色素细胞肿瘤中不会表达。实际上在这类病损中的确很少检测到它们表达。即使观察到，也只有在表现出奇异性肌纤维母细胞分化的梭形细胞黑色素瘤中检测到[2]。

细胞膜蛋白

与细胞膜有关的许多蛋白在恶性黑色素瘤的鉴别诊断中起重要作用。虽然如此，大致可分为两类：与上皮细胞有关的蛋白、与造血细胞成分有关的蛋白。

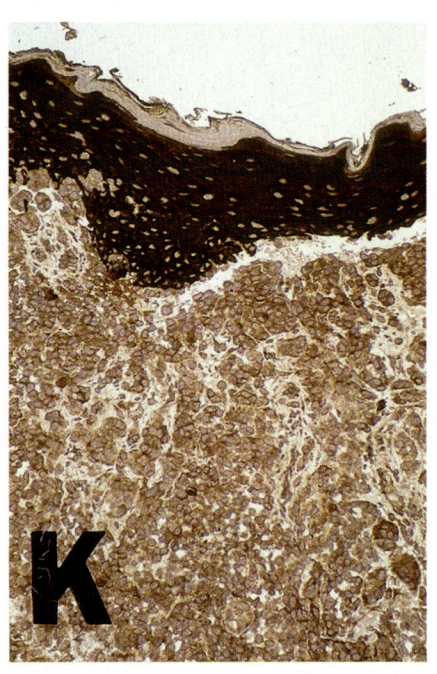

图6.6 在常规制作的标本中，极少数黑色素瘤显示角蛋白（K）阳性表达（此处显示）

上皮性抗原决定簇

EMA：EMA属于与乳脂球蛋白有关的糖蛋白家族，表达于多种体腔上皮及其肿瘤[10]。其阴性表达的肿瘤包括生殖细胞瘤、肾上腺皮质增生和肝细胞肿瘤等[11, 12]。在所选择的淋巴和浆细胞肿瘤中有一半可观察到EMA表达[10, 11]。另一方面，黑色素细胞增生时此标记物均为阴性[10-12]。在黑色素瘤坏死区周边可能见到令人吃惊的细胞膜灶性假阳性分布，此为人工假象，不能视为阳性。只有细胞浆阳性的EMA染色同样不能完全相信。

CEA：CEA也属于细胞膜糖蛋白家族，主要存在于内胚层起源或分化的组织和肿瘤的细胞膜中。在过去，黑色素瘤中也能观察到CEA[13]，但是，最近的研究显示[14]，出现这种结果看来是由于技术不完善和免疫组化时使用不吸收的异血清抗体造成的。这样的试剂还可以识别除了CEA之外的许多蛋白（例如非特异性交叉反应性抗原、胆汁糖蛋白等），许多并不是严格的上皮细胞特异。如果利用只是针对CEA抗原决定簇的特异性单克隆抗体，黑色素肿瘤不会有CEA的表达[15]。

肿瘤相关糖蛋白72 [TAG72 (CA72-4)] /BerEP4抗原/MOC-31抗原：TAG72（CA72-4）（被单克隆抗体B72.3识别）、BerEP4和MOC-31都是细胞膜糖蛋白，多数均由上皮细胞合成[16]。但是也有少数情况例外，例如，在某些上皮样血管瘤中也有TAG72出现，但是这并不包括黑色素细胞肿瘤[15]。因此，本组辅助性上皮标记物免疫染色比其他上皮标记如角蛋白、EMA、CEA在区别恶性黑色素瘤和上皮性肿瘤中更有帮助。可以肯定地说，实际上所有的体细胞肿瘤都对至少一种上述列举的膜抗原决定簇有反应，包括角蛋白。相反，有些罕见的黑色素瘤可有角蛋白的表达，而缺乏其他类似的上皮细胞分化的证据。

PLAP：PLAP是肿瘤性生殖细胞和部分体腔上皮细胞性恶性肿瘤经常合成的一种异构酶[17]。因此是性腺肿瘤的一个有用的筛选标记物，例如精原细胞瘤、癌胚性癌、卵黄囊瘤，这些都需要与恶性黑色素瘤作鉴别诊断。比较而言，黑色素细胞增生通常PLAP阴性。然而，需要注意的一点是，这个抗原决定簇位于细胞膜上，因此在免疫组织学的标本中（包括黑色素瘤）只出现细胞浆PLAP着色并不能认为是真正的阳性反应。

"造血系统"标记

与造血细胞和肿瘤有关的一些细胞表面抗原，也有可能在黑色素细胞和肿瘤中见到。它们包括CD10、CD44、CD56、CD57、CD59、CD68、CD74、CD99、CD117（c-kit蛋白）、CD146、Ⅱ型主要组织相容性抗原 [MHC2A (HLA-DR、HLA-DP、HLA-DQ)]、β2微球蛋白（B2M）、bcl-2蛋白[18-26]。作者已经观察了所有这些标记物在一些Spitz痣（上皮样细胞和梭形细胞）、结构紊乱痣（发育不良痣）、黑色素瘤中的表达。相反，黑色素细胞一致缺乏可以对恶性黑色素瘤进行鉴别诊断的造血细胞抗原决定簇，例如末端脱氧核苷转移酶Ⅻa因子、myeloperoxidase、CD15、CD35、CD43、CD45、CD138[27]。

MHC2A和B2M在黑色素细胞增生中的表达，可以出现于从一般的炎性痣或错构痣到恶性黑色素瘤中[28]。临床医生对于应用免疫疗法治疗黑色素瘤很有兴趣，因此经常需要免疫组织学研究此类肿瘤合成这些标记物的情况。有趣的是，有报道发现，随着时间的延长，也许是通过相应的基因复合体突变或其他的机制，恶性黑色素瘤降低了B2M和组织相容性抗原的表达，"逃脱"免疫监视[26]。由于黑色素细胞病变中的MHC2A和B2M的免疫表型的异质性，此类抗原决定簇不能用于鉴别诊断。

黑色素肿瘤可以表达bcl-2蛋白和CD10、CD68、

CD56、CD57和CD99，以及CD117，使得其可能与淋巴瘤、组织细胞病变、原始神经外胚层肿瘤和神经内分泌肿瘤、胃肠间质瘤相混淆。通常，谨慎的选择抗体组合，制订恰当的诊断方案，会避免产生这些错误。

NB84

NB84是在神经母细胞瘤中发现的抗细胞膜的单克隆抗体。在石蜡切片中有活性，不但可以标记神经母细胞瘤，还可以标记原始神经外胚层肿瘤[29]。黑色素细胞增生对此标记物无反应，此现象在小细胞黑色素瘤与起源于大的先天性痣或神经嵴错构瘤的神经母细胞或神经外胚层肿瘤的鉴别诊断中是有用的[30]。

钙结合蛋白

一些蛋白质与细胞内钙的新陈代谢有关，包括膜联蛋白Ⅵ、ｃａｐ-ｇ、膜联蛋白Ⅴ、钙调蛋白（calmodulin）、calretinin和S-100蛋白，这些都可以见于黑色素细胞增生[31]。在此将讨论其中两个具有确定的诊断意义的标记物。

S-100蛋白

在恶性黑色素瘤中首选的、也是最持久的标记物是S-100蛋白。其21kD部分在中枢神经系统的胶质细胞中首次被检测出来，如此命名是因为其在饱和的硫酸铵溶液中的溶解度为100%[32]。在1981年，Gaynor等发现在人黑色素细胞中也存在S-100蛋白，使得其成为一个广泛应用的诊断性指标（图6.7、6.8）。

关于S-100蛋白的功能从未被确切地下过定论，可能有细胞内钙的运输或微管集合功能，或者在两者中都起作用[34, 35]。另外，它还与另一种钙流出蛋白——钙调蛋白有些生理学联系[31]。S-100蛋白有两种亚单位α和β产生三种二聚体：α-α、α-β、β-β[36]，黑色素细胞只合成第一种。S-100蛋白的阳性表现应同时呈现胞核和胞浆的着色。免疫电镜研究证实了此种蛋白存在于正常和肿瘤性黑色素细胞内[37]。

现在，开发了许多S-100蛋白抗体，其中有些是二聚体特异性单克隆产品[38]。但是在一般的应用中，许多临床实验室依然应用该蛋白的所有三种同种型全部识别的异体抗血清，使得此种试剂成为高度敏感的筛选工具。因而，有的作者的经验是，无论何种组织亚型，大于98%的恶性黑色素瘤表达S-100蛋白。Smoller[39]对有关的文献进行分析校订，得出一个稍微低些的数据是97.4%。需要与黑色素病变鉴别的其他

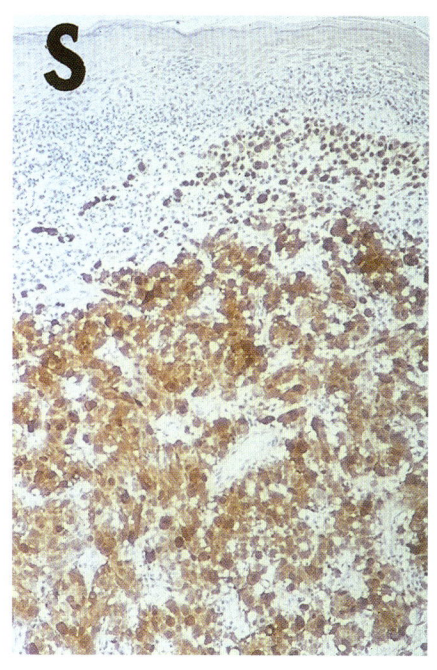

图6.7 在原发性皮肤上皮样黑色素瘤中，S-100蛋白（S）呈现胞核与胞质的强阳性表达

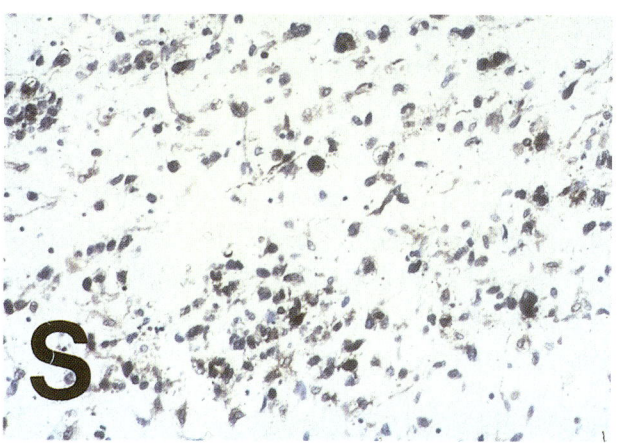

图6.8 黏液样/肉瘤样黑色素瘤中S-100蛋白（S）在胞核和胞浆着色

的S-100蛋白阳性的肿瘤，包括各种低分化癌、部分组织细胞增生症、恶性神经胶质细胞瘤、外周神经鞘肿瘤，以及朗格汉斯细胞病变[37, 39-43]。显然，与作为此类肿瘤的特异性标记物相比，S-100蛋白作为黑色素肿瘤的初始筛选指标更有价值。

最近，许多S-100蛋白的亚型（A2、A6、A8/A9和A12）被认为对于不同的黑色素细胞病变有诊断意义。Ribe和McNutt[44]认为S-100蛋白在Spitz痣和黑色素瘤中的表达有差异，所有的Spitz痣均为A6阳性，而只有33%的黑色素瘤呈现阳性反应。另外，还观察了标记范围的差异，Spitz痣呈弥漫性A6着色，而黑色素瘤呈弱的灶性阳性。这个观测结果能否应用

于实际工作的鉴别诊断中还有待进一步观察。

calretinin

calretinin是分子量为31kD的胞浆蛋白，最初由中枢神经系统组织中分离出来[45,46]，在皮肤以及其他地方的周围神经也可以发现[47]。另外，这种多肽的分布相当局限，至今只在间皮[46]、卵巢的生发上皮[46]、某些部位的腺癌（特别是结肠和直肠的亚类）[48]中检测出，黑色素瘤并不在calretinin阳性表达的肿瘤之列。

黑色素细胞-"特异性"单克隆抗体

自20世纪80年代初开始，由于实用单克隆抗体技术的需要，就开始寻找"黑色素瘤-特异性"试剂，其不但可以适用于诊断，而且可以用于治疗[49]。这项研究持续了已有20多年，但至今还没有最终的结果。

许多抗黑色素细胞杂交瘤产物已被报道，但只有少数可以应用于石蜡切片和常规制作的组织标本中。Smoller[39]先前已经对此作过总结。活性仅局限于冰冻组织的包括PAL-M1、PAL-M2、691-13-17、691-15-Nu4B，以及"MEL"系列抗体1～4。相反，HMSA-2、2-139-1、6-26-3、KBA62、1C11、7H11、MEL-CAM、MEL-5和SM5-1在福尔马林固定的石蜡包埋标本中有免疫活性[39,50,51]。总的来说，上述标记物并未或不继续在诊断病理中应用，因为它们要求特殊的组织处理过程，不利于商业化运作，或对恶性黑色素细胞病变缺少特异性和敏感性。下面的章节将对已经应用于临床的指标进行讨论。

gp100/PMel 17 相关单克隆抗体

现在有几个针对糖蛋白类抗原组的单克隆抗体，它们只局限于黑色素细胞系。此类抗原被命名为"gp100"，其相应的cDNA已被克隆出来[52,53]。该核酸序列编码两种蛋白——gp100本身（分子量为100kD）和gp10（分子量为10kD）[53]。gp100-C1 cDNA相关转录产物是非常相似的，但是不完全一致。另一种黑色素蛋白命名为PMel17[54]。两者均定位于1、2、3型黑色素前体的膜内，它们都可能成为细胞毒性T淋巴细胞的作用靶点，可能与MHC2A有关[55]。事实上，此组标记物之一MART-1是特别据此特性命名的（T细胞-1识别的黑色素瘤抗原），它可被两种单克隆抗体识别，A103和M2-7C10，因此被称为"melan-A"（图6.9）[56-67]。Adema等进行了核酸序列分析，显示gp100和PMel17的cDNA出自同一基因，

是两者剪接而成[53]。他们又发现在非肿瘤性和肿瘤性黑色素细胞群中都伴有gp100和PMel17的表达，这个发现进一步证实了他们的结论[68]。Chiamenti和同事提出相反的意见，认为HMB-45的靶蛋白是黑色素前体相关多肽，但是这种想法并没有被其他的学者所证实。

有趣的是，gp100的转录产物对黑色素细胞并无特异性，而且有许多不同的组织亚型[52]。但是，其mRNA的翻译产物确实只存在于黑色素细胞中。这个发现有力地支持了免疫组织学是评估gp100作为一个黑色素细胞标记的最实用的技术方法，同时以核酸为基础的试验方法（例如原位杂交、PCR）有可能解决gp100在黑色素制造细胞中的特异性低的问题。

gp100/PMel17组中的抗体包括NKI-β、NKI/C3、HMB-45、HMB-50和MART-1/melan-A（图6.10、6.11）[53,54,56-68,70-88]。与其他细胞谱系和肿瘤类型相比，这些抗体对黑色素细胞、痣及黑色素瘤的特异性和敏感性文献报道多有不同。实际应用中，HMB-45和MART-1更常用，用于进一步证实S-100蛋白阳性的肿瘤确实为黑色素细胞来源。

HMB-45的商业运作中存在不合理性。作者有机会对HMB-45克隆的原始上清液进行评估，这是在20世纪80年代中期来自于Allen Gown博士（此抗体的开发者之一）的慷慨惠赠。在已发表的关于此评价的文章中，我们的研究小组发现，HMB-45对黑色素瘤的敏感性大于95%，对非梭形细胞恶性肿瘤的特异性基本上达到100%[78]。其后，HMB-45被卖于商业公司，不纯的杂交瘤产物进入市场，其特异性降低了很多，而且除了黑色素瘤还可以标记许多其他的肿

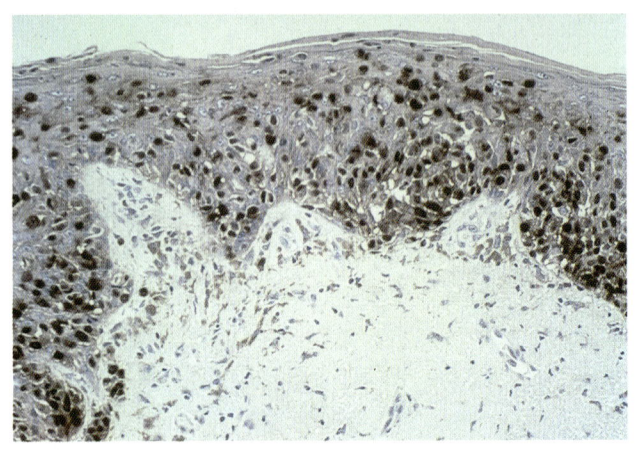

图6.9 在此表浅扩散型黑色素瘤中，MART-1/melan-A蛋白染色呈全胞浆阳性反应

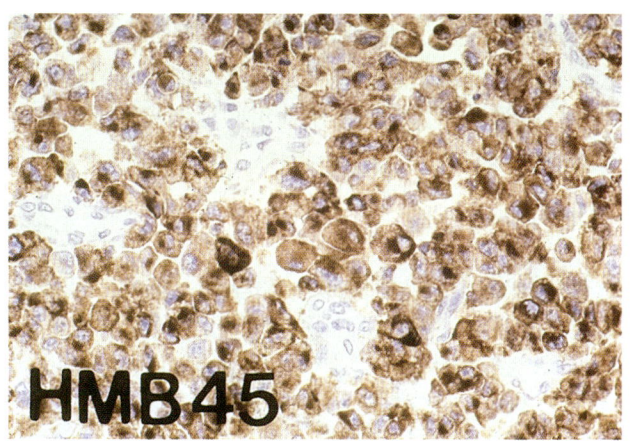

图 6.10　上皮性黑色素瘤转移至淋巴结，可见 HMB-45 呈胞浆强阳性

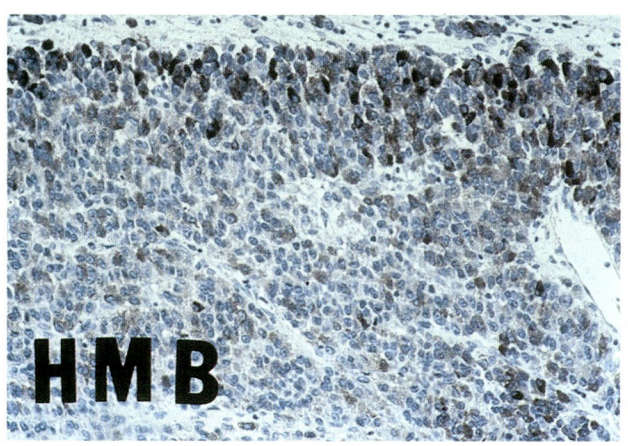

图 6.11　上皮性黑色素瘤转移至淋巴结，可见 HMB-50（HMB）呈不同的胞浆表达

瘤[37, 89-92]。随后，当其他公司经销 HMB-45 时，它的特异性又"恢复"了。然而，为了牟取最大利益，许多公司将提供给使用者的"纯"抗体预先稀释了，因此最后结果是其总的敏感性不超过 60%。

另一些关于 HMB-45、HMB-50、MART-1 和其他 gp100 相关反应物的观察资料普遍而且错误地认为与非黑色素细胞存在"交叉反应"，这些抗体可以标记血管平滑肌脂肪瘤、淋巴管血管平滑肌瘤病、肺或其他器官的"糖"瘤（透明细胞肌黑色素瘤），以及其他的表现出血管周上皮样细胞增生特征的增生性病变（图6.12）[93-99]。这些病变的超微结构确实显示黑色素前体的合成，因此至少有部分黑色素细胞分化[94, 95]。因此，gp100 相关抗体在标记这些肿瘤时，并不能认为其显示交叉反应。这种免疫亲和力只是显示了它们对黑色素前体相关蛋白识别特异性的一种生物学拓展。

关于上一个说法确实存在一个例外，MART-1/melan-A（但不是 HMB-45、NKI-β 或 HMB-50）可以标记一些肾上腺皮质肿瘤和生殖腺的性索肿瘤（图6.13）[62, 100]。在这些肿瘤中并未发现黑色素细胞分化的证据，因此推测 MART-1 抗体识别这些生成类固醇的增生性改变中所表达的抗原决定簇，这些抗原决定簇还可以为 gp100 和 PMel17 分子所识别。

综上所述，此章节中没有一个抗体对于标记小部分（<10%）的梭形细胞/促纤维增生性/神经样黑色素瘤有效[63, 78, 79]。这个"缺点"的结果可以反映出这样的事实：在这些肿瘤中存在典型的克隆进化，从黑色素细胞表型到纤维母细胞或施万细胞为主，在这个过程中，逐渐失去了合成黑色素前体和这些细胞器相关蛋白的能力。

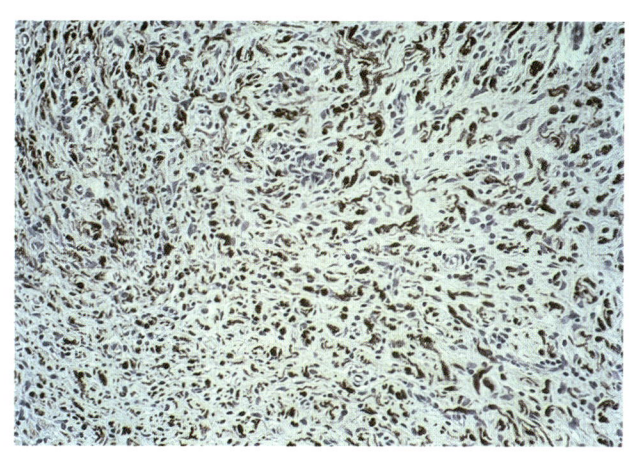

图6.12　肾富于梭形细胞的血管平滑肌脂肪瘤中，HMB-45呈多灶性阳性反应

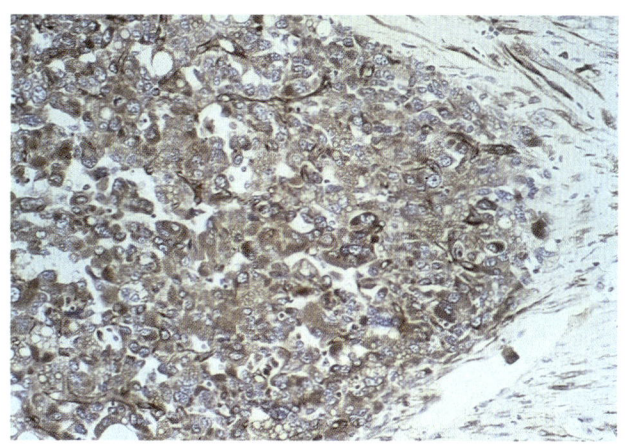

图6.13　肾上腺皮质癌中 MART-1/melan-A（抗体克隆系 A103）的弥漫染色

诊断要点：gp100 抗体
1. HMB-45 和 melan-A 对黑色素细胞高度特异，敏感度在 60%～80%。
2. gp100 抗体通常在血管平滑肌脂肪瘤和上皮样血管周细胞瘤细胞中有反应。
3. Melan-A 可以标记肾上腺皮脂腺癌和卵巢的性索肿瘤。
4. 少部分促纤维增生性/梭形细胞黑色素瘤对 gp100 抗体组有免疫反应。

酪氨酸酶相关抗体

在正常黑色素生成过程中，酪氨酸被羟化形成 3,4-二羟基苯丙氨酸（"多巴"），然后被氧化形成多巴醌，多巴醌聚合形成黑色素。随后，黑色素蛋白聚合形成稳定的复合物，包含黑色素前体和黑色素小体[101]。酪氨酸酶在这个过程中起重要作用，在上述反应的第一步中起催化作用[102]。因此，它是鉴别黑色素细胞分化特异性的标记物。而且，酪氨酸酶基因转录严格局限于黑色素生成细胞中，进一步证明了其特异性。

T311 和 MAT-1 是两个在外科病理学中分析较多的抗酪氨酸酶单克隆抗体[104-113]。MAT-1 是 IgG 反应物，它是利用与人酪氨酸酶羧基末端相对应的合成肽作为免疫原而产生的[131]。在所有的恶性肿瘤中，这两种抗体对非梭形细胞黑色素瘤都表现出高度的敏感性（>80%）和几乎绝对的特异性（图6.14）。有趣的是，有研究认为许多病例中，痣对 MAT-1 并无免疫反应，非肿瘤性黑色素细胞也是如此[110]。因此，对抗原

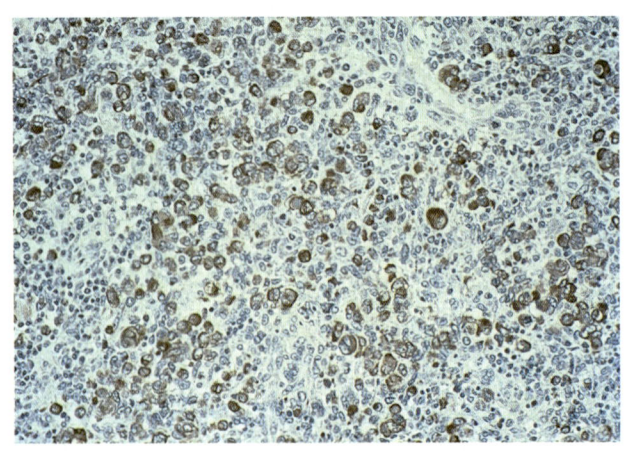

图 6.14　肝转移性上皮样黑色素瘤中，酪氨酸酶呈多灶性强阳性

决定簇的识别可能与黑色素细胞的成熟以及分化有关。考虑到这些发现，以及抗酪氨酸酶抗体极好的特异性，在诊断中将它们搭配使用应是比较合理的方法（也叫做"鸡尾酒"法）。

小眼转录因子蛋白

小眼基因（microphthalmia gene）编码的转录因子是胚胎发生中黑色素细胞存活和生长必需的转录因子[114]。小眼转录因子蛋白（MTFP）是胞核碱性螺旋-环-螺旋亮氨酸链结构，与 PAX3 和 MSG1 基因产物一起，上调磷酸腺苷酸通路，可以控制黑色素生成酶的活性[115-117]。（还有另一个相关基因 TFE 也有类似的特性，其转录因子也有可能成为黑色素细胞的辅助标记[117]。）

虽然关于 MTFP 抗体的免疫反应的研究只是初步的，但是这些抗体在鉴定黑色素细胞增生中表现出较好的敏感性和特异性[118-121]。事实上，在其他多数标记物中除了 S-100 蛋白外，MTFP 可以标记多数非肉瘤样黑色素细胞病变，但除外一小部分梭形细胞/促纤维结缔组织黑色素瘤[118,119,121]。由于已经清楚它在细胞内的定位，因此只有 MTFP 核着色时才能认为是真正的阳性[120]。有趣的是，血管平滑肌脂肪瘤、淋巴血管平滑肌瘤病、"糖"瘤也有和恶性黑色素瘤同样的免疫反应，进一步证明了其部分为黑色素细胞的本质。

PNL2

2003 年，Rochaix 等[124]描述了一种新的单克隆抗体 PNL2 的临床应用，这种抗体是抗耐固定的黑色素抗原所产生的。在一项包括良性和恶性黑色素细胞病变的研究中，这些学者发现在真皮的平常痣细胞中表达较少，而在交界痣细胞中 PNL2 阳性。除了促纤维组织增生型的肿瘤，所有的黑色素瘤也呈阳性。PNL2 至今未在非黑色素肿瘤中广泛测试，但是在初步的研究中表现出了良好特异性，其临床应用价值值得进一步评估。

黑色素细胞病变中的神经内分泌标记物

由于黑色素细胞和神经内分泌增生与神经外胚层在理论上存在联系，因此，此两类肿瘤可能表现出显

著的免疫组织学同源性。随着研究不断深入，现在已经明确发现两者之间既有相似之处，又有一定的差别。

蛋白质仅存在于解剖学上的神经内分泌颗粒和神经突触囊泡中，如嗜铬素和突触素，在"纯粹的"黑色素细胞肿瘤中一般不存在[127-131]。然而，比较明显的是，有部分病例，即诊断为神经内分泌肿瘤或非黑色素细胞神经外胚层肿瘤（例如神经内分泌癌、副神经节瘤、原始神经外胚层肿瘤、外周神经鞘瘤），有可能呈现出程度不同的异源性黑色素细胞分化。这种现象造成了许多如"色素性类癌"[132, 133]、"色素性副神经节瘤"[134]、"黑色素性神经外胚层肿瘤"[135, 136]和"黑色素性施万细胞瘤"[137]（包括良性和恶性）的诊断（图6.15）。在这些病变中，"小部分"的黑色素细胞成分表现出与皮肤痣或恶性黑色素瘤细胞相同的免疫表型（如，S-100蛋白+、HMB-45+、MART-1+、酪氨酸酶+）。但是其他成分是单一分化的上皮、神经或施万细胞组织，它们不表达黑色素细胞标记，因而，出现相互独立的免疫表型。

在黑色素瘤中也可以见到其他的"神经内分泌"抗原决定簇，事实上它们是在多种细胞中合成的。包括但不仅限于黑色素细胞、神经内分泌上皮细胞和施万细胞，上述这些标记物主要包括神经特异性烯醇化酶、神经细胞黏附分子（CD56）、CD57和CD99（MIC2蛋白）[138-143]。除CD99外，它们比较常见于具有神经样特征的黑色素细胞增生中，例如神经性皮内痣和"嗜神经性"黑色素瘤[141]。因此，很明显这些指标不能用于鉴别真正的神经内分泌肿瘤和黑色素肿瘤。

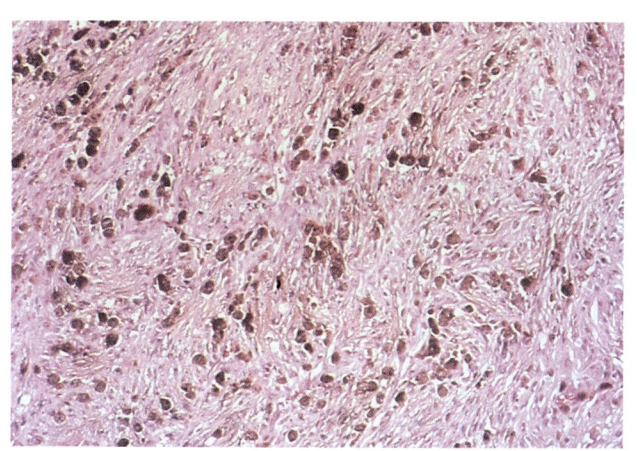

图6.15 "黑色素性"施万细胞瘤，大部分肿瘤细胞表现出黑色素细胞的歧异性分化

转移性黑色素瘤的"前哨"淋巴结活检

在过去的十年中，外科医师对"前哨"淋巴结活检（SLNB）的热情十分高涨，认为可以用来评价黑色素瘤患者有无转移灶[144]。此技术的核心概念就是，SLNB没有发现黑色素瘤，就不用局部清扫淋巴结。而如果发现转移灶，无论淋巴结大小，也要尽快完成淋巴结切除。这个论题与我们的讨论有关，是因为现在的指导性的病理学书籍认为，用SLNB标本作广泛的免疫组化检查，对发现黑色素瘤的"微小"转移灶是很有帮助的[145, 146]。事实上，已经设计出多种"鸡尾酒"抗体应用于淋巴结活检，以使免疫组化的敏感性得到最大的发挥[147]。

在Medalie和Ackerman[148]关于SLNB应用于黑色素瘤的专著中，他们提出了许多概念性的问题。最重要的一点是，许多事先设计好的黑色素瘤淋巴清扫的随机实验并没有提高总的生存率。另外，目前对于此种肿瘤尚无有效的辅助治疗。第三，SLNB阳性对黑色素瘤的预后意义，尤其是"微小"转移灶，具有很大的个体差异。因此，在作者看来，无需继续讨论SLNB以及免疫组化的应用[146, 149]。当然，也不能成为"标准化"操作。

判断黑色素瘤预后的标记物

在过去的十年里，许多出版物都探讨过对恶性黑色素瘤形态学以外的有预后意义的辅助指标。包括突变型p53蛋白（细胞程序性死亡相关蛋白）、Ki-67、增殖细胞核抗原、Ki-S5（细胞周期相关性增生指标）、热休克蛋白（细胞复制的标记或"应激"细胞）、bcl-2蛋白（凋亡抑制蛋白）、VLA-4和α-v/β-3整合素（细胞内黏附分子，与黑色素瘤进入直线生长期有关联）、CD26/二肽氨肽酶IV（细胞膜相关蛋白酶，与肿瘤细胞侵袭有关）、cyclin D1、cyclin D3、Trk-A和p16INK4-α（CDKN2A）基因产物（细胞周期调节因子）[150-156]。另外提出一种方法，利用内皮性标记物（例如von Willebrand因子、CD31和CD34）进行免疫组化染色来评估处于结节状垂直生长期的黑色素瘤间质的血管状态，从而推测过多增生的血管与预后不良的关系[157, 158]。总的来说，前面提到的指标并未在临床展开应用，因为关于其意义的解释存在不同意见，另外，其方法学也有争议。

需重点指出的是，通过上述分析技术的研究，不良的预后与黑色素瘤处于垂直生长期密切相关。这个事实反映出，从黑色素瘤的水平式放射状生长期过渡到垂直生长期的"恶性潜伏"期中，伴随着许多生物学行为的变化。这些可能包括在垂直生长期黑色素瘤的（VGMs）自分泌，有丝分裂生长因子的增多，垂直生长期黑色素瘤肿瘤细胞中凋亡率的下降，在垂直生长期对生长抑制因子获得性抵抗，垂直生长期黑色素瘤细胞过多的血管增生，c-kit（CD117）基因产物（具有酪氨酸酶活性）的丢失等[159, 160]。在细胞遗传学水平，从水平期到垂直生长期的过渡中，与获得的基因复制数量相关，按照频率从高到低，发生在染色体7、8、6p、1q、20、17和2[161]。

现在，利用非形态学技术判断恶性黑色素瘤的预后只能作为科学研究，不能作为常规的临床应用。所有必要的病理学指标，如肿瘤的发病部位、大小、深度、是否伴有溃疡形成、核分裂象数目和生长期等，仍然必须依靠恶性黑色素瘤的HE染色来获得。

诊断要点：几种病变的鉴别诊断

黑色素瘤与各种黑色素细胞痣

不少文章讨论过免疫组织化学在区别各类良性和恶性黑色素肿瘤中的应用。具体如下，关于Spitz痣和黑色素瘤的鉴别诊断在参考文献中已讨论过多次，它们与突变型p16和p53蛋白、Ki-67、Ki-S5、S100P-A6以及其他的与细胞转化和增殖有关的标记物的表达有关[44, 162-166]。虽然这些分析结果得出了一般的趋势，但是黑色素细胞痣和黑色素瘤的免疫表型统计结果中有许多重叠，因此在个别的病例中使用的意义不是很大。

黑色素细胞肿瘤和组织细胞增生

在皮肤或其他部位，从组织学上鉴别无黑色素的黑色素病变和组织细胞增生比较困难，比如上皮样组织细胞瘤、缺乏泡沫细胞的黄肉芽肿、非典型性纤维黄瘤和网状组织细胞瘤（病）[167-169]。尽管有时组织细胞肿瘤可能标记S-100蛋白，但是一般HMB-45、HMB-50、MART-1、抗-酪氨酸酶和抗-MTFP阴性。相比之下，组织细胞瘤和黑色素瘤都与ⅩⅢa因子和CD68有免疫反应，这两者曾被错误地认为是"组织细胞标记"[23, 170-172]。

梭形和肉瘤样恶性黑色素瘤的识别

之所以挑选梭形和肉瘤样黑色素瘤（包括促纤维组织增生型、黏液型、嗜神经型和骨软骨样型等亚型）进行讨论分析，是因为它们在相当一部分病例中表现出抗原缺失和畸变。实际上，作者遇见的第一例梭形黑色素瘤是转移性的，呈现角蛋白阳性，而S-100蛋白阴性，患者过去曾有黑色素瘤病史。根据作者的经验，这些特殊的恶性黑色素细胞肿瘤的亚型约有20%的病例失去了对S-100蛋白、HMB-45、MART-1、酪氨酸酶的免疫反应性，而约有1%~3%的病例获得了角蛋白和desmin的阳性表达[2, 173-175]。因此一个广泛的、包括所有基本的黑色素细胞标记的试剂组合，对于更加正确地识别梭形黑色素瘤是有必要的。

肉瘤样黑色素瘤一般S-100蛋白阳性。但是，只有3%~10%的可以标记其他更特异的黑色素细胞标记物（图6.16）[78, 118, 119, 121, 176]。因为有相当一部分此类病变转变为增生的梭形细胞，伴异源性的细胞类型，CD56、CD57阳性，也有可能检测到神经生长因子受体、desmin和actin（图6.17）[2, 138-143]。在没有黑色素瘤病史的时候，尤其要留意这些奇特的免疫表型，提示需要鉴别诊断，从而避免误诊。

无黑色素的黑色素瘤和其他上皮性恶性肿瘤

外科病理学家曾提出过一个比较经典的鉴别诊断，就是关于黑色素瘤和低分化癌、大细胞非霍奇金淋巴瘤或"合体细胞性"霍奇金淋巴瘤的鉴别[177, 178]。这是在淋巴结真实存在的一类肿瘤，以前并不知道其恶性病史。

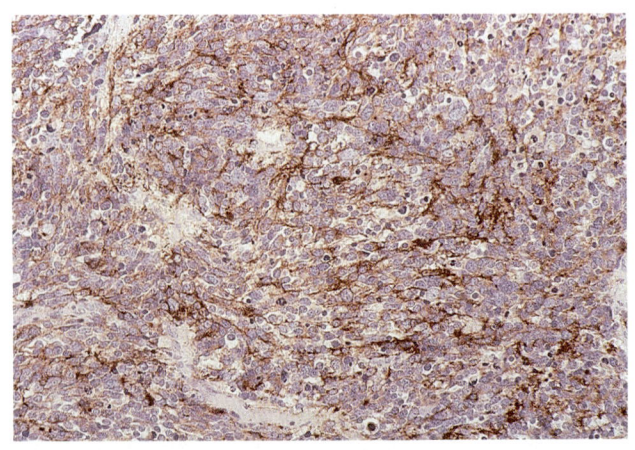

图6.16　肉瘤样黑色素瘤中酪氨酸酶标记；除了S-100蛋白，<10%的病例不同程度对黑色素细胞标记着色

6 黑色素细胞肿瘤的免疫组织化学

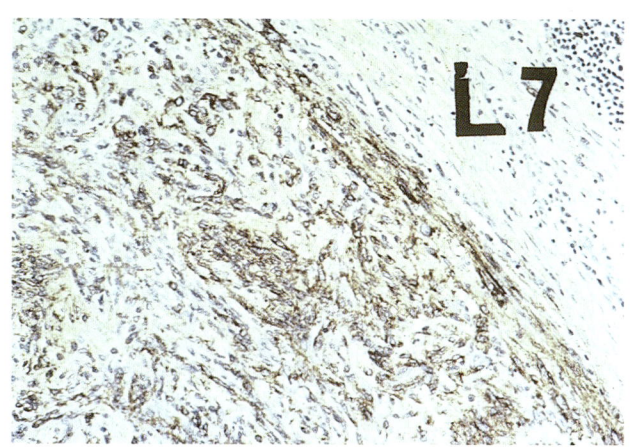

图 6.17　在肉瘤样/促纤维增生恶性黑色素瘤中 CD57/Leu (L7) 阳性，显示出神经样分化

在这种情况下，使用的抗体组合应该包括角蛋白、EMA、vimentin、S-100蛋白、HMB-45、酪氨酸酶、MART-1、CD15、CD30 和 CD45。图 6.18 显示了所考虑的特定肿瘤的预期结果。

同样的基本方法可以用于鉴别浆膜转移性黑色素瘤和恶性间皮瘤，除了上述抗体外，还应包括 calretinin、血栓调节素和 HBME-1。大部分的间皮瘤对于后三种抗体即使不是全部表达，至少会表达其中的一种。而恶性黑色素瘤对这些都没有反应[179-181]。

神经内分泌癌可以用角蛋白阳性与恶性黑色素瘤区别，同时嗜铬素（CgA）和突触素（Syn）阳性[131]。如前所述，黑色素细胞病变缺乏后两种标记的表达，而 50% 以上的神经内分泌上皮性肿瘤至少会表达其中一种。在神经内分泌肿瘤中，角蛋白呈现圆点状、胞浆内核周着色[182]，有小部分恶性黑色素瘤也可表达角蛋白，但是，上述阳性构型还没有发现过。

转移性黑色素瘤和恶性胶质瘤

在中枢神经系统中，转移性无黑色素的黑色素瘤在显微镜下与高级别的恶性胶质瘤极其相似。由于两种病变对 S-100 蛋白都有同样的免疫反应，而且小部分黑色素瘤也有可能表达 GFAP，所以两者的鉴别就更为复杂[21]。因此，其他的黑色素细胞标记物例如 HMB-45、抗-酪氨酸酶和 MART-1 对这个鉴别诊断十分重要。这些抗原在单纯的神经胶质肿瘤中都不存在[184, 185]。

黑色素瘤和软组织肉瘤

黑色素瘤与各种软组织肉瘤具有相似性是有据可查的[186]。包括恶性外周神经鞘瘤、胃肠道间质瘤、上皮样血管瘤、横纹肌样瘤、骨肉瘤和原始神经外胚层肿瘤等，不再一一列举[187]。这些病变的详细免疫表型特征在此章已有描述。但上述肿瘤都不具有 gp100 相关黑色素细胞标记物或酪氨酸酶的反应活性，因而，这些标记物在鉴别诊断中十分必要。

除了上述典型的病变，透明细胞肉瘤（软组织黑色素瘤）是软组织肉瘤的一个例外，它真正地呈现出黑色素细胞分化[188-190]。因为此肿瘤的免疫组化谱和恶性黑色素瘤有重叠[190]，因此当临床诊断不确定时，需要做其他的专业研究进行鉴别。尤其是透明细胞肉瘤一般有 t（12；22）染色体易位，而在黑色素瘤中不存在[191, 192]。

原始神经外胚层肿瘤也可能显示黑色素细胞分

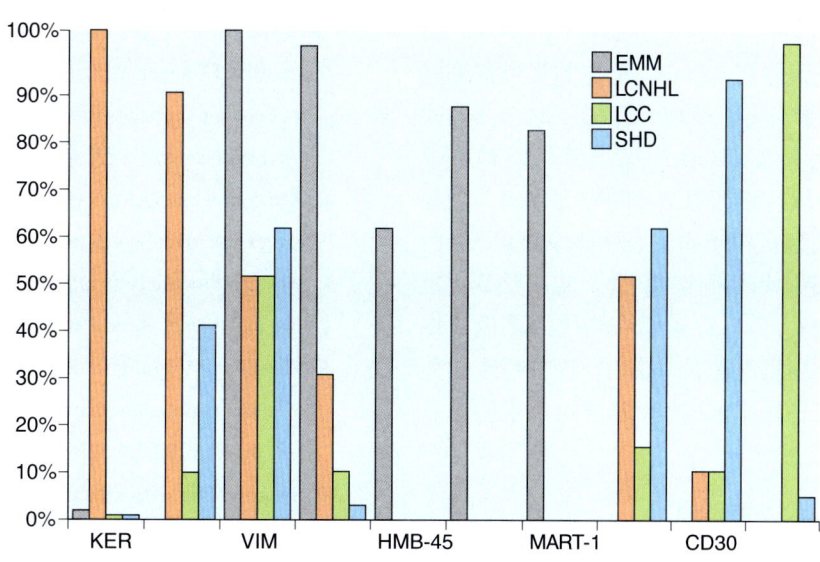

图 6.18　大细胞未分化恶性肿瘤的免疫反应模式

化，但较少见，因此与小细胞性恶性黑色素瘤有相似之处[2,127,135,136]。此外，两者都有可能表达CD56、CD57和CD99。S-100蛋白、gp100相关蛋白或MTFP的弥漫阳性表达强烈支持黑色素瘤的诊断。相反，FLI-1蛋白的阳性表达局限于原发性神经外胚层肿瘤（PNETs）[193]。此外，在这种情况下也可以应用细胞遗传学，因为PNETs有t（11；22）染色体易位[194]。

此章节中最困难的鉴别诊断是肉瘤样恶性黑色素瘤和表浅恶性外周神经鞘瘤（SMPNST）。事实上两者在许多方面都很相似[195]。很明显，在这种情况下，曾经有黑色素瘤的病史是相当重要的信息，如果没有，作者一般将SMPNST解释为是与大神经或以前存在的神经纤维瘤有密切关系的病变，或发生于系统性神经纤维瘤病的患者[196]。

原位黑色素瘤和色素性日光性角化病

皮肤病理诊断学医师有一个较普遍的问题，就是如何鉴别细胞学特征温和的原位黑色素瘤（MIS）和色素性日光性角化病（PAK）。Shabrawi-Caelen等特别论述了此种鉴别诊断，使用的抗体包括S-100蛋白、HMB-45、MART-1和酪氨酸酶[197]。研究结果表明，免疫组化对鉴别诊断的确有帮助，但是他也发现MART-1过于敏感，在色素性日光性角化病的病例中也有意想不到的表达。作者的经验不同于Shabrawi-Caelen，而是倾向于后一种观点。事实上，在鉴别原位黑色素瘤和色素性日光性角化病时，比起其他的抗体，作者更常用MART-1，因为它的敏感度较高，染色背景干净。

先天性痣的增生性真皮结节和黑色素瘤

在比较大的先天性复合痣中，增生的黑色素细胞结节（PNs）发生于真皮，呈现"克隆"形态，因此须警惕继发性黑色素瘤。Herron等[198]系统地检查了一系列带有增生的黑色素细胞结节的先天性痣，发现这种病变的肿瘤细胞自相矛盾地表达突变型p53蛋白和bcl-2蛋白（两者皆为抗凋亡蛋白），也表达Bax蛋白（一种凋亡蛋白）。CD117通常在增生的黑色素细胞结节中表达，而在黑色素瘤中缺乏。这种特定的免疫谱系对鉴别先天性痣中的PNs和恶性黑色素瘤是有帮助的。

原发性和转移性皮内黑色素瘤

皮肤黑色素瘤有较强的向皮肤内迁移的能力。一旦发生迁移，肿瘤有可能表现出明显的交界真皮-表皮生长，或表皮内"派杰样"扩散。因此没有可靠的形态学特征来鉴别原发性和转移性的"噬表皮"黑色素瘤。Guerriere-Kovach等[199]研究了一组两种诊断都可能成立的病例，使用的抗体包括bcl-2蛋白、突变型p53蛋白、Ki-67、增殖性核抗原（PCNA）、α-异构肌动蛋白和CD117（c-kit蛋白）。转移性黑色素瘤中突变型p53蛋白和Ki-67表达较强，CD117反应下降。尽管有这个倾向，但是这种表现并不总是一致。因此，在处理这个问题中，目前的免疫组化还不是很可靠。

参考文献

1. Nakhleh RE, Wick MR, Rocamora A, et al. Morphologic diversity in malignant melanomas. Am J Clin Pathol 1990; 93:731–740.
2. Banerjee SS, Harris M. Morphologic and immunophenotypic variation in malignant melanoma. Histopathology 2000; 36: 387–402.
3. Reed RJ, Martin P. Variants of melanoma. Semin Cutan Med Surg 1997; 16:137–158.
4. Battifora H. Clinical application of the immunohistochemistry of filamentous proteins. Am J Surg Pathol 1988; 12(Suppl): 24–42.
5. Osborn M. Intermediate filaments as histologic markers: an overview. J Invest Dermatol 1983; 81(Suppl 1):104s–109s.
6. Ramaekers FCS, Puts JJ, Moesker O, et al. Intermediate filaments in malignant melanomas: identification and use as a marker in surgical pathology. J Clin Invest 1983; 71:635–643.
7. Caselitz J, Janner M, Breitbart E, et al. Malignant melanomas contain only the vimentin type of intermediate filaments. Virchows Arch A 1983; 400:43–51.
8. Zarbo RJ, Gown AM, Nagle RB, et al. Anomalous cytokeratin expression in malignant melanoma: one-and two-dimensional Western blot analysis and immunohistochemical survey of 100 melanomas. Mod Pathol 1990; 3:494–502.
9. Miettinen M, Franssila K. Immunohistochemical spectrum of malignant melanoma: the common presence of keratins. Lab Invest 1989; 61:623–628.
10. Swanson PE. Monoclonal antibodies to human milk fat globule proteins. In: Wick MR, Siegal GP, eds. Monoclonal antibodies in diagnostic immunohistochemistry. New York:

Dekker; 1988:227–284.

11. Pinkus GS, Kurtin PJ. Epithelial membrane antigen – a diagnostic discriminant in surgical pathology. Hum Pathol 1985; 16:929–940.

12. Sloane JP, Ormerod MG. Distribution of epithelial membrane antigen in normal and neoplastic tissues and its value in diagnostic tumor pathology. Cancer 1981; 47:1786–1795.

13. Selby WL, Nance KV, Park KH. Carcinoembryonic antigen–immunoreactivity in metastatic malignant melanoma. Mod Pathol 1992; 5:415–419.

14. Ravindranath MH, Shen P, Habal N, et al. Does human melanoma express carcinoembronic antigen? Anticancer Res 2000; 20:3083–3092.

15. Ben-Izhak B, Levy R, Weill S, et al. Anorectal malignant melanoma: a clinicopathology study, including immunohistochemistry and DNA flow cytometry. Cancer 1997; 79:18–25.

16. Muraro R, Kuroki M, Wunderlich D, et al. Generation and characterization of B72.3 second generation monoclonal antibodies reactive with the tumor associated glycoprotein-72 antigen. Cancer Res 1988; 48:4588–4596.

17. Wick MR, Swanson PE, Manivel JC. Placental alkaline phosphatase-like reactivity in human tumors: an immunohistochemical study of 520 cases. Hum Pathol 1987; 18:946–954.

18. Chorvath B, Hunakova L, Turzova M, et al. Monoclonal antibodies to two adhesive cell surface antigens (CD43 and CD59) with different distribution on hematopoietic and non-hematopoietic tumor cell lines. Neoplasma 1992; 39:325–329.

19. Radka SF, Charron DJ, Brodsky FM. Class II molecules of the major histocompatibility complex considered as differentiation markers. Hum Immunol 1986; 16:390–400.

20. Carrel S, Schmidt-Kessen A, Mach JP, et al. Expression of common acute lymphoblastic leukemia antigen (CALLA) on human malignant melanoma cell lines. J Immunol 1983; 130: 2456–2460.

21. Herbold KW, Zhou J, Haggerty JG, et al. CD44 expression on epidermal melanocytes. J Invest Dermatol 1996; 106:1230–1235.

22. Sarlomo-Rikala M, Kovatich AJ, Barusevicius A, et al. CD117: a sensitive marker for gastrointestinal stromal tumors that is more specific than CD34. Mod Pathol 1998; 11:728–734.

23. Pernick NL, DaSilva M, Gangi MD, et al. 'Histiocytic' markers in melanoma. Mod Pathol 1999; 12:1072–1077.

24. Tang NE, Luyten GP, Mooy CM, et al. HNK-1 antigens on uveal and cutaneous melanoma cell lines. Melanoma Res 1996; 6:411–418.

25. Weidner N, Tjoe J. Immunohistochemical profile of monoclonal antibody O13. Am J Surg Pathol 1994; 18:486–494.

26. Tron VA, Krajewski S, Klein-Parker H, et al. Immunohistochemical analysis of *bcl*-2 protein regulation in cutaneous melanoma. Am J Pathol 1995; 146:643–650.

27. Chu PG, Arber DA, Weiss LM. Expression of T/NK-cell and plasma-cell antigens in nonhematopoietic epithelioid neoplasms: an immunohistochemical study of 447 cases. Am J Clin Pathol 2003; 120:64–70.

28. Ruiter DJ, Bhan AK, Harrist TJ, et al. Major histocompatibility antigens and mononuclear inflammatory infiltrate in benign nevomelanocytic proliferations and malignant melanoma. J Immunol 1982; 129:2808–2815.

29. Miettinen M, Chatten J, Paetan A, et al. Monoclonal antibody NB84 in the differential diagnosis of neuroblastoma and other small round cell tumors. Am J Surg Pathol 1998; 22: 327–332.

30. Mezebish D, Smith K, Williams J, et al. Neurocristic cutaneous hamartoma: a distinctive dermal melanocytosis with an unknown malignant potential. Mod Pathol 1998; 11:573–578.

31. Van Ginkel PR, Gee RL, Walker TM, et al. The identification and differential expression of calcium-binding proteins associated with ocular melanoma. Biochim Biophys Acta 1998; 1448:290–297.

32. Ludwin SK, Kosek JC, Eng LF. The topographical distribution of S100 protein and GFA protein in the adult rat brain: an immunohistochemical study using horseradish peroxidase-labeled antibodies. J Comp Neurol 1976; 165:197–208.

33. Gaynor R, Irie R, Morton D, et al. S100 protein: a marker for human malignant melanomas? Lancet 1981; 1:869–871.

34. Baudier J, Briving C, Deinum J, et al. Effect of S100 protein and calmodulin on calcium-induced disassembly of brain microtubule proteins in vitro. FEBS Lett 1982; 147:165–168.

35. Stefansson K, Wollmann R, Jerkovic M. S100 protein in soft tissue tumors derived from Schwann cells and melanocytes. Am J Pathol 1982; 106:261–268.

36. Takahashi K, Isobe T, Ohtsuki Y, et al. Immunohistochemical study on the distribution of alpha and beta subunits of

S100 protein in human normal and neoplastic tissues. Virchows Arch B 1984; 45 385–396.

37. Herrera GA, Pena JR, Turbat-Herrera EA, et al. The diagnosis of melanoma: current approaches addressing tumor differentiation. Pathol Annu 1994; 29(Part 1):233–260.

38. Loeffel SC, Gillespie GY, Mirmiram SA, et al. Cellular immunolocalization of S100 protein within fixed tissue sections by monoclonal antibodies. Arch Pathol Lab Med 1985; 109:117–122.

39. Smoller BR. Immunohistochemistry in the diagnosis of melanocytic neoplasms. Pathol State Art Rev 1994; 2:371–383.

40. Kindblom LG, Lodding P, Rosengren L, et al. S100 protein in melanocytic tumors. Acta Pathol Microbiol Scand 1984; 92:219–230.

41. Nakajima T, Watanabe S, Sato Y, et al. An immunoperoxidase study of S100 protein distribution in normal and neoplastic tissues. Am J Surg Pathol 1982; 7:715–727.

42. Cochran AJ, Lu HF, Li PX, et al. S100 protein remains a practical marker for melanocytic and other tumors. Melanoma Res 1993; 3:325–330.

43. Swanson PE, Wick MR. Immunohistochemistry of cutaneous tumors. In: Applied immunohistochemistry for the surgical pathologist. Cambridge, UK: Edward Arnold; 1993:269–308.

44. Ribe A, McNutt NS. S100A6 protein expression is different in Spitz nevi and melanomas. Mod Pathol 2003; 16:505–511.

45. Rogers J, Khan M, Ellis J. Calretinin and other calcium binding proteins in the nervous system. Adv Exp Med Biol 1990; 269:195–203.

46. Tos AP, Doglioni C. Calretinin: a novel tool for diagnostic immunohistochemistry. Adv Anat Pathol 1998; 5:61–66.

47. Schulze E, Witt M, Fink T, et al. Immunohistochemical detection of human skin nerve fibers. Acta Histochem 1997; 99:301–309.

48. Gotzos V, Wintergerst ES, Musy JP, et al. Selective distribution of calretinin in adenocarcinomas of the human colon and adjacent tissues. Am J Surg Pathol 1999; 23:701–711.

49. Nance KV, Siegal GP. The use of monoclonal antibodies in the search for tumor-specific antigens. In: Wick MR, Siegal GP, eds. Monoclonal antibodies in diagnostic immunohistochemistry. New York: Dekker; 1988:593–622.

50. Shih IM, Nesbit M, Herlyn M, et al. A new MEL-CAM (CD146)-specific monoclonal antibody, MN-4, on paraffinembedded tissue. Mod Pathol 1998; 11:1098–1106.

51. Trefzer U, Rietz N, Chen Y, et al. SM5-1: a new monoclonal antibody which is highly sensitive and specific for melanocytic lesions. Arch Dermatol Res 2000; 292:583–589.

52. Brouwenstijn N, Slager EH, Bakker AB, et al. Transcription of the gene encoding melanoma-associated antigen gp10 tissues and cell lines other than those of the melanocytic lineage. Br J Cancer 1997; 76:1562–1566.

53. Adema GJ, deBoer AJ, Vogel AM, et al. Molecular characterization of the melanocyte lineage-specific antigen gp100. J Biol Chem 1994; 269:20126–20133.

54. Adema GJ, Bakker AB, deBoer J, et al. PMel17 is recognized by monoclonal antibodies NKI-beteb, HMB-45, HMB-50, and by anti-melanoma cytotoxic T-cells. Br J Cancer 1996; 73:1044–1048.

55. Kawakami Y, Nishimura MI, Restifo NP, et al. T-cell recognition of human melanoma antigens. J Immunother 1993; 14: 88–93.

56. Chen YT, Stockert E, Jungbluth A, et al. Serological analysis of Melan-A (MART-1), a melanocyte-specific protein homogeneously expressed in human melanomas. Proc Natl Acad Sci USA 1996; 93:5916–5919.

57. Kawakami Y, Battles JK, Kobayashi T, et al. Production of recombinant MART-1 proteins and specific anti-MART-1 polyclonal and monoclonal antibodies: use in the characterization of the human melanoma antigen MART-1. J Immunol Methods 1997; 202:13–25.

58. Kageshita T, Kawakami Y, Hirai S, et al. Differential expression of MART-1 in primary and metastatic melanoma lesions. J Immunother 1997; 20:460–465.

59. Nicotra MR, Nistico P, Mangoni A, et al. Melan-A/MART-1 antigen expression in cutaneous and ocular melanomas. J Immunother 1997; 20:466–469.

60. Pierard-Franchimont C, Letawe C, Nikkels AF, et al. Patterns of the immunohistochemical expression of melanoma-associated antigens and density of CD45R0+ activated T-lymphocytes and L1-protein-positive macrophages in primary cutaneous melanomas. Int J Mol Med 1998; 2:721–724.

61. Fetsch PA, Marincola FM, Filie A, et al. Melanoma associated antigen recognized by T-cells (MART-1): the advent of a preferred immunocytochemical antibody for the diagnosis of metastatic malignant melanoma with fine needle aspiration.

Cancer 1999; 87:37–42.

62. Busam KJ, Jungbluth AA. Melan-A, a new melanocytic differentiation marker. Adv Anat Pathol 1999; 6:12–18.

63. Orosz Z. Melan-A/MART-1 expression in various melanocytic lesions and in non-melanocytic soft tissue tumors. Histopathology 1999; 34:517–525.

64. Yu LL, Flotte TJ, Tanabe KK, et al. Detection of microscopic melanoma metastases in sentinel lymph nodes. Cancer 1999; 86:617–627.

65. Anichini A, Molla A, Mortarini R, et al. An expanded peripheral T-cell population to a cytotoxic T-lymphocyte (CTL)-defined, melanocyte-specific antigen in metastatic melanoma patients impacts on generation of peptide specific CTLs but does not overcome tumor escape from immune surveillance in metastatic lesions. J Exp Med 1999; 190:651–667.

66. Bergman R, Azzam H, Sprecher E, et al. A comparative immunohistochemical study of MART-1 expression in Spitz nevi, ordinary melanocytic nevi, and malignant melanomas. J Am Acad Dermatol 2000; 42:496–500.

67. Heegaard S, Jensen OA, Prause JU. Immunohistochemical diagnosis of malignant melanoma of the conjunctiva and uvea: comparison of the novel antibody against Melan-A with S100 protein and HMB-45. Melanoma Res 2000; 10:350–354.

68. Adema GJ, deBoer AJ, VantHullenaar R, et al. Melanocyte lineage-specific antigens recognized by monoclonal antibodies NKI-beteb, HMB-50, and HMB-45 are encoded by a single cDNA. Am J Pathol 1993; 143:1579–1585.

69. Chiamenti AM, Vella F, Bonetti F, et al. Anti-melanoma monoclonal antibody HMB-45 on enhanced chemiluminescence- Western blotting recognizes a 30–35 kDa melanosome-associated sialated glycoprotein. Melanoma Res 1996; 6:291–298.

70. Esclamado RM, Gown AM, Vogel AM. Unique proteins defined by monoclonal antibodies specific for human melanoma. Am J Surg 1986; 152:376–385.

71. Gown AM, Vogel AM, Hoak DH, et al. Monoclonalantibodies specific for melanocytic tumors distinguish subpopulations of melanocytes. Am J Pathol 1986; 123:195–203.

72. Schaumburg-Lever G, Metzler G, Kaiserling E. Ultrastructural localization of HMB-45 binding sites. J Cutan Pathol 1991; 18:432–435.

73. Palazzo JP, Duray PH. Congenital agminated Spitz nevi: immunoreactivity with a melanoma-associated monoclonal antibody. J Cutan Pathol 1988; 15:166–170.

74. Smoller BR, McNutt NS, Hsu A. HMB-45 staining of dysplastic nevi: support for a spectrum of progression toward melanoma. Am J Surg Pathol 1989; 13:680–684.

75. Skelton HG III, Smith KJ, Barrett TL, et al. HMB-45 staining in benign and malignant melanocytic lesions: a reflection of cellular activation. Am J Dermatopathol 1991; 131:543–550.

76. Wick MR. HMB-45: a clue to the biology of malignant melanoma? J Cutan Pathol 1991; 18:307–308.

77. Smoller BR, Hsu A, Krueger J. HMB-45 monoclonal antibody recognizes an inducible and reversible melanocyte cytoplasmic protein. J Cutan Pathol 1991; 18:315–322.

78. Wick MR, Swanson PE, Rocamora A. Recognition of malignant melanoma by monoclonal antibody HMB-45: an immunohistochemical study of 200 paraffin-embedded cutaneous tumors. J Cutan Pathol 1988; 15:201–207.

79. Blessing K, Sanders DS, Grant JJ. Comparison of immunohistochemical staining of the novel antibody melan-A with S100 protein and HMB-45 in malignant melanoma and melanoma variants. Histopathology 1998; 32:139–146.

80. Vogel AM, Esclamado RM. Identification of a secreted Mr 95,000 glycoprotein in human melanocytes and melanomas by a melanocyte specific monoclonal antibody. Cancer Res 1988; 48:1286–1294.

81. Kim RY, Wistow GJ. The cDNA RPE1 and monoclonal antibody HMB-50 define gene products preferentially expressed in retinal pigment epithelium. Exp Eye Res 1992; 55:657–662.

82. Bar H, Schlote W. Malignant melanoma in the CNS: subtyping and immunocytochemistry. Clin Neuropathol 1997; 16:337–345.

83. Barrett AW, Bennett JH, Speight PM. A clinicopathological and immunohistochemical analysis of primary oral mucosal melanoma. Eur J Cancer B Oral Oncol 1995; 31B:100–105.

84. Fernando SS, Johnson S, Bate J. Immunohistochemical analysis of cutaneous malignant melanoma: comparison of S100 protein, HMB-45 monoclonal antibody, and NKI/C3 monoclonal antibody. Pathology 1994; 26:16–19.

85. Bishop PW, Menasce LP, Yates AJ, et al. An immunophenotypic survey of malignant melanomas. Histopathology 1993; 23:159–166.

86. Mackie RM, Campbell I, Turbitt M. Use of NKI/C3 mono-

clonal antibody in the assessment of benign and malignant melanocytic lesions. J Clin Pathol 1984; 37:367–372.

87. Yaziji H, Gown AM. Immunohistochemical markers of melanocytic tumors. Int J Surg Pathol 2003; 11:11–15.

88. Mangini J, Li N, Bhawan J. Immunohistochemical markers of melanocytic lesions: a review of their diagnostic usefulness. Am J Dermatopathol 2002; 24:270–281.

89. Friedman HD, Tatum AH. HMB-45 positive malignant lymphoma: a case report with literature review of aberrant HMB-45 reactivity. Arch Pathol Lab Med 1991; 115:826–830.

90. Hancock C, Allen BC, Herrera GA. HMB-45 detection in adenocarcinomas. Arch Pathol Lab Med 1991; 115:886–890.

91. Unger PD, Hoffman K, Thung SN, et al. HMB-45 reactivity in adrenal pheochromocytomas. Arch Pathol Lab Med 1992; 116:151–153.

92. Zimmer CM, Gottschalk J, Goebel S, et al. Melanoma associated antigens in tumors of the nervous system: an immunohistochemical study with the monoclonal antibody HMB-45. Virchows Arch A 1992; 420:121–126.

93. Eble JN, Amin MB, Young RH. Epithelioid angiomyolipoma of the kidney: a report of five cases with prominent and diagnostically confusing epithelioid smooth muscle component. Am J Surg Pathol 1997; 21:1123–1130.

94. Fetsch PA, Fetsch JF, Marincola FM, et al. Comparison of melanoma antigen recognized by T-cells (MART-1) to HMB-45: additional evidence to support a common lineage for angiomyolipoma, lymphangiomyomatosis, and clear cell sugar tumor. Mod Pathol 1998; 11:699–703.

95. Ribalta T, Lloreta J, Munne A, et al. Malignant pig-mented clear cell epithelioid tumor of the kidney: clear cell ('sugar') tumor versus malignant melanoma. Hum Pathol 2000; 31: 516–519.

96. Zamboni G, Pea M, Martignoni G, et al. Clear cell 'sugar' tumor of the pancreas: a novel member of the family of lesions characterized by the presence of perivascular epithelioid cells. Am J Surg Pathol 1996; 20:722–730.

97. Bonetti F, Pea M, Martignoni G, et al. Clear cell ('sugar') tumor of the lung is a lesion strictly related to angiomyolipoma – the concept of a family of lesions characterized by the presence of the perivascular epithelioid cells (PEC). Pathology 1994; 26:230–236.

98. Tanaka Y, Ijiri R, Kato K, et al. HMB-45/Melan-A and smooth muscle actin-positive clear-cell epithelioid tumor arising in the ligamentum teres hepatis: additional example of clear-cell 'sugar' tumors. Am J Surg Pathol 2000; 24:1295–1299.

99. Gaffey MJ, Mills SE, Zarbo RJ, et al. Clear cell tumor of the lung: immunohistochemical and ultrastructural evidence of melanogenesis. Am J Surg Pathol 1991; 15:644–653.

100. Busam KJ, Iversen K, Coplan KA, et al. Immunoreactivity for A103, an antibody to melan-A (MART-1) in adrenocortical and other steroid tumors. Am J Surg Pathol 1998; 22:57–63.

101. Lerner AB, Fitzpatrick TB. Biochemistry of melanin formation. Physiol Rev 1950; 30:91–126.

102. Fitzpatrick TB, Miyomato M, Iskikawa K. The evolution of concepts of melanin biology. Arch Dermatol 1967; 96:305–323.

103. Pellegrino D, Bellina CR, Manca G, et al. Detection of melanoma cells in peripheral blood and sentinel lymph nodes by RT-PCR analysis: a comparative study with immunohistochemistry. Tumori 2000; 86:336–338.

104. Orchard GE. Comparison of immunohistochemical labeling of melanocyte differentiation antibodies melan-A, tyrosinase, and HMB-45 with NKI/C3 and S100 protein in the evaluation of benign nevi and malignant melanoma. Histochem J 2000; 32:475–481.

105. Jungbluth AA, Iversen K, Coplan K, et al. T311 – an antityrosinase monoclonal antibody for the detection of melanocytic lesions in paraffin embedded tissues. Pathol Res Pract 2000; 196:235–242.

106. DeVries TJ, Trancikova D, Ruiter DJ, et al. High expression of immunotherapy candidate proteins gp100, MART-1, tyrosinase, and TRP-1 in uveal melanoma. Br J Cancer 1998; 78:1156–1161.

107. Kaufmann O, Koch S, Burghardt J, et al. Tyrosinase, melan-A, and KBA62 as markers for the immunohistochemical identification of metastatic amelanotic melanomas on paraffin sections. Mod Pathol 1998; 11:740–746.

108. Blaheta HJ, Schittek B, Breuninger H, et al. Lymph node micrometastases of cutaneous melanoma: increased sensitivity of molecular diagnosis in comparison to immunohistochemistry. Int J Cancer 1998; 79:318–323.

109. Cormier JN, Abati A, Fetsch P, et al. Comparative analysis of the in vivo expression of tyrosinase, MART-1/Melan-A, and gp100 in metastatic melanoma lesions: implications for

immunotherapy. J Immunother 1998; 21:27–31.
110. Sato N, Suzuki S, Takimoto H, et al. Monoclonal antibody MAT-1 against human tyrosinase can detect melanogenic cells on formalin-fixed paraffin-embedded sections. Pigment Cell Res 1996; 9:72–76.
111. Takimoto H, Suzuki S, Masui S, et al. MAT-1, a monoclonal antibody that specifically recognizes human tyrosinase. J Invest Dermatol 1995; 105:764–768.
112. Chen YT, Stockert E, Tsang S, et al. Immunophenotyping of melanomas for tyrosinase: implications for vaccine development. Proc Natl Acad Sci USA 1995; 92:8125–8129.
113. Clarkson KS, Sturdgess IC, Molyneux AJ. The usefulness of tyrosinase in the immunohistochemical assessment of melanocytic lesions: comparison of the novel T311 antibody (anti-tyrosinase) with S100, HMB-45, and A103 (MART-1; Melan-A). J Clin Pathol 2001; 54:196–200.
114. Takeda K, Yasumoto K, Takada R, et al. Induction of melanocyte-specific microphthalmia-associated transcription factor by Wnt-3a. J Biol Chem 2000; 275:14013–14016.
115. Vachtenheim J, Novotna H. Expression of genes for microphthalmia isoforms, Pax3 and MSG1, in human melanomas. Cell Mol Biol 1999; 45:1075–1082.
116. Galibert MD, Yavuzer U, Dexter TJ, et al. Pax3 and regulation of the melanocyte-specific tyrosinase-related protein-1 promoter. J Biol Chem 1999; 274:26894–26900.
117. Verastegui C, Bertolotto C, Bille K, et al. TFE3, a transcription factor homologous to microphthalmia, is a potential transcriptional activator of tyrosinase and TyrpI genes. Mol Endocrinol 2000; 14:449–456.
118. Koch MB, Shih IM, Weiss SW, et al. Microphthalmia transcription factor and melanoma cell adhesion molecule expression distinguish desmoplastic/spindle-cell melanoma from morphologic mimics. Am J Surg Pathol 2001; 25:58–64.
119. King R, Googe PB, Weilbaecher KN, et al. Microphthalmia transcription factor expression in cutaneous benign and malignant melanocytic, and nonmelanocytic tumors. Am J Surg Pathol 2001; 25:51–57.
120. King R, Weilbaecher KN, McGill G, et al. Microphthalmia transcription factor: a sensitive and specific melanocyte marker for melanoma diagnosis. Am J Pathol 1999; 155:731–738.
121. Miettinen M, Fernandez M, Franssila K, et al. Microphthalmia transcription factor in the immunohistochemical diagnosis of metastatic melanoma: comparison with four other melanoma markers. Am J Surg Pathol 2001; 25:205–211.
122. Zavala-Pompa A, Folpe AL, Jimenez RE, et al. Immunohistochemical study of microphthalmia transcription factor and tyrosinase in angiomyolipoma of the kidney, renal cell carcinoma, and retroperitoneal sarcomas: comparative evaluation with traditional diagnostic markers. Am J Surg Pathol 2001; 25:65–70.
123. Folpe AL, Goodman ZD, Ishak KG, et al. Clear cell myomelanocytic tumor of the falciform ligament/ligamentum teres: a novel member of the perivascular epithelioid cell family of tumors with a predilection for children and young adults. Am J Surg Pathol 2000; 24:1239–1246.
124. Rochaix P, Lacroix-Triki M, Lamant L, et al. PNL2, a new monoclonal antibody directed against a fixative-resistant melanocyte antigen. Mod Pathol 2003; 16:481–490.
125. Busam KJ. The use and application of special techniques in assessing melanocytic tumors. Pathology 2004; 36:462–469.
126. Busam KJ, Kucukgol D, Sato E, et al. Immunohistochemical analysis of novel monoclonal antibody PNL2 and comparison with other melanocyte differentiation markers. Am J Surg Pathol 2005; 29:400–406.
127. Wick MR, Stanley SJ, Swanson PE. Immunohistochemical diagnosis of sinonasal melanoma, carcinoma, and neuroblastoma with monoclonal antibodies HMB-45 and antisynaptophysin. Arch Pathol Lab Med 1988; 112:616–620.
128. Franquemont DW, Mills SE. Sinonasal malignant melanoma: a clinicopathologic and immunohistochemical study of 14 cases. Am J Clin Pathol 1991; 96:689–697.
129. Wiedenmann B, Franke WW, Kuhn C, et al. Synaptophysin: a marker protein for neuroendocrine cells and neoplasms. Proc Natl Acad Sci USA 1986; 83:3500–3504.
130. Lloyd RV, Wilson BS. Specific endocrine tissue marker defined by a monoclonal antibody. Science 1983; 222:628–630.
131. Kontochristopoulos GJ, Stavropoulos PG, Krasagakis K, et al. Differentiation between Merkel cell carcinoma and malignant melanoma: an immunohistochemical study. Dermatology 2000; 201:123–126.
132. Klemm KM, Moran CA, Suster S. Pigmented thymic carcinoids: a clinicopathological and immunohistochemical study of two cases. Mod Pathol 1999; 12:946–948.
133. Gal AA, Koss MN, Hochholzer L, et al. Pigmented pulmonary carcinoid tumor: an immunohistochemical and ultrastruc-

tural study. Arch Pathol Lab Med 1993; 117:832–836.

134. Moran CA, Albores-Saavedra J, Wenig BM, et al. Pigmented extraadrenal paragangliomas: a clinicopathologic and immunohistochemical study of five cases. Cancer 1997; 79:398–402.

135. Pettinato G, Manivel JC, d'Amore ESG, et al Melanotic neuroectodermal tumor of infancy: a reexamination of a histogenetic problem based on immunohistochemical, flow cytometric, and ultrastructural study of 10 cases. Am J Surg Pathol 1991; 15:233–245.

136. Kapadia SB, Frisman DM, Hitchcock CL, et al. Melanotic neuroectodermal tumor of infancy: clinicopathological, immunohistochemical, and flow cytometric study. Am J Surg Pathol 1993; 17:566–573.

137. Mennemeyer RP, Hallman KO, Hammar SP, et al. Melanotic schwannoma: clinical and ultrastructural studies of three cases with evidence of intracellular melanin synthesis. Am J Surg Pathol 1979; 3:3–10.

138. Orchard GE, Wilson-Jones E. Immunocytochemistry in the diagnosis of malignant melanoma. Br J Biomed Sci 1994; 51:44–56.

139. Springall DR, Gu J, Cocchia D, et al. The value of S100 immunostaining as a diagnostic tool in human malignant melanomas: a comparison using S100 and neuron-specific enolase antibodies. Virchows Arch A 1983; 400:331–343.

140. Dhillon AP, Rode J, Leathem A. Neuron-specific enolase: an aid to the diagnosis of melanoma and neuroblastoma. Histopathology 1982; 6:81–92.

141. Reed JA, Finnerty B, Albino AP. Divergent cellular differentiation pathways during the invasive stage of cutaneous malignant melanoma progression. Am J Pathol 1999; 155:549–555.

142. Sangueza OP, Requena L. Neoplasms with neural differentiation: a review. Part II: Malignant neoplasms. Am J Dermatopathol 1998; 20:89–102.

143. Mooy CM, Luyten GP, DeJong PT, et al. Neural cell adhesion molecule distribution in primary and metastatic uveal melanomas. Hum Pathol 1995; 26:1185–1190.

144. Cochran AJ, Roberts A, Wen DR, et al. Update on lymphatic mapping and sentinel node biopsy in the management of patients with melanocytic tumors. Pathology 2004; 36:478–484.

145. Prieto VG, Clark SH. Processing of sentinel lymph nodes for detection of metastatic melanoma. Ann Diagn Pathol 2002; 6:257–264.

146. Spanknebel K, Coit DG, Bieligk SC, et al. Characterization of micrometastatic disease in melanoma sentinel lymph nodes by enhanced pathology: recommendations for standardizing pathologic analysis. Am J Surg Pathol 2005; 29:305–317.

147. Shidham VB, Komorowski R, Macias V, et al. Optimization of an immunostaining protocol for the rapid intraoperative evaluation of melanoma sentinel lymph node imprint smears with the 'MCW melanoma cocktail.' Cytojournal 2004; 1:2.

148. Medalie N, Ackerman AB. Sentinel lymph node biopsy has no benefit for patients with primary cutaneous melanoma: an assertion based on comprehensive, critical analysis. 2nd edn. New York: Ardor Scribendi Press; 2004:1–95.

149. Abrahamsen HN, Hamilton-Dutoit SJ, Larsen J, et al. Sentinel lymph nodes in malignant melanoma: extended histopathologic evaluation improves diagnostic precision. Cancer 2004; 100:1683–1691.

150. Wick MR. Prognostic factors for cutaneous melanoma. Am J Clin Pathol 1998; 110:713–718.

151. Moretti S, Spallanzani A, Chiarugi A, et al. Correlation of Ki-67 expression in cutaneous primary melanoma with prognosis in a prospective study: different correlation according to thickness. J Am Acad Dermatol 2001; 44:188–192.

152. Florenes VA, Faye RS, Maelandsmo GM, et al. Levels of cyclin D1 and D3 in malignant melanoma: deregulated cyclin expression is associated with poor clinical outcome in superficial melanomas. Clin Cancer Res 2000; 6:3614–3620.

153. Straume O, Sviland L, Akslen LA. Loss of nuclear p16 protein expression correlates with increased tumor proliferation (Ki-67) and poor prognosis in patients with vertical growth phase melanoma. Clin Cancer Res 2000; 6:1845–1853.

154. Kaleem Z, Lind AC, Humphrey PA, et al. Concurrent Ki-67 and p53 immunolabeling in cutaneous melanocytic neoplasms: an adjunct for recognition of the vertical growth phase in malignant melanomas? Mod Pathol 2000; 13 217–222.

155. Henrique R, Azevedo R, Bento MJ, et al. Prognostic value of Ki-67 expression in localized cutaneous malignant melanoma. J Am Acad Dermatol 2000; 43:991–1000.

156. Florenes VA, Maelandsmo GM, Holm R, et al. Expression of activated Trk-A protein in melanocytic tumors: relationship to cell proliferation and clinical outcome. Am J Clin Pathol 2004; 122:412–420.

157. Graham CH, Rivers J, Kerbel RS, et al. Extent of vascularization as a prognostic indicator in thin (<0.76 mm) malignant melanomas. Am J Pathol 1994; 145:510–514.

158. Vlaykova T, Talve L, Hahka-Kemppinen M, et al. MIB-1 immunoreactivity correlates with blood vessel density and survival in disseminated malignant melanoma. Oncology 1999; 57:242–252.

159. Kerbel RS, Kobayashi H, Graham CH, et al. Analysis and significance of the malignant 'eclipse' during the progression of primary cutaneous human melanomas. J Invest Dermatol Symp Proc 1996; 1:183–187.

160. Gutman M, Singh RK, Radinsky R, et al. Intertumoral heterogeneity of receptor-tyrosinase kinase expression in human melanoma cell lines with metastatic capabilities. Anticancer Res 1994; 14:1759–1765.

161. Elder D. Tumor progression, early diagnosis, and prognosis of melanoma. Acta Oncol 1999; 38:535–547.

162. Nagasaka T, Lai R, Medeiros LJ, et al. Cyclin D1 overexpression in Spitz nevi: an immunohistochemical study. Am J Dermatopathol 1999; 21:115–120.

163. Kanter-Lewensohn L, Hedblad MA, Wedje J, et al. Immunohistochemical markers for distinguishing Spitz nevi from malignant melanomas. Mod Pathol 1997; 10:917–920.

164. Bergman R, Shemer A, Levy R, et al. Immunohistochemical study of p53 protein expression in Spitz nevi as compared with other melanocytic tumors. Am J Dermatopathol 1995; 17:547–550.

165. Penneys NS, Seigfried E, Nahass G, et al. Expression of proliferating cell nuclear antigen in Spitz nevus. J Am Acad Dermatol 1995; 32:964–967.

166. Takahashi H, Maeda K, Maeda K, et al. Immunohistochemical characterization of Spitz's nevus: differentiation from common melanocytic nevi, dysplastic melanocytic nevus, and malignant melanoma. J Dermatol 1987; 14:533–541.

167. Glusac EJ, McNiff JM. Epithelioid cell histiocytoma: a simulant of vascular and melanocytic neoplasms. Am J Dermatopathol 1999; 21:1–7.

168. Busam KJ, Granter SR, Iversen K, et al. Immunohistochemical distinction of epithelioid histiocytic proliferations from epithelioid melanocytic nevi. Am J Dermatopathol 2000; 22:237–241.

169. Busam KJ, Rosai J, Iversen K, et al. Xanthogranulomas with inconspicuous foam cells and giant cells mimicking malignant melanoma: a clinical, histologic, and immunohistochemical study of three cases. Am J Surg Pathol 2000; 24:864–869.

170. Ma CK, Zarbo RJ, Gown AM. Immunohistochemical characterization of atypical fibroxanthoma and dermato-fibrosarcoma protuberans. Am J Clin Pathol 1992; 97:478–483.

171. Diaz-Cascajo C, Borghi S, Bonczkowitz M. Pigmented atypical fibroxanthoma. Histopathology 1998; 33:537–541.

172. Gloghini A, Rizzo A, Zanette I, et al. KP1/CD68 expression in malignant neoplasms including lymphomas, sarcomas, and carcinomas. Am J Clin Pathol 1995; 103:425–431.

173. Suster S. Tumors of the skin composed of large cells with abundant eosinophilic cytoplasm. Semin Diagn Pathol 1999; 16:162–177.

174. Borek BT, McKee PH, Freeman JA, et al. Primary malignant melanoma with rhabdoid features: a histologic and immunocytochemical study of two cases. Am J Dermatopathol 1998; 20:123–127.

175. Laskin WB, Knittel DR, Frame JN. S100 protein and HMB-45-negative 'rhabdoid' malignant melanoma: a totally dedifferentiated malignant melanoma? Am J Clin Pathol 1995; 103:772–773.

176. Anstey A, Cerio R, Ramnarain N, et al. Desmoplastic malignant melanoma: an immunocytochemical study of 25 cases. Am J Dermatopathol 1994; 16:14–22.

177. Gatter KC, Alcock K, Heryet A, et al. The differential diagnosis of routinely-processed anaplastic tumors using monoclonal antibodies. Am J Clin Pathol 1984; 82:33–43.

178. Strickler JG, Michie SA, Warnke RA, et al. The 'syncytial' variant of nodular sclerosing Hodgkin's disease. Am J Surg Pathol 1986; 10:470–477.

179. Ritter JH, Mills SE, Gaffey MJ, et al. Clear cell tumors of the alimentary tract and abdominal cavity. Semin Diagn Pathol 1997; 14:213–219.

180. Ordonez NG. Role of immunohistochemistry in differentiating epithelial mesothelioma from adenocarcinoma. Am J Clin Pathol 1999; 112:75–89.

181. Mizutani H, Ohyanagi S, Hayashi T, et al. Functional thrombomodulin expression on epithelial skin tumors as a differentiation marker for suprabasal keratinocytes. Br J Dermatol 1996; 135:187–193.

182. Battifora H, Silva EG. The use of antikeratin antibodies in the immunohistochemical distinction between neuroendocrine (Merkel cell) carcinoma of the skin, lymphoma, and oat cell

183. Clark HB. Immunohistochemistry of nervous system antigens: diagnostic applications in surgical neuropathology. Semin Diagn Pathol 1984; 1:309–316.

184. Zimmer C, Gottschalk J, Goebel S, et al. Melanomaassociated antigens in tumors of the nervous system: an immunohistochemical study with monoclonal antibody HMB-45. Virchows Arch A 1992; 420:121–126.

185. Gottschalk J, Jautzke G, Schreiner C. Epithelial and melanoma antigens in gliosarcoma: an immunohistochemical study. Pathol Res Pract 1992; 188:182–190.

186. Lodding P, Kindblom LG, Angervall L. Metastases of malignant melanoma simulating soft tissue sarcoma: a clinicopathological, light- and electron microscopic and immunohistochemical study of 21 cases. Virchows Arch A 1990; 417:377–388.

187. Banerjee SS, Coyne JD, Menasce LP, et al. Diagnostic lessons of mucosal melanoma with osteocartilaginous differentiation. Histopathology 1998; 33:255–260.

188. Swanson PE, Wick MR. Clear cell sarcoma: an immunohistochemical analysis of six cases and comparison with other epithelioid neoplasms of soft tissue. Arch Pathol Lab Med 1989; 113:55–60.

189. Mechtersheimer G, Tilgen W, Klar E, et al. Clear cell sarcoma of tendons and aponeuroses: case presentation with special reference to immunohistochemical findings. Hum Pathol 1989; 20:914–917.

190. Almeida MM, Nunes AM, Frable WJ. Malignant melanoma of soft tissue: a report of three cases with diagnosis by fine needle aspiration cytology. Acta Cytol 1994; 38:241–246.

191. Stenman G, Kindblom LG, Angervall L. Reciprocal translocation t(12;22)(q13;q13) in clear-cell sarcoma of tendons and aponeuroses. Genes Chromosomes Cancer 1992; 4:122–127.

192. Langezaal SM, Graadt van Roggen JF, Gleton-Jansen AM, et al. Malignant melanoma is genetically distinct from clear cell sarcoma of tendons and aponeuroses (malignant melanoma of soft parts). Br J Cancer 2001; 84:535–538.

193. Folpe AL, Hill CE, Parham DM, et al. Immunohistochemical detection of FLI-1 protein expression: a study of 132 round cell tumors with emphasis on mimics of Ewing's sarcoma/primitive neuroectodermal tumor. Am J Surg Pathol 2000; 24:1657–1662.

194. Winters JL, Geil JD, O'Connor WN. Immunohistology, cytogenetics, and molecular studies of small round cell tumors of childhood: a review. Ann Clin Lab Sci 1995; 25:66–78.

195. Swanson PE, Scheithauer BW, Wick MR. Peripheral nerve sheath neoplasms: clinicopathologic and immunochemical observations. Pathol Annu 1995; 30(Pt. 2):1–82.

196. Wick MR. Malignant peripheral nerve sheath tumors of the skin. Mayo Clin Proc 1990; 65:279–282.

197. Shabrawi-Caelen LE, Kerl H, Cerroni L. Melan-A: not a helpful marker in distinction between melanoma in-situ on sun-damaged skin and pigmented actinic keratosis. Am J Dermatopathol 2004; 26:364–366.

198. Herron MD, Vanderhoof SL, Smock K, et al. Proliferative nodules in congenital melanocytic nevi: a clinicopathologic and immunohistochemical analysis. Am J Surg Pathol 2004; 28:1017–1025.

199. Guerriere-Kovach PM, Hunt EL, Patterson JW, et al. Primary melanoma of the skin and cutaneous melanomatous metastases: comparative histologic features and immunophenotypes. Am J Clin Pathol 2004; 122:70–77.

# 7 不明来源转移癌的免疫组织化学

原作者：David J. Dabbs
译　者：孟　斌
审校者：郭成浩，高　鹏

目　录

引言	183
临床表现	183
未知原发灶肿瘤的诊断策略	185
抗原/抗体生物学	185
第一步和第二步：细胞角蛋白——概述	186
联合（成组）抗体法解决诊断问题	195
第三步：伴波形蛋白共表达的癌	195
第四步：备选的组织系标志物	196
第五步：肿瘤分化抗原——细胞特异性产物	200
激素受体（雌激素/孕激素）	210
Paget 病	210
小结	211

引　言

免疫组化技术（IHC）对外科病理学家的影响十分巨大，尤其是在研究未知原发部位的恶性肿瘤时最能感受其带来的帮助。绝大多数医院的实验室都开展了免疫组化技术，而且操作常常是自动化、短周期的，作为一个物有所值的工具，IHC能提供给病理学家所期望的所有特性。用于诊断的抗体数量每年都呈指数式增加，充分说明了该领域正在进行的研究的重要性。自从本书第一版出版以来，各类重要抗体都有了实质性的增加，这些抗体对于未知原发部位的转移性恶性肿瘤的明确诊断非常有用。但即使有如此大量的抗体，仍只有极少数特异抗体能对病例作出"100%的明确诊断"。确实有这样一种说法：不管抗体宣称的如何特异，在肿瘤病理鉴别诊断中主要依赖某一种标记物的免疫组化结果作出诊断可能是危险的[1]。这个说法强调了以组织病理形态改变作为外科病理诊断基础的重要性。当单独依赖形态学不足以作出诊断时，标准组织切片则作为解决问题的起始点，而IHC也许是在石蜡切片中获得更多信息的最好方法。

即使是最特异的抗体［如抗甲状腺球蛋白和前列腺特异性抗原（PSA）抗体］也不是完全部位特异性的，因此我们需要借助于成套或一组抗体所给出的统计学意义来加强形态学诊断。基于免疫组化研究所获得的信息，相应的诊断性的抗体组也很快发生着变化，可以预期有关抗体敏感性和特异性的新数据将持续不断融入，这种缓慢的不断变化的状况虽然让人心烦，但这种变化常常促进了IHC的不断提高。目前对不明来源转移性恶性肿瘤的基本分类原则是将其分为癌、黑色素瘤、淋巴瘤、生殖细胞肿瘤和肉瘤几大类，这种分类方式已经经历了时间的验证。

临床表现

未知原发病灶转移癌（metastatic carcinoma of unknown primary，MCUP）是指虽然经过详细的询问病史、体检、放射影像学和生化或组织学检查，仍未发现有明确的原发病灶。对肿瘤病人的研究表明，MUCP病人占所有恶性肿瘤患者的5%～15%[2-5]，近来放射影像学的发展使此类病人的百分比降低到5%～7%[6,7,8]。

对于这些病人的临床检查过程还没有从经济学角度给予广泛研究。

关于 IHC 在外科病理学中的成本与效益方面的数据很少。Putti 及其同事在对186例病人的回顾性研究中发现，IHC对于18%未分化肿瘤的明确诊断是必需的，对于40%病例的诊断起支持作用，为其余的病例提供了预后判断信息[9]。Schapira和Jerrett[5]对一组199例病人的临床诊断过程进行了分析和总结，其中为寻找原发病灶平均花费17 973美元，但只有19.6%的病人存活期超过1年。Raab[10]的研究显示IHC可用于预后判断或者得出一个更加精确的诊断以指导治疗。在应用了几种不同的方法后，Rabb认为IHC的价值可能被低估了，对于MCUP的诊断研究来说IHC是一项成本与效益合算的策略。

对于此类病人的诊断，放射学单独的作用有限，而且对预后判断没用[11, 12]。由于原发灶体积小、广泛扩散或治疗后退化，有些病人即使死后进行尸体解剖也很难发现其原发病灶[13]。

1988年，Le-Chevalier及其同事对302例MCUP病人的尸检标本进行了研究[14]，其中27%的病人在死前确定了原发灶，50%的病人通过尸检确诊，仍有16%的病人未找到原发灶[14]。此次研究中最常见的原发肿瘤部位包括胰腺、肺、肾、结直肠，其中包括了男、女两性发病率最高的两类恶性肿瘤。病人的预后只与转移灶的多少有关，而死前是否发现原发灶与病人的生存期并不相关[14]。

Kirsten及其同事研究了286例MCUP病人的生存状况，发现病人的预期生存因素包括淋巴结转移情况、身体状况以及体重下降小于10%[15]。Van der Gaast及其同事[16]对41例MCUP病人应用一系列抗体来确定肿瘤的分化，认为应用免疫组化成组抗体的方法确定肿瘤的起源，对病人选择恰当的治疗是有益的，尤其是能从联合化疗中获益[17]。

其他研究者发现肿瘤分化差的组织学特征对生存期没有影响[18]。应用免疫组化技术能明确少至5%多至70% MCUP病人的肿瘤起源[19]。大多数研究者得出了同一结论：对病人的个体治疗而言，最好能找出肿瘤的来源，这对病人的化疗是有利的。

要根据病人的临床症状、年龄、病史、性别以及找到原发灶的可能性来确定合适的寻找原发灶的检查方法。临床医师还要考虑到大量临床检查的经济问题和给病人带来的不便与不适[20]。MCUP病人的预后很差，中位生存时间只有6～12个月[21, 22]，因此确立原发肿瘤的起源从而指导激素疗法、化疗、放疗等治疗干预是非常重要的[23]。

目前的临床研究是试图去确定预后相对较好的几组MCUP病人，以使其能得到适当的治疗[2, 24-27]。这些肿瘤包括白血病/淋巴瘤、生殖细胞肿瘤、小细胞肺癌以及来自乳腺、卵巢、子宫内膜、肾上腺、甲状腺和前列腺的癌[15, 28, 29]。如有可能应将区域转移与远处转移区分开，因为局限性病变更适合治疗[3, 30]。已报道的另外一些有利的临床特征包括位于腹膜后或外周淋巴结的肿瘤、局限于1～2个转移部位的肿瘤、无吸烟史以及年轻[3]。

成人大多数MCUP是腺癌和未分化癌，但依据性别和年龄，其相对数各有不同[31, 32]。Huebner及其同事对343例病人的研究发现40%为腺癌、28%为未分化癌、14%为鳞癌、3%为小细胞癌，其余的难以确定类型[33]。有膈肌以下脏器转移的病人预后差并且对化疗反应差[34]。在一些研究中，腺癌占不明来源癌的48%～60%[4, 21, 35-37]。对有淋巴结转移的病人，淋巴结的解剖位置可能是肿瘤原发灶的一个线索。

虽然胃肠道和前列腺的腺癌偏好于转移到左颈部，但对于颈部有转移性腺癌的病人，检查原发灶应从肺（男性）或乳腺（女性）开始[38, 39]。

头颈部淋巴结转移癌最常见的来源是头颈部的未分化癌[4]，其大部分为鳞状上皮黏膜起源。这类病人的预后很大程度上取决于淋巴结的转移状况，N3期病人预后差[40]。淋巴结活检加上全上消化道内镜检查可以发现30%病人的隐匿原发灶，从而使其接受合适的治疗，预后相对较好[41]。

在女性腋窝出现的转移性腺癌，其原发瘤最常见于同侧乳腺[42]。女性出现腹腔恶性渗出物，其原发瘤多位于卵巢、子宫内膜和宫颈；而在男性，典型的原发部位为胃肠道，尤其是结肠、直肠或胃[43]。非妇科来源的腹膜转移癌最常来自于胃、结肠或胰腺，中位生存期为3个月[44]。

对于胸腔出现恶性渗出液的病人，原发灶最常见的部位，在女性为乳腺，在男性为肺癌。恶性淋巴瘤则见于男、女两性[45]。

腹股沟淋巴结转移癌，如果是位于股三角淋巴结，则可能来自下肢；如果位于股内侧淋巴结则转移可能来自肛门、直肠或女性生殖系统器官肿瘤[4]。

骨转移病人的原发瘤多来自肺、乳腺、肾或泌尿生殖系统，影像学检查对明确原发肿瘤特别有用[46]。

肝是各种类型恶性肿瘤发生转移的最大的单一脏器之一，尤其是癌。最常见的肝转移性恶性肿瘤来自胃肠道，其中结直肠癌占第一位，肺癌和乳腺癌以及胰胆管癌也常发生肝转移。所有转移性腺癌的形态可以与肝的原发性胆管癌相似，有些可以与肝细胞癌相像，特别是低分化的肝细胞癌。尽管前列腺癌肝转移不常见，但一旦转移则可能和胆管癌相混淆。因此，就未知原发肿瘤的肝转移来说，在女性首先考虑来自于结直肠癌、乳腺癌和肺癌；而在男性，则把结直肠癌、肺癌和前列腺癌放在首位。恶性黑色素瘤转移到肝并非少见，其中最常见的是眼黑色素瘤的肝转移[3]。

Pisharodi 及其同事[47]对200例肝恶性肿瘤的细针穿刺活检标本进行研究发现，32%的病例是肝细胞癌，49.5%很容易诊断为转移癌，有18.5%诊断困难。在最后一组里应用 IHC 使一半病例得到明确诊断。

虽然确定转移瘤的来源可能比较困难，尤其是原发灶隐匿未知时，但在大脑将转移性腺癌或低分化癌与胶质瘤区分开还是比较容易的[48-51]。肺癌是中枢神经系统（CNS）最可能的转移来源，其次是乳腺癌、肾癌、甲状腺癌和胃肠道癌。其他腺癌如卵巢癌、前列腺癌和胰胆管癌很少有脑转移，因为这些部位的恶性肿瘤在脑转移之前几乎都已有广泛的播散。仍有5%的病人癌的原发部位不明[53]。大部分脑转移病人的生存期为3～11个月[34, 54, 55]。

和肝一样，肺也是癌转移的主要脏器，尤其是腺癌。对于外科病理医师来说，鉴别肺内腺癌的起源是一项经常性的、有难度并富于挑战性的工作，因为腺癌不仅是肺最常见的原发肿瘤，而且也是肺最常见的转移性肿瘤。在一些小的活检材料中，如支气管活检或细针吸取活检（fine needle aspiration biopsy, FNAB），区别这些肿瘤类型可能更具挑战性。对这些癌的鉴别很重要，以便确定是采用化学疗法还是激素疗法，或者两者都用，特别是对于转移性乳腺癌或前列腺癌。

未知原发灶肿瘤的诊断策略

外科病理医师的目标是确定肿瘤的分化倾向以及是否属于"可治疗"范围内的肿瘤，即乳腺癌、前列腺癌、卵巢癌、子宫内膜癌、甲状腺癌和肾上腺癌，以及生殖细胞肿瘤和神经内分泌癌[2]。激素及抗激素治疗对于乳腺癌、前列腺癌和肾上腺癌有效。化疗药物可抑制神经内分泌癌、甲状腺癌和生殖细胞癌。其他癌对治疗的反应则较少肯定[32]，但如有可能仍应确定癌的类型，这样有助于对此类病人确定更有效的治疗措施。近来研究表明多达三分之一的MCUP病人对基于紫杉醇（taxane-based therapies）的疗法敏感[56, 57]。

获取组织是对来源未明肿瘤进行检查的第一步。实践中常通过细针吸取活检（FNAB）或芯针组织活检（core tissue biopsy）法来获取组织。对266例浅表淋巴结的研究显示，FNAB对转移癌的敏感性为96.5%，没有发现假阳性结果，但有9例假阴性[58]。对同一种研究方式来说，选用FNAB还是芯针活检应根据具体情况确定。对恶性渗出物进行免疫组化研究也有很大价值，恶性渗出液可通过治疗性抽液获得，因此常常是所能得到的病人的第一份标本[59-65]。无论通过何种方法获取组织，理想的状态是能够监控这一过程，以便能获取足够的组织，根据需要解决的问题对组织进行适当分配，也就是说根据需要将标本分别用于免疫组化、电镜、流式细胞仪或其他研究。

可以通过冷冻切片、FNAB组织现场观察或组织印片等方法对组织获取过程进行监控。除了获取组织，病理医生还必须了解病人的年龄、性别、已知风险因素、症状持续时间以及临床和放射学检查结果，根据这些信息和肿瘤的形态学表现，开始对肿瘤起源进行探索。

在外科病理学和细胞学上，分化差的癌可大致分为大细胞未分化癌、小细胞未分化癌和梭形细胞癌。标准的苏木精-伊红染色或巴氏染色切片是诊断研究的起始点，不应低估组织形态学在获得明确诊断中的重要性，形态学是解释所有免疫组化结果的基础。

对于IHC方法来说，根据细胞的分化倾向选择能正确鉴别肿瘤的合适抗体是第一步。一旦将肿瘤归类为癌、淋巴瘤、肉瘤或黑色素瘤，便可以通过特异性的细胞成熟标记物或组织特异性标记物，如不同的细胞角蛋白（CK）、造血系统的特异性标记物等，来获取关于细胞分化的进一步信息。另外，特异性的细胞产物（如神经内分泌颗粒）也可用于鉴别，有一系列成熟标记物的表达可资鉴别（如L26和CD43在小细胞淋巴瘤共表达），或者可通过证实肿瘤性胚胎抗原的表达进行鉴别。关于 IHC/超微结构方法联合用于诊断，读者可参考 Hammar 的一篇专题综述[35]。

在本章中，着重强调了诊断性 IHC 在 MCUP 诊断中的作用，尤其是发生在肝、肺、脑和淋巴结的MCUP。提供了一些表格以帮助发生于特殊解剖部位的肿瘤的鉴别诊断。关于电镜超微结构与IHC联合在MCUP病人诊断中的作用已有讨论[35]。

抗原/抗体生物学

对 MCUP 的广泛研究始于对未知原发灶转移

性肿瘤的研究。由于事实上所有的癌均显示细胞角蛋白（CK）阳性，因此当肿瘤CK阳性就很容易表明其具有癌分化。单一的和广谱的CK是检测癌分化首先选择的抗体，然后就可以应用各种部位特异性CK和直接针对细胞产物的不同抗体对肿瘤来源进行更特异的亚分类。对肿瘤的分类来说，这些细胞抗原的联合检测可能是一个成本-效益相称的方法。

对MCUP病人的有效明确诊断可遵循以下五个序列步骤：

1. 确定细胞的分化方向，应用包括角蛋白、淋巴样、黑色素瘤和肉瘤标记物在内的主要系标记物。

2. 确定CK的类型或其在肿瘤细胞内的分布类型，因为某些肿瘤类型具有独特的CK亚型。

3. 确定是否有波形蛋白的共表达。

4. 确定是否有备选的上皮性或生殖细胞源性抗原的表达，即是否有癌胚抗原（CEA）、上皮细胞膜抗原（EMA）或胎盘碱性磷酸酶（PLAP）的表达。

5. 确定是否有细胞特异性产物、细胞特异性结构、具有细胞类型独特标志的转录因子或受体的表达，例如：神经内分泌颗粒、肽类激素、甲状腺球蛋白、PSA、前列腺特异性膜抗原、抑制素（inhibin）、GCDFP（gross cystic disease fluid protein）、绒毛素（villin）、uroplakin、甲状腺转录因子1（TTF-1）或转录因子CDX-2。

第一步和第二步：细胞角蛋白——概述

软性上皮角蛋白中间丝由大约30种角蛋白多肽中的大约20种不同的角蛋白多肽组成[66-68]，1到20号多肽包括Ⅱ型（碱性）角蛋白和Ⅰ型（酸性）角蛋白（表7.1）。在免疫组化诊断中，该中间丝家族对于鉴别癌分化和确定癌的亚型起关键作用。

角蛋白丝是由两种不同角蛋白的四聚体组成的，其中2个来自Ⅰ型，2个来自Ⅱ型，以保持细胞的电荷呈中性。绝大部分角蛋白由酸型和碱型配对形成，很少有例外。角蛋白的分类和编号系统是以Moll及其同事的分类为基础[69]。

有12个呈偏酸性等电点的角蛋白形成Ⅰ型（酸性）角蛋白，8个偏碱性等电点的角蛋白形成Ⅱ型（碱中性）角蛋白[70]。角蛋白是两个基因家族的产物：编码Ⅱ型角蛋白的大部分基因位于12号染色体，编码Ⅰ型角蛋白的基因位于17号染色体[71-73]。在每一组内，CK的编号是连续的，组内的分子量则从高到低排列。大部分低分子量角蛋白（low molecular weight，LMW）典型地位于除鳞状上皮以外的所有上皮细胞，而高分子量角蛋白（high molecular weight，HMW）则典型地位于鳞状上皮[69]。

最初鉴定组织中不同的角蛋白类型依赖于繁冗的

表7.1　最常见的软角蛋白及其分布

Ⅱ型（碱性）角蛋白			Ⅰ型（酸性）角蛋白	
角蛋白	分子量（kD）	在正常组织中的典型分布	角蛋白	分子量（kD）
CK1	67	手掌和脚掌的表皮	CK9	64
		角化的鳞状上皮表皮	CK10	56.5
CK2	65	上皮细胞，所有部位	CK11	56
CK3	63	角膜	CK12	55
CK4	59	非角化的鳞状上皮细胞	CK13	51
CK5	58	鳞状上皮和腺上皮的基底细胞、肌上皮、间皮细胞	CK14	50
		鳞状上皮	CK15	50
CK6	56	鳞状上皮，尤其是增生的	CK16	48
CK7	54	单层上皮	CK17	46
CK8	52	腺上皮的基底细胞、肌上皮细胞	CK18	45
		单层上皮、大部分腺上皮和鳞状上皮（基底细胞）	CK19	40
		胃肠的单层上皮、Merkel细胞	CK20	46

（引自Quinlan RA，Schiller DL，Hatzfeid M，et al. Patterns of expression and organization of cytokeratin intermediate filaments. Ann NY Acad Sci 1985; 455:282-306）

生化方法，这些方法主要由 Franke 和 Moll 及其同事创立[69,74]。最近，由于大量的角蛋白特异性单克隆抗体的出现，使得角蛋白的分型鉴别大大加速[66,68,69,75]。这些发展对于简化角蛋白分型至关重要，对外科病理医生也非常有用。

在伴有广泛坏死的肿瘤中可通过检测角蛋白来确定肿瘤的癌分化。Judkins等[76]对少量伴有坏死的肿瘤进行了研究，包括癌、黑色素瘤和肉瘤，通过一组抗体的检测，发现在坏死区域有78%的癌至少有一种抗角蛋白抗体阳性，并具有100%的特异性。

角蛋白抗原在组织中的分布

单层上皮细胞角蛋白

单层上皮细胞角蛋白是胚胎发育中最先出现的角蛋白，实际上在所有单层（非复层）、导管和假复层上皮组织中均表达[68,69]。由于它们分布广泛，因此可以用做上皮分化的鉴定。除了鳞状细胞癌，几乎所有的间皮瘤和癌[68,69]都含有单层上皮角蛋白8和18。一些内脏器官如肝只含有角蛋白8和18。

尽管许多角蛋白抗体能识别多种角蛋白多肽（如广谱角蛋白抗体AE1和AE3），但CAM5.2和35βH11对角蛋白8和18的识别却几乎是特异性的（图7.1）。在外科病理诊断中，对证实单层上皮角蛋白该组抗体或许是最常用的。由于单层上皮角蛋白在大部分癌中广泛存在，因此，它们的抗体在初步确定癌分化方面极为有用（表7.2；并参照表7.1）。

CK19　CK19是分子量最小的角蛋白，属于单层上皮角蛋白，其分布与角蛋白8和18相似，也出现在黏膜鳞状上皮的基底层，还可见于表皮的基底细胞[77]。由于CK19在单层上皮细胞和许多鳞状上皮组织中广泛存在，因此是上皮性肿瘤的一个很好的筛选标记物。单克隆抗体AE1（Boehringer-Mannheim，Indianapolis，IN）与CK19的反应和AE1/AE3混合抗体（Boehringer-Mannheim）相同，单克隆抗体CK19-

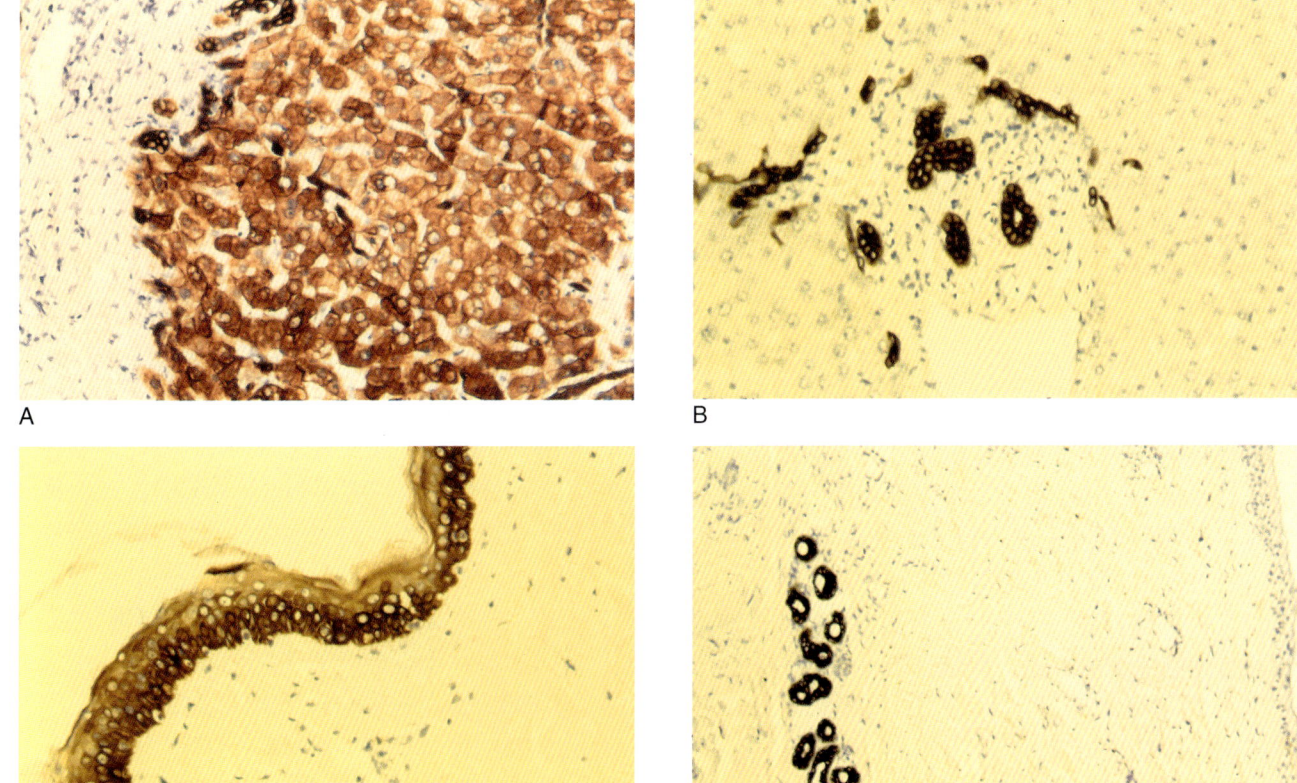

图7.1　(A) CAM5.2在肝细胞和相邻的胆管着色，而角蛋白903（K903）在胆管（B）和皮肤的角质层（C）着色。(D) CAM5.2和35βH11只在汗腺管着色，表皮不着色

表7.2　角蛋白抗原及其抗体

CK抗原	单克隆抗体	注　释
CK8	35βH11	单层上皮细胞来源的癌
CK8	CAM5.2	单层上皮细胞来源的癌
Pan-keratin	AE1/AE3	单层上皮和复层上皮来源的癌
CK1/10	34B4	鳞状细胞癌
CK7	OV-TL 12/30	非胃肠道来源的癌 某些胃肠道癌的极少细胞
CK20	K20	大部分胃肠道癌、黏液性的卵巢癌、胆管、移行上皮以及Merkel细胞癌
CK19	RCK 108	大部分癌，多种伴有鳞状上皮成分的癌，肌上皮细胞
CK1/10/5/14	34βE12	前列腺的基底细胞，大部分导管上皮来源的癌
CK18/19	PKK1	大部分癌
CK10/11/13/14/15/16/19	AE1	大部分鳞癌和多种癌
CK8/14/15/16/18/19	MAK-6	大部分癌

RCK108（DAKO，Carpinteria，CA）还能用于福尔马林固定的组织[78]。在肝肿瘤CK19大部分为阴性，极少数呈灶状阳性[78]。

CK7　CK7分子量54kD，为Ⅱ型单层上皮角蛋白，同角蛋白8和18相比，分布较局限。

在单层、假复层以及导管上皮和间皮细胞中CK7同角蛋白8和18的分布相似。文献中关于CK7的许多资料都是基于抗体OV-TL 12/30（DAKO，Carpinteria，CA）在福尔马林固定、石蜡包埋组织中的反应模式。OV-TL 12/30抗体和CK7的免疫反应活性与RCK105相同，RCK105是一种用于冰冻切片的抗体（表7.3）[79, 80]。

OV-TL12/30抗体需要蛋白酶预消化或抗原热修复（heat-induced epitope retrieval，HIER）。CK7在有些组织如结肠上皮、肝细胞和前列腺腺泡组织中缺乏或极少分布，此点有利于诊断[79-82]。此种抗体能识别移行细胞上皮，但不识别鳞状上皮[64]。CK7的局限性分布在鉴别腺癌来源时非常有用，如CK7在大部分乳腺[75]、肺[64]、卵巢[83-89]、胰胆管[64]和移行细胞癌[64]中表达，在结直肠、肾和前列腺癌中不表达或极少表达[64, 67, 69, 70, 90, 91]（表7.4、7.5及图7.2）。在宫颈鳞癌和非典型增生的鳞状细胞中有CK7的表达。在用于诊断时CK7有一个陷阱，即在正常软组织中的内皮细胞以及小肠黏膜、子宫外宫颈和淋巴样组织中的小静脉和淋巴管的内皮细胞中CK7表达阳性[92]。

重要的是要记住，在某些肿瘤中CK7的表达可

> **CK7的诊断应用**
>
> CK7特异性的诊断应用基于3种主要的免疫染色类型[93]：
>
> 1. 特征性的弥漫强阳性肿瘤包括唾液腺、肺、乳腺、卵巢、子宫内膜、膀胱和胸腺肿瘤以及间皮瘤、神经内分泌肿瘤、胰胆管腺癌和肝癌的纤维板层变型（fibrolamellar variant of hepatoma）[94]。
>
> 2. 在多数胆管和胃肿瘤细胞中CK7呈不同程度染色。
>
> 3. 几乎总是阴性但偶尔极少数细胞可显示阳性的癌有肝癌、十二指肠壶腹癌、结肠癌和肾上腺皮质肿瘤。在与肛周Paget病无关的直肠腺癌中20%~50%的细胞可表达CK7，而在乳腺和乳腺外的Paget细胞则典型表达CK7[95]。对诊断来说，淋巴结、肝或者脑转移癌CK7免疫染色强阳性提示其可能来源于肺、乳腺、卵巢、子宫内膜、膀胱或神经内分泌系统。CK7弥漫强阳性是诊断癌的一个有价值的标记物，可被用做进行进一步免疫组化研究的起始点。
>
> CK7阳性的肺转移癌必须应用多种抗体与肺原发癌进行鉴别，免疫组化检查要根据病人的年龄、性别和已有的检查结果综合分析应用。

不明来源转移癌的免疫组织化学 7

表7.3　细胞角蛋白免疫组化			
抗原	克隆	方法	来源
CK7	OV-TL 12/30	A,B	Boehringer Mannheim, Indianapolis, IN
CK8	CAM5.2	C	Becton, Dickinson and Co., Franklin Lakes, NJ
CK17	E3	B	Novocastra, Newcastle on Tyne, UK
CK19	RCK 108	B	DAKO, Carpinteria, CA
PAN	AE1/AE3	A	Boehringer Mannheim, Indianapolis, IN

A，Sigma 蛋白酶Ⅷ型，Sigma Diagnostics Inc.，St. Louis，MO
B，在缓冲液中经微波炉两个循环，Ventana Medical Systems, Tucson, AZ
C，Pepsin-Crude Pepsin

表7.4　CK7/CK20 在所选肿瘤中的主要免疫表达谱
CK7+/CK20+
移行细胞癌
胰腺癌
卵巢黏液性癌
CK7+/CK20-
非小细胞肺癌
小细胞肺癌
乳腺癌，导管和小叶
非黏液性卵巢癌
子宫内膜腺癌
间皮瘤
宫颈鳞状细胞癌
CK7-/CK20+
结直肠腺癌
Merkel 细胞癌
CK7-/CK20-
鳞状细胞癌，肺
前列腺腺癌
肾细胞癌
肝癌
胸腺

(引自Wang MP, Zee S, Zarbo RJ, et al. Coordinate expression of cytokeratin 7 and 20 defines unique subsets of carcinomas. Appl Immunohistochem 1995; 3: 99-107 and Chu P, Wu E, Weiss L. Cytokeratin 7 and cytokeratin 20 expression in epithelial neoplasms. A survey of 435 cases. Mod Pathol 2000; 13:962-972)

表7.5　CK7：肿瘤表达百分率	
肿瘤	表达百分率
肺，腺癌	100
肺，小细胞癌	43
卵巢，腺癌	100
唾液腺，所有肿瘤	100
子宫，内膜癌	100
甲状腺，所有肿瘤	98
乳腺，导管/小叶癌	96
肝，胆管癌	93
胰腺，腺癌	92
膀胱，移行细胞癌	88
宫颈，鳞癌	87
间皮瘤	65
神经内分泌癌	56
胃，腺癌	38
头颈部，鳞状细胞癌	27
食管，鳞状细胞癌	21
肾，腺癌	11
生殖细胞，癌	7
结肠，腺癌	5
肾上腺，癌	0
前列腺，癌	0
胸腺，胸腺瘤	0

(摘自 Chu P, Wu E, Weiss L. Cytokeratin 7 and cytokeratin 20 expression in epithelial neoplasms. A survey of 435 cases. Mod Pathol 2000; 13:962-972)

> **诊断要点**：CK7（见表7.3至7.5）
>
> 1. 在大部分唾液腺、肺、乳腺、卵巢、子宫内膜、膀胱、胸腺、腮腺、胰腺、神经内分泌癌和间皮瘤以及纤维板层肝癌呈弥漫强阳性表达。
> 2. 在结直肠及其他胃肠道癌、肝癌、前列腺和肾细胞癌、鳞癌（除了宫颈）和小细胞癌中大多为阴性表达，偶尔有极少数阳性细胞。
> 3. 正常组织的内皮细胞能被染色。

> **CK7 用于鉴别诊断**
>
> 1. 移行细胞癌（+），而鳞状细胞癌（-）。
> 2. 结直肠癌（R~N），而肺、乳腺、胸腺和卵巢癌阳性（大部分阳性）。
> 3. 子宫内膜和胰腺癌染色阳性，神经内分泌肿瘤可能为阳性或阴性。

能并不多见（表7.5）[96]。一般来说，在原发癌和转移癌中 CK7 的表达具有高保真性[96]。

CK20　CK20 分子量 46kD，是一种低分子量角蛋白，由 Moll 及其同事发现[97]。CK20 的组织分布主

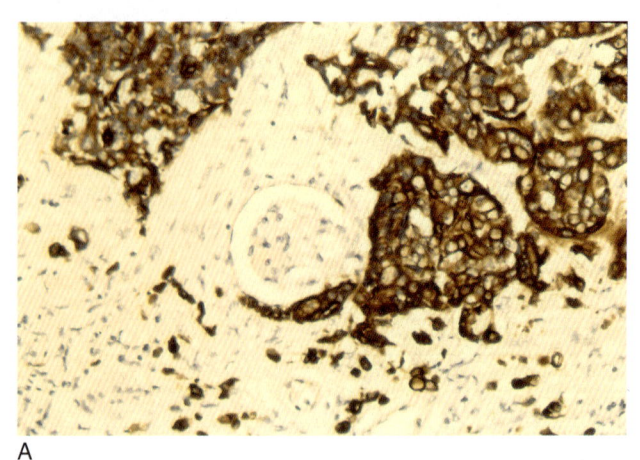

图 7.2 肾移行细胞癌 CK7（A）和 CK20（B）的免疫组化染色

要局限于胃肠道上皮及其来源肿瘤、卵巢的黏液性肿瘤和 Merkel 细胞肿瘤[84-86, 98-100]，从而使 CK20 可用于结直肠癌、胰腺和胆囊癌、Merkel 细胞癌以及移行细胞癌的原发灶甚至转移灶的明确诊断[63, 100, 101]。CK20 在这些肿瘤中大部分呈弥漫强阳性分布，此点对鉴别很重要。如与其他具有特异性组织分布的角蛋白如 CK7 联合应用，可以用于鉴定肺转移性结肠癌、鉴别肺小细胞癌与 Merkel 细胞癌[102, 103]、区别移行细胞癌和其他鳞癌及低分化癌。在其他一些肿瘤仅可见少数 CK20+ 细胞，约 10% 的原发性肺腺癌（非特殊类型或黏液性细支气管肺泡型）可显示高达 25% 的 CK20+ 细胞[104, 105]。另外，在有争议的肺原发性黏液癌（"胶样癌"，杯状细胞亚型），约 50% 的病例显示 CK20 染色阳性，并伴有胃肠道特异性标志物 CDX2 核阳性表达[106]。乳腺的乳头状癌或黏液性癌也可显示 CK20 阳性表达[107]。

据临床结果显示，联合应用 CK7 和 CK20 预测结直肠癌或肝源性胰胆管癌发生的转移癌的阳性预测值接近 0.9[108]。

不论是中心起源还是外周起源的肝的胆管癌，几乎都呈弥漫强阳性表达，但中心起源的（大胆管）胆管癌除了 CK7 外，对 CK20 更可能有一个高的阳性指数[109]。

需记住在某些肿瘤中 CK20 可能很少表达（表 7.6）[96, 110]。总的来说，CK20 在原发灶和转移灶中的表达具有高保真性[96]。

CK7、CK8、CK18 和 CK19 在胆管癌表达，在肝癌 CK7 或 AE1/AE3 抗体的免疫染色不确定，据此可对肝癌和胆管癌进行鉴别[111-113]。

肝内的上皮样血管内皮瘤（EH）可能与癌相似，尤其是其对 AE1/AE3 或 CAM5.2 可以呈不同程度的阳性[114]。应用血管标记物 CD31 和 VIII 因子对鉴别诊断非常关键。

尽管 CKs 的明显表达是上皮分化的基本要素，但是特异性标志物在其他组织的偶尔表达可能会使人对组织起源产生疑问。例如在非上皮组织中发现角蛋白（见下），以及偶尔在一些未分化癌或神经内分泌癌中观察到白细胞共同抗原（CD45）的表达、在胚胎性癌中 CD30 的表达[116]。应用成组抗体并结合免疫染色的分布和强度对解决这些易混淆的问题极为重要。

> **诊断要点：单层上皮角蛋白**
>
> 1. CAM5.2 和 AE1/AE3：癌分化的组织有广泛表达。
> 2. CK7（+）：间皮瘤，移行细胞、神经内分泌和胸腺癌，乳腺、肺、卵巢、子宫内膜和胰腺腺癌，纤维板层型肝癌。
> 3. CK7（R~N）：肾、前列腺、鳞状细胞（除宫颈）和小细胞癌，肝癌。
> 4. CK20（+）：结直肠、胰腺、卵巢黏液性、Merkel 细胞和移行细胞癌，在乳腺癌（尤其是乳头状和黏液癌）和肺腺癌中呈局灶阳性。
> 5. CK20（N）：肝和肾、前列腺、鳞状细胞以及小细胞癌，大多数唾液腺癌，低于 10% 的非小细胞肺癌有少量灶性染色。
> 6. 诊断陷阱——在未分化癌和神经内分泌癌中偶见 CD45 胞膜着色。

单层上皮角蛋白：鉴别诊断抗体组（见表 7.7 小结）。

表7.6 CK20：肿瘤表达百分率

肿 瘤	表达百分率
结肠，腺癌	100
皮肤，Merkel 细胞	78
胰腺，腺癌	62
胃，腺癌	50
肝，胆管癌	43
膀胱，移行细胞癌	29
肺，腺癌	10
肝，肝细胞癌	9
胃肠道，类癌	6
头颈部，鳞状细胞癌	6
卵巢，腺癌	4
肾上腺，癌	0
乳腺，导管/小叶癌	0
宫颈，鳞状细胞癌	0
食管，鳞状细胞癌	0
生殖细胞，癌	0
肾，癌	0
间皮瘤	0
前列腺，腺癌	0
唾液腺，所有肿瘤	0
甲状腺，所有肿瘤	0
胸腺，胸腺瘤	0
子宫，子宫内膜癌	0
肺，类癌	0
肺，小细胞癌	0
肺，鳞状细胞癌	0

（摘自 Chu P, Wu E, Weiss L. Cytokeratin 7 and cytokeratin 20 expression in epithelial neoplasms. A survey of 435 cases. Mod Pathol 2000; 13:962-972）

表7.7 小结：角蛋白在所选肿瘤（癌和间皮瘤）中的免疫染色

	AE1/3	CAM5.2	CK7	CK20	CK5
肝细胞癌	R~N	+	N	N	N
纤维板层型肝癌	R~N	+	+	N	N
肝的转移性癌	+	+	S	S	S
胆管癌	+	+	S	S	S
上皮样血管内皮瘤	S	S	N	N	N
肺，非小细胞癌	+	+	+	R~N	S
间皮瘤	+	+	+	N	+
肺，小细胞癌	+	+	+	N	N
鳞状细胞癌	+	S	R~N	N	+
移行细胞癌	+	+	+	+	+
前列腺癌	+	+	N	N	N
肾细胞癌	+	+	N	N	N
子宫内膜癌	+	+	+	N	N
结肠癌	+	+	R~N	+	N
胰腺，胆管癌	+	+	S	S	R~N
卵巢浆液性癌	+	+	+	N	S
卵巢黏液性癌	+	+	+	+	R~N
乳腺癌	+	+	+	R	N
Merkel 细胞癌	+	+	R~N	+	N

+，阳性；S，有时阳性；R，极少阳性；N，阴性

肝细胞癌与转移性癌（图 7.3）

1. 肝细胞癌：AE1/AE3（R~N），CK7（N），CK20（N），CAM5.2+，35βH11+。
2. 纤维板层型肝癌变型：CK7+。
3. 转移性癌：AE1/AE3+，CAM5.2+，35βH11+，CK7、CK20 不确定。

肝细胞癌与胆管癌（图 7.4）

1. 肝细胞癌：AE1/AE3（R~N），CK7（N），CK20（N），CAM5.2+，35βH11+。
2. 胆管癌：AE1/AE3+，CK7+，CK20+，CAM5.2+，35βH11+。

肝细胞癌与上皮样血管内皮瘤（EH）

1. 肝细胞癌：AE1/AE3（R~N）；EH：AE1/AE3（S）。
2. EH：CD34/CD31/Ⅷ因子肿瘤细胞有时阳性。
3. 肝细胞癌：窦细胞而非肿瘤细胞 CD34+。

肺腺癌与转移性结直肠 - 胰腺腺癌

1. 肺腺癌：CK7+，不到 10% 的肺腺癌呈局灶性 CK20+。
2. 结直肠腺癌：CK20+，CK7-，或极少数CK7+。
3. 胰腺腺癌：CK20+，CK7+，不确定

肺鳞状细胞癌与转移性移行细胞癌

1. 鳞状细胞癌：K903+，CK7-，CK20-。
2. 移行细胞癌：K903+/-，CK7+，CK20+。

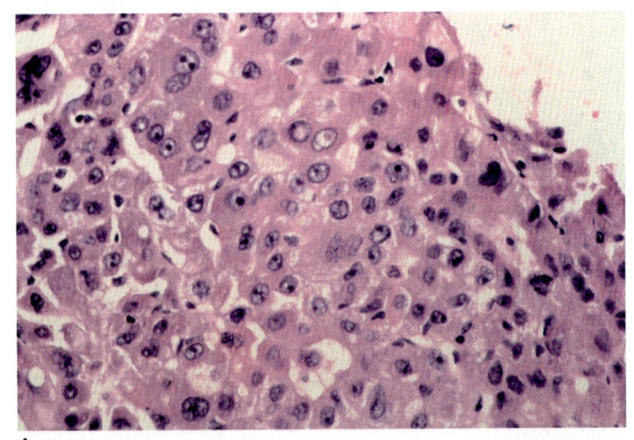
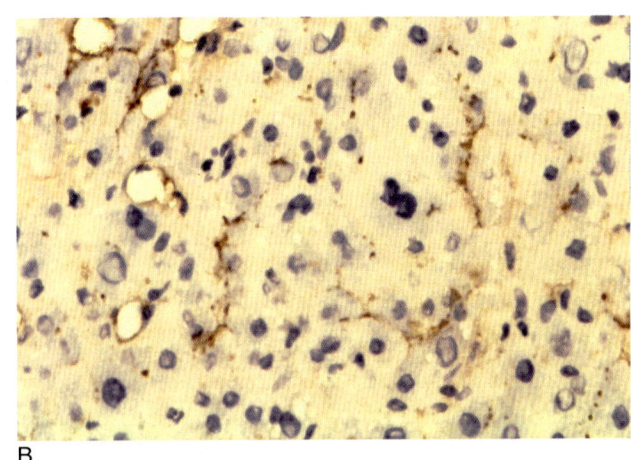
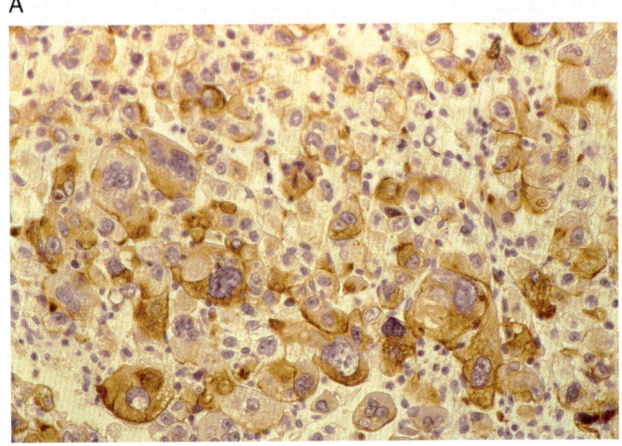

图 7.3 肝细胞癌（A）可以显示小管型多克隆癌胚抗原（pCEA）（B）及 CAM5.2（C）免疫染色阳性

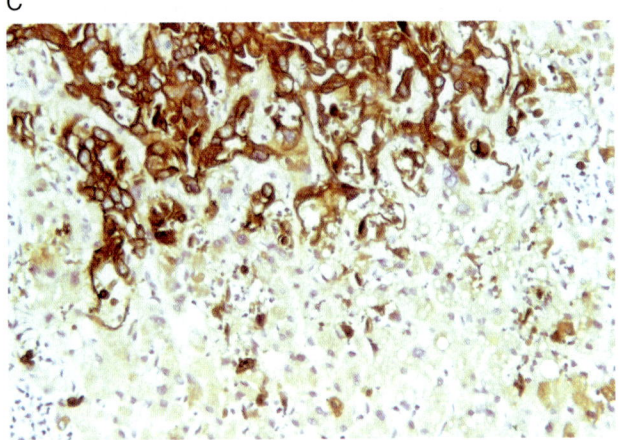

图 7.4 胃肠道来源的转移癌常呈 CK20+，但肝实质细胞呈 CK20-

复层上皮角蛋白：复合性角蛋白

高分子量（HMW）角蛋白见于复层上皮，单层内脏型上皮一般不出现。前列腺基底细胞以及导管和腺组织的肌上皮细胞也含有丰富的 HMW Ⅱ 型角蛋白和 LMW Ⅰ 型角蛋白。34βE12 或角蛋白 903（K903）抗体[117-119]能识别多种角蛋白包括 Moll Ⅰ、Ⅱ、Ⅴ、Ⅹ、Ⅺ 和 ⅩⅣ/ⅩⅤ 型，在实际诊断中应用这种表达形式来鉴别相应器官中的基底细胞和肌上皮细胞。在前列腺组织中，用 K903（34βE12）标记基底细胞可以排除浸润癌[117-119]，虽然在前列腺基底细胞中用该抗体染色阴性支持癌的诊断，但考虑到其他相应的形态学数据，染色阴性还不能作为诊断癌的唯一证据。同样，在腺器官如乳腺中，肌上皮细胞的标记对区别良恶性病变也是非常重要的。例如，在导管原位癌或硬化性腺病中，肌上皮细胞标记阳性可以确定病灶为非浸润性[119]。复层上皮型角蛋白典型的也出现在鳞状上皮中，可以用 K903 抗体检测，对在分化差的鳞状细胞癌中确定鳞状细胞分化来说，K903 是一个不错的抗体。

HMW 角蛋白也常见于导管来源的上皮（乳腺、胰腺、胆管、肺）和移行上皮、卵巢及间皮组织[117-119]。HMW 角蛋白抗体在这些组织中的免疫染色呈典型的弥漫强阳性，此特征有助于诊断，因为 HMW 角蛋白在内脏型上皮组织如结肠、胃、肾和肝中的染色呈局灶状[94-96]。

CK14 是一个敏感而特异的嗜酸细胞标记物，是由 LL002 抗体克隆（YLEM，Avezzano，Italy）确定的[120]。作为一个与线粒体有效反应的抗体，该抗体能识别正常及肿瘤性甲状腺组织中的嗜酸细胞。对其他器官的嗜酸细胞和嗜酸细胞性肿瘤中是否会出现同样的结果尚需进一步研究。

> **诊断要点**：复合性角蛋白抗体
>
> 1. 证实前列腺基底细胞的存在（图 7.5）。
> 2. 证实导管及腺组织中肌上皮细胞的存在。
> 3. 在复层上皮及鳞状上皮的基底细胞层呈阳性。
> 4. 在鳞状上皮分化中呈弥漫强阳性。
> 5. 在各种导管来源的癌和间皮瘤，以及超微结构证实有弹力原纤维的大多数肿瘤中呈阳性。
> 6. CK14用于鉴别嗜酸细胞性肿瘤中的嗜酸细胞。

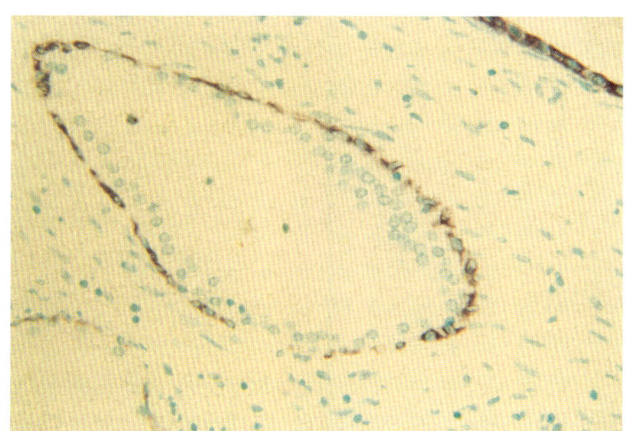

图7.5 前列腺切片，用K903显示的基底细胞清晰可见。K903亦可显示肌上皮细胞

CK5 CK5在胸膜转移癌和上皮型间皮瘤的鉴别诊断中很有用。在所有的上皮型间皮瘤中CK5都呈强阳性，而最多只有30%的肺腺癌呈不同程度的局灶性阳性（图7.6）[121]。

在几乎所有的鳞状细胞癌、半数移行细胞癌和许多未分化大细胞癌中CK5染色阳性[122, 123]。在分化差的癌中CK5对鉴定鳞状分化具有极高的敏感性和特异性[124, 125]。p63在鳞状细胞癌和移行细胞癌中也具有很高的阳性率，因此p63与CK5/6抗体联合应用对鳞状分化具有高敏感性和特异性[125, 126]。

乳腺的肌上皮细胞、前列腺的腺上皮和基底细胞都表达CK5[124]。卵巢来源的一些癌也可表达CK5[100]。

在胸腔或子宫颈旁淋巴结窦内偶尔会发现增生的间皮细胞[127]，此时需要与转移癌进行鉴别。在这些细胞巢中CK5/CK6呈弥漫强阳性有助于确定其为间皮来源。

对所选择肿瘤的角蛋白免疫染色情况总结于表7.8。

> **诊断要点**：CK5
>
> 1. 鳞状细胞及移行细胞分化的良好标记物。
> 2. 肺间皮瘤与腺癌鉴别的良好标记物。
> 3. 在腺体的肌上皮细胞和前列腺基底细胞中阳性。

非上皮细胞中的角蛋白

在没有上皮分化形态学证据的几种肿瘤中，经IHC[128-134]、免疫印迹[135]和PCR[136]证实有角蛋白存在，这种角蛋白的免疫染色被称为是异常的、畸变的、假的和出乎意料的[109, 137, 138]。

在这些非上皮间叶组织或黑色素细胞病变中最常发现的角蛋白是CK8和CK18，少见的有CK19。已证实检测这些LMW角蛋白的抗体在各种福尔马林固定、石蜡包埋的间叶组织肿瘤中染色呈阳性，这些肿瘤包括平滑肌肉瘤（21%～25%）[104, 139, 140]、纤维肉瘤

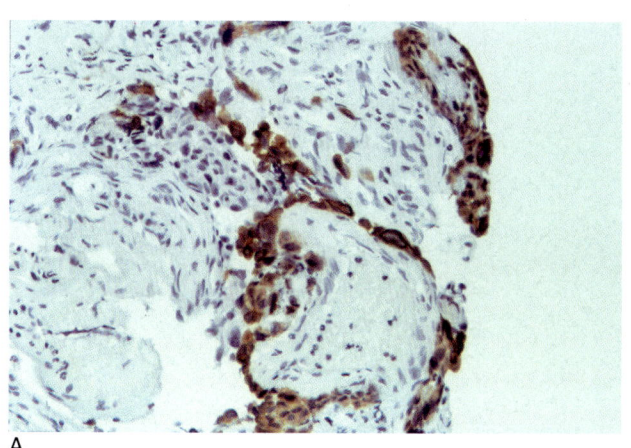

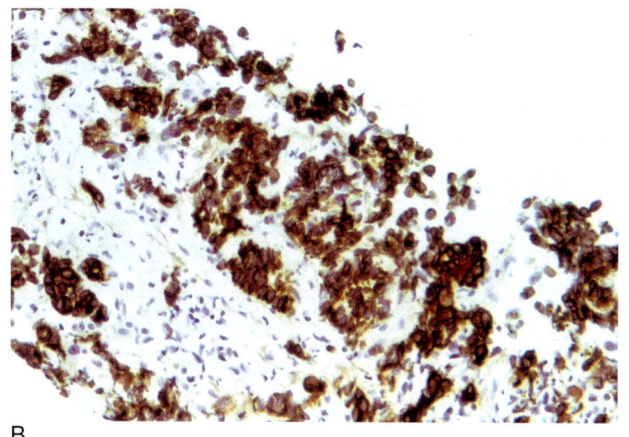

图7.6 在胸膜活检中的间皮细胞（A）和上皮型间皮瘤细胞（B）CK5/CK6呈强阳性反应

表 7.8　CK5/6：在肿瘤中表达的百分率

肿瘤	表达百分率
皮肤，鳞状细胞癌	100
皮肤，基底细胞癌	100
胸腺，胸腺瘤	100
唾液腺，所有肿瘤	93
间皮瘤	76
膀胱，移行细胞癌	62
子宫，子宫内膜癌	50
胰腺，癌	38
乳腺，癌	31
卵巢，癌	25
肝，胆管癌	14
胃肠道，类癌	10
肺，腺癌	5
肝，肝细胞癌	4
肾上腺，癌	0
结肠，腺癌	0
生殖细胞，癌	0
肾，癌	0
前列腺，癌	0
胃，腺癌	0
甲状腺，所有肿瘤	0

(摘自 Chu P, Weiss LM. Expression of CK 5/6 in epithelial neoplasms: An immunohistochemical study of 509 cases. Mod Pathol 2002; 6:6-10)

骨组织肿瘤中，角蛋白不同程度分布于预期的上皮样区域。此类肿瘤包括滑膜肉瘤、上皮样肉瘤、脊索瘤、恶性外周神经鞘瘤及长骨的造釉细胞瘤[156-162]。尽管一些软组织肿瘤在形态上与转移癌类似，但散在的细胞免疫着色却与在癌组织中看到的弥漫强阳性染色不同，特别是应用覆盖广的抗体检测时。冰冻切片是在丙酮或酒精中固定，包括酒精固定的细胞学标本，会产生更多的角蛋白阳性细胞，这可能使诊断混乱，尤其是细胞学标本，因为酒精固定是细针穿刺标本的标准固定剂[133]。

恶性黑色素瘤CK8和CK18免疫组化染色也可呈阳性，但在福尔马林固定、石蜡包埋组织中，仅有1%左右的阳性病例，肿瘤细胞呈局灶性着色[163-166]。实际上在冰冻切片及酒精固定的黑色素瘤标本中阳性细胞数要比福尔马林固定的标本多，认识到这一点对避免将黑色素瘤误诊为癌非常重要，尤其是对酒精固定的细胞学标本[109, 133, 167]。对非上皮样肉瘤及黑色素瘤中角蛋白免疫染色的一致观点认为，尽管通过分子生物技术和更敏感的免疫组化方法（冷冻切片、酒精固定）检测角蛋白确实存在，但在这些肿瘤的福尔马林固定组织中并没有观察到角蛋白的表达，此点从有益于诊断的角度更合乎人们意愿。

已有报道在人的神经胶质及一些星形细胞瘤中有真正的"假性"角蛋白免疫反应活性存在，尤其是使用AE1和34βE12抗体时[140, 168]。另外，AE1/AE3混合抗体可与正常及肿瘤性星形细胞发生交叉反应[141, 169]。假性角蛋白的免疫反应活性可能是与胶质细胞所含的胶质原纤维酸性蛋白的交叉反应所致[142]。通过免疫学或分子生物学技术尚未证实在星形细胞中有角蛋白的存在，这是造成误诊为脑转移癌的一个明显陷阱。CAM5.2抗体与星形胶质细胞不发生反应，因此最好

(4%)、脂肪肉瘤 (21%)、横纹肌肉瘤[141]、恶性外周神经鞘瘤 (5%)、一些恶性纤维组织细胞瘤 (5%)[142]、胃肠间质瘤 (50%)、极少数胸膜孤立性纤维瘤[143]、血管肉瘤 (33%)[144-146]、子宫内膜间质肉瘤[147]和原始神经外胚层肿瘤 (50%)[119, 146, 148-154]。在这些传统的福尔马林固定、石蜡包埋的肿瘤中角蛋白通常呈散在细胞着色，而在癌及肉瘤样癌中染色强而弥漫（图7.7）[155]。另外，在角蛋白阳性伴有部分上皮样分化的软组织和

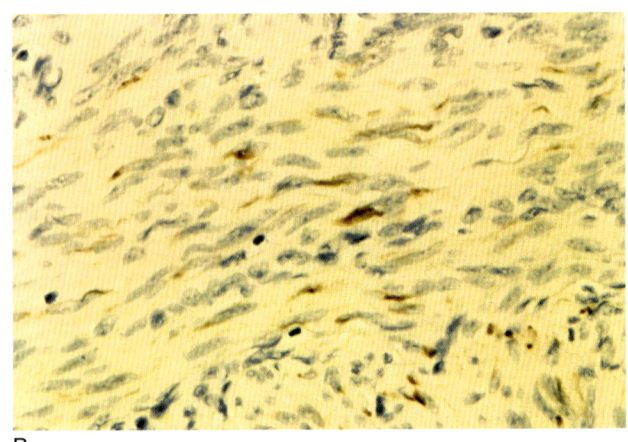

图 7.7　(A，B) 平滑肌肿瘤显示散在的CAM5.2阳性细胞，见于各种间叶组织肿瘤的典型的灶状角蛋白免疫组化染色模式

使用该抗体来检测中枢神经系统中肿瘤的癌分化。

脑膜瘤，尤其是"分泌型"脑膜瘤，可有多达三分之一的病例表达角蛋白[170-173]。

淋巴结内可见模拟上皮分化区，在副皮质区的纤维母细胞性网状细胞LMW角蛋白阳性（图7.8）[174-182]。这些树突状细胞的CAM5.2免疫染色阳性，少数AE1/AE3着色，显示了在淋巴结、扁桃体和脾内广泛的滤泡外树突状细胞突起网络[153, 183]。这些角蛋白阳性细胞对转移癌的诊断是一个陷阱，因为常规看法认为在淋巴结内出现角蛋白阳性细胞即等同于转移癌，这个陷阱是双重的。

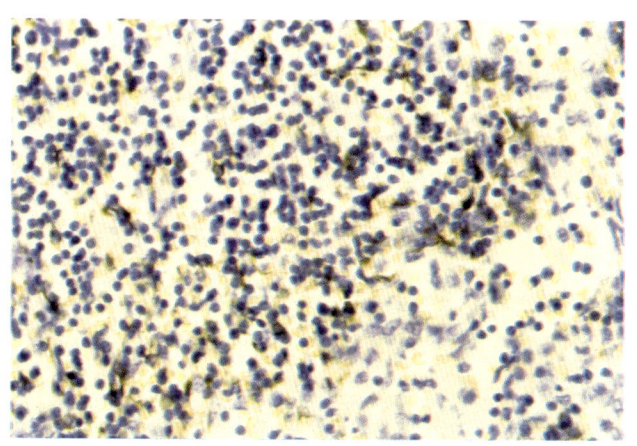

图7.8　此为正常淋巴结，其中滤泡间树突状细胞 CAM5.2+

在乳腺癌病人寻找角蛋白阳性的微小转移灶时，必须对癌细胞与淋巴结边缘窦内成簇的树突状细胞进行鉴别[2]。在淋巴结细针吸取活检和淋巴结印片标本中也可能含有角蛋白阳性细胞而并非转移癌；因此一定要注意角蛋白阳性细胞的形态学特点[150-152, 154]。

已有报道在浆细胞、浆细胞瘤和K-1间变性大细胞淋巴瘤中可见角蛋白阳性反应[183-190]。在间变性大细胞淋巴瘤，可有多达30%的病例检测到角蛋白，同时还伴有一些EMA阳性的间变性淋巴瘤细胞，可能使最终诊断产生混乱。然而，在大部分这些淋巴瘤中角蛋白的广谱抗体仅呈灶状着色。浆细胞瘤同样需要用广谱角蛋白抗体以及包括CD138和κ/λ轻链在内的一组抗体进行染色。

大多数角蛋白免疫染色是用福尔马林固定、石蜡包埋的组织进行的，如要对角蛋白免疫过氧化物酶染色技术进行优化，则福尔马林固定的时间是一个关键因素。固定时间与所需的酶预消化时间紧密相关[156, 191]。通常，如果组织在10%福尔马林中固定时间超过2天，就需要更长的酶预消化时间，而短时固定的组织（数小时）则需要较少的预消化时间。绝大多数角蛋白抗体，如果不是全部的话，都需要抗原修复（依赖于抗体和固定时间），以优化角蛋白抗体的反应（表7.3）。

> **诊断要点：** 非上皮性肿瘤中的角蛋白
>
> 1. 在许多肉瘤中呈灶状阳性（见文中所述）。
> 2. 在黑色素瘤中呈少数灶状阳性。
> 3. 在浆细胞中常见；其他淋巴样肿瘤中少见。
> 4. 在淋巴结树突状细胞中常见。
> 5. 在星形细胞瘤中 AE1/AE3 抗体可能会出现假阳性。

联合（成组）抗体法解决诊断问题

当CK7、CK20、CK5或其他角蛋白抗体与针对其他中间丝（如波形蛋白）的抗体、备选的上皮抗原（如CEA、EMA）抗体或特异性细胞产物（如神经内分泌颗粒）抗体联合应用时，就可以更特异地确定细胞类型。

第三步：伴波形蛋白共表达的癌

正常情况下，间叶和内皮细胞都有波形蛋白的免疫染色，这为免疫反应活性的质量控制提供了一个内对照[192]，如果在血管或间质细胞没有波形蛋白的免疫染色，就说明组织抗原受到严重损害或者染色的其他步骤出错。

在癌性渗液标本中，波形蛋白染色全部呈阳性（可能是活体体液所致），因此没有诊断价值[165]。

开始认为中间丝局限于间叶细胞，现在在各种不同肿瘤包括各种癌内都已发现有波形蛋白的存在（表7.9）。在所有的梭形细胞肿瘤，包括间叶梭形细胞肿瘤和肉瘤样癌，波形蛋白都呈阳性染色。波形蛋白在一些癌中常规表达并较明显，可在成组抗体中用来缩小鉴别诊断的范围。在细胞内波形蛋白常在核周呈带状染色，尤其在子宫内膜样腺癌。波形蛋白共表达阳性率高（超过50%~60%）而且强（超过25%的细胞）的癌包括梭形细胞癌、肾细胞癌（嫌色细胞癌除外）、子宫内膜的内膜样腺癌和恶性混合性苗勒瘤、浆液性卵巢癌、唾液腺多形性腺瘤及滤泡性甲状腺癌[193, 194]。上皮性和肉瘤样间皮瘤也常规表达波形蛋白[195]。有些癌可能也有波形蛋白表达，但阳性率低（10%~20%）、强度小（<10%的细胞），这些癌包括结直肠腺癌、肺腺癌、乳腺癌、前列腺癌及非浆液性卵巢癌。

因此，在转移癌中发现波形蛋白共表达，可有助于缩小鉴别诊断的范围并增加抗体组中其他抗体的价值（图7.9）。

在子宫刮除标本中，波形蛋白共表达对鉴别子宫内膜内膜样腺癌和宫颈管腺癌包括宫颈管腺癌的子宫内膜样变型非常有用。子宫内膜的内膜样癌波形蛋白免疫染色强而宫颈管腺癌很少着色（在宫颈管腺癌中最高只有13%的病例呈灶状弱阳性）[196, 197]。

> **诊断要点**：波形蛋白共表达的癌
>
> 1. 常表达于肾癌、子宫内膜癌、浆液性卵巢癌、唾液腺癌、滤泡性甲状腺癌和肉瘤样（梭形细胞）癌以及恶性混合性苗勒瘤中的上皮和间质成分。
> 2. 在结直肠、肺、乳腺、前列腺和非浆液性卵巢腺癌中可有10%~20%的灶状细胞阳性。
> 3. 在体腔渗液中无诊断价值。
> 4. 在上皮性及肉瘤样间质瘤中通常为阳性。
> 5. 在任何组织中都可作为评价抗原的重要内对照。

第四步：备选的组织系标志物

当缺乏组织系特异性标志物时，这些备选标志物在某些组织类型中具有特征性的免疫染色模式，因而可作为成组抗体的一部分用于证实诊断。

癌胚抗原（CEA）和 HepPar-l

CEA 是一个180kD的糖蛋白，50%为碳水化合

表 7.9 CK/波形蛋白在癌中共表达的主要形式

常见共表达（>50%）	少见共表达（<10%）
子宫内膜腺癌	宫颈管腺癌
肾细胞癌	结直肠腺癌
唾液腺癌	乳腺导管-小叶癌
梭形细胞癌	肺非小细胞癌
甲状腺滤泡癌	前列腺腺癌

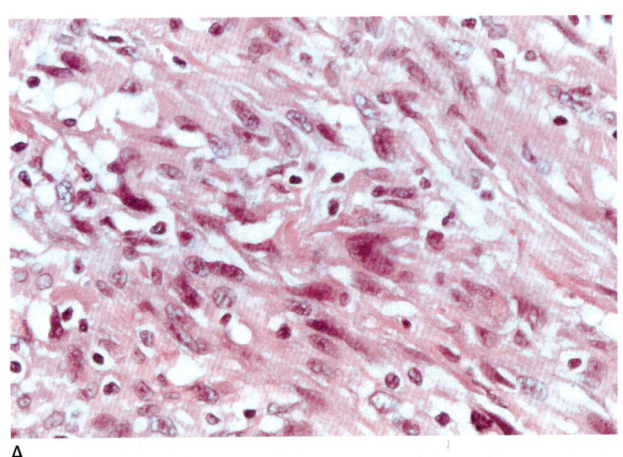

A

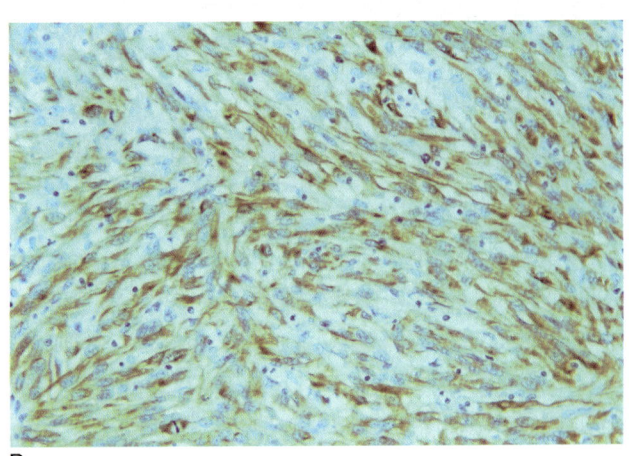

B

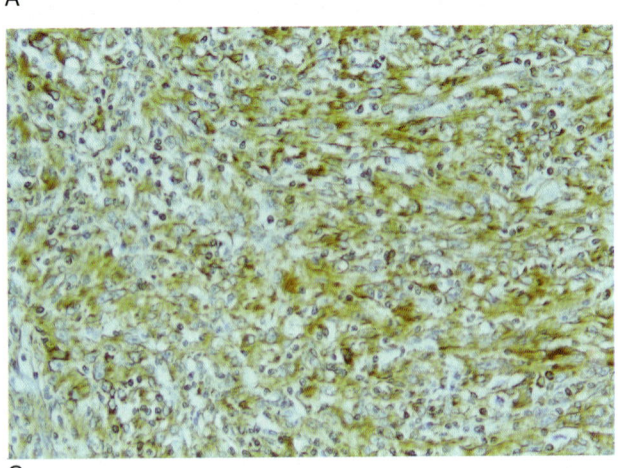

C

图7.9 肺的肉瘤样癌（A）呈丰富的CAM5.2（B）和波形蛋白（C）共表达。肺和上呼吸消化道（upper aerodigestive tract）的绝大部分该类型的癌是肉瘤样鳞状细胞癌

物[198]。针对不同的CEA抗原决定簇有多种CEA抗体，多克隆抗体常与组织非特异性交叉反应抗原及胆管糖蛋白Ⅰ发生交叉反应[199-202]。较老的CD66e系列的CEA抗体在乳腺导管癌以及肺和结直肠癌中呈典型的弥漫强阳性反应。尽管CEA是一个敏感的标志物，但由于其特异性低，所以不能将结直肠原发腺癌与肺腺癌或乳腺导管癌区分开。

肺原发性腺癌典型的呈CK7+、CK20-、CEA+，而结直肠癌呈CK7-、CK20+、CEA+；乳腺导管癌和小叶癌呈CK7+、CK20-、CEA常为+；卵巢癌CK7+、CK20+/-、CEA-[80, 83, 86-88, 203-207]。对大部分CEA抗体呈典型强阳性的肿瘤包括肺、结肠、胃、胆道系统、胰腺、膀胱、宫颈管、鼻窦、汗腺及乳腺腺癌（表7.10、7.11）[177, 208, 209]。当与角蛋白联合应用时，CEA的用途是用于证实CEA的预期染色，无论是阳性还是阴性。

对大部分CEA抗体基本呈阴性反应的肿瘤包括前列腺、肾、肾上腺和子宫内膜腺癌，以及浆液性卵巢肿瘤和间皮瘤[208]。肝细胞来源的肿瘤对单克隆CEA抗体无反应，但对多克隆CEA抗体呈独特的胆小管周围着色，这是因为多克隆抗体与肝胆小管的胆管糖蛋白Ⅰ有交叉反应[210-212]。来源于肺、胃肠道、胸腺、宫颈管和胰胆管的腺癌对CEA抗体典型的呈胞浆强阳性，尽管染色强度可有不同。在86%的肝细胞肝癌中也可见到CD10抗体的小管型免疫染色，而在其他一些癌中尤其是肾细胞癌CD10是在胞浆或胞膜着色[213, 214]。绒毛素（villin）抗体与多克隆CEA抗体相似，在肝细胞肿瘤中也呈胆小管型着色[215]。

在肝CEA的免疫染色类型非常有意义。肝的上皮样血管内皮瘤（EH）可以与癌非常相似，如果证实CD31/CD34及Ⅷ因子阳性，再加上不同的角蛋白染色（常为灶性，有时为弥漫性）和缺乏CEA染色，则可以将肝上皮样血管内皮瘤与癌及肝细胞癌区分开[112]。已证实肿瘤性肝窦状隙有CD34表达，此与正常肝组织不同，可用于原发性肝癌与转移性癌和非肿瘤性肝组织的鉴别诊断，尤其是小的活检标本（图7.10）[216]。

HepPar-1抗体检测的是肝细胞内一个未知功能的蛋白，对肝细胞分化的特异性为79%，并且敏感性高[215, 217, 218]。已有报道真正的肝细胞癌分化（多克隆CEA+、HepPar-1+、窦样细胞CD34+）偶尔可作为来自膀胱和胃的一些腺癌的成分[219, 220]，卵巢肿瘤中肝样癌成分常规表达HepPar-1[221]。

HepPar-1在胃的印戒细胞癌（SRCC）通常呈弥漫性胞浆染色，而乳腺或结直肠SRCC HepPar-1为阴性[222]。

MOC-31抗体（DAKO，Carpinteria，CA）检测一种含量丰富、位于上皮细胞及癌细胞表面的糖蛋白，Morrison等证实，联合应用HepPar-1、CEA和MOC-31能区分99%的肝转移癌和肝细胞癌[218, 223, 224]。

原发性肝癌与转移性腺癌的鉴别

> **诊断要点**：肝癌与转移性肿瘤
>
> 1. 肝癌：多克隆CEA抗体（抗胆管糖蛋白Ⅰ）小管型分布；86%的病例绒毛素及CD10小管型分布；CAM5.2+、AE1/AE3-、CK7/CK20-、窦状隙CD34+、HepPar-1+、MOC-31-、胞浆型TTF-1（71%）（见下面）[225]。
> 2. 胃肠道、肺、乳腺、胸腺、宫颈管、原发性胆管癌：CEA+、AE1/AE3+、CK7/CK20不同程度免疫染色、MOC-31+。
> 3. 非精原细胞瘤性生殖细胞肿瘤：AE1/AE3+、PLAP+。
> 4. 乳腺癌：CEA（S）、CK7+、GCDFP-15+。
> 5. 前列腺、肾、子宫内膜、肾上腺及浆液性卵巢癌和间皮瘤：CEA-。
> 6. 肝上皮样血管内皮瘤：CD31/CD34+、Ⅷ因子+、CAM5.2（S）、CEA-。

上皮细胞膜抗原（EMA）

EMA由位于1号染色体的*MUC1*基因编码并衍化形成，为乳腺黏蛋白复合物，是一个跨膜糖蛋白，在癌细胞中表达增加[226-228]。在正常乳腺，EMA表达于顶端细胞膜，而在肿瘤细胞，EMA环绕整个细胞膜分布[227]。肿瘤细胞大分子量糖蛋白的增加干扰了

表7.10 癌胚抗原在腺癌中的免疫染色	
癌胚抗原（+）	癌胚抗原（-）
鼻窦	前列腺
肺	肾
结肠	肾上腺
胃	子宫内膜
胆管*	卵巢浆液性
胰腺	
汗腺	
乳腺	

* 多克隆抗体呈小管周型染色

表 7.11　CK/CEA 与癌的鉴别诊断

肿瘤	K903	CAM5.2	AE1/AE3	CK7	CK20	CEA	CK17	TTF-1
Merkel 细胞	N	+	+	R~N	+	N	N	R~N
小细胞癌	N	+	+	+	N	S	N	+
肺腺癌	S	+	+	+	R~N	+	S	S
乳腺	S	+	+	+	N	R~N	S	N
精原细胞瘤	N	R~N	R~N	N	N	N	N	N
子宫内膜	S	+	+	+	N	S	S	N
膀胱	S	+	+	+	+	R~N	+	N
腮腺	S	+	+	+	N	N	N	N
神经内分泌系统	N	+	+	+	N	S	S	N
胰腺	S	+	+	S	S	+	S	N
胆管	S	+	+	+	S	+	S	N
胃	N	+	+	S	+	+	N	N
结直肠	N	+	+	R~N	+	+	N	N
前列腺	N	+	+	S	N	N	R~N	N
肾癌	N	+	+	N	N	N	N	N
生殖细胞癌	N	+	+	+	N	N	N	N
肝细胞*	N	+	N	R~N	N	+	N	N
卵巢黏液性	N	+	+	+	+	+	N	N
卵巢非黏液性	N	+	+	+	N	+	S	N
甲状腺	S	+	+	S	S	S	S	+
肾上腺	N	N	N	N	N	N	N	N
胸腺	S	+	+	N	N	S	N	N
宫颈管	R~N	+	+	+	N	+	N	N

* 多克隆 CEA 围绕小管分布

+，阳性；S，有时阳性；R，少数细胞阳性；N，阴性

细胞与细胞和细胞与基质之间的黏附作用[229]。

EMA 抗体作为 CK 的补充用于检测上皮性分化。梭形细胞、小细胞和大细胞肿瘤可偶尔表达 EMA，但 CK 可能仅呈灶状阳性[230-232]。

有几种 EMA 抗体可用，每一种抗体针对该大分子糖蛋白抗原的不同抗原决定簇，包括 MAM-6[233]、episialin[234]、CA15-3[236]、DF3 抗原[237]，以及乳腺上皮黏蛋白[238,239]。对于肿瘤性上皮分化，绝大多数抗体有 85% 的敏感性和 89% 的特异性[240]。

EMA抗体在皮肤及其附属器、乳腺、肺、胆管、胰腺、唾液腺、尿路上皮、子宫内膜和宫颈管、前列腺导管、甲状腺、间皮以及来自这些组织的肿瘤中染色阳性（表 7.12）。许多肉瘤样癌以及上皮样和肉瘤样间皮瘤也呈阳性[61,63,240]。与间皮瘤浓厚的膜染色相比，反应性的间皮细胞膜染色较弱[241,242]。很多类型的腺癌EMA染色阳性，因此在渗出液中必须与间皮细胞相鉴别，可应用成组抗体包括CK5/CK6、CEA、LeuM1 和 BerEP4[61,121,243]。

正常和肿瘤性造血细胞的部分亚群表达 EMA，包括浆细胞和有核红细胞[190,244]，肿瘤性细胞包括淋巴细胞为主型霍奇金淋巴瘤中的 L&H 细胞（60% 的病例）[245-247]、5% 的 B 细胞淋巴瘤[31,248,249]、18% 的 T 细胞淋巴瘤[250-253]以及大约 60% 的间变性大细胞淋巴瘤[254,258]。EMA抗体对癌没有绝对的敏感性和特异性，因此总是与成组的CKs和其他证实性抗体如白细胞共同抗原一起应用[213,240]。

除了上皮性肿瘤，许多肉瘤、中枢神经系统肿瘤、小圆细胞肿瘤和一些生殖细胞肿瘤EMA也可阳性[240]。这些肿瘤包括恶性神经鞘瘤、滑膜肉瘤、平滑肌肉瘤、恶性纤维组织细胞瘤、上皮样肉瘤和脊索瘤[206]。除了上面提到的最后两种肿瘤，其他肿瘤 EMA 免疫染色都呈局灶性。

脉络丛肿瘤和脑膜瘤的细胞膜 EMA 呈强阳性[240]。除了在绒毛膜癌和畸胎瘤中有不同程度的 EMA 染色，大部分生殖细胞肿瘤 EMA 阴性，而在肾母细胞瘤和肝母细胞瘤这些上皮性小圆细胞肿瘤的大部分病例中 EMA 为阳性[240,259]。

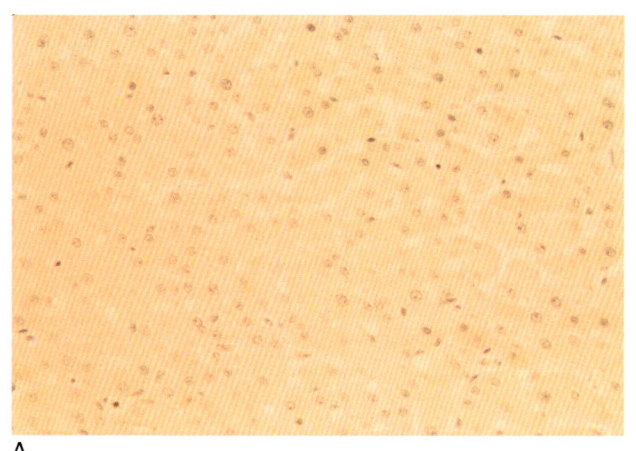
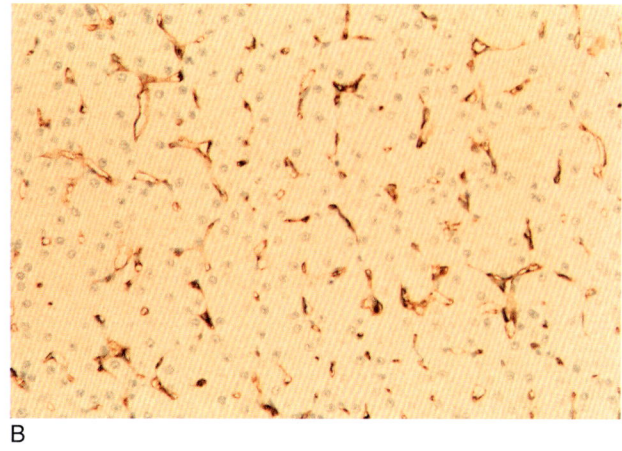
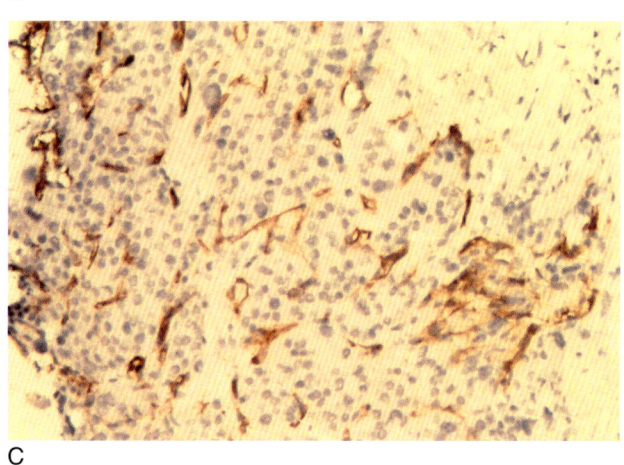

图7.10　正常肝组织（A）窦状隙CD34不表达，而在肝腺瘤（B）和肝细胞癌（C）的窦状隙CD34常为阳性；这对在针吸或活检标本中确定肝原发性肿瘤非常有用

表7.12　EMA在癌和非上皮组织中的免疫染色		
典型阳性	绝大多数阴性	非上皮组织灶状阳性
皮肤及附属器	除绒毛膜癌/畸胎瘤以外的生殖细胞肿瘤	浆细胞
乳腺		有核红细胞
肺		霍奇金淋巴瘤的L&H细胞
胆管		非霍奇金淋巴瘤的少数细胞
胰腺		间变性大细胞淋巴瘤
唾液腺		恶性神经鞘瘤
尿路上皮		滑膜肉瘤
子宫内膜		平滑肌肉瘤
宫颈内管		恶性纤维组织细胞瘤
前列腺导管		
甲状腺		
间皮瘤		
肉瘤样癌		
脑膜瘤		

诊断要点：上皮细胞膜抗原（EMA）

1. 作为备选标记用于上皮性肿瘤的鉴别诊断，因为CKs在未分化癌中可能呈少量灶状阳性或阴性。
2. EMA免疫染色可在胞膜或胞浆，或两者都有。
3. 恶性黑色素瘤为阴性。
4. 除了绒毛膜癌和畸胎瘤以外的生殖细胞肿瘤为阴性。
5. EMA在浆细胞、60%的间变性大细胞淋巴瘤、霍奇金淋巴瘤的L&H细胞和部分T细胞、B细胞淋巴瘤表达。
6. 在恶性间皮瘤和一些反应性增生的间皮细胞呈强阳性，在正常间皮细胞呈弱阳性或阴性。

生殖细胞肿瘤

对生殖细胞肿瘤的正确诊断非常重要，因为即使是在进展期其对治疗的反应也非常好[5,29]。它们的原发灶可能不明确，包括精原细胞瘤及其变型、胚胎性癌、内胚窦瘤和绒毛膜癌。联合应用单层CKs、EMA、PLAP、AFP 和 HCG 抗体可以对大多数病例作出正确诊断。

据文献资料抗PLAP抗体包括M2A、43-9F和TRA-1-60[260-262]。CAM5.2 在除精原细胞瘤外的生殖细胞肿瘤中呈弥漫阳性，大部分精原细胞瘤主要呈阴性但可有极少的灶状着色[263]。在精原细胞瘤中如果角蛋白染色范围超过灶状，就应怀疑其有胚胎性癌的成分。

在经典的精原细胞瘤，PLAP 在细胞膜皱褶和胞浆呈强阳性染色，而在精母细胞变型为阴性[264,265]，在胚胎性癌、卵黄囊瘤和绒毛膜癌呈不同程度的阳性[265,271]。PLAP 对生殖细胞肿瘤并非 100% 的特异，有 10%~15% 的非生殖细胞癌也呈阳性，包括苗勒癌、胃肠道、肺、少数乳腺及肾癌[272,273]，但在这些癌中EMA为阳性而生殖细胞肿瘤为阴性。

除了绒癌所有生殖细胞肿瘤EMA都呈阴性，约 50% 的绒癌 EMA 呈阳性[263,265,274]。AFP 在绝大多数卵黄囊瘤中呈斑片状分布，而在胚胎性癌仅有部分病例呈灶状分布[263,265,274-276]。

生殖细胞肿瘤中的肝样分化，尤其是卵黄囊瘤，典型的呈AFP阳性，但并不显示真正的肝细胞分化的免疫组化谱，即多克隆 CEA 胆管型免疫染色。

OCT4是由POU5F1基因编码的转录因子，参与多潜能细胞和胚系细胞的发育和分化。OCT4抗体对精原细胞瘤/无性细胞瘤和胚胎性癌具有高敏感性和特异性[277-279]。OCT4着色部位在细胞核，典型的在精原细胞瘤/无性细胞瘤和胚胎性癌中有90%的细胞核着色。部分卵巢透明细胞癌OCT4可呈阳性，但其他类型的生殖细胞瘤和癌阴性。混合性生殖细胞肿瘤若伴有精原细胞瘤成分则呈阳性。

> **诊断要点：生殖细胞肿瘤**
>
> 1. 精原细胞瘤：CAM5.2（R~N），PLAP+，OCT4+，EMA-。
> 2. 胚胎性癌：CAM5.2+，PLAP+，OCT4+，EMA（N），AFP（R~N），CD30+。
> 3. 卵黄囊瘤：CAM5.2+，PLAP+，EMA-，AFP+，OCT4-。
> 4. 绒毛膜癌：CAM5.2+，PLAP+/-，EMA-/+，HCG+，OCT4-。
> 5. PLAP 在 10%~15% 的非生殖细胞癌中呈阳性，但其 EMA 也呈阳性。

第五步：肿瘤分化抗原——细胞特异性产物

即使联合应用 CKs、CEA、EMA 和 vimentin 抗体可以查明大多数转移性肿瘤的组织来源，但仍有一部分肿瘤难以鉴定其来源。另外有一些针对细胞特异性产物的抗体，这些抗体对某些组织具有非常高的特异性，在绝大多数病例中，应用这些抗体可以使病理学家更精准地寻找转移癌的来源。

在这里讨论了部分此类抗体，包括嗜铬素A、突触素、甲状腺球蛋白、前列腺特异性抗原、抑制素、melan-A、TTF-1、CDX2、GCDFP-15、绒毛素。

神经内分泌抗体

针对神经内分泌细胞成分的抗体通常被用于鉴别发生在某些器官的肿瘤的细胞类型，如肺、甲状腺、结肠和肾上腺。此类抗体一般不作为对未分化肿瘤一开始的筛选检测，因此关于这方面的文献很少[280]。联合应用下列的成组抗体是非常重要的，因为没有哪一个单一的抗体具有完美的特异性和敏感性。

众所周知，在各种类型的癌中应用IHC都可能显示一些"神经内分泌细胞"，但这并不能诊断"神经内分泌癌"，只有在综合了临床表现、影像学、组织学及免疫组织化学检查后才能作出诊断。

嗜铬素（chromogranin，Cg）

嗜铬素（A、B和C型）是一组单体蛋白，是神经内分泌细胞神经分泌颗粒中可溶性蛋白的主要组成成分；嗜铬素A（CgA）分子量为75kD，分布最广泛。嗜铬素细胞的免疫染色质量与电镜下神经内分泌型分泌颗粒的数量高度相关[281]。

LK2H10 是一个单克隆抗体，在文献中报道最多[281-284]。随着细胞分化程度的降低，免疫染色的强度也降低。LK2H10的特异性接近100%，但敏感性只接近75%[285]。

LK2H10 对典型类癌的敏感性最低（约50%），但类癌的组织学识别是非常容易的。

突触素（Syn）

突触素是一种糖蛋白，是神经内分泌细胞分泌颗粒膜的组成部分[280,286]，在各种神经内分泌肿瘤中可被单克隆抗体（SY38）识别。突触素是一个广谱的神经内分泌标志物[287]，其敏感性高但特异性比嗜铬素抗体低。据报道，SY38的免疫染色在鉴别神经内分泌类型转移癌中最有效[280]。单独的突触素免疫染色尚不足以作为"神经内分泌"肿瘤的标记。若结合适当的形态学特征，突触素对于确定神经内分泌特征是很有用的。

大细胞未分化神经内分泌癌（LCNEC）可表现为MCUP，如果不应用合适的神经内分泌标志物标记极易误诊。LCNEC的正确诊断具有重要意义，因为不论是肺还是胃肠道LCNEC与小细胞癌具有同样差的预后[288, 289]。在LCNEC，突触素可能是阳性率最高的标志物[289]。

有一项研究，在小细胞肺癌中可有多达79%的病例突触素呈阳性，而嗜铬素为47%~60%，铃蟾肽为45%，NSE为33%~60%[290]。在非小细胞癌中，突触素的阳性率为8%[291]。

Leu7

自人的T细胞系CD57抗原产生了一个单克隆抗体（HNK-1），此T细胞系分化抗原是自然杀伤细胞活性的标记物[292, 293]。CD57抗体还能识别中枢及周围神经系统髓磷脂中的髓磷脂相关糖蛋白。在肠嗜铬细胞、胰腺胰岛细胞、胰岛细胞瘤、类癌、嗜铬细胞瘤和小细胞肺癌中也发现CD57呈阳性反应[294-297]。CD57缺乏像嗜铬素和突触素那样的敏感性及特异性，因此应当与包括这些抗体在内的成组抗体联合应用。

神经特异性烯醇化酶（NSE）

烯醇化酶由五种不同的形式组成，每一种都由三个同二聚体和两个杂合体组成。在各种正常和肿瘤性神经内分泌细胞中都发现有NSE，但以大脑中占优势[298-301]。起初认为NSE是神经内分泌分化的特异性标志物，后来发现实际上在任何类型的肿瘤中都可能有NSE表达，因此NSE抗体对于神经内分泌分化的筛选来说并不好。虽然如此，若与其他更具特异性的抗体如嗜铬素和突触素联合使用，对适当的神经内分泌形态的鉴定和证实还是有用的。

肽类激素

在正常情况下，肽类激素产生于独特的、隔离的组织，并且一般情况下同样的激素产物可以在肿瘤中重现。除少数病例外，内分泌肿瘤都有其特征性的组织形态，因此关于激素产物的研究常常只是出于学术兴趣。

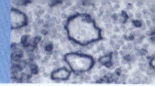

不明来源转移癌的免疫组织化学 7

分化差的内分泌肿瘤，依其原发部位不同，可以产生特征性的肽类激素。这些低分化的神经内分泌肿瘤和它们的激素产物包括胰岛细胞瘤（胰岛素、胰高血糖素、生长抑素、胃泌素）、肺小细胞癌（45%的病例产生铃蟾肽）[290]、甲状腺髓样癌（降钙素）。

神经内分泌肿瘤的CK表达谱多少有些特征，实际上所有的神经内分泌肿瘤角蛋白8和18均呈阳性（如CAM5.2），有时CK7阳性，但CK20和高分子量角蛋白（如K903）阴性。Merkel细胞癌特征性的CK20阳性（67%的病例）、CK7阴性，与小细胞肺癌的免疫染色正好相反（CK7+、CK20-）。

> **诊断要点**：神经内分泌分化
>
> 1. 典型的神经内分泌细胞角蛋白表达谱：CAM 5.2+，CK7（S）。
> 2. 嗜铬素和突触素相互补充作为成组诊断性抗体的一部分。
> 3. 特异性多肽（铃蟾肽、胰高血糖素等）可作为诊断过程的补充。
> 4. 部分周围神经内分泌癌可以呈TTF-1+（见下述）。
> 5. 部分胃肠道的神经内分泌癌可以呈CDX-2+（见下述）。

甲状腺球蛋白

甲状腺球蛋白是一个分子量为670kD的重糖基化蛋白，为甲状腺素的产生提供碘化位点，是甲状腺滤泡上皮的独特产物。绝大部分甲状腺癌的甲状腺球蛋白免疫染色为阳性，尽管大多数阳性病例很容易诊断为滤泡性或乳头状癌，但未分化间变性癌可能只有极少数阳性细胞。甲状腺癌对单克隆CEA抗体几乎总是呈阴性，这点有助于鉴别诊断。在髓样癌中，甲状腺球蛋白阳性细胞呈散在分布，相反，在分化差的滤泡性癌中可看到降钙素阳性细胞[303-305]。在10%~25%的白血病病人的骨髓白血病母细胞中可见到有甲状腺球蛋白[306]。

> **诊断要点**：甲状腺球蛋白
>
> 1. 几乎所有的甲状腺癌均呈阳性，在分化差及间变性甲状腺癌中阳性减弱或散在分布。
> 2. 对甲状腺癌高度特异，在一些白血病母细胞中有少数细胞阳性。

甲状腺转录因子-1（TTF-1）

TTF-1是一个核组织特异性蛋白转录因子，仅发现于甲状腺和甲状腺肿瘤（任何组织学类型），以及肺癌包括腺癌（75%）、非小细胞癌（63%）、神经内分泌癌和小细胞癌（>90%）及鳞状细胞癌（10%）[307-312]。在胚胎发育期的甲状腺、间脑和呼吸道上皮中TTF-1选择性表达，TTF-1结合并激活Clara细胞产生的表面活性剂蛋白因子[313, 314]。在肺或甲状腺以外的癌中极少看到TTF-1表达（图7.11）[315-317]。肺的神经内分泌肿瘤，包括典型和非典型类癌以及大细胞神经内分泌癌TTF-1几乎总是阳性，说明了其与小细胞癌的亲缘关系[316]。肺外器官来源的小细胞和大细胞神经内分泌癌 TTF-1 也常常呈阳性[318]。这些部位包括前列腺、膀胱、宫颈、胃肠道、甲状腺和乳腺[318, 319]。

在鉴别原发癌和转移癌，尤其是在肺或胸性渗液中，TTF-1的使用使其变得简单明了[320, 321]。CK7和CK20联合TTF-1和CEA是区别原发性肺癌和转移性肺癌的最佳抗体组合。在Roh[332]的研究中，TTF-1对淋巴结转移性肺癌的敏感性为69%。

Chang等人[323]最近证实了TTF-1对肺癌的特异性。在肝细胞癌中，有71%的病例TTF-1可呈胞浆染色，但没有核染色[225]。

> **诊断要点：TTF-1**
>
> 1. 在甲状腺来源的任何组织学类型的肿瘤中均呈核染色。
> 2. 在大多数肺癌中呈核染色——腺癌（66%）、大细胞癌和小细胞癌（95%）。
> 3. 其他部位的小细胞癌（胃肠道、膀胱、子宫颈、前列腺）虽然少见，但常常呈TTF-1阳性。

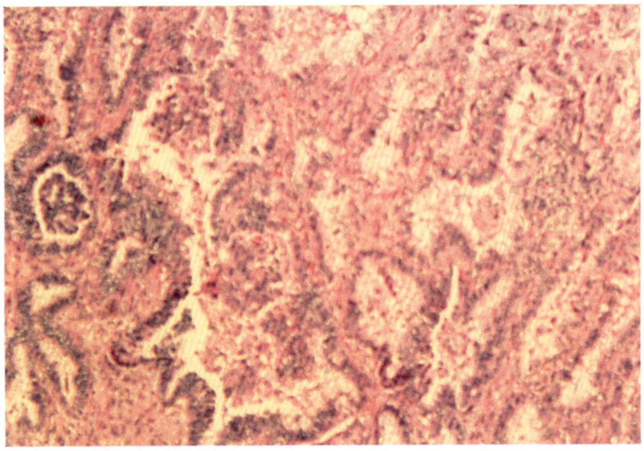

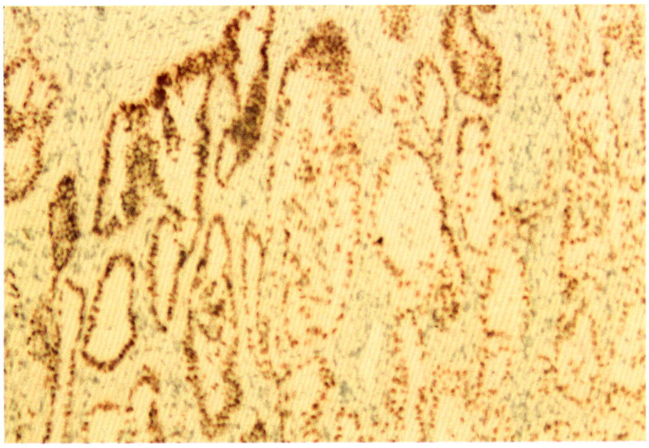

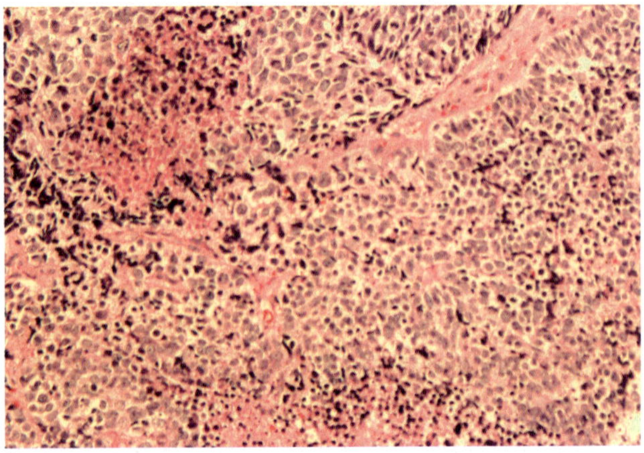

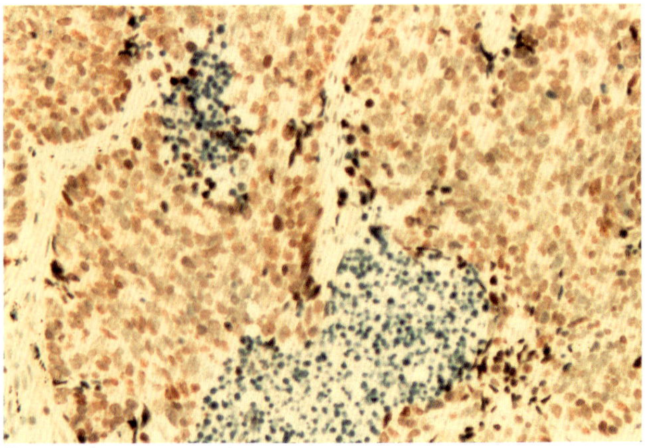

图7.11 甲状腺转录因子-1（TTF-1）抗体可以鉴别60%~70%的肺腺癌（A，B）和95%的肺小细胞癌（C，D）

不明来源转移癌的免疫组织化学 7

联合应用TTF-1的鉴别诊断

原发性肺癌与转移性乳腺癌：
1. *肺：TTF-1+，CK7+，CEA+。
2. *乳腺：TTF-1-，CK7+，CEA+，GCDFP15（S），ER/PR（S）。

原发性肺腺癌与恶性上皮样间皮瘤：
1. 肺：TTF-1+，CK7+，Bg8+，MOC-31+，BerEP4+，CEA+，CK5/CK6（R~N），calretinin（R）。
2. 间皮瘤：TTF-1（N），CK5/CK6+，CK7+，CK20（R~N），BerEP4（N），Bg8（N），CEA（N），calretinin+，mesothelin+，WT-1+。

原发性肺癌与所有类型的转移性甲状腺癌：
1. 肺：TTF-1+，CEA+，甲状腺球蛋白（N）。
2. 甲状腺：TTF-1+，CEA（N），甲状腺球蛋白（S）。

原发性肺癌与非肺源转移性癌：
1. 肺：TTF-1+。
2. 其他部位的癌：TTF-1（N）。
3. 其他适用的特异性抗体。

绒毛素（villin）

绒毛素是一种钙依赖性肌动蛋白结合骨架蛋白，见于小肠的刷状缘及近端肾小管上皮。刷状缘是结直肠癌的特征，在超微结构水平表现为微绒毛，是由一个致密的微丝核心、核根及表面的多糖组成。有多达33%的肺腺癌可在超微结构水平观察到微绒毛根，它们的出现与绒毛素的免疫染色密切相关[324-327]。绒毛素抗体可用于识别绒毛蛋白分子的存在，几乎所有结直肠癌及超过90%的肺癌有微绒毛根[281-284]。CKs是鉴别肺癌和结直肠癌抗体组合的必需部分，90%的肺腺癌CK20-，而结直肠腺癌CK20+。绒毛素与多克隆CEA相似，在肝细胞肿瘤中呈胆小管型分布[215]。

CDX2

CDX2是编码一种转录蛋白因子的同源异形盒基因，该蛋白因子引导从十二指肠区到直肠肠上皮细胞的发育[328]。CDX2是在1983年发现的，其编码的蛋白被称为同源域（homeodomains），在很多多细胞生物体的发育过程中非常重要。同源异形盒是一段保守的DNA序列，其编码的蛋白作为转录因子通过与DNA特定区域结合而起控制其他基因的作用。CDX2的缺失对胚胎的发育是致死性的，而其杂合子则导致胃肠道发育异常[329-332]。

Barbareschi等人发现用CDX2-88克隆检测结直肠癌的特异性和敏感性都非常高，同时发现其他的胃肠道腺癌和卵巢黏液性肿瘤也有CDX2表达[333]。通过对石蜡包埋组织和细胞学标本的研究，他们得出结论：CDX2对肠分化有高度敏感性和特异性（表7.13）。其他研究证实了CDX2对肠源性腺癌的高特异性，包括胃、十二指肠、胃食管、胰腺和胆道系统[334, 335]。在结直肠和十二指肠腺癌CDX2倾向于在大部分细胞核中呈弥漫性分布，而来自其他肠道部位的腺癌倾向于在少部分细胞中染色。在一项研究中发现，肠源性神经内分泌癌只有42%的病例呈灶状核阳性[335]。在Barbareschi等人的研究中，在回肠/阑尾分化好的神经内分泌癌CDX2的表达最强，而直肠和上消化道则表达较低。另外，在39%的胃肠道外神经内分泌肿瘤CDX2呈低表达，包括膀胱、乳腺、子宫、涎腺、前列腺和肺[336]。

毫不奇怪，就像膀胱中的脐尿管囊肿一样，来源于肠脐尿管的膀胱腺癌也常为CDX2+（图7.12）。

Wang等人研究了原发性膀胱腺癌和结直肠腺癌累及膀胱之间免疫组化的不同[337]。能够区别这些肿瘤的关键抗体是β-catenin（克隆14，Transduction Labs，Lexington，KY）、CK7和血栓调节素（thrombomodulin）。全部的结直肠癌呈β-catenin核阳性（膀胱阴性），CK7及血栓调节素阴性；而膀胱腺癌血栓调节素全部为阳性，CK7呈不同程度阳性。

重要的是，具有肠上皮形态特征的其他黏液性肿瘤如有杯状细胞的肺"胶样"癌（100%）和部分卵巢黏液性癌（64%）为CDX2阳性[335]。由于大多数肺胶样癌TTF-1为阳性，因此可将其与转移性结直肠黏液腺癌区别开。卵巢黏液性癌可通过CK7对卵巢肿瘤的

表7.13　CDX2与绒毛素免疫染色（2~3+）* 在不同部位腺癌的百分率

癌	CDX2	绒毛素
结直肠	99	82
十二指肠	100	100
胃	70	42
食管	67	78
胰腺	32	40
胆管	25	60
卵巢黏液性	64	64
膀胱	100	100
甲状腺	4	0
前列腺	4	0

* 摘自 Werling et al. Am J Surg Pathol 2003;27（3):303-310

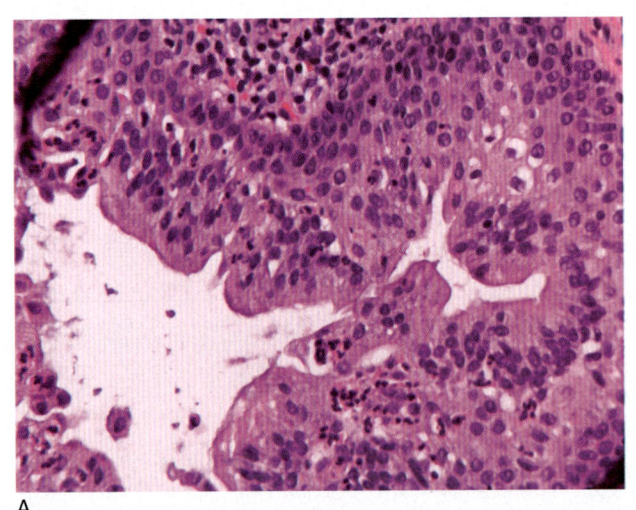 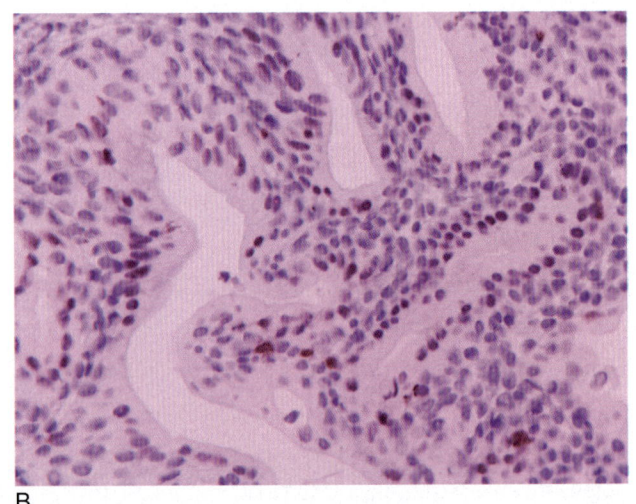

图 7.12　脐尿管囊肿（A，HE）；(B) CDX2 在膀胱穹隆部脐尿管残余中核阳性证实了这种囊肿的胃肠来源

典型免疫染色与胃肠黏液性癌区别开。有肠分化特征的子宫颈腺癌 CDX2 与 CK20 均为阴性[338]。

在前列腺或甲状腺癌中CDX2很少阳性，可呈局灶性染色[335]。同时应用绒毛素抗体可增加对肠分化的特异性。虽然在一些非肠源性癌中可以见到CDX2，但这些肿瘤中绒毛素为阴性[335]。在肝、肝细胞癌、肾癌、乳腺癌、肺癌、宫颈癌（伴肠分化）或唾液腺癌无 CDX2 免疫染色[338]。由于 CDX2 在上消化道癌中也可为阳性，因此可同时应用CK20+/CK7-来增强CDX2对结直肠癌肝转移诊断的特异性[339]。子宫或卵巢的子宫内膜样癌可与结直肠癌相似，也可显示 CDX2 核染色，在这种情况下，需要用包括绒毛素、波形蛋白和雌激素受体在内的一组抗体与结直肠癌进行鉴别（图 7.13）。

> **诊断要点**：CDX2
>
> 1. 对肠分化具有高度敏感性和特异性。
> 2. 膀胱腺癌为CDX2+，血栓调节素+，CK7+；而结直肠癌血栓调节素和CK7为阴性，β-catenin核阳性。
> 3. 肺胶样癌 TTF-1+，卵巢黏液性癌为 CDX2+。
> 4. 卵巢黏液性癌 CK7+，结肠癌 CK7-。
> 5. 绒毛素能增加对肠分化的特异性。
> 6. 卵巢和子宫的子宫内膜样腺癌 25% 的病例为 CDX2+（图 7.13）。

在"最低分化"的结肠癌中 CDX2 表达显著降低，并且常与 DNA 错配修复基因有关[340]。

前列腺癌抗原

前列腺特异性抗原

总起来说，前列腺特异性抗原（PSA）和前列腺酸性磷酸酶（PAP）能标记出95%以上的前列腺癌，但有一些需要注意之处。随着Gleason分级的提高，这两种抗体在肿瘤细胞的免疫染色下降，并且PAP在很多其他类型的肿瘤中也有表达，包括后肠类癌[341]。已经发现 PSA 在一些唾液腺导管癌、1/3的乳腺癌和汗腺肿瘤、两性尿道旁腺、膀胱的腺性膀胱炎、脐尿管残余及某些肛门腺中呈斑片状染色[342-350]。然而，PSA对前列腺组织还是有高度特异性的，其功能为精液丝氨酸蛋白酶[351, 352]，并可显示某些肿瘤的组织学亚型，包括黏液性、印戒细胞和子宫内膜样癌[353-355]。转移的前列腺癌在转移部位（包括淋巴结）可有不同程度的PSA染色[356-358]。短时脱钙不会使 PSA 免疫活性消失。

已发现 PSA 在来自皮肤的恶性黑色素瘤及其转移灶的肿瘤细胞中呈散在阳性[359]。这不应引起诊断困难，因为前列腺癌的 LMW 角蛋白抗体如 CAM5.2 呈弥漫强阳性，这也再一次说明了使用成组抗体检测肿瘤的必要性。

涎腺导管癌PSA和PAP常呈斑片状分布，并有雄激素受体（AR）的强阳性染色[360]，PSA+、PAP+、AR+ 与涎腺导管癌临床表现密切相关，已为诊断所必需。

前列腺特异性膜抗原

前列腺特异性膜抗原（PSMA）与转铁蛋白受体

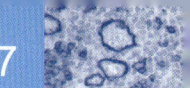

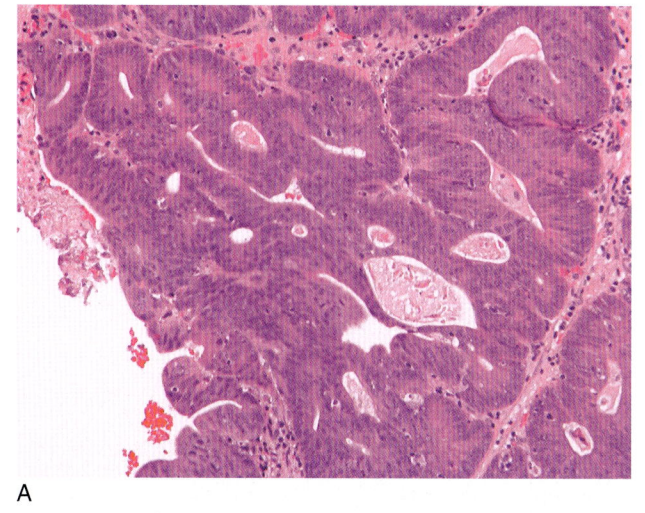

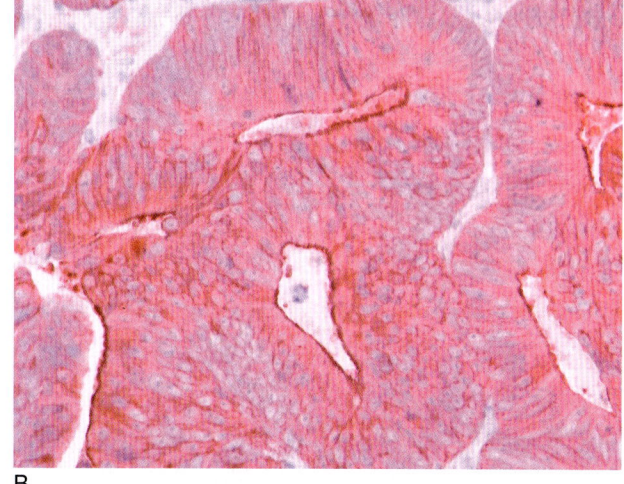

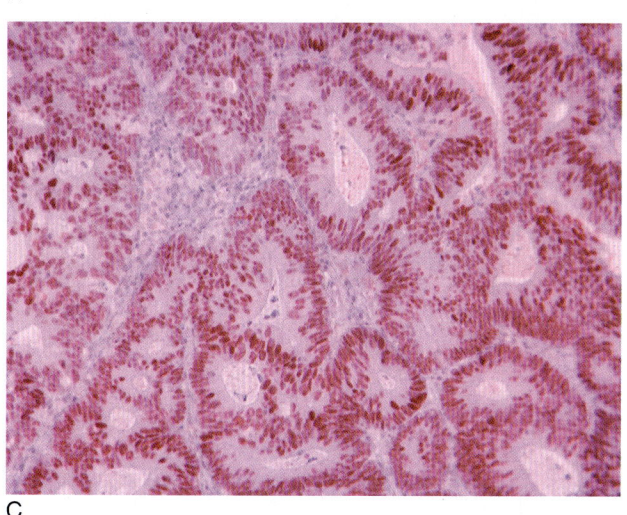

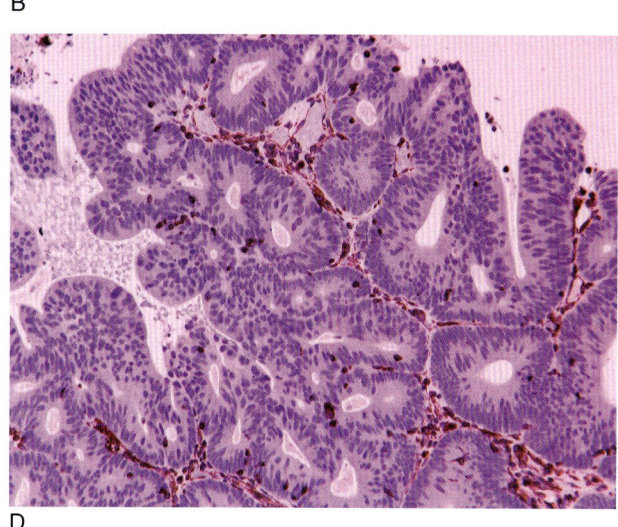

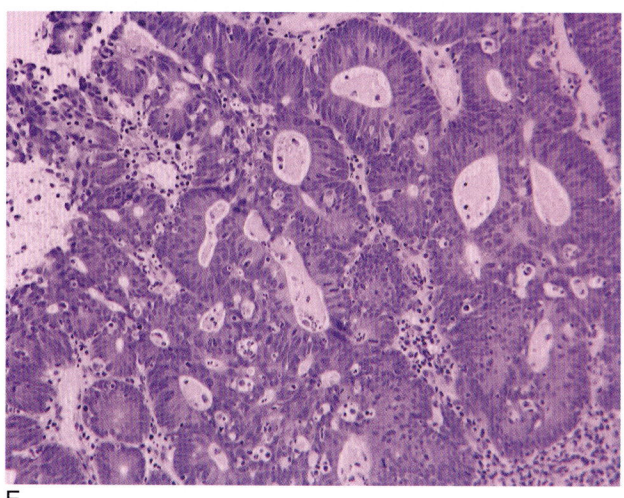

图7.13 侵入阴道的子宫内膜样癌的形态学（A，HE切片）；（B）绒毛素+，（C）CDX2+，（D）波形蛋白-，（E）ER受体-，证实为转移的结肠癌

有部分同源性，对前列腺细胞高度特异[361-364]。与PAP不同，PSMA在前列腺癌时表达上调，因此在高级别前列腺癌中染色更强[362,363,365]。PSMA也有前列腺外表达，见于结肠神经内分泌细胞、乳腺和唾液腺[305,306,309]。文献中引用的抗体为7E11-C5.3[366,367]和3F5.4G6[368]。对来源不明的转移性肿瘤，PSMA对前列腺癌有高度特异性（见第14章）。

α-甲基脂酰辅酶A消旋酶

α-甲基脂酰辅酶A消旋酶（α-methylacyl-CoA racemase, AMACR）（*P504S*基因编码）是线粒体过氧化物酶，催化羧基辅酶A硫酯的α-甲基的消旋作用，出现在前列腺组织和各种癌组织（结直肠、卵巢、乳腺、膀胱、肺、肾细胞）、黑色素瘤和淋巴瘤[369]。虽然对于前列腺癌转移灶不是特异的，但对前列腺穿刺活检需与癌鉴别时 AMACR 却十分有用。Zhou[369]运用多克隆抗体发现，大多数前列腺癌（83%）AMACR 为阳性，但在高级别 PIN 中也呈阳性（64%），在萎缩的腺体 36% 为阳性[369, 370]。

Jiang 用针对 P504S 的单克隆抗体（13H4 克隆）也发现在各种正常组织和肿瘤中有免疫活性[370]。然而，单克隆抗体在前列腺癌中 100% 阳性，而在良性腺体只有 12% 阳性，在萎缩腺体中没有着色。对于前列腺尿道部的肾源性腺瘤是一个诊断陷阱，因为这个部位的病灶常呈弥漫性阳性且缺乏基底细胞存在的证据[371]。

Beach 等认为 AMACR 有 18% 的假阴性率，并且偶尔对前列腺良性病变染色，因此建议 AMACR 用于前列腺时需联合应用基底细胞抗体 p63 和 K903。他们认为很重要的一点是，腺腔及腔下圆周型免疫着色对癌是高度特异的。

肾细胞癌抗原

肾细胞癌抗原（RCC）是一个 200kD 的糖蛋白，称为 gp200，存在于各种正常组织的细胞表面和胞浆，包括肾近端小管的刷状缘、乳腺腺泡的表面、附睾、甲状旁腺和甲状腺组织[372]。McGregor 等研究了一些非肾肿瘤发现 29% 的乳腺肿瘤、28% 的胚胎性癌及所有的甲状旁腺腺瘤 RCC 都呈阳性[373]。80% 的原发性肾细胞癌 RCC 阳性（透明细胞癌 84%，乳头状癌 96%，嫌色细胞癌 45%，肉瘤样癌 25%，集合管癌 0%），其中 93% 的病例其阳性细胞超过 10%。其他原发性肾肿瘤无阳性表达，包括嗜酸细胞瘤（oncocytomas）。有 67% 的转移性肾癌 RCC 阳性，只有 2% 的非肾转移癌 RCC 阳性（绝大多数是转移的乳腺癌）。RCC 抗体对肾细胞癌特异性高而敏感性相对较低，特别是在小的活检标本中可能只有少数肿瘤细胞免疫染色阳性。

肾、肾上腺与透明细胞癌　α-抑制素是一种二聚体糖蛋白，功能上与 TGF-β 相似，在卵巢（颗粒细胞）、睾丸（Sertoli 细胞）、肾上腺皮质、胎盘及垂体都有发现[374, 375]。α-抑制素可用于卵巢性索间质肿瘤的诊断，也可用于肾上腺皮质腺瘤和腺癌与肾细胞癌和肾上腺转移癌的鉴别诊断，并具有较高的特异性和敏感性[375]。

抗体 A103 是肾上腺皮质肿瘤较好的标志物。A103 可以识别黑色素细胞中由 MART-1 基因编码的抗原。除了肾上腺皮质肿瘤和恶性黑色素瘤，其他肿瘤 A103 很少阳性，因此 A103 对于区别肾上腺皮质肿瘤与肾肿瘤及转移癌非常有用[376, 377]。

Ad4BP，又称为类固醇因子-1，是一个转录因子，在所有的肾上腺皮质癌中阳性，而在肾、肝细胞癌及嗜铬细胞瘤为阴性。转录因子 Ad4BP 可作为肾上腺皮质恶性肿瘤的标记物。

透明细胞癌在转移部位总是个问题，在大多数病例需要鉴别的原发部位包括肾、肾上腺、肺、肝以及卵巢的透明细胞癌。转移到胸膜的透明细胞癌也是个问题。最有可能区分这些肿瘤的抗体组包括RCC、A103、CD10、CKs、抑制素、波形蛋白和HepPar-1[214, 378-381]。

> **诊断要点**：透明细胞癌与肾细胞癌的鉴别诊断
>
> 1. 肾细胞：RCC+、A103-、波形蛋白+、CD10+，抑制素-、HepPar-1-、CK7（R~N）、CAM5.2+。
> 2. 肾上腺皮质：Ad4BP+、RCC-、A103+、波形蛋白+、CD10-、抑制素+、HepPar-1-、CK7（R~N）、CAM5.2-。
> 3. 肺：RCC-、波形蛋白（S）、CD10-、抑制素-、A103-、HepPar-1-、TTF-1+、CK7+。
> 4. 卵巢：RCC（R）、波形蛋白+、CD10-、抑制素-、A103-、HepPar-1-、CK7+、ER（S）。
> 5. 肝透明细胞癌：RCC-、A103-、波形蛋白-、CD10+（小管型）、抑制素-、CK7-。
> 6. 间皮瘤：calretinin+、间皮素（mesothelin）+、WT-1+、CK5/6+、CK7+、CD10（S）、RCC-、MOC-31-。

前列腺作为不明来源转移癌的原发部位

实际上，联合应用 PSA、PAP 和 PSMA 可以诊断所有非前列腺部位（转移性）的前列腺癌。

非前列腺组织也可以对这些抗体着色，因此必须根据临床情况在抗体组中增加相关的验证抗体。

较为常见的对 PSA 和 PSMA 免疫着色的非前列腺病变包括乳腺癌（男性罕见）、唾液腺肿瘤、胰腺及肛门腺癌。罕见的情况下，转移的黑色素瘤可见到 PSA 免疫染色。

Pro-PSA（pPSA）是 PSA 前体的抗体，出现在良性、癌前病变及恶性的前列腺上皮细胞，并且在高级别癌中染色没有减弱。抗体 PS2P446（Beckman Coulter, San Diego, CA）可用于检测转移部位的高级别前列腺癌[382,383]。

Uroplakin Ⅲ （URO Ⅲ）

泌尿道移行上皮伞细胞独特的不对称单位膜上含有移行上皮特有的跨膜蛋白。在至今仍在进行的研究中发现，uroplakins 对移行上皮具有高度特异性和中度敏感性[384,385]，在鳞状上皮中未发现。

Parker 等人研究证明 URO Ⅲ 的敏感性达 57%，特异性近乎完美[386]。

考虑到 URO Ⅲ 的中度敏感性，用于尿路上皮癌检测时，通常需要使用一组抗体以提高阳性率。用于鉴别尿路上皮癌同其他盆腔器官肿瘤如结直肠癌、前列腺癌、肾细胞癌或卵巢移行细胞癌的最佳抗体组合包括 URO Ⅲ、血栓调节素（TM）、p63、K903 和 CK7/20[386-389]。检测尿路上皮癌敏感性最高的抗体是 p63（90%）、K903（88%）、TM（70%~90%）以及 CK20（48%）[386,387]。

卵巢癌的移行细胞成分与尿路上皮癌的免疫组化染色不同[390]。

卵巢移行细胞癌呈少量、局灶性表达 TM（18%）和 URO Ⅲ（6%），同时也表达 WT-1（82%）和 CK7，但不表达 CK20；而尿路上皮癌 WT-1-、CK7/20+（50%）、TM+（76%）及 URO Ⅲ +（50%）[390-392]。卵巢 Brenner 瘤和尿路上皮肿瘤有相似的免疫组化谱。

> **诊断要点：局部盆腔肿瘤**
>
> 1. 尿路上皮癌：URO Ⅲ+、TM+、P63+、K903+、CK7/20+、WT-1-。
> 2. 卵巢移行细胞癌：WT-1+、CK7+、CK20-、URO Ⅲ-、TM-、p63-。
> 3. 前列腺癌：PSA+、PAP+、CK7/20-、URO Ⅲ-、WT-1-、TM-、p63-。
> 4. 结直肠癌：CDX2+、CK20+、CK7-、URO Ⅲ-、WT-1-、TM-、p63-。

巨囊病囊液蛋白（GCDFP）和乳球蛋白

最初由 Pearlman 及其同事[393]和 Haagensen 及其助手[394]描述，由 Murphy 及其同事[395]发现的催乳素诱导蛋白具有与 GCDFP-15 相同的氨基酸序列，在乳腺囊液中含量丰富并在具有顶浆分泌的任何类型细胞均可发现[396-398]。后者除了乳腺，还包括唾液腺的腺泡结构、顶浆分泌腺、汗腺、皮肤 Paget 病、女性外阴和前列腺[399-403]。除了这些部位，其他绝大多数癌没有明显可见的免疫染色[324]。

GCDFP-15 的阳性预测值和特异性均为 99%[403]。据报道，单克隆抗体 D6 克隆（Cambridge Research Laboratories, Cambridge, MA）的敏感性高达 74%[403]，但其他实验报道为 40%~50%[399]。采取抗原热修复后敏感性可提高到 80%。用 BRST-2 抗体的研究结果相似（Signet Laboratories, Inc., Dedham, MA）。

由于 GCDFP 抗体对乳腺癌的高度特异性，因而常被用做筛选有相应临床表现的病人，如患有未知原发肿瘤的女性患者或有乳腺癌病史肺部出现新肿块的病人。其他病例也证实 GCDFP-15 抗体对鉴别乳腺癌肺转移是有效和特异的[404,405]。

乳球蛋白基因编码含有 93 个氨基酸的蛋白，主要表达于乳腺组织。Han 等人研制了针对乳球蛋白的抗体并发现其对鉴别乳腺癌的淋巴结转移具有很高的敏感性（84.3%）和特异性（85%）[406]。在他们的研究中 GCDFP-15、BRST-2 表达的敏感性和特异性为 44.3% 和 97.9%，免疫染色为胞浆弥漫性分布。有一个研究发现，乳球蛋白在 15% 的非乳腺癌肿瘤中表达，包括胃、肺、结肠、肝胆管、甲状腺、尿路上皮、卵巢和涎腺癌，但在这些肿瘤往往呈局灶性弱表达。

> **诊断要点：转移性乳腺癌**
>
> 1. GCDFP-15 对乳腺癌具有 99% 的特异性、60%~70% 的敏感性。
> 2. 乳球蛋白对乳腺癌具有高敏感性，但特异性尚未深入研究。
> 3. 乳腺癌肺转移：
>   乳腺：GCDFP-15+，TTF-1（N）、CEA（S）、ER/PR（S）。
>   肺癌：GCDFP-15（N），TTF-1+、CEA+、ER/PR（N）。

肾上腺皮质肿瘤中的 melan-A 和抑制素

Melan-A 是 *MART-1* 基因的产物，是抗体 A103 识别的一个抗原，尽管最初是用于鉴别黑色素瘤细胞的，但也可被用于鉴别半数以上的肾上腺皮质肿瘤，尤其是癌[407-411]。同抑制素一样，melan-A 也在一些性索间质肿瘤中表达[363]。由于 A103 抗体不与其他癌发生反应，因此对肾上腺皮质肿瘤更特异，而抑制素更敏感[410]。抑制素抗体对肾上腺癌的反应还需要更多的研究。但是如果排除黑色素瘤的可能性，A103免疫染色阳性强烈支持诊断肾上腺皮质癌[409]。

CD5

CD5是一分子量67kD的糖蛋白受体，可能表达于各种T淋巴细胞及套区淋巴细胞[412]。Hishima及其同事[413]发现胸腺癌表达CD5，随后的报道证实并扩展了这一发现。在已公布的研究中，使用的抗体克隆包括NCL-CD5（CD5/54/B4）[404, 415]，其对胸腺癌的敏感性为29%~67%[414, 416]；NCL-CD5-4C7克隆的敏感性为62%~100%[416, 417]。对于纵隔肿瘤，通常需要鉴别诊断的包括转移性鳞癌以及其他分化差的转移性肺癌和生殖细胞肿瘤，这些肿瘤对NCL-CD5-4C7克隆抗体均不着色[337]。尽管胃肠道、乳腺及泌尿道部位的一些正常上皮和癌可与该克隆抗体反应，但事实上这些部位的肿瘤大部分与纵隔无关[417]。虽然有些非典型胸腺瘤和发生于胸腺瘤内的胸腺癌也呈阳性，但CD5阳性的纵隔肿瘤对胸腺癌的诊断是一个很强的证据[417, 418]。梭形细胞癌与CD5抗体无反应[419]。

> **诊断要点：CD5**
> 1. 除了梭形细胞亚型，绝大部分组织学类型的大部分胸腺癌呈阳性反应。
> 2. 胸腺梭形细胞癌为阴性。
> 3. 肺癌大部分CD5为阴性。

胸膜转移癌和上皮样间皮瘤

正如本章开篇之言，转移性肿瘤的解剖部位是探究肿瘤起源的良好起始点。胸膜转移癌最多来自肺癌，但也可起源于其他解剖部位。远处肿瘤转移至胸膜更多是由于病人有更长的生存时间，因此，胸膜恶性上皮性肿瘤的鉴别诊断包括转移性肺癌、转移性非肺源性癌和恶性间皮瘤。

用于鉴别肺癌和间皮瘤的最好的单一抗体是TTF-1，该抗体对肺癌具有高敏感性和极高的特异性，特别是腺癌、非小细胞癌和小细胞癌[309, 311, 313]。另外，CK5/CK6主要局限于间皮瘤细胞，鳞状细胞癌、肺癌及非肺癌可呈局灶状染色。下面讨论用于这些肿瘤鉴别诊断的抗体组合。

B72.3

B72.3抗体与肿瘤相关糖蛋白发生反应。这种糖蛋白常在腺癌中广泛表达，有些研究发现，只有2%~5%的间皮瘤呈局灶性反应[420-425]。

据Ordonez的一项大型研究，84%的癌表达B72.3，但60例上皮样间皮瘤均为阴性[426]。

癌胚抗原

除了前列腺、肾、乳腺和肝癌，高达95%的肺癌和非肺癌对CEJO65T和A5B7抗体克隆呈阳性反应[427]。

Bg8

Bg8是一个抗Lewis（y）抗体，由Jordon及其同事[428]在1989年报道，主要与腺癌反应，在上皮性间皮瘤呈局灶性/弱阳性。Riera及其合作者[424]进一步研究证实，93%的肺腺癌Bg8免疫染色阳性，只有9%的上皮样间皮瘤呈局灶或弱阳性。

Ordonez发现88%的癌和7%的间皮瘤Bg8阳性[426]。

BerEP4

单克隆抗体BerEP4用于鉴别肺腺癌和间皮瘤存在一些争议，这是由于对其阳性结果的解释有很多差异[429-431]。近期研究发现[431]，92%~100%的肺腺癌呈弥漫阳性。Ordonez发现癌100%表达，而间皮瘤只有8%呈局灶性染色[426, 432]。

在腹腔积液中用于鉴别卵巢癌与间皮增生和间皮瘤时，BerEP4是一个关键抗体（图7.14）。

间皮素

间皮素（mesothelin）是一个细胞表面抗原，在间皮细胞中强表达。研究表明，虽然其对间皮细胞和间皮瘤的敏感性达100%，但特异性却不高[433, 434]。各种癌都可表达间皮素，包括50%的肺腺癌。间皮素的价值在于当应用其他抗体没有得到明确结果时用于帮助鉴别诊断。由于间皮素对间皮瘤的敏感性为100%，因此在这些病例中如果其为阴性，则可以排除间皮瘤[433, 434]。

Wilms瘤抑癌基因（WT-1）

此抑癌基因产物的免疫染色为核阳性。对间皮细胞和卵巢上皮癌尤其是浆液性癌，WT-1具有高度敏感性和特异性[435]。

在卵巢浆液性肿瘤、间皮的增生和肿瘤中WT-1呈弥漫强阳性，因此WT-1可用于鉴别这些肿瘤（图7.15）。对于盆腹腔积液，BerEP4可用于鉴别间皮增生（阴性）和卵巢浆液性癌（阳性）。

MOC-31

MOC-31与一分子量为38kD的膜糖蛋白反应，在89%~100%各种来源的腺癌中呈典型的强阳性染色[436-441]，在一项研究中只有5%的间皮瘤呈局灶或弱阳性[441]，另一项研究为8%阳性[426]。

calretinin

calretinin是分子量为29kD的细胞内钙结合蛋白，存在于多种细胞中包括神经元、类固醇激素生成细胞、肾曲小管、外分泌腺、胸腺角化细胞和间皮细胞[442, 443]。不同抗体的免疫染色结果有所不同，其中Zymed克隆特异性较高[444]。calretinin在来自不同部位的腺癌中只有8%呈阳性表达，而且几乎均呈局灶性或弱阳性[426]。

总而言之，对胸膜转移性腺癌和上皮性间皮瘤的鉴别具有最高特异性和敏感性的抗体组合包括间皮瘤阳性标志组（calretinin、CK5/CK6、WT-1和间皮素）和间皮瘤阴性标志组（MOC-31、Bg8、BerEP4）[426, 433, 434, 445, 446]。腺癌的阳性标志物包括MOC-31、Bg8、BerEP4[123, 447]。其他的有用抗体如TTF-1对鉴别肺癌特异（表7.14）。

在其他抗体不能作出明确诊断时联合应用B72.3和CEA可以帮助诊断。另外，在其他抗体免疫染色结果均不能确定诊断时，间皮素阴性则可以排除间皮瘤[426]。

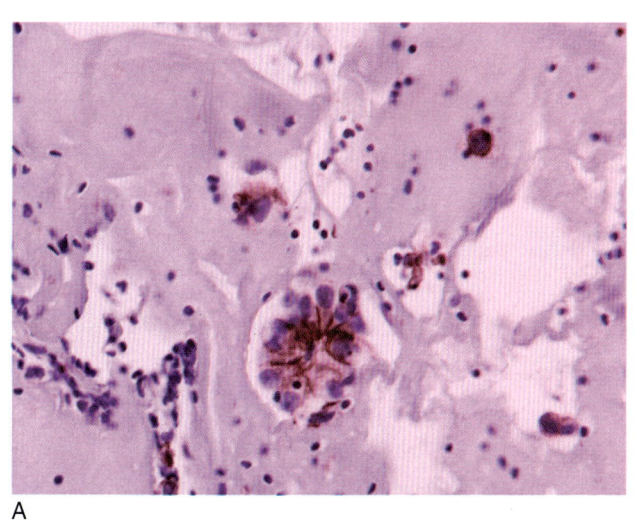
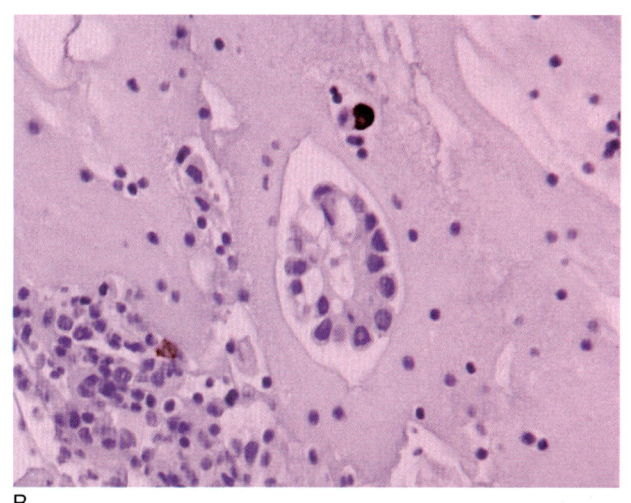

图7.14 （A）BerEP4+，卵巢癌盆腔冲洗液中细胞膜染色；(B) calretinin 阴性

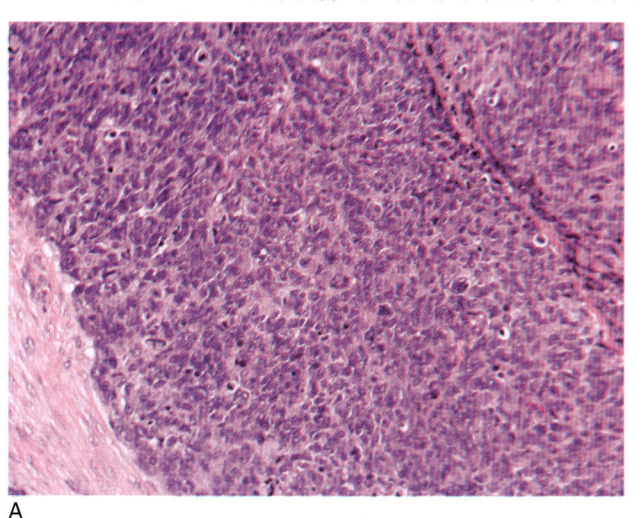
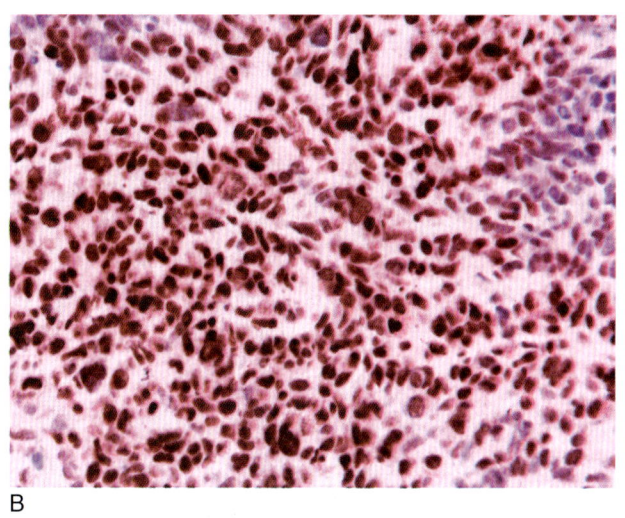

图7.15 （A）一位老年妇女来源不明的实体癌浸润肠壁；(B) WT-1+证实其为卵巢来源（同时CK7+、BerEP4+，未图示）

表7.14 抗体组合：间皮瘤与肺癌

	间皮瘤	肺癌
Calretinin	+	R
WT-1	+	N
Mesothelin	+	N
CK5	+	S
Bg8	N	+
BerEP4	N	+
MOC-31	N	+

+，阳性；S，部分阳性；R，少数细胞染色；N，阴性

> **诊断要点**：胸膜／腹膜转移癌与上皮样间皮瘤
>
> 1. 在肺癌中TTF-1+，在其他癌和间皮瘤中TTF-1（N）。
> 2. 上皮样间皮瘤CK5/CK6+、肺癌CK5/CK6（S）、其他癌CK5/CK6（S）——主要是鳞癌、移行细胞癌和卵巢癌。
> 3. 间皮瘤阳性标志物：calretinin、CK5/CK6、WT-1、间皮素。
> 4. 间皮瘤阴性标志物：CEA、MOC-31、B72.3、Bg8、BerEP4。
> 5. 卵巢浆液性乳头状癌：WT-1+、BerEP4+、MOC-31+、Bg8+、B72.3+、CK5/6+、calretinin（R）；腹膜间皮瘤：WT-1+、BerEP4-、MOC-31-、Bg8-、B72.3-、CK5/6+、calretinin+。

激素受体（雌激素／孕激素）

直觉上，雌／孕激素受体（ER/PR）似乎应只局限于性激素反应组织如乳腺，但最近的文献对此却提出争议。尽管一些研究者认为ER/PR只在部分乳腺癌、卵巢癌和子宫内膜癌中出现[404,448,449]，但其他一些研究已在肺癌[450-454]、胃癌和甲状腺癌中观察到ER（多见）和PR（少见）的存在。

Vargas及其同事[454]用免疫组化证实在98%的非小细胞肺癌中存在雌激素相关蛋白p29，提示雌激素轴在这类恶性肿瘤中可能是重要的。Vargas及其助手在实验中对同一组肿瘤用商业化抗体ER1D5（DAKO，Carpinteria，CA）进行检测却均显示为阴性，该组病人男女之间的生存时间也存在差异，提示可能存在性别特异性p29相关因子的影响。

Dabbs等用6F11抗体克隆（Ventana，Tucson，AZ）和HIER观察了肺腺癌中的ER[455]，发现67%的肺腺癌，包括支气管肺泡癌，有细胞核雌激素受体表达，但用ER1D5抗体克隆（DAKO，Carpinteria，CA）检测则为阴性。因此，该作者对用抗体ER6F11检测肺腺癌中的ER作为乳腺癌转移的证据并不太赞成。考虑到在研究MCUP时ER的低特异性，其他研究者也得出同样的结论[448]。结合CK的表达，对于性激素靶肿瘤如乳腺癌的鉴别诊断ER可能有所帮助[456]。

Paget病

Paget病分为乳腺Paget病和乳腺外Paget病，乳腺Paget病几乎总是潜在乳腺癌的预兆[457-459]，而乳腺外Paget病可能预示着转移癌。

乳腺Paget病表现为CK7+恶性细胞在乳头的表皮内浸润，恶性细胞很醒目，呈"散弹样"浸润，体积大、胞浆丰富、印戒样，有时黏液染色阳性。表皮角细胞CK7阴性，而大多数Paget细胞CK7+、GCDFP-15+及CEA+，具有乳腺癌的特征，但偶尔可为CK7-（图7.16）。Toker细胞CK7+，可能出现在正常乳头的皮肤，但一般来说与Paget细胞相比，这些细胞不那么醒目[460]，而且由于Toker细胞温和，在正常上皮中很难看到，因此不会造成诊断上的困难。

乳头表皮内出现CK7阳性细胞并不等同于Paget病，包括乳头良性病变如乳头腺瘤。表皮内若出现良性形态的CK7阳性细胞，则可能是输乳管细胞扩展而来或乳头上皮良性增生进入表皮所致[461]。

可以用ER[462]或neu-oncoprotein[463]检测Paget细胞。

乳腺外Paget病主要发生在女性外阴或肛周区，但也可发生在男性及其他部位。

原发性外阴Paget病是起源于汗腺导管的局限性癌，可为原位癌或发生浸润；组织学上，由富于胞浆的大细胞组成，黏蛋白阳性，并呈广泛性的CK7+和GCDFP-15+[395]。

肛周区的外阴外Paget病可能是由直肠、宫颈或膀胱等部位的癌转移而来[395]。因此，外阴外Paget病的组织学诊断问题是鉴别Paget病是来自于皮肤附属器肿瘤还是来自于直肠、宫颈或膀胱的转移癌。

表现为Paget病的结直肠癌细胞常呈印戒样、黏蛋白阳性，且腔内可见"污秽"样坏死物[399]；免疫组化GCDFP-15-、CEA+、CK20强阳性，CK7虽然大部分为阴性但也可呈局灶性或弱阳性[395-402]。

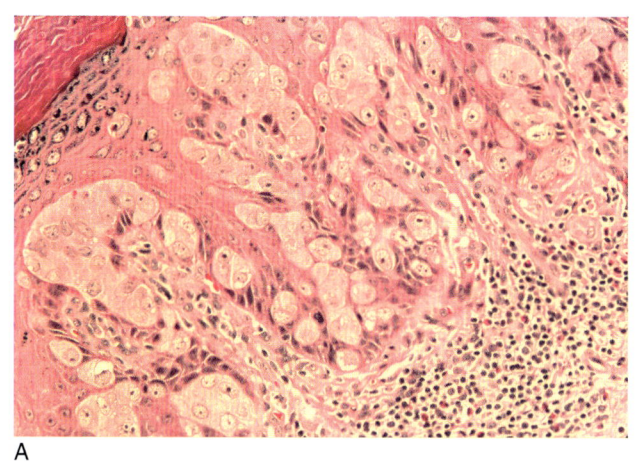
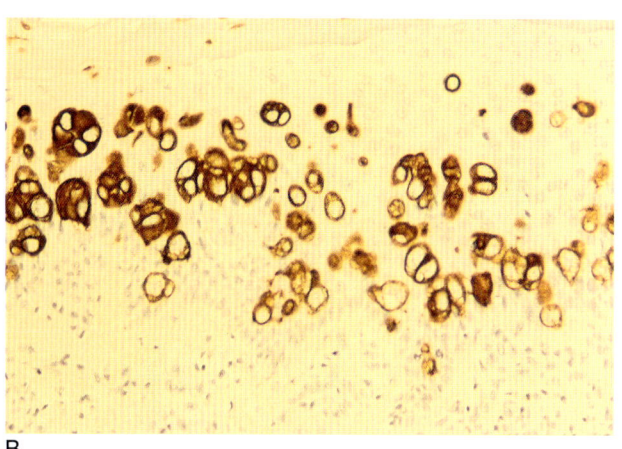
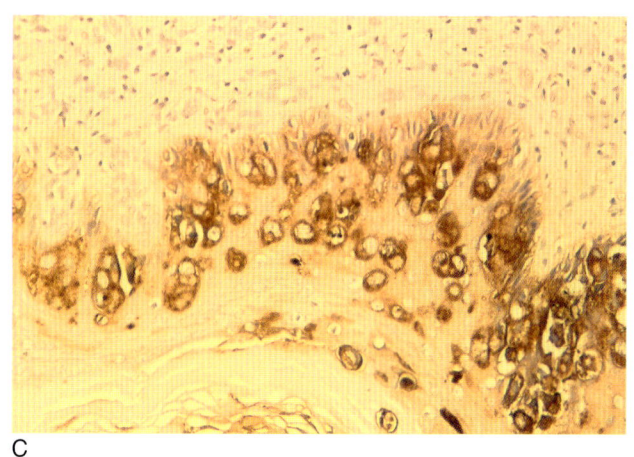
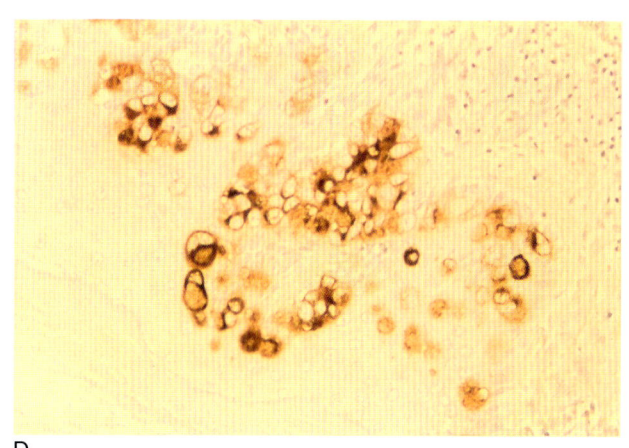

图 7.16　一例典型的原发性会阴 Paget 病（A），呈 CK7+（B）、CEA+（C）、GCDFP-15+（D）

移行细胞癌 CK7 和 CK20 均呈典型强阳性，但 GCDFP-15-，并且缺少印戒样细胞或黏蛋白，uroplakin 抗体免疫染色可能阳性。

> **诊断要点**：Paget 病
>
> 1. 乳腺 Paget 病人：CK7+、GCDFP-15+、CEA+、CEA（S）。
> 2. Paget 样鳞癌：p16+、CK7-。
> 3. 外阴 Paget 病、原发附件癌：CK7+，GCDFP-15+，CEA+。
> 4. 表现为肛周-外阴 Paget 病的转移性结直肠癌：CK7（N）、CK20+、CDX2+、CEA+、GCDFP-15（N）。
> 5. 表现为肛周-外阴 Paget 病的转移性移行细胞癌：CK7+、CK20+、GCDFP-15（N）、CEA（S）、uroplakin（S）。

小　结

通过与临床医师的密切合作，详细了解病人的临床病史，并根据肿瘤部位和/或放射学医生对肿瘤的评估，病理医生应该能得出一个可进行下一步工作的鉴别诊断来。这个初步诊断对于应用 IHC 是非常关键的，对病人的治疗来说 IHC 是一个物有所值的工具。表 7.15、7.16，图 7.17 总结了检测 MCUP 诊断抗体组的联合应用。

表7.15 诊断性抗体的组合应用

病变部位	抗 体			病变部位	抗 体		
		肺原发	肝原发			肺原发	肝原发
乳腺				精原细胞瘤			
CK7	+	+	N	CAM5.2	N~R	+	+
AE1/AE3	+	+	R~N	AE1/AE3	N	+	N~R
mCEA	S	+	N	PLAP	+	N	N
GCDFP-15	+	N	N	EMA	N	+	S
TTF-1	N	+	N	CD30	N~R	N	N
结肠				胚胎生殖细胞			
CK7	R~N	+	N	AE1/AE3	+	+	N~R
CK20	+	R~N	N	TTF-1	N	+	N
TTF-1	N	+	N	CK7	+/−	+	N
CDX2	+	R~N	N	PLAP	+	N	N
Villin	+	S	N	CD30	+	N	N
胰胆管				甲状腺			
CK7	+	+	N	TTF-1	+	+	N
CK20	+	N	N	mCEA	N	+	N
mCEA	+	+	N	胸腺			
CDX2	S!	N	N	CD5	S	S	N
Villin	S	S	N	TTF-1	N	+	N
前列腺				CEA	S	+	N
PSA	+	N	N	子宫内膜			
PSMA	+	N	N	CEA	N	+	N
mCEA	N	+	N	Vimentin	+	N	N
pCEA	N	+	S*	AE1/AE3	+	+	N~R
肾细胞				ER/PR	+	N	N
AE1/AE3	+	+	N~R	子宫颈内膜			
CEA	N	+	N	mCEA	N	+	N
TTF-1	N	+	N	AE1/AE3	+	+	R~N
Renal Cell Ag	+!	N	N	pCEA	S	+	S*
膀胱移行细胞癌				ER/PR	S	N	N
CK7	+	+	N				
CK20	+	N	N				
Uroplakin	+!	N	N				
	非肺源性				非肺源性		
	小细胞肺癌	小细胞肿瘤	Merkel细胞		小细胞肺癌	小细胞肿瘤	Merkel细胞
CK7	+	+	N	Chromogranin	S	S	S
CK20	N	N	+	CEA	S	S	N
TTF-1	+	R~N	N	NSE	+	+	+
Synaptophysin	+	+	+				

* 小管型；−，低敏感性；+，几乎总为阳性；S，有时阳性；R，很少阳性；N，阴性
GCDFP-15, gross cystic disease fluid protein fraction 15; TTF-1, thyroid transcription factor 1; CEA, carcinoembryonic antigen; PSA, prostate-specific antigen; PSMA, prostate-specific membrane antigen; pCEA, polyclonal carcinoembryonic antigen; PLAP, placenta-like alkaline phosphatase; EMA, epithelial membrane antigen; NSE, neuron-specific enolase

不明来源转移癌的免疫组织化学 7

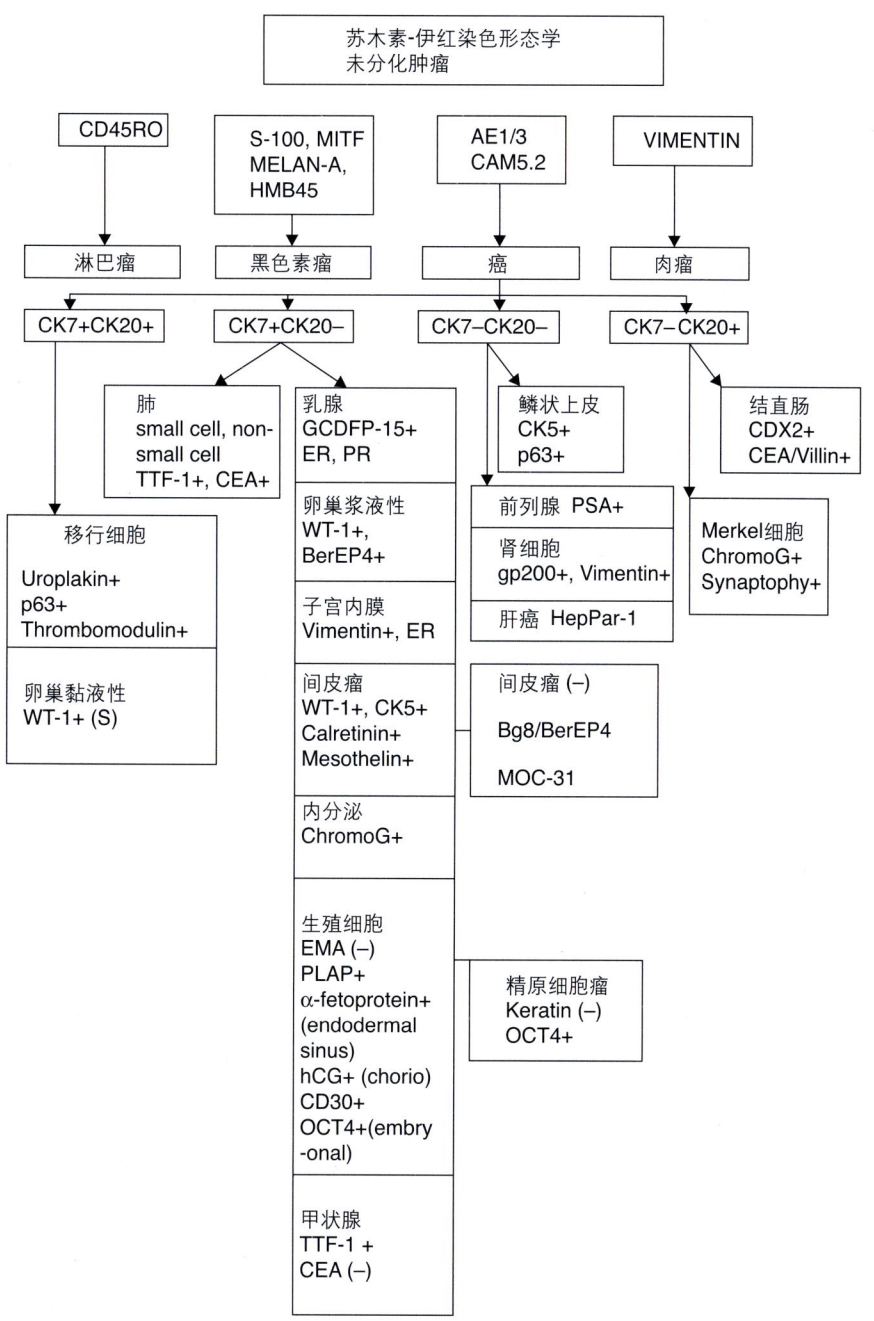

图 7.17　未分化肿瘤苏木精-伊红染色图示

表7.16　未分化恶性肿瘤的主要筛选抗体

	CAM5.2	EMA	S-100	LCA	PLAP	CD30
癌	+	+	S	N	S	N
黑色素瘤	R~N	N	+	N	N	N
淋巴瘤	N	R~N	N	+	N	S
非精原细胞生殖细胞肿瘤	+	N	N	N	+	+
精原细胞瘤	R~N	N	N	N	+	R~N

213

参考文献

1. Rosai J. Author's response to letter. Am J Surg Pathol 1999; 23:491.
2. Greco F, Hainsworth J. The management of patients with adenocarcinoma of unknown primary site. Semin Oncol 1989; 6(Suppl 6):116–122.
3. Haskel CM, Cochran AJ, Barsky SH. Metastasis of unknown origin. Curr Probl Cancer 1988, 12:5–58.
4. Krementz ET, Cerise EJ, Foster DS, et al. Metastases of undetermined source. Curr Probl Cancer 1979; 4:4–37.
5. Schapira DV, Jerrett AR. The need to consider survival, outcome, and expense when evaluating and treating patients with unknown primary carcinoma. Arch Intern Med 1995; 155:2050–2054.
6. van de Wouw AJ, Jansen RL, Griffioen AW, et al. Clinical and immunohistochemical analysis of patients with unknown primary tumour. A search for prognostic factors in UPT. Anticancer Res 2004; 24:297–301.
7. Blaszyk H, Hartmann A, Bjornsson J. Cancer of unknown primary: clinicopathologic correlations. APMIS 2003; 111: 1089–1094.
8. Pavlidis N, Briasoulis E, Hainsworth J, et al. Diagnostic and therapeutic management of cancer of an unknown primary. Eur J Cancer 2003; 39:1990–2005.
9. Putti T, Win K, Choi Y, et al. Cost effectiveness of immunohistochemistry in surgical pathology. Am J Clin Pathol 1998; 110:512A.
10. Dabbs D. Diagnostic immunohistochemistry. Philadelphia, PA: Churchill Livingstone; 2002:641.
11. Steckel RJ, Kagan AR. Metastatic tumors of unknown origin. Cancer 1991; 67:1242–1244.
12. Kagan AR, Steckel RJ. The limited role of radiologic imaging in patients with unknown primary tumor. Semin Oncol 1991; 18:170–173.
13. Jonk A, Kroon BB, Rumke P, et al. Lymph node metastasis from melanoma with unknown primary site. Br J Surg 1990; 77:665–666.
14. Le-Chevalier T, Cvitkivic E, Caille P, et al. Early metastatic cancer of unknown primary origin at presentation: A clinical study of 302 consecutive autopsy patients. Arch Intern Med 1988; 148:2035–2039.
15. Kirsten FC, Leary JA, et al. Metastatic adeno- or undifferentiated carcinoma from an unknown primary site – natural history and guidelines for identification of treatable subsets. Q J Med 1987; 62:143–161.
16. Van der Gaast A, Verwei J, Plantane AS, et al. The value of immunocytochemistry in patients with poorly differentiated adenocarcinomas and undifferentiated carcinomas of unknown primary. J Cancer Res Clin Oncol 1996; 122:181–185.
17. Greco FA, Hainsworth JD. Poorly differentiated carcinoma or adenocarcinoma of unknown primary site: Long term results with cisplatin based chemotherapy. Semin Oncol 1994; 21:77–82.
18. Greco FA, Hainsworth JD. The management of patients with adenocarcinoma and poorly differentiated carci-noma of unknown primary site. Semin Oncol 1989; 16:116–122.
19. Matthews P, Ellis IO. Use of immunocytochemistry in a diagnosis of metastatic carcinoma. Ann Med 1996; 28:38–44.
20. Mackay B, Ordonez NG. Pathologic evaluation of neoplasms with unknown primary tumor site. Semin Oncol 1993; 20: 206–228.
21. Hess KR, Abbruzzese MC, Lenzi R, et al. Classification and regression tree analysis of 1000 consecutive patients with unknown primary carcinoma. Clin Cancer Res 1999; 5:3403–3410.
22. Song SY, Kim WS, Lee HR, et al. Adenocarcinoma of unknown primary site. Korean J Intern Med 2002; 17:234–239.
23. Osteen RT, Kopf G, Wilson RE. In pursuit of the unknown primary. Am J Surg Pathol 1978; 135:494.
24. Ayoub JP, Hess KR, Abbruzzese MC, et al. Unknown primary tumors metastatic to liver. J Clin Oncol 1998; 16:2105–2112.
25. Guthrie T. Treatable carcinoma of unknown origin. Am J Med 1989; 298:74–78.
26. Hainsworth JD, Greco FA. Managing carcinomas of unknown primary site. Oncology (Williston Park) 1988; 2:439–524.
27. Lenzi R, Hess KR, Abbruzzese MC, et al. Poorly differentiated carcinoma and poorly differentiated adenocarcinoma of unknown origin: Favorable subsets of patients with unknown primary carcinoma. J Clin Oncol 1997; 15:2056–2066.
28. Perchalski JE, Hall KL, Dewar MA. Metastasis of unknown origin. Prim Care 1992; 19:747–757.
29. Haskell CM, Cochran AJ, Barski SH, et al. Current problems in cancer. Cancer 1991; 2:5–58.

30. Jakobsen JH, Johanssen J, Jurgensen KE. Neck lymph node metastases from an unknown primary tumor. Ugeskr Laeger 1991; 153:428–430.

31. Hainsworth JD, Greco FA. Poorly differentiated carcinoma and poorly differentiated adenocarcinoma of unknown primary tumor site. Semin Oncol 1993; 20:279–286.

32. Hainsworth JD, Wright EP, Johnson DH, et al. Poorly differentiated carcinoma of unknown primary site: Clinical usefulness of immunoperoxidase staining. J Clin Oncol 1991; 9: 1931–1938.

33. Huebner G, Tamme C, Schouber C, et al. Prognostically different subgroups in patients with carcinoma of unknown primary. J Chemother Infect Dis Malig 1989; 1:816.

34. Kambhu SA, Kelsen DP, Fiore J, et al. Metastatic adenocarcinomas of unknown primary site: Prognostic variables and treatment results. Am J Clin Pathol 1990; 13:55–60.

35. Hammer SP. Metastatic adenocarcinoma of unknown primary origin. Hum Pathol 1998; 29:1393–1402.

36. Gil GM, Vadell NC, Fabregat X, et al. Yield of diagnostic tests in neoplasms of unknown origin: A retrospective study. Rev Clin Esp 1990; 186:252–258.

37. Romeu J, Texido A, Rosell R, et al. Carcinoma of unknown origin: Diagnostic study of 48 cases and its clinical yield. Med Clin (Barc) 1989; 92:201–206.

38. Renshaw AA, Pinkus GS, Corson JM. CD34 and AE1/AE3 diagnostic discriminates in a distinction of solitary fibrous tumor of the pleura from sarcomatoid mesothelioma. Appl Immunohistochem 1994; 2:94–102.

39. Cho KR, Epstein JI. Metastatic prostatic carcinoma to supradiaphragmatic lymph nodes: A clinicopathologic and immunohistochemical study. Am J Surg Pathol 1987; 11:457–463.

40. Nguyen C, Shenouda G, Black MJ, et al. Metastatic squamous cell carcinoma to cervical lymph nodes from unknown primary mucosal sites. Head Neck 1994; 16:58–63.

41. Haas I, Hoffmann TK, Engers R, et al. Diagnostic strategies in cervical carcinoma of an unknown primary (CUP). Eur Arch Otorhinolaryngol 2002; 259:325–333.

42. Willis D, Brown PW, Roger A. Adenocarcinoma from an unknown primary presenting in women with an axillary mass. Clin Oncol(R Coll Radiol) 1990; 2:189–192.

43. Ringenberg QS, Doll DC, Loy TS, et al. Malignant ascites of unknown origin. Cancer 1989; 64:753–755.

44. Sadeghi B, Arvieux C, Glehen O, et al. Peritoneal carcinomatosis from non-gynecologic malignancies: results of the EVOCAPE 1 multicentric prospective study. Cancer 2000; 88:358–363.

45. Sears D, Hajdu SI. The cytologic diagnosis of malignant neoplasms in pleura and peritoneal effusions. Acta Cyto 1987; 31:85–97.

46. Rougraff BT, Kneisl JS, Simon MA. Skeletal metastases of unknown origin: A prospective study of a diagnostic strategy. J Bone Joint Surg Am 1993; 75:1276–1281.

47. Pisharodi LR, Lavoie R, Bedrossian CW. Differential diagnostic dilemmas in malignant fine needle aspirates of liver: A practical approach to final diagnosis. Diagn Cytopathol 1995; 12:364–371.

48. Perry A, Parisi JE, Kurtin PJ. Metastatic adenocarcinoma to the brain: An immunohistochemical approach. Hum Pathol 1997; 28:938–943.

49. Perry A, White C. Colon biopsies of metastatic neoplasms in central nervous system: The surgical pathologist's prospective. Brain Pathol 1994; 4:435.

50. Debevec M. Management of patients with brain metastases of unknown origin. Neoplasma 1990; 37:601–606.

51. Merchutt MP. Brain metastases from undiagnosed systemic neoplasms. Arch Intern Med 1989; 149:1076–1080.

52. Nussbaum ES, Djalilian A, Cho KH, et al. Brain metastases: Histology, multiplicity, surgery and survival. Cancer 1996; 15:1781–1788.

53. Bartelt S, Lutterbach J. Brain metastases in patients with cancer of unknown primary. J Neurooncol 2003; 64:249–253.

54. Nguyen LN, Maor MH, Oswald MJ. Brain metastases as the only manifestation of an undetected primary tumor. Cancer 1998; 15:2181–2184.

55. Lagerwaard FJ, Levendag PC, Nowak PJ, et al. Identification of prognostic factors in patients with brain metastases: A review of 1292 patients. Int J Radiat Oncol Biol Phys 1999; 1:793–803.

56. Greco FA, Gray J, Burris HA, 3rd, et al. Taxane-based chemotherapy for patients with carcinoma of unknown primary site. Cancer J 2001; 7:203–212.

57. Mukai H, Watanabe T, Ando M, et al. Unknown primary carcinoma: a feasibility assessment of combination chemotherapy with cisplatin and docetaxel. Int J Clin Oncol 2003; 8:23–25.

58. Martelli G, Pilotti S, Lepara P, et al. Fine needle aspiration

cytology and superficial lymph nodes: Analysis of 266 cases. Eur J Surg Oncol 1989; 15:13–16.

59. Lai CR, Pan CC, Tsay SH. Contribution of immunocytochemistry in routine diagnostic cytology. Diagn Cytopathol 1996; 14:221–225.

60. DiBonito L, Falconieri G, Colautti I, et al. The positive peritoneal effusion: A retrospective study of cytopathologic diagnoses with autopsy confirmation. Acta Cytol 1993; 37:483–488.

61. Bedrossian CW. Special stains: The old and the new: The impact of immunocytochemistry in effusion cytology. Diagn Cytopathol 1998; 18:141–149.

62. Longatto FA, Bisi H, Alves VA, et al. Adenocarcinoma in females detected in serous effusions: Cytomorphologic aspects and immunocytochemical reactivity to cytokeratins 7 and 20. Acta Cytol 1997; 41:961–971.

63. Lidang JM, Johansen P. Immunocytochemical staining of serous effusions: An additional method in the routine cytology practice? Cytopathology 1994; 5:93–103.

64. Bonnefoi H, Smith IE. How should cancer presenting as a malignant pleural effusion be managed? Br J Cancer 1996; 74:832–835.

65. Ascoli V, Taccogna S, Scalzo CC, et al. Utility of cytokeratin 20 in identifying the origin of metastatic carcinomas and effusions. Diagn Cytopathol 1995; 12:303–308.

66. Moll R. Cytokeratins in the histological diagnosis of malignant tumors. Int J Biol Markers 1994; 9:63–69.

67. Miettinin M. Keratin immunohistochemistry: Update of applications and pitfalls. Pathol Annu 1993; 1:113–143.

68. Quinlan RA, Schiller DL, Hatzfeld M, et al. Patterns of expression and organization of cytokeratin intermediate filaments. Ann NY Acad Sci 1985; 455:282–306.

69. Moll R, Franke WW, Schiller DL, et al. The catalog of human cytokeratins: Patterns of expression in normal epithelia, tumors and cultured cells. 1982; 31:11–24.

70. Schaafsma HE, Ramaekers FCS. Cytokeratin subtyping in normal and neoplastic epithelium: Basic principles in diagnostic applications. Pathol Annu 1994; 29(Part 1):21–62.

71. Rosenberg M, Fuchs E, LeBeau M, et al. Three epidermal and one simple epithelial type II keratin genes mapped to human chromosome 12. Cytogenet Cell Genet 1991; 57:33–38.

72. Rosenberg M, Chaudhury A, Shows TB, et al. A group of type I keratin genes on human chromosome 17: Characterization and expression. Mol Cell Biol 1988; 8:722–726.

73. Romano V, Bosco P, Rocchi M, et al. Chromosomal assignments of human type I and type II cytokeratin genes to different chromosomes. Cytogenet Cell Genet 1988; 48:148–153.

74. Franke WW, Schmidt E, Schiller DL, et al. Differentiation related patterns of expression of proteins of intermediate size in tissues and cultured cells. Cold Spring Harbor Symp Quant Biol 1982; 46:431–445.

75. Wang MP, Zee S, Zarbo RJ, et al. Coordinate expression of cytokeratin 7 and 20 defines unique subsets of carcinomas. Appl Immunohistochem 1995; 3:99–107.

76. Judkins AR, Montone KT, LiVolsi VA, et al. Sensitivity and specificity of antibodies on necrotic tumor tissue. Am J Clin Pathol 1998; 110:641–646.

77. Stasik PC, Purkis PE, Laigh IN, et al. Keratin 19: Predicted amino acid sequence and broad tissue distribution suggest evolution from keratinocyte keratins. J Invest Dermatol 1989; 92:707.

78. Bartek JB, Taylor-Papadimitriou J, et al. Differential expression of keratin 19 in normal human epithelial tissues revealed by monospecific monoclonal antibodies. Histochem J 1986; 18:656.

79. Van Niekerk CC, Jap PHK, Ramakers FCS, et al. Immunohistochemical demonstration of keratin 7 in routinely fixed paraffin embedded human tissues. J Pathol 1991; 165:145–152.

80. Ramakers F, Van NiekerkC, Poels L, et al. Use of monoclonal antibodies to keratin 7 and the differential diagnosis of adenocarcinomas. Am J Pathol 1990; 136:641–655.

81. Loy TS, Calaluce RD. Utility of cytokeratin immuno-staining in separating pulmonary adenocarcinomas from colonic adenocarcinomas. Am J Clin Pathol 1994; 102:764–767.

82. Van de Molengraft FJJM, Van Niekerk CC, Jap PHK, et al. OV-TL 12/30 (keratin 7 antibody) is a marker of glandular differentiation in lung cancer. Histopathology 1993; 22:35–38.

83. Prayson RA, Hart WR, Petras RE. Pseudomyxoma peritonei: A clinicopathologic study of 19 cases with emphasis on site of origin and nature of associated ovarian tumors. Am J Surg Pathol 1994; 18:591–603.

84. Ronnett BM, Shmookler BM, Diener-West M, et al. Immunohistochemical evidence supporting the appendiceal origin of

pseudomyxoma peritonei in women. Int J Gyn Pathol 1997; 16:1–9.
85. Ronnett BM, Kurman RJ, Shmookler BM, et al. The morphologic spectrum of ovarian metastases of appendiceal adenocarcinomas: A clinicopathologic and immunohistochemical analysis of tumors often misinterpreted as primary ovarian tumors or metastatic tumors. Am J Surg Pathol 1997; 21:1144–1155.
86. Loy TS, Calaluce RD, Keeney GL. Cytokeratin immunostaining in differentiating primary ovarian carcinoma from metastatic colonic adenocarcinoma. Mod Pathol 1996; 9:1040–1044.
87. Guerrieri C, Franlund B, Boeryd B. Expression of cytokeratin 7 in simultaneous mucinous tumors of the ovary and appendix. Mod Pathol 1995; 8:573–576.
88. Berezowski K, Stastny J, Kornstein MJ. Cytokeratin 7 and 20 and carcinoembryonic antigen in ovarian and colonic carcinoma. Mod Pathol 1996; 9:426–429.
89. Ueda G, Sawada M, Ogawa H, et al. Immunohistochemical study of cytokeratin 7 for the differential diagnosis of adenocarcinomas in the ovary. Gynecol Oncol 1993; 51:219–223.
90. Ramakers F, Huysmans A, Schaart G, et al. Tissue distribution of keratin 7 as monitored by a monoclonal antibody. Exp Cell Res 1987; 170:235–249.
91. Osborne M, VanLessen G, Weber K, et al. Methods in laboratory investigation: Differential diagnosis of gastro-intestinal carcinomas by using monoclonal antibody specific for individual keratin polypeptides. Lab Invest 1986; 55:497.
92. Miettinen MFJ. Keratin 7 reactivity in endothelial cells: A potential pitfall in diagnostic immunohistochemistry. Appl Immunohistochem 1997; 5:229–233.
93. Chu P, Wu E, Weiss LM. Cytokeratin 7 and cytokeratin 20 expression in epithelial neoplasms: a survey of 435 cases. Mod Pathol 2000; 13:962–972.
94. VanEyken P, Brock B, et al. Abundant expression of cytokeratin 7 in fibrolamellar carcinoma of the liver. Histopathology 1990; 17:101–106.
95. Ramalingam P, Hart WR, Goldblum JR. Cytokeratin subset immunostaining in rectal adenocarcinoma and normal anal glands. Arch Pathol Lab Med 2001; 125:1074–1077.
96. Tot T. Cytokeratins 20 and 7 as biomarkers: usefulness in discriminating primary from metastatic adenocarcinoma. Eur J Cancer 2002; 38:758–763.
97. Moll R SD, Franke WW. Identification of protein IT of the intestinal cytoskeleton as a novel type I cytokeratin with unusual properties and expression patterns. J Cell Biol 1990; 111:567.
98. Miettinen M. Keratin 20: Immunohistochemical marker for gastrointestinal, urothelial and Merkel cell carcinomas. Mod Pathol 1995; 8:384–388.
99. Moll R, Goldschmidt MD, et al. The human gene in coding cytokeratin 20 and its expression during fetal development and in gastrointestinal carcinomas. Differentiation 1993; 53:75–93.
100. Moll R, Lowe A, Laufer J, et al. Cytokeratin 20 in human carcinomas: A new histodiagnostic marker detected by monoclonal antibodies. Am J Pathol 1992; 140:427–447.
101. Tot T. Adenocarcinomas metastatic to the liver: The value of cytokeratins 20 and 7 in the search for unknown primary tumors. Cancer 1999; 85:171–177.
102. Moll I, Kuhn C, Moll R. Cytokeratin 20 is a general marker of cutaneous Merkel cells while certain neuronal proteins are absent. J Invest Dermatol 1995; 104:910–915.
103. Chan JK, Suster S, Wenig BM, et al. Cytokeratin 20 immunoreactivity distinguishes Merkel cell (primary cutaneous neuroendocrine) carcinomas and salivary gland small cell carcinomas from small cell carcinomas of various sites. Am J Surg Pathol 1997; 21:226–234.
104. Goldstein NS, Thomas M. Mucinous and nonmucinous bronchioloalveolar adenocarcinomas have distinct staining patterns with thyroid transcription factor and cytokeratin 20 antibodies. Am J Clin Pathol 2001; 116:319–325.
105. Lau SK, Desrochers MJ, Luthringer DJ. Expression of thyroid transcription factor-1, cytokeratin 7, and cyto-keratin 20 in bronchioloalveolar carcinomas: an immuno-histochemical evaluation of 67 cases. Mod Pathol 2002; 15:538–542.
106. Rossi G, Murer B, Cavazza A, et al. Primary mucinous (so-called colloid) carcinomas of the lung: a clinicopathologic and immunohistochemical study with special reference to CDX-2 homeobox gene and MUC2 expression. Am J Surg Pathol 2004; 28:442–452.
107. Delgado Y, Melamed J, Feiner H. Expression of cytokeratins 7 and 20 in 87 breast cancers. Am J Clin Pathol 1998; 110:517A
108. Tot T, Samii S. The clinical relevance of cytokeratin phenotyping in needle biopsy of liver metastasis. Apmis 2003,

111:1075–1082

109. Rullier A, Le Bail B, Fawaz R, et al. Cytokeratin 7 and 20 expression in cholangiocarcinomas varies along the biliary tract but still differs from that in colorectal carcinoma metastasis. Am J Surg Pathol 2000; 24:870–876.

110. Nikitakis NG, Tosios KI, Papanikolaou VS, et al. Immunohistochemical expression of cytokeratins 7 and 20 in malignant salivary gland tumors. Mod Pathol 2004; 17:407–415.

111. Fischer HP, Wilber K, et al. Keratin polypeptides in malignant epithelial liver tumors: Differential diagnosis and histogenetic aspects. Am J Pathol 1987; 127:530.

112. VanEyken P, Sciot R, Paterson A, et al. Cytokeratin expression in hepatocellular carcinoma: An immunohistochemical study. Hum Pathol 1988; 19:562.

113. Kim M-K, Park CK. Variable cytokeratin 7/20 profiles in carcinomas involving the liver. Appl Immunohistochem Mol Morphol 1999; 7:52–57.

114. Makhlouf HR, Ishak KG, Goodman ZD. Epithelioid hemangioendothelioma of the liver: A clinicopathologic study of 137 cases. Cancer 1999; 85:562–582.

115. Nandedkar MA, Abbondanzo SL, et al. CD45 (leukocyte common antigen) immunoreactivity in metastatic undifferentiated and neuroendocrine carcinoma: A potential diagnostic pitfall. Mod Pathol 1998; 11:1204–1210.

116. Millward C. CD 30 (Ber-H2) expression in non-hemopoietic tumors. Appl Immunohistochem 1998; 6:164–168.

117. Gown AM, Vogel AM. Anti-intermediate filament monoclonal antibodies: Tissue specific tools in tumor diagnosis. Surv Synth Pathol 1984; 3:369–385.

118. Gown AM, Vogel AM. Monoclonal antibodies to human intermediate filament proteins. II: Distribution of filament proteins in normal human tissues. Am J Pathol 1984; 114:309–321.

119. Gown AM, Vogel AM. Monoclonal antibodies to human intermediate filament proteins. III: Analysis of tumors. Am J Clin Pathol 1985; 84:413–424.

120. Santeusanio GD, D'Alfonso V, Lafrte E, et al. Antibodies to cytokeratin 14 specifically identify oncocytes (Hürthle cells) in thyroid lesions and tumors. Appl Immunohisto-chem 1997; 5:223–228.

121. Cover J, Oates J, Edwards C. Anti-cytokeratin 5-6: A positive marker for epithelioid mesothelioma. Histopathology 1997; 31:140–143.

122. Gotzos V, Fogt P, Celio MR. The calcium binding protein calretinin is a selective marker for malignant pleural mesotheliomas of the epithelial type. Pathol Res Pract 1996 192:137–147.

123. Ordonez NG. Value of cytokeratin 5/6 immunostaining in distinguishing epithelial mesothelioma of the pleura from lung adenocarcinoma. Am J Surg Pathol 1998; 22:1215–1221.

124. Reis-Filho JS, Simpson PT, Martins A, et al. Distribution of p63, cytokeratins 5/6 and cytokeratin 14 in 51 normal and 400 neoplastic human tissue samples using TARP-4 multi-tumor tissue microarray. Virchows Arch 2003; 443:122–132.

125. Kaufmann O, Fietze E, Mengs J, et al. Value of p63 and cytokeratin 5/6 as immunohistochemical markers for the differential diagnosis of poorly differentiated and undifferentiated carcinomas. Am J Clin Pathol 2001; 116:823–830.

126. Chu PG, Weiss LM. Expression of cytokeratin 5/6 in epithelial neoplasms: an immunohistochemical study of 509 cases. Mod Pathol 2002; 15:6–10.

127. Argani P, Rosai J. Hyperplastic mesothelial cells in lymph nodes: Report of 6 cases of a benign process that can simulate metastatic involvement by mesothelioma or carcinoma. 1998; Hum Pathol 29:339–346.

128. Miettinen M. Keratin subsets in spindle cell sarcomas: Keratins are widespread but synovial sarcoma contains a distinctive keratin polypeptide pattern and desmoplakins. Am J Pathol 1991; 138:505–513.

129. Miettinen M. Keratin immunohistochemistry: Update of applications and pitfalls. Pathol Annu 1993; 28:113–143.

130. Miettinen M. Immunoreactivity for cytokeratin and epithelial membrane antigen in leiomyosarcomas. Arch Pathol Lab Med 1988; 112:637–640.

131. Litzky LA, Brooks J. Cytokeratin immunoreactivity in malignant fibrous histiocytoma and spindle cell tumors: Comparison between frozen and paraffin embedded tissues. Mod Pathol 1992; 5:30–34.

132. Rosenberg AE, O'Connell J, Dickerson GR, et al. Expression of epithelial markers in malignant fibrous histiocytoma of the musculoskeletal system: An immunohistochemical and electron microscopic study. Hum Pathol 1993; 24:284–293.

133. Hazelbag HM, Mooi WJ, Fleuren GJ, et al. Chain specific keratin profile of epithelioid soft tissue sarcomas: An immunohistochemical study on synovial sarcoma and epithelioid sarcoma. Appl Immunohistochem 1996; 4:176–183.

134. Alobeid B, Brooks JJ, Zhang PJ. Cytokeratin subset immunoreactivity in sarcomas using a large panel of cyto-keratin subset antibodies. Appl Immunohistochem 1998; 6:154–157.

135. Zarbo RJ, Gown AM, Nagel RB, et al. Anomalous cyto-keratin expression in malignant melanoma: One and two dimensional Western blot analysis and immunohistochemical survey of 100 melanomas. Mod Pathol 1990; 3:494–501.

136. Traweek ST, Liu J, Battifora H. Keratin gene expression in non-epithelial tissues: Detection with polymerase chain reaction. Am J Pathol 1993; 142:1111–1118.

137. Swanson PE. Heffalumps, jagulars and cheshire cats. Am J Clin Pathol 1991; 95:S2–S7.

138. Alobeid B, Brooks, JJ, Zhang PJ. Aberrant cytokeratin subset immunoreactivity in sarcomas using a large panel of cytokeratin subset antibodies. Appl Immunohistochem 1998; 6:154–157.

139. Rizeq MN, Van De Rijn M, Hendrickson MR, et al. A comparative immunohistochemical study of uterine smooth muscle neoplasms with emphasis on the epithelioid variant. Hum Pathol 1994; 25:671–677.

140. Brown DC, Theaker JM, Banks PM, et al. Cytokeratin expression in smooth muscle and smooth muscle tumors. Histopathology 1987; 11:477.

141. Miettinen M, Rapola J. Immunohistochemical spectrum of rhabdomyosarcoma and rhabdomyosarcoma-like tumors: Expression of cytokeratin and the 68 kD neurofilament protein. Am J Surg Pathol 1989; 13:120–126.

142. Hirose T, Kudo E, Hasegawa T, et al. Expression of intermediate filaments in malignant fibrous histiocytomas. Hum Pathol 1989; 20:871–877.

143. Jones HJ, Anthony PP. Metastatic prostatic carcinoma presenting as left-sided cervical lymphadenopathy: A series of 11 cases. Histopathology 1992; 21:149–154.

144. Fletcher CD, Beham A, Bekir S, et al. Epithelioid angiosarcoma of deep soft tissue: A distinctive tumor readily mistaken for an epithelial neoplasm. Am J Surg Pathol 1991; 15:915–922.

145. Eusebi V, Carangiu ML, Dina R, et al. Keratin positive epithelioid angiosarcoma of thyroid: A report of four cases. Am J Surg Pathol 1990; 14:737.

146. Meis-Kindblom JM, Kindblom LG. Angiosarcoma of soft tissue: A study of 80 cases. Am J Surg Pathol 1998; 22:683–697.

147. Aubry MC, Myers JL, Colby TV, et al. Endometrial stromal sarcoma metastatic to the lung: a detailed analysis of 16 patients. Am J Surg Pathol 2002; 26:440–449.

148. Kwaspen FH, Smedts FM, Broos A, et al. Reproducible and highly sensitive detection of the broad spectrum epithelial marker keratin 19 in routine cancer diagnosis. Histopathology 1997; 31:503–516.

149. McCluggage WG, Clarke R, Toner PG. Cutaneous epi-thelioid angiosarcoma exhibiting cytokeratin positivity. Histopathology 1995; 27:291–294.

150. Jochum W, Schroder S, Risti B, et al. Cytokeratin positive angiosarcoma of the adrenal gland. Pathologe 1994; 15:181–186.

151. Goldblum J, Weiss TW. Epithelioid angiosarcoma of the pulmonary artery. Hum Pathol 1995; 26:1275–1277.

152. Hasegawa T, Fujii Y, Seki K, et al. Epithelioid angiosarcoma of bone. Hum Pathol 1997; 28:985–989.

153. Gown AM, Boyd H, Chang Y, et al. Smooth muscle cells can express cytokeratins of simple epithelium: Immunocytochemical and biochemical studies in vitro and in vivo. Am J Pathol 1988; 132:223.

154. Knapp AC, Franke WW. Spontaneous losses of control of cytokeratin gene expression in transformed nonepithelial human cells occurring at different levels of regulation. Cell 1989; 59:67.

155. Frisman DM, McCarthy WF, Schleiff P, et al. Immunocytochemistry in the differential diagnosis of effusions: Use of logistic regression to select the panel of antibodies to distinguish adenocarcinomas from mesothelial proliferations. Mod Pathol 1993; 6:179–184.

156. Ordonez NG, Tornos C. Malignant peripheral nerve sheath tumor of the pleura with epithelial and rhabdo-myoblastic differentiation: Report of a case clinically simulating mesothelioma. Am J Surg Pathol 1997; 21:1395–1398.

157. Banks DR, Jansen JF, Oberle E, et al. Cytokeratin positivity in fine needle aspirates of melanomas and sarcomas. Diagn Cytopathol 1995; 12:230–233.

158. Rosai J PG. Immunohistochemical demonstration of epithelial differentiation in adamantinoma of the tibia. Am J Surg Pathol 1982; 6:427.

159. Heikinheimo K, Persson S, Kindblom L-G, et al. Expression of different cytokeratin subclasses in human chordoma. J Pathol 1991; 164:145.

160. Gerharz CD, Moll R, Meister P, et al. Cytoskeletal heterogeneity of an epithelioid sarcoma with expression of vimentin, cytokeratins and neurofilaments. Am J Surg Pathol 1990; 14: 274.

161. Battifora H ed. Diagnostic uses of antibodies to keratins: a review and immunohistochemical comparison of 7 monoclonal and 3 polyclonal antibodies. Philadelphia: Field and Wood; 1988.

162. Smith KJ, Skelton HG 3rd, Morgan AM, et al. Spindle cell neoplasms coexpressing cytokeratin and vimentin. J Cutan Pathol 1992; 19:286–293.

163. Mooi WJ, Deenik W, Peterse JL, et al. Keratin immuno-reactivity in melanoma of soft parts (clear cell sarcoma). Histopathology 1995; 27:61–65.

164. Ben-Izhak A, Stark P, Lebi R, et al. Epithelial markers in malignant melanoma: A study of primary lesions and their metastases. Am J Dermatopathol 1994; 16:241–246.

165. Gatter KC, Ralkliaer E, Skinner JM, et al. An immunocytochemical study of malignant melanoma and its differential diagnosis from other malignant tumors. J Clin Pathol 1985; 38:1353–1357.

166. Miettinin M, Franssila K. Immunohistochemical spectrum of malignant melanoma: The common presence of keratin. Lab Invest 1989; 61:623–629.

167. Cosgrove M, Fitzgibbon P, Scherrod A, et al. Intermediate filament expression in astrocytic neoplasms. Am J Surg Pathol 1989; 13:144–145.

168. Krihl VK, Yang H, Moskal JR, et al. Keratin expression in astrocytomas: An immunofluorescence and biochemical reassessment. Virchows Arch 1997; 431:139–147.

169. Bacchi C, Zarbo R, Jiang JJ, et al. Do glioma cells express cytokeratin? Appl Immunohistochem 1995; 3:45–53.

170. Probst-Cousin S, Villagran Lillo R, Lahl R, et al. Secretory meningioma: Clinical, histologic, and immunohistochemical findings in 31 cases. Cancer 1997; 79:2003–2015.

171. Meis J, Ordonez N, Bruner JM. Meningiomas: An immunohistochemical study of 50 cases. Arch Pathol Lab Med 1986; 110:934.

172. Artleich A, Schmidt D. Immunohistochemical profile of meningiomas and their histologic subtypes. Hum Pathol 1990; 21:843.

173. Radley MG, DiSant'agnese P, Eskin TA, et al. Epithelial differentiation in meningiomas: An immunohistochemical, histochemical and ultrastructural study – with review of the literature. Am J Clin Pathol 1989; 92:26–31.

174. Gould VE, Bloom K, Franke WW, et al. Increased numbers of cytokeratin positive interstitial reticulum cells in reactive, inflammatory and neoplastic lymphadenopathies: Hyperplasia or induced expression? Virchows Arch 1995; 425:617–629.

175. Lasota J, Hyjek E, Koo CH, et al. Cytokeratin positive large cell lymphomas of B-cell lineage: A study of five phenotypically unusual cases verified by polymerase chain reaction. Am J Surg Pathol 1996; 20:346–354.

176. Cho J, Gong C, Choe G, et al. Extrafollicular reticulum cells in pathologic lymph nodes. J Korean Med Sci 1994; 9:9–15.

177. Zoltowska A. Immunohistochemical comparative investigations of lymphoid tissue in reactive processes, myasthenic thymuses and Hodgkin's disease. Arch Immunol Ther Exp 1995; 43:15–22.

178. Ramaekers F, Haag D, Rap P, et al. Immunochemical demonstration of keratin and vimentin in cytologic aspirates. Acta Cytol 1984; 28:385–392.

179. Iuzzolino P, Bontempini L, Doglioni C, et al. Keratin immunoreactivity in extrafollicular reticular cells of the lymph node. Am J Clin Pathol 1989; 91:239–240.

180. Franke WW, Moll R. Cytoskeletal components of lymphoid organs. I: Synthesis of cytokeratins 8 and 18 and desmin in subpopulations of extrafollicular reticulum cells of human lymph nodes, tonsils and spleen. Differentiation 1987; 36: 145–163.

181. Doglioni C, Dell'Orto P, Zanetti G, et al. Cytokeratin immunoreactive cells of lymph nodes and spleen in normal and pathologic conditions. Virchows Arch (A) 1990; 416:479–490.

182. Carbone A, Manconi R, Poletti A, et al. Heterogeneous immunostaining patterns of follicular dendritic reticulum cells in human lymphoid tissue with selected antibodies reactive with different cell lineages. Hum Pathol 1988; 19:51–56.

183. Xu X, Roberts SA, Pasha TL, et al. Undesirable cytokeratin immunoreactivity of native nonepithelial cells in sentinel lymph nodes from patients with breast carcinoma. Arch Pathol Lab Med 2000; 124:1310–1313.

184. Battifora H, Kapinski M. The influence of protease digestion and duration of fixation on the immunostaining of keratins: A comparison of formalin and ethanol fixation. J Histochem

Cytochem 1986; 34:1095–1099.
185. Frierson HF, Bellafiore F, Gaffey MJ, et al. Cytokeratin in anaplastic large cell lymphoma. Mod Pathol 1994; 7:317–321.
186. Kolarik J, Rejtthar A, Lauerova L, et al. Monoclonal antibodies against individual cytokeratins in the detection of metastatic spread. Int J Cancer 1988; 3:50.
187. Petruch U, Homy H-P, Keiserling E. Frequent expression of hemopoietic and nonhemopoietic antigens by neoplastic plasma cells: An immunohistochemical study using formalin-fixed paraffin embedded tissue. Histopathology 1992; 20:35.
188. Watherspoon AC, Norton A, Isaacson PG. Immunoreactive cytokeratins in plasmacytomas. Histopathology 1989; 14:141.
189. Gastmann C, Altmannberger M, Osborne M, et al. Cyto-keratin expression and vimentin content in large cell anaplastic lymphomas and other non-Hodgkin's lymphomas. Am J Pathol 1991; 138:1413.
190. Delsol G, AlSaati T, Gatter KC, et al. Coexpression of epithelial membrane antigen (EMA), Ki-1 and interleukin-2 receptor by anaplastic large cell lymphomas. Am J Pathol 1988; 130:59.
191. Miettenin M. Immunostaining of intermediate filament proteins in paraffin sections: Evaluation of optimal protease treatment to improve the immunoreactivity. Pathol Res Pract 1989; 184:431–435.
192. Battifora H. Assessment of antigen damage in immunohistochemistry: The vimentin internal control. Am J Clin Pathol 1991; 96:669–671.
193. Ramakers FCS, Haag D, Kant A, et al. Co-expression of keratin and vimentin-type intermediate filaments in human metastatic carcinoma cells. Proc Natl Acad Sci USA 1983; 80:2618–2622.
194. McNutt MA, Bolen J, Gown AM, et al. Co-expression of intermediate filaments in human epithelial neoplasms. Ultrastruct Pathol 1985; 9:31–43.
195. Geisinger K, Dabbs DJ, Marshall RB. Malignant mixed mullerian tumors and ultrastructural and immunohistochemical analysis with histogenetic considerations. Cancer 1987; 59:1781–1790.
196. Dabbs D, Geisinger K, Norris HT. Intermediate filaments in endometrial and endocervical carcinoma: The diagnostic utility of vimentin patterns. Am J Surg Pathol 1986; 10:568–576.
197. Dabbs D, Sturtz K, Zaino RJ. The immunohistochemical discrimination of endometrioid adenocarcinoma. Hum Pathol 1996; 27:172–177.
198. Pritchard D, Todd CW, Eghan ML. Chemistry of carcinoembryonic antigen. Methods Cancer Res 1978; 14:55–85.
199. Buchegger F, Schreyer M, Correl S, et al. Monoclonal antibodies identify a CEA cross-reacting antigen of 95 KD (MCA-95) distinct in antigenicity and tissue distribution from the previously described MCA 55 KD. Int J Cancer 1984; 33:643–649.
200. Nach J, Pusztaszeri G. Carcinoembryonic antigen: Demonstration of a partial identity between CEA and a normal glycoprotein. Immunochemistry 1972; 9:1031–1033.
201. Svenberg T. Carcinoembryonic antigen-like substances of human bile: Isolation and partial characterization. Int J Cancer 1976; 17:588–596.
202. Nagora H, Tsusumi Y, Watanabe K, et al. Immunohistochemistry of carcinoembryonic antigen, secretory component and lysozyme in benign and malignant common bile duct tissues. Virchows Arch (Pathol Anat) 1984; 403:271–280.
203. Maeda T, Kajiyama K, Adachi E, et al. The expression of cytokeratin 7, 19 and 20 in primary and metastatic carcinomas of the liver. Mod Pathol 1996; 9:901–909.
204. Osborne M, VanLessen G, Weber K, et al. Differential diagnosis of gastrointestinal carcinomas by using monoclonal antibodies specific for individual keratin polypeptides. Lab Invest 1986; 55:497–504.
205. Ferrandez-Izquierdo A, Llombart-Bosch A. Immunohistochemical characterization of 130 cases of primary hepatic carcinomas. Pathol Res Pract 1987; 182:783–791.
206. Chedid A CG, Eichorst M, et al. Antigenic markers of hepatocellular carcinoma. Cancer 1990; 65:84–87.
207. Ronnett BM, Kurman R, Zahn C, et al. Pseudomyxoma peritonei in women: A clinicopathologic analysis of 30 cases with emphasis on site of origin, prognosis and relationship to ovarian mucinous tumors of low malignant potential. Hum Pathol 1995; 26:509–524.
208. Wick M, Siegal G. Monoclonal antibodies to carcinoembryonic antigen in diagnostic immunohistochemistry. In: Wick MR, Siegal GP, eds. Monoclonal antibodies in diagnostic immunohistochemistry. New York: Marcel Dekker; 1988.

209. Sheahan K, O'Brian M, Burke D, et al. Differential reactivities of carcinoembryonic antigen and CEA-related monoclonal and polyclonal antibodies in common epithelial malignancies. Am J Clin Pathol 1990; 94:157–164.

210. Ma C, Zarbo R, Frierson H, et al. Comparative immunohistochemical study of primary and metastatic carcinomas of the liver. Am J Clin Pathol 1993; 99:551–557.

211. Balaton A, Nehama-Sibony M, Gotheil C, et al. Distinction between hepatocellular carcinoma, cholangiocarcinoma and metastatic carcinoma based on immunohistochemical staining for carcinoembryonic antigen and for cytokeratin 19 on paraffin sections. J Pathol 1988; 156:305–310.

212. Gottschalk-Sabag S, Ron N, Glick T. Use of CD-34 and factor VIII to diagnose hepatocellular carcinoma on fine needle aspirates. Acta Cytol 1998; 42:691–696.

213. Thomas P, Battifora H. Keratins versus epithelial membrane antigen in tumor diagnosis: an immunohistochemical comparison of five monoclonal antibodies. Hum Pathol 1987; 18:728–734.

214. Avery AK, Beckstead J, Renshaw AA, et al. Use of antibodies to RCC and CD10 in the differential diagnosis of renal neoplasms. Am J Surg Pathol 2000; 24:203–210.

215. Lau SK, Prakash S, Geller SA, et al. Comparative immunohistochemical profile of hepatocellular carcinoma, cholangiocarcinoma, and metastatic adenocarcinoma. Hum Pathol 2002; 33:1175–1181.

216. Cui S, Hanno H, Sakata A, et al. Enhanced CD-34 expression of sinusoid-like vascular endothelial cells in hepatocellular carcinoma. Pathol Int 1996; 46:751–756.

217. Wennerberg A, Nalesnik M, Coleman WB. Hepatocyte paraffin 1: A monoclonal antibody that reacts with hepatocytes and can be used for differential diagnosis of hepatic tumors. Am J Pathol 1993; 143:1050–1056.

218. Morrison C, Marsh W Jr, Frankel WL. A comparison of CD10 to pCEA, MOC-31, and hepatocyte for the distinction of malignant tumors in the liver. Mod Pathol 2002; 15:1279–1287.

219. Sinard J, Macleay L, Melamed J. Hepatoid adenocarcinoma in the urinary bladder: Unusual localization of a newly recognized tumor type. Cancer 1994; 73:1919–1925.

220. Ishikura H, Fukasawa Y, Ogasawara K, et al. An AFP-producing gastric carcinoma with features of hepatic differentiation: A case report. Cancer 1985; 56:840–848.

221. Pitman MB, Triratanachat S, Young RH, et al. Hepatocyte paraffin 1 antibody does not distinguish primary ovarian tumors with hepatoid differentiation from metastatic hepatocellular carcinoma. Int J Gynecol Pathol 2004; 23:58–64.

222. Chu PG, Weiss LM. Immunohistochemical characterization of signet-ring cell carcinomas of the stomach, breast, and colon. Am J Clin Pathol 2004; 121:884–892.

223. Porcell AI, De Young BR, Proca DM, et al Immunohistochemical analysis of hepatocellular and adenocarcinoma in the liver: MOC31 compares favorably with other putative markers. Mod Pathol 2000; 13:773–778.

224. Siddiqui MT, Saboorian MH, Gokaslan ST, et al. Diag-nostic utility of the HepPar1 antibody to differentiate hepatocellular carcinoma from metastatic carcinoma in fine-needle aspiration samples. Cancer 2002; 96:49–52.

225. Wieczorek TJ, Pinkus JL, Glickman JN, et al. Comparison of thyroid transcription factor-1 and hepatocyte antigen immunohistochemical analysis in the differential diagnosis of hepatocellular carcinoma, metastatic adenocarcinoma, renal cell carcinoma, and adrenal cortical carcinoma. Am J Clin Pathol 2002; 118:911–921.

226. Hilkens J, Buijs F, Hilgers J, et al. Monoclonal antibodies against human milk-fat globule membrane detecting differentiation antigens of the mammary gland and its tumors. Int J Cancer 1984; 34:197–206.

227. McGuckin M, Walsh M, Hohn B, et al. Prognostic significance of MUC1 epithelial mucin expression in breast cancer. Hum Pathol 1996; 26:432–439.

228. Zoretsky J, Weiss M, Tsafaty I, et al. Expression of genes coding of PS2, C-erB2 estrogen receptor and the H23 breast tumor associated antigen: A comparative analysis in breast cancer. FEBS Lett 1990; 265:46–50.

229. Hilkens J, Ligtenberg MJL, Vos HL, et al. Cell membrane associated mucins and their adhesion property. Trends Biochem Sci 1992; 17:359–363.

230. Pinkus G, Etheridge C, O'Connor E. Are keratin proteins a better tumor marker than epithelial membrane antigen? A comparative immunohistochemical study of various paraffin-embedded neoplasms using monoclonal and polyclonal antibodies. Am J Clin Pathol 1986; 85:269–277.

231. Gatter K, Alcock C, Heryet A, et al. The clinical importance of analyzing tumors of uncertain origin by immunohistological techniques. Lancet 1985; 1:1302–1305.

232. Wick MR, Swanson PE, eds. Immunohistochemical findings in tumors of the skin. New York: Marcel Dekker; 1989.

233. Hilkens J, Buijs F. Biosynthesis of NAM-6, an epithelial sialomucin. J Biol Chem 1988; 263:4215–4222.

234. Hilkens J, Buijs F, Ligtenberg M. Complexity of MAM-6, an epithelial sialomucin associated with carcinomas. Cancer Res 1989; 49:786–793.

235. Gendler S, Taylor-Papadimitriou J, Duhig T, et al. Immunogenic region of a human polymorphic epithelial mucin expressed by carcinomas is made up of tandem repeats. J Biol Chem 1988; 263:12820–12823.

236. Hayes DF, Zurawski V, Kufe DW. Comparison of circulating CA15-3 and carcinoembryonic antigen levels in patients with breast cancer. J Clin Oncol 1986; 4:1532–1550.

237. Kufe D, Inghirami G, Abe M, et al. Differential reactivity of a novel monoclonal antibody (DF3) with human malignant vs benign breast tumors. Hybridoma 1984; 3:223–232.

238. Peterson JA, Zava DT, Duwe A, et al. Biochemical and histological characterization of antigens preferentially expressed on the surface and cytoplasm of breast carcinoma cells identified by monoclonal antibodies against a human milk fat globule. Hybridoma 1990; 9:221–235.

239. Peterson J, Couto J, Taylor M, et al. Selection of tumor-specific epitopes on target antigens for radioimmuno-therapy. Cancer Res 1995; 55:5847S–5851S.

240. Swanson P, ed. Monoclonal antibodies to human milk fat globule proteins. New York: Marcel Dekker; 1988.

241. Al-Naffussi A, Carder PJ. Monoclonal antibodies in the cytodiagnosis of serous effusions. Cytopathology 1990; 1:119–128.

242. Leong A-Y, Parkinson R, Milios J. 'Thick' cell mem-branes revealed by immunocytochemical staining: A clue to the diagnosis of mesothelioma. Diagn Cytopathol 1990; 6:9–13.

243. Singh HK, Silverman JF, Burns L, et al. Significance of epithelial membrane antigen in the workup of problematic serous effusions. Diagn Cytopathol 1995; 13:3–7.

244. Delsol G, Gatter KC, Stein H, et al. Human lymphoid cells express epithelial membrane antigen. Lancet 1984; 2:1124–1129.

245. Chittal SM, Delsol G. The interface between Hodgkin's disease and anaplastic large cell lymphoma. Cancer Surv 1997; 30:87–105.

246. Stein H, Hansmann M-L, Lennert K, et al. Reed-Sternberg and Hodgkin's cells in lymphocyte predominant Hodgkin's disease of nodular subtype contain J-chain. Am J Clin Pathol 1986' 86:292–297.

247. Chittal SM, Caveriviere P, Schwarting R, et al. Mono-clonal antibodies in the diagnosis of Hodgkin's disease: The search for a rational panel. Am J Surg Pathol 1988; 12:9–21.

248. Gatter K, Abdulaziz Z, Beverly P, et al. Use of monoclonal antibodies for the histopathological diagnosis of human malignancy. J Clin Pathol 1982; 35:1253–1267.

249. Sarkar AB, Akagi T, Yoshino T, et al. Expression of vimentin and epithelial membrane antigen in malignant lymphomas. Acta Pathol Jpn 1990; 40:581–587.

250. Hall PA, D'Ardenne J, Stansfeld A. Paraffin section of immunohistochemistry. I: Non-Hodgkin's lymphoma. Histopathology 1988; 13:149–160.

251. Strickler JG, Weiss LM, Copenhaver CM, et al. Monoclonal antibodies reactive in routinely processed tissue sections of malignant lymphoma, with emphasis on T-cell lymphomas. Hum Pathol 1987; 18:808–814.

252. Fujimoto J, Hata J, Ishii E, et al. Ki1 lymphomas in childhood: Immunohistochemical analysis and the significance of epithelial membrane antigen (EMA) as a new marker. Virchows Arch A Pathol Anat Histopathol 1988; 412:307–314.

253. Al Saati T, Caveriviere P, Gorguet B, et al. Epithelial antigen in hemopoietic neoplasms [letter]. Hum Pathol 1986; 17:533–534.

254. Leocini L, Del Vecchio MT, Kraft R, et al. Hodgkin's disease and CD30 positive anaplastic large cell lymphomas – a continuous spectrum of malignant disorders. Am J Pathol 1990; 137:1047–1057.

255. Carbone A, Gloghini A, Volpe R. Paraffin section immunohistochemistry in the diagnosis of Hodgkin's disease and anaplastic large cell (CD30+) lymphomas. Virchows Arch A Pathol Anat Histopathol 1992; 420:527–532.

256. Piris M, Brown D, Gatter K, et al. CD30 expression in non-Hodgkin's lymphoma. Histopathology 1990; 17:211–218.

257. Chott A, Kasere K, Augustin I, et al. Ki-1 positive large cell lymphoma: A clinicopathologic study of 41 cases. Am J Surg Pathol 1990; 14:439–448.

258. Pilieri S, Bocchia M, Baroni C, et al. Anaplastic large cell lymphoma (CD30+/Ki-1+): Results of a prospective clinicopathologic study of 69 cases. Br J Haematol 1994; 86:513–523.

259. Shek T, Yuen S, Luk I, et al. Germ cell tumor as a diagnostic pitfall of metastatic carcinoma. J Clin Pathol 1996; 49:223.

260. Giwercman A, Marks A, Bailey D, et al. M2A – a monoclonal antibody as a marker for carcinoma in-situ germ cells of the human adult testis. Acta Pathol Microbiol Immunol Scand (A) 1988; 96:667–670.

261. Jacobson G, Norgaard-Pedersen D. Placental alkaline phosphatase in testicular germ cell tumors and carcinoma in situ of the testis: An immunohistochemical study. Acta Pathol Microbiol Immunol Scand (A) 1984; 92:323–329.

262. Giwercman A, Andrews P, Jorgensen M, et al. Immunohistochemical expression of embryonal marker TRA-1-60 in carcinoma in-situ and germ cell tumors of the testis. Cancer 1993; 72:1308–1314.

263. Fogel M, Lifschitz-Nercer B, Moll R. Heterogeneity of intermediate filament expression in human testicular seminomas. Differentiation 1990; 45:242–249.

264. Burke A, Mostofi FK. Placental alkaline phosphatase immunohistochemistry of intratubular malignant germ cells and associated testicular germ cell tumors. Hum Pathol 1988; 19:663–670.

265. Cummings OW, Ulbright TM, Eble JM, et al. Spermatocytic seminoma: An immunohistochemical study. Hum Pathol 1994; 25:54–59.

266. Niehans GA, Nanibel JC, Copland GT, et al. Immunohistochemistry of germ cell and trophoblastic neoplasms. Cancer 1988; 62:1113–1123.

267. Nanibel JC, Jessuran J, Wick MR, et al. Placental alkaline phosphatase immunoreactivity in testicular germ cell tumors. Am J Surg Pathol 1987; 11:21–29.

268. Uchiba T, Shimoda T, Miyata H, et al. Immunoperoxidase study of alkaline phosphatase in testicular tumors. Cancer 1981; 48:1455–1462.

269. Hustin J, Collettee J, Franchimont P. Immunohistochemical demonstration of placental alkaline phosphatase in various states of testicular development and in germ cell tumors. Int J Androl 1987; 10:29–35.

270. Wick M, Swanson P, Manivel J. Placental-like alkaline phosphatase reactivity in human tumors: An immuno-histochemical study of 520 cases. Hum Pathol 1987; 18:946–954.

271. Bailey D, Marks A, Stratis M, et al. Immunohistochemical staining of germ cell tumors and intratubular malignant germ cells of the testis using antibody to placental alkaline phosphatase and a monoclonal antiseminoma antibody. Mod Pathol 1991; 4:167–171.

272. Lles RK, Ind TE, Chard T. Production of placenta-like alkaline phosphatase and PLAP-like material in epithelial germ cell and non-germ cell tumors in vitro. Br J Cancer 1994; 69:274–278.

273. Watanabe H, Tokuyama H, Ohta H, et al. Expression of placental alkaline phosphatase in gastric and colorectal cancers: An immunohistochemical study using the prepared monoclonal antibody. Cancer 1990; 66:2575–2582.

274. Mostofi FK, Sesterhenn RA, David CJJ. Immunopathology of germ cell tumors of the testis. Semin Diagn Pathol 1987; 4:320–341.

275. Jacobsen GK, Jacobsen M. Alpha-fetoprotein (AFP) and human chorionic gonadotropin in testicular germ cell tumors: A prospective immunohistochemical study. Acta Pathol Microbiol Immunol Scand (A) 1983; 91:165–176.

276. Eglen D, Ulbright T. The differential diagnosis of yolk sac tumor and seminoma: Usefulness of cytokeratin, alpha-fetoprotein and alpha-1-antitrypsin immunoperoxidase reactions. Am J Clin Pathol 1987; 88:328–332.

277. Hattab EM, Tu PH, Wilson JD, et al. OCT4 immunohistochemistry is superior to placental alkaline phosphatase (PLAP) in the diagnosis of central nervous system germinoma. Am J Surg Pathol 2005; 29:368–371.

278. Cheng L, Thomas A, Roth LM, et al. OCT4: a novel biomarker for dysgerminoma of the ovary. Am J Surg Pathol 2004; 28:1341–1346.

279. Jones TD, Ulbright TM, Eble JN, et al. OCT4 staining in testicular tumors: a sensitive and specific marker for seminoma and embryonal carcinoma. Am J Surg Pathol 2004; 28:935–940.

280. Wiedemann MB, Kuhn C, Schwechheimer K, et al. Synaptophysin identified by metastases of neuroendocrine tumors by immunocytochemistry and immunoblotting. Am J Clin Pathol 1987; 88:560–569.

281. Wilson BS, Lloyd R. Detection of chromogranin in neuroendocrine cells with a monoclonal antibody. Am J Pathol 1984; 115:458–468.

282. Lloyd RV, Wilson BS. Specific endocrine marker defined by a monoclonal antibody. Science 1983; 222:628–630.

283. DeStephano DV, Lloyd RV, Pike AM, et al. Pituitary adenomas: An immunohistochemical study of hormone pro-

duction and chromogranin localization. Am J Pathol 1984; 116:464–472.

284. Lloyd R, Mervak T, Schmidt K, et al. Immunohistochemical detection of chromogranin and neuron-specific enolase in pancreatic endocrine neoplasms. Am J Surg Pathol 1984; 8:607–614.

285. Wick MR, Siega GP, eds. Monoclonal antibodies to chromogranin: characterization and comparison with other neuroendocrine markers. New York: Marcel Dekker; 1988.

286. Wiedemann B, Franke WW. Identification and localization of synaptophysin, an integral membrane glycoprotein of MW 38,000 characteristic of presynaptic vesicles. Cell 1985; 41:1017–1028.

287. Thomas L, Hartung K, Langosch D, et al. Identifica-tion of synaptophysin as a hexomeric channel protein of the synaptic vesicle membrane. Science 1988; 242:1050–1053.

288. Staren ED, Gould VE, Warren WH, et al. Neuroendocrine carcinomas of the colon and rectum: A clinicopathologic evaluation. Surgery 1988; 104:1080–1089.

289. Piehl M, Gould V, Warren W, et al. Immunohistochemical identification of exocrine and neuroendocrine subsets of large cell carcinomas. Pathol Res Pract 1988; 183:675–682.

290. Guinee DG Jr, Fishback MF, Koss MN, et al. The spectrum of immunohistochemical staining of small cell lung carcinoma and specimens from transbronchial and open lung biopsies. Am J Clin Pathol 1994; 102:406–414.

291. Kayser K, Schmid W, Ebert W, et al. Expression of neuroendocrine markers (neuron specific enolase, synaptophysin and bombesin) in carcinoma of the lung. Pathol Res Pract 1988; 183:412–417.

292. Abel T, Balch CM. The differentiation antigen of human NK and K-cells identified by a monoclonal antibody (HNK-1). J Immunol 1981; 127:1024–1029.

293. Mechtersheimer G. Towards the phenotyping of soft tissue tumors by cell surface molecules. Virchows Arch A Pathol Anat Histopathol 1991; 419:7–28.

294. Baylon SB, Jackson RD, Goodwin G, et al. Neuroendocrine-related biochemistry in the spectrum of human lung cancers. Exp Lung Res 1982; 3:209–223.

295. Caillaud JM, Benjelloun S, Bosq J, et al. HNK-1 defined antigen detected in paraffin embedded neuroectodermal tumors and those derived from cells of the amine precursor uptake and decarboxylation system. Cancer Res 1984; 44:4432–4439.

296. Shioda Y, Nagura H, Tsutsumi Y, et al. Distribution of Leu-7 (HNK-1) antigen in human digestive organs: An immunohistochemical study with monoclonal antibody. Histochem J 1984; 16:843–854.

297. Cole SP, Mirski A, McGarry RC, et al. Differential expression of the Leu-7 antigen on human lung tumor cells. Cancer Res 1985; 45:4285–4290.

298. Battifora H, Silva E. The use of antikeratin antibodies in the immunohistochemical distinction between neuroendocrine (Merkel cell) carcinoma of the skin, lymphoma and oat cell carcinoma. Cancer 1986; 58:1040–1046.

299. Osborne M, Dirk T, Kaser H. et al. Immunohistochemical localization of neurofilaments and neuron-specific enolase in 29 cases of neuroblastoma. Am J Pathol 1986; 122:437–442.

300. Tsokos M, Linnoila RI, Chandra RS, et al. Neuron-specific enolase in the diagnosis of neuroblastoma and other small round cell tumors in children. Hum Pathol 1984; 15:575–584.

301. Vinores SA, Bonnin JN, Rubenstein LJ, et al. Immunohistochemical demonstration of neuron specific enolase in neoplasms of the CNS and other tumors. Arch Pathol Lab Med 1984; 108:536–540.

302. Nicholson SA, McDermott MB, Swanson PE, et al. CD99 and cytokeratin-20 in small-cell and basaloid tumors of the skin. Appl Immunohistochem Mol Morphol 2000; 8:37–41.

303. Jiang C, Tan Y, Li E. Histopathological and immunohistochemical studies on medullary thyroid carcinoma. Chung Hua Ping Li Hsueh Tsa Chih 1996; 25:332–335.

304. Kargi A, Yorukoglu A, Aktas S. Neuroendocrine differentiation in non-neuroendocrine thyroid carcinoma. Thyroid 1996; 6:207–210.

305. Kovacs CS, Mase RM, Kovacs K, et al. Thyroid medullary carcinoma with thyroglobulin immunoreactivity in sporadic multiple endocrine neoplasia type 2-B. Cancer 1994; 74:928–932.

306. Ruck P, Horny HP, Greschniok A, et al. Non-specific immunostaining of blast cells of acute leukemia by antibodies against non-hemopoietic antigens. Hematol Pathol 1995; 9:39–56.

307. DiLoreto C, Pglisi F, DiLauro V, et al. Immunocytochemical expression of tissue specific transcription factor-1 in lung carcinoma. J Clin Pathol 1997; 50:30–32.

308. DiLoreto C, Pglisi F, DiLauro V, et al. TTF-1 protein expression in pleural malignant mesotheliomas and adenocarcinomas of the lung. Cancer Lett 1998; 124:73–78.

309. Fabbro D, DiLoreto C, Stamerra O, et al. TTF-1 gene expression and human lung tumors. Eur J Cancer 1996; 32A: 512–517.

310. Bejarno PA, Baughman RP, Biddinger PW, et al. Surfactant proteins and thyroid transcription factor 1 in pulmonary and breast carcinomas. Mod Pathol 1996; 9:445–452.

311. Lazzaro D, Price M, DeFelice M, et al. The transcription factor TTF-1 is expressed at the onset of thyroid and lung morphogenesis and in restricted regions of the fetal brain. Development 1991; 113:1093–1104.

312. Stahlman MT, Gray ME, Whitsett JA. Expression of thyroid transcription factor-1 (TTF-1) and fetal and neo-natal human lung. J Histochem Cytochem 1996; 44:673–678.

313. Anwar F, Schmidt RA. Thyroid transcription factor-1 (TTF-1) distinguishes mesothelioma from pulmonary adenocarcinoma. Lab Invest 1997; 79:181A.

314. Guazzi S, Price M, DeFelice M, et al. Thyroid nuclear factor 1 (TTF-1) contains a homeodomain and displays a novel DNA binding specificity. Endo J 1990; 9:3631–3639.

315. Khoor A, Whitsett JA, Stahlman MT, et al. Utility of surfactant protein B precursor and thyroid transcription factor-1 in differentiating adenocarcinoma from malignant mesothelioma. Hum Pathol 1999; 30:695–700.

316. Folpe AL, Gown AM, Lamps LW, et al. Thyroid transcription factor-1 immunohistochemical evaluation of pulmonary neuroendocrine tumors. Mod Pathol 1999; 12:5–8.

317. Holzinger A, Dingle S, Bejarano PA, et al. Monoclonal antibody to thyroid transcription factor-1: Production, characterization and usefulness in tumor diagnosis. Hybridoma 1996; 15:49–53.

318. Kaufmann O, Dietel M. Expression of thyroid transcription factor-1 in pulmonary and extrapulmonary small cell carcinomas and other neuroendocrine carcinomas of various primary sites. Histopathology 2000; 36:415–420.

319. Ordonez NG. Value of thyroid transcription factor-1 immunostaining in distinguishing small cell lung carcinomas from other small cell carcinomas. Am J Surg Pathol 2000; 24:1217–1223.

320. Afify AM, al-Khafaji BM. Diagnostic utility of thyroid transcription factor-1 expression in adenocarcinomas presenting in serous fluids. Acta Cytol 2002; 46:675–678.

321. Jang KY, Kang MJ, Lee DG, et al. Utility of thyroid transcription factor-1 and cytokeratin 7 and 20 immunostaining in the identification of origin in malignant effusions. Anal Quant Cytol Histol 2001; 23:400–404.

322. Roh MS, Hong SH. Utility of thyroid transcription factor-1 and cytokeratin 20 in identifying the origin of metastatic carcinomas of cervical lymph nodes. J Korean Med Sci 2002; 17:512–517.

323. Chang YL, Lee YC, Liao WY, et al. The utility and limitation of thyroid transcription factor-1 protein in primary and metastatic pulmonary neoplasms. Lung Cancer 2004; 44:149–157.

324. Tan J, Sidhu G, Greco A, et al. Villin, cytokeratin 7 and cytokeratin 20 expression in pulmonary adenocarcinoma with ultrastructural evidence of microvilli with rootlets. Hum Pathol 1998; 29:390–396.

325. Nambu Y, Iannettoni MD, Orringer MB, et al. Unique expression patterns and alterations in the intestinal protein villin in primary and metastatic pulmonary adenocarcinomas. Mol Carcinog 1998; 23:233–242.

326. Sharma S, Tan J, Sidhu G, et al. Lung adenocarcinomas metastatic to the brain with and without ultrastructural evidence of rootlets: An electron microscopic and immunohistochemical study using cytokeratins 7 and 20 and villin. Ultrastruct Pathol 1998; 22:385–391.

327. Bacchi CE, Gown AM. Distribution and pattern of ex-pression of villin, a gastrointestinal-associated cytoskeletal protein in human carcinomas: A study employing paraffin-embedded tissue. Lab Invest 1991; 64:418–424.

328. Drummond F, Putt W, Fox M, et al. Cloning and chromosome assignment of the human CDX2 gene. Ann Hum Genet 1997; 61(Pt 5):393–400.

329. Mallo GV, Rechreche H, Frigerio JM, et al. Molecular cloning, sequencing and expression of the mRNA encoding human Cdx1 and Cdx2 homeobox. Down-regulation of Cdx1 and Cdx2 mRNA expression during colorectal carcinogenesis. Int J Cancer 1997; 74:35–44.

330. Beck F, Chawengsaksophak K, Waring P, et al. Reprogramming of intestinal differentiation and intercalary regeneration in Cdx2 mutant mice. Proc Natl Acad Sci USA 1999; 96: 7318–7323.

331. Chawengsaksophak K, James R, Hammond VE, et al.

Homeosis and intestinal tumours in Cdx2 mutant mice. Nature 1997; 386:84–87.

332. Tamai Y, Nakajima R, Ishikawa T, et al. Colonic hamartoma development by anomalous duplication in Cdx2 knockout mice. Cancer Res 1999; 59:2965–2970.

333. Barbareschi M, Murer B, Colby TV, et al. CDX-2 homeobox gene expression is a reliable marker of colorectal adenocarcinoma metastases to the lungs. Am J Surg Pathol 2003; 27:141–149.

334. Bai YQ, Yamamoto H, Akiyama Y, et al. Ectopic expression of homeodomain protein CDX2 in intestinal metaplasia and carcinomas of the stomach. Cancer Lett 2002; 176:47–55.

335. Werling RW, Yaziji H, Bacchi CE, et al. CDX2, a highly sensitive and specific marker of adenocarcinomas of intestinal origin: an immunohistochemical survey of 476 primary and metastatic carcinomas. Am J Surg Pathol 2003; 27:303–310.

336. Barbareschi M, Roldo C, Zamboni G, et al. CDX-2 homeobox gene product expression in neuroendocrine tumors: its role as a marker of intestinal neuroendocrine tumors. Am J Surg Pathol 2004; 28:1169–1176.

337. Wang HL, Lu DW, Yerian LM, et al. Immunohistochemical distinction between primary adenocarcinoma of the bladder and secondary colorectal adenocarcinoma. Am J Surg Pathol 2001; 25:1380–1387.

338. Raspollini MR, Baroni G, Taddei A, et al. Primary cervical adenocarcinoma with intestinal differentiation and colonic carcinoma metastatic to cervix: an investigation using Cdx-2 and a limited immunohistochemical panel. Arch Pathol Lab Med 2003; 127:1586–1590.

339. Tot T. Identifying colorectal metastases in liver biopsies: the novel CDX2 antibody is less specific than the cytokeratin 20+/7- phenotype. Med Sci Monit 2004; 10:BR139–143.

340. Hinoi T, Tani M, Lucas PC, et al. Loss of CDX2 expression and microsatellite instability are prominent features of large cell minimally differentiated carcinomas of the colon. Am J Pathol 2001; 159:2239–2248.

341. Lowe FC, Trauzzi SJ. Prostatic acid phosphatase in 1993: Its limited clinical utility. Urol Clin North Am 1993; 20:589–596.

342. Komoshida S, Tsutsumi Y. Extraprostatic localization of prostatic acid phosphatase and prostate specific antigen: Distribution in cloacogenic glandular epithelium and sex dependent expression. Hum Pathol 1990; 21:1108–1115.

343. Kote RJ, Taylor CR. Prostate, bladder, and kidney. Philadelphia: WB Saunders; 1994.

344. Frazier HA, Humphrey PA, Burchette JL, et al. Immunoreactive prostate specific antigen in male periurethral glands. J Urol 1992; 147:246–250.

345. Elgamaol A, van de Voorde W, van Poppel W, et al. Immunohistochemical localization of prostate-specific markers within the accessory periurethral glands of Calper, Lattre and Morgagni. Urology 1994; 434:84–90.

346. Nowels K, Kent E, Ranshl K. Prostate specific antigen and acid phosphatase-reactive cells in cystitis cystica and glandularis. Arch Pathol Lab Med 1988; 112:734–738.

347. Golz R, Shubert GE. Prostate specific antigen: Immuno-reactivity in urachal remnants. J Urol 1989; 141:1480–1484.

348. Van Krieken J. Prostate marker immunoreactivity in salivary gland neoplasms – a rare pitfall in immunohistochemistry. Am J Surg Pathol 1993; 17:410–414.

349. Alanen KA, Kuopio T, Koskinen PJ, et al. Immunohistochemical labeling for prostate specific antigen in non-prostatic tissues. Pathol Res Pract 1996; 192:233–237.

350. Bostwick DG. Prostate specific antigen: Current role in diagnostic pathology of prostate cancer. Am J Clin Pathol 1994; 102:(Suppl):S31–S37.

351. Kuriyama J, Wang M, Lee C, et al. Multiple marker evaluation in human prostate cancer with use of tissue specific antigens. J Natl Cancer Inst 1982; 68:99–105.

352. Nadji J, Tabei SZ, Castro A, et al. Prostatic origin of tumors: An immunohistochemical study. Am J Clin Pathol 1980; 73:735–739.

353. Millar EA, Sharma MK, Lessells AM. A clinicopathologic study of 16 cases. Ductal (endometrioid) adenocarcinoma of the prostate. Histopathology 1996; 29:11–19.

354. Lee SS. Endometrioid adenocarcinoma of the prostate: A clinicopathologic and immunohistochemical study. J Surg Onco 1994; 55:235–238.

355. Leong FJ, Leong AS, Swift J. Signet ring carcinoma of the prostate. Pathol Res Pract 1996; 192:1232-1238.

356. Kremer S, Farnham RJ, Glen JF, et al. Comparative morphology of primary and secondary deposits of prostatic adenocarcinoma. Cancer 1981; 38:271–273.

357. Bovenberg SA, Vanderzvet CJJ, Vanderkrast T, et al. Prostate specific antigen expression in prostate cancer and its metastasis. J Urol Pathol 1993; 1:55–62.

358. Estabon JN, Battifora H. Tumor immunophenotype: Comparison between primary neoplasm and its metastases. Mod Pathol 1990; 3:192–196.

359. Bodey B, Birdie B, Kaiser H. Immunocytochemical detection of prostate specific antigen expression in human primary and metastatic melanomas. Anticancer Res 1997; 17:2343–2346.

360. Fan CY, Wang J, Barnes EL. Expression of androgen receptor and prostatic specific markers in salivary duct carcinoma: an immunohistochemical analysis of 13 cases and review of the literature. Am J Surg Pathol 2000; 24:579–586.

361. Horoszewicz JS, Kawinski E, Murphy GP. Monoclonal antibodies to a new antigenic marker in epithelial prostatic cells and serum prostatic cancer patients. Anticancer Res 1987; 7:927–936.

362. Wright GLJ, Haley C, Beckett NO, et al. Expression of prostate-specific membrane antigen in normal, benign and malignant tissues. Urol Oncol 1995; 1:18–28.

363. Silver DA, Pellicer I, Fair WR, et al. Prostate-specific membrane antigen expression in normal and malignant human tissues. Clin Cancer Res 1997; 3:81–85.

364. Murphy GP, Elgamal A-A, Su SL, et al. Current evaluation of the tissue localization and diagnostic utility of prostate specific membrane antigen. Cancer 1998; 83:2259–2269.

365. Bostwick DG, Pacelli A, Blute M, et al. Prostate specific membrane antigen expression in prostatic intraepithelial neoplasia and adenocarcinoma: A study of 184 cases. Cancer 1998; 82:2256–2261.

366. Murphy GP, Barren RJ, Erickson SJ, et al. Evaluation and comparison of two new prostate carcinoma markers: Free-prostate specific antigen and prostate specific membrane antigen. 1996; 78:809–818.

367. Troyer J, Beckett ML, White GLJ. Location of prostate-specific membrane antigen in the LNCaP prostate carcinoma cell line. Prostate 1997; 30:232–242.

368. Murphy G, Teno W, Holmes E, et al. Measurement of prostate-specific membrane antigen in the serum with a new antibody. Prostate 1996; 28:266–271.

369. Zhou M, Chinnaiyan AM, Kleer CG, et al. Alpha-methylacyl-CoA racemase: a novel tumor marker over-expressed in several human cancers and their precursor lesions. Am J Surg Pathol 2002; 26:926–931.

370. Jiang Z, Fanger GR, Woda BA, et al. Expression of alpha-methylacyl-CoA racemase (P504s) in various malignant neoplasms and normal tissues: a study of 761 cases. Hum Pathol 2003; 34:792–796.

371. Skinnider BF, Oliva E, Young RH, et al. Expression of alpha-methylacyl-CoA racemase (P504S) in nephrogenic adenoma: a significant immunohistochemical pitfall compounding the differential diagnosis with prostatic adenocarcinoma. Am J Surg Pathol 2004; 28:701–705.

372. Yoshida SO, Imam A. Monoclonal antibody to a proximal nephrogenic renal antigen: immunohistochemical analysis of formalin-fixed, paraffin-embedded human renal cell carcinomas. Cancer Res 1989; 49:1802–1809.

373. McGregor DK, Khurana KK, Cao C, et al. Diagnosing primary and metastatic renal cell carcinoma: the use of the monoclonal antibody 'Renal Cell Carcinoma Marker'. Am J Surg Pathol 2001; 25:1485–1492.

374. Meunier H, Rivier C, Evans RM, et al. Gonadal and extragonadal expression of inhibin alpha, beta A, and beta B subunits in various tissues predicts diverse functions. Proc Natl Acad Sci USA 1988; 85:247–251.

375. Cho EY, Ahn GH. Immunoexpression of inhibin alpha-subunit in adrenal neoplasms. Appl Immunohistochem Mol Morphol 2001; 9:222–228.

376. Loy TS, Phillips RW, Linder CL. A103 immunostaining in the diagnosis of adrenal cortical tumors: an immunohistochemical study of 316 cases. Arch Pathol Lab Med 2002; 126:170–172.

377. Shin SJ, Hoda RS, Ying L, et al. Diagnostic utility of the monoclonal antibody A103 in fine-needle aspiration biopsies of the adrenal. Am J Clin Pathol 2000; 113:295–302.

378. Murakata LA, Ishak KG, Nzeako UC. Clear cell carcinoma of the liver: a comparative immunohistochemical study with renal clear cell carcinoma. Mod Pathol 2000; 13:874–881.

379. Fetsch PA, Powers CN, Zakowski MF, et al. Antialpha-inhibin: marker of choice for the consistent distinction between adrenocortical carcinoma and renal cell carcinoma in fine-needle aspiration. Cancer 1999; 87:168–172.

380. Cameron RI, Ashe P, O'Rourke DM, et al. A panel of immunohistochemical stains assists in the distinction between ovarian and renal clear cell carcinoma. Int J Gynecol Pathol 2003; 22:272–276.

381. Ghorab Z, Jorda M, Ganjei P, et al. Melan A (A103) is expressed in adrenocortical neoplasms but not in renal cell and

hepatocellular carcinomas. Appl Immunohistochem Mol Morphol 2003; 11:330–333.

382. Chan TY, Mikolajczyk SD, Lecksell K, et al. Immunohistochemical staining of prostate cancer with monoclonal antibodies to the precursor of prostate-specific antigen. Urology 2003; 62:177–181.

383. Beach R, Gown AM, De Peralta-Venturina MN, et al. P504S immunohistochemical detection in 405 prostatic specimens including 376 18-gauge needle biopsies. Am J Surg Pathol 2002; 26:1588–1596.

384. Moll R, Wu X, Lin J, et al. Uroplakins, specific membrane proteins of urothelial umbrella cells, as histologic markers of metastatic transitional cell carcinoma. Am J Pathol 1995; 147:1383–1397.

385. Wu R, Osman I, Wu X, et al. Uroplakin II gene is expressed in transitional cell carcinoma but not in Bilharzial bladder squamous cell carcinoma: Alternative pathways of bladder epithelial differentiation and tumor formation. Cancer Res 1998; 58:1291–1297.

386. Parker DC, Folpe AL, Bell J, et al. Potential utility of uroplakin III, thrombomodulin, high molecular weight cyto-keratin, and cytokeratin 20 in noninvasive, invasive, and metastatic urothelial (transitional cell) carcinomas. Am J Surg Pathol 2003; 27:1–10.

387. Ordonez NG. Value of thrombomodulin immunostaining in a diagnosis of mesothelioma. Histopathology 1997; 31:25–30.

388. Langner C, Ratschek M, Tsybrovskyy O, et al. P63 immunoreactivity distinguishes upper urinary tract transitional-cell carcinoma and renal-cell carcinoma even in poorly differentiated tumors. J Histochem Cytochem 2003; 51:1097–1099.

389. Jiang J, Ulbright TM, Younger C, et al. Cytokeratin 7 and cytokeratin 20 in primary urinary bladder carcinoma and matched lymph node metastasis. Arch Pathol Lab Med 2001; 125:921–923.

390. Logani S, Oliva E, Amin MB, et al. Immunoprofile of ovarian tumors with putative transitional cell (urothelial) differentiation using novel urothelial markers: histogenetic and diagnostic implications. Am J Surg Pathol 2003; 27:1434–1441.

391. Ordonez NG. Transitional cell carcinomas of the ovary and bladder are immunophenotypically different. Histopathology 2000; 36:433–438.

392. Mhawech P, Uchida T, Pelte MF. Immunohistochemical profile of high-grade urothelial bladder carcinoma and prostate adenocarcinoma. Hum Pathol 2002; 33:1136–1140.

393. Pearlman WH, Giueriguian JD, Sawyer ME. A specific progesterone-binding component of human breast cyst fluid. J Biol Chem 1973; 248:5736–5741.

394. Haagensen DE Jr, Mazoujian G, Holder WD Jr, et al. Evaluation of a breast cyst fluid protein detectable in the plasma of breast carcinoma patients. Ann Surg 1977; 185:279–285.

395. Murphy LC, Lee-Wing M, Goldenberg GJ, et al. Expression of the gene encoding a prolactin-inducible protein by human breast cancers in vivo. Cancer Res 1987; 47:4160–4164.

396. Eusebi V, Magalhaes F, Azzopardi JG. Pleomorphic lobular carcinoma of the breast: An aggressive tumor showing apocrine differentiation. Hum Pathol 1992; 23:655–662.

397. Mazoujian G, Parish TH, Haagensen DEJ. Immunoperoxidase location of GCDFP-15 with mouse monoclonal antibodies versus rabbit antiserum. J Histochem Cytochem 1988; 36:377–382.

398. Losi L, Lorenzini RL, Eusebi V, et al. Aprocrine differentiation in invasive carcinoma of the breast: Comparison of monoclonal and polyclonal gross cystic disease fluid protein-15 antibodies with prolactin-inducible protein mRNA gene expression. Appl Immunohistochem 1995; 3:91–98.

399. Mazoujian G, Pinkus GS, David S, et al. Immunohistochemistry of a breast gross cystic disease fluid protein (GCDFP-15): A marker of apocrine epithelium and breast carcinomas with apocrine features. Am J Pathol 1983; 110:105–112.

400. Mazoujian G, Margolis R. Immunohistochemistry of gross cystic disease fluid protein (GCDFP-15) in 65 benign sweat gland tumors of the skin. Am J Dermatopathol 1988; 10:28–35.

401. Swanson PE, Pettinato G, Lillemoe TJ, et al. Gross cystic disease fluid protein-15 in salivary gland tumors. Arch Pathol Lab Med 1991; 115:158–163.

402. Viacava P, Naccarato AG, Bevilacqua G. Spectrum of GCDFP-15 expression in human fetal and adult normal tissues. Virchows Arch 1998; 432:255–260.

403. Wick MR, Lillemoe TJ, Copland GT, et al. Gross cystic disease fluid protein-15 as a marker for breast cancer: Immunohistochemical analysis of 690 human neoplasms and comparison with alpha-lactalbumin. Hum Pathol 1989; 20:281–287.

404. Raab S, Berg SC, Swanson PE, et al. Adenocarcinoma in lung in patients with breast cancer: A prospective analysis of the discriminatory value of immunohistology. Am J Clin Pathol 1993; 100:27–35.

405. Kufmann O, Deidesheimer T, Muehlenberg M, et al. Immunohistochemical differentiation of metastatic breast carcinomas from metastatic adenocarcinomas of other common sites. Histopathology 1996; 29:233–240.

406. Han JH, Kang Y, Shin HC, et al. Mammaglobin expression in lymph nodes is an important marker of metastatic breast carcinoma. Arch Pathol Lab Med 2003; 127:1330–1334.

407. Busam KJ, Jungbluth AA. Melan-A, a new melanocytic differentiation marker. Adv Anat Pathol 1996; 6:12–18.

408. Jungbluth AA, Busam KJ, Gerald WL, et al. A103: An anti-melan-A monoclonal antibody for the detection of malignant melanoma in paraffin-embedded tissues. Am J Surg Pathol 1998; 22:595–602.

409. Busam KJ, Iverson K, Coplin KA, et al. Immunoreactivity for A103, an antibody to melan-A (Mart-1) in adrenal cortical and other steroid tumors. Am J Surg Pathol 1998; 1:57.

410. Renshaw AA, Granter SR. A comparison of A103 and inhibin reactivity in adrenal cortical tumors: Distinction from hepatocellular carcinoma and renal tumors. Mod Pathol 1998; 3:1160–1164.

411. Hofbauer GF, Kamarashev J, Geertsen R. Melan-A/MART-1 immunoreactivity in formalin-fixed paraffin-embedded primary and metastatic melanoma: Frequency and distribution. Melanoma Res 1998; 8:337–343.

412. Arber DA, Weiss LM. CD5: A review. Appl Immunohistochem 1995; 3:1–22.

413. Hishima T, Fukayama M, Fujisawa M, et al. CD5 expression in thymic carcinoma. Am J Pathol 1994; 145:268–275.

414. Dorfman DM, Shahsafaei A, Chan JK. Thymic carcinomas, but not thymomas and carcinomas of other sites, show CD5 immunoreactivity. Am J Surg Pathol 1997; 21:936–940.

415. Berezowski K, Grimes MM, Gal A, et al. CD5 immunoreactivity of epithelial cells in thymic carcinoma and CASTLE using paraffin-embedded tissue. Am J Clin Pathol 1996; 106:483–486.

416. Kornstein MJ, Rosai J. CD5 labeling of thymic carcinomas and other non-lymphoid neoplasms. Am J Clin Pathol 1998; 109:722–726.

417. Tateyama H, Eimoto T, Tada T, et al. Immunoreactivity of a new CD5 antibody with normal epithelium and malignant tumors including thymic carcinoma. Am J Clin Pathol 1999; 111:235–240.

418. Kuo TT, Chan JK. Thymic carcinoma arising in thymoma is associated with alterations in immunohistochemical profile. Am J Surg Pathol 1998; 22:1474–1481.

419. Suster S, Moran CA. Spindle cell thymic carcinoma: Clinicopathologic and immunohistochemical study of a distinctive variant of primary thymic epithelial neoplasm. Am J Surg Pathol 1999; 23:691–700.

420. Johnston WW. Applications of monoclonal antibodies in clinical cytology as exemplified by studies with monoclonal antibody B72.3. Acta Cytol 1987; 31:537–566.

421. Johnson VG, Schlom J, Paterson AJ, et al. Analysis of a human tumor-associated glycoprotein (TAG-72) identified by monoclonal antibody B72.3. Cancer Res 1986; 46:850–857.

422. Ordonez NG. The immunohistochemical diagnosis of mesothelioma: Differentiation of mesothelioma and lung adenocarcinoma. Am J Surg Pathol 1989; 13:276–291.

423. Garcia-Prats MD, Ballestin C, Sotelo T, et al. A comparative evaluation of immunohistochemical markers for the differential diagnosis of malignant pleural tumors. Histopathology 1998; 32:462–472.

424. Riera JR, Astengo-Osuna C, Longmate JA, et al. The immunohistochemical diagnostic panel for epithelial mesothelioma: A re-evaluation after heat induced epitope retrieval. Am J Surg Pathol 1997; 21:1409–1419.

425. Szpak CA, Johnston WW, Roggli V, et al. The diagnostic distinction between malignant mesothelioma of the pleura and adenocarcinoma of the lung as defined by a monoclonal antibody (B72.3). Am J Pathol 1986; 122:252–260.

426. Ordonez NG. The immunohistochemical diagnosis of mesothelioma: a comparative study of epithelioid mesothelioma and lung adenocarcinoma. Am J Surg Pathol 2003; 27:1031–1051.

427. Wick MR, Loy T, Mills SE, et al. Malignant epithelioid pleural mesothelioma versus peripheral pulmonary adenocarcinoma: A histochemical, ultrastructural and immunohistologic study of 103 cases. Hum Pathol 1990; 21:759–766.

428. Jordon D, Jagirdar J, Kaneko M. Blood group antigens, Lewis x and Lewis y, in the diagnostic discrimination of malignant mesothelioma versus adenocarcinoma. Am J Pathol 1989;

135:931–937.

429. Gaffey MJ, Mills SE, Swanson PE, et al. Immunoreactivity for Ber-EP4 in adenocarcinomas, adenomatoid tumors and malignant mesotheliomas. Am J Surg Pathol 1992; 16:593–599.

430. Sheibani K, Shin S, Kezirian J, et al. Ber-EP4 antibody as a discriminant in a differential diagnosis of malignant mesothelioma versus adenocarcinoma. Am J Surg Pathol 1991; 15: 779–784.

431. Ordonez NG. Value of the Ber-EP4 antibody in differentiating epithelial pleural mesothelioma from adenocarcinoma: The MD Anderson experience and a critical review of the literature. Am J Clin Pathol 1998; 109:85–89.

432. Ordonez NG. The diagnostic utility of immunohistochemistry in distinguishing between mesothelioma and renal cell carcinoma: a comparative study. Hum Pathol 2004; 35:697–710.

433. Ordonez NG. Value of mesothelin immunostaining in the diagnosis of mesothelioma. Mod Pathol 2003; 16:192–197.

434. Miettinen M, Sarlomo-Rikala M. Expression of calretinin, thrombomodulin, keratin 5, and mesothelin in lung carcinomas of different types: an immunohistochemical analysis of 596 tumors in comparison with epithelioid mesotheliomas of the pleura. Am J Surg Pathol 2003; 27:150–158.

435. Hwang H, Quenneville L, Yaziji H, et al. Wilms tumor gene product: sensitive and contextually specific marker of serous carcinomas of ovarian surface epithelial origin. Appl Immunohistochem 2004; 12:122–126.

436. Leers MP, Aarts MM, Theunissen, PH. E-Cadherin and calretinin: A useful combination of immunochemical markers for differentiation between mesothelioma and metastatic adenocarcinoma. Histopathology 1998; 32:209–216.

437. Ruitenbeek T, Gouw AS, Poppema S. Immunocytology of body cavity fluids: MOC-31, a monoclonal antibody discriminating between mesothelial and epithelial cells. Arch Pathol Lab Med 1994; 118:265–269.

438. Delahaye M, Hoogsteden HC. Vanderkwast TH. Immunocytochemistry of malignant mesothelioma: OV632 as a marker of malignant mesothelioma. J Pathol 1991; 165:137–143.

439. Edwards C, Oates J. OV632 and MOC31 in a diagnosis of mesothelioma and adenocarcinoma: An assessment of their use in formalin-fixed and paraffin wax embedded material. J Clin Pathol 1995; 48:626–630.

440. Sosolik RC, McGaughey VR, DeYoung BR. Anti-MOC-31: A potential addition to the pulmonary adenocarcinoma vs. mesothelioma immunohistochemistry panel. Mod Pathol 1997; 10:716–719.

441. Ordonez NG. Value of the MOC-31 monoclonal antibody in differentiating epithelial pleural mesothelioma from lung adenocarcinoma. Hum Pathol 1998; 29:166–169.

442. Andressen C, Blumcke I, Celio MR. Calcium binding proteins: Selective markers of nerve cells. Cell Tissue Res 1993; 271:181–208.

443. Doglioni C, Tos A, Laurino L, et al. Calretinin: A novel immunocytochemical marker for mesothelioma. Am J Surg Pathol 1996; 20:1037–1046.

444. Ordonez NG. Value of calretinin immunostaining in differentiating epithelial mesothelioma from lung adenocarcinoma. Mod Pathol 1998; 11:929–933.

445. Carella R, Deleonardi G, D'Errico A, et al. Immunohistochemical panels for differentiating epithelial malignant mesothelioma from lung adenocarcinoma: a study with logistic regression analysis. Am J Surg Pathol 2001; 25:43–50.

446. Ordonez NG. Value of thyroid transcription factor-1, Ecadherin, BG8, WT1, and CD44S immunostaining in distinguishing epithelial pleural mesothelioma from pulmonary and nonpulmonary adenocarcinoma. Am J Surg Pathol 2000; 24:598–606.

447. Ordonez NG. Value of antibodies 44-3A6 SM3 HBME-1 and thrombomodulin in differentiating epithelial pleural mesothelioma from lung adenocarcinoma: A comparative study with other commonly used antibodies. Am J Surg Pathol 1997; 21:1399–1408.

448. Deamant FT, Pombo MT, Battifora H. Estrogen receptor immunohistochemistry as a predictor of site of origin in metastatic breast cancer. Appl Immunohistochem 1993; 1:188–192.

449. Bacchi CE, Garcia RL, Gown AM. Immunolocalization of estrogen and progesterone receptors in neuroendocrine tumors of the lung, skin, gastrointestinal and female genital tracts. Appl Immunohistochem 1997; 5:17–22.

450. Cagle PT, Mody DR. Estrogen and progesterone receptors in bronchogenic carcinoma. Cancer Res 1990; 50:632–635.

451. Su JM, Shu HK, Chang H, et al. Expression of estrogen and progesterone receptors in non-small cell lung cancer: Immunohistochemical study. Anticancer Res 1996; 16:3803–3806.

452. Kaiser U, Hofmann J, Schilli M, et al. Steroid hormone receptors in cell lines and tumor biopsies of human lung cancer. Int J Cancer 1996; 67:357–364.

453. Beattie CW, Hansen NW, Thomas PA. Steroid receptors in human lung cancer. Cancer Res 1985; 45:4206–4214.

454. Vargas SO, Leslie KO, Vacek PM, et al. Estrogen receptor related protein P29 in primary non-small cell carcinoma: Pathologic and prognostic correlations. Cancer 1998; 82:1495–1500.

455. Dabbs DJ, Landreneau RJ, Liu Y, et al. Detection of estrogen receptor by immunohistochemistry in pulmonary adenocarcinoma. Ann Thorac Surg 2002; 73:403–405; discussion 406.

456. Tot T. The role of cytokeratins 20 and 7 and estrogen receptor analysis in separation of metastatic lobular carcinoma of the breast and metastatic signet ring cell carcinoma of the gastrointestinal tract. APMIS 2000; 108:467–472.

457. Ashikari R, Park K, Huvos AG, et al. Paget's disease of the breast. Cancer 1970; 26:680–685.

458. Kister SJ, Haagensen CD. Paget's disease of the breast. Am J Surg Pathol 1977; 119:606–609.

459. Salvadori BG, Saccozzi R. Analysis of 100 cases of Paget's disease of the breast. Tumori 1976; 62:529–536.

460. Lundquist K, Kohler S, Rouse R. Intraepidermal cytokeratin 7 expression is not restricted to Paget cells but is also seen in Toker cells and Merkel cells. Am J Surg Pathol 1999; 23:212–219.

461. Yao DX, Hoda SA, Chiu A, et al. Intraepidermal cytokeratin 7 immunoreactive cells in the non-neoplastic nipple may represent interepithelial extension of lactiferous duct cells. Histopathology 2002; 40:230–236.

462. Tani EM, Skoog L. Immunocytochemical detection of estrogen receptors in mammary Paget cells. 1988; 23:825–828.

463. Meissner K, Riviere A, Haupt G, et al. Study of neuroprotein expression in mammary Paget's disease with and without underlying breast carcinoma and in extramammary Paget's disease. Am J Pathol 1990; 137:1305–1309.

8 头颈部肿瘤的免疫组织化学

原作者：Jennifer L. Hunt and Leon Barnes
译　者：高　鹏
审校者：李劲松，甄军晖

目　录

引言	233
抗原/抗体生物学	233
鳞状上皮增生性病变	233
鼻腔和鼻旁窦	237
鼻咽部	244
口腔和口咽部	245
咽喉部	246
涎腺	247
耳－颞骨	252
副神经节瘤和恶性副神经节瘤	254
转移性肿瘤	255
预测性和预后性标记	256
新型预测性或预后性抗体	256

引　言

头颈部范围包括锁骨到蝶鞍，是一个高度器官化、解剖结构复杂的区域，包括多种类型的组织，如黏膜、软组织、周围和中枢神经组织成分、骨、软骨、涎腺、淋巴组织、牙源性组织、副神经节、内分泌器官和皮肤。

由于起源于以上组织的一些肿瘤在本书的其他章节有讨论，本章节主要介绍头颈部常见或特发病变中免疫组化的诊断或预后价值，那些通过HE切片可作出诊断的肿瘤在本节中不作介绍。

抗原/抗体生物学

头颈部不同器官来源的肿瘤可表达许多共同的肿瘤抗原。诊断应用的大多数角蛋白抗体为检测范围较广的种类，如AE1/AE3、CAM5.2和广谱角蛋白（CK），CK5/6和p63对于检测鳞状细胞分化是很好的选择。神经内分泌分化最好使用突触素（Syn）、嗜铬素A（CgA）共同检测，有时也要用神经特异性烯醇化酶（NSE）。血管标记物（CD31、CD34、Ⅷ因子）和黑色素标记物（S-100、HMB-45、melan-A、MITF）在头颈部肿瘤的研究中也有较特异性的作用。常用抗体如表8.1所示。

鳞状上皮增生性病变

反应性改变

鳞状上皮在外源性损伤因子如酶性分泌物、咀嚼、义齿、吸入性化学毒物、吸烟、酒精等的作用下可发生反应或肿瘤性病变。

反应性上皮改变可出现一系列组织学改变并可见细胞异型性。细胞核的改变不包括非典型增生中常见的核染色质增多、病理核分裂象或核异型性。细胞核可见核仁，通常界限清楚、不拥挤。结构上，表面上皮细胞分化很成熟。免疫组化染色不能鉴别细胞反应性增生。假上皮瘤样增生是一种特殊的反应性增生，在颗粒细胞瘤表面可以出现。由于该肿瘤在切除不完全时易复发，有必要充分认识该肿瘤。该肿瘤会出现

表8.1 头颈部标本中应用的抗体

抗体	来源	稀释度	抗体	来源	稀释度
雄激素受体	Biogenex	1:2000	CK20	DAKO	1:40
bcl-2	DAKO	1:200	CK903	Sigma	1:20
β-catenin	BD Transduction Labortatories		Ki-67	AMAC	1:200
Calponin	DAKO	1:200	Laminin	Sigma	1:20
Calretinin	Zymed	1:750	LCA	DAKO	1:20
CD31	DAKO	1:40	Melan-A	Novocastro	1:40
CD34	DAKO	1:800	Microphthalmic transcription factor	Neomarkers	1:40
CD99	DAKO	1:20			
CDX2	Biogenex	1:50			
CEA	Boehringer-Mannheim	1:4000	Muscle specific actin(HHF-35)	Enzo	1:8000
Chromogranin	Boehringer-Mannheim	1:4000			
Desmin	Biogenex	1:2000	MUC2	Novocastro	1:100
EMA	DAKO	1:400	MUC5	Novocastro	1:150
FLI-1	Santa Cruz	1:40	Myogenin	Novocastro	1:30
GFAP	DAKO	1:300	Neuron-specific enolase	Bio Genes	1:450
Her 2-neu	DAKO	1:100			
HMB-45	Biogenex	1:60	Pit-1	Santa Cruz	
角蛋白			p53	Oncogene	1:160
AE1/AE3	Boehringer-Mannheim	1:100	p63	Neomarkers	1:200
CAM5.2	Becton-Dickinson	1:200	S-100 protein	DAKO	1:1000
CK4	Novocastro	1:100	Smooth muscle actin	DAKO	1:80
CK5/6	Roche	1:20			
CK7	Biogenex	1:800	Synaptophysin	Boehringer-Mannheim	1:40
CK8	Novocastro	1:60	Thyriod transcription factor	Neomarkers	1:50
CK10	Novocastro	1:50			
CK13	DAKO	1:100	Tyrosinase	Novocastro	1:20
CK14	Novocastro	1:40	Vimentin	Biogenex	1:20
CK19	Novocastro	1:50			

特征性的S-100阳性,同时出现PAS阳性、淀粉酶阴性的胞浆颗粒[1]。该种上皮反应性增生的病因不清,但认为本身不是肿瘤性的[2],可能与生长因子或肿瘤细胞分泌的其他物质有关[3]。

异型增生和经典的鳞状细胞癌

鳞状细胞癌（SCC）是头颈部最常见的恶性肿瘤[4-5]。绝大多数病例的致癌因素与吸烟和酒精有关[6-8]。浸润性鳞状细胞癌患者年龄大于60岁,男性多见。

鳞状细胞癌的致癌物最常见的是烟草中的毒性物质。许多研究显示,这些化学性毒物作用于上呼吸道黏膜不仅导致早期肿瘤的形态学改变,而且会出现肿瘤的分子水平突变。无烟烟草和其他咀嚼性含烟草制品,如betal-nut-quid,也可作为鳞状细胞癌特别是口腔鳞状细胞癌的病因[9-10]。

病毒在头颈部鳞状细胞癌中的致病作用尚有争议。EB病毒当然与某些肿瘤有关（参见"鼻咽癌"）,头颈部肿瘤与人乳头状瘤病毒（HPV）的相关性有更大的争议。不同的研究显示,0%～90%的头颈部肿瘤中存在HPV感染。据报道,基底细胞样鳞状细胞癌和口咽环周围组织（扁桃体、舌根、鼻咽）起源肿瘤的感染率较高[11-14]。鳞状细胞癌中HPV感染率的差异可能与检测方法有关。HPV的免疫组化检测是可行的。原位杂交可检测整合的HPV基因组,这对病因有重要的提示作用[12]。PCR分析通常只检测HPV DNA的存在,该技术高度敏感（可能过度敏感,有假阳性）[15]。

鳞状黏膜的肿瘤性转化可经典地分为4类：低度异型性增生、中度异型性增生、重度异型性增生（含原位癌，CIS）和浸润癌。异型性增生的细胞学和组织学具有相当的特征性。细胞核染色质增多，核增大，呈基底细胞样外观，细胞核不规则，有多形性，核分裂增多。在结构上，异型性增生上皮拥挤、结构紊乱、基底层出现异常核分裂。

头颈部异型性增生的分类不像子宫颈病变那样明确，但大多数病理学家使用同样的分级标准。低级别异型性增生显示局限于基底层下1/3的核异型性和结构紊乱，中度异型性增生显示的异型改变不超过中1/3，重度异型性增生则达到上1/3[4, 16-18]。

异型性增生到鳞状细胞癌转化的机制尚不十分清楚，涉及多个细胞途径。主要涉及抑癌基因的失活和癌基因的激活[19-20]。许多致癌途径可检测到蛋白产物，已有多项研究涉及鳞状细胞癌的免疫组化染色。但目前仍没有可实际应用于异型性增生诊断的免疫组化染色。经典鳞状细胞癌通常有特征性的组织形态，高分化者不需额外染色，而低分化者特别是转移病灶，有时需要CK染色。典型的头颈部鳞癌AE1/AE3和广谱CK阳性。

许多头颈部鳞癌需要切除原发病灶并可能需要颈部淋巴结清扫[21-23]。转移性病变可能需要应用免疫组化染色，特别是如放疗后的淋巴结等困难的病例。临床应用PET/CT扫描可较敏感地确定治疗后的残留肿瘤，但这些孤立的病灶有时仅见肉芽组织或坏死组织，没有组织特异性的肿瘤。对于这些病例，CK染色对于确定坏死物质沉积的病因有帮助，前哨淋巴结切除对于头颈外科尚属新鲜事物。目前尚无使用免疫组化检测前哨淋巴结的标准操作（将在"新型标记物"中讨论）。

诊断要点：鳞状细胞癌

1. 鳞状细胞癌通常均对CK呈阳性染色。
2. CK染色有助于检测转移病灶，特别是治疗后的淋巴结病变。

基底细胞样鳞状细胞癌

基底细胞样鳞状细胞癌（BSCC）是一种不常见的、组织学特征明显的鳞状细胞癌。在上消化道，它好发于舌根、咽喉，也可见于腭、扁桃体、颊黏膜、口底、鼻咽、鼻窦[24-26]。

基底细胞样鳞状细胞癌多见于男性（82%），平均发病年龄63岁（27~88岁）[27]。症状因原发部位不同而有差异，但最常见的症状包括吞咽困难、声嘶、疼痛、耳痛、咳嗽、咯血、颈部包块和体重下降。

烟草和酒精可能是基底细胞样鳞状细胞癌的主要原因，多数患者有大量吸烟和酗酒的病史。人类乳头状瘤病毒和基底细胞样鳞状细胞癌的关系尚有争议。有作者发现HPV高发生率与基底细胞样鳞状细胞癌之间没有关系[11, 12, 29-30]。部分差异由检测手段不同导致，如免疫组化和高敏感PCR。HPV在这些肿瘤中的致病作用仍有待证实。

组织学上，基底细胞样鳞状细胞癌有双相性表现，以基底细胞样成分为主，但也可见经典鳞癌成分[31]。基底样成分通常呈小叶状、大巢状或小梁条索状生长，也可见小簇甚至单细胞排列。在少数的肿瘤，可见囊腔甚至发育不良的导管分化。基底样细胞的小叶常可见中央的粉刺样坏死。细胞学上，基底样肿瘤细胞有圆形至椭圆形的细胞核，染色深，核浆比例升高。小叶周边的细胞核栅栏状排列。基底细胞样成分可见显著的核分裂和凋亡小体[27, 32, 33]。经典鳞癌成分可有浸润癌或原位癌，可见于独立的病灶或出现于基底细胞样成分中。

基底细胞样鳞状细胞癌的鉴别诊断较广泛，特别在活检的小标本中识别所有的组织成分较困难，最需要与之鉴别的是腺样囊性癌和小细胞神经内分泌癌[27]，鉴别诊断可能需要免疫组化染色（表8.2）。

表8.2 基底细胞样鳞癌和腺样囊性癌、小细胞神经内分泌癌的鉴别

抗体标记	肿瘤类型		
	基底细胞样鳞癌	腺样囊性癌	小细胞神经内分泌癌
CK	+	+	+
CgA	N	N	+
S-100	S	+	N
p53	+	S	+
Ki-67	高	低	高
c-kit	S	+	S

+，阳性；S，部分阳性；N，阴性

基底细胞样鳞状细胞癌的染色模式已有多项研究[34-37]，大多数肿瘤 AE1/AE3 和上皮细胞膜抗原（EMA）阳性，53% 的病例癌胚抗原（CEA）阳性，39% 的病例 S-100 阳性[34, 36, 38]，75% 的基底细胞样鳞癌可见 NSE 的弥漫性弱表达，但通常 Syn、CgA、肌动蛋白和 GFAP 阴性表达，这些染色有助于区别神经内分泌癌。c-kit 在绝大多数腺样囊性癌呈阳性表达，但这对于区别基底细胞样鳞状细胞癌可能用处不大，有些基底细胞样鳞状细胞癌也表达 c-kit[40]。但 p53 对此有帮助，基底细胞样鳞状细胞癌通常呈 p53 强阳性表达，而只有去分化的腺样囊性癌会显示 p53 表达[29, 38, 41, 42]。

> **诊断要点：基底细胞样鳞状细胞癌**
>
> 1. 基底细胞样鳞状细胞癌的鉴别诊断包括腺样囊性癌和小细胞神经内分泌癌。
> 2. 基底细胞样鳞状细胞癌呈 CK 阳性表达，而对大多数神经内分泌标记和 S-100 通常为阴性。
> 3. 腺样囊性癌通常 S-100 阳性，而小细胞神经内分泌癌通常神经内分泌标记呈阳性。

疣状癌和乳头状鳞状细胞癌

疣状癌（VC）和乳头状鳞状细胞癌（PSCC）是最常见于口腔和咽的外生性肿瘤。疣状癌是一种局部浸润而不发生转移的鳞状细胞癌变型，而乳头状鳞状细胞癌是具有转移潜能的浸润性肿瘤。烟草是导致这些肿瘤的主要因素，口腔卫生状况差和人类乳头状瘤病毒也与其发生有关[43]。

疣状癌的角状的乳头状上皮巢没有不典型性或异型性。肿瘤和间质的交界处有特征性的推进式边缘，呈球根状[44]。细胞学的异型性提示合并有经典鳞癌（混合型）或乳头状鳞状细胞癌[45]。乳头状鳞状细胞癌呈乳头状生长，伴有乳头状的纤维血管轴心[46]。乳头状结构表面的上皮细胞显示细胞学异型性[47]。乳头状表面成分下面的浸润部分可呈现经典鳞癌的表现或作为乳头状鳞状细胞癌基底部深面的浸润性鳞癌成分[48]。

良性乳头状增生病变、疣状癌和乳头状鳞状细胞癌之间的鉴别可以十分困难，尤其在小的活检标

> **诊断要点：疣状癌和乳头状鳞状细胞癌**
>
> 1. 疣状癌和乳头状鳞状细胞癌有相似的大体外观，但疣状癌有推进式的边缘，没有异型性，而乳头状鳞状细胞癌有细胞异型性和典型的浸润。
> 2. 免疫组化标记物对鉴别疣状癌和乳头状鳞状细胞癌没有帮助。

本，主要依赖组织学图像，免疫组化对鉴别诊断没有帮助。

梭形细胞癌

梭形细胞癌（SPCC）是另一种少见的鳞癌变型，以前有假性癌、肉瘤样癌和癌肉瘤等不同的名称。平均年龄 64 岁（31～81 岁），男性显著多见。常见的原发部位包括声门和咽，其他部位也可发生。烟草和酒精是主要风险因素[49]。

肿瘤的肉眼观察常为息肉状，生长迅速。组织学上，梭形细胞癌的诊断十分困难，特别是活检标本。绝大多数肿瘤由梭形细胞成分构成，细胞异型性和细胞密度变化不一。确认存在鳞状细胞肿瘤成分如高度异型的上皮细胞或浸润性鳞癌对于诊断很关键，但梭形细胞癌中出现以上成分者不足 50%。

免疫组化在此是很必要的，但特异性或敏感性可能不高。梭形细胞成分呈波形蛋白强阳性。CK 染色的变化较大（图 8.1、8.2）[49, 51, 52]，所以证明其上皮

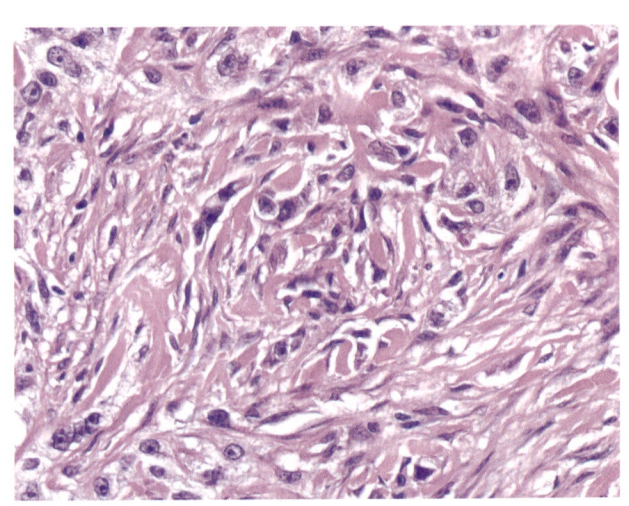

图 8.1　梭形细胞癌中显示梭形细胞形态（HE，×200）

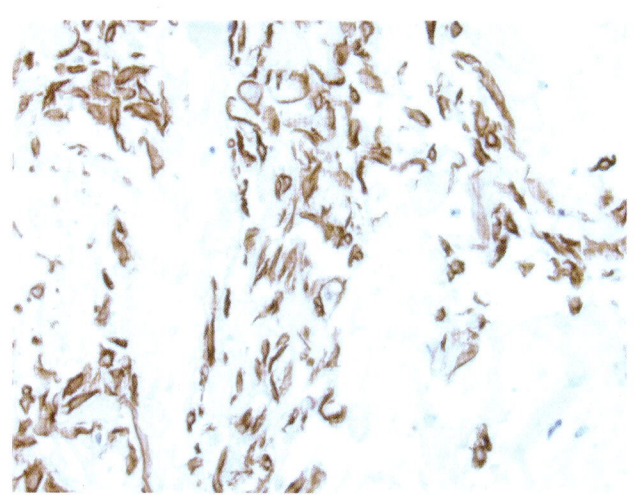

图 8.2 梭形细胞癌显示 CK 强染色 (CAM 5.2，×200)

起源可能较困难。CK 在 70% 的肿瘤呈梭形细胞阳性表达，但染色为灶性且使用多种上皮抗体是必要的。高达 36% 的梭形细胞癌中 CK 可以完全缺失[49]。其他的间叶性标记物如平滑肌肌动蛋白、肌肉特异性肌动蛋白和结蛋白在梭形细胞成分中的阳性较低（大约 1%~30%）。

梭形细胞癌的主要鉴别诊断包括反应性和良性肿瘤的间质细胞增生，偶见于黏膜部位的原发肉瘤。良性病变包括肉芽组织、脓性肉芽肿、梭形细胞肌上皮瘤、平滑肌瘤、纤维瘤病和其他良性间质病变。需鉴别的恶性肿瘤包括滑膜肉瘤和其他表型肉瘤。免疫组化有助于区分梭形细胞癌和其中某些上述病变，但由于组织学和免疫表型重叠，最终诊断依赖组织学特征和合适的免疫标记。有研究者认为缺乏上皮性免疫标记可能提示该类患者预后不良[50]。

> **诊断要点：梭形细胞癌**
> 1. 诊断梭形细胞癌要求证实梭形细胞中存在鳞癌成分或上皮性分化。
> 2. 梭形细胞成分可能需多种 CK 和上皮标记显示阳性。但最高可达 30% 的梭形细胞癌中的梭形细胞呈 CK 阴性。

鼻腔和鼻旁窦

许多鼻腔和鼻窦肿瘤归入圆形细胞肿瘤[53-56]，包括嗅神经母细胞瘤、鼻腔未分化癌、恶性黑色素瘤、神经内分泌癌/小细胞神经内分泌癌、恶性淋巴瘤、髓外浆细胞瘤、浸润性/异位垂体腺瘤、横纹肌肉瘤和 Ewing 肉瘤/外周神经外胚层肿瘤（表 8.3）。

嗅神经母细胞瘤

嗅神经母细胞瘤（ONB）是鼻腔的原发圆细胞肿瘤。发病人群年龄广泛（平均 40~45 岁），男女比例相当，好发于鼻腔近筛板处，常为息肉状，临床表现主要为鼻衄和鼻腔阻塞[57-58]。

嗅神经母细胞瘤的细胞浆界限不清，细胞形态较圆且相当一致，核染色质轻度变深，偶见核仁但不清楚。细胞呈小叶状，弥漫型或混合型分布（图 8.3）。可见 Rosettes 花环样结构，但坏死和凋亡不常见。间质血管丰富并常见神经原纤维。

肿瘤细胞呈 Syn 和 NSE 阳性，偶尔 CgA 阳性（图

表 8.3 鼻道小圆细胞肿瘤的免疫组化染色								
肿瘤	CK[a]	EMA[a]	LCA[a]	Synaptophysin	HMB-45	Desmin	Vimentin	CD99
SNUC[b]	+	+	N	N	N	N	N	N
ONB[b]	S	N	N	+	N	N	N	N
NPC[b]	+	+	N	N	N	N	N	N
淋巴瘤	N	N	+	N	N	N	N	N
黑色素瘤	N	N	N	N	+	N	+	N
横纹肌肉瘤	N	N	N	N	N	+	+	S
SCNEC[b]	+	+	N	S	N	N	N	N
ES/PNET[b]	S	N	N	S	N	N	+	+

[a] CK，细胞角蛋白；EMA，上皮细胞膜抗原；LCA，白细胞共同抗原
[b] SNUC，鼻窦未分化癌；ONB，嗅神经母细胞瘤；NPC，鼻咽癌；SCNEC，小细胞神经内分泌癌；ES/PNET，Ewing 肉瘤/外周神经外胚层肿瘤
+，阳性；S，部分阳性；N，阴性

8.4），高达30%的病例可呈CAM5.2阳性，但所有病例EMA、S-100、CD99及肌肉标记为阴性，所谓支持细胞或施万细胞呈S-100和GFAP阳性（图8.5，表8.3、8.4、8.5）。

> **诊断要点：嗅神经母细胞瘤**
>
> 1. 嗅神经母细胞瘤由小圆细胞组成，轻度深染，常呈小叶状或弥漫分布。
> 2. 肿瘤细胞呈神经内分泌标记阳性，高达30%的病例呈CK阳性。

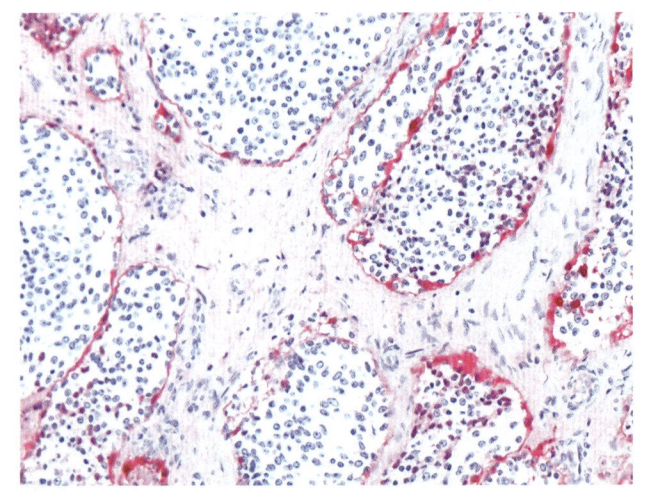

图8.5 神经母细胞瘤中的支持细胞染色（S-100，×200）

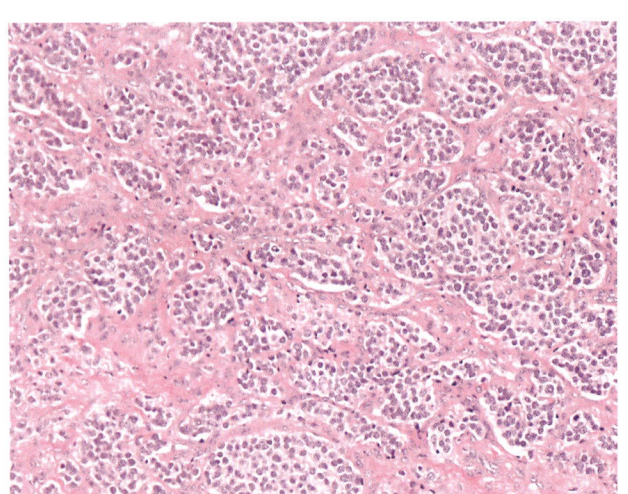

图8.3 嗅神经母细胞瘤显示小叶状的生长模式和细胞核神经内分泌特征（HE，×100）

表8.4 嗅神经母细胞瘤(ONB)与鼻窦未分化癌(SNUC)对比

特征	嗅神经母细胞瘤	鼻窦未分化癌
年龄	40~45	58
位置	鼻腔顶部	多部位
预后/生存	60%~80% 5年	中位数为18
视神经	偶见	常见
异型性	偶见	常见
核分裂	不确定	多见
坏死	偶见	显著
血管浸润	偶见	显著
神经纤维间质	常见	缺乏
H-W花环	常见	缺乏
角蛋白	25%~35%*	90%
EMA	0%	65%
NSE	80%~100%	50%
S-100	60%	0%~15%
Syn	100%（支持细胞）	0%
神经内分泌颗粒	多见	罕见

*ONB通常是CK阴性但偶尔可呈低分子量CK局灶性表达

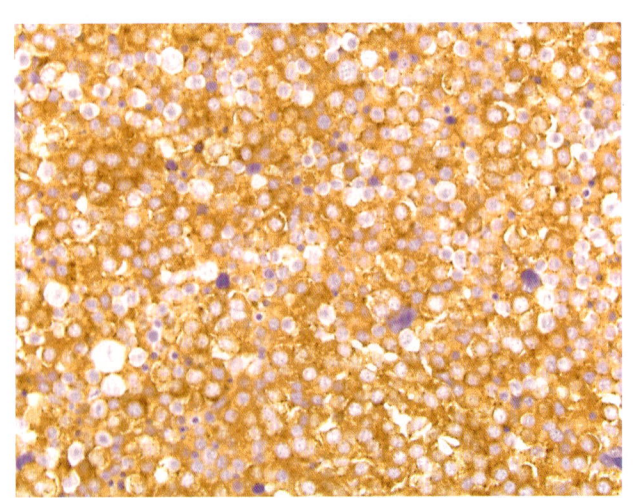

图8.4 嗅神经母细胞瘤的免疫染色（Syn，×200）

表8.5 角蛋白在鼻窦肿瘤中的表达*

肿瘤	CK4	CK5	CK7	CK8	CK13	CK14	CK19
SCC(n=10)	30%	90%	60%	90%	90%	80%	90%
NKSCC(n=10)		90%		90%	80%	80%	90%
NPTC(n=5)		80%		80%		80%	100%
SNUC(n=6)				50%	100%		50%

* 数据来源于 Franchi, et al. Am J Surg Pathol 2002;26:1597-1604
SCC，鳞状细胞癌；NKSCC，非角化鳞癌；NPTC，鼻咽型未分化癌；SNUC，鼻腔未分化癌

鼻窦未分化癌

鼻窦未分化癌（SNUC）是一种侵袭性肿瘤，男性比女性发病率高2~3倍，发病年龄广泛（平均55~60岁）。发生于鼻腔的肿瘤多位于鼻窦，但仅发生于上述单一部位的肿瘤不常见。更常见的情况是在诊断时肿瘤已广泛累及鼻腔、鼻窦、眶部或颅骨。

显微镜下，鼻窦未分化癌由小至中等的多边形细胞组成，呈片状、巢状、粗条索状或条带状分布。细胞核呈圆形、卵圆形、染色质多、轻至中度异型，偶尔可见透明核。核仁大小变化不一。细胞浆呈轻-中度异型，嗜酸性或双嗜性。核分裂、脉管浸润和坏死很显著（图8.6）。

鼻窦未分化癌通常呈CK系列抗体阳性表达（图8.7）。通常情况下为CK8阳性，半数病例为CK7和CK19阳性。而CK4、5/6、10、13和14为阴性表达（表8.5）[59]。可以出现EMA、NSE和p53阳性表达。有些病例也可出现CD99阳性，染色主要在胞浆而不是细胞膜[60]。Syn、CgA和CEA阴性表达也是其特性（表8.3~8.7）。美国的患者病毒检测为阴性，而亚洲患者其发病与EB病毒有关[60, 61]。

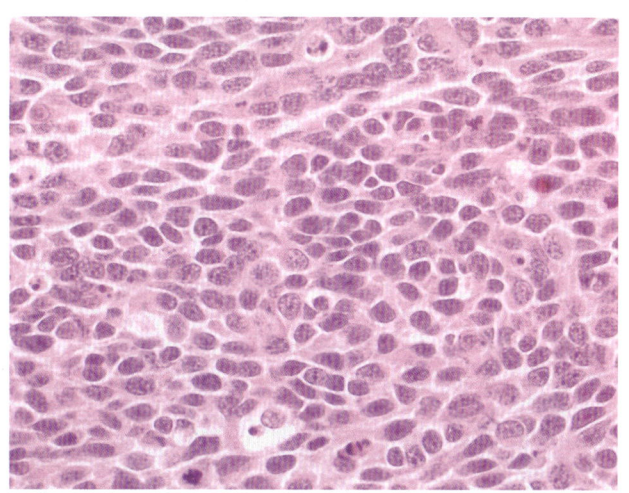

图8.6　鼻窦未分化癌（HE, ×200）

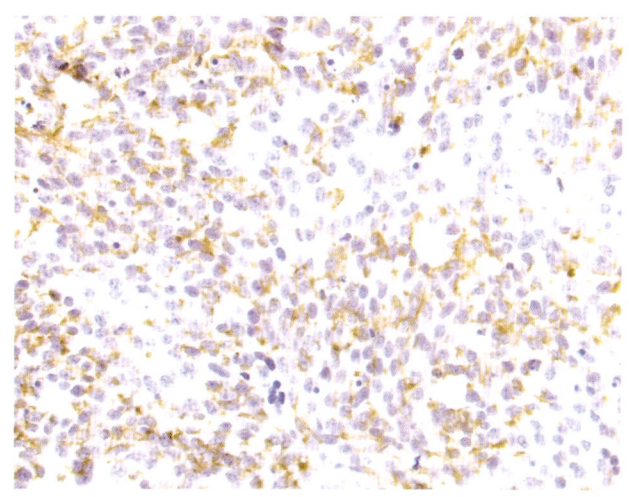

图8.7　鼻窦未分化癌免疫染色（CAM5.2, ×200）

> **诊断要点**：鼻窦未分化癌
> 1. 鼻窦未分化癌由高级别、小至中等大小的细胞构成，有明显的核分裂和坏死。
> 2. 肿瘤细胞呈CK阳性表达，并可呈EMA、NSE和p53阳性。

表8.6　鼻窦未分化癌(SNUC)与小细胞神经内分泌癌(SCNEC)对比

特征	SNUC	SCNEC
梭形细胞	N	+
核仁	S	N
核型改变	N	+
DNA 包被	N	+
异型性	S	N
Syn	N	S
TTF	N	+
点状 CK 阳性	N	S

+, 阳性；S, 部分阳性；N, 阴性

恶性黑色素瘤

恶性黑色素瘤（MM）发生于鼻窦并不常见，主要见于50岁以上人群，绝大多数发生于鼻前隔或靠近中鼻甲或前鼻甲，尽管肿瘤可以原发于鼻窦，但鼻腔原发而鼻窦继发的情况更常见。

鼻窦的恶性黑色素瘤常见出血、坏死，连接经常缺乏且对于诊断不是必需的。但当连接缺乏且伴有黑色素缺乏（10%~30%的恶性黑色素瘤）和细胞形态的多样化（上皮样、梭形、浆细胞样、横纹肌

表 8.7　鼻窦未分化癌（SNUC）与未分化鼻咽癌（UNPC）对比

特征	SNUC	UNPC
部位	鼻腔	鼻咽
临床特点	原发灶较大，有时伴淋巴转移	原发灶较小，伴颈部淋巴结转移
X 线	显著破坏，由原发灶向周围扩散	很少破坏或向周围扩散
生长	条索状、巢状、片状	合体细胞状
细胞	染色质可多可少，核仁可有可无	细胞核大、透明、核仁显著
核分裂	非常显著	不明显
坏死	非常显著	不明显
血管浸润	非常显著	不明显
淋巴细胞	缺乏或少量	大量浸润
EB 病毒（USA）	N	+
CK5/6&13	N	+
CK7	S	N

+，阳性；S，部分阳性；N，阴性

样、未分化型）及排列方式的多形性（腺样、乳头状、外皮瘤样、实性）时，处理这类肿瘤必须高度警惕（图 8.8）[62, 63]。

恶性黑色素瘤诊断应用的 5 种标准标记物中，S-100 阳性率 91%～95%，HMB-45 阳性率 76%～98%，酪氨酸酶阳性率 78%～100%，melan-A 阳性率 65%～100%，小眼（microphthalmic）转录因子阳性率 57%～91%（图 8.9、8.10）[63, 64]。

恶性黑色素瘤对波形蛋白总呈阳性表达，这在诊断无色素性梭形细胞恶性黑色素瘤时易将其误诊为软组织肉瘤，作为常规，在未排除恶性黑色素瘤、梭形细胞癌和恶性肌上皮瘤的情况下，不应该作出鼻窦软

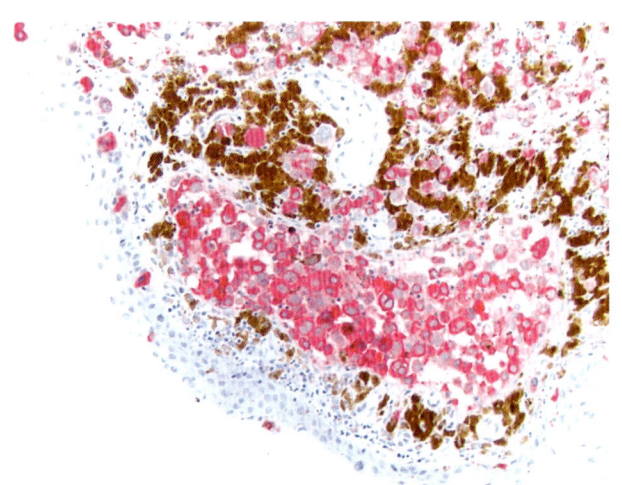

图 8.9　黏膜恶性黑色素瘤呈红色染色（酪氨酸酶，×200）

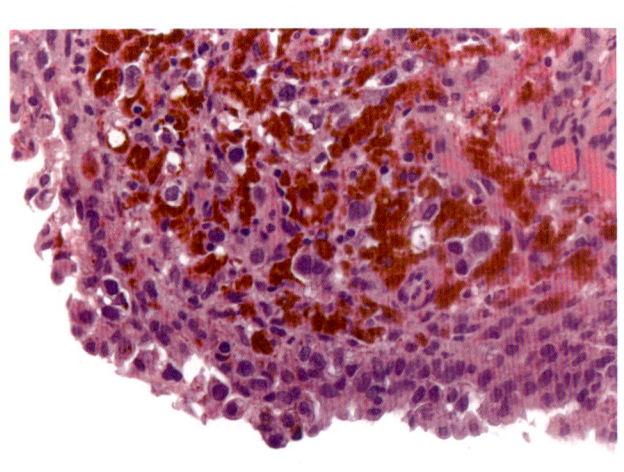

图 8.8　黏膜恶性黑色素瘤伴严重色素沉积（HE，×200）

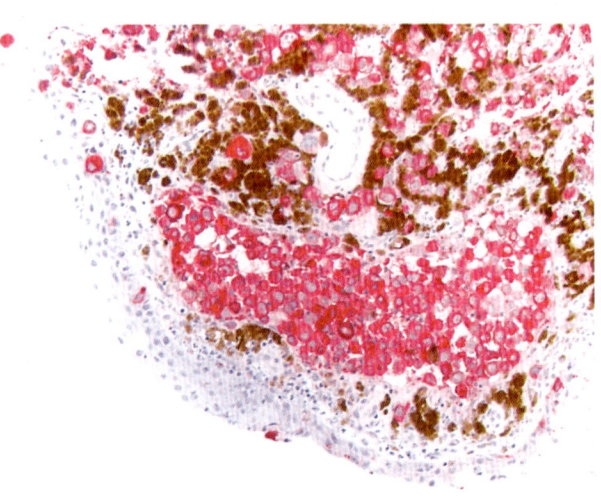

图 8.10　黏膜恶性黑色素瘤呈红色染色（HMB-45，×200）

组织肉瘤的诊断。偶尔，恶性黑色素瘤可呈CAM5.2和EMA局灶性阳性。这在处理上皮样恶性黑色素瘤时可能会是个问题。

神经内分泌癌——小细胞神经内分泌癌

鼻腔和鼻窦的神经内分泌癌这个名词在没有进一步界定的情况下易使人困惑或没有实际意义，不应当作为特异性诊断应用[66,67]。在过去甚至当前，这个名词包括不同的群体如嗅神经母细胞瘤、小细胞神经内分泌癌、类癌、不典型类癌、副神经节瘤，可能还包括鼻窦未分化癌。当上述肿瘤排除后，仍有少量不能进一步分类的肿瘤。这些应诊断为非特异性神经内分泌癌，随后可分级为中分化或低分化。

发生于肺的类似的小细胞神经内分泌癌（SCNEC、燕麦细胞癌、小细胞未分化癌）罕见于鼻腔和鼻窦。男女发病比例相当，发病年龄广泛（38～68岁）[68]。可起源于鼻腔和鼻窦，特别是筛骨和上颌骨。肿瘤可限于上述部位或扩散到眶部、筛状板或颅腔。

显微镜下，小细胞神经内分泌癌的形态学与发生于肺的同类病变一致，由圆形、短梭形细胞构成，细胞浆少，染色质深，没有核仁，核异型、核分裂和坏死常见。

肿瘤几乎总是呈CAM5.2和AE1/AE3（偶尔呈点状图像）、Syn、CgA、NSE阳性。CK20、S-100和NF呈阴性表达[68-69]。约半数肿瘤可呈甲状腺转录因子（TTF）阳性，并可呈CD99阳性（表8.3、8.6）[68-69]，偶尔可表达激素（降钙素、肾上腺皮质激素、β黑色素细胞刺激素、5-羟色胺、甲状旁腺激素）[70]。源于肺的SCNEC转移应作为鉴别诊断之一。

恶性淋巴瘤

大约1.5%的非霍奇金淋巴瘤发生于鼻道，占该部位所有恶性肿瘤的6%[71-72]。在美国，B细胞淋巴瘤的发生率高于T细胞淋巴瘤，而在亚洲则相反[73-76]。

不同资料中，淋巴瘤在鼻腔和鼻窦的分布不同。在一组120例鼻周淋巴瘤的研究中，53%发生于鼻腔，33%发生于鼻窦，12%两者均被累及，4%无法分类[71]。在另一组70例患者中，69%发生于上颌窦，20%发生于鼻腔，1%发生于筛窦[74]。

通常，鼻腔淋巴瘤倾向于T细胞起源，而B细胞淋巴瘤在鼻窦更常见，大多数肿瘤呈弥漫分布，中等级别。大细胞型、伴免疫母细胞特征的大细胞和大小细胞混合型是最常见的类型。

髓外浆细胞瘤

髓外浆细胞瘤（EMP）可发生于软组织但不常见，由单克隆增生的浆细胞组成。

大约80%的EMP发生于上呼吸道和上消化道，特别是鼻旁区，20%发生于其他部位[77]。所有患者中，80%是原发，在确诊时没有多发性骨髓瘤的证据。另外20%为继发，诊断时伴有多发性骨髓瘤[78]。

髓外浆细胞瘤患者男女发病比例为（2～3）：1，几乎所有患者年龄均超过40岁[77,79]。5%～10%的EMP患者伴有颈部淋巴结受累。治疗后，15%～20%的患者会局部复发，15%～30%患者通常在24个月内最终发展为多发性骨髓瘤[77,78]。

髓外浆细胞瘤在细胞浆表达单一类型的免疫球蛋白，缺乏细胞膜免疫球蛋白表达，绝大多数为IgG表达，偶见IgA表达，而IgD、IgE和IgM表达罕见。半数患者可出现κ和λ轻链限制性表达。

有证据显示，浆细胞的增殖率（由PCNA反映）可能与肿瘤分化程度和预后有关[79]。PCNA阳性率低于10%者通常分化好且预后好，而PCNA阳性率11%～75%者为中分化，阳性率大于75%者为低分化。PCNA阳性率越高预后越差。

浸润性/异位垂体腺瘤

发生于鼻腔、鼻旁（特别是筛骨）和鼻咽的垂体腺瘤十分少见，可分为浸润性和异位两种类型[80-82]。浸润性鼻旁区垂体腺瘤可继发于原发性鞍区肿瘤。这种现象见于2%的鞍区肿瘤[81]。异位腺瘤起源于垂体的胚胎发育畸形。

病理学上，该肿瘤没有什么特殊的，但由于活检标本通常较小且有挤压，诊断发生于异常部位的该类肿瘤需要考虑临床病史、实验室检查和查体结果。

该类肿瘤呈Syn、CgA和NSE阳性，并可表达不同的激素（生长激素、催乳素、TSH、ACTH、FSH）。部分病例呈激素表达阴性，诊断为裸细胞腺瘤，几乎所有病例呈CAM5.2阳性，可为局灶性或弥漫性，半数病例呈AE1/AE3阳性[83]。CK7、19、20和S-100均呈阴性表达。垂体转录因子-1可选择性地表达于分泌生长因子、催乳素和TSH的肿瘤[84]。

鉴别诊断可包括嗅神经母细胞瘤、副神经节瘤和类癌。表8.8有助于区分这些肿瘤。

横纹肌肉瘤

横纹肌肉瘤（RMS）是儿童最常见的软组织肉瘤，在这个年龄组约1/3的横纹肌肉瘤发生于头颈部，特别是眶部、中耳、鼻咽和鼻道。相反，发生于成人的横纹肌肉瘤在头颈部较少见。当该肿瘤发生于成人时，最常见的发生部位是鼻道。

尽管多种免疫标记可以鉴定横纹肌肉瘤，但我们较常使用结蛋白和成肌素。结蛋白是胞浆着色，在80%的横纹肌肉瘤石蜡切片中可见表达[87]。但是，一些其他的非横纹肌源性的软组织肿瘤（纤维瘤、恶性横纹肌样瘤、PNET）也可见表达。成肌素为细胞核着色，对于横纹肌肉瘤来说敏感性较高。在Cessna等的研究中，所有的32例横纹肌肉瘤均呈阳性表达（图8.11、8.12）[88]。通常情况下，腺泡状横纹肌肉瘤的染色比胚胎性横纹肌肉瘤强。成肌素偶尔可在一些其他软组织肿瘤局灶性阳性表达，包括硬纤维瘤、先天性肌纤维瘤病、先天性纤维肉瘤和滑膜肉瘤[88]。如不能确诊，则两种抗体均应使用。

Ewing肉瘤和外周神经外胚层肿瘤

尽管外周神经外胚层肿瘤（PNET）和Ewing肉瘤（ES）分别在1918年和1921年就首先被报道，但直到最近免疫组化和遗传分子学研究才揭示这两种疾病属于同一肿瘤家族。这些肿瘤构成一个谱系，区别仅在于有无神经外胚层分化。

ES/PNET可发生于骨、软组织和多种间叶性器官（肺、胰腺、肾），也可见于头颈部，与神经纤维瘤病无关。大多数患者为青少年或青年，通常小于30岁（中位数10~22岁）。但年龄大的人也可发生。男性患者稍多一些（男女比例为1.4∶1），罕见于非洲裔美国人。仅2%~10%的ES/PNET发生于

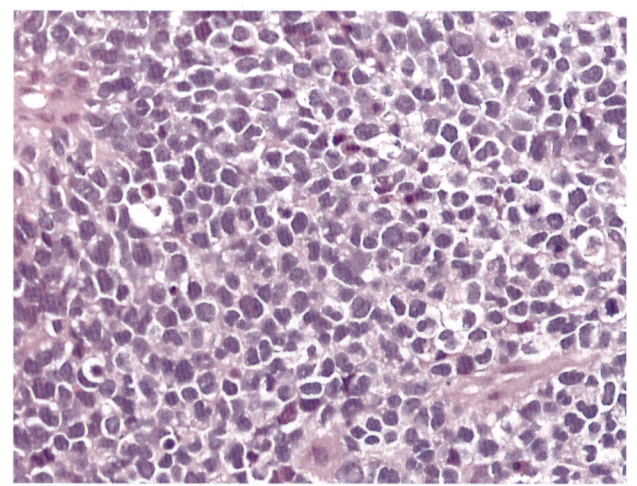

图8.11　鼻道横纹肌肉瘤（HE, ×100）

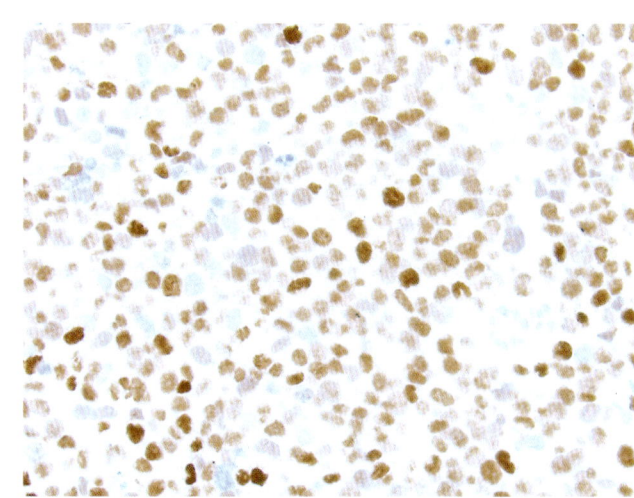

图8.12　鼻道横纹肌肉瘤免疫染色（myogenin, ×100）

表8.8　浸润性/异位垂体腺瘤的鉴别诊断

特征	垂体腺瘤	嗅神经母细胞瘤	副神经节瘤	类癌
Syn	+	+	+	+
CAM5.2	+	S	N	S
S-100（支持细胞）	N	+	+	R
激素	+	N	N	S
Pit-1	+	不明	不明	不明

+, 阳性；S, 部分阳性；R, 罕见阳性；N, 阴性

头颈部[89,90]。

光镜下，ES/PNET由一致的圆形细胞组成，常呈分叶状图像（图8.13）。细胞核直径为10～15μm，染色质分散，有时核仁不清楚。胞浆较少，界限不清，经常由于富含糖原而淡染。Homer-Wright（H-W）花环结构，偶尔Flexner-Wintersteiner（F-W）花环结构均可出现。核分裂多少不一。有些肿瘤可出现类似恶性神经鞘瘤的局灶性梭形细胞。

ES/PNET 呈糖原（PAS 染色）、波形蛋白和CD99（图 8.14）阳性。有些也可表达 Syn、CgA、NSE、Leu-7、PGP9.5 和 NB-84。最高 20% 的比例可呈 AE1/AE3、CAM5.2 局灶性或弥漫性表达，偶尔也可出现结蛋白表达。

过去，研究者根据神经分化区分 ES 和 PNET。如果肿瘤显示明确的 H-W 花环或 F-W 花环，有两种以上神经标记呈阳性或超微结构显示神经分化，则可诊断 PNET，如果无上述特征则考虑 ES。显示 PNET 特征的肿瘤预后较差。后来的研究显示有无神经分化对预后无影响。当 ES 和 PNET 是同一临床分期且治疗相同时，两者的预后一致。

ES/PNET 与两种特征的染色体易位有关，它导致 EWS 基因与 ETS 转录因子家族融合。大约 85%～90% 的肿瘤可见 t (11; 22) (q24; q12) 易位，涉及 22 号染色体的 EWS 基因和 11 号染色体的 FLI-1 基因融合，产生异常的基因产物 EWS-FLI-1[92]。

另有 5%～10% 的 ES/PNET 出现 t (2; 22) (q22; q12) 易位，导致 EWS-ERG 特异基因。

现在已有FLI-1蛋白表达的免疫组化检测，对ES/PNET 的敏感性为 71%，特异性为 92%[93]。

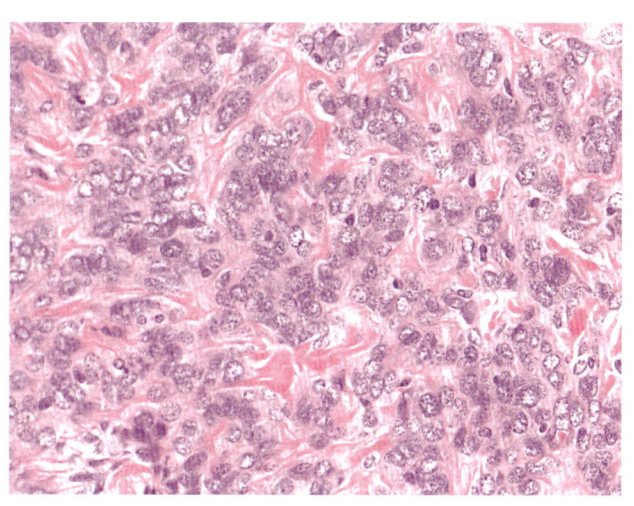

图 8.13　鼻道 ES/PNET（HE，×200）

> **诊断要点**：ES/PNET
>
> 1. ES/PNET由一致的圆形细胞构成，呈分叶状图像。
> 2. 肿瘤细胞呈 CD99 和波形蛋白阳性。
> 3. 有些呈神经内分泌标记（Syn 和 CgA）阳性，最多 20% 可呈 CK 阳性。

肠型腺癌

肠型腺癌（ITAC）是鼻道罕见的肿瘤，其组织学与结肠的腺癌十分相似，有时像绒毛状腺瘤[94]。有些甚至可能像正常小肠黏膜。有些病例发生与职业性接触木屑有关，而其余为特发性。

男性患者较常见，男女发病比例4∶1，发病年龄跨度较大，平均年龄58岁[94]。

可出现 5 种组织学生长模式：乳头型、结肠型、黏液型、实体型和混合型（以上两种以上混合）。在不认识这些肿瘤的情况下，可能会将它们与转移的结肠腺癌混淆。表8.9对于区分两者有帮助[95-100]。

鼻窦型血管外皮瘤

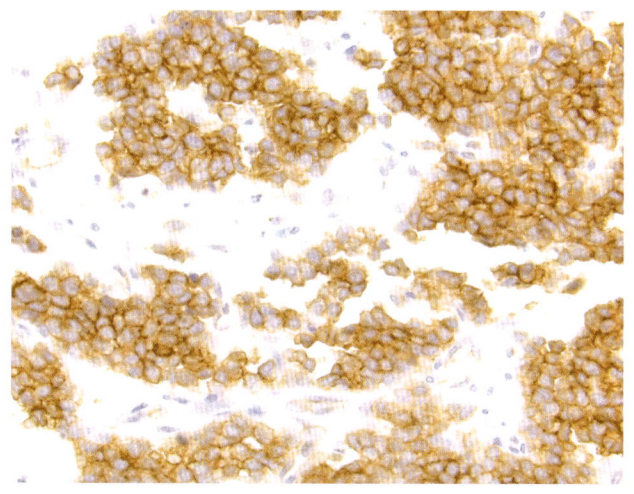

图 8.14　鼻道 ES/PNET 免疫染色（CD99，×200）

鼻窦型血管外皮瘤（SNTHPC）是一种不常见的

表8.9　结肠肠型腺癌与转移性结肠癌对比

	CK7	CK20	CEA	CDX2	CgA	MUC2	MUC5
ITAC	S	+	S	+	S	+	R-N
结肠	N	+	+	+	R	+	R-N

+ 阳性；S, 部分阳性；R, 罕见阳性；N, 阴性

肿瘤，鼻腔发生者多于鼻窦。男性患者稍多，发病年龄范围广，平均发病年龄 63 岁[63]。显微镜下，肿瘤由短梭形或上皮样细胞组成。核染色质较多，胞浆透亮或嗜酸性，血管丰富。

该肿瘤与软组织血管外皮瘤的关系以及血管外皮瘤是一个特殊的整体还是仅作为其他肿瘤的一种结构模式出现一直是一个有争议的问题。最近的研究提示鼻窦型血管外皮瘤与血管球瘤有密切关系，血管球外周细胞瘤这个名词可能更合适[63, 101-104]。

在一组 104 例鼻窦型血管外皮瘤的病例研究中，Thompson 等观察到 98% 呈波形蛋白阳性，92% 为 SMA 阳性，78% ⅩⅢa 阳性，77%MSA 阳性，52% 层粘连蛋白阳性，8%CD34阳性，3%S-100阳性，3%bcl-2 阳性，所有病例均呈结蛋白阴性。

尽管有数据提示鼻窦外软组织血管外皮瘤与孤立性纤维性肿瘤有关系，反映了同一整体的不同谱系，鼻窦型血管外皮瘤与孤立性纤维组织则没有关系。与鼻窦型血管外皮瘤不同的是，孤立性纤维性肿瘤呈 CD34 弥漫阳性，对 bcl -2 和 CD99 的染色反应不一。而对肌动蛋白、结蛋白、S-100 则呈阴性表达。

鼻咽部

鼻咽癌

鼻咽癌（NPC）被 WHO 定义为起源于鼻咽黏膜具有轻度鳞状细胞分化或超微结构上有鳞状细胞分化的癌。它包含鳞状细胞癌、非角化癌（去分化或未分化）和基底细胞样鳞癌。不包括腺癌和涎腺型癌[104]。

世界范围内均可发生该肿瘤，但呈明显的种族和地理性分布，在东南亚、北非和爱斯基摩人中更常见，所有年龄组均可发生，包括儿童。男性发病率是女性的 2~3 倍。鼻咽癌的病因是多因素的。相关因素包括种族（特别是中国人）、遗传环境因素和EB病毒（EBV）。

WHO 将鼻咽癌划分为3类（表8.10）。鳞状细胞癌的名词应用于有多数区域呈明确鳞状分化的肿瘤（细胞间桥、角化），与促纤维增生反应有关，可以将其分为高分化、中分化和低分化。其与 EBV 的关联度不强，倾向于局部生长，对放疗反应不一，40岁以下人群罕见发生。

表 8.10　鼻咽癌的 WHO 分类

1	鳞状细胞癌
2	非角化癌
	A 分化型非角化癌
	B 未分化癌
3	基底细胞样鳞癌

[引自 Barnes L, Eveson JW, Reichart PA, Sidnansky O. Pathology and genetics of head and neck tumours, WHO（104）]

分化型非角化癌正如其名称一样没有角化的证据。细胞呈层状，具有同膀胱移行细胞癌相似的表现。细胞边界清楚，间质和上皮间分界明显。该肿瘤与 EBV 关系密切，倾向于向周边播散，通常对放疗较敏感。

未分化癌（也称淋巴上皮癌、淋巴上皮瘤）由界限不清的细胞构成，核圆形或卵圆形，核仁明显（图 8.15）。细胞倾向于合体生长，而不是层状外观。有些病例，肿瘤形成界限清楚的上皮团，易确定为癌。有些病例由界限不清的细胞条索、小团或单个细胞混合淋巴细胞组成，给人恶性淋巴瘤的印象。但是，淋巴样成分不是恶性的，有时在转移性病灶中也可观察到该成分。未分化癌是儿童中最常见的类型。它与 EBV 有密切关系（图 8.16），有扩散倾向，对放疗敏感。

与未分化型鼻咽癌同样的肿瘤也可起源于鼻咽以外的部位，特别是鼻腔周围，喉、咽和涎腺[105, 106]。它们与鼻咽癌的区别仅在于部位不同。同样，EBV 也

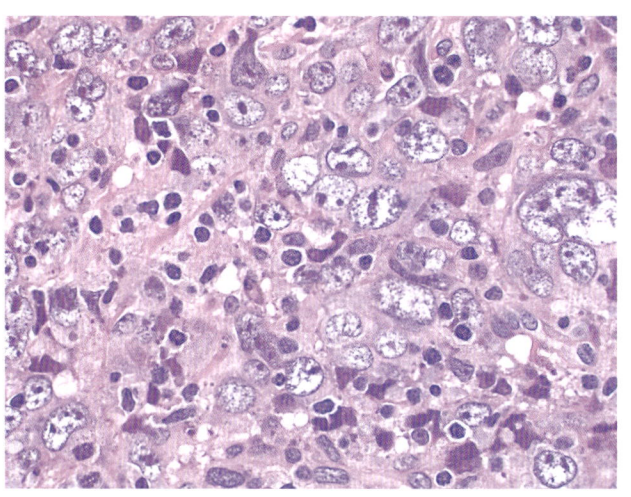

图8.15 鼻咽癌，未分化型，显示合体细胞群、透明细胞核和浸润的淋巴细胞（HE，×200）

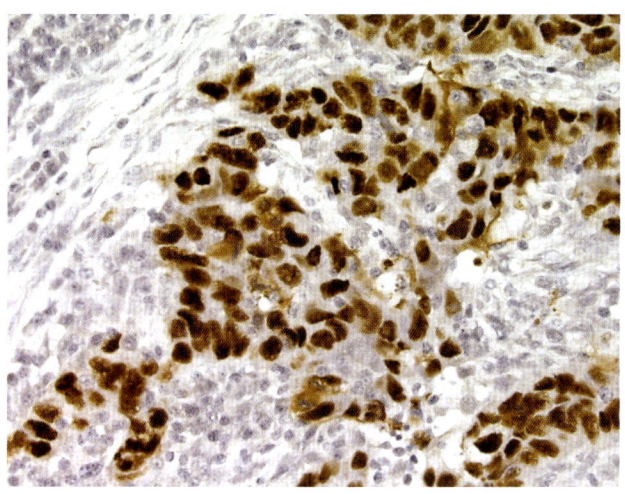

图8.16 未分化型鼻咽癌的原位杂交（EBER原位杂交，×200）

不仅在NPC中出现。在东南亚地区患者中，该病毒在鼻咽多种组织类型肿瘤中均可发现[107]。

鼻咽基底细胞样鳞癌很少见，仅有少部分报道，主要来源于中国香港。有些病例与EBV有关。

未分化鼻咽癌呈广谱CK、CK5/6、8、13、19强阳性，CK4、7、10和14则为阴性（表8.5）[59]。鼻咽癌经常出现p53阳性，偶尔c-kit阳性，而HER-2和LCA则阴性表现[108, 109]。淋巴细胞由B和T细胞混合组成，其中间夹杂有多克隆的浆细胞。S-100阳性的树突状细胞也可出现。

角化型鼻咽癌（鳞状细胞癌）易于辨认，与身体其他部位的鳞癌相似。而非角化亚型可能问题较

多，有时可能与许多鼻腔周围的其他小圆细胞肿瘤如恶性淋巴瘤、恶性黑色素瘤、嗅神经母细胞癌、髓外浆细胞瘤和横纹肌肉瘤混淆（表8.3）。鼻窦未分化癌（SNUC）经常与未分化鼻咽癌混淆。表8.7显示了有助于区分这两个肿瘤的特征。其他的小圆细胞肿瘤通常可以使用一系列免疫标记排除（如LCA、S-100、HMB-45、Syn、IgG、λ和κ轻链、成肌素等）（表8.3）。

鼻咽血管纤维瘤

鼻咽血管纤维瘤（NAF）是一种血管丰富、组织形态良性的肿瘤，但有时有局灶侵袭性，几乎均见于男性，10～20岁多见。

肿瘤由血管和纤维性间质两种成分组成。血管具有特征性的大管腔，常呈"鹿角状"外观，另有些可呈毛细血管状或血窦样。尽管典型的血管没有平滑肌，但偶尔可见所有血管有不均匀的平滑肌围绕的鼻咽血管纤维瘤。间质为致密的纤维性细胞，主要是纤维母细胞，偶尔有肌纤维母细胞。细胞核圆形、梭形或角状，有时可见小核仁。

间质细胞呈波形蛋白强阳性，CK34阴性[110, 111]。有些细胞可呈SMA局灶性阳性。大多数鼻咽血管纤维瘤中，可见纤维母细胞的胞核呈β-catenin阳性，而上皮细胞无此现象[112]。

该肿瘤是否表达激素受体特别是雌激素受体仍有争议。Hwang等使用免疫组化研究了24例鼻咽血管纤维瘤中睾酮受体（AR）、雌激素受体（ER）、孕激素受体（PR）表达，显示18例（75%）出现AR阳性，2例（8.3%）呈PR阳性。上皮和间质可出现阳性。而所有病例均呈ER阴性。

最近，Montag等研究了10例鼻咽血管纤维瘤中AR、ER和PR表达[114]。其中4例（40%）AR仅限于间质细胞。所有病例的间质和上皮细胞呈ER-β阳性而ER-α阴性。1例（10%）PR仅限于间质细胞。这提示不同研究中ER表达的差异可能与抗体的性质有关。

口腔和口咽部

颗粒细胞瘤

颗粒细胞瘤（GCT）是一种起源于施万细胞的少见肿瘤，肿瘤突起于皮肤和黏膜表面，好发于舌，多

数为良性，少数为恶性。

肿瘤呈S-100、NSE、α-1-抗胰岛素、CD68、波形蛋白、抑制素-α、蛋白质基因产物9.5、calretinin阳性，偶见CD57阳性[115-118]。对于CK、MAC387、SMA、MSA和结蛋白呈阴性。

Fanburgh-Smith等在一组73例恶性颗粒细胞瘤的研究中认为，恶性的特征有：坏死、梭形细胞、大核仁的透明细胞核、核分裂增多（＞2/10HPF）、核浆比升高、异型性[116]。满足以上3个标准者判定为恶性（n=46），满足1个或2个标准为不典型颗粒细胞瘤(n=21)，仅显示局灶异型性而没有以上特征则判定为良性（n=6）。14/25（56%）的恶性颗粒细胞瘤的Ki-67增殖指数为10%~50%，其余则小于10%。Le等在一组27例的良性颗粒细胞瘤研究中显示Ki-67增殖指数为1%~20%[118]。他们认为Ki-67染色在区分良性和不典型颗粒细胞瘤、恶性颗粒细胞瘤中的作用并不可靠，而组织学图像更可靠一些。

先天性牙龈瘤（CE，先天性颗粒细胞瘤）

先天性颗粒细胞瘤（CE）是一种不常见的良性软组织肿瘤，几乎均发生于新生儿。肿瘤表现为女性患者的一个突起性肿块，好发于中线偏后，与侧切牙和犬牙发育有关。上颌骨常被累及，与腭骨的发病率之比为（2~3）：1。

尽管先天性颗粒细胞瘤组织学上与颗粒细胞瘤相似，但没有颗粒细胞瘤中常见的表面上皮假上皮瘤样增生。它呈S-100和NSE阴性，因此不是施万细胞起源的[115]。但该肿瘤呈波形蛋白、α-1-抗胰岛素和CD68阳性。

咽喉部

该部位目前最常见的恶性肿瘤是鳞状细胞癌及其变型。涎腺型肿瘤可起源于喉黏膜腺体，此处也可发生间质肿瘤。咽喉部的特发良性病变包括声带结节和呼吸道乳头状瘤病。喉的神经内分泌肿瘤相对不常见。

声带结节

声带结节几乎总与声带过度使用有关，发生于真性声带，通常发生于游离边缘。声带结节有5种不同的组织类型：黏液型、纤维素型、血管型、纤维型和混合型。该病变没有任何特异免疫组化标记物，鉴别诊断仅用于将其与其他良性病变区分开。如可使用S-100染色将纤维型声带结节与神经纤维瘤区别。

呼吸道乳头状瘤病

呼吸道乳头状瘤病有两种分布模式：儿童起源型和成人起源型。病变与HPV感染有密切关系，主要是HPV6型和11型，可用免疫组化检测到[119]。

神经内分泌癌谱系

尽管头颈部的神经内分泌癌分类有争议[120]，WHO将该肿瘤分为4类：类癌、不典型类癌、小细胞神经内分泌癌和副神经节瘤，随后将分别讨论。鉴别诊断中，免疫组化对于区分这4者作用不大，但在将该肿瘤与其他肿瘤相鉴别时有帮助。其免疫表达状况如表8.11所示。喉的副神经节瘤将在头颈部副神经节瘤部分讨论[121]。

表8.11 应用于副神经节瘤鉴别诊断的免疫组化染色模式

染色	类癌	副神经节瘤	甲状腺髓样癌	黑色素瘤	肾细胞癌	小细胞肺癌
CgA	+	+	+	N	N	S
Syn	+	+	S	N	N	S
CK7	S	N	N	N	S	+
CK20	S	N	N	N	N	R
CEA	S	不明	+	N	S	+
S-100	N	+（支持细胞）	N	+	N	N
钙黏素	+/-	N	+	N	N	N
TTF-1	S	N	+	N	N	+

+ 阳性；S，部分阳性；R，罕见阳性；N，阴性

典型类癌

该肿瘤较罕见，在喉神经内分泌癌中的比例不足3%。组织学上，小的、一致的细胞可呈不同的生长模式，包括小的巢状、条索状、大的片状、腺样、假菊形团样。细胞核具有典型的神经内分泌细胞特点，染色质较细。间质血管丰富，也可出现间质一定程度的纤维化或玻璃样变。核分裂罕见或没有，无坏死。

不典型类癌

该类型在喉神经内分泌肿瘤中最常见的，约占54%[123]。肿瘤常见于喉声门上部，男性多见。不典型类癌呈浸润性生长，有多种不同的形态模式。细胞与典型类癌相比，细胞体积较大，可见核仁，偶见核分裂。而且可见坏死和血管或神经浸润。

小细胞神经内分泌癌（SCNEC）很少见，占所有喉癌的比例不足1%[124]。其分类与肺肿瘤相似，分为燕麦细胞癌、中间型和复合型。前两者有典型的神经内分泌分化，与发生于肺者组织学形态相似。肿瘤由小到中等大小的细胞组成，坏死、凋亡、核异型、血管和外周神经浸润均较显著。复合型除神经内分泌癌以外还可见到传统的鳞癌或腺癌。

免疫组化

喉的这3种类型的神经内分泌癌均可显示典型的神经内分泌标记阳性，如CgA、Syn、NSE[125]。有时CEA或EMA也可呈阳性。不典型类癌和小细胞神经内分泌癌也可显示其他的神经内分泌标记。如血清素、降钙素和生长抑素[126]。TTF-1在区别肺转移的小细胞癌和原发于头颈部的同类肿瘤中可能没有帮助，约有50%的肺外小细胞癌呈TTF-1阳性[127]。

喉类癌和不典型类癌的鉴别诊断包括副神经节瘤、黑色素瘤和甲状腺髓样癌。副神经节瘤呈CK阴性，并可出现特征性的支持细胞S-100阳性。TTF-1、降钙素和CEA在甲状腺髓样癌为阳性。HMB-45和酪氨酸酶在黑色素瘤为阳性，而两者在神经内分泌癌为阴性。

小细胞神经内分泌癌还必须与基底细胞样鳞癌、恶性淋巴瘤及肺的转移癌相鉴别。基底细胞样鳞癌通常不显示神经内分泌分化。恶性淋巴瘤出现典型的造血系统标记如CD20、CD3/CD43和LCA。头颈部原发和肺转移的神经内分泌癌的鉴别较困难，CK7、CK20，有时TTF-1的表达有重叠，应借助临床表现和影像学检查。

> **诊断要点**：神经内分泌癌
>
> 1. 神经内分泌癌的3种类型（类癌、不典型类癌和小细胞神经内分泌癌）的区分主要依靠组织学表现。
> 2. 这些肿瘤的免疫表型包括神经内分泌标记和CK阳性。
> 3. TTF-1在肺外小细胞癌中可阳性表达。

涎 腺

涎腺的大多数肿瘤可以通过常规HE切片诊断。免疫组化作用有限，但在以下情况时可能有帮助：①确定肌上皮细胞的存在，②区分原发和继发的涎腺肿瘤，③区分反应性和恶性淋巴组织浸润，④确定神经和血管、淋巴管浸润，⑤评估肿瘤的增殖率，⑥确定肿瘤中有诊断、预后或治疗意义的特征。

多形性腺瘤

多形性腺瘤（PA，良性混合瘤）是最常见的涎腺肿瘤。各年龄段均可发生，女性多见，大、小涎腺均可发生。发生于大涎腺者通常有包膜，而发生于小涎腺者无包膜。

显微镜下，多形性腺瘤由不同比例的上皮和肌上皮细胞组成，间质可呈黏液样、玻璃样变和软骨样。

尽管该肿瘤在完整切除时通常易于辨认，而在小的活检标本中很难与其他肿瘤如多形性低度恶性腺癌和腺样囊性癌区分。表8.12显示的特征对于鉴别有帮助[128-132]。

多形性低度恶性腺癌

多形性低度恶性腺癌（PLGA，末梢导管癌、小叶癌）最初于1983年由Freedman、Lumerman和Batasakis等分别描述。正如其名，该肿瘤是一种低级别、生长缓慢的肿瘤，大多数起源于口腔小涎腺，特别是腭部。另外也可发生于腮腺、多形性腺瘤或其他非口腔小黏液-浆液腺。

女性患者发病2倍于男性，发病年龄广泛（23～49岁），平均55～60岁[130]。

多形性低度恶性腺癌的组织学标志有多形性的生长模式、细胞学形态一致和浸润性生长。肿瘤由一致的、形态较温和的细胞组成，呈上皮样、立方形、柱状或梭形，肿瘤排列呈实性、腺管状、筛状、梁状囊形、滤泡状或局灶乳头状结构。细胞具有轻到中度的嗜酸或嗜碱性胞浆，核圆形，较一致，染色质稀疏透明。细胞核经常呈毛玻璃样，与甲状腺乳头状癌的细胞核相似。核仁缺乏，核分裂少见，无坏死。有些肿瘤可局灶出现透明或嗜酸胞浆。肌上皮细胞散在分布或缺乏。

间质呈黏液样、玻璃样变性或纤维血管状不等，没有软骨。偶尔可见腺腔含有黏液，但胞浆内黏液不常见。有些肿瘤可见腺管间砂粒体样的钙化。

肿瘤没有包膜，向周围组织浸润。神经周围浸润常见并且有特征性。

鉴别诊断包括多形性腺瘤和腺样囊性癌（ACC）。GFAP免疫组化染色对区分多形性低度恶性腺癌和多形性腺瘤有帮助。多形性腺瘤的间质，有时包括上皮呈典型的GFAP阳性，而多形性低度恶性腺癌中上述成分通常为阴性[129]。上皮细胞膜抗原（EMA）在区分多形性低度恶性腺癌和ACC中可能有帮助。多形性低度恶性腺癌中90%以上的细胞呈EMA阳性，而腺样囊性癌中仅有腔内衬细胞出现EMA阳性，而非腔内衬细胞和假囊性内衬细胞为阴性[135]。表8.12中列出了对鉴别以上肿瘤有帮助的其他指标。

> **诊断要点**：多形性低度恶性腺癌
> 1. 多形性低度恶性腺癌主要是发生于口腔小涎腺的肿瘤。
> 2. 该肿瘤GFAP呈阴性而EMA通常弥漫阳性。

腺样囊性癌

腺样囊性癌（ACC）几乎无例外的均是低度恶性肿瘤，特征是反复局部复发，后期可出现转移，最终生存期为5～15年。多发生于女性，发病年龄广泛，20岁以下人群较少见。

病理学上，肿瘤由不同程度的上皮细胞和肌上皮细胞组成，排列呈腺管状、筛状或实性结构，常伴有黏液样或透明变性圆环（图8.17）。上皮细胞可出现不同程度的CK系列标记（AE1/AE3，CK1、5、7、8、10、14、18和19）[131,136]。肌上皮细胞较具特征性，细胞较小、染色深、角状，可呈一系列肌上皮标记表达（表8.13）。当肿瘤分化较低时，肌上皮成分

表8.13　用于鉴别肌上皮瘤的免疫组化染色

AE1/AE3	S-100蛋白	CD10
CAM5.2	Calponin	Maspin
CK5/6	SMA	Metallothionein
CK14	Smooth muscle myosin heavy chain	GFAP
34βE12	p63	

表8.12　多形性腺瘤（PA）、多形性低度恶性腺癌（PLGA）和腺样囊性癌（ACC）的鉴别诊断

特征	PA	PLGA	ACC
部位	大涎腺或小涎腺	主要在口内特别是上腭	大涎腺或小涎腺
包膜	±	N	N
软骨	±	N	N
周围神经	N	±	+
Ki-67	<5%	<5%	>20%
S-100	强	强	强
bcl-2	弱至中等强度	弱至中等强度	强
GFAP	+	R	R
SMA	+	R～N	+
肌上皮细胞	+	R	+
c-kit	19%	25%	94%

+，阳性；S，部分阳性；R，罕见阳性；N，阴性

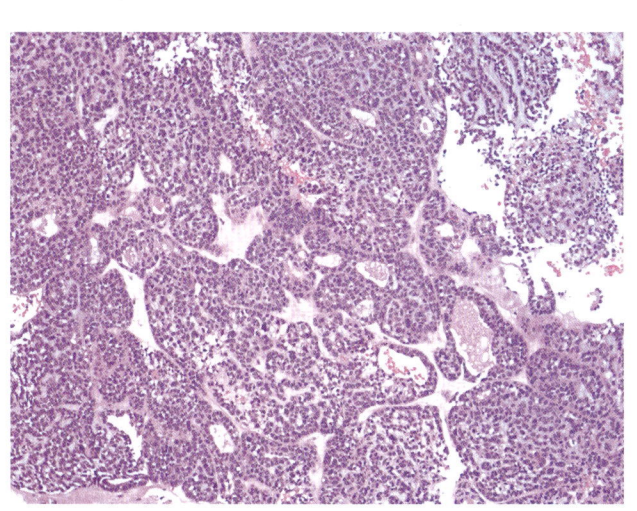

图 8.17　腺样囊性癌（HE,×200）

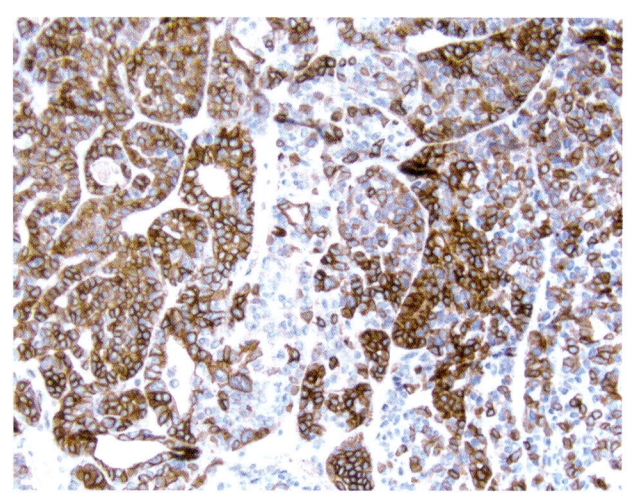

图 8.18　腺样囊性癌的免疫染色（c-kit,×200）

减少而上皮成分较明显[136]。

最初，c-kit 表达被认为在腺样囊性癌中是唯一的，可用于活检标本与其他类似的涎腺肿瘤鉴别。经验显示，c-kit 也可见于其他涎腺肿瘤，如多形性低度恶性腺癌和基底细胞腺癌等[132]。但多形性低度恶性腺癌中 c-kit 的染色范围和强度通常超过其他肿瘤，因此有一定程度的诊断意义（图 8.18）。该表达在 ACC 中仅见于上皮细胞，肌上皮细胞不表达。

多形性低度恶性腺癌通常不难识别，但在小的活检标本中可能出现问题（表 8.12）。

肌上皮瘤

尽管肌上皮细胞在多种涎腺肿瘤中均可出现，特别是多形性腺瘤，但完全或几乎完全由肌上皮细胞构成的肿瘤不常见，其被诊断为肌上皮瘤[137, 138]。

该肿瘤男女发病平均，发病年龄广泛，平均 40～50 岁[139]。大、小涎腺均可发生。发生于前者通常有包膜，而在后者出现时没有包膜。

肌上皮细胞可出现多种表现亚型，包括浆细胞型、梭形细胞型、透明或上皮细胞型，相应形成梭形细胞肌上皮瘤、透明细胞肌上皮瘤等（图 8.19）。

对应于组织学的多样性，肌上皮瘤可以表现出免疫表达的差异。有多种免疫标记可以鉴别肌上皮瘤，它们的敏感度和特异性有差别（表 8.13）。在怀疑肌上皮瘤时，不应该仅依靠一种标记而应使用一组标

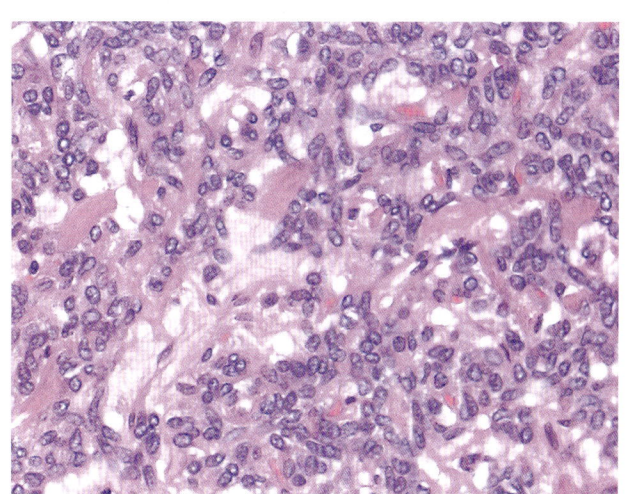

图 8.19　呈梭形细胞外观的肌上皮瘤（HE,×200）

记。我们选择使用 AE1/AE3、S-100、p63、calponin 和波形蛋白（图 8.20）。

由于该肿瘤相对不常见，伴有组织形态的多样性，肌上皮瘤有时难以诊断。

例如梭形细胞肌上皮瘤经常与平滑肌瘤和神经鞘瘤混淆。CK 和 S-100 阳性可将其与平滑肌瘤区分。神经鞘瘤也有包膜且 S-100 阳性，但呈 CK 阴性。

浆细胞变型可能与髓外浆细胞瘤混淆，但后者 CK 阴性而且免疫球蛋白呈阳性。

透明细胞肌上皮瘤没有导管而上皮/肌上皮瘤有导管，这有助于两者鉴别。其他的鉴别诊断还包括透

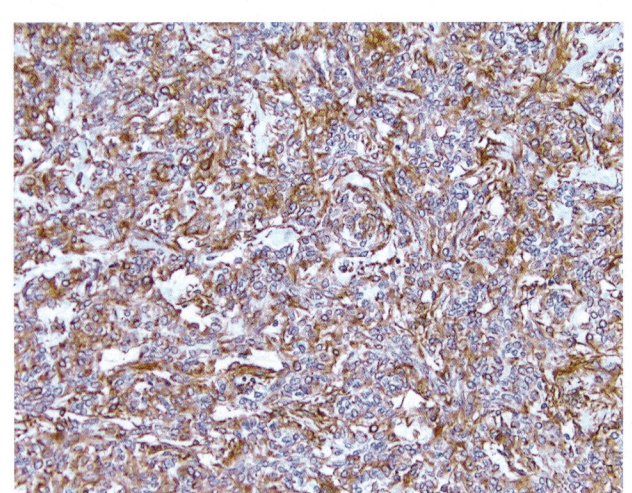

图 8.20　肌上皮瘤的免疫染色（vimentin，×200）

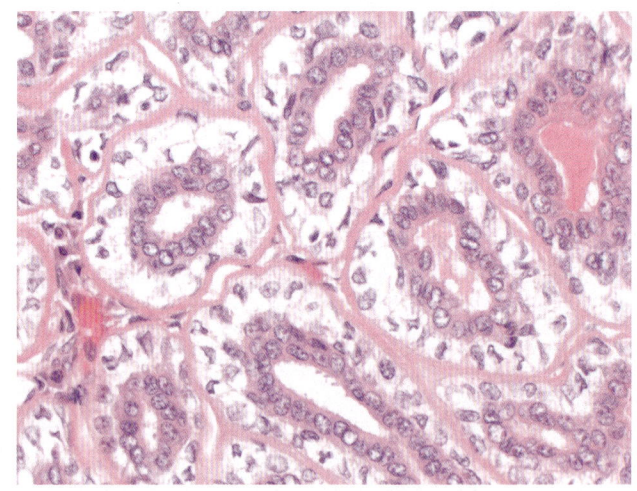

图 8.21　上皮/肌上皮癌显示两种细胞成分及致密的基底膜（HE，×200）

明细胞癌和转移的肾细胞癌，但上述两种肿瘤缺乏肌上皮细胞。

尽管大多数肌上皮瘤呈良性，但仍有些可为恶性。它们可能起源于多形性腺瘤，常显示浸润、多形性、坏死和核分裂等恶性特征。Nagao等认为肿瘤中出现核分裂大于7/10HPF、Ki-67指数大于10%及p53强表达的可能为恶性[140]。

在一组25例的恶性肌上皮瘤研究中，Savera等观察到100%呈AE1/AE3、53%呈CK14、100%呈calponin、50%呈SMA、31%呈GFAP阳性[141]。

上皮/肌上皮癌

上皮/肌上皮癌（EMC）是一种叶间导管起源的低度恶性双相分化涎腺肿瘤，占所有涎腺肿瘤的1%~2%。Donath及其合作者在1972年的研究引起对该肿瘤的关注[142]。

肿瘤最常见于腮腺（占75%），也可发生于小涎腺，女性多见（55%~67%），患者平均年龄59岁（范围13~83岁）[143]。

肿瘤有部分包膜或没有包膜，低倍镜下呈弥漫或多结节排列。肿瘤由小导管组成，围绕一层或多层透明细胞（肌上皮细胞），间杂一层厚的嗜酸性基底膜（图8.21）。导管内衬细胞呈立方形，粉红色胞浆，细胞核在中央或基底部。透明细胞呈立方形、卵圆形、梭形不等，有稀疏到中等染色的染色质。有些导管含有嗜酸性分泌物质，黏液染色阳性，但细胞浆内见不到黏液。透明细胞含有丰富糖原。免疫组化方面，导管细胞呈CK强阳性而S-100或其他肌上皮标记在透明细胞中阳性（表8.13；图8.22、8.23）。

肿瘤中即使同一病例的组织学表现也不同。有些病例主要由透明细胞组成，仅有少量散在分布的导管，而另一些可以主要由导管构成。亲神经性和乳头状/囊状区域可以出现，但坏死和核分裂很少或没有。

上皮/肌上皮癌中PCNA的免疫组化研究显示肌上皮细胞而不是上皮细胞是主要的增殖成分[144]。没有HER-2的过表达，DNA倍体的初步检测显示其在上皮/肌上皮癌中没有预后意义[143, 145]。

鉴别诊断时偶尔要考虑透明细胞癌和透明细胞肌

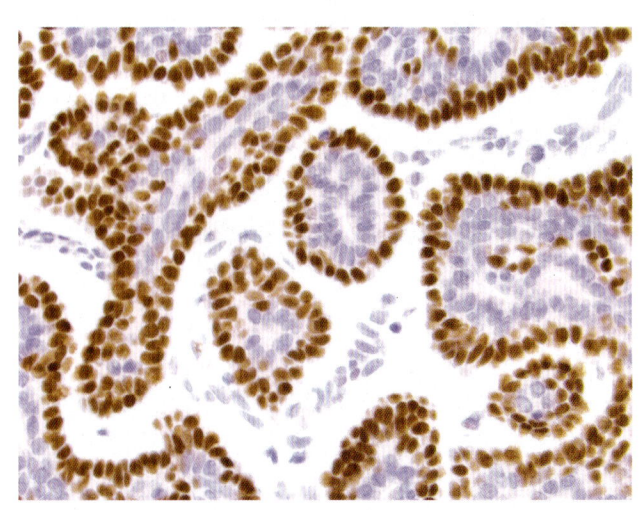

图 8.22　上皮/肌上皮癌中显示肌上皮细胞（p63，×200）

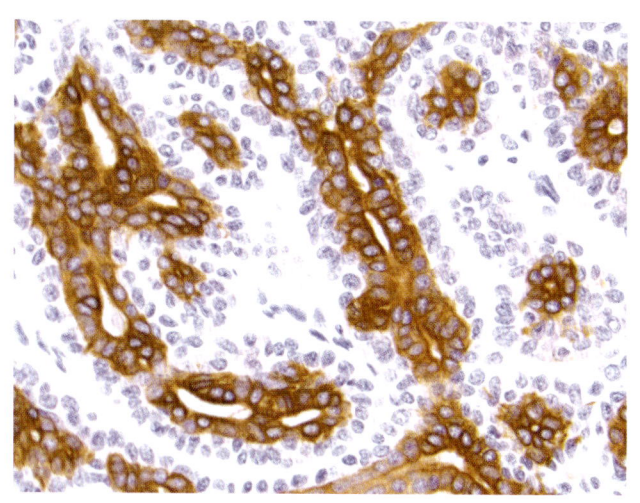

图 8.23 上皮/肌上皮癌中显示上皮腺腔细胞（AE1/AE3,×200）

上皮瘤，但这些肿瘤缺乏显著的导管成分。

腺样囊性癌（特别是腺管变型）有时也应作为鉴别诊断。存在筛状结构和缺乏显著透明细胞（肌上皮细胞）成分提示是腺样囊性癌。

多形性腺瘤可出现局灶性上皮/肌上皮癌样结构，这些区域的出现对其生物学行为没有影响，可以忽略。

透明细胞癌

有许多涎腺和非涎腺肿瘤可含有透明细胞，包括黏液表皮癌、涎泡细胞癌、嗜酸细胞癌、肾细胞癌、牙龈癌等[146-147]。如果有足够的切片并且认真观察细节，大多数病例均可诊断、分类，但仍存在一组无法进一步分类的肿瘤，这些称为透明细胞癌。

透明细胞癌，也称玻璃样变透明细胞癌，主要起源于口腔和口咽的小涎腺。在 Ellis 和 Auclair 总结的 60 个病例中 28% 发生于腮腺，12% 发生于颌下腺，其余 60% 为小涎腺起源[148]。

女性发病稍高，是男性的 1.6 倍，平均发病年龄 53 岁（范围 1～86 岁）[149]。大多数表现为黏膜下 0.5～3.5cm 的灰白肿块。

透明细胞癌由圆形至多边形细胞组成，细胞核相对一致，核仁不清楚。胞浆由于有糖原沉积而透明，没有显著的细胞异型性，核分裂罕见。肿瘤细胞呈实性巢状、条索状或梁状生长，周围经常有玻璃样变的结缔组织分割。周围神经浸润常见。细胞呈黏蛋白阴性，而 CK、EMA，有时还有 CEA 呈阳性，肌上皮标记为阴性（S-100、肌动蛋白、GFAP、p63 等）。

由于透明细胞癌中没有肌上皮成分，因此该肿瘤可以与透明细胞肌上皮癌和上皮/肌上皮癌相区分[149,150]。而且，该肿瘤也没有上皮/肌上皮癌中所含有的导管结构。肾细胞癌呈肾细胞癌抗原和波形蛋白阳性，高分子量的 CK903（CK1、5、10、11）为阴性[151]。而透明细胞癌 CK903 阳性，波形蛋白和肾细胞癌抗原均阴性。

涎腺导管癌

涎腺导管癌（SDC）是一种相对不常见、临床上有侵袭性的腺癌，起源于涎腺，组织学上与乳腺癌无法区分。

1994 年 Barner 等总结了 104 个病例，结果显示该肿瘤在男性中的发病率是女性的 3 倍，多数患者大于 50 岁（范围 22～91 岁）[152]。肿瘤主要发生于腮腺（占 88%），颌下腺（占 8%）和小涎腺（占 4%）均不多见。肿瘤可以起源于多形性腺瘤（多形性腺瘤恶变）。

显微镜下，涎腺导管癌中可见特征性的导管内癌和浸润性导管癌。肿瘤呈乳头状、筛状或实体生长，中央有坏死（图 8.24）。有些病例可似乳腺的硬癌，在促纤维增生性间质反应中可见小导管状或条索状的浸润癌。肿瘤细胞胞浆由嗜碱性到粉红色，细胞大，多形性明显，核较透明，核仁显著，有些可见充满大汗腺样顶浆分泌。核分裂，淋巴管、血管和周围神经浸润十分常见。有时可见营养不良性钙化，甚至影像学中也可看为假性结石。

肿瘤细胞岛周围可见一层形态一致的细胞，呈 CK14 和 p63（肌上皮细胞）阳性，这有助于确定肿瘤中的原位成分（导管内癌）。

Lewis 等研究了 25 例该肿瘤，观察到 EMA 100% 阳性，AE1/AE3 有 88% 阳性，GCDFP 有 76% 阳性，CEA 72% 阳性[153]。与乳腺癌中 ER、PR 常呈阳性不同，涎腺导管癌除少数外对这些受体均呈阴性。但 90% 以上的涎腺导管癌呈雄激素受体阳性（图 8.25）[154]。令人感到矛盾的是，有些病例可出现前列腺特异性抗原（PSA）和前列腺酸性磷酸酶（PA）阳性，在伴有雄激素受体阳性的情况下，可能与前列腺癌转移混淆[155]。

25%～88% 的涎腺导管癌中可出现 HER-2（c-erbB-2）过表达（图 8.26）[156]。但其是否有预后意义尚有争议。在关于涎腺导管癌和 HER-2 的一项较好的研究中，Skalova 等观察到 11 例中有 8 例出现细胞膜强表达（3+），其余 3 例为 1+ 或 2+[157]。FISH 结果显示，10 例中有 4 例出现 HER-2 基因扩增。但是出现基因扩增的肿瘤患者和未出现者的预后没有差别。

Felix 等的研究显示，58% 的涎腺导管癌中出现 p53 阳性，但与临床进展没有关系[156]。

耳 - 颞骨

神经胶质组织

中枢神经系统（CNS）之外的神经胶质组织（ENGT）不常见，但在头颈部的多个位置可以发生。最常见的两个位置是鼻（鼻胶质瘤）和中耳-颞骨[158-160]。ENGT 不应与脑膨出混淆，脑膨出与 CNS 有联系，而 ENGT 没有。

ENGT 呈灰色，可局限或弥漫分布，有时完全出现在意想不到的部位。经常与胆脂瘤或肉芽组织有关。ENGT 可伴有或不伴炎症存在，脑脊膜常缺失。显微镜下与肉芽组织难以区分，但 ENGT 呈 GFAP 阳性而肉芽组织为阴性。

中耳腺瘤

中耳腺瘤（MEA，类癌、神经内分泌腺瘤）是罕见的肿瘤。男女发病均等，发病年龄广泛（14～80岁）[161-162]。最常见的并发症是单侧听力丧失、耳鸣。耳漏和疼痛不常见。影像学上，肿瘤位于骨外，没有骨质破坏的证据。

大体上，肿瘤呈灰白色、棕红或黄色，可部分或全部占据中耳，经常包住耳小骨。显微镜下，中耳腺瘤结构呈多样性，细胞呈一致性。有些病例由腺样结构、细胞条索、小的细胞团块、梁状结构或多种结构混合（图 8.27）。细胞呈圆形、立方形、柱状，细胞核位于中央或偏位。胞浆粉红色或嗜碱性。没有核分裂和坏死。间质血管丰富，纤维组织疏松。炎细胞很少。

在一组 48 例标本的研究中，Torske 观察到 90%AE1/AE3 阳性，90%CK7 阳性，6%CK20 阳性，81%CAM5.2 阳性，88%CgA 阳性，31%Syn 阳性，25% 血清素阳性，84% 人胰腺多肽阳性，100% 波形蛋白阳性。

中耳腺瘤和类癌是独立疾病还是相关联的整体尚

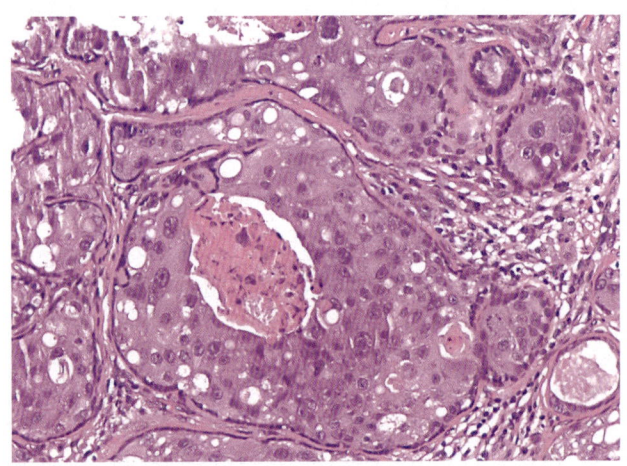

图 8.24　涎腺导管癌显示中央粉刺样坏死（HE，×200）

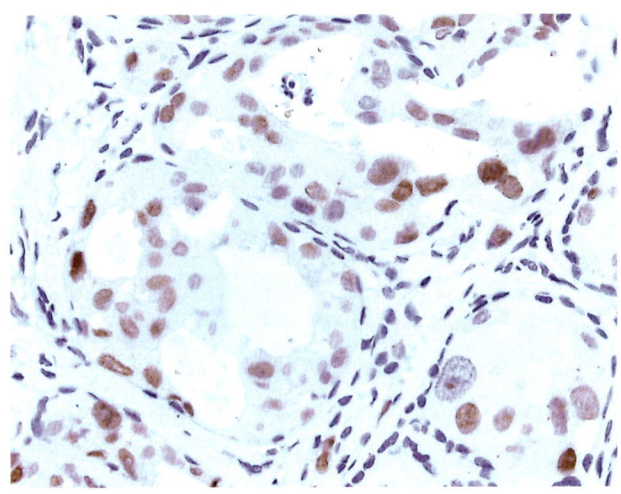

图 8.25　涎腺导管癌中雄激素受体表达（雄激素受体，×200）

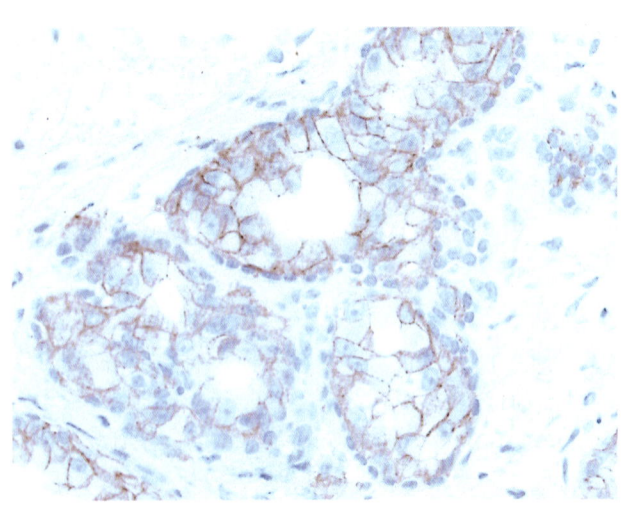

图 8.26　涎腺导管癌显示细胞染色模式（HER-2/neu，×100）

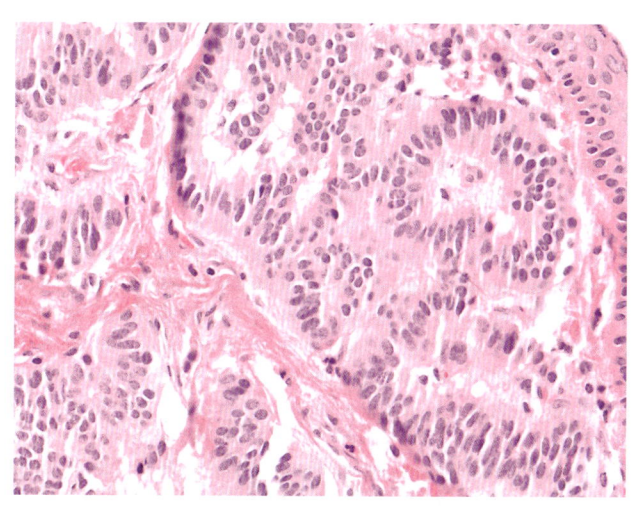

图8.27 中耳腺瘤的腺样模式（HE，×100）

存在争议。目前的观点认为它们代表同一种肿瘤中具有不同程度神经内分泌分化的群体。

鉴别诊断包括具有腺样分化的中耳炎（OMGD）、耵聍腺腺瘤、颈静脉窦副神经节瘤（JTPG）、内淋巴囊肿瘤（ELST）和颞骨转移癌。与中耳腺瘤不同，具有腺样分化的中耳炎中的腺体排列不紧密，而是在炎性背景中疏松排列，而且腺体呈神经内分泌标记阴性。耵聍腺肿瘤仅靠组织学就可排除。该肿瘤仅见于外耳道，而不发生于中耳，其神经内分泌标记也呈阴性。颈静脉窦副神经节瘤缺乏腺体，呈条带状生长，CK表达阴性。内淋巴囊肿瘤具有特征性的乳头状图像，而这在中耳腺瘤中见不到。乳腺癌、肺癌、肾癌是颞骨最常见的转移癌。转移是血源性的，主要为骨转移，而中耳腺瘤总是位于骨外。而且转移癌通常有细胞多形性和异常核分裂。转移瘤通常神经内分泌标记阴性，而中耳腺瘤为阳性。

内淋巴囊肿瘤

内淋巴囊肿瘤（endolymphatic sac tumor, ELST；侵袭性乳头状中耳肿瘤，乳头状腺瘤，低级别乳头状腺癌，Heffner肿瘤）罕见，是一种发生于淋巴内囊、生长缓慢、局部侵袭生长的肿瘤，特征性地累及中耳-颞骨和小脑脑桥角[163-164]。

同中耳腺瘤一样，内淋巴囊肿瘤发病年龄广泛（平均40岁），男女发病均等。单侧听力丧失、耳鸣和眩晕是最常见的临床表现，偶尔伴有面部神经麻痹。

查体可以正常或表现为鼓膜后蓝色或红色团块。双耳发病均等。双侧病变同时或先后发生也有报道，但很少见。应怀疑是否是von Hippel-Lindau病（VHLD）。初步数据显示至少15%的内淋巴囊肿瘤与VHLD有关，内淋巴囊肿瘤是与该综合征有关的另一系列病变[165]。

组织学上，肿瘤由乳头状/囊状成分组成，乳头血管丰富，被覆单层立方上皮，胞浆透明或粉红色，核圆形，大小一致，细胞多形性和核分裂缺乏。囊腔内含有特征性的粉红胶样物质，似甲状腺外观。这些分泌物质呈高碘酸-雪夫反应强阳性，黏液反应阴性。可见腺管密集排列区及纤维化、出血和胆固醇结晶。上皮细胞含糖原但没有胞浆内黏液。与中耳腺瘤不侵犯骨质不同，内淋巴囊肿瘤中常有骨质侵犯。

由于该病罕见，内淋巴囊肿瘤的免疫表型仍待研究[164, 166, 167]。初步研究显示100%出现CK阳性（AE1/AE3，CAM5.2），100%呈波形蛋白阳性，86%呈NSE阳性，61%呈S-100阳性，0%～20%呈GFAP阳性[166]。甲状腺转运蛋白和甲状腺球蛋白均呈阴性。

内淋巴囊肿瘤最常与转移的甲状腺乳头状癌（PTC）和绒毛膜网状乳头状瘤（CPP）混淆。甲状腺乳头状癌呈甲状腺球蛋白阳性，绒毛膜网状乳头状瘤呈甲状腺转运蛋白、GFAP阳性，而内淋巴囊肿瘤通常上述标记均为阴性[166, 168]。

异位脑膜瘤

颅外的脑膜瘤不常见，好发于中耳/乳突和鼻腔/鼻咽，诊断时应先排除原发于颅内脑膜瘤的继发转移。

中耳/乳突的真性异位脑膜瘤好发于女性，男女比例为1：2，发病年龄10～80岁（平均为50岁）[169]。偶尔可在胆脂瘤和中耳炎患者中意外发现，与脑膜瘤相比，更像脑膜细胞巢，但有些肿瘤可较大（最大4.5cm），可导致听力丧失、头痛、头晕、耳鸣、耳痛。

在一组36例标本的研究中，Thompson等观察到25例发生于中耳，4例发生于外耳道，2例发生于颞骨（骨内），5例为多灶性[169]。

组织学上，它们与颅内脑膜瘤相似，免疫组化呈波形蛋白阳性，EMA和孕激素受体通常为弱的或局灶性阳性（图8.28、8.29）。

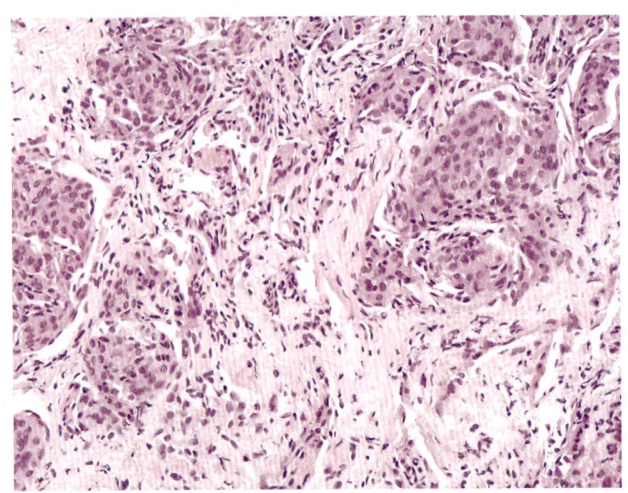

图 8.28 乳突脑膜瘤的巢状模式（HE，×100）

呈不同的生长模式，包括巢状、梁状，梭形细胞罕见（图 8.30）[173]。胞浆透明、嗜酸性、颗粒状，也可呈嗜碱性。细胞核通常较小而淡，但可出现多形性。核分裂罕见，坏死不明显。但术后行栓塞治疗者可出现大片的地图状坏死区。

坏死和核分裂增多是可疑恶性的特征。出现包膜、血管和周围神经浸润不是恶性的证据，这些特征也可出现于良性病变[174]。

副神经节瘤的染色模式具有特征性，几乎所有肿瘤均呈 CgA、Syn 和其他神经内分泌标记如 NSE、Leu7 阳性[173]。肿瘤细胞呈 CK 阴性。肿瘤巢周围的支持细胞总是呈 S-100 和 GFAP 阳性（图 8.31）[175]。当使用 S-100 诊断时，阳性部位应在肿

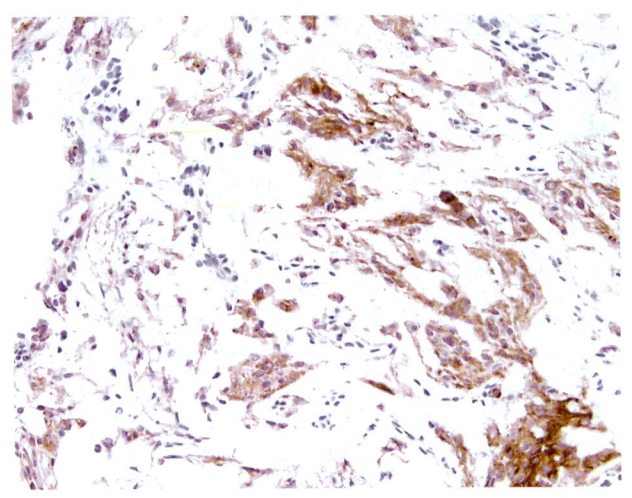

图 8.29 乳突脑膜瘤的免疫染色（EMA，×200）

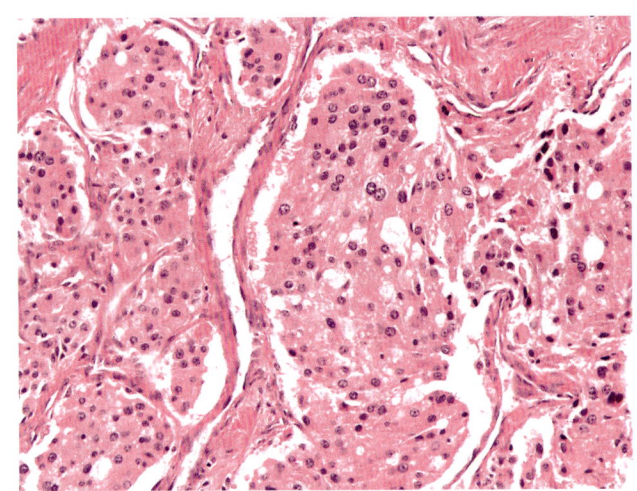

图 8.30 副神经节瘤（HE，×100）

副神经节瘤和恶性副神经节瘤

头颈部的副神经节瘤可发生于许多位置，最常见于颈部，常与颈动脉体有关，或见于中耳（颈静脉窦副神经节瘤）[170, 171]。副神经节瘤罕见于咽、鼻腔、鼻旁窦、口腔等其他部位[126, 170]。肿瘤的症状与解剖位置有关，患者可出现跳动的肿块。所有部位的副神经节瘤有相似的组织学和免疫学表型。

恶性副神经节瘤难以诊断，主要依靠查找转移病灶[172]。尽管有些组织学和细胞学特征被认为与恶性有关，但没有一种能作为预后差的指标。

组织学上，副神经节瘤由不同大小的细胞组成，

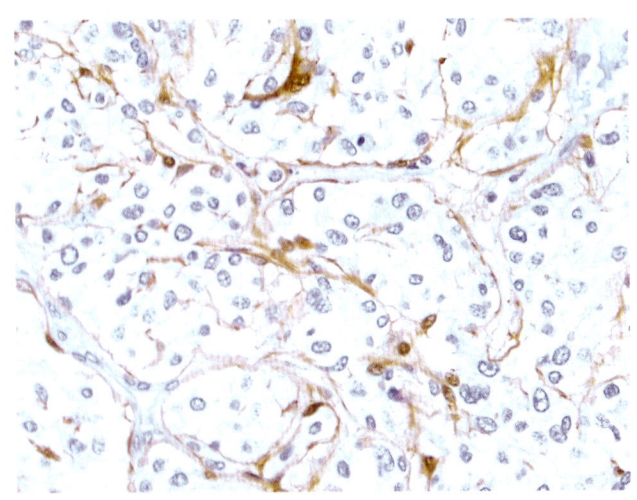

图 8.31 副神经节瘤中显示支持细胞（S-100，×200）

瘤巢周围，在支持细胞所处的纤维血管支持网中。有研究提示恶性副神经节瘤可出现S-100表达缺失或表达降低[176,177]。

副神经节瘤的鉴别诊断依据所处位置不同而有差别。颈静脉窦副神经节瘤的鉴别诊断包括中耳腺瘤、类癌、脑膜瘤[162,169,178]。通常依据组织学特征来鉴别它们，但相应的免疫组化组合也有帮助。中耳腺瘤可出现神经内分泌标记，但CK也呈阳性。类癌也显示同样的神经内分泌标记，但不会出现支持细胞S-100阳性的染色模式[178,179]。脑膜瘤通常EMA阳性而神经内分泌标记为阴性[169]。

颈部常见或不常见部位的副神经节瘤必须与其他上皮性神经内分泌肿瘤如类癌、不典型类癌、小细胞神经内分泌癌和甲状腺髓样癌相鉴别[126]。神经内分泌章节将讨论鉴别这些肿瘤的免疫组化组合（表8.11）。

> **诊断要点**：副神经节瘤
> 1. 头颈部副神经节瘤发生于相当特殊的部位。
> 2. 肿瘤细胞CgA、Syn阳性，CK阴性。
> 3. 支持细胞-间质细胞呈S-100阳性。
> 4. 单独组织学特征不能预测恶性，只有转移才能作为肿瘤恶性的证据。

转移性肿瘤

任何类型的肿瘤均可转移到头颈部，在不清楚原发灶的情况下，鉴别诊断中所有位置均应考虑到。当然，头颈部肿瘤最常累及颈淋巴结。

转移性前列腺癌

头颈部转移灶中，一种不常见但重要的肿瘤是前列腺癌[180]。这些肿瘤可出现不同的组织学特征，但通常出现前列腺癌的显著核仁特征。头颈部转移性前列腺癌的诊断有助于原发肿瘤的诊断。转移癌与原发前列腺癌的免疫染色模式类似，但一些低分化者可丧失PSA表达[180]。由于转移癌与涎腺导管癌（参见涎腺肿瘤）在PSA、AR、PSAP染色中有重叠表达，两者的鉴别有困难，这时需要依靠临床和影像学相关表现。

转移性肾细胞癌

转移性肾细胞癌可表现为没有原发肾细胞癌病史[181]。组织学上，肿瘤通常有典型肾细胞癌中出现的透明、嗜酸细胞及纤细的血管网。鉴别诊断依赖于解剖部位，包括嗜酸细胞瘤和具有透明细胞分化的肿瘤如透明细胞玻璃样癌和透明细胞肌上皮瘤。免疫组化组合有助于上述肿瘤的鉴别（表8.14）。

肺癌

肺癌转移到头颈部的情况较少见，特别是低位的颈部淋巴结通常与肺原发肿瘤的免疫表型相同。可用于鉴别诊断的典型染色包括CK7、CK20和TTF-1。

但可惜的是大多数肺鳞状细胞癌呈TTF-1阴性。因此，当病理学家遇到不明原发灶的颈部鳞癌转移时，鉴别诊断应包括最常见的情况：头颈部鳞癌和可能性更小的转移性肺癌。临床和影像学检查常常是区别两者的唯一方法。

表8.14 透明细胞肿瘤的免疫染色鉴别诊断

染色	肾细胞癌	嗜酸细胞瘤	玻璃样变透明细胞癌	透明细胞肌上皮瘤
EMA	+	N	+	+
CD10	+	N	不明	S
Vimentin	+	+	不明	+
RCC	S	N	不明	不明
CEA	N	不明	+	N
S-100	S	不明	N	+
SMA	N	不明	N	+
GFAP	N	不明	N	+

+，阳性；S，部分阳性；R，罕见阳性；N，阴性

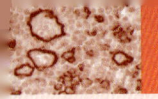

> **诊断要点：转移性肿瘤**
>
> 1. 转移性肿瘤最常见于原发于头颈部肿瘤的转移，但原发于锁骨以下部位也有可能。
> 2. 依赖于组织学指导的免疫组化组合有时有助于确定肿瘤类型。
> 3. 即使借助免疫组化，有时确定头颈部转移癌的来源通常很困难或不可能，经常需要临床和影像学的相关资料。

预测性和预后性标记

表皮生长因子

表皮生长因子（EGFR）已经成为多种不同肿瘤的重要生物标记，主要原因是有几种使用该受体进行药物靶向性治疗的药物已获得FDA批准[182]。使用抗EGFR药物较有效的主要肿瘤有肺癌、头颈癌和转移性结肠癌[183-189]。肺癌中的最新证据提示DNA水平的某种突变可提高对治疗的反应性，但不存在这些突变的患者也可出现部分反应[190-192]。

免疫组化已显示头颈部鳞癌中存在EGFR过表达[189]。头颈部鳞癌的抗EGFR治疗是否有益尚不清楚，但目前正在进行临床试验，在不久的将来可能提供结果。

p53

头颈部鳞癌的p53突变和过表达十分常见，大约50%~60%的肿瘤显示p53异常[193, 194]。p53在蛋白和基因水平的改变对预后的影响已被广泛研究，结果之间有冲突[195]。有几项研究显示p53过表达与预后差有关，而其他研究显示没有相关性[196]。另有证据提示鳞癌中p53状态与化疗和放疗的反应性有关[197]。

根据作者的经验，p53染色在异型增生中可作为一个预后标记。在与增殖性标记Ki-67联合使用时，大多数异型增生显示上皮细胞p53的染色与异型增生程度有相关性。

其他标记

从抑癌基因到癌基因，从细胞因子、生长因子到病毒相关基因，头颈部鳞癌中许多其他分子标记都已有评估。鳞癌中，许多体细胞突变事件相当常见。但目前尚没有在诊断和评估预后方面使用这些。目前的标准仍然是借助TNM分期、肿瘤边缘、神经浸润、淋巴结转移灶的包膜外侵犯等传统形态学预后因素。

前哨淋巴结评估

在乳腺癌、恶性黑色素瘤等几种肿瘤的外科治疗中，前哨淋巴结切除已成为一种标准治疗方式，并已成为外科医生治疗头颈肿瘤的一种手段。正如其他器官一样，病理学通常联合应用HE切片和免疫组化染色来决定处理这些特殊标本的最好方式[198]。对于头颈部肿瘤没有标准的治疗指南。任何免疫组合在应用于肿瘤类型的确定时需要分析，例如鳞癌会出现不同于涎腺腺癌的免疫染色。甲状腺和涎腺病变中区分淋巴结的良性上皮成分和恶性成分总是很困难。

新型预测性或预后性抗体

在头颈部病理中新型标记物在诊断或预后中可能有用。目前已知头颈部肿瘤中存在许多癌基因和抑癌基因改变。p63是一种近期认知的一种抗体，在几乎所有头颈部鳞癌的细胞核中表达，但在许多其他类型细胞中也表达[199]。它在肌上皮和基底细胞中阳性表达，这在头颈部病变中有用处（参见涎腺章节）。

另有几种潜在标记物在检测和确定鳞状细胞异型增生分级中也有帮助，包括p16、p53和Ki-67[200-203]。这些指标在头颈鳞状细胞异型增生中均有望应用[204, 205]。由于在异型增生的诊断和分级方面争议较多，应用这些标记物有可能提高我们辨别异型增生病变的能力。

> **诊断要点：新型预测性或预后性抗体**
>
> 1. 目前头颈癌预后相关的免疫染色尚未在临床病理中应用。
> 2. 新型标记物包括p53、Ki-67和p16的联合应用，有助于将异型增生与正常或反应性鳞状上皮区分开。
> 3. p63在头颈部肿瘤中有帮助但不是特异性标记物，它在正常和肿瘤性鳞状上皮和肌上皮细胞均可表达。

参考文献

1. Simons JP, Hunt JL, Johnson JT. Pathology quiz case. Granular cell tumor of the tongue, with extensive overlying pseudoepitheliomatous hyperplasia. Arch Otolaryngol Head Neck Surg 2003; 129:127-128.
2. Lassaletta L, Alonso S, Granell J, et al. Synchronous glottic granular cell tumor and subglottic spindle cell carcinoma. Arch Otolaryngol Head Neck Surg 1998; 124:1031–1034.
3. Barkan GA, Paulino AF. Are epidermal growth factor and transforming growth factor responsible for pseudoepitheliomatous hyperplasia associated with granular cell tumors? Ann Diagn Pathol 2003; 7:73-77.
4. Wenig BM. Squamous cell carcinoma of the upper aero-digestive tract: precursor and problematic variants. Mod Pathol 2002; 15:229–254.
5. van Oijen MG, Leppers Vd Straat FG, Tilanus MG, et al. The origins of multiple squamous cell carcinomas in the aerodigestive tract. Cancer 2000; 88:884-893.
6. Sturgis EM, Wei Q. Genetic susceptibility – molecular epidemiology of head and neck cancer. Curr Opin Oncol 2002; 14:310-317.
7. Crowe DL, Hacia JG, Hsieh CL, et al.. Molecular pathology of head and neck cancer. Histol Histopathol 2002; 17:909-914.
8. van Oijen MG, Slootweg PJ. Oral field cancerization: carcinogen-induced independent events or micrometastatic deposits? Cancer Epidemiol Biomarker Prevent 2000; 9:249–256.
9. Jacob BJ, Straif K, Thomas G, et al. Betel quid without tobacco as a risk factor for oral precancers. Oral Oncol 2004; 40:697–704.
10. Sharma DC. Betel quid and areca nut are carcinogenic without tobacco. Lancet Oncol 2003; 4:587.
11. Herrero R, Castellsague X, Pawlita M, et al. Human papillomavirus and oral cancer: the International Agency for Research on Cancer multicenter study. J Natl Cancer Inst 2003; 95:1772–1783.
12. Hafkamp HC, Speel EJ, Haesevoets A, et al. A subset of head and neck squamous cell carcinomas exhibits integration of HPV 16/18 DNA and overexpression of p16INK4A and p53 in the absence of mutations in p53 exons 5-8. Int J Cancer 2003; 107:394–400.
13. Ha PK, Pai SI, Westra WH, et al. Real-time quantitative PCR demonstrates low prevalence of human papillomavirus type 16 in premalignant and malignant lesions of the oral cavity. Clin Cancer Res 2002; 8:1203–1209.
14. Gillison ML, Shah KV. Human papillomavirus-associated head and neck squamous cell carcinoma: mounting evidence for an etiologic role for human papillomavirus in a subset of head and neck cancers. Curr Opin Oncol 2001; 13:183–188.
15. Hesselink AT, van den Brule AJ, Brink AA, et al. Comparison of hybrid capture 2 with in situ hybridization for the detection of high-risk human papillomavirus in liquid-based cervical samples. Cancer 2004; 102:11–18.
16. McGregor F, Muntoni A, Fleming J, et al. Molecular changes associated with oral dysplasia progression and acquisition of immortality: potential for its reversal by 5-azacytidine. Cancer Res 2002; 62:4757–4766.
17. Sudbo J, Lippman SM, Lee JJ, et al. The influence of resection and aneuploidy on mortality in oral leukoplakia. [see comment]. N Engl J Med 2004; 350:1405–1413.
18. Lydiatt WM, Anderson PE, Bazzana T, et al. Molecular support for field cancerization in the head and neck. Cancer 1998; 82:1376–1380.
19. Saunders JR Jr. The genetic basis of head and neck carcinoma. Am J Surg 1997; 174:459–461.
20. Fiedler W, Hoppe C, Schimmel B, et al. Molecular characterization of head and neck tumors by analysis of telomerase activity and a panel of microsatellite markers. Int J Molec Med 2002; 9:417–423.
21. Vartanian JG, Pontes E, Agra IM, et al. Distribution of metastatic lymph nodes in oropharyngeal carcinoma and its implications for the elective treatment of the neck. Arch Otolaryngol Head Neck Surg 2003; 129:729–732.
22. Slootweg PJ, Hordijk GJ, Schade Y, et al. Treatment failure and margin status in head and neck cancer. A critical view on the potential value of molecular pathology. Oral Oncol 2002; 38:500–503.
23. Hoffman HT. Surgical treatment of cervical node metastases from squamous cell carcinoma of the upper aerodigestive tract: evaluation of the evidence for modifications of neck dissection. Head Neck 2001; 23:907–915.
24. Paulino AF, Singh B, Shah JP, et al. Basaloid squamous cell carcinoma of the head and neck. Laryngoscope 2000; 110:1479–1482.

25. Erdamar B, Suoglu Y, Cuhadaroglu C, et al. Basaloid squamous cell carcinoma of the supraglottic larynx. Eur Arch Oto-Rhino-Laryngol 2000; 257:154–157.

26. Winzenburg SM, Niehans GA, George E, et al. Basaloid squamous carcinoma: a clinical comparison of two histologic types with poorly differentiated squamous cell carcinoma. Otolaryngol Head Neck Surg 1998; 119:471–475.

27. Barnes L, Ferlito A, Altavilla G, et al. Basaloid squamous cell carcinoma of the head and neck: clinicopathological features and differential diagnosis. Ann Otol Rhinol Laryngol 1996; 105:75–82.

28. Ferlito A, Altavilla G, Rinaldo A, et al. Basaloid squamous cell carcinoma of the larynx and hypopharynx. Ann Otol Rhinol Laryngol 1997; 106:1024–1035.

29. Poetsch M, Lorenz G, Bankau A, et al. Basaloid in contrast to nonbasaloid head and neck squamous cell carcinomas display aberrations especially in cell cycle control genes. Head Neck 2003; 25:904–910.

30. Gillison ML, Koch WM, Capone RB, et al. Evidence for a causal association between human papillomavirus and a subset of head and neck cancers. J Natl Cancer Inst 2000; 92:709–720.

31. Muller S, Barnes EL. Basaloid squamous cell carcinoma of the head and neck with a spindle cell component. An unusual histologic variant. Arc Pathol Lab Med 1995; 119:181–182.

32. Ide F, Shimoyama T, Horie N, et al. Basaloid squamous cell carcinoma of the oral mucosa: a new case and review of 45 cases in the literature. Oral Oncol 2002; 38:120–124.

33. Raslan WF, Barnes L, Krause JR, et al. Basaloid squamous cell carcinoma of the head and neck: a clinicopathologic and flow cytometric study of 10 new cases with review of the English literature. Am J Otolaryngol 1994; 15:204–211.

34. Klijanienko J, el-Naggar A, De Brand F, et al. Basaloid squamous carcinoma of the head and neck. Immunohistochemical comparison with adenoid cystic carcinoma and squamous cell carcinoma. Arch Otolaryngol Head Neck Surg 1993; 119:887–890.

35. Coletta RD, Cotrim P, Almeida OP, et al. Basaloid squamous carcinoma of oral cavity: a histologic and immunohistochemical study. Oral Oncol 2002; 38:723–729.

36. Banks ER, Frierson HF Jr, Mills SE, et al. Basaloid squamous cell carcinoma of the head and neck. A clinicopathologic and immunohistochemical study of 40 cases. Am J Surg Pathol 1992; 16:939–946.

37. Morice WG, Ferreiro JA. Distinction of basaloid squamous cell carcinoma from adenoid cystic and small cell undifferentiated carcinoma by immunohistochemistry. Human Pathol 1998; 29609–612.

38. Tsubochi H, Suzuki T, Suzuki S, et al. Immunohistochemical study of basaloid squamous cell carcinoma, adenoid cystic and mucoepidermoid carcinoma in the upper aerodigestive tract. Anticancer Res 2000; 20:1205–1211.

39. Holst VA, Marshall CE, Moskaluk CA, et al. KIT protein expression and analysis of c-kit gene mutation in adenoid cystic carcinoma. Mod Pathol 1999; 12:956–960.

40. Mino M, Pilch BZ, Faquin WC. Expression of KIT (CD117) in neoplasms of the head and neck: an ancillary marker for adenoid cystic carcinoma. Mod Pathol 2004; 16:1224–1231.

41. Kiyoshima T, Shima K, Kohayashi I, et al. Expression of p53 tumor suppressor gene in adenoid cystic and mucoepidermoid carcinomas of the salivary glands. Oral Oncol 2001; 37:315–322.

42. Owonikoko T, Loberg C, Gabbert HE, et al. Comparative analysis of basaloid and typical squamous cell carcinoma of the oesophagus: a molecular biological and immunohistochemical study. J Pathol 2001; 193:155–161.

43. Kroch BB, Trask DK, Hoffman HT. National survey of head and neck verrucous carcinoma: Patterns of presentation, care and outcome. Cancer 2001; 92:110–120.

44. Barnes EL, Hunt JL. Squamous cell carcinoma of the oral cavity and oropharynx: A review of current data. Selected Readings in Oral and Maxillofacial Pathology 2003; 11:1–60.

45. Medina JE, Dichtel W, Luna MA. Verrucous-squamous carcinomas of the oral cavity. A clinicopathologic study of 104 cases. Arch Otolaryngol 1984; 110:437–440.

46. Ishiyama A, Eversole LR, Ross DA, et al. Papillary squamous neoplasms of the head and neck. Laryngoscope 1994; 104:1446–1452.

47. Suarez PA, et al. Papillary squamous cell carcinomas of the upper aerodigestive tract: a clinicopathologic and molecular study. Head Neck 2000; 22:360–368.

48. Thompson LD, Wenig BM, Heffner DK, et al. Exophytic and papillary squamous cell carcinomas of the larynx: A clinicopathologic series of 104 cases. Otolaryngol Head Neck Surg 1999; 120:718–724.

49. Thompson LD, Wieneke JA, Miettinen M, et al. Spindle cell (sarcomatoid) carcinomas of the larynx: a clinico-pathologic study of 187 cases. Am J Surg Pathol 2002; 26:153–170.

50. Olsen KD, Lewis JE, Suman VJ. Spindle cell carcinoma of the larynx and hypopharynx. Otolaryngol Head Neck Surg 1997; 116:47–52.

51. Lewis JE, Olsen KD, Sebo TJ. Spindle cell carcinoma of the larynx: review of 26 cases including DNA content and immunohistochemistry. Hum Pathol 1997; 28:664–673.

52. Thompson LD. Diagnostically challenging lesions in head and neck pathology. Eur Arch Oto-Rhino-Laryngol 1997; 254: 357–366.

53. Mills SE, Fechner RE. 'Undifferentiated' neoplasms of the sinonasal region: differential diagnosis based on clinical, light microscopic, immunohistochemical, and ultrastructural features. Sem Diagn Pathol 1989; 6:316–328.

54. Devaney K, Wenig BM, Abbondanzo SL. Olfactory neuroblastoma and other round cell lesions of the sinonasal region. Mod Pathol 91996; :658–663.

55. Meis-Kindblom JM, Stenman G, Kindblom LG. Differential diagnosis of small round cell tumors. Sem Diagn Pathol 1996; 13:213–241.

56. Devoe K, Weidner N. Immunohistochemistry of small round-cell tumors. Sem Diagn Pathol 2000; 17:216–224.

57. Broich G, Pagliari A, Ottaviani F. Esthesioneuroblastoma: a general review of the cases published since the discovery of the tumour in 1924. Anticancer Res 1997; 17:2683–2706.

58. Dulguerov P, Allal AS, Calcaterra TC. Esthesioneuroblastoma: a meta-analysis and review. Lancet Oncol 2001; 2:683–690.

59. Franchi A, Moroni M, Massi D, et al. Sinonasal undifferentiated carcinoma, nasopharyngeal-type undifferentiated carcinoma, and keratinizing and nonkeratinizing squamous cell carcinoma express different cytokeratin patterns. Am J Surg Pathol 1597; 26:1597–1604.

60. Cerilli LA, Holst VA, Brandwein MS, et al. Sinonasal undifferentiated carcinoma: immunohistochemical profile and lack of EBV association. Am J Surg Pathol 2001; 25:156–163.

61. Lopategui JR, Gaffey MJ, Frierson HF Jr, et al. Detection of Epstein-Barr viral RNA in sinonasal undifferentiated carcinoma from Western and Asian patients. Am J Surg Pathol 1994; 18:391–398.

62. Nakhleh RE, Wick MR, Rocamora A, et al. Morphologic diversity in malignant melanomas [see comment]. Am J Clin Pathol 1990; 93:731–740.

63. Thompson LD, Miettinen M, Wenig BM. Sinonasal-type hemangiopericytoma: a clinicopathologic and immunophenotypic analysis of 104 cases showing perivascular myoid differentiation. Am J Surg Pathol 2003; 27:737–749.

64. Prasad ML, Jungbluth AA, Iversen K, et al. Expression of melanocytic differentiation markers in malignant melanomas of the oral and sinonasal mucosa. Am J Surg Pathol 2001; 25: 782–787.

65. Franquemont DW, Mills SE. Sinonasal malignant melanoma. A clinicopathologic and immunohistochemical study of 14 cases. Am J Clin Pathol 1991; 96:689–697.

66. Silva EG, Butler JJ, Mackay B. Neuroblastomas and neuroendocrine carcinoma of the paranasal sinuses. A morphological and endocrinological study. Cancer 1980; 45:330–339.

67. Fitzek MM, Thoraton AF, Uarvares M, et al. Neuroendocrine tumors of the sinonasal tract. Results of a prospective study incorporating chemotherapy, surgery, and combined proton-photon radiotherapy. Cancer 2002; 94:2623–2634.

68. Perez-Ordonez B, Caruana SM, Huvos AG, et al. Small cell neuroendocrine carcinoma of the nasal cavity and paranasal sinuses. Hum Pathol 1998; 29:826–832.

69. Cheuk W, Kwan MY, Suster S, et al. Immunostaining for thyroid transcription factor 1 and cytokeratin 20 aids the distinction of small cell carcinoma from Merkel cell carcinoma, but not pulmonary from extrapulmonary small cell carcinomas. Arch Pathol Lab Med 2001; 125:228–231.

70. Mineta H, Miura K, Takebayashi S, et al. Immunohistochemical analysis of small cell carcinoma of the head and neck: a report of four patients and a review of sixteen patients in the literature with ectopic hormone production. Ann Otol Rhinol Laryngol 2001; 110:76–82.

71. Abbondanzo SL, Wenig BM. Non-Hodgkin's lymphoma of the sinonasal tract. A clinicopathologic and immunophenotypic study of 120 cases. Cancer 1995; 75: 1281–1291.

72. Vidal RW, Devaney K, Ferlito A, et al. Sinonasal malignant lymphomas: a distinct clinicopathological category. Ann Otol Rhinol Laryngol 1999; 108:411–419.

73. Arber DA, Weiss LM, Albujar PF, et al. Nasal lymphomas in Peru. High incidence of T-cell immunophenotype and Epstein-

Barr virus infection [see comment]. Am J Surg Pathol 1993; 17:392–399.

74. Logsdon MD, Ha CS, Kavadi VS, et al. Lymphoma of the nasal cavity and paranasal sinuses: improved outcome and altered prognostic factors with combined modality therapy. Cancer 1997; 80:477–488.

75. Cuadra-Garcia I, Proulx GM, Wu CL, et al. Sinonasal lymphoma: a clinicopathologic analysis of 58 cases from the Massachusetts General Hospital. Am J Surg Pathol 1999; 23:1356–1369.

76. Gaal K, Sun NC, Hernandez AM, et al. Sinonasal NK/T-cell lymphomas in the United States. Am J Surg Pathol 2000; 24:1511–1517.

77. Alexiou C, Kau RJ, Dietzfelbirger H, et al. Extramedullary plasmacytoma: tumor occurrence and therapeutic concepts [see comment]. Cancer 1999; 85:2305–2314.

78. Kapadia SB, Desai U, Cheng VS. Extramedullary plasmacytoma of the head and neck. A clinicopathologic study of 20 cases. Medicine 1982; 61:317–329.

79. Aquilera NS, Kapadia SB, Nalesnik MA, et al. Extramedullary plasmacytoma of the head and neck: use of paraffin sections to assess clonality with in situ hybridization, growth fraction, and the presence of Epstein-Barr virus. Mod Pathol 1995; 8:503–508.

80. Lloyd RV, Chandler WF, Kovacs K, et al. Ectopic pituitary adenomas with normal anterior pituitary glands. Am J Surg Pathol 1986; 10:546–552.

81. van der Mey AG, van Seters AP, van Krieken JH, et al. Large pituitary adenomas with extension into the nasopharynx. Report of three cases with a review of the literature. Ann Otol Rhinol Laryngol 1989; 98:618–624.

82. Luk IS, Chan JK, Chow SM, et al. Pituitary adenoma presenting as sinonasal tumor: pitfalls in diagnosis. Hum Pathol 1996; 27:605–609.

83. O'Hara BJ, Paetau A, Miettinen M. Keratin subsets and monoclonal antibody HBME-1 in chordoma: immunohistochemical differential diagnosis between tumors simulating chordoma. Hum Pathol 1998; 29:119–126.

84. Asa SL, Puy LA, Lew AM, et al. Cell type-specific expression of the pituitary transcription activator pit-1 in the human pituitary and pituitary adenomas. J Clin Endocrinol Metabol 1993; 77:1275–1280.

85. Mauer HM, et al. The Intergroup Rhabdomyosarcoma Study-I. A final report. Cancer 1988; 61:209–220.

86. Callender TA, Weber RS, Janjan N, et al. Rhabdomyosarcoma of the nose and paranasal sinuses in adults and children. Otolaryngol Head Neck Surg 1995; 112:252–257.

87. Parham DM, Webber B, Holt H, et al. Immunohistochemical study of childhood rhabdomyosarcomas and related neoplasms. Results of an Intergroup Rhabdomyosarcoma study project. Cancer 1991; 67:3072–3080.

88. Cessna MH, Zhou H, Perkins SL, et al. Are myogenin and myoD1 expression specific for rhabdomyosarcoma? A study of 150 cases, with emphasis on spindle cell mimics. Am J Surg Pathol 2001; 25:1150–1157.

89. Jones JE, McGill T. Peripheral primitive neuroectodermal tumors of the head and neck. Arch Otolaryngol Head Neck Surg 1995; 121:1392–1395.

90. Nikitakis NG, Salama AR, O'Malley BW Jr, et al. Malignant peripheral primitive neuroectodermal tumor-peripheral neuroepithelioma of the head and neck: a clinicopathologic study of five cases and review of the literature. Head Neck 2003; 25:488–498.

91. Gu M, Antonescu CR, Guiter G, et al. Cytokeratin immunoreactivity in Ewing's sarcoma: prevalence in 50 cases confirmed by molecular diagnostic studies [see comment]. Am J Surg Pathol 2000; 24:410–416.

92. de Alava E, Gerald WL. Molecular biology of the Ewing's sarcoma/primitive neuroectodermal tumor family. J Clin Oncol 2000; 18:204–213.

93. Folpe AL, Hill CE, Parham DM, et al. Immunohistochemical detection of FLI-1 protein expression: a study of 132 round cell tumors with emphasis on CD99-positive mimics of Ewing's sarcoma/primitive neuroectodermal tumor. Am J Surg Pathol 2000; 24:1657–1662.

94. Barnes L. Intestinal-type adenocarcinoma of the nasal cavity and paranasal sinuses. Am J Surg Pathol 1986; 10:192–202.

95. McKinney CD, Mills SE, Franquemont DW. Sinonasal intestinal-type adenocarcinoma: immunohistochemical profile and comparison with colonic adenocarcinoma. Mod Pathol 1995; 8:421–426.

96. Krane JF, O'Connel JT, Pilch BZ, et al. Sinonasal adenocarcinoma: Evidence for histogenetic divergence of the enteric and nonenteric phenotypes (Abstract). Mod Pathol 2000; 17:139A.

97. Choi HR, Sturgis EM, Rashid A, et al. Sinonasal

adenocarcinoma: evidence for histogenetic divergence of the enteric and nonenteric phenotypes. Hum Patholo 2003; 34: 1101–1107.

98. Bashir AA, Robinson RA, Benda JA, et al. Sinonasal adenocarcinoma: immunohistochemical marking and expression of oncoproteins. Head Neck 2003; 25:763–771.

99. Franchi A, Massi D, Baroni G, et al. CDX-2 homeobox gene expression [comment]. Am J Surg Pathol 2003; 27:1390–1391.

100. Amre R, Ghali V, Elmberger G, et al. Sinonasal 'intestinal-type' adenocarcinomas (SNITAC): An immunohistochemical (IHC) study of 22 cases (Abstract). Mod Pathol 2004; 17: 221A.

101. Chu PG, Chang KL, Wu AY, et al. Nasal glomus tumors: report of two cases with emphasis on immunohistochemical features and differential diagnosis. Hum Pathol 1999; 30: 1259–1261.

102. Watanabe K, Saito A, Suzuki M, et al. True hemangiopericytoma of the nasal cavity. Arch Pathol Lab Med 2001; 125: 686–690.

103. Tse LL, Chan JK. Sinonasal haemangiopericytoma-like tumour: a sinonasal glomus tumour or a haemangiopericytoma? Histopathology 2002; 40:510–517.

104. Barnes L, Eveson JW, Reichert PA, Sindransky D. Pathology and genetics of head and neck tumours. World Health Organization Lyons, France, IARC Press, 2005.

105. Dubey P, Ha CS, Ang KK, et al. Nonnasopharyngeal lymphoepithelioma of the head and neck. Cancer 1998; 82:1556–1562.

106. Jeng YM, Sung MT, Fang CL, et al. Sinonasal undifferentiated carcinoma and nasopharyngeal-type undifferentiated carcinoma: two clinically, biologically, and histopathologically distinct entities. Am J Surg Pathol 2002; 26:371–376.

107. Leung SY, et al. Epstein-Barr virus is present in a wide histological spectrum of sinonasal carcinomas. Am J Surg Pathol 1995; 19:994–1001.

108. Sheu LF, Chen A, Tseng HH, et al. Assessment of p53 expression in nasopharyngeal carcinoma. Hum Pathol 1995; 26: 380–386.

109. Bar-Sela G, Kuten A, Ben-Eliezer S, et al. Expression of HER2 and C-KIT in nasopharyngeal carcinoma: implications for a new therapeutic approach. Mod Pathol 2003; 16:1035–1040.

110. Beham A, Kainz J, Stammberger H, et al. Immunohistochemical and electron microscopical characterization of stromal cells in nasopharyngeal angiofibromas. Eur Arch Oto Rhino Laryngol 1997; 254:196–199.

111. Beham A, Regauer S, Beham-Schmid C, et al. Expression of CD34-antigen in nasopharyngeal angiofibromas. Int J Pediatr Otorhinolaryngol 1998; 44:245–250.

112. Abraham SC, Montgomery EA, Giardiello FM, et al. Frequent beta-catenin mutations in juvenile nasopharyngeal angiofibromas. Am J Pathol 2001; 158:1073–1078.

113. Hwang HC, Mills SE, Patterson K, et al. Expression of androgen receptors in nasopharyngeal angiofibroma: an immunohistochemical study of 24 cases. Mod Pathol 1998; 11: 1122–1126.

114. Montag AG, Richardson MS, Tretiakova M. Nasopharyngeal angiofibromas: Consistent expression of estrogen receptor beta (abstract). Mod Pathol 2004; 17:228A.

115. Filie AC, Lage JM, Azumi N. Immunoreactivity of S100 protein, alpha-1-antitrypsin, and CD68 in adult and congenital granular cell tumors. Mod Pathol 1996; 9:888–892.

116. Fanburg-Smith JC, Meis-Kindblom JM, Fante R, et al. Malignant granular cell tumor of soft tissue: diagnostic criteria and clinicopathologic correlation. [erratum appears in Am J Surg Pathol 1999; 23(1):136]. Am J Surg Pathol 1998; 22: 779–794.

117. Fine SW, Li M. Expression of calretinin and the alpha-subunit of inhibin in granular cell tumors. Am J Clin Pathol 2003; 119:259–264.

118. Le BH, Boyer PJ, Lewis JE, et al. Granular cell tumor: immunohistochemical assessment of inhibin-alpha, protein gene product 9.5, S100 protein, CD68, and Ki-67 proliferative index with clinical correlation. Arch Pathol Lab Med 2004; 128: 771–775.

119. Steinberg BM, DiLorenzo TP. A possible role for human papillomaviruses in head and neck cancer. Cancer Metastasis Rev 1996; 15:91–112.

120. Mills SE. Neuroectodermal neoplasms of the head and neck with emphasis on neuroendocrine carcinomas. Mod Pathol 2002; 15:264–278.

121. Barnes EL. Paraganglioma of the larynx: A critical review of the literature. Ann Otol Rhinol Laryngol 1991; 53:220–234.

122. el Naggar A, Batsakis JG. Carcinoid tumors of the larynx. A critical review of the literature. Ann Otol Rhinol Laryngol

1991; 53:185–187.

123. Woodruff JM, Senie RT. Atypical carcinoid tumor of the larynx. Ann Otol Rhinol Laryngol 1991; 53:194–209.

124. Gnepp DR. Small cell neuroendocrine carcinoma of the larynx: A critical review of the literature. Ann Otol Rhinol Laryngol 1991; 53:210–219.

125. Milroy CM, Ferlito A. Immunohistochemical markers in the diagnosis of neuroendocrine neoplasms of the head and neck. Ann Otol Rhinol Laryngol 1995; 104:413–418.

126. Woodruff JM, Huvos AG, Erlandson RA, et al. Neuroendocrine carcinomas of the larynx. A study of two types, one of which mimics thyroid medullary carcinoma. Am J Surg Pathol 1985; 9:771–790.

127. Oliveira AM, Tazelaar HD, Myers JL, et al. Thyroid transcription factor-1 distinguishes metastatic pulmonary from well-differentiated neuroendocrine tumors of other sites. Am J Surg Pathol 2001; 25:815–819.

128. Vargas V, Sudilovsky D, Kaplan MJ, et al. Mixed tumor, polymorphous low-grade adenocarcinoma and adenoid cystic carcinoma of the salivary gland: pathogenic implications and differential diagnosis by Ki-67 (Mib1), Bcl 2 and S-100 immunohistochemistry. Appl Immunohistochemist 1997; 5:8–16.

129. Gnepp DR, el-Mofty S. Polymorphous low-grade adenocarcinoma: glial fibrillary acidic protein staining in the differential diagnosis with cellular mixed tumors. Oral Surg Oral Med Oral Pathol Oral Radiol Endodontic 1997; 83:691–695.

130. Castle JT, Thompson LD, Frommelt RA, et al. Polymorphous low grade adenocarcinoma: a clinicopathologic study of 164 cases. Cancer 1999; 86:207–2019.

131. Darling MR, Schneider JW, Phillips VM. Polymorphous low-grade adenocarcinoma and adenoid cystic carcinoma: a review and comparison of immunohistochemical markers. Oral Oncol 2002; 38:641–645.

132. Mino M, Pilch BZ, Faquin WC. Expression of KIT (CD117) in neoplasms of the head and neck: an ancillary marker for adenoid cystic carcinoma. Mod Pathol 1224; 16:1224–1231.

133. Freedman PD, Lumerman H. Lobular carcinoma of intraoral minor salivary gland origin. Report of twelve cases. Oral Surg Oral Med Oral Pathol 1983; 56:157–166.

134. Batsakis JG, Pinkston GR, Luna MA, et al. Adenocarcinomas of the oral cavity: a clinicopathologic study of terminal duct carcinomas. J Laryngol Otol 1983; 97:825–835.

135. Gnepp DR, Chen JC, Warren C. Polymorphous low-grade adenocarcinoma of minor salivary gland. An immunohistochemical and clinicopathologic study. Am J Surg Pathol 1988; 12:461–468.

136. Nagao T, et al. Dedifferentiated adenoid cystic carcinoma: a clinicopathologic study of 6 cases. Mod Pathol 2003; 16:1265–1272.

137. Prasad AR, Savera AT, Gown AM, et al. The myoepithelial immunophenotype in 135 benign and malignant salivary gland tumors other than pleomorphic adenoma. Arch Pathol Lab Med 1999; 123:801–806.

138. Savera AT, Zarbo RJ. Defining the role of myoepithelium in salivary gland neoplasia. Adv Anatomic Pathol 2004; 11:69–85.

139. Barnes L, Appel BN, Perez H, et al. Myoepithelioma of the head and neck: case report and review. J Surg Oncol 1985; 28:21–28.

140. Nagao T, et al. Salivary gland malignant myoepithelioma: a clinicopathologic and immunohistochemical study of ten cases. Cancer 1998; 83:1292–1299.

141. Savera AT, Sloman A, Huvos AG, et al. Myoepithelial carcinoma of the salivary glands: a clinicopathologic study of 25 patients. Am J Surg Pathol 2000; 24:761–774.

142. Donath K, Seifert G, Schmitz R. [Diagnosis and ultrastructure of the tubular carcinoma of salivary gland ducts. Epithelial-myoepithelial carcinoma of the intercalated ducts]. Virchows Archiv A: Pathol Pathologische Anatomie. 1972; 356:16–31.

143. Cho KJ, el-Naggar AK, Ordonez NG, et al. Epithelial-myoepithelial carcinoma of salivary glands. A clinicopathologic, DNA flow cytometric, and immunohistochemical study of Ki-67 and HER-2/neu oncogene. Am J Clin Pathol 1995; 103:432–437.

144. Fronseca I, Soares J. Proliferating cell nuclear antigen immunohistochemistry in epithelial-myoepithelial carcinoma of the salivary glands. Arch Pathol Lab Med 1993; 117:993–935.

145. Rosa JC, Felix A, Fonseca I, et al. Immunoexpression of c-erbB-2 and p53 in benign and malignant salivary neoplasms with myoepithelial differentiation. J Clin Pathol 1997; 50:661–663.

146. Seifert G. Classification and differential diagnosis of clear

and basal cell tumors of the salivary glands. Sem Diagn Pathol 1996; 13:95–103.
147. Ellis GL. Clear cell neoplasms in salivary glands: clearly a diagnostic challenge. Ann Diagn Pathol 1998; 2:61–78.
148. Ellis GL, Auclair PL. Malignant epithelial tumors. In: Ellis GL, Auclair PL, Gnepp DR, eds. Surgical pathology of the salivary glands. Philadelphia: WB Saunders; 1991:379–389.
149. Wang B, Brandwein M, Gordon R, et al. Primary salivary clear cell tumors – a diagnostic approach: a clinicopathologic and immunohistochemical study of 20 patients with clear cell carcinoma, clear cell myoepithelial carcinoma, and epithelial-myoepithelial carcinoma. Arch Pathol Lab Med 2002; 126:676–685.
150. Michal M, Skalova A, Simpson RH, et al. Clear cell malignant myoepithelioma of the salivary glands. Histopathology 1996; 28:309–315.
151. Rezende RB, Drachenburg CB, Kumar D, et al. Differential diagnosis between monomorphic clear cell adenocarcinoma of salivary glands and renal (clear) cell carcinoma. Am J Surg Pathol 1999; 23:1532–1538.
152. Barnes L, Rao U, Knausse J, et al. Salivary duct carcinoma. Part I. A clinicopathologic evaluation and DNA image analysis of 13 cases with review of the literature. Oral Surg Oral Med Oral Pathol 1994; 78:64–73.
153. Lewis JE, McKinney BC, Weiland LH, et al. Salivary duct carcinoma. Clinicopathologic and immunohistochemical review of 26 cases. Cancer 1996; 77:223–230.
154. Kapadia SB, Barnes L. Expression of androgen receptor, gross cystic disease fluid protein, and CD44 in salivary duct carcinoma. Mod Pathol 1998; 11:1033–1038.
155. Fan CY, Wang J, Barnes EL. Expression of androgen receptor and prostatic specific markers in salivary duct carcinoma: an immunohistochemical analysis of 13 cases and review of the literature. Am J Surg Pathol 2000; 24:579–586.
156. Felix A, el-Naggar, Press MF, et al. Prognostic significance of biomarkers (c-erbB-2, p53, proliferating cell nuclear antigen, and DNA content) in salivary duct carcinoma. Hum Pathol 1996; 27:561–566.
157. Skalova A, Starck I, Vanecek T, et al. Expression of HER-2/neu gene and protein in salivary duct carcinomas of parotid gland as revealed by fluorescence in-situ hybridization and immunohistochemistry [see comment]. Histopathology 2003; 42:348–356.
158. Tashiro Y, Sueishi K, Nakao K. Nasal glioma: an immunohistochemical and ultrastructural study. Pathol Int 1995; 45: 393–398.
159. Francis HW, Nager GT, Holliday MJ, et al. Association of heterotropic neuroglial tissue with an arachnoid cyst in the internal auditory canal. Skull Base Surg 1995; 5:37–49.
160. Glasscock ME 3rd, Dickins JR, Jackson CG, et al. Surgical management of brain tissue herniation into the middle ear and mastoid. Laryngoscope 1979; 89:1743–1754.
161. Mills SE, Fechner RE. Middle ear adenoma. A cytologically uniform neoplasm displaying a variety of architectural patterns. Am J Surg Pathol 1984; 8:677–685.
162. Torske KR, Thompson LD. Adenoma versus carcinoid tumor of the middle ear: a study of 48 cases and review of the literature. Mod Pathol 2002; 15:543–555.
163. Gaffey MJ, Mills SE, Fechner RE, et al. Aggressive papillary middle-ear tumor. A clinicopathologic entity distinct from middle-ear adenoma [see comment]. Am J Surg Pathol 1988; 12:790–797.
164. Heffner DK. Low-grade adenocarcinoma of probable endolymphatic sac origin A clinicopathologic study of 20 cases. Cancer 1989; 64:2292–2302.
165. Gaffey MJ, Mills SE, Boyd JC. Aggressive papillary tumor of middle ear/temporal bone and adnexal papillary cystadenoma. Manifestations of von Hippel-Lindau disease. Am J Surg Pathol 1994; 18:1254–1260.
166. Megerian CA, Pilch BZ, Bhan AK, et al. Differential expression of transthyretin in papillary tumors of the endolymphatic sac and choroid plexus. Laryngoscope 1997; 107:216–221.
167. Horiguchi H, Sano T, Toi H, et al. Endolymphatic sac tumor associated with a von Hippel-Lindau disease patient: an immunohistochemical study. Mod Pathol 2001; 14:727–732.
168. Gyure KA, Morrison AL. Cytokeratin 7 and 20 expression in choroid plexus tumors: utility in differentiating these neoplasms from metastatic carcinomas. Mod Pathol 2000; 13: 638–643.
169. Thompson LD, Bouffard JP, Sandberg GD, et al. Primary ear and temporal bone meningiomas: a clinicopathologic study of 36 cases with a review of the literature. Mod Pathol 2003; 16:236–245.
170. Erickson D, et al. Benign paragangliomas: clinical presentation and treatment outcomes in 236 patients. J Clin Endocrinol Metabol 2001; 86:5210–5216.

171. Sennaroglu L, Sungur A. Histopathology of paragangliomas. Otol Neurotol 2002; 23:104–105.
172. Lam KY, Lo CY, Wat NM, et al. The clinicopathological features and importance of p53, Rb, and mdm2 expression in phaeochromocytomas and paragangliomas. J Clin Pathol 2001; 54:443–448.
173. Martinez-Madrigal F, Bosq J, Micheau C, et al. Paragangliomas of the head and neck. Immunohistochemical analysis of 16 cases in comparison with neuroendocrine carcinomas. Pathol Res Pract 1991; 187:814–823.
174. Barnes EL, Taylor S. Carotid body paragangliomas: a clinicopathologic and DNA analysis of 13 tumors. Arch Otolaryngol 1991; 116:447–453.
175. Min KW. Diagnostic usefulness of sustentacular cells in paragangliomas: immunocytochemical and ultrastructural investigation. Ultrastruct Pathol 1998; 22:369–376.
176. Achilles E, Padberg BC, Holl K, et al. Immunocytochemistry of paragangliomas – value of staining for S100 protein and glial fibrillary acidic protein in diagnosis and prognosis. Histopathology 1991; 18:458.
177. Kliewer KE, Wen DR, Cancilla PA. Paragangliomas: assessment of prognosis by histologic, immunohistochemical, and ultrastructural techniques. Hum Pathol 1989; 20:29–39.
178. Mooney EE, Dodd LG, Oury TD, et al. Middle ear carcinoid: an indolent tumor with metastatic potential. Head Neck 1999; 21:72–77.
179. Mandigers CM, van Gils AP, Derksen J, et al. Carcinoid tumor of the jugulo-tympanic region. J Nuclear Med 1996; 37:270–272.
180. Hunt JL, Tomaszewski JE, Montone KT. Prostatic adenocarcinoma metastatic to the head and neck and the workup of an unknown epithelioid neoplasm. Head Neck 2004; 26:171–178.
181. Ozolek JA, Bastacky S, Myers E, et al. Immunohistochemical staining characteristics of oncocytomas of major salivary glands: comparison to conventional renal cell carcinoma. Laryngoscope 2005; 115:1097–1100.
182. Khalil MY, Grandis JR, Shin DM. Targeting epidermal growth factor receptor: novel therapeutics in the management of cancer. Expert Review of Anticancer Therapy 2003; 3:367–380.
183. Iqbal S, Lenz HJ. Integration of novel agents in the treatment of colorectal cancer. Cancer Chemother Pharmacol 2004; 54:S32–S39.
184. Diaz-Rubio E. New chemotherapeutic advances in pancreatic, colorectal, and gastric cancers. Oncologist 2004; 9:282–294.
185. Resnick MB, Routhier J, Konkin T, et al. Epidermal growth factor receptor, c-MET, beta-catenin, and p53 expression as prognostic indicators in stage II colon cancer: a tissue microarray study. Clin Cancer Res 2004; 10:3069–3075.
186. Kondo Y, Hollingsworth EF, Kondo S. Molecular targeting for malignant gliomas (review). Int J Oncology 2004; 24:1101–1109.
187. Li B, Chang CM, Yuan M, eet al. Resistance to small molecule inhibitors of epidermal growth factor receptor in malignant gliomas. Cancer Res 2003; 63:7443–7450.
188. Nadal A, Cardesa A. Molecular biology of laryngeal squamous cell carcinoma. Virchows Archiv 2003; 442:1–7.
189. Ford AC, Grandis JR. Targeting epidermal growth factor receptor in head and neck cancer. Head Neck 2003; 25:67–73.
190. Paez JG, Janne PA, Lee JC, et al. EGFR mutations in lung cancer: correlation with clinical response to gefitinib therapy. Science 2004; 304:1497–1500.
191. Lynch TJ, Bell DW, Sordella R, et al. Activating mutations in the epidermal growth factor receptor underlying responsiveness of non-small-cell lung cancer to gefitinib. N Engl J Med 2004; 350:2129–2139.
192. Yaziji H, Gown AM. Testing for epidermal growth factor receptor in lung cancer: have we learned anything from HER-2 testing? J Clin Oncol 2004; 22:3646–3648
193. Gasco M, Crook T. The p53 network in head and neck cancer. Oral Oncol 2003; 39:222–231.
194. Blons H, Laurent-Puig P. TP53 and head and neck neoplasms. Hum Mutation 2003; 21:252–257.
195. van Houten VM, Tabor MP, van den Brekel MW, et al. Mutated p53 as a molecular marker for the diagnosis of head and neck cancer. J Pathol 2002; 198:476–486.
196. Vielba R, Bilbao J, Ispizua A, et al. p53 and cyclin D1 as prognostic factors in squamous cell carcinoma of the larynx. Laryngoscope 2003; 113:167–172.
197. Smith BD, Haffty BG. Molecular markers as prognostic factors for local recurrence and radioresistance in head and neck squamous cell carcinoma. Radiation Oncol Investigat 1999; 7:125–144.
198. Hunt JL, Baloch ZW, LiVolsi VA. Sentinel lymph node evaluation for tumor metastasis. Sem Diagn Pathol 2002; 19:263–

277.
199. Sniezek JC, Matheny KE, Westfall MD, et al. Dominant negative p63 isoform expression in head and neck squamous cell carcinoma. Laryngoscope 2004; 114:2063–2072.
200. Fregonesi PA. P16INK4A immunohistochemical over-expression in premalignant and malignant oral lesions infected with human papillomavirus. J Histochem Cytochem 2003; 51: 1291–1297.
201. Namazie A, Alavi S, Olopade OI, et al. Cyclin D1 amplification and p16(MTS1/CDK4I) deletion correlate with poor prognosis in head and neck tumors. Laryngoscope 2002; 112: 472–481.
202. Schoelch ML, et al. Cell cycle proteins and the development of oral squamous cell carcinoma. Oral Oncol 1999; 35:333–342.
203. Oliver RJ, MacDonald DG, Felix DH. Aspects of cell proliferation in oral epithelial dysplastic lesions. J Oral Pathol Med 2000; 29:49–55.
204. Kresty LA, Mallery SR, Knobloch TJ, et al. Alterations of p16(INK4a) and p14(ARF) in patients with severe oral epithelial dysplasia. Cancer Res 2002; 62:5295–5300.
205. Ambrosch P, Schlott T, Hilmes D, et al. p16 alterations and retinoblastoma protein expression in squamous cell carcinoma and neighboring dysplasia from the upper aero-digestive tract. Virchows Archiv 2001; 438:343–349.

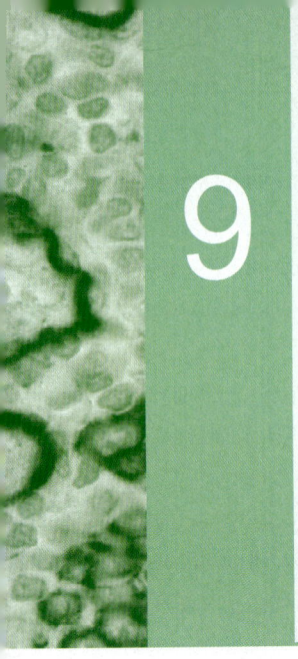

9 内分泌肿瘤的免疫组织化学

原作者：Ronald A. DeLellis and Sandra J. Shin

译　者：刘志艳

审校者：甄军晖，张建平

目　录

引言　　　　　　　　　　　　　　　　266
抗原/抗体生物学　　　　　　　　　　　266
特殊部位肿瘤　　　　　　　　　　　　269

引　言

免疫组化方法对内分泌系统及其各种疾病的理解及各种疾病的阐述具有深刻影响。尤其是使内分泌肿瘤的功能性分类得以发展，使其成为传统形态分类的补充，并部分取代了传统的形态学分类。根据激素表达形式和各种其他标记，内分泌病理应用免疫组化方法，对认识新的肿瘤、确定转移性肿瘤的原发部位、评估肿瘤预后等十分重要。而且，这些方法在认识内分泌肿瘤前期病变、阐明由增生至肿瘤形成的系列过程中起着十分重要的作用。本章旨在总结现在内分泌肿瘤中常用的免疫组化标记及其在特定内分泌肿瘤诊断中的应用。

抗原/抗体生物学

激　素

内分泌肿瘤的诊断和分类依赖于它们激素的检测[1,2]。可以通过用抗体标记成熟的激素和激素前体的方式来实现。也可以通过一项新技术——原位杂交技术（原位杂交组织化学）对特定激素信使RNA（mRNA）进行检测，其最新进展在几篇综述中均有详细介绍[3,4]。几乎所有的激素（小的肽类、大的多肽类激素、固醇类、氨类）以及激素受体，都可用免疫组化的方法显现出来[2,5]。随着微波抗原修复法的应用，大量的免疫组化产品均可用于福尔马林固定、石蜡包埋的标本。但激素类产品不能用做种系特定标记[6]。如生长激素抑制素表达于胰岛的D细胞，胃肠道和支气管、肺的内分泌细胞，胸腺内分泌细胞，甲状腺C细胞及其相关肿瘤。因此，生长激素抑制素自身的表达并不能确定其为原发灶还是转移。激素将在特定内分泌细胞及其相关肿瘤一节讨论。

酶

肽类激素和胺类生物合成和加工活化酶类是内分泌细胞的重要标记[6]。如左旋芳香氨基酸脱羧酶，在神经内分泌细胞广泛阳性[7]。相反，酪氨酸羟化酶、多巴胺-β-羟化酶和儿茶酚胺N-甲基转化酶等组织分布比较局限，仅位于已知的儿茶酚胺生物合成部位[8]。这些酶的免疫组化定位，使我们可以推断出石蜡标本中的儿茶酚胺合成能力。但这些酶的免疫反应，并不一定表明其处于功能状态[6]。

从前体分子活化为激活状态的肽类需要大量位于高尔基转化区和神经内分泌细胞的颗粒中的肽链内切酶和羧肽酶。包括激素原转化酶（prohormone convertase, PC）PC1/PC3、PC2，及羧肽酶H、E[9,10]。这些转化酶原广泛分布于神经内分泌细胞及其相关肿瘤中，而其他类型内分泌细胞（甲状腺滤泡细胞、甲状旁腺主细胞、肾上腺皮质细胞和睾丸）中则为阴性[10]。具有神经表型的神经内分泌细胞（如肾上腺髓质细胞）为PC2优势型，而上皮型神经内分泌细胞含PC1/PC3优势型。除甲状旁腺细胞外，PC1/

PC3的存在与嗜铬素和分泌素相关。PC2和PC1/PC3存在于正常垂体和垂体腺瘤，促肾上腺皮质激素（ACTH）腺瘤为PC1/PC3优势型，其他腺瘤为PC2优势型[9]。甘氨肽-α-酰胺化单氧酶和多肽-α-羟基甘氨酸裂解酶存在于神经内分泌颗粒中[11]。这些酶负责肽类激素C-末端的α-酰胺化，这对肽类的生物活性功能至关重要。

神经特异性烯醇化酶（neuron-specific enolase，NSE）是另外一种研究比较广的神经内分泌细胞标记酶[12]。其对神经内分泌肿瘤的标记与细胞内神经内分泌颗粒无关，即使去除神经内分泌颗粒的细胞NSE也呈阳性表达。NSE是糖分解烯醇化酶的酸性同工酶，既可表达于神经元，也可表达于神经内分泌细胞[12]。烯醇化酶是α、β和γ三个遗传基因座的产物。非神经性烯醇化酶（α-α）型以不同形式存在于胚胎组织、神经胶质细胞，以及成人的许多非神经内分泌组织内。肌肉性烯醇化酶是β-β型烯醇化酶，神经性烯醇化酶是γ-γ型烯醇化酶。杂合型烯醇化酶可见于巨核细胞和多种其他细胞。NSE（γ-γ）型在神经元移动和分化过程中替代了非神经性烯醇化酶。该同工酶的出现，预示着神经突触及其电兴奋性的形成。尽管许多早期研究把NSE作为神经内分泌细胞的特异性标记，但更多最新研究表明，应用多克隆抗血清的NSE特异性较差[13, 14]。

Seshi及其合作者报道了应用抗单克隆抗NSE（γ-γ）抗体特异性强[15]。一些NSE单克隆抗体主要是神经纤维阳性，而其他抗体为细胞核周阳性或细胞核周及相关性神经纤维阳性。与多克隆抗血清相比，单克隆抗体标记神经元的选择性更好。部分单克隆NSE抗体可标记肾上腺髓质细胞及各种胰腺神经内分泌细胞。由于多克隆血清的低特异性，一般认为NSE并不能作为神经内分泌标记物，尤其不能单独用做神经内分泌分化的标记物。

蛋白基因产物9.5（PGP9.5）泛素化羧基末端水解酶，在催化降解变性的异常蛋白过程中发挥作用。因此大量的神经元、神经纤维和神经内分泌细胞均可表达PGP9.5，但正常消化道的神经内分泌细胞并不表达PGP9.5。相反，类癌和一些其他内分泌肿瘤可表达PGP9.5。NSE和PGP9.5的表达形式在某种程度上是一样的。两者均弥漫表达于细胞浆内，且与其所产生的激素类型和细胞分化程度均无关联[19]。然而对照研究表明，一些神经内分泌细胞可表达PGP9.5而不表达NSE，另一些表达NSE而不表达PGP9.5。抗PGP9.5的抗体主要用于标记神经元及向神经元分化的细胞。一些无神经内分泌分化的肿瘤，如胰腺外分泌肿瘤，也可表达PGP9.5[20]。

组胺酶（二胺氧化酶）也被用做神经内分泌细胞及其肿瘤的标记物。该酶在甲状腺髓样癌中高表达，有报道称也可表达于肺小细胞癌及其他神经内分泌肿瘤。妊娠期间血清组胺酶水平增高，免疫组化研究也表明，蜕膜细胞中存在组胺酶。

免疫组化方法可以有效地检测类固醇激素生物合成过程中的酶类。它们分别为P450$_{SCC}$（胆固醇副链裂解酶）、3α-羧基类固醇脱氢酶、21-羟化酶、17α-羟化酶、11β-羟化酶等[22-24]。然而迄今为止，针对这些酶的相应诊断性抗体试剂的研究尚且不多。

嗜铬素、分泌素和其他颗粒蛋白

嗜铬素（chromogranins，Cg）和分泌素（secretogranins）代表了神经内分泌颗粒的主要成分[25-29]。3种主要的嗜铬素蛋白分别为嗜铬素A、B和分泌素Ⅱ，其他颗粒分别为分泌素Ⅲ、Ⅳ和Ⅴ。嗜铬素和分泌素蛋白含大量二碱基残基，是内源性蛋白水解酶最终分解其为小分子肽类的作用位点[30]。如，CgA含439个氨基酸，其中10对氨基酸是蛋白酶如激素原转化酶的潜在裂解点。合成的肽类包括嗜铬素抑制蛋白（chromostatin）、胰抑制素（pancreastatin）、旁抑制素（parastatin）和血管抑制因子（vasostatin）。这些小分子肽类的功能包括细胞内激素结合、对其他激素分泌的抑制及抗细菌和抗真菌作用。许多神经内分泌细胞含有所有主要粒蛋白，而其他的则表现出与嗜铬素不同的分布形式。

由Lloyd和Wilson提出的单克隆抗体LK2H10直接作用于CgA，是近来最常用的嗜铬素抗体[25]。嗜铬素位于神经内分泌细胞的分泌颗粒内。因此，肿瘤的分泌颗粒越丰富，其嗜铬素免疫反应就越强；肿瘤的分泌颗粒越少，其嗜铬素免疫反应就越弱。大量研究表明，CgA是广泛应用的、唯一的、最为特异的神经内分泌分化的标记物。CgB、分泌素Ⅱ抗体虽有效，但应用较少。

神经内分泌肿瘤中嗜铬素的典型表达具有组织特异性和相应的表达率。例如，Cg A主要表达于胃肠道类癌，阑尾及回肠类癌主要表达5-羟色胺。相反，CgB、分泌素Ⅱ主要在直肠的神经内分泌肿瘤（类癌和小细胞癌）和催乳素瘤中呈强表达，而CgA阴性[31, 32]。

HISL-19 和 PHE5 也是用于研究神经内分泌肿瘤的单克隆抗体。HISL-19 为抗人胰岛细胞抗体,并与 CgA、CgB、分泌素 II 截然不同的蛋白发生反应。在正常胰岛内,高血糖素细胞的反应强于其他胰岛细胞。HISL-19 既表达于高尔基体又表达于分泌颗粒[19,35]。该抗体也可标记其他神经内分泌细胞及其相关肿瘤。PHE5 为抗人嗜铬细胞瘤抗体,并与大量正常和肿瘤性神经内分泌细胞反应[34]。

突触素及其他突触小泡蛋白

突触素(synaptophysin,Syn)是一种钙结合糖蛋白(38 000kD),是构成神经元突触小泡的最丰富的完整的膜蛋白[36],也可见于广谱的神经内分泌细胞及其相关肿瘤。典型的 Syn 阳性反应点状分布于神经元突触区,或弥漫分布于神经内分泌细胞的胞浆内。超微结构显示,Syn 位于突触小泡内,而嗜铬素位于分泌颗粒内。这些不同表明,嗜铬素和 Syn 是两种互补的神经内分泌细胞标记物。Syn 免疫反应还可见于肾上腺皮质细胞,因而并非特异性神经内分泌细胞抗体[37]。

突触小泡蛋白2(SV2)可表达于中枢神经系统、周围神经系统及大量神经内分泌细胞。研究表明 SV2、Syn、CgA 在神经内分泌肿瘤中分布完全一致,仅后肠神经内分泌肿瘤弱表达 Syn,不表达 CgA,高表达 SV2。

小泡单氨基酸转移子(VMATs)介导氨基酸向神经元及神经内分泌细胞中的转移,VMAT1 和 VMAT2 在胃肠道各型神经内分泌肿瘤中的表达各不相同[39]。如产生 5-羟色胺的神经内分泌肿瘤高表达 VMAT1,而生成组胺的神经内分泌肿瘤(胃类癌)几乎只表达 VMAT2。生成肽类激素的胃肠道肿瘤(直肠类癌)及胰腺内分泌肿瘤,VMAT1 或 VMAT2 阳性细胞却很少[39]。

突触结合蛋白(p65)属钙结合蛋白家族,在神经递质释放过程中发挥作用,而突触结合蛋白 I 是神经细胞突触囊泡上的一个膜整合蛋白。在胰岛内,突触结合蛋白与胰岛素表达于同一部位,但其作为神经内分泌肿瘤的标记物尚未完全开发[40,41]。

突触小泡相关膜蛋白(vesicle-associated membrane proteins,VAMPs;或突触小泡蛋白,synaptobrevin)有 3 种异构体,是锚定于细胞浆内的突触小泡膜和分泌颗粒上的蛋白。VAMP2 和 3 见于胰岛 B 细胞,但其作为神经内分泌肿瘤的标记物尚未被广泛研究[42]。

与突触素和其他突触小泡蛋白不同,SNAP-25(25kD 突触后的末端蛋白)和突触融合蛋白位于细胞浆和细胞膜。

CD57

CD57 抗原表达于各种 T 细胞和自然杀伤细胞[43-45]。其抗体可与施万细胞、少突胶质细胞及大量神经和上皮性神经内分泌细胞反应。此外还可阳性表达于前列腺、肾和胸腺皮质上皮细胞。抗 CD57 的抗体可与部分神经肿瘤,包括神经鞘瘤、神经纤维瘤、神经瘤、颗粒细胞瘤发生反应。CD57 在神经内分泌肿瘤中的应用比较广泛,如可表达于 100% 的嗜铬细胞瘤、85% 的肾上腺外副神经节瘤、50% 的支气管源性小细胞癌、85% 的多器官来源的类癌。而其表达并不局限于神经内分泌肿瘤,因为 95% 以上的甲状腺乳头状癌,近 70% 的甲状腺滤泡癌也可表达 CD57[46]。一些非神经内分泌肿瘤,如前列腺癌、胸腺瘤,及大量小圆蓝细胞肿瘤也可表达 CD57。以上结果表明 CD57 不宜单独用做神经内分泌肿瘤的特异性标记物。

神经细胞黏附分子(CD56)

神经细胞黏附分子(NCAMs)是一大类糖蛋白,在细胞结合、移动和分化过程中发挥重要作用[47]。NCAMs 包括 3 个组成部分,由免疫球蛋白超基因选择性剪切后的 RNA 序列,通过磷酸化、糖基化和硫酸化完成转化后分子的修饰生成。NCAMs 的同嗜性结合特性受多聚唾液酸的不同表达来调节。尽管初期研究表明 NCAM 局限表达于神经内分泌系统,更多最新研究表明其分布比较广泛,包括肾上腺髓质和皮质(球状带)、心肌、甲状腺滤泡上皮、肾近曲小管上皮、肝细胞、胃壁细胞、朗格汉斯细胞岛等。肿瘤中的甲状腺乳头状癌、滤泡性癌、肾细胞癌、肝细胞癌 NCAMs 均呈阳性表达[48]。Leu7 抗原,为 HNK-1 单克隆抗体所识别,现在认为是 NCAM 和其他黏附分子的碳水化合物性抗原决定簇。绝大多数神经内分泌细胞及其肿瘤的神经内分泌颗粒中都含有 NCAM 的 mRNA 及其蛋白[49]。在 NCAM 中发现的长链多聚唾液酸(polySia)抗体已用于研究正常或肿瘤性 C 细胞以及肺神经内分泌肿瘤[50,51]。

中间丝

细胞角蛋白（CK）是除类固醇生成细胞外的其他神经内分泌细胞的主要中间丝。这些蛋白是细胞骨架蛋白中间丝（10nm）超家族的成员[52]。与其他骨架纤维在大小和理化功能上均有所不同。微丝（5~15 nm）含有肌动蛋白，而25 nm的微管含有微管蛋白。其他位于内分泌细胞及其支持组织的各型中间丝包括波形蛋白、胶质原纤维酸性蛋白（GFAP）和神经细丝蛋白。CK是最大、最复杂的中间丝，由至少30多种分子量在40~68kD之间的蛋白组成。其中Ⅱ型碱性角蛋白包含8种蛋白（CK1~CK8），Ⅰ型角蛋白为酸性蛋白，包括CK9~CK20共11种上皮角蛋白。碱性和酸性型成对表达于上皮细胞增殖、分化的不同时期，可用广谱CK抗体标记所有具有相同抗原决定簇的角蛋白，或用链特异性单克隆抗体标记各型角蛋白。CK在各组织中的分布具有特异性。原发肿瘤趋于表达与其来源细胞相同的角蛋白[53-55]。有些病例，CK表达趋于简单，而某些病例则较为复杂。波形蛋白（57 kD）与CK可同时表达于一些正常和肿瘤性内分泌细胞。在类固醇形成细胞，波形蛋白是主要的中间丝蛋白。

神经丝由3种分子量分别为70kD、170 kD、195 kD的杂聚亚单位组成，相应为低（L）、中（M）、高（H）分子量亚单位[56]。这3种亚单位按照不同比例发生磷酸化。神经丝是成熟、未成熟神经元、副神经节细胞和几种正常神经内分泌细胞的重要中间丝，也可表达于一些具有神经分化的肿瘤和不同程度地表达伴有CK表达的上皮型神经内分泌肿瘤。大多数正常上皮型神经内分泌细胞（胰岛、Merkel细胞）神经丝表达呈阴性，但其相关神经内分泌肿瘤往往呈阳性，而且呈典型的点状表达于高尔基体区域。Perez及其合作者研究表明，神经丝亚型的表达不同与肿瘤部位有关[57]。GFAP（50kD）是纤维及原浆型星形细胞的主要中间丝，也可见于无鞘施万细胞、垂体前叶和副神经节的支持细胞及许多癌中。GFAP还可见于皮肤和涎腺混合瘤、神经鞘膜肿瘤和脊索瘤。

转录因子

转录因子（transcription factor，TF）是DNA启动子和增强子调节元件的结合蛋白，可促进或抑制基因表达及蛋白质合成[58]。转录因子可以是组织特异性的，也可见于各种不同组织。一些所谓的组织特异性转录因子也并不限于一种组织。如甲状腺转录因子-1（TTF-1）既可见于甲状腺滤泡，也可见于肺内；肾上腺4位/类固醇生成因子（ad4BP/SF-1）可见于类固醇生成细胞及几种垂体前叶细胞；垂体转录因子（pit-1）可见于腺垂体的各种细胞及胎盘。转录因子的定位及免疫组化应用将于后述部分讨论。

生长抑素受体

生长抑素通过特异性受体发挥作用，其受体是7个跨膜配对G蛋白超家族成员之一。生长抑素受体（somatostatin receptor，sst）分为sst1~5五个亚型，对激素分泌的抑制作用由sst2介导；sst1、2、5介导对细胞生长的抑制；sst2、3介导其凋亡。sst的免疫组化研究用于判定神经内分泌肿瘤及sst类似物[59]。

细胞周期标记物

在内分泌病例中细胞周期标记物开始时被用做判断良、恶性肿瘤的辅助抗体[60-62]。总的来说，恶性肿瘤的阳性指数比良性肿瘤要强，正如Ki-67（MIB-1）抗体的评估结果。但良、恶性肿瘤的增殖指数标记会有所重叠。周期蛋白依赖性激酶抑制子p27在恶性内分泌肿瘤中的表达比良性肿瘤减少。有些病例中Ki-67和p27抗体组合更为有效[60]。

特殊部位肿瘤

腺垂体

根据HE染色，腺垂体细胞可分为嗜酸性细胞、嗜碱性细胞和嫌色性细胞。应用复杂的组织化学标记，这3种细胞仍可细分，如嗜酸性细胞分为橘黄-G阳性胎盘阳性细胞、赤藓红阳性的生长激素生成细胞；而嗜碱性细胞可根据高碘酸-雪夫反应（PAS）阳性结果进行分类。免疫组化标记使其可根据特定激素类型进行分类[63]。主要细胞及其相关产物包括：生长激素细胞（生长激素）、催乳素生成细胞（催乳素）、催乳素生长激素细胞（催乳素、生长激素）、促甲状腺激素细胞（促甲状腺激素）、促肾上腺皮质激素细胞（促肾上腺皮质激素、β-内啡肽、促黑素细胞生成激素）、促性腺激素细胞（促滤泡激素、黄体生成素）。生长激素细胞主要位于侧翼，约占腺垂体细胞总数的50%；催乳素生成细胞主要位于后外侧，约占15%~25%；促肾上腺皮质细胞主要位于中央黏液样楔形区，约占15%～25%；促甲状腺激素细胞位于腺垂体前内侧，约占细胞总数的5%；促性腺激素细胞弥漫分布于腺体前叶，约占细胞总数的5%。

除激素生成细胞外，存在于正常腺体中的第二大类细胞为滤泡状树突细胞[64]。该细胞呈树突状，通常环绕在激素阳性细胞周围。免疫组化染色S-100呈阳性，GFAP呈不同程度阳性。

垂体腺瘤根据其所分泌激素的不同的分类见表9.1（图9.1、9.2）。也可根据转录因子和CK抗体反应性的不同分为不同的类型。90%以上的垂体腺瘤表达CK8，在稀疏颗粒生长激素腺瘤，其阳性结果呈球形表达，与纤维小体的存在有关。核周阳性表达是密集型颗粒性生长激素腺瘤和催乳素生长激素腺瘤的特点。近50%的腺瘤阳性表达CK AE1/AE3混合抗体，而CK19和CK7的阳性表达率为7%～10%（图9.3）[54]。

垂体腺瘤神经内分泌标记呈典型阳性，包括CgA（100%）、Syn（92%）、NSE（80%）[32, 65, 66]。这些肿瘤的激素成分可被垂体前叶特异性单克隆抗体和激素前体成分所标记（表9.1）。

与正常垂体前叶不同，在垂体腺瘤中S-100呈阳性的滤泡状树突细胞往往少见[67]。

垂体腺癌罕见，其诊断必须依据转移来确定。这

表9.1 垂体腺瘤的分类及免疫组化

类型	发病率（%）	免疫组化
稀疏颗粒催乳素腺瘤	27	PRL（核周），α-su（很少），pit-1，ER局灶性阳性
致密颗粒催乳素腺瘤	0.4	PRL（弥漫），pit-1
稀疏颗粒生长激素腺瘤	7.6	GH（弱），α-su（弱），pit-1
致密颗粒生长激素腺瘤	7.1	GH（强），α-su（≈50%），pit-1
混合性生长激素催乳素腺瘤	3.5	GH、PRL在不同细胞中表达
催乳素生长激素腺瘤	1.2	GH、PRL共同表达于同一细胞，pit-1，ER局灶性阳性
促肾上腺皮质激素腺瘤	9.6	ACTH，β-end，β-LPH，神经链D1，pit-1
促甲状腺激素腺瘤	1.1	β-TSH，α-su（各不相同）
促性腺激素腺瘤	9.8	β-FSH，β-LH，α-su，SF-1
无功能性促肾上腺皮质激素腺瘤（Ⅰ型）	2.0	ACTH，β-end（β-end＞ACTH）
无功能性促肾上腺皮质激素腺瘤（Ⅱ型）	1.5	ACTH（局灶性），β-end（β-end＞ACTH）
无功能性腺瘤（Ⅲ型）	1.4	GH，PRL，α-su
裸细胞腺瘤	12.4	激素往往呈阴性，在有些病例阳性表达β-FSH、α-su，SF-1
嗜酸细胞腺瘤	13.4	同裸细胞腺瘤
未分类的	8.8	

ACTH，促肾上腺皮质激素；α-su，α-亚单位；β-end，β-内啡肽；β-FSH，β-卵泡刺激素；β-LH，β-黄体生成素；β-LPH，β-亲脂激素；β-TSH，β-促甲状腺素；ER，雌激素受体；GH，生长激素；pit-1，垂体-1转录因子

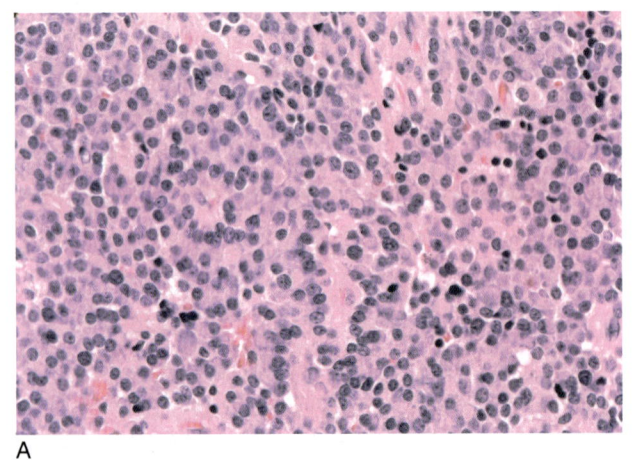

A

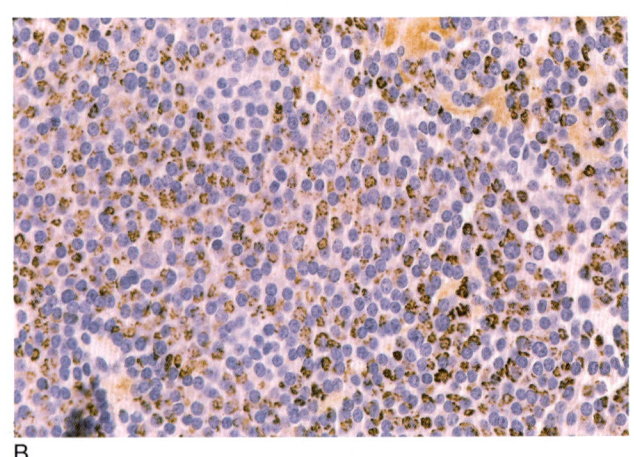

B

图9.1 垂体腺瘤。（A）HE染色；（B）PRL免疫过氧化物酶染色。位于细胞浆内，颗粒状，弱阳性（稀疏颗粒催乳素腺瘤）

内分泌肿瘤的免疫组织化学 9

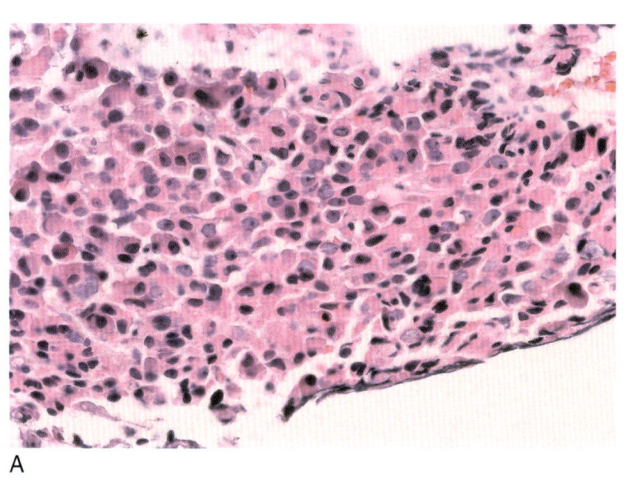
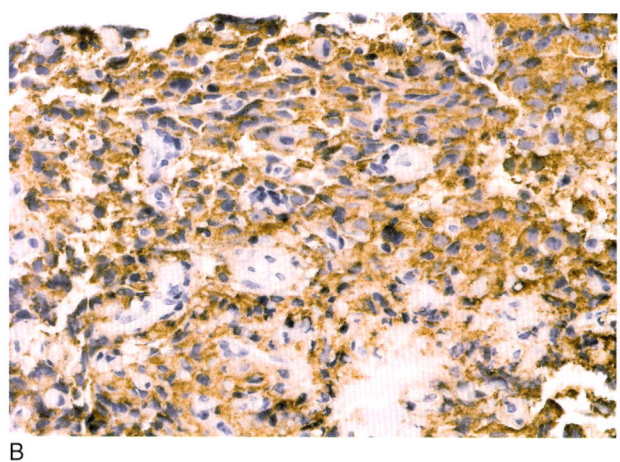

图9.2 垂体腺瘤。(A) HE染色；(B) GH免疫过氧化物酶染色。所有细胞均呈阳性表达

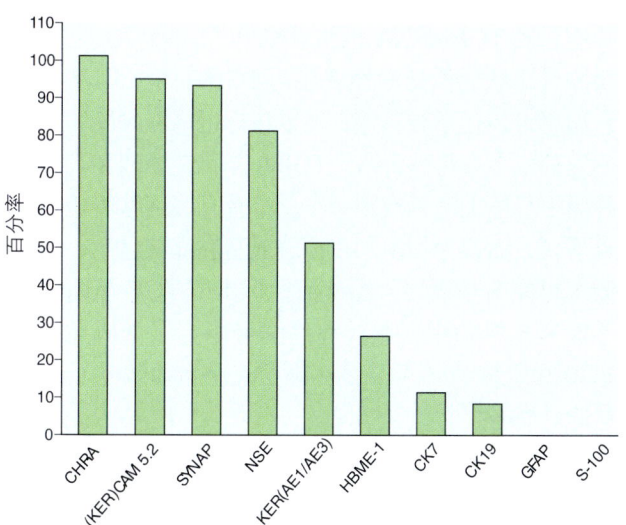

图9.3 垂体腺瘤标记物分布图。[CHR-A，嗜铬素A；(KER) CAM5.2，用单抗CAM5.2检测的CK；SYNAP，突触素；NSE，神经特异性烯醇化酶；KER (AE1/AE3)，用单抗AE1/AE3检测的CK；HBME-1；CK7；CK19；GFAP，胶质纤维酸性蛋白；S-100]

些肿瘤一般的神经内分泌标记呈典型阳性，并可表达一种或几种垂体前叶激素。其中最常见的合成激素为催乳素和ACTH，而生长激素、TSH、FSH/LH产物则罕见[68]。在没有转移的情况下区分腺瘤和腺癌十分困难。

MIB-1阳性指数在腺瘤、侵袭性腺瘤、腺癌中明显不同，但3个指数之间存在重叠。在一些腺癌中的表达范围与腺瘤中相同[69]。Thappar及其合作者报道，p53表达率分别为0%、15%、100%（腺瘤、侵袭性腺瘤、腺癌），但要除外泛染病例[70]。

松果体

松果体原发性肿瘤大多起源于松果体细胞，它是像视网膜光觉受体细胞一样的一种修饰的神经元[71]。松果体肿瘤包括生殖细胞源性及胶质源性的。松果体瘤呈典型的NSE、Syn、神经丝蛋白、T形蛋白和微管结合蛋白-2（MAP2）阳性（图9.4）[71-73]。GFAP和S-100分别阳性表达于75%和83%的病例。S-抗原定位于光觉受体细胞的一种蛋白，表达于28%的松果体瘤和50%的松果体母细胞瘤[74,75]。与生殖细胞肿瘤不同，松果体瘤PLAP、hCG和α-FP均呈阴性[71]。

甲状腺

甲状腺上皮细胞包括滤泡细胞和C细胞。滤泡细胞内含甲状腺球蛋白（TGB）、T_3、T_4，可表达于冰冻切片、福尔马林固定的石蜡切片。C细胞的主要产物是降钙素。

滤泡细胞及其肿瘤

TGB、T_3、T_4和TTF-1

TGB是660kD的糖蛋白。沉降系数为19S。免疫组化也可定位检测高、低沉淀系数的碘蛋白[76]。正常甲状腺组织中TGB表达可有不同。正常腺体立方细胞和柱状细胞TGB免疫活性较腺体内充满胶体而受压的扁平（萎缩的）的滤泡细胞要强。胶体着色的变化也很明显。增生性细胞TGB着色强，萎缩的滤泡细胞着色较弱或呈阴性。Grave病和增生型桥本甲状腺炎TGB着色由温和至强烈。

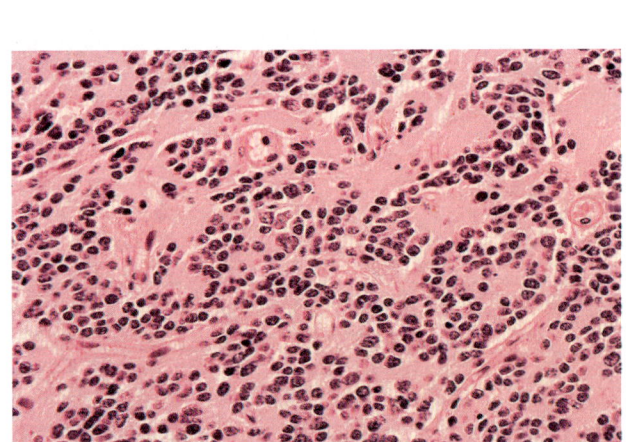
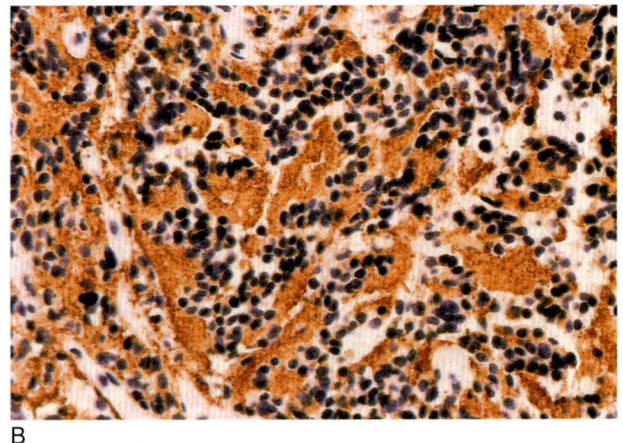

图9.4 松果体瘤。(A) HE 染色;(B) Syn 免疫过氧化物酶染色,所有细胞均呈强阳性表达

滤泡性腺瘤TGB呈阳性表达,其强弱随细胞成分功能状态的不同而各异[76]。动能亢进的腺瘤TGB呈强阳性,巨滤泡腺瘤则相应减弱以至呈阴性。正常滤泡性腺瘤TGB中等表达,而结构更为致密的腺瘤其TGB表达减弱。

玻璃样小梁状肿瘤TGB呈典型阳性,也可表达一些神经内分泌标记物,包括CgA和激素肽(神经降压素、内啡肽类)[77]。研究表明,玻璃样小梁状肿瘤对单克隆抗体 MIB-1 呈细胞膜和细胞浆表达。

甲状腺癌 TGB 阳性率与分化程度和组织学亚型有关。总而言之,低分化癌 TGB 表达弱于分化好的肿瘤,其TGBmRNA 也相对减少[79]。95%以上的甲状腺乳头状癌及滤泡性癌表达 TGB(图 9.5、9.6)。TGB也可表达于转移癌,所以该标记物在判断转移癌原发部位上有特殊价值。TGB在分化性滤泡和乳头状肿瘤中总体上呈不规则分布。尽管有些细胞着色弥漫且均匀,而其他细胞却呈顶端或基底部着色。一些肿瘤也可完全呈阴性。因此活检标本中 TGB 呈阴性并不能完全排除甲状腺转移癌的可能。罕见情况下,TGB 单克隆抗体可与多克隆位点结合而表达于非甲状腺转移癌[80]。

岛状型低分化甲状腺癌 TGB 既表达于胶质又可见于肿瘤细胞,细胞内着色常呈局灶性弱阳性[81]。未分化(间变型)甲状腺癌 TGB 阴性表达。在Ordonez及其合作者的系列研究中,应用单克隆抗体、多克隆抗血清标记,32例间变型癌中的5例(15.6%)少数

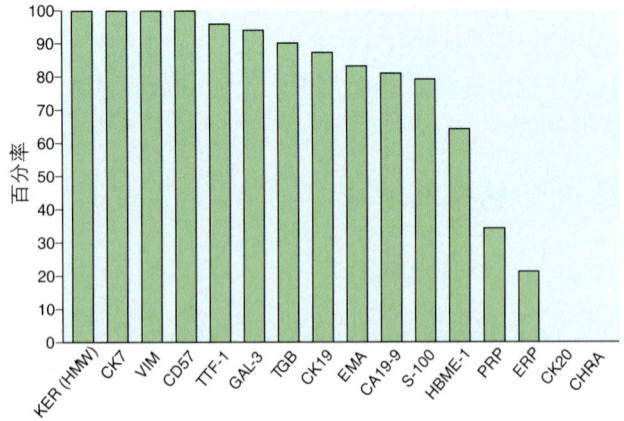

图9.5 甲状腺乳头状癌标记物分布图。[KER(HMW),高分子量CK;CK7;VIM,波形蛋白;TTF-1,甲状腺转录因子-1;GAL-3,galectin-3;TGB,甲状腺球蛋白;CK19;EMA,上皮细胞膜抗原;CA19-9;S-100;HBME-1;PRP,孕激素受体蛋白;ERP,雌激素受体蛋白;CK20;CHR-A,嗜铬素A]

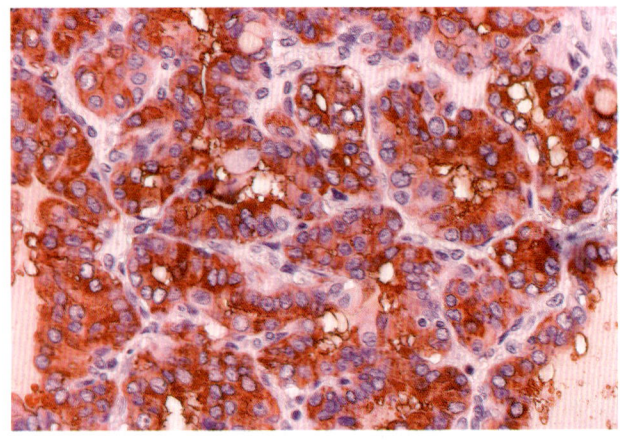

图9.6 甲状腺乳头状癌。高分化肿瘤细胞内TGB呈一致阳性(TGB 免疫过氧化物酶染色)

细胞表达TGB[82]。该研究中，8例巨细胞型中3例呈阳性，4例梭形细胞型中1例呈阳性，6例鳞状细胞型全为阴性，13例混合变异型也全为阴性。这些病例的连续切片研究并未发现有陷入的正常滤泡细胞或分化好的甲状腺癌灶。而其他作者在间变型甲状腺癌未找到任何TGB的表达。即使在残留的分化性甲状腺癌中也未发现[83]。

T_3、T_4抗体在甲状腺癌研究中应用较TGB为少。Kawaoi及其合作者报道95%的甲状腺乳头状癌、54%的甲状腺滤泡性癌T_4呈阳性，但间变性甲状腺癌呈阴性[84]。66%的甲状腺乳头状癌、81%的甲状腺滤泡性癌、45%的间变性甲状腺癌 T_3 呈阳性[84]。T_4阴性时，T_3阳性表达的统计学意义尚不明了。

TTF-1是一包含同源结构域的转录因子，存在于甲状腺、间脑和肺。甲状腺内TTF-1调节甲状腺氧化酶、TGB基因的表达。肺内TTF-1在表面活性剂A、B、C及Clara细胞分泌蛋白的特异性表达中发挥重要作用[85,86]。96%的甲状腺乳头状癌、100%的甲状腺滤泡性癌、20%的Hürthle细胞、100%的岛状癌、90%的髓样癌均可表达TTF-1，而未分化（间变性）癌则呈阴性（图9.7）[86]。在肺内，72.5%的腺癌、10%的鳞状细胞癌、26%大细胞癌、75%大细胞神经内分泌癌、>90%的小细胞癌、100%肺泡细胞癌均可表达TTF-1，相反286例非肺非甲状腺性腺癌中只有2例表达TTF-1。

Kaufmann和Dietel在对甲状腺癌、肺癌的研究中报道，7例甲状腺癌中有3例灶性表达肺表面活性蛋白A[87]。Byrd-Gloster等报道TTF-1在区分肺小细胞癌及Merkel细胞癌中发挥作用[88]。其研究表明：97%支气管源性小细胞癌TTF-1呈阳性表达；21例Merkel细胞癌均呈阴性。然而，也有人报道TTF-1可表达于肺外小细胞癌，如前列腺、膀胱、子宫颈等（表9.4）[89]。

中间丝

有大量关于中间丝在正常及肿瘤性滤泡细胞中分布的报道（表9.2）[90-101]。广谱角蛋白抗体可在正常和增生的滤泡细胞、慢性甲状腺炎的滤泡细胞和几乎所有甲状腺上皮源性恶性肿瘤表达。而在同一研究中高分子量角蛋白可表达于8%的正常滤泡细胞、44%的增生性腺体和几乎所有的甲状腺炎，并表达于100%的甲状腺乳头状癌、6%的甲状腺滤泡性癌、20%间变性癌[91]。Schelfhout及其合作者研究表明，CK19在甲状腺乳头状癌中100%表达，与广谱角蛋白抗体一

表9.2 甲状腺乳头状癌和滤泡性癌CK分布情况**

CK 类型	乳头状癌（%）	滤泡性癌（%）
8	100	100
18	100	100
7	100	100
19	98*	84*
1, 5, 10, 11/14	97	22
5, 6	68	8
17	40	15
13	30	0
20	26	12
14	11	10
4	24	0

* 尽管CK19既可表达于甲状腺乳头状癌又可表达于滤泡性癌，但通常在乳头状癌中的着色程度较强
** 数据源于Schelfhout[93]、Raphael[94]、Fonseca[95]、Baloch[97]、Kragsterman[98]和Lieberman[101]等的研究报道

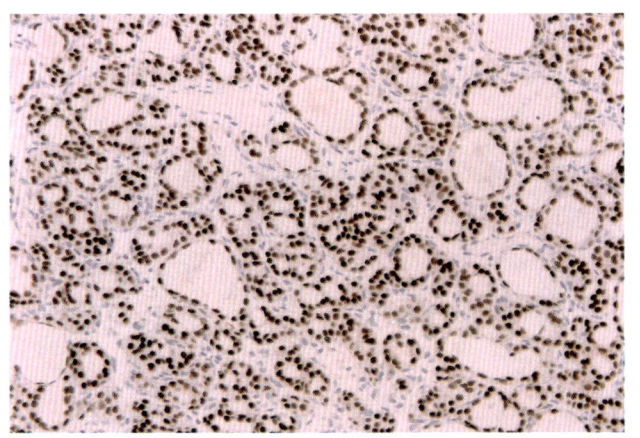

图9.7 高分化甲状腺滤泡性癌。TTF-1 免疫过氧化物酶染色，呈典型的细胞核阳性

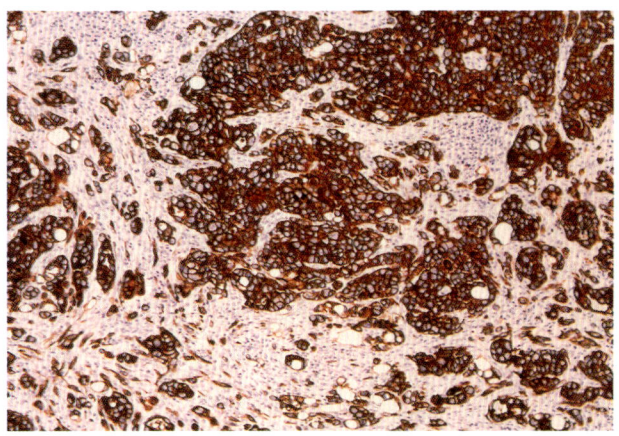

图9.8 甲状腺乳头状癌。CK19免疫过氧化物酶染色，呈细胞浆强阳性

致[93]（图9.8）。CK19灶性阳性（<5%的肿瘤细胞中）可见于80%的甲状腺滤泡性癌和90%滤泡腺瘤，而在90%的胶体结节中的50%以下的细胞呈弥漫阳性。Raphael及其合作者证实了这一结论[94]。

更多最新研究表明，正常甲状腺强表达单层上皮角蛋白CK7、CK18，其次是CK8、CK19，但不表达复层上皮角蛋白[95]。同样结果可见于淋巴细胞性甲状腺炎，但其CK19的表达更强。CK7、CK8、CK18、CK19的免疫反应既可见于甲状腺乳头状癌也可见于甲状腺滤泡性癌。其中CK19在乳头状癌中的表达广泛而强烈，在所有滤泡性癌中或多或少都有表达，有的呈局灶性。复层上皮角蛋白（CK5/CK6、CK13）在乳头状癌中分别为41例中的27例（66%）、41例中的14例表达（34%），但这些蛋白在其他类型肿瘤中均不表达。Miettinen及其合作者观察到，CK19表达于所有甲状腺乳头状癌及近50%滤泡性癌，而CK5/CK6在甲状腺乳头状癌中仅呈局灶性表达[96]。Kragsterman及其合作者得出结论，CK19在常规组织病理学诊断中的应用价值比较局限，但其表达增加了乳头状癌的可疑度[98]。

Baloch等对经典型及滤泡亚型乳头状癌各种CK的表达作了系列研究，包括CK5/CK6/CK18、CK18、CK10/CK13、CK20、CK17和CK19[97]。研究表明，包括滤泡亚型在内的所有乳头状癌均表达CK19（图9.9）。滤泡亚型具有乳头状癌特征区域的核呈强阳性，而其他区域呈中到强阳性。滤泡亚型乳头状癌周围紧邻的正常甲状腺实质也呈阳性，而常见亚型癌旁正常甲状腺组织呈阴性。滤泡性腺瘤、滤泡癌和增生结节CK19呈阴性表达。CK19在滤泡性肿瘤和其他肿瘤中的不同表达的原因尚未阐明。

根据CK19的表达，甲状腺玻璃样小梁状肿瘤的归属问题尚有争议。Fonseca等报道CK19表达于所有玻璃样小梁状肿瘤，认为可能是乳头状癌的特殊包裹性变型。而Hirokawa等却没有或极少发现阳性表达的CK19病例[100]。

Liberman和Weidner用单克隆抗体34βE12（CK1、CK5、CK10、CK14）及外皮蛋白（一种角质层机构蛋白）抗体研究高分子量CK在甲状腺乳头状癌和滤泡性癌中的表达[101]。高分子量CK抗体表达于91%的包括滤泡亚型在内的甲状腺乳头状癌、20%的滤泡性肿瘤（滤泡性腺瘤、腺癌）。总的来说，乳头状癌中着色强而不规则；滤泡性肿瘤中则较弱。外皮蛋白表达于72.5%的乳头状癌和29%的滤泡性肿瘤。CK34βE12的这种表达方式最好解释为CK1上的抗原决定簇的存在，或是存在一种不能被CK5、CK10、CK14抗体所识别的抗原决定簇[101]。

用AE1/AE3、35βH11、CAM5.2抗体标记的CK，可表达于70%~75%的间变性癌中，其中近30%可与CK34βE12反应（图9.10）[82,83]。低分化癌广谱CK阳性率可达100%[66]。

波形蛋白在大量正常及肿瘤性甲状腺组织中与CK同时表达[91]。Miettinen等的研究表明，滤泡、乳头状肿瘤中，50%以上的细胞可表达波形蛋白。与CK弥漫表达在细胞浆不同，波形蛋白多表达在细胞基底部。94%的间变性甲状腺癌可表达波形蛋白。

HBME-1和galectin-3

单克隆抗体HBME-1广泛应用于间皮瘤的诊断。也用于评价其在穿刺活检（包括直接涂片或细胞涂片）和组织切片中辨别良、恶性甲状腺病变的功效[102]。

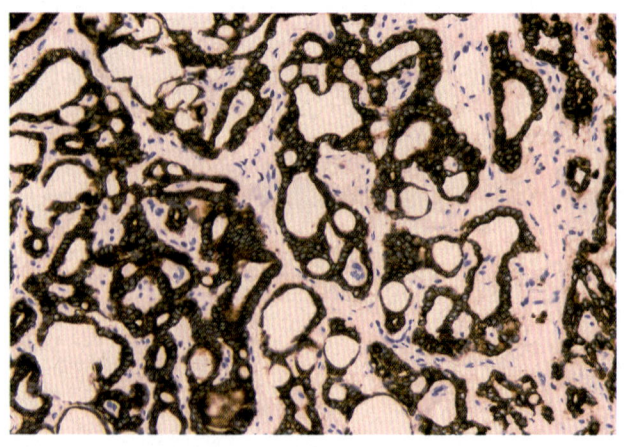

图9.9　甲状腺乳头状癌，滤泡亚型。CK19免疫过氧化物酶染色，呈细胞浆强阳性

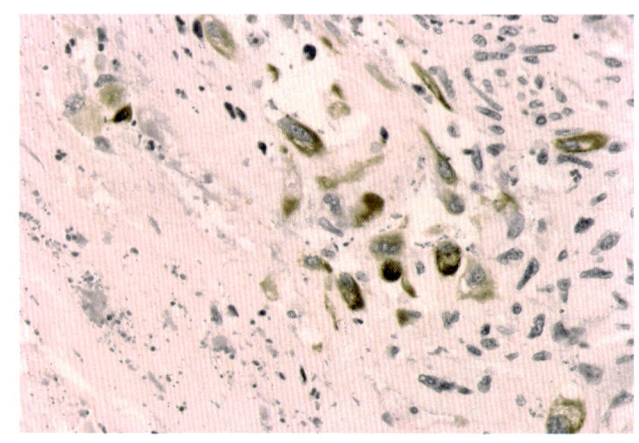

图9.10　间变性（未分化）甲状腺癌。广谱CK（AE1/AE3）免疫过氧化物酶染色，呈细胞浆强阳性

Miettinen 和 Kerkkainen 证明，乳头状癌（145/145）和滤泡性癌（27/27）阳性率为100%，而良性肿瘤呈阴性或有30%表现为局灶性阳性[103]。Mase 等的更多最新研究证明阳性率分别为腺瘤性甲状腺肿13%，腺瘤27%，滤泡癌84%和乳头状癌97%（图9.11）[104]。在滤泡性肿瘤中，阳性表达的敏感率为84.6%，而特异性、阳性预测值、总准确性分别为72.6%、66%和77.2%。HBME-1也可用于细胞学标本[102]。Sack等作出结论：细针穿刺上的HBME-1呈阳性即可判定为癌，但阴性结果并不能排除癌的可能。该标记物是区别乳头状增生和乳头状癌的有效指标，但根据阳性结果并能诊断为恶性肿瘤[105]。髓样癌和未分化癌HBME-1均呈阴性。

galectin-3是大量表达在正常和肿瘤组织的β-半乳糖苷结合样凝集素[106]。1995年，Xu等对少量甲状腺肿瘤中的galectin-1、3的表达作了系列研究，结果表明它们可表达于乳头状癌、滤泡性癌，而不表达于腺瘤、结节性甲状腺肿或正常甲状腺组织。由此他们得出结论，galectin在区分良、恶性肿瘤中发挥作用。随之，依次报道了一系列与之大致相同的galectin-3的研究结论（图9.12）[107-109]。Bartolazzi等对1000多例良、恶性甲状腺肿瘤中galectin-3和CD44v6的表达作了回顾性和前瞻性研究[110]。其前瞻性区别良、恶性肿瘤的敏感性、特异性、阳性预测值、诊断准确性分别为88%、98%、91%和97%。

当galectin-3在同一实验组中表达时，其敏感性、特异性分别为99%、98%，阳性预测值、诊断准确性分别为92%、99%。这些结果表明galectin-3是诊断低级别甲状腺癌的有效指标。但需要注意的是，最新

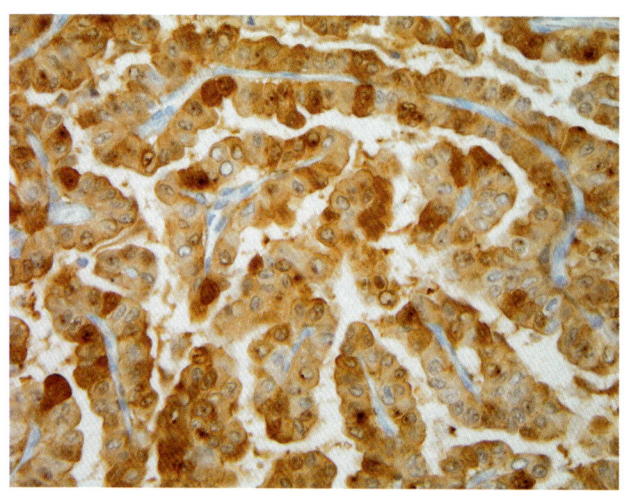

图9.12　甲状腺乳头状癌。galectin-3免疫过氧化物酶染色，呈阳性

研究比较了它在一系列乳头状癌、乳头状增生中的表达，两者之间有一定的重叠[105]。

galectin-3和HBME-1均被用做区分瘤细胞或者癌细胞。galectin-3标记癌细胞尤其是乳头状变型时，其敏感性可达95%，而HBME-1只有53%。两者合用，其敏感性可达99%，而两者的特异性均为88%[111]。

癌胚抗原及其相关标记物

非髓样甲状腺癌不表达癌胚抗原（CEA）。Dasovic-Knezevic及其同事应用6种不同的单克隆CEA抗体研究发现，10例乳头状癌、10例滤泡性癌、8例间变性癌CEA均为阴性[112]。Ordonez等用一种单克隆抗体发现其表达于9%的间变性癌[82]。

近30%的乳头状癌表达CD15。Schroder及其同事研究表明，CD15更易表达于晚期肿瘤[113]。因此，CD15可作为判断这些肿瘤预后的标记。Ghali及其合作者报道，100%的乳头状癌、滤泡癌CD57呈强阳性；25%的胶样型甲状腺肿、21%的滤泡型腺瘤呈局灶性阳性[46]。而其他作者对CD57作为甲状腺恶性肿瘤标记物的特异性表示质疑[114, 115]。

CA15-3、CA19-9在甲状腺滤泡性肿瘤中的表达各不相同。CA15-3阳性表达于100%的甲状腺滤泡性癌；CA19-9阳性表达于70%乳头状癌，但在滤泡性癌肿并无表达[116]。据报道近40%的乳头状癌可表达CA125[80]。黏蛋白相关抗原在甲状腺肿瘤中的分布也有所研究[117]。结果表明，MUC1在高分化甲状腺癌蛋白质糖基化过程中发挥重要作用，而黏蛋白在甲状腺乳头状癌、滤泡性癌中的表达并无稳定差异。

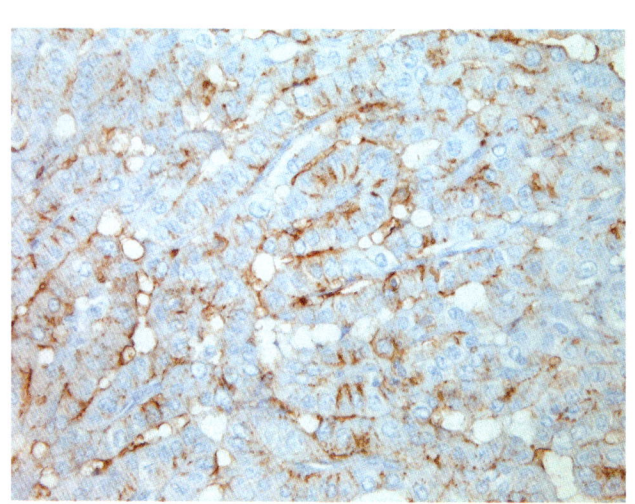

图9.11　甲状腺乳头状癌。HBME-1免疫过氧化物酶染色，肿瘤细胞细胞浆和细胞膜呈阳性

癌基因及肿瘤抑制基因

有人研究了p53在甲状腺癌中的分布。在Soares及其合作者的系列报道中，14例甲状腺肿及腺瘤、12例乳头状癌均未表达p53；20%滤泡性癌（尤其是弥漫浸润型）、16%低分化癌、67%未分化癌均表达p53[118]。Holm和Nesland报道，32例乳头状癌中的6例(19%)、29例滤泡性癌中的5例(17%)、24例未分化癌中的18例(75%)均表达p53。相反，RB(视网膜母细胞瘤)基因产物则可见于所有甲状腺癌[119]。

ret癌基因蛋白可表达于甲状腺乳头状癌及一部分玻璃状小梁状肿瘤[120-122]。但ret抗体作为判定甲状腺乳头状癌特异性指标的敏感性和特异性还需进一步研究。

t (2; 3)、(q13; p25)染色体易位见于部分甲状腺滤泡性癌，可导致甲状腺转录因子PAX8的DNA结合区域融合，形成过氧化物酶体增殖剂激活受体(PPAR)γ1的A-F区域。PCR、免疫组化研究表明，PPARγ阳性的滤泡性癌多广泛浸润，缺乏PPARγ重组的肿瘤PPARγ呈阴性[125]。乳头状癌和桥本甲状腺炎呈阴性，但也有报道滤泡性癌和腺瘤均呈阳性者[126, 127]。Volante等报道，PPARγ表达于10%的嗜酸细胞癌，而嗜酸细胞腺瘤呈阴性[111]。

其他标记物

类固醇激素受体在甲状腺癌中不同程度表达。Bur等报道雌激素受体在39例乳头状癌中有8例(21%)表达，5例滤泡性肿瘤中(3例腺瘤、2例癌)无一例表达。15例桥本甲状腺炎呈阴性[128]。孕激素受体在39例乳头状癌中有13例(33%)表达，5例滤泡性肿瘤中有2例(1/3为腺瘤、1/2为癌)(40%)表达。15例Hurthle细胞肿瘤中有8例(53%)表达。肿瘤ER、PR状态与性别、年龄或侵袭性行为等无显著相关性。

S-100蛋白在甲状腺肿瘤中的表达：McLaren和Cossar报道，100%甲状腺乳头状癌，75%的滤泡性癌、37.5%的滤泡性腺瘤、28.5%的乳头状增生S-100呈阳性[129]。

抗线粒体抗原抗体在辨认具有Hürthle嗜酸细胞的甲状腺肿瘤中发挥作用[130]。其典型阳性部位在细胞浆内线粒体区域(图9.13)。

p63是p53的同源基因，可在多种细胞中表达。如鳞状上皮的基底细胞、乳腺和涎腺的肌上皮细胞、前列腺基底细胞等。在甲状腺内，选择性表达于实性细胞(后鳃体残留物)巢。在甲状腺肿瘤中表达于可能来源于后鳃体残留物的硬化型嗜酸性粒细胞增多性黏液表皮样癌[132]。乳头状癌和间变性癌p63阳性罕见。

> **诊断要点：甲状腺癌**
>
> 1. TGB和TTF-1表达于95%以上的分化型甲状腺癌。
> 2. CK19常表达于乳头状癌，但也可见于其他甲状腺恶性肿瘤。
> 3. 大多数甲状腺肿瘤同时表达波形蛋白和CK。
> 4. HBME-1和glactin-3是诊断分化型甲状腺癌有效但并不完全特异的标记物。
> 5. 未分化(间变性)甲状腺癌TGB、TTF-1典型阴性，但常表达CK。

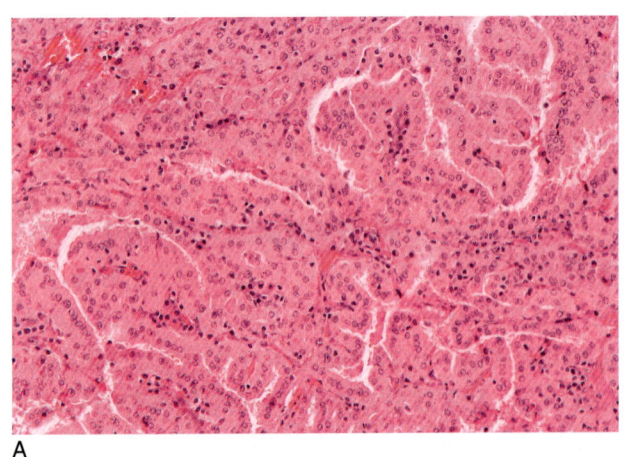
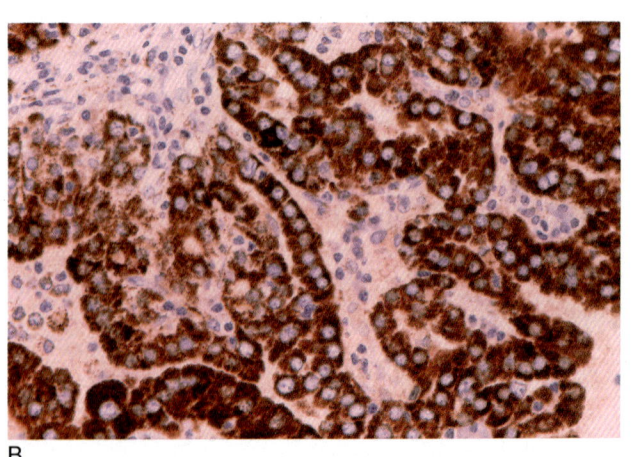

图9.13 甲状腺乳头状癌，嗜酸细胞型。(A)HE染色；(B)免疫过氧化物酶染色，线粒体抗体MITO-113表达于细胞浆内，呈颗粒状，强阳性

内分泌肿瘤的免疫组织化学 9

C 细胞及甲状腺髓样癌

C 细胞是甲状腺中的第二大类主要内分泌细胞，是降钙素合成和最初储存的部位。这些细胞还可合成一些其他调节产物，包括生长抑素、胃泌素释放肽和胺类[133, 134]。可通过降钙素和一般性神经内分泌细胞标记物包括 NSE、嗜铬素 A、Syn 对 C 细胞和滤泡细胞进行区分。

C 细胞在正常腺体中位于滤泡内，集中位于上叶和中叶交界处[133]。在多发性内分泌肿瘤综合征 2 型（multiple endocrine neoplasia, type 2）(MEN2) C 细胞增生被认为是甲状腺髓样癌的前期病变。详细的免疫组化研究表明，C 细胞增生表现为腺体同一区域滤泡内 C 细胞数量增多并成为主要细胞（图 9.14）。这种关联多存在于 C 细胞增生更加明显的区域，C 细胞往往呈环形取代中央的滤泡上皮。结节状增生是指滤泡腔完全闭塞，代以增生的 C 细胞。最早期的甲状腺髓样癌的标志为 C 细胞侵犯滤泡基底膜。这种情况除见于 MEN2 病例外，也见于高钙血症和高胃泌素血症及滤泡或乳头状肿瘤周围组织。与 MEN2 中的 C 细胞增生（原发性或肿瘤性增生）不同，该型 C 细胞增生被称为继发性增生[135]。

95% 以上的甲状腺髓样癌降钙素呈阳性（图 9.15、9.16）[134, 136, 137]。少数降钙素肽阴性的病例，原位杂交技术可检测出其 mRNA[138]。罕见发生类似于燕麦细胞癌的小细胞癌，其降钙素及相应的 mRNA 也呈阴

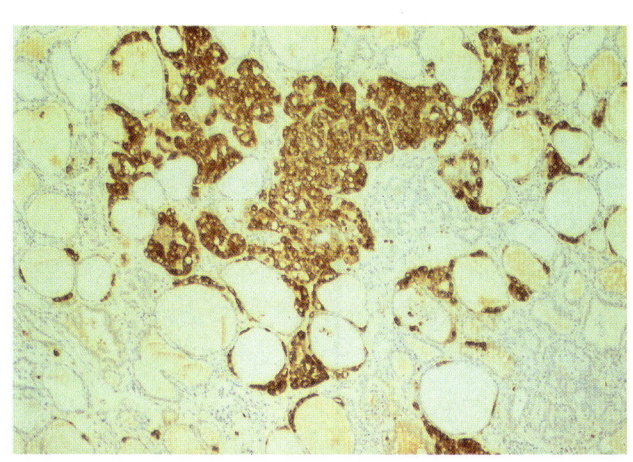

图 9.14 一例 2A 型多发性内分泌肿瘤中的 C 细胞增生。免疫过氧化物酶染色，增生的 C 细胞降钙素呈强阳性，而滤泡细胞呈阴性。该图中央显示了早期局灶性甲状腺髓样癌

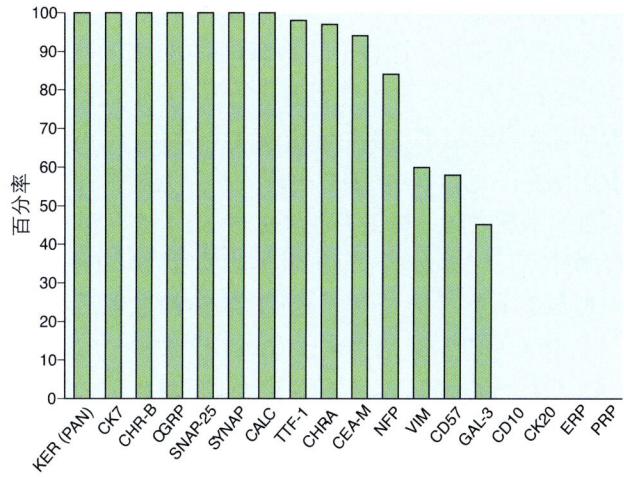

图 9.15 甲状腺髓样癌中标记物的表达。[KER (PAN)，广谱 CK；CK7；CHR-B，嗜铬素 B；CGRP，降钙素基因相关蛋白；SNAP-25，突触素相关蛋白-25；CALC，降钙素；TTF-1，甲状腺转录因子-1；CHR-A，嗜铬素 A；CEA-M，单克隆 CEA；NFP，神经细丝蛋白；VIM，波形蛋白；CD57；GAL-3, galectin-3；CD10；CK20；ERP，雌激素受体蛋白；PRP，孕激素受体蛋白]

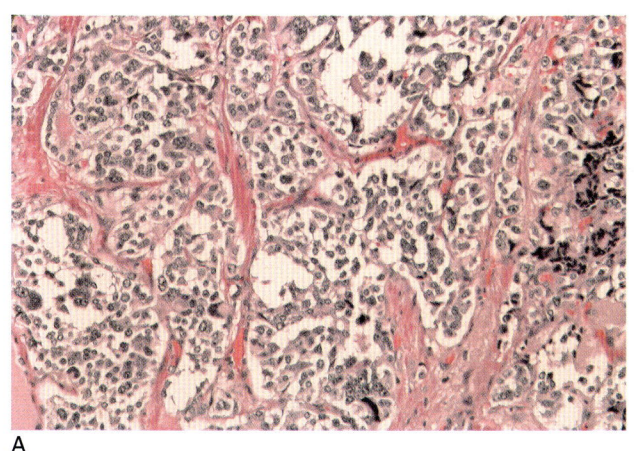

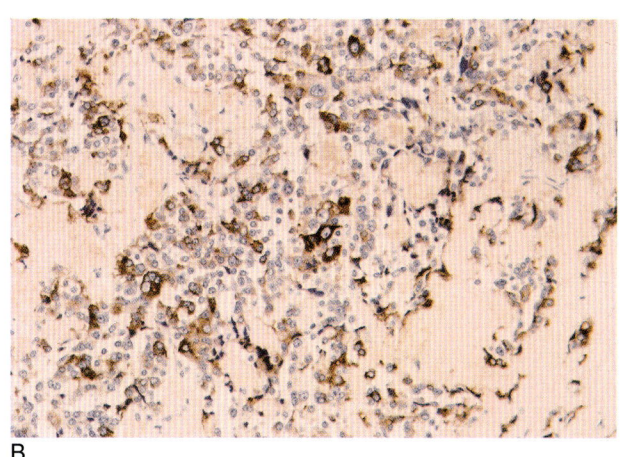

图 9.16 甲状腺髓样癌。(A) HE 染色；(B) 免疫过氧化物酶染色，降钙素在单个肿瘤细胞细胞浆内呈不同程度表达

性[139]。一些研究表明，降钙素表达情况对判断肿瘤预后有重要作用，其水平越低，肿瘤侵袭性越强。Franc等的单变量分析表明，降钙素表达率低于50%比高于50%的患者生存率低[140]。除了降钙素，正常和肿瘤性C细胞还含有降钙素基因相关肽（CGRP）[141]。CGRP由原始降钙素基因转录子交替选择性剪接而成。正常甲状腺主要表达降钙素，而CGRP最早发现在中枢和周围神经系统。在甲状腺髓样癌中，降钙素和CGRP合成表达一致[142]。

免疫组化方法也检测到许多其他肽类，并被相应肿瘤萃取物的放射免疫测定法（RIA）证实。生长抑素和胃泌素释放肽在甲状腺髓样癌中也比较常见[143,144]。Scopsi等用抗血清对4种不同部位的前生长抑素抗血清免疫组化染色，阳性率高达100%（33/33）[143]。但并非全部的生长抑素阳性细胞其降钙素都呈阳性。生长抑素阳性细胞多呈单个分布或几个一组，仅占所有肿瘤细胞不足5%。该细胞呈树突状，突起延伸至相邻肿瘤细胞之间。胃泌素释放肽表达于近30%的甲状腺髓样癌[144]。该肿瘤表达的其他肽类包括ACTH、前阿黑皮素肽类、神经降压素、P物质和血管活性肽[136]。46%（17/37）病例表达α-hCG[145]。

儿茶酚胺和5-羟色胺均表达于甲状腺髓样癌。Uribe及其合作者报道了5-羟色胺可见于70%（20例中的14例）的病例[137]，多表达于树突状细胞，与生长抑素阳性细胞一致。

甲状腺髓样癌TTF-1呈典型阳性[86]。甲状腺球蛋白（TGB）可表达于包绕陷入的滤泡内、单个滤泡细胞或细胞外沉积（图9.17）。该现象多发生于肿瘤交界处、邻近的甲状腺实质或是沿脉管间隙。一项研究中近60%的原发性甲状腺肿瘤表达TGB，但转移性甲状腺髓样癌并不表达TGB[146]。具有C细胞和滤泡特征的混合性肿瘤也有报道（图9.18）[147,148]。这些肿瘤的存在可以解释为何少数甲状腺髓样癌病例可吸收放射性碘。

混合具有甲状腺髓样癌和滤泡特征的肿瘤的可能来源尚有争议。Volante及其合作者提出了两种起源假说[149]。根据其假说，C细胞的肿瘤性转化，随肿瘤生长为甲状腺髓样癌包绕陷入的正常滤泡，并刺激受累滤泡导致其增生，最终形成滤泡（或乳头状）肿瘤（俘获假说）。肿瘤性C细胞和滤泡细胞均有转移能力，因此可以解释远处转移灶中及滤泡成分的肿瘤性C细胞的存在。

甲状腺髓样癌中的多种常用神经内分泌癌标记物均呈阳性，包括NSE、嗜铬素A、Syn和组胺[133,136]（图9.15）。因为NSE也表达于一些非C细胞肿瘤，所以不可能作为诊断甲状腺髓样癌的独立指标。除嗜铬素A外，甲状腺髓样癌还可稳定表达嗜铬素B和分泌素Ⅱ[150]。钙结合蛋白calbindin-D_{28K}也是一种广泛的神经内分泌癌标记物，可表达于95%（19例中的18例）的甲状腺髓样癌。

NCAM多聚唾液酸在甲状腺髓样癌中也可稳定表达。Komminoth及其合作者发现NCAM在33例甲状腺髓样癌中100%呈阳性，而在其他肿瘤中则呈阴性[105]。多聚唾液酸在所有原发性C细胞增生的病例中均呈强阳性，而在多数正常C细胞和继发性C细胞增生的病例中则呈阴性。

bcl-2表达于79%（33例中的26例）甲状腺髓样癌[152]。在Viale等的研究报道中，bcl-2表达缺失的患者生存期较短（$P=0.0001$）[152]。在大量变量分析中，bcl-2表达缺失可作为独立的预后较差的指标。Viale等还报道p53在33例甲状腺髓样癌中12%（4例）表达p53[152]。Holm和Nesland报道其表达率为13%（46例中的6例）[119]。

用单克隆抗体、多克隆抗血清检测CEA，多数甲状腺髓样癌均呈阳性[153]。CEA特异性单克隆抗体可与近50%的甲状腺髓样癌病例反应，但不与其他各型反应[154]。可与抗原决定簇及非特异性交叉反应点反应的CEA抗体可表达于几乎90%的甲状腺髓样癌病例，但也可与其他各型反应。也有研究表明，一些失去合成和分泌降钙素能力，但仍具有产生CEA能力的甲状腺髓样癌具有侵袭性[155]。Franc等认为CEA阳性率大于50%、降钙素阳性率小于50%的甲状腺髓样癌病例预后较差[140]。

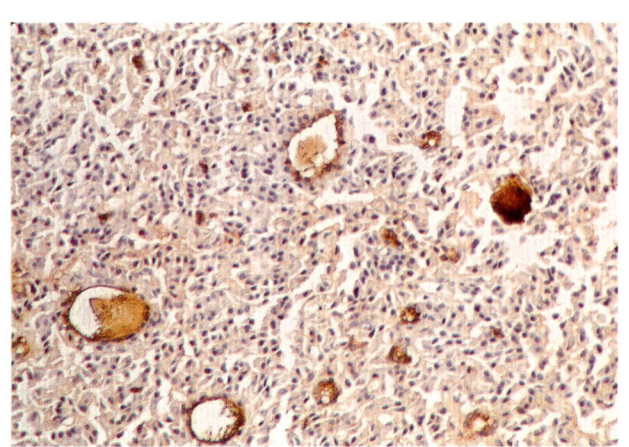

图9.17 甲状腺髓样癌。免疫过氧化物酶染色，甲状腺球蛋白在受累滤泡中呈强阳性表达

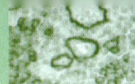

内分泌肿瘤的免疫组织化学 9

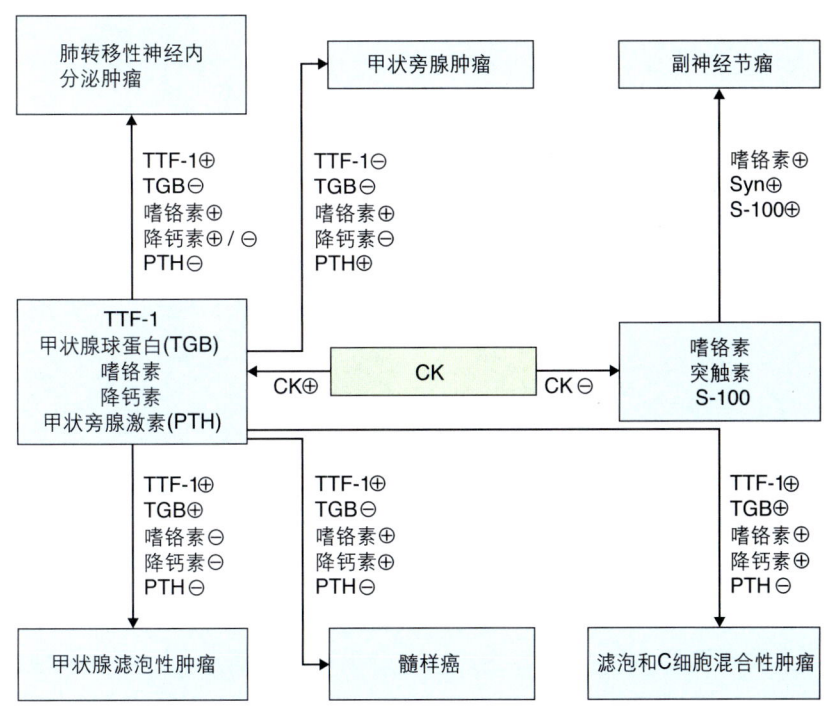

图9.18 头颈部内分泌肿瘤免疫组化特征

低分子量CK呈典型阳性的甲状腺髓样癌，近60%表达波形蛋白，而神经细丝蛋白表达为85%（12例中有10例）[156]。正常C细胞不表达神经细丝蛋白，特征性表达低分子量CK，而波形蛋白阳性率变化较大。

> **诊断要点：甲状腺髓样癌**
> 1. 滤泡内可出现正常C细胞，并表达降钙素。
> 2. 95%的甲状腺髓样癌降钙素呈阳性表达，也可表达其他肽类。
> 3. CEA表达于大多数甲状腺髓样癌，其他甲状腺癌不表达。
> 4. 一般性神经内分泌癌标记物均呈阳性，如NSE、Syn、嗜铬素A、嗜铬素B和分泌素Ⅱ。
> 5. TTF-1呈阳性表达，TGB呈阴性。
> 6. 真正的C细胞和滤泡混合性肿瘤少见。

甲状旁腺

Miettinen等研究了正常和肿瘤性甲状旁腺中中间丝的结构。正常和肿瘤性腺体均阳性表达CK8、CK18和CK19，而波形蛋白仅表达于间质细胞（图9.19）[157]。正常腺体主细胞不表达神经细丝蛋白，而33%的腺瘤可表达神经细丝蛋白，也可表达CK。与甲状腺滤泡细胞TGB、TTF-1呈阳性不同，正常和肿瘤性主细胞均呈阴性。

甲状旁腺激素（parathyroid hormone，PTH）的免疫组化研究比较困难，因为既缺乏合适的抗体，其主细胞中的激素含量又比较低[158]。而抗原修复技术的应用，大大易化了PTH在福尔马林固定、石蜡包埋标本中的定位[159]（图9.20）。已证明PTH和CgA可表达于大量正常的、增生性的和肿瘤性的甲状旁腺组织

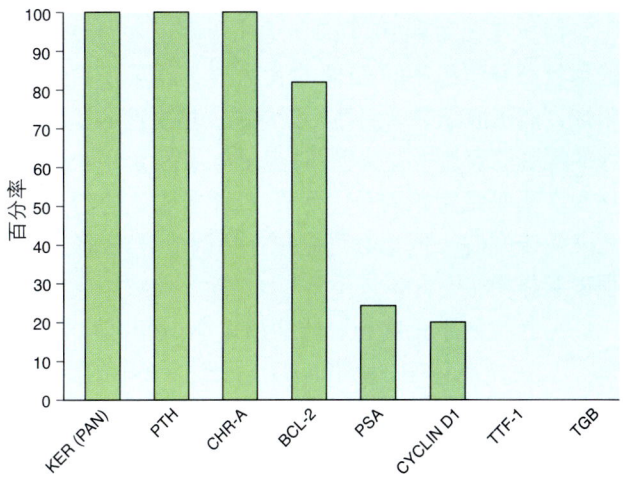

图9.19 甲状旁腺腺瘤标记物的表达。[KER（PAN），广谱CK；PTH，甲状旁腺激素；CHR-A，CgA；BCL-2，bcl-2；PSA，前列腺特异性抗原；cyclin D1，周期素D1；TTF-1，甲状腺转录因子-1；TGB，甲状腺球蛋白]

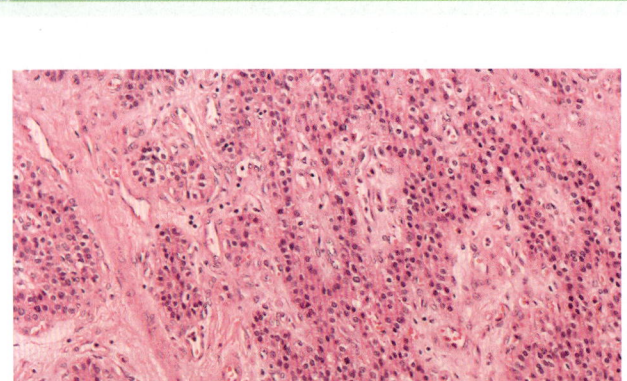
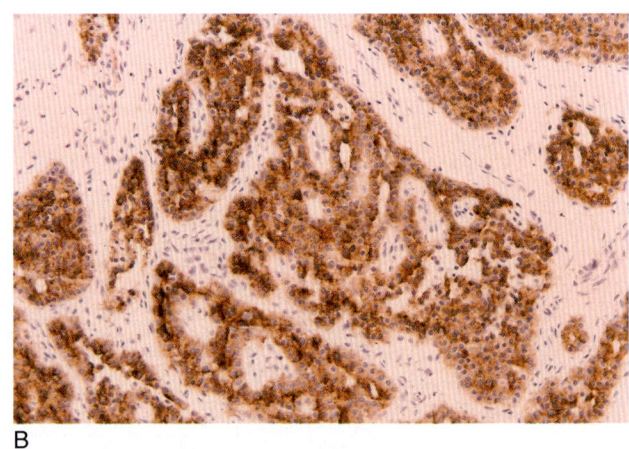

图 9.20 甲状腺内甲状旁腺瘤。(A，B) 免疫过氧化物酶染色，甲状旁腺激素呈强阳性表达于主细胞的细胞浆内

中（图9.19）。在正常腺体内CgA、PTH的表达比瘤细胞中更为强烈，增生性的腺体着色相对减弱，腺瘤中的表达较正常的和增生性的又弱一些。总而言之，肿瘤边缘的旁腺组织较瘤内组织着色要强[159]。甲状旁腺mRNA探针的原位杂交结果与之一致[122]。Tomita报道了一系列PTH阳性，而CgA并无阳性的甲状旁腺癌[160]。PTH的表达形式与PTH提取物的水平一致，即正常腺体中最高，而腺瘤性腺体中最低[161]。除PTH外，PTH相关蛋白也用免疫组化方法得以论证[162]。

Schmid等证明，14%（86例中的12例）的增生性甲状旁腺CgB呈灶性阳性表达，这12例中有10例在同一部位表达降钙素[163]。表达降钙素的10例中有4例降钙素阳性细胞中的一小部分表达CGRP。该研究结果表明，CGRP可合成并储存于增生的旁腺主细胞中。其他相关研究证实了这一结论[164]。

用抗-Leu3a和OKT4D抗体来检测正常的和异常的甲状旁腺组织中的CD4的表达[165]，结果仅主细胞阳性，而嗜酸细胞为阴性。正常的、增生性的和肿瘤性的细胞的表达主要位于细胞表面。相反，甲状旁腺癌则主要是细胞浆着色。尽管CD4类表达的功能及意义尚未知晓，但半数可能是在钙调节PTH释放过程中起作用。

另外检测了正常和肿瘤性腺体中cyclin D1的分布[166]。正常腺体中，cyclin D1只表达于6%的病例。相反则表达于11例甲状旁腺癌中的10例（91%）、38例甲状旁腺腺瘤中的11例（39%）、18例增生性甲状旁腺腺体中的11例（61%）。这些研究还证实cyclin D1在腺瘤和腺癌中高表达，同时高表达的情况可见于增生性疾病[166]。

甲状旁腺腺瘤与腺癌的鉴别有时极其困难，有研究用MIB-1来辅助其鉴别诊断。Abbona及其合作者报道了腺癌（侵袭性和非侵袭性）与腺瘤在MIB-1评分上有显著差异[167]。而在非侵袭性腺癌与腺瘤之间则无显著差异。相反，临床上侵袭性腺癌核分裂率和MIB-1评分明显高于腺瘤。Vargas等报道，如1000个细胞中有40个以上的MIB-1指数呈阳性，则极可能为恶性肿瘤[168]。p27（Kip1）在甲状旁腺增生、腺瘤和腺癌中也有表达[60]。p27标记指数为腺瘤56.8 ± 3.4，腺癌13.9 ± 2.6，而MIB-1标记指数腺癌明显高于腺瘤。这些结果表明，p27和MIB-1抗体组合可区分甲状旁腺腺瘤与腺癌。

RB（视网膜母细胞瘤）蛋白相应抗体的应用是另一个区分甲状旁腺腺瘤与腺癌的可能方法。Cryns及其合作者报道了一小组的腺癌中RB蛋白表达缺失，而腺瘤中呈阳性表达[169]。但Vargas等证明，腺瘤中RB的阳性率为100%而腺癌中为80%[168]。最近Farnebo等认为RB作为区分甲状旁腺腺瘤与腺癌的指标尚不成熟[170]。

p53在正常、增生、瘤性甲状旁腺组织中均有表达。Kayath及其同事研究表明，36%（28例中的10例）的腺瘤、42%（12例中的5例）的原发性增生、72%（18例中的13例）的弥漫性增生及40%（5例中的2例）的腺癌p53均呈阳性表达[171]。结果表明，用免疫组化方法分析p53，无助于鉴别甲状旁腺的各种增生状态。

肾上腺

皮质

鉴定肾上腺皮质的标记物包括类固醇生成酶、单克隆抗体D11、肾上腺结合蛋白4（Ad4BP）、A103（melan-A）、calretinin和抑制素A（图9.21）。Sasano等的研究表明，Cushing综合征病人束状带和网状带P450$_{17a}$的表达均呈强阳性[22-24]。皮质醇增多性皮质腺瘤P450$_{17a}$呈强阳性表达，而邻近的网状带着色弱，与正常腺体受抑制相一致。

单克隆抗体D11识别几个可与载脂蛋白E相结合的59kD蛋白[172,173]。近80%肾上腺皮质腺瘤D11呈核阳性。100%的肝细胞癌、60%的肺癌，偶尔在肾癌D11呈细胞浆阳性[174]。Ad4BP，也叫类固醇因子1（steroid factor，SF-1），是调节类固醇生成性细胞色素P450基因表达的转录子，可表达于100%的肾上腺皮质腺癌，而肾细胞癌、肝细胞癌和其他各型肿瘤（包括嗜铬细胞瘤）呈阴性[175]。

单克隆抗体A103（melan-A）最初用于诊断恶性黑色素瘤（图9.22）。该抗体可与类固醇生成细胞上的抗原决定簇交叉反应，其中包括肾上腺皮质细胞。Busam及其合作者报道，A103表达于100%的肾上腺皮质腺癌，而肾细胞癌、肝细胞癌、嗜铬细胞瘤和其他上皮性肿瘤均不表达[176]。Renshaw和Granter的小样本研究表明，4例肾上腺皮质癌中有2例cyclin D1呈阳性[177]。Loy及其合作者对A103在肾上腺皮质肿瘤鉴别诊断中的作用作了广泛研究[178]。结果发现，21例肾上腺皮质肿瘤均呈阳性，而16例来自肺、肾、乳腺、肝、食管的转移癌及几例嗜铬细胞瘤均呈阴性。此外他们还对来源于肺、乳腺、肾、胰腺、肝、食管、胃、卵巢、肠、胆管、膀胱、喉和胆囊等各个部位的269例肾上腺外肿瘤作了研究，其中只发现1例卵巢浆液性癌A103呈阳性[178]。Ghorab等的另1项研究发现，32例肾上腺皮质肿瘤（21例腺瘤、11例癌）中有31例A103呈阴性[179]。86例肾细胞癌（67例透明细胞癌，10例乳头状癌，4例嫌色细胞癌，4例肉瘤，1例集合管癌）和57例肝细胞肝癌（25例高分化，25例中分化，7例低分化）中，除1例肾透明细胞癌A103呈阳性外，其余均为阴性[179]。这些研究强调了A103在判定肾上腺皮质原发性肿瘤、区分包括髓质在内的其他肿瘤上的应用局限性[180]。

抑制素A抗体也可用于类固醇生成细胞的鉴定[181]。Fetsch及其合作者用抑制素A来鉴定肾上腺皮质肿瘤的细胞学标本[182]。并报道肾上腺皮质肿瘤全部呈阳性，而肾细胞癌全部呈阴性。Renshaw和Granter证明，抑制素A和A103可用于肾上腺皮质肿瘤的鉴定。其中A103特异性比较强，抑制素A敏感性稍强一些[177]。

随后研究得出相同结论。总之，抑制素A在肾上腺皮质肿瘤中的阳性率为71%～100%，腺癌为75%～100%；而在转移癌中则很少，如肾细胞癌（0%～20%）、肝细胞癌（0%～4%）、嗜铬细胞瘤（0%～14%）[171,181-188]。

腹膜后或右上腹部肿瘤细针吸取标本或细针穿刺标本往往小且局限。而且获取标本的过程中难免会横断其他组织（如肝），导致混有其他组织或无肿瘤细胞，造成诊断困难。从形态学上，即使正常细胞也可形似其他部位的恶性肿瘤。如，肝的细针穿刺标本可含有非典型的、反应性的肝细胞，而容易怀疑为转移性的腺癌、肾细胞癌或肾上腺皮质癌。而这些部位肿瘤的诊断也有相应的困难。因此，正确的组织病理学诊断日益依赖于免疫组化手段。

诊断的主要困难在于区分肾上腺皮质和髓质肿瘤（即嗜铬细胞瘤），区分是肾上腺内原发的，还是转移性肿瘤（即转移癌或邻近部位的原发癌——如原发性肝癌或原发性肾癌）。

肾上腺皮质癌有神经内分泌分化，已证实的有Syn、神经细丝蛋白、NSE（图9.22C）[37,189]。与嗜铬细胞瘤相反，肾上腺皮质癌嗜铬素呈阴性表达。在一系列研究中，60%肾上腺皮质癌表达低分子量神经细丝蛋白，80%表达Syn，60%表达NSE[189]。这些发现

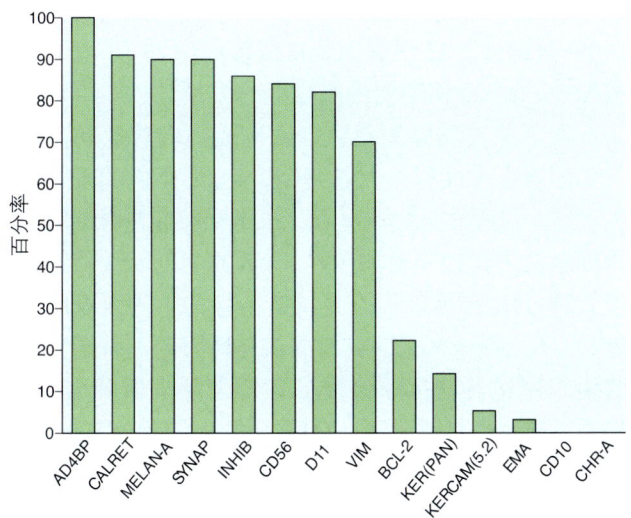

图9.21 肾上腺皮质肿瘤中标记物的表达。[AD4BP，肾上腺结合蛋白4；CALRET，calretinin；MELAN-A，A103；SYNAP，突触素；INHIB，抑制素；CD56；D11；VIM，波形蛋白；BCL-2，bcl-2；KER（PAN），广谱CK；KER（CAM5.2），单克隆抗体CAM5.2检测的角蛋白；EMA，上皮细胞膜抗原；CD10；CHR-A，嗜铬素A]

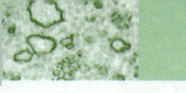

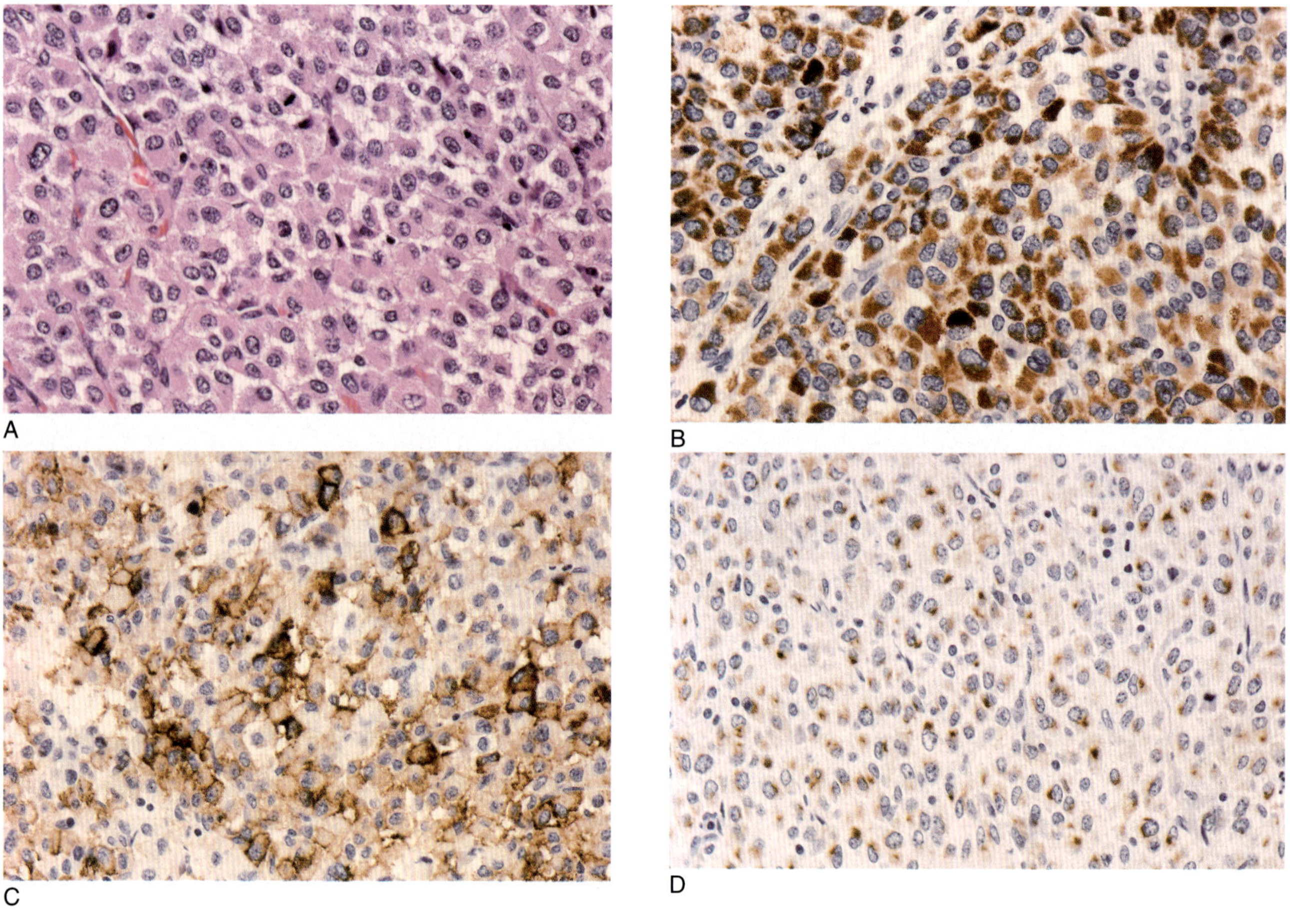

图9.22 肾上腺皮质癌。（A）HE染色；（B）免疫过氧化物酶染色，melan-A（A103）呈颗粒状阳性；（C）免疫过氧化物酶染色，Syn呈明显细胞浆阳性；（D）免疫过氧化物酶染色，角蛋白CAM5.2局灶性细胞浆阳性

对判断肾上腺皮质癌起源的重要性尚未明了。除了嗜铬素可作为区分要点外，嗜铬细胞瘤通常不表达角蛋白，尽管也有报道其阳性率可达29%[190, 191]。

更多最新研究关注于区别肾上腺皮质腺瘤与腺癌的其他标记物，如bcl-2、降钙素。bcl-2通常表达于正常肾上腺皮质各层细胞内，而髓质不表达。Fogt等报道bcl-2 100%表达于23例肾上腺皮质腺瘤及腺癌，而11例嗜铬细胞瘤中仅1例表达[192]。该研究表明，bcl-2可用于区分皮质、髓质肿瘤。但Zhang等的另一最新研究与该结论不一致[193]，15例肾上腺皮质腺瘤中有2例（13%）、10例肾上腺皮质腺癌中仅3例（30%）阳性表达bcl-2。更令人惊异的是，大多数嗜铬细胞瘤（14例中的12例，86%）表达bcl-2。作者最终认为，这种矛盾现象的出现可能与抗原修复方法的不同有关。

calretinin，一种钙结合蛋白，一般用于标记神经的、间皮的及卵巢性索间质肿瘤。最近发现73%的肾上腺皮质肿瘤也可表达calretinin[194]。Zhang等的研究证实了这一结论。他们发现16例肾上腺皮质腺瘤100%呈阳性，12例肾上腺皮质腺癌中11例（92%）呈阳性，而20例嗜铬细胞瘤无一阳性[193]。

肾上腺皮质腺癌与肾上腺皮质内转移癌的区别尤为困难。中间丝，尤其是CK和波形蛋白的研究易化了这一过程。正常情况下，正常和腺瘤性肾上腺皮质细胞波形蛋白呈典型阳性；CK的免疫活性随组织预处理（固定/冰冻）及其抗体活性的不同而有所差异[195, 196]。新鲜冰冻组织和福尔马林固定、石蜡包埋的组织用微波法抗原修复后，肾上腺皮质肿瘤CK阳性反应可由灶性上升为60%，尤其是CAM5.2（图9.22D）。肾上腺皮质腺癌的中间丝表达应为：波形蛋白呈不同程度阳性，而CK反应普遍较弱[197, 198]。肾上腺皮质内转移癌却相反，CK反应较强，CEA、CD15及EMA（上皮细胞膜抗原）往往也呈阳性，而肾上腺皮质腺癌这些指标均呈阴性。

肾上腺免疫组化染色需要注意的几点是：S-100阳性需排除恶性黑色素瘤，肾上腺髓质的支持细胞也可呈典型阳性。标记恶性黑色素瘤的HMB-45，偶尔在嗜铬细胞瘤呈阳性[199, 200]。肾上腺皮质腺瘤、嗜铬细胞瘤Syn均呈阳性。抑制素A在其他生成类固醇的肿瘤（如卵巢来源的）也可呈阳性。

肾上腺髓质及肾上腺外副神经节

肾上腺髓质的主细胞和肾上腺外副神经节包括儿茶酚胺合成细胞和支持细胞[201, 202]。应用免疫荧光技术、免疫过氧化物酶技术对福尔马林固定的上述细胞中儿茶酚胺及其合成酶进行测定[8, 201-203]。结果儿茶酚胺合成细胞多种常用神经内分泌细胞标记物呈典型阳性。几种肽类激素则呈不同程度阳性。支持细胞S-100呈阳性[201]。

肾上腺髓质细胞、肾上腺外副神经节细胞及其肿瘤呈典型神经纤维阳性型、波形蛋白阳性型（图9.23）[56, 195, 204]。CK则相反，Kimura及其合作者报道，广谱CK抗体在45例嗜铬细胞瘤中有13例（29%）呈阳性[191]。其阳性结果普遍稀疏，但有时也呈小组或小簇出现。与嗜铬细胞瘤呈阳性相反，肾上腺外副神经节细胞瘤CK呈阴性。然而其他作者未能阐述嗜铬细胞瘤和肾上腺外副神经节细胞瘤CK的表达[190]。Chetty及其合作者检测了18例肾上腺外副神经节细胞瘤和7例嗜铬细胞瘤中CK AE1/AE3、CAM5.2及34βE12经抗原微波修复后的表达情况[190]。结果表明，AE1/AE3和CAM5.2在3例肾上腺外副神经节细胞瘤（马尾、迷走神经内及眼眶内）中阳性表达，而在嗜铬细胞瘤中均呈阴性。其他上皮标记物，如EMA，两者均呈典型阴性。

NSE实际上可表达于所有的嗜铬细胞瘤和肾上腺外副神经节细胞瘤[201]。Syn100%阳性，嗜铬素A表达率在95%以上[201, 205, 206]。概言之，嗜铬素在正常细胞中的表达比副神经节瘤组织中要强（图9.24A）。其表达呈独特的颗粒状，而NSE在细胞浆中呈弥漫性阳性。Syn100%阳性，其他神经内分泌标记，如PGP9.5，在已报道病例中的表达率接近80%[207]，S-100只在支持细胞中表达。

正常肾上腺内，CD56表达于髓质及球状带[48]。其在嗜铬细胞瘤呈典型的强阳性。Komminoth及其合作者用在NCAM上发现的可与多聚唾液酸（polySia）特异性结合的单克隆抗体来研究并证实染色仅限于人类正常肾上腺髓质[37]。100%的嗜铬细胞瘤的多聚唾液酸表达呈弥漫性阳性，而28例肾上腺皮质癌中只有8例（28%）呈灶性阳性。

除儿茶酚胺外，5-羟色胺表达于近80%的嗜铬细胞瘤中[205]。嗜铬细胞瘤和肾上腺外副神经节细胞瘤还表达肽类激素，包括神经肽Y（64%）、P物质（36%）、降钙素（21%）及亮氨酸脑啡肽（leu-enkephalin）和甲硫啡肽（met-enkephalin）（70%）[205, 207]。一些研究还表明，血循环神经肽Y水平的测定，有助于此类肿瘤的诊断和调节。Hellman及其合作者还证明，神经肽YmRNA表达于所有良性嗜铬细胞瘤，恶性嗜铬细胞瘤仅有30%阳性[208]。

尽管α-抑制素被认为是肾上腺皮质肿瘤的特异性标记物，Pelkey及其合作者曾经报道了19例嗜铬细胞瘤中2例呈阳性[181]。

Clarke及其合作者用大量标记物来辅助鉴别良、恶性嗜铬细胞瘤[209]。结果表明，MIB-1指数大于3%者诊断恶性嗜铬细胞瘤中的特异性为100%、敏感性为50%。August合作组的研究中，其所研究的肿瘤中有85%的病例MIB-1阳性指数大于5%者与恶性行为有关[210]。他们还指出，若CD44-S呈阴性，肿瘤更易发生转移。前面研究表明，S-100阳性对诊断良性肿瘤有统计意义但非线性相关，且S-100表达缺失者肿瘤较大。良、恶性肿瘤均可表达组织蛋白酶B、D，IV型胶原，c-met、bcl-2和碱性纤维母细胞生长因子。

神经母细胞瘤是小圆蓝细胞肿瘤，可发生于肾上腺及多种肾上腺外组织。其鉴别诊断范围较广，包括横纹肌母细胞瘤、尤文肉瘤/原始神经外胚层肿瘤

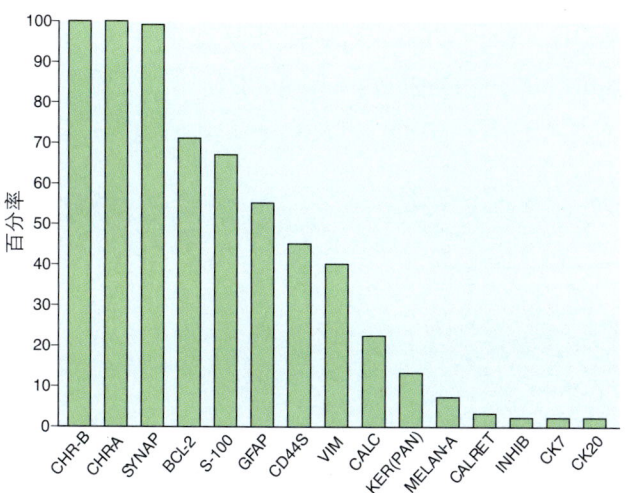

图9.23　嗜铬细胞瘤中标记物分布图。[CHR-B，嗜铬素B；CHR-A，嗜铬素A；SYNAP，突触素；BCL-2，bcl-2；S-100；GFAP，胶质纤维酸性蛋白；CD44S；VIM，波形蛋白；CALC，降钙素；KER（PAN），广谱CK；MELAN-A，A103；CALRET，calretinin；INHIB，抑制素；CK7；CK20]

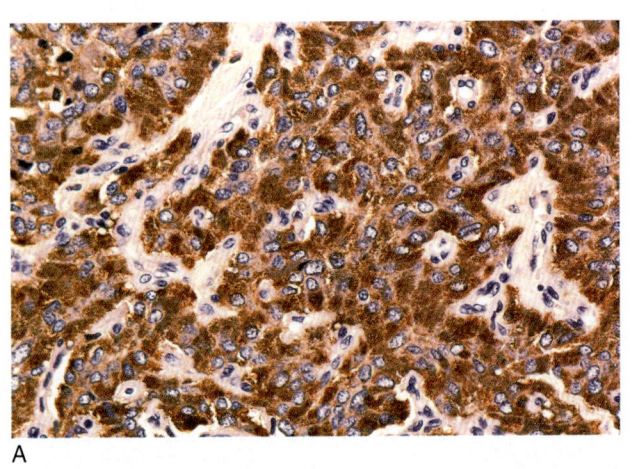
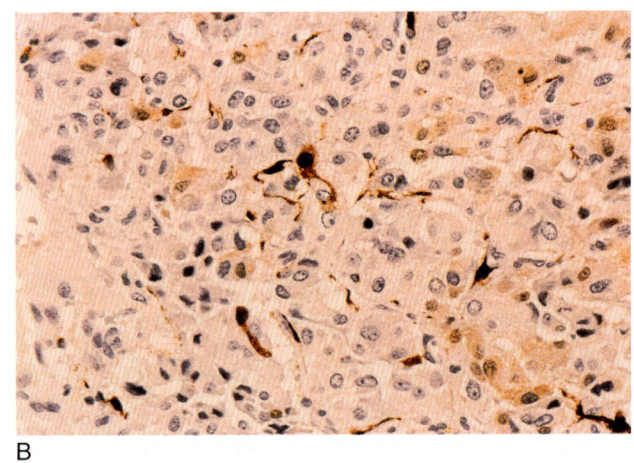

图 9.24　肾上腺嗜铬细胞瘤。（A）免疫过氧化物酶染色，嗜铬素 A 呈细胞浆强阳性着色；（B）免疫过氧化物酶染色，S-100 蛋白支持细胞呈阳性表达

（ES/PNETS）、髓母细胞瘤、小细胞骨肉瘤、淋巴母细胞性淋巴瘤、胚胎性 Wilms 瘤、促纤维组织增生性小圆细胞肿瘤（见第 15 章）。大量标记物被用于神经母细胞瘤的诊断，包括：神经内分泌标记物、细胞骨架蛋白、儿茶酚胺合成酶和神经母细胞瘤特异性抗体（图 9.25）[211-217]。其中大多数抗体单用缺乏特异性或敏感性，或者两者都缺乏，所以必须抗体组合应用。

85%～100% 的神经母细胞瘤 NSE 呈阳性，PGP9.5 阳性率同样比较高（图 9.26）[215]。但两种指标均可表达于其他小圆蓝细胞肿瘤。据 Wirnsberger 及其合作者报道，抗嗜铬素及其相关蛋白抗体中，HISL-19 可 100% 表达于神经母细胞瘤，其次是 CgA（52%）、CgA 和 CgB（45%）（图 9.27A）[215]。神经细丝蛋白阳性率为 80%，定位于细胞突起或神经纤维，Syn 表达于 75% 的病例；多巴胺 β- 羟化酶阳性率为 75%。总之，这些指标在高分化神经母细胞瘤中的表达比低分化的要好[215]。在肽类激素，VIP 表达于 30% 的病例，而神经肽 Y 表达于 10% 的病例；神经母细胞瘤不表达 CD57，但 7 例节细胞神经瘤均呈阳性[215]。微管相关蛋白（MAP-1）、MAP-2 和 β- 微管蛋白表达于 100% 的病例，但迄今为止研究的病例数尚少[216, 217]。S-100 局限表达于支持细胞内（图 9.27B）。

图 9.25　神经母细胞瘤中标记物的表达。[CD56；NB84；PGP9.5，蛋白基因产物 9.5；NSE，神经非特异性烯醇化酶；NFP，神经细丝蛋白；CHR-A，嗜铬素 A；VIM，波形蛋白；SYNAP，突触素；CD117；CEA-P，多克隆 CEA；S-100；WT-1，Wilms 瘤；CD57；KER（AE1/AE3），单克隆抗体 AE1/AE3 检测的角蛋白；KER（CAM5.2），CAM5.2 检测的角蛋白；CD99]

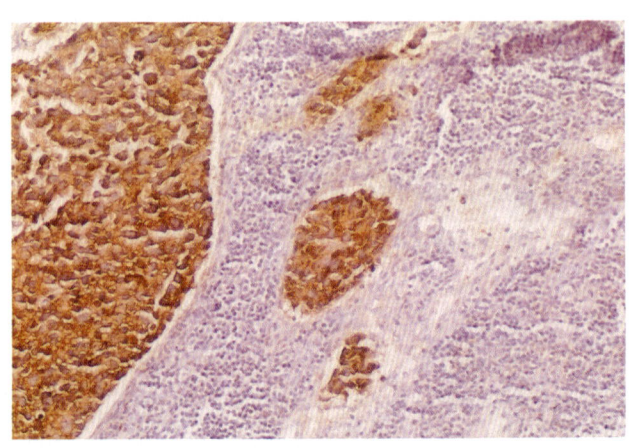

图 9.26　淋巴结中转移的神经母细胞瘤。免疫过氧化物酶染色，NSE 表达局限于肿瘤细胞

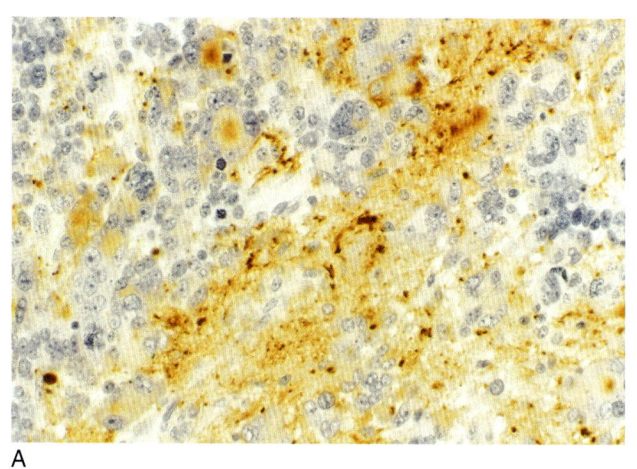 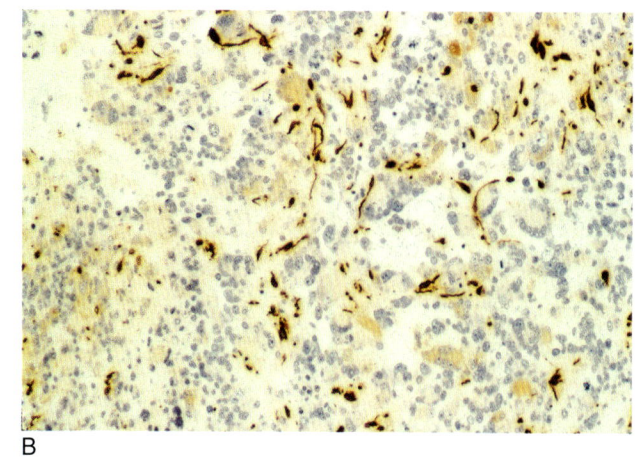

图9.27 肾上腺外神经母细胞瘤。(A)免疫过氧化物酶染色，进展型区域嗜铬素A呈颗粒状着色;(B)免疫过氧化物酶染色，S-100蛋白支持细胞呈阳性表达

CD99在区别神经母细胞瘤和其他小圆蓝细胞肿瘤中比较实用[218-222]。至今对100多例神经母细胞瘤的CD99研究结果均呈阴性。相反，几乎100%的ES/PNET CD99呈阳性表达。抗β2微球蛋白是另一种在神经母细胞瘤中不表达而在大约75%的ES/PNET中呈阳性的标记物[223]。

值得注意的是另一种标记神经母细胞瘤的单克隆抗体NB84[223]。Miettnen及其合作者研究了22例未分化型神经母细胞瘤及83例分化型神经母细胞瘤（共105例），发现21例（95.5%）未分化型、83例（100%）分化型（共计99%，105例中的104例）NB84呈阳性反应[224]。此外，5例ES/PNET中有4例（80%）、3例纤维组织增生性小圆细胞肿瘤中全部（100%）阳性表达NB84。相反，39例ES中有7例（17.9%）、14例胚胎性Wilms瘤中仅1例（7.1%）NB84呈阳性表达。腺泡性和胚胎性横纹肌母细胞瘤（RMS）、淋巴母细胞性淋巴瘤和肺小细胞癌均呈阴性[224]。而Folpe及其合作者报道了13例横纹肌母细胞瘤中有3例、11例髓母细胞瘤中有10例、9例感觉神经母细胞瘤中有1例、3例小细胞骨肉瘤中有2例NB84均呈阳性[225]。抗体组合NB84、CD99、CK、淋巴系统及肌肉特异性标记物可用于神经母细胞瘤的鉴别诊断。

> **诊断要点：肾上腺肿瘤**
>
> 1. 肾上腺皮质癌波形蛋白呈典型阳性，角蛋白在福尔马林固定标本中呈可疑、较弱或局灶性阳性。
> 2. 肾上腺内的上皮转移癌角蛋白几乎总是弥漫性强阳性表达，且CEA、EMA、CD15也常呈阳性表达。
> 3. melan-A（A-103）、抑制素、calretinin在区分肾上腺皮质癌和其他肿瘤中最为有效。
> 4. 肾上腺皮质癌Syn、NSE、神经纤维呈阳性表达，但CgA呈阴性。嗜铬素可用于鉴别肾上腺皮质癌（均呈阴性表达）和嗜铬细胞瘤（大多数呈阳性表达）。

胃肠内分泌细胞

胃肠道类癌根据其胚胎性起源主要分为3型：前肠、中肠、后肠的衍生物。其起源部位与肽类、胺类激素的分布有着密切关联。如5-羟色胺可见于89%的中肠类癌、30%的前肠类癌和40%的后肠类癌（表9.3）[226]。

表9.3 胃肠道类癌激素表达情况

产物	前肠(%+)	中肠(%+)	后肠(%+)
5-羟色胺	30	89	13
生长抑素	80	4	63
P物质	10	41	0
胰多肽	0	0	88
胰高血糖素	10	0	50
降钙素	0	11	0
促肾上腺皮质激素	20	4	0
胃泌素	30	0	0

类癌中CK呈典型阳性，其中CAM5.2呈100%阳性，而其他广谱CK80%阳性[227,228]。CK20阳性表达于30%病例[229]。波形蛋白表达于近25%病例，神经细丝蛋白的阳性率易变。类癌可广泛表达于各种神经内分泌标记物。NSE阳性表达于近80%病例，PGP阳性表达率近90%[16]。其他神经内分泌标记物的表达随肿瘤起源而不同[230]。Syn100%阳性表达于所有部位的类癌，嗜铬素A表达于88%～100%的前肠型、100%中肠型、24%～40%的后肠型类癌（图9.28、9.29）。而嗜铬素B100%表达于后肠型类癌[31,231]。甘氨肽-α-乙酰化单氧酶则表达于14%胃类癌、100%回肠类癌、100%直肠类癌[231]。NCAM表达于76%的前肠型、58%中肠型、20%的后肠型类癌。NCAM抗体可同时标记瘤细胞和支持细胞[231]。S-100阳性表达于41%的前肠型类癌、50%的中肠和后肠型肿瘤，其着色形式和NCAM一样，可同时标记瘤细胞和支持细胞。

用单克隆抗体、多克隆抗血清检测CEA表达于近40%的类癌，而CD15表达于30%的类癌[232-234]。单克隆抗体CA15.3可辨认碳水化合物和肽类决定簇（MUC1型黏蛋白），与75%类癌反应，可与唾液酸Lewis抗原反应的CA19.9则呈阴性[116]。

还对CDX2作了研究。Moskaluk及其合作者研究表明，73%的中肠型、44%的后肠型类癌CDX2呈弥漫阳性着色[235]。

前列腺酸性磷酸（PAP）也见于一些类癌的表达。对33例前肠、中肠和后肠来源的类癌研究表明，5例后肠类癌均呈阳性表达，而其他各型均呈阴性[236]。而前列腺特异性抗原均呈典型的阴性。α-hCG在类癌中有不同程度的表达，Heiz及其合作者研究表明，其表达于46%的前肠型、25%的后肠型，但在35例中肠型类癌中均不表达[145]。28 000kD的钙结合蛋白分布于中枢及周围神经系统的各级分支内、肾腺管状细胞末梢及肠神经内分泌细胞。免疫组化研究证实钙结合蛋白表达于少量神经内分泌细胞内，尤其是阑尾和

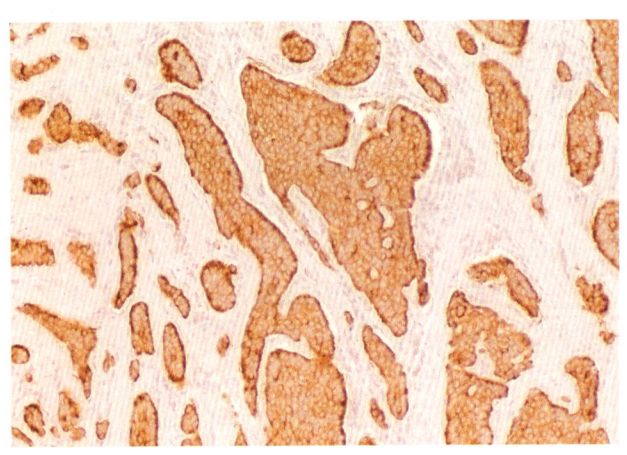

图9.28 小肠类癌。免疫过氧化物酶染色，嗜铬素A在肿瘤细胞中呈阳性表达

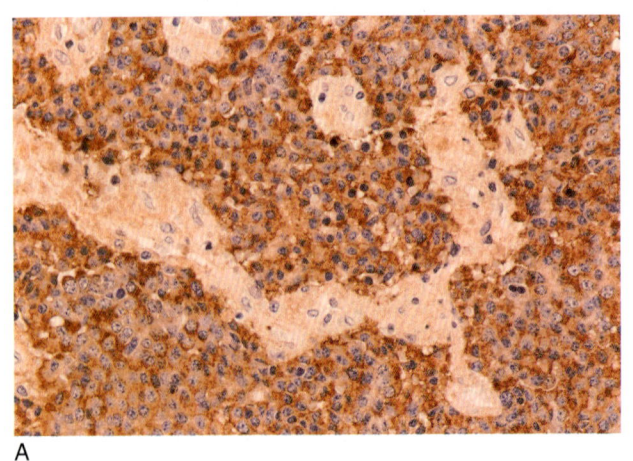

A

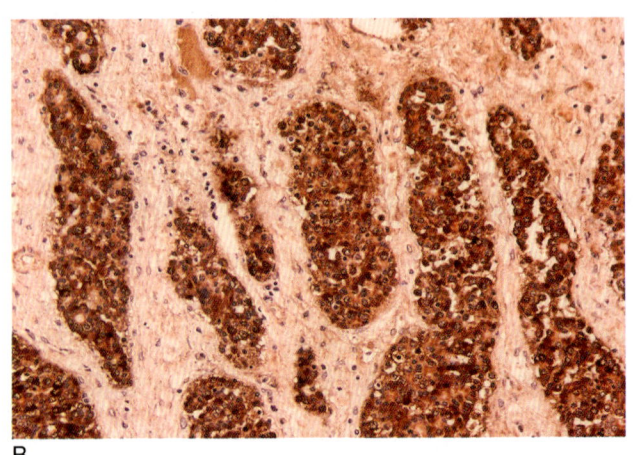

B

图9.29 肝内转移的类癌。（A）免疫过氧化物酶染色，CgA在肿瘤细胞中呈强阳性着色；（B）肝内转移的类癌。免疫过氧化物酶染色，5-羟色胺在肿瘤细胞中呈强阳性着色

小肠，100%的中肠和前肠（胃）内类癌[151]。而在1例后肠类癌的病例中并未表达。

胰腺神经内分泌细胞

广谱CK抗体表达于正常胰腺神经内分泌细胞及近90%的胰腺神经内分泌肿瘤，而CK20仅表达于12.5%病例（图9.30）[53, 57, 156, 229, 237]。波形蛋白的表达不定，只有近25%呈明确的细胞浆着色。神经纤维表达于50%以上的病例。神经内分泌标记物NSE和Syn表达于所有正常胰腺神经内分泌细胞及其神经内分泌肿瘤[238]。CgA表达于近75%的胰腺内分泌肿瘤。总体上，其着色范围与神经内分泌颗粒多少有关，如在肽类激素染色标本中明显[238]。曾有报道两例胰岛素瘤钙结合蛋白均呈阳性反应。CD99表达于5例胰腺神经内分泌肿瘤中的2例[220]。

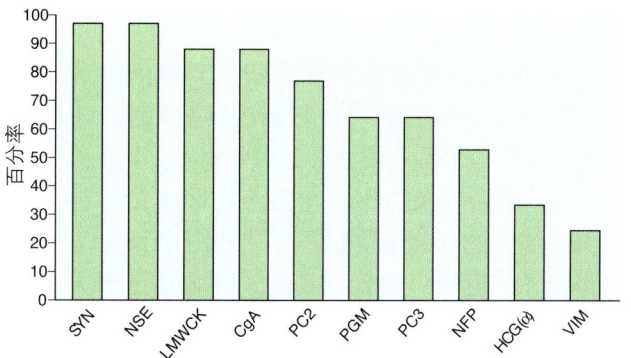

图9.30 胰腺神经内分泌肿瘤标记物的分布。[SYN，突触素；NSE，神经特异性烯醇化酶；LMWCK，低分子量细胞角蛋白；CgA；PC2，转化酶原2；PGM，甘氨肽-α-乙酰化单氧酶；PC3，转化酶原3；NFP，神经细丝蛋白；HCG（α），人类促绒毛膜性腺激素α链；VIM，波形蛋白]

正常朗格汉斯岛包括4种主要细胞[239]：生成胰岛素的B细胞，占胰腺中央部细胞的60%~70%、胰头后部的20%~30%；生成高血糖素的A细胞，占胰腺中央部细胞的15%~20%、胰头后部的5%；分泌胰多肽（PP）的细胞，占胰头后部的70%、其他胰岛细胞的2%~5%。近10%的胰腺内分泌细胞分布在外分泌部的小管细胞或副管腺泡细胞周围。偶见出现在大导管的生长抑素生成细胞，胰腺类癌大多数起源于该细胞。

胰岛素瘤可典型表达胰岛素和胰岛素原，其中包括标准组织化学染色呈阴性的病例[239, 240]。近50%的胰岛素瘤分泌多种激素并含有阳性表达胰高血糖素、生长抑素、PP、胃泌素、ACTH或降钙素的细胞。胰岛素的阳性结果可有所不同，超微结构上含大量颗粒的细胞免疫组化着色最强。胰高血糖素瘤诊断依赖于胰高血糖素的免疫组化染色。胰高血糖素前体和高血糖素类似肽也呈典型阳性，还可表达与高血糖素原无关的激素，包括生长抑素和胰岛素。

生长抑素瘤根据生长抑素阳性结果来判定[239]。该类肿瘤也可表达降钙素、ACTH、胃泌素。相同的组织形态和免疫组化反应模式也可发生在十二指肠。PP生成性肿瘤通常归为无功能性肿瘤，虽然偶尔伴有WDHA综合征（水泻、低钾血症和胃酸缺乏）。除了PP外，这些肿瘤内还散在分布着一些分泌其他肽类激素的细胞。

胃泌素瘤可不同程度地表达胃泌素；但也有些肿瘤不表达（图9.31）[239, 240]。应用抗胃泌素分子N-、C-末端部分不同区域的抗体标记，后者也可呈阳性。一些胃泌素呈阳性的胃泌素瘤，原位杂交技术可检测出胃泌素的mRNA[241]。与其他胰腺内分泌肿瘤

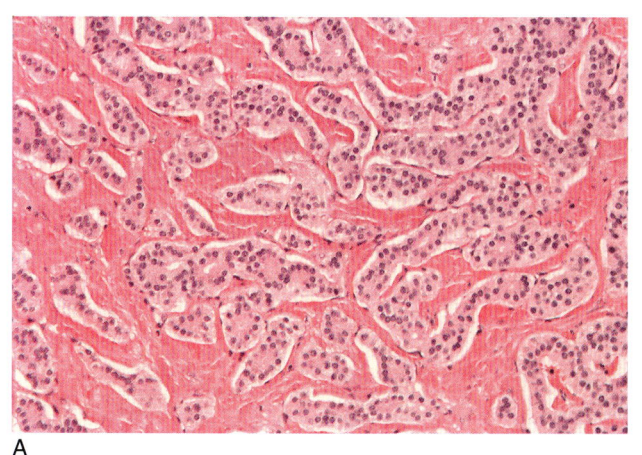
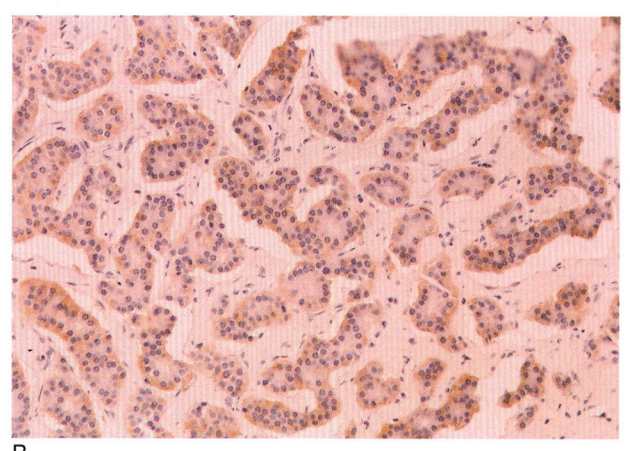

图9.31 胰腺胃泌素瘤。（A）HE染色；（B）免疫过氧化物酶染色，胃泌素在细胞浆内呈弱阳性表达

一样，胃泌素瘤内散在分布着一些可分泌高血糖素、PP、胰岛素、生长抑素、5-羟色胺或ACTH的细胞[242]。胃泌素瘤也可发生于包括十二指肠在内的一些胰腺外部位。

VIP生成性肿瘤与WDHA综合征有关。Solcia及其同事研究的28例VIP生成性肿瘤中87%表达VIP，57%表达肽组蛋氨酸。生长激素释放激素和PP表达率分别为50%和53%[243]。除胰腺内分泌肿瘤外，神经节瘤、节细胞神经母细胞瘤也可出现WDHA综合征。

胰腺内罕见真正的类癌，这些肿瘤可表达5-羟色胺。其他原发性胰腺内分泌肿瘤可分泌生长激素释放激素（肢端肥大症）、ACTH（库欣综合征）和PTH或PTH样肽（高钙血症）。

无功能性胰腺内分泌肿瘤内有散在的细胞阳性表达几种激素，最为常见的是PP和高血糖素（图9.32）。

α链hCG被认为是恶性胰腺内分泌肿瘤的标记物，可表达于近70%的病例（图9.33）[244]。更多最新研究表明，α链hCG也可表达于其他良性胰腺内分泌肿瘤[245]。胰腺内分泌肿瘤也可表达孕激素受体蛋白[246]。

肺内分泌细胞

肺内分泌细胞多单个存在，或呈小簇存在，称为神经上皮小体[247]。现认为神经上皮小体可能有化学感受器功能，而单个神经内分泌细胞可能是旁分泌成分。包括5-羟色胺、胃泌素释放肽和降钙素在内的多种调节产物，都既可表达于单个神经内分泌细胞，也可表达于神经上皮小体。而亮氨酸脑啡肽只表达于单个神经内分泌细胞（图9.34）[247]。肺神经内分泌细胞在受刺激或暴露于致癌因子后，会经历一系列增生性改变。通常，增生性神经内分泌细胞仍具有正常细胞的分泌调节产物的功能。重度增生和非典型增生可同时生成具有抗原决定簇的产物，包括VIP和不同分子形式的ACTH。

肺神经内分泌肿瘤根据组织形态和免疫组化特点可分为4个主要类型[248]，包括经典型类癌、不典型类癌、小细胞癌和大细胞神经内分泌癌。其免疫组化表达情况总结在图9.35～9.38。近85%的肺神经内分泌肿瘤表达低分子量CK[248,249]。根据Travis等的系列报道，广谱CK（AE1/AE3）抗体表达于56%的经典型类癌、40%的不典型类癌、100%的小细胞癌和大细胞神经内分泌癌[248]。82%的小细胞癌CK7、CK20呈阴性[55]。

TTF-1见于正常肺神经内分泌细胞，是鉴别肺神经内分泌肿瘤的有效指标。Oliveira等的研究表明，

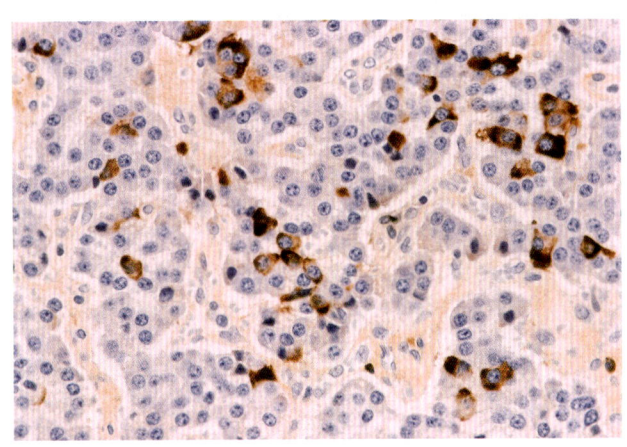

图9.32　无功能性胰腺内分泌肿瘤。免疫过氧化物酶染色，胰多肽在肿瘤细胞中呈散在阳性

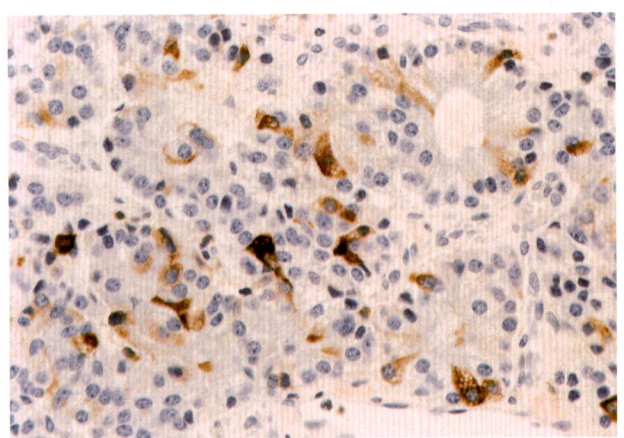

图9.33　无功能性胰腺内分泌肿瘤。免疫过氧化物酶染色，α链hCG有少数几个细胞呈阳性

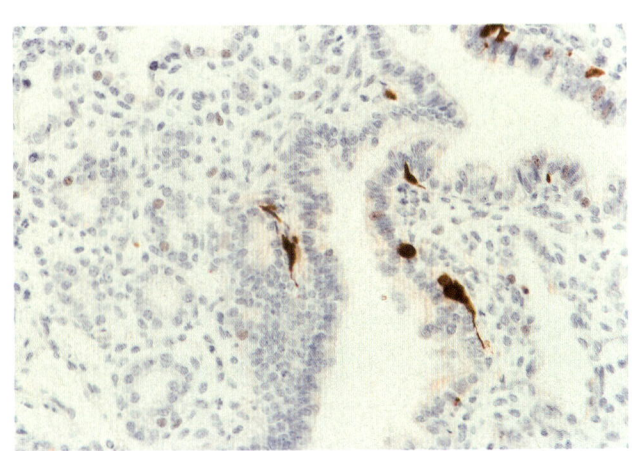

图9.34　胎肺。免疫过氧化物酶染色，胃泌素释放肽呈单个细胞阳性

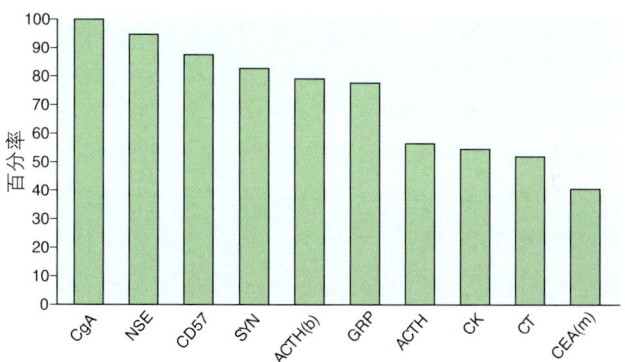

图9.35 经典型肺类癌标记物分布图。[CgA；NSE，神经特异性烯醇化酶；SYN，突触素；ACTH（b），大促肾上腺皮质激素；GRP，胃泌素释放肽；ACTH，促肾上腺皮质激素；CK，细胞角蛋白；CT，降钙素；CEA（m），单克隆癌胚抗原]

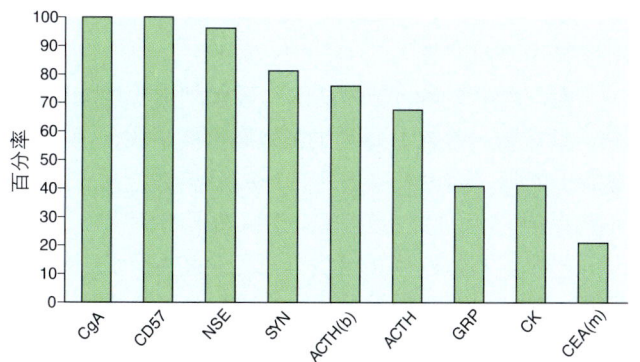

图9.36 不典型肺类癌标记物分布图。[CgA，嗜铬素A；NSE，神经特异性烯醇化酶；SYN，突触素；ACTH（b），大促肾上腺皮质激素；ACTH，促肾上腺皮质激素；GRP，胃泌素释放肽；CK，细胞角蛋白；CEA（m），单克隆癌胚抗原]

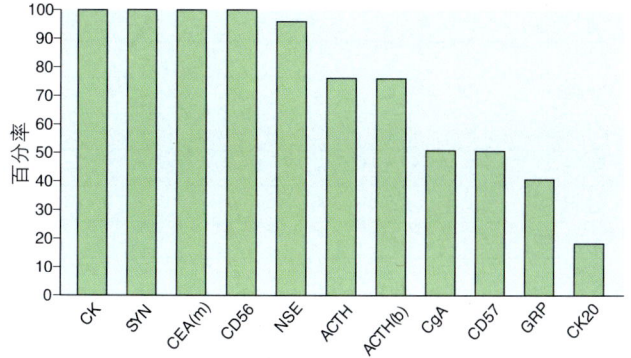

图9.37 小细胞癌标记物分布图。[CK，细胞角蛋白；SYN，突触素；CEA（m），单克隆癌胚抗原；NSE，神经特异性烯醇化酶；ACTH，促肾上腺皮质激素；ACTH（b），大促肾上腺皮质激素；CgA，嗜铬素A；GRP，胃泌素释放肽]

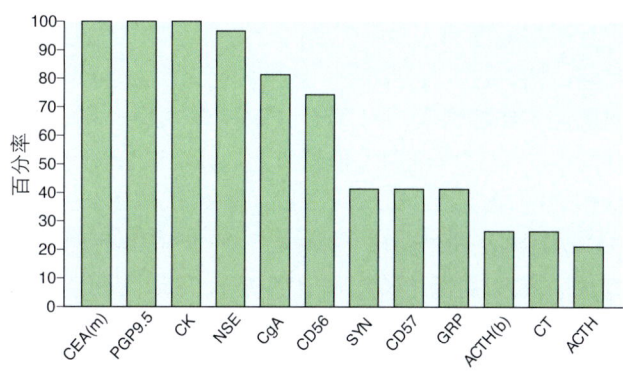

图9.38 大细胞神经内分泌癌标记物分布图。[CEA（m），单克隆癌胚抗原；PGP9.5，蛋白基因产物9.5；CK，细胞角蛋白；NSE，神经特异性烯醇化酶；CgA，嗜铬素A；SYN，突触素；GRP，胃泌素释放肽；ACTH（b），大促肾上腺皮质激素；CT，降钙素；ACTH，促肾上腺皮质激素]

20例高分化肺神经内分泌肿瘤（包括经典型类癌、不典型类癌）中有19例（95%）以及10例转移癌中的8例（80%）表达TTF-1[250]。相反，他们还报道了所有小肠神经内分泌肿瘤均不表达TTF-1。罕见情况下可表达于胃肠及胰腺神经内分泌瘤[251]。支气管源性小细胞神经内分泌癌TTF-1常呈阳性。

所有类型的肺神经内分泌肿瘤中95%以上表达NSE[248]。依赖抗原修复技术和灵敏的检测方法，CgA表达于100%的经典型、不典型类癌，80%的大细胞神经内分泌癌，50%以上的小细胞癌。Syn表达于84%的经典型、80%的不典型类癌，40%的大细胞神经内分泌癌，100%的小细胞癌。CD57表达于89%的经典型、100%的不典型类癌，40%的大细胞神经内分泌癌，50%的小细胞癌。肺微神经内分泌瘤（tumorlet）CD57也呈阳性表达（图9.39）。单克隆CEA100%表

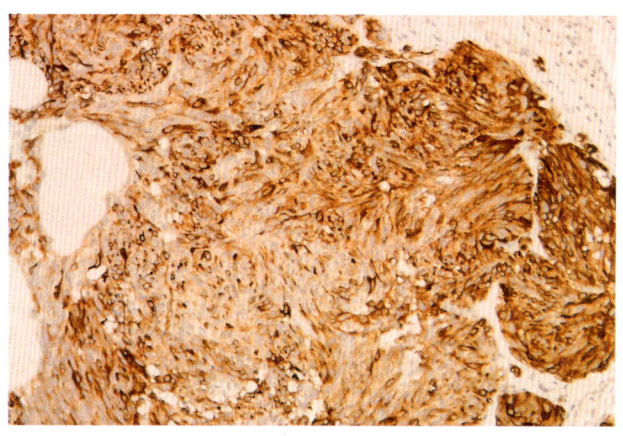

图9.39 肺微神经内分泌瘤。免疫过氧化物酶染色Leu7在病变细胞中呈阳性表达

达于小细胞癌和大细胞神经内分泌癌，42%的经典型类癌、20%的不典型类癌。这些肿瘤还表达多种不同的肽类，如降钙素、ACTH、胃泌素释放肽。Jiang及其同事[252]也对大细胞癌作了研究，证实了Travis及其合作者的发现[248]。此外，Jiang报道了PGP49.5可100%阳性表达，TuJ1（神经特异性Ⅲβ微管蛋白）表达于82%病例，NCAM阳性率为73%[252]。

其他部位神经内分泌肿瘤

子宫颈

类癌、小细胞癌和大细胞神经内分泌癌都可原发于子宫颈[253-255]。子宫颈所有小细胞癌CK均呈阳性表达；EMA阳性率大于90%。多聚抗血清CEA反应活性为77%。CK20、TTF-1分别表达于14.3%、20%的肿瘤[256-258]。至于神经内分泌标记物，NSE95%阳性，Syn46%阳性，CgA43%阳性，CD5730%阳性（图9.39）。更多最新研究与该结果一致[259-261]。这些肿瘤还可表达肽类和胺类激素，包括5-羟色胺（31%）、ACTH（23%）、生长抑素（8%）。

Stoler及其合作者对18型人类乳头状瘤病毒（HPV18）研究表明，78%的伴神经内分泌分化的子宫颈小细胞癌HPV18呈阳性[262]。更多最新研究证实了这类肿瘤中HPV18的高发率[260,263]。而且，一种与HPV感染有关的周期蛋白酶依赖性激酶抑制子——p16，其过表达的情况几乎在所有的病例均很显著（31例中的30例，96.8%）[260,263]。极少数情况下也有HPV16表达[260]。

所有子宫颈大细胞神经内分泌肿瘤均可表达CgA[255]。该研究中，Syn的阳性率为66%，NSE为50%

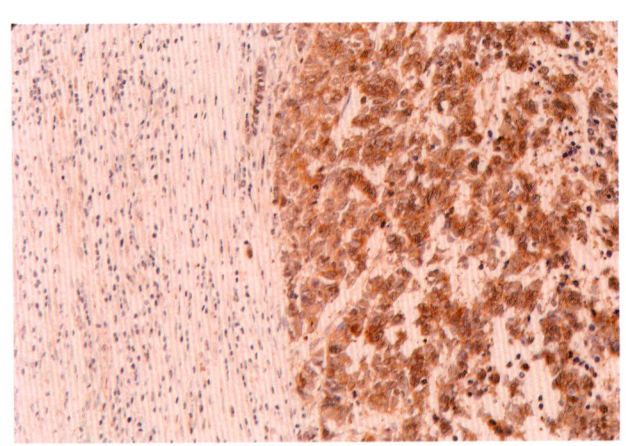

图9.40 子宫颈大细胞（神经内分泌）癌。免疫过氧化物酶染色，NSE在肿瘤细胞中呈阳性表达

（图9.40）。50%的病例可查见少数5-羟色胺阳性表达的细胞，37%的病例可查见生长抑素阳性表达的细胞。其他报道与之相似[264]。75%的病例表达CEA单克隆抗体。与小细胞癌不同，子宫颈大细胞神经内分泌癌与HPV16感染有关。Grayson及其合作者研究的12例中有7例HPV16呈阳性；另有2例HPV18呈阳性[265]。最近，Matthews-Greer等报道了另外两例HPV16呈阳性的大细胞神经内分泌癌[266]。

前列腺

正常前列腺上皮有一小部分神经内分泌细胞可用NSE、嗜铬素、肽激素和5-羟色胺来识别[267-269]。伴有神经内分泌分化的前列腺肿瘤包括类癌、小细胞癌和常见腺癌伴有少量神经内分泌细胞。纯粹的神经内分泌癌如类癌、小细胞癌罕见，只占前列腺恶性肿瘤的不足5%[270-277]。前列腺小细胞癌TTF-1近50%呈阳性（表9.4）[257,276]。

而225例Gleason分级高的一般前列腺腺癌均呈阴性[273]。尽管一些报道猜测小细胞癌可能来源于前列腺多能干细胞，因为其既表达神经内分泌标记又表达前列腺特异性标记物，但其真正来源尚不明了[271,274,275]。

一般前列腺癌伴神经内分泌分化可见于近10%的病例，至少会出现灶性或明显的神经内分泌细胞[270]。神经内分泌分化在判断非雄激素依赖性肿瘤和转移癌上较之于激素敏感性及局部复发性肿瘤更为重要[268]。

表9.4 各个部位小细胞癌的免疫组化表达情况*
（参考文献89, 274, 275, 298, 299a）

解剖部位/起源	TTF-1	CK-7	CK20	ER/PR	PSA	PAP
肺	+	S	S	-	-	-
前列腺	S	S	S	-	S	S
膀胱	S	-	-	-	-	-
乳腺	S	+	-	S	-	-
甲状腺**	S	?	?	-	-	-
胃肠	S	?	S	-	-	-
涎腺	S	?	S	-	-	-
子宫颈	S	?	S	?	-	-
皮肤（Merkel细胞）	-	-	+	-	-	-

+，几乎总是阳性；S，有时阳性；-，阴性
*神经内分泌特异性抗体，如嗜铬素和突触素在所有部位肿瘤中均有不同程度表达，因此不作此用
** 除髓样癌TTF-1典型阳性外，其他非髓性甲状腺小细胞癌也可阳性TTF-1，甲状腺转录因子；CK，细胞角蛋白；ER，雌激素受体；PR，孕激素受体；PSA，前列腺特异性抗原；PAP，前列腺酸性磷酸酶

伴神经内分泌分化的腺癌，54%5-羟色胺呈阳性表达，46%NSE呈阳性表达，65%嗜铬素呈阳性表达，22%hCG呈阳性表达（图9.41）。生长抑素、降钙素、ACTH的阳性率均不足5%[277]。Schmid及其合作者认为嗜铬素的分布形式与肿瘤分级有关[269]。Ⅰ级CgA、CgB、分泌素Ⅱ呈阳性，3种标记物表达于大部分神经内分泌细胞的同一部位。相反，Ⅱ级、Ⅲ级中主要表达CgB颗粒。88%的前列腺高级别上皮内瘤变中查见散在的神经内分泌细胞[277]。其中大部分表达5-羟色胺（73%）、NSE（67%）、嗜铬素（62%）、hCG（30%）。

皮肤

皮肤Merkel细胞（神经内分泌）癌（Merkel cell carcinoma）并不常见，最先由Toker误认为梁状癌[278]。这些肿瘤一致表达广谱CK；97%的病例CK20呈点状阳性（图9.42，表9.4）[229, 279]。许多其他研究证实了CK20的高表达率[280-283]。其他表达CK20的小细胞恶性肿瘤包括支气管源性小细胞癌（0.03%）、子宫颈小细胞癌（9%）和涎腺源性小细胞癌（60%）（表9.4）。Nagoa及其合作者报道起源于涎腺的15例小细胞癌中有11例（73%）CK20呈阳性，几乎都表现为核周的点状阳性[284]。Cheuk等报道了许多部位的小细胞癌不表达CK20，包括胃肠道、胰腺、前列腺、膀胱、胸腺和眼眶，除了2例子宫颈/阴道源性病例表达[281]。Merkel细胞癌CK7阳性率为25%，但13例病例CK5/6、CK17均呈阴性[285]，78%的病例EMA呈阳性[286]，还可表达微管相关蛋白[287]，但TTF-1呈阴性[89]。

事实上所有的Merkel细胞癌均表达NSE[288]。CgB、CgA分别表达于100%、72%的肿瘤。起源于分泌素Ⅱ的分泌神经素表达于22%的病例，Syn表达于39%的病例[289]。CD99呈不同程度阳性。Nicholson及其合作者的系列研究中，30例中有12例（40%）CD99呈阳性表达[283]。9例临床表现为Merkel细胞癌的病例，CD99呈阳性，CK20呈阴性表达[283]。CD117（c-kit）也呈不同程度阳性。也有研究报道c-kit阳性病例高达95.5%（22例中的21例），另有报道呈低表达59.0%（22例中的13例）[290-292]。肺小细胞癌c-kit呈阳性表达[290]。还有报道上皮钙黏素表达于Merkel细胞癌的细胞核，有助于该肿瘤的诊断[293, 294]。

乳腺

乳腺神经内分泌肿瘤包括类癌及小细胞性神经内分泌癌（图9.43A）[295-297]。小细胞癌CK呈典型的阳性，包括CK AE1/AE3（91%）、CAM5.2（82%）、CK7（78%）和CK19（78%），而CK20呈阴性表达（表9.4）[298]。这些肿瘤的神经内分泌表达并不典型，且各种标记物的表达都有所不同。但需要强调的是，与其他部位小细胞神经内分泌癌一样，根据免疫组化结果来判定乳腺癌神经内分泌分化并非偶然[298]。在神经内分泌标记物中，NSE表达于90%的病例，而Syn、Cg分别为56%和41%（图9.43B）。CD56和CD57分别表达于78%和43%的病例。

降钙素表达见于27%的病例，而胃泌素释放肽和5-羟色胺分别表达于39%和14%的病例，雌激素和孕激素受体阳性表达率分别为54%和45%。bcl-2呈恒定阳性，而HER-2/neu呈阴性[298]。CD99在3例小细胞癌中均阳性表达，而12例中有11例（92%）上皮钙黏素呈细胞膜阳性[299-301]。TTF-1阳性表达于近20%的病例[299a]。

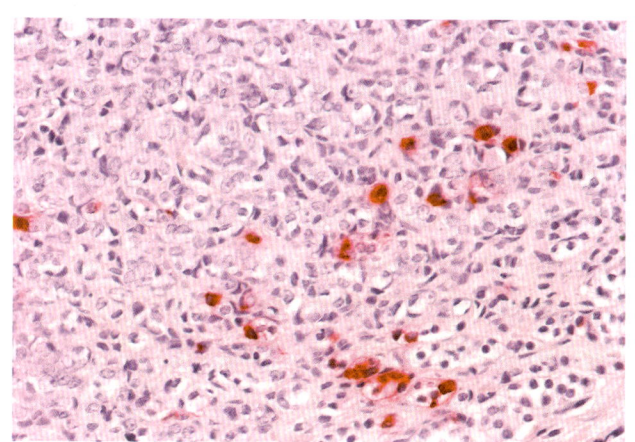

图9.41　含神经内分泌细胞的前列腺转移癌。免疫过氧化物酶染色，CgA在少数肿瘤细胞呈阳性表达

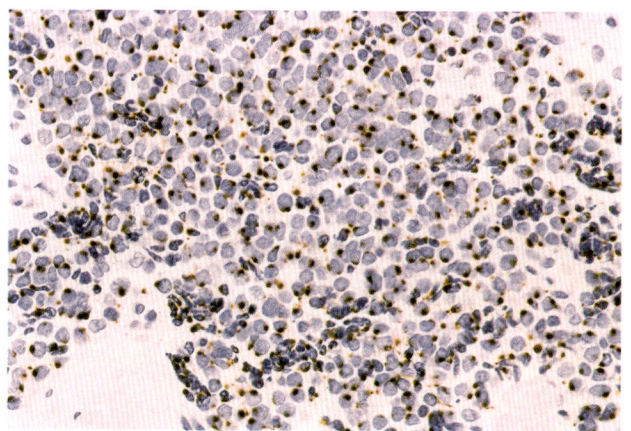

图9.42　Merkel细胞癌。免疫过氧化物酶染色，CK20着色呈点状

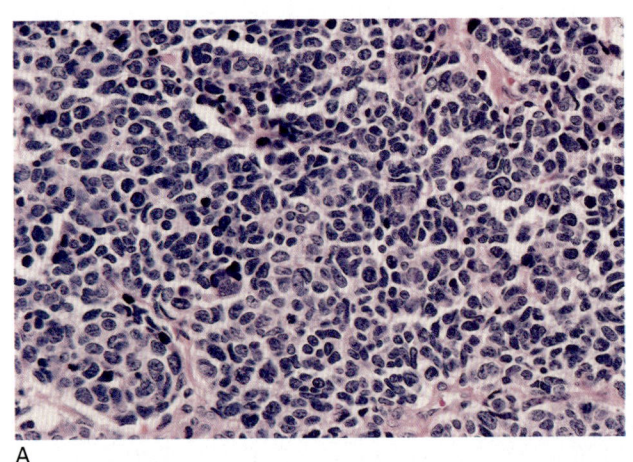
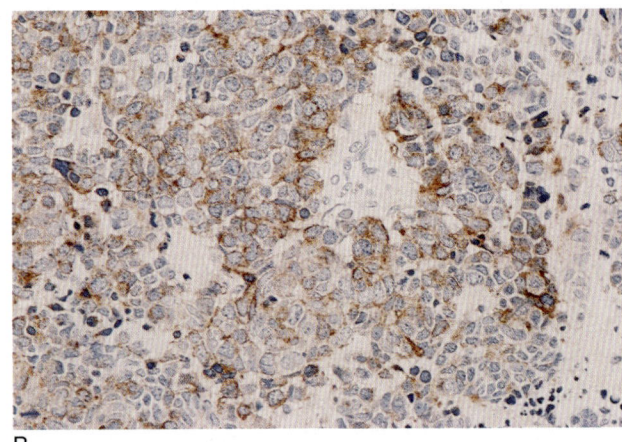

图9.43 乳腺小细胞（神经内分泌）癌。（A）HE染色；（B）免疫过氧化物酶染色，CgA在细胞浆内呈中等强度表达

胸腺

胸腺神经内分泌肿瘤包括类癌、非典型类癌和小细胞癌。从组织形态学上，单个肿瘤往往具有从类癌到小细胞癌的综合特征[303, 304]。肿瘤均可典型表达CK（AE1/AE3和CAM5.2），并阳性表达NSE（100%）、Syn（81%）、Cg（75%）和CD57（67.5%）等大量神经内分泌标记物，也可表达α链hCG（100%）、β链hCG（37.5%）、生长抑素（33%）、ACTH（30%）、CGRP（25%）、胆囊收缩素（17%）、降钙素（10%）和5-羟色胺（5%）等糖蛋白、肽类激素和胺[304-311]。与肺神经内分泌肿瘤相反，胸腺神经内分泌肿瘤TTF-1呈阴性。

致谢

谨向助手Dennis Frisman表示感谢，并感谢其网站ImmunoHistoQuery所提供的图表中的大量数据！

谨向Joanne Harker女士在手稿整理过程中的辛勤劳动表示衷心的感谢！

参考文献

1. DeLellis RA, Wolfe HJ. Contributions of immunohistochemical and molecular biological techniques to endocrine pathology. J Histochem Cytochem 1987; 35:1347–1351.
2. DeLellis RA. Endocrine tumors. In: Colvin RB, Bhan AK, McCluskey RT, eds. Diagnostic immunopathology. New York: Raven Press; 1995:551–578.
3. DeLellis RA, Wolfe HJ. Analysis of gene expression in endocrine cells. In: Fenoglio-Preiser CM, Williman CL, eds. Molecular diagnostics in pathology. Baltimore: Williams & Wilkins; 1991:299–323.
4. Lloyd RV, Jin L, Kulig E, et al. Molecular approaches for the analysis of chromogranins and secretogranins. Diagn Mol Pathol 1992; 1:2–15.
5. Portela-Gomes GM, Stridsberg M, Grimelius L, et al. Expression of five different somatostatin receptor subtypes in endocrine cells of the pancreas. Appl Immunohistochem 2000; 8:126–132.
6. DeLellis RA, Tischler AS. The dispersed neuroendocrine cell system. In: Kovacs K, Asa SL, eds. Functional endocrine pathology. Oxford, Blackwell Science; 1998:529–549.
7. Lauweryns JM, Van Ranst L. Immunocytochemical localization of aromatic l-amino acid decarboxylase in human, rat and mouse bronchopulmonary and gastrointestinal endocrine cells. J Histochem Cytochem 1988; 36:1181–1186.
8. Lloyd RV, Sisson JC, Shapiro B, et al. Immunohistochemical localization of epinephrine, norepinephrine, catecholamine-synthesizing enzymes and chromogranin in neuroendocrine cells and tumors. Am J Pathol 1986; 125:45–54.
9. Lloyd RV, Jin L, Qian X, et al. Analysis of the chromogranin A post-translational cleavage product pancreastatin and the prohormone convertases PC2 and PC3 in normal and neoplastic human pituitaries. Am J Pathol 1995; 146:1188–1198.
10. Scopsi L, Gullo M, Rilke F, et al. Proprotein convertases (PC1/PC3 and PC2) in normal and neoplastic tissues: Their use as markers of neuroendocrine differentiation. J Clin Endocrinol Metab 1995; 80:294–301.
11. Scopsi L, Lee R, Gullo M, et al. Peptidylglycine, an amidating monooxygenase in neuroendocrine tumors: Its identification, characterization, quantification and relation to the grade of

12. morphologic differentiation, amidated peptide content and granin immunocytochemistry. Appl Immunohistochem 1998: 6:120–132.

12. Schmechel D, Marangos PJ, Brightman M. Neurone-specific enolase is a molecular marker for peripheral and central neuroendocrine cells. Nature 1978; 276:834–836.

13. Haimoto H, Takahashi Y, Koshikawa T, et al. Immunohistochemical localization of gamma enolase in normal human tissues other than nervous and neuroendocrine tissue. Lab Invest 1985; 52:257–263.

14. Schmechel DE. Gamma submit of the glycolytic enzyme enolase: Nonspecific or neuron specific? Lab Invest 1985; 52:239–242.

15. Seshi B, True L, Carter D, et al. Immunohistochemical characterization of a set of monoclonal antibodies to human neuron-specific enolase. Am J Pathol 1988; 131: 258–269.

16. Rode J, Dillon AP, Doran JF, et al. PGP 9.5, a new marker for human neuroendocrine tumors. Histopathology 1985; 9: 147–158.

17. Li GL, Farooque M, Holtz A, et al. Expression of the ubiquitin carboxyl-terminal hydrolase PGP 9.5 in axons following spinal cord compression trauma. APMIS 1997; 105:384–390.

18. Wilson PO, Barber PC, Hamid QA, et al. The immuno-localization of protein gene product 9.5 using rabbit polyclonal and mouse monoclonal antibodies. Br J Exp Pathol 1988; 69: 91–104.

19. Bordi C, Pilato FP, D'Adda T. Comparative study of several neuroendocrine markers in pancreatic endocrine tumors. Virchows Arch A Pathol Anat Histopathol 1988; 413:387–398.

20. Tezel E, Hibi K, Nagasaka T, et al. PGP9.5 as a prognostic factor in pancreatic cancer. Clin Cancer Res 2000; 6:4764–4767.

21. Mendelsohn G. Histaminase localization in medullary thyroid carcinoma and small cell lung carcinoma. In: DeLellis RA, ed. Diagnostic immunohistochemistry. New York: Masson; 1981:299–312.

22. Sasano H, Mason JI, Sasano N. Immunohistochemical analysis of cytochrome P450 17 alpha in human adrenocortical disorders. Hum Pathol 1989; 20:113–117.

23. Sasano H, Okamoto M, Sasano N. Immunohistochemical study of cytochrome P-450 11b hydroxylase in human adrenal cortex with mineralo- and glucocorticoid excess. Virchows Arch A Pathol Anat Histopathol 1988; 413:313–318.

24. Sasano H, Okamoto M, Mason JI, et al. Immunohistochemical studies of steroidogenic enzymes (aromatase, 17 alpha-hydroxylase and cholesterol side chain cleavage cytochrome P450) in sex cord stromal tumors of the ovary. Hum Pathol 1989; 20:452–457.

25. Lloyd RV, Wilson BS. Specific endocrine tissue marker defined by a monoclonal antibody. Science 1983; 222:628–630.

26. O'Connor DT, Burton D, Deftos LJ. Chromogranin A: Immunohistology reveals its universal occurrence in normal polypeptide hormone producing endocrine glands. Life Sci 1983; 33:1657–1663.

27. Wilson BS, Lloyd RV. Detection of chromogranin in neuroendocrine cells with a monoclonal antibody. Am J Pathol 1984; 115:458–468.

28. Hagn C, Schmid KW, Fischer-Colbrie R, et al. Chromogranin A, B, and C in human adrenal medulla and endocrine tissues. Lab Invest 1986; 55:405–411.

29. Huttner WB, Gerdes H-H, Rosa P. Chromogranins/secretogranins – widespread constituents of the secre-tory granule matrix in endocrine cells and neurons. In: Langley K, Gratzl M, eds. Markers for neural and endocrine cells: molecular and cell biology. Weinhein, VCH, 1991.

30. Portela-Gomes MG, Hacker GW, Weitgasser R. Neuroendocrine cell markers for pancreatic islets and tumors. Appl Immunohistochem Mol Morphol 2004; 12:183–192.

31. Fahrenkamp AG, Wibbeke C, Winde G. Immunohistochemical distribution of chromogranins A and B and secretogranin II in neuroendocrine tumors of the gastrointestinal tract. Virchows Arch 1995; 426:361–367.

32. Schmid KW, Kroll M, Hittmair A, et al. Chromogranin A and B in adenomas of the pituitary: An immunohistochemical study of 42 cases. Am J Surg Pathol 1991; 15:1072–1077.

33. Buffa R, Pelagi M, Siccardi AG, et al. Identification of the endocrine cells detected by the monoclonal antibody HISL-19 in human tissues. Basic Appl Histochem 1990; 34:259–268.

34. Riddel K, Tippens D, Gown AM. PHE5: A new monoclonal antibody to a unique neuroendocrine granule protein. Lab Invest 1987; 56:64A.

35. Krisch K, Horvat G, Krisch I, et al. Immunochemical characterization of a novel secretory protein (defined by monoclonal antibody HISL-19) of peptide hormone producing cells

which is distinct from chromogranin A, B and C. Lab Invest 1988; 58:411–420.

36. Gould VE, Lee I, Wiedenmann B, et al. Synaptophysin: A novel marker for neurons, certain neuroendocrine cells and their neoplasms. Hum Pathol 1986; 17:979–983.

37. Komminoth P, Roth J, Schroder S, et al. Overlapping expression of immunohistochemical markers and synaptophysin mRNA in pheochromocytomas and adrenocortical carcinomas: Implications for the differential diagnosis of adrenal gland tumors. Lab Invest 1995; 72:424–431.

38. Portela-Gomes GM, Lukinius GM, Grimelius L. Synaptic vesicle protein 2: A new neuroendocrine cell marker. Am J Pathol 2000; 157:1299–1309.

39. Jakobsen AM, Anderson P, Saglik G, et al. Differential expression of vesicular monoamine transporter (VMAT) 1 and 2 in gastrointestinal endocrine tumors. J Pathol 2001; 195: 463–472.

40. Gut A, Kiraly CE, Fukuda M, et al. Expression and localization of synaptotagmin isoforms in endocrine beta cells: their function in insulin exocytosos. J Cell Sci 2001; 114;1709–1716.

41. Adolfsen B, Saraswati S, Yoshihara M, et al. Synaptotagmins are trafficked to distinct subcellular domains including the postsynaptic compartment. J Cell Bol 2004; 166:249–260.

42. Regazzi R, Wolheim CB, Lang J, et al. VAMP-2 and cellubrevin are expressed in pancreatic beta cells and are essential for Ca(2+) but not for GTP gamma S-induced insulin secretion EMBO J 1995; 14:2723–2730.

42a. Wiedenmann B, John M, Ahnert-Hilger G, Riecken E-O. Molecular and cell biological aspects of neuroendocrine tumors of the gastrointestinal tract. J Mol Med 1998; 76:637–647.

43. Arber DA, Weirs LM. CD57: A review. Appl Immunohistochem 1995; 3:137–152.

44. McGarry RC, Helfand SL, Quarles RH, et al. Recognition of the myelin associated glycoprotein by the monoclonal antibody HNK-1. Nature 1983; 306:376–378.

45. Tischler AS, Mobtaker H, Mann K, et al. Anti-lymphocyte antibody Leu 7 (HNK-1) recognizes a constituent of neuroendocrine granule matrix. J Histochem Cytochem 1986; 34: 1213–1216.

46. Ghali VS, Jimenez EJS, Garcia RL. Distribution of Leu 7 antigen (HNK-1) in thyroid tumors: Its usefulness as a diagnostic marker for follicular and papillary carcinomas. Hum Pathol 1992; 23:21–25.

47. Langley K, Gratzl M. Neural cell adhesion molecule (NCAM) in neural and endocrine cells. In: Langley K, Gratzl M, eds. Markers for neural and endocrine cells: molecular and cell biology. diagnostic applications. Weinheim VCH, 1991:133–177.

48. Shipley WR, Hammer RD, Lennington WJ, et al. Paraffin immunohistochemical detection of CD56, a useful marker for neural cell adhesion molecule in normal and neoplastic fixed tissues. Appl Immunohistochem 1997; 5:87–93.

49. Jin L, Hemperly JJ, Lloyd RV. Expression of neural cell adhesion molecule in normal and neoplastic human neuroendocrine tissues. Am J Pathol 1991; 138:961–969.

50. Komminoth P, Roth J, Saremaslani P, et al. Polysialic acid of the neural cell adhesion molecule in the human thyroid: A marker for medullary thyroid carcinoma and primary C-cell hyperplasia: An immunohistochemical study on 79 thyroid lesions. Am J Surg Pathol 1994; 18:399–411.

51. Komminoth P, Roth J, Lackie PM, et al. Polysialic acid of the neural cell adhesion molecule distinguishes small cell lung carcinoma from carcinoids. Am J Pathol 1991; 139:297–304.

52. Fuchs E, Weber K. Intermediate filaments: Structure, dynamics, function and disease. Ann Rev Biochem 1994; 63: 345–382.

53. Hoefler H, Denk H, Lackinger E, et al. Immunocytochemical demonstration of intermediate filament cytoskeleton proteins in human endocrine tissues and (neuro-) endocrine tumors. Virchows Arch A Pathol Anat Histopathol 1986; 409: 609–626.

54. O'Hara BJ, Paetau A, Miettinen M. Keratin subsets and monoclonal antibody to HBME-1 in chordoma: Immunohistochemical differential diagnosis between tumors simulating chordoma. Hum Pathol 1998; 29:119–126.

55. Wang NP, Zee S, Zarbo RJ, et al. Coordinate expression of cytokeratins 7 and 20 defines unique subsets of carcinomas. Appl Immunohistochem 1995; 3:99–107.

56. Trojanowski JQ, Lee VM, Schlaepfer WW. An immunohistochemical study of human central and peripheral nervous system tumors, using monoclonal antibodies against neurofilaments and glial filaments. Hum Pathol 1984; 15: 248–257.

57. Perez MA, Saul SH, Trojanowski JQ. Neurofilament and

chromogranin expression in normal and neoplastic neuroendocrine cells of the human gastrointestinal tract and pancreas. Cancer 1990; 65:1219–1227.
58. Kulig E, Lloyd RV. Transcription factors and endocrine disease. Endocr Pathol 1996; 1:245–250.
59. Reubi JC, Kappeler A, Waser B, et al. Immunohistochemical localization of somatostatin receptors sst2A in human tumors. Am J Pathol 1998; 153:233–245.
60. Erickson LA, Jin L, Wollen P, et al. Parathyroid hyperplasia, adenomas and carcinomas: differential expression of p27 Kip1 protein. AM J Surg Pathol 1999; 23:288–295.
61. LaRosa S, Sessa F, Capella C, et al. Prognostic criteria in non-functioning pancreatic endocrine tumors. Virchows Arc 1996; 429:323–333.
62. DeLellis RA. Proliferation markers in neuroendocrine tumors: useful or useless? A critical reappraisal. Verh Dtsch Ges Pathol 1997; 81:53–61.
63. Asa SL. Atlas of tumor pathology: tumors of the pituitary gland. Washington, DC: Armed Forces Institute of Pathology; 1998.
64. Girod C, Trouillar J, Dubois MP. Immunocytochemical localization of S100 protein in stellate cells (folliculo-stellate cells) of the anterior lobe of the normal human pituitary. Cell Tissue Res 1985; 241:505–511.
65. Lloyd RV, Cano M, Rosa P, et al. Distribution of chromogranin A and secretogranin I (chromogranin B) in neuroendocrine cells and tumors. Am J Pathol 1988; 130:296–304.
66. Erickson LA, Lloyd RV. Practical markers used in the diagnosis of endocrine tumors. Adv Anat Pathol 2004; 11:175–189.
67. Hofler H, Walter GF, Denk H. Immunohistochemistry of folliculo-stellate cells in normal human adenohypophyses and in pituitary adenomas. Acta Neuropathol (Berl) 1994; 65:35–40.
68. DeLellis RA, Lloyd RV, Heitz P, et al. Tumours of the endocrine organs. WHO Classification of Tumours. 2004.
69. Thappar K, Kovacs K, Scheithauer BW, et al. Proliferative activity and invasiveness among pituitary adenomas and carcinomas: an analysis using the MIB-1 antibody. Neurosurg 1996; 38:99–106.
70. Thappar K, Schaithauer BW, Kovacs K, et al. p53 expression in pituitary adenomas and carcinomas: correlation with invasiveness and tumor growth fractions. Neurosurg 1996; 38:765–771.
71. Burger PC, Scheithauer BW. Atlas of tumor pathology: tumors of the central nervous system. Third Series. Washington, DC: Armed Forces Institute of Pathology; 1994.
72. Coca S, Vaquero J, Escandon J, et al. Immunohistochemical characterization of pineocytomas. Clin Neuropathol 1992; 11: 298–303.
73. Hayashi K, Hoshida Y, Horie Y, et al. Immunohistochemical study on the distribution of α and β subunits of S100 protein in brain tumors. Acta Neuropathol (Berl) 1991; 81:657–663.
74. Korf HW, Klein DC, Zigler JS, et al. S-antigen-like immunoreactivity in a human pineocytoma. Acta Neuropathol (Berl) 1986; 69:165–167.
75. Perentes E, Rubinstein LJ, Herman MM, et al. S-antigen immunoreactivity in human pineal glands and pineal parenchymal tumors: A monoclonal antibody study. Acta Neuropathol (Berl) 1986; 71:224–227.
76. Bocker W, Dralle H, Dorn G. Thyroglobulin: An immunohistochemical marker in thyroid disease. In: DeLellis RA, ed. Diagnostic immunohistochemistry. New York: Masson; 1981:37–60.
77. Sambade C, Franssila K, Cameselle-Teijeiro J, et al. Hyalinizing trabecular adenoma: A misnomer for a peculiar tumor of the thyroid gland. Endocr Pathol 1991; 2:83–91.
78. Hirokawa M, Carney JA. Cell membrane and cytoplasmic staining for MIB-1 in hyalinizing trabecular adenoma of the thyroid. Am J Surg Pathol 2000; 24:575–578.
79. Berge-Lefranc JL, Cartouzou G, DeMicco C, et al. Quantification of thyroglobulin messenger RNA by in-situ hybridization in differentiated thyroid cancers: Difference between well-differentiated and moderately differentiated histologic types. Cancer 1985; 56:345–350.
80. Keen CE, Szakacs S, Okon E, et al. CA125 and thyroglobulin staining in papillary carcinomas of thyroid and ovarian origin is not entirely specific for site of origin. Histopathology 1999; 34:113–117.
81. Carcangiu ML, Zampi G, Rosai J. Poorly differentiated ('insular') thyroid carcinoma: A reinterpretation of Langhans' 'wuchernde Struma.' Am J Surg Pathol 1984; 8:655–668.
82. Ordonez NG, El-Naggar AK, Hickey RC, et al. Anaplastic thyroid carcinoma: Immunocytochemical study of 32 cases. Am J Clin Pathol 1991; 96:15–24.

83. Carcangiu ML, Steeper T, Zampi G, et al. Anaplastic thyroid cancer: A study of 70 cases. Am J Clin Pathol 1985; 83:135–158.

84. Kawaoi A, Okano T, Nemoto N, et al. Simultaneous detection of thyroglobulin (T_g), thyroxine (T_4) and tri-iodothyronine (T_3) in nontoxic thyroid tumors by the immunoperoxidase method. Am J Pathol 1982; 108:39–49.

85. Lau SK, Luthringer DJ, Eisen RN. Thyroid transcription factor-1: a review. Appl Immunohistochem Mol Morphol 2002; 10:97–102.

86. Ordonez NG. Thyroid transcription factor 1 is a marker of lung and thyroid carcinomas. Adv Anat Pathol 2000; 7:123–127.

87. Kaufmann O, Dietel M. Thyroid transcription factor-1 is the superior immunohistochemical marker for pulmonary adenocarcinomas and large cell carcinomas compared to surfactant proteins A and B. Histopathology 2000; 36:8–16.

88. Byrd-Gloster AL, Khoor A, Glass LF, et al. Differential expression of thyroid transcription factor-1 in small cell lung carcinoma and Merkel cell tumor. Hum Pathol 2000; 31:58–62.

89. Agoff SN, Lamps LW, Philip AT, et al. Thyroid transcription factor-1 is expressed in extrapulmonary small cell carcinomas but not in other extrapulmonary neuroendocrine tumors. Mod Pathol 2000; 13:238–242.

90. Henzen-Logmans SC, Mullink H, Ramaekers FC, et al. Expression of cytokeratins and vimentin in epithelial cells of normal and pathologic thyroid tissue. Virchows Arch A Pathol Anat Histopathol 1987; 410:347–354.

91. Miettinen M, Franssila K, Lehto V-P, et al. Expression of intermediate filament proteins in thyroid gland and thyroid tumors. Lab Invest 1984; 50:262–270.

92. Viale G, Dell'Orto P, Coggi G, et al. Co-expression of cytokeratins and vimentin in normal and diseased thyroid glands: Lack of diagnostic utility of vimentin immunostaining. Am J Surg Pathol 1989; 13:1034–1040.

93. Schelfhout LJDM, van Muijen GN, Fleuren GJ. Expression of keratin 19 distinguishes papillary thyroid carcinoma from follicular carcinomas and follicular thyroid adenoma. Am J Clin Pathol 1989; 92:654–658.

94. Raphael SJ, McKeown-Eyssen G, Asa SL. High molecular weight cytokeratin and cytokeratin 19 in the diagnosis of thyroid tumors. Mod Pathol 1994; 7:295–300.

95. Fonseca E, Nesland JM, Hoie J, et al. Pattern of expression of intermediate cytokeratin filaments in the thyroid gland: An immunohistochemical study of simple and stratified epithelial-type cytokeratins. Virchows Arch 1997; 430:239–245.

96. Miettinen M, Kovatich AJ, Karkkainen P. Keratin subsets in papillary and follicular thyroid lesions: A paraffin section analysis with diagnostic implications. Virchows Arch 1997: 431:407–413.

97. Baloch ZW, Abraham S, Roberts S, et al. Differential expression of cytokeratins in follicular variant of papillary carcinoma: An immunohistochemical study and its diagnostic utility. Hum Pathol 1999; 30:1166–1171.

98. Kragsterman B, Grimelius L, Wallin G, et al. Cytokeratin 19 expression in papillary thyroid carcinoma. Appl Immunohistochem 1999; 7:181–185.

99. Fonseca E, Nesland J, Sobrinho-Simoes M. Expression of stratified epithelial cytokeratins in hyalinizing trabecular adenoma supports their relationship with papillary carcinoma of the thyroid. Histopathology 1997; 31:330–335.

100. Hirokawa M, Carney JA, Ohtsuki Y. Hyalinizing trabecular adenoma and papillary carcinoma of the thyroid express different cytokeratin patterns. Am J Surg Pathol 2000; 24:877–881.

101. Liberman E, Weidner N. Papillary and follicular neoplasms of the thyroid gland: Differential immunohistochemical staining with high molecular weight keratin and involucrin. Appl Immunohistochem 2000; 8:42–48.

102. Sack MJ, Astengo-Osuna C, Lin BT, et al. HBME-1 immunostaining in thyroid fine needle aspirations: A useful marker in the diagnosis of carcinoma. Mod Pathol 1997; 10: 668–674.

103. Miettinen M, Karkkainen P. Differential HBME-1 reactivity in benign vs. malignant thyroid tissue is helpful in the diagnosis of thyroid tumors [abstract]. Mod Pathol 1996; 5:50A.

104. Mase T, Funahashi H, Koshikawa T, et al. HBME-1 immunostaining in thyroid tumors, especially in follicular neoplasms. Endocr J 2003; 50:173–177.

105. Casey MB, Lohse CM, Lloyd RV. Distinction between papillary thyroid hyperplasia and papillary thyroid carcinoma by immunohistochemical staining for cytokeratin 19, galectin-3 and HBME-1. Endocr Pathol 2003; 14:55–60.

106. Xu XC, el-Nagger AK, Lotan R. Differential expression of galectin-1 and galectin-3 in thyroid tumors. Potential diag-

nostic implications. Am J Pathol 1995; 147:815–822.
107. Fernandez PL, Merino MJ, Gomez M, et al. Galectin-3 and laminin expression in neoplastic and non-neoplastic thyroid tissue. J. Pathol 1997; 181:80–86.
108. Orlandi F, Saggiorato E, Pivano G, et al. Galectin-3 is a presurgical marker of human thyroid carcinoma. Cancer Res 1998; 58:3015–3020.
109. Herrmann ME, LiVolsi VA, Pasha TL, et al. Immunohistochemical expression of galectin 3 in benign and malignant lesions. Arch Pathol Lab Med 2002; 126:710–713.
110. Bartolazzi A, Gasbarri A, Papotti M, et al. Application of an immunodiagnostic method for improving preoperative diagnosis of nodular thyroid lesions. Lancet 2001; 357:1644–1650.
111. Volante M, Bozzala-Cassione F, DePompa R, et al. Galectin-3 and HBME-1 expression in oncocytic cell tumors of the thyroid. Virchows Arch 2004; 445:183–188.
112. Dasovic-Knezevic M, Bormer O, Holm R, et al. Carcinoembryonic antigen in medullary thyroid carcinoma: An immunohistochemical study applying six novel monoclonal antibodies. Mod Pathol 1989; 2:610–617.
113. Schroder S, Schwarz W, Rehpenning W, et al. Prognostic significance of Leu M1 immunostaining in papillary carcinomas of the thyroid gland. Virchows Arch A Pathol Anat Histopathol 1987; 411:435–439.
114. Loy TS, Darkow GV, Spollen LE, et al. Immunostaining for Leu 7 in the diagnosis of thyroid carcinoma. Arch Pathol Lab Med 1994; 118:172–174.
115. Ostrowski ML, Brown RW, Wheeler TM, et al. Leu 7 immunoreactivity in cytologic specimens of thyroid lesions with an emphasis on follicular neoplasms. Diagn Cytopathol 1995; 12:297–302.
116. Gatalica Z, Miettinen M. Distribution of carcinoma antigens CA19-9 and CA15-3: An immunohistochemical study of 400 tumors. Appl Immunohistochem 1994; 2:205–211.
117. Alves P, Soares P, Fonseca E, et al. Papillary thyroid carcinoma overexpresses fully and underglycosylated mucins together with native and sialylated simple mucin antigens and histo-blood group antigens. Endocrine Pathol 1999; 10:315–324.
118. Soares P, Cameselle-Teijeiro J, Sobrinho-Simoes M. Immunohistochemical detection of p53 in differentiated, poorly differentiated and undifferentiated carcinomas of the thyroid. Histopathology 1994; 24:205–210.
119. Holm R, Nesland JM. Retinoblastoma and p53 tumor suppressor gene protein expression in carcinomas of the thyroid gland. J Pathol 1994; 172:267–272.
120. Tallini G, Santoro M, Helie M, et al. RET/PTC oncogene activation defines a subset of papillary thyroid carcinomas lacking evidence of progression to poorly differentiated or undifferentiated tumor phenotypes. Clin Cancer Res 1998; 4:287–294.
121. Papotti M, Volante M, Guiliano A, et al. RET/PTC activation in hyalinizing trabecular tumors of the thyroid. Am J Surg Pathol 2000; 24:1615–1621.
122. Cheung CC, Boerner SL, MacMillan CM, et al. Hyalinizing trabecular tumor of the thyroid: A variant of papillary carcinoma proved by molecular genetics. Am J Surg Pathol 2000; 24:1622–1626.
123. LiVolsi VA. Hyalinizing trabecular tumor of the thyroid: Adenoma, carcinoma, or neoplasm of uncertain malignant potential? Am J Surg Pathol 2000; 24:1683–1684.
124. Kroll TG, Sarraf P, Pecciarini L, et al. PAX8-PPAR gamma 1 fusion oncogene in human thyroid carcinoma. Science 2000; 289:1357–1360.
125. Nikiforova MN, Biddinger PW, Candill CM, et al. PAX8-PPAR gamma rearrangement in thyroid tumors: RT-PCR and immunohistochemical analyser. Am J Surg Pathol 2002; 26:1016–1023.
126. Marques AR, Espadinha C, Catarino AL, et al. Expression of PAX8-PPAR gamma rearrangements in both follicular thyroid carcinoma and adenoma. J Clin Endocrinol Metab 2002; 87:3947–3952.
127. Cheung L, Messina M, Gill A, et al. Detection of the PAX8-PPAR gamma fusion oncogene in both follicular thyroid carcinomas and adenomas. J Clin Endocrinol Metab 2003; 88:354–357.
128. Bur M, Shiraki W, Masood S. Estrogen and progesterone receptor detection in neoplastic and non-neoplastic thyroid tissue. Mod Pathol 1993; 6:469–472.
129. McLaren KM, Cossar DW. The immunohistochemical localization of S-100 in the diagnosis of papillary carcinoma of the thyroid. Hum Pathol 1996; 27:633–636.
130. Papotti M, Gugliotta P, Forte G, et al. Immunocytochemical identification of oxyphilic mitochondrion rich cells. Appl Immunohistochem 1994; 2:261–267.
131. Nylander K, Vojtesek B, Nenutil R, et al. Differential expres-

sion of p63 isoforms in normal tissues and neoplastic cells. J Pathol 2002; 198:417–427.
132. Hunt JL, LiVolsi VA, Barnes EL. p63 expression in sclerosing mucoepidermoid carcinomas with eosinophilia arising in the thyroid. Mod Pathol 2004; 17:526–529.
133. DeLellis RA, Wolfe HJ. The pathology of the human calcitonin C- cell. Pathol Annu 1981; 16:25–52.
134. Sikri KL, Varndell IM, Hamid QA, et al. Medullary carcinoma of the thyroid: An immunocytochemical and histochemical study of 25 cases using 8 separate markers. Cancer 1985; 56:2481–2491.
135. Perry A, Molberg K, Albores-Saavedra J. Physiologic versus neoplastic C-cell hyperplasia of the thyroid: Separation of distinct histologic and biologic entities. Cancer 1996; 77:750–756.
136. Holm R, Sobrinho-Simoes M, Nesland JM, et al. Medullary carcinoma of the thyroid gland: An immunocytochemical study. Ultrastruct Pathol 1985; 8:25–41.
137. Uribe M, Fenoglio-Preiser CM, Grimes M, et al. Medullary carcinoma of the thyroid gland: Clinical, pathological and immunohistochemical features with a review of the literature. Am J Surg Pathol 1985; 9:577–594.
138. Zajac JD, Penschow J, Mason T, et al. Identification of calcitonin and calcitonin gene related peptide messenger RNA in medullary thyroid carcinoma by hybridization histochemistry. J Clin Endocrinol Metab 1986; 62:1037–1043.
139. Eusebi V, Damiani S, Riva C, et al. Calcitonin-free oat cell carcinoma of the thyroid gland. Virchows Arch A Pathol Anat Histopathol 1990; 417:267–271.
140. Franc B, Rosenberg-Bourgin M, Caillou B, et al. Medullary thyroid carcinoma: Search for histological predictors of survival (109 proband case analysis). Hum Pathol 1998; 29:1078–1084.
141. Steenbergh PH, Hoppener JW, Zandberg J, et al. Calcitonin gene related peptide coding sequence is conserved in the human genome and is expressed in medullary thyroid carcinoma. J Clin Endocrinol Metab 1984; 59:358–360.
142. Komminoth P, Roth J, Saremaslani P, et al. Polysialic acid of the neural cell adhesion molecule in the human thyroid: A marker for medullary thyroid carcinoma and primary C-cell hyperplasia: An immunohistochemical study on 79 thyroid lesions. Am J Surg Pathol 1994; 18:399–411.
143. Scopsi L, Ferrari C, Pilotti S, et al. Immunocytochemical localization and identification of prosomatostatin gene products in medullary carcinoma of human thyroid gland. Hum Pathol 1990; 21:820–830.
144. Sunday ME, Wolfe HJ, Roos BA, et al. Gastrin releasing peptide gene expression in developing, hyperplastic and neoplastic thyroid C-cells. Endocrinology 1988; 122:1551–1558.
145. Heitz PU, von Herbay G, Kloppel G, et al. The expression of subunits of human chorionic gonadotropin (hCG) by nontrophoblastic, nonendocrine and endocrine tumors. Am J Clin Pathol 1987; 88:467–472.
146. DeLellis RA, Moore FM, Wolfe HJ. Thyroglobulin immunoreactivity in human medullary thyroid carcinoma. Lab Invest 1983; 48:20A.
147. Holm R, Sobrinho-Simoes M, Nesland JM, et al. Concurrent production of calcitonin and thyroglobulin by the same neoplastic cells. Ultrastruct Pathol 1986; 10:241–248.
148. Ljungberg O, Bondeson L, Bondeson AG. Differentiated thyroid carcinoma, intermediate type: A new tumor entity with features of follicular and parafollicular cell carcinomas. Hum Pathol 1984; 15:218–228.
149. Volante M, Papotti M, Roth J, et al. Mixed medullary follicular thyroid carcinoma: Molecular evidence for a dual origin of tumor components. Am J Pathol 1999; 155:1499–1509.
150. Schmid KW, Fischer-Colbrie R, Hagn C, et al. Chromogranin A and B and secretogranin II in medullary carcinomas of the thyroid. Am J Surg Pathol 1987; 11:551–556.
151. Katsetos CD, Jami MM, Krishna L, et al. Novel immunohistochemical localization of 28000 molecular weight (Mr) calcium binding protein (Calbindin-D_{28k}) in enterochromaffin cells of the human appendix and neuroendocrine tumors (carcinoids and small cell carcinomas) of the midgut and foregut. Arch Pathol Lab Med 1994; 118:633–639.
152. Viale G, Roncalli M, Grimelius L, et al. Prognostic value of bcl-2 immunoreactivity in medullary thyroid carcinoma. Hum Pathol 1995; 26:945–950.
153. DeLellis RA, Rule AH, Spiler I, et al. Calcitonin and carcinoembryonic antigen as tumor markers in medullary thyroid carcinoma. Am J Clin Pathol 1978; 70:587–594.
154. Schroder S, Kloppel G. Carcinoembryonic antigen and nonspecific cross-reacting antigen in thyroid cancer: An immunocytochemical study using polyclonal and monoclonal antibodies. Am J Surg Pathol 1987; 11:100–108.
155. Mendelsohn G, Wills SA Jr, Baylin SB. Relationship of tis-

sue carcinoembryonic antigen and calcitonin to tumor virulence in medullary thyroid carcinoma: An immunohistochemical study in early, localized and virulent disseminated stages of disease. Cancer 1984; 54:657–662.

156. Kimura N, Nakazato Y, Nagura H, et al. Expression of intermediate filaments in neuroendocrine tumors. Arch Pathol Lab Med 1990; 114:506–510.

157. Miettinen M, Clark R, Lehto VP, et al. Intermediate filament proteins in parathyroid glands and parathyroid adenomas. Arch Pathol Lab Med 1985; 109:986–989.

158. Futrell JM, Roth SI, Su SP, et al. Immunocytochemical localization of parathyroid hormone in bovine parathyroid glands and human parathyroid adenomas. Am J Pathol 1979; 94:615–622.

159. Tomita T. Immunocytochemical staining patterns for parathyroid hormone and chromogranin in parathyroid hyperplasia, adenoma and carcinoma. Endocr Pathol 1999; 10:145–156.

160. Stork PJ, Herteaux C, Frazier R, et al. Expression and distribution of parathyroid hormone and parathyroid hormone messenger RNA in pathological conditions of the parathyroid gland. Lab Invest 1992; 61:169–174.

161. Weber CJ, Russell J, Chryssochoos JT, et al. Parathyroid hormone content distinguishes true normal parathyroids from parathyroids of patients with primary hyperpara-thyroidism. World J Surg 1996; 20:1010–1015.

162. Danks JA, Ebeling PR, Hayman J, et al. Parathyroid hormone related protein: Immunohistochemical localization in cancers and in normal skin. J Bone Miner Res 1989; 4:273–278.

163. Schmid KW, Morgan JM, Baumert M, et al. Calcitonin and calcitonin gene related peptide mRNA detection in a population of hyperplastic parathyroid cells, also expressing chromogranin B. Lab Invest 1995; 73:90–95.

164. Kahn A, Tischler AS, Patwardhan NA, et al. Calcitonin immunoreactivity in neoplastic and hyperplastic para-thyroid glands. Endocr Pathol 2003; 14:249–250.

165. Hellman P, Karlsson-Parra A, Klareskog L, et al. Expression and function of a CD4-like molecule in parathyroid tissue. Surgery 1996; 120:985–992.

166. Vasef MA, Brynes RK, Sturm M, et al. Expression of cyclin D1 in parathyroid carcinomas, adenomas and hyperplasias: A paraffin immunohistochemical study. Mod Pathol 1999; 12:412–416.

167. Abbona GC, Papotti M, Gasparri G, et al. Proliferative activity in parathyroid tumors as detected by Ki-67 immunostaining. Hum Pathol 1995; 26:135–138.

168. Vargas MP, Vargas HI, Kleiner DE, et al. The role of prognostic markers (MIB-1, RB, bcl-2) in the diagnosis of parathyroid tumors. Mod Pathol 1997; 10:12–17.

169. Cryns VL, Thor A, Xu H-J, et al. Loss of the retinoblastoma tumor suppressor gene in parathyroid carcinoma. N Engl J Med 1994; 330:757–761.

170. Farnebo F, Auer G, Farnebo LO, et al. Evaluation of retinoblastoma and Ki-67 immunostaining as diagnostic markers of benign and malignant parathyroid disease. World J Surg 1999; 23:68–74.

171. Kayath MJ, Martin LC, Vieira JG, et al. A comparative study of p53 immunoexpression in parathyroid hyperplasias secondary to uremia, primary hyperplasias, adenomas and carcinomas. Eur J Endocrinol 1998; 139:78–83.

172. Schroder S, Niendorf A, Achilles E, et al. Immunocytochemical differential diagnosis of adrenocortical neoplasms using the monoclonal antibody D11. Virchows Arch A Pathol Anat Histopathol 1990; 417:89–96.

173. Schroder S, Padberg BC, Achilles E, et al. Immunocytochemistry in adrenocortical tumors: A clinicopathological study of 72 neoplasms. Virchows Arch A Pathol Anat Histopathol 1992; 420:65–70.

174. Tartour E, Caillou B, Tenenbaum F, et al. Immunohistochemical study of adrenocortical carcinoma: Predictive value of the D11 monoclonal antibody. Cancer 1993; 72:3296–3303.

175. Sasano H, Shizawa S, Suzuki T, et al. Transcription factor adrenal 4 binding protein as a marker of adrenocortical malignancy. Hum Pathol 1995; 26:1154–1156.

176. Busam KJ, Iversen K, Coplan KA, et al. Immunoreactivity for A103, an antibody to melan-A (Mart-1) in adrenocortical and other steroid tumors. Am J Surg Pathol 1998; 22:57–63.

177. Renshaw AA, Granter SR. A comparison of A103 and inhibin reactivity in adrenal cortical tumors: Distinction from hepatocellular carcinoma and renal tumors. Mod Pathol 1998; 11: 1160–1164.

178. Loy TS, Phillips RW, Linder CL. A103 immunostaining in the diagnosis of adrenal cortical tumors: an immunohistochemical study of 316 cases. Arch Pathol Lab Med 2002; 126:170–172.

179. Ghorab Z, Jorda M, Ganjei P, et al. Melan-A (A103) is expressed in adrenocortical neoplasms but not in renal cell and

hepatocellular carcinomas. Appl Immunohistochem Mol Morphol 2003; 11:330–333.
180. Shin SJ, Hoda RS, Ying L, et al. Diagnostic utility of the monoclonal antibody A103 in fine-needle aspiration biopsies of the adrenal. Am J Clin Pathol 2000; 113: 295–302.
181. Pelkey TJ, Frierson HF, Mills SE, et al. The a submit of inhibin in adrenal cortical neoplasia. Mod Pathol 1998; 11:516–524.
182. Fetsch PA, Powers CN, Zakowski M, et al. Anti-alpha inhibin: Marker of choice for the consistent distinction between adrenocortical carcinoma (ACC) and renal cell carcinoma (RCC) in fine needle aspirations (FNA). Cancer 1999; 87: 168–172.
183. McCluggage WG, Maxwell P, Patterson A, et al. Immunohistochemical staining of hepatocellular carcinoma with monoclonal antibody against inhibin. Histopathology 1997; 30:518–522.
184. Munro LM, Kennedy A, McNicol AM. The expression of inhibin/activin subunits in the human adrenal cortex and its tumors. J Endocrinol 1999; 161:341–347.
185. McCluggage WG, Maxwell P. Adenocarcinoma of various sites may exhibit immunoreactivity with anti-inhibin antibodies. Histopathology 1999; 35:216–220.
186. Brown FM, Gaffey TA, Wold LE, et al. Myxoid neoplasms of the adrenal cortex: a rare histologic variant. Am J Surg Pathol 2000; 24:396–410.
187. Arola J, Liu J, Heikkila P, et al. Expression of inhibin alpha in adrenocortical tumors reflects the hormonal status of the neoplasm. J Endocrinol 2000; 165:223–229.
188. Cho EY, Ahn GH. Immunoexpression of inhibin α-subunit in adrenal neoplasms. Appl Immunohistochem Mol Morphol 2001; 9:222–228.
189. Miettinen M. Neuroendocrine differentiation in adrenocortical carcinoma: New immunohistochemical findings supported by electron microscopy. Lab Invest 1992; 66:169–174.
190. Chetty R, Pillay P, Jaichand V. Cytokeratin expression in adrenal phaeochromocytomas and extra-adrenal paragangliomas. J Clin Pathol 1998; 51:477–478.
191. Kimura N, Nakazato Y, Nagura H, et al. Expression of intermediate filaments in neuroendocrine tumors. Arch Pathol Lab Med 1990; 114:506–510.
192. Fogt F, Vortmeyer AO, Poremba C, et al. Bcl-2 expression in normal adrenal glands and in adrenal neoplasms. Mod Pathol 1998; 11:716–720.

193. Zhang PJ, Genega EM, Tomaszewski JE, et al. The role of calretinin, inhibin, melan-A, bcl-2, and c-kit in differentiating adrenal cortical and medullary tumors: an immuno-histochemical study. Mod Pathol 2003; 16:591–597.
194. Jorda M, De Madeiros B, Nadji M. Calretinin and inhibin are useful in separating adrenocortical neoplasms from pheochromocytomas. Appl Immunohistochem Mol Morphol 2002; 10:67–70.
195. Miettinen M, Lehto V-P, Virtanen I. Immunofluorescence microscopic evaluation of the intermediate filament expression of the adrenal cortex and medulla and their tumors. Am J Pathol 1985; 118:360–366.
196. Gaffey MJ, Traweek ST, Mills SE, et al. Cytokeratin expression in adrenocortical neoplasia: An immunohistochemical and biochemical study with implications for the differential diagnosis of adrenocortical, hepatocellular and renal cell carcinoma. Hum Pathol 1992; 23:144–153.
197. Wick MR, Cherwitz DL, McGlennen RC, et al. Adreno-cortical carcinoma: An immunohistochemical comparison with renal cell carcinoma. Am J Pathol 1986; 122:343–352.
198. Cote RJ, Cardon-Cardo C, Reuter VE, et al. Immunopathology of adrenal and renal cortical tumors: Coordinated change in antigen expression is associated with neoplastic conversion in the adrenal cortex. Am J Pathol 1990; 136:1077–1084.
199. Unger PD, Hoffman K, Thung SN, et al. HMB-45 reactivity in adrenal pheochromocytomas. Arch Pathol Lab Med 1992; 116:151–153.
200. Caya JG. HMB-45 reactivity in adrenal pheochromocytomas. Arch Pathol Lab Med 1994; 118:1169.
201. Lloyd RV, Shapiro B, Sisson JC, et al. An immunohistochemical study of pheochromocytomas. Arch Pathol Lab Med 1984; 108:541–544.
202. Lloyd RV, Blaivas M, Wilson BS. Distribution of chromogranin and S100 protein in normal and abnormal adrenal medullary tissues. Arch Pathol Lab Med 1985; 109:633–635.
203. Verhofstad AAJ, Steinbusch HWM, Joosten JWJ, et al. Immunocytochemical localization of nonadrenaline, adrenaline and serotonin. In: Polak JM, Van Noordens S, eds. Immunohistochemistry: practical applications in pathology and biology. Bristol, England: Wright-PSG; 1983:143–168.
204. Trojanowski JQ, Lee VM. Expression of neurofilament antigens by normal and neoplastic human adrenal chromaffin

cells. N Engl J Med 1985; 313:101–104.
205. Grignon DJ, Ro JY, Mackay B, et al. Paraganglioma of the urinary bladder: Immunohistochemical, ultrastructural and DNA flow cytometric studies. Hum Pathol 1991; 22:1162–1169.
206. Johnson TL, Zarbo RJ, Lloyd RV, et al. Paragangliomas of the head and neck: Immunohistochemical neuroendocrine and intermediate filament typing. Mod Pathol 1988; 1:216–223.
207. Salim SA, Milroy C, Rode J, et al. Immunocytochemical characterization of neuroendocrine tumors of the larynx. Histopathology 1993; 23:69–73.
208. Helman LJ, Cohen PS, Averbuch SD, et al. Neuropeptide Y expression distinguishes malignant from benign pheochromocytoma. J Clin Oncol 1989; 7:720–725.
209. Clarke MR, Weyant RJ, Watson CG, et al. Prognostic markers in pheochromocytoma. Hum Pathol 1998; 29:522–526.
210. August C, August K, Schroeder S, et al. CGH and CD44/MIB-1 immunohistochemistry are helpful to distinguish metastasized sporadic pheochromocytomas. Mod Pathol 2004; 17:1119–1128.
211. Triche TJ, Askin F. Neuroblastoma and the differential diagnosis of small, round, blue cell tumors. Hum Pathol 1983; 14:569–595.
212. Hachitanda Y, Tsuneyoshi M, Enjoji M. An ultrastructural and immunohistochemical evaluation of cytodifferentiation in neuroblastic tumors. Mod Pathol 1989; 2:13–19.
213. Pagani A, Forni M, Tonini GP, et al. Expression of members of the chromogranin family in primary neuroblastomas. Diagn Mol Pathol 1992; 1:16–24.
214. Carter RL, Al-sams SZ, Corbett RP, et al. A comparative study of immunohistochemical staining for neuron-specific enolase, protein gene product 9.5 and S-100 in neuro-blastoma, Ewing's sarcoma and other round cell tumors in children. Histopathology 1990; 16:461–467.
215. Wirnsberger GH, Becker H, Ziervogel K, et al. Diagnostic immunohistochemistry of neuroblastic tumors. Am J Surg Pathol 1992; 16:49–57.
216. Franquemont DW, Mills SE, Lack EE. Immunohistochemical detection of neuroblastomatous foci in composite adrenal pheochromocytoma-neuroblastoma. Am J Clin Pathol 1994; 102:163–170.
217. Argani P, Erlandson RA, Rosai J. Thymic neuroblastoma in adults: Report of three cases with special emphasis on its association with the syndrome of inappropriate secretion of antidiuretic hormone. Am J Clin Pathol 1997; 108:537–543.
218. Fellinger EJ, Garin-Chesa P, Triche TJ, et al. Immunohistochemical analysis of Ewing's sarcoma cell surface antigen p30/32 MIC2. Am J Pathol 1991; 39:317–325.
219. Stevenson AJ, Chatten J, Bertoni F, et al. CD99 (p30/32MIC2) neuroectodermal/Ewing's sarcoma antigen as an immunohistochemical marker: Review of more than 600 tumors and the literature experience. Appl Immunohistochem 1994; 2:231–240.
220. Weidner N, Tjoe J. Immunohistochemical profile of monoclonal antibody 013: Antibody that recognizes glycoprotein p 30/32MIC2 and is useful in diagnosing Ewing's sarcoma and peripheral neuroepithelioma. Am J Surg Pathol 1994; 18:486–494.
221. Scotlandi K, Serra M, Manara MC, et al. Immunostaining of the p30/32MIC2 antigen and molecular detection of EWS rearrangements for the diagnosis of Ewing's sarcoma and peripheral neuroectodermal tumor. Hum Pathol 1996; 27:408–416.
222. Hess E, Cohen C, DeRose PB, et al. Nonspecificity of p30/32MIC2 immunolocalization with the 013 monoclonal antibody in the diagnosis of Ewing's sarcoma: Application of an algorithmic immunohistochemical analysis. Appl Immunohistochem 1997; 5:94–103.
223. Pappo AS, Douglass ED, Meyer WH, et al. Use of HBA 71 and anti-B2-microglobulin to distinguish peripheral neuroepithelioma from neuroblastoma. Hum Pathol 1993; 24:880–885.
224. Miettinen M, Chatten J, Paetau A, et al. Monoclonal antibody NB84 in the differential diagnosis of neuroblastoma and other small round cell tumors. Am J Surg Pathol 1998; 22:327–332.
225. Folpe AL, Patterson K, Gown AM. Antineuroblastoma antibody NB-84 also identifies a significant subset of other small blue round cell tumors. Appl Immunohistochem 1997; 5:239–245.
226. Dayal Y. Endocrine cells of the gut and their neoplasms. In: Norris HT, ed. Pathology of the colon, small intestine and anus. New York: Churchill Livingstone; 1991:305–366.
227. Moll R, Franke WW. Cytoskeletal differences between human neuroendocrine tumors: A cytoskeletal protein of molecular weight 46000 distinguishes cutaneous from pulmo-

nary neuroendocrine tumors. Differentiation 1985; 30:165–175.
228. Burke AP, Sobin LH, Federspiel BH, et al. Appendiceal carcinoids: Correlation of histology and immunohistochemistry. Mod Pathol 1989; 2:630–637.
229. Miettinen M. Keratin 20: Immunohistochemical marker for gastrointestinal, urothelial, and Merkel cell carcinomas. Mod Pathol 1995; 8:384–388.
230. Al-Khafaji B, Noffsinger AE, Miller MA, et al. Immunohistologic analysis of gastrointestinal and pulmonary carcinoid tumors. Hum Pathol 1998; 29:992–999.
231. Kimura N, Pilichowska M, Okamoto H, et al. Immunohistochemical expression of chromogranins A and B, prohormone convertases 2 and 3, and amidating enzyme in carcinoid tumors and pancreatic endocrine tumors. Mod Pathol 2000; 13:140–146.
232. Thomas RM, Baybick JH, Elsayed AM, et al. Gastric carcinoids: An immunohistochemical and clinicopathologic study of 104 patients. Cancer 1994; 73:2053–2058.
233. Machlouf HR, Burke AP, Sobin LH. Carcinoid tumors of the ampulla of Vater: A comparison with duodenal carcinoid tumors. Cancer 1999; 85:1241–1249.
234. Sheibani K, Battifora H, Burke JS, et al. Leu-M1 antigen in human neoplasms: An immunohistologic study of 400 cases. Am J Surg Pathol 1986; 10:227–236.
235. Moskaluk CA, Zheng H, Powell SM, et al. CDX2 protein expression in normal and malignant human tissue: an immunohistochemical survey using tissue microarrrays. Mod Pathol 2003; 16:913–919.
236. Azumi N, Traweek ST, Battifora H. Prostatic acid phosphatase in carcinoid tumors: Immunohistochemical and immunoblot studies. Am J Surg Pathol 1991; 15:785–790.
237. Shah IA, Schlageter M-O, Netto D. Immunoreactivity of neurofilament proteins in neuroendocrine neoplasms. Mod Pathol 1991; 4:215–219.
238. Chejfec G, Falkmer S, Grimelius L, et al. Synaptophysin: A new marker for pancreatic neuroendocrine tumors. Am J Surg Pathol 1987; 11:241–247.
239. Solcia E, Capella C, Kloppel G. Atlas of tumor pathology: tumors of the pancreas. Washington, DC: Armed Forces Institute of Pathology; 1997.
240. Heitz PU, Kasper M, Polak JM, et al. Pancreatic endocrine tumors: Immunocytochemical analysis of 125 tumors. Hum Pathol 1982; 13:263–271.
241. Perkins PL, McLeod MK, Jin L, et al. Analysis of gastrinomas by immunohistochemistry and in-situ hybridization histochemistry. Diagn Mol Pathol 1992; 1:155–164.
242. Le Bodic M-F, Heyman M-F, Lecomete M, et al. Immunohistochemical study of 100 pancreatic tumors in 28 patients with multiple endocrine neoplasia type I. Am J Surg Pathol 1996; 20:1378–1384.
243. Solcia E, Capella C, Riva C, et al. The morphology and neuroendocrine profile of pancreatic epithelial VIPomas and extrapancreatic VIP producing neurogenic tumors. Ann NY Acad Sci 1988; 527:508–517.
244. Heitz PU, Kasper M, Kloppel G, et al. Glycoprotein-hormone alpha-chain production by pancreatic endocrine tumors: A specific marker for malignancy: Immunocytochemical analysis of tumors of 155 patients. Cancer 1983; 51:277–282.
245. Graeme-Cook F, Nardi G, Compton CC. Immunocytochemical staining for human chorionic gonadotropin subunits does not predict malignancy in insulinomas. Am J Clin Pathol 1990; 93:273–276.
246. Viale G, Doglioni C, Gambacorta M, et al. Progesterone receptor immunoreactivity in pancreatic endocrine tumors: An immunocytochemical study of 156 neuroendocrine tumors of the pancreas, gastrointestinal and respiratory tracts and skin. Cancer 1992; 70:2268–2277.
247. Gould VE, Linnoila RI, Memoli VA, et al. Neuroendocrine components of the bronchopulmonary tract: Hyperplasias, dysplasias and neoplasias. Lab Invest 1983; 49:519–537.
248. Travis WD, Linnoila ID, Tsokos MG, et al. Neuroendocrine tumors of the lung with proposed criteria for large cell neuroendocrine carcinoma: An ultrastructural, immunohistochemical and flow cytometric study of 35 cases. Am J Surg Pathol 1991; 15:529–553.
249. Blobel GA, Gould VE, Moll R, et al. Co-expression of neuroendocrine markers and epithelial cytoskeletal proteins in bronchopulmonary neuroendocrine neoplasms. Lab Invest 1985; 52:39–51.
250. Oliveira AM, Tazelaar HD, Myers JL, et al. Thyroid transcription factor-1 distinguishes metastatic pulmonary from well differentiated neuroendocrine tumors of other sites. Am J Surg Pathol 2001; 25:815–819.
251. Cai YC, Banner B, Glickman J, et al. Cytokeratin 7 and 20 and thyroid transcription factor-1 can help distinguish pul-

monary from gastrointestinal carcinoid and pancreatic endocrine tumors. Hum Pathol 2001; 32:1087–1093.
252. Jiang S-X, Kameya T, Shoji M, et al. Large cell neuroendocrine carcinoma of the lung: A histological and immunohistochemical study of 22 cases. Am J Surg Pathol 1998; 22: 526–537.
253. Gersell DJ, Mazoujian G, Mutch DG, et al. Small cell undifferentiated carcinoma of the cervix: A clinicopathologic, ultrastructural and immunocytochemical study of 15 cases. Am J Surg Pathol 1988; 12:684–698.
254. Abeler VM, Holm R, Nesland JM, et al. Small cell carcinoma of the cervix: A clinicopathologic study of 26 patients. Cancer 1994; 73:672–677.
255. Gilks CB, Young RH, Gersell DJ, et al. Large cell neuroendocrine carcinoma of the uterine cervix: A clinicopathologic study of 12 cases. Am J Surg Pathol 1997; 21:905–914.
256. Chan JK, Suster S, Wenig B, et al. Cytokeratin 20 immunoreactivity distinguishes Merkel cell (primary cutaneous neuroendocrine) carcinomas and salivary gland small cell carcinomas from small cell carcinomas of various sites. Am J Surg Pathol 1997; 21(2):226–234.
257. Agoff SN, Lamps LW, Philip AT, et al. Thyroid transcription factor-1 is expressed in extrapulmonary small cell carcinomas but not in other extrapulmonary neuroendocrine tumors. Mod Pathol 2000; 13:238–242.
258. Ordonez NG. Value of thyroid transcription factor-1 immunostaining in distinguishing small cell lung carcinomas from other small cell carcinomas. Am J Surg Pathol 2000; 24:1217–1223.
259. Straughn JM, Richter HE, Conner MG, et al. Predictors of outcome in small cell carcinoma of the cervix – a case series. Gynecol Oncol 2001; 83:216–220.
260. Masumoto N, Fujii T, Ishikawa M, et al. p16 overexpression and human papillomavirus infection in small cell carcinoma of the uterine cervix. Hum Pathol 2003; 34:778–783.
261. Conner MG, Richter H, Moran CA, et al. Small cell carcinoma of the cervix: a clinicopathologic and immunohistochemical study of 23 cases. Ann Diagn Pathol 2002; 6:345–348.
262. Stoler MH, Mills SE, Gersell DJ, et al. Small cell neuroendocrine carcinoma of the cervix: A human papillomavirus 18 associated cancer. Am J Surg Pathol 1991; 15:28–32.
263. Wang HL, Lu DW. Detection of human papillomavirus DNA and expression of p16, RB, and p53 proteins in small cell carcinomas of the uterine cervix. Am J Surg Pathol 2004; 28: 901–908.
264. Sato Y, Shimamoto T, Amada S, et al. Large cell neuroendocrine carcinoma of the uterine cervix: a clinicopathological study of six cases. Int J Gynecol Pathol 2003; 22:226–230.
265. Grayson W, Rhemtula HA, Taylor LF, et al. Detection of human papillomavirus in large cell neuroendocrine carcinoma of the uterine cervix: a study of 12 cases. J Clin Pathol 2002; 55:108–114.
266. Matthews-Greer J, Dominguez-Malagon H, Herrera GA, et al. Human papillomavirus typing of rare cervical carcinomas. Arch Pathol Lab Med 2004; 128:553–556.
267. diSant'Agnese PA, de Mesy Jensen KL, Churukian CJ, et al. Human prostatic endocrine-paracrine (APUD) cells: Distributional analysis with a comparison of serotonin and neuron specific enolase immunoreactivity and silver stains. Arch Pathol Lab Med 1985; 109:607–612.
268. diSant'Agnese PA. Neuroendocrine differentiation in prostatic carcinoma: An update. Prostate (Suppl) 1998; 8:74–79.
269. Schmid KW, Helpap B, Totsch M, et al. Immunohistochemical localization of chromogranins A and B and secretogranin II in normal, hyperplastic and neoplastic prostate. Histopathology 1994; 24:233–239.
270. di Sant'Agnese PA, Divergent neuroendocrine differentiation in prostatic carcinoma. Sem Diagn Pathol 2000; 17:149–161.
271. Ghannoum JE, DeLellis RA, Shin SJ. Primary carcinoid tumor of the prostate with concurrent adenocarcinoma: a case report. Int J Surg Pathol 2004; 12(2):167–170.
272. Azumi N, Shibuya H, Ishikura M. Primary prostatic carcinoid with intracytoplasmic prostatic acid phosphatase and prostate specific antigen. Am J Surg Pathol 1984; 8:545–550.
273. Goldstein NS. Immunophenotypic characterization of 225 prostate adenocarcinomas with intermediate or high Gleason scores. Am J Clin Pathol 2002; 117:471–477.
274. Kawai S, Hiroshima K, Tsukamoto Y, et al. Small cell carcinoma of the prostate expressing prostate-specific antigen and showing syndrome of inappropriate secretion of anti-diuretic hormone: an autopsy case report. Pathol Int 2003; 53:892–896.
275. Azumi N, Shibuya H, Ishikura M. Primary prostatic carcinoid tumor with intracytoplasmic prostatic acid phosphatase and prostate-specific antigen. Am J Surg Pathol 1984; 8:545–

550.

276. Ordóñez NG. Value of thyroid transcription factor-1 immunostaining in distinguishing small cell lung carcinomas from other small cell carcinomas. Am J Surg Pathol 2000; 24(9):1217–1223.

277. Bostwick DG, Dousa MK, Crawford BG, et al. Neuroendocrine differentiation in prostatic intraepithelial neoplasia and adenocarcinoma. Am J Surg Pathol 1994; 18:1240–1246.

278. Gould VE, Moll R, Moll I, et al. Neuroendocrine (Merkel) cells of the skin: Hyperplasias, dysplasias and neoplasms. Lab Invest 1985; 52:334–353.

279. Chan JKC, Suster S, Wenig BM, et al. Cytokeratin 20 immunoreactivity distinguishes Merkel cell (primary cutaneous neuroendocrine) carcinomas and salivary gland small cell carcinomas from small cell carcinomas of various sites. Am J Surg Pathol 1997; 21:226–234.

280. Leech SN, Kolar AJO, Barrett PD, et al. Merkel cell carcinoma can be distinguished from metastatic small cell carcinoma using antibodies to cytokeratin 20 and thyroid transcription factor 1. J Clin Pathol 2001; 54:727–729.

281. Cheuk W, Kwan MY, Suster S, et al. Immunostaining for thyroid transcription factor 1 and cytokeratin 20 aids the distinction of small cell carcinoma from Merkel cell carcinoma, but not pulmonary from extrapulmonary small cell carcinomas. Arch Pathol Lab Med 2001; 125:228–231.

282. Hanly AJ, Elgart GW, Jorda M, et al. Analysis of thyroid transcription factor-1 and cytokeratin 20 separates Merkel cell carcinoma from small cell carcinoma of lung. J Cutan Pathol 2000; 27:118–120.

283. Nicholson SA, McDermott MB, Swanson PE, et al. CD99 and cytokeratin 20 in small cell and basaloid tumors of the skin. Appl Immunohistochem Mol Morphol 2000; 8:37–41.

284. Nagao T, Gaffey TA, Olsen KD, et al. Small cell carcinoma of the major salivary glands: clinicopathologic study with emphasis on cytokeratin 20 immunoreactivity and clinical outcome. Am J Surg Pathol 2004; 28(6):762–770.

285. Jensen K, Kohler S, Rouse RV. Cytokeratin staining in Merkel cell carcinoma: an immunohistochemical study of cytokeratins 5/6, 7, 17, and 20. Appl Immunohistochem Mol Morph 2000; 8:310–315.

286. Drijkoningen M, de Wolf-Peeters C, van Limbergen E, et al. Merkel cell tumor of the skin: An immunohistochemical study. Hum Pathol 1986; 17:301–307.

287. Liu Y, Mangini J, Saad R, et al. Diagnostic value of microtubule-associated protein-2 in Merkel cell carcinoma 2003; 11:326–329.

288. Sibley RK, Dahl D. Primary neuroendocrine (Merkel cell?) carcinoma of the skin. II: An immunohistochemical study of 21 cases. Am J Surg Pathol 1985; 9:109–116.

289. Brinkschmidt C, Stolze P, Fahrenkamp AG, et al. Immunohistochemical demonstration of chromogranin A, chromogranin B and secretoneunin in Merkel cell carcinoma of the skin: An immunohistochemical study suggesting two types of Merkel cell carcinoma. Appl Immunohistochem 1995; 3:37–44.

290. Yang DT, Holden JA, Florell SR. CD117, CK20, TTF-1, and DNA topoisomerase II-a antigen expression in small cell tumors. J Cutan Pathol 2004; 31:254–261.

291. Su LD, Fullen DR, Lowe L, et al. CD117 (kit receptor) expression in Merkel cell carcinoma. Am J Dermatopathol 2002; 24:289–293.

292. Strong S, Shalders K, Carr R, et al. KIT receptor (CD117) expression in Merkel cell carcinoma. Br J Dermatol 2004; 150:384–385.

293. Han AC, Soler AP, Tang C-K, et al. Nuclear localization of E-cadherin expression in Merkel cell carcinoma. Arch Pathol Lab Med 2000; 124:1147–1151.

294. Tanaka Y, Sano T, Qian ZR, et al. Expression of adhesion molecules and cytokeratin 20 in Merkel cell carcinomas. Endocr Pathol 2004; 15:117–129.

295. Maluf HM, Koerner FC. Carcinomas of the breast with endocrine differentiation: A review. Virchows Arch 1994; 425:449–457.

296. Papotti M, Gherardi G, Eusebi V, et al. Primary oat cell (neuroendocrine) carcinoma of the breast: Report of four cases. Virchows Arch A Pathol Anat Histopathol 1992; 420:103–108.

297. Francois A, Chatikhine VA, Chevallier B, et al. Neuroendocrine primary small cell carcinoma of the breast: Report of a case and review of the literature. Am J Clin Oncol 1995; 18:133–138.

298. Shin SJ, DeLellis RA, Ying BA, et al. Small cell carcinoma of the breast: A clinico-pathological and immunohistochemical study of 9 patients. Am J Surg Pathol 2000; 24:1231–1238.

299. Bergman S, Hoda SA, Geisinger KR, et al. E-cadherin-nega-

tive primary small cell carcinoma of the breast: report of a case and review of the literature. Am J Clin Pathol 2004; 121: 117–121.

299a. Shin SJ, Detellis RA, Rosen PP. Small cell carcinoma of the breast – Additional immunohistochemical studies. Am J Surg Pathol 2001; 25:831–832.

300. Hoang MP, Maitra A, Gazdar AF, et al. Primary mammary small cell carcinoma: a molecular analysis of 2 cases. Human Pathol 2001; 32:753–757.

301. Yamasaki T, Shimazaki H, Aida S, et al. Case report: primary small cell (oat cell) carcinoma of the breast: report of a case and review of the literature. Pathol Int 2000; 50:914–918.

302. Klemm KM, Moran CA. Primary neuroendocrine carcinoma of the thymus. Semin Diagn Pathol 1999; 16:32–41.

303. Moran CA, Suster S. Thymic neuroendocrine carcinomas with combined features ranging from well-differentiated (carcinoid) to small cell carcinoma: A clinicopathologic and immunohistochemical study of 11 cases. Am J Clin Pathol 2000; 113:345–350.

304. De Montpreville VT, Macchiarini P, Dulmet E. Thymic neuroendocrine carcinoma (carcinoid): A clinicopathologic study of fourteen cases. J Thorac Cardiovasc Surg 1996; 111:134–141.

305. Du EZ, Goldstraw P, Zacharias J, et al. TTF-1 expression in specific for lung primary in typical and atypical carcinoids: TTF-1-positive carcinoids are predominantly in peripheral location. Hum Pathol 2004; 25:825–831.

306. Oliveira AM, Tazelaar HD, Myers JL, et al. Thyroid transcription factor-1 distinguishes metastatic pulmonary from well-differentiated neuroendocrine tumors of other sites. Am J Surg Pathol 2001; 25:815–819.

307. Kaufmann O, Dietel M. Expression of thyroid transcription factor-1 in pulmonary and extrapulmonary small cell carcinomas and other neuroendocrine carcinomas of various primary sites. Histopathology 2000; 36:415–420.

308. Moran CA, Suster S. Neuroendocrine carcinomas (carcinoid tumor) of the thymus. A clinicopathologic analysis of 80 cases. Am J Clin Pathol 2000; 114:100–110.

309. Hishima T, Fukayama M, Hayashi Y, et al. Neuroendocrine differentiation in thymic epithelial tumors with special reference to thymic carcinoma and atypical thymoma. Hum Pathol 1998; 29:330–338.

310. Kimura N, Pilichowska M, Okamoto H, et al. Immunohistochemical expression of chromogranins A and B, prohormone convertases 2 and 3, and amidating enzyme in carcinoid tumors and pancreatic endocrine tumors. Mod Pathol 2000; 13: 140–146.

311. Goto K, Kodama T, Matsuno Y, et al. Clinicopathologic and DNA cytometric analysis of carcinoid tumors of the thymus. Mod Pathol 2001; 14:985–994.

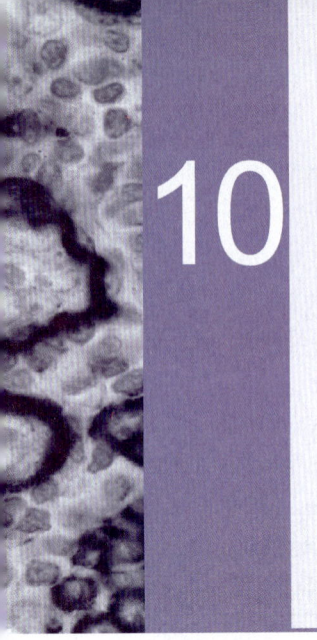

10 纵隔的免疫组织化学

原作者：Mark R.Wick
译　者：郝春燕
审校者：周庚寅，张翠娟

目录

引言	306
抗原/抗体生物学	306
纵隔疾病的免疫组化流程	306
纵隔特殊疾病中的免疫组化发现	307

引　言

纵隔是一个相对局限的解剖部位，但却可以发生多种不同种类的疾病，不仅有非肿瘤性的，也有肿瘤性的，还包括上皮细胞、淋巴细胞、间叶组织以及生殖细胞的增生性病变。纵隔内镜检查或者体外针穿活检已经成为诊断纵隔疾病的常规诊断方法[1-6]，面对这些微小的活检标本，纵隔外科病理学家感受到了巨大的挑战，他们经常需要对这些活检标本进行免疫组化检测，以获得有意义的诊断。本章只是给出了适用于特定纵隔疾病的简要的免疫组化信息，并不想做成包含所有纵隔疾病，或者是包含所有用于诊断纵隔疾病的免疫组化反应物的百科全书，而是侧重于鉴别诊断以及在鉴别过程中的免疫组化应用原则。

抗原/抗体生物学

不管是肿瘤性还是非肿瘤性增生，纵隔部位的细胞增生很少是特异性的，因而应用于这个部位的免疫反应物，与在其他章节曾经提到过的有明显的重叠，我们对各种中间丝亚型、上皮细胞与造血细胞合成的各种膜糖蛋白，以及胞质分化相关蛋白的生物学特性也不会再详细描述。读者可参考其他章节有关癌、淋巴造血系统疾病及间叶组织特异性增生等病变的讨论，然而，还是有少量的标记物被特异地应用于纵隔疾病，或者在那些疾病里有独特的表现形式。

胸腺"激素"：有几种"激素样"蛋白可能是由胸腺上皮分泌的，被认为可以对机体发育及免疫功能起到远程调节作用，其中包括促胸腺生成素、胸腺激素因子、胸腺素、facteur thymique serique，胸腺因子"X"、胸腺血浆再循环因子、胸腺毒素、thymulin和胸腺激素[7]。其中只有胸腺素在人体肿瘤主要是胸腺瘤中曾被用于免疫组化检测，阳性率为80%[8]。但是，现在还没有系统地研究过胸腺"激素"的鉴别诊断效用（或者没有作用），它们在外科病理实验室中的实际应用也不为人知。

角蛋白各亚型：与其他器官一样，角蛋白各亚型在正常胸腺及胸腺起源的肿瘤中已被检测和分析过[9,10]，特别是角蛋白7、13和18在这些组织中的表达，角蛋白13局限于胸腺髓质中的上皮细胞，也表达于各型胸腺瘤中的上皮细胞[9]。事实上，角蛋白7和18在胸腺的肿瘤性增生中更容易看到。

纵隔疾病的免疫组化流程

目前，在外科病理实践中可以用大量的抗体进行疾病诊断，但令人担忧的是，漫无目的地滥用免疫组化越来越普遍。从法医学责任的考虑，推动人们"用尽"所有试剂以评估疑难病例。然而已经发表的极具特性的操作流程和抗体使用经验使这些尝试变得没有必要。事实上，现在有充分的有关抗体特异性和敏感性的资料，我们可以把它们归纳成一个流程表。

辅助性的流程式诊断具有几个优点：它提供了解决组织病理学常见问题的可重复策略；预先界定的抗体染色结果可相互补充，便于进行综合分析；实际上没有任何疾病可以用单个抗体进行诊断。在这三条中最后一条是非常重要的，因为它较普遍地被大家所接受，对单个试剂的特异性提出了挑战。

在安全有效地使用这个免疫组化诊断流程之前，有几点说明需要引起重视：

1. 使用者（病理学家）必须严格控制实验室中所有组织的处理过程，如果标本的固定时间和条件明显改变，抗体的反应形式也会改变。

2. 使用者（不是生产商或者销售商）必须确定个人的最佳抗体稀释浓度，单一地接受商业建议是不明智的，公开发表的有关该试剂的论文对于实际操作是非常有用的。

3. 对于本实验室处理或研究的大量病理组织或者肿瘤，使用者必须积累所有的抗体反应数据，如果不能做到这一点，病理学家就必须严格采用公认的要求条件，固定、处理标本及染色。

4. 在应用选定的病理鉴别诊断指标时，流程表必须建立在对特异性、敏感性及贝氏P值规范性地统计分析基础之上。

5. 对一组免疫染色结果进行分析，应采用相关统计学方法，从最特异到最不特异或者从最强阳性到最弱阳性进行统计分析。

6. 使用前述的原理时，必须明确形态学分类，例如，作者一般在形态学上把纵隔的不确定的和未分化的肿瘤分为三大类：小细胞肿瘤、大多角形细胞肿瘤及梭形细胞/多形细胞肿瘤。

7. 免疫组化结果必须在全面的形态学分析及合理的组织学诊断的基础上应用，免疫组化只是辅助诊断手段，不能取代苏木精-伊红染色切片的作用，一个低水平的组织学诊断医生可能是一个更拙劣的免疫组织化学专家。因此，必须把临床资料、组织学诊断及免疫组化结果有机地结合起来。

8. 诊断流程是可变的，随着特性更适宜的新试剂的出现，它们会被补充进流程表格，取代或补充原来的抗体。

本章中给出的诊断流程举例是在作者的实验室中使用的，用于构建诊断流程的标本统计数据是多年内积累起来的，这些标本都是经10%中性福尔马林固定，一抗4℃孵育16~18小时，使用的是Elite®亲和素-生物素-过氧化物酶免疫检测法（Vector实验室，Burlingame，CA），抗体试剂见表10.1。

纵隔特殊疾病中的免疫组化发现

囊性胸腺瘤与囊性精原细胞瘤相比

在很多方面，在形态上囊性胸腺瘤与胸腺囊肿非常相似[11-13]。而事实上，它们也可以和具有明显囊性变特征的胸腺内精原细胞瘤混淆[14-15]。显微镜下足以将这些病变区别开来，因为典型的囊性精原细胞瘤细胞核比胸腺瘤具有更大的异型性，但小的活检标本这个特征可能不明显。PAS染色可以显示典型的精原细胞瘤内含有糖原，同时也可以用来筛选聚集的瘤细胞。同样，胎盘碱性磷酸酶（PLAP）和众多的角蛋白单克隆抗体免疫组化染色也有助于鉴别这两种肿瘤，精原细胞瘤PLAP阳性（细胞膜着色），但是只有<15%角蛋白阳性[14-16]，相反，胸腺瘤角蛋白广泛阳性但是不表达PLAP[17,18]。

各型胸腺瘤的鉴别诊断

根据镜下图像将胸腺瘤分为以下几类：淋巴细胞为主型（淋巴细胞>66%）、上皮细胞为主型（上皮细胞>66%）、淋巴上皮混合型（上皮细胞34%~66%）和梭形细胞型（上皮细胞为主型的一个亚型，具有特有的纺锤形瘤细胞）[17,19-22]。然而必须说明的是，为了使鉴别流程具有临床价值，这些胸腺瘤在细胞形态上必须是温和的上皮型肿瘤。该流程虽起不到判断预后的作用，但却可以对上述4种的主要胸腺瘤组织学类型提供鉴别诊断线索。关于胸腺瘤各亚型的特殊诊断问题将在后面给出，胸腺瘤和胸腺癌（偶尔可能由胸腺瘤转化而来）的鉴别在稍后的讨论中也会涉及。

淋巴细胞为主型胸腺瘤与淋巴组织增生相比

在临床外检中，对于患有重症肌无力的病人，经常会被问及区分胸腺组织增生和胸腺瘤的问题[23]。一般来说，胸腺瘤内不会出现淋巴滤泡，但淋巴滤泡在胸腺组织增生中也很少见。在这种情况下，就需要借助角蛋白免疫组化染色，胸腺瘤中淋巴细胞间上皮细胞呈树枝状网状连接(图10.1)，而这种现象不见于胸腺增生，以资鉴别[18,19,24]。

淋巴细胞为主型胸腺瘤与淋巴瘤相比

淋巴细胞为主型胸腺瘤中浸润性的淋巴细胞，大

表10.1 纵隔疾病中免疫组化使用的抗体

抗原	抗体（克隆）	来源	稀释度	抗原	抗体（克隆）	来源	稀释度
Cytokeratins	AE1	Boehringer-Mannheim	1:100	Placental alkaline phosphatase	Polyclonal	DAKO	1:800
	AE1/AE3	Boehringer-Mannheim	1:150	Alpha fetoprotein	C3	BioGenex	1:40
	CAM5.2	Becton-Dickinson	1:150	CD31	JC/70A	DAKO	1:40
	MAK6	Triton BioSciences	1:40	CD34	MyI 0	DAKO	1:800
CK20	ITKs20.8	DAKO	1:40	CD45	PD7/26-2B11	DAKO	1:80
Vimentin	V9	BioGenex	1:2000	CD3	Polyclonal	DAKO	1:40
Desmin	033	BioGenex	1:2000	CD5	CD5/54/B4	Vector	1:4
Epithelial membrane antigen	E29	DAKO	1:400		4C7	Vector	1:100
Carcinoembryonic antigen	NG	Boehringer-Mannheim	1:4000	CD43	MT1	BioGenex	1:50
'Epithelial antigen'	BerEP4	DAKO	1:200		DF-T1	DAKO	1:50
Calretinin	Polyclonal	Zymed	1:750	CD45RO	UCHL-1	DAKO	1:120
Neuron-specific enolase	Polyclonal	BioGenex	1:450	CD20	L26	DAKO	1:200
Chromogranin A	LK2H10	Boehringer-Mannheim	1:4000	'Membrane-bound MB2 B-cell antigen'		BioGenex	1:80
Synaptophysin	SY38	Boehringer-Mannheim	1:40	CD74	LN2	BioGenex	1:8
CD57	Leu7	Becton-Dickinson	1:20	CD15	LeuM1	Becton-Dickinson	1:150
S-100 protein	Polyclonal	DAKO	1:300	CD30	BerH2	DAKO	1:40
'Antimelanoma'	HMB-45	BioGenex	1:60	'Anti-Hodgkin's disease'	BLA.36	DAKO	1:200
Tyrosinase	T311	Novocastra	1:20	'Anti-large cell lymphoma'	BNH9	DAKO	1:200
MART-1	A103	BioGenex	1:25	Lysozyme	Polyclonal	DAKO	1:400
Muscle-specific actin	HHF-35	BioGenex	1:400	Cathepsin B	Polyclonal	ICN Biomed	1:800
Alpha-isoform actin	1A4	BioGenex	1:2	'Myeloid/Histiocyte Antigen'	MAC387	DAKO	1:800
Myogenin	F5D	DAKO	1:10	CD68	KP1	DAKO	1:800
Myo-D1	AntiMyoD1	DAKO	1:10	Myeloperoxidase	Polyclonal	DAKO	1:250
				Ki-67	MIB-1	AMAC	1:200
				PCNA	PC10	Novocastra	1:400
				p53	DO1	Oncogene Sci	1:160
					DO7	DAKO	1:240

NG,制造商未给出

大增加了其与淋巴母细胞淋巴瘤（LL）的相似性，细胞核扭曲，核浆比增大及活跃的核分裂，就像在典型的淋巴母细胞淋巴瘤中看到的一样。而且，胸腺瘤中淋巴细胞的免疫表型与淋巴母细胞淋巴瘤中的极为类似。两者都标记CD1a、CD2、CD3、CD5、CD43、CD99（MIC-2）[25-27]和bcl-2[27-29]以及末端脱氧核苷酸转移酶[26, 27, 30-36]，因此，用免疫组化的方法鉴别这两种肿瘤必须十分谨慎。

鉴别这两种肿瘤最有用的免疫组化染色（通过作者的一次失误偶然发现的）是评估角蛋白的反应活性，上皮细胞的相互连接是淋巴细胞为主型胸腺瘤的特征表现，而在淋巴母细胞淋巴瘤中则无此特征。在鉴别诊断中这种模式十分必要，因为在淋巴母细胞淋巴瘤和其他胸腺淋巴瘤中，可以看见角蛋白着色的非瘤性胸腺上皮细胞（散在分布且并不相互连接）[5, 37]。

梭形细胞为主型胸腺瘤与纤维组织细胞瘤和血管外皮瘤相比

用普通的组织学方法，很难把由梭形细胞构成的上皮细胞为主型胸腺瘤（PET）与纤维组织细胞瘤（FH）或血管外皮瘤（HPC）区分开来[19]，免疫组化是一个很好的最终鉴别手段，尤其是当只能获取小的活检标本的时候。假间叶细胞胸腺瘤通常呈角蛋白阳性，波形蛋白阴性[18]，而纤维组织细胞瘤和血管外皮瘤正好相反[38]。另外，血管外皮瘤通常表达CD34（图10.2）[39]，而胸腺瘤不表达。

> **诊断要点**：胸腺
> 1. 胸腺瘤中可见角蛋白阳性的网状胸腺上皮，但不见于胸腺增生和淋巴瘤。
> 2. 血管外皮瘤中的梭形细胞CD34+，而在胸腺瘤中的梭形细胞CD34-。

良性外周神经鞘瘤和神经节细胞瘤

后纵隔发生的绝大部分肿瘤在性质上来说是神经源性的[40-42]，因而，这些肿瘤往往在组织形态上具有相似性，从而导致诊断上的困难。尤其是施万细胞瘤（神经鞘瘤，PNST）通常根据它们与多发性神经纤维瘤病的关系及恶变的危险程度[42-45]，将其分为神经纤维瘤和神经鞘瘤（施万细胞瘤），该种肿瘤必须要与神经节细胞瘤区分[41,46]。所有这些病变都一致呈波形蛋白和S-100蛋白阳性，这三个诊断中任何一个S-100阴性都应给予高度怀疑。Fine等[47]发现，calretinin在绝大多数施万细胞瘤中阳性，但只在少数神经纤维瘤中阳性，这使得这个标记物在鉴别两者时具有潜在的使用价值。Syn（一种突触相关蛋白）是一个经典的神经和神经内分泌疾病的标记物[48]，可以帮助标记节细胞瘤中的节细胞（可以是局灶性或者弥漫的）。

纤维性和肌纤维母细胞性增生

纵隔有4种细胞形态温和的梭形细胞增生会被混淆，分别是：孤立性纤维性肿瘤（SFT）[49-51]、促纤维增生型纤维瘤病、硬化性纵隔炎和炎症性肌纤维母细胞瘤（炎性假瘤）。孤立性纤维性肿瘤[51-55]免疫表型的特征是波形蛋白和CD34阳性，而角蛋白、EMA、S-100蛋白、结蛋白和肌动蛋白阴性。

相反的是，纤维瘤病和炎性假瘤表达波形蛋白、肌特异性肌动蛋白或α-异构肌动蛋白，表达或不表达结蛋白（图10.3）[56-58]。因此区分后两者只有依靠形态学特征。硬化性纵隔炎（SM）的梭形细胞只表达波形蛋白，然而在考虑为硬化性纵隔炎时必须时刻警惕，那就是要排除恶性淋巴瘤（尤其是闭塞性完全硬化性霍奇金淋巴瘤[14,59]）、转移癌，或者促纤维增生的间皮瘤，它们都可以在纵隔的软组织或淋巴结内产生致密的纤维性反应，肿瘤细胞在这些病变中较稀疏，且细胞学上异常温和，因此可能被漏诊，导致错误的诊断（图10.4）[60-62]，因此，在给出硬化性纵隔炎的诊断时要常规做角蛋白、CD15、CD20、CD30和CD45染色。

恶性小细胞纵隔肿瘤

表10.2、10.3，图10.5~10.8。

纵隔小细胞神经内分泌癌
（神经内分泌癌Ⅲ级，小细胞型）

几乎所有的纵隔小细胞神经内分泌癌（SCNC）都是转移来的[63]，通常是来自肺或食管。小细胞神经内分泌癌典型的免疫组化表型常常是点状的核周角蛋白染色阳性（图10.9）[18]，角蛋白是小细胞肿瘤中神经内分泌癌的特异性标记物。少数情况下，肿瘤还可以表达一种或几种神经内分泌标记，如CgA、Syn、CD57或者特异性的神经肽[64-69]。目前没有可靠的标准用来区别原发的（胸腺的）和继发的纵隔小细胞神经内分泌癌。甲状腺转录因子-1（TTF-1）在85%~95%的肺神经内分泌肿瘤中表达[70-71]，但是在原发胸腺的神经内分泌肿瘤中，缺少该标记物表达的有价值的参考资料。

纵隔基底细胞样鳞状细胞癌

基底细胞样鳞状细胞癌（BSCC）可以原发于胸腺[68,72,73]，也可以继发于咽、咽喉、喉或者是肛门直肠区[73]，基底细胞样鳞状细胞癌通常呈角蛋白胞浆弥漫阳性，也可表达EMA、CK5/6及p63[19,71,73,74]，依作者的经验，基底细胞样鳞状细胞癌中通常不表达神经内分泌标记物。

纵隔的神经母细胞瘤

典型的神经母细胞瘤（NBL）发生于儿童[42,75]，通常位于后纵隔[76,77]。然而，也有少数报道该种肿瘤或同类肿瘤可以发生于成年人的前纵隔[78,79]。神经母细胞瘤对波形蛋白和NF的反应不一，部分病例缺乏这两种蛋白表达，神经特性通常表现为CD56、CD57和Syn阳性（图10.10）[41,81]。神经母细胞瘤通常缺乏肌源性分化（结蛋白、肌动蛋白、Myo-D1、成肌素）、淋巴造血标记（CD45）和上皮特征（角蛋白、上皮细胞膜抗原）的标记物[52,78]，NB84是一种单克隆抗体，可以提高对神经母细胞瘤的特异性，然

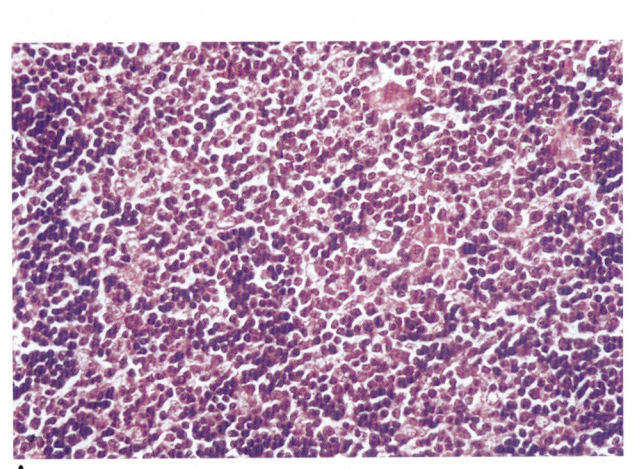
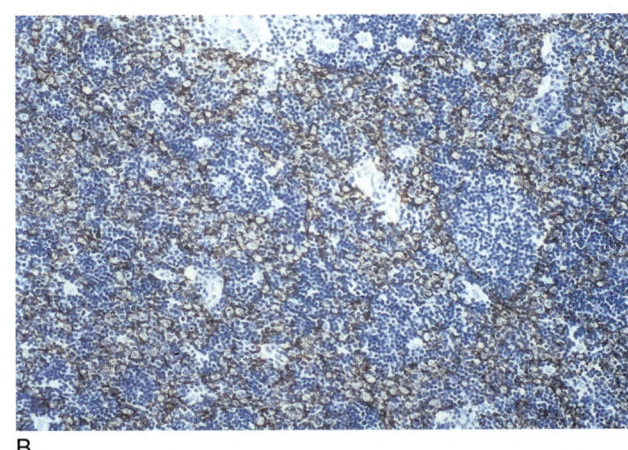

图 10.1　淋巴细胞为主型胸腺瘤中角蛋白染色（A），呈纤细的"连锁式"的反应模式（B）

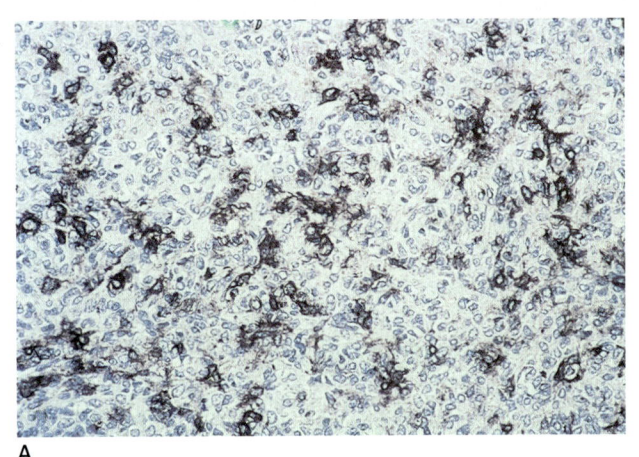
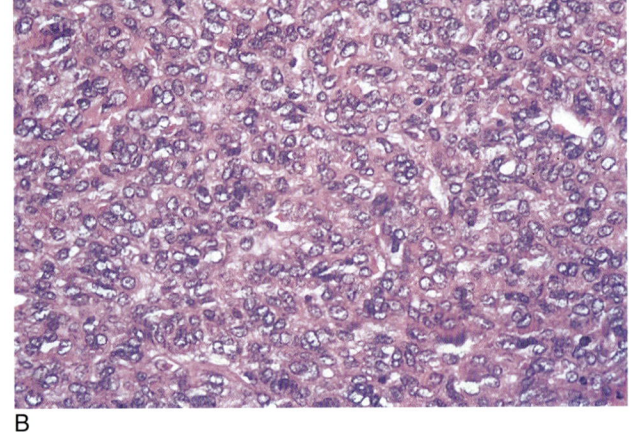

图 10.2　CD34（A）在纵隔血管外皮细胞瘤（B）中阳性

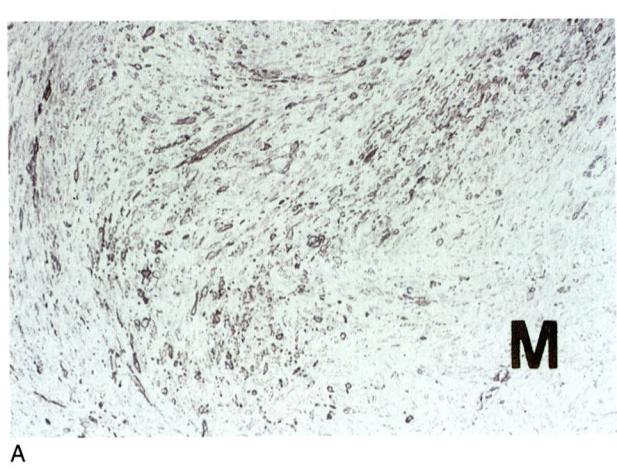
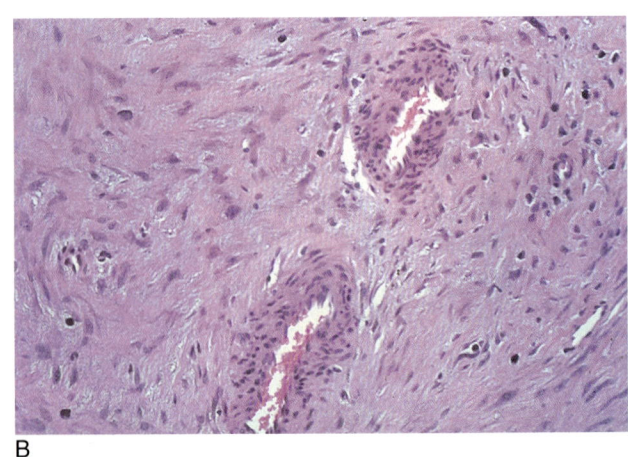

图 10.3　MSA（M）（A）在纵隔促纤维增生型纤维瘤病（B）增生的细胞中阳性

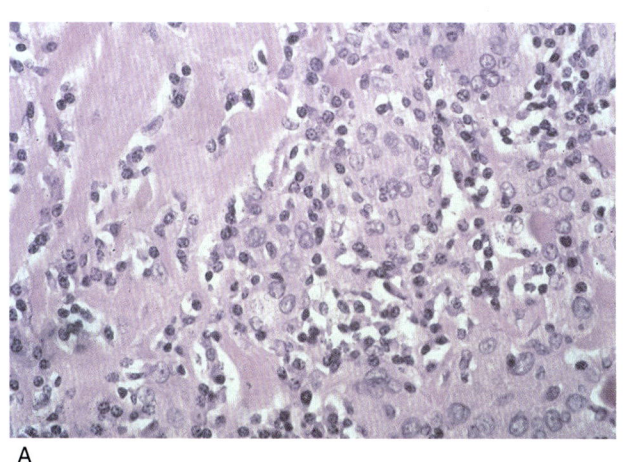 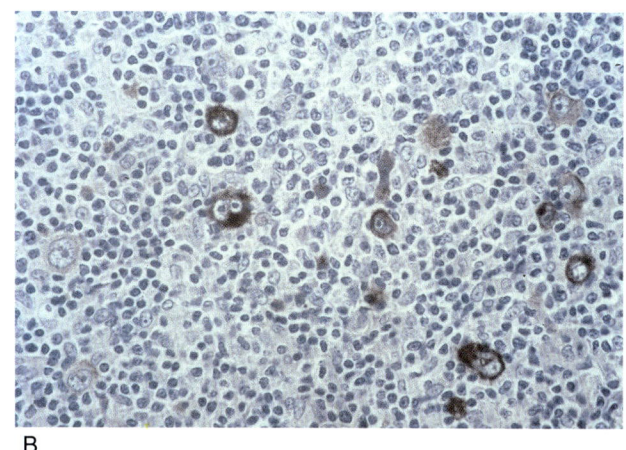

图 10.4 （A）这个纵隔的致密的纤维炎性包块呈现"瘤样纤维炎性病变"（纤维性纵隔炎）的外观，然而邻近的淋巴结活检（B）却显示出典型的 R-S 细胞（CD30 阳性），确诊为"完全闭塞的"结节硬化型霍奇金病

而它并不是这种肿瘤的特异性抗体，可见于绝大多数神经母细胞性肿瘤。

纵隔的原始神经外胚层肿瘤

原始神经外胚层肿瘤（PNET）很少发生于纵隔，不管是前纵隔还是后纵隔[83]，原始神经外胚层肿瘤的免疫表型与神经母细胞瘤相似，但是前者对波形蛋白的反应更一致，并且只偶尔标记NF[38]。另外，CD99[p30/32 (MIC-2)]和MB2抗原及β2微球蛋白在原始神经外胚层肿瘤中恒定阳性，但在神经母细胞瘤为阴性（图 10.11）[84-87]。Syn、CD56和CD57在很多原始神经外胚层肿瘤的病例中也可以检测到。具有多向分化的原始神经外胚层肿瘤，还可以检测到局灶性的角蛋白、波形蛋白和肌动蛋白阳性[38, 88]，这类病变也被命名为"腹膜促纤维增生性小细胞肿瘤"、"软组织横纹肌肉瘤样小细胞肿瘤"及"外胚层间叶瘤"。在一定程度上，区分一个MIC-2阳性的实体小圆细胞横纹肌肉瘤（见后）和一个具有横纹肌母细胞分化，特别是Syn表达缺如的原始神经外胚层肿瘤是很困难的。在这种情况下，就必须依赖细胞遗传学信息，借助于查找小圆细胞横纹肌肉瘤特征性的t(2;13)或t(1;13)染色体易位，或原始神经外胚层肿瘤的t(11;22)染色体易位。另外可能的区分方法是做FLT-1的免疫染色，FLT-1是一种在大多数原始神经外胚层肿瘤中表达的核转录因子，组织学上与原始神经外胚层肿瘤相似的横纹肌肉瘤无 FLI-1 表达[89]。

纵隔的横纹肌肉瘤

纵隔横纹肌肉瘤（RMS）几乎总是发生在儿童和青少年[41, 90, 91]，表现为胚胎性或腺泡性特征（见第 15 章），几乎所有的横纹肌肉瘤都表达结蛋白（图 10.12）和肌特异性肌动蛋白及波形蛋白。肌球蛋白只在大细胞的分化成熟的横纹肌肉瘤中表达，因此在纯粹的小细胞类型的横纹肌肉瘤中不是一个特别有效的标记物，横纹肌肉瘤不表达突触素，但是有些病例可以表达 CD56、CD57 或者 MIC-2[38, 52, 85, 86, 92]。结蛋白和肌动蛋白诊断横纹肌肉瘤的特异性受到挑战，因为在平滑肌肿瘤中它们也阳性，尽管如此，对作者来说，这种讨论看上去也是多余的，因为平滑肌肉瘤的

表10.2 免疫组化在纵隔不确定小细胞和未分化肿瘤鉴别诊断中的应用
Keratin (monoclonal mixture)
Epithelial membrane antigen
Vimentin
Desmin
Muscle-specific actin
Myo-D1
Myogenin
Neuron-specific enolase
Synaptophysin
Chromogranin A
CD15
CD45
CD99 (MIC-2 protein)
BerEP4
S-100 protein
HMB-45
MART-1
Tyrosinase

表10.3 纵隔具有不确定或未分化特征的恶性小细胞肿瘤所选标记物的免疫组化反应率

Tumor	KER	EMA	VIM	DES	MSA	MYO-D1	MYOGN	S-100	HMB-45	TYR	MART-1	NSE	SYN	CGA	BER-EP4	CD45	CD15	CD99
ES/PNET	10	0	87	1	3	3	3	10	0	0	0	91	74	0	70	0	0	81
RMS	0	0	91	93	97	91	92	7	0	0	0	37	0	0	0	0	0	20
LL/TAL*	0	0	23	0	0	0	0	10	0	0	0	11	0	0	0	90/78	85/52	10
SCMM	1	3	100	0	0	0	0	97	50	86	87	70	0	0	0	0	0	7
PNBL	0	0	56	0	0	0	0	37	0	0	0	99	65	71	0	0	0	0
MSCSCC	100	83	35	0	0	0	0	52	0	0	0	50	40	0	60	0	0	0
MSCADCA	100	99	12	0	0	0	0	5	0	0	0	44	15	0	92	0	69	0
SCNC	99	73	0	0	0	0	0	0	0	0	0	70	35	40	100	0	18	20
SCUS	0	0	100	0	0	0	0	0	0	0	0	10	0	0	0	0	0	0

* 除非特别注明,所给出的反应百分率适用于所有实体肿瘤

KER,角蛋白(单克隆抗体混合物);EMA,上皮细胞膜抗原;VIM,波形蛋白;DES,结蛋白;MSA,肌特异性肌动蛋白;MYOGN,成肌素;S-100,S-100蛋白;TYR,酪氨酸酶;NSE,神经特异性(γ二聚体)烯醇化酶;SYN,突触素;CGA,嗜铬素A;PNET,原始神经外胚层肿瘤;ES,尤文瘤;RMS,横纹肌肉瘤;LL,淋巴母细胞瘤;TAL,急性髓性白血病;SCMM,小细胞恶性黑色素瘤;PNBL,外周神经母细胞瘤;MSCSCC,转移的小细胞鳞状细胞癌;MSCADCA,转移的小细胞腺癌;SCNC,小细胞神经内分泌癌;SCUS,小细胞未分化肉瘤

(数据摘自 Frisman D. Immunoquery. 网站 http://www.immunoquery.com,以及作者的经验)

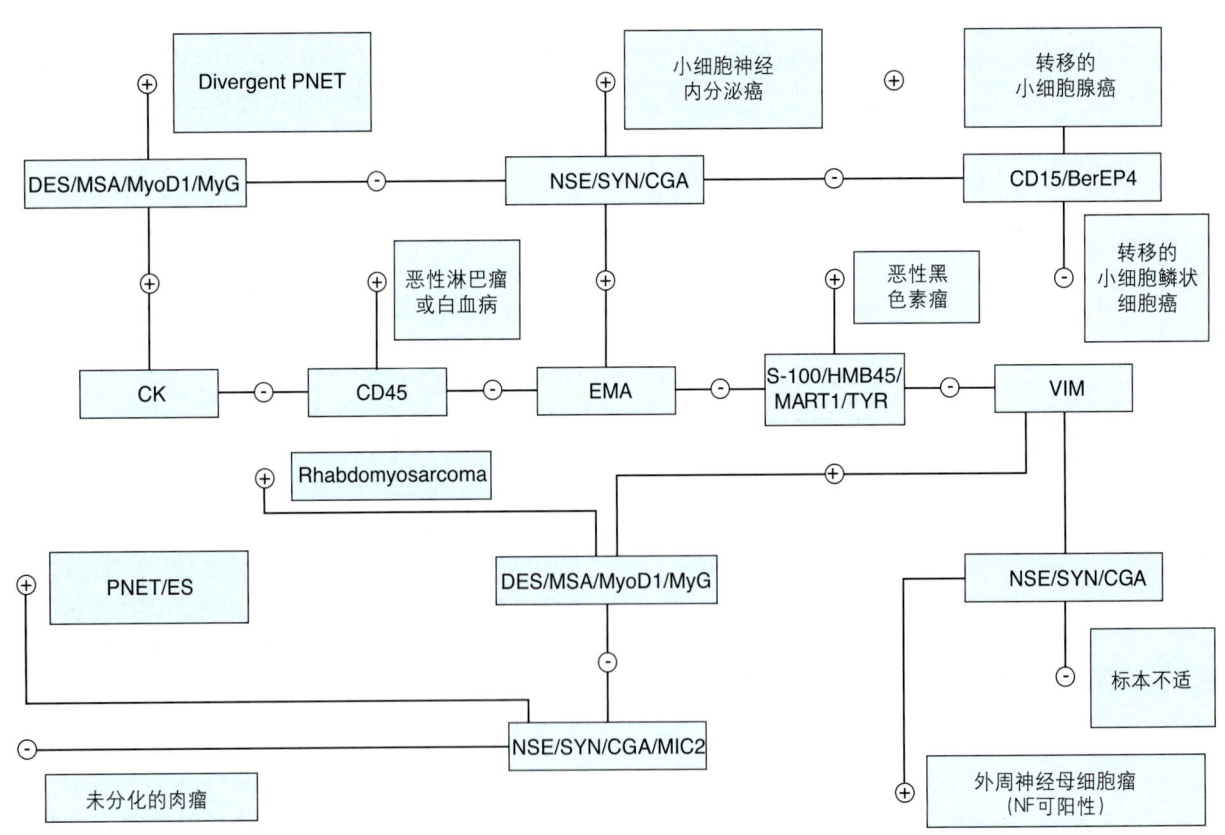

图10.5 纵隔恶性小细胞肿瘤的免疫组化分析流程

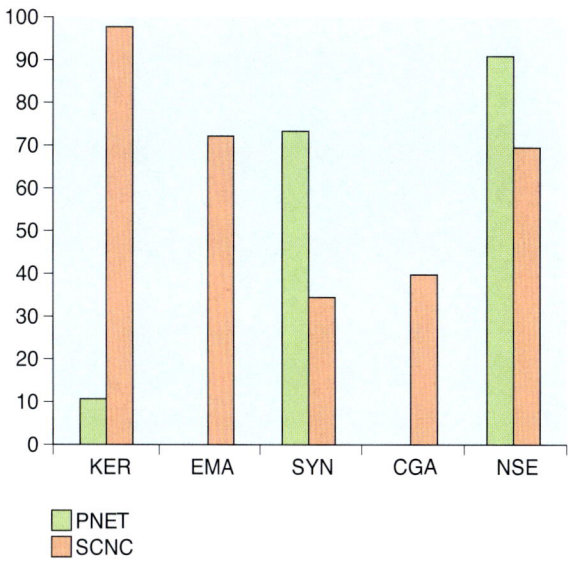

图10.6 纵隔原始神经外胚层肿瘤（PNET）与小细胞神经内分泌癌（SCNC）用于鉴别诊断的标记物

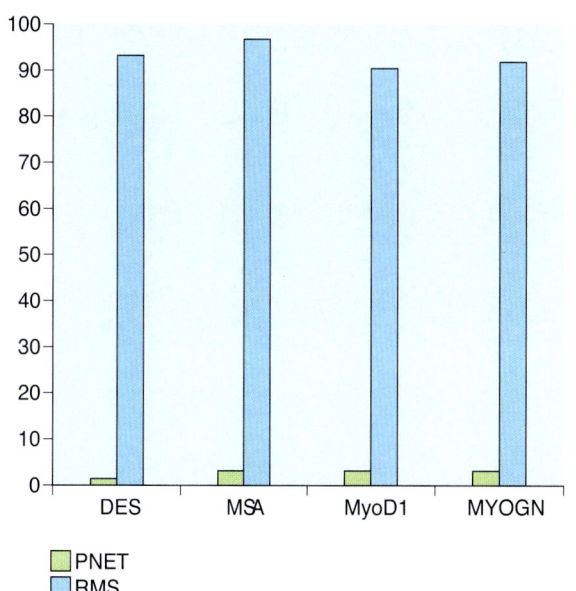

图 10.7 纵隔原始神经外胚层肿瘤（PNET）与横纹肌肉瘤（RMS）用于鉴别诊断的标记物

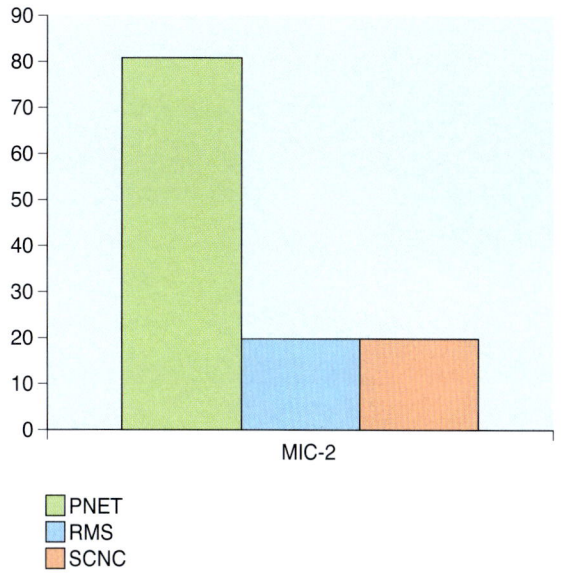

图10.8 CD99（MIC-2）在纵隔原始神经外胚层肿瘤（PNET）与横纹肌肉瘤（RMS）及小细胞神经内分泌癌（SCNC）中的阳性率比较

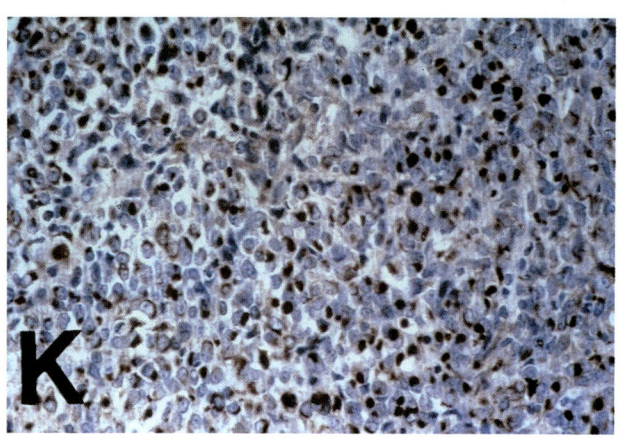

图 10.9 典型的核周"点"状角蛋白染色是纵隔小细胞神经内分泌癌的证据。

小细胞变型根本就不存在。在任何情况下，限定于横纹肌的核蛋白，Myo-D1 和成肌素[92,93]，可以用于疑难病例的鉴别诊断。

纵隔小细胞恶性淋巴瘤

少数小细胞非霍奇金淋巴瘤（SCNHL）可以原发于纵隔，包括淋巴母细胞淋巴瘤（LL）[94-96]（参见前文），小无裂细胞（Burkitt/非Burkitt）淋巴瘤（SNCL）[97,98]和0（MALT 淋巴瘤)[99,100]。

免疫组化分析对于区分这些肿瘤的诊断是很有帮助的，它们通常表达CD45（白细胞共同抗原），但是淋巴母细胞淋巴瘤的某些病例并不表达，淋巴母细胞淋巴瘤通常表达 CD43 系列（L60、Leu22、MT-1），CD99 系列抗体如 HBA-71、O13 或 12E7，抗-CD10（急性淋巴母细胞白血病共同抗原），及 bcl-2 和 TdT 的抗体（图 10.13）[27]，SNCL 表达 CD20，表达或不表达bcl-2[27]。MALT淋巴瘤表达CD20和CD79a，但是不表达 CD10、CD43、CD99、bcl-2 和 TdT。在 3 种 SCNHL 中，CD5 表达不一，但角蛋白、CD56、CD57、Syn、结蛋白、肌动蛋白、Myo-D1和成肌素均不表达。约 50% 表达波形蛋白[104]。

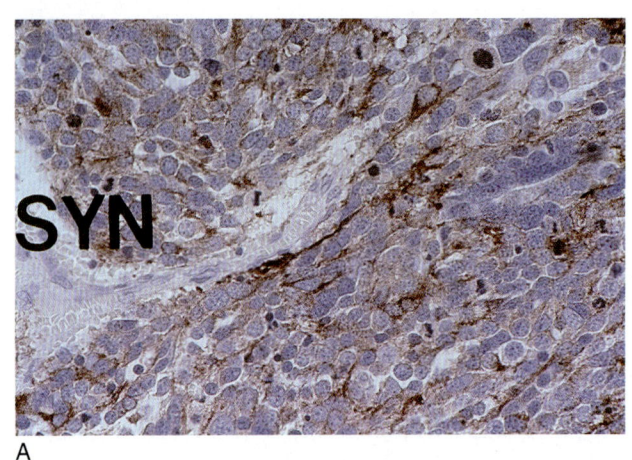

图 10.10　突触素（SYN）(A) 在纵隔神经母细胞瘤（B）中弥漫阳性

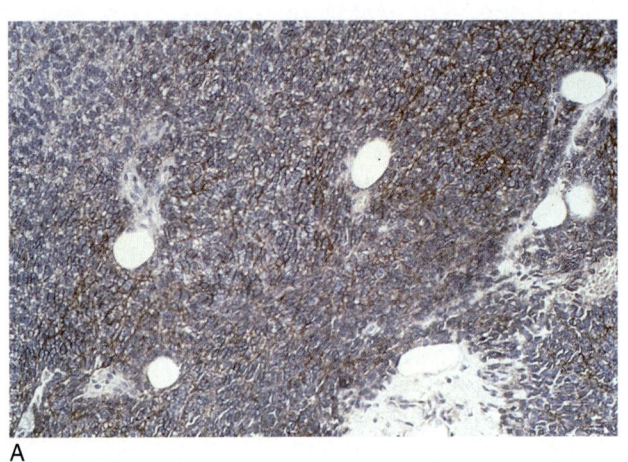

图 10.11　CD99 (MIC-2)(A)在纵隔原始神经外胚层肿瘤（B）中阳性

其他小细胞纵隔肿瘤

除了前面讲过的小细胞肿瘤，其他一些转移性肿瘤也可以累及纵隔。包括小细胞骨肉瘤及骨的 Ewing 肉瘤以及小细胞恶性黑色素瘤，除了小细胞恶性黑色素瘤以外，其他肿瘤都有明确的原发灶，毫无疑问不会来自胸腔。然而，黑色素瘤在未找到明确原发灶的前提下，依然可以发生远处转移。而且，它们可以模仿小细胞肿瘤的形态，与小细胞神经内分泌癌极为相似[105]。小细胞黑色素瘤免疫组化的特点是 S-100、酪氨酸酶、MART-1 和 HMB-45 阳性[105, 106]，这些标记在纵隔其他的小细胞肿瘤中都不表达。

纵隔大多角形细胞肿瘤

表 10.4、10.5，图 10.14～10.18。

原发的胸腺癌

原发的胸腺癌（PTC）是一个令人兴奋的诊断，因为它太少见了，但是应该记住，大多数认为是原发的胸腺癌最终会被证实为转移来的。原发的胸腺癌免疫组化较一致地表达角蛋白和 p63[107]，很多病例也表达上皮细胞膜抗原（EMA）。癌胚抗原、分泌因子、Bg8、MOC-31、calretinin、HBME-1、BerEP4 和 TAG-72 也有不同程度的表达，尤其是在局灶或弥漫的腺样分化的肿瘤中。但是，波形蛋白、血栓调节素、WT-1

10 纵隔的免疫组织化学

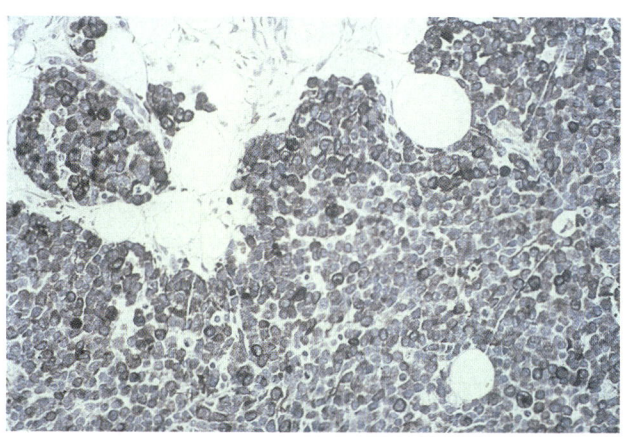

图 10.12　纵隔横纹肌肉瘤中结蛋白的免疫反应

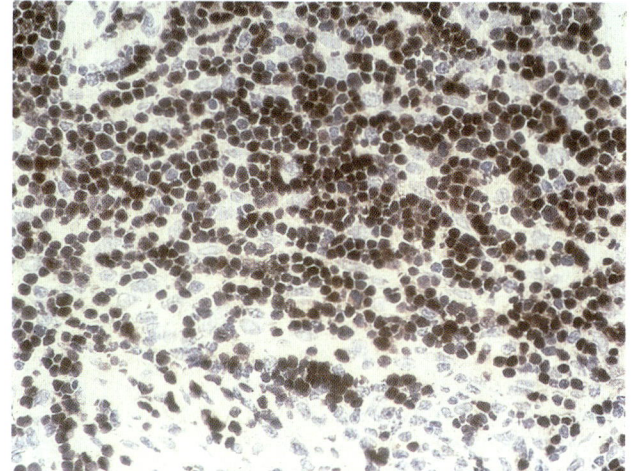

图10.13　胸腺淋巴母细胞淋巴瘤中末端脱氧核甘酸转移酶细胞核着色。

表10.4　免疫组化在纵隔不确定的大细胞或未分化肿瘤鉴别诊断中的应用
Keratin (monoclonal mixture)
Vimentin
Synaptophysin
Chromogranin A
CD15
CD30
CD45
Placenta-like alkaline phosphatase
Carcinoembryonic antigen
BerEP4
Calretinin
S-100 protein
HMB-45
Tyrosinase
MART-1

和 TTF-1 在原发的多角形细胞胸腺癌变型中不表达[18, 104, 107, 108]。可能存在的陷阱是原发的胸腺癌的"肝细胞样"变型，由成片的、体积较大的嗜酸性瘤细胞构成，看起来很像转移的肝细胞肝癌（MHCC）[109]。事实上，肝细胞样胸腺癌和肝细胞肝癌都表达 Hep-PAR1，通常被认为是一种肝细胞标记物[110]。

有报道称胸腺癌的上皮细胞表达 CD5 而普通胸腺瘤中的上皮细胞则不表达（图 10.19）[104-106,111]，对

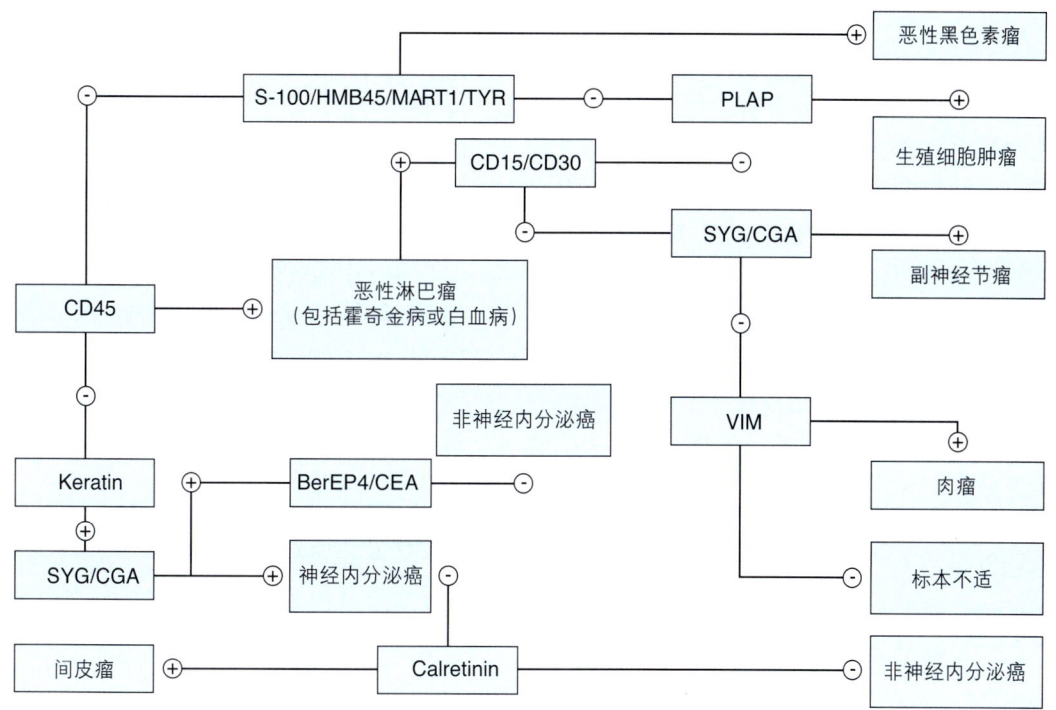

图 10.14　恶性纵隔大多角形细胞肿瘤的免疫组化分析流程

表10.5 纵隔不确定或未分化大多角形细胞肿瘤相关标记物的免疫组化反应率

Tumor	KER	CMA	VIM	CALRET	PLAP	S-100	HMB-45	TYR	MART-1	SYN	CGA	BER-EP4	CD45	CD15	CD30
PTADCA	100	70	5	67	0	0	0	0	0	40	20	70	0	65	0
MADCA	100	75	12	10	10	10	0	0	0	3	5	90	0	70	0
PNEC	100	40	20	0	0	6	0	0	0	80	90	90	0	85	0
MNEC	100	62	20	0	0	10	0	0	0	80	75	90	0	20	0
LCL/TAL*	0	0/50	65	0	0	3	0	0	0	0	0	0	99/85	3/85	23/3
ALCL	0	0	100	0	0	10	0	0	0	0	0	0	90	13	99
SYNHD	0	0	50	0	0	0	0	0	0	0	0	0	6	90	90
MELAN	1	0	100	0	0	97	50	86	90	0	0	0	0	0	0
SEMIN	12	0	70	0	93	0	0	0	0	0	0	0	0	0	3
EMBCA	100	0	17	0	90	0	0	0	0	0	0	0	0	0	80
YST	100	0	50	0	50	0	0	0	0	0	0	0	0	0	20
EPSARCS[a]	V	0	100	V	0	V	0	0	0	0	0	V	0	0	0
PSCC	100	40	5	0	3	0	0	0	0	40	20	50	0	20	0
MSCC	100	50	30	33	10	10	0	0	0	20	3	50	0	20	0
LELCT	100	0	50	0	0	0	0	0	0	40	20	10	0	0	0
MESOTH	100	0	54	90	3	7	0	0	0	0	2	10	0	1	0
PARAGANG	2	0	40	0	0	40	0	0	0	100	100	0	0	0	0

* 除非特别注明，给出的反应百分率适用于所有实体肿瘤

[a] 上皮样滑膜肉瘤，角蛋白100%阳性，BerEP4 90%阳性；上皮样恶性外周神经鞘瘤 S-100 蛋白80%阳性

V，可变的，通常阳性

KER，角蛋白（单克隆抗体混合物）；CEA，癌胚抗原；VIM，波形蛋白；CALRET，calretinin；PLAP，胎盘碱性磷酸酶；S-100，S-100蛋白；TYR，酪氨酸酶；SYN，突触素；CGA，嗜铬素 A；PTADCA，原发的胸腺癌；MADCA，转移的腺癌；PNEC，原发的神经内分泌癌；MNEC，转移的神经内分泌癌；LCL，大细胞淋巴瘤；TAL，急性髓性白血病；ALCL，间变性大细胞淋巴瘤；SYNHD，合体细胞型霍奇金病；MELAN，恶性黑色素瘤；SEMIN，精原细胞瘤；EMBCA，胚胎性癌；YST，卵黄囊瘤；EPSARCS，具有上皮样分化的肉瘤；PSCC，原发的胸腺梭形细胞癌；MSCC，转移的鳞状细胞癌；LELCT，胸腺的淋巴上皮样癌；MESOTH，间皮瘤；PARAGANG，恶性副神经节瘤。

（数据摘自 Frisman D.Immunoquery.网站 http://www.immunoquery.com，以及作者的经验）

于这种说法必须有所保留，因为不典型上皮为主型胸腺瘤（也就是说上皮细胞的异型性不足以作出恶性诊断）也有40%的病例表达CD5[106]。Saud等[108]也发现大多数原发的、分化较差的肺癌也表达CD5（原发的胸腺癌最重要的鉴别诊断对象）。

文献介绍突变的p53在某种程度上可以作为区别胸腺瘤和胸腺癌的另一个潜在标记物[112-114]。一般来说，胸腺癌比胸腺瘤更容易出现抗突变的p53蛋白的抗体 DO1 和 DO3 免疫染色阳性，因此，这两个抗体可以作为区分这两者的辅助指标。类似的标记物还有Mcl-1蛋白[115]和Fas抗原[116]，但是有关它们在胸腺肿瘤中的资料甚少。

其他的胸腺原发的恶性肿瘤，如生殖细胞肿瘤和淋巴瘤，CD5呈典型的阴性[105, 106, 111]。该发现是否经得住时间考验，需要将来作更多的研究判定。另一方面，现在发现胸腺大多数的原发的胸腺癌和转移癌中缺少MIC-2阳性的淋巴细胞，说明CD99在区别这些肿瘤时没有作用。

另一个需要提及的方面是原发的胸腺癌的神经内分泌"潜能"，尽管缺乏明显的神经内分泌的组织学特征，但是Syn、CgA、CD56或CD57免疫染色阳性（图10.20）[117]。这些发现的生物学意义目前还不确定，但是也还不足以把目前的诊断分型变成"神经内分泌癌"。

> **诊断要点：原发性胸腺癌**
>
> 1. 角蛋白和p63阳性，CD5呈典型阳性。
> 2. TTF-1 和 WT-1 均阴性。

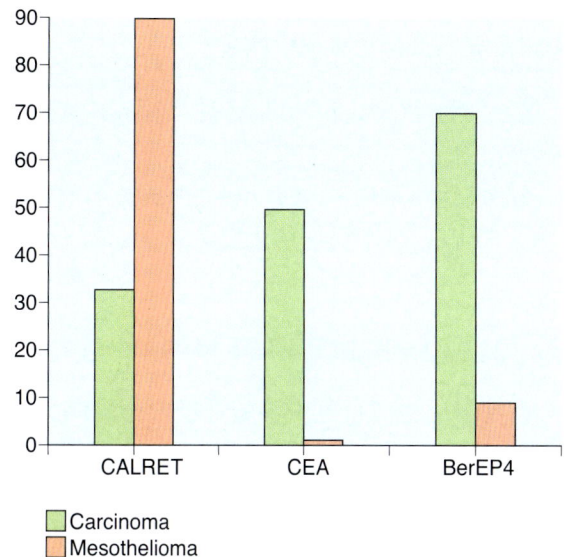

图 10.15 纵隔的癌和间皮瘤用于鉴别诊断的标记物

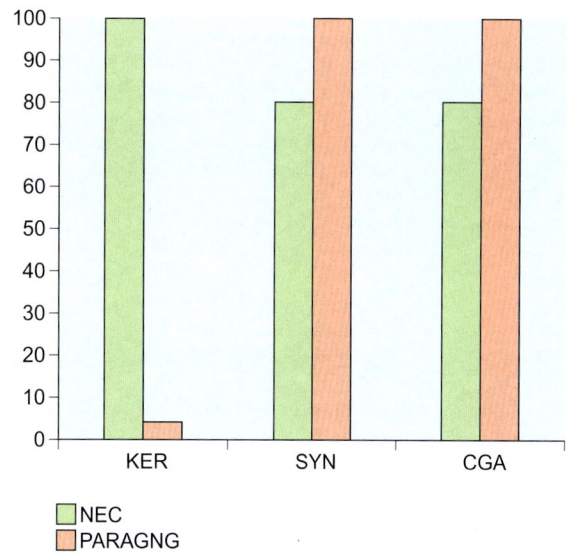

图10.17 纵隔神经内分泌癌和恶性副神经节瘤免疫反应对比图

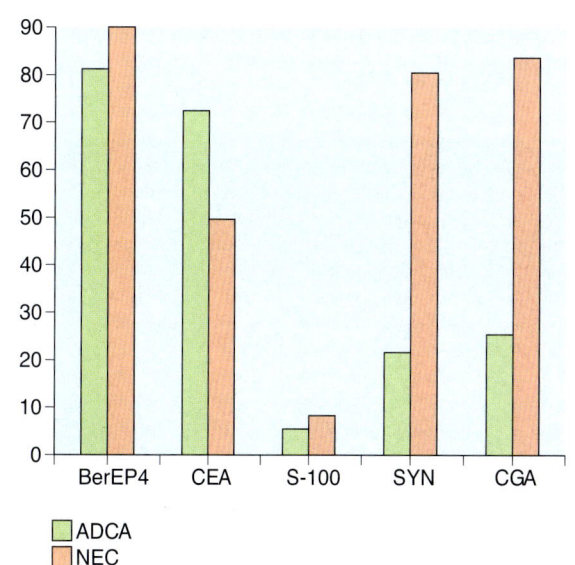

图10.16 纵隔低分化腺癌和神经内分泌癌用于鉴别诊断的标记物

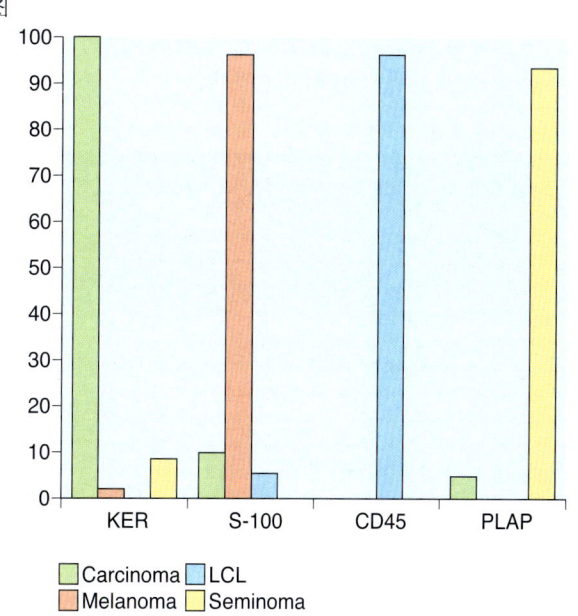

图10.18 纵隔的癌与转移性恶性黑色素瘤、大细胞非霍奇金淋巴瘤及精原细胞瘤用于鉴别诊断的标记物

纵隔的甲状旁腺癌

甲状旁腺癌（PAC）可以发生在胸腺或者前上纵隔的软组织。有些病例与胸腺的神经内分泌癌相似，副神经节瘤也需要与其鉴别[118-120]。恶性甲状旁腺病变可以导致溶骨性的血钙增高，因此具有典型的临床表现。然而，无分泌功能的甲状旁腺癌或许需要免疫组化来明确诊断，这可以通过检测细胞内的甲状旁腺激素来实现（图 10.21）[121]。除此以外，甲状旁腺癌的免疫表型与其他神经内分泌癌大致相同[120]。

恶性纵隔生殖细胞肿瘤

单纯的或者混合的纵隔生殖细胞肿瘤，如精原细胞瘤、胚胎性癌、内胚窦瘤和滋养细胞肿瘤都可以在纵隔发生或者是转移到纵隔[15, 16, 122-126]，对于这些肿瘤的确诊，免疫组化经常是必需的，尤其是标本组织有限的时候。精原细胞瘤典型的免疫表型是肿瘤细胞角蛋白和EMA阴性，细胞膜CD117和PLAP阳性（图10.22）[16, 127, 128]。然而，将近10%~15%的这种病例确实局限性地表达角蛋白[16]。胚胎性癌和卵黄囊癌与

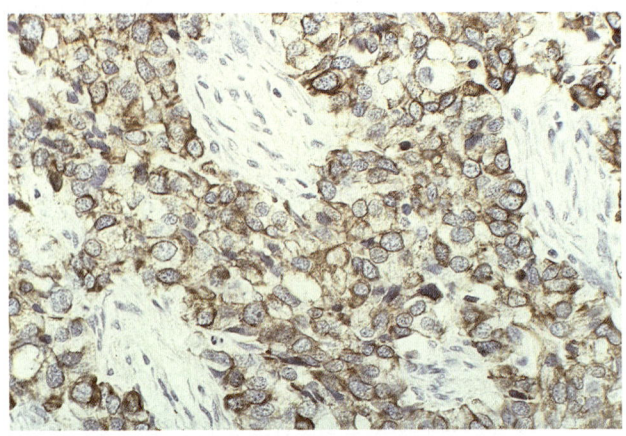

图 10.19 原发性胸腺癌中 CD5 弥漫性染色

> **诊断要点：纵隔生殖细胞肿瘤**
>
> 1. 精原细胞瘤 CD117+、PLAP+、角蛋白-（少数灶性+）。
> 2. 胚胎性癌角蛋白+、CD30+，卵黄囊瘤角蛋白+、AFP+，绒毛膜癌角蛋白+。

精原细胞瘤的区别在于弥漫的角蛋白阳性和潜在的α-甲胎蛋白（AFP）染色阳性[16, 125, 129]。另外，胚胎性癌反常地标记 CD30（图 10.23）[130]，CD30 被看做是典型的造血系统标记物。绒毛膜癌角蛋白阳性，其典型的免疫表现是 EMA 和 β-hCG 阳性[16, 131]。

纵隔"类癌"（神经内分泌癌 I 和 II 级）

免疫组化检测可见胸腺的神经内分泌癌呈角蛋白、NSE、Syn、CD56、CD57 和 CgA 阳性[18, 132-135]。而且，即使没有出现明显的内分泌临床症状，也可以在细胞水平检测到特异的神经肽表达[136-138]。

纵隔副神经节瘤

胸内副神经节瘤（PG）可以发生在前纵隔、主肺动脉根部或者椎旁组织[135,139,140]，向神经方向分化，

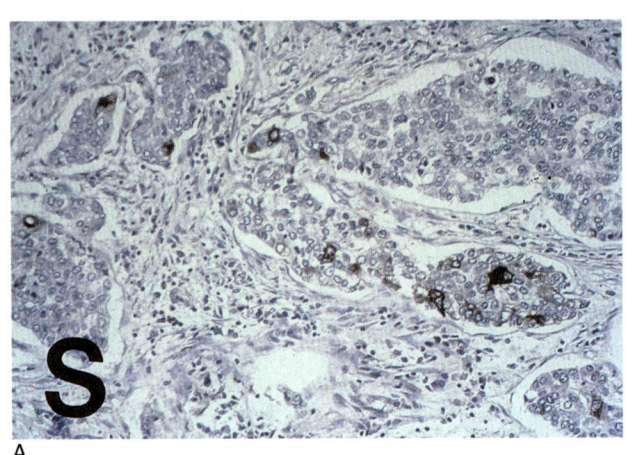
A

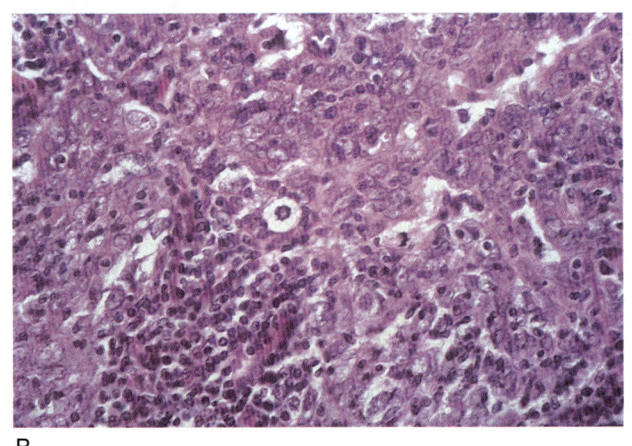
B

图 10.20 突触素（S）(A) 在一例缺乏神经内分泌癌典型形态特征的原发性胸腺癌（B）中的免疫染色

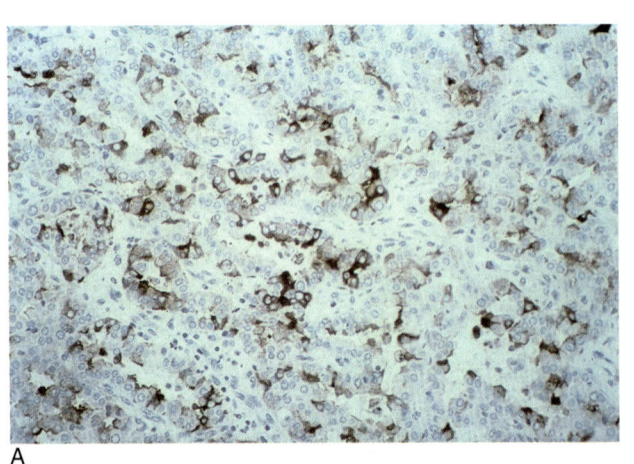
A

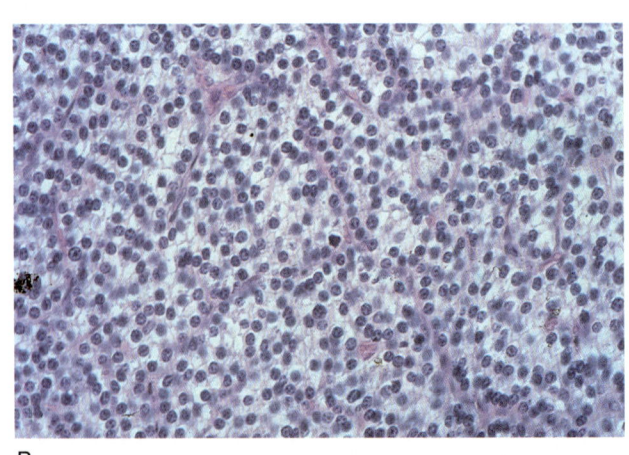
B

图 10.21 甲状旁腺激素（PTH）(A) 在原发于纵隔的甲状旁腺癌（B）中的免疫染色

纵隔的免疫组织化学

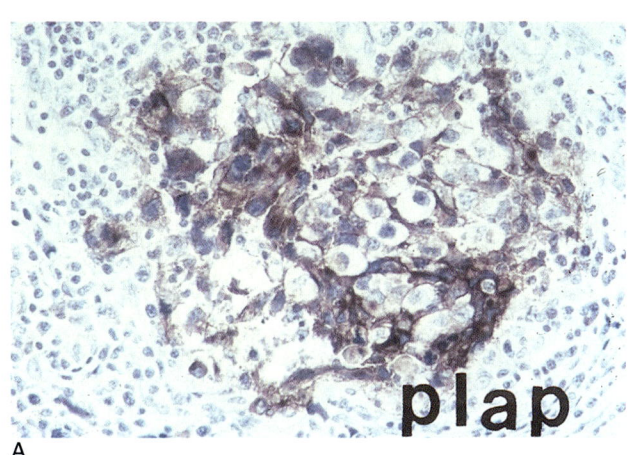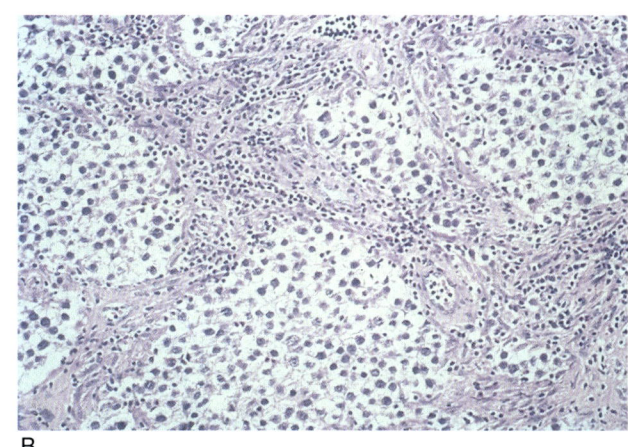

图 10.22　胎盘碱性磷酸酶 PLAP（A）在原发于纵隔的精原细胞瘤（B）中细胞膜染色阳性

所以不表达角蛋白和 EMA 而表达 NF 蛋白，表达或不表达波形蛋白，与神经母细胞瘤相似[115]。S-100蛋白可以标记副神经节瘤肿瘤细胞巢周围的支持细胞（图 10.24）[141]，瘤细胞本身通常会含有一种神经肽[142]。CgA 标记瘤细胞普遍阳性。

纵隔大细胞非霍奇金淋巴瘤

见表 10.6，图 10.25。

继霍奇金淋巴瘤之后，大细胞非霍奇金淋巴瘤（LCNHL）是又一个容易在纵隔原发的恶性肿瘤[104]。所有的大细胞非霍奇金淋巴瘤细胞膜都表达 CD45[37, 104, 143-146]。然而，有个别报道在此部位可见"Ki-1+"（CD30+）的大细胞间变性淋巴瘤[147]，其中有些CD45阴性。因此当CD30阳性，在考虑大细胞非霍奇金淋巴瘤的可能性时要谨慎地分析。如果同时角蛋白阴性，那么CD30对诊断淋巴瘤来说是一个特异性标记[104]。大多数纵隔的大细胞非霍奇金淋巴瘤标记CD20、PAX-5 和 CD79a，加上其间变的特征都支持它们的 B 细胞分化（图 10.26）[145, 146, 148, 149]。T 细胞或"真正的组织细胞样"分化的大细胞非霍奇金淋巴瘤在纵隔非常罕见，但在纵隔已有报道[104]。

"合体细胞型"纵隔霍奇金病

霍奇金淋巴瘤（HL）是最常见的纵隔恶性肿瘤[104]。它不仅发生在胸腺及胸腺旁淋巴结，还可以通过直接蔓延的方式累及邻近的组织[150-152]。大多数HL不需要借助免疫组化就可以诊断，但是有一个变型，即合体细胞型霍奇金淋巴瘤，其中的单核R-S细胞成片排列，非常像癌或者是大细胞非霍奇金淋巴瘤[153]。几乎所有大细胞非霍奇金淋巴瘤中的 R-S 细胞 CD45 染

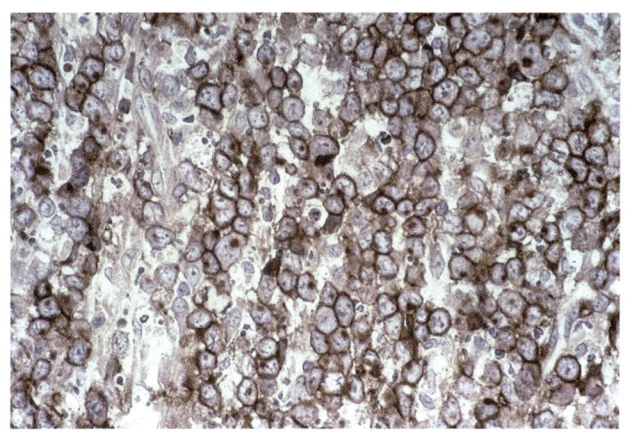

图 10.23　胸腺胚胎性癌中 CD30 弥漫阳性

表10.6　免疫组化在纵隔造血系统疾病鉴别诊断中的应用

Keratin
HMB-45
MART-1
Tyrosinase
Placenta-like alkaline phosphatase
CD3
CD15
CD20
CD30
CD43
CD45
CD45RO
CD68
CD74
MB2
BLA.36
BNH9
Cathepsin-B
Lysozyme
Myeloperoxidase

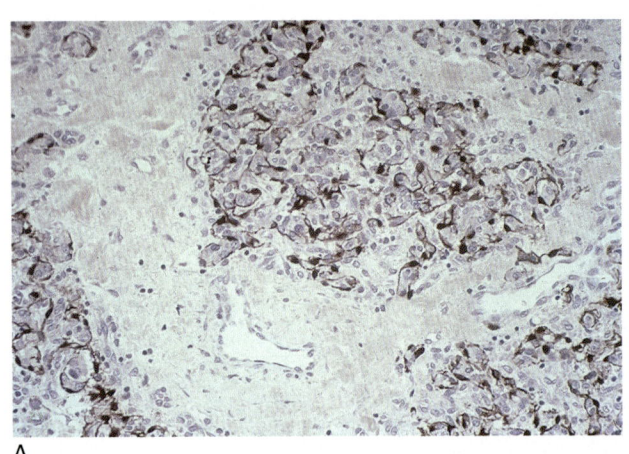

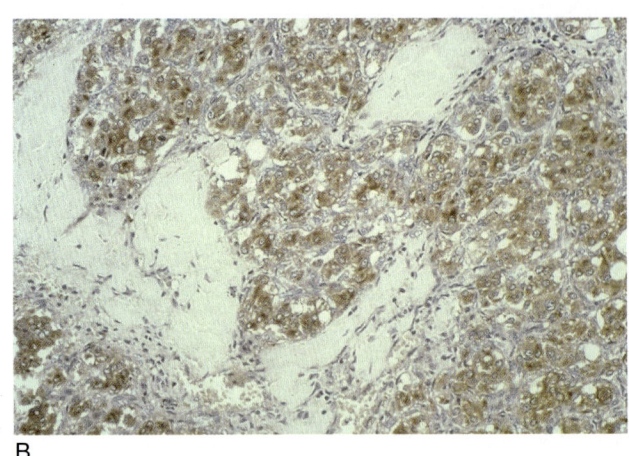

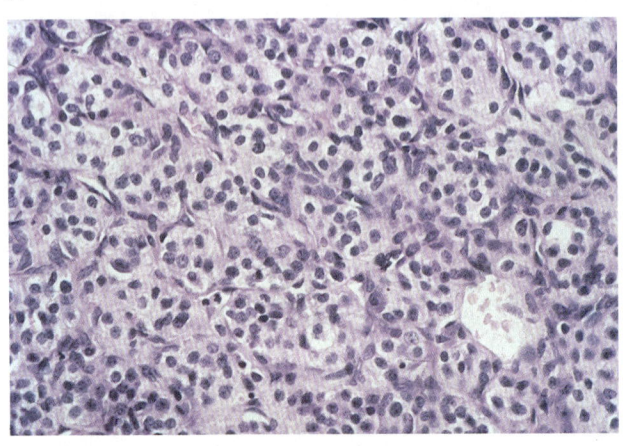

图10.24　S-100（A）和CgA（B）在纵隔副神经节瘤支持细胞（C）中染色阳性，当肿瘤具有明显的恶性生物学行为时S-100阴性

色阳性，与HL中R-S细胞CD45染色阴性截然相反[18,104]。另一方面，合体细胞型HL中的R-S细胞同时表达CD15和CD30（图10.27）。CD15在大多数大细胞非霍奇金淋巴瘤中都不表达，因此可以作为这些肿瘤的鉴别标记。然而，必须知道霍奇金淋巴瘤和CD30+的大细胞非霍奇金淋巴瘤是有一部分重叠的。细胞遗传学研究可查见5q35位点的异常，是"Ki-1+"大细胞淋巴瘤的特征性表现[154,155]。不像恶性上皮性肿瘤那样，合体细胞型HL角蛋白阴性，可以用来与发生在纵隔的癌鉴别。

其他的纵隔造血系统肿瘤

可以发生在纵隔的另外两个造血系统肿瘤是粒细胞肉瘤（髓外的髓性白血病）[156,157]和骨外的浆细胞瘤（EPM）[158,159]，粒细胞肉瘤CD15、CD33、CD34、CD68、MPO染色阳性而大细胞非霍奇金淋巴瘤阴性（图10.28）[160-162]。纵隔的骨外浆细胞瘤在镜下与神经内分泌肿瘤非常相似[158,159]，有时与大细胞淋巴瘤也难以鉴别。但是骨外浆细胞瘤表达轻链免疫球蛋白（图10.29）、CD38和CD138（syndecan-1）[163]，而不

表达角蛋白、CgA和Syn[164]。应特别注意该肿瘤的诊断陷阱，因为它具有表达EMA的潜能，如果不警惕的话，这种结果就会支持一个错误的神经内分泌肿瘤的诊断。

恶性纵隔上皮样间皮瘤

尽管恶性间皮瘤通常被认为是发生在胸膜和腹膜的肿瘤，但是它们也可以发生在纵隔，可能是发生在胸膜表面肺门反折的部位，所有组织学类型的间皮瘤，包括单一上皮样型都呈角蛋白免疫染色阳性，同样，calretinin也是阳性[166]。约50%的间皮瘤共表达波形蛋白，也可异质性表达HBME-1[167]和血栓调节素等此类标记物（并不十分特异）[168]。癌性分化的特异性标记物，如CEA、CD15、p63、TTF-1，血型组抗原（如A、B、H和Lewis）及CA72-4抗原（被B72.3抗体识别）在间皮瘤中都不表达[169-171]。

纵隔转移的癌和黑色素瘤

如前所述，纵隔的绝大部分非造血系统恶性病变，在诊断为其他疾病之前，要首先考虑转移的可能性，免疫组化只是某种程度上证实转移癌的起源部位，如果发现标记物与原发性胸腺癌无关，如TTF-1、甲状腺球蛋白、PSA、S-100、PLAP、CA19-9（一种肠癌标记物），或者CA125（浆膜和苗勒管标记物）

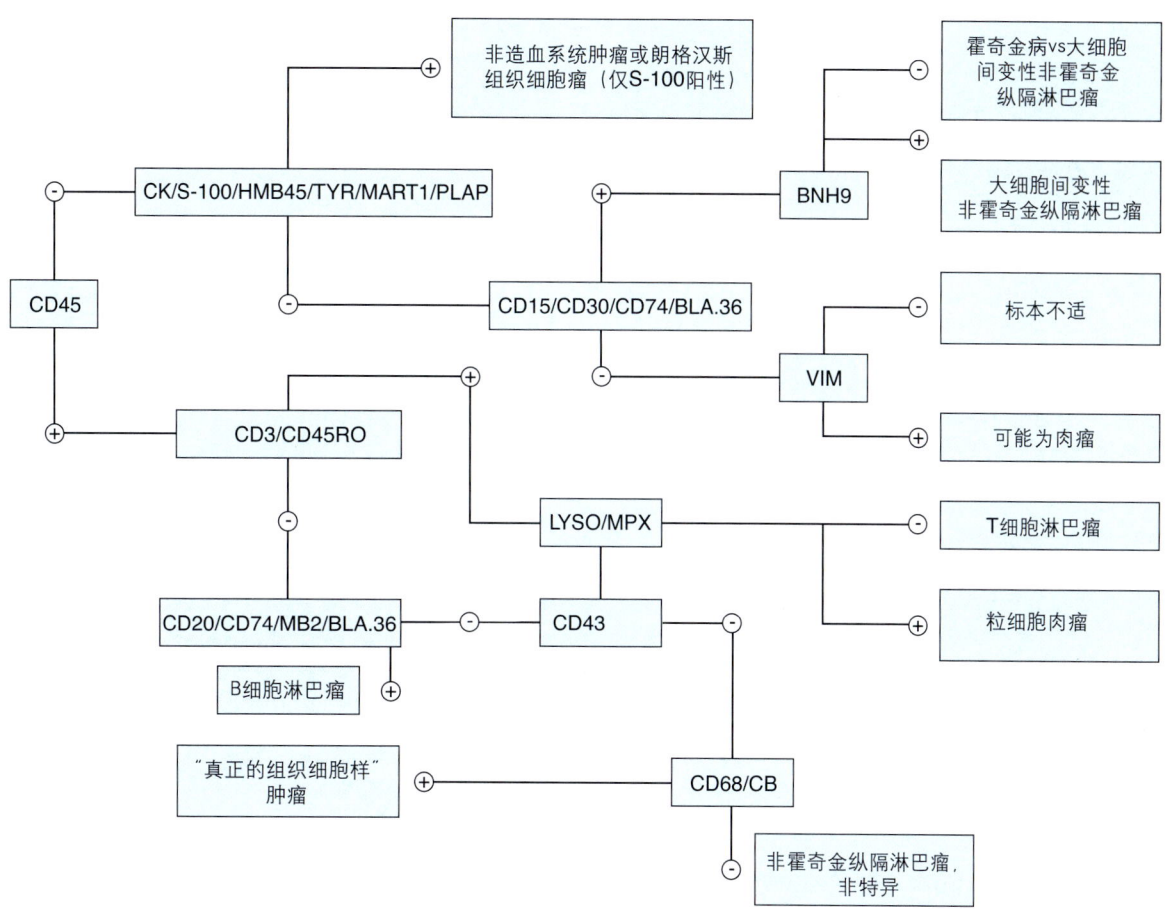

图10.25 纵隔造血系统肿瘤免疫组化分析流程

[172]标记阳性，则很可能是转移性的。相反，如果表达CK5/6、p63和CD5，那至少可以推测，这个肿瘤可能原发于胸腺[111]。

纵隔转移的无色素性恶性黑色素瘤很少表现出它的初始症状[173]，在面部没有明显的皮肤的或者黏膜的病变。在这种情况下，就需要与包括原发的或者转移的癌、恶性生殖细胞肿瘤和淋巴瘤鉴别。免疫组化研究发现转移的纵隔大细胞黑色素瘤不表达角蛋白、EMA、PLAP、CD15、CD30和CD45，相反，它们表达波形蛋白、S-100蛋白、酪氨酸酶、MART-1和HMB-45[106, 172, 174]。

混合性小细胞和大细胞恶性病变

混合性大细胞和小细胞非霍奇金淋巴瘤

当与大细胞非霍奇金淋巴瘤区别时，混合性大细胞和小细胞非霍奇金淋巴瘤（MNHL）的命名仍有争议。大细胞不超过30%即可诊断混合性非霍奇金淋巴瘤的标准比较主观。免疫组化可区分混合性大细胞和小细胞非霍奇金淋巴瘤与其他纵隔恶性混合性肿瘤，混合性大细胞和小细胞非霍奇金淋巴瘤所有的瘤细胞CD45都阳性，B细胞肿瘤CD20阳性，T细胞肿瘤CD3、CD43或者CD45RO阳性[175]，角蛋白通常为阴性，但某些非霍奇金淋巴瘤的变型可能会或多或少地表达p63类的标记物[176]。

混合细胞型霍奇金淋巴瘤

混合细胞型霍奇金淋巴瘤在组织学上和混合性大细胞和小细胞非霍奇金淋巴瘤非常相似，但是前者的大细胞（R-S细胞）不表达CD45。另外，它们也缺乏CD3、CD20、CD43和CD45RO的标记，但CD15染色阳性，CD30表达或不表达，染色部位在高尔基体区和细胞膜[104, 15, 177]。有些混合细胞型霍奇金病可以表达EMA，但是不表达角蛋白[177]。

淋巴上皮样癌

胸腺的淋巴上皮样癌（LELC）由体积较大的上皮样细胞和小淋巴细胞混合组成，和典型的鼻咽癌类似，所有的淋巴上皮样癌免疫组化均表达角蛋白（图10.30）、p63和EMA，相反的是，这些大的瘤细胞不

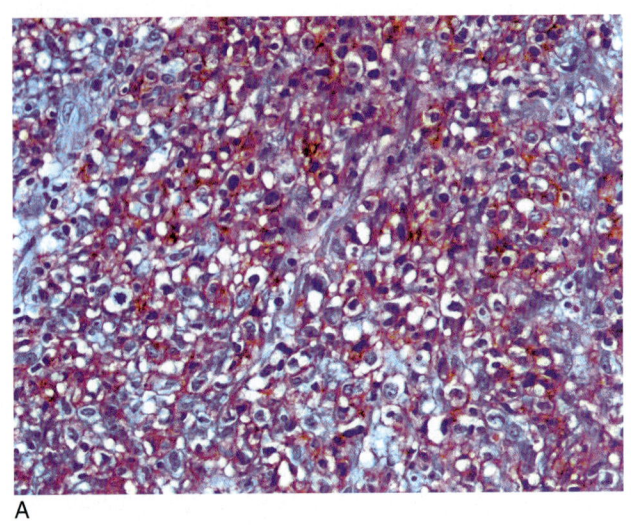

图 10.26　CD45（A）和 CD20（B）在原发于胸腺的大细胞淋巴瘤（C）中的染色

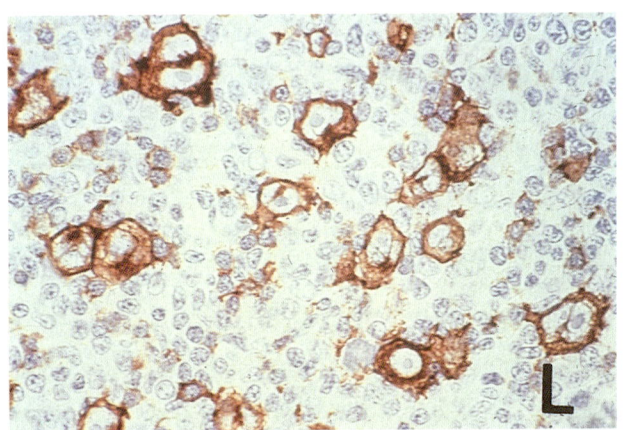

图 10.27　CD15 在纵隔霍奇金淋巴瘤 R-S 细胞中典型的胞膜和高尔基体着色（L=LeuM1）

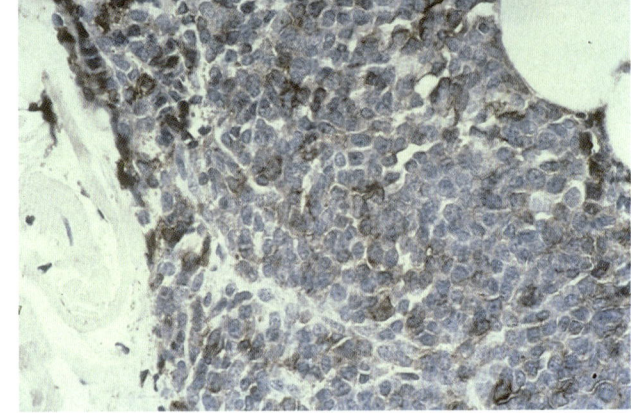

图 10.28　纵隔粒细胞肉瘤中髓过氧化物酶细胞浆弥漫着色

表达PLAP、CD3、CD15、CD20、CD30、CD43、CD45 和 CD45RO[18,69]。

恶性梭形细胞纵隔肿瘤

表 10.7、10.8，图 10.31 ~ 10.33。

肉瘤样胸腺癌

肉瘤样胸腺癌（STC）的报告相对较少[69, 178-180]。镜下，这种病变具有特征性的、成簇的梭形或多形性瘤细胞，很少有一定的组织结构。然而，有些病例由相互黏附的、局灶性的上皮样细胞巢和梭形细胞成分

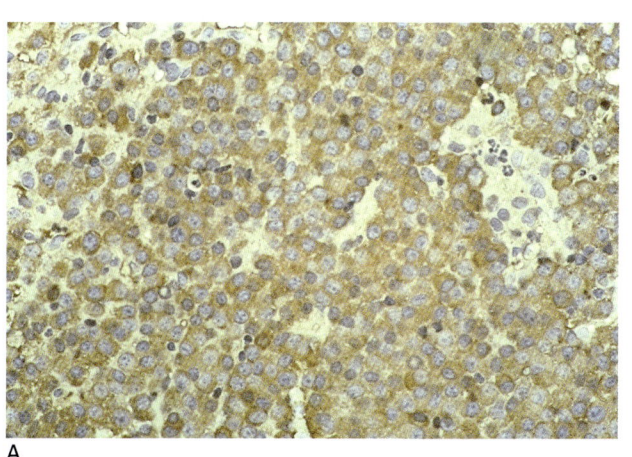

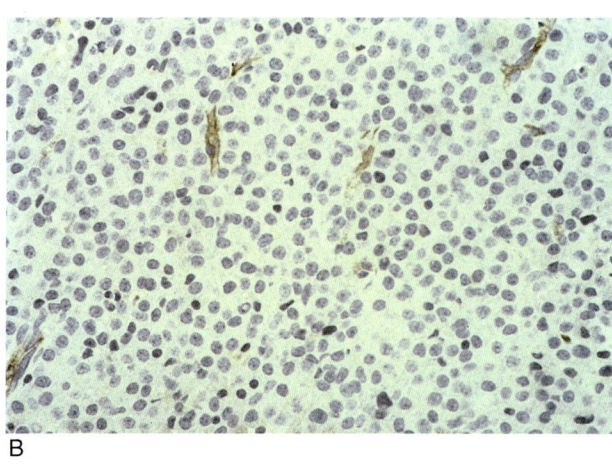

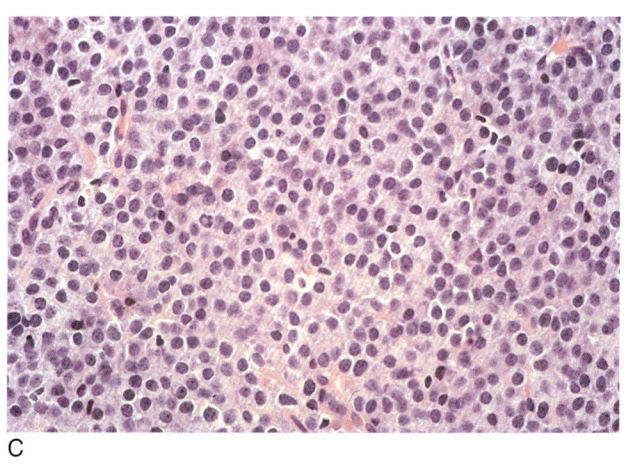

图10.29 纵隔原发的浆细胞瘤（C）中λ轻链免疫球蛋白（A）单型性染色而κ轻链（B）不着色

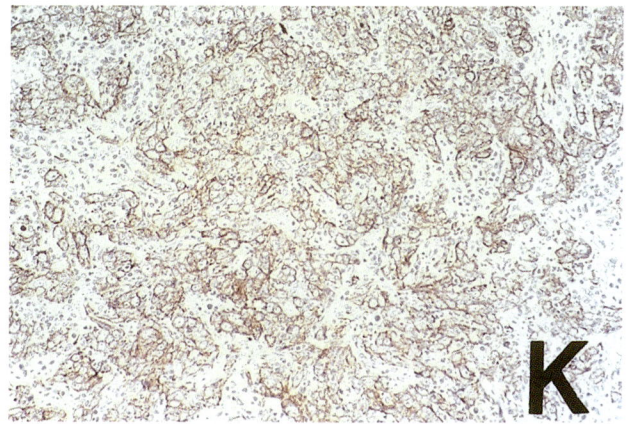

图10.30 角蛋白（K）在原发的淋巴上皮样胸腺癌中呈纤细的"连锁式"染色

表10.7	免疫组化在纵隔不确定的梭形细胞或未分化肿瘤中的应用
Keratin (monoclonal mixture)	
Epithelial membrane antigen	
Calretinin	
Vimentin	
Desmin	
Muscle-specific actin	
Alpha fetoprotein	
Synaptophysin	
Chromogranin A	

混合在一起[72]。具有双相分化的肉瘤样胸腺癌也有报告[181]，Snove 等[72]报告了一例含有界限清楚的灶性横纹肌样分化的肉瘤样胸腺癌，胞浆内有典型的横纹。有些人倾向于把该病变定义为"癌肉瘤"[182]，但是作者认为它们实际上还是上皮性的，就像化生的或肉瘤样癌[183]。

肉瘤样胸腺癌的梭形和多形性瘤细胞免疫组化表达波形蛋白，角蛋白和EMA也有表达，但可能是局灶性的（图 10.34）[19, 183]。这个发现提示大家，应该考虑到由于取材的限制而使小的活检标本不能表达任何上皮性标记物的可能性。具有多种成分的肿瘤，如肌原性成分，通常表达结蛋白、肌动蛋白、肌球蛋白、Myo-D1 或者成肌素[69, 72]。显然，有限的组织样本增加了诊断肉瘤样胸腺癌的困难性。

一个特别让人头痛的鉴别诊断是原发于纵隔的滑膜肉瘤和原发性胸腺癌，因为它们的临床表现、电镜

表10.8 纵隔不确定或未分化的恶性小细胞肿瘤相关标记物免疫组化的反应率

Tumor	KER	EMA	VIM	CALRET	DES	MSA	AFP	SYN	CGA
MESOTH	100	3	86	100	20	90	0	0	0
SCYST	100	10	50	0	0	0	80	0	0
LMS	3	0	89	0	70	90	0	0	0
SPCCA	86	67	96	0	3	10	0	0	0
SYNSC	80	85	100	67	0	0	0	0	0
SPCNC	100	80	3	0	0	0	10	80	75
FS/MFH	1	1	100	0	0	0	0	0	0

KER,角蛋白（单克隆抗体混合物）；EMA,上皮细胞膜抗原；VIM,波形蛋白；CALRET, calretinin；DES, 结蛋白；MSA, 肌特异性肌动蛋白；AFP, 甲胎蛋白；SYN, 突触素；CGA, 嗜铬素A；MESOTH, 间皮瘤；SCYST, 梭形细胞卵黄囊瘤；LMS, 平滑肌肉瘤；SPCCA, 梭形细胞癌（原发的或转移的）；SYNSC, 滑膜肉瘤；SPCNC, 梭形细胞神经内分泌癌；FS, 纤维肉瘤；MFH, 恶性纤维组织细胞瘤
（数据摘自 Frisman D.Immunoquery. 网站 http://www.immunoquery.com，以及作者的经验）

量反应性增生的胸腺瘤[186]。在组织学上双相分化，这两种病变成分表现出相互排斥的免疫表型，角蛋白和波形蛋白分别阳性，因此，表面上的"癌肉瘤样"的病变很多，只有通过观察平淡无奇的细胞学图像才能避免诊断错误。

胸腺的梭形细胞类癌

1976年，Levine和Rosai[187]首先报道了胸腺类癌的梭形细胞变型，但是它看起来是一个非常少见的变型，随后也只有很有限的病例被发现[188]。从应用的角度来说，这种肿瘤的免疫表型与前文提到的多角形细胞神经内分泌癌是相同的。

肉瘤样纵隔恶性间皮瘤

除了梭形的和多形性的肿瘤细胞成分以外，肉瘤样纵隔间皮细胞瘤在超微结构和免疫表型方面与上皮样和双相分化的间皮瘤也不一样，它们更接近于前述的肉瘤样癌的病理特征，间皮瘤与后者的区别在于，间皮瘤 WT-1 和 calretinin 都阳性，而肉瘤样癌均阴性。

肉瘤样胸腺卵黄囊癌

Moran和Suster[189]报告了一例特殊的原发性纵隔卵黄囊瘤变型（MYST），尽管具有以梭形细胞为主的

及免疫组化特征都非常相似。荧光原位杂交和传统的细胞遗传学分析都已证明，滑膜肉瘤的t(X;18)染色体易位[184]。显然，间皮瘤也应在鉴别诊断的范围之内，它和肉瘤样原发性胸腺癌及滑膜肉瘤一样，都表达calretinin，然而，这其中只有间皮瘤表达WT-1蛋白[185]。

肉瘤样胸腺癌另一个诊断陷阱是梭形间质细胞大

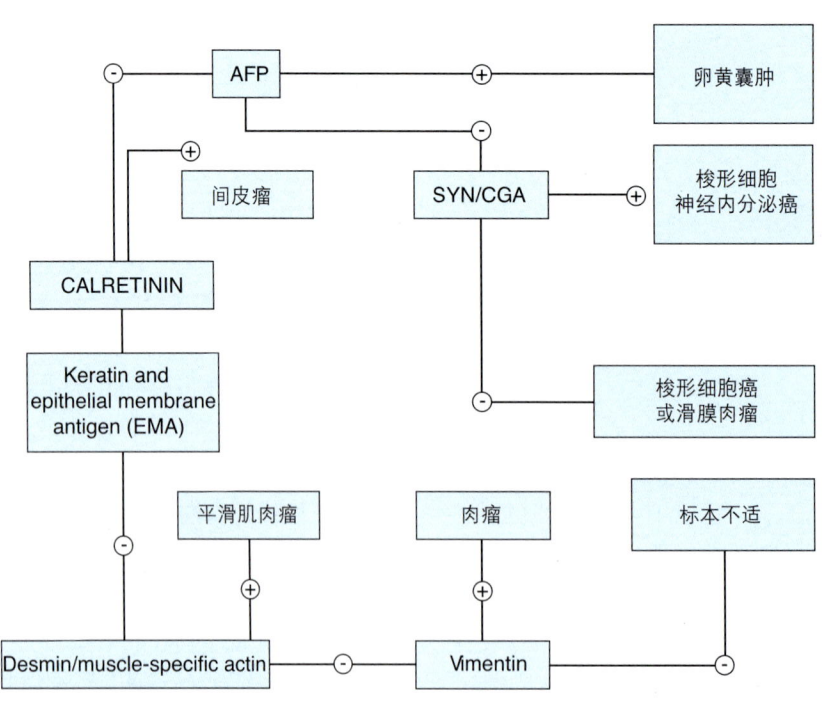

图 10.31　纵隔恶性梭形细胞肿瘤免疫组化分析流程

纵隔的免疫组织化学 10

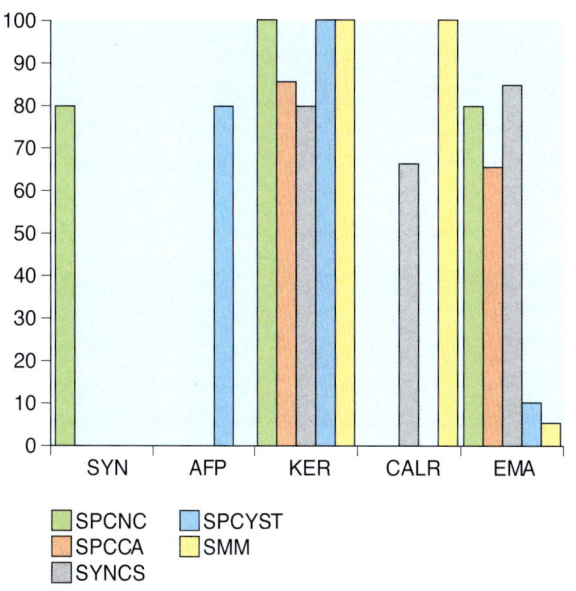

图10.32 纵隔恶性上皮样梭形细胞肿瘤用于鉴别诊断的标记物

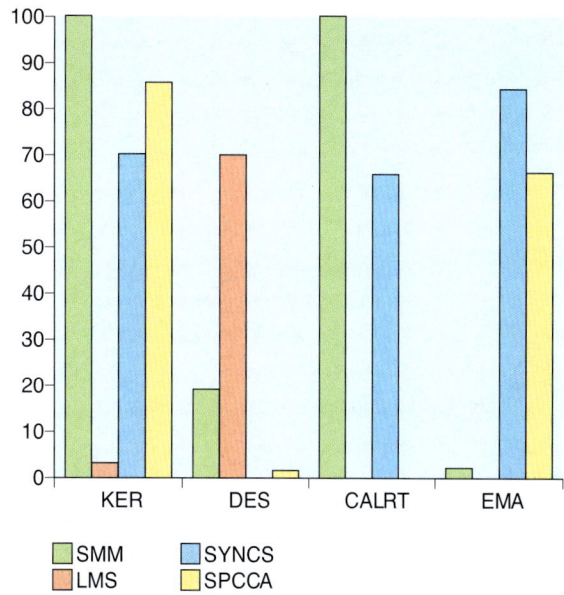

图10.33 纵隔平滑肌肉瘤与恶性上皮样梭形细胞肿瘤用于鉴别诊断的抗体

形态特征，易于与本章提到的其他肿瘤混淆，但是肉瘤样纵隔卵黄囊瘤的免疫表型与"传统的"内胚窦肿瘤相同（参见前面）。在梭形细胞纵隔卵黄囊瘤中，角蛋白和AFP阳性，第二个抗体还可以用来与肉瘤样胸腺癌鉴别，肉瘤样胸腺癌 AFP 是阴性的[178-180, 189]。

纵隔平滑肌肉瘤

Moran[190]等报告了原发性纵隔平滑肌肉瘤，既可以发生在前纵隔也可以发生在后纵隔，这些梭形肿瘤细胞一致地表达结蛋白（图10.35）、MSA、α-异构肌动蛋白、钙调素结合蛋白和calponin[191]，可能也表达波形蛋白。相反，EMA、角蛋白、Myo-D1、肌红蛋白、成肌素和S-100蛋白在平滑肌肉瘤中不表达[38]。

纵隔肿瘤的"预后性"标记物

现已使用核增殖抗原（PCNA）和Ki-67借助免疫组化半定量地检测肿瘤细胞的增殖率[192-194]，以及用免疫印迹及探针的方法检测bcl-2、Fas或者p53基因产物的异常表达[28, 29, 11, 116, 195]，试图预测胸腺瘤的生物学行为。总体来说，这些方法都不能给出一致的可重复的结果，类似的情况还有 E-钙黏素免疫组化表达的分析应用[196, 197]。同样，目前还没有"分子"标记物可以预测其他纵隔肿瘤的预后。因此，作者认为，目前有关判断预后的免疫组化应用已超出了外科病理学实际应用的要求。

参考文献

1. Sterrett G, Whitaker D, Shilkin KB, et al. The fine needle aspiration cytology of mediastinal lesions. Cancer 1983; 51: 127–135.
2. Gherardi G, Marveggio C, Placidi A. Neuroendocrine carcinoma of the thymus: aspiration biopsy, immunocytochemistry, and clinicopathologic correlates. Diagn Cytopathol 1995; 35: 158–164.
3. Heilo A. Tumors in the mediastinum: ultrasound-guided histologic core-needle biopsy. Radiology 1993; 189:143–146.
4. Powers CN, Silverman JF, Geisinger KR, et al. Fine needle aspiration biopsy of the mediastinum: a multiinstitutional analysis. Am J Clin Pathol 1996; 105:168–173.
5. Yu GH, Salhany KE, Gokaslan ST, et al. Thymic epithelial cells as a diagnostic pitfall in the fine needle aspiration diagnosis of primary mediastinal lymphoma. Diagn Cytopathol 1997; 16: 460–465.
6. Shin HJ, Katz RL. Thymic neoplasia as represented by fine needle aspiration biopsy of anterior mediastinal masses: a practical approach to the differential diagnosis. Acta Cytol 1998; 42:855–864.
7. Wick MR, Rosai J. The endocrine thymus. In: Kovacs K, Asa SL, eds. Functional endocrine pathology. 2nd edn. Oxford: Blackwell; 1998:869–894.
8. Hirokawa K, Utsuyama M, Moriizumi E, et al. Immunohis-

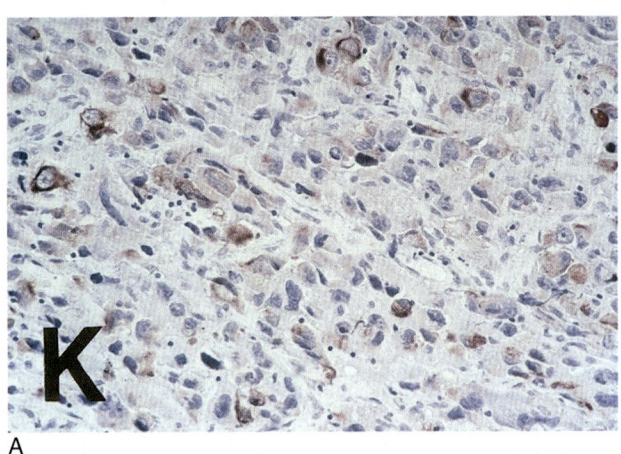
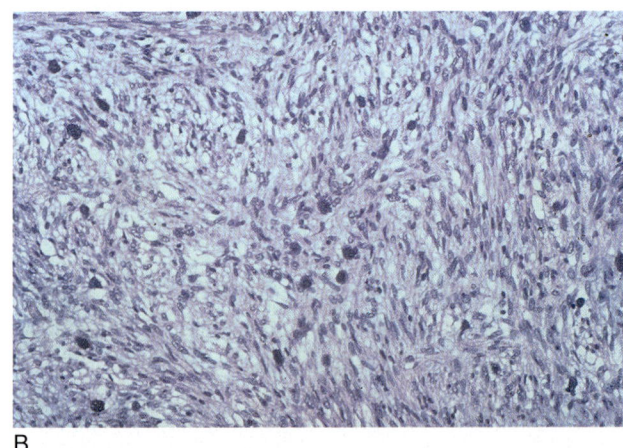

图 10.34　角蛋白（K）（A）在胸腺原发的肉瘤样癌（B）中局灶性免疫染色

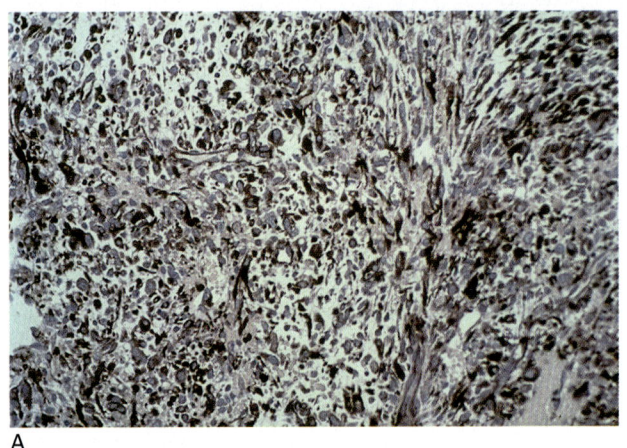
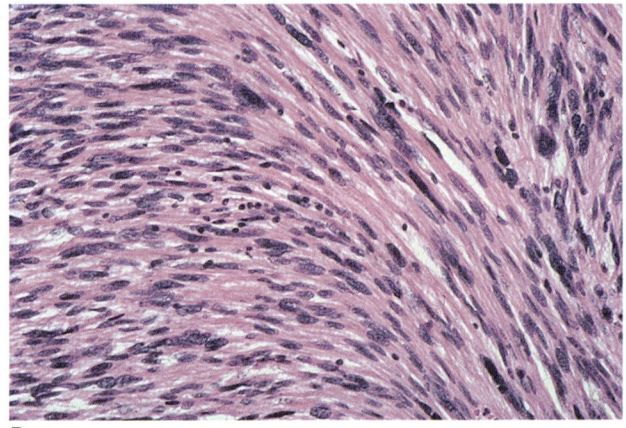

图 10.35　结蛋白（A）在纵隔平滑肌肉瘤（B）中的染色

tochemical studies in human thymomas: localization of thymosin and various cell markers. Virchows Arch B Cell Pathol 1988; 55:371–380.

9. Fukai I, Masaoka A, Hashimoto T, et al. Cytokeratins in normal thymus and thymic epithelial tumors. Cancer 1993; 71: 99–105.

10. Fukai I, Masaoka A, Hashimoto T, et al. Differential diagnosis of thymic carcinoma and lung carcinoma with the use of antibodies to cytokeratins. J Thorac Cardiovasc Surg 1995; 110:1670–1675.

11. Wick MR. Mediastinal cysts and intrathoracic thyroid tumors. Semin Diagn Pathol 1990; 7:285–294.

12. Sabiston D, Scott HW. Primary neoplasms and cysts of the mediastinum. Ann Surg 1961; 136:777–797.

13. LeRoux BT, Kallichurum S, Shama DM. Mediastinal cysts and tumors. Curr Probl Surg 1984; 21:1–77.

14. Suster S, Moran CA. Malignant thymic neoplasms that may mimic benign conditions. Semin Diagn Pathol 1995; 12:98–110.

15. Moran CA, Suster S. Mediastinal seminomas with prominent cystic changes: a clinicopathologic study of 10 cases. Am J Surg Pathol 1995; 25:1047–1053.

16. Niehans GA, Manivel JC, Copland GT, et al. Immunohistochemistry of germ cell and trophoblastic neoplasms. Cancer 1988; 62:1113–1123.

17. Suster S, Moran CA. Primary thymic epithelial neoplasms: spectrum of differentiation and histological features. Semin Diagn Pathol 1999; 16:2–17.

18. Wick MR, Simpson RW, Niehans GA, et al. Anterior mediastinal tumors: a clinicopathologic study of 100 cases, with emphasis on immunohistochemical analysis. Prog Surg Pathol 1990; 11:79–119.

19. Wick MR, Rosai J. Epithelial tumors. In: Givel JC, ed. Surgery of the thymus. Berlin: Springer-Verlag; 1990:79–107.

20. Walker AN, Mills SE, Fechner RE. Thymomas and thymic carcinomas. Semin Diagn Pathol 1990; 7:250–265.

21. Lewis JE, Wick MR, Scheithauer BW, et al. Thymoma: a clinicopathologic review. Cancer 1987; 60:2727–2743.
22. Rosai J, Sobin LH, Caillaud JM, et al. WHO classification of thymic tumors. Geneva: World Health Organization; 1999: 1–25.
23. Rice HE, Flake AW, Hori T, et al. Massive thymic hyperplasia: characterization of a rare mediastinal mass. J Pediatr Surg 1994; 29:1561–1564.
24. Battifora H, Sun TT, Bahu RM, et al. The use of antikeratin antiserum as a diagnostic tool: thymoma versus lymphoma. Hum Pathol 1980; 11:635–641.
25. Chan JKC, Tsang WY, Seneviratne S, et al. The MIC2 antibody O13: practical application for the study of thymic epithelial tumors. Am J Surg Pathol 1995; 19:1115–1123.
26. Robertson PB, Neiman RS, Worapongpaiboon S, et al. O13 (CD99) positivity in hematologic proliferations correlates with TdT positivity. Mod Pathol 1997; 10:277–282.
27. Soslow RA, Bhargava V, Warnke RA. MIC2, TdT, bcl-2, and CD34 expression in paraffin-embedded high-grade lymphoma/acute lymphoblastic leukemia distinguishes between distinct clinicopathologic entities. Hum Pathol 1997; 28:1158–1165.
28. Brocheriou I, Carnot F, Briere J. Immunohistochemical detection of bcl-2 protein in thymoma. Histopathology 1995; 27:251–255.
29. Chen FF, Yan JJ, Jin YT, et a. Detection of bcl-2 and p53 in thymoma: expression of bcl-2 as a reliable marker of tumor aggressiveness. Hum Pathol 1996; 27:1089–1092.
30. Chan WC, Zaatari GS, Tabei S, et al. Thymoma: an immunohistochemical study. Am J Clin Pathol 1984; 82:160–166.
31. Knowles DM II. Lymphoid cell markers: their distribution and usefulness in the immunopathologic analysis of lymphoid neoplasms. Am J Surg Pathol 1985; 9(Suppl):85–108.
32. Weiss LM, Bindl JM, Picozzi VJ, et al. Lymphoblastic lymphoma: an immunophenotypic study of 26 cases with comparison to T-cell acute lymphoblastic leukemia. Blood 1986; 67:474–478.
33. Picker LJ, Weiss LM, Medeiros LJ, et al. Immunophenotypic criteria for the diagnosis of non-Hodgkin's lymphoma. Am J Pathol 1987; 128:181–201.
34. Berrih-Aknin S, Safar D, Cohen-Kaminsky S. Analysis of lymphocyte phenotype in human thymomas. Adv Exp Med Biol 1988; 237:369–374.
35. Ito M, Taki T, Mihaye M, et al. Lymphocyte subsets in human thymoma studied with monoclonal antibodies. Cancer 1988; 61:284–287.
36. Perrone T, Frizzera G, Rosai J. Mediastinal diffuse large-cell lymphoma with sclerosis: a clinicopathologic study of 60 cases. Am J Surg Pathol 1986; 10:176–191.
37. Wick MR, Swanson PE, Manivel JC. Immunohistochemical analysis of soft tissue sarcomas: comparisons with electron microscopy. Appl Pathol 1988; 6:169–196.
38. Nappi O, Ritter JH, Pettinato G, et al. Hemangiopericytoma: histopathological pattern or clinicopathologic entity? Semin Diagn Pathol 1995; 12:221–232.
39. Shimosato Y, Mukai K. Tumors of the mediastinum. In: Rosai J, ed. Atlas of tumor pathology, series 3, fascicle 21. Washington, DC: Armed Forces Institute of Pathology; 1997: 33–273.
40. Swanson PE. Soft tissue neoplasms of the mediastinum. Semin Diagn Pathol 1991; 8:14–34.
41. Marchevsky AM. Mediastinal tumors of peripheral nervous system origin. Semin Diagn Pathol 1999; 16:65–78.
42. Chaves-Espinosa JI, Chaves-Fernandez JA, Hoyer OH, et al. Endothoracic neurogenic neoplasms: analysis of 30 cases. Rev Interamer Radiol 1980; 5:49–54.
43. Gale AW, Jelihovsky T, Grant AF, et al. Neurogenic tumors of the mediastinum. Ann Thorac Surg 1974; 17:434–443.
44. Davidson KG, Walbaum PR, McCormack RJM. Intrathoracic neural tumors. Thorax 1978; 33:359–367.
45. Young DG. Thoracic neuroblastoma/ganglioneuroma. J Pediatr Surg 1983; 18:37–41.
46. Gould VE, Wiedenmann B, Lee I, et al. Synaptophysin expression in neuroendocrine neoplasms as determined by immunocytochemistry. Am J Pathol 1987; 126:243–257.
47. Fine SW, McClain SA, Li M. Immunohistochemical staining for calretinin is useful for differentiating schwannomas from neurofibromas. Am J Clin Pathol 2004; 122:552–559.
48. Witkin GB, Rosai J. Solitary fibrous tumor of the mediastinum: a report of 14 cases. Am J Surg Pathol 1989; 13:547–557.
49. Balassiano M, Reichert N, Rosenman Y, et al. Localized fibrous mesothelioma of the mediastinum devoid of pleural connections. Postgrad Med J 1989; 65:788–790.
50. Hanau CA, Miettinen M. Solitary fibrous tumor: histological and immunohistochemical spectrum of benign and malignant

variants presenting at different sites. Hum Pathol 1995; 26: 440–449.

51. Wick MR, Manivel JC, Swanson PE. Contributions of immunohistochemistry to the diagnosis of soft tissue tumors. Prog Surg Pathol 1988; 8:197–249.

52. England DM, Hochholzer L, McCarthy MJ. Localized benign and malignant fibrous tumors of the pleura: a clinicopathologic review of 223 cases. Am J Surg Pathol 1989; 13: 640–658.

53. Swanson PE, Wick MR. Immunohistochemical diagnosis of soft tissue tumors. In: Colvin R, Bhan A, McCluskey R, eds. Diagnostic immunopathology. 2nd edn. New York: Raven Press; 1995:599–632.

54. Dines DE, Payne WS, Bernatz PE, et al. Mediastinal granulomas and fibrosing mediastinitis. Chest 1979; 75:320–324.

55. Coffin CM, Watterson J, Priest JR, et al. Extrapulmonary inflammatory myofibroblastic tumor (inflammatory pseudotumor): a clinicopathologic and immunohistochemical study of 84 cases. Am J Surg Pathol 1995; 19:859–872.

56. Lukes RJ, Butler JJ, Hicks EB. Natural history of Hodgkin's disease as related to its pathologic picture. Cancer 1966; 19: 317–344.

57. Matsubara O, Mark EJ, Ritter JH. Pseudoneoplastic lesions of the lungs, pleural surfaces, and mediastinum. In: Wick MR, Humphrey PA, Ritter JH, eds. Pathology of pseudo-neoplastic lesions. Philadelphia: Lippincott-Raven; 1997:97–129.

58. Crotty TB, Colby TV, Gay PC, et al. Desmoplastic malignant mesothelioma masquerading as sclerosing mediastinitis: a diagnostic dilemma. Hum Pathol 1992; 23:79–82.

59. Ritter JH, Humphrey PA, Wick MR. Malignant neoplasms capable of simulating inflammatory (myofibroblastic) pseudotumors and tumefactive fibroinflammatory lesions: pseudopseudotumors. Semin Diagn Pathol 1998; 15:111–132.

60. Rosai J, Levine GD, Weber WR, et al. Carcinoid tumors and oat cell carcinomas of the thymus. Pathol Annu 1976; 11: 201–226.

61. Wick MR, Rosai J. Neuroendocrine neoplasms of thethymus. Pathol Res Pract 1988; 183:188–199.

62. Kuo TT, Chang JP, Lin FJ, et al. Thymic carcinomas:histopathological varieties and immunohistochemical study. Am J Surg Pathol 1990; 14:24–34.

63. Truong LD, Mody DR, Cagle PT, et al. Thymic carcinoma: a clinicopathologic study of 13 cases. Am J Surg Pathol 1990; 14:151–166.

64. Shimizu J, Hayashi Y, Morita K, et al. Primary thymic carcinoma: a clinicopathological and immunohistochemical study. J Surg Oncol 1994; 56:159–164.

65. Suster S, Rosai J. Thymic carcinoma: a clinicopathologic study of 60 cases. Cancer 1991; 67:1025–1032.

66. Ritter JH, Wick MR. Primary carcinomas of the thymus gland. Semin Diagn Pathol 1999; 16:18–31.

67. Snover DC, Levine GD, Rosai J. Thymic carcinomas: five distinctive histological variants. Am J Surg Pathol 1982; 6: 451–470.

68. Iezzoni JC, Nass LB. Thymic basaloid carcinoma: a case report and review of the literature. Mod Pathol 1996; 9:21–25.

69. DeLorimier AA, Bragg KU, Linden G. Neuroblastoma in childhood. Am J Dis Child 1969; 118:441–450.

70. Ordonez NG. Value of thyroid transcription factor-1immunostaining in distinguishing small cell carcinomas from other small cell carcinomas. Am J Surg Pathol 2000;24:1217–1223.

71. Kaufmann O, Fietze E, Mengs J, et al. Value of p63 and cytokeratin 5/6 as immunohistochemical markers for the differential diagnosis of poorly differentiated and undifferentiated carcinomas. Am J Clin Pathol 2001; 116:823–830.

72. Salter JE Jr, Gibson D, Ordonez NG, et al. Neuroblastoma of the anterior mediastinum in an 80 year old woman. Ultrastruct Pathol 1995; 19:305–310.

73. Hachitanda Y, Hata J. Stage IVS neuroblastoma: a clinical, histological, and biological analysis of 45 cases. Hum Pathol 1996; 27:1135–1138.

74. Jerome-Marson V, Mazieres J, Groussard O, et al. Expression of TTF-1 and cytokeratins in primary and secondary epithelial lung tumors: correlation with histological type and grade. Histopathology 2004; 45:125–134.

75. Argani P, Erlandson RA, Rosai J. Thymic neuroblastoma in adults: report of three cases with special emphasis on its association with the syndrome of inappropriate secretion of antidiuretic hormone. Am J Clin Pathol 1997; 108:537–543.

76. Asada Y, Marutsuka K, Mitsukawa T, et al. Ganglioneuroblastoma of the thymus: an adult case with the syndrome of inappropriate secretion of antidiuretic hormone. Hum Pathol 1996; 27:506–509.

77. Wirnsberger GH, Becker H, Ziervogel K, et al. Diagnostic immunohistochemistry of neuroblastic tumors. Am J Surg

Pathol 1992; 16:49–57.

78. Dehner LP. Peripheral and central primitive neuroectodermal tumors: a nosologic concept seeking a consensus. Arch Pathol Lab Med 1986; 110:997–1005.
79. Fellinger EJ, Garin-Chesa P, Su SL, et al. Biochemical and genetic characterization of the HBA71 Ewing's sarcoma cell surface antigen. Cancer Res 1991; 51:336–340.
80. Dehner LP. Primitive neuroectodermal tumor and Ewing's sarcoma. Am J Surg Pathol 1993; 17:1–13.
81. Gluer S, Zense M, Radtke E, eet al. Polysialylated neural cell adhesion molecule in childhood ganglioneuroma and neuroblastoma of different histological grade and clinical stage. Langenbecks Arch Surg 1998; 383:340–344.
82. Miettinen M, Chatten J, Paetau A, et al. Monoclonal antibody NB84 in the differential diagnosis of neuroblastoma and other small round cell tumors. Am J Surg Pathol 1998; 22:327–332.
83. Leong ASY, Wick MR, Swanson PE. Immunohistology and electron microscopy of anaplastic and pleomorphic tumors. Cambridge, UK: Cambridge Press; 1997:109–208.
84. Parham DM, Dias P, Kelly DR, et al. Desmin positivity in primitive neuroectodermal tumors of childhood. Am J Surg Pathol 1992; 16:483–492.
85. Pachter MR, Lattes R. Mesenchymal tumors of the mediastinum. I. Tumors of fibrous tissue, adipose tissue, smooth muscle, and striated muscle. Cancer 1963; 16:74–94.
86. Suster S, Moran CA, Koss MN. Rhabdomyosarcomas of the anterior mediastinum: report of four cases unassociated with germ cell, teratomatous, or thymic carcinomatous components. Hum Pathol 1994; 25:349–356.
87. Tsokos M. The diagnosis and classification of childhood rhabdomyosarcoma. Semin Diagn Pathol 1994; 11:26–38.
88. Cui S, Hano H, Harada T, et al. Evaluation of new monoclonal anti-MyoD1 and anti-myogenin antibodies for the diagnosis of rhabdomyosarcoma. Pathol Int 1999; 49:62–68.
89. Rossi S, Orvieto E, Furlanetto A, et al. Utility of theimmunohistochemical detection of FLI-1 expression in round cell and vascular neoplasms using a monoclonal antibody. Mod Pathol 2004; 17:547–552.
90. Nathwani BN, Kim H, Rappaport H. Malignant lymphoma, lymphoblastic. Cancer 1976; 38:964–983.
91. Nathwani BN, Diamond LW, Winberg CD, et al. Lymphoblastic lymphoma: a clinicopathologic study of 95 patients. Cancer 1981; 48:2347–2357.
92. Shikano T, Arioka H, Kobayashi R, et al. Acute lymphoblastic leukemia and non-Hodgkin's lymphoma with mediastinal mass – a study of 23 children; different disorders or different stages? Leuk Lymphoma 1994; 13:161–167.
93. Trump DL, Mann RB. Diffuse large cell and undifferentiated lymphomas with prominent mediastinal involvement: a poor prognostic subset of patients with non-Hodgkin's lymphoma. Cancer 1982; 50:277–282.
94. Majolino I, Marceno R, Magrin S, et al. Burkitt's cell leukemia with mediastinal mass and unusually good prognosis. Haematologica 1983; 68:287–288.
95. Isaacson PG, Chan JKC, Tang C, et al. Low-grade B-cell lymphoma of mucosa-associated lymphoid tissue arising in the thymus: a thymic lymphoma mimicking myoepithelial sialadenitis. Am J Surg Pathol 1990; 14:342–351.
96. Takagi N, Nakamura S, Yamamoto K, et al. Malignant lymphoma of mucosa-associated lymphoid tissue arising in the thymus of a patient with Sjögren's syndrome: a morphologic, phenotypic, and genotypic study. Cancer 1992; 69:1347–1355.
97. Ozdemirli M, Fanburg-Smith JC, Hartmann DP, et al. Precursor B-lymphoblastic lymphoma presenting as a solitary bone tumor and mimicking Ewing's sarcoma: a report of four cases and review of the literature. Am J Surg Pathol 1998; 22:795–804.
98. Zukerberg LR, Medeiros LJ, Ferry JA, et al. Diffuse lowgrade B-cell lymphomas: four clinically distinct subtypes defined by a combination of morphologic and immunophenotypic features. Am J Clin Pathol 1993; 100:373–385.
99. Banks PM, Isaacson PG. MALT lymphomas in 1997. Am J Clin Pathol 1999; 111(Suppl 1):S75–S83.
100. Strickler JG, Kurtin PJ. Mediastinal lymphoma. Semin Diagn Pathol 1991; 8:2–13.
101. Nakhleh RE, Wick MR, Rocamora A, et al. Morphologic diversity in malignant melanomas. Am J Clin Pathol 1990; 93:731–740.
102. Fetsch PA, Marincola FM, Abati A. The new melanoma markers: MART-1 and Melan-A. Am J Surg Pathol 1999; 23:607–610.
103. Matsuno Y, Mukai K, Noguchi M, et al. Histochemical and immunohistochemical evidence of glandular differentiation in thymic carcinomas. Acta Pathol Jpn 1989; 39:433–438.

104. Kuo TT, Chan JKC. Thymic carcinoma arising in thymoma is associated with alterations in immunohistochemical profile. Am J Surg Pathol 1998; 22:1474–1481.

105. Berezowski K, Grimes MM, Gal A, et al. CD5 immunoreactivity of epithelial cells in thymic carcinoma and CASTLE using paraffin-embedded tissue. Am J Clin Pathol 1996; 106:483–486.

106. Hishima T, Fukayama M, Fujisawa M, et al. CD5 expression in thymic carcinoma. Am J Pathol 1994; 145:268–275.

107. Pan CC, Chen PC, Chou TY, et al. Expression of calretinin and other mesothelioma-related markers in thymic carcinoma and thymoma. Hum Pathol 2003; 34:1155–1162.

108. Saad RS, Landreneau RJ, Liu Y, et al. Utility of immunohistochemistry in separating thymic neoplasms from germ cell tumors and metastatic lung cancer involving the anterior mediastinum. Appl Immunohistochem Molec Morphol 2003; 11:107–112.

109. Franke A, Strobel P, Fackeldey V, et al. Hepatoid thymic carcinoma: report of a case. Am J Surg Pathol 2004; 28:250–256.

110. Lugli A, Tornillo L, Mirlacher M, et al. Hepatocyte paraffin-1 expression in human normal and neoplastic tissues: tissue microarray analysis on 3,940 tissue samples. Am J Clin Pathol 2004; 122:721–727.

111. Kornstein MJ, Rosai J. CD5 labeling of thymic carcinomas and other non-lymphoid neoplasms. Am J Clin.Pathol 1998; 109:722–726.

112. Tateyama H, Eimoto T, Tada T, et al. p53 protein expression and p53 gene mutation in thymic epithelial tumors: an immunohistochemical and DNA sequencing study. Am J Clin Pathol 1995; 104:375–381.

113. Stefanaki K, Rontogianni D, Kouvidou CH, et al. Expression of p53, mdm2, p21/waf1, and bcl-2 proteins in thymomas. Histopathology 1997; 30:549–555.

114. Weirich G, Schneider P, Fellbaum C, et al. p53 alterations in thymic epithelial tumors. Virchows Arch A 1997; 431:17–23.

115. Chen FF, Yan JJ, Chang KC, et al. Immunohistochemical localization of Mcl-1 and bcl-2 proteins in thymic epithelial tumors. Histopathology 1996; 29:541–547.

116. Tateyama H, Eimoto T, Tada T, et al. Apoptosis, bcl-2 protein, and Fas antigen in thymic epithelial tumors. Mod Pathol 1997; 10:983–991.

117. Lauriola L, Erlandson RA, Rosai J. Neuroendocrine differentiation is a common feature of thymic carcinoma. Am J Surg Pathol 1998; 22:1059–1066.

118. Clark OH. Mediastinal parathyroid tumors. Arch Surg 1988; 123:1096–1100.

119. Nathaniels EK, Nathaniels AM, Wang CA. Mediastinal parathyroid tumors: a clinical and pathological study of 84 cases. Ann Surg 1970; 171:165–170.

120. Murphy MN, Glennon PG, Diocee MS, et al. Nonsecretory parathyroid carcinoma of the mediastinum. Cancer 1986; 58:2468–2476.

121. Ordonez NG, Ibanez ML, Samaan NA, et al. Immunoperoxidase study of uncommon parathyroid tumors. Am J Surg Pathol 1983; 7:535–542.

122. Dehner LP. Germ cell tumors of the mediastinum. Semin Diagn Pathol 1990; 7:266–284.

123. Wick MR, Ritter JH, Humphrey PA, et al. Clear cell neoplasms of the endocrine system and thymus. Semin Diagn Pathol 1997; 14:183–202.

124. Knapp RH, Hurt RD, Payne WS, et al. Malignant germ cell tumors of the mediastinum. J Thorac Cardiovasc Surg 1985; 89:82–89.

125. Truong LD, Harris L, Mattioli C, et al. Endodermal sinus tumor of the mediastinum: a report of seven cases and review of the literature. Cancer 1986; 58:730–739.

126. Weidner N. Germ cell tumors of the mediastinum. Semin Diagn Pathol 1999; 16:42–50.

127. Moran CA, Suster S, Przygodzki RM, et al. Primary germ cell tumors of the mediastinum: II. Mediastinal seminomas–a clinicopathologic and immunohistochemical study of 120 cases. Cancer 1997; 80:691–698.

128. Przygodzki RM, Hubbs AE, Zhao F, et al. Primary mediastinal seminomas: evidence of single and multiple KIT mutations. Lab Invest 2002; 82:1369–1375.

129. Moran CA, Suster S. Hepatoid yolk sac tumors of the mediastinum: a clinicopathologic and immunohistologic study of four cases. Am J Surg Pathol 1997; 21:1210–1214.

130. Suster S, Moran CA, Dominguez-Malagon H, et al. Germ cell tumors of the mediastinum and testis: a comparative immunohistochemical study of 120 cases. Hum Pathol 1998; 29:737–742.

131. Moran CA, Suster S. Primary mediastinal choriocarcinomas: a clinicopathologic and immunohistochemical study of eight

cases. Am J Surg Pathol 1997; 21:1007–1012.

132. Klemm KM, Moran CA. Primary neuroendocrine carcinomas of the thymus. Semin Diagn Pathol 1999; 16:32–41.

133. DeMontpreville VT, Macchiarini P, Dulmet E. Thymic neuroendocrine carcinoma (carcinoid): a clinicopathologic study of fourteen cases. J Thorac Cardiovasc Surg 1996; 111:134–141.

134. Caceres W, Baldizon C, Sanchez J. Carcinoid tumor of the thymus: a unique neoplasm of the mediastinum. Am J Clin Oncol 1998; 21:82–83.

135. Wick MR, Rosai J. Neuroendocrine neoplasms of the mediastinum. Semin Diagn Pathol 1991; 8:35–51.

136. Valli M, Fabris GA, Dewar A, et al. Atypical carcinoid tumor of the thymus: a study of eight cases. Histopathology 1994; 24:371–375.

137. Wick MR, Scheithauer BW. Thymic carcinoid: a histologic, immunohistochemical, and ultrastructural study of 12 cases. Cancer 1984; 53:475–484.

138. Herbst WM, Kumner W, Hofmann W, et al. Carcinoid tumors of the thymus: an immunohistochemical study. Cancer 1987; 60:2465–2470.

139. Odze R, Begin LR. Malignant paraganglioma of the posterior mediastinum. Cancer 1990; 65:564–569.

140. Olson JL, Salyer WR. Mediastinal paraganglioma (aortic body tumor): a report of four cases, and a review of the literature. Cancer 1978; 41:2405–2412.

141. Schroder HD, Johannsen L. Demonstration of S100 protein in sustentacular cells of phaeochromocytomas and paragangliomas. Histopathology 1986; 10:1023–1033.

142. DeLellis RA, Tischler AS, Lee AK, et al. Leu-enkephalin-like immunoreactivity in proliferative lesions of the human adrenal medulla and extra-adrenal paraganglia. Am J Surg Pathol 1983; 7:29–37.

143. Lamarre L, Jacobson JO, Aisenberg AC, et al. Primary large cell lymphoma of the mediastinum: a histologic and immunophenotypic study of 29 cases. Am J Surg Pathol 1989; 13:730–739.

144. Suster S. Primary large-cell lymphomas of the mediastinum. Semin Diagn Pathol 1999; 16:51–64.

145. Davis RE, Dorfman RF, Warnke RA. Primary large-cell lymphoma of the thymus: a diffuse B-cell neoplasm presenting as primary mediastinal lymphoma. Hum Pathol 1990; 21:1262–1268.

146. Al-Sharabati M, Chittal S, Duga-Neulat, et al. Primary anterior mediastinal B-cell lymphoma: a clinicopathologic and immunohistochemical study of 16 cases. Cancer 1991; 67:2579–2587.

147. Suster S, Moran CA. Pleomorphic large cell lymphomas of the mediastinum. Am J Surg Pathol 1996; 20:224–232.

148. Addis BJ, Isaacson PG. Large-cell lymphoma of the mediastinum: a B-cell tumor of probable thymic origin. Histopathology 1986; 10:379–390.

149. Torlakovic E, Torlakovic G, Nguyen PL, et al. The value of anti-PAX-5 immunostaining in routinely fixed and paraffin-embedded sections: a novel pan pre-B and B-cell marker. Am J Surg Pathol 2002; 26:1343–1350.

150. Fechner RE. Hodgkin's disease of the thymus. Cancer 1969; 23:16–23.

151. Katz A, Lattes R. Granulomatous thymoma or Hodgkin's disease of thymus? A clinical and histologic study and a re-evaluation. Cancer 1969; 23:1–15.

152. Lazzarino M, Orlandi E, Paulli M, et al. Treatment outcome and prognostic factors for primary mediastinal (thymic) Bcell lymphoma: a multicenter study of 106 patients. J Clin Oncol 1997; 15:1646–1653.

153. Strickler JG, Michie SA, Warnke RA, et al. The 'syncytial variant" of nodular sclerosing Hodgkin's disease. Am J Surg Pathol 1986; 10:470–477.

154. Frizzera G. The distinction of Hodgkin's disease from anaplastic large cell lymphoma. Semin Diagn Pathol 1992; 9:291–296.

155. Menestrina F, Chilosi M, Scarpa A. Nodular lymphocyte predominant Hodgkin's disease and anaplastic large cell (CD30+) lymphoma: distinct entities or nonspecific patterns? Semin Diagn Pathol 1995; 12:256–269.

156. Kubonishi I, Ohtsuki Y, Machida K, et al. Granulocytic sarcoma as a mediastinal mass. Am J Clin Pathol 1984; 83:730–734.

157. Chubachi A, Miura I, Takahashi N, et al. Acute myelogenous leukemia associated with a mediastinal tumor. Leuk Lymphoma 1993; 12:143–146.

158. Niwa K, Tanaka T, Mori H, et al. Extramedullary plasmacytoma of the mediastinum. Jpn J Clin Oncol 1987; 17:95–100.

159. Miyazaki T, Kohno S, Sakamoto A, et al. A rare case of extramedullary plasmacytoma in the mediastinum. Intern Med 1992; 31:1363–1365.

160. Meis JM, Butler JJ, Osborne BM, et al. Granulocytic sarcoma in nonleukemic patients. Cancer 1986; 58:2697–2709.

161. Quintanilla-Martinez L, Zukerberg LR, Ferry JA, et al. Extramedullary tumors of lymphoid or myeloid blasts: the role of immunohistology in diagnosis and classification. Am J Clin Pathol 1995; 104:431–443.

162. Goldstein NS, Ritter JH, Argenyi ZB, et al. Granulocytic sarcoma: potential diagnostic clues from immunostaining patterns seen with anti-lymphoid antibodies. Int J Surg Pathol 1995; 2:199–206.

163. Aref S, Goda T, El-Sherbiny M. Syndecan-1 in multiple myeloma: relationship to conventional prognostic factors. Hematology 2003; 8:221–228.

164. Tong AW, Lee JC, Stone MJ. Characterization of a monoclonal antibody having selective reactivity with normal and neoplastic plasma cells. Blood 1987; 69:238–245.

165. Petruch UR, Horny HP, Kaiserling E. Frequent expression of haematopoietic and non-haematopoietic antigens by neoplastic plasma cells: an immunohistochemical study using formalin-fixed, paraffin-embedded tissue. Histopathology 1992; 20:35–40.

166. Ordonez NG. Role of immunohistochemistry in differentiating epithelial mesothelioma from adenocarcinoma: review and update. Am J Clin Pathol 1999; 112:75–89.

167. Kennedy AD, King G, Kerr KM. HBME-1 and antithrombomodulin in the differential diagnosis of malignant mesothelioma of pleura. J Clin Pathol 1997; 50:859–862.

168. Ordonez NG. Value of thrombomodulin immunostaining in the diagnosis of mesothelioma. Histopathology 1997; 31:25–30.

169. Wick MR, Loy T, Mills SE, et al. Malignant epithelioid pleural mesothelioma versus peripheral pulmonary adenocarcinoma: a histochemical, ultrastructural, and immunohistologic study of 103 cases. Hum Pathol 1990; 21:759–766.

170. Riera JR, Astengo-Osuna C, Longmate JA, et al. The immunohistochemical diagnostic panel for epithelial mesothelioma: a reevaluation after heat-induced epitope retrieval. Am J Surg Pathol 1997; 21:1409–1419.

171. Khoor A, Whitsett JA, Stahlman MT, et al. Utility of surfactant protein B precursor and thyroid transcription factor 1 in differentiating adenocarcinoma of the lung from malignant mesothelioma. Hum Pathol 1999; 30:695–700.

172. Wick MR. Immunohistochemistry in the diagnosis of 'solid' malignant tumors. In: Jennette JC, ed. Immunohistology in diagnostic pathology. Boca Raton: CRC Press;1989:161–191.

173. Feldman L, Kricun ME. Malignant melanoma presenting as a mediastinal mass. JAMA 1979; 241:396–397.

174. Kaufmann O, Koch S, Burghardt J, et al. Tyrosinase, melan-A, and KBA62 as markers for the immunohistochemical identification of metastatic amelanotic melanomas on paraffin sections. Mod Pathol 1998; 11:740–746.

175. Andrade RE, Wick MR, Frizzera G, et al. Immunophenotyping of hematopoietic malignancies in paraffin sections. Hum Pathol 1988; 19:394–402.

176. Nylander K, Vojtesek B, Nenutil R, et al. Differential expression of p63 isoforms in normal tissues and neoplastic cells. J Pathol 2002; 198:417–427.

177. Said JW. The immunohistochemistry of Hodgkin's disease. Semin Diagn Pathol 1992; 9:265–271.

178. Suster S, Moran CA. Spindle cell thymic carcinoma: a clinicopathologic and immunohistochemical study of a distinctive variant of primary thymic epithelial neoplasm. Am J Surg Pathol 1999; 23:691–700.

179. Suster S, Moran CA. Thymic carcinoma: spectrum of differentiation and histologic types. Pathology (Australasian) 1998; 30:111–122.

180. Moran CA, Suster S. Primary thymic carcinomas. Pathology (American) 1996; 4:141–153.

181. Kuo TT. Carcinoid tumor of the thymus with divergent sarcomatoid differentiation: report of a case with histogenetic considerations. Hum Pathol 1994; 25:319–323.

182. Suarez-Vilela D, Salas-Valien JS, Gonzalez-Moran MA, et al. Thymic carcinosarcoma associated with a spindle cell thymoma: an immunohistochemical study. Histopathology 1992; 21:263–268.

183. Wick MR, Swanson PE, Carcinosarcomas – current perspectives and a historical review of nosological concepts. Semin Diagn Pathol 1993; 10:118–127.

184. DeLeeuw B, Suijkerbuijk RF, Olde-Weghuis D, et al. Distinct Xp11.2 breakpoint regions in synovial sarcoma revealed by metaphase and interphase FISH: relationship to histologic subtypes. Cancer Genet Cytogenet 1994; 73:89–94.

185. Miettinen M, Limon J, Niezabitowski A, et al. Calretinin and other mesothelioma markers in synovial sarcoma: analysis

of antigenic similarities and differences with malignant mesothelioma. Am J Surg Pathol 2001; 25:610–617.

186. Suster S, Moran CA, Chan JKC. Thymoma with pseudosarcomatous stroma: report of an unusual histologic variant of thymic epithelial neoplasm that may simulate carcinosarcoma. Am J Surg Pathol 1997; 21:1316–1323.

187. Levine GD, Rosai J. A spindle-cell variant of thymic carcinoid tumor: a clinical, histologic, and fine structural study with emphasis on its distinction from spindle-cell thymoma. Arch Pathol Lab Med 1976; 100:293–300.

188. Moran CA, Suster S. Spindle-cell neuroendocrine carcinomas of the thymus (spindle-cell thymic carcinoid): a clinicopathologic and immunohistochemical study of seven cases. Mod Pathol 1999; 12:587–591.

189. Moran CA, Suster S. Yolk sac tumors of the mediastinum with prominent spindle cell features: a clinicopathologic study of three cases. Am J Surg Pathol 1997; 21:1173–1177.

190. Moran CA, Suster S, Perino G, et al. Malignant smooth muscle tumors presenting as mediastinal soft tissue masses: a clinicopathologic study of 10 cases. Cancer 1994; 74:2251–2260.

191. Hisaoka M, Wei-Qi S, Jian W, et al. Specific but variable expression of H-caldesmon in leiomyosarcomas: an immunohistochemical reassessment of a new myogenic marker. Appl Immunohistochem Molec Morphol 2001; 9:302–308.

192. Yang WI, Efird JT, Quintanilla-Martinez L, et al. Cell kinetic study of thymic epithelial tumors using PCNA (PC10) and Ki-67 (MIB-1) antibodies. Hum Pathol 1996; 27:70–76.

193. Pan CC, Ho DM, Chen WY, et al. Ki-67 labeling index correlates with stage and histology but not significantly with prognosis in thymoma. Histopathology 1998; 33:453–458.

194. Yang WI, Efird JT, Quintanilla-Martinez L, et al. Cell kinetic study of thymic epithelial tumors using PCNA (PC10) and Ki-67 (MIB-1) antibodies. Hum Pathol 1996; 27:70–76.

195. Tateyama H, Eimoto T, Tada T, et al. Apoptosis, bcl-2 protein, and fas antigen in thymic epithelial tumors. Mod Pathol 1997; 10:983–991.

196. Yang WI, Yang KM, Hong SW, et al. E-cadherin expression in thymomas. Yonsei Med J 1998; 39:37–44.

197. Pan CC, Ho DM, Chen WY, et al. Expression of E-cadherin and alpha- and beta-catenins in thymoma. J Pathol 1998; 184:207–211.

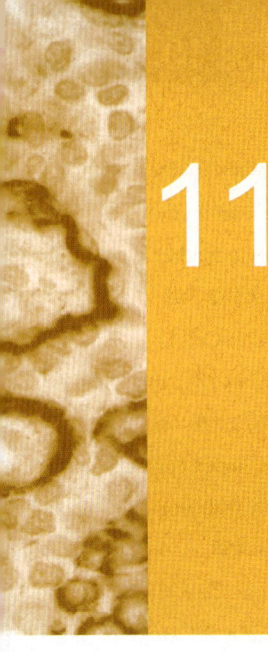

11 肺和胸膜肿瘤的免疫组织化学

原作者：Samuel P. Hammar
译　者：吴晓娟，张翠娟
审校者：张庆慧，张廷国，郭成浩，吴晓娟

目　录

引言	334
原发性肺癌	334
抗原/抗体生物学	335
肺的神经内分泌肿瘤	339
原发性肺癌的罕见类型	344
肺的转移性癌	360
肺肿瘤的其他标记物和诊断难点	361
胸膜肿瘤	366
不常见/罕见的胸膜肿瘤	381
总结/结论	388

引　言

免疫组化是诊断肺、胸膜原发性和转移性肿瘤的有效而常用的辅助技术。由于此种方法简单易行，特异性强，目前在诊断肺和胸膜肿瘤方面已大范围地取代了黏蛋白组织化学和电镜技术。但在某些情况下，电镜在诊断上要优于免疫组化；而在某些特定肿瘤，免疫组化和电镜均不易明确诊断。

自本书第一版出版以来，已积累了许多关于肺和胸膜肿瘤免疫组化特点的重要的新资料。正如所预期的那样，某些标记物的特异性和敏感性已经改变（提高），新的、高敏感性、高特异性的标记物逐渐被发现。最初认为在某些特定肿瘤表达的标记，现在已证实，它们在其他肿瘤亦有表达，而过去认为这些肿瘤是不表达这些标记的。现在，有些抗体可以用于确定肿瘤的分化程度以及作为判断肿瘤预后的指标[1-7]。

如 Pelosi[6]等的研究发现，fascin 是预测典型和非典型类癌淋巴结转移的重要指标，fascin 是肌动蛋白结合蛋白，它可诱导上皮细胞膜伸出伪足，以增加正常细胞以及转化细胞的运动性，这在典型和非典型类癌，有助于预测淋巴结转移。研究人员还发现，在典型类癌和非典型类癌，fascin 的免疫反应性与淋巴结转移密切相关，而在高级别神经内分泌肿瘤却没有这种相关性。fascin 的表达与细胞增殖活性增高（Ki-67）亦密切相关。Pelosi[7]在其另一篇文献中指出，fascin 的免疫反应性是评价Ⅰ期非小细胞肺癌的指标，其在浸润性和侵袭性高的非小细胞肺癌中表达上调，它可以作为临床预后不良的独立指标。他们还提出可以将 fascin 通路作为治疗的靶点。

绝大多数原发性肺癌仅仅通过组织学特点即可确诊。肺癌分化程度越低，其临床表现也就越复杂，而免疫组化技术则常被用于确诊或排除某个病理诊断。此外，其他组织起源的肿瘤，在形态学上可以与肺和胸膜的原发性肿瘤相似，这时免疫组化则是进行鉴别诊断的最有效方法。

原发性肺癌

肺的原发性肿瘤种类很多，主要可以分为四大类：腺癌、鳞状细胞癌、小细胞癌和大细胞未分化癌，约占肺的原发性肿瘤的85%～90%[8]。在美国，目前腺癌是肺的原发性肿瘤中最常见的类型[9,10]，通常位于胸膜下（周围型），偶见于中央和支气管内；鳞状细胞癌居第二位，主要位于中央，起源于主支气管和叶支气管，另有10%的鳞状细胞癌呈周围型；小细胞肺癌多为中央型，起源于主支气管或叶支气管的神经内分泌细胞，但约有10%的小细胞肺癌呈周围型；大细胞肺癌约占肺的原发性肿瘤的8%~10%，它可以发生于肺的任何部位。

有几个抗体有益于确诊或排除原发性肺癌，而这些抗体的应用要根据肿瘤的类型和临床情况的需要。常用于检测、确诊或排除原发性肺癌的抗体见表11.1（不包括神经内分泌癌，其见后文）。

抗原/抗体生物学

用于检测非神经内分泌肺癌的抗体

角蛋白属多肽家族，已按分子量和（碱性或酸性）等电点将其区分开来。Moll等[11,12]按分子种类对其进行分类，共有20个类型。CK7表达于肺的上皮细胞，但在其他上皮细胞和许多肺外肿瘤中亦有表达[13]。CK7是原发性肺癌中最常见的一个CK分子类型。CK5主要见于鳞状细胞癌。有腺样结构时，CK7常与CK20和非角蛋白抗体联合应用于诊断。除小细胞肺癌（仅表达低分子量角蛋白）外，绝大多数原发性肺癌可表达多种CK。

Chu等[14]应用CK7和CK20两项指标对435例不同组织来源的上皮性肿瘤进行了免疫组化研究，结果发现，除大肠癌、前列腺癌、肾癌和胸腺癌、肺和胃肠道的类癌以及皮肤的Merkel细胞癌CK7呈阴性表达外，绝大多数的癌CK7呈阳性表达。许多不同组织起源的鳞状细胞癌CK7呈阴性表达，但在宫颈的鳞状细胞癌CK7呈阳性表达。CK20几乎在所有的结直肠癌和Merkel细胞癌中均有表达。在62%的胰腺癌、50%的胃癌、43%的胆管细胞癌和29%的移行细胞癌中有CK20的表达。如表11.2所示，CK7表达的阳性率，在原发性肺腺癌中为100%（10/10），小细胞肺癌为43%（3/7），类癌为22%（2/9），肺鳞状细胞癌CK7的表达为0%（0/15）；CK20表达的阳性率，在肺腺癌为10%（1/10），类癌为0%（0/9），小细胞肺癌为0%（0/7），鳞状细胞癌亦为0%（0/15）。

CDX2是一个以同源序列盒为主体的转录因子，在小肠的分化过程中起重要作用。Kaimaktchiev等[15]研究了CDX2在一系列腺癌中的表达。CDX2在85.7%的结直肠癌和97.9%的结直肠腺瘤中表达。39例原发性肺腺癌、10例细支气管肺泡癌、48例肺原发性大细胞未分化癌和48例小细胞肺癌均无CDX2的表达。

p63是p53家族成员之一，其表达在上皮细胞分化过程中以及在鳞状细胞癌中均起重要作用。Au等[16]在两个不同的实验室，应用组织芯片技术，对408例肺癌p63的表达进行了研究。在两个实验室中p63的表达情况见表11.3。正如预测，在绝大多数鳞状细胞癌、大部分大细胞神经内分泌癌和小细胞肺癌均有p63的表达。p63的表达是用于判断神经内分泌癌预后的重要指标，如高级别神经内分泌癌与低级别神经内分泌癌相比较，前者更易于表达p63。从实际工作的角度，Au还将p63作为鳞状细胞分化的一个指标（图11.1）。

Sheikh等[17]应用免疫组化技术，对33例腺癌、43例纤维化和化生性肺良性病变、5例非典型性腺瘤样增生、5例腺鳞癌和3例鳞状细胞癌p63的表达进行了研究。肺的良性病变主要包括普通型间质性肺炎、肺实质瘢痕、隐源性机化性肺炎和弥漫性肺泡损伤。在正常的肺组织，大小气道的储备细胞有p63的表达，偶尔在终末小叶单位的细胞亦有表达。在纤维化过程中，大气道的基底细胞、细支气管上皮以及鳞化的上皮内均可见到核着色。在急性肺损伤中，p63的免疫反应性较低。在1/33例肺腺癌和2/5例非典型腺瘤样增生，绝大多数细胞呈p63的强阳性表达。而在3例肺腺癌中，仅有少数癌细胞呈强阳性表达。因此作者得出结论，细支气管肺泡病变部位不同，p63的表达亦有明显差异，p63有助于鉴别肺的反应性腺体增生和肿瘤性腺体增生。

β-钙黏素是一种多功能蛋白，其在介导细胞黏附和信号转导过程中起重要作用。该膜蛋白的下调在人类的多种肿瘤发病机制中起重要作用。其在结直肠癌的癌变过程中也起着重要作用。

Nakatani等[18]应用β-钙黏素染色，研究了9例以前诊断为双相性（分化的）肺母细胞瘤，在4例典型的肺母细胞瘤中，在上皮样分化和间叶样分化成分中的细胞核/细胞浆内均有β-钙黏素的异常表达，尤其是在腺体出芽部分以及小巢状的细胞中呈强阳性表达。其余5例肺母细胞瘤的母细胞样区，细胞核/细胞浆有β-钙黏素表达。其中向上皮分化的成分中胞核/胞浆均无表达；而向间叶分化的成分中也无表达或仅有灶性表达。由此作者推测，β-钙黏素基因突变，可能在经典型肺母细胞瘤癌变过程中起重要作用。

表 11.1　肺肿瘤鉴别诊断的常用抗体（神经内分泌癌除外）

抗原	克隆	抗原的特征	免疫原	制造商	稀释度	抗原修复
CK	AE1/AE3	AE1-酸性亚家族 40、48、50、56.5kD AE3-碱性亚家族 52、56、58、59、64、65~67kD	人表皮角蛋白	DAKO	1：200	HIER
CK	5D3	CK8、CK18	结直肠癌细胞株	BioGenex	1：100	HIER
CK	MAK6	CK8、CK14~CK16、CK18、CK19	来自 MCF 组织培养和足底表皮的细胞外抗原	Zymed	1：100	HIER
CK	35bH11	CK8-54kD	Hep3B 肝癌细胞株	DAKO	1：50	HIER
CK	34bE12	CK-Moll1、5、10 和 14	人角质层角蛋白	DAKO	1：100	HIER
CK5/6	D5/16B4	中间纤维 CK5/CK6 和少量 CK4	纯化的 CK5	Biocare Medical	1：100	HIER
CK7	OV-TL12/30	MollCK7-54kD	OTN11 卵巢癌细胞株	Cell Marque	NA	HIER
CK20	Ks20.8	Moll CK20	从人十二指肠黏膜获得的细胞骨架蛋白	Cell Marque	NA	HIER
Vimentin	Vim3B4	中间纤维 -57kD	牛晶状体的波形蛋白	DAKO	1：100	HIER
EMA	E29	糖蛋白 -250~400kD	人乳脂提取物	Ventana	NA	HIER
人乳脂球蛋白 -2（HMFG-2）	115D8	MAM-6 黏液糖蛋白 > 400kD	纯化的人乳脂球蛋白	BioGenex	1：25	HIER
多克隆癌胚抗原（pCEA）		抗体识别 CEA 和 CEA 样蛋白，包括非特异性交叉反应物和胆汁糖蛋白	从转移性结肠癌分离的人 CEA	Ventana	NA	HIER
CD15（LeuM1）	C3D-1	3-岩藻糖 -N-乙酰乳糖胺	正常人外周血纯化的中性粒细胞	Ventana	NA	HIER
肿瘤相关糖蛋白	B72.3	各种腺癌中的糖蛋白	转移性乳腺癌的膜浓缩碎片	Cell Marque	NA	HIER
人上皮抗原	VU-ID9	除鳞状上皮、肝细胞和壁细胞外，所有上皮细胞表面和胞浆的 34 和 49kD 糖蛋白	MCF-7 细胞株	Ventana	NA	HIER
甲状腺转录因子 -1（TTF-1）	8G7G3/1	NKx2 家族同源功能区转录因子	鼠腹水	Cell Marque	NA	HIER
S-100 蛋白		S-100 蛋白 A 和 B	牛脑分离获得的 S-100 蛋白	DAKO	1：3000	HIER
表面活性脂蛋白 A（SP-A）	PE-10	表面活性物质 A	从肺泡蛋白沉积症病人肺泡冲洗液中分离的表面活性物质脂蛋白	DAKO	1：100	HIER
CDX2	CDX2-88	调节肠上皮增殖、分化的肠特异性转录因子同源序列家族	全长 CDX2	BioGenex	NA	HIER
p63	4A4	人 p63 蛋白，p53 家族成员	鼠单克隆抗体	Cell Marque	1：100	HIER
fascin	55K-2	55kD 激动蛋白结合蛋白	HeLa 细胞纯化的 fascin	DAKO	1：1000	HIER

表 11.2A　上皮性肿瘤 CK7 的表达

器官	肿瘤的类型	总例数	阳性例数	百分比
肺	腺癌	10	10	100
卵巢	腺癌	24	24	100
唾液腺	所有肿瘤	9	9	100
子宫	内膜癌	10	10	100
甲状腺	所有肿瘤	55	54	98
乳腺	导管和小叶癌	26	25	96
肝	胆管细胞癌	14	13	93
胰腺	腺癌	13	12	92
膀胱	移行细胞癌	24	21	88
子宫颈	鳞癌	15	13	87
间皮	恶性间皮瘤	17	11	65
肺、肝、小肠	神经内分泌癌	9	5	56
肺	小细胞癌	7	3	43
胃	腺癌	8	3	38
头颈部	鳞癌	30	8	27
肺	类癌	9	2	22
食管	鳞癌	14	3	21
胃肠道	类癌	15	2	13
肾	癌	19	2	11
肝	肝癌	11	1	9
生殖细胞	生殖细胞肿瘤	14	1	7
大肠	腺癌	20	1	5
肾上腺	皮质癌	10	0	0
肺	鳞癌	15	0	0
前列腺	腺癌	18	0	0
皮肤	Merkel 细胞肿瘤	9	0	0
胸腺	胸腺瘤	8	0	0
软组织	上皮样肿瘤	12	0	0

（引自 Chu P, Wu E, Weiss LM. Cytokeratin 7 and cytokeratin 20 expression in epithelial neoplasms: A survey of 435 cases. Mod Pathol 2000; 13:962-972）

波形蛋白是一种 58kD 的中间丝，主要存在于间叶细胞中。但波形蛋白在绝大多数梭形细胞癌中有表达[19]，部分报道其表达的阳性率在肺腺癌中亦很高[20]。

原发性肺癌，尤其是肺腺癌可有一系列上皮细胞性标记的表达。这些标记物主要包括癌胚抗原（CEA）、人乳脂球蛋白-2（HMFG-2）、上皮细胞膜抗原（EMA）、LeuM1(CD15)、B72.3 和 BerEP4 表面蛋白。这些标记绝大多数是非特异性的，通常用于肺间皮瘤与肺及肺外腺癌（见下）的鉴别，以及组织起源不明的腺癌的诊断（见第 7 章）[21]。

甲状腺转录因子 -1（TTF-1）是一种 38～40kD 的转录因子，属于 NKx2 家族的同源核转录因子。主要表达于甲状腺上皮和肺的上皮细胞中[22,23]。TTF-1 可与 Clara 细胞分泌蛋白、肺表面活性蛋白 A、B 和 C 结合，并活化这些蛋白的启动子[24,25]。文献中报道和作者研究观察到，60%～75% 肺腺癌细胞核 TTF-1 呈阳性表达[26-29]，在绝大多数的小细胞肺癌、非典型类癌、大细胞神经内分泌癌以及约 35% 的典型类癌亦有 TTF-1 的阳性表达[36]。

图 11.2 为普通型非神经内分泌肺肿瘤的直方图图示，肺肿瘤其他抗原的表达情况见表 11.4[14,31-38]。

表11.2B 上皮性肿瘤CK20的表达

器官	肿瘤的类型	总例数	阳性例数	百分比
大肠	腺癌	20	20	100
皮肤	Merkel 细胞癌	9	7	78
胰腺	腺癌	13	8	62
胃	腺癌	8	4	50
肝	胆管上皮癌	14	6	43
膀胱	移行细胞癌	24	7	29
肺	腺癌	10	1	10
肝	肝细胞癌	11	1	9
胃肠道	类癌	15	1	7
头颈部	鳞状细胞癌	30	2	6
卵巢	腺癌	24	1	4
肾上腺	皮质癌	10	0	0
乳腺	小叶和导管癌	26	0	0
子宫颈	鳞状细胞癌	15	0	0
食管	鳞状细胞癌	14	0	0
生殖细胞	生殖细胞癌	14	0	0
肾	癌	19	0	0
肺、肝、小肠	神经内分泌癌	9	0	0
肺	类癌	9	0	0
肺	小细胞癌	7	0	0
肺	鳞状细胞癌	15	0	0
间皮	恶性间皮瘤	17	0	0
前列腺	腺癌	18	0	0
唾液腺	所有肿瘤	9	0	0
软组织	上皮样癌	12	0	0
甲状腺	所有肿瘤	55	0	0
胸腺	胸腺瘤	8	0	0
子宫	内膜癌	10	0	0

(引自 Chu P,Wu E,Weiss LM. Cytokeratin 7 and cytokeratin 20 expression in epithelial neoplasms: A survey of 435 cases. Mod Pathol 2000; 13:962-972)

> **诊断要点**：肺的非神经内分泌肿瘤
>
> 1. 典型者 CK7+/CK20。
> 2. 除部分胶样癌外（见后），CDX2通常呈阴性表达。
> 3. p63 于良性和恶性鳞状上皮病变、气道储备细胞和部分远端小叶上皮呈阳性表达；在腺癌很少表达。
> 4. 在梭形细胞癌中，常有波形蛋白与CK的共同表达。
> 5. 75%腺癌、绝大多数肺小细胞癌、大细胞神经内分泌癌、非典型类癌及35%的类癌有TTF-1的表达。大约5%～10%的鳞状细胞癌可有TTF-1的表达。

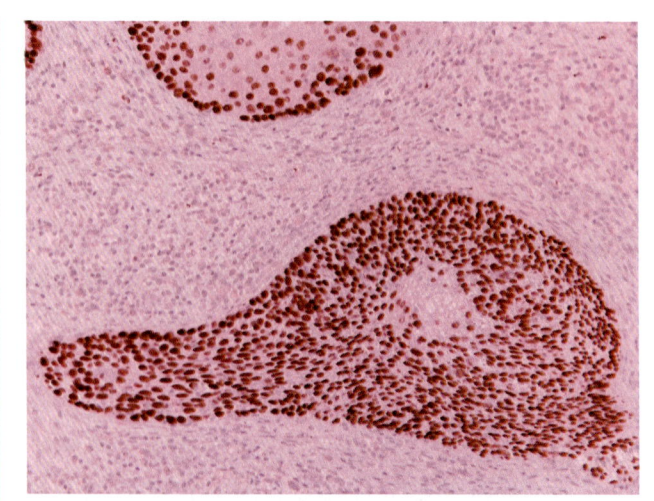

图11.1 肺的低分化鳞状细胞癌细胞核有 p63 的表达（×100）

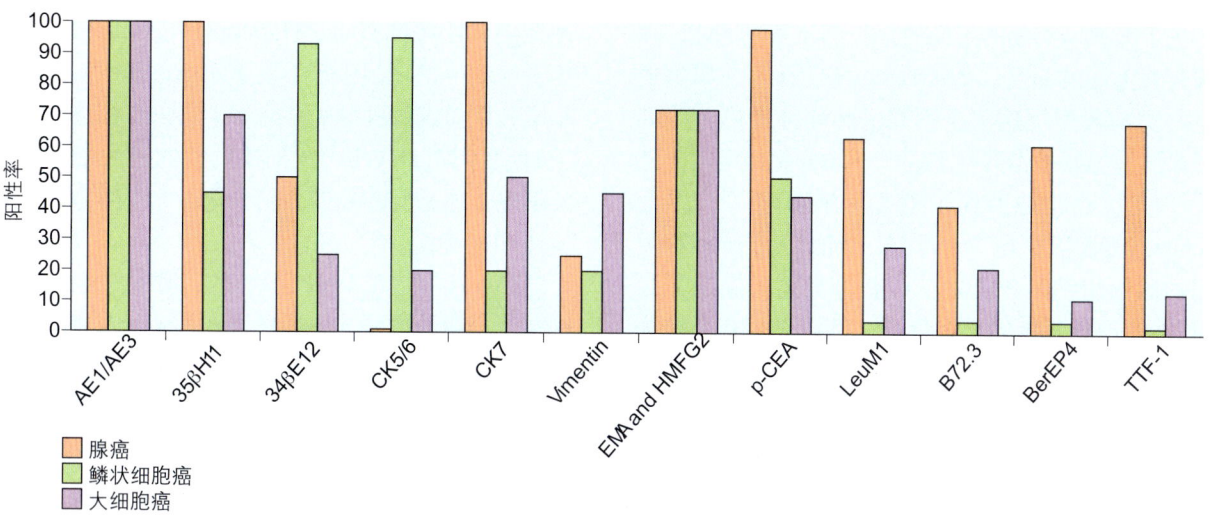

图 11.2　除小细胞肺癌外，常见原发性肺癌的直方图（腺癌、鳞癌、大细胞癌）

表11.3　p63在肺癌中的表达

肿瘤类型	免疫组化结果（PhenoPath Laboratory）				
	阴性	弱阳性	强阳性	无法解释	% 阳性率
鳞状细胞癌	3	1	93	26	96.9
腺癌	56	14	10	13	30.0
大细胞癌	34	5	15	14	37.0
经典型类癌	51	1	0	16	1.9
非典型类癌	18	4	4	5	30.8
大细胞神经内分泌癌	4	3	1	3	50.0
小细胞癌	3	5	5	1	76.9
肿瘤类型	免疫组化结果				
	阴性	弱阳性	强阳性	无法解释	阳性率
鳞状细胞癌	4	11	89	19	96.2
腺癌	74	2	5	12	8.6
大细胞癌	42	3	10	13	23.6
经典型类癌	57	0	1	10	1.7
非典型类癌	23	1	3	4	14.8
大细胞神经内分泌癌	9	0	0	2	0
小细胞癌	9	2	2	1	30.8

（引自Au NHC, Gown AM, Cheang M, et al.p63 expression in lung carcinoma: a tissue microarray study of 408 cases.Appl Immunohistochem Mol Morphol 2004; 12: 240-247）

肺的神经内分泌肿瘤

小细胞癌是肺组织最常见的神经内分泌癌[39,40]。目前已将以往所划分的亚型（如淋巴细胞样、多角形/梭形细胞癌）归纳为小细胞癌[41]。

WHO 将小细胞癌定义为"由小细胞构成的恶性上皮性肿瘤，肿瘤细胞胞浆稀少，边界不清，核染色质呈细颗粒状，无核仁或核仁不明显。瘤细胞可以呈圆形、卵圆形及梭形，核明显，核分裂象较多。"混合型小细胞肺癌是"小细胞肺癌的一个变异型，组织学上由小细胞癌与其他任意一种非小细胞癌组织类型成分构成，通常为腺癌、鳞状细胞癌或大细胞癌，少见的有梭形细胞癌和巨细胞癌"。

其他肺的原发性神经内分泌肿瘤包括：典型类癌、非典型类癌和大细胞神经内分泌癌。WHO 将典型类癌定义为"具有类癌的组织学形态，直径≥0.5cm，无坏死，核分裂≤2/10HPF($2mm^2$)的肿瘤"。

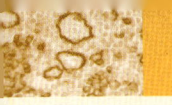

关于非典型类癌的定义尚存在部分易混淆处，该肿瘤有着不同的命名。如Arrigoni等[42]认为非典型类癌是一类与典型类癌完全不同的肺的神经内分泌肿瘤。非典型类癌是指恶性类癌[43]、高分化神经内分泌癌[44]、与类癌相似的周围型小细胞肺癌[45]，以及Kulchitzky细胞癌Ⅱ型[46]。目前，WHO关于肺和胸膜肿瘤的国际组织学分类中[47]，将非典型类癌定义为"具有神经内分泌癌的形态特征，且有2～10个核分裂/10HPF和/或灶性点状坏死，或二者兼有"。

另有文献，将肺的典型类癌和非典型类癌进行了对比[48-49]。Thomas等[48]指出，有局部淋巴结转移的非典型类癌，如果单纯手术切除，该肿瘤术后易复发，其预后比有胸腔淋巴结转移的典型类癌患者差。

1978年Gould和Chejfec[50]首次提出了肺大细胞神经内分泌癌的概念，Hammond和Sause[51]在1985年、Neal等[52]在1986年及Barbareschi等[53]在1989年又分别对这种肿瘤的存在作了进一步描述。但是关于1981年McDavell[54]所描述的肿瘤是大细胞神经内分泌癌，还是有神经内分泌分化的非小细胞肺癌，目前还不能确定。

Travis等[55]在1991年对35例肺的神经内分泌癌进行了报道，其中包括5例大细胞神经内分泌癌。他们对大细胞神经内分泌癌的诊断标准包括：①光镜下，肿瘤具有神经内分泌癌的形态特点，如癌细胞呈器官样、小梁状、栅栏状或菊形团样排列；②大细胞的直径大于淋巴细胞核直径的3倍；③癌细胞多角形，核/浆比较小，细颗粒状嗜酸性胞浆，核染色质粗大，核仁易见；④每10个高倍视野，核分裂多于

表11.4 原发性肺肿瘤中CK、TTF-1和SP-A的表达

参考文献	研究病例数	肺癌的组织类型	CK5	CK7	Cam5.2 CK8	CK20	TTF-1	SP-A
Chu P et al.[14]	10	腺癌	ND	10(100%)	ND	1(10%)	ND	ND
Mod Pathol	15	鳞癌	ND	0(0%)	ND	0(0%)	ND	ND
2000；13：962-972	7	小细胞癌	ND	3(43%)	ND	0(0%)	ND	ND
	9	典型类癌	ND	2(22%)	ND	0(0%)	ND	ND
Amin et al.[31] Am J Sur Pathol 2002；26：358-364	15	微乳头腺癌	ND	14(93%)	ND	2(13%)	12(80%)	ND
Nakamural N et al.[32]	52	腺癌	ND	ND	ND	ND	50(96.2%)	38(73.1%)
Mod Pathol 2002；	19	高分化	ND	ND	ND	ND	19(100%)	17(89.5%)
15：1058-1067	29	中分化	ND	ND	ND	ND	27(93%)	18(62%)
	4	低分化	ND	ND	ND	ND	4(10%)	2(50%)
	26	鳞癌	ND	ND	ND	ND	0(0%)	0(0%)
	18	小细胞癌	ND	ND	ND	ND	16(88.9%)	0(0%)
	8	大细胞未分化癌	ND	ND	ND	ND	0(0%)	0(0%)
Lau SK et al.[33]	67	细支气管肺泡：						
Mod Pathol	48	非黏液癌	ND	46(96%)	ND	0(0%)	36(75%)	ND
2002；15：538-542	12	黏液癌	ND	10(83%)	ND	3(25%)	0(0%)	ND
	7	混合癌	ND	7(100%)	ND	0(0%)	6(86%)	ND
Simsir A et al.[34]	16	细支气管肺泡：						
Am J Clin Pathol	6	黏液癌	ND	4(67%)	ND	4(67%)	0(0%)	ND
2004；121：350-357	4	非黏液癌	ND	4(100%)	ND	0(0%)	2(50%)	ND
	6	混合癌	ND	6(100%)	ND	6(100%)灶性+	5(83%)	ND
Johansson L.[35]	12	鳞癌	12(100%)	3(25%)	12(100%)	0(0%)	0(0%)	ND
Ann Diagn Pathol	13	小细胞癌	0(0%)	13(100%)	13(100%)	0(0%)	13(100%)	ND
2002；8：259-267	11	腺癌	0(0%)	11(100%)	11(100%)	0(0%)	11(100%)	ND
	9	大细胞多形性癌	0(0%)	5(55%)	9(100%)	0(0%)	5(55%)	ND
Yatabe Y et al.[36] Am J Surg Pathol 2002；26：767-773	64	腺癌	ND	ND	ND	ND	54(84.4%)	41(64.1%)

续表

参考文献	研究病例数	肺癌的组织类型	CK5	CK7	Cam5.2 CK8	CK20	TTF-1	SP-A
Chang Y et al.[37]	99	鳞癌	ND	ND	ND	ND	4(4%)	ND
Lung Cancer	176	腺癌	ND	ND	ND	ND	169(96%)	ND
2004；44：149-157	12	腺鳞癌	ND	ND	ND	ND	12(100%)	ND
	0	鳞癌						
	36	小细胞癌	ND	ND	ND	ND	19(53%)	ND
		大细胞未分化癌	ND	ND	ND	ND	0(0%)	ND
	23	多形性癌						
	25	淋巴上皮癌						
	8	典型类癌	ND	ND	ND	ND	0(0%)	ND
	3	非典型类癌	ND	ND	ND	ND	0(0%)	ND
	44	硬化性血管内皮瘤	ND	ND	ND	ND	39(89%)	ND
	1	间皮瘤	ND	ND	ND	ND	0(0%)	ND
	1	假间皮瘤	ND	ND	ND	ND	0(0%)	ND
	83	转移性*肺肿瘤					5	
	125	非肺的转移性肿瘤	ND	ND	ND	ND	0(0%)	ND
Saad RS et al.[38]	50	"传统的"腺癌 细支气管肺泡癌	ND	ND	ND	ND	30(60%)	ND
Hum Pathol								
2004；35：3-7	32	非黏液癌	ND	ND	ND	ND	20(62.5%)	ND
	18	黏液癌	ND	ND	ND	ND	4(22.2%)	ND

ND,没有做；* 阳性——所有甲状腺癌

10个；⑤坏死；⑥免疫组化和/或电镜技术检测，可见神经内分泌特征。

WHO肿瘤的国际组织学分类指出，大细胞神经内分泌癌是指，大细胞癌在形态上可以表现为癌细胞呈器官样、巢状、小梁状、菊形团样或栅栏状排列，这些排列方式往往提示肿瘤向神经内分泌方向分化，并可通过免疫组化或电镜技术所证实。

作者在1989年[56]的一篇文献中即指出，肺的神经内分泌癌分化的差异很大，并且，有一部分神经内分泌癌并不适宜归入到某一特定的类型。

关于大细胞神经内分泌癌的报道还有很多[57-62]，这些文章中均指出肺的大细胞神经内分泌癌是一种侵袭性肿瘤。Peng等[63]指出，肺的大细胞神经内分泌癌与小细胞肺癌具有相似的免疫组化标记，但它与有神经内分泌特征的大细胞肺癌具有不同的生物学行为。然而，在大细胞神经内分泌癌，具有神经内分泌特征的大细胞癌和小细胞癌均有3p的杂合性丢失。因此，作者指出：在肺的大细胞癌，具有神经内分泌分化的形态学特征，并不等同于其具有神经内分泌分化的生物学行为。

用于检测肺神经内分泌癌的抗体

人体的许多器官和组织均有神经内分泌细胞，这些细胞被Pearse[64]称为弥散性神经内分泌系统,而被Gould和DeLellis称为散在的神经内分泌系统[65]。不难想象，神经内分泌细胞和具有神经内分泌分化的肿瘤细胞应具有相似的免疫组化特征。主要包括一些生物源性胺、肽类激素、神经递质等，这些物质均可用生物化学或免疫组化技术检测出来[66]。免疫组化标记可以验证肿瘤具有神经内分泌分化，但通常不是特异性的。表11.5列出了常用的用于显示有神经内分泌分化的抗体。

突触素（Syn）是分子量38kD的糖蛋白，由牛神经元分离出的突触前囊泡成分[67,68]。作者认为，Syn是神经内分泌肿瘤最敏感、最具特异性的抗体。本章后面还将探讨，在肺的非神经内分泌癌和非小细胞癌偶尔也可有Syn的表达。

嗜铬素（CgA），是一组含有高浓度谷氨酸的酸性蛋白家族，存在于正常和肿瘤性神经内分泌细胞神经内分泌颗粒基质中[69,70]。Banks和Helle在1965年

表11.5 检测肺神经内分泌肿瘤的常用抗体

抗原	克隆	抗原特性	免疫原	制造商	稀释度	抗原修复
Syn		38kD 突触囊泡膜成分	与清蛋白结合的合成型人 Syn	DAKO	1:100	HIER
CgA	DAK-A3	位于神经内分泌颗粒内由14号染色体编码的439氨基酸蛋白	C-末端 20kD CgA 片段	DAKO	1:100	HIER
NSE		46kDγ-γ烯醇酶同工酶	人脑分离获得的 NSE	DAKO	1:400	HIER
Leu7 CD57	NK-1	110kD 人骨髓细胞相关的表面糖蛋白	抗原由人自然杀伤细胞获得	BioGenex	1:20	HIER
神经细胞黏附分子(NCAM)	UJ13A	125kD 唾液酸糖蛋白	16周胎牛脑组织匀浆	DAKO	1:20	HIER
TTF-1	8G7G3/1	肺和甲状腺 NKx2 家族同源功能区转录因子中 40kD 成分	鼠腹水	Cell Marque	NA	HIER
CD117		145kD 跨膜受体结合区	兔	DAKO	1:400	HIER
Ki-67		Ki-67 增殖细胞核抗原	鼠单克隆抗体	Ventana	NA	HIER

首次于肾上腺髓质细胞发现了 CgA。抗 CgA 抗体是正常和肿瘤性神经内分泌细胞最具特异性的标记。通常情况下，在某个肿瘤中嗜铬素的表达与胞浆内神经内分泌颗粒的数量相关，内分泌颗粒的数量是可以通过电镜进行判断的。

神经特异性烯醇化酶（NSE）催化糖酵解通路中2-磷酸甘油酸和磷酸烯醇丙酮酸之间的相互转换。烯醇化酶是由α、β、γ三种亚单位组成的二聚体，NSE 含有高浓度γ-烯醇化酶，通常在神经元和神经内分泌细胞中浓度较高。但是，NSE 并不是神经元或神经内分泌细胞所特有的。NSE 在很多非神经元或非神经内分泌细胞中均可存在，如平滑肌细胞、肌上皮细胞、肾上皮细胞、浆细胞以及巨核细胞等[72,73]。NSE 常被称为非特异性烯醇化酶。尽管它的特异性很低，但它仍是肿瘤性神经内分泌细胞的一个高敏感性标记。

另有其他一些神经内分泌标记偶尔也可用于肺的正常神经内分泌细胞和肿瘤性神经内分泌细胞的鉴别，如神经丝[74]、神经细胞黏附分子（NCAM）[75,76]和 Leu7[77]。表11.6 中列出了肺的神经内分泌肿瘤中常见的神经肽、神经胺和激素。TTF-1 在小细胞癌、非典型类癌和大细胞神经内分泌癌中阳性表达率也很高，但它在典型类癌中的表达<50%。

CD117（c-kit）是一种跨膜酪氨酸激酶受体，存在于多种肿瘤细胞，尤其是在胃肠道间质瘤。c-kit是

表11.6 肺的神经内分泌肿瘤中常见的神经肽、神经胺和激素

铃蟾肽
降钙素
促肾上腺皮质激素(ACTH)
亮氨酸-脑啡肽（Leu-enkephalin）
胃泌素
生长抑制激素
血管活性肠多肽
神经降压素
精氨酸加压素
5-羟色胺

胃肠道间质瘤相对特异性和敏感性的免疫组化标记。如果某个胃肠道间质瘤表达CD117，通常情况下可用格列卫（Gleevec）®治疗。对 CD117 在肺和胸膜肿瘤的表达情况已经进行研究[78-80]。Lanarelo 等[78]应用两种抗体，在应用和未应用抗原热修复的情况下，对原发性肺癌和间皮瘤c-kit的表达进行了评价。c-kit的阳性反应主要见于小细胞肺癌，偶尔在其他类型的癌中也有阳性表达。应用DAKO抗体，在33例间皮瘤中，7例有c-kit的免疫表达。作者认为c-kit在小细胞肺癌中的表达提示其在肿瘤的恶性生物学行为中起着重要的作用，可将c-kit的亚单位作为靶点，应用c-kit抑制剂对患者进行治疗。Pelosi 等[79]报道，88例腺癌中的19例（22%）和113例鳞状细胞癌中的15例

（13％）CD117呈膜阳性。28例腺癌和8例鳞状细胞癌为胞浆阳性。在CD117膜阳性的肿瘤中，免疫反应性强与肿瘤的高增殖性活性和肿瘤生物学行为不良的指标有关，如高分期、体积大、高级别，以及临床症状和其他改变等。阳性表达的肿瘤表现为bcl-2、cyclin E、Her-2/neu、p27和fascin水平升高。作者认为，在Ⅰ期肺腺癌和鳞状细胞癌，CD117的免疫反应性由其特有的亚单位决定，这个亚单位往往与病人的预后有关。他们还指出，将CD117通路作为治疗靶点可能是治疗原发性肺癌亚型的新策略。由于在小细胞肺癌有c-kit的表达，并且其与预后呈负相关，因此Casali等[80]研究了c-kit蛋白在大细胞神经内分泌癌的过度表达。他们应用抗c-kit多克隆抗体对33例术后曾经接受放射治疗的病人进行了研究，结果为，在33例病人中，有c-kit表达的肿瘤患者1年、3年、5年存活率分别为79％、58％和51％。生存率分析表明，除CD117免疫染色外，其他临床病理特征在不同病例之间无差异性。CD117阴性大细胞神经内分泌癌，患者1年、3年存活率分别为91％、82％，而CD117阳性者分别为72％、44％。CD117的表达与复发率的升高有关（CD117阳性和CD117阴性的大细胞神经内分泌癌复发率分别为60％和23％）。由此作者认为c-Kit蛋白在大细胞神经内分泌癌常有表达，并且是一个代表预后差的指标。Butnor等[81]应用抗c-kit多克隆抗体对61例病例进行了研究，其中小细胞癌11例，大细胞神经内分泌癌4例，鳞状细胞癌22例，腺癌23例，肺典型类癌11例，胸膜恶性间皮瘤19例，胸膜局限性纤维性肿瘤6例。小细胞癌c-kit的阳性率为82％，并且几乎所有病例均为中等强度至强阳性表达。大细胞神经内分泌癌c-kit的阳性率为25％，鳞状细胞癌中9％为灶性阳性，腺癌中17％为灶性阳性，肺典型类癌无反应性。50％的胸膜局限性纤维性肿瘤呈中度强度阳性，95％的胸膜恶性间皮瘤无反应性。因此作者认为，c-kit在小细胞肺癌的高表达，对其治疗有重要提示。

组胺脱羧酶（histidine decarboxylase），是一种属于摄取胺前体脱羧系统的酶，存在于肥大细胞和肠嗜铬样细胞。Matsuki等[82]提出假说认为，该酶是神经内分泌分化的一个标记。他们发现大多数小细胞肺癌抗组胺脱羧酶抗体免疫组化呈阳性（18/23，敏感性0.78），而在非神经内分泌肺癌则几乎无反应性（2/44，特异性0.95）。其反应与CD56染色结果相似。12例大细胞神经内分泌癌中的6例和7例胃肠道小细胞癌中的4例中，组胺脱羧酶有阳性表达。因此，他们得出结论，组胺脱羧酶可用于小细胞肺癌和非神经内分泌性肺癌的鉴别，并可证实肿瘤具有神经内分泌分化。

文章作者用于确定神经内分泌分化肺肿瘤的抗体包括：抗低分子量角蛋白、高分子量角蛋白、Syn、CgA、TTF-1和白细胞共同抗原（LCA）抗体。肺的神经内分泌肿瘤偶尔表达CEA[83]，而几乎所有肺的神经内分泌肿瘤均表达NSE。图11.3为肺神经内分泌肿瘤免疫组化染色特征性的直方图图示。

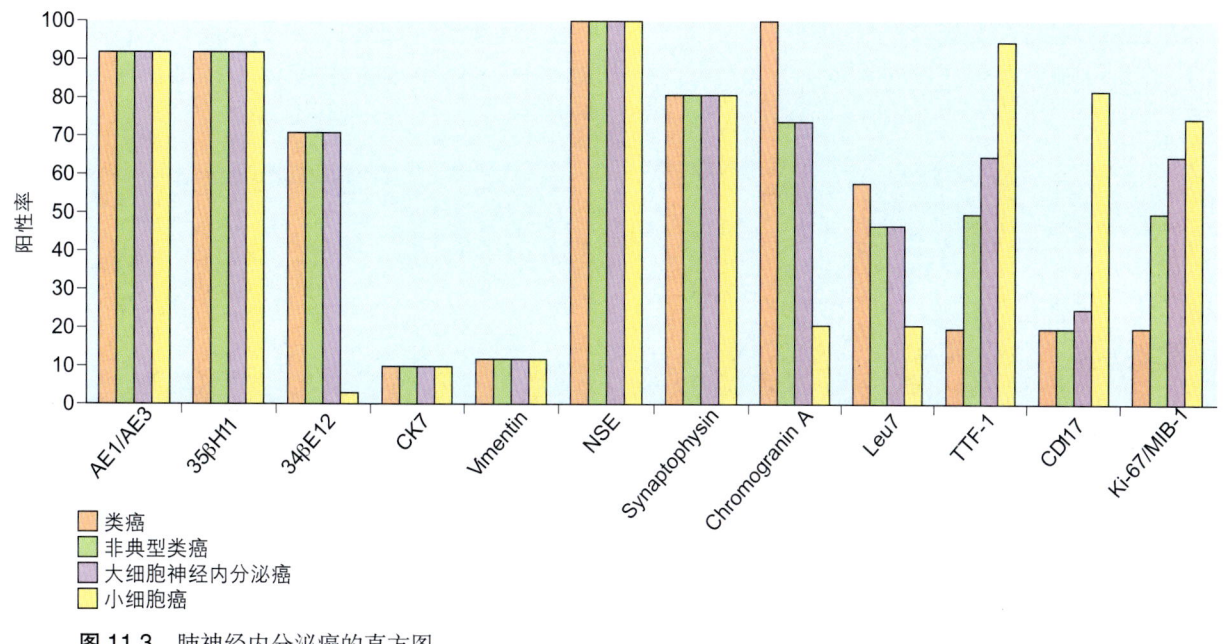

图11.3　肺神经内分泌癌的直方图

小细胞肺癌，约占肺原发性肿瘤的20%～25%，免疫组化示，低分子量角蛋白（CAM5.2、35βH11）阳性，高分子量角蛋白阴性，而Syn、NSE、CEA免疫组化染色均呈阳性（图11.4），CgA免疫组化结果不一，而TTF-1通常为核阳性（图11.5）。且低分子量角蛋白和CgA通常为点状着色（图11.6、11.7）。依本文作者的经验，虽然CgA的表达有赖于肿瘤细胞胞浆中神经内分泌颗粒的数量，但是绝大多数小细胞癌是不表达CgA的。而电镜研究则发现，偶尔在小细胞癌胞浆中含相当数量的神经内分泌颗粒（图11.8）。

典型类癌、非典型类癌和大细胞神经内分泌癌特征性地表达低分子量角蛋白、高分子量角蛋白、Syn和CgA。非典型类癌和大细胞神经内分泌癌通常可表达TTF-1。免疫组化染色对确定肿瘤是否具有神经内分泌功能有一定帮助，但对肿瘤类型的鉴别诊断却没有特异性。在典型类癌，CgA的着色最强（图11.9），这与其胞浆中具有多数神经内分泌颗粒有关。

> **诊断要点**：神经内分泌癌
>
> 1. NSE、Syn和CgA对神经内分泌分化检测的敏感性依次降低，而其特异性与之相反（即特异性依次升高）。
> 2. CD117在小细胞癌和非小细胞癌的某些亚型中有膜阳性。要确定其与临床的关系还需进一步研究。

原发性肺癌的罕见类型

病理学家偶尔会遇到一些罕见类型的原发性肺肿瘤，它可能会给诊断带来一定困难，但均不常见，包括肉瘤样癌（癌肉瘤、梭形细胞癌）、肺母细胞瘤、恶性血管内皮瘤（血管内细支气管肺泡肿瘤，IVBAT）、肉瘤、淋巴组织增生性病变、肺朗格汉斯组织细胞增多症、Kaposi肉瘤、透明细胞肿瘤（糖原瘤，

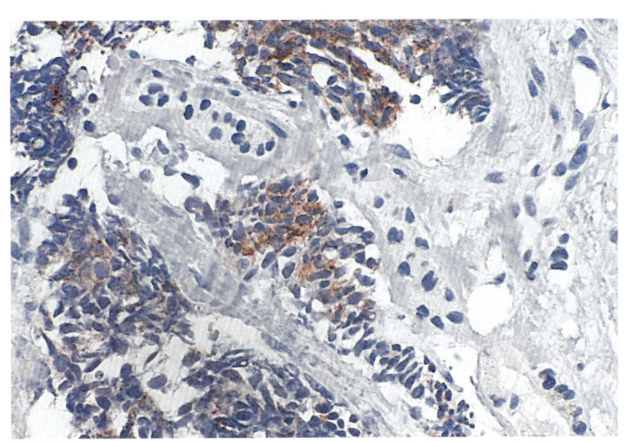

图 11.4　许多小细胞肺癌表达 CEA（×200）

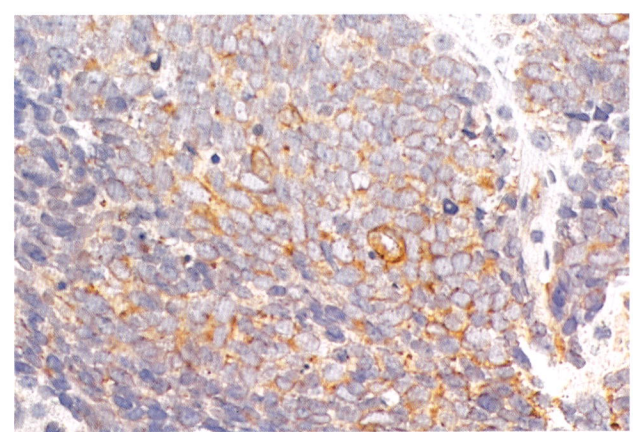

图 11.6　多数肺小细胞癌有低分子量角蛋白的点状表达（×400）

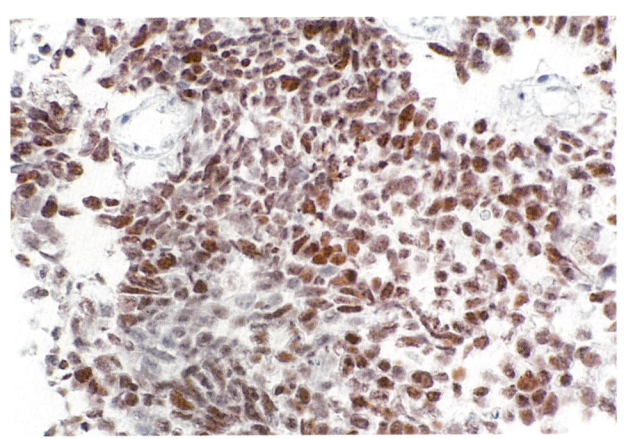

图 11.5　肺小细胞的免疫组化示，癌细胞核 TTF-1 呈强阳性表达（×200）

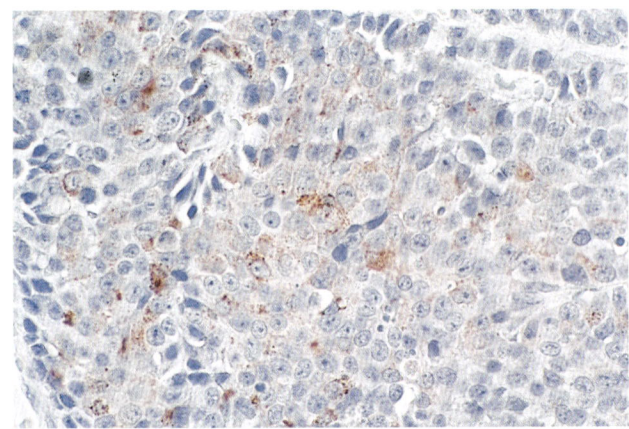

图 11.7　如图所示，肺小细胞癌 CgA 呈点状阳性表达（×400）

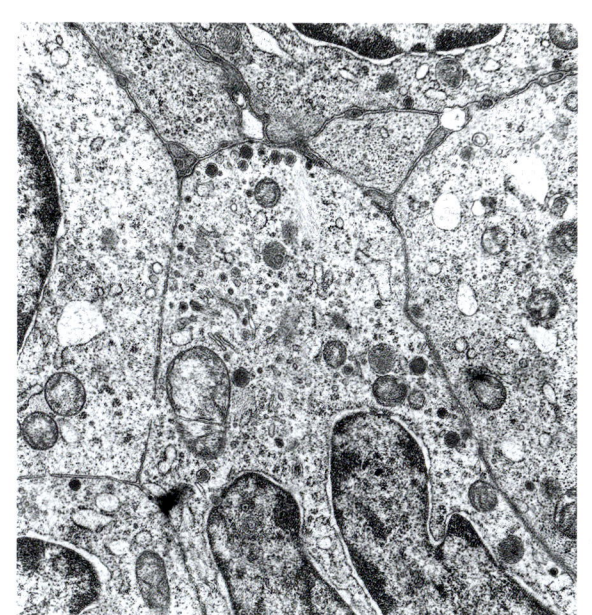

图11.8　电镜示，肺小细胞癌的癌细胞胞浆内有中等数量致密的神经内分泌颗粒（×16 000）

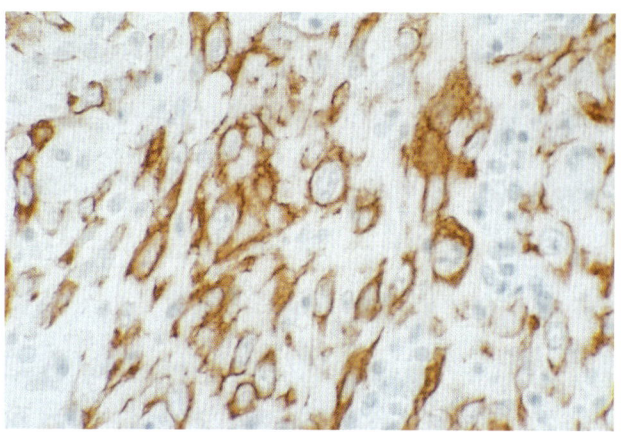

图11.10　示肉瘤样癌区梭形细胞的低分子量CK免疫组化呈阳性（×400）

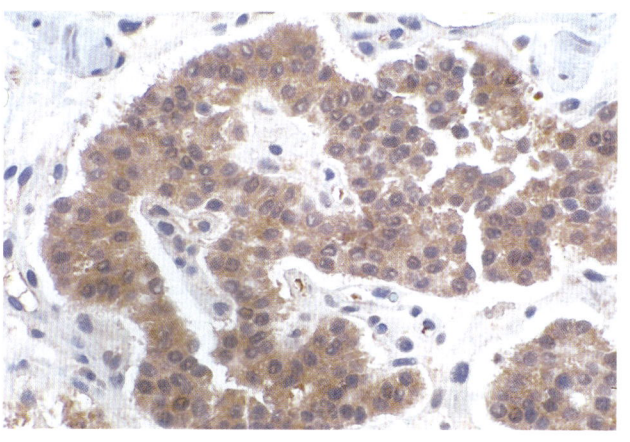

图11.9　典型类癌，免疫组化显示胞浆内CgA呈强阳性表达（×400）

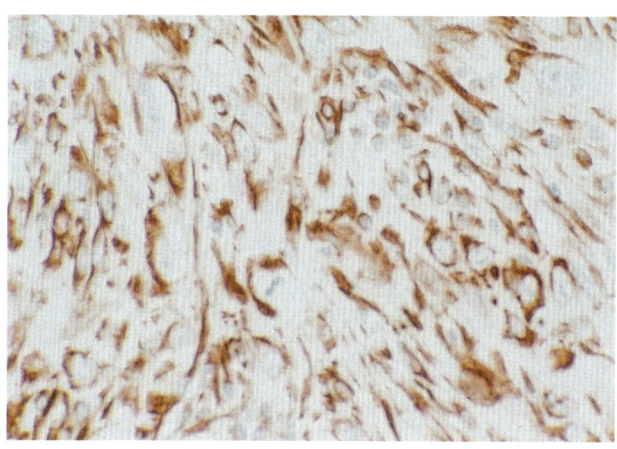

图11.11　与图11.10为同一个肿瘤，肿瘤性梭形细胞波形蛋白免疫组化呈强阳性（×400）

PEComa）、横纹肌样瘤、硬化性血管瘤和炎性假瘤[84]。

肉瘤样癌

肉瘤样癌又称癌肉瘤、梭形细胞癌、母细胞瘤和畸胎癌，它是上皮起源但具有不同分化的肿瘤。Wick和Swanson[85]从概念上对肉瘤样癌进行了回顾。在许多研究中，应用抗角蛋白（CK）抗体和/或电镜对肉瘤样癌进行研究，结果发现肿瘤中的梭形细胞为上皮性起源[86-90]。绝大多数的病例，梭形细胞既表达CK又表达波形蛋白（图11.10、11.11），偶尔情况下，CK与其他中间丝如结蛋白（desmin）或肌动蛋白（actin）共同表达。

多形性癌

Fishback等[91]将多形性癌定义为，主要见于成年人，由梭形细胞和大的多形巨细胞构成的肿瘤。作者发现，在78例病例中，8%有灶性鳞状上皮分化，25%为大细胞未分化癌，45%为腺癌，其余22%为由梭形细胞和巨细胞构成的肿瘤。通常情况下，肿瘤性梭形细胞仅表达波形蛋白肿瘤细胞中上皮性成分的免疫组化染色有赖于其分化方向。

Pelosi等[92]研究了31例肺多形性癌，用CK、EMA、CEA、波形蛋白、S-100蛋白、平滑肌肌动蛋白（smooth muscle actin, SMA）、结蛋白，显示肿瘤性上皮细胞、梭形细胞和/或巨细胞成分，并探讨其周期调控和凋亡（p53、p21Waf1、p27Kip1、FHIT）、肿瘤的生长（Ki-67抗原评价增殖活性，CD34免疫着色评价微血管密度）和肿瘤的运动性（fascin）。作者发现，肿瘤的上皮成分对CK、EMA、CEA、细胞周期抑制因子和肿瘤抑制基因的表达有着一定反应性，而肉瘤样成分，无论肿瘤分期和大小如何，其对波形蛋白、fascin和微血管密度免疫组化染色的反应性更强些。作者提出建立一个肿瘤发生的模型，这样多形性细胞的间叶表型就可以被选择性诱导激活，继而分离出与细胞分化、周期调控、肿瘤细胞生长和运动性有关的分子。

肺母细胞瘤

肺母细胞瘤由上皮和梭形细胞两种成分构成，其中上皮细胞成分形成腺样结构，腺体类似子宫内膜腺体或胎儿腺体。上皮性肿瘤细胞偶尔呈鳞状细胞（桑葚胚）排列。Koss[93]和Yousem[94]报道肺母细胞瘤可以多向分化，并且有时呈神经内分泌分化。有腺样结构形成的上皮细胞，免疫组化CK、CEA和EMA呈阳性。而梭形细胞则可表达波形蛋白，并且依赖于肉瘤样成分的分化类型，可伴有结蛋白、肌动蛋白和S-100蛋白的表达。具有神经内分泌成分的肿瘤细胞，还可伴有神经内分泌细胞标记的表达。前面我们已提及，具有上皮性成分的肺母细胞瘤还可以表达β-钙黏素。

原发性肉瘤

肺的原发性肉瘤比较罕见，而且类型多样。肺肉瘤瘤细胞的免疫表型与发生在软组织和其他器官的肉瘤（见第3章）在形态上基本一致。Etienne-Mastroianni等[95]对12例肺的原发性肉瘤进行了临床病理学研究。组织学上已诊断为肉瘤的这12例肿瘤，又经过免疫组化进一步确诊。其中7例为平滑肌肉瘤，2例为单相性滑膜肉瘤，恶性外周神经鞘瘤、上皮样肉瘤和恶性纤维组织细胞瘤各1例。12例病人中9例进行了手术，其中6例进行了肺叶切除，在这6例中又有2例进行了更进一步的手术，其余3例进行了全肺切除。4例病人接受了化疗，2例病人接受了放疗。对这12例病例进行了随访，他们的生存期为3～144个月，平均为42个月。其中5例生存期达到3年。所有病例中5年存活率为38%。由此此文作者得出结论，肺的原发性肉瘤是一种罕见而且有侵袭性的肿瘤，其治疗和预后与其他软组织肉瘤没有不同。

Kaposi 肉瘤

在获得性免疫缺陷综合征患者，Kaposi肉瘤较常见，并且多数肺Kaposi肉瘤是转移性肿瘤[96-105]。Kaposi肉瘤经淋巴循环转移至肺，因而常有淋巴结受累。肿瘤细胞呈梭形（图11.12），波形蛋白和内皮细胞标记如CD31免疫组化染色阳性（图11.13）。

血管内皮细胞瘤

恶性血管内皮细胞瘤，又称血管内细支气管肺泡瘤（intravascular bronchioloalveolar tumor, IVBAT），通常见于年轻女性，累及双侧肺，表现为大量的小结节充满肺泡腔，这些小结节可以有变性、坏死和钙化[84]。最初，认为这种肿瘤起源于肺泡上皮细胞。组织学上，瘤细胞圆形、多角形，呈上皮样（图11.14）。肿瘤细胞可特征性地表达内皮细胞标记如CD31、CD34和Ⅷ因子抗原，并且波形蛋白免疫组化呈阳性。在极少数情况下，上皮样血管内皮瘤

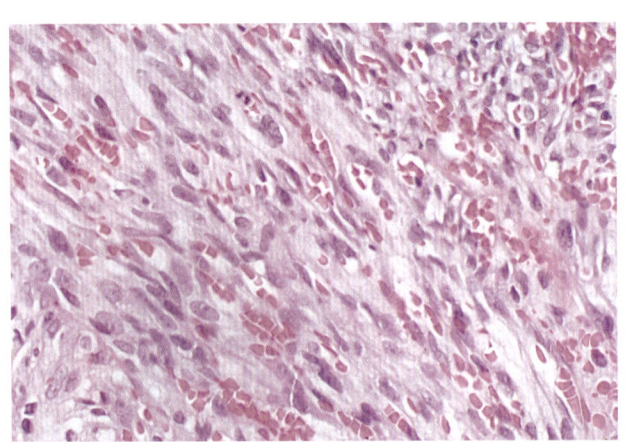

图11.12　Kaposi肉瘤的瘤细胞呈梭形，在淋巴管内分布（×400）

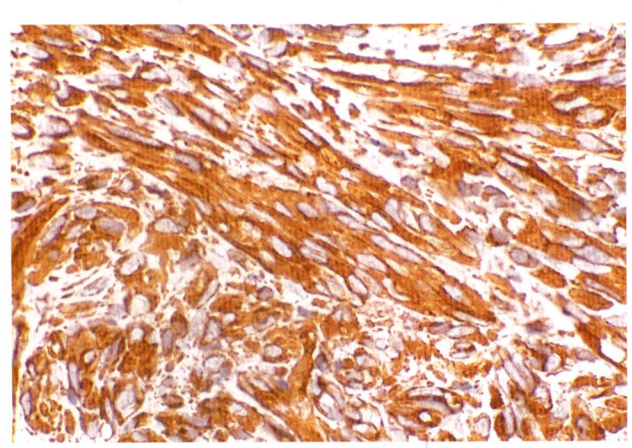

图11.13　Kaposi肉瘤的瘤细胞表达血管源性标记，如CD31（×400）

还可表达CK（图11.15）。超微结构示，肿瘤细胞包含有Weibel-Palade小体，此乃内皮细胞的特征性标记（图11.16）。

> **诊断要点**：肺的血管内细支气管肺泡瘤
>
> 1. 是一种恶性血管内皮细胞瘤。
> 2. 血管标记物阳性，如：CD31、CD34、Ⅷ因子。
> 3. 有些情况下表达单一性角蛋白。

血管肉瘤

原发性血管肉瘤罕见，它可以表现为没有明显血管腔形成的去分化状态，肿瘤细胞的免疫组化染色与恶性血管内皮瘤相似。Adem等[106]报道了7例转移性血管肉瘤的病例，这些病例表现为弥漫性肺出血。7例中，男性6例，女性1例，年龄31～73岁，其中6例病例临床表现为咯血，所有病人X线片均有肺的弥漫性病变。这些病例的临床诊断包括：肺出血综合征（2例）、急性肺功能衰竭（1例）和感染（1例）。其中1例病人的鉴别诊断中包括了转移性疾病，所有病例既往均无恶性肿瘤病史，所有的活检均显示：肺出血与肺内由非典型上皮样细胞和梭形细胞形成的相互吻合的血管腔有关，这些血管腔样结构可在淋巴管和动脉内分布。肿瘤细胞Ⅷ因子相关蛋白和CD31免疫染色阳性。对3例病人进行了随访，这3例病人均死于该种疾病。对他们进行尸检发现，其原发病灶均位于肺外。其中2例血管肉瘤发生于心脏，1例发生于骨盆软组织。心脏超声检查示：1例病人原发部位可能在右心房。该文章作者认为，在对弥漫性肺出血的鉴别诊断中应将血管肉瘤考虑在内，尤其在青年人病例中更应引起注意。作者还见过一个相似的病例，瘤细胞呈上皮样，肺内有多发病灶，但原发部位却未被找到（图11.17）。

肺的淋巴组织增生性病变

许多类型的非肿瘤性和肿瘤性淋巴组织增生性病变均可累及肺（见第4、5章）。随着分子生物学和遗传学研究的不断深入，关于淋巴增生性肺疾病的分类也有了明显的变化。几年前还被认为是非肿瘤性的病变，目前研究已证实它们可能是低级别淋巴瘤。

支气管相关淋巴样组织

支气管相关淋巴样组织（bronchial-associated

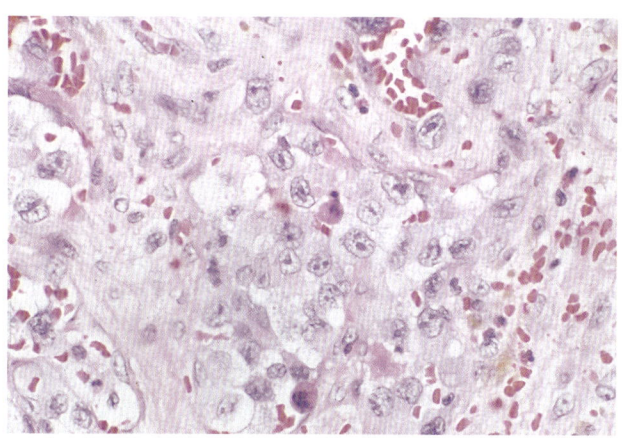

图 11.14 恶性上皮样血管内皮瘤，肿瘤性细胞呈上皮样排列，易与癌相混淆（×400）

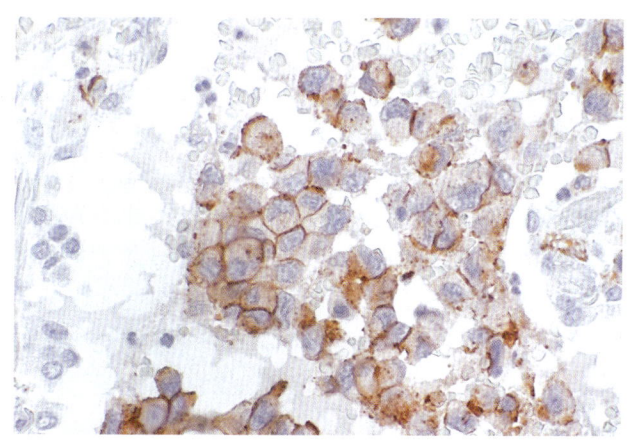

图 11.15 偶尔在上皮样血管内皮瘤的瘤细胞胞浆内可有CK的表达（×400）

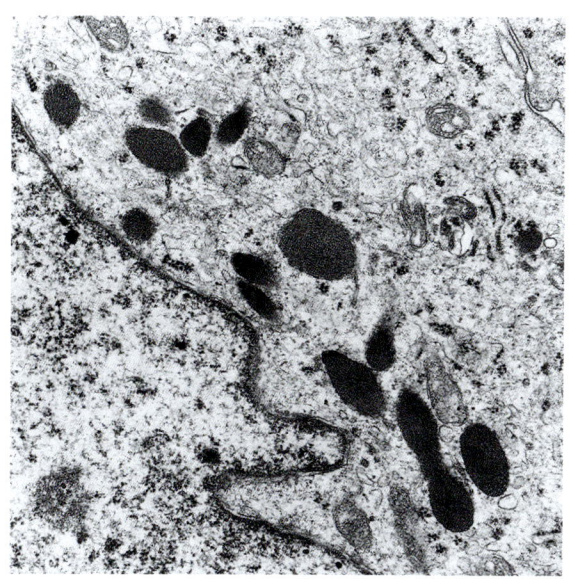

图11.16 在本病例中，上皮样血管内皮瘤的瘤细胞胞浆内含有Weibel-Palade小体（×20 000）

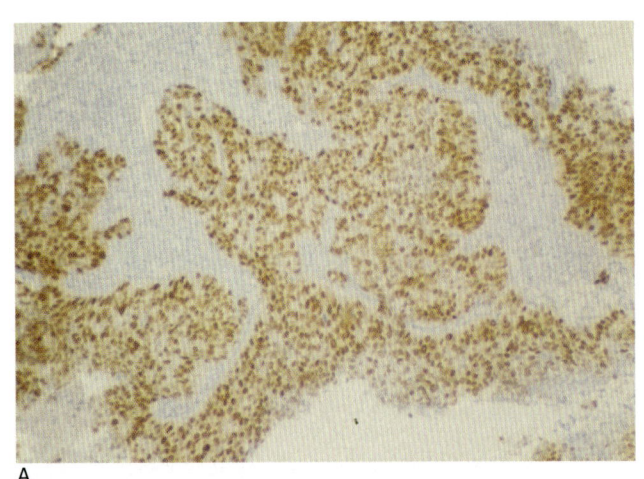
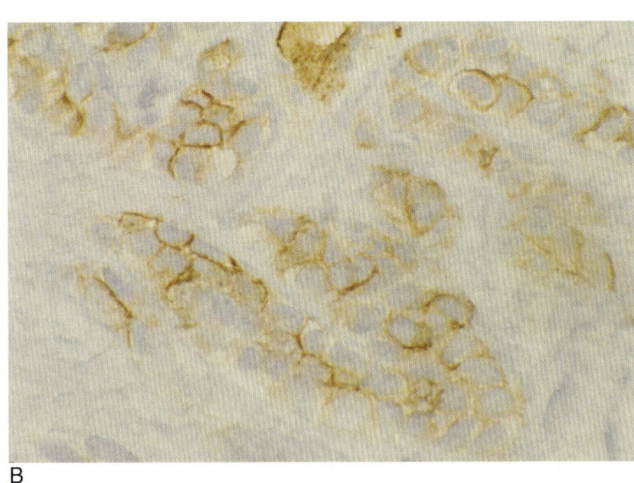

图 11.17　肺的血管肉瘤(A)HE；(B)CD31 免疫染色

lymphoid tissue, BALT）在大多数正常成人的肺是不明显或缺如的。关于在成人肺组织内是否存在有支气管相关淋巴样组织，曾存在很多的争议[107]。多种外源性或内源性抗原性刺激作用于人体，肺组织内就会出现淋巴样组织，而绝大多数情况下，这些淋巴样组织是出现在相对特定的解剖部位，也就是与支气管和细支气管密切相关的部位。这些淋巴样组织也就是所提及的"支气管相关淋巴样组织（BALT）"。在非吸烟成人中，肺内几乎见不到淋巴样组织，但在支气管分支处以及邻近呼吸性细支气管的部位则有少量淋巴样组织。在吸烟者，BALT明显增多，偶尔还可见到较大的淋巴滤泡，部分淋巴滤泡内还可见生发中心[108]。

Swigris 等[109]在新近的综述中指出，BALT 属黏膜相关淋巴组织（MALT），在正常人肺不易见到，但在其他哺乳动物，如鼠、兔、羊等则比较容易见到。目前，人们对淋巴样组织知之甚少，认为它们是在小支气管周围和支气管区的一些淋巴细胞的集合。有些淋巴细胞就位于支气管黏膜层的上皮细胞之间。这些淋巴细胞位于这些区域，其作用是与细胞表面的归巢受体相接触，如整合素、特异性肺内血管的黏附分子，正如在毛细血管后微静脉血管内皮细胞所见到的黏附分子一样。大约60%的 BALT 由 B 淋巴细胞构成，其余为T淋巴细胞。BALT在抵御吸入性病原微生物方面起着重要作用，并且它还是淋巴细胞分化的场所，在这里淋巴细胞与吸入性抗原接触，继而转化成为抗原特异性的记忆细胞或效应细胞。当受到抗原刺激时，这些细胞就会通过BALT进入循环，并停留于肺实质，准备与暴露的抗原发生免疫反应。在此过程中还有其他细胞的参与，如树突状细胞（Langerhans 细胞）。被覆于BALT表面的呼吸性上皮通常仅含有少量的杯状细胞和纤毛细胞。而 BALT 相关的上皮表面则布满微绒毛。在这些上皮内有 CD8 阳性细胞为主的淋巴细胞浸润，偶尔也有CD4阳性淋巴细胞。按照 Swigris 等[109]观点，BALT 不表达分泌性抗体 IgA，并且它与其他黏膜相关淋巴组织，如胃肠道黏膜相关淋巴组织有所不同。Bienenstock 等[110, 111]，首次就 BALT 的形态学和功能特点提出了新见解。

肺内的绝大多数非肿瘤性和肿瘤性淋巴样细胞的浸润与BALT有关。在肿瘤形成中，BALT增殖可以解释绝大多数肺的肿瘤性淋巴样疾病。前面已提到，对病理学家来说，要将肿瘤性和非肿瘤性淋巴样病变鉴别开来常常有一定的困难。在多数情况下，分子生物学技术，如基因重排、T细胞的分子生物学检测对确诊其恶性行为是必要的[112, 113]。

许多肺的良性病变都有散在的淋巴细胞浸润。此类情况可见于普通型间质性肺炎、脱屑性间质性肺炎、部分胶原血管相关性疾病的肺病变、非特异性间质性肺炎的细胞期、局限性过敏性肺炎、结节病早期、Wegner 肉芽肿、Churg-Strauss 肉芽肿性、镜下结节性多动脉炎以及某些药物性（如柳氮磺胺吡啶）的淋巴细胞浸润。参考文献114～119是介绍关于肺的淋巴细胞增殖性疾病的具体文献。

绝大多数肺的淋巴组织病变表明是 BALT 的增生，而肿瘤性淋巴组织异常增殖也来源于 BALT。Kradin 和Mark[120]首次丢弃"假性淋巴瘤和淋巴样间质性肺炎"这两个术语，而代之以"结节性和弥漫性BALT增生"。正如Koss等[119]所详细讨论的，局限性BALT增生也称为滤泡性支气管炎/细支气管炎，由于BALT的增生主要位于小支气管和细支气管区。在很多临床疾病中都可以看到淋巴样增生，如慢性感染、先天性免疫缺陷综合征、阻塞性肺疾病和胶原血管病。其病理特征是，在支气管周围区/细支气管周围区，出现增生的淋巴滤泡，伴有或不伴有生发中心存在。

BALT结节性淋巴组织增生已取代了假性淋巴瘤这一名词，特点是淋巴组织反应性增生，其特征性表现为肺内可见到大量淋巴滤泡形成，这些淋巴滤泡往往有一个较大的生发中心，主要见于中年人，绝大多数无自觉症状。大约10%～15%的结节性淋巴组织增生患者有胶原血管病，如系统性红斑狼疮，或病因不明的免疫性疾病，并且常有多克隆丙种球蛋白病。多形性浆细胞比较常见。标记物研究发现，增生的淋巴组织由CD4阳性和CD8阳性T细胞混合而成。绝大多数病例表现为多个结节，约15%的病例手术切除后复发。

淋巴细胞性间质性肺疾病/肺炎

目前认为，淋巴细胞性间质性肺疾病/肺炎（lymphocytic interstitial pneumonia/pneumonitis, LIP）是支气管相关淋巴组织的一种弥漫性增生[121]。这是对多种刺激的一种反应。这些刺激包括：各种自身免疫性疾病，系统性免疫性缺陷，同种异体骨髓移植，肺泡微结石病，及某些少见感染性疾病，如军团菌肺炎、结核病、支原体肺炎、衣原体肺炎，服用苯妥英钠和肺泡蛋白沉积症。LIP患者多为40～70岁女性。他们可表现出一系列症状，如发热、咯血、关节痛、体重减轻、胸膜痛。有些可表现为Sjögren综合征或重症肌无力。胸片示，弥漫性网状或网状结节状浸润，偶尔有结节性病变。部分病人会有高丙种球蛋白血症，还有10%的病人可有低丙种球蛋白血症。如果LIP患者是单克隆丙种球蛋白病，那么通常患者同时患有淋巴瘤。多数LIP患者对类固醇有反应性，但还有30%～50%患者5年内会死亡，他们往往死于感染性并发症，有些是治疗所致。部分病人会发展成为淋巴瘤和免疫母细胞性肉瘤。

性质未定的结节性淋巴细胞浸润

肺内存在一些病因不明的结节性淋巴细胞病变。如浆细胞性肉芽肿、肺玻璃样变肉芽肿以及良性淋巴细胞性血管炎和肉芽肿性炎（benign lymphocytic angiitis and granulomatosis, BLAG）。

浆细胞性肉芽肿又称为肌纤维母细胞瘤或炎性假瘤，主要发生于年轻人的肺内，但在许多器官和组织内均可见到这类病变，如气管、甲状腺、心脏、胃、肝、胰腺、脾、淋巴结、肾、腹膜后、肠系膜、膀胱、盆腔软组织、乳腺、脑脊髓膜和眼眶[84]。肉芽肿这个名词容易引起误导，除非我们能认识到肉芽肿这个名词已经被广义地用于描述有肿块形成的炎症性病变，正如Wegener肉芽肿和淋巴瘤样肉芽肿一样。在组织学上，这些结节由以浆细胞为主的大量炎细胞浸润，并有肌纤维母细胞增殖。有些研究指出，浆细胞肉芽肿是肿瘤性疾病。炎性假瘤将在后面详细介绍。

肺的玻璃样变肉芽肿多数情况为单发，偶尔为多发性结节。部分患者无临床症状，部分患者有咳嗽、呼吸急促、胸痛或体重减轻等症状。组织学上，主要由互相平行的薄到致密胶原束构成，伴有淋巴细胞浸润，主要分布于支气管周围。

Saldana等[122]及Israel等[123]在1977年对良性淋巴细胞性血管炎和肉芽肿进行了描述。这个疾病较Wegener肉芽肿和淋巴瘤样肉芽肿少见，好发于中年人，主要表现为肺部的多结节性病变。组织学上，结节由致密淋巴细胞浸润而形成，偶尔可见巨细胞，包括组织性多核巨细胞，但没有界限清楚的肉芽肿形成。淋巴细胞主要在动脉和静脉周围浸润，可以浸润血管壁，偶尔可阻塞血管腔。当病变为多发性时，应与淋巴细胞性淋巴瘤和淋巴瘤样肉芽肿相鉴别。

肺的淋巴瘤

淋巴瘤比任何一种肿瘤都强调分类及对亚型的分类。组织学/细胞学、免疫组织化学、流式细胞术和其他分子生物学技术均被广泛应用于淋巴瘤的分型。近来发表了不少关于淋巴瘤的处理、分类和报道的文章[124]，对诊断淋巴瘤的免疫组化标准近来也有详细报道[125]。

肺的非霍奇金淋巴瘤

绝大多数发生于肺的非霍奇金淋巴瘤都是低级别B细胞淋巴瘤，往往来源于BALT。如前所述，在鉴别低级别B细胞淋巴瘤和非肿瘤性疾病时往往有一定的困难。常规免疫组化标记如κ、λ轻链在鉴别肿瘤和非肿瘤性疾病时偶尔有一定价值。对于疑难病例可用流式细胞仪和PCR来帮助诊断。低级别B细胞淋巴瘤临床预后较好。

肺内也可发生T细胞淋巴瘤，但远较B细胞淋巴瘤少见[126]。偶尔，肺的原发性淋巴瘤以浆细胞分化为主[127]。

诊断肺的原发性非霍奇金淋巴瘤的主要标准包括：①累及肺、肺叶或主支气管，单侧或双侧，伴或不伴纵隔淋巴结受累；②在诊断时或诊断后3个月，未发现胸廓外淋巴瘤[128]。肺的原发性非霍奇金淋巴瘤患者通常年龄在60岁以上，50%病人无临床症状。多数病人胸部X线片可见有异常。有症状的患者常有"B"型症状：发热、夜间出汗、体重下降，偶有呼气性呼吸困难、咳嗽、胸痛，绝大多数肺非霍奇金淋巴瘤患者的发病与von Willebrand综合征、结节性红斑或Sjögren综合征有关。

肺的原发性淋巴瘤在所有肺原发性肿瘤中所占比例<1%，小细胞淋巴瘤占所有肺原发性淋巴瘤的80%~90%，而这些小细胞淋巴瘤中，90%以上都是边缘区B细胞淋巴瘤。

黏膜相关淋巴组织型边缘区B细胞淋巴瘤

MALT型边缘区B细胞淋巴瘤（marginal zone B-cell lymphoma of MALT type, MZBCL/MALT）为低级别结外淋巴瘤，由边缘区B淋巴细胞表型的小B样细胞构成。尽管这种淋巴瘤可见于儿童，但是绝大多数边缘区B细胞淋巴瘤患者为成人，尤其是那些感染了HIV的人群。尽管有学者怀疑多数MALT淋巴瘤是慢性抗原刺激的结果，如胃MALT淋巴瘤与幽门螺杆菌有关，但未发现肺边缘区B细胞瘤与特异性致病因素有关。绝大多数病人表现为非特异性肺部症状，并且可见直径<5cm的肿块或多发性肿块。几乎见不到肺门淋巴结肿大，有一小部分病人还可在身体的其他部位同时发生MALT型淋巴瘤。较大的肿瘤往往由小淋巴细胞构成，这些小淋巴细胞与淋巴引流通路中周边区的细胞有相似性。支气管淋巴细胞的浸润通常与淋巴上皮性病变有关。在近支气管处的肿瘤内或周边区可见到反应性生发中心。肿瘤性成分可以取代生发中心，增宽边缘区。在细胞学上，肿瘤性细胞主要为小淋巴细胞，通常为圆形或淋巴浆细胞样。有些细胞可以看到透明的胞浆，被称为单核样细胞。也可见到散布的浆细胞。边缘区淋巴瘤的淋巴细胞可以特征性地表达pan-B标记，如CD20、PAX5和CD79a（表11.7），肿瘤细胞CD5、CD10、CD23、bcl-6和bcl-1/cyclin D1均为阴性。约50%的病人可有CD43的表达，并且可有核bcl-10的表达。在大约25%病人的浆细胞可以看到轻链限制性表达。

慢性淋巴细胞性白血病/小细胞淋巴细胞性淋巴瘤

慢性淋巴细胞性白血病/小细胞淋巴细胞性淋巴瘤（chronic lymphocytic leukemia/small cell lymphocytic lymphoma, CLL-SLL）累及肺，通常见于CLL-SLL病史较长的患者。多数病例不需要做活检，因为从临床的角度就可以对其进行诊断。病人常表现为进行性呼吸困难，咳嗽，胸片有间质浸润。部分病人可有支气管腔阻塞。绝大多数患者年龄超过50岁，男女发病比例约2:1。组织学特征为致密的淋巴样细胞浸润，沿支气管血管束和/或以支气管为中心分布，周围肺组织病变不明显。浸润的细胞以小圆形淋巴细胞为主，这些淋巴细胞核染色质较成熟。有时可见大的瘤细胞，假如大细胞成片出现，那

表11.7 肺原发性淋巴瘤的免疫组化特征

淋巴瘤的类型	抗原													单克隆轻链
	CD20	PAX5	CD79a	CD43	CD5	CD10	CD23	CD15	CD30	Cyclin D1	bcl-2	BCL10	EBV	
边缘区B细胞淋巴瘤	+	+	+	S	N	N	N	N	N	N	N	S	N	S
慢性淋巴细胞性白血病/小淋巴细胞淋巴瘤	+	+	+	S	S	N	N	N	N	+	S	N	N	S
套细胞淋巴瘤	+	+	+	S	S	N	N	N	N	S	S	N	N	S
滤泡性淋巴瘤	+	+	+	N	N	S	N	N	N	N	+	N	N	S
霍奇金淋巴瘤	S	S	S	N	N	N	N	+	+	N	N	N	S	N
淋巴瘤样肉芽肿病	S	U	U	N	N	N	N	N	N	N	N	N	U	N
血管内淋巴瘤	+	+	+	R	S	U	N	N	N	N	S	U	U	U
原发性渗出性淋巴瘤	N	N	N	N	N	N	N	N	+	N	N	U	U	U
脓胸相关性淋巴瘤	+	+	+	N	N	N	N	N	N	U	U	U	U	S

反应性：+，弥漫性强阳性；S，有时阳性；R，少数细胞阳性；N，阴性；U，不确定

么提示可能合并有弥漫性大 B 细胞淋巴瘤。CLL-SLL 的细胞属 B 系，表达 B 细胞标记，如 CD20、PAX5 和 CD79a（表 11.7），常同时共表达 CD5、CD43、CD23 和 bcl-2，而 CD10、bcl-6、bcl-1、cyclin D1 则为阴性表达。通常 Ki-67 阳性率低（约 10%～20%）。分子研究显示免疫球蛋白重链或轻链的单克隆性。这些细胞常有核型异常。

套细胞淋巴瘤

即使是进展期的套细胞淋巴瘤，一般也不累及肺。肿瘤由单一形态、小至中等大小的淋巴细胞构成，细胞核轻度或明显不规则，染色质相对成熟，核仁不明显。偶尔可见上皮样巨噬细胞，其与肿瘤性淋巴细胞有一定关系，但不聚集形成肉芽肿。约有 10% 的病例染色质较细，称为母细胞样亚型，这类肿瘤与淋巴母细胞性淋巴瘤相似。套细胞淋巴瘤的瘤细胞与小 B 细胞淋巴瘤相似，表达 pan-B 的标记，如 CD20、PAX5 和 CD79a（表 11.7），通常也表达 CD5、CD43、bcl-2、bcl-1 和 cyclin D1，而 CD10、CD23、和 bcl-6 为阴性。约 20%～50% 的肿瘤细胞 Ki-67 阳性表达。多数病例有 bcl-2 基因的 t(14;18) 易位。

滤泡性淋巴瘤

滤泡性淋巴瘤累及到肺者罕见，病变常分布广泛，临床上常常诊断为感染。在肺内见到的病变与滤泡性淋巴瘤累及淋巴结时所见的滤泡样结构相同。肿瘤性淋巴细胞表达 pan-B 细胞标记如 CD20、PAX5、CD79a、bcl-2、bcl-6 和 CD10，但不表达 CD5、CD43 和 CD23。分子研究表明，免疫球蛋白的重链和/或轻链为克隆性的，大约 90% 的病例有 bcl-2 基因的 t(14;18) 易位。

肺的原发性霍奇金淋巴瘤

肺的原发性霍奇金淋巴瘤不常见，其形态上与淋巴结的霍奇金淋巴瘤相似。肺的原发性霍奇金淋巴瘤常被误诊为炎性疾病或机化性肺炎。1990 年，Radin[129] 报道了 61 例原发性肺的霍奇金淋巴瘤。在这些病例中，36 例为女性，25 例为男性，平均年龄 42.5 岁，总的年龄介于 12～82 岁。最常见的霍奇金淋巴瘤的组织类型为结节硬化型，其次为混合细胞型。肺原发性霍奇金淋巴瘤的诊断标准为病变原发于肺实质，肺门和纵隔淋巴结轻度增大或不增大。在确诊前最常见的症状为咳嗽、体重减轻、胸痛、呼吸困难、咯血、乏力、皮疹、夜间出汗和喘鸣。体检常正常。61 例病例中 35 例进行了支气管镜检查，结果 18 例正常，17 例异常。影像学检查示，61 例病例中 45 例肺内有结节样肿块，13 例有肺炎样的浸润。在诊断肺的原发性霍奇金淋巴瘤时，医生应想到此病，确诊的标准与累及淋巴结的霍奇金淋巴瘤的组织学标准相同。免疫组化有助于诊断，CD15、CD30 在 Reed-Sternberg 细胞常阳性，且偶尔可表达 CD20（表 11.7）。

肺/胸腔罕见型原发性淋巴瘤

肺内有几种罕见淋巴瘤，其中最值得重视的就是淋巴瘤样肉芽肿。其他罕见类型还包括：血管内淋巴瘤、原发性渗出性淋巴瘤、脓胸相关淋巴瘤、继发性淋巴瘤及白血病。

淋巴瘤样肉芽肿病

Liebow 等[130] 首次报道了淋巴瘤样肉芽肿病（LYG），他们在论文中对该病进行了详尽的病理描述。他们对 40 个病例进行了研究，其中半数病人有 "B" 症状，而这些病人常伴发有淋巴瘤。半数以上病人在确诊后 1 年内死亡。1979 年，Katzenstein 等[131] 对淋巴瘤样肉芽肿病的临床病理特征作了一个综述，结果显示年龄小于 25 岁，有白细胞升高、神经系统异常、肝脾肿大、非典型淋巴细胞浸润的病例，均预后不良。在之后的几年，对该病有了新认识，认为它是一种血管中心性淋巴瘤；在免疫组化研究的基础上，认为它是一种血管中心性 T 细胞淋巴瘤。Guinee 等[132] 对 10 例淋巴瘤样肉芽肿病采用免疫组化和原位杂交技术进行 CD20 和 EB 病毒研究，并且应用 PCR 技术对 IgG 重链基因重排进行了研究。结果发现，所有病例中，小淋巴细胞和中等大小淋巴细胞均为 CD45RO 阳性 T 细胞。少数异型的大细胞是 CD20 阳性 B 细胞。联合应用免疫组化和原位杂交检测发现在 CD20 阳性的 B 细胞内有 EB 病毒。因此作者得出结论，在淋巴瘤样肉芽肿病中，这些增生的细胞是大 B 细胞，并且该病可能与 EB 病毒感染有关。对临床医生和病理学家来说，该病的本质和临床病程仍是一个谜。尽管有些患者对 Cytoxan 治疗敏感，但多数患者病程快速进展，短期内即死亡[133]。病理学上，LYG 病变由明显的结节构成，结节内可见多种淋巴细胞浸润。其中夹杂大的非典型淋巴样细胞（图 11.18）。并且这些细胞浸润肺静脉引起坏死。淋巴瘤样肉芽肿病中的大细胞表达 B 细胞的抗原 CD20，见图 11.19。

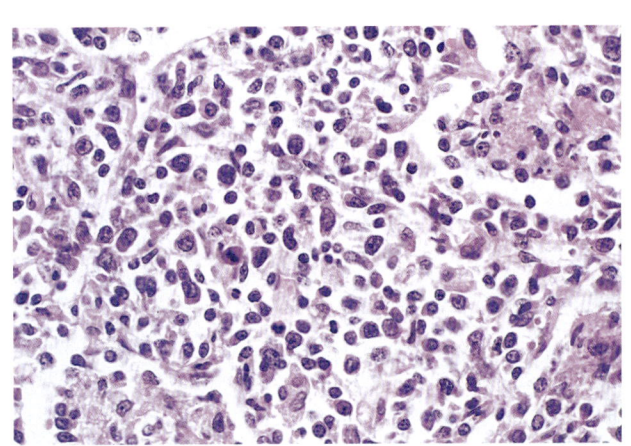

图11.18 淋巴瘤样肉芽肿病中，有不同的淋巴样细胞浸润（×100）

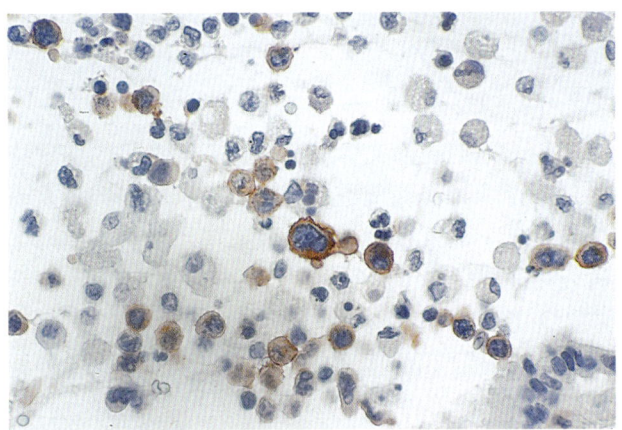

图11.19 淋巴瘤样肉芽肿病中，大的异型细胞可表达B细胞抗原CD20（×400）

血管内淋巴瘤

血管内淋巴瘤是发生于淋巴结外的一种大B细胞性肿瘤，其特征是肿瘤细胞位于小血管腔，尤其是毛细血管管腔内，以往称之为增生性血管内皮病[134-140]。肿瘤的血管内生长模式被认为是由于肿瘤细胞归巢受体有缺陷引起的继发性改变所致。研究表明，肿瘤性B细胞缺乏黏附分子。血管内淋巴瘤常累及中枢神经系统和皮肤，但也可原发于肺。除非很有把握，否则这将是一个非常有挑战性的诊断。免疫组化染色对诊断是必需的。

原发性渗出性淋巴瘤

原发性渗出性淋巴瘤（primary effusion lymphoma, PEL）属于大B细胞淋巴瘤，表现为以浆液渗出为主，而在身体其他部位无明显肿块形成[141-144]。现在认为，它与人类疱疹病毒8型和Kaposi肉瘤疱疹病毒感染有关，常见于获得性免疫缺陷综合征（AIDS）患者。典型的PEL患者表现为胸膜腔渗出而缺乏淋巴和脏器的病变。在所有患者的肿瘤性细胞中，都可以检测到人类疱疹病毒8/Kaposi肉瘤疱疹病毒。肿瘤细胞CD45阳性而B细胞性标记阴性，细胞表面免疫球蛋白亦为阴性。肿瘤细胞常表达CD30、CD38或CD138。

脓胸相关性淋巴瘤

脓胸相关性淋巴瘤（pyothorax-associated lymphoma, PAL）是淋巴瘤的一种罕见类型，发生于慢性脓胸患者，通常在胸膜损伤后数十年发病[145-147]。该病在日本首次被报道，并且最大的病例数也源于日本。临床主要表现为渗出、胸痛、体重减轻和呼吸困难。通常男性发病多于女性。典型患者无HIV感染史和免疫抑制史。脓胸常由结核病所致，其发病机制可能与胃的MALT相似，是由于慢性抗原刺激作用的结果。大体上，肿瘤呈实体肿块，直径约10cm，甚至更大，并且与胸膜纤维化关系密切，可以直接浸润周围肺组织，肿瘤细胞为体积较大的B淋巴母细胞性细胞。少数病例肿块可由淋巴浆细胞性细胞构成。尸检发现，半数以上患者病变局限于胸腔，其余半数可扩展至胸腔外。肿瘤细胞特征性地表达CD45、CD20、CD79a，少数细胞可表达CD138，多数细胞CD3阴性。

肺的继发性淋巴瘤和白血病浸润肺

确诊肺的淋巴瘤，必须考虑是否有肺外淋巴瘤存在。如果有，还必须对比肺内、肺外两个部位淋巴瘤的形态。有时淋巴瘤可以发生转化，这就给诊断肺原发性淋巴瘤还是转移性淋巴瘤带来一定困难。慢性淋巴细胞性白血病是白血病中最容易浸润肺的一个类型，并且它难以与原发性或继发性小淋巴细胞性淋巴瘤区分。当霍奇金淋巴瘤累及肺时，通常沿支气管血管浸润，肿瘤细胞围绕于血管周围。尸检发现25%～64%的白血病患者有肺浸润，但这些人在生前很少被发现。急性白血病和非淋巴细胞性白血病较急性淋巴细胞性白血病更容易浸润肺。

肺朗格汉斯细胞组织细胞增生症X（肺的组织细胞增生症X、肺的嗜酸性肉芽肿）

对肺朗格汉斯细胞组织细胞增生症X的概念理解，是在对正常朗格汉斯细胞理解的基础上形成的[148]。这些细胞于1869年首次被Paul朗格汉斯确认，它们占表皮细胞的3%~8%。这种细胞可以出现在许多组织中，包括表皮、食管、肛管/直肠、宫颈、胸腺、淋巴结，偶尔见于正常肺组织。在肺组织内的朗格汉斯细胞与BALT有关，常位于上皮细胞之间。1961年，Michael Birbeck医生首次在朗格汉斯细胞内发现了少见的细胞内包涵体并将其命名为Birbeck颗粒或朗格汉斯细胞颗粒。正常的朗格汉斯细胞是体积较大的树突状细胞，其功能为处理抗原，继而将抗原递呈给T细胞。

朗格汉斯细胞组织细胞增生症X无一例外地发生于吸烟人群，年轻人较老年人易发。单个组织细胞较正常的朗格汉斯细胞小，并且突起少。朗格汉斯组织细胞增生症中，典型的朗格汉斯细胞胞浆含朗格汉斯细胞颗粒，免疫组化示S-100蛋白（图11.20）、CD1A、CD68和CD31阳性。病变首先发生于支气管分布区，并可以从细胞期进入纤维化期。有些纤维化期的病例，朗格汉斯细胞较少，这为诊断带来一定困难。朗格汉斯组织细胞增生症患者可以无症状，也可以表现出一些比较严重的症状，如红细胞沉降率增快、发热、体重减轻，胸部X线示肺内有结节，偶尔，结节体积大到提示为转移性癌。尽管多数病例表现为除肺下叶以外的多发性、散在性结节，罕见病例也可表现为单个结节。病变常有囊性变，高分辨CT扫描常会考虑到该病的诊断。有时，较小的支气管穿刺标本就足够诊断该病。但多数病例开胸取活检是非常必要的。朗格汉斯细胞组织细胞增生症的结节常由组织细胞增多症X细胞，掺杂着不同量的淋巴细胞、浆细胞、嗜酸性粒细胞、中性粒细胞和含炭末的巨噬细胞共同构成。组织细胞增多症X细胞较成熟的肺泡巨噬细胞和成熟的朗格汉斯细胞体积小，组织细胞增多症X细胞呈明显的曲核（图11.21）。

透明细胞瘤/糖瘤/PEComa

发生在肺的透明细胞瘤没有包膜结节状，又称为糖瘤，属PEComa家族，PEComa是一个肿瘤家族，包括血管平滑肌脂肪瘤、淋巴血管平滑肌瘤病、肺的透明细胞糖瘤、圆韧带/镰状韧带的透明细胞黑色素细胞性肿瘤和腹部盆腔的上皮样血管外周细胞瘤[150]。这些肿瘤同时表达HMB-45和肌源性标记。组织学上，肿瘤常由大小、形状、核形态较一致的细胞构成（图11.22），但有时细胞也可呈多形性（图11.23）。其特征为肿瘤细胞的胞浆内含有大量的糖原，电镜

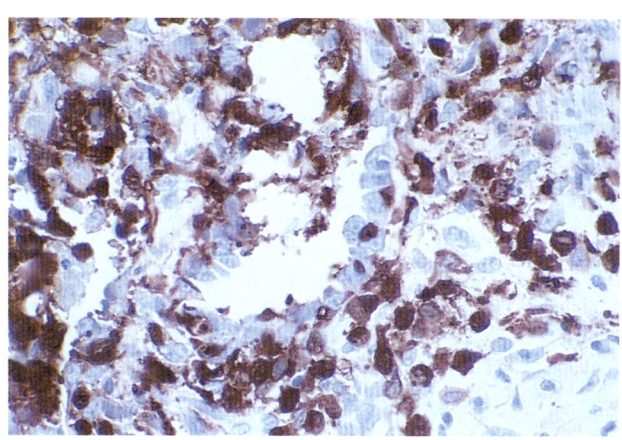

图11.20 免疫组化示朗格汉斯细胞核与胞浆S-100蛋白阳性表达（×400）

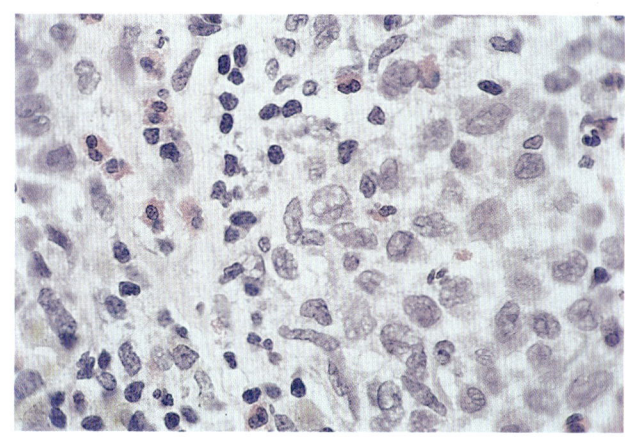

图11.21 肺朗格汉斯细胞肉芽肿的结节，朗格汉斯细胞较成熟的肺泡巨噬细胞小，核高度扭曲，胞浆淡染且较少。注意相关的炎细胞（×400）

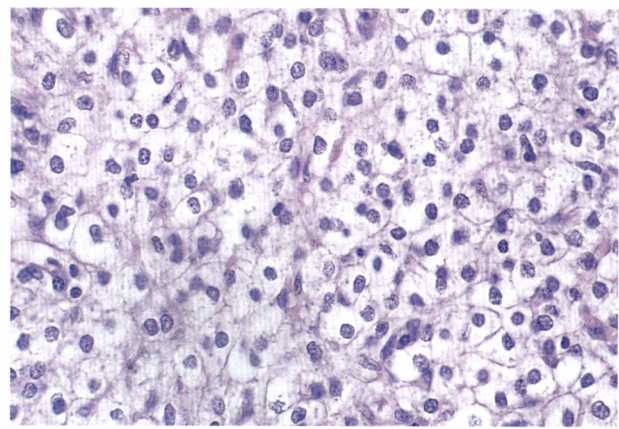

图11.22 肺的透明细胞肿瘤由形态较一致的细胞构成，胞浆因含糖原而透明（×400）

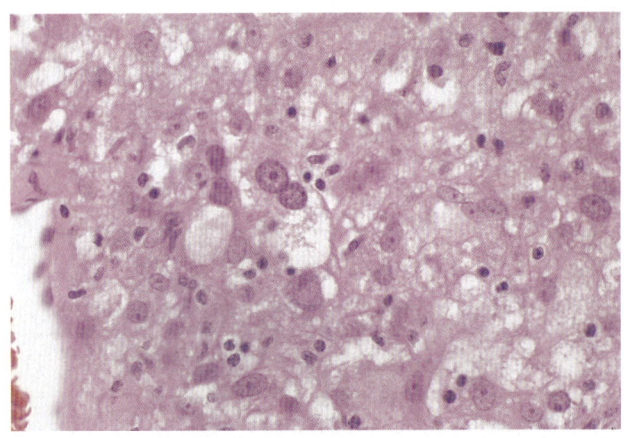

图 11.23 该肺透明细胞肿瘤由比图 11.22 多形性明显的细胞构成（×400）

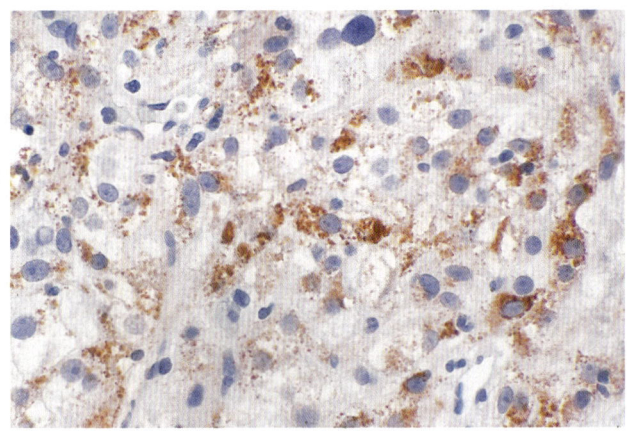

图 11.24 肺透明细胞肿瘤的瘤细胞表达 HMB-45（×400）

示，这些糖原为膜结合糖原。肿瘤细胞示波形蛋白阳性，且 HMB-45（图 11.24）和 S-100 蛋白常有表达。有些病例，肿瘤性细胞可表达 NSE、Leu7、Syn 和 HMB-50，CK 常阴性。新近报道，Myo-D1 亦可有表达[151]。Gaffey 等[152] 报道，电镜显示有些肿瘤细胞胞浆内含黑色素小体（图 11.25）。

淋巴血管平滑肌瘤病

淋巴血管平滑肌瘤病是一种罕见、增生性、非肿瘤性肺疾病，在此对该病作简要介绍，因为该病可表达 HMB-45[153, 154]。该病主要见于育龄期妇女，其特征为在淋巴管和血管周围由增生的非典型平滑肌细胞围绕，伴有囊腔形成。这些细胞可以表达肌动蛋白、波形蛋白、雌激素受体蛋白（ER）、孕激素受体蛋白（PR）和 HMB-45。淋巴血管平滑肌瘤病患者常伴发肾血管平滑肌脂肪瘤。

硬化性血管瘤

硬化性血管瘤属于在肺的罕见肿瘤中研究最广泛、最深入的类型之一，该肿瘤常为胸膜下圆形或卵圆形孤立结节[155, 156]，主要见于青年女性[157]。硬化性血管瘤组织学上成分多样，可有细胞区、大小不等的腔隙，其内偶尔含有血液、硬化和乳头状结构。在实性细胞区内，肿瘤细胞呈圆形、卵圆形或略呈梭形（图 11.26）。腔隙区常被覆立方上皮或柱状上皮，这些上皮形态似上皮细胞，与周围肿瘤细胞截然不同。许多硬化性血管瘤中都含有不同类型和不同量的炎细胞，尤其是肥大细胞。有一些对硬化性血管瘤的免疫组化研究，Dail[84] 对其进行了综述，对实性区肿瘤细胞免疫组化的阳性和阴性结果

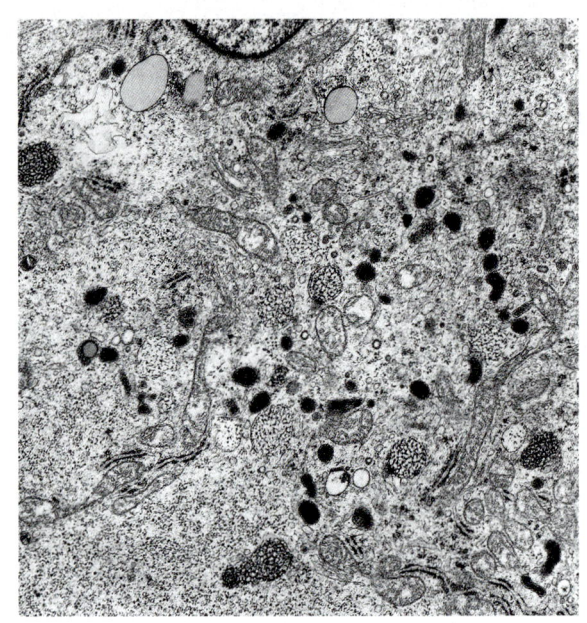

图 11.25 肺透明细胞肿瘤的瘤细胞含有黑色素小体（×16 000）

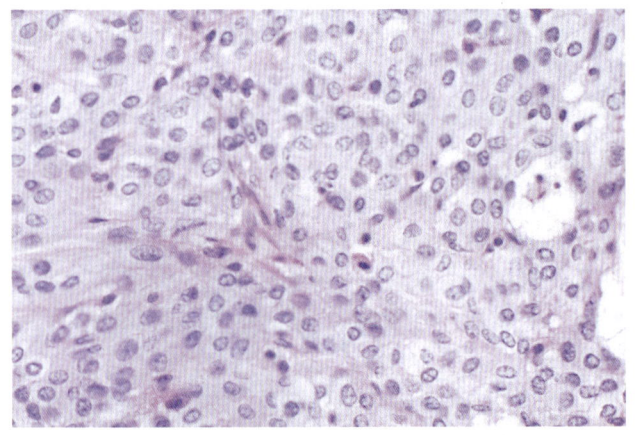

图 11.26 硬化性血管瘤的实性区，多数肿瘤细胞呈圆形、卵圆形，偶尔略呈梭形（×400）

肺和胸膜肿瘤的免疫组织化学 11

与被覆上皮细胞的免疫组化结果作了一个对比，结果见表11.8。这位作者在新近的研究中还指出，实性区被覆细胞和肿瘤细胞对EMA免疫组化反应呈强阳性（图11.27），中等强度的胞浆波形蛋白阳性。偶尔，被覆细胞对CK呈弱阳性表达。被覆细胞和实性区的肿瘤细胞对肌动蛋白、结蛋白、S-100、HMB-45、CD31和Ⅷ因子抗原呈阴性表达。电镜示，实性区肿瘤细胞有"上皮样"特征，如短小的微绒毛突起和较小的细胞间连接（图11.28）。

新近研究表明，硬化性血管瘤的瘤细胞也可表达TTF-1（图11.29）[158]。在一种支气管内的变型中[159]，有的患者可有淋巴结转移[160]。

横纹肌样瘤

1978年Beckwith和Palmer[161]首次报道了肾的恶性横纹肌样瘤，它是发生于婴幼儿和儿童的高度恶性肿瘤。起初认为它是Wilms瘤的一个变型。成年人，亦有肾外相似肿瘤的病例报道[162-175]。那些与肾的横纹肌样瘤形态相似但发生于肾外的肿瘤，我们称之为假横纹肌样瘤。尽管假横纹肌样瘤可表达波形蛋白，并且多数可同时表达波形蛋白和CK，但是它们与横纹肌样瘤免疫表型不同[162-175]。

1996年Cavazza等[176]报道了6例肺的横纹肌样瘤。这些肿瘤主要由大而圆的细胞构成，细胞核呈卵圆形，其中可见一大核仁。胞浆内含有较大的圆形嗜酸性包涵体，可将核挤向细胞的一侧（图11.30）。对这6例肺原发性横纹肌样瘤的免疫组化进行了分析，其中5例用了17种抗体，1例用了8种抗体。在所有病例中肿瘤的横纹肌样瘤成分均有波形蛋白的着色反应，且常为较强的阳性反应。6例中5例的胞浆嗜酸性包涵体EMA和NSE阳性反应；6例中3例有嗜铬素和广谱CK的着色；6例中2例CAM5.2CK阳性；

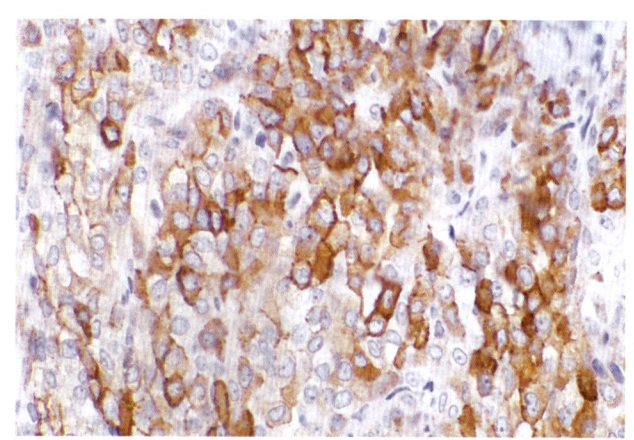

图11.27 硬化性血管瘤由上皮细胞膜抗原强阳性表达的细胞构成（×400）

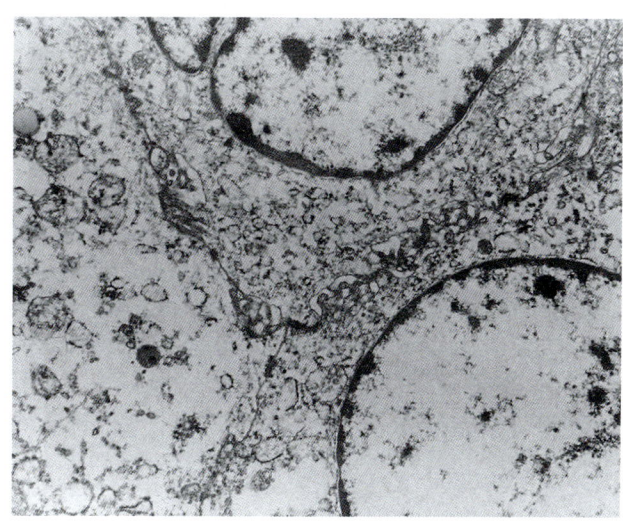

图11.28 超微结构示，硬化性血管瘤中央细胞有"上皮样"特征，即短小的微绒毛突起和小的细胞间连接（×10 000）

2/6例有神经丝（NF）着色；1/6例Leu7、胶质细丝酸性蛋白（GFAP）呈阳性；3/6例Syn呈灶性阳性；1/6例CD34阳性，但球形包涵体为阴性。1例有肌球蛋白弥漫性颗粒性胞浆阳性，肿瘤细胞的Ⅷ因子抗

表11.8 肺硬化性血管瘤免疫组化染色结果

肿瘤实性区的细胞		肿瘤被覆上皮区的细胞	
阳性	阴性	阳性	阴性
波形蛋白	CK	CK	波形蛋白
EMA	S-100蛋白	波形蛋白	S-100蛋白
CK（很少）		EMA	
		表面脂蛋白	
		Clara细胞抗原	
		CEA	
		TTF-1	

EMA，上皮细胞膜抗原；CEA，癌胚抗原；TTF-1，甲状腺转录因子-1

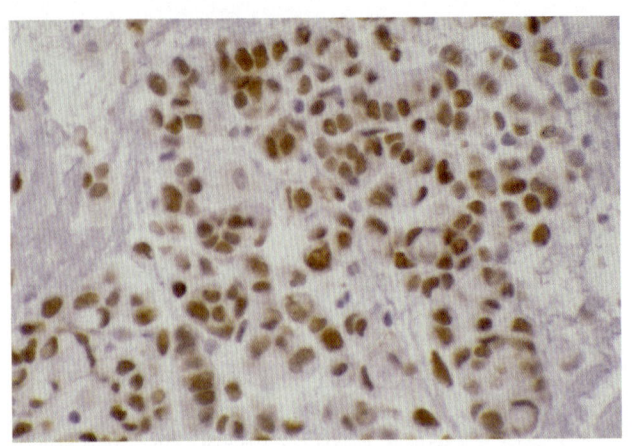

图 11.29　硬化性血管瘤的瘤细胞特征性地表达 TTF-1

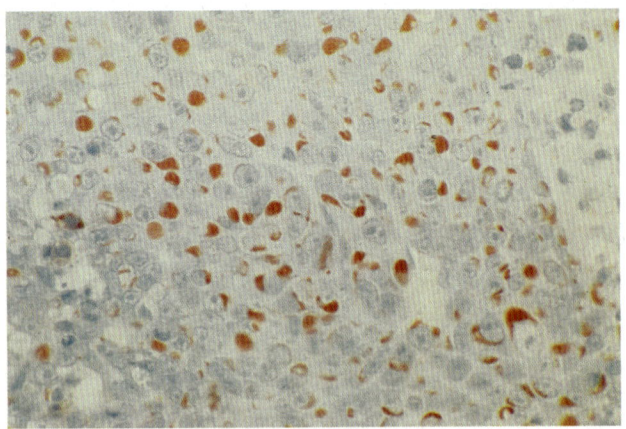

图 11.31　肺的原发性横纹肌样瘤免疫组化示，胞浆包涵体波形蛋白呈强阳性表达（×200）

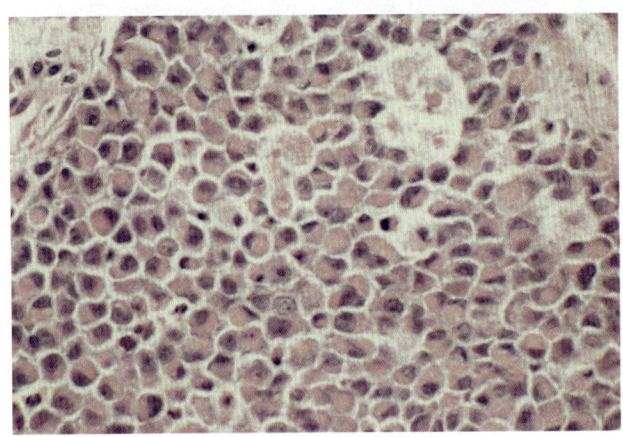

图 11.30　肺的原发性横纹肌样瘤由较大的细胞构成，胞浆内含有球形嗜酸性包涵体（×400）

原、肌动蛋白、结蛋白、S-100、HMB-45 和轻链免疫球蛋白均呈阴性（仅观察 1 例）。在该作者的实验中，6 例原发性肺的横纹肌样瘤中，5 例有波形蛋白的阳性反应（图 11.31），1 例既有波形蛋白又有 CK 的阳性表达。Miyagi 等[177]报道了 3 例肺的原发性横纹肌样瘤，这 3 个病例都与腺癌有一定关系。因此作者认为，3 例中的横纹肌样瘤代表了腺癌的去分化成分。

炎性假瘤

肺的炎性假瘤，又称为肺的浆细胞肉芽肿，在所有肺肿瘤中所占比例不超过 1%[178]。其发病多见于 40 岁以下人群，15% 可见于 1～10 岁儿童[179, 180]。该病引发的症状/体征主要有：咳嗽、胸痛、呼吸困难、咯血、杵状指和发热。胸部 X 线示肺内界限清楚的阴影，但有时形状不规则。大体观，病变呈灰黄色，界限清楚，可以浸润周围正常肺组织，并可引起肺组织的破坏。组织学上，炎性假瘤主要由成熟的浆细胞、巨噬细胞、多核巨细胞、淋巴细胞、肥大细胞、中性粒细胞和梭形细胞构成。炎性假瘤须与以下病变进行鉴别：硬化性血管瘤、恶性纤维组织细胞瘤、恶性浆细胞瘤和反应性淋巴细胞增生。免疫组化染色示，浆细胞轻链免疫球蛋白为多克隆表达。梭形细胞染色与肌纤维母细胞一样，可表达波形蛋白和肌动蛋白，在极少数病例，梭形细胞可同时表达 CK。炎性假瘤可以是浸润性的，类似于低级别肉瘤[181, 182]。尽管肿瘤抑制性基因产物 p53 对鉴别某些炎性疾病和肿瘤尚存在争议，如对纤维性胸膜炎和促结缔组织增生性间皮瘤的鉴别，但是其对鉴别炎性假瘤和肉瘤还是有帮助的。新近报道，肺的炎性假瘤有细胞基因性克隆的改变[184]。Yousem 等[185]指出肺的炎性假瘤存在染色体的异常，其报道的 9 例病例中有 3 例有 2p23 和间变性淋巴瘤激酶（anaplastic lymphoma kinase, ALK）基因区的变化。他们还指出，用免疫组化技术检测 ALK 可能对判断炎性假瘤的生物学行为有帮助。Freeman 等[186]也指出检测 ALK-1 的表达有助于炎性假瘤的诊断。

促结缔组织增生性小圆细胞肿瘤

促结缔组织增生性小圆细胞肿瘤主要发生于腹腔[187]。肿瘤可以特征性地表达结蛋白（点状）、WT-1、CK、NSE、CD99 和肌动蛋白。还可表现为 EWS-WT-1 基因融合转录。Syed 等[188]首次报道了肺的原发性促结缔组织增生性小圆细胞肿瘤。电镜示：肿瘤细胞胞浆内有旋涡状排列的中间丝，这些纤维可能为结蛋白。促结缔组织增生性小圆细胞肿瘤作为原发性肿瘤，发生于胸膜的病例亦有报道[189]。

上皮性/肌上皮性肿瘤

上皮性/肌上皮性肿瘤可以原发于肺[190-193]。该肿瘤内层上皮细胞CK、CEA和EMA呈阳性，而外层细胞肌上皮细胞S-100和肌动蛋白免疫着色呈阳性。

颗粒细胞肿瘤

颗粒细胞肿瘤可能来源于施万细胞，在肺表现为孤立性的肿瘤结节[194]。肿瘤细胞特征性地表达S-100、NSE、波形蛋白和肌动蛋白。

唾液腺肿瘤

唾液腺肿瘤在肺内比较罕见。由于这种肿瘤与发生在唾液腺的肿瘤有相似的免疫表型[195]，因此认为它可能起源于支气管黏膜的微小涎腺。

原发性肺内胸腺瘤

Moran等[196]报道了8例原发性肺内胸腺瘤，在这8例中，影像学和手术均未发现纵隔肿块。肿块直径0.5~10cm，其中5例靠近肺门，3例位于胸膜下。肿物由淋巴细胞、上皮细胞构成。淋巴细胞和上皮细胞由纤维分隔。上皮细胞免疫组化呈CK和EMA阳性。

肺脑膜上皮结节——脑膜瘤

微小肺脑膜上皮样结节（minute pulmonary meningothelial-like nodules, MPMN），以前又被称为微小化学感受器瘤样小体。多数情况下，该肿瘤是被偶然发现的。肿瘤由梭形细胞构成，以小静脉为中心形成结节。Ionescu等[197]报道了16例，有33个MPMN和10例脑膜瘤。在所有MPMN病例中，免疫组化示：波形蛋白的阳性率为96.6%，EMA33.3%，S-100蛋白3%。CK和Syn均为阴性反应。研究人员还发现MPMN缺乏突变性损伤，这与MPMN是一种反应性改变是一致的。相反，4例多发性MPMNs（微小肺脑膜上皮瘤病）中，发现了基因型改变，提示多发性MPMNs是一种介于反应性和肿瘤性转化之间的一种改变。10例脑膜瘤均发现了基因高频率的杂合性缺失。

肺胎盘绒毛异位

在此简单介绍一下肺胎盘绒毛异位。它常与脂肪瘤病和大泡性肺气肿有一定关系[199]，在肺实质内可见胎盘绒毛样结构。多数情况下，胎盘样结构表面被覆的上皮免疫组化示TTF-1阳性。间质细胞表达波形蛋白，而对TTF-1无反应性。间质内常可见到肥大细胞。

变化和陷阱

肺的鳞状细胞癌组织形态多样，有时可以分化很差。肺的小细胞鳞癌容易与小细胞神经内分泌癌相混淆。两种肿瘤的对比见表11.9。两者的主要差别为小细胞鳞癌不表达神经内分泌标记，而是常表达高分子量CK，免疫组化示TTF-1阴性而小细胞神经内分泌癌可特征性地表达神经内分泌标记，免疫组化示高分子量CK阴性，低分子量CK灶性阳性，且TTF-1的阳性表达率较高。小细胞鳞癌p63常呈阳性，而小细胞神经内分泌癌常呈阴性。

鳞癌有时可呈梭形细胞分化特征。肿瘤性梭形鳞状细胞同时表达CK和波形蛋白。有些梭形细胞鳞癌可以表达波形蛋白为主，而表达CK成分相对较少。

肺的肿瘤中，基底细胞样癌是相对少见的肺肿瘤[200]，这种肿瘤容易与神经内分泌癌相混淆。基底细胞样癌主要由体积较小的未分化细胞呈巢状排列而构成，癌组织中坏死常见，在癌巢周围细胞呈栅栏样排列（图11.32）。尽管其分化程度低，但它们还是可以向鳞癌和腺癌方向分化。其中腺样成分由小细胞构成。基底细胞样癌容易与小细胞癌、非典型类癌和大细胞神经内分泌癌相混淆。基底细胞样癌常表达低、高分子量CK，不表达神经内分泌标记。Sturm等[201]对基底细胞样癌和大细胞神经内分泌癌的TTF-1和34βE12（CK1、5、10和14）的表达情况进行了研究。在基底细胞样癌无TTF-1的表达，而高分子量角蛋白（34βE12）仅在1例大细胞神经内分泌癌有表

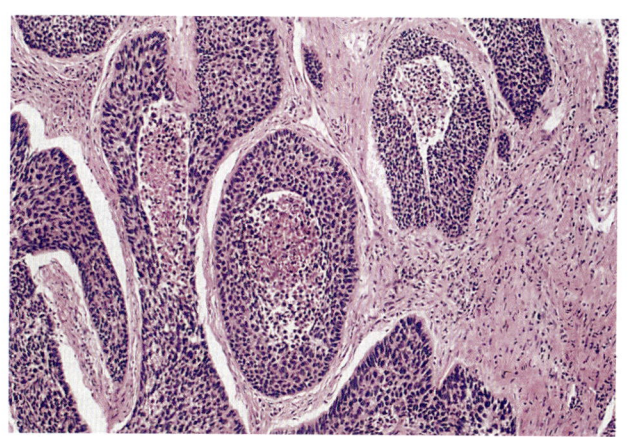

图11.32 肺的基底细胞样癌由未分化的小细胞构成，似肺原发性神经内分泌癌（×200）

表11.9　肺的小细胞鳞癌和小细胞神经内分泌癌的免疫组化特征

肿瘤类型	抗体检测的抗原								
	低分子量CK	高分子量CK	CK5/CK6	CK7	CK20	Syn	CgA	TTF-1	p63
小细胞鳞癌	S	S	S	N	R	N	N	N	S
小细胞神经内分泌癌	+*	N	N	R	R	+	S+	+	S

* 应用抗体35βH11，染色模式常呈点状
+ 染色模式常呈点状
反应性：+，几乎总是弥漫性强阳性；S，有时阳性；R，少数细胞阳性；N，几乎总是阴性

达。基底样细胞癌与小细胞癌、非典型类癌和大细胞癌的对比见表11.10。

目前，肺腺癌是原发性肺癌中为最常见的一种[9,10]，并且其分化具有多样性。多数情况下，肺腺癌可有一种以上的组织类型。原发性肺腺癌中，可有几种黏液型存在。如囊性黏液腺癌和印戒细胞癌。组织学上，难以将原发性黏液腺癌与来自胃肠道如结肠的转移性黏液腺癌相区分，电镜也不可能对两种肿瘤的起源进行区分。肺腺癌和转移性结肠性腺癌的免疫组化的特点对比见表11.11。一般来讲，原发性肺腺癌可特征性地表达CK7和TTF-1，而不表达CK20。转移性结肠性腺癌可特征地表达CK20和CDX2，而不表达CK7和TTF-1。前面已讲过，TTF-1是区分原发性肺腺癌和转移性腺癌最具有特异性的标志。约60%~75%的原发性肺腺癌可表达TTF-1。

然而，我们必须明了TTF-1在其他肿瘤细胞胞浆亦可有免疫着色。Bejarano和Mousavi[202]对起源于29个组织的361例肿瘤进行的研究，包括原发性和转移性肿瘤。23例（6.3%）胞浆有TTF-1的阳性表达。在这23例中有13例肿瘤的起源组织是可以确定的：7例肺癌（3例原发性肺癌，1例肺大细胞癌，1例转移至肝的小细胞癌，1例转移至颈部淋巴结的腺癌和1例转移至股部软组织的腺癌）；3例结肠性腺癌（2例转移至脊椎，1例转移至肺）；1例乳腺导管癌转移至股骨；1例喉鳞状细胞癌转移至肝；1例脑膜癌累及眶骨。作者认为，在几种不同类型的肿瘤胞浆中，偶尔可见TTF-1的免疫着色，但是并不具有特异性，对此在诊断时可以忽略不计。

随着时间的推移，许多免疫组化已失去了特异性。Leu等[33]对48例非黏液性、12例黏液性和7例混合型细支气管肺泡癌的TTF-1、CK7和CK20的表达进行了研究。12例黏液性细支气管肺泡癌TTF-1呈阴性表达，并且在混合型细支气管肺泡癌中，其黏液性成分的TTF-1也有呈阴性表达的趋势。67例中有

表11.10　肺的基底细胞样癌与小细胞癌、非典型类癌和大细胞神经内分泌癌对比的免疫组化特征

肿瘤类型	抗体检测的抗原								
	低分子量CK(35βH11)	高分子量CK(34βE12)	CK5/CK6	CK7	CK20	Syn	CgA	CEA	TTF-1
基底细胞样癌	S	S	S	S	R	N	N	S	R
小细胞癌	+	N	N	R	N	+	S	S	+
非典型类癌	S	S	S	R	N	S	+	S	S
大细胞神经内分泌癌	S	R	R	R	N	S	+	S	S

TTF-1，甲状腺转录因子-1
反应性：+，总是弥漫性强阳性；S，有时阳性；R，少数细胞阳性；N，几乎总是阴性

表11.11　原发性肺黏液腺癌与转移性大肠腺癌免疫组化特征的比较

肿瘤类型	抗体检测的抗原						
	CK5/CK6	CK7	CK20	CEA	表面脂蛋白A	TTF-1	CDX2
原发性肺黏液性肿瘤	R	S	S	+	S	S	R
转移性大肠黏液腺癌	N	S	S	+	N	N	S

TTF-1，甲状腺转录因子-1
反应性：+总是弥漫性强阳性；S，有时阳性；R，少数细胞阳性；N，几乎总是阴性

63例（94%）细支气管肺泡癌CK7呈阳性，并且在各种亚型之间其表达无差异。3例细支气管肺泡癌组织学呈黏液性图像，其CK20呈阳性。结果提示，有些黏液性细支气管细胞癌TTF-1呈阴性表达，但它们可以表达CK20。

Simsir等[34]研究了6例黏液性细支气管肺泡癌、4例非黏液性细支气管肺泡癌和6例伴灶性黏液分化者。6例黏液性细支气管肺泡癌中4例（67%）CK7阳性、CK20阳性、TTF-1阴性。所有4例非黏液性细支气管肺泡癌均有CK7阳性、CK20阴性。4例中2例TTF-1阳性。6例混合型细支气管肺泡癌中，CK7呈弥漫阳性，CK20呈灶性阳性；其中5例（83%）有TTF-1的阳性表达。作者得出结论，黏液性和混合型细支气管肺泡癌与普通的肺腺癌具有不同的免疫表型。

CDX2转录因子在胃肠道腺癌中特异表达[15]。Rossi等[203]应用免疫组化技术，对13例肺的原发性黏液性（胶样）癌进行了研究。其中11例杯状细胞型黏液腺癌有CDX2和MUC2的强阳性表达。8例中有TTF-1的表达，6例中有CK20表达，9例有CK7表达，2例有MUC-5AC表达。2例印戒细胞黏液癌有TTF-1、CK7和MUC-5AC的表达，但CDX2和CK20则呈阴性表达。作者认为，由于杯状细胞型黏液癌有CDX2、MUC2和CK20的强阳性表达，这就给与转移性结肠癌的鉴别带来一定的困难，也就更需要与临床紧密联系。

Mazziotta等[204]研究了多种腺癌的CDX2的表达，其中84例为肺腺癌。84例中10例可见CDX2免疫组化染色强阳性区，其中7例为肺腺癌，3例为肺大细胞癌。7例腺癌中3例及1例大细胞癌有TTF-1和CK7阳性表达，而CK20则呈阴性表达，8例中有7例可确认有CDX2的基因表达。该文章作者认为，CDX2在伴有肠上皮分化的肿瘤中，是一个具有特征性的标记，这表明在某些原发性肺腺癌、大细胞癌和卵巢的黏液腺癌中，均可见CDX2的表达。

少数肺原发性腺癌的免疫组化示S-100蛋白呈弱阳性[205]。然而，在肺原发性腺癌，尤其是非黏液性细支气管肺泡癌中，免疫组化染色示肿瘤细胞之间掺杂的树突状细胞的S-100蛋白阳性更为常见（图11.33）[206]。这些S-100蛋白阳性的细胞代表的是朗格汉斯细胞（图11.34）。这提示，腺癌可分泌趋化因子，吸引朗格汉斯细胞[207]。然而，在许多肿瘤和非肿瘤性的疾病中都可见朗格汉斯细胞[208]。

非黏液性细支气管肺泡癌核内包涵体并不少见，

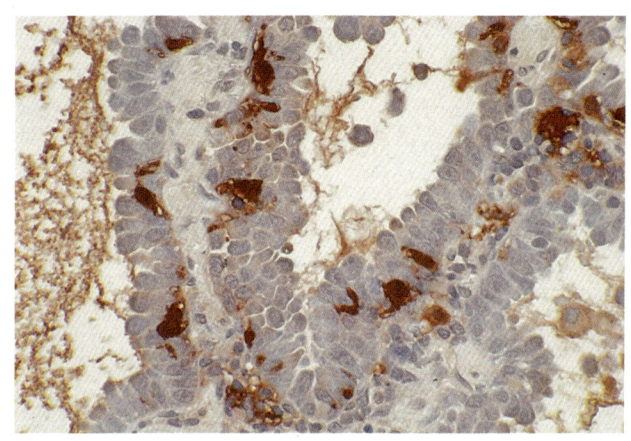

图11.33 非黏液性细支气管肺泡癌，大量S-100蛋白呈阳性表达的树突状细胞掺杂在肿瘤细胞之间（×400）

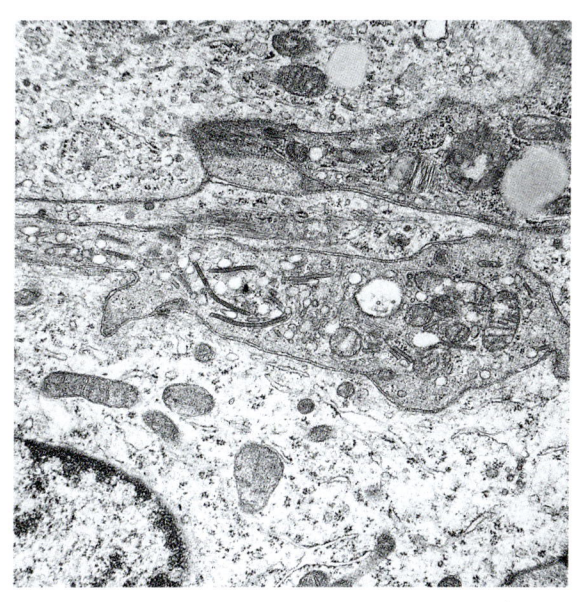

图11.34 超微结构示，S-100蛋白阳性细胞代表朗格汉斯细胞。朗格汉斯细胞为递呈并处理抗原的巨噬细胞，其胞浆内含有特征性颗粒——朗格汉斯细胞颗粒或Birbeck颗粒（×20 000）

这种包涵体PAS-淀粉酶消化阳性（图11.35）[209-212]。免疫组化示，PAS阳性的核内包涵体为肺表面活性物质的脂蛋白成分（图11.36）。电镜示这些核内包涵体由直径为45nm的小管构成，这些小管黏附于核膜内侧（图11.37）。

现在，在美国已经可以购买到商品化的抗表面活性物质抗体，并被用于分析其在肺腺癌诊断中的作用。对能够产生表面活性物质的肺腺癌，抗表面活性物质抗体并非100%有特异性。Bejarano等[26]用免疫组化标记物来鉴别原发性非小细胞肺癌和转移性乳腺癌。他们研究了57例原发性非小细胞癌，其中46例

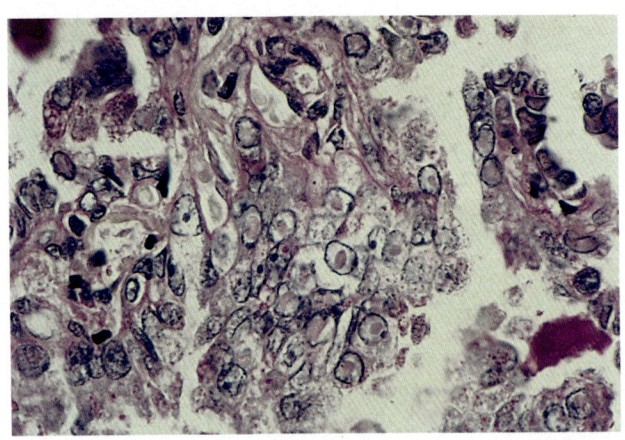

图 11.35 非黏液性细支气管肺泡癌 PAS 阳性的核内包涵体 (×400)

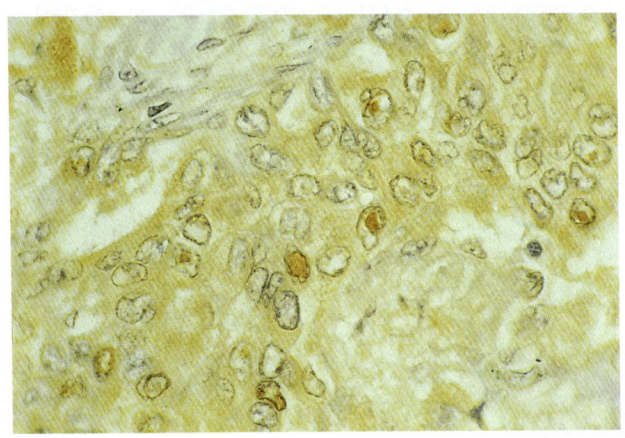

图 11.36 非黏液性细支气管肺泡癌核内包涵体，免疫组化表面活性物质 A 脂蛋白成分呈阳性 (×400)

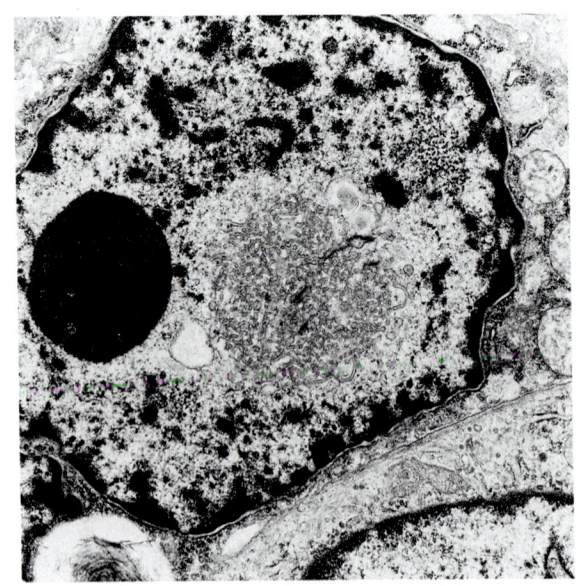

图 11.37 超微结构示，核内包涵体由与核膜内侧相连的直径为 45nm 的小管构成 (×20 000)

腺癌和 51 例乳腺癌，结果表面活性物质蛋白 A、表面活性物质蛋白 B 和 TTF-1 在非小细胞肺癌的阳性表达率分别为 49%、53% 和 63%；在原发性肺腺癌的阳性表达率分别为 54%、63% 和 76%。肺鳞癌几乎不表达这些抗原。51 例乳腺癌中有 4 例表面活性物质 A 免疫组化呈阳性，而 TTF-1 和表面活性物质 B 则呈阴性表达。

由表 11.4 可见，大量新近研究显示，有 TTF-1 表达的原发性肺癌，通常也有 SP-A 的表达，这并不意外，因为在原发性肺腺癌中，TTF-1 是表面活性物质的转录因子。

> **诊断要点**：原发性肺癌
>
> 1. 胞浆 TTF-1 的免疫组化着色不具特异性，在许多肿瘤中都可见到。
> 2. 黏液性细支气管肺泡癌特异性的 TTF-1-，但其 CK20+。
> 3. 非黏液性细支气管肺泡癌倾向于 TTF-1+，CK20-。
> 4. 在肺腺癌/大细胞癌，尤其是原发性胶样癌罕见 CDX2 阳性。

肺的转移性癌

(参见第 7 章)

肺是多种肿瘤转移的部位，病理学家必须对此心中有数[213, 214]。肺的转移性癌较原发性癌更为常见。由于肺的原发性和转移性肿瘤往往具有相似的组织学图像，因此必须对原发性肺癌和转移性癌加以鉴别。腺癌是对原发性和转移性肿瘤鉴别中最具有困难的一种，当诊断原发性肺癌时，即便是一个孤立的肺部结节，也要考虑是否有转移癌的可能。

正如本书作者[21]和其他研究者[215]所讨论的，尽管不具有特异性，抗 CK7 和 CK20 抗体对鉴别原发性和转移性癌还是有帮助作用的，许多胃肠道癌、部分肾细胞癌、妇科肿瘤和膀胱肿瘤均可表达 CK7。TTF-1 对诊断肺腺癌最具有特异性，但仍有 25%～40% 的肺腺癌不表达 TTF-1。如前所述，免疫标记表达还存在不一致之处，尤其在产生黏液的肺腺癌、黏液性细支气管肺泡癌和原发性黏液腺癌杯状细胞变型中。有些原发性肺癌，尤其是能产生黏液的癌，还可表达 CK20 和 CDX2。

乳腺癌常可在诊断数年后，转移至肺和胸膜[214]。Ollayos等[216]检测了诊断明确的结肠、胰腺和肺的腺癌中ER表达的敏感性。43例结肠腺癌和18例胰腺癌细胞核无ER表达，而42例原发性肺腺癌中有3例ER表达。

Canver等[217]研究了64例非小细胞癌雌激素受体表达情况。标本应用丙酮固定。在正常肺组织内，无性激素受体的表达，而在64例非小细胞肺癌中有62例可见核的ER呈阳性表达，在50例（78%）标本中孕激素受体呈阴性表达，有14例（22%）PR呈弱阳性。Bacchi等[218]报道了ER和PR在肺类癌和小细胞癌的表达情况。Dinunno等[219]研究了248例Ⅰ期、Ⅱ期非小细胞肺癌连续性病例，组织用福尔马林固定，石蜡包埋，而后观察ER、PR的表达情况。结果并未发现胞核/胞浆ER和PR的表达。因此，作者认为，ER、PR的表达是肺外肿瘤转移至肺的标记。与之相对应，Dabbs等[220]研究了45例手术切除的肺原发性肺腺癌，其中25例为非黏液型细支气管肺泡癌，20例为非特殊性中分化腺癌，组织用福尔马林固定，石蜡包埋，应用两个不同的单克隆抗体（6F11克隆和1D5克隆）观察其ER、PR表达情况，结果应用克隆6F11抗体组，56%非黏液性细支气管肺泡癌和80%原发性非特殊性肺腺癌有ER的核阳性表达，应用1D5克隆抗体组无ER表达。两种肿瘤中均无PR的表达，作者认为，6F11克隆抗ER抗体的性质、临床作用，及其雌激素受体的衍生物在肺腺癌中的作用等问题尚需作进一步研究。

肺肿瘤的其他标记物和诊断难点

Selvaggi等[221]分析了130例原发性肺癌中（60例鳞状细胞癌、48例腺癌和22例大细胞未分化癌）HER-2/neu的表达情况，发现60例鳞状细胞癌中的6例、48例腺癌中的6例和22例大细胞未分化癌中的3例表达HER-2/neu。多因素分析表明，HER-2/neu的表达及肿瘤的大小与生存期无关。肿瘤细胞中HER-2/neu阳性率高于5%的病人的中位生存时间（85周对179周）和总体生存率显著降低。

本文作者通过免疫组化热抗原修复法在75例原发性非小细胞肺癌中并未发现ER和PR的表达。部分小细胞肺癌中发现存在核ER和PR蛋白表达。

大细胞未分化肺肿瘤的免疫表型无法预测，大部分大细胞未分化肿瘤是癌并且共表达CK和波形蛋白，但有些只表达波形蛋白。有一些大细胞未分化肿瘤看起来像癌而实际上并不是，还有一些容易混淆的如非神经内分泌癌和非小细胞癌，可以通过一些神经内分泌的标记物来区分。我们后面将讨论这部分内容。

淋巴上皮样癌是原发性大细胞未分化癌的一种亚型，可以是肺原发性的，主要由大间变细胞构成，与淋巴瘤和其他肿瘤难以鉴别[222]。大部分淋巴上皮样癌表达低分子量和高分子量CK，并具有上皮分化的超微结构特点，如可以见到桥粒和细胞内张力丝。还有一些表达EB病毒和bcl-2[223]。

巨细胞肺癌是大细胞未分化癌的一种亚型，至少40%的细胞直径超过40μm[224]，通常共表达CK和波形蛋白，必须与转移的肉瘤和恶性黑色素瘤鉴别。部分巨细胞肺癌癌细胞胞浆中CEA染色阳性。

一些大细胞间变性淋巴瘤呈上皮样并表达角蛋白[225]。大部分Ki-1（CD30）阳性的间变性淋巴瘤表达EMA[226]。一些大细胞间变性淋巴瘤的超微结构呈现上皮分化特征[227]。

表11.12示不同种类的大细胞未分化肿瘤及其免疫表型。

Chu等[228]最近报道发现了大量的非造血上皮样肿瘤表达T/NK细胞抗原，但对诊断没有重要价值（表11.13）。

外科病理医师都知道，恶性黑色素瘤呈现分化多样化，几乎所有恶性黑色素瘤均可表达S-100蛋白和波形蛋白，近50%存在HMB-45阳性表达，极少数可以表达角蛋白[229]，给病理诊断带来困惑。

纵隔可以发生包括生殖细胞来源的多种肿瘤，所以区分是肺原发的肿瘤浸润到纵隔，还是纵隔原发的肿瘤浸润到肺是非常困难的。另外，胸腺癌也表现为分化多样性，如有些病例呈生殖细胞分化。据报道某些肺原发性癌也可以表达生殖细胞的标记物，这就使诊断更加困难。Yoshimoto等[230]报道了1例原发性低分化黏液性肺肿瘤可以同时表达CEA、AFP和人促绒毛膜性腺激素（human chorionic gonadotropin, hCG）。尸检组织表明这些抗原物质也可以存在于不同的肿瘤细胞中，对此现象，该作者认为在肺癌中至少存在3种不同表型的癌细胞克隆。Kuida等[231]发现在11例原发性肺癌中有4例表达hCG。TTF-1可能会对区分肿瘤是原发于肺还是原发于纵隔有所帮助。

为了分析肺癌中滋养层细胞性抗原的表达情况，有实验对40例神经内分泌肺肿瘤、29例原发性肺腺

表11.12 侵及肺的不同类型大细胞未分化肿瘤的免疫组化特征

肿瘤类型	一抗													
	AE1/AE3	低分子量CK	高分子量CK	CK7	CK20	波形蛋白	EMA	CEA	S-100	HMB-45	CD30	CD20	NSE	SYN	CGA
肺大细胞未分化癌	+	+	S	S		S	S	S	R	N	N	N	S	R	R
肺巨细胞癌	+	+	S	S		S	S	S	R	N	N	N	S	R	R
肺淋巴上皮样癌	S	S	S	S		S	S	S	R	N	N	N	R	R	R
大细胞神经内分泌癌	S	S	S	R		+	R	R	S	S	N	N	+	+	S
恶性间皮瘤	R	R	R	R		S	S	R	R	S	R	N	S	R	R
间变型淋巴瘤	R	R	R	N	N	S	S	N	R	N	S	S	R	N	N

CEA, 癌胚抗原; SYN, 突触素; CGA, 嗜铬素A
反应性: +, 几乎总是弥漫强阳性; S, 有时候阳性; R, 少数细胞阳性; N, 几乎总是阴性

表11.13 CD2、CD3、CD4、CD5、CD7、CD8、CD56和CD138在447例具有上皮样特征的非造血性肿瘤中的表达情况

肿瘤类型	总数	CD2	CD3	CD4	CD5	CD7	CD8	CD56	CD138
肺									
肺腺癌	21	0	0	0	2	8	0	1	11
小细胞癌	6	0	0	0	0	0	0	6	0
胃肠道									
结肠癌	10	0	0	0	5	6	0	0	9
胰腺癌	13	0	0	0	6	9	0	0	4
胃腺癌	15	0	0	0	0	3	0	0	2
肝细胞癌	25	0	0	0	0	0	0	0	15
胆管癌	14	0	0	0	12	13	0	3	13
生殖泌尿道									
前列腺癌	18	0	0	0	4	0	0	1	6
肾细胞癌	19	0	0	0	1	0	0	2	12
过渡型细胞癌	24	0	0	0	5	9	0	0	22
女性生殖系统									
乳腺（导管和小叶）	26	0	0	0	7	3	0	1	18
卵巢癌	24	0	0	0	3	8	0	2	10
子宫内膜腺癌	10	0	0	0	0	3	0	1	9
皮肤									
鳞状细胞癌	25	0	0	0	0	2	0	0	25
基底细胞癌	20	0	0	0	0	2	0	0	14
甲状腺肿瘤									
滤泡腺瘤	24	0	0	0	0	0	0	17	10
乳头状腺癌	9	0	0	0	0	0	0	9	2
髓样癌	17	0	0	0	0	0	0	15	2
神经内分泌肿瘤									
肾上腺皮质肿瘤	20*	0	0	0	2	1	0	18	7
神经内分泌癌	9	0	0	0	0	0	0	9	3
类癌	10	0	0	0	0	0	0	9	2
Merkel细胞癌	9	0	0	0	0	0	0	9	2
其他									
胸腺瘤	8	0	0	0	0	0	0	0	0
生殖细胞肿瘤	14	0	0	0	0	0	0	0	0
恶性黑色素瘤	20	0	0	0	2	8	0	1	1
涎腺肿瘤	11	0	0	0	1	1	0	0	3
恶性间皮瘤	16#	0	0	0	2	4	0	0	0
上皮样肉瘤	10	0	0	0	3	7	0	2	0
总数	447	0(0.0)	0(0.0)	0(0.0)	55(12.3%)	87(19.5%)	0(0.0)	106(23.7%)	202(45.2%)

* 另外还研究了10例肾上腺皮质癌中CD56的表达情况。总共30例肾上腺皮质癌中，25例呈CD56阳性。
# 另外还研究了5例恶性间皮瘤中CD138的表达情况。总共22例恶性间皮瘤中，1例呈CD138阳性。
（引自Chu PG, Arber DA, Weiss LM. Expression of T/NK-cell and plasma cell antigens in nonhematopoietic epitheliod neoplasm：an immunohistochemical study of 447 cases. Am J Clin Pathol 2003; 120: 64-70）

癌、20例鳞状细胞癌和1例腺鳞癌中hCG及其衍生物、黄体生成素（LH，LHβ）、卵泡刺激素（FSH，FSHβ）、胎盘催乳素（PL）和生长激素（GH-227）[232]的表达情况进行了研究，结果发现所有90例肺癌中有28例（31%）表达滋养层细胞激素，但主要是在典型的类癌中表达。

某些罕见的类似肝细胞肝癌的肺肿瘤可以有AFP的强阳性表达和异常凝血酶原（prothrombin）的表达[233]。

病理医师和临床医师继续大规模地分析了神经内分泌肿瘤。Cooper等[234]回顾性地分析了77例手术切除的肿瘤，其中有50例典型类癌、5例非典型类癌、9例大细胞神经内分泌癌、4例混合型大细胞/小细胞神经内分泌癌和9例小细胞神经内分泌癌。77例病例中有62例进行了平均38.1个月（2～132个月）的随访，13例死亡病例中有8例死于肺肿瘤：4例死于大细胞神经内分泌癌；2例死于小细胞神经内分泌癌；1例死于非典型类癌；1例死于混合型大细胞/小细胞神经内分泌癌。神经内分泌肿瘤患者的平均无瘤时间是：典型类癌，41.3个月；非典型类癌，20个月；大细胞神经内分泌癌，25个月；小细胞神经内分泌癌，48个月。该作者承认此研究的局限性及高级别神经内分泌癌手术治疗的争议性。

Lyda和Weiss[235]检测了142例原发性肺癌中的B72.3、34βE12（CK 1、5、10、14）、CK7、CK17、Syn和CgA的表达情况，以分析神经内分泌标记物和上皮标记物在诊断原发性肺癌中的价值。84%（37/44）的大细胞和小细胞神经内分泌癌CgA表达阳性；64%（21/36的小细胞癌和6/6的大细胞神经内分泌癌）Syn表达阳性；5%（2/43）角蛋白34βE12表达阳性；9%（4/44）CK7表达阳性；5%（2/37）的小细胞癌和50%（3/6）的大细胞神经内分泌癌B72.3表达阳性。在98例非神经内分泌肺癌中，5%（5/98）CgA表达阳性，3%（3/98）Syn表达阳性，97%（95/98）34βE12或CK7表达阳性，99%（97/98）34βE12、CK7或B72.3表达阳性。一组抗体CK7、34βE12、CgA和Syn联合检测可以将94%（132/141）的肿瘤区分开来，本文作者认为有比Lyda和Weiss提出的更好的抗体组合可将神经内分泌和非神经内分泌原发性肺肿瘤区分开来。

Sturm等[236]分析了227例神经内分泌增生性病变以及肿瘤中TTF-1（调节肺形态发生和分化的因子）的表达情况。结果发现，在55例小细胞肺癌中有47例（85.5%）、64大细胞癌中有31例（49%）存在表达；15例神经内分泌性增生中，23例微小肿瘤、27例典型类癌和23例非典型类癌中均无表达（0%）。在20例混合性小细胞肺癌和大细胞神经内分泌癌中，19例（95%）TTF-1在肿瘤中的神经内分泌和非神经内分泌成分中都有表达。这些发现对神经内分泌肿瘤的范畴提出质疑，并提出小细胞肺癌和非小细胞肺癌属于同一起源的假说。但对本文作者来说，Sturm等的结论很难被接受，因为在不同的神经内分泌肺肿瘤中存在着生物化学、组织化学和超微结构等各个方面的种种不同。另外，在前面我们也讨论过，其他学者也发现TTF-1在典型类癌和非典型类癌中都有表达。

最后，Lin等[237]用增殖抗原标记物MIB-1/Ki-67来区分低级别和高级别神经内分泌癌。该作者指出，一旦MIB-1表达阳性，则阳性率低于25%的可以认为是低级别神经内分泌肿瘤，而阳性率高于50%的可以认为是高级别神经内分泌肿瘤。

该结论被Pelosi等[238]进一步作了补充。他们在支气管活检标本中发现7例典型或非典型类癌被过诊为小细胞肺癌。他们连续研究了9例支气管活检的小细胞肺癌病人，并进行了组织学和免疫组化（CK、CgA、Syn、Ki-67、MIB-1和TTF-1）的检测，发现类癌为中央型或周围型，核染色质呈颗粒状或粗块状，CgA和Syn高表达，而Ki-67/MIB-1低表达（<20%），肿瘤间质中含有薄壁血管。小细胞癌为中央型，核染色质细而均匀，CgA和Syn低表达，Ki-67/MIB-1高表达（>50%）。该作者认为在小的、被挤压的支气管活检标本中把类癌过诊为小细胞肺癌仍然是个很大的问题，并且指出，仔细观察HE切片及联合检测Ki-67和MIB-1是目前能够正确诊断的最有用的手段。

本文作者最近发现了3例此类病例，其中2例起初被诊断为小细胞癌。这3例病人都不吸烟。第1例病人是一个67岁的老年男性，有石棉接触史并存在石棉肺，起初被诊断为小细胞肺癌。肿瘤位于右肺上叶并已手术切除，肿瘤直径3cm，界限清楚，细胞单一，圆形或梭形，核分裂象每50个高倍视野小于1个，免疫组化CgA和Syn表达强阳性，TTF-1表达阴性。Ki-67表达小于20%。

第2例病人是一个71岁的老年女性，支气管活检发现有局灶性的挤压细胞（图11.38），起初被诊断为小细胞肺癌。总的来讲，肿瘤细胞呈圆形或梭形，染色质均一，核分裂不活跃，肿瘤细胞胞浆呈CgA和

Syn表达强阳性（图11.39），TTF-1表达阴性，Ki-67表达小于20%（图11.40）。

第3例病人是一个70岁的老年男性，支气管活检发现瘤细胞形态单一并伴有局灶性的挤压假象，但没有坏死或核分裂活跃。肿瘤细胞TTF-1表达阴性而CgA和Syn表达阳性，Ki-67表达小于20%。

非小细胞原发性肺肿瘤可以表现神经内分泌分化，如果被分析的肿瘤在组织学上呈现出非神经内分泌肿瘤的图像，这一点可能会给诊断带来困惑。Visscher等[239]用抗CgA、Syn、S-100、CK、波形蛋白、NF抗原的单克隆抗体分析了56例低分化非小细胞肺肿瘤。这些肿瘤没有神经内分泌分化的组织学特征。用未固定的冷冻组织切片，发现17例大细胞未分化癌中的5例（29%）和19例腺癌中的4例（21%）呈CgA或Syn染色阳性，在2例大细胞未分化癌和1例低分化腺癌中Syn呈弥漫强阳性。20例低分化鳞状细胞癌中有1例（5%）Syn表达阳性。有趣的是，17例大细胞未分化癌中的10例（58.8%）和19例低分化腺癌中的10例（52.6%）都表达波形蛋白或NF抗原。该作者认为在大量的大细胞未分化癌和低分化腺癌中都存在着神经内分泌分化的免疫组织学证据并伴有异源性中间丝的表达。该作者并未分析NF在未分化或低分化原发性肺癌中的表达情况，但这些肿瘤超过半数都共表达角蛋白和波形蛋白，它们甚至在免疫组化中并不呈现神经内分泌分化。

Linnoila等[240]在福尔马林固定、石蜡包埋的标本中用抗CgA、Leu7、NSE、5-羟色胺、铃蟾肽（bombesin）、降钙素、ACTH、血管加压素、神经紧张素（neurotensin）、CEA、角蛋白、波形蛋白和NF抗体分析了113例手术切除的原发性肺肿瘤病例，发

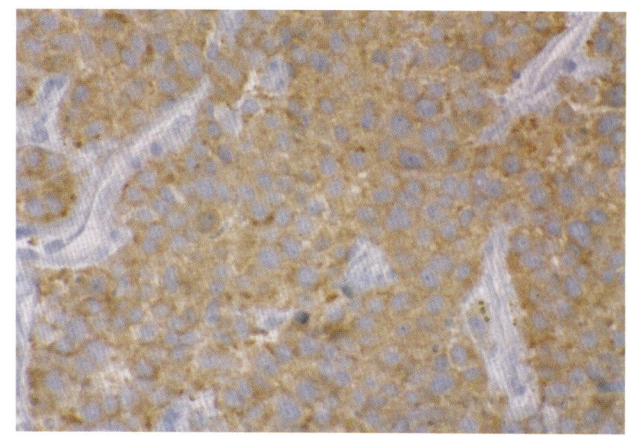

图11.39 免疫组化染色，肿瘤细胞呈CgA强阳性表达

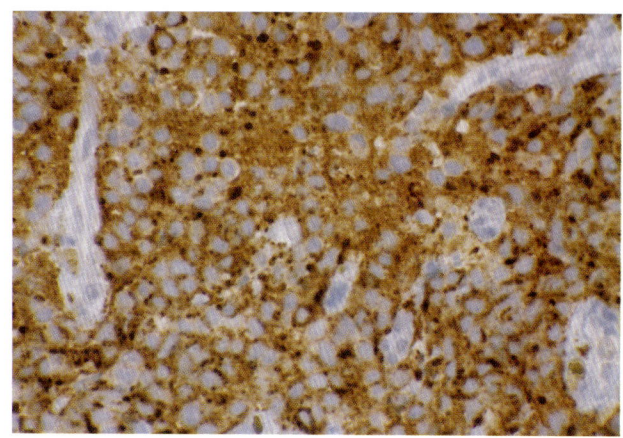

图11.40 Ki-67染色，不到20%的肿瘤细胞呈核染色阳性

现大多数类癌和小细胞癌中相当一部分肿瘤细胞表达多种神经内分泌标记物，约50%的非小细胞肺癌也有部分肿瘤细胞表达神经内分泌标记物。少数情况下，免疫组化难以区分非小细胞肺癌和小细胞癌。另外，他们还发现，神经内分泌标记物在大细胞未分化癌和腺癌中的表达率要高于鳞状细胞癌。

Mooi等[241]分析了11例手术切除的原发性肺肿瘤，组织学类型为大细胞癌或鳞状细胞癌，但显微镜下与支气管类癌和小细胞癌有些许的相似之处。所有病例NSE和蛋白基因产物9.5阳性，该作者认为这表明该肿瘤有神经内分泌分化。铃蟾肽和CgA在2例病例中表达阳性，C-末端肽在5例病例中表达阳性。电镜下观察，7例病例中有6例发现存在致密的神经内分泌颗粒。根据发表在杂志上的肿瘤图片，可能会有人对报道的所谓混合性神经内分泌/非神经内分泌肿瘤提出质疑。

Wick及其同事[242]比较了12例具有神经内分泌分化的肺大细胞癌和15例没有神经内分泌分化的肺大

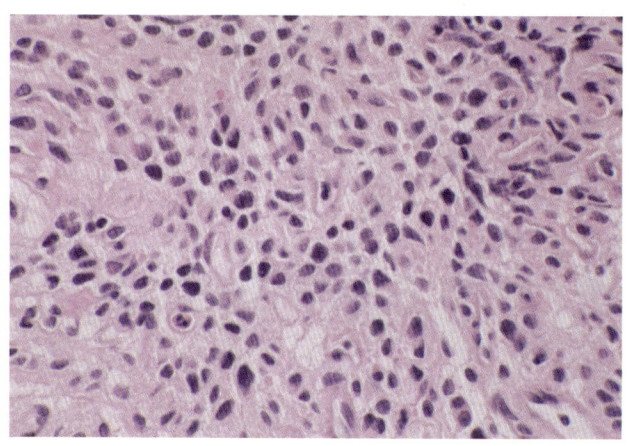

图11.38 该例支气管活检标本最初被诊断为小细胞肺癌（×400）

细胞肿瘤。数据显示，具有神经内分泌分化的大细胞肿瘤按照Travis及其同事的分类标准应该是大细胞神经内分泌癌，而不是具有局部神经内分泌分化的大细胞未分化癌。有趣且重要的是，具有神经内分泌分化的大细胞肿瘤预后远远差于没有神经内分泌分化的肿瘤。该作者指出，免疫组化和电镜观察对诊断这种肿瘤是必需的，而且，很可能即使运用这些手段也不足以诊断。一些肿瘤学家建议，所有的肺大细胞癌都应分析其是否具有神经内分泌分化，因为是否具有神经内分泌分化在化疗方案选择上可能会存在差异。至于这个建议是否合适，可以参考下面我们要讨论的研究进行分析。

Loy等[243]分析了66例已进行了超微结构检测的肺肿瘤中神经内分泌标记物的表达情况，包括NSE、CgA、Leu7和Syn，同时还检测了非神经内分泌标记物B72.3的表达情况。他们研究了11例小细胞癌、4例低级别神经内分泌癌（非典型类癌？）、2例具有神经内分泌分化的大细胞癌（大细胞神经内分泌癌？）、26例腺癌、10例鳞状细胞癌及11例大细胞未分化癌，发现10例鳞状细胞癌中有4例、26例腺癌中有3例、11例大细胞未分化癌中有1例呈CgA表达阳性。10例鳞状细胞癌均不表达Leu7，26例腺癌中有4例表达，11例大细胞未分化癌均无表达。10例鳞状细胞癌中有6例、26例腺癌中有15例、11例大细胞未分化癌中有7例表达NSE。10例鳞状细胞癌中有6例、26例腺癌中有16例、11例大细胞未分化癌中有7例表达Syn。总的来讲，47例没有神经内分泌分化特征的癌中有34例（79%）至少表达一种神经内分泌免疫组化标记物。19例神经内分泌癌中有19例（100%）至少表达一种神经内分泌标记物。

Schleusener等[244]分析了107例ⅢA、ⅢB和Ⅳ期非小细胞肺癌（62例腺癌、22例鳞状细胞癌、18例大细胞癌、5例腺鳞癌）病人中角蛋白、Syn、Leu7和CgA的免疫组化表达情况。角蛋白作为对照在99.1%的病例中表达阳性。35%的腺癌、41%的鳞状细胞癌和33%的大细胞癌至少表达一种神经内分泌标记物。令人意外的发现是表达一种或多种神经内分泌标记物的病人生存期延长，但是，神经内分泌标记物与对化疗的反应之间没有发现相关性。

总的来说，按组织学分类标准并未划分为神经内分泌肿瘤的肺肿瘤，免疫组化染色可以表达神经内分泌标记物。图11.41总结了这些研究中CgA、Syn、NSE和Leu7的阳性表达率。

胸膜肿瘤

胸膜肿瘤是相对常见的肿瘤，且胸膜转移瘤要比胸膜原发的肿瘤更为常见[214, 245]。用免疫组化将胸膜原发性肿瘤和转移瘤区分开来是被广泛关注的一大领域，在某种程度上这要归功于对浆膜生物学以及间皮瘤病理学/病理生物学不断深入的了解。

胚胎形成过程中，体腔的发育相对较早，并通过膜的分割产生了胸膜腔、腹膜腔和心包腔[246]。间皮瘤来源于体腔的浆膜。除了Selikoff等[247]研究的孤立群体（石棉肺患者群体），胸膜间皮瘤大约占所有间皮瘤的90%。

胸膜的间皮瘤组织学分化复杂多样，主要分为4个亚型：①上皮型，②肉瘤样型（纤维性、肉瘤性），③混合型，④促结缔组织增生型（肉瘤样型间皮瘤的一种亚型）。

免疫组化是准确诊断间皮瘤的最主要手段，并能将其与浸润到胸膜的原发性肺癌、转移到胸膜的原发性肺癌及胸腔外肿瘤区分开来。胸膜间皮瘤的4种主要组织学类型实际上是一种非常简化的分型，比如

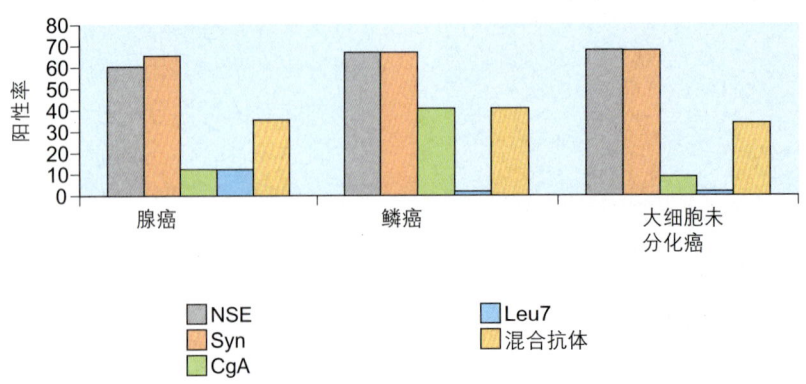

图11.41 组织学上诊断为非神经内分泌肿瘤中神经内分泌标记物的表达情况。阳性表达通常是局灶、弱阳性的

说，上皮型间皮瘤中又有很多亚型，包括小管乳头状型、组织细胞样型、腺型、微囊型、囊腺型、肾小球样型、胎盘样型、印戒型、透明细胞型、实体型、小细胞型、大细胞型以及由相对多形性大细胞构成的间皮瘤。分化较好的乳头状间皮瘤主要在腹膜腔和胸膜腔，由于它们不同于其他间皮瘤，而通常在临床上呈良性或低度恶性潜能，所以将该型区分开来是很重要的[248-250]。另外，浆膜组织非常活跃，当受到损伤时细胞形态变化较大，很容易被误诊为恶性肿瘤[251]。免疫组化通常无法区分非典型反应的浆膜和恶性肿瘤，但可以帮助区分这些细胞是上皮型间皮细胞还是胸膜的梭形细胞[252]。

正常胸膜的生物学和形态学已被广泛研究，在静止状态下，胸膜由一层相对扁平的上皮型间皮细胞构成，基底膜将其与其下的结缔组织分开（图11.42）。基底膜下的细胞为梭形细胞并与弹性组织和胶原有关，在弹性组织染色的切片中可以清楚看到弹性组织和胶原。上皮型间皮细胞和胸膜梭形细胞都对损伤有强烈反应，主要表现为细胞变大、数量增加（图11.43）。有趣的是，胸膜梭形细胞免疫组化染色表达角蛋白、波形蛋白、肌动蛋白和calretinin（图11.44），并且其超微结构显示具有肌纤维母细胞的特征（图11.45）。1986年，我和同事们[253]对胸膜及其对损伤的反应作了大量研究，并阐述了间皮瘤和反应性胸膜细胞的组织学、免疫组织化学以及超微结构特征，尽管仍有许多疑问，但已有证据表明上皮型间皮细胞是由基底膜下的梭形细胞增殖、分化而来的，我们把这些细胞命名为多潜能性浆膜下细胞。

很多抗体已经被用来研究和帮助诊断间皮瘤。可以把这些抗体分为3种主要类型：①对间皮细胞和间皮瘤相对特异性的抗体，在间皮瘤中表达阳性，可以作为间皮瘤阳性标记物。②对间皮细胞或间皮瘤没有反应的抗体，在间皮瘤中表达阴性，可以作为间皮瘤阴性标记物。③对间皮细胞和间皮瘤均有所反应的抗体，但相对不特异。

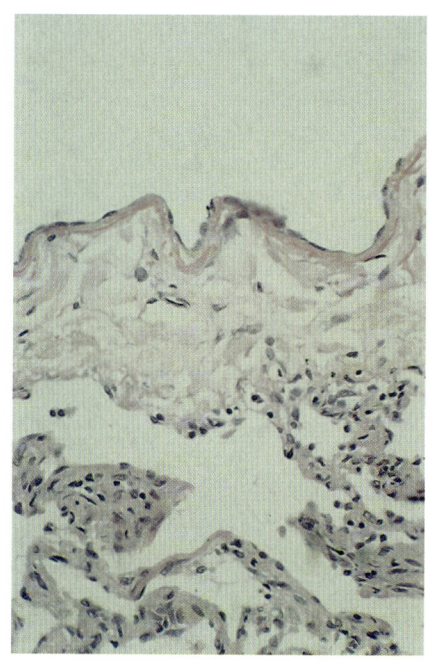

图11.42 在静止状态下，正常胸膜由一层略呈扁平的间皮细胞及其下方的梭形细胞、胶原和弹性组织构成（×200）

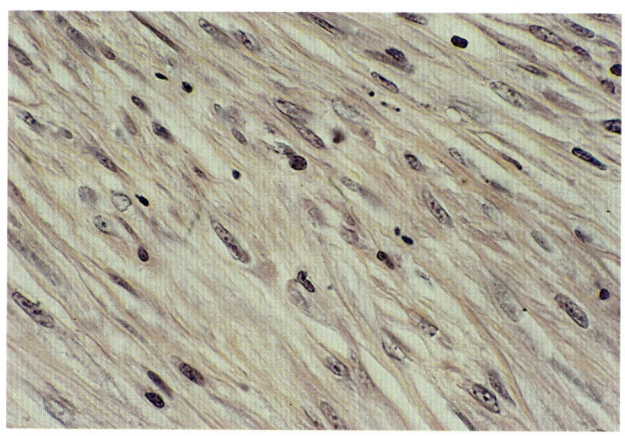

图11.43 胸膜在受到损伤后，其扁平的间皮细胞肥大增生，下方的梭形细胞也随之增生，呈现肌纤维母细胞的图像（×400）

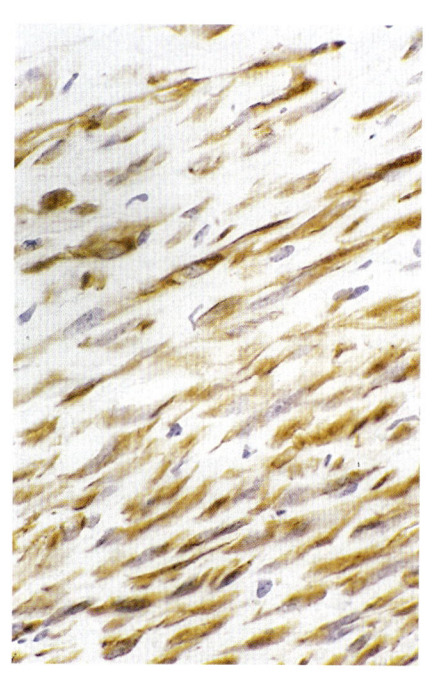

图11.44 胸膜增生的肌纤维母细胞呈角蛋白、波形蛋白、肌动蛋白和calretinin染色阳性。本图片显示的是calretinin染色（×400）

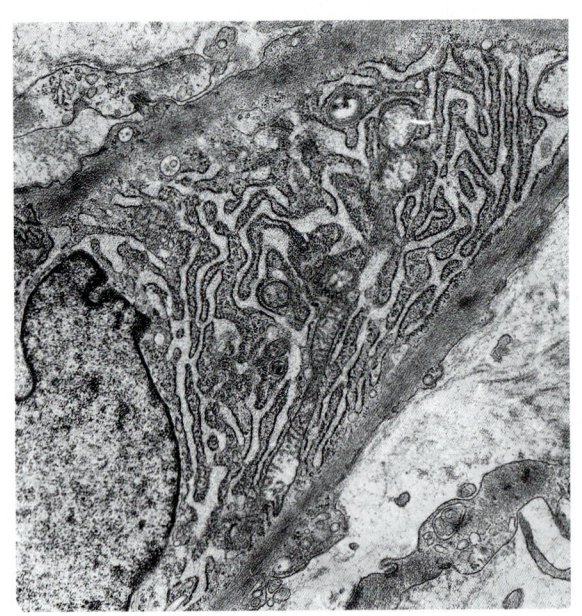

图11.45 增生的梭形细胞具有肌纤维母细胞的超微结构特点（×40 000）

如上所述，间皮瘤的组织学特征复杂，分化多样。诊断间皮瘤抗体的选择主要根据其所呈现的分化类型。表11.14总结了诊断间皮瘤的常用抗体及抗体特征。

阳性标记物

几乎100%的间皮瘤都表达角蛋白，角蛋白抗体主要用来确定肿瘤性间皮细胞，判断可疑间皮瘤的浸润，诊断肉瘤样型间皮瘤以及区分肉瘤样型间皮瘤、肉瘤、胸膜局灶性纤维性肿瘤和其他角蛋白常为阴性的肿瘤。在大部分间皮瘤中都可检测到低分子量和高分子量角蛋白，尤其是低分子量角蛋白，可用CAM5.2和35βH11抗体进行检测。该作者用AE1/AE3角蛋白作为广谱角蛋白。CK在间皮瘤中的表达情况已由Henderson等[254]和Ordonez[255]进行了总结。

1985年，Blobel等[256]曾报道，正常的和肿瘤性的间皮细胞都表达CK7、CK8、CK18和CK19，而这些标记物在单层上皮细胞和腺癌细胞中都经常见到。他们发现一些上皮型间皮瘤表达CK4、CK14、CK16和CK17。在以前发表过的研究中[257]，腺癌表达CK7、CK8、K18和CK19，而鳞状细胞癌表达的CK谱更为复杂，包括单层上皮型CK（CK7、CK8、CK18和CK19）和复层上皮型CK，尤其是CK5/6。1989年，Moll等[258]用AE14抗体证明在13例上皮型和混合型间皮瘤中有12例表达CK5，而在21例肺间皮瘤中均不表达。他们由此得出结论，CK5是区分肺腺癌和上皮-混合型间皮瘤的一个有用的标记物。遗憾的是，AE14抗体不能用于石蜡标本，直到1997年，Clover等[259]用商业化的单克隆抗体D5/16B4来检测福尔马林固定、石蜡包埋组织中CK5和CK6的表达，发现在23例（100%）上皮型间皮瘤中全部呈阳性表达，27例肺腺癌中有5例（18.5%）表达阳性。在5例肺腺癌中有4例（90%）为弱阳性或可疑阳性。在1例标本中呈局灶阳性。Ordonez等[255]与Clover等[259]用同样的抗体发现，在40例上皮型间皮瘤（100%）和15例肺鳞状细胞癌（100%）中全部呈阳性表达，而在30例肺腺癌中均为阴性。在93例非肺腺癌中有14例（15.1%）为局灶性或弱阳性表达，具体的讲，在30例卵巢腺癌中有10例（33.3%）、10例子宫内膜腺癌中有2例（20%）、18例乳腺癌中有1例（5.6%）、7例甲状腺癌中有1例（14.3%）存在局灶性或弱阳性表达，而10例肾癌、10例结肠腺癌和8例前列腺癌均为阴性。CK在上皮型间皮瘤、肺腺癌和肺鳞状细胞癌中的表达比较见表11.15。

Kahn及其同事[260]报道了良恶性间皮细胞与腺癌之间角蛋白分布模式的区别。他们发现，在间皮细胞中角蛋白细丝在核周或核的外围分布，而在腺癌中则呈分支状分布。继Kahn及其同事的报道[260]之后又有学者作了大量的研究[261]，用抗角蛋白的3种单克隆抗体和3种多克隆抗体分析了10例腺癌、10例类癌和4例间皮瘤中角蛋白中间丝的分布。当用二氨基联苯胺显色将显色时间缩短在2分钟之内时，发现在腺癌中阳性分布呈网络样模式，在类癌中呈斑点构成的新月体模式，在间皮瘤中呈核周染色模式。角蛋白中间丝的核周分布模式在上皮型间皮瘤中常见，但并不是出现在所有的病例中，而且一些肺腺癌中也出现角蛋白核周分布模式。该作者并未诊断性地应用角蛋白"分布模式"。

尽管100%的上皮型间皮瘤表达角蛋白，但文献报道肉瘤样型间皮瘤角蛋白的表达却并不一致。Montag等[262]发现16例肉瘤样型间皮瘤均表达角蛋白（100%），Battifora证实了这一结果[263]，他检测了20多例肉瘤样型间皮瘤，发现100%存在角蛋白表达。相反，一些研究发现超过40%的肉瘤样型间皮瘤并不表达角蛋白[264-271]。美国-加拿大（US-Canadian）间皮瘤小组也发现了很多角蛋白阴性的肉瘤样型间皮瘤。根据本作者的经验，在大量的固定良好的尸检组织中，肉瘤样型间皮瘤的角蛋白表达可以高度多样化。用广谱角蛋白抗体（AE1/AE3）和低分子量角蛋

表11.14 用于诊断、排除和分类间皮瘤的抗体

一抗	克隆	抗原特征	免疫原	厂家	稀释度	抗原修复类型
角蛋白	AE1/AE3	角蛋白-分子序号1~5、6、8、9、10、14~16、18	人表皮的角蛋白	DAKO	1:200	HIER
角蛋白	MAK-6	角蛋白-分子序号8、14~16、18、19	MCF-组织培养和人单层表皮的细胞外抗原	Zymed	1:100	HIER
角蛋白	5D3	角蛋白-分子序号8、18	结肠癌细胞株	BioGenex	1:100	HIER
角蛋白	35βH11	角蛋白-分子序号8	Hep3B肝癌细胞株	DAKO	1:50	HIER
角蛋白	34βE11	角蛋白-分子序号1、5、10、14	人角质层角蛋白	DAKO	1:100	HIER
CK5/CK6	D5/16B4	角蛋白-分子序号5、6，少数为角蛋白4	纯化的CK5	Biocare Medical	1:100	HIER
CK7	OV-TL 12/30	角蛋白-分子序号7	OTN II型卵巢癌细胞株	Cell Marque	NA	HIER
CK20	K_s20.8	角蛋白-分子序号20	人十二指肠黏膜绒毛	Cell Marque	NA	HIER
波形蛋白	Vim3B4	中间丝57kD	牛眼晶状体波形蛋白	DAKO	1:100	HIER
α-肌动蛋白	IA4	α-平滑肌肌动蛋白	人α-平滑肌肌动蛋白的N-末端十肽	Cell Marque	NA	HIER
肌肉特异性肌动蛋白	HHF-35	分子量为42kD纯化的骨骼肌肌动蛋白以及动脉、子宫、膜性组织和心脏的提取物	用SDS从人心肌组织里提取的蛋白成分	Cell Marque	NA	HIER
结蛋白	NCL-DE-R-11	肌细胞中53kD中间丝，识别18kD杆状分子片段	猪胃中纯化的结蛋白	Ventana	NA	HIER
calretinin		29kD的钙结合蛋白	人重组calretinin	Cell Marque	NA	HIER
间皮瘤抗原	HBME-1	间皮细胞膜上的抗原	恶性上皮型间皮瘤中的间皮细胞悬浮液	DAKO	1:400	HIER
血栓调节素	1009	75kD跨膜糖蛋白，含6个与表皮生长因子同源的重复结构域	重组血栓调节素	DAKO	1:50	HIER
EMA	E29	乳脂球蛋白家族中250~400kD的糖蛋白	人乳脂提取物的稀释液	Ventana	NA	HIER
人乳脂糖蛋白-2 (HMFG-2)	115D8	见于上皮细胞多糖外被>400kD的MAM-6黏糖蛋白	纯化的人乳脂糖蛋白	BioGenex	1:25	HIER

一抗	克隆	抗原特征	免疫原	厂家	稀释度	抗原修复类型
N-钙黏素	389	钙依赖性细胞黏附中的转膜糖蛋白	鸡N-钙黏素的细胞内结构域	Zymed	1∶100	HIER
多克隆癌胚抗原（CEA）		CEA和CEA样蛋白，包括非特异性交叉反应物质和胆汁糖蛋白	从转移性结肠腺癌里分离的人CEA	Ventana	NA	HIER
CD15（LeuM1）	C3D-1	3-岩藻糖-N-乙酰乳糖胺	从正常人外周血中纯化的中性粒细胞	Ventana	NA	HIER
肿瘤相关糖蛋白	B72.3	多种类型的人腺癌肿瘤相关糖蛋白	转移性乳腺癌的膜丰富区域	Cell Marque	NA	HIER
人上皮型抗原	VU-1D9	大部分上皮细胞（除了鳞状上皮、肝细胞和体腔细胞）表面和细胞浆里的34&49 kD糖蛋白	MCF-7细胞株	Ventana	NA	HIER
甲状腺球蛋白	2H11+6E1	甲状腺球蛋白	人甲状腺腺体的甲状腺球蛋白	Cell Marque	NA	HIER
甲状腺转录因子-1（TTF-1）	8G7G3/1	同源结构域转录因子NKx2家族的40kD成员	小鼠腹水	Cell Marque	NA	HIER
前列腺特异性抗原（PSA）	ER-PR8	33kD前列腺特异性抗原	纯化的人前列腺特异性抗原	Ventana	NA	HIER
前列腺酸性磷酸酶（PAP）	PASE/4LJ	52kD人前列腺酸性磷酸酶	从人精液中纯化的前列腺酸性磷酸酶	Ventana	NA	HIER
人上皮型相关抗原	MOC-31	大部分正常和恶性上皮细胞中的40kD跨膜糖蛋白	神经酰胺酶处理的小细胞癌细胞株细胞	DAKO	1∶50	HIER
Lewis Y抗原	BG8-F3	2型血型寡糖中的二聚岩藻糖四糖	SK-LU-3肺癌细胞株	Signet	1∶40	HIER
E-钙黏素	4A2C7	钙依赖性细胞黏附素中的跨膜糖蛋白	重组人E-钙黏素	Ventana	NA	HIER
Gross cystic disease fluid protein-15（BRST-2）	D6	乳腺病理性分泌物构成的数个糖蛋白，包括15kD单体蛋白	Gross cystic disease fluid protein-15	Signet	1∶50	HIER
雌激素受体蛋白	1D5	66kD的具有配体激活转录因子功能的核激素蛋白成员	重组人雌激素受体蛋白	Ventana	NA	HIER
c-erb-B2癌蛋白		c-erb-B2癌基因190kD蛋白产物	合成人c-erb-B2癌蛋白多肽	DAKO	1∶500	HIER
人白细胞抗原CD45	DAKO-LCA	大多数人白细胞表面的5个或5个以上高分子量糖蛋白	维持T细胞生长因子的人外周血淋巴细胞	Ventana	NA	HIER

续表

一抗	克隆	抗原特征	免疫原	厂家	稀释度	抗原修复类型
CD20，人B淋巴细胞抗原	L26	33kD 非糖基化的跨膜蛋白	人扁桃体B淋巴细胞	Ventana	NA	HIER
CD3，人T淋巴细胞抗原		CD3抗原的胞浆内成分	合成人CD3多肽	Ventana	NA	HIER
CD30 Ki-1抗原	Ber-H2	120kD 跨膜糖蛋白	Co细胞株细胞	Ventana	NA	HIER
bcl-2癌蛋白	124	线粒体内抑制凋亡的25kD 整数倍蛋白	bcl-2蛋白的合成多肽序列氨基酸41~54	Ventana	NA	HIER
NSE		烯醇化酶的γ-球蛋白亚基	从人脑中分离的NSE	DAKO	1:400	HIER
CgA	DAK-A3	内分泌和神经元细胞分泌腺蛋白中的的分泌粒蛋白和嗜铬素蛋白成员	CgA C-末端的20kD 片段	Ventana	NA	HIER
Syn		神经突触小泡中的38kD 膜成分	合成人Syn多肽偶联卵清蛋白	Cell Marque	NA	HIER
S-100		S-100蛋白A和B	牛脑中分离的S-100蛋白	Ventana	NA	HIER
黑色素瘤抗原	HMB-45	不成熟黑色素小体复合糖对神经氨酸酶敏感的寡糖侧链	淋巴结中转移的恶性黑色素瘤中的色素提取物	DAKO	1:200	HIER
CD34	My10	人造血干细胞相关的105~120kD 单链跨膜糖蛋白	CD34抗原	Ventana	NA	HIER
CD31	JC/70A	内皮细胞中的100kD 糖蛋白和血小板中的130kD 糖蛋白	毛细胞白血病病人脾中的膜性标本	Cell Marque	NA	HIER
Ⅷ因子抗原		人von Willebrand因子	从人血浆中分离的von Willebrand因子	Cell Marque	NA	HIER
间皮素	5B2	间皮素分子的氨基酸	小鼠骨髓瘤	Novo Castra	NA	HIER
WT-1	6F-H2	染色体11p13上的肿瘤抑制基因	小鼠组织培养上清液中的抗体	Cell Marque	NA	HIER
D2-40	D2-40	癌胚抗原M2A	小鼠腹水	Signet	NA	HIER
表面活性脂蛋白A(SP-A)	PE-10	表面活性剂A	肺泡蛋白沉积症病人肺冲洗液中分离的表面活性脂蛋白	DAKO	1:100	HIER
CDX2	CDX2-88	调节肠上皮细胞增生和分化的肠特异性转录因子同源家族	全长CDX2	BioGenex	NA	HIER
p63	4A4	人p63蛋白，p53蛋白家族成员	小鼠单克隆抗体	Cell Marque	1:100	HIER

表 11.15　上皮型间皮瘤、肺腺癌和鳞状细胞癌中的 CK 表达情况

肿瘤类型	CK 的分子序列号、分子量和等电 pH																			
	1	2	3	4	5	6	7	8	9	10	11	12	13	14	15	16	17	18	19	20
	68 kD	65.5 kD	63 kD	59 kD	58 kD	56 kD	54 kD	52.5 kD	64 kD	56.5 kD	56 kD	55 kD	54 kD	50 kD	50 kD	48 kD	46 kD	45 kD	40 kD	46 kD
	7.8	7.8	7.5	7.3	7.4	7.8	6.0	6.1	5.4	5.3	5.3	4.9	5.1	5.3	4.9	5.1	5.1	5.7	5.2	5.2
原发性肺腺癌	N	N	N	N	N	N	S	S	N	N	N	N	N	N	N	N	N	N	S	R
上皮型间皮瘤	N	N	N	N	S	S	S	S	N	N	N	N	N	N	N	S	N	N	S	R
原发性肺鳞状细胞癌	N	N	N	S	S	S	R	S	N	N	N	N	N	N	S	S	S	S	S	R

反应性：+，几乎总是弥漫强阳性；S，有时候阳性；R，少数细胞阳性；N，几乎总是阴性

表 11.16　组织学类型不同的间皮瘤免疫组化阳性比率

	Pan-CK	CK5/6	calretinin	WT-1	血栓调节素	SMA
上皮型间皮瘤	100	100	100	69	81	50
混合型间皮瘤/上皮样成分	100	40	90	60	90	20
混合型间皮瘤/肉瘤样成分	90	10	60	20	50	60
肉瘤样间皮瘤	70	0	70	10	70	60
肉瘤和肺肉瘤样癌的免疫组化阳性比例						
肉瘤	17	4	17	4	38	58
肉瘤样癌	90	0	60	0	40	10

（引自Lucas Dr, Pass HI, Madan NV, et al. Sarcomatoid mesothelioma and its histological mimics：a comparative immunohistochemical study. Histopathology 2003; 42: 270-279)

白（35βH11、CAM5.2）抗体发现，在同一例肉瘤样型间皮瘤中，某些区域可以染色很强，而另一些区域可以没有任何染色。

Lucas 等[272]检测了 20 例具有肉瘤样成分的间皮瘤（10例混合型和10例肉瘤样型）中广谱CK、CK5/6、calretinin、WT-1、血栓调节素和SMA的表达情况，并比较了这些肿瘤与 24 例高级别肉瘤、10 例肺肉瘤样癌和16例上皮型间皮瘤的免疫表型。在 10 例肺肉瘤样癌中还检测了 TTF-1 的表达情况。结果见表 11.16，简单总结如下：①肉瘤样型间皮瘤中的上皮和间皮抗原决定簇减少；②肉瘤样型间皮瘤、肉瘤和肉瘤样癌之间存在较广的免疫表型重叠；③CK 和 calretinin是区分肉瘤样型间皮瘤和肉瘤的最有价值的标记物；④除了 SMA，其他所有标记物在肉瘤样型间皮瘤和肉瘤样癌中分布相似，包括在这两种肿瘤中都高表达的calretinin和血栓调节素；⑤由于CK在肉瘤样型间皮瘤中可以不表达，所以其与肉瘤的表达差异具有较大的主观性；⑥免疫组化在区分肉瘤样肿瘤和上皮样肿瘤中有很大的局限性，应该将肿瘤的大体、显微镜下图像及免疫组化结果相联系进行诊断。

Attanoos 等[273]用CK、血栓调节素、calretinin 和 CK5/6 抗体分析了 31 例肉瘤样型间皮瘤和一系列其他梭形细胞肿瘤，发现 31 例肉瘤样型间皮瘤中有 24 例（77%）表达CK，9 例（29%）表达calretinin，12 例（39%）表达血栓调节素，12 例（39%）表达CK5/6。9 例肉瘤有 2 例（非特殊性肉瘤）（22%）表达广谱CK和血栓调节素，1 例（11%）表达CK5/6。正如我们所推测的，100% 的滑膜肉瘤表达广谱CK但不表达血栓调节素、calretinin 和 CK5/6。在 3 例血管肉瘤中有 2 例（67%）表达血栓调节素，此结果并不奇怪，因为血栓调节素在正常的内皮细胞中就可以表达。此作者认为将广谱CK和calretinin联用可以提高诊断肉瘤样型间皮瘤的敏感性（77%表达 AE1/AE3）和特异性（100%表达calretinin）。他们指出间皮标记物血栓调节素和CK5/6单独使用对诊断肉瘤样型间皮瘤没有价值。他们的研究也提示3%的肉瘤样型间皮

瘤不表达广谱CK，这同样支持存在CK阴性的肉瘤样型间皮瘤的论点。

本文作者没有发现Lucas等[272]所报道的肉瘤中存在广谱角蛋白（AE1/AE3角蛋白）表达，也没有发现肉瘤样型间皮瘤、肉瘤或肉瘤样癌中存在同样程度的calretinin表达。本文作者的经验是，肉瘤中仅有不到1%表达广谱角蛋白，calretinin在肉瘤样型间皮瘤中的阳性率不会超过20%，在肉瘤或肉瘤样癌中是不表达的。其他学者免疫组化结果与之相似（见下面）。

波形蛋白是58kD的中间丝蛋白，主要在间叶来源的细胞中表达。尽管早在20世纪70年代末80年代初就发现波形蛋白可以帮助区分癌和肉瘤，但最近发现，在正常上皮细胞和各种类型的癌中都表达波形蛋白[274-277]。本文作者的经验是，所有的肉瘤样型间皮瘤都表达波形蛋白，通常都是强阳性，在大多数未分化和过渡型间皮瘤中也表达波形蛋白。Churg[278]报道了2例酒精固定的上皮型间皮瘤中都表达波形蛋白，其中1例为小管乳头型。Jasani等[279]发现44例恶性间皮瘤中75%都有波形蛋白表达，而24例肺腺癌中46%也被证实存在波形蛋白表达。Mullink等[280]发现上皮型间皮瘤比肺腺癌更常见到角蛋白和波形蛋白共表达，该作者还发现30%～45%的上皮型间皮瘤可共表达角蛋白和波形蛋白。

就本文作者来说，calretinin抗体是一种特异性和可重复性都很好的上皮型间皮瘤抗体，跟S-100蛋白相似，也是一种钙结合蛋白[281,282]，分子量为29kD，在中枢和周围神经系统以及相当范围的非神经细胞，包括卵巢和睾丸的产类固醇的细胞、脂肪细胞、肾小管上皮细胞、外分泌腺细胞、胸腺上皮细胞和间皮细胞中都存在表达。Gotzos等[283]发现7例上皮型间皮瘤（100%）和15例混合型间皮瘤（100%）中的上皮成分全部表达calretinin，而在混合型间皮瘤中的肉瘤样成分和1例肉瘤样型间皮瘤中没有发现存在calretinin表达，在4例肺腺癌中也呈阴性表达。Doglioni等[284]发现44例（100%）上皮型间皮瘤全部表达calretinin，294例不同来源的腺癌中有28例（9.5%）呈局灶性阳性，在3例肉瘤样型间皮瘤（100%）和5例混合型间皮瘤的肉瘤样成分中都呈阳性表达。Barberis等[285]研究了浆液中的细胞，发现8例上皮型间皮瘤（100%）全部存在calretinin阳性表达，13例腺癌中有3例（23.1%）呈弱阳性表达。Leers等[286]发现20例上皮型间皮瘤（100%）全部呈calretinin阳性表达，21例腺癌（4.8%）中只有1例呈弱阳性表达。

Ordonez[287]比较了两种商业化calretinin抗体，发现Zymed实验室的抗体在38例上皮型间皮瘤中有8例（21.1%）呈阳性表达，155例不同类型的腺癌中有14例（9%）呈局灶性弱阳性表达。而CHEMICON公司的抗体在38例上皮型间皮瘤中有28例（73.1%）、155例腺癌中有6例（3.8%）呈阳性表达。作者使用了Biocare的calretinin抗体进行实验，发现210例上皮型间皮瘤中有198例（94%）呈calretinin阳性表达，像S-100蛋白一样，阳性部位在胞浆和胞核（图11.46）。应该注意的是，反应性的多潜能胸膜下梭形细胞也表达calretinin。

其他研究也表明[288-291]calretinin是一种区分上皮型间皮瘤和肺腺癌以及其他上皮样肿瘤的高度特异性和敏感性抗体。

ME1抗体的作用最初被O'Hara等[292]在1990年报道。ME1是从SPC111细胞系中分离出来的一种单克隆抗体，在正常间皮细胞和恶性上皮型间皮瘤中表达。此抗体仅能在冰冻切片中使用，并在40例上皮型间皮瘤（100%）中全部表达。19例高分化和中分化原发性肺腺癌不表达ME1，而在1例低分化肺腺癌中呈强阳性表达。经Sheibani等[293]总结，Battifora公司生产的ME1单克隆抗体，命名为HBME-1，可以在福尔马林固定、石蜡包埋的切片中应用。许多作者报道，该抗体在上皮型间皮瘤阳性率较高，主要于细胞膜着色（图11.47），就该作者的经验，每例标本之间的阳性强度存在差异。DAKO公司产品说明书提到19例上皮型间皮瘤中有17例（89.5%）呈HBME-1阳性表达，但该抗体在50例腺癌中也有19例（38%）呈阳性表达。说明书推荐的稀释度为1∶100，

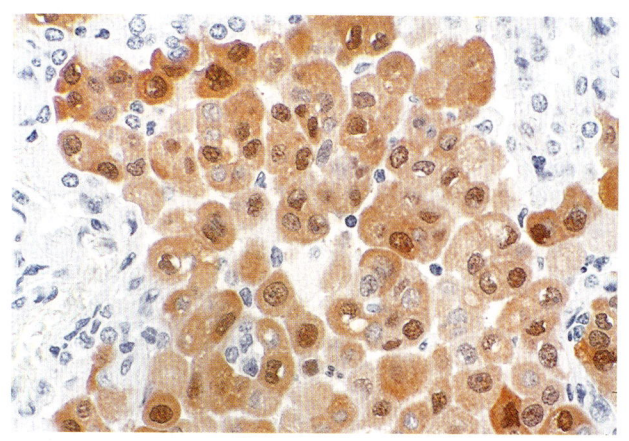

图11.46 大部分高至中高分化上皮型间皮瘤和少数肉瘤样间皮瘤的胞浆和胞核呈calretinin阳性表达（×400）

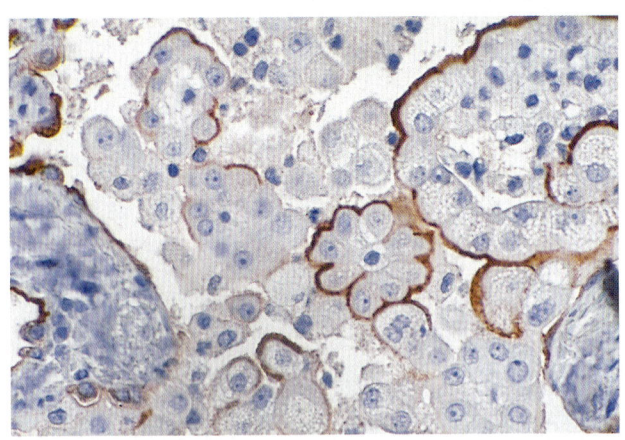

图11.47 大部分高至中高分化上皮型间皮瘤的胞膜呈HBME-1强阳性表达（×400）

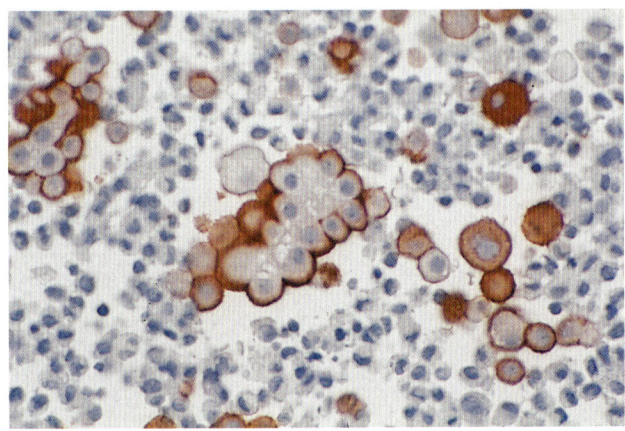

图11.48 大部分高至中高分化上皮型间皮瘤呈EMA厚胞膜阳性染色（×400）

本文作者的经验是，应该使用更大的稀释度（本文作者实验室使用的是1:7500）。这与Henderson等[254]报道的稀释度相似，他们使用的稀释度在1:5000到1:15 000之间。他们发现，当使用更低稀释度的时候，许多间皮瘤和相当一部分的腺癌都表达阳性，这些结果提示HBME-1应该使用高稀释度才能更有效地区分上皮型间皮瘤和其他肿瘤。该作者没有发现HBME-1在诊断肉瘤样型间皮瘤中有何帮助，在腺癌中也几乎不见阳性表达。有趣的是，HBME-1在呼吸性上皮中可以表达，偶尔也可以在原发性肺鳞状细胞癌的细胞膜上表达。

EMA和人乳脂糖蛋白（HMFG-2）都属于高分子量（250～400kD）糖蛋白，并以乳糖蛋白为大家所熟知。这些糖蛋白存在于乳脂中并在肿瘤性上皮细胞中或多或少的存在。抗EMA和HMFG-2抗体可以用来诊断上皮型间皮瘤，阳性部位主要在胞膜（目前仅能得到抗EMA抗体），而大部分的腺癌和其他癌阳性部位主要在胞浆。我们[294]检测到在64例上皮型间皮瘤中有50例（78.1%）、60例腺癌中有37例（61.7%）、19例鳞状细胞癌中有8例（42%）表达EMA。Walz和Koch[295]报道在44例上皮型间皮瘤中有33例表达EMA。Wick等[296]发现在51例上皮型间皮瘤中有43例（84%）呈EMA阳性表达。如前所述，抗原主要集中在细胞膜上，而间皮瘤细胞的表面有大量的微绒毛，所以大部分高分化和中分化的上皮型间皮瘤都出现"厚"的胞膜反应（图11.48）。Henderson等[297]证实在上皮型间皮瘤中呈现细胞表面EMA的强阳性表达，一些淋巴样细胞膜上也可见到阳性表达。根据该作者的经验，大部分反应性（良性）的上皮样间皮细胞不表达EMA和HMFG-2。该作者还发现在某些非黏液性细支气管肺泡细胞癌和肾乳头状腺癌中可见相对较强的EMA和HMFG-2阳性染色。

血栓调节素是一种浆膜相关性糖蛋白，有很强的抗凝血作用。存在于多种细胞中，包括系膜细胞、滑膜细胞、间皮细胞、内皮细胞、巨噬细胞和一些鳞状上皮细胞。Fink等[298]证实在8例上皮型间皮瘤和2例间皮细胞株中存在血栓调节素表达，这些细胞株的原位杂交结果表明细胞内存在血栓调节素的mRNA。相反，15例腺癌中有14例（93.3%）呈血栓调节素阴性表达，仅1例呈局灶性阳性。Collins等[299]发现31例上皮型间皮瘤（100%）和48例肺腺癌中的4例（8.3%）表达血栓调节素。相反，Brown等[300]仅在60%的上皮型和混合型间皮瘤中发现存在血栓调节素阳性表达，而在58%的肺腺癌中存在阳性表达。Ascoli等[301]证实在33例上皮型间皮瘤（100%）、35例反应性渗出的间皮细胞以及57/145例（39.3%）渗出的癌细胞中都发现存在血栓调节素阳性表达。他们报道在良性反应性间皮细胞、恶性上皮型间皮瘤和癌中的血栓调节素表达模式不同，良性反应性间皮细胞的阳性反应呈细线型，恶性上皮型间皮瘤呈膜着色且较厚，而大多数癌呈胞浆染色。

钙黏素是一个黏附蛋白家族，在特异的组织形态分类过程中起重要作用[302, 303]。钙黏素家族包括上皮（E）钙黏素、神经（N）钙黏素、视网膜（R）钙黏素、成骨细胞（OB）钙黏素和胎盘（P）钙黏素。N-钙黏素是一个在神经细胞、分化的肌细胞和间皮细胞中发现的分子量为135 000kD的蛋白[304]。Peralta-Soler等[305]用13A9抗N-钙黏素单克隆抗体在冰冻切片中发现，19例上皮型间皮瘤全部（100%）呈强阳性表达，16例肺腺癌中有3例（18.8%）呈局灶弱阳性。

Han等[306]用抗原修复法在石蜡包埋切片中发现，13例上皮型间皮瘤中有12例（92.3%）、14例肺腺癌中有1例（7.1%）呈N-钙黏素阳性表达。

Ordonez[307]分析了31例上皮型间皮瘤和29例肺腺癌中5H9、HECD-1和克隆36抗E-钙黏素抗体以及3B9和克隆32抗N-钙黏素抗体的表达情况，发现68%、52%和19%的上皮型间皮瘤分别表达E-钙黏素克隆36、克隆HECD-1和克隆5H9；74%和71%的上皮型间皮瘤分别表达N-钙黏素克隆3B9和克隆32；93%、90%和90%的肺腺癌分别表达E-钙黏素克隆36、克隆HECD-1和克隆5H9；45%和34%的肺腺癌分别表达N-钙黏素克隆32和克隆3B9。Ordonez总结说，只有5H9抗E-钙黏素抗体在区分胸膜的上皮型间皮瘤和肺腺癌中是有帮助的。

Wilms瘤抑制基因（WT-1）位于11p13染色体，其失活可易感Wilms肿瘤。该基因主要存在于中胚层来源的组织中。Amin等[308]用冰冻组织切片发现21例恶性间皮瘤中有20例（95.2%）核呈阳性表达，而在26例肺非间皮肿瘤（包括20例原发性非小细胞癌）中无一例表达。Kumar-Singh等[309]用可以用于福尔马林固定、石蜡包埋切片的抗体发现，42例间皮瘤中的39例（92.9%）、2例卵巢乳头状癌（100%）和1例肾细胞癌（100%）全部呈WT-1蛋白强阳性表达。12例肺腺癌、4例肺鳞状细胞癌、8例乳腺转移腺癌和3例结肠转移腺癌中不表达WT-1蛋白。由此可见，该抗体在诊断间皮瘤中具潜在价值。用分子生物学技术发现，26个间皮瘤细胞株中的23个（88.5%）和8例人恶性间皮瘤中的5例（62.5%）表达WT-1转录产物，而在非小细胞肺癌细胞株和少数活检标本中未发现存在WT-1转录产物表达。

间皮素是一个分子量为40kD的糖蛋白，其具体作用尚不清楚，主要在间皮细胞、卵巢的浆液细胞和胰腺的胆管细胞中高表达。Ordonez[311]用单克隆抗体5B2发现在正常间皮细胞、间皮瘤、非黏液性卵巢癌中都存在间皮素阳性表达，偶尔在其他肿瘤中也可见到表达（见Ordonez文章中的表1）。Ordonez最后总结说，尽管14例卵巢癌、14例胰腺胆管腺癌中的12例、12例促结缔组织增生型小圆细胞肿瘤中的7例和9例滑膜肉瘤都表达间皮素，该抗体（5B2）仍可以用来帮助诊断间皮瘤，但在使用时要注意正确分析。

D2-40是最近报道的一种商业化抗M2A抗体，分子量为40 000kD，属于唾液酸糖蛋白，主要存在于生殖细胞和淋巴内皮。Chu等[312]分析了53例间皮瘤、28例反应性胸膜组织、30例肺腺癌、35例肾细胞癌、26例卵巢浆液性癌、16例浸润性乳腺癌、11例前列腺腺癌和7例尿路上皮癌中D2-40的表达情况，发现，53例间皮瘤中有51例（96%）、28例反应性胸膜组织中有27例（96%）、26例卵巢浆液性癌中有17例（65%）存在D2-40阳性表达，而在其他肿瘤中未发现D2-40表达。肿瘤细胞的阳性表达部位在细胞膜上。

> **诊断要点**：阳性间皮标记物
> 1. 可以用于诊断的有：calretinin、WT-1、CK5/6、HBME-1、EMA、血栓调节素。
> 2. D2-40尚处于初期研究阶段。

阴性标记物

在所有用于诊断上皮型间皮瘤的排除性抗体中，多克隆CEA是最常用的。CEA是一种分子量将近200kD的糖蛋白，含有约50%碳水化合物[313-316]，它是一个由29个基因编码的家族，其中有18个基因表达，7个属于CEA亚群，11个属于妊娠特异性亚群。

虽然是一个癌胚抗原，CEA在正常成人组织和多种上皮型肿瘤中也有表达，其亚群包括胆汁性糖蛋白和非特异交叉反应性物质。该作者用的抗体是多克隆性的，免疫原CEA来自转移到肝的结肠腺癌。该抗体与非特异交叉反应性物质和胆汁糖蛋白反应。非特异交叉反应性物质在粒细胞和单核细胞中表达，胆汁糖蛋白在大量正常上皮细胞和粒细胞、淋巴细胞中表达，内皮细胞也可能会表达胆汁糖蛋白。因此，大部分组织切片可以作为多克隆CEA的阳性内对照。

大部分上皮型间皮瘤不表达多克隆CEA[318-320]，相反，在肺腺癌中阳性表达率（85%~100%）却很高。Henderson等[297]从21个独立报道中分析了598例弥漫性恶性间皮瘤，发现58例（9.7%）存在CEA表达，且在大多数阳性表达的病例中，主要是局灶性和弱阳性表达。而在404例肺腺癌中发现有359例（88.9%）表达CEA。该作者观察到CEA阳性的间皮瘤是罕见的，主要是在"黏液素"阳性的上皮型间皮瘤中表达，该黏液素可能与产生大量透明质酸或蛋白多糖有关。据该作者的经验，多克隆CEA是最好的间皮瘤阴性标记物。

LeuM1是一种抗骨髓单核细胞3-岩藻糖-N-乙酰乳糖胺的单克隆抗体。其抗原又称为CD15或X-半抗原。LeuM1在大部分霍奇金淋巴瘤的Reed-Sternberg

细胞中表达。1985 年，Sheibani 和 Battifora[321]报道了一例转移性低分化肺腺癌表达 LeuM1。1986 年，Sheibani 等[322]用免疫组化法检测了 400 例恶性肿瘤中 LeuM1 的表达，发现 179 例腺癌中有 105 例（58.7%）呈 LeuM1 阳性表达，18 例上皮型间皮瘤中未见表达。他们随后[323]又研究了 50 例原发性肺腺癌和 28 例胸膜上皮型间皮瘤，发现 50 例肺腺癌中有 47 例（94%）呈阳性表达，28 例上皮型间皮瘤中未见表达。在另一项研究中，Sheibani 等[324]报道在 127 例恶性间皮瘤中没有发现 LeuM1 的阳性表达。Wick 及其同事[296]也证实 52 例肺腺癌全部（100%）表达 LeuM1，而 51 例上皮型间皮瘤全部呈阴性表达。相反，Otis 等[325]则发现仅有 50% 的肺腺癌表达 LeuM1，而上皮型间皮瘤中也可以表达 LeuM1。Battifora 和 McCaughey 等[248]发现上皮型间皮瘤中 LeuM1 呈局灶性表达。本文作者观察了数例 LeuM1 阳性的上皮型间皮瘤，也发现阳性多为局灶性，与目前文献报道相反的是，不管是否应用抗原热修复，本文作者仅在大约 50% 的原发性肺腺癌中发现存在 LeuM1（CD15）的阳性反应。

B72.3 抗体是一种能识别高分子量糖蛋白复合体的肿瘤相关糖蛋白 72（TAG-72），来源于人转移性乳腺癌的富于膜的片段。Szpak 等[326]和 Ordonez 等[327]报道在 45 例肺腺癌中有 38 例（84.4%）呈 B72.3 阳性表达，38 例上皮型间皮瘤中仅有 1 例（2.6%）呈阳性表达。Wick 等[296]报道 52 例肺腺癌中有 43 例（82.6%）表达 B72.3，而在 51 例上皮型间皮瘤中未见表达。Bollinger 等在腹膜间皮瘤和腹膜浆液性乳头状腺癌的研究中发现 46 例浆液性乳头状腺癌中有 43 例（93.4%）呈 B72.3 阳性表达，8 例上皮型间皮瘤均为阴性。Ordonez[255]列表显示了文献报道的 684 例上皮型间皮瘤中有 69 例（10.1%）呈 B72.3 阳性表达（0%～48%），607 例腺癌中有 578 例（95.2%）呈阳性表达（47%～100%），上皮型间皮瘤 B72.3 呈阳性表达时，通常只有一小部分细胞染色阳性。Henderson 等[254]报道上皮型间皮瘤中 B72.3 的阳性表达更多的是出现在胞浆中，他还描述了 1 例与胞浆内糖蛋白超微结构相关的新月形阳性染色的病例。

BerEP4 是一种能识别人上皮细胞 2、34 和 39kD 糖多肽半抗原决定簇的单克隆抗体。Latza 等[329]发现 144 例不同部位的腺癌中有 142 例（98.6%）呈 BerEP4 阳性反应，而在 14 例上皮型间皮瘤中均为阴性。Sheibani 等[330]发现 115 例上皮型间皮瘤中有 1 例（0.86%）、83 例不同位点的腺癌中有 72 例（86.7%）呈 BerEP4 阳性表达，25 例乳腺癌中的 8 例以及 3 例肾细胞癌为阴性表达。Gaffey 等[331]的结果有所不同，他们发现在 120 例腺癌中有 103 例（83%）呈 BerEP4 阳性反应，而 49 例上皮型间皮瘤中的 10 例（20%）和 9 例腺瘤样肿瘤中的 2 例（22%）也呈阳性反应。Gaffey 等[331]报道了 1 例上皮型间皮瘤 BerEP4 呈弥漫阳性。BerEP4 的阳性表达部位一般在胞膜上。对这些不同结果的可能解释是，Sheibani 等[330]在 BerEP4 染色之前用 14 型蛋白酶进行了预消化，而 Gaffey 等[331]则在染色前用 0.4% 的胃蛋白酶预消化了 30 分钟。目前我们用热修复抗原法发现约 20% 的上皮型间皮瘤细胞膜呈弱阳性染色。Ordonez[255]总结了已发表的上皮型间皮瘤和不同种类的腺癌中 BerEP4 的阳性表达情况，发现在 611 例上皮型间皮瘤中有 76 例（12.4%）（0%～88%）、1399 例腺癌中有 940 例（67.2%）（35%～100%）呈阳性表达。

MOC31 是一种能与小细胞肺癌的 38kD 上皮相关跨膜糖蛋白反应的单克隆抗体，又被称为上皮型糖蛋白-2[330, 332]。DeLejj 等[333]报道 MOC31 在所有肺癌中呈阳性表达，包括 28 例腺癌（100%）。正常间皮细胞和肿瘤性上皮型间皮细胞不表达该抗体。1991 年，Delahaye 等[334]研究了浆液的细胞学，发现在 24 例上皮型间皮瘤中有 2 例（8.3%）、31 例不同组织来源的腺癌中有 18 例（58.1%）存在 MOC31 的阳性表达。Riutenbeek 等[335]发现 63 例腺癌中有 62 例（98.4%）表达 MOC31，而 5 例上皮型间皮瘤中均无阳性反应。Ordonez 等[336]报道 40 例肺腺癌（100%）、11 例结肠腺癌（100%）、21 例卵巢腺癌中的 20 例（95.2%）、10 例乳腺癌中的 9 例（90%）和 13 例肾腺癌中的 5 例（38.5%）都呈 MOC31 强阳性表达。在 38 例上皮型间皮瘤中也发现 2 例（5.3%）呈 MOC31 阳性反应，但反应呈局灶性，阳性细胞数不超过 10%。Ordonez 等[255]总结了发表过的上皮型间皮瘤和不同类型腺癌中 MOC31 的阳性反应情况，发现在 333 例腺癌中有 307 例（92.2%）（58%～100%），158 例上皮型间皮瘤中有 23 例（14.6%）呈 MOC31 阳性表达（0%～88%）。

单克隆抗体 Bg8 在 SK-LU-3 肺癌细胞中呈阳性表达，能够识别血型抗原 Lewis^y。Jordon 等[337]报道在 18 例肺腺癌（100%）和 30 例上皮型间皮瘤中的 7 例（23.3%）都表达 Bg8。间皮瘤中 Bg8 表达通常呈局灶性，只有少数细胞呈阳性反应，而在肺腺癌中通常为弥漫强阳性反应。Riera 等[338]发现 123 例肺腺癌中的114例（92.7%）、57例上皮型间皮瘤中的5例（8.8%）呈Bg8阳性表达，上皮型间皮瘤中的染色常为局灶弱阳性。

E-钙黏素是一种在上皮细胞中表达、分子量为120kD的细胞黏附分子[302, 339]。E-钙黏素失表达与多种癌（包括肺癌）浸润及恶性潜能增高密切相关[340]。Peralta-Sler等[305]报道E-钙黏素在16例肺腺癌中全部（100%）呈强阳性表达，19例上皮型间皮瘤中有8例（42.1%）也存在E-钙黏素阳性表达，但通常只有少数细胞阳性。用热修复抗原法在福尔马林固定的标本中发现，14例肺腺癌中有13例（92.9%）E-钙黏素呈阳性表达，而13例上皮型间皮瘤无一例表达。Leers等[341]报道21例不同组织来源的腺癌中有20例（95.2%），20例上皮型间皮瘤中有3例（15%）表达E-钙黏素。Ordonez[255]用商品化5H9抗E-钙黏素抗体在福尔马林固定、石蜡包埋的切片中发现，18例肺腺癌中有15例（83.3%）呈阳性表达，17例上皮型间皮瘤中为阴性表达。当Ordonez用抗E-钙黏素单克隆抗体克隆36（Transduction Laboratory, Lexington, Kentucky）时，发现6例上皮型间皮瘤全部（100%）呈强阳性表达。这提示大家对该抗体要谨慎使用，而5H9抗E-钙黏素抗体是可以放心使用的。如前所述，Ordonez等[307]认为在区分上皮型间皮瘤和肺腺癌中只有5H9克隆抗E-钙黏素抗体是有帮助的。

血型相关抗原表达已经被用来分析间皮瘤和肺腺癌。Wick等[296]发现52例腺癌中有35例（67.3%）表达ABH同种抗原，而51例上皮型间皮瘤中均为阴性表达。Kawai等[342]用ABH血型相关抗原（BGRA-g）抗体和Helix pomotia凝集素（HPAgg）分析了20例上皮型、3例混合型、6例肉瘤样型间皮瘤和5例反应性间皮病变以及38例高分化肺腺癌，发现反应性间皮病变和间皮瘤不表达BGRA-g和HPAgg，并跟血型无关；40例（83%）血型相同的腺癌病人A、B或H血型相关抗原呈阳性表达。17例A型血中的16例（94.1%）和所有AB型血的病人都表达HPAgg；5例B型血中的4例（80%）和12例O型血中的4例（33.3%）表达HPAgg。

Riera等[338]用热抗原修复研究了268例石蜡包埋、福尔马林固定的肿瘤标本，其中包括57例上皮型间皮瘤和211例不同组织来源的腺癌，经统计学分析发现，在所使用的一系列抗体中，CEA、BerEP4和Bg8是鉴别腺癌和上皮型间皮瘤最好的标记物。间皮瘤相关抗体HBME-1、calretinin和血栓调节素尽管在某些病例的诊断中有帮助，但其敏感性和特异性要差一些。他们观察了所有的腺癌和间皮瘤，发现角蛋白均呈强阳性，两者在染色模式上没有明显区别。在57例间皮瘤中有46例（81.5%）、211例腺癌中有66例（31.2%）都表达波形蛋白。间皮瘤中波形蛋白表达的强度和分布都要强于腺癌。211例腺癌中有175例（82.9%）表达CEA，而间皮瘤中未见表达。卵巢和乳腺腺癌CEA的阳性率分别为44.8%和79.3%。63.7%的腺癌BerEP4呈局灶性阳性，间皮瘤呈阴性表达。88.6%的腺癌Bg8呈阳性，而57例间皮瘤有5例（8.7%）也发现Bg8呈阳性，间皮瘤中的肿瘤细胞仅为局灶性阳性且强度相对要低。211例腺癌中的170例（80.5%）和57例间皮瘤中的2例（3.5%）呈B72.3阳性表达，在间皮瘤中，阳性为局灶性但强度很高。211例腺癌中的159例（75.3%）和123例肺腺癌中的104例（84.5%）LeuM1呈胞浆颗粒状着色。57例间皮瘤中的2例（3.5%）主要为局灶性胞膜阳性。211例腺癌中的180例（85.3%）和57例间皮瘤中的16例（28.1%）呈BerEP4弥漫中等强度的胞浆染色阳性，大部分腺癌主要为胞浆染色，相反，57例上皮型间皮瘤中有33例（57.8%）为胞膜染色，而胞浆通常不着色。在少数病例中，其强的胞膜染色模式跟HBME-1非常相似。

至于间皮瘤相关抗原，在57例上皮型间皮瘤中有28例（49.1%）呈血栓调节素染色阳性，211例腺癌中有13例（6.1%）染色阳性，其中7例为肺腺癌。57例上皮型间皮瘤中有45例（78.9%）呈HBME-1阳性反应，通常是胞膜一周都呈强或中等强度的阳性反应，211例腺癌中有83例（39.3%）通常是在胞膜顶端呈弱阳性反应。211例腺癌中有19例（9%）在胞膜顶端呈强的胞膜染色。在57例上皮型间皮瘤中有24例（42.1%）呈calretinin染色阳性，22例为胞浆颗粒状弥漫性阳性，2例为局灶性阳性，在211例腺癌中有13例（6.1%）呈弱或中等强度的阳性。

Riera等[338]总结的腺癌和间皮瘤标记物的敏感性和特异性分别见表11.17和11.18。

Riera等[338]的研究提供了大量的实践资料。在这些研究中颇为有趣的是，他们使用的HBME-1抗体的稀释度是1∶40，而其他学者用1∶7500，Henderson[254]用的是1∶5000～1∶15 000。本文作者发现在上皮型间皮瘤中calretinin的阳性率（约95%）要高于Riera等[338]的结果。

表11.17 用于诊断腺癌的免疫组化标记物的敏感性和特异性*

抗体	1		2		3	
	敏感性	特异性	敏感性	特异性	敏感性	特异性
CEA-I	83	100	79	100	75	100
CEA-D			75	100	64	100
Bg8-I	89	91	82	91	50	96
Bg8-D			75	100	42	100
BerEP4-I	64	100	64	100	39	100
BerEP4-D			55	100	29	100
B72.3-I	81	96	77	96	68	96
B72.3-D			50	98	19	98
LeuM1-I	75	96	71	96	55	96
LeuM1-D			55	100	33	100
HMFG-2-CI	85	72	64	79	19	89
HMFG-2-CD		72	73	77	40	89

*必要时用 HIER（热抗原修复）
I, 染色强度；D, 染色部位

（引自 Riera JR, Astengo-Osuna C, Longmate JA, et al. The immunohistochemical diagnostic panel for epithelial mesothelioma: a re-evaluation after heat-induced epitope retrieval. Am J Surg Pathol 1997; 21:1409-1419）

表11.18 用于诊断间皮瘤的免疫化标记物的敏感性和特异性*

评分	1		2		3	
	敏感性	特异性	敏感性	特异性	敏感性	特异性
calretinin-I	42	94	31	96	8	100
calretinin-D	49	94	39	97	16	98
血栓调节素 -I	49	94	46	95	35	97
血栓调节素 -D	49	94	32	96	32	96
HBME-1-I†	79	61	74	72	53	91
HBME-2-D†	79	61	65	73	39	89

*必要时用 HIER（热抗原修复）；†仅细胞膜阳性
I, 染色强度；D, 染色部位

（引自 Riera JR, Astengo-Osuna C, Longmate JA, et al. The immunohistochemical diagnostic panel for epithelial mesothelioma: a re-evaluation after heat-induced epitope retrieval. Am J Surg Pathol 1997; 21:1409-1419）

> **诊断要点**：间皮瘤阴性标记物
>
> 1. BerEP4、B72.3、多克隆CEA、LeuM1、MOC-31、Bg8。
> 2. E-钙黏素、克隆 5H9。

其他类型的抗体

肿瘤抑制基因p53的表达产物被认为可以用来鉴别间皮瘤和反应性间皮增生[343, 344]。Ramael等[344]分析了40例非肿瘤反应性胸膜间皮增生性病例和36例上皮型间皮瘤 p53 的表达情况。用 DO-7 和 CM-1 抗体发现在25%的间皮瘤中存在p53的表达，而用PAb240抗体未见阳性反应。p53在间皮瘤的各种组织学分型中表达没有显著差异。Mayall 等[343]用 DO-7 和 CM-1 抗体分析了p53在胃蛋白酶消化的组织切片中的表达情况，发现 16 例上皮型间皮瘤中有 10 例（62.5%）、19 例混合型间皮瘤中有 9 例（47.4%）、12 例肉瘤样型间皮瘤中有 2 例（16.7%）存在 p53 表达，20 例反应增生性间皮细胞中未见表达。研究者们发现，在石棉导致的间皮瘤和非石棉导致的间皮瘤中p53表达没有差异，说明石棉并不是 p53 基因突变的原因。

Hurlimann[346]在福尔马林固定、石蜡包埋的组织切片中发现，16 例间皮瘤中有 9 例（8 例上皮型、1 例混合型）（56.3%）表达结蛋白，阳性染色呈局灶性，极少数肿瘤细胞表达用热修复抗原之后，阳性表达明显提高。16 例间皮瘤中有 4 例（3 例上皮型、1 例混合型）（25%）表达NSE，5例（31.3%）表达CgA（4例上皮型、1例混合型），5例（均为上皮型）（31.3%）表达S-100，极少数肿瘤细胞表达神经上皮性标记物。

Azumi等[347]用免疫组化方法检测了33例上皮型间皮瘤（32例位于胸膜，1例位于腹膜；其中18例为上皮型，10例为混合型，4例为肉瘤样型，1例组织学类型为促结缔组织增生型）和37例腺癌中的透明质酸盐（hyaluronate）表达情况。37例腺癌中的3例（8.1%）和所有的间皮瘤呈透明质酸盐阳性表达，30例间皮瘤呈膜染色阳性，21例呈胞浆阳性，19例呈胞浆和胞膜均阳性。33例间皮瘤中有27例（81.8%）呈中等或更强的阳性反应。因此作者作出总结，透明质酸可以联合其他的标记物以及电镜用来诊断上皮型间皮瘤。

在胸水中检测多聚透明质酸（hyaluronan）已经被看做诊断间皮瘤的一种方法[348]。在13例胸水病人中，多聚透明质酸超过225mg/L的病人只考虑间皮瘤，而不考虑其他诊断。多聚透明质酸超过75mg/L诊断为间皮瘤的特异性为96%，超过225mg/L的特异性为100%。

最近，Martensson等[349]分析了19例男性间皮瘤患者胸水中的多聚透明质酸情况，并用透射CT扫描测量肿瘤体积。发现19例病人中有13例（68.4%）胸水中多聚透明质酸浓度超过7100mg/L，胸水中多聚透明质酸的浓度与血清中的浓度存在明显相关性。在多聚透明质酸导致的间皮瘤中，胸水中多聚透明质酸的浓度与肿瘤的体积呈明显正相关，而与非多聚透明质酸导致的间皮瘤无相关性。

Thylen等[350]分析了多聚透明质酸和非多聚透明质酸导致的恶性间皮瘤中几种免疫组化标记物的表达情况。在多聚透明质酸导致的上皮型间皮瘤中，EMA和CAM5.2角蛋白的表达显著高于非多聚透明质酸导致的恶性间皮瘤，而波形蛋白的表达则低于非多聚透明质酸导致的恶性间皮瘤。两类肿瘤CEA都为阴性。本文作者与Thylen等[350]的结果不同，认为过表达多聚透明质酸或黏多糖的间皮瘤更容易"黏液素"染色阳性，并表达上皮型间皮瘤的阴性标记物如CEA、LeuM1和B72.3。

CA125是胚胎发育和女性生殖系统肿瘤形成过程中在体腔上皮细胞膜上表达的一种糖蛋白[351-354]。在组织切片中用来检测CA125的抗体中，OC-125最初被认为只能在冰冻切片中使用，但后来发现也适用于酶消化或热抗原修复的福尔马林固定、石蜡包埋的切片。很快又发现，OC-125表达不仅限于女性生殖系统肿瘤，在乳腺肿瘤[356]、肺肿瘤[357,358]、胸膜及腹膜肿瘤中都可检测到[359,360]。

第二代CA125抗体M-11比OC-125的染色更强[361]。M-11在6~14周妊娠自发流产标本的间皮细胞中呈阳性反应[362]。本文作者仅发现少数几例上皮型间皮瘤的细胞膜低表达OC-125。

在罕见的情况下，用免疫组化可以发现间皮瘤中出现不常见物质。Okamoto等[363]报道了2例原发性胸膜间皮瘤的间变瘤巨细胞中含有hCG，并可用免疫组化检测。

McAuley等[364]分析了1例伴有高钙血症和血清甲状旁腺样激素过多的恶性间皮瘤病人，他们分析了9例上皮型间皮瘤中甲状旁腺样多肽的表达情况，发现在8例标本中均存在大量肿瘤细胞阳性染色，在正常和反应性上皮型间皮细胞增生中甲状旁腺样多肽也呈阳性反应。

Tateyama等[365]报道胸腺癌、非典型胸腺瘤以及13例间皮瘤中的9例（5例上皮型、3例混合型、1例肉瘤样）（69.2%）都表达CD5，所有CD5阳性的间皮瘤阳性部位都在胞浆。13例肺腺癌中的8例（61.5%）呈低到中等程度的阳性染色，阳性部位主要在胞膜。大多数的间皮瘤呈现多种CD抗原阳性，如CD30、CD56和CD99。

诊断要点

本文作者用了一系列抗体来分析间皮增生性病变（包括反应性增生和肿瘤性增生）。除了CK5/6，角蛋白抗体基本上不能用来区分间皮瘤和其他肿瘤或反应性增生病变，但可以用来分析肿瘤性或反应性间皮细胞增生的程度。在作者所用的抗体中，AE1/AE3 CK、CK5/6、CK7、CK20、波形蛋白、EMA、HBME-1、calretinin、间皮素、WT-1、CEA、LeuM1、B72.3、BerEP4和TTF-1可以用来鉴别高分化或中至高分化上皮型间皮瘤和肺腺癌或非肺腺癌。

图11.49用直方图总结了高至中高分化的上皮型间皮瘤中各抗体的表达情况。高至中高分化上皮型间皮瘤和肺腺癌的免疫组化比较见表11.19。

大部分肉瘤样型间皮瘤表达角蛋白（通常是低分子量角蛋白）、波形蛋白和肌肉特异性肌动蛋白。根据本文作者的经验，一小部分（10%~15%）的肉瘤样型间皮瘤可以表达calretinin，大部分的肉瘤样型间皮瘤不表达CK5/6，约30%的肉瘤样型间皮瘤表达

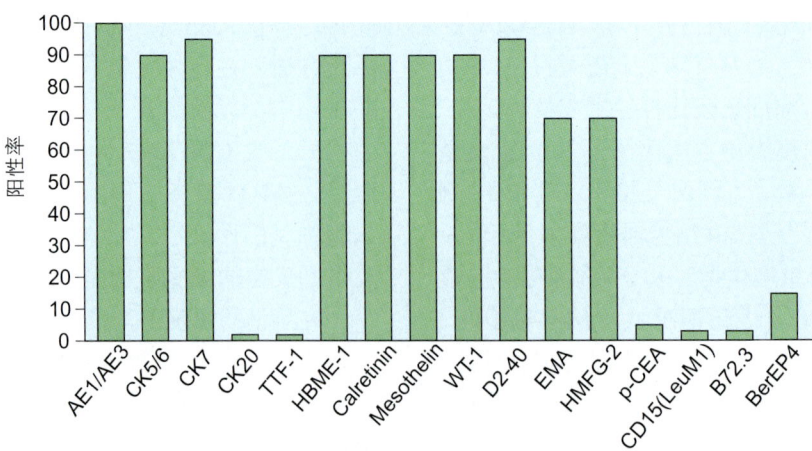

图11.49　高至中高分化上皮型间皮瘤免疫组化柱状图

表11.19　高至中高分化上皮型间皮瘤和高至中高分化肺腺癌免疫组化对比

肿瘤类型	一抗								
	AE1/AE3	低分子量角蛋白 (35βH11)	高分子量角蛋白 (34βE12)	CK5/6	CK7	CK20	波形蛋白	HBME-1	calretinin
高至中高分化上皮型间皮瘤	+	+	+	S	+	S	S	S*	S**
高至中高分化肺腺癌	+	+	S	R	+	S	S	R	R
肿瘤类型	一抗								
	EMA	CEA	CD15 (LeuM1)	BerEP4	B72.3	TTF-1	WT-1	间皮素	D2-40	HMEG-2
高至中高分化上皮型间皮瘤	S*	R	R	S	R	N	+	+	+	S
高至中高分化肺腺癌	S†	+	S	S	S	S	N	N	N	S†

*阳性部位在细胞膜；**阳性部位在核和胞浆；†阳性部位在胞浆
反应性：+ 几乎总是弥漫强阳性；S，有时候阳性；R，少数细胞阳性；N，几乎总是阴性

CK7，有时候可以呈中等强度的表达。根据本文作者的经验，肉瘤样型间皮瘤以及一些可以与之混淆的肿瘤都不表达高或中高分化上皮型间皮瘤的"阴性"标记物，这些抗体包括CEA、LeuM1、B72.3、BerEP4、Bg8和TTF-1。因此，作者在总结可以用于诊断胸膜的恶性梭性细胞增生性病变的抗体时，不会将这些抗体列进来。图11.50用直方图显示了肉瘤样型间皮瘤中各抗体的表达情况。肉瘤样型间皮瘤的免疫组化中最重要的发现就是共表达角蛋白和波形蛋白。

一些分化很低的间皮瘤，像我们[253]所说的"过渡型"，通常只表达广谱CK和波形蛋白。

转移到胸膜的肿瘤要比原发性肿瘤更为常见，任何浸润到胸膜的肿瘤都必须考虑到转移瘤的可能性，并用免疫组化加以鉴别。因此，病人的临床资料就显得非常重要，并可能对免疫组化的选择有很大影响，但病理诊断是建立在客观发现而不是临床病史的基础上。

不明原发灶的转移瘤在第3章里已进行了讨论，这些肿瘤也可以浸润到胸膜。我们和其他的研究人员提供了不明原发灶可疑转移瘤的一些非常有效的病理诊断方法，包括免疫组化和电镜[366,367]。这类肿瘤的组织学图像可以指导选择抗体。病理医师应该熟记间皮

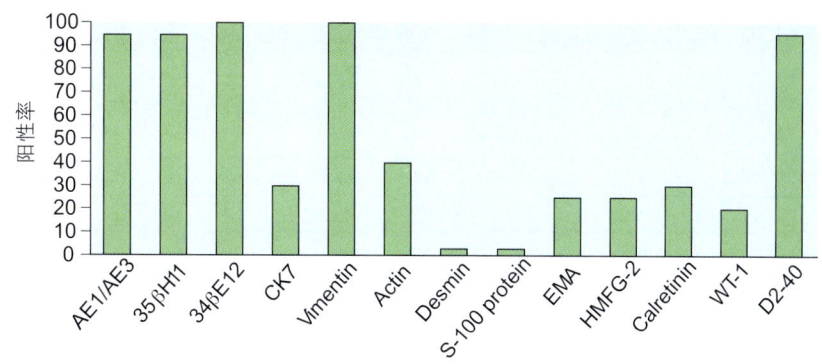

图 11.50　一例肉瘤样型间皮瘤免疫组化柱状图

瘤各种组织学图像，以免将一些不常见的间皮瘤误诊为转移瘤。对于一些可疑的胸膜间皮瘤，临床资料可能会有些帮助：X线证明肿瘤包绕肺组织，在其他器官或组织内未查见肿瘤都可证实为间皮瘤。某些恶性间皮瘤[368]是局灶性的，但有些可能已经发生了弥漫性浸润，而目前的放射技术如CT、MRI尚不能分辨。

不常见 / 罕见的胸膜肿瘤

胸膜的孤立性纤维性肿瘤

胸膜的孤立性局灶性纤维性肿瘤是一种不常见肿瘤，被认为主要来源于胸膜下的结缔组织细胞[369-371]。该肿瘤发生于肺的脏层胸膜下区域，在胸腔内有一细蒂与胸膜相连（通常是脏层胸膜），或者位于壁层胸膜上。该肿瘤体积可以很大，并伴随着某些不常见的临床体征，如低血糖。组织学上，该肿瘤由梭形细胞构成，细胞数量可多可少，并有不同程度的细胞外胶原成分。恶性孤立性局灶性纤维性肿瘤的诊断是很困难的，其恶性指征包括：每10个高倍视野超过4个核分裂象、出血、坏死以及浸润肺和胸壁组织[371]。100%的胸膜局灶性纤维性肿瘤表达波形蛋白，而角蛋白均为阴性，约75%~80%表达CD34，有更高比例的瘤细胞表达抗凋亡蛋白bcl-2[374]，极少数可以表达肌动蛋白[371]。胸膜局灶性纤维性肿瘤与肉瘤样型间皮瘤和肉瘤的比较见表 11.20。

肺的假间皮瘤样癌

某些肺的罕见原发性肿瘤在一定程度上与间皮瘤相似。Babolini 和 Blasi[375]在1956年报道了5例这样的肿瘤，Harwood 等[376]在1976年报道了6例，并提出了"假间皮瘤样癌"的概念。1992年，Koss 等[377]报道了30例肺的假间皮瘤样腺癌，其中15例是已经发表的文献回顾，15 例来源于 Armed Forces 病理研究所的资料。Hartman 和 Schutz[378]报道了72 例，并把这些肿瘤命名为胸膜间皮瘤样肿瘤。后来 Koss 又描述了29例肺的假间皮瘤样腺癌。我们[380]以摘要形式报道了17例，目前正在准备一篇150多例的报道，其中包括一些罕见病例。Attanoos 和 Gibbs[381]在最近也报道了 53 例假间皮瘤样癌。

这些肿瘤在肉眼形态上跟间皮瘤没有差别（图11.51），根据 Koss 等[377, 379]的报道以及我们[380]的经验，大多数肺假间皮瘤样肿瘤是腺癌，而且大部分组织学类型是我们所说的管状促结缔组织增生性假间皮瘤样腺癌（图11.52）。假间皮瘤样肺腺癌通常黏液染色阳性，并表达肺腺癌的免疫组化标记物。偶尔，这些肿瘤也表现出鳞状细胞和小细胞神经内分泌分化，一些为大细胞未分化癌表现，还有一些为低分化癌表现，与低分化间皮瘤很难鉴别。这些低分化假间皮瘤样癌通常共表达角蛋白和波形蛋白，而不表达一些特异性的癌或间皮瘤标记物，有时候几乎不可能与间皮瘤区分开来。Koss 等[377, 379]报道了2例混合型变型，我们报道了1例。

肺的假间皮瘤样腺癌的免疫组化检测与原发性肺腺癌一样，正如我们[380]和Koss等[377, 379]报道的，相当比例的肺假间皮瘤样腺癌发生在接触石棉的病人，在这些病人的肺组织中石棉的含量高于正常人。

假间皮瘤样上皮型血管内皮瘤

极少数由内皮细胞构成的肿瘤跟间皮瘤非常相似，通常指的是假间皮瘤样上皮型血管内皮瘤或上皮型血管内皮瘤样间皮瘤[382, 383]。本文作者提供了1例病例作为Lin等系列[383]研究的补充。该病例是一个50岁的男性，20 岁时在五金店工作，有潜在的石棉接触

表11.20 胸膜的局灶性纤维性肿瘤、肉瘤样间皮瘤和软组织肉瘤的免疫组化比较

肿瘤类型	一抗									
	AE1/AE3	低分子量角蛋白	高分子量角蛋白	CK7	波形蛋白	肌动蛋白	结蛋白	S-100蛋白	CD34	bcl-2
肉瘤样间皮瘤	S	S	S	S	+	S	R	R	R	R
局灶性纤维性肿瘤	N	N	N	N	+	S	N	N	+	+
软组织肉瘤	R	R	R	R	+	S*	S*	S*	R*	R

* 阳性反应取决于软组织肿瘤的类型
反应性：+ 几乎总是弥漫强阳性；S，有时候阳性；R，少数细胞阳性；N，几乎总是阴性

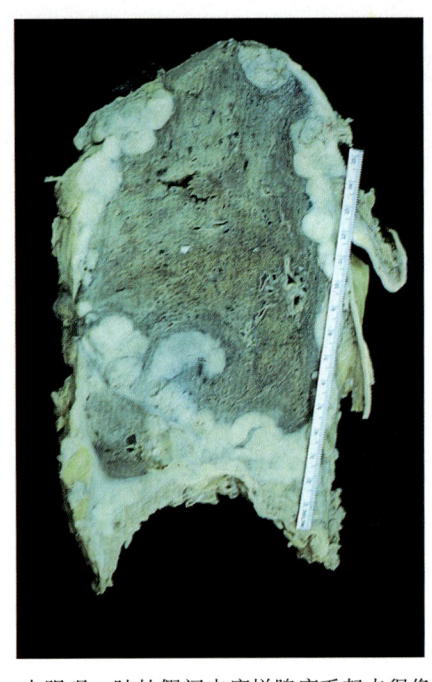

图11.51 肉眼观，肺的假间皮瘤样腺癌看起来很像弥漫性恶性间皮瘤

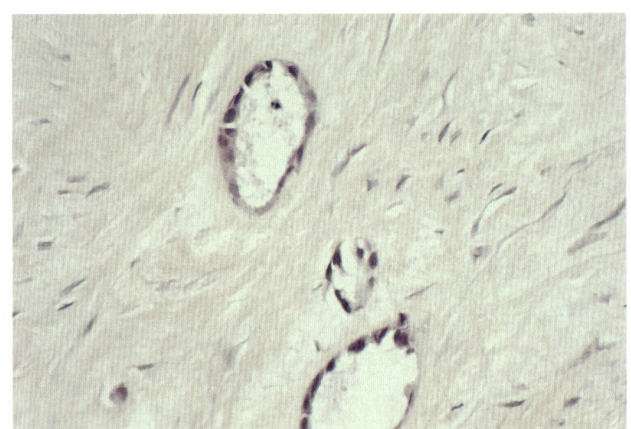

图11.52 假间皮瘤样腺癌的最常见组织学图像是呈管状促结缔组织增生性模式（×400）

史，右侧胸膜有渗出物，肿瘤包绕右肺。最初的活检被值班病理医师诊断为腺癌，另一个病理医师诊断为上皮型间皮瘤。该作者在病历中提到波形蛋白，而且免疫组化染色的表现也令人迷惑：该肿瘤细胞表达低分子量（35βH11）和高分子量（34βE12）角蛋白、波形蛋白、CD31、Ⅷ因子抗原（图11.53）和CD34。该肿瘤细胞的超微结构特点与内皮细胞相似，胞浆内含有Weibel-Palade小体（图11.54）。有报道表明在正常内皮细胞和血管源性肿瘤中都可表达角蛋白[384]。

胸膜的钙化纤维性假瘤

胸膜的钙化纤维性假瘤是最近才被认识的一种胸膜纤维性软组织肿瘤，主要发生于青年人，X线上表现为胸膜的块状阴影[385]。患有此肿瘤的病人通常伴有胸痛和/或咳嗽以及隐约的胸部不适感。该肿瘤为界限清楚但无包膜的肿块，含有致密的玻璃样变的胶原，并伴有淋巴浆细胞浸润和钙盐沉积，很多可以形成砂粒体样结构。本文作者观察了4例此类病变，其梭形细胞免疫组化呈波形蛋白阳性，而角蛋白、α-肌动蛋白、结蛋白、S-100蛋白、CD34、bcl-2和CD117阴性。

胸膜的原发性硬纤维瘤

该肿瘤与其他部位的硬纤维瘤相似，表现为肥胖的梭形细胞向邻近的脂肪和骨骼肌内浸润[386]。免疫组化染色发现，肿瘤性的梭形细胞呈波形蛋白、结蛋白、SMA和肌特异性肌动蛋白阳性表达，S-100蛋白和角蛋白呈阴性表达。超微结构方面，肿瘤细胞与肌纤维母细胞相似。

胸膜原发性胸腺瘤

胸腺瘤可以发生在胸膜并容易与间皮瘤相混淆[387-390]，主要易与伴有大量淋巴细胞浸润的肉瘤样型间皮瘤或淋巴组织细胞瘤样间皮瘤相混淆。

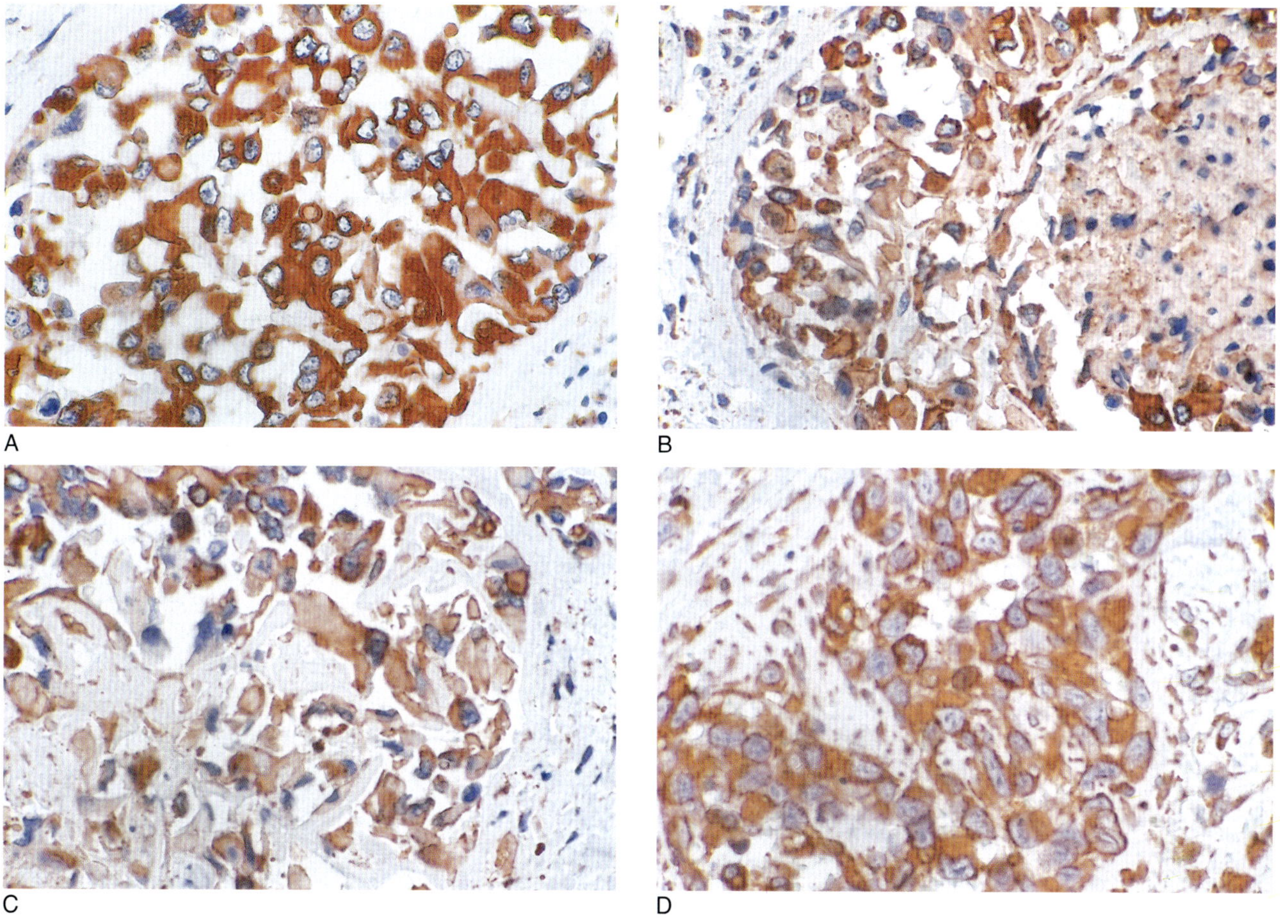

图 11.53 该例假间皮瘤上皮样血管内皮瘤起初被诊断为腺癌，后又诊断为上皮型间皮瘤。在该病例中，肿瘤细胞表达角蛋白、内皮细胞标记物 CD31、Ⅷ因子抗原和波形蛋白（×400）

Moran 等[387]提供了一些 X 线下未发现纵隔肿瘤的病例，6 例组织学图像为"混合型"（淋巴细胞/上皮型）胸腺瘤。这些肿瘤性胸腺上皮细胞表达角蛋白和 CD5。

滑膜肉瘤

滑膜肉瘤可以是胸膜的原发肿瘤，组织学上容易跟混合型和肉瘤样型间皮瘤混淆[391-394]，肿瘤性的上皮细胞表达角蛋白并呈腺样分化。细胞形成腺样结构并常表达 CEA 和 BerEP4，并且中性黏液染色阳性，而在上皮型间皮瘤中多不具有这些特征。在超微结构中，滑膜肉瘤中的肿瘤性上皮细胞跟上皮型间皮瘤明显不同，有很多短小的微绒毛和糖原小体[395]。单相滑膜肉瘤与肉瘤样型间皮瘤区分甚为困难，肉瘤样型滑膜肉瘤通常都表达 bcl-2 和 CD99。Colwell 等[393]和 Yano 等[394]报道在滑膜肉瘤中用荧光原位杂交检测到 SYT 和 SYX 基因融合。胸腔中还可以发生其他的一些肉瘤[393]。

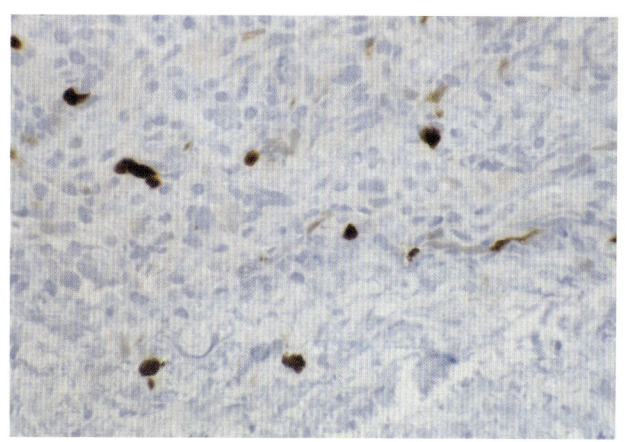

图 11.54 电镜下，该例假间皮瘤上皮样血管内皮瘤的很多肿瘤细胞中含有 Weibel-Palade 小体

胸膜肺母细胞瘤

胸膜肺母细胞瘤是比较罕见的肿瘤，主要发生于婴儿和儿童，并常侵及肺和/或胸膜[396-397]，成人罕见[398]。该肿瘤多为囊性，被覆良性化生的上皮，有时可

以有纤毛。恶性成分由已分化的和/或间变型肉瘤成分构成，包括纤维肉瘤、软骨肉瘤、胚胎性横纹肌肉瘤以及这些成分的混合成分，其免疫组化结果据肉瘤分化的类型不同而异。

结果的可变性及缺点

当前诊断间皮瘤的一个主要缺点是病理医师不能正确认识上皮型和肉瘤样型间皮瘤复杂多样的组织学图像。大部分的免疫组化资料都是讨论上皮型间皮瘤，尤其是高分化和中高分化的上皮型间皮瘤。大部分的抗体也都用来区分高分化和中高分化的间皮瘤与腺癌。一旦当间皮瘤呈低分化时，很多相对特异的阳性标记物如HBME-1、calretinin和CK5/6都呈阴性反应，低分化的间皮瘤特征性地表达低分子量角蛋白和波形蛋白，偶尔也表达高分子量角蛋白。绝对诊断该种间皮瘤是不可能的，有时候只能根据组织学和免疫组化结果与低分化间皮瘤相一致来进行诊断。胸膜肿瘤的"临床"（弥漫性）分布可以帮助间皮瘤的诊断。

目前已有文章探讨了用免疫组化方法来鉴别上皮型间皮瘤和肺腺癌及其他癌[399-404]，Ordonez等[404-406]对此作了大量的文献回顾。Ordonez[406]在最近的综述中分析了一系列抗体（表11.21A）在60例诊断明确的上皮型间皮瘤和50例肺腺癌中的表达情况，结果分析见表11.21B。Ordonez发表的关于不同免疫组化检测的研究结果列于其文章中的表4至表17，总结的结果见表11.22。根据其敏感性和特异性，Ordonez总结认为，calretinin、CK5/6和WT-1是最好的阳性标记物，calretinin和CK5/6比WT-1的敏感性要高。血栓调节素的敏感性和特异性都要低于calretinin、CK5/6和WT-1。间皮素是上皮型间皮瘤的一个高度敏感标记物，但特异性不高。HBME-1、N-钙黏素和CD44S被认为对诊断上皮型间皮瘤没有帮助。CEA、MOC31、BerEP4、Bg8和B72.3是高度特异和敏感的上皮型间皮瘤的阴性标记物。TTF-1、LeuM1（CD15）和CA19-9具有高度特异性，但敏感性不高。Ordonez[406]总结说，从经验来讲，可以用4个抗体（2个阳性、2个阴性）来区分上皮型间皮瘤和肺腺癌。Ordonez[406]推荐的阳性标记物是calretinin和CK5/6（或WT-1），阴性标记物是CEA和MOC31（或B72.3，BerEP4，Bg8），并指出要注意，阳性标记物WT-1在肺腺癌中不表达，但在浆液性卵巢癌中高表达。其他一些学者[407]在选择阳性和阴性标记物中有些许的差别。有报道calretinin在非间皮肿瘤中

存在不同的表达[408-411]，在其他一些肿瘤中也发现存在WT-1的表达[412-415]。另外，神经生长因子受体TfkA和p75的表达也有报道[416]。

根据Henderson等[251]的报道，胸膜的非肿瘤性反应性增生病变与间皮瘤非常相似。这个"领域"是"诊断性胸膜病理"最为困难的领域。困难主要来自纤维性胸膜炎和促结缔组织增生型间皮瘤之间的鉴别，以及表浅的浸润性上皮型间皮瘤和反应性间皮细胞增生的鉴别。根据本文作者的经验，肿瘤性间皮细胞EMA和HMFG-2胞膜染色阳性，而反应性非肿瘤间皮细胞通常不表达这些抗原，但这并不是绝对的，所以需要非常小心。

这里还要提一下不常见类型的间皮瘤，因为这些肿瘤可以引起诊断上的混淆。黏液染色阳性的上皮型间皮瘤并不少见，1%～5%的中高分化至高分化的上皮型间皮瘤呈黏液卡红和/或PAS-淀粉酶染色（图11.55）。该作者深入地描述了其黏液染色模式[417]。那些黏液染色阳性的上皮型间皮瘤经常表达一些一般上皮型间皮瘤中呈阴性而肺腺癌中呈阳性的免疫组化标记物（如CEA、LeuM1、B72.3、BerEP4）。黏液阳性的上皮型间皮瘤表达calretinin和HBME-1，并呈EMA和HMFG-2胞膜阳性。在超微结构中，黏液素阳性的上皮型间皮瘤的细胞内新生管腔、肿瘤细胞形成的腺样腔隙内，或细胞外通常都含有结晶体（图11.56），这种结晶体是上皮型间皮瘤所特有的。

一些间皮瘤由小细胞构成，可能会与小细胞肺癌混淆[418]。Mayall和Gibbs[418]报道了13例小细胞间皮瘤具有"非典型"上皮型间皮瘤的图像。其中7例90%的肿瘤细胞为小细胞。Mayall等[419]报道在48例间皮瘤中有46例（96%）呈NSE阳性，20例间皮瘤中有14例（70%）呈Leu7阳性。跟Hurlimann[346]报道不同的是，间皮瘤不表达CgA和铃蟾肽。Falconieri等[420]报道了4例假胸膜瘤样小细胞肺癌，该肿瘤可能会与小细胞间皮瘤相混淆。该作者认为最好的区分假间皮瘤样小细胞肺癌和小细胞间皮瘤的方法是染TTF-1（小细胞肺癌90%阳性，间皮瘤为阴性）、CEA（约30%～50%的小细胞肺癌呈阳性，小细胞间皮瘤为阴性）和Syn（小细胞肺癌90%阳性，大部分小细胞间皮瘤为阴性）。

淋巴组织细胞瘤样间皮瘤[421]是肉瘤样型间皮瘤的一种罕见类型，组织学上给人的第一印象是淋巴瘤。这种间皮瘤由大的类圆细胞构成，与大量的炎细胞混杂在一起，很容易被误诊为大细胞淋巴细胞性

表11.21A Ordonez[406] 研究中使用的抗体

抗体	公司	型号	稀释度	抗原修复
calretinin	Zymed (South San Francisco, CA)	PAb (rabbit)	1:20	是（枸橼酸盐）
CK5/6	Boehringer-Mannheim (Indianapolis, IN)	D5/16B4 MAb	1:25	是（枸橼酸盐）
WT-1	DAKO Corporation (Carpinteria, CA)	6F-H2 MAb	1:40	是（Tris-EDTA）
血栓调节素	DAKO Corporation	1005 MAb	1:50	是（枸橼酸盐）
间皮素	Novocastra (Newcastle-upon-Tyne, UK)	5B2 MAb	1:30	是（Tris-EDTA）
N-钙黏素	Zymed	3B9 MAb	1:20	是（Tris-EDTA）
HBME-1	DAKO Corporation	MAb	1:50	是（枸橼酸盐）
CD44S	Vector Laboratories (Burlingame, CA)	F10-44.2 MAb	1:75	是（枸橼酸盐）
MOC-31	DAKO Corporation	MAb	1:50	是（枸橼酸盐）
E-钙黏素	Zymed	HECD-1 MAb	1:20	是（枸橼酸盐）
Bg8 (Lewis^y)	Signet (Dedham, MA)	Bg8 MAb	1:50	是（枸橼酸盐）
TTF-1	DAKO Corporation	BG7G3/1 MAb	1:25	是（枸橼酸盐）
CEA	NeoMarkers (Fremont, CA)	PAb (rabbit)	1:175	否
B72.3	BioGenox (San Ramon, CA)	B72.3	1:300	否
Leu-M1 (CD15)	Becton-Dickinson (Mountainview, CA)	LeuM1 (MAb)	1:40	是（Tris-EDTA）
BerEP4	DAKO Corporation	MAb	1:30	是（酶消化）
CA19-9	DAKO Corporation	MAb	1:50	是（枸橼酸盐）
EMA	DAKO Corporation	E29 MAb	1:20	是（枸橼酸盐）
波形蛋白	DAKO Corporation	V9 MAb	1:500	是（枸橼酸盐）

CEA，癌胚抗原；EMA，上皮细胞膜抗原；TTF-1，甲状腺转录因子-1
（引自Ordonez NG. The immunohistochemical diagnosis of mesothelioma: a comparative study of epithelioid mesothelioma and lung adenocarcinoma. Am J Surg Pathol 2003; 27:1031-1051）

表11.21B 上皮型间皮瘤和肺腺癌的免疫组化结果

抗体	上皮型间皮瘤阳性反应分级 ($n=60$) +例数(%)	痕量	1+	2+	3+	4+	肺腺癌阳性反应分级 ($n=50$) +例数(%)	痕量	1+	2+	3+	4+
calretinin	60 (100%)	0	0	0	15	45	4 (8%)	2	2	0	0	0
细胞角蛋白5/6	60 (100%)	2	3	7	16	32	1 (2%)	0	1	0	0	0
WT-1	56 (93%)	0	4	9	16	27	0 (0%)	0	0	0	0	0
血栓调节素	46 (77%)	0	10	16	16	3	7 (14%)	2	5	0	0	0
间皮素	60 (100%)	0	11	4	17	28	19 (38%)	0	8	5	5	1
N-钙黏素	44 (73%)	1	5	13	14	11	15 (30%)	2	4	3	6	0
HBME-1	51 (85%)	0	7	11	14	28	34 (68%)	0	4	5	9	16
CD44S	44 (73%)	5	7	4	11	17	24 (48%)	0	14	7	2	1
MOC-31	5 (8%)	2	3	0	0	0	50 (100%)	0	3	7	19	21
E-钙黏素	24 (40%)	0	14	5	2	3	44 (88%)	0	9	8	20	7
Bg8 (Lewis^y)	4 (7%)	2	2	0	0	0	48 (96%)	1	6	7	15	21
TTF-1	0 (0%)	0	0	0	0	0	37 (74%)	0	4	10	15	8
CEA	0 (0%)	0	0	0	0	0	44 (88%)	0	3	8	17	16
B72.3 (TAG-72)	0 (0%)	0	0	0	0	0	42 (84%)	0	7	12	15	8
LeuM1 (CD15)	0 (0%)	0	0	0	0	0	36 (72%)	0	4	9	13	7
BerEP4	11 (18%)	2	9	0	0	0	50 (100%)	0	0	0	13	37
CA19-9	0 (0%)	0	0	0	0	0	24 (48%)	0	6	10	6	2
EMA	56 (93%)	0	7	9	19	21	50 (100%)	0	3	12	10	25
波形蛋白	33 (55%)	1	28	4	0	0	19 (38%)	1	16	2	0	0

（引自Ordonez NG. The immunohistochemical diagnosis of mesothelioma: a comparative study of epithelioid mesothelioma and lung adenocarcinoma. Am J Surg Pathol 2003; 27:1031-1051）

表11.22 Ordonez[404]研究中的免疫组化结果总结

抗原	上皮型间皮瘤			原发性肺腺癌			总结			
	例数	阳性例数	阳性百分率范围	阳性百分率平均值	例数	阳性例数	阳性百分率范围	阳性百分率平均值	有用	无用	有时有用	不能应用	没有结论

抗原	例数	阳性例数	阳性百分率范围	阳性百分率平均值	例数	阳性例数	阳性百分率范围	阳性百分率平均值	有用	无用	有时有用	不能应用	没有结论
calretinin	805	648	50~100	86.2	238	74	0~70	9.5	16	8	2		
CK5/6	309	286	64~100	90.1	183	16	0~19	6.2	未提供				
WT-1	298	231	43~95	77.7	154	8	0~20	10	未提供				
血栓调节素	637	501	30~100	51.4	430	109	5~77	21.9	未提供				
HBME-1	613	516	57~100	86.2	249	175	55~100	71.7	5	9	1		
CD44S	495	336	47~100	72	159	100	15~57	54	未提供				
MOC-31	265	34	0~88	19.5	173	167	90~100	97.5	未提供				
E-钙黏素	224	101	0~100	51.9	123	116	84~100	96.2	3	6		1	1
Bg8 (Lewis^y)	316	34	6~24	13.2	108	105	96~100	98	未提供				
CEA	1392	68	0~45	5.0	1023	840	25~100	81.6	未提供				
B72.3	797	68	0~48	8.0	490	412	35~100	82.1	未提供				
LeuM1 (CD15)	1423	173	0~33	5.0	693	521	44~100	84.6	未提供				
BerEP4	1055	139	0~88	10.5	222	210	57~100	93.8	未提供				
波形蛋白	715	418	16~100	60.3	354	73	0~50	19.5	6	9			2

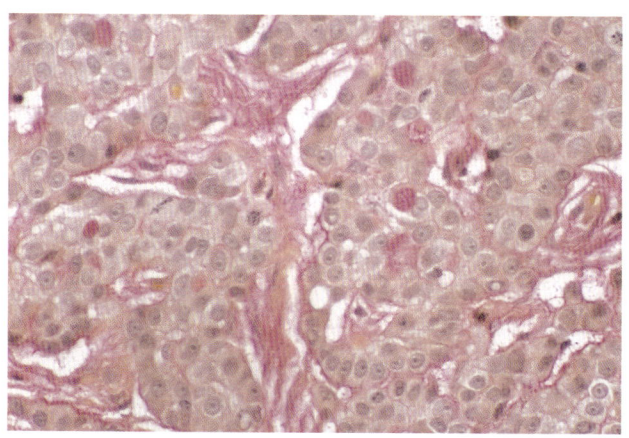

图11.55 该例黏液阳性的上皮型间皮瘤呈细胞内黏液卡红染色，可能会被误诊为产生黏液的腺癌（×400）

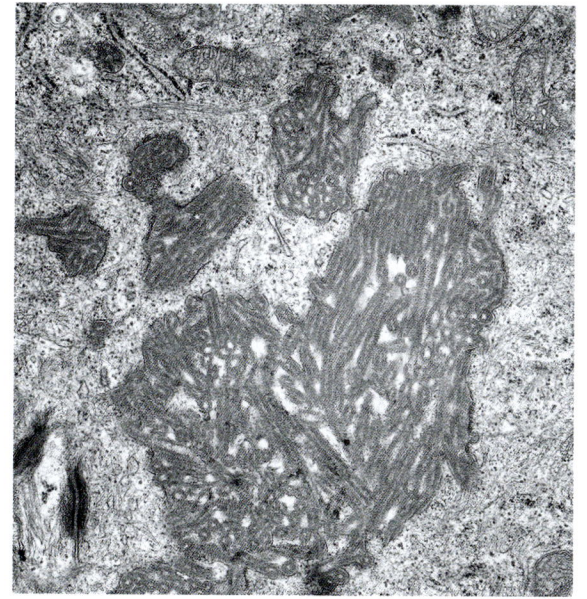

图11.56 该例黏液阳性的上皮型间皮瘤，在肿瘤细胞构成的腺腔中和新生管腔细胞内可见结晶体（×20 000）

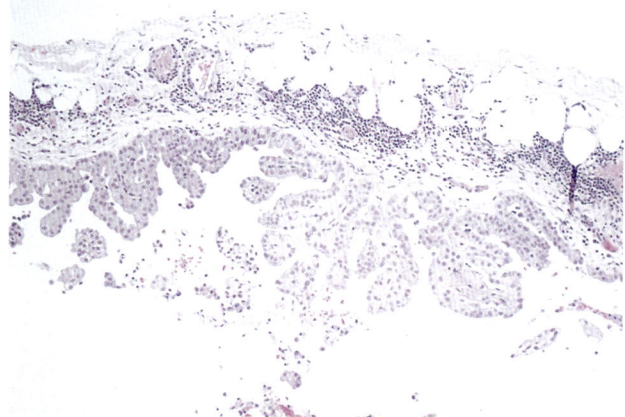

图11.57 该例浸润到胸膜的高分化乳头状上皮型间皮瘤呈现乳头分化，并由小而均匀一致的立方细胞构成。该类型的间皮瘤通常在临床上呈良性表现（×200）

淋巴瘤。肿瘤细胞特征性地表达低分子量角蛋白，偶尔也表达高分子量角蛋白和波形蛋白。大多数淋巴组织细胞瘤样间皮瘤calretinin、HBME-1和EMA阴性。在超微结构上，肿瘤细胞存在细胞间连接和细胞内张力丝。

高分化乳头状上皮型间皮瘤常常因为一些病理医师对此不熟悉而导致诊断混淆[248-250, 422]。尽管是在胸膜中报道的，但大部分病例是发生在年轻女性（20～30岁）的腹腔。大体上看，在浆膜表面有多数结节，主要侵及网膜、肠系膜、盆腔和胸膜。结节直径从数微米到几厘米不等。组织学上，表现为管状乳头状分化，由高分化的相对一致的立方细胞构成（图11.57）。免疫组化大体上是"典型"的高分化上皮型间皮瘤模式，对大多数病例该作者显示了细胞膜EMA或HMFG-2染色。这些肿瘤与"典型"的上皮型间皮瘤又有所不同，通常预后较好，进展不快，但有的病例进展很快，发生浸润并导致死亡。

一些上皮型间皮瘤由均匀一致的立方间皮细胞围成的小囊构成，并含有大量的血管（图11.58）。这种类型的间皮瘤可能会与血管肿瘤难以区分。上皮型间皮细胞胞浆内含有含铁血黄素（图11.59）。该种肿瘤的免疫表型与其他的上皮型间皮瘤相同，其血管增生与肿瘤性间皮细胞产生的内皮生长因子有关[424]。

腺瘤样瘤属于良性间皮增生，常发生于附睾和子宫角[425]。肾上腺[426]和胰腺[427]中已经发现腺瘤样肿瘤。该肿瘤由形态一致的小立方细胞构成，具有侵袭性。肿瘤细胞表达角蛋白和间皮细胞的其他标记物，并具有间皮细胞特征性的超微结构。腺瘤样肿瘤在胸膜中也有报道。

在纵隔淋巴结内可能发现增生的间皮细胞，与转移的间皮瘤或腺癌非常相似[428, 429]。这些非典型的间皮细胞常发生于皮质窦且主要在被膜下窦内，可能会与巨噬细胞混淆，实际上，Ordonez等[430]报道了一些被认为是由反应性增生的间皮细胞构成而实际上是由巨噬细胞构成的病变。这些间皮细胞通常表达上皮型间皮细胞表达的"阳性"标记物，上皮型间皮瘤特征性的阴性标记物在这些间皮细胞中也不表达。有一点必须注意，在淋巴结中也可以出现不明原发灶的转移性上皮型间皮瘤。

高分化的上皮型间皮瘤和高分化乳头状上皮型间皮瘤需要与浆膜的原发性乳头状浆液癌鉴别，后者几乎所有的都发生在妇女的腹腔[432-441]，男性中仅有1例报道[442]。极少数病例可以累及胸腔[254]。组织学上，这

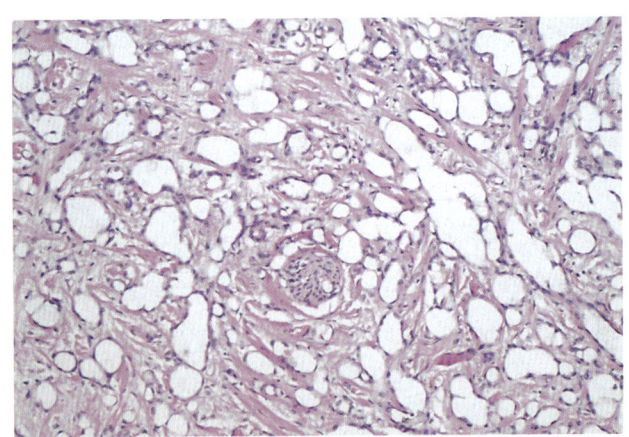

图11.58 该例上皮型间皮瘤由小囊腔和丰富的血管构成（×200）

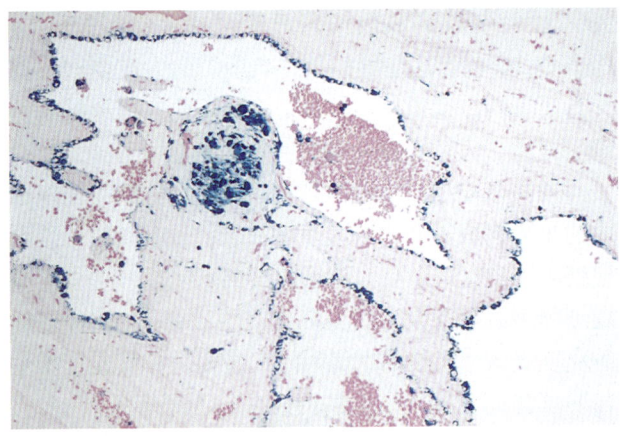

图11.59 在普鲁士蓝铁染色切片中，肿瘤性间皮细胞的胞浆内出现丰富的含铁血黄素颗粒（×200）

些肿瘤呈高分化并呈现乳头结构，原发性乳头状腺癌比乳头状上皮型间皮瘤更常见砂粒体，尽管在乳头状上皮型间皮瘤中偶尔可见到砂粒体，但其数量远远不如原发性乳头状腺癌。原发性浆液性乳头状腺癌通常黏液染色和PAS-淀粉酶阴性，其免疫组化染色模式跟上皮型间皮瘤相似。但Khoury等[443]发现浆液性乳头状肿瘤表达CEA、LeuM1（CD15）和TAG-72（B72.3）中的至少一种抗原。用胃蛋白酶消化组织切片，20例中有17例存在阳性表达，7例表达单克隆CEA，6例表达LeuM1，13例表达B72.3。在超微结构中，原发性乳头状浆液性腺癌可以出现纤毛、整齐的刷状缘和相对较短的多糖蛋白包被的微绒毛，有时候微绒毛可以较长并有分支。

肉瘤样肾细胞癌可以转移到胸膜，其大体分布跟间皮瘤尤其是肉瘤样型间皮瘤非常相似[444]。该肿瘤可以认为是一种假间皮样癌，但不是肺原发的假间皮瘤样癌。其免疫组化染色模式跟肉瘤样型间皮瘤相同。由于肉瘤样型间皮瘤可以转移到肾，可能会使诊断更为复杂。如果已经知道病人患有肉瘤样肾细胞癌并且有胸膜的梭形细胞肿瘤，必须要考虑转移性肉瘤样肾细胞癌的可能性。如果肿瘤是透明细胞和肉瘤样模式，很有可能就是转移性肉瘤样肾细胞癌，尽管间皮瘤也可以表现为透明细胞模式。

总结 / 结论

免疫组化是一种准确诊断肺和胸膜原发性及转移性肿瘤非常有价值的技术。跟其他的辅助诊断病理技术一样，免疫组化的结果必须与组织学、组织化学、超微结构观察以及临床结果相结合。

参考文献

1. Han H, Landreneaux RJ, Santucci TS, et al. Prognostic value of immunohistochemical expression of p53, HER-2-neu and bcl-2 in stage I non-small cell lung cancer. Hum Pathol 2002; 33:105–110.

2. Minami K, Saito Y, Imamura H, et al. Prognostic significance of p53, Ki67, VEGF and GLUT-1 in resected stage I adenocarcinoma of the lung. Lung Cancer 2002; 38:51–57.

3. Nakanishi K, Kawai T, Kumaki F, et al. Survivin expression in atypical adenomatous hyperplasia of the lung. Am J Clin Pathol 2003; 120:712–719.

4. Yamaguchi NH, Lichetenfels AJ, Demarchi LMM, et al. Cox-2, MMP-9 and Noguchi classification provide additional prognostic information about adenocarcinomas of the lung: a study of 117 patients from Brazil. Am J Clin Pathol 2004; 121:78–86.

5. Saad RS, Liu Y, Han H, et al. Prognostic significance of HER2/neu, p53 and vascular endothelial growth factor expression in early stage conventional adenocarcinoma and bronchioloalveolar carcinoma of the lung. Mod Pathol 2004; 17:1234–1242.

6. Pelosi G, Pasini F, Fraggetta F, et al. Independent value of fascin immunoreactivity for predicting lymph node metastases in typical and atypical pulmonary carcinoids. Lung Cancer 2003; 42:203–213.

7. Pelosi G, Pastorini O, Pasini F, et al. Independent prognostic value of fascin immunoreactivity in stage I nonsmall cell lung cancer. Br J Cancer 2003; 88:537–547.

8. Hammar SP. Common neoplasms. In: Dail DH, Hammar SP,

eds. 2nd edn. Pulmonary pathology. New York: Springer-Verlag; 1994:1487–1579.

9. Dodds L, Davis S, Polissar L. A population-based study of lung cancer incidence by histological type. J Natl Cancer Inst 1986; 76:21–29.

10. Thun MJ, Lally CA, Flannery JT, et al. Cigarette smoking and changes in the histopathology of lung cancer. J Natl Cancer Inst 1997; 89:1580–1586.

11. Moll R, Franke WW, Schiller DL, et al. The catalog of human cytokeratins: Patterns of expression in normal epithelia, tumors and cultured cells. Cell 1982; 31:11–24.

12. Moll R, Lowe A, Laufer J, et al. Cytokeratin 20 in human carcinomas. A new histodiagnostic marker detected by monoclonal antibodies. Am J Surg Pathol 1992; 140:427–447.

13. Ramaekers F, Huysmans A, Schaart G, et al. Tissue distribution of keratin 7 as monitored by a monoclonal antibody. Exp Cell Research 1987; 170:235–249.

14. Chu P, Wu E, Weiss LM. Cytokeratin 7 and cytokeratin 20 expression in epithelial neoplasms: A survey of 435 cases. Mod Pathol 2000; 13:962–972.

15. Kaimaktchiev V, Terracciano L, Tornillo L, et al. The homeobox intestinal differentiation factor CDX2 is selectively expressed in gastrointestinal carcinomas. Mod Pathol 2004; 17:1392–1399.

16. Au NHC, Gown AM, Cheang M, et al. p63 expression in lung carcinomas: A tissue microarray study of 408 cases. Appl Immunohistochem Mol Morphol 2004; 12:240–247.

17. Sheikh HA, Fuhrer K, Cieply K, et al. p63 expression in assessment of bronchioloalveolar proliferations of the lung. Mod Pathol 2004; 17:1134–1140.

18. Nakatani Y, Miyagi Y, Takemura T, et al. Aberrant nuclear/cytoplasmic localization and gene mutation of beta-catenin in classic pulmonary blastoma: beta-catenin immunostaining is useful in distinguishing between classic pulmonary blastoma and a blastomatoid variant carcino-sarcoma. Am J Surg Pathol 2004; 28:921–927.

19. Hammar SP, Hallman KO. Unusual primary lung neoplasms: spindle cell and undifferentiated carcinomas expressing only vimentin. Ultrastruct Pathol 1990; 14:407–422.

20. Upton MP, Hirohashi S, Tome Y, et al. Expression of vimentin in surgically resected adenocarcinomas and large cell carcinomas of lung. Am J Surg Pathol 1986; 10:560–567.

21. Hammar SP. Metastatic adenocarcinoma of unknown primary origin. Hum Pathol 1998; 29:1393–1402.

22. Guazzi S, Price M, DeFelice M, et al. Thyroid transcription factor-1 (TTF-1) contains a homeodomain and displays a novel DNA-binding specificity. EMBO J 1990; 9:3631–3639.

23. Lazzaro D, Price M, DeFelice M, et al. The transcription factor TTF-1 expressed at the onset of thyroid and lung morphogenesis and in the restricted regions of the foetal brain. Development 1991; 113:1093–1094.

24. Bohinski RJ, DiLauro R, Whitsett JA. The lung specific surfactant protein B promoter is a target for thyroid transcription factor-1 and hepatocyte nuclear factor 3, indicating common factors for organ-specific gene expression along the foregut axis. Mol Cell Biol 1994; 14:5671–5678.

25. Bohinski RJ, Huffman JA, Whitsett JA, et al. Cis-active elements controlling lung cell-specific expression of human pulmonary surfactant B gene. J Biol Chem 1993; 268:11160–11166.

26. Bejarano PA, Baughman RP, Biddinger PW, et al. Surfactant proteins and thyroid transcription factor-1 in pulmonary and breast carcinomas. Mod Pathol 1996; 9:445–452.

27. Fabbro D, DiLoreto C, Stamerra O, et al. TTF-1 gene expression in human lung tumors. Eur J Cancer 1996; 32A:512–573.

28. DiLoreto C, DiLauro V, Puglisi F, et al. Immunohistochemical expression of tissue specific transcription factor-1 in lung carcinoma. J Clin Pathol 1997; 50:30–32.

29. Holzinger A, Dingle S, Bejarano PA, et al. Monoclonal antibody to thyroid transcription factor-1: Production, characterization and usefulness in tumor diagnosis. Hybridoma 1996; 15:49–53.

30. Folpe AL, Gown AM, Lamps LW, et al. Thyroid transcription factor-1: Immunohistochemical evaluation in pulmonary neuroendocrine tumors. Mod Pathol 1999; 12:5–8.

31. Amin MB, Tamboli P, Merchant SH. Micropapillary component in lung adenocarcinoma: a distinctive histologic feature with possible prognostic significance. Am J Surg Pathol 2002; 26:358–364.

32. Nakamura N, Miyagi E, Murata S, et al. Expression of thyroid transcription factor-1 in normal and neoplastic lung tissues. Mod Pathol 2002; 15:1058–1067.

33. Lau SK, Desrochers MJ, Luthringer DJ. Expression of thyroid transcription factor-1, cytokeratin 7 and cytokeratin 20 in bronchioloalveolar carcinomas: an immunohistochemical

evaluation of 67 cases. Mod Pathol 2002; 15:538–542.

34. Simsir A, Wei XJ, Yee H, et al. Differential expression of cytokeratins 7 and 20 and thyroid transcription factor-1 in bronchioloalveolar carcinoma: an immunohistochemical study in fine needle aspiration biopsy specimens. Am J Clin Pathol 2004; 11:350–357.

35. Johansson L. Histopathologic classification of lung cancer: relevance of cytokeratin and TTF-1 immunophenotyping. Ann Diagn Pathol 2004; 8:259–267.

36. Yatabe Y, Mitsudomi T, Takahashi T. TTF-1 expression in pulmonary adenocarcinomas. Am J Surg Pathol 2002; 26:767–773.

37. Chang Y, Lee Y, Lia W, et al. The utility and limitation of thyroid transcription factor-1 protein in primary and metastatic pulmonary neoplasms. Lung Cancer 2004; 44:149–157.

38. Saad RS, Liu YL, Han H, et al. Prognostic significance of thyroid transcription factor-1 expression in both early-stage conventional adenocarcinoma and bronchioloalveolar carcinoma of the lung. Hum Pathol 2004; 35:3–7.

39. Yesner R. Small cell tumors of the lung. Am J Surg Pathol 1983; 7:775–785.

40. Carter D. Small-cell carcinoma of the lung. Am J Surg Pathol 1983; 7:787–795.

41. Yesner R. Classification of lung cancer histology. N Engl J Med 1985; 312:652–653.

42. Arrigoni MG, Woolner LB, Berantz PE. Atypical carcinoid tumors of the lung. J Thorac Cardiovasc Surg 1972; 64:413–421.

43. Leschke H. Über nur regionär bösartige und über krebsig entartete Bronchusadenome bzw. Carcinoide. Virch Arch [Pathol Anat] 1956; 328:635–657.

44. Warren WH, Memoli VA, Gould VE. Immunohistochemical and ultrastructural analysis of bronchopulmonary neuroendocrine neoplasms: II. Well-differentiated neuroendocrine carcinomas. Ultrastruct Pathol 1984; 7:185–199.

45. Mark EJ, Ramirerz JF. Peripheral small-cell carcinoma of the lung resembling carcinoid tumor: a clinical and pathologic study of 14 cases. Arch Pathol Lab Med 1985; 109:263–269.

46. Paladugu RR, Benfield JR, Pak HY, et al. Broncho-pulmonary Kulchitzky cell carcinomas. Cancer 1985; 55:1303–1311.

47. Travis WD, Colby TV, Corrin B, et al. Histological typing of lung and pleural tumors. New York: Springer-Verlag; 1999.

48. Thomas CF, Tazelaar HD, Jett JR. Typical and atypical pulmonary carcinoids: outcome in patients presenting with regional lymph node involvement. Chest 2001; 119:1143–1150.

49. Slodkowska J, Langfort R, Rudzinski P, et al. Typical and atypical pulmonary carcinoids – pathologic and clinical analysis of 77 cases. Pneumonol Alergol Pol 1998; 66:297–303.

50. Gould VE, Chejfec G. Ultrastructural and biochemical analysis of pulmonary 'undifferentiated' carcinomas. Hum Pathol 1978; 9:377–384.

51. Hammond ME, Sause WT. Large cell neuroendocrine tumors of the lung: Clinical significance and histological definition. Cancer 1985; 56:1624–1629.

52. Neal MH, Kosinki R, Cohen P, et al. Atypical endocrine tumors of the lung: A histologic, ultrastructural and clinical study of 19 cases. Hum Pathol 1986; 17:1264–1277.

53. Barbareschi M, Mariscotti C, Barberis M, et al. Large cell neuroendocrine of the lung. Tumor 1989; 75:583–588.

54. McDowell EM, Wilson TS, Trump BF. Atypical endocrine tumors of the lung. Arch Pathol Lab Med 1981; 105:20–28.

55. Travis WD, Linnoila I, Tsokos MG, et al. Neuroendocrine tumors of the lung with proposed criteria for large cell neuroendocrine carcinoma: an ultrastructural, immunohistochemical and flow cytometric study of 35 cases. Am J Surg Pathol 1991; 15:529–533.

56. Hammar S, Bockus D, Remington F, et al. The unusual spectrum of neuroendocrine lung neoplasms. Ultra Pathol 1989; 13:515–560.

57. Jiang SX, Kameya T, Shoji M, et al. Large cell neuroendocrine carcinoma of the lung: a histologic and immunohistochemical study of 22 cases. Am J Surg Pathol 1998; 22:526–537.

58. Sturm N, Lantuejoul S, Laverriere MH, et al. Thyroid transcription factor-1 and cytokeratins 1, 5, 10, 14 (34bE12) expression in basaloid and large cell neuroendocrine carcinomas of the lung. Hum Pathol 2001; 32:918–925.

59. Jung KJ, Lee KS, Han J, et al. Large cell neuroendocrine carcinoma of the lung: clinical, CT and pathologic findings in 11 patients. J Thorac Imaging 2001; 16:156–162.

60. Mazieres J, Daste G, Molinier L, et al. Large cell neuro-endocrine carcinoma of the lung: pathological study and clinical outcome of 18 resected cases. Lung Cancer 2002; 37:287–292.

61. Paci M, Cavazza A, Annessi V, et al. Large cell neuro-endo-

crine carcinoma of the lung: a 10 year clinicopathologic retrospective study. Ann Thorac Surg 2004; 77:1163–1167.

62. Doddoli C, Barlesi F, Chetaille B, et al. Large cell neuroendocrine carcinoma of the lung: an aggressive disease potentially treatable with surgery. Ann Thorac Surg 2004; 77: 1168–1172.

63. Peng WX, Sano T, Oyama T, et al. Large cell neuroendocrine carcinoma of the lung: a comparison with large cell carcinoma with neuroendocrine morphology and small cell carcinoma. Lung Cancer 2005; 47:225–233.

64. Pearse AGE. The diffuse neuroendocrine system: an extension of the APUD concept. In: Taylor S, ed. Endocrinology. London: Heinemann; 1972:145–222.

65. Gould VE, DeLellis RA. The neuroendocrine cell system: its tumors, hyperplasias and dysplasias. In: Silverberg SG, ed. Principles and practice of surgical pathology. New York: John Wiley; 1983:1488–1501.

66. Hammar SP, Gould VE. Neuroendocrine neoplasms. In: Azar HA, ed. Pathology of human neoplasms: an atlas of diagnostic electron microscopy and immunohistochemistry. New York: Raven Press; 1988:333–404.

67. Jahn B, Schibler W, Ouimet C, et al. A 38,000 dalton membrane protein (p38) present in synaptic vesicles. Proc Natl Acad Sci USA 1985; 82:4137–4141.

68. Wiedenmann B, Franke WW. Identification and localization of synaptophysin, an integral membrane glycoprotein of Mr 38,000 characteristic of presynaptic vesicles. Cell 1985; 41: 1017–1028.

69. Carmichael SW, Winkler H. The adrenal chromaffin cell. Sci Am 1985; 253:40–49.

70. O'Connor DT, Frigon RP. Chromogranin A, the major catecholamine storage vesicle protein. J Biol Chem 1984; 259: 3237–3247.

71. Banks P, Helle K. The release of protein from the stimulated adrenal medulla. Biochem J 1965; 97:40C–41C.

72. Haimoto H, Takahashi V, Koshikawa T, et al. Immunohistochemical localization of gamma-enolase in normal human tissues other than nervous and neuroendocrine tissues. Lab Invest 1985; 52:257–263.

73. Pahlman S, Esscher T, Nilsson K. Expression of gamma-subunit of enolase, neuron-specific enolase in human non-neuroendocrine tumors and derived cell lines. Lab Invest 1986; 54:554–560.

74. Leoncini P, DeMarco EB, Bognoli M, et al. Expression of phosphorylated and non-phosphorylated neurofilament subunits and cytokeratins in neuroendocrine lung tumors. Pathol Res Pract 1989; 185:848–855.

75. Komminoth P, Roth J, Lackie PM, et al. Polysialic acid of the neural cell adhesion molecule distinguishes small cell carcinoma from carcinoids. Am J Pathol 1991; 139:297–304.

76. Kibbelaar RE, Moolenaar CEC, Michalides RJAM, et al. Expression of the embryonal neural cell adhesion molecule N-CAM in lung carcinoma: diagnostic usefulness of monoclonal antibody 735 for the distinction between small cell lung cancer and non-small cell lung cancer. J Pathol 1989; 159:23–28.

77. Bunn P, Linnoila I, Minna J, et al. Small-cell lung cancer, endocrine cells of the fetal bronchus and other neuroendocrine cells express Leu-7 antigenic determinant present on natural killer cells. Blood 1985; 65:764–768.

78. Lonardo F, Pass HI, Lucas DR. Immunohistochemistry frequently detects c-Kit expression in pulmonary small cell carcinoma and may help select clinical subsets for a novel form of chemotherapy. Appl Immunohist Mol Morphol 2003; 11: 51–55.

79. Pelosi G, Barisella M, Pasini F, et al. CD117 immunoreactivity in stage I adenocarcinoma and squamous carcinoma of the lung: relevance to prognosis in a subset of adenocarcinoma patients. Mod Pathol 2004; 17:711–721.

80. Casali C, Stefani A, Rossi G, et al. The prognostic role of c-Kit protein expression in resected large cell neuroendocrine carcinoma of the lung. Ann Thorac Surg 2004; 77:252–253.

81. Butnor KJ, Burchette JL, Sporn TA, et al. The spectrum of Kit (CD117) immunoreactivity in lung and pleural tumors: a study of 96 cases using a single-source antibody with a review of the literature. Arch Pathol Lab Med 2004; 128: 538–543.

82. Matsuki Y, Tanimoto A, Hamada T, et al. Histidine decarboxylase expression as a new sensitive and specific marker for small cell lung carcinoma. Mod Pathol 2003; 16:72–78.

83. Gibbs AR, Whimster WF. Tumors of the lung and pleura. In: Fletcher CDM, ed. Diagnostic histopathology of tumors. Edinburgh: Churchill Livingstone; 1995:127–150.

84. Dail DH. Uncommon neoplasms. In Dail DH, Hammar SP eds. Pulmonary pathology. 2nd ed. New York: Springer-Verlag; 1994:1279–1461.

85. Wick MR, Swanson PE. Carcinosarcomas: current perspective and a historical review of nosologic concepts. Semin Diag Pathol 1993; 10:118–127.
86. Addis BJ, Corrin B. Pulmonary blastoma, carcinosarcoma and spindle cell carcinoma: an immunohistochemical study of keratin intermediate filaments. J Pathol 1985; 147:291–301.
87. Zarbo RJ, Crissman JD, Venkat H, et al. Spindle cell carcinoma of the upper aerodigestive tract mucosa: an immunohistologic and ultrastructural study of 18 biphasic tumors and comparison with seven monophasic spindle cell tumors. Am J Surg Pathol 1986; 10:741–753.
88. Humphrey PA, Scroggs MW, Roggli VL, et al. Pulmonary carcinomas with a sarcomatoid element: an immunohistochemical and ultrastructural analysis. Hum Pathol 1988; 19:155–165.
89. Colby TV, Bilbao JE, Battifora H, et al. Primary osteosarcoma of the lung: a re-appraisal following immunohistologic study. Arch Pathol Lab Med 1989; 113:1147–1150.
90. Nappi O, Glasner SD, Swanson PE, et al. Biphasic and monophasic sarcomatoid carcinomas of the lung: a re-appraisal of 'carcinosarcomas' and 'spindle cell carcinomas.' Am J Clin Pathol 1994; 102:331–340.
91. Fishback NF, Travis WD, Moran CA, et al. Pleomorphic (spindle/giant cell) carcinoma of the lung. Cancer 1994; 73:2936–2945.
92. Pelosi G, Fraggetta F, Nappi O, et al. Pleomorphic carcinomas of the lung show a selective distribution of gene products involved in cell differentiation, cell cycle control, tumor growth and tumor cell motility: a clinicopathologic and immunohistochemical study of 31 cases. Am J Surg Pathol 2003; 27:1203–1215.
93. Koss MN, Hochholzer L, O'Leary T. Pulmonary blastomas. Cancer 1983; 73:265–294.
94. Yousem SA, Wick MR, Randhawa P, et al. Pulmonary blastoma: an immunohistochemical analysis and comparison with fetal lung in its pseudoglandular stage. Am J Clin Pathol 1990; 93:167–175.
95. Etienne-Mastroianni B, Falchero L, Chalabreysse L, et al. Primary sarcomas of the lung: a clinicopathologic study of 12 cases. Lung Cancer 2002; 38:283–290.
96. Ognibene FP, Steis RG, Macher AM, et al. Kaposi's sarcoma causing pulmonary infiltrates and respiratory failure in the acquired immunodeficiency syndrome. Ann Intern Med 1985; 102:471–475.
97. Garay SM, Belenko M, Fazzini E, et al. Pulmonary manifestations of Kaposi's sarcoma. Chest 1987; 91:39–43.
98. White DA, Matthay RA. Noninfectious pulmonary complications of infection with the human immunodeficiency virus. Am Rev Respir Dis 1989; 140:1763–1787.
99. McLoud TC, Naidich DP. Thoracic disease in the immunocompromised patient. Radiol Clin North Am 1992; 30:525–554.
100. Ognibene FP, Shelhamer JH. Kaposi's sarcoma. Clin Chest Med 1988; 9:459–465.
101. Heitzman ER. Pulmonary neoplastic lymphoproliferative disease in AIDS: a review. Radiology 1990; 177:347–351.
102. Purdy LJ, Colby TV, Yousem SA, et al. Pulmonary Kaposi's sarcoma. Premortem histologic diagnosis. Am J Surg Pathol 1986; 10:301–311.
103. Hymes KB, Cheung T, Greene JB, et al. Kaposi's sarcoma in homosexual men: a report of eight cases. Lancet 1981; 2:598–600.
104. Kaposi's sarcoma and Pneumocystis pneumonia in homosexual men – New York City and California. MMWR 1981; 30:305–308.
105. Gottlieb GJ, Ackerman AB. Kaposi's sarcoma: an extensively disseminated form in young homosexual men. Hum Pathol 1982; 13:882–892.
106. Adem C, Aubry MC, Tazelaar HD, et al. Metastatic angiosarcoma masquerading as diffuse pulmonary hemorrhage: clinicopathologic analysis of 7 new patients. Arch Pathol Lab Med 2001; 125:1562–1565.
107. Tschernig T, Pabst R. Bronchus-associated lymphoid tissue (BALT) is not present in the normal adult lung but in different disease. Pathobiology 2000;68:1–8.
108. Richmond I, Pritchard GE, Ashcroft T, et al. Bronchus associated lymphoid tissue (BALT) in human lungs: Its distribution in smokers and nonsmokers. Thorax 1993; 48:1130–1134.
109. Swigris JJ, Berry GJ, Raffin TA, et al. Lymphoid interstitial pneumonia. A narrative review. Chest 2002; 122:2150–2164.
110. Bienenstock J, Johnston N, Perey DYE. Bronchial lymphoid tissue. I. Morphologic characteristics. Lab Invest 1973; 28:686–692.
111. Bienenstock J, Johnston N, Perey DYE. Bronchial lymphoid tissue II. Functional characteristics. Lab Invest 1973; 28:693–

698.

112. Pisani RJ, Witzit TE, Li CY, et al. Confirmation of lymphomatous pulmonary involvement by immunophenotypic and gene rearrangement analysis of broncho-alveolar lavage fluid. Mayo Clin Proc 1990; 65:651–656.

113. Kuroso K, Yumo T, Rom WN, et al. Oligoclonal T cell expansions in pulmonary lymphoproliferative disorders: Demonstration of the frequent occurrence of oligoclonal T cells in human immunodeficiency virus-related lymphoid interstitial pneumonia. Am J Respir Crit Care Med 2002; 165:254–259.

114. Colby TV. Lymphoproliferative diseases. In: Dail DH, Hammar SP, Colby TV, eds. Pulmonary pathology tumors. New York: Springer Verlag; 1995:343–368.

115. Lymphoproliferative disorders and leukemia. Fraser RS, Pare PD, Muller NL, eds. Diagnosis of diseases of the chest, 4th edn. Philadelphia: WB Saunders; 1999:1269–1330.

116. Jaffe ES, Harris NL, Stein H, et al. Genetics of tumours of hematopoietic and lymphoid tissues. Lyon: IARC Press; 2001.

117. Nicholson AG. Lymphoproliferative lung disease. In: Corrin B. ed. Pathology of lung tumors. New York: Churchill Livingstone; 1997:213–223.

118. Yousem SA. Lung tumors in the immunocompromised host. Corrin B, ed. Pathology of lung tumors. New York: Churchill Livingstone; 1997:189–212.

119. Koss MN. Pulmonary lymphoid disorders. Sem Diagn Pathol 1995; 12:158–171.

120. Kradin RL, Mark EG. Benign lymphoid disorders of the lung with a theory regarding their development. Human Pathol 1983; 14:857–867.

121. Colby TV. Lymphoproliferative diseases. In: Dail DH, Hammar SP, eds. Pulmonary pathology. 2nd edn. New York: Springer-Verlag; 1994:1097–1122.

122. Saldana MJ, Patchfsky AS, Israel HL, et al. Pulmonary angiitis and granulomatosis. The relationship between histologic features, organ involvement and response to treatment. Hum Pathol 1977; 8:391–409.

123. Israel HL, Patchfsky AS, Saldana MJ. Wegener's granulomatosis, lymphomatoid granulomatosis, and benign lymphocytic angiitis and granulomatosis of lung. Recognition and treatment. Ann Intern Med 1977; 87:691–699.

124. Jaffe ES, Banks PM, Natwhani B, et al. Recommendations for reporting of lymphoid neoplasms: A report from the association of directors of anatomic and surgical pathology. The ad hoc committee of reporting of lymphoid neoplasms. Hum Pathol 2002; 33:1064–1068.

125. His ED, Yegaptan S. Lymphoma immunophenotyping: A new era in paraffin-sectioned immunohistochemistry. Adv Anatom Pathol 2001; 8:218–239.

126. Rosenow C, Wilson WR, Cockerill FR. Pulmonary disease in the immunocompromised host. Mayo Clin Proc 1985; 60:473–487.

127. Lin Y, Rodriguez GD, Turner JF, et al. Plasmablastic lymphoma of the lung: Report of a unique case and review of the literature. Arch Pathol Lab Med 2001; 125:282–285.

128. L'Hoste RJ, Filippa DA, Lieberman PH, et al. Primary pulmonary lymphomas: a clinicopathologic analysis of 36 cases. Cancer 1984; 54:1397–1406.

129. Radin AI. Primary pulmonary Hodgkin's disease. Cancer 1990; 65:550–563.

130. Liebow AA, Carrington CB, Friedman PJ. Lymphomatoid granulomatosis. Hum Pathol 1972; 3:457–558.

131. Katzenstein AL, Carrington CB, Liebow AA. Lymphomatoid granulomatosis: a clinicopathologic study of 152 cases. Cancer 1979; 43:360–373.

132. Guinee D, Kingma D, Fishback N, et al. Pulmonary lesions with features of lymphomatoid granulomatosis/angiocentric immunoproliferative lesion (LYT/AIL); evidence for Epstein-Barr virus within B lymphocytes. 1994; USCAP Abstract #881.

133. Fauci AS, Haynes BF, Costa J, et al. Lymphomatoid granulomatosis: prospective, clinical and therapeutic experience over 10 years. N Engl J Med 1982; 306:68–74.

134. Demirer T, Dail DH, Aboulafia DM. Four varied cases of intravascular lymphomatosis and a literature review. Cancer 1994; 73:1738–1745.

135. Tan TB, Spaander PJ, Blaisse M, et al. Angiotropic large cell lymphoma presenting as interstitial lung disease. Thorax 1988; 43:578–579.

136. Snyder LS, Harmon KR, Estensen RD. Intravascular lymphomatosis (malignant angioendotheliomatosis) presenting as pulmonary hypertension. Chest 1989; 96:1199–1200.

137. Yousem SA, Colby TB. Intravascular lymphomatosis presenting in the lung. Cancer 1990; 65:349–353.

138. Pellicone JT, Goldstein HB. Pulmonary malignant angio-endotheliomatosis: presentation with fever and syndrome of inappropriate anti-diuretic hormone. Chest 1990; 98:1292–

1294.

139. Takamura K, Nasuhara Y, Mishina T, et al. Intravascular lymphomatosis diagnosed by transbronchial lung biopsy. Eur Respir J 1997; 10:955–957.

140. Walls JG, Hong YG, Cox JE, et al. Pulmonary intravascular lymphomatosis: presentation with dyspnea and air trapping. Chest 1999; 115:1207–1210.

141. Ansari MQ, Dawson DB, Nador R, et al. Primary body cavity-based AIDS-related lymphomas. Am J Clin Pathol 1996; 105:221–229.

142. Banks PM, Warnke RA. Primary effusion lymphoma. In: WHO classification of tumors of hematopoietic and lymphoid tissues. Lyon: IARC Press; 2001:179–180.

143. Banks PM, Harris NL, Warnke RA. Primary effusion lymphoma. In: Travis WD, Brambilla E, eds. WHO classification of tumors of the lung, pleura and mediastinum. Lyon: IARC Press; 2004.

144. Cesarman E, Chang Y, Moore PS, et al. Kaposi's sarcoma-associated herpes virus-like DNA sequencing in age-related body cavity lymphoma. N Engl J Med 1995; 332:1186–1191.

145. Aozasa K, Ohsaw AM, Kanno H. Pyothorax-associated lymphoma: a distinctive type of lymphoma strongly associated with Epstein-Barr virus. Adv Anat Pathol 1997; 4:58–63.

146. Gaulard P, Harris NL. Pyothorax-associated lymphoma. In: Travis WD, Brambilla E, eds. WHO classification of tumors of the lung, pleura and mediastinum. Lyon: IARC Press; 2004.

147. Ibuka T, Fukayama M, Hayashi Y, et al. Pyothorax-associated pleural lymphoma. Cancer 1994; 73:738–744.

148. Hammar SP. Pulmonary histiocytosis-X (Langerhans cell granulomatosis). In: Dail DH, Hammar SP, eds. Pulmonary pathology, 2nd edn. New York: Springer-Verlag; 1994:567–596.

149. Carter D, Patchefsky AS, Mountain CF. Clear cell lesions. In: Carter D, Patchefsky AS, eds. Tumors and tumor-like lesions of the lung. Philadelphia: WB Saunders; 1998:271–274.

150. Bonetti F, Pea M, Martigoni G, et al. Clear cell ('sugar tumor') of the lung is a lesion strictly related to angiomyo-lipoma – the concept of a family of lesions characterized by the presence of the perivascular epithelioid cells (PEC). Pathology 1994; 26:230–236.

151. Panizo-Santos A, Sola I, de Alava E, et al. Angiomyolipoma and PEComa are immunoreactive for MyoD1 in cell cytoplasmic staining pattern. Appl Immunohistochem Mol Morphol 2003; 11:156–160.

152. Gaffey M, Mills S, Zarbo R, et al. Clear cell tumor of the lung: Immunohistochemical and ultrastructural evidence of melanogenesis. Am J Surg Pathol 1991; 15:644–653.

153. Sullivan EJ. Lymphangioleiomyomatosis: a review. Chest 1998; 114:1689–1703.

154. Johnson S. Lymphangioleiomyomatosis: clinical features, management and basic mechanism. Thorax 1999; 54:254–264.

155. Liebow AA, Hubbell DS. Sclerosing hemangioma (histocytoma, xanthoma) of the lung. Cancer 1956; 9:53–75.

156. Sogio K, Yokoyama H, Kanedo S, et al. Sclerosing hemangioma of the lung: radiographic and pathologic study. Ann Thorac Surg 1992; 53:295–300.

157. Katzenstein A-LA, Gmelich JT, Carrington CB. Sclerosing hemangioma of the lung: a clinicopathologic study of 51 cases. Am J Surg Pathol 1982; 4:343–356.

158. Devouassoux-Shisheboran M, Hayashi T, Linnoila RI, et al. A clinicopathologic study of 100 cases of pulmonary sclerosing hemangioma with immunohistochemical studies: TTF-1 is expressed in both round and surface cells, suggesting an origin from primitive respiratory epithelium. Am J Surg Pathol 2000; 24:906–916.

159. Devouassoux-Shisheboran M, de la Fouchardiere A, Thivolet-Bejui F, et al. Endobronchial variant of sclerosing hemangioma of the lung: histological and cytological features on endobronchial material. Mod Pathol 2004; 17:252–257.

160. Miyagawa-Hayashino A, Tazelaar HD, Langel DJ, et al. Pulmonary sclerosing hemangioma with lymph node metastases: report of 4 cases. Arch Pathol Lab Med 2003; 127:321–325.

161. Beckwith JB, Palmer NF. Histopathology and prognosis of Wilms' tumor: results from the first national Wilms' tumor study. Cancer 1978; 55:2850–2853.

162. Small EJ, Gordon GJ, Dahms BB. Malignant rhabdoid tumor of the heart in an infant. Cancer 1985; 55:2850–2853.

163. Balaton AJ, Vaury P, Videgrain M. Paravertebral malignant rhabdoid tumor in an adult: a case report of immunocytochemical study. Pathol Res Pract 1987; 182:713–718.

164. Harris M, Eyden BP, Joglekar VM. Rhabdoid tumour of the bladder: a histological, ultrastructural and immunohistochemical study. Histopathology 1987; 11:1083–1089.

165. Biggs PJ, Garren PD, Posers JM, et al. Malignant rhabdoid

tumor of the central nervous system. Hum Pathol 1987; 18: 332–337.
166. Dervan PA, Cahalane SF, Kneafsey P, et al. Malignant rhabdoid tumor of soft tissue: an ultrastructural and immunohistological study of a pelvic tumour. Histopathol 1987; 11:183–190.
167. Parham DM, Peiper S, Robicheaux G, et al. Malignant rhabdoid tumor of the liver: evidence for epithelial differentiation. Arch Pathol Lab Med 1988; 112:61–64.
168. Jakate SM, Mardsen HB, Ingram L. Primary rhabdoid tumour of the brain. Virch Arch [A]. 1988; 412:393–397.
169. Uchida H, Yokoyama S, Nakayama I, et al. An autopsy case of malignant rhabdoid tumor arising from soft parts in the left inguinal region. Acta Pathol Jpn 1988; 38:1087–1096.
170. Patron M, Palacious J, Rodriguez-Peralto JL, et al. Malignant rhabdoid tumor of the tongue: a case report with immunohistochemical and ultrastructural findings. Oral Surg Oral Med Oral Path 1988; 65:67–70.
171. Carter RL, McCarthy KP, al-Sam SZ, et al. Malignant rhabdoid tumour of the bladder with immunohistochemical and ultrastructural evidence suggesting histiocytic origin. Histopathology 1989; 14:179–190.
172. Jsujimura T, Wasa A, Kawano K, et al. A case of malignant rhabdoid tumor arising from soft parts of the prepubic region. Acta Pathol Jpn 1989; 37:677–682.
173. Cho KR, Rosenshein NB, Epstein JI. Malignant rhabdoid tumor of the kidney and soft tissues: evidence for a diverse morphological and immunocytochemical phenotype. Arch Pathol Lab Med 1989; 113:115–120.
174. Tsokos M, Kouraklis G, Chandra RS, et al. Malignant rhabdoid tumor of the uterus. Int J Gynecol Pathol 1989; 8:381–387.
175. Molenaar WM, DeJong B, Dam-Meiring A, et al. Epithelioid sarcoma or malignant rhabdoid tumor of soft tissue. Epithelioid immunophenotype and rhabdoid karyotype. Hum Pathol 1989; 20:347–351.
176. Cavazza A, Colby TV, Tsokos M, et al. Lung tumors with a rhabdoid phenotype. Am J Clin Pathol 1996; 105:182–188.
177. Miyagi J, Tsuhako K, Kinjo T, et al. Rhabdoid tumor of the lung is a dedifferentiated phenotype of pulmonary adenocarcinoma. Histopathology 2000; 37:37–44.
178. Bahadori H, Liebow AA. Plasma cell granuloma of the lung. Cancer 1973; 31:191–208.
179. Lane JD, Krohn S, Kolozzi W, et al. Plasma cell granuloma of the lung. Dis Chest 1955; 27:216–221.
180. Berardi RS, Lee SS, Chen HP, et al. Inflammatory pseudotumors of the lung. Surg Gynecol Obstet 1983; 156:89–96.
181. Tang TT, Segura AD, Oechler HW, et al. Inflammatory myofibrohistiocytic proliferation simulating sarcoma in children. Cancer 1990; 65:1626–1634.
182. Tan-Liu NS, Matsubara MD, Grillo HC, et al. Invasive fibrous tumor of the tracheobronchial tree: clinical and pathological study of seven cases. Hum Pathol 1989; 20:180–184.
183. Ledet SC, Brown RW, Cagle PT. p53 immunostaining of the differentiation of inflammatory pseudotumor from sarcoma involving the lung. Mod Pathol 1995; 8:282–286.
184. Snyder CS, Dell-Aquila M, Haghighi P, et al. Clonal changes in inflammatory pseudotumor of the lung. Cancer 1995; 76:1545–1549.
185. Yousem SA, Shaw H, Cieply K. Involvement of 2p23 pulmonary inflammatory pseudotumors. Hum Pathol 2001; 32:428–433.
186. Freeman A, Geddes N, Munson P, et al. Anaplastic lymphoma kinase (ALK 1) staining and molecular analysis in inflammatory myofibroblastic tumors of the bladder: a preliminary clinicopathologic study of nine cases and review of the literature. Mod Pathol 2004; 17:765–771
187. Lae ME, Roche PC, Jin L, et al. Desmoplastic small round cell tumor: a clinicopathologic, immunohistochemical and molecular study of 32 tumors. Am J Surg Pathol 2002; 26:823–835.
188. Syed S, Hague AK, Hawkins HK, et al. Desmoplastic small round cell tumor of the lung. Arch Pathol Lab Med 2002; 126:1226–1228.
189. Ostoros G, Orosz Z, Kovacs G, et al. Desmoplastic small round cell tumor of the pleura: a case report with unusual follow-up. Lung Cancer 2002; 36:333–336.
190. Tsuji N, Tateishi R, Ishigoro S, et al. Adenomyoepithelioma of the lung. Am J Surg Pathol 1995; 19:956–962.
191. Veeramechaneni R, Gulic J, Halldorsson AO, et al. Benign myoepithelioma of the lung: a case report and review of the literature. Arch Pathol Lab Med 2001; 125:1494–1496.
192. Pelosi G, Fraggetta F, Maffini F, et al. Pulmonary epithelial-myoepithelial tumor of unproven malignant potential: report of a case and review of the literature. Mod Pathol 2001; 14:

521–526.

193. Ro K, Srivastava A, Tischer AS. Bronchial epithelial-myoepithelial carcinoma. Arch Pathol Lab Med 2004; 128:92–94.

194. Dearers M, Guinee D, Koss MN, et al. Granular cell tumors of the lung: clinicopathologic study of 20 cases. Am J Surg Pathol 1995; 19:627–635.

195. de Araujo VC, de Sousa SOM, Carvalho YR, et al. Application of immunohistochemistry to the diagnosis of salivary gland tumors. Appl Immunohist Mol Morphol 2000; 8:195–202.

196. Moran CA, Suster S, Fishback NF, et al. Primary intrapulmonary thymoma: a clinicopathologic and immunohistochemical study of eight cases. Am J Surg Pathol 1995; 19: 304–312.

197. Ionescu DN, Sasatomi E, Aldeeb D, et al. Pulmonary meningothelial-like nodules: a genotypic comparison with meningiomas. Am J Surg Pathol 2004; 28:207–214.

198. Hochholzer L, Moran CA, Koss MN. Pulmonary lipomatosis: a variant of placental transmogrification. Mod Pathol 1997; 10:846–849.

199. Fidler ME, Koomen M, Sebek B, et al. Placental transmogrification of the lung, a histologic variant of giant bullous emphysema. Am J Surg Pathol 1995; 19:563–570.

200. Brambilla E. Basaloid carcinoma of the lung. In: Corrin B, ed. Pathology of lung tumors. New York: Churchill Livingstone; 1997:71–82.

201. Sturm N, Lantuejoul S, Laverriere M, et al. Thyroid transcription factor-1 and cytokeratins 1, 5, 10 and 14 (34bE12) expression in basaloid and large-cell neuroendocrine carcinomas of the lung. Hum Pathol 2001; 32:918–925.

202. Bejarano PA, Mousavi F. Incidence and significance of cytoplasmic thyroid transcription factor-1 immunoreactivity. Arch Pathol Lab Med 2003; 127:193–195.

203. Rossi G, Murer B, Cavazza A, et al. Primary mucinous (so-called colloid) carcinomas of the lung: a clinicopathologic and immunohistochemical study with special reference to CDX2 homeobox gene and MUC2 expression. Am J Surg Pathol 2004; 28:442–452.

204. Mazziotta RM, Borczuk AC, Powell CA, et al. CDX2 immunostaining as a gastrointestinal marker: expression in lung carcinomas is a potential pitfall. Appl Immunohistochem Mol Morphol 2005; 13:55–60.

205. Herrera GA, Turbat-Herrera EA, Lott RL. S100 protein expression by primary and metastatic adenocarcinoma. Am J Clin Pathol 1988; 89:168–176.

206. Hammar SP, Bockus D, Remington F, et al. Langerhans cells and serum precipitating antibodies against fungal antigens in bronchioloalveolar cell carcinomas: Possible association with eosinophilic granuloma. Unltrastruct Pathol 1980; 1:19–37.

207. Colasante A, Castrilli G, Aiello FB, et al. Role of cytokines in the distribution of dendritic cells/Langerhans cell lineage in human primary carcinomas of the lung. Hum Pathol 1995; 26:866–872.

208. Hammar SP, Bockus D, Remington F, et al. The widespread distribution of Langerhans cells in pathologic tissues: An ultrastructural and immunohistochemical study. Hum Pathol 1986; 17:894–905.

209. Torikata C, Ishiwata K. Intranuclear tubular structures observed in the cells of alveolar cell carcinomas of the lung. Cancer 1977; 40:1194–1201.

210. Singh G, Katyal SL, Torikata C. Carcinoma of type II pneumocytes: Immunodiagnosis of a subtype of bronchioloalveolar carcinoma. Am J Pathol 1981; 102:195–208.

211. Singh G, Katyal SL, Torikata C. Carcinoma of type II pneumocytes: PAS staining as a screening test for nuclear inclusions of surfactant-specific apoprotein. Cancer 1982; 50: 946–948.

212. Ghadially FN, Harawi S, Khan W. Diagnostic ultrastructural markers in alveolar cell carcinoma. J Submicrosc Cytol 1985; 17:269–278.

213. Abrams HJ, Spiro R, Goldstein N. Metastases in carcinoma, analysis of 1000 autopsied cases. Cancer 1950; 3:74–85.

214. Dail DH. Metastases to and from the lung. In: Dail DH, Hammar SP, Colby TV, eds. Pulmonary tumors. New York: Springer-Verlag; 1995:369–403.

215. Wang NP, Zee S, Zarbo RJ, et al. Coordinate expression of cytokeratins 7 and 20 defines unique subsets of carcinomas. Appl Immunohist 1995; 3:99–107.

216. Ollayos CW, Riordan P, Rushin JM. Estrogen receptor detection in paraffin section of adenocarcinoma of colon, pancreas and lung. Arch Pathol Lab Med 1994; 118:630–632.

217. Canver CC, Memoli VA, Vanderveer PL, et al. Sex hormones in non-small cell lung cancer in human beings. J Thorac Cardiovasc Surg 1994; 108:153–157.

218. Bacchi CE, Garcia RL, Gown AM. Immunolocalization of

estrogen and progesterone receptors in neuroendocrine tumors of lung, skin, gastrointestinal and female genital tracts. Appl Immunohist 1997; 5:17–22.

219. DiNunno LD, Larsson LG, Rinehart JJ, et al. Estrogen and progesterone receptors in non-small cell lung cancer in 248 consecutive patients who underwent surgical resection. Arch Pathol Lab Med 2000; 124:1467–1470.

220. Dabbs DJ, Landreneau RJ, Liu Y, et al. Detection of estrogen receptor by immunohistochemistry in pulmonary adenocarcinoma. Ann Thorac Surg 2002; 73:403–406.

221. Selvaggi G, Scagliotti GV, Torri V, et al. HER-2/neu overexpression in patients with radically resected nonsmall cell lung carcinoma: impact on long-term survival. Cancer 2002; 94:2669–2674.

222. Butler AE, Colby TV, Weiss L, et al. Lymphoepithelioma-like carcinoma of lung. Am J Surg Pathol 1989; 13:632–639.

223. Chen F, Yan J, Lai W, et al. Epstein-Barr virus-associated nonsmall cell lung carcinoma: undifferentiated 'lymphoepithelioma-like' carcinomas as a distinct entity with better prognosis. Cancer 1998; 82:2334–2342.

224. Ginsberg SS, Buzaid AC, Stern H, et al. Giant cell carcinoma of the lung. Cancer 1992; 70:606–610.

225. Gustmann C, Altmannsberger M, Osborn M, et al. Cytokeratin expression and vimentin content in large cell anaplastic lymphoma and other non-Hodgkin's lymphoma. Am J Pathol 1991; 38:1413–1422.

226. Delsol G, AlSaati T, Gatter KC, et al. Coexpression of epithelial membrane antigen (EMA), Ki-1 and interleukin-2 receptor by anaplastic large cell lymphomas. Diagnostic value in so-called malignant histiocytosis. Am J Pathol 1988; 130:59–70.

227. Osborne BM, Mockay B, Butler JJ, et al. Large cell lymphoma with microvillus-like projections: an ultrastructural study. Am J Clin Pathol 1983; 79:433–450.

228. Chu PG, Arber DA, Weiss LM. Expression of T/NK-cell and plasma cell antigens in nonhematopoietic epithelioid neoplasms. Am J Clin Pathol 2003; 120:64–70.

229. Bishop PW, Menasce LP, Yates AJ, et al. An immunophenotypic survey of malignant melanomas. Histopathology 1993; 23:159–166.

230. Yoshimoto T, Higashino K, Hada T, et al. A primary lung carcinoma producing alpha-fetoprotein, carcinoembryonic antigen and human chorionic gonadotropin. Cancer 1987; 60:2744–2750.

231. Kuida CA, Braunstein GD, Shintaku P, et al. Human chorionic gonadotropin expression in lung, breast and renal carcinomas. Arch Pathol Lab Med 1988; 112:282–285.

232. Dirnhofer S, Freund M, Rogatsch H, et al. Selective expression of trophoblastic hormones by lung carcinoma: neuroendocrine tumors produce human chorionic gonadotropin alpha-subunit (hCGa). Hum Pathol 2000; 31:966–972.

233. Nasu M, Soma T, Fukushima H, et al. Hepatoid carcinoma of the lung with production of alpha fetoprotein and abnormal prothrombin: an autopsy case report. Mod Pathol 1997; 10:1054–1058.

234. Cooper WA, Thourani VH, Gal AA, et al. The surgical spectrum of pulmonary neuroendocrine neoplasms. Chest 2001; 119:14–18.

235. Lyda MH, Weiss LM. Immunoreactivity for epithelial and neuroendocrine antibodies are useful in the differential diagnosis of lung carcinomas. Hum Pathol 2000; 31:980–987.

236. Sturm N, Rossi G, Lantuejoul S, et al. Expression of thyroid transcription factor-1 in the spectrum of neuroendocrine cell lung proliferations with special interest in carcinoids. Hum Pathol 2002; 33:175–182.

237. Lin O, Olgac S, Green I, et al. Immunohistochemical staining of cytologic smears with MIB-1 helps distinguish low-grade from high-grade neuroendocrine neoplasms. Am J Clin Pathol 2003; 120:209–216.

238. Pelosi G, Rodriguez J, Viale G, et al. Typical and atypical pulmonary carcinoid tumor overdiagnosed as small cell carcinoma on biopsy specimens: a major pitfall in the management of lung cancer patients. Am J Surg Pathol 2005; 29:179–187.

239. Visscher DW, Zarbo RJ, Trojanowski JQ, et al. Neuroendocrine differentiation in poorly differentiated lung carcinomas: a light microscopic and immunohistochemical study. Mod Pathol 1990; 3:508–512.

240. Linnoila RI, Mulshine JL, Steinberg SM, et al. Neuroendocrine differentiation in endocrine and nonendocrine lung carcinomas. Am J Clin Pathol 1988; 90:641–652.

241. Mooi WJ, Dewar A, Springall D, et al. Non-small cell lung carcinomas with neuroendocrine features: a light microscopic, immunohistochemical and ultrastructural study of 11 cases. Histopathology 1988; 13:329–337.

242. Wick MR, Berg LC, Hertz MI. Large cell carcinoma of the

lung with neuroendocrine differentiation: a comparison with large cell 'undifferentiated' pulmonary tumors. Am J Clin Pathol 1992; 97:796–805.

243. Loy TS, Darkow GVD, Quesenberry JT. Immunostaining in the diagnosis of pulmonary neuroendocrine carcinomas: an immunohistochemical study with ultrastructural correlations. Am J Surg Pathol 1995; 19:173–182.

244. Schleusener JT, Tazelaar HD, Jung S, et al. Neuroendocrine differentiation is an independent prognostic factor in chemotherapy-treated non-small cell lung carcinoma. Cancer 1996; 77:1284–1291.

245. Hammar SP. Pleural diseases. In: Dail DH, Hammar SP, Colby TV, eds. Pulmonary pathology tumors. New York: Springer-Verlag; 1995:405–530.

246. Davies J. Human developmental anatomy. New York: Roland Press; 1963:51–52.

247. Selikoff IJ, Seidman H. Asbestos-associated deaths among insulation workers in the United States and Canada, 1967–1987. Annl NY Acad Sci 1991; 643:1–14.

248. Battifora H, McCaughey WTE. Tumors of the serosal membranes. Washington DC: Armed Forces Institute of Pathology; 1995:17–88.

249. Butnor KJ, Sporn TA, Hammar SP, et al. Well-differentiated papillary mesothelioma. Am J Surg Pathol 2001; 25:1304–1309.

250. Galateau-Salle F, Vignaud J, Burke L, et al. Well-differentiated papillary mesothelioma of the pleura: a series of 24 cases. Am J Surg Pathol 2004; 28:534–540.

251. Henderson DW, Shilkin KB, Whitaker D. Reactive mesothelial hyperplasia vs. mesothelioma, including mesothelioma in situ: a brief review. Am J Clin Pathol 1998; 110:397–404.

252. US-Canadian Mesothelioma Reference Panel: Churg A, Colby TV, Cagle P, et al. The separation of benign and malignant mesothelial proliferations. Am J Surg Pathol 2000; 24:1183–1200.

253. Bolen JW, Hammar SP, McNutt MA. Reactive and neoplastic serosal tissue: a light-microscopic, ultrastructural and immunocytochemical study. Am J Surg Pathol 1986; 10:34–47.

254. Henderson DW, Comin CE, Hammar SP, et al. Malignant mesothelioma of the pleura: current surgical pathology. In: Corrin B, ed. Pathology of lung tumors. New York: Churchill Livingstone; 1997:241–280.

255. Ordonez NG. The immunohistochemical diagnosis of epithelial mesothelioma. Hum Pathol 1999; 30:313–323.

256. Blobel GA, Moll R, Franke WW, et al. The intermediate filament cytoskeleton of malignant mesothelioma and its diagnostic significance. Am J Pathol 1985; 121:235–247.

257. Blobel GA, Moll R, Franke WW, et al. Cytokeratins in normal lung and lung carcinomas. I. Adenocarcinomas, squamous cell carcinomas and cultured cell lines. Virchows Arch A Cell Pathol 1984; 45:407–429.

258. Moll R, Dhovailly D, Sun T-T. Expression of keratin 5 as a distinctive feature of epithelial and biphasic mesotheliomas: an immunohistochemical study using monoclonal antibody AE14. Virchows Archiv B Cell Pathol 1989; 58:129–145.

259. Clover J, Oates J, Edwards C. Anti-cytokeratin 5/6: a positive marker for epithelial mesothelioma. Histopathology 1997; 31:140–143.

260. Kahn HJ, Thorner PS, Yeager H, et al. Immunohistochemical localization of pre-keratin filaments in benign and malignant cells in effusions: comparison with intermediate filament distribution by electron microscopy. Am J Pathol 1982; 109:206–214.

261. Kahn HJ, Thorner PS, Yeger H, et al. Distinct keratin patterns demonstrated by immunoperoxidase staining of adenocarcinomas, carcinoids and mesotheliomas using polyclonal and monoclonal keratin antibodies. Am J Clin Pathol 1986; 86:566–574.

262. Montag AG, Pinkus GS, Corson JM. Keratin protein reactivity immunoreactivity of sarcomatoid and mixed types of diffuse malignant mesotheliomas: an immunoperoxidase study of 30 cases. Hum Pathol 1988; 19:336–342.

263. Battifora H. The pleura. In: Sternberg SS, ed. Diagnostic surgical pathology, Vol. I. New York: Raven Press; 1989:829–855.

264. Roggli VL, Kolbeck J, Sanfilippo F, et al. Pathology of human mesothelioma: etiologic and diagnostic considerations. Pathol Ann 1987; 22(pt 2):91–131.

265. Al-Izzi M, Thurlow NP, Corrin B. Pleural mesothelioma of connective tissue type, localized fibrous tumour of the pleura and reactive submesothelial hyperplasia: an immunohistochemical comparison. J Pathol 1989; 157:41–44.

266. Blobel GA, Moll R, Franke WW, et al. The intermediate filament cytoskeleton of malignant mesotheliomas and its diagnostic significance. Am J Pathol 1985; 121:235–247.

267. Mayall FG, Goddard H, Gibbs AR. Intermediate filament

expression in mesotheliomas: leiomyoid mesotheliomas are not uncommon. Histopathology 1992; 21:453–457.
268. Yousem SA, Hochholzer L. Malignant mesotheliomas with osseous and cartilaginous differentiation. Arch Pathol Lab Invest 1987; 111:62–66.
269. Wirth PR, Legler J, Wright GL. Immunohistochemical evaluation of seven monoclonal antibodies for differentiation of pleural mesothelioma from lung adenocarcinoma. Cancer 1991; 67:655–662.
270. Carter D, Otis CN. Three types of spindle cell tumors of pleura: Fibroma, sarcoma and sarcomatoid mesothelioma. Am J Surg Pathol 1988; 12:747–753.
271. Azumi N, Battifora H, Carlson G, et al. Sarcomatous (spindle-cell) mesothelioma of pleura: Immunohistochemical study. Lab Invest 1989; 60:4A.
272. Lucas DR, Pass HI, Madan SK, et al. Sarcomatoid mesothelioma and its histologic mimics. Histopathology 2003; 42:270–279.
273. Attanoos RL, Dojcinov SD, Webb R, et al. Anti-mesothelial markers in sarcomatoid mesothelioma and other spindle cell neoplasms. Histopathology 2000; 37:224–231.
274. McNutt MA, Bolen JW, Gown AM, et al. Coexpression of intermediate filaments in human epithelial neoplasms. Ultrastruct Pathol 1985; 9:31–43.
275. Upton MP, Hirohashi S, Tome Y, et al. Expression of vimentin in surgically resected adenocarcinomas and large cell carcinomas of lung. Am J Surg Pathol 1986; 10:560–567.
276. Azumi N, Battifora H. The distribution of vimentin and keratin in epithelial and non-epithelial neoplasms. A comprehensive study on formalin and alcohol-fixed tumors. Am J Clin Pathol 1987; 88:286–296.
277. Raymond WA, Leong AS-Y. Vimentin – a new prognostic marker in breast carcinoma. J Pathol 1989; 158:107–114.
278. Churg A. Immunohistochemical staining for vimentin and keratin in malignant mesothelioma. Am J Surg Pathol 1985; 9:360–365.
279. Jasani B, Edwards RE, Thomas ND, et al. The use of vimentin antibodies in the diagnosis of malignant mesothelioma. Virch Arch A Pathol Anat 1985; 406:441–448.
280. Mullink H, Henzen-Logmans SC, Alons-van Kordelaan JJM, et al. Simultaneous immunoenzyme staining of vimentin and cytokeratins with monoclonal antibodies as an aid in the differential diagnosis of malignant meso-thelioma from pulmonary adenocarcinoma. Virch Arch B Pathol Anat 1986; 42:55–65.
281. Andersen C, Blumcke I, Celio MR. Calcium-binding proteins: selective markers of nerve cells. Cell Tissue Res 1993; 271:181–208.
282. Schwaller B, Buchwald P, Blucke I, et al. Characterization of a polyclonal antiserum against the purified human recombinant calcium binding protein calretinin. Cell Calcium 1993; 14:639–648.
283. Gotzos V, Schwaller B, Hertzel N, et al. Expression of the calcium binding protein calretinin in Wi Dr cells and its correlation to their cell cycle. Exp Cell Res 1992; 202:292–302.
284. Doglioni C, Dei Tos AP, Laurino L, et al. Calretinin: a novel immunocytochemical marker for mesothelioma. Am J Surg Pathol 1996; 20:1037–1046.
285. Barberis MCP, Faleri M, Veronese S, et al. Calretinin: a selective marker of normal and neoplastic mesothelial cells in serous effusions. Acta Cytol 1997; 41:1757–1761.
286. Leers MPG, Aarts MMJ, Theunissen PHMH. E-cadherin and calretinin: a useful combination of immunochemical markers for differentiation between mesothelioma and metastatic adenocarcinoma. Histopathol 1998; 32:209–216.
287. Ordonez NG. Value of calretinin immunostaining in differentiating epithelial mesothelioma from lung adenocarcinoma. Mod Pathol 1998; 10:929–933.
288. Chenard-Neu MP, Kabou A, Mechine A, et al. Immunohistochemistry in the differential diagnosis of mesothelioma and adenocarcinoma: evaluation of 5 new and 6 traditional antibodies. Ann Pathol 1998; 18:460–465.
289. Cury PM, Butcher DN, Fisher C, et al. Value of mesothelium-associated antibodies thrombomodulin, cytokeratin 5/6, calretinin and CD44H in distinguishing epithelioid mesothelioma from adenocarcinoma metastatic to the pleura. Mod Pathol 2000; 13:107–112.
290. Oates J, Edwards C. HBME-1, MOC-31, WT1 and calretinin: an assessment of recently described markers for mesothelioma and adenocarcinoma. Histopathology 2000; 36:341–347.
291. Chhieng DC, Yee H, Schaefer D, et al. Calretinin staining pattern aids in the differentiation of mesothelioma from adenocarcinoma in serous effusions. Cancer 2000; 25:194–200.
292. O'Hara CJ, Corson JM, Pinkus GS, et al. ME1: a monoclonal antibody that distinguishes epithelial-type mesothelioma from pulmonary adenocarcinoma and extrapulmonary

malignancies. Am J Pathol 1990; 136:421–428.

293. Sheibani K, Esteban JM, Bailey A, et al. Immunopathologic and molecular studies as an aid to the diagnosis of malignant mesothelioma. Hum Pathol 1992; 23:107–116.

294. Hammar SP, Bolen JW, Bockus D, et al. Ultrastructural and immunohistochemical features of common lung tumors: an overview. Ultrastruct Pathol 1985; 9:283–318.

295. Walz R, Koch HK. Malignant pleural mesotheliomas: some aspects of epidemiology, differential diagnosis and prognosis. Histological and immunohistochemical evaluation and follow-up of mesotheliomas diagnosed from 1964 to January 1985. Pathol Res Pract 1990; 186:124–134.

296. Wick MR, Loy T, Mills SE, et al. Malignant epithelioid pleural mesothelioma versus peripheral pulmonary adenocarcinoma: a histochemical, ultrastructural and immunohistologic study of 103 cases. Hum Pathol 1990; 21:759–766.

297. Henderson DW, Shilkin KB, Whitaker D, et al. The pathology of mesothelioma, including immunohistology and ultrastructure. In: Henderson DW, Shilkin KB, Langlois SL, et al., eds. Malignant mesothelioma. New York: Hemisphere; 1992:69–139.

298. Fink L, Collins CL, Schaefer R, et al. Thrombomodulin expression can be used to differentiate between mesotheliomas and adenocarcinomas. Lab Invest 1992; 66:113A.

299. Collins CL, Ordonez NG, Schaefer R, et al. Thrombomodulin expression and pulmonary adenocarcinoma. Am J Pathol 1992; 141:827–833.

300. Brown RW, Clark GM, Tandon AK, et al. Multiple-marker immunohistochemical phenotypes distinguishing malignant pleural mesothelioma from pulmonary adenocarcinoma. Hum Pathol 1993; 24:347–354.

301. Ascoli V, Scalzo CC, Taccogna S, et al. The diagnostic value of thrombomodulin immunolocalization in serous effusions. Arch Pathol Lab Med 1995; 119:1136–1140.

302. Geiger B, Ayalon O. Cadherins. Annu Rev Cell Biol 1992;8: 307–332.

303. Takeichi M. Cadherin cell adhesion receptors as a morphogenetic regulator. Science 1991; 251:1451–1455.

304. Hatta K, Takagi S, Fujisawa H, et al. Spatial and temporal expression pattern of N-cadherin cell adhesion molecules correlated with morphogenetic processes of chicken embryos. Dev Biol 1987; 120:215–227.

305. Peralta-Soler A, Knudsen KA, Jaurand MC, et al. The differential expression of N-cadherin, E-cadherin distinguished pleural mesotheliomas from lung adenocarcinomas. Hum Pathol 1995; 26:1363–1369.

306. Han AC, Peralta-Soler A, Knudsen KA, et al. Differential expression of N-cadherin in pleural mesotheliomas and E-cadherin in lung adenocarcinomas in formalin-fixed, paraffin-embedded tissues. Hum Pathol 1997; 28:641–645.

307. Ordonez NG. Value of E-cadherin and N-cadherin immunostaining in the diagnosis of mesothelioma. Hum Pathol 2003; 34:749–755.

308. Amin KM, Litzky LA, Smythe WR, et al. Wilms' tumor 1 susceptibility (WT1) gene products are selectively expressed in malignant mesothelioma. Am J Pathol 1995; 146:344–356.

309. Kumar-Singh S, Segers K, Rodeck O, et al. WT1 mutation in malignant mesothelioma and WT1 immunoreactivity in relation to p53 growth factor expression, cell-type transition and prognosis. J Pathol 1997; 181:67–74.

310. Walker C, Rutlen F, Yuan X, et al. Wilms' tumor suppressor gene expression in rat and human mesothelioma. Cancer Res 1994; 54:1301–1306.

311. Ordonez NG. Application of mesothelin immunostaining in tumor diagnosis. Am J Surg Pathol 2003; 27:1418–1428.

312. Chu AY, Litzky LA, Pasha TL, et al. Utility of D2-40, a novel mesothelial marker, in the diagnosis of malignant mesothelioma. Mod Pathol 2005; 18:105–110.

313. Shivley JE, Beatty JD. CEA-related antigens: molecular biology and clinical significance. CRC Crit Rev Oncol Hematol 1985; 2:355–399.

314. Thompson J, Grunert F, Zimmermann W. Carcinoembryonic antigen gene family: molecular biology and clinical perspectives. J Clin Labor Anal 1991; 5:344–366.

315. Hammarstrom S, Khan WN, Teglund S, et al. The carcinoembryonic antigen family. In: Van Regenmortel MHV, ed. Structure of antigens. Boca Raton: CRC Press; 1993:341–376.

316. Hammarstrom S, Olsen A, Teglund S, et al. The nature and expression of the human CEA family. In: Stanners C, ed. Cell adhesion and clinical perspectives. Amsterdam: Harwood Academic Publishers; 1997:1–30.

317. Hammarstrom S. The carcinoembryonic antigen (CEA) family: structures, suggested functions and expression in normal and malignant tissues. Cancer Biol 1999; 9:67–81.

318. Wang N-S, Huang S-N, Gold P. Absence of carcinoembryonic antigen-like material in mesothelioma: an immunohistochemical differentiation from other lung cancers. Cancer 1979; 44: 437–443.

319. Whitaker D, Shilkin KB. Carcinoembryonic antigen in the tissue diagnosis of malignant mesothelioma. Lancet 1981; 1: 1369–1370.

320. Whitaker D, Sterret GF, Shilkin KB. Detection of tissue CEA-like substance as an aid in the differential diagnosis of malignant mesothelioma. Pathology 1982; 14:255–258.

321. Sheibani K, Battifora H. Leu-M1 positivity is not specific for Hodgkin's disease. Am J Clin Pathol 1985; 84:682.

322. Sheibani K, Battifora H, Burke JS, et al. Leu-M1 in human neoplasms: An immunohistologic study of 400 cases. Am J Surg Pathol 1986; 10:227–236.

323. Sheibani K, Battifora H, Burke J. Antigenic phenotype of malignant mesotheliomas and pulmonary adeno-carcinomas: an immunohistologic analysis demonstrating the value of Leu-M1 antigen. Am J Pathol 1986; 123:212–219.

324. Sheibani K, Azumi N, Battifora H. Further evidence demonstrating the value of LeuM1 antigen in differential diagnosis of malignant mesothelioma and adenocarcinoma: an immunohistologic evaluation of 395 cases. Lab Invest 1988; 58: 84A.

325. Otis CN, Carter O, Cole S, et al. Immunohistochemical evaluation of pleural mesothelioma and pulmonary adenocarcinoma. Am J Surg Pathol 1987; 11:445–456.

326. Szpak CA, Johnston WW, Roggli V, et al. The diagnostic distinction between malignant mesothelioma and adenocarcinoma of the lung as defined by a monoclonal antibody (B72.3). Am J Pathol 1986; 122:252–260.

327. Ordonez NG. The immunohistochemical diagnosis of mesothelioma: Differentiation of mesothelioma and lung adenocarcinoma. Am J Surg Pathol 1989; 13:276–291.

328. Bollinger DJ, Wick MR, Dehner LP, et al. Peritoneal malignant mesothelioma versus serous papillary adenocarcinoma: A histochemical and immunohistochemical comparison. Am J Surg Pathol 1989; 13:659–670.

329. Latza V, Niedobitek G, Schwarting R, et al. Ber-EP4: new monoclonal antibody which distinguishes epithelia from mesothelia. J Clin Pathol 1990; 43:213–219.

330. Sheibani K, Shin SS, Kezirian J, et al. Ber-EP4 antibody as a discriminant in the differential diagnosis of malignant mesothelioma versus adenocarcinoma. Am J Surg Pathol 1991; 15:779–784.

331. Gaffey MJ, Mills SE, Swanson PE, et al. Immunoreactivity for Ber-EP4 in adenocarcinomas, adenomatoid tumors and malignant mesotheliomas. Am J Surg Pathol 1992; 16:593–599.

332. Souhami RL, Beverly PCL, Bobrow LG. Antigens of small cell lung cancer. First International Workshop. Lancet 1987; 2:325–326.

333. DeLeij L, Broers J, Ramaekers F, et al. Monoclonal antibodies in clinical and experimental pathology of lung cancer. In: Roiter DJ, Fleuren GJ, Warner SO, eds. Applications of monoclonal antibodies in tumor pathology. Dordrecht: Martinus Nijhoff; 1987:191–210.

334. Delahaye M, Hoogsteden HC, van der Kwast TH. Immunocytochemistry of malignant mesothelioma: OV 632 as a marker of malignant mesothelioma. J Pathol 1991; 165:137–143.

335. Riutenbeek T, Gouw ASH, Poppema S. Immunocytology of body cavity fluids: MOC-31, a monoclonal antibody discriminating between mesothelial and epithelial cells. Arch Pathol Lab Med 1994; 118:265–269.

336. Ordonez NG. Value of MOC-31 monoclonal antibody in differentiating epithelial pleural mesothelioma from lung adenocarcinoma. Hum Pathol 1998; 29:166–169.

337. Jordon D, Jagirdar J, Kaneko M. Blood group antigens Lewis x and Lewis y in the diagnostic discrimination of malignant mesothelioma versus adenocarcinoma. Am J Pathol 1989; 135:931–937.

338. Riera JR, Astengo-Osuna C, Longmate JA, et al. The immunohistochemical diagnostic panel for epithelial mesothelioma. A reevaluation after heat-induced epitope retrieval. Am J Surg Pathol 1997; 21:1409–1419.

339. Kinsella AR, Green B, Lepts GC, et al. The role of cell–cell adhesion molecule E-cadherin in large bowel tumour cell invasion and metastasis. Br J Cancer 1993; 67:904–909.

340. Williams CL, Hayes VY, Hummel AM, et al. Regulation of E-cadherin mediated adhesion by muscarinic acetylcholine receptor in small cell lung carcinoma. J Cell Biol 1993; 121: 643–654.

341. Leers MPG, Aarts MMJ, Theunissen PTMH. E-Cadherin and calretinin: a useful combination of immunochemical markers for differentiation between mesothelioma and metastatic

adenocarcinoma. Histopathology 1998; 32:209–216.

342. Kawai T, Suzuki M, Torikata C, et al. Expression of blood group-related antigens and Helix pomatia agglutinin in malignant pleural mesothelioma and pulmonary adenocarcinoma. Hum Pathol 1991; 22:118–124.

343. Mayall FG, Goddard H, Gibbs AR. p53 immunostaining in the distinction between benign and malignant mesothelial proliferations using formalin-fixed paraffin sections. J Pathol 1992; 168:377–381.

344. Ramael M, Lemmens G, Eerdekens C, et al. Immunoreactivity for p53 protein in malignant mesothelioma and non-neoplastic mesothelium. J Pathol 1992; 168:371–375.

345. Mayall FG, Goddard H, Gibbs AR. The frequency of p53 immunostaining in asbestos-associated mesotheliomas. Histopathology 1993; 22:383–386.

346. Hurlimann J. Desmin and neural marker expression in mesothelial cells and mesotheliomas. Hum Pathol 1994; 25:753–757.

347. Azumi N, Underhill CB, Kagan E, et al. A novel biotinylated probe specific for hyaluronate. Am J Surg Pathol 1992; 16:116–121.

348. Thylen A, Wallin J, Martensson G. Hyaluronan in serum as an indicator of progressive disease in hyaluronan-producing malignant mesothelioma. Cancer 1999; 86:2000–2005.

349. Martensson G, Thylen A, Lindquist U, et al. The sensitivity of hyaluronan analysis of pleural fluid from patients with malignant mesothelioma and a comparison of different methods. Cancer 1994; 73:1406–1410.

350. Thylen A, Levin-Jacobsen AM, Hjerpe A, et al. Immunohistochemical differences between hyaluronan and non-hyaluronan-producing malignant mesothelioma. Eur Respir J 1997; 10:404–408.

351. Kabawat SE, Bast RC, Bhan AK, et al. Immunopathologic characterization of a monoclonal antibody that recognizes common surface antigens of human ovarian tumors of serous, endometrioid and clear cell types. Am J Clin Pathol 1983; 79:98–104.

352. Kabawat SE, Blast RC, Bhan AK, et al. Tissue distribution of celomic epithelium related antigen recognized by monoclonal antibody OC-125. Int J Gynecol Pathol 1983; 2:275–285.

353. Dabbs DJ, Geisinger KR. Selective application of immunohistochemistry in gynecological neoplasms. Pathol Ann 1993; 28(Pt 1):329–353.

354. Bast RC, Freeney M, Lazarus H, et al. Reactivity of a monoclonal antibody with human ovarian carcinoma. J Clin Invest 1981; 68:1331–1337.

355. Koelma IA, Nap M, Rodenburg CJ, et al. The value of tumor marker CA-125 in surgical pathology. Histopathology 1987; 11:287–294.

356. Nanbu Y, Fujii S, Konishi I, et al. Immunohistochemical localization of CA-130 in fetal tissue and in normal and neoplastic tissues of the female genital tract. Asia Oceania J Obstet Gynecol 1990; 16:379–387.

357. Tamura S, Yamaguchi K, Terada M, et al. Immunohistochemical analysis of CA19-9, SLX and CA-125 in adenoidcystic carcinoma of trachea and bronchus. Nippon Kyobu Shikkan Gakkai Zasshi 1992; 3:407–411.

358. Zhou J, Iwasa Y, Konishi I, et al. Papillary serous carcinoma of the peritoneum in women: A clinicopathologic and immunohistochemical study. Cancer 1995; 76:429–436.

359. Nouwen EJ, Pollet DE, Eerdekens MW, et al. Immunohistochemical localization of placental alkaline phosphatase, carcinoembryonic antigen and cancer antigen 125 in normal and neoplastic human lung. Cancer Res 1986; 46:866–876.

360. Bateman AC, al-Talib RK, Newman T, et al. Immunohistochemical phenotype of malignant mesothelioma: predictive value of CA-125 and HBME-1 expression. Histopathology 1997; 30:49–56.

361. Nap M. Immunohistochemistry of CA-125: unusual expression in normal tissues, distribution in the human fetus and questions around its application in diagnostic pathology. Int J Biol Markers 1998; 13:210–215.

362. O'Brien TJ, Raymond LM, Bannon GA, et al. New monoclonal antibodies identify the glycoprotein carrying the CA-125 epitope. Am J Obst Gynecol 1991; 61:1857–1864.

363. Okamoto H, Matsuno Y, Noguchi M, et al. Malig-nant pleural mesothelioma producing chorionic gonadotropin: report of two cases. Am J Surg Pathol 1992; 16:969–974.

364. McAuley P, Asa SL, Chiv B, et al. Parathyroid hormone-like peptide in normal and neoplastic mesothelial cells. Cancer 1990; 66:1975–1979.

365. Tateyama H, Eimoto T, Tada T, et al. Immunoreactivity of a new CD5 antibody with normal epithelium and malignant tumors including thymic carcinoma. Am J Clin Pathol 1999; 111:235–240.

366. Hammar SP, Bockus D, Remington F. Metastatic tumors of

unknown origin: an ultrastructural analysis of 265 cases. Ultrastruct Pathol 1987; 11:209–250.

367. Gaber AO, Rice P, Eaton C, et al. Metastatic malignant disease of unknown origin. Am J Surg Pathol 1983; 145:493–497.

368. Crotty TB, Myers JL, Katzenstein AL, et al. Localized malignant mesothelioma: a clinicopathologic and flow cytometric study. Am J Surg Pathol 1994; 18:357–363.

369. Briselli M, Mark EJ, Dickersin GR. Solitary fibrous tumors of the pleura: eight new cases and review of 360 cases in the literature. Cancer 1981; 47:2678–2689.

370. Doucet J, Dardick I, Srigley JR, et al. Localized fibrous tumour of serosal surfaces. Virch Arch Pathol Anat 1986; 409:349–363.

371. England DM, Hochholzer L, McCarthy MJ. Localized benign and malignant fibrous tumors of the pleura. A clinicopathologic review of 223 cases. Am J Surg Pathol 1989; 13:640–658.

372. van de Rijn M, Lombard CM, Rouse RV. Expression of CD34 by solitary fibrous tumors of the pleura, mediastinum and lung. Am J Surg Pathol 1994; 18:814–820.

373. Flint A, Weiss SW. CD-34 and keratin expression distinguishes solitary fibrous tumor (fibrous mesothelioma) of pleura from desmoplastic mesothelioma. Hum Pathol 1995; 26:428–431.

374. Hasegawa T, Matsuno Y, Shimoda T, et al. Frequent expression of bcl-2 protein in solitary fibrous tumors. Jpn J Clin Oncol 1998; 28:86–91.

375. Babolini G, Blasi A. The pleural form of primary cancer of the lung. Dis Chest 1956; 29:314–323.

376. Harwood TR, Gracey DR, Yokoo H. Pseudomesotheliomatous carcinoma of the lung. Am J Clin Pathol 1976; 65:159–167.

377. Koss M, Travis W, Moran C, et al. Pseudomesotheliomatous adenocarcinoma: a reappraisal. Semin Diagn Pathol 1992; 9:117–123.

378. Hartman C-A, Schutze H. Mesothelioma-like tumors of the pleura: a review of 72 cases. Cancer Res Clin Oncol 1994; 120:331–347.

379. Koss MN, Fleming M, Przygodzki RM, et al. Adenocarcinoma simulating mesothelioma: a clinicopathologic and immunohistochemical study of 29 cases. Ann Diagn Pathol 1998; 2:93–102.

380. Robb JA, Hammar SP, Yokoo H. Pseudomesotheliomatous carcinoma of lung. Lab Invest 1993; 68:134A.

381. Attanoos RL, Gibbs AR. 'Pseudomesotheliomatous' carcinomas of the pleura: a 10-year analysis of cases from the Environmental Lung Disease Research Group, Cardiff. Histopathology 2003; 43:444–452.

382. Battifora H. Epithelioid hemangioendothelioma imitating mesothelioma. Appl Immunohistochem 1993; 1:220–221.

383. Lin BT-Y, Colby T, Gown AM, et al. Malignant vascular tumors of the serous membranes mimicking mesothelioma: A report of 14 cases. Am J Surg Pathol 1996; 20:1431–1439.

384. Gray MH, Rosenberg AE, Dickersin GR, et al. Cytokeratin expression in epithelioid vascular neoplasms. Hum Pathol 1990; 21:212–217.

385. Pinkard NB, Wilson RW, Lawless N, et al. Calcifying fibrous pseudotumor of pleura: A report of three cases of a newly described entity involving the pleura. Am J Clin Pathol 1996; 105:189–194.

386. Wilson RW, Galateau-Salle F, Moran CA. Desmoid tumors of the pleura: a clinicopathologic mimic of localized fibrous tumor. Mod Pathol 1999; 12:9–14.

387. Moran CA, Travis WD, Rosada-de-Christenson M, et al. Thymomas presenting as pleural tumors: report of eight cases. Am J Surg Pathol 1992; 16:138–144.

388. Payne CB Jr, Morningstar WA, Chester EH. Thymoma of the pleura masquerading as diffuse mesothelioma. Am Rev Respir Dis 1966; 94:441–446.

389. Honma K, Shimada K. Metastasizing ectopic thymoma arising in the right thoracic cavity and mimicking diffuse pleural mesothelioma: An autopsy study of a case with review of the literature. Wien Klin Wschr 1986; 98:14–20.

390. Shih D, Wang J, Tseng H, et al. Primary pleural thymoma. Arch Pathol Lab Med 1997; 121:79–82.

391. Gaertner E, Zeren H, Fleming MV, et al. Biphasic synovial sarcomas arising in the pleural cavity: a clinicopathologic study of five cases. Am J Surg Pathol 1996; 20:36–45.

392. Nicholson AG, Goldstraw P, Fischer C. Synovial sarcoma of the pleura and its differentiation from other primary pleural tumors: a clinicopathological and immunohistochemical review of three cases. Histopathology 1998; 33:508–513.

393. Colwell AS, D'Cunha J, Vargas SO, et al. Synovial sarcoma of the pleura: a clinical and pathologic study of three cases. J Thorac Cardiovasc Surg 2002; 124:828–832.

394. Yano M, Toyooka S, Tsukuda K, et al. SYT-SSX fusion genes

in synovial sarcoma of the thorax. Lung Cancer 2004; 44: 391–397.

395. Ordonez NG, Mahfouz SM, Mackay B. Synovial sarcoma: an immunohistochemical and ultrastructural study. Hum Pathol 1990; 21:733–749.

396. Hachitanda Y, Aoyama C, Sato JK, et al. Pleuropulmonary blastoma in childhood. A tumor of divergent differentiation. Am J Surg Pathol 1993; 17:382–391.

397. Priest JR, McDermott MB, Bhatia S, et al. Pleuropulmonary blastoma: a clinicopathologic study of 50 cases. Cancer 1997; 80:147–161.

398. Hill DA, Sadeghi S, Schultz MZ, et al. Pleuropulmonary blastoma in an adult: an initial case report. Cancer 1999; 85:2368–2374.

399. Fetsch PA, Abati A, Hijazi YM. Utility of the antibodies CA-19-9, HBME-1 and thrombomodulin in the diagnosis of malignant mesothelioma and adenocarcinoma in cytology. Cancer 1998; 84:101–108

400. Khoor A, Whitsett JA, Stahlman MT, et al. Utility of surfactant protein B precursor and thyroid transcription factor-1 in differentiating adenocarcinoma of the lung from malignant mesothelioma. Hum Pathol 1999; 30:695–700.

401. Curry PM, Butcher DN, Fisher C, et al. Value of the mesothelium associated antibodies thrombomodulin, cytokeratin 5/6, calretinin and CD44H in distinguishing epithelioid pleural mesothelioma from adenocarcinoma metastatic to the pleura. Mod Pathol 2000; 13:107–112.

402. Oates J, Edwards C. HBME-1, MOC-31, WT-1 and calretinin: an assessment of recently described markers for mesothelioma and adenocarcinoma. Histopathology 2000; 36: 341–342.

403. Chieng DC, Yee H, Schaefer D, et al. Calretinin staining pattern aids in the differentiation of mesothelioma from adenocarcinoma in serous effusions. Cancer 2000; 25:194–200.

404. Ordonez NG. Role of immunohistochemistry in differentiating epithelial mesothelioma from adenocarcinoma: review and update. Am J Clin Pathol 1999; 112:75–89.

405. Ordonez NG. Immunohistochemical diagnosis of epithelioid mesotheliomas: a critical review of old markers, new markers. Hum Pathol 2002; 33:953–967.

406. Ordonez NG. The immunohistochemical diagnosis of mesothelioma: a comparative study of epithelioid mesothelioma and lung adenocarcinoma. Am J Surg Pathol 2003; 27: 1031–1051.

407. Commin CE, Novelli L, Boddi V, et al. Calretinin, thrombomodulin, CEA and CD15: a useful combination of immunohistochemical markers for differentiating pleural epithelial mesothelioma from peripheral pulmonary adenocarcinoma. Hum Pathol 2001; 32:529–536.

408. Zhang PJ, Genega EM, Tomaszewski JE, et al. The role of calretinin, inhibin, melan-A, BCL-2 and C-kit in differentiating adrenal cortical and medullary tumors: an immunohistochemical study. Mod Pathol 2003; 16:591–597.

409. Laskin WB, Miettinen M. Epithelioid sarcoma: new insights based on an extended immunohistochemical analysis. Arch Pathol Lab Med 2003; 127:1161–1168.

410. Pan C, Chen DC, Choo T, et al. Expression of calretinin and other mesothelioma-related markers in thymic carcinoma and thymoma. Hum Pathol 2003; 34:1155–1162.

411. Fine SW, McClain SA, Li M. Immunohistochemical staining for calretinin is useful for differentiating schwannomas from neurofibromas. Am J Clin Pathol 2004; 122:552–559.

412. Bergmann L, Maurer U, Weidmann E. Wilms tumor gene expression in acute myeloid leukemias. Leuk Lymphoma 1997; 25:435–443.

413. Sugiyama H. Wilms tumor gene (WT1) as a new marker for the detection of minimal residual disease in leukemia. Leuk Lymphoma 1998; 30:55–61.

414. Hwang H, Quenneville L, Yaziji H, et al. Wilms tumor gene product: sensitive and contextually specific marker of serous carcinoma of ovarian surface epithelial origin. Appl Immunohistochem Mol Morphol 2004; 12:122–126.

415. Carpentieri DF, Nichols K, Chou PM, et al. The expression of WT-1 in the differentiation of rhabdomyosarcoma from other pediatric small round blue cell tumors. Mod Pathol 2002; 15:1080–1086.

416. Davidson B, Reich R, Lazarovici P, et al. Expression of the nerve growth factor receptor TrkA and p75 in malignant mesothelioma. Lung Cancer 2004; 44:159–165.

417. Hammar SP, Bockus DE, Remington FL, et al. Mucin-positive epithelial mesotheliomas: a histochemical, immunohistochemical and ultrastructural comparison with mucin-producing pulmonary adenocarcinomas. Ultra Pathol 1996; 20: 293–325.

418. Mayall FG, Gibbs AR. The histology and immunohistochemistry of small cell mesothelioma. Histopathology 1992; 20:

47–51.
419. Mayall FG, Jasani B, Gibbs AR. Immunohistochemical positivity for neuron specific enolase and Leu 7 in malignant mesotheliomas. J Pathol 1992; 165:325–328.
420. Falconieri G, Zanconati F, Bussani R, et al. Small cell carcinoma of lung simulating mesothelioma. Pathol Res Pract 1995; 191:1147–1151.
421. Henderson DW, Atwood HD, Constance TJ, et al. Lymphohistiocytoid mesothelioma: a rare lymphomatoid variant of predominantly sarcomatoid mesothelioma. Ultrastruct Pathol 1988; 12:367–384.
422. Daya D, McCaughey WTE. Well-differentiated papillary mesothelioma of the peritoneum: a clinicopathologic study of 22 cases. Cancer 1990; 65:292–296.
423. Yesner R, Hurwitz A. Localized pleural mesothelioma of epithelial type. J Thorac Surg 1953; 26:325–329.
424. Thickett DR, Armstrong L, Millar AB. Vascular endothelial growth factor (VEGF) in inflammatory and malignant pleural effusions. Thorax 1999; 54:707–710.
425. Golden A, Ash J. Adenomatoid tumors of genital tract. Am J Pathol 1990; 14:63–80.
426. Isotalo PA, Keeney GL, Sebo TJ, et al. Adenomatoid tumor of the adrenal gland: a clinicopathologic study of five cases and review of the literature. Am J Surg Pathol 2003; 27:969–977
427. Overstreet K, Wixum C, Shabaik A, et al. Adenomatoid tumor of the pancreas: a case report with comparison of histology and aspiration cytology. Mod Pathol 2003; 16:613–617.
428. Argani P, Rosai J. Hyperplastic mesothelial cells in lymph nodes. Report of six cases of a benign process that simulates metastatic involvement by mesothelioma or carcinoma. Am J Surg Pathol 1998; 29:339–346.
429. Brooks JSJ, LiVolsi VA, Pietra GG. Mesothelial cell inclusions in mediastinal lymph nodes mimicking metastatic carcinoma. Am J Clin Pathol 1990; 93:741–748.
430. Ordonez NG, Ro JY, Ayal AG. Lesions described as nodular mesothelial hyperplasia are primarily composed of histiocytes. Am J Surg Pathol 1998; 22:285–292.
431. Sussman J, Rosai J. Lymph node metastasis as the initial manifestation of malignant mesothelioma: Report of six cases. Am J Surg Pathol 1990; 14:819–828.
432. Kannerstein M, Churg J, McCaughey WTE, et al. Papillary tumors of the peritoneum in women: mesothelioma or papillary carcinoma. Am J Obstet Gynecol 1977; 127:306–314.
433. Foyle A, Al-Jabi M, McCaughey WTE. Papillary peritoneal tumors in women. Am J Surg Pathol 1981; 5:241–249.
434. Mills SE, Andersen WA, Fechner RE, et al. Serous surface papillary carcinomas: a clinicopathologic study of 10 cases and comparison with stage III–IV ovarian serous carcinoma. Am J Surg Pathol 1988; 12:827–834.
435. Bollinger DJ, Wick MR, Dehner LP, et al. Peritoneal malignant mesothelioma versus serous papillary adenocarcinoma. A histochemical and immunohisto-chemical comparison. Am J Surg Pathol 1989; 13:659–670.
436. Raju U, Fine G, Greenwald KA, et al. Primary papillary serous neoplasia of the peritoneum: a clinicopathologic and ultrastructural study of eight cases. Hum Pathol 1989; 20:426–436.
437. Bell DA, Scully RE. Benign and borderline serious lesions of the peritoneum in women. Pathol Ann 1989; 24(Pt 2):1–21.
438. Rutledge ML, Silva EG, McLemore D, et al. Serous surface carcinoma of the ovary and peritoneum: A flow cytometric study. Pathol Ann 1989; 24(Pt 2):227–235.
439. Bell DA, Scully RE. Serous boderline tumors of the peritoneum. Am J Surg Pathol 1990; 14:230–239.
440. Truong LD, Maccato ML, Awalt H, et al. Serous surface carcinoma of the peritoneum: a clinicopathologic study of 22 cases. Hum Pathol 1990; 21:99–110.
441. Biscotti CV, Hart WR. Peritoneal serous micropapillomatosis of low malignant potential (serous borderline tumors of the peritoneum): A clinicopathologic study of 17 cases. Am J Surg Pathol 1992; 16:467–475.
442. Shah IA, Jayram L, Gani OS, et al. Papillary serous carcinoma of the peritoneum in a man. Cancer 1998; 82:860–866.
443. Khoury N, Raju R, Crissman JD, et al. A comparative immunohistochemical study of peritoneal and ovarian tumors, and mesotheliomas. Hum Pathol 1990; 21:811–819.
444. Taylor DR, Page W, Huges D, et al. Metastatic renal cell carcinoma mimicking pleural mesothelioma. Thorax 1987; 42:901–902.
445. Ordonez NG, Myhre M, Mackay B. Clear cell mesothelioma. Ultrastruct Pathol 1996; 20:331–336.

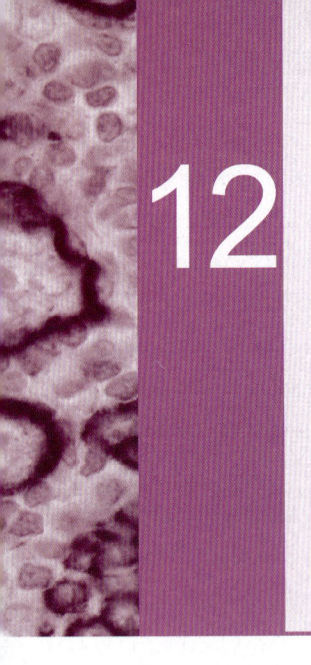

12 皮肤肿瘤的免疫组织化学

原作者：Mark R. Wick, Paul E. Swanson and James W. Patterson
作　者：牟　坤，李　丽
审校者：李　丽，牟　坤，高　鹏

目　录

引言	406
皮肤上皮来源肿瘤	406
皮肤淋巴造血组织病变	415
皮肤间叶来源肿瘤	421
皮肤的特殊免疫组织化学标记物	429

引　言

皮肤是一个复杂的微环境体系。表皮、真皮和皮肤附属器无论是在结构还是功能上都比较复杂，所以由不同结构发生的皮肤疾病也就多种多样。皮肤疾病可以是全身系统性疾病的一部分，或者是与其他器官的病变相伴发生的，例如淋巴网状组织疾病和间叶来源的肿瘤，这些疾病的诊断和免疫组织化学特点在其他章节已有介绍，本章仅介绍发生在皮肤的病变。最后需要指出的是，本章所涉及的抗原表型均为商业化抗体在石蜡标本中可以检测到的。

皮肤上皮来源肿瘤

皮肤上皮组织及附属器具有不同的分化特征，因此皮肤肿瘤的命名和分类也就比较混乱。从实际工作角度出发，免疫组化主要用于以下5种基本形态的诊断：表皮、汗腺、皮脂腺、毛发、内分泌腺。

表皮肿瘤

具有一定分化的表皮肿瘤是皮肤最常见的上皮来源肿瘤，其中最重要的是鳞状细胞癌和基底细胞癌。

鳞状细胞癌（SCC）的肿瘤细胞一般是由相对一致的具有角化物质的多角形细胞组成，诊断相对不难。但某些亚型的镜下改变有时与皮肤腺上皮或间叶来源的肿瘤相似，这些亚型包括腺样（皮肤棘层松解）型、多形型、小细胞型和梭形细胞型[1-3]。由于各亚型细胞的多样性，所以掌握鳞状细胞癌的一般免疫组织化学特点对于皮肤肿瘤的鉴别诊断非常重要。除极少数情况外，所有类型SCC的抗原表型都基本相似。

SCC肿瘤细胞内含有大量分子量40～68kD的角化中间丝蛋白[4-7]。高分化的SCC能够合成高分子量细胞角蛋白（CK），而分化较差的肿瘤则表达低分子量的CK。CK和波形蛋白双表达是梭形细胞、多形性、部分腺样鳞癌的特点（图12.1）[3,8]。

肉瘤样癌有时也可非常局灶地表达角蛋白，采用多种CK单克隆抗体组合能有效识别肉瘤样癌。角蛋白5/6是一个较特异的指标，因其仅在鳞状细胞中表达[7]。

SCC表达的另一个上皮源性标记物是上皮细胞膜抗原（EMA）。尽管几乎所有的SCC均可不同程度地表达EMA[9]，但笔者观察到EMA弥漫性阳性只在分化差的SSC中出现（Broders 3～4级）。SCC还可表达癌胚抗原（CEA）[10]，但据我们的经验，这种情况非常少见。p63属于p53多肽家族，其成员包括p53、p63和p73，在皮肤的鳞癌、基底细胞癌和附属器恶性肿瘤中均可见到p63呈核阳性表达（图12.2）[5]。

所有的皮肤鳞癌均不表达S-100蛋白、嗜铬素（Cg）、突触素（Syn）、CD99、CD15和CD57，也不表达HMB-45和抗黑素A（anti-melan-A）。但许

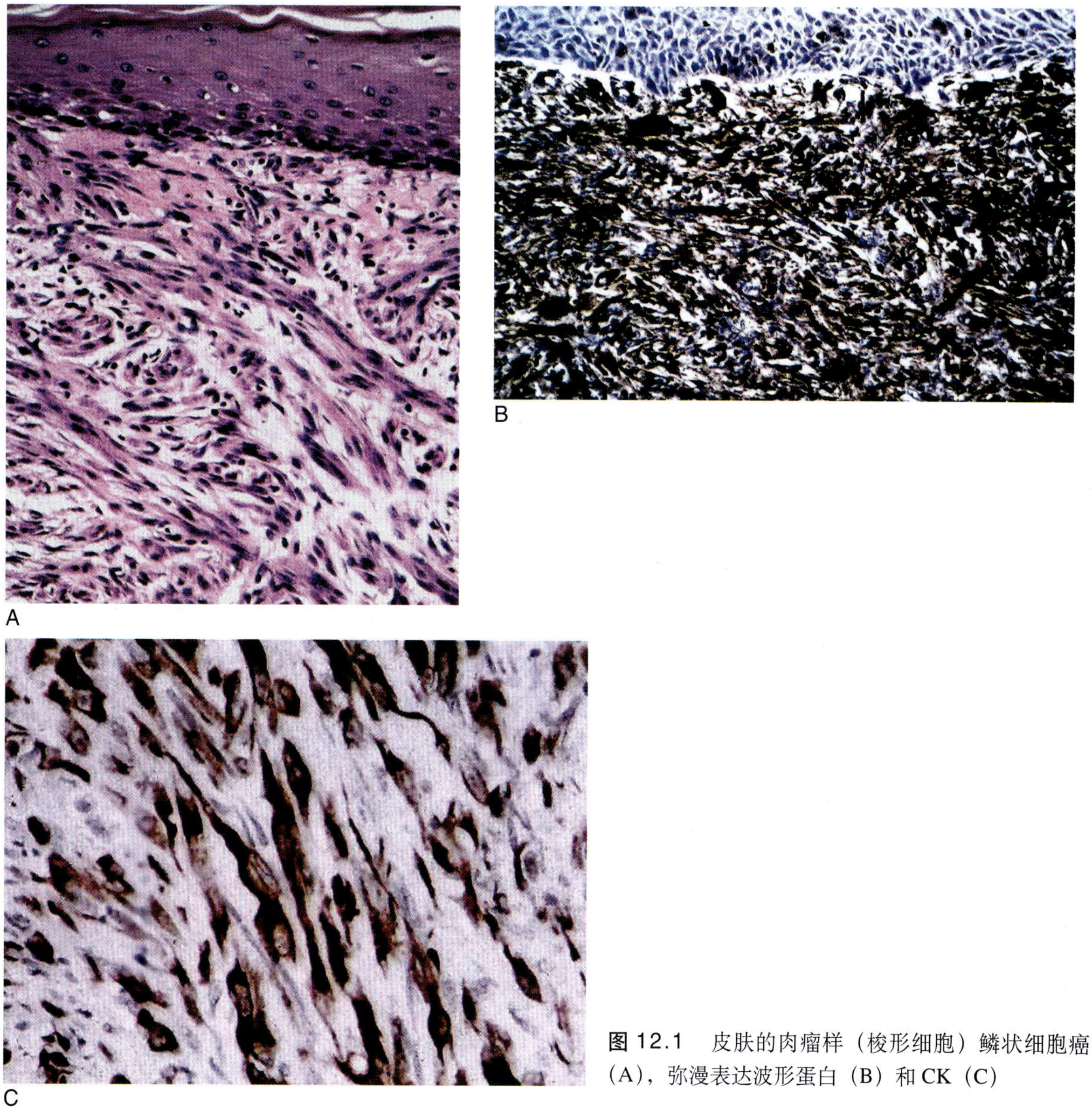

图 12.1 皮肤的肉瘤样（梭形细胞）鳞状细胞癌（A），弥漫表达波形蛋白（B）和 CK（C）

多梭形细胞鳞癌多能表达结蛋白和肌特异性标记物肌动蛋白[8]。

遗憾的是，没有有效的免疫组化标记物能检测上皮细胞的分化程度。中间丝（filaggrin）和外皮蛋白（involucrin）[11-15]，与上皮角化有关，在 SCC 中有表达，有时被当做角化上皮恶性增生的标志，但还没有被认可。笔者认为没有一种标记物能很好地区别皮肤良、恶性肿瘤，例如中间丝和外皮蛋白，两者在各种上皮良性肿瘤和增生性疾病中都有表达[13,16]。中间丝和外皮蛋白对于鉴别 SCC 和基底细胞癌有帮助，但不能区别 SCC 和皮肤附属器来源的肿瘤[12,17]，尤其是来源于毛发的肿瘤。所以尽管两者能说明肿瘤细胞有角

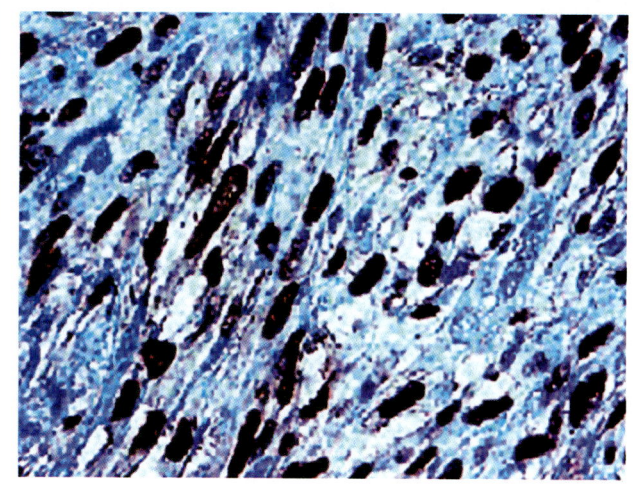

图 12.2 皮肤低分化鳞状细胞癌 p63 阳性

化功能，但对于实际工作意义不大。

基底细胞癌（BCC）同SCC一样，有许多不同亚型，需注意鉴别诊断。其中了解比较多的亚型包括：硬皮病样型、腺样型、透明细胞型、角化型和异型型（鳞状上皮样）[18]。

总的来说，基底细胞癌表达的抗原较少，同SCC一样，BCC可以表达CK，但这些中间丝的分子量一般小于50kD。与SCC不同，BCC各亚型均不表达EMA（图12.3）[9, 20, 21]。

少数的BCC可以表达HMB-45，还有少数病例可表达内分泌相关多肽，如CD56、突触素（Syn）和嗜铬素A（CgA）[22-24]。需要注意的是，大多数BCC并不表达这些抗原。BCC的一个显著特征是能表达一些特殊的分化标记物，如α-肌动蛋白（α-actin）[25]，因此有观点认为该肿瘤细胞具有表皮干细胞特征。然而BCC不表达波形蛋白、CEA、S-100、CD57和CD15[26]，这些证据又不支持上述观点。BCC可以向不同方向分化，如"小汗腺上皮瘤"[27]、"大汗腺上皮瘤"[28]、"基底皮脂腺样上皮瘤"[18]，在这些具有不同分化的区域，可以表达EMA、CEA或者CD15。

BerEP4是另一个能在大多数BCC中表达的糖蛋白，其抗体能与人类皮肤上皮细胞的两个抗原决定簇（分子量分别为34kD和39kD）结合（图12.4）[29]。BerEP4不仅在BCC中有表达，在Paget病、Merkel细胞癌和某些附属器肿瘤中也有表达。BerEP4对于鉴别异型型（鳞状上皮样）BCC和基底细胞样SCC最有帮助，后者BerEP4阴性[30]。这一指标对于某些部位的肿瘤的诊断非常关键，如肛门和肛周皮肤。

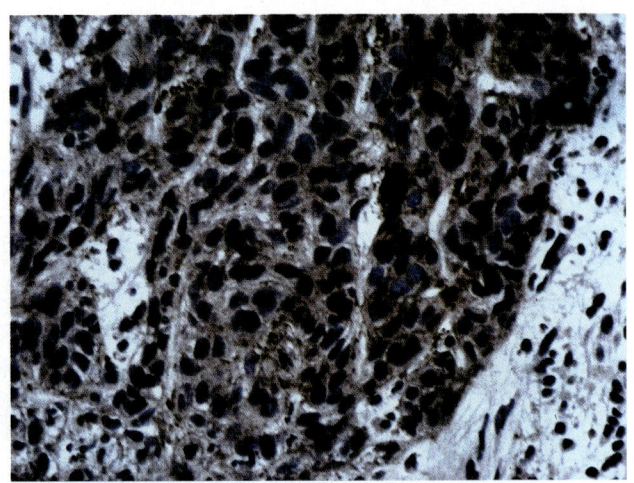

图12.4　基底细胞癌BerEP4弥漫阳性

> **诊断要点：上皮性肿瘤**
>
> 1. 鳞状上皮细胞癌（SCC）各亚型：腺样（皮肤棘层松解）型、多形型、小细胞型和梭形细胞型，基底细胞癌也包括许多亚型。
> 2. SCC表达AE1/AE3、K903、CK5/6。
> 3. 低分化SCC表达CAM5.2、AE1/AE3。
> 4. SCC：EMA+、p63+、BerEP4-。
> 5. BCC：EMA-、BerEP4+。

汗腺肿瘤

皮肤的汗腺组织主要由小汗腺和大汗腺组成。由这些结构起源的肿瘤，组织学特点多样[31]，但能表达一些相同的抗原。所有这些肿瘤均表达CK，部分表达CEA、肿瘤相关糖蛋白72（TAG-72，又称作CA72.4）（图12.5）、EMA、CD15和p63[32, 33]。后三者在汗腺瘤或汗腺癌中均有不同程度的表达，EMA阳性在汗腺恶性肿瘤中较良性肿瘤更常见，事实上，小汗腺来源的良性肿瘤，如螺旋腺瘤和圆柱瘤，并不表达EMA。无论何种生物学行为，CEA和CD15在大约70%~80%的所有小汗腺和大汗腺肿瘤中均有表达[20, 32, 34, 35]。CA72.4在大汗腺肿瘤中表达，而在小汗腺肿瘤中通常不表达[36, 37]，有助于鉴别汗腺来源的肿瘤和皮肤其他腺样或上皮性肿瘤，也有助于显示少数皮肤淋巴上皮样癌的汗腺分化成分，该肿瘤分化低，与鼻咽部的淋巴上皮癌相似[38]。

小汗腺来源肿瘤和大汗腺来源肿瘤的抗原表型有所不同，这对诊断有帮助。大约50%的小汗腺肿瘤表达S-100蛋白，而大汗腺肿瘤，包括侵袭性乳腺外

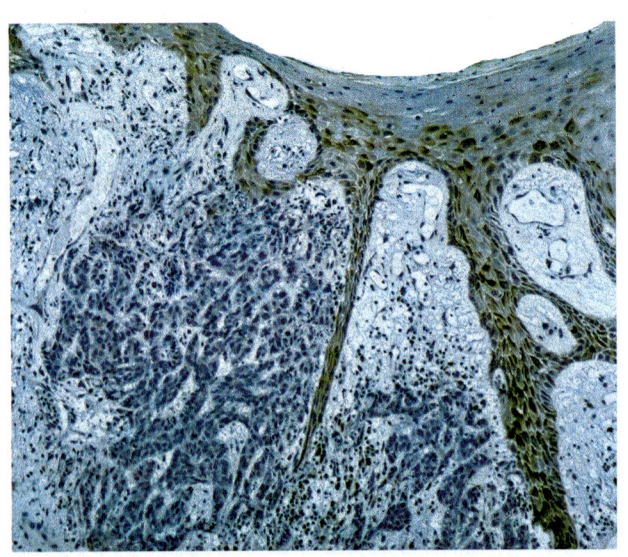

图12.3　基底细胞癌不表达EMA，其被覆的表皮表达EMA

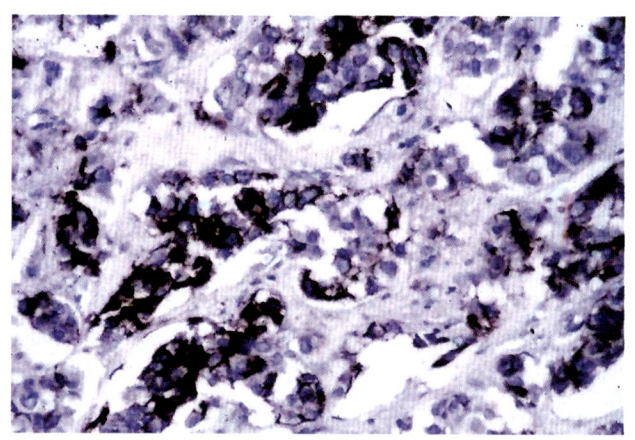

图 12.5　汗腺癌 CD72.4（抗体 B72.3）阳性

Paget 病（EPD），通常不表达 S-100[39]。囊泡病液体蛋白 15（GCDFP-15）在大汗腺细胞及其来源的肿瘤中选择性表达（图 12.6）[32, 40]，其他阳性标记物还有 CA72.4、CK7 及 BerEP4。这些指标有助于区别 EPD 和浅表扩散性恶性黑色素瘤及 Paget 病样鲍温病（上皮内鳞癌），因为只有前者表达上述标记物[41-43]。CK20 在会阴部 EPD 或伴有附近脏器癌（如直肠癌或子宫颈内膜癌）[44-46]的肛周 EPD 中表达。在以上需要鉴别的肿瘤中只有鲍温病表达高分子量角蛋白（这也是其他 SCC 的典型特征）[47]，仅黑色素瘤表达 HMB-45、MART-1 和 S-100 蛋白（见第 6 章）[39]。

GCDFP-15 并不是大汗腺细胞的特异性标记物，笔者的实验室证实部分小汗腺来源肿瘤也可以表达该抗原[32]。然而 GCDFP-15 在诊断一些良性汗腺肿瘤时还是有帮助的。例如，尽管有少数小汗腺来源的汗腺瘤能散在地表达 GCDFP-15，但只有在有大汗腺分化特征的肿瘤中才有稳定的表达[40]。良性混合性肿瘤（软骨样汗管瘤）以前被认为是一种小汗腺肿瘤，然而在一些病例中，管状成分能一致地表达 GCDFP-15，故目前认为该肿瘤既有小汗腺又有大汗腺的特征[40]。其他囊泡病液体蛋白，包括 GCDFP-24 和锌-α-2- 糖蛋白特异性不高[48]。

有资料表明小汗腺肿瘤可选择性地表达一些特殊 CK 及其他细胞标记物，如"EKH5"、"EKH6"、"IKH-4"[49, 50]，但由于对这些指标在皮肤和皮外肿瘤中表达的系统性研究较少，故它们的特异性还不明确。

汗腺癌的一个诊断难点是与皮肤转移性腺癌鉴别（图 12.7）[51]。目前最好的鉴别方法还是依靠临床病史。皮肤原发附属器肿瘤多为孤立性肿块，生长缓慢；而转移性腺癌为多个肿块，生长迅速。有研究表明 p63 对于鉴别两者有帮助[33]，在绝大多数汗腺癌中 p63 阳性表达，而几乎所有的转移性腺癌不表达。

> **诊断要点：汗腺肿瘤**
>
> 1. 表达 CK、CEA、CA72.4、CD15、p63。
> 2. EMA 在汗腺恶性肿瘤中表达多为阳性。
> 3. 小汗腺癌：S-100+；大汗腺癌：S-100-，GCDFP-15+。
> 4. Paget 病：CK7+，GCDFP-15+、BerEP4+、CA72.4+。
> 5. 恶性黑色素瘤：Paget 病标记物阴性，HMB-45+、melan-A+、S-100+。
> 6. 鲍温病：AE1/AE3、K903+、Paget 病和黑色素瘤标记物阴性。

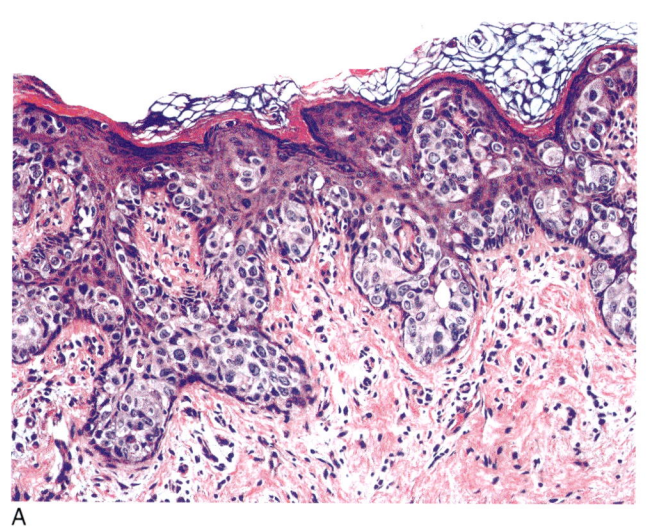

A

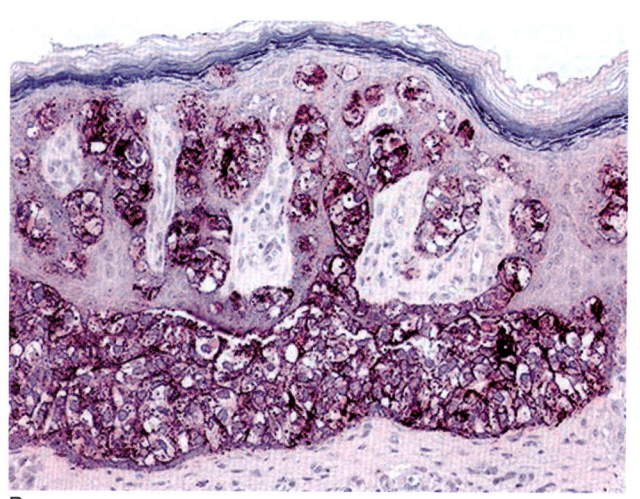

B

图 12.6　皮肤乳外 Paget 病（A）通常表达 GCDFP-15（B）

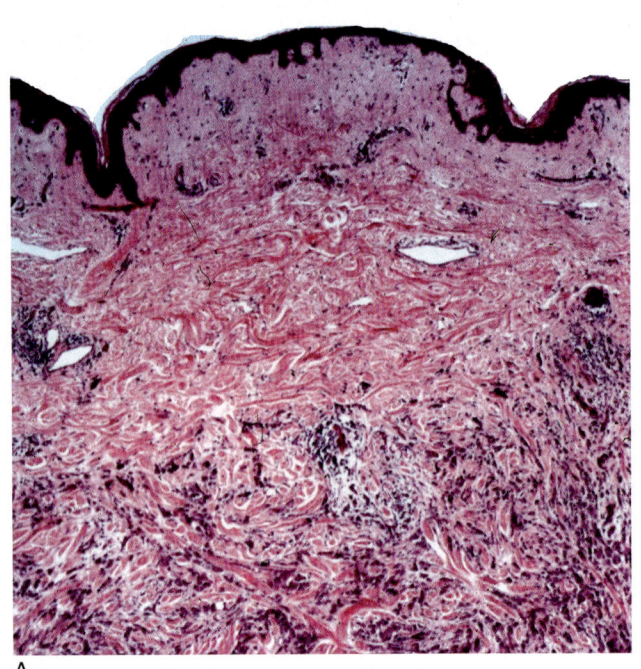 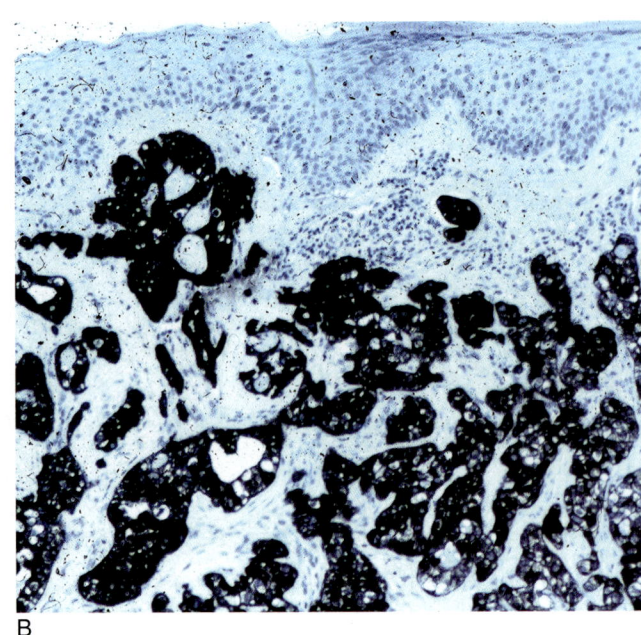

图12.7 皮肤转移的腺癌（A），弥漫性表达癌胚抗原CEA（B）。皮肤原发性和转移的腺癌除此以外，还共同表达其他一些标记物

皮脂腺肿瘤

尽管皮脂腺具有腺样结构，但无论从局部解剖学上，还是个体发生上，都与毛囊关系密切。因此，该肿瘤表达的抗原成分介于外毛鞘峡部和皮脂腺出芽性基底样细胞之间，也就不足为奇了。同样，基底皮脂腺和毛鞘成分也可混合出现在同一肿瘤中（如伴有皮脂腺分化的浅表上皮瘤和"皮脂腺瘤"）。毛发和皮脂腺来源的肿瘤都可以同时表达高分子量和低分子量角蛋白，但绝大多数汗腺来源的肿瘤不表达，同样说明前两者具有共同的细胞起源[51]。就组织结构来说，皮脂腺来源的肿瘤与毛发来源的肿瘤较汗腺肿瘤更相似，免疫组化研究也发现许多汗腺肿瘤标记物，如S-100蛋白、CA72.4、GCDFP-15、CEA在皮脂腺肿瘤中不表达。

EMA及其相关产物在皮脂腺肿瘤中多有表达[52]，呈一种独特的表达方式。无论是良性还是恶性皮脂腺上皮增生，类似于成熟皮脂腺细胞的微囊状或泡沫状胞浆的特点都可以见到（图12.8）。由于EMA包绕细胞浆内脂滴呈膜状表达，所以能将肿瘤性和非肿瘤性增生的皮脂腺细胞很好区别开。即使在分化较差的皮脂腺癌中，EMA染色也可以将不明显的多泡状胞浆的特点显示出来[53]。

尽管皮脂腺肿瘤和汗腺肿瘤都表达CD15和BerEP4[29, 35]，但在大多数情况下，对EMA、S-100、CEA的不同表达还是能将两者很好地区别开。到目前为止，还没有很好的皮脂腺肿瘤的特异性标记物[52]。有研究认为细胞核雄激素受体蛋白（ARP）能很好地选择性标记皮脂腺细胞及其来源的肿瘤。但对于该标记物学者们研究结果不同，Bayer-Garner等人[54]认为所有皮脂腺肿瘤均表达ARP，而Shikata及其同事[55]却认为皮脂腺肿瘤并不表达ARP。Bayer-Garner等人还发现低分化的皮脂腺癌缺少胞浆多泡状的EMA阳性特点。其他研究发现免疫球蛋白A、脂肪酶、乳脂肪球相关（卵巢癌相关）皮脂样抗原OV-2以及OKM5（CD36）可能在皮脂腺肿瘤中选择性表达[52]。但对于这些指标还缺少在皮外病变表达的系统性研究。

> **诊断要点：皮脂腺肿瘤**
>
> 1. 不表达S-100、CA72.4、GCDFP-15、CEA，而汗腺肿瘤这些指标阳性。
> 2. 皮脂腺和汗腺肿瘤均表达CD15和BerEP4。
> 3. EMA呈胞浆特征的泡沫状阳性表达。

毛发肿瘤

由于毛发有不同分化方向，因而毛发来源的良性肿瘤形态多种多样，诊断也就比较复杂[56]。遗憾的是

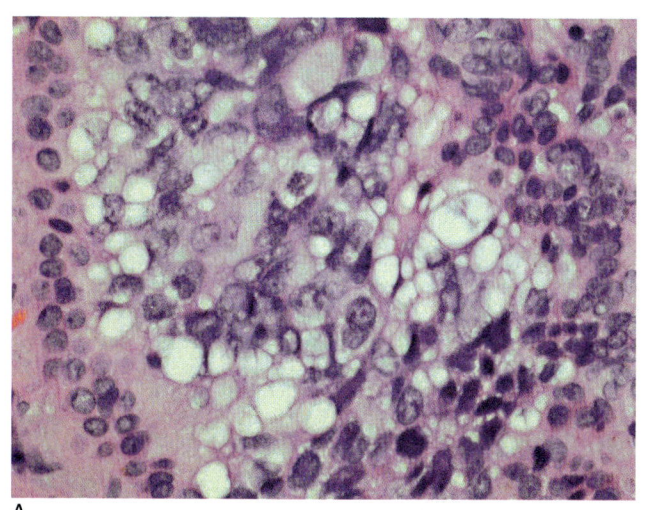

图 12.8 皮脂腺癌（A）通常弥漫性表达 EMA（B），细胞浆呈特征性的泡沫状

几乎所有的商业化抗体都不能将毛发来源的各种肿瘤区分开，例如来源于生毛基、毛皮质、内毛鞘、外毛鞘以及毛囊漏斗的病变。事实上所有的毛发良性肿瘤表达的抗原基本相似，包括 BerEP4、p63 及分子量 50kD 以上的CK[4, 5, 57]，除了个别增生性毛发肿瘤表达外，一般不表达EMA[57]，其他不表达的抗原还包括：CEA、S-100、CD15、CA72.4、HMB-45 和 GCDFP-15。由此可见，毛发来源腺瘤的免疫表型与BCC相似。

不少研究认为经典毛发上皮瘤（CTE）与 BCC 有很多概念上的不同，因此也在积极寻找区别两者的免疫组化标记物。有观点认为用bcl-2标记上皮细胞（图12.9）及用CD34标记瘤周组织可以鉴别BCC和 CTE[58, 59]。Lum 和 Binder[60]发现 Ki-67 指数大于 25% 和 p21 蛋白阳性支持 BCC 的诊断。许多学者[61]在鉴别两种肿瘤上的研究并未得出有用结论，总之，我们认为区别 BCC 和 CTE 不能只依靠免疫组化，因为 CTE 很可能是一种高分化 BCC。已经有越来越多的研究证实CTE"转化"为BCC[62-66]，两种肿瘤在基因表达上的相同改变（均有染色体 9q22.3 片段的缺失）[67]就是一个很好的证据。

促结缔组织增生性毛发上皮瘤（DTE）和浸润性基底细胞癌（IBCC）的小组织活检标本在组织学上有些相似，因此关于如何鉴别两者的研究也很多。较 IBCC 来说，DTE 的上皮细胞更常表达 EMA 和表现出神经内分泌分化（多灶性表达 CD56、嗜铬素 A 和角蛋白 20）（图 12.10）[68, 69]。而 IBCC 的瘤周间质细胞多表达间质水解酶 -3（一种蛋白水解酶），DTE 则不表达[70]。

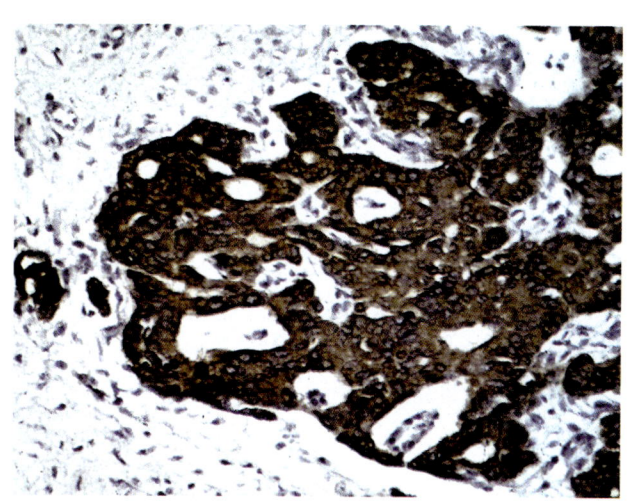

图 12.9 基底细胞癌 bcl-2 阳性

在对毛发和表皮肿瘤的某些研究显示，角蛋白的表达方式对于诊断毛囊病变有帮助[71, 72]。最有趣的发现是，在有毛母质分化的细胞，用抗体AE12和AE13染色后可以显示出"硬角化珠"的特点。毛母质瘤作为毛母质来源肿瘤的代表，弥漫表达 AE13，而对于毛囊瘤，AE13 仅在缩小的或残余的毛囊细胞中表达。伴有毛根鞘分化的肿瘤，例如增生性毛发肿瘤和外毛根鞘瘤 AE13 阴性，但 AE14 阳性（图 12.11）。AE14 是一种单克隆抗体，可以同时识别毛皮质的含硫部分和一种低分子量角蛋白[72]。这种小分子量角蛋白普遍表达于大多数附属器上皮和上皮基底细胞，因此，AE14不如AE13有意义。有趣的是在促结缔组织增生性毛发上皮瘤中，少数小角化巢表达 AE13，而经典的毛发上皮瘤一致不表达AE13。在微囊状附属器癌中，小角化巢也恒定表达 AE13，说明该肿瘤有

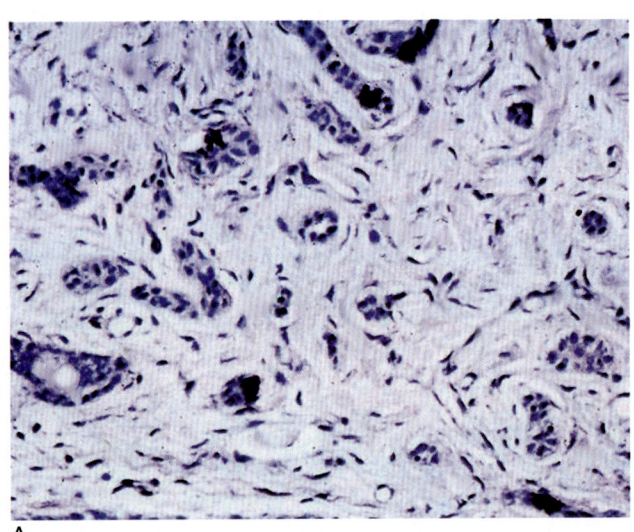
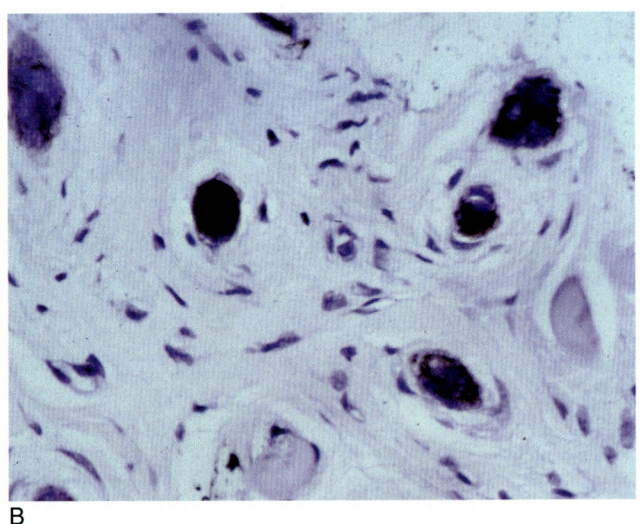

图12.10 嗜铬素A（A）和CK20（B）在结缔组织增生性毛发上皮瘤散在的细胞巢中阳性表达。这些指标在硬化性基底细胞癌（主要的鉴别肿瘤）中一般不表达

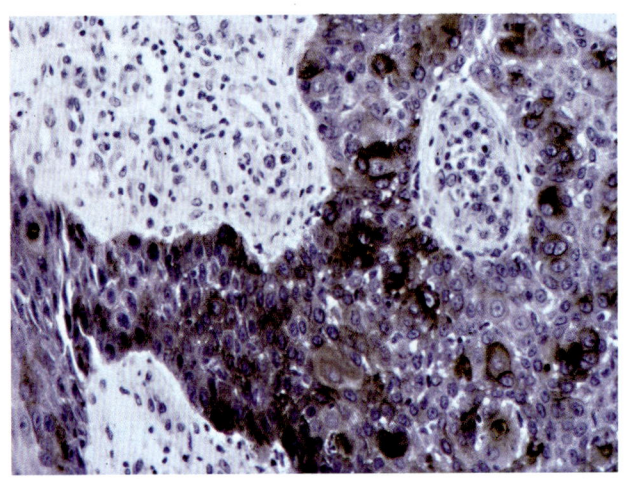

图12.11 AE14染色显示低度恶性的增生性毛发肿瘤的"毛发型"角化现象

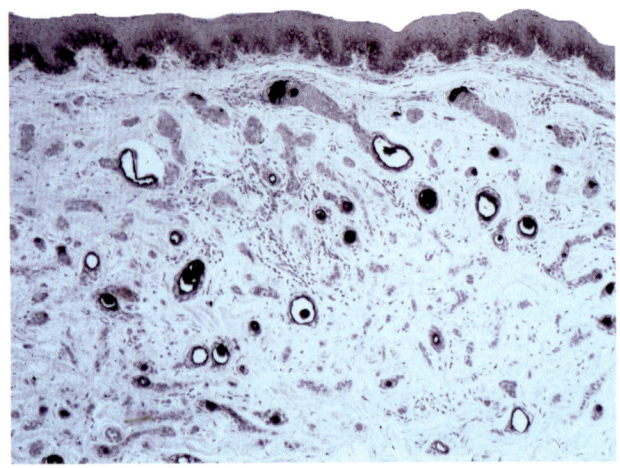

图12.12 AE13在皮肤微囊性腺癌中呈多灶性表达。其抗体可用于识别毛囊相关的角化亚型癌

部分毛发分化特征（图12.12）[73]。

标记角蛋白的抗体HKN5、HKN6、HKN7[71]和抗人毛发角蛋白（HHK）抗体[74]阳性说明有毛发方向分化。HKN6/7表达仅见于表皮、毛皮质、内毛鞘细胞，而HKN5还可以标记外毛鞘细胞。毛母质瘤特异性表达HKN6/7和HHK抗原[74]，HHK阳性还可见于恶性毛母质瘤，而绝大多数毛发其他肿瘤、BCC和其他表皮增生性病变不表达HKN6/7和HHK抗原。毛发肿瘤和BCC均可表达HKN5，但脂溢性角化病不表达。"Borst-Jadassohn"（克隆）型上皮内癌的部分病例可以表达HKN5、HKN6和HKN7，说明这些病变具有毛发分化的一些特征[71]。

随着恶性转化，毛发肿瘤的免疫表型在一定程度也变得越来越复杂。毛发癌[增生性毛发肿瘤发展而来的鳞癌样肿瘤（高级别恶性的增生性毛发肿瘤）][75]多表达EMA，外毛根鞘癌（一种在组织结构和细胞形态上都与外毛根鞘瘤相似的肿瘤）能局灶性表达CEA和S-100[76]。除了一部分CK和p63外，毛发和汗腺肿瘤缺少相同的免疫标记物。

> **诊断要点：** 毛发来源肿瘤
>
> 1. 毛发腺瘤的免疫表型与皮肤BCC相似，不表达EMA、CEA、S-100、CD15、CA72.4。
> 2. DTE同IBCC相比表达EMA、CD15、嗜铬素和CK20，而上述指标大多在IBCC阴性。
> 3. IBCC间质细胞表达间质水解酶-3。

内分泌肿瘤

皮肤原发性神经内分泌癌（PCNC）最早被称为"皮肤小梁癌"，现在公认称作"Merkel细胞癌"。30年来，PCNC的生物学和免疫组织化学特点一直吸引着学者的兴趣。一些学者推测PCNC同正常皮肤和口腔黏膜的Merkel细胞一样[77]，具有神经方向分化的特点，但是缺少证据支持或否定这一假设。非肿瘤性Merkel细胞表达CK20、CG、MOC-31、神经丝、CD56、甲硫氨酸脑啡肽、血管活性肠肽（VIP）和血型抗原Pr（h），但总的来说缺乏其他内分泌标记物的表达[78-83]。绝大多数（但不是所有的）PCNC表达广谱角蛋白、CK20、MOC-31抗原、BerEP4抗原、嗜铬素A、降钙素、生长抑素、促肾上腺皮质激素、VIP、胰多肽和P物质[84-88]。

有观点认为PCNC与汗腺癌关系密切[89]。但作者研究了200例以上的Merkel细胞癌，却没有发现任何一例表达CEA、S-100、CA72.4或GCDFP-15，而这些指标在汗腺肿瘤中均有表达。

PCNC肿瘤细胞较小、一致，细胞连接不紧密，呈弥漫性或髓样生长，因此有时被误认为是真皮内的淋巴瘤。免疫组化容易鉴别，淋巴瘤CD45阳性而PCNC阴性。CK在Merkel细胞癌中多在细胞核周围环状聚集，染色后呈特征性的圆点状（图12.13）[90]。这种图像如果出现在皮肤小细胞肿瘤中，即使该肿瘤不表达嗜铬素、突触素或CD56，也说明其具有上皮和神经内分泌分化特点。

单凭组织学图像，不能区分PCNC和转移到皮肤的肺或其他脏器的小细胞神经内分泌癌，CEA、CK20和甲状腺转录因子-1（TTF-1）对鉴别诊断有帮助。支气管的小细胞神经内分泌癌能特异性表达CEA或TTF-1（图12.14），或者同时表达两者，但不表达CK20[91, 92]。同皮外的神经内分泌癌不同[88]，CK20在PCNC中多有表达。尽管有以上免疫组化鉴别方法，但在完全排除转移癌前，还是应该进行全面的临床检查，尤其是进行细致的胸腔影像学检查。

皮肤深部的PCNC要考虑与皮下的原发性尤文肉瘤/原始神经外胚层肿瘤（ES/PNET）鉴别[93-98]。两者均表达CD56、CD57、FLI-1、Syn和CD99（图12.15），但广谱角蛋白在PNET中少见表达，该肿瘤也不表达CK20和EMA[95, 96, 98-101]；波形蛋白在绝大多数PNET有表达，在PCNC中不表达。

单凭形态学图像，有时可将某些PCNC误诊为BCC，有研究认为BCC有向神经内分泌分化的潜能，但远不及PCNC普遍，而且与Merkel细胞癌不同，BCC不表达CK20和EMA，也没有PCNC中见到的核周角蛋白阳性现象。

各种皮肤上皮性肿瘤的免疫表型特点见图12.15B。

> **诊断要点：内分泌肿瘤**
>
> 1. PCNC阳性指标：CK20（核周圆点状）、神经丝、CD15、CD56、CD57、嗜铬素及多种神经内分泌激素，不表达波形蛋白。
> 2. 皮肤转移的肺小细胞癌：CEA+、TIF-1+、CK-，而PCNC的免疫组化表型与其相反。
> 3. 皮肤的尤文肉瘤或PNET：CK如有表达多呈局灶性，波形蛋白+、CK20-、EMA-。

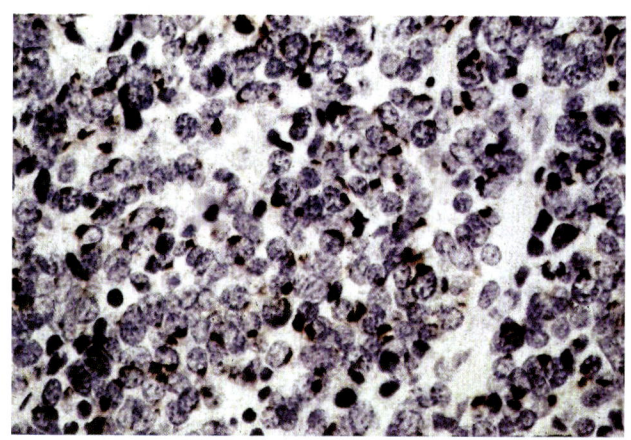

图12.13 角蛋白在Merkel细胞癌中呈核周"点状"阳性，这种着色方式说明该肿瘤具有上皮和神经内分泌分化的特征

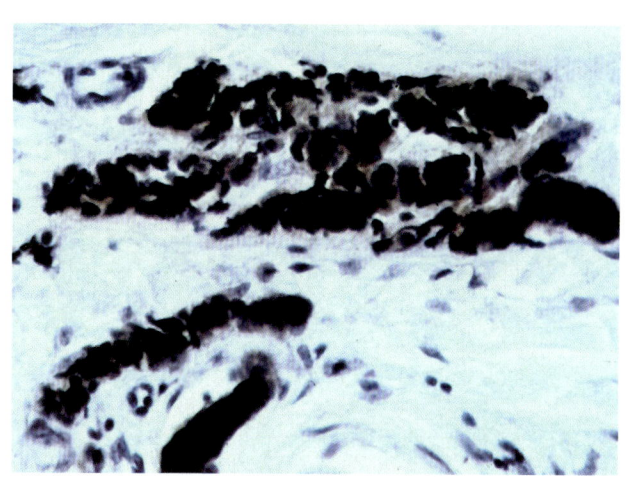

图12.14 甲状腺转录因子-1在转移到皮肤的肺小细胞神经内分泌癌中呈弥漫性核阳性染色，在Merkel细胞癌中通常不表达

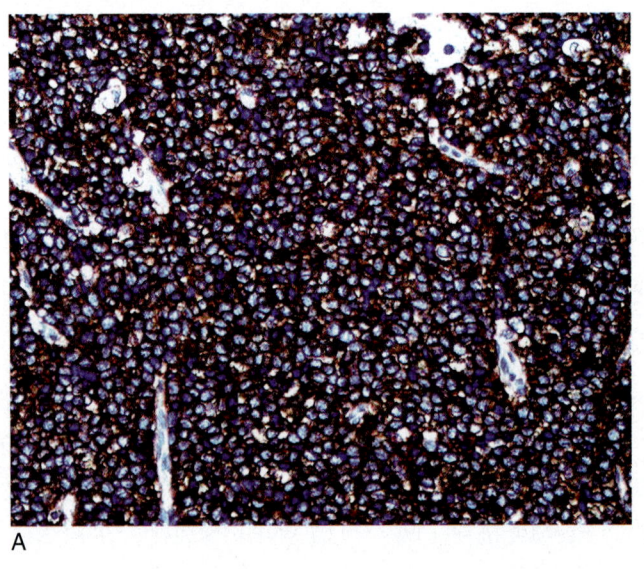

图 12.15　CD99 在皮下原始神经外胚层肿瘤中表达（A），这一指标在 Merkel 细胞癌中也有表达。各种皮肤癌的免疫组化表型（B）（SCC，鳞状细胞癌；BCC，基底细胞癌；SGC，汗腺癌；SBC，皮脂腺癌；PC，毛发癌；NEC，神经内分泌癌；CK5/6，角蛋白5/6；AE13，AE14，毛发相关角蛋白；PER CK，角蛋白核周点状阳性；EMA，上皮细胞膜抗原；CEA，癌胚抗原；S-100，S-100 蛋白；ARP，雄激素受体蛋白；CA72.4，TAG-72，肿瘤相关糖蛋白-72；CGA，嗜铬素 A；SYN，突触素）

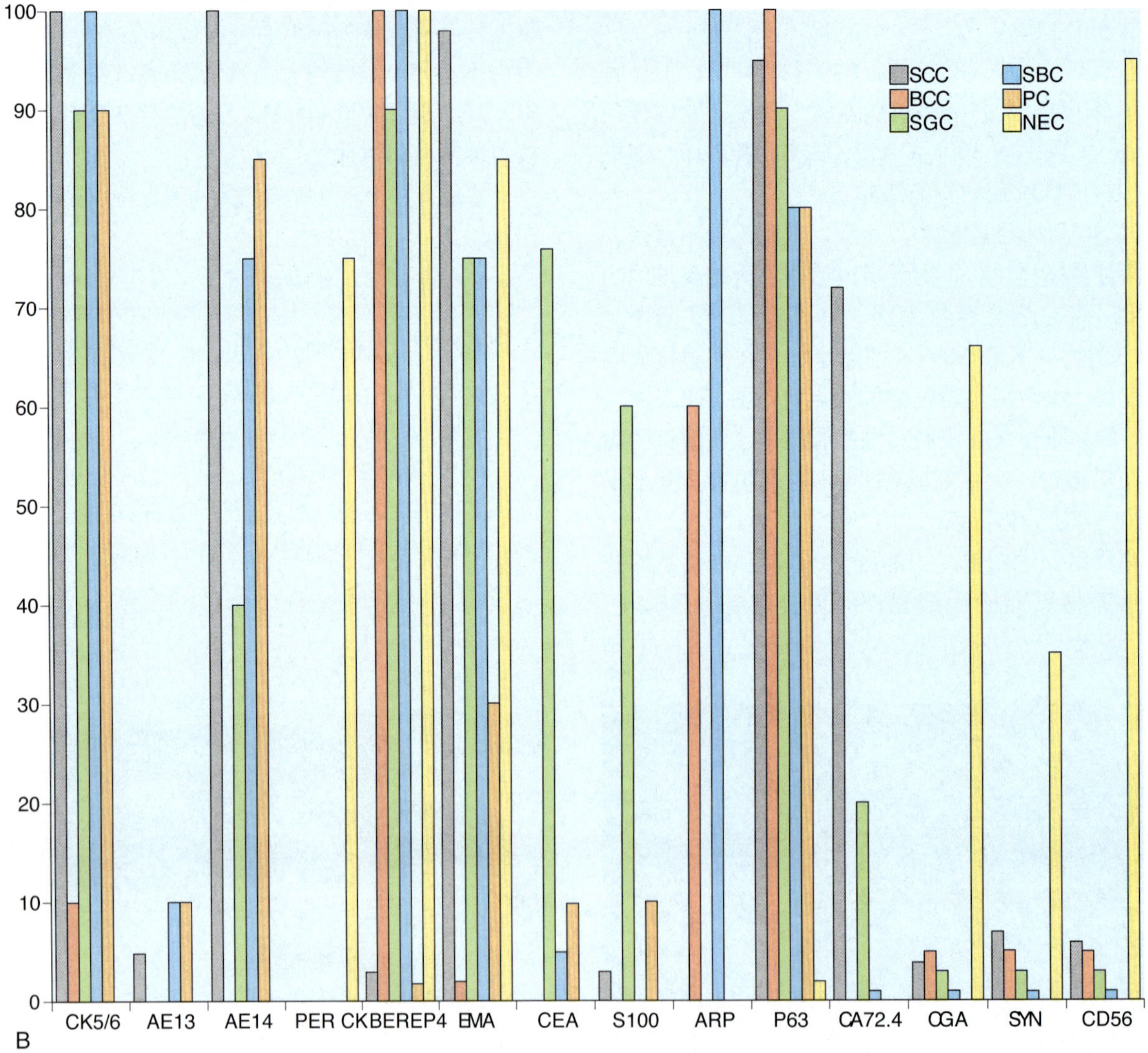

皮肤淋巴造血组织病变

由于皮肤的T淋巴细胞、B淋巴细胞和组织细胞的增生性病变多种多样，所以不可能在这一章中对每一种病变都能详细介绍，第4章和第5章对血液系统疾病的免疫组化特点已有详细的介绍。区别良、恶性淋巴网状增生性病变的组织学指标，尽管不是全部，但还是同样能用于皮肤淋巴病变的诊断。单凭形态学图像和临床病史常常很难对淋巴细胞类型作出判断，本章主要介绍对皮肤淋巴造血组织病变诊断有帮助的免疫组化特点。

皮肤淋巴瘤和白血病

针对淋巴细胞不同抗原的各种有效抗体已经应用于皮肤活检标本的淋巴造血组织疾病的诊断[102-117]。事实上皮肤所有淋巴瘤和白血病的石蜡标本均能表达CD45[118]，借此可排除其他组织图像相似的其他非造血组织增生性疾病。不同细胞选择性表达不同种系抗原的特点也可用于诊断。T细胞标记物包括：CD3、CD4、CD5、CD7、CD8、CD43和CD45RO；B细胞标记物包括：CD20、4KB5 CD45R、CD79α、PAX-5、CD179和cyclin D1；单核组织细胞标记物包括：CD68、MAC387、Ⅷα因子和组织蛋白酶B。CD30和ALK-1是原发性和继发性间变性大细胞淋巴瘤的标记物（图12.16）[102-117, 119]。皮肤的霍奇金淋巴瘤非常罕见[120]，本章不作介绍。

上述标记物大多只在相应的种系细胞中表达，然而CD43却在B细胞病变、T细胞浸润和髓样增生性疾病中均有表达[121]。髓样增生性疾病尤其值得注意，皮内浸润的髓单核细胞CD43阳性，但CD45一般仅为弱阳性[122]。通过检测其他粒细胞和单核细胞标记物如髓过氧化物酶、CD117和组织蛋白酶B，对于仅CD43阳性的病例，可作出真皮髓样白血病（髓

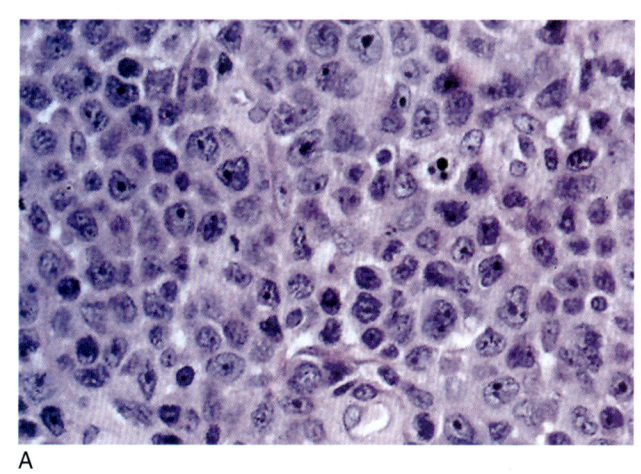

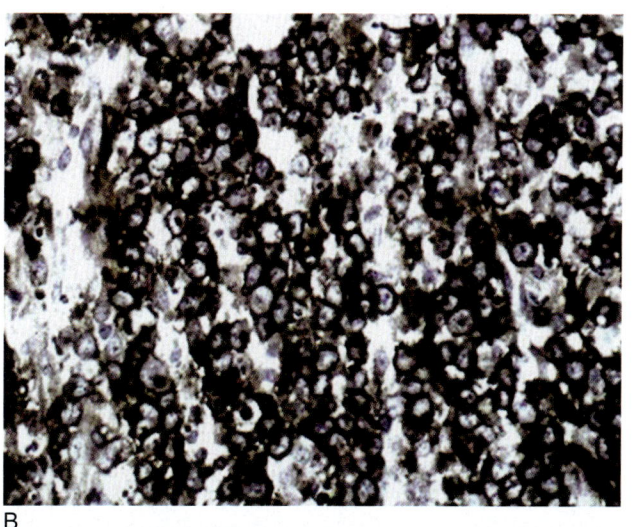

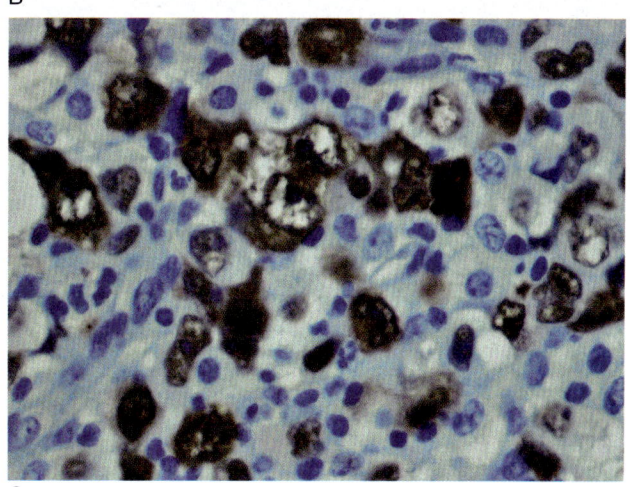

图12.16 皮肤间变性大细胞淋巴瘤（A）通常表达CD30（B）。全身性淋巴瘤累及皮肤也会表达 ALK-1 蛋白（C）

外髓样瘤、粒细胞肉瘤)的诊断(图12.17)[111, 112, 117]。小儿皮肤的淋巴母细胞白血病/淋巴瘤也可以仅表达CD43,但如果CD10、CD99、PAX-5、末端脱氧核糖核酸转移酶(图12.18)和CD179阳性[108, 123, 124],有助于淋巴母细胞白血病/淋巴瘤的诊断。

石蜡切片免疫表型分析用于诊断的一个限制因素是这些标记物不能区分正常浸润细胞和恶性增生的淋巴细胞。Southern杂交和PCR可以很好地区分这两种病变[125, 126]。然而近年来的研究发现皮肤的淋巴样增生和皮肤淋巴瘤可能是一组连续的病变,而不是毫无关联、各自独立的[127, 128]。因此即使采用分子生物学手段,有时也不能完全区分两种病变。

尽管不容易区分,但如果看到完整的、免疫表型成熟的淋巴滤泡和复杂的炎细胞背景还是更支持皮肤良性B淋巴细胞增生,而不是B细胞淋巴瘤的诊断。许多皮肤B细胞淋巴瘤胞膜或胞浆单独表达免疫球蛋白轻链κ或λ[114]。κ和λ的商业化抗体在石蜡组织中表达很差,但在冰冻切片或细胞悬浮液中有很好的敏感性和特异性。原位杂交检测肿瘤细胞的单克隆属性对于石蜡切片淋巴瘤的诊断有帮助[129],另外一个有效手段是检测免疫球蛋白重链或轻链的单克隆性基因重排[126, 130]。

目前还没有发现检测T淋巴细胞单克隆性增生的有效标记物。但T细胞活化过程中免疫表型的细微改变对部分病例的诊断还是有帮助的。皮肤T细胞淋巴瘤(CTCL)的免疫表型较特殊,可表现为缺少

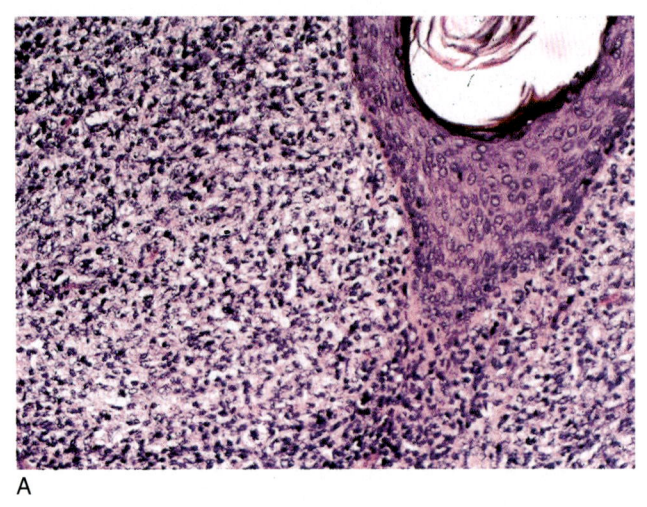
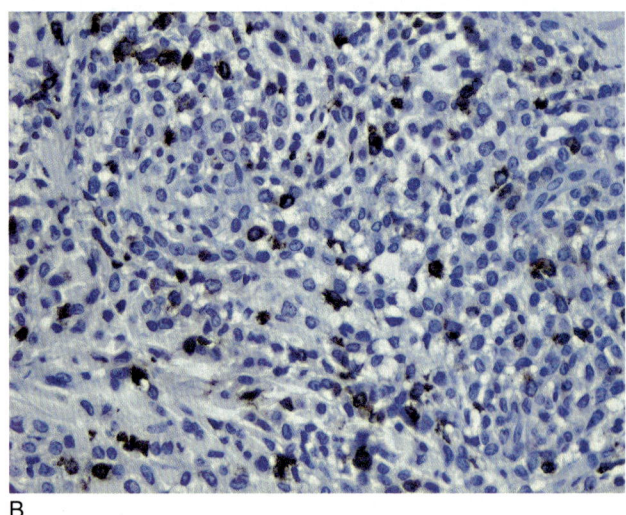

图12.17 皮肤的髓外髓样瘤(真皮髓样白血病、粒细胞肉瘤)(A),髓过氧化物酶呈多灶性阳性(B)

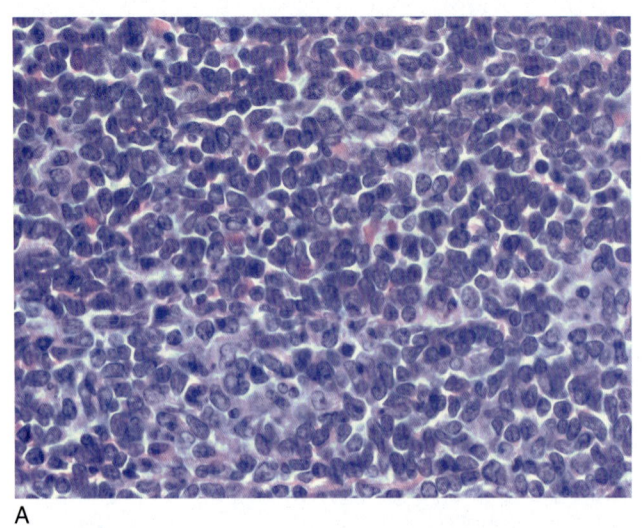
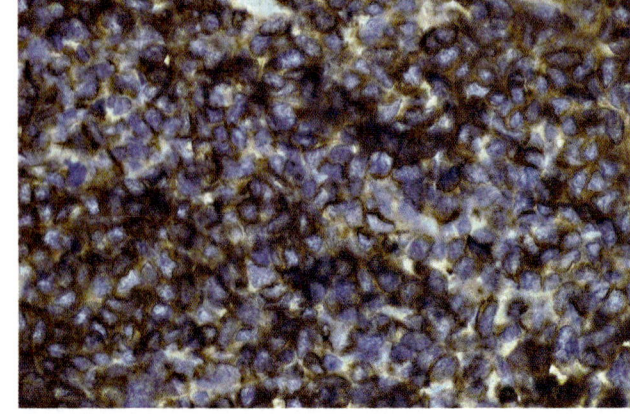

图12.18 皮肤淋巴母细胞性淋巴瘤(A),CD10弥漫阳性(B)

全T细胞标记物CD3、CD5、CD43和CD7（尤其是CD7）的表达，或者表现为同时表达CD4和CD8或者同时缺失（图12.19）[131, 132]。这种表达缺失在成熟的反应性增生的T淋巴细胞中一般不出现[103, 133, 134]。遗憾的是一些CTCL的免疫表型无上述特点，因此这一特征在鉴别淋巴瘤和富于T细胞的良性病变中并不一定可行[103, 133]。同时，一些良性浸润的T淋巴细胞也可出现淋巴瘤样的异常表型[132]。故诊断T细胞淋巴瘤更主要还是靠T细胞受体基因重排的检测[125, 135]。

B细胞免疫表型的一些异常也可用于诊断。最主要的就是B淋巴细胞CD5（或CD43）与CD20的共同表达[103, 136]，这种改变与免疫球蛋白轻链的单克隆性表达相符合。

在下文中，我们只对困扰诊断的皮肤的淋巴细胞浸润性病变进行介绍，与之相关的皮肤淋巴造血组织肿瘤的免疫组化特点在本书的其他章节可以找到[137-139]。

特殊类型的皮肤假瘤性淋巴样病变

蕈样霉菌病样亲表皮性浸润

在组织形态上与蕈样霉菌病（MF）相似的病变主要有药物引起的假淋巴瘤样浸润、慢性苔藓样皮炎、棘层松解性皮炎和光化性类网状细胞增多症[133, 140-142]。这些病变也表现为表皮和真皮间质的淋巴细胞聚集，而且这些淋巴细胞至少表现有中等程度的活化和核异型。同MF增生的细胞一样，这些细胞几乎都是T淋巴细胞[133, 141]。

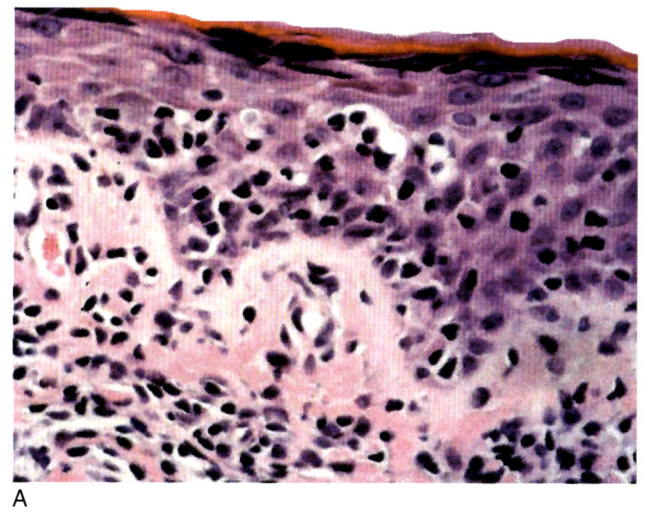

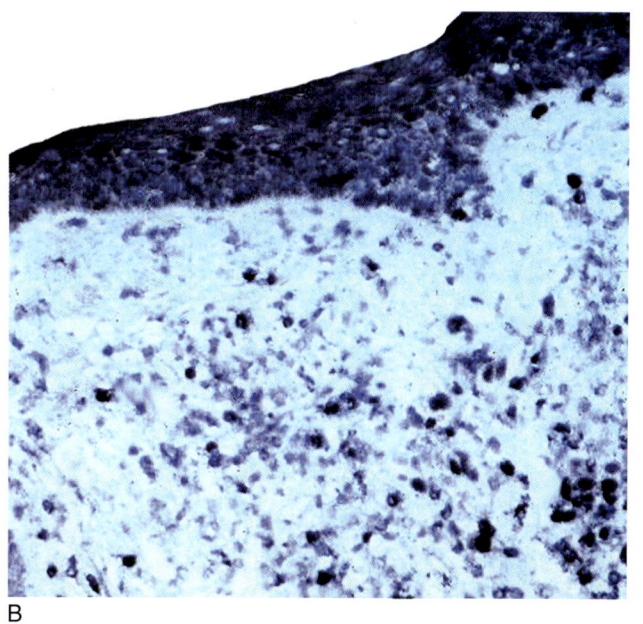

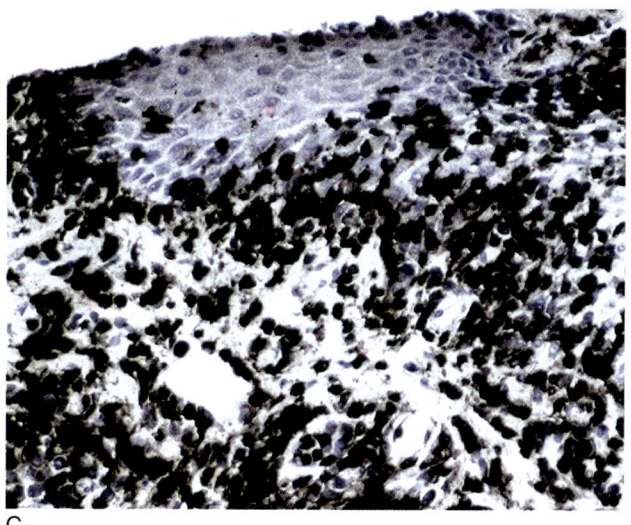

图12.19 蕈样霉菌病（A）的肿瘤性淋巴样细胞通常部分或全部不表达CD7（B），而CD4呈弥漫阳性（C）

如果可能的话,可以检测冰冻组织中细胞是否具有异常的T细胞免疫表型。如前面所述,异常的T细胞表型指缺少一种或更多的全T细胞标记物(CD2、3、5、7),或者同时表达几种通常不在一起表达的抗原(如CD4和CD8在同一细胞中表达)[103, 144]。CD7作为CD4+细胞增生的特异指标[103, 131],是MF中最常缺失的一个全T细胞标记物。然而并不是所有的皮肤T细胞淋巴瘤都有此特征,在一些良性炎性疾病中也发现有上述改变[132]。光化性类网状细胞增多症和大多数其他皮肤慢性炎性疾病通常表达全T细胞标记物。药物引起的假性MF可有和慢性皮肤棘层松解性皮炎相似的免疫表型,或者与MF表型相似[103, 141]。然而令人遗憾的是,药物引起的假性MF和MF的T细胞受体的基因重排结果也是一致的[145]。最后的结论是,在某种程度上,密切的临床随访观察是唯一有效的区别假性MF和真性皮肤T细胞淋巴瘤(CTCL)的方法。

石蜡切片的免疫组化分析能够用于区别皮肤良、恶性T细胞浸润病变。如前所述,笔者发现CD4-为主的上皮内淋巴细胞浸润,如CD3、CD5、CD7、CD43或CD45RO同时阴性,更多见于MF,而非皮肤的良性T细胞浸润病变。

类似于小细胞或混合性B细胞淋巴瘤的深部淋巴细胞浸润

一般来说,真皮和皮下深部出现大片浸润的淋巴细胞更有可能是B细胞淋巴瘤,而不是CTCL或外周T细胞淋巴瘤[146]。有些CTCL和外周T细胞淋巴瘤容易被误诊为良性病变,因为肿瘤主要由T淋巴细胞或者数量大致相同的T细胞和B细胞组成。易被混淆的病变包括Jessner浸润、活动性皮肤红斑狼疮和皮肤炎性假瘤[103]。然而,有些病变如皮肤淋巴腺瘤、皮肤淋巴细胞瘤和滤泡性皮肤淋巴组织增生(CLH),浸润的细胞主要由B淋巴细胞构成,诊断较困难[103, 139, 147-149]。

冰冻切片或原位杂交如能检测到B淋巴细胞限制性表达免疫球蛋白轻链κ或λ,对诊断很有帮助[150]。但κ或λ的表达差别必须大于10倍以上才有意义。

对于石蜡标本,一些指标也能有效区分B细胞淋巴瘤和各种类型的皮肤淋巴组织增生(CLH)。当CD20和CD43在肿瘤细胞中同时表达,且大于75%的浸润细胞是B淋巴细胞,其中超过30%的细胞PCNA或Ki-67阳性[136],则支持B细胞淋巴瘤的诊断。这一结论与Ngan等人对皮外淋巴病变的研究结果一致[151]。

另一指标bcl-2蛋白(BCLP)已被用于许多皮肤淋巴增生性病变的研究。BCLP是一种凋亡抑制因子,在有t(14;18)染色体易位的恶性淋巴瘤细胞中过表达[152],这种染色体易位是滤泡性淋巴瘤的特征改变(图12.20)。但BCLP对于鉴别皮肤淋巴增生性病变的帮助不大,一些皮肤CLH、CTCL和各种B细胞淋巴瘤均表达BCLP。必须牢记的是该指标只有在明显增生的滤泡中表达才有意义。滤泡性CLH不表达BCLP,但BCLP在皮肤滤泡性淋巴瘤中也不一定总是阳性[153-159]。

类似于大细胞淋巴瘤的皮肤大细胞淋巴组织增生

偶尔有些滤泡性CLH中有大量活化的免疫母细胞,镜下表现与结节性B细胞淋巴瘤大细胞型相似[146]。川崎病——一种少见的良性淋巴组织增生性病变,亚洲人较美国多见,镜下由大的异型的淋巴细胞组成,有时可被误认为是恶性病变[160-163]。

其实,采用多组常规免疫组化指标就有助于诊断富于滤泡性CLH。免疫组化发现增生的大细胞主要是B淋巴细胞,还可以观察到正常滤泡套区、富于T细胞的滤泡间区、滤泡中心Ki-67高表达。这些所见同淋巴结增生的图像相同。还要注意的是CD30,一种与

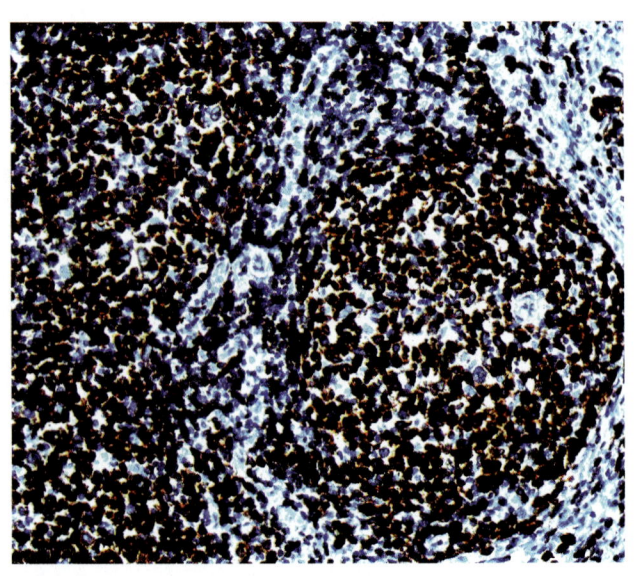

图12.20 bcl-2仅在皮肤原发性滤泡性淋巴瘤时有表达,主要见于低度恶性肿瘤

特定大细胞淋巴瘤相关的标记物[164]，在皮肤和其他部位的良性免疫母细胞增生性病变中也可以阳性[165, 166]。因此，不能单凭这一指标诊断为恶性病变。

川琦病（KD）表现为真皮内大的异型单核细胞浸润，同时伴有中性粒细胞浸润和坏死带，因此与间变性大细胞淋巴瘤（ALCL）相似[160-163]。事实上，KD是一种真正的组织细胞增生症，可以用单克隆抗体MAC387和CD68组的抗体（如KP-1）标记，但不表达CD20和全T细胞标记物[167]。由于新的疾病分类已经不包括恶性组织细胞增生症[164]，所以上述标记物对于诊断良性病变很有帮助。

朗格汉斯细胞组织细胞增生症（组织细胞增生症X）

朗格汉斯细胞组织细胞增生症（LCH）同皮肤其他造血组织浸润性病变一样，在临床病理表现典型的情况下，容易作出诊断[168]。LCH一般见于儿童，表现为皮肤多发的斑点样或丘疹样的突起。镜下由具有特征性核皱褶或核沟的组织细胞样细胞组成，排列成结节状或者边界不清。LCH通常在发病之前（或同时）出现皮外的相同病变，偶尔也表现为孤立的皮肤肿块。也有少数局限性皮肤LCH发生在成人[169-171]。上述情况均应从临床上和形态学上和以下疾病鉴别：皮肤淋巴瘤、恶性黑色素瘤、低分化的上皮和间叶肿瘤。

不管LCH在皮肤表现为何种形态，都具有一致的免疫表型。同上皮内非肿瘤性朗格汉斯组织细胞一样，LCH常常表达S-100、fascin、CD1α和CD31（图12.21）[172-175]，石蜡切片即可检测到，在其他标记物如CD21和melan-A都不表达的情况下，上述标记物对诊断很有帮助[172, 176]。S-100在少数非LCH的组织细胞浸润中也有表达，包括网状细胞增生和结外皮肤窦组织细胞增生伴巨大淋巴结病（Rosai-Dorfman病）[177, 178]。电镜观察到Birbeck颗粒进一步证实有朗格汉斯细胞的分化特征，但不是在所有的LCH中都能见到该包涵体[177]。

发生在儿童的其他皮肤组织细胞增生症的诊断并不难，包括所谓的先天性自限性网状组织细胞增生症（CSHR）[179, 180]和良性头部组织细胞增生症（BCH）[181-183]。CSHR是一种明确的朗格汉斯细胞增生症，具有与LCH全部相同的免疫表型和超微结构改变[179]。事实上，CSHR被普遍认为是一种局限型LCH。BCH同样来源于组织细胞，表达S-100，但与LCH的临床表现和组织图像却很少相似。BCH组织轮廓较清，局限在真皮浅层，缺少朗格汉斯细胞核的特点，不表达CD1α，无Birbeck颗粒[183]。

> **诊断要点：** 假瘤性淋巴组织增生性疾病
>
> 1. 上皮内浸润的CD4+淋巴细胞，如同时CD3、CD5、CD7、CD43或CD45RO阴性，更有可能是蕈样霉菌病，而不是其他良性病变。
> 2. CD20和CD43在某肿瘤中同时表达，且大于75%的浸润细胞是B淋巴细胞，其中超过30%的细胞Ki-67阳性，支持B细胞淋巴瘤的诊断。
> 3. 川崎病中增生的细胞是真正的组织细胞：不表达B细胞和T细胞的标志物，CD68和MAC387阳性。
> 4. 朗格汉斯细胞组织细胞增生症表达S-100、fascin、CD1α和CD31。

皮肤"假性假淋巴瘤"

皮肤所有的淋巴血液病变中，那些容易复发的病例往往是诊断的难点。其中两种病变：所谓的退行性非典型组织细胞增生症/皮肤间变性大细胞淋巴瘤（ALCL）和淋巴瘤样丘疹病，在组织学上被认为是皮肤良性增生性病变（假淋巴瘤），但临床评估和免疫表型分析却发现两者具有恶性肿瘤的特征。因此可认为两种病变是"假性假淋巴瘤"。

1982年Flynn等人[184]描述了一种特殊的皮肤病变，该病表现为真皮和皮下出现间变性、多形性的大淋巴样细胞。尽管有间变性大细胞的浸润，但患者一开始的临床表现却较好，皮肤病变可自行消退，有一段较长时间的缓解期。故退行性非典型组织细胞增生症（RAH），就是强调该病的惰性特征。然而遗憾的是，很多当初缓解的RAH患者会最终发展为皮肤和皮外的侵袭性淋巴细胞增生，具有"Ki-1"（CD30+）ALCL的特征性免疫表型[185-188]。

RAH/ALCL石蜡切片免疫组化特点：CD3、CD5、CD45、CD30、CD43和CD45RO常阳性（图12.22）[185, 188-193]，提示大多数病变（大约80%）是T细胞肿瘤。其他病例具有"无标记淋巴细胞"分化特征。皮肤原发性ALCL一般ALK-1蛋白阴性，而全身性ALCL累及皮肤时则ALK-1阳性。

与RAH/ALCL不同，淋巴瘤样丘疹病（LYP）多呈一致的更加惰性的发展经过，因此，对于这一病变

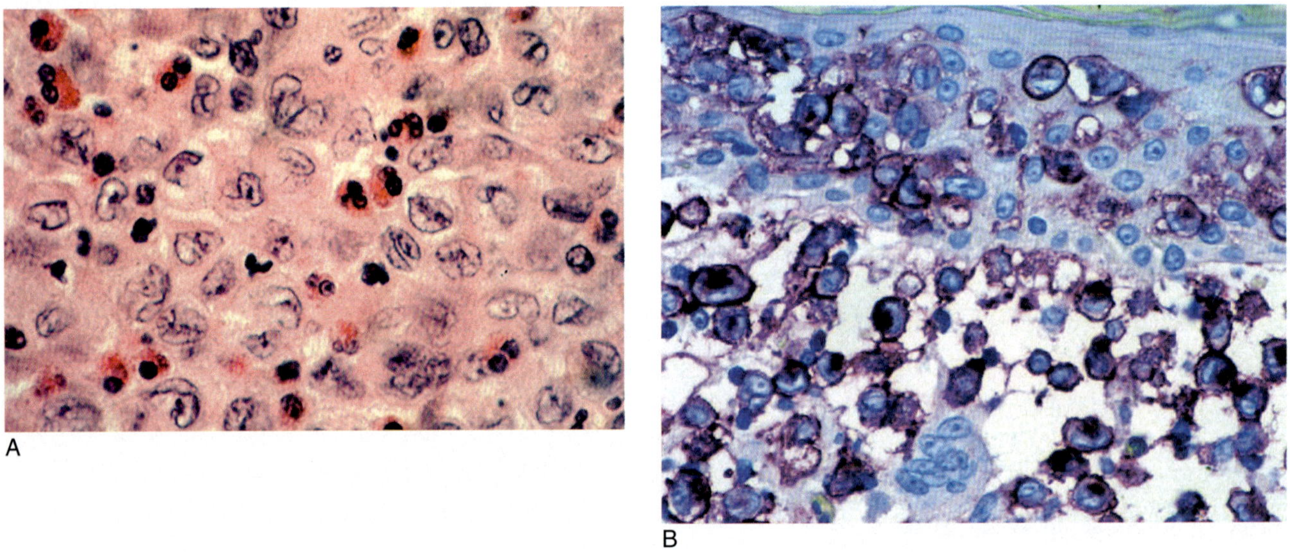

图 12.21 皮肤朗格汉斯细胞组织细胞增生症（组织细胞增生症 X）(A)，表达 CD1α (B)

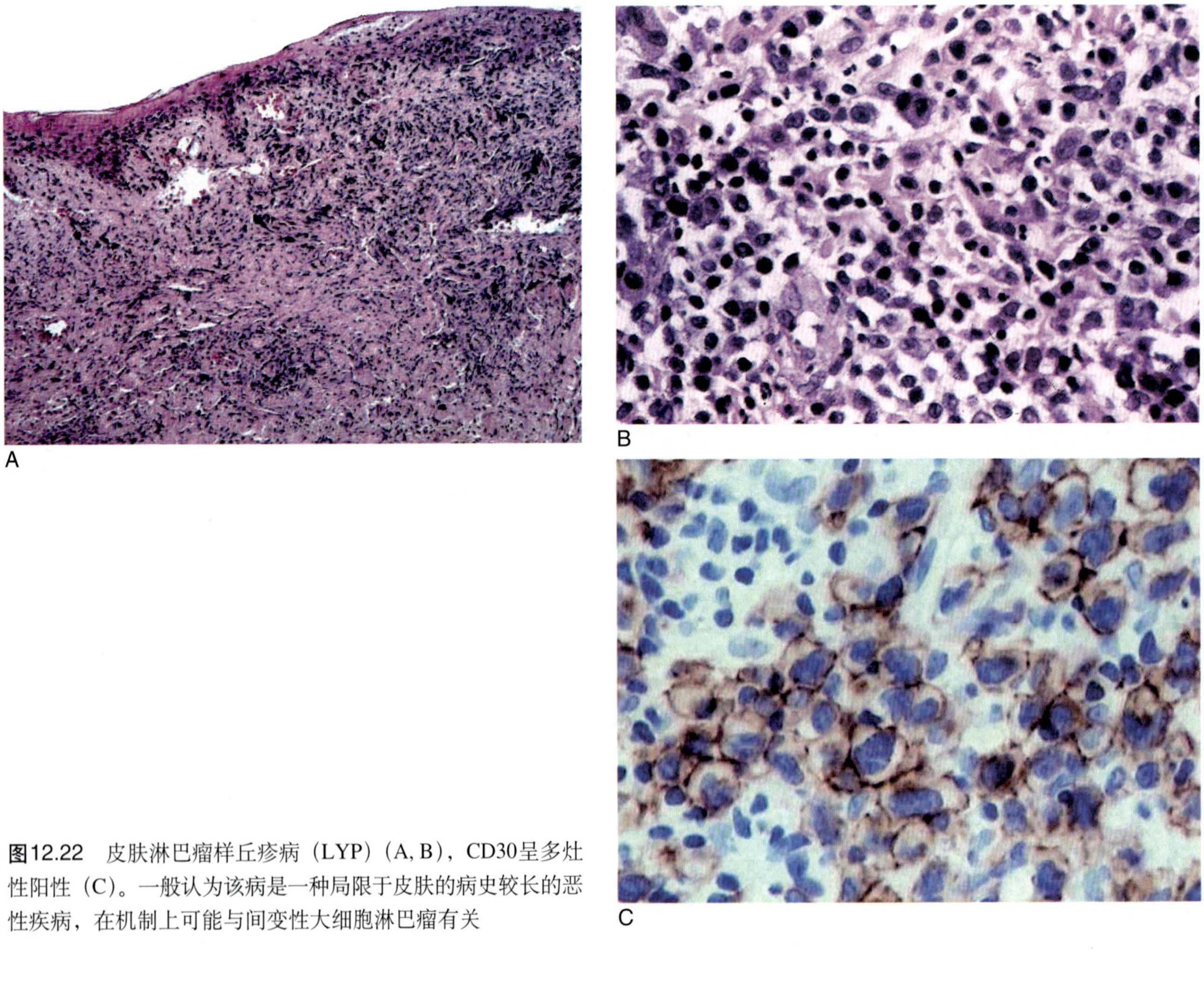

图 12.22 皮肤淋巴瘤样丘疹病（LYP）(A, B)，CD30 呈多灶性阳性 (C)。一般认为该病是一种局限于皮肤的病史较长的恶性疾病，在机制上可能与间变性大细胞淋巴瘤有关

的恶性特性还有争议[194-196]。尽管身体中轴部位更常见，但LYP可以发生在任何部位的皮肤和黏膜表面。典型病变为小的丘疹，在自愈前，中心可有出血和坏死。一些病例可始终没被发现，局部和远处复发常见[197]。

组织学上，LYP可表现为表浅部位、深部血管周以及间质的浸润，浸润通常呈楔形，真皮浅层浸润呈苔藓样。覆盖的表皮多有棘细胞层水肿及不全角化。浸润的细胞较杂，其淋巴细胞通常较ALCL的小。然而，有少部分肿瘤细胞具有高度异型性，一部分病例甚至可见到多核细胞和病理性核分裂。这种异型改变多见于活动性病变，在好转或愈合的病例中很少见到[189,192,193]。在一些少见的情况下，LYP中的大细胞形成肿瘤性结节或片状，对于这些病例，尽管其临床表现为LYP的特征，但是诊断ALCL还是更合适些。

大多数学者认为LYP是一种由宿主免疫反应引起的局限于皮肤的丘疹样T细胞淋巴瘤[189,195,198]。免疫组化分析也支持这一观点，因为在大多数病例可以检测到与ALCL相似的异常表型[192,199,200]。CD4阳性在LYP和ALCL中都很常见。T细胞受体克隆性基因重排的结果进一步证实LYP的恶性特性[135,198]，因为这一结果在良性活化的T细胞浸润中不常见。最终有大约10%~20%的LYP患者后来发展成全身性淋巴瘤[192,201,202]。

皮肤间叶来源肿瘤

发生在皮肤的向间叶方向分化的肿瘤同深部软组织的间叶肿瘤一样，有多种类型。发生于真皮和皮下的原发肿瘤可来源于：纤维母细胞或肌纤维母细胞、"纤维组织细胞"、肌肉、神经、上皮、血管。同深部软组织的病变一样，单凭组织学图像很难作出正确诊断，因此，免疫组化对皮肤间叶来源肿瘤的诊断很有帮助，根据肿瘤细胞免疫表型的不同可以区别皮肤的梭形细胞、多边形细胞、上皮样细胞和小细胞肿瘤。

纤维母细胞/肌纤维母细胞肿瘤

总的来说，肿瘤细胞只单纯表现出纤维母细胞或肌纤维母细胞分化的情况较少。只有以下3种皮肤肿瘤增生性病变属于这种情况：复发性指纤维瘤（指纤维瘤病）[203-206]、皮肤纤维肉瘤[207,208]和先天性表浅血管外皮细胞瘤[209,210]。复发性指纤维瘤（指纤维瘤病）一般发生于小儿手部，常为多灶性。超微结构显示指纤维瘤（DF）由肌纤维母细胞构成[203]，因此一致表达波形蛋白和肌特异性指标肌动蛋白。尽管其他学者有异议[211]，但据笔者的经验，可以有结蛋白的表达。超微结构观察和生化指标检测证实肌纤维母细胞中有与平滑肌细胞一样的收缩单位。另一个特征是细胞内包涵体，免疫组化证实该包涵体是聚集的肌动蛋白[204-206]。

皮肤纤维肉瘤（FS）被报道多发生在烧伤瘢痕、手术瘢痕、牛痘疫苗瘢痕及其他注射部位[208]。这种非常少见的肿瘤仅由纤维母细胞组成，因此仅波形蛋白阳性，不表达其他任何与纤维母细胞分化无关的间叶特异性标记物（图12.23）。很多情况下，皮肤的纤维肉瘤是由隆突性皮肤纤维肉瘤（DFSP，后面有介绍）去分化（克隆性演变）发展而来的。

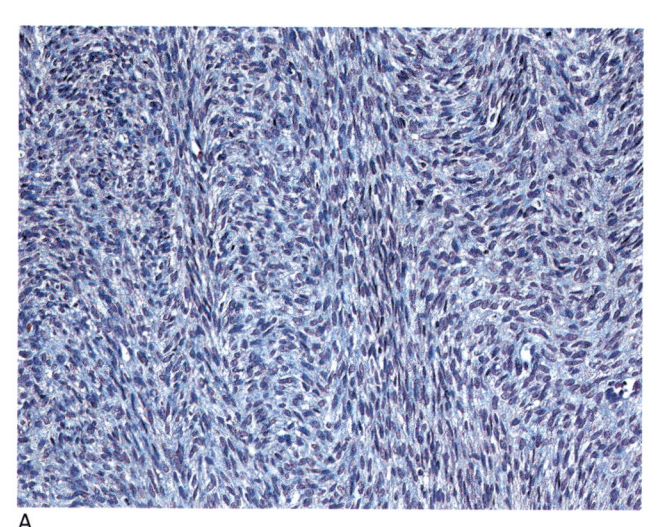 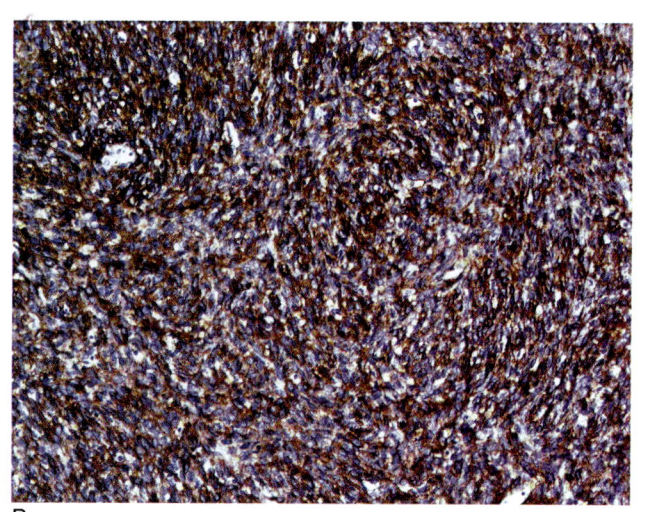

图12.23　真皮和皮下的纤维肉瘤（A），波形蛋白呈弥漫阳性（B）

先天性血管外皮细胞瘤发生于小儿，具有特征性的"鹿角样"血管结构，因此得名。该肿瘤与小儿肌纤维瘤病和成人孤立性肌纤维瘤具有相似的临床表现和组织学图像[212-214]。与真正的血管外皮瘤不表达肌源性指标肌动蛋白不同，先天性血管外皮细胞瘤肌动蛋白通常呈弥漫阳性（图12.24）[214]。

"纤维组织细胞"肿瘤

这一组肿瘤如非典型纤维黄色瘤（AFX）、恶性纤维组织细胞瘤（MFH）和皮肤隆突性纤维肉瘤（DFSP）均表现出"纤维组织细胞"的形态学特点，有观点认为这组肿瘤仅是一个相似的形态学称谓，而非统一的实体。仅少数该肿瘤能表达特异性的造血细胞标记物，如骨髓来源的单核细胞和组织细胞相关的标记物CD14、CD16、CD18、CD36、CD43、CD68[215,216]，对此还有不同观点[215]。有报道发现MFH能表达HLA-DR[215]，但其他软组织恶性肿瘤也可以表达该种人类组织相容性抗原Ⅱ[217,218]。

同样的，细胞蛋白酶如α-1-抗糜蛋白酶和组织蛋白酶-B也不仅只在AFX、MFH、DFSP中表达[219]，在皮肤其他的梭形细胞肿瘤也均有表达[176,216]。抗原L1（相应抗体MAC387）是针对功能成熟的单核细胞和巨噬细胞的特异性胞浆标志物，在AFX、MFH、DFSP的多核细胞中有表达，但在梭形细胞中表达较少。事实上MAC387能在皮肤的任何一种恶性肿瘤表达[220]。XⅢα因子作为一种凝血因子，在纤维母细胞和"皮肤的树突状细胞"中有表达，在皮肤纤维瘤（图12.25）AFX和MFH也阳性，但同样情况也见于其他肉瘤、颗粒细胞瘤和神经纤维瘤[221-225]。

与期望的一致，波形蛋白在AFX、MFH、DFSP弥漫阳性[226]。肌源性特异性指标肌动蛋白和钙调素结合蛋白在上述某些肿瘤也有表达，尤其是AFX[227,228]。CD34在DFSP中呈弥漫性阳性（图12.26），可以将其与其他真皮和皮下的梭形细胞肿瘤区分开来，但不能与部分外周神经鞘膜肿瘤和梭形细胞脂肪瘤区别[229-234]。巨细胞纤维母细胞瘤、巨细胞血管纤维瘤、皮肤孤立性纤维性肿瘤在生物学特性上与DFSP相似，因此具有一些与DFSP相同的免疫组化表型[235-242]。很多情况下，CD34对于诊断DFSP并非必需，但对于小的结构不完整的活检标本，CD34染色就很有帮助。还要注意的是，皮肤纤维瘤有时虽肿瘤中心CD34阴性，但瘤周组织CD34阳性（图12.27），这时不要把良性病变诊断为恶性。DFSP的另一个特性是部分病例有灶性肌样分化的能力，呈肌动蛋白、结蛋白灶性阳性[243-247]，这种情况在某些皮肤纤维瘤中也能见到。

具有纤维肉瘤成分的DFSP是皮肤纤维肉瘤的一种特殊类型。该组合肿瘤具有两者的免疫表型：可以弥漫性表达CD34，或者其中的纤维肉瘤成分呈阴性，说明具有双相分化的肿瘤成分[244-251]。

CD34染色对于诊断DFSP的一个亚型——萎缩型很有帮助。该肿瘤缺少DFSP特征性的粗大隆起的结节，取而代之的是皮下阶梯状梭形细胞增生（图12.28）[252]。CD34弥漫阳性能够避免将该肿瘤诊

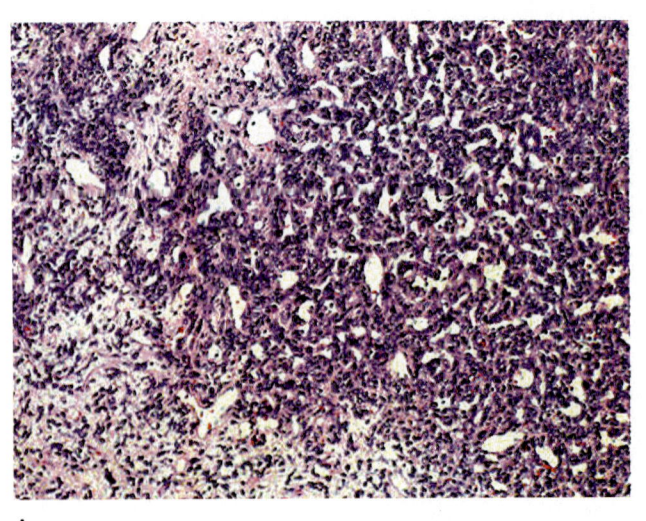

A

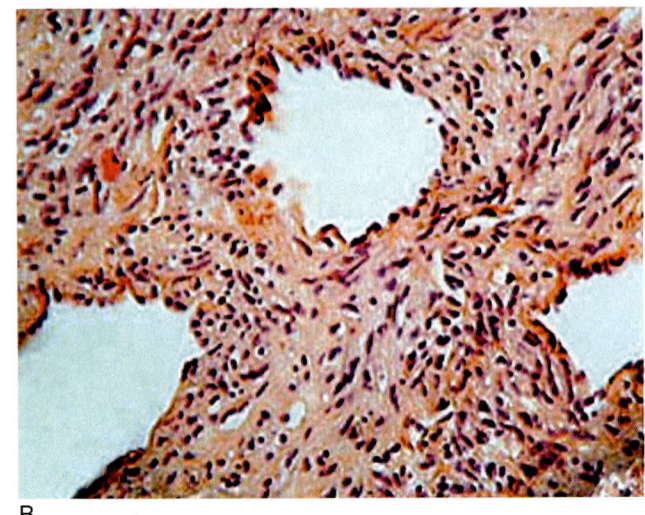

B

图12.24 真皮和皮下的血管外皮细胞瘤（A），目前被认为是一种肌纤维瘤病，因此肌动蛋白表达阳性（B）

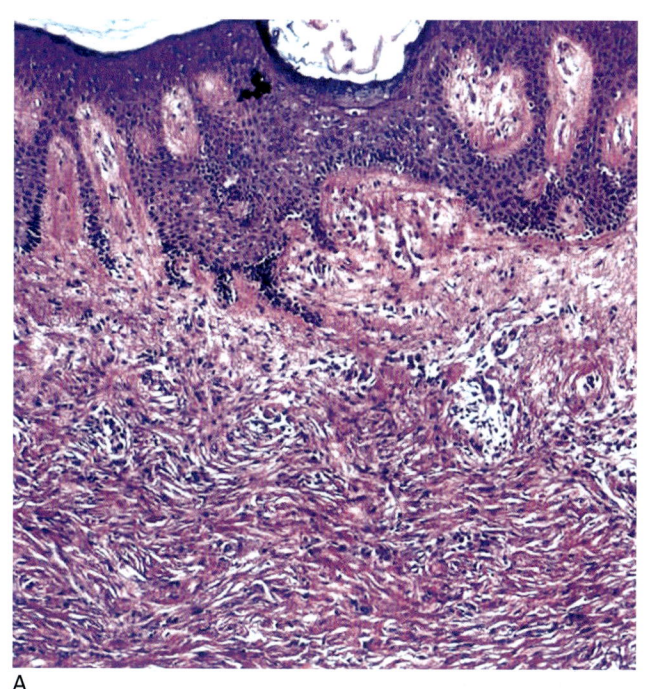
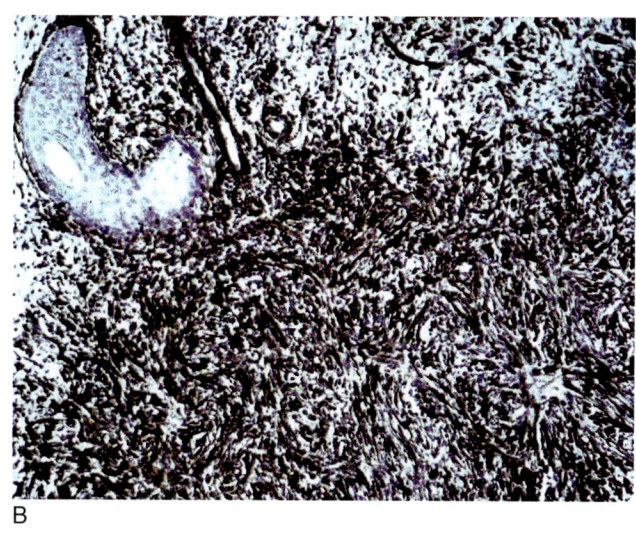

图 12.25　皮肤纤维瘤（A）通常弥漫性表达 XIIIα 因子（B）

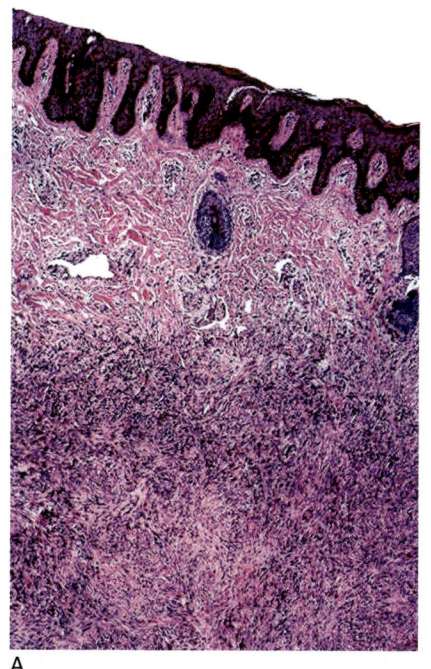
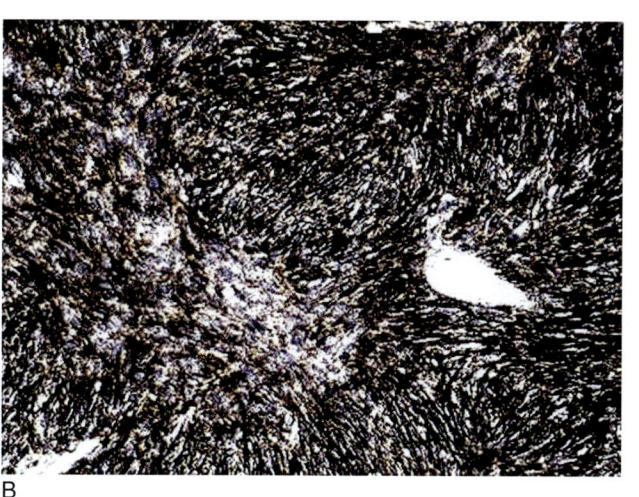

图 12.26　皮肤隆突性纤维肉瘤（A）特征性弥漫表达 CD34

断为良性病变。

　　皮肤或其他部位的 MFH 很可能不是一组统一的病变，而是多种间叶肿瘤向某一共同方向分化的同一组织学表现，这一观点首先得到 Brooks 的支持[253]。因此，MFH 样改变和其他间叶肿瘤图像可以出现在同一肿瘤中，被认为是肿瘤克隆性演化的结果。对于一个多形性的恶性肿瘤，如果仅表达波形蛋白，而缺少上皮性、肌源性、神经和内皮标记物的表达，尽管不能明确，仍可暂时诊断为 MFH。目前还没有针对该肿瘤的有效的标记物。

　　笔者认为 AFX 是 MFH 发生在浅表部位的一种特殊类型，因此具有 MFH 的特征。有些学者认为 CD99

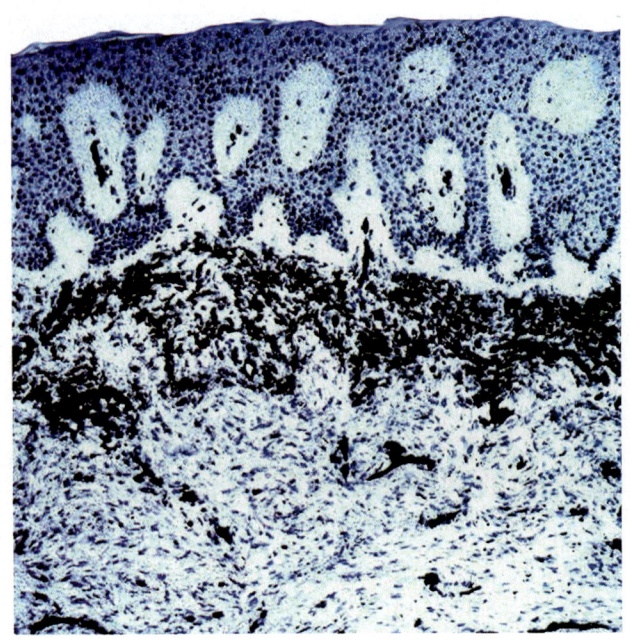

图12.27 同皮肤纤维肉瘤不同，如果皮肤纤维瘤表达CD34，也仅限于肿瘤边缘细胞

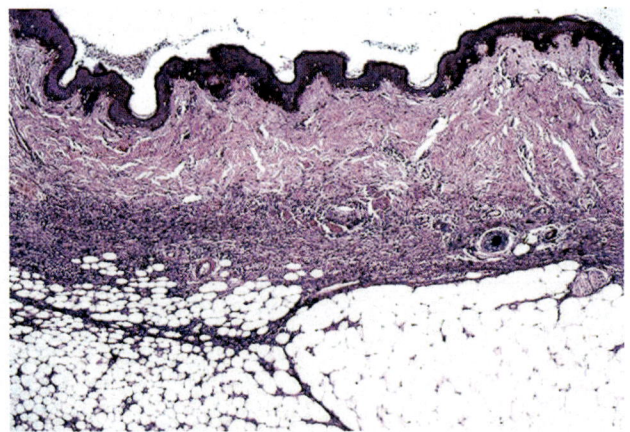

图12.28 "退行性"皮肤纤维肉瘤，向真皮下不规则长入，较难诊断。CD34对诊断很有帮助

是AFX的一个有帮助的标记物[254]，但笔者的研究并不支持该观点。我们发现许多AFX不表达CD99，而在DFSP、孤立性纤维瘤，甚至是梭形细胞黑色素瘤中CD99都可以有表达。

皮肤纤维瘤及其特殊类型（如结节性组织细胞瘤、黄色肉芽肿、移行性组织细胞瘤、结节性皮下纤维瘤、动脉瘤样皮肤纤维组织细胞瘤、栅栏样纤维组织细胞瘤、上皮样组织细胞瘤）均可表达波形蛋白、XIIIα因子和CD68[255]。形态学差别已经足以区分这些肿瘤，因此免疫组化检查也就没有必要了。

> **诊断要点：纤维组织细胞肿瘤**
>
> 1. DFSP呈弥漫性CD34+、XIIIα因子-；皮肤纤维瘤CD34-、XIIIα因子+；皮肤纤维瘤的肿瘤边缘可表达CD34+。
> 2. MFH和AFX缺少特异性免疫标记物。

平滑肌肿瘤

同皮外平滑肌瘤和平滑肌肉瘤一样，皮肤的平滑肌肿瘤也弥漫表达波形蛋白、结蛋白、钙调素结合蛋白、肌动蛋白（图12.29）[256-261]。然而，值得注意的是皮肤平滑肌肿瘤的免疫表型不具有特异性。肌纤维母细胞增生性疾病，包括细胞性瘢痕、损伤后梭形细胞结节、结节性筋膜炎都可以表达肌源性标记物。

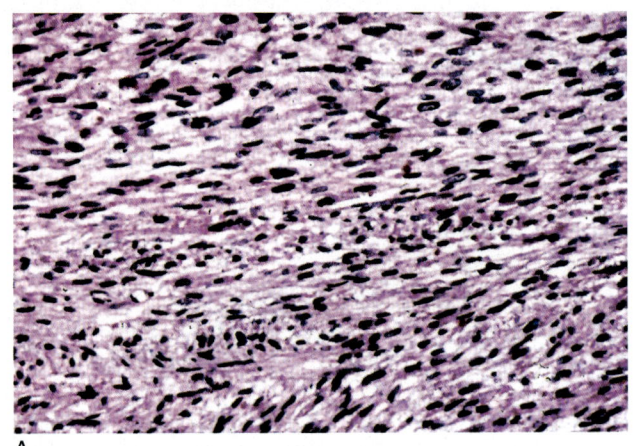

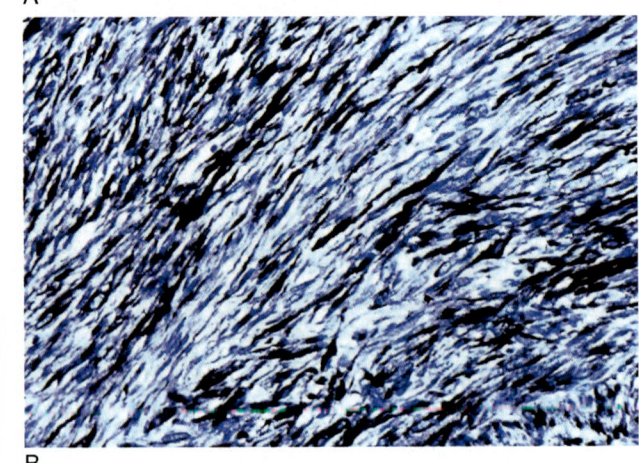

图12.29 皮下平滑肌肉瘤（A），结蛋白呈弥漫阳性（B）

因此，最后的诊断要结合免疫组化和形态学图像综合分析。

皮肤的平滑肌肿瘤还是有一些特殊的免疫组化特点的。大约30%的皮肤平滑肌瘤和平滑肌肉瘤S-100阳性，皮下该病变CD57阳性亦为30%[256]。以上结果表明这些病变具有分别向立毛肌和血管平滑肌分化的能力，这在鉴别诊断中很有意义，因为皮肤平滑肌肿瘤和皮肤外周神经鞘膜肿瘤有某些共同的免疫表型，但外周神经鞘膜肿瘤很少表达肌源性的指标。

另一个争论的问题是皮肤平滑肌瘤异常表达CK和EMA的情况。尽管有的学者报道，无论发生于何种部位，总体来说，该肿瘤可以高表达CK和EMA[262]，但作者的经验表明发生于皮肤的平滑肌瘤和平滑肌肉瘤很少表达上述上皮性标记物。

血管球瘤、球血管瘤和血管球肉瘤也属于平滑肌来源的肿瘤，因为它们显示向特定的血管周平滑肌（外皮性）分化的特征[263-266]。但是与其他肌源性肿瘤不同，上述肿瘤一般不表达结蛋白。过去有观点认为血管球细胞肿瘤应该归入血管来源的肿瘤，但作者认为该观点并不正确，因为其缺少内皮细胞标记物的表达。但是，血管球肿瘤偶尔也会表达CD34[267]。

神经鞘肿瘤

最常见的皮肤神经鞘肿瘤是神经纤维瘤。该肿瘤一般多发，由von Recklinghausen神经纤维瘤病发展而来。其他肿瘤还包括：神经鞘瘤（施万细胞瘤）、颗粒细胞瘤、神经束膜瘤、神经鞘黏液瘤[268]。皮肤恶性外周神经鞘膜肿瘤较罕见[269-272]，大多数原发于真皮或皮下，也有少数可能是皮下深部组织的恶性病变累及皮肤。

诊断外周神经鞘肿瘤（PNST）常用的免疫组化指标有：波形蛋白、S-100、CD56、CD57（图12.30）[269, 273-275]。在所有肌源性和上皮性标记物都阴性的情况下，单独或联合使用后3种标记物对于诊断PNST很有帮助。神经鞘瘤总是弥漫强阳性表达S-100，但神经纤维瘤的免疫组化较复杂，缺乏一致性[274]。在PNST中能检测到的其他指标还包括：胶质纤维酸性蛋白、神经特异性烯醇化酶和神经生长因子受体[274, 276]。

普遍认为大多数颗粒细胞瘤（GCT）具有施万细胞分化的特征[277]，但是某些平滑肌瘤、平滑肌肉瘤、基底细胞癌和血管肉瘤也可具有颗粒细胞瘤的特点[278, 279]。绝大多数（但不是所有）颗粒细胞瘤S-100[280]、CD56、CD57阳性。GCT和神经纤维瘤（不是神经鞘瘤）一样能表达XIIIα因子[221]，还可表达蛋白基因产物9.5、calretinin、抑制素（图12.31）[281]。皮肤的恶性GCT非常罕见，同良性GCT一样，大多数具有神经鞘膜分化特征。

皮肤神经束膜瘤是不常见的一种特殊类型的PNST[282-294]，其形态学图像多样，部分肿瘤呈梭形一致细胞，向心性排列；另一些类似于皮肤纤维瘤，呈孤立的纤维性肿瘤或车辐状胶原瘤。该肿瘤的典型特征是缺少与施万细胞有关的标记物，不表达角蛋白，EMA总是阳性（图12.32）[288, 292]。这些免疫组化特征与非肿瘤性外周神经纤维母细胞相同。皮肤的脑膜上皮性增生与神经束膜瘤的免疫表型相似，两者的鉴别主要依靠形态学图像和超微结构改变[287]。Folpe等

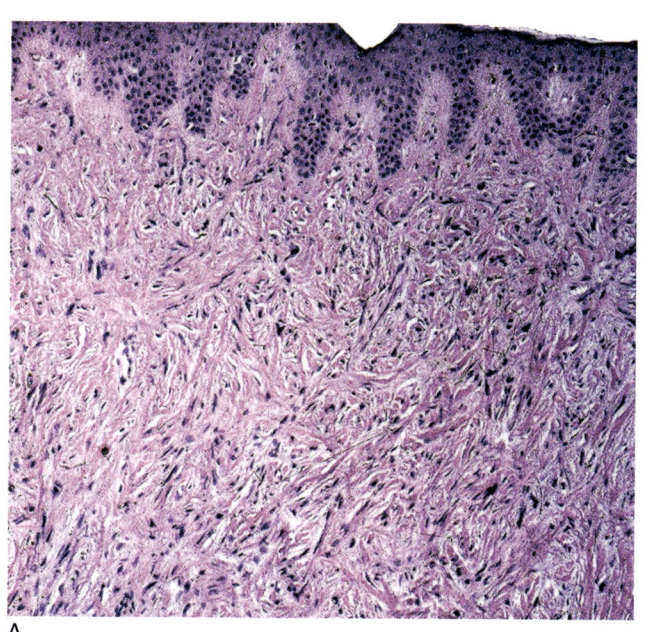
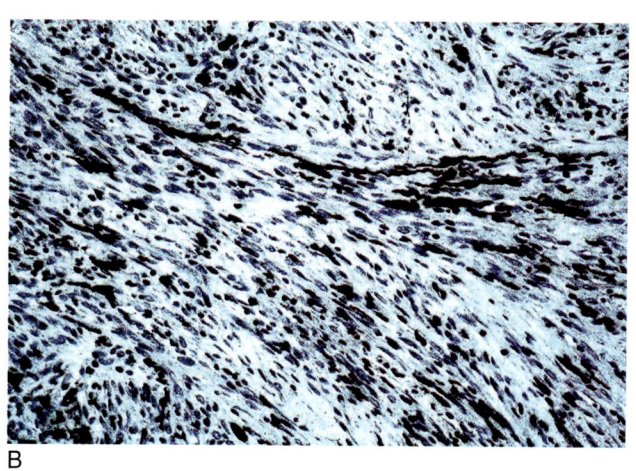

图12.30 神经纤维瘤病患者真皮内恶性外周神经鞘瘤（A），肿瘤细胞S-100多灶性阳性（B）

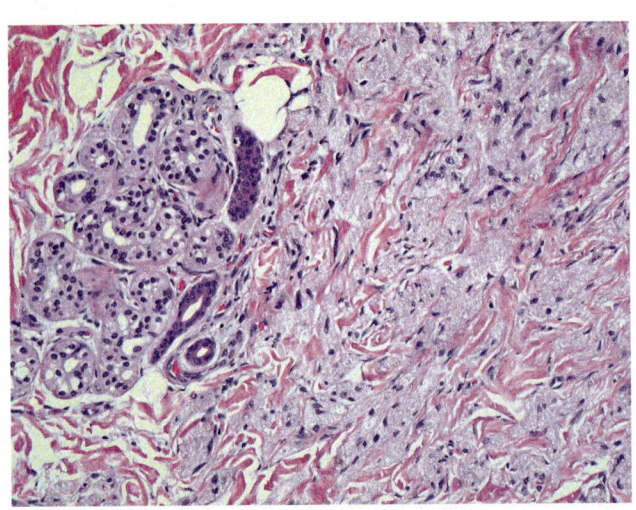
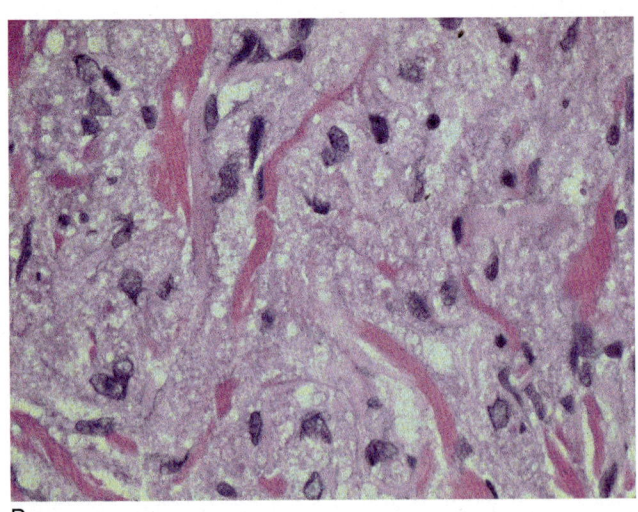
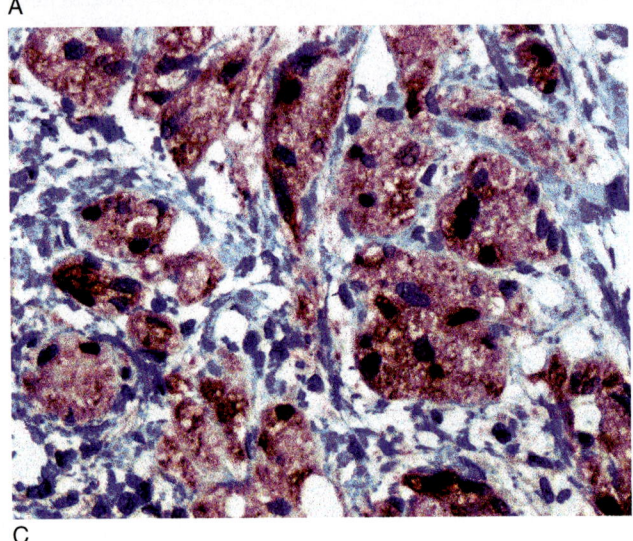

图12.31 皮肤颗粒细胞瘤（A，B），显示胞核和胞浆calretinin阳性（C）

人曾将claudin-1（一种紧密连接相关蛋白）用于神经束膜细胞瘤的诊断[295]。

笔者认为神经鞘黏液瘤（NTK）是一种仅见于皮肤的、异质性的特殊类型肿瘤。该肿瘤可分为以下3种类型："传统NTK"、"真皮神经鞘黏液瘤"、"细胞性NTK"[268, 296]。传统NTK表达施万细胞和神经外胚层的一些标记物[291, 296, 297]；皮肤神经鞘黏液瘤特异性地表达波形蛋白和S-100（图12.33）[298]；细胞性NTK具有肌源性和组织细胞的一些特征（表达肌动蛋白和CD68），而缺少神经来源的特征[299, 300]。

血管肿瘤

发生于皮肤的血管肿瘤形态学图像多种多样，所以其免疫组化特点备受关注[301]，就此意义来讲，有多种内皮分化标记物可供临床使用，但其中大多都需要与其他指标联合才能作出最后的诊断。因为肿瘤性内皮细胞可表达一些非肿瘤性血管内皮细胞不表达的蛋白，且这些抗原也可见于非血管源性肿瘤，尤其是恶性肿瘤。某些血管瘤也可表达一些特殊的免疫组化指标。在此不再一一介绍每种皮肤血管肿瘤[302]，而是将把它们作为一个整体来讨论，并对部分肿瘤稍作介绍。

与血管内皮分化相关的指标包括Ⅷ因子相关抗原（von Willebrand factor，vWF）、CD31、CD34、CD141（thrombomodulin）、FLI-1和富含岩藻糖细胞膜荆豆凝集素1（Ulex europaeus I lectin，UEL）结合位点

> **诊断要点：外周神经鞘肿瘤**
> 1. S-100的表达分布取决于肿瘤类型。
> 2. 通常CD56+、CD57+。
> 3. 颗粒细胞瘤和神经纤维瘤阳性指标：XIIIα因子+、calretinin+、抑制素+。
> 4. 神经束膜瘤EMA+，其他标记物阴性。

皮肤肿瘤的免疫组织化学 12

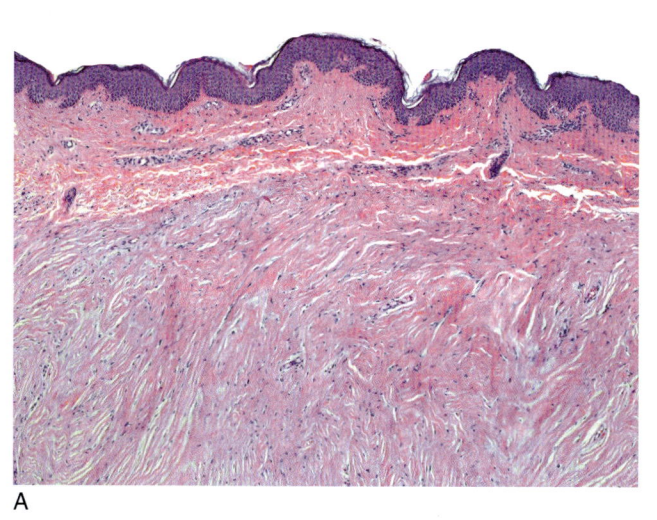
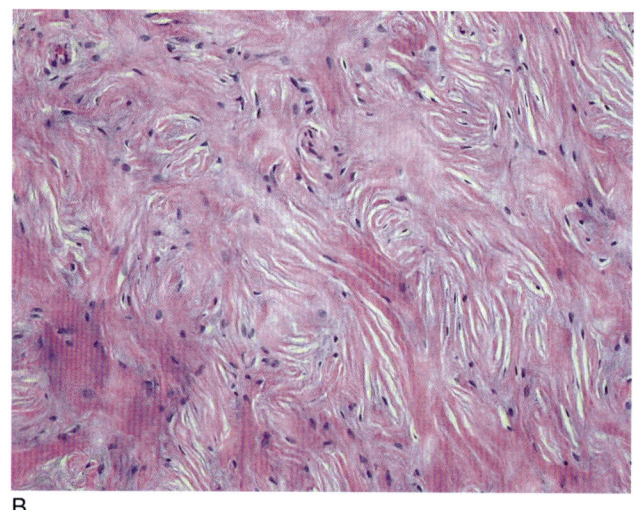
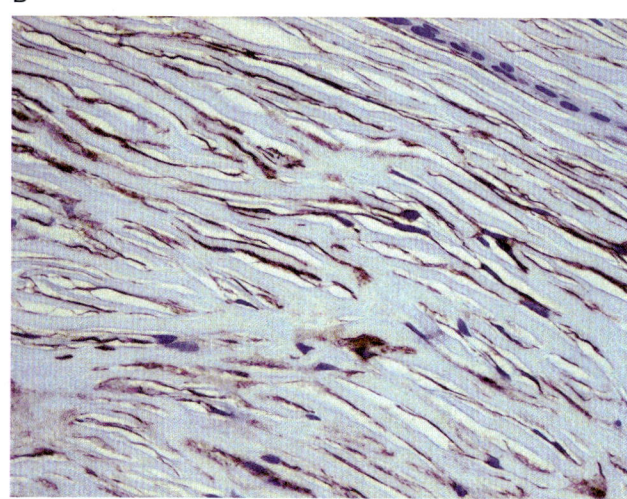

图12.32　皮肤神经束膜瘤（A，B），弥漫性表达EMA（C）

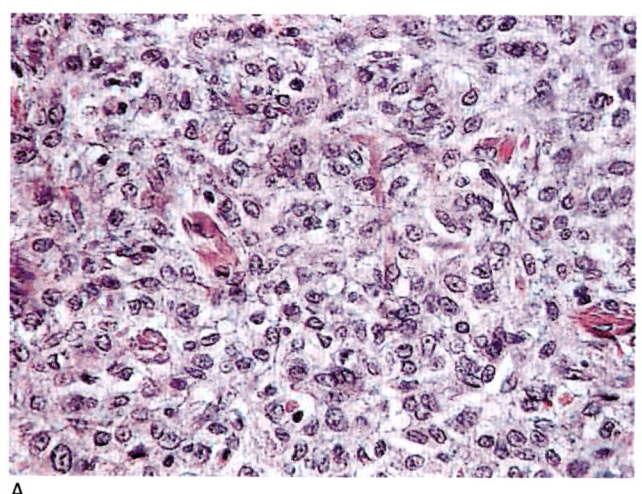
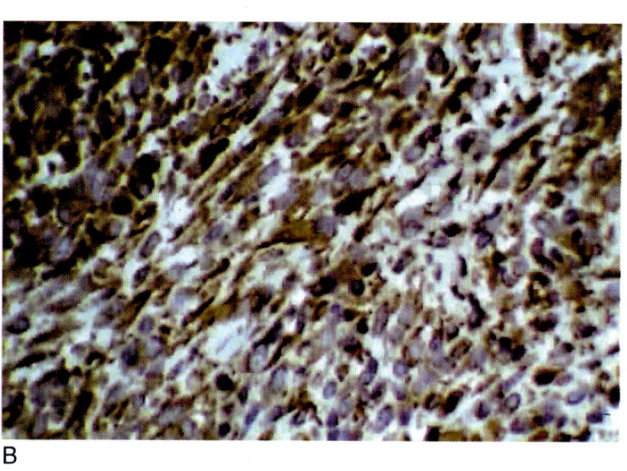

图12.33　细胞性神经鞘黏液瘤（A）镜下呈组织细胞样，CD68弥漫阳性（B），缺乏其他神经标记物表达

（图12.34）[303-309]。其中，后4个指标对于诊断足够敏感，vWF则不然。另一个让人感兴趣的问题是内皮来源肿瘤其内皮究竟显示血管内皮还是淋巴管内皮分化，作者认为这对于实用皮肤病理并不重要，将不作进一步讨论。

区别血管肿瘤最常用的方法是选用一组内皮相关抗原与几种上皮源性及肌源性相关抗原联合检测，因为部分内皮肿瘤图像与癌或有肌肉分化的肉瘤相像（反之亦然）。此外，上皮样血管肿瘤能异常合成角蛋白[310, 311]，因此，在作出最终诊断前，应该把上皮分化的其他标记物（如EMA、p63、E-钙黏素和desmoplakin）与CD31、CD34、CD141、FLI-1或UEL结合位点结合起来分析。

直到最近，免疫组化在诊断Kaposi肉瘤（最常见的血管恶性肿瘤之一）中的应用依然很少。因为在其"红斑"期，仅依靠组织学便很容易诊断Kaposi肉瘤，而梭形细胞期或"结节"期，肿瘤细胞则失去内皮相关抗原。然而，现在多组研究表明，人类疱疹病毒8型隐匿型核抗原-1（HH8LNA）对Kaposi肉瘤，无论何种组织学形态，均具有高度选择性（图12.35）。绝大多数Kaposi肉瘤HH8LNA阳性，而其他形态相似的肿瘤无一阳性[312-314]。

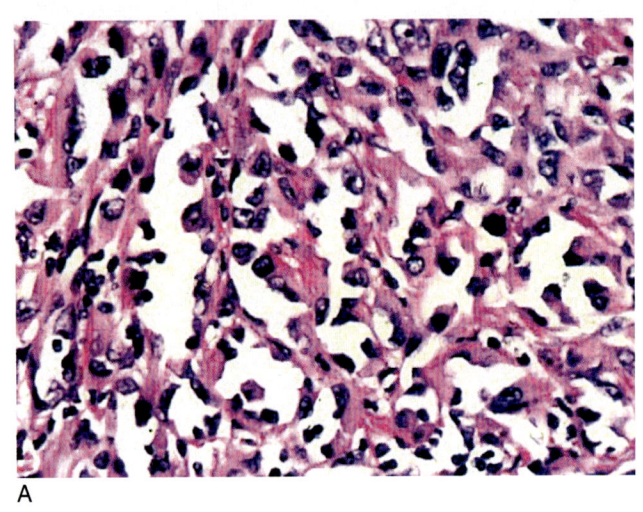
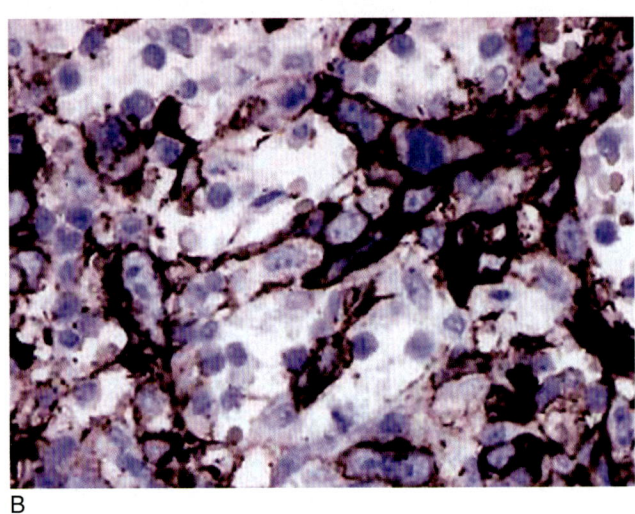

图12.34 皮肤血管肉瘤（A）呈CD31阳性（B）

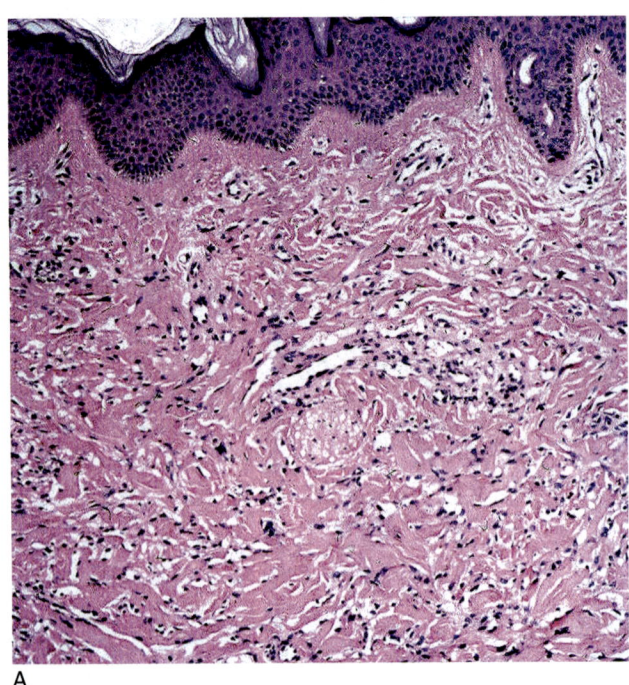
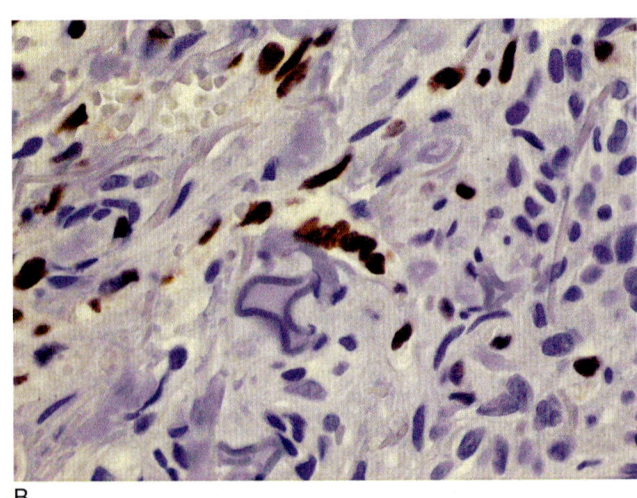

图12.35 皮肤Kaposi肉瘤（A）显示HH8LNA核阳性着色（B）

血管内皮细胞瘤被划分到交界性血管内皮肿瘤的范畴，近年来发病率上升[315-318]。其免疫表型与其他血管肿瘤相似，但有例外——Billings等曾描述过一种特殊的肿瘤，光镜下图像与上皮样肉瘤（详见下一节）非常相似[319]，因此命名为上皮样肉瘤样血管内皮瘤（图12.36）。实际上，该肿瘤与真正的上皮样肉瘤一样，角蛋白和波形蛋白阳性，但不表达CD34（而在上皮样肉瘤[320]和大多其他血管内皮瘤均为阳性），此外CD31、FLI-1在上皮样肉瘤样血管内皮瘤表达阳性。

> **诊断要点：血管肿瘤**
>
> 1. 最好的免疫组化指标包括CD31、CD141、CD34和FLI-1或Ulex。
> 2. 上皮样血管肉瘤多同时表达AE1/AE3和CAM5.2两种角蛋白，特别注意的是要同时使用血管标记物以避免诊断错误。
> 3. HH8LNA抗体对Kaposi肉瘤高度敏感和特异。
> 4. 上皮样肉瘤样血管内皮瘤表达CD31、FLI-1，但CD34阴性，而上皮样肉瘤CD34+。

上皮样肉瘤

上皮样肉瘤是一种发生于真皮和皮下的由多边形细胞构成的肿瘤，镜下图像多变[321]，因此容易与其他病变混淆。当肿瘤呈实性生长时，容易误认为转移癌或恶性黑色素瘤；当肿瘤呈肉芽肿样生长时，肿瘤细胞围绕坏死组织呈栅栏状排列，又容易与坏死的肉芽肿混淆（如风湿结节、深部环状肉芽肿）。上皮样肉瘤的假性血管瘤性区很可能造成与血管内皮瘤鉴别困难[319, 321-323]。

在浅表软组织上皮样间叶组织肿瘤中，只有上皮样肉瘤总是角蛋白阳性（图12.37）[321, 324-327]，这种现象也可见于单相性滑膜肉瘤，但后者多位于深部软组织。在前一节还介绍了上皮样血管肿瘤角蛋白也为阳性[328]。70%~80%的上皮样肉瘤出现上皮细胞膜抗原阳性，注意与转移癌鉴别[321-323]。所有上皮样肉瘤均呈现CD34阳性[320]，而该标记物在癌组织很少阳性。相反，Lin等[329]和Laskin与Miettinende[327]的研究表明SCC对CK5/6和p63恒定阳性，但是大多数上皮样肉瘤则相反。同样的现象也见于E-钙黏素的表达[327-330]。鉴别上皮样肉瘤与黑色素瘤或透明细胞肉瘤（软组织恶性黑色素瘤）则比较简单，只有不到15%的上皮样肉瘤S-100阳性，且HMB-45、酪氨酸酶或MART-1均为阴性，而在黑色素细胞来源肿瘤这些指标呈阳性[321]。

如前所述，鉴别上皮样肉瘤与上皮样肉瘤样血管内皮瘤主要依靠后者表达特异性内皮抗原，其中CD31和FLI-1最有鉴别价值[319]。实际上，这同样适用于所有血管肿瘤与上皮样肉瘤的鉴别诊断。

小圆细胞间叶肿瘤

皮肤和皮下小细胞肿瘤包括Merkel细胞癌、小细胞鳞状细胞癌、小细胞小汗腺癌、小细胞黑色素瘤、外周原始神经外胚层肿瘤/骨外Ewing肉瘤（PNET/ES）、淋巴瘤及横纹肌肉瘤（图12.38）[100, 331]，其中间叶来源肿瘤在该组肿瘤中仅占少数。横纹肌肉瘤恒定表达结蛋白、成肌素和肌特异性肌动蛋白，不表达角蛋白，而PNET/ES则一致表达CD99，另外CD56、CD57和突触素也可能阳性，角蛋白呈局灶阳性[95-100]。上述肿瘤上皮细胞膜抗原、CD45、S-100蛋白、癌胚抗原及HMB-45均为阴性。

皮肤的特殊免疫组织化学标记物

雌激素受体与孕激素受体

这些激素受体最初是作为小汗腺癌与组织学图像相似的转移乳腺癌之间的鉴别诊断指标[332]，然而并

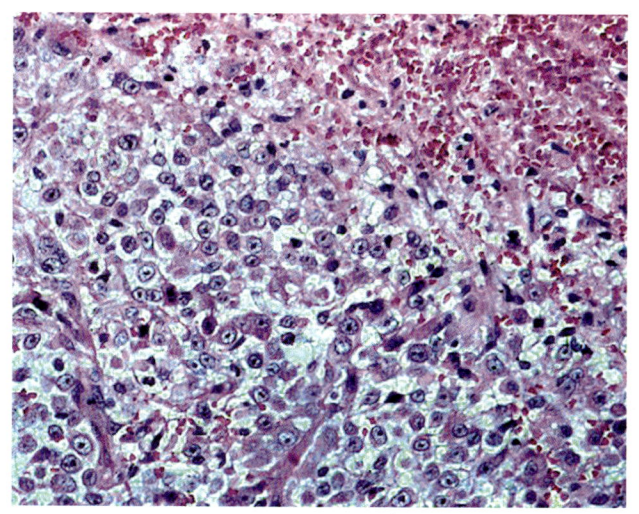

图12.36 发生于皮下组织的上皮样肉瘤样血管内皮瘤，该肿瘤为一种特殊的内皮肿瘤，因其角蛋白总呈阳性，但CD34阴性，CD31通常阳性

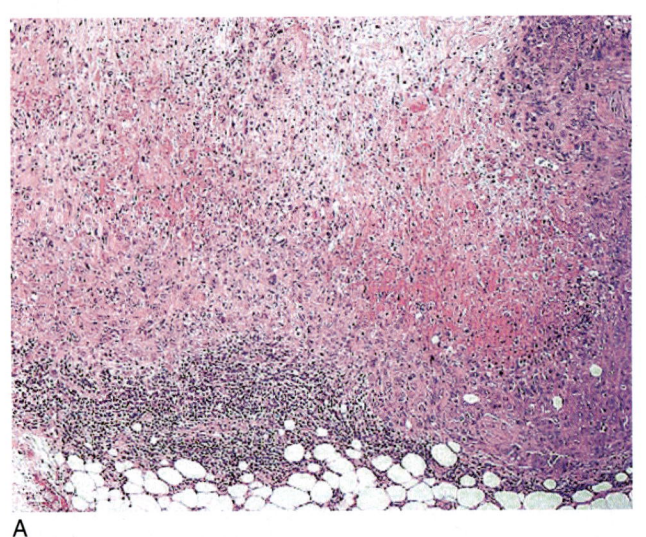

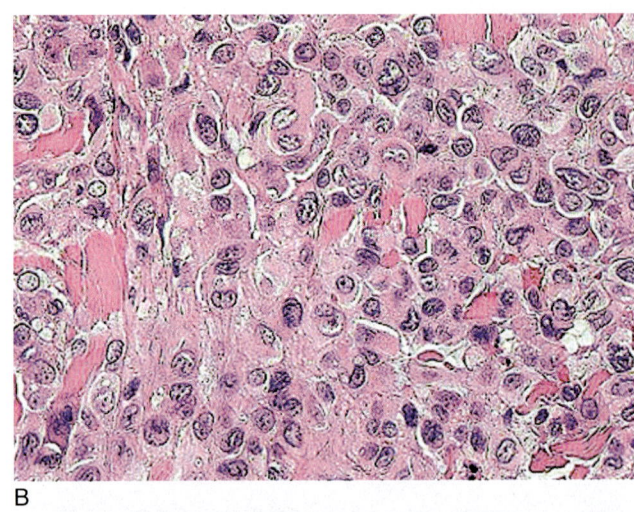

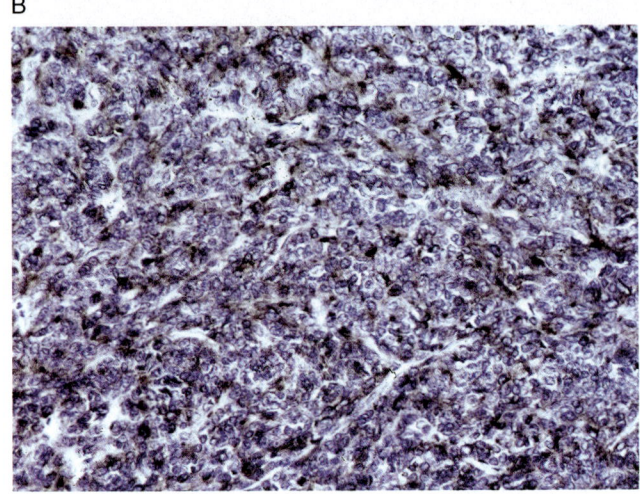

图 12.37 皮下上皮样肉瘤（A，B）显示肿瘤细胞普遍表达角蛋白（C）

没有达到预期目的。多组分析表明雌激素受体（estrogen receptor protein，ERP）在某些良性大汗腺肿瘤（尤其乳头状汗腺腺瘤）以及小汗腺癌中普遍阳性（图12.39）[333-336]，孕激素受体（progesterone receptor protein，PRP）在一些小汗腺腺癌中也可阳性[336-337]。这些发现对于预后或免疫组化阳性患者治疗的意义还不明确，因为尚没有利用激素拮抗剂进行汗腺腺癌全身治疗的试验。有意思的是，大汗腺腺癌或乳腺外Paget病通常ERP或PRP阴性[332, 333]。

癌基因和其他预后相关指标

癌基因在皮肤肿瘤生长的激发与调节中的作用是一个非常有意思的领域，但是尚未更多地应用于实际工作中。对于皮肤，已经有两种研究得很细致的癌基因，即表皮生长因子受体（EGFR）和c-erbB-2（neu）。后者为一种分子量为185kD、有酪氨酸激酶活性、在功能和结构上与分子量175kD的EGFR基因产物相关的跨膜糖蛋白，尽管其在细胞分化和增殖中的确切作用尚不确定，但当其生理性表达时发挥生长因子受体的作用。正常分化和生长的细胞表达野生型EGFR和c-erbB-2，但在某些上皮肿瘤中，二者可发生结构改变或者过度表达。

EGFR在鳞状细胞癌中表达不足为奇（图12.40）[339, 340]，但是并无证据表明EGFR受体分子野生型或突变型的表达或表达数量与鳞状细胞癌分级或临床行为相关。有研究发现EGFR在BCC也有表达，但只见于不足50%的病例[339, 340]。除了皮肤附属器癌，EGFR在良性角化细胞增生也有表达，包括软垂疣和脂溢性角化病[336, 341]。在妊娠、摄入外源性雌激素或孕激素或合并发育不良痣综合征的皮肤附属器癌患者，EGFR表达增强[341]。

尽管c-erbB-2在部分侵袭性乳腺癌过表达，但却不能说明该指标与恶性汗腺肿瘤预后不良有关。在我们对小汗腺癌的研究中，27%的病例c-erbB-2免疫组化阳性，所有阳性肿瘤均为中低级，无转移或复发（Swanson PE，Wick MR；尚未发表）。相反，Hasebe

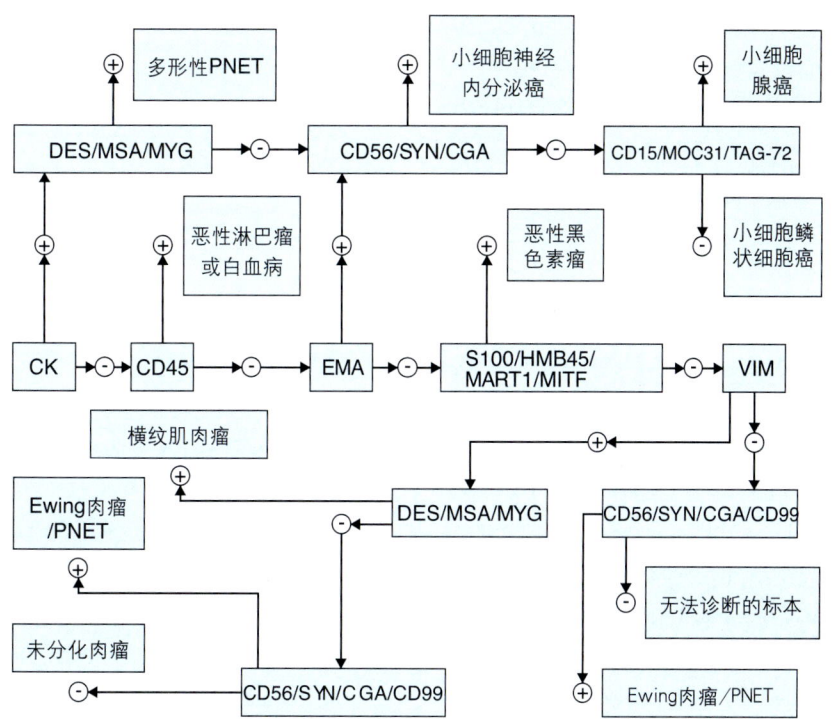

图 12.38　皮肤和皮下小细胞未分化肿瘤诊断有关的免疫组化表型

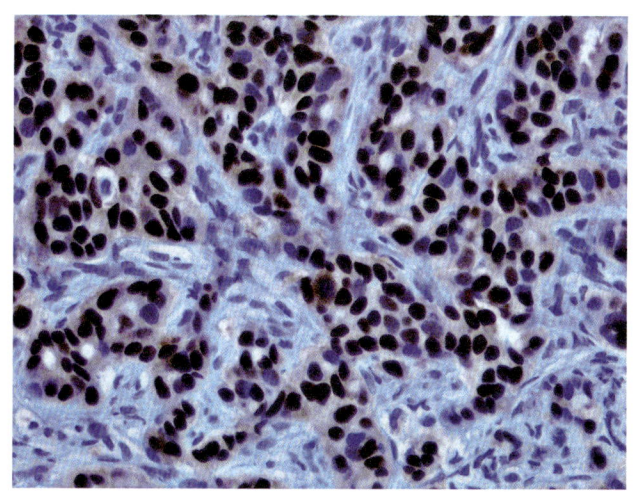

图 12.39　雌激素受体在皮肤原发性小汗腺癌呈阳性表达

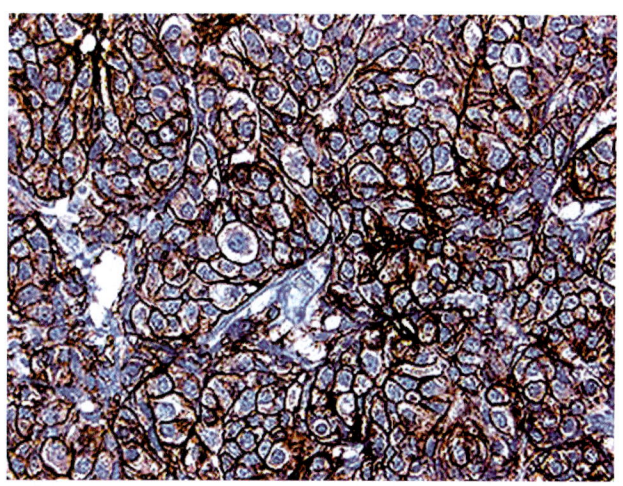

图 12.40　上皮生长因子受体在皮肤低分化鳞状细胞癌呈弥漫阳性

等人报道了 c-erbB-2 表达和汗腺癌预后相关[342]。乳腺外 Paget 病同样 c-erbB-2 阳性[343]。

CD44 是一种细胞表面蛋白，与细胞间及细胞与基质之间黏附性及淋巴细胞归巢有关。在表皮角化细胞、毛囊、皮脂腺细胞和小汗腺细胞中有表达[344,345]。有人报道 CD44 异常表达见于多种肿瘤，CD44 阳性与高侵袭性相关。与鳞状细胞癌和转移的腺癌不同，基底细胞癌 CD44 阴性，而前两者几乎 100% 的阳性[346]。Merkel 细胞癌 CD44 阳性也与高转移风险相关[347]。

目前，我们还不知道很多单一癌基因如何以及在何种程度下激发或调节细胞内级联事件，进而导致细胞的生长失控。尽管某些癌基因产物可以使细胞永生化或者维持培养细胞的转化表型，但体外这种效果的最终意义还不清楚。可以说皮肤肿瘤各种特异性肿瘤性多肽过度表达与肿瘤侵袭性相关。但是其中任何一种多肽都不可能单独作为提示肿瘤生物学行为的指标。就像病理医师这时需要借助一组有帮助的免疫组化指标一样，将来关于癌基因表达与组织病理学或临床的关系的研究也应该同时分析多种癌基因产物。

参考文献

1. Lohmann CM, Solomon AR. Clinicopathologic variants of cutaneous squamous cell carcinoma. Adv Anat Pathol 2001; 8:27–36.
2. Petter G, Haustein UF. Histologic subtyping and malignancy: assessment of cutaneous squamous cell carcinoma. Dermatol Surg 2000; 26:521–530.
3. Nappi O, Pettinato G, Wick MR. Adenoid (acantholytic) squamous cell carcinoma of the skin. J Cutan Pathol 1989; 16:114–121.
4. van Muijen GNP, Ruiter DJ, Ponec M, et al. Monoclonal antibodies with different specificities against cytokeratins: an immunohistochemical study of normal tissues and tumors. Am J Pathol 1984; 114:9–17.
5. Reis-Filho JS, Simpson PT, Martins A, et al. Distribution of p63, cytokeratins 5/6 and cytokeratin 14 in 51 normal and 400 neoplastic human tissue samples using TARP-4 multi-tumor tissue microarray. Virchows Arch 2003; 443:122–132.
6. Suo Z, Holm R, Nesland JM. Squamous cell carcinomas: an immunohistochemical study of cytokeratins and involucrin in primary and metastatic tumors. Histopathology 1993; 23:45–54.
7. Sigel JE, Skacel M, Bergfeld WF, et al. The utility of cytokeratin 5/6 in the recognition of cutaneous spindle cell squamous cell carcinoma. J Cutan Pathol 2001; 28:520–524.
8. Wick MR, Fitzgibbon JF, Swanson PE. Cutaneous sarcomas and sarcomatoid neoplasms of the skin. Semin Diagn Pathol 1993; 10:148–158.
9. Pinkus GS, Kurtin PJ. Epithelial membrane antigen: a diagnostic discriminant in surgical pathology. Hum Pathol 1985; 16:929–940.
10. Egawa K, Honda Y, Ono T, et al. Immunohistochemical demonstration of carcinoembryonic antigen and related antigens in various cutaneous keratinous neoplasms and verruca vulgaris. Br J Dermatol 1998; 139:178–185.
11. Dale BA, Gown AM, Fleckman P, et al. Characterization of two monoclonal antibodies to human epidermal keratohyaline: reactivity with filaggrin and related proteins. J Invest Dermatol 1987; 88:306–313.
12. Hashimoto T, Inamato N, Nakamura K, et al. Involucrin expression in skin appendage tumors. Br J Dermatol 1987; 117:325–332.
13. Klein-Szanto AJP, Barr RJ, Reiners JJ, et al. Filaggrin distribution in keratoacanthomas and squamous cell carcinomas. Arch Pathol Lab Med 1984; 108:888–890.
14. Said JW, Sassoon AF, Shintaku JP, et al. Involucrin in squamous and basal cell carcinomas of the skin: an immunohistochemical study. J Invest Dermatol 1984; 82:449–452.
15. Smoller BR, Kwan TH, Said JW. Keratoacanthoma and squamous cell carcinoma of the skin: immunohistochemical localization of involucrin and keratin proteins. J Am Acad Dermatol 1986; 14:225–236.
16. Murphy CF, Flynn RC, Rice RH, et al. Involucrin expression in normal and neoplastic human skin: a marker for keratinocyte differentiation. J Invest Dermatol 1984; 82:453–457.
17. Kanitakis J, Zambruno G, Viae J, et al. Involucrin expression in adnexal skin tumors: an immunohistochemical study. Virchows Archiv A 1986; 408:527–540.
18. Strutton GM. Pathological variants of basal cell carcinoma. Australas J Dermatol 1997; 38(Suppl 1):S31–S35.
19. Shimizu N, Ito M, Tazawa T, et al. Immunohistochemical study of keratin expression in certain cutaneous epithelial neoplasms. Basal cell carcinoma, pilomatricoma, and seborrheic keratosis. Am J Dermatopathol 1989; 11:534–540.
20. Heyderman E, Graham RM, Chapman DV, et al. Epithelial markers in primary skin cancer: an immunoperoxidase study of the distribution of epithelial membrane antigen (EMA) and carcinoembryonic antigen (CEA) in 65 primary skin carcinomas. Histopathology 1984; 8:423–434.
21. Wick MR, Swanson PE. Primary adenoid cystic carcinoma of the skin: a clinical, histologic, and immunohistochemical comparison with adenoid cystic carcinoma of salivary glands,

and adenoid basal cell carcinoma. Am J Dermatopathol 1986; 8:2–13.
22. George E, Swanson PE, Wick MR. Neuroendocrine differentiation in basal cell carcinoma: an immunohistochemical study. Am J Dermatopathol 1989; 11:131–135.
23. Foschini MP, Eusebi V. Divergent differentiation in endocrine and nonendocrine tumors of the skin. Semin Diagn Pathol 2000; 17:162–168.
24. Collina G, Macri L, Eusebi V. Endocrine differentiation in basocellular carcinoma. Pathologica 2001; 93:208–212.
25. Tsukamoto H, Hayashibe K, Mishima Y, et al. The altered expression of alpha-smooth muscle actin in basal cell epithelioma and its surrounding stroma, with special reference to proliferating cell nuclear antigen expression and adenoid differentiation. Br J Dermatol 1994; 130:189–194.
26. Grando SA, Schofield OM, Skubitz AP, et al. Nodular basal cell carcinoma in vivo vs. in vitro. Establishment of pure cell cultures, cytomorphologic characteristics, ultrastructure, immunophenotype, biosynthetic activities, and generation of antisera. Arch Dermatol 1996; 132:1185–1193.
27. Sanchez NP, Winkelmann RK. Basal cell tumor with eccrine differentiation (eccrine epithelioma). J Am Acad Dermatol 1982; 6:514–518.
28. Sakamoto F, Ito M, Sato S, et al. Basal cell tumor with apocrine differentiation: apocrine epithelioma. J Am Acad Dermatol 1985; 13:355–363.
29. Jimenez FJ, Burchette JL Jr, Grichnik JM, et al. Ber-EP4 immunoreactivity in normal skin and cutaneous neoplasms. Mod Pathol 1995; 8:854–858.
30. Swanson PE, Fitzpatrick MM, Ritter JH, et al. Immunohistologic differential diagnosis of basal cell carcinoma, squamous cell carcinoma, and trichoepithelioma in small cutaneous biopsy specimens. J Cutan Pathol 1998; 25:153–159.
31. Urso C, Bondi R, Paglierani M, et al. Carcinomas of sweat glands: report of 60 cases. Arch Pathol Lab Med 2001; 125: 498–505.
32. Swanson PE, Cherwitz DL, Neumann MP, et al. Eccrine sweat gland carcinoma: a histologic and immunohistochemical study of 32 cases. J Cutan Pathol 1987; 14:65–86.
33. Qureshi HS, Ormsby AH, Lee MW, et al. The diagnostic utility of p63, CK5/6, CK7, and CK20 in distinguishing primary cutaneous adnexal neoplasms from metastatic carcinomas. J Cutan Pathol 2004; 31:145–152.
34. Metze D, Grunert F, Neumaier M, et al. Neoplasms with sweat gland differentiation express various glycoproteins of the carcinoembryonic antigen (CEA) family. J Cutan Pathol 1996; 23:1–11.
35. Ansai S, Koseki S, Hozumi Y, et al. An immunohistochemical study of lysozyme, CD15 (Leu-M1), and gross cystic disease fluid protein-15 in various skin tumors: assessment of the specificity and sensitivity of markers of apocrine differentiation. Am J Dermatopathol 1995; 17:249–255.
36. Tsubura A, Senzaki H, Sasaki M, et al. Immunohisto-chemical demonstrated of breast-derived and/or carcinoma-associated glycoproteins in normal skin appendages and their tumors. J Cutan Pathol 1992; 19:73–79.
37. Santos-Juanes J, Bernaldo-de Quiros JF, Galache-Osuna C, et al. Apocrine carcinoma, adenopathies, and raised TAG-72 serum tumor marker. Dermatol Surg 2004; 30:566–569.
38. Wick MR, Swanson PE, LeBoit PE, et al. Lymphoepithelioma-like carcinoma of the skin with adnexal differentiation. J Cutan Pathol 1991; 18:93–102.
39. Ramachandra S, Gillette CE, Millis RR. A comparative immunohistochemical study of mammary and extramammary Paget's disease and superficial spreading melanoma, with particular emphasis on melanocytic markers. Virchows Arch A 1996; 429:371–376.
40. Mazoujian G, Margolis R. Immunohistochemistry of gross cystic disease fluid protein (GCDFP-15) in 65 benign sweat gland tumors of the skin. Am J Dermatopathol 1988; 10:28–35.
41. Battles OE, Page DL, Johnson JE. Cytokeratins, CEA, and mucin histochemistry in the diagnosis and characterization of extramammary Paget's disease. Am J Clin Pathol 1997; 108:6–12.
42. Hitchcock A, Topham S, Bell J, et al. Routine diagnosis of mammary and extramammary Paget's disease: a modern approach. Am J Surg Pathol 1992; 16:58–61.
43. Mazoujian G, Pinkus GS, Haagensen DE Jr. Extramammary Paget's disease – evidence for an apocrine origin: an immunoperoxidase study of gross cystic disease fluid protein-15, carcinoembryonic antigen, and cytokeratin proteins. Am J Surg Pathol 1984; 8:43–50.
44. Nowak MA, Guerriere-Kovach P, Pathan A, et al. Perianal Paget's disease: distinguishing primary and secondary lesions using immunohistochemical studies including gross cystic

disease fluid protein-15 and cytokeratin 20 expression. Arch Pathol Lab Med 1998; 122:1077–1081.

45. Ohnishi T, Watanabe S. The use of cytokeratins 7 and 20 in the diagnosis of primary and secondary extramammary Paget's disease. Br J Dermatol 2000; 142:243–247.

46. Haga R, Suzuki H. Rectal carcinoma associated with pagetoid phenomenon. Eur J Dermatol 2003; 13:93–94.

47. Raju RR, Goldblum JR, Hart WR. Pagetoid squamous cell carcinoma in situ (Pagetoid Bowen's disease) of the external genitalia. Int J Gynecol Pathol 2003; 22:127–135.

48. Mazoujian G. Immunohistochemistry of GCDFP-24 and zinc-alpha-2-glycoprotein in benign sweat gland tumors. Am J Dermatopathol 1990; 12:452–457.

49. Hashimoto K, Eto H, Matsumoto M, et al. Antikeratin antibodies: production, specificity, and applications. J Cutan Pathol 1983; 10:529–539.

50. Ishihara M, Mehregan OR, Hashimoto K, et al. Staining of eccrine and apocrine neoplasms and metastatic adenocarcinoma with IKH-4, a monoclonal antibody specific for the eccrine gland. J Cutan Pathol 1998; 25:100–105.

51. Ormsby AH, Snow JL, Su WPD, et al. Diagnostic immunohistochemistry of cutaneous metastatic breast carcinoma: a statistical analysis of the utility of gross cystic disease fluid-protein-15 and estrogen receptor protein. J Am Acad Dermatol 1995; 32:711–716.

52. Latham JA, Redfern CP, Thody AJ, et al. Immunohistochemical markers of human sebaceous gland differentiation. J Histochem Cytochem 1989; 37:729–734.

53. Swanson PE. Monoclonal antibodies to human milk fat globule proteins. In: Wick MR, Siegal GP, eds. Monoclonal antibodies in diagnostic immunohistochemistry. New York: Marcel Dekker; 1988:227–283.

54. Bayer-Garner IB, Givens V, Smoller BR. Immunohistochemical staining for androgen receptors: a sensitive marker of sebaceous differentiation. Am J Dermatopathol 1999; 21:426–431.

55. Shikata N, Kurokawa I, Andachi H, et al. Expression of androgen receptors in skin appendage tumors: an immunohistochemical study. J Cutan Pathol 1995; 22:149–153.

56. Headington JT. Tumors of the hair follicle: a review. Am J Pathol 1976; 85:480–505.

57. Manivel JC, Wick MR, Mukai K. Pilomatrix carcinoma: an immunohistochemical comparison with benign pilomatrixoma and other benign cutaneous lesions of pilar origin. J Cutan Pathol 1986; 13:22–29.

58. Basarab TG, Orchard R, Russell-Jones R. The use of immunostaining for bcl-2 and CD34 and the lectin peanut agglutinin in differentiating between basal cell carcinoma and trichoepithelioma. Am J Dermatopathol 1998; 20:448–452.

59. Kirchmann TT, Prieto VG, Smoller BR. CD34 staining pattern distinguishes basal cell carcinoma from trichoepithelioma. Arch Dermatol 1994; 21:332–336.

60. Lum CA, Binder SW. Proliferative characterization of basal cell carcinoma and trichoepithelioma in small biopsy specimens. J Cutan Pathol 2004; 31:550–554.

61. Poniecka AW, Alexis JB. An immunohistochemical study of basal cell carcinoma and trichoepithelioma. Am J Dermatopathol 1999; 21:332–336.

62. Hunt SJ, Abell E. Malignant hair matrix tumor ('malignant trichoepithelioma') arising in the setting of multiple hereditary trichoepithelioma. Am J Dermatopathol 1991; 13:275–281.

63. Johnson SC, Bennett RG. Occurrence of basal cell carcinoma among multiple trichoepitheliomas. J Am Acad Dermatol 1993; 28:322–326.

64. Wallace ML, Smoller BR. Trichoepithelioma with an adjacent basal cell carcinoma: transformation or collision? J Am Acad Dermatol 1997; 37:343–345.

65. Yamamoto N, Gonda K. Multiple trichoepitheliomas with basal cell carcinoma. Ann Plast Surg 1999; 43:221–222.

66. Martinez CA, Priolli DG, Piovesan H, et al. Nonsolitary giant perianal trichoepithelioma with malignant transformation into basal cell carcinoma: report of a case and review of the literature. Dis Colon Rectum 2004; 47:773–777.

67. Harada H, Hashimoto K, Toi Y, et al. Basal cell carcinoma occurring in multiple familial trichoepithelioma: detection of loss of heterozygosity in chromosome 9q. Arch Dermatol 1997; 133:666–667.

68. Hartschuh W, Schulz T. Merkel cells are integral constituents of desmoplastic trichoepithelioma: an immunohistochemical and electron microscopic study. J Cutan Pathol 1995; 22:413–421.

69. Abesamis-Cubillan E, El-Shabrawi-Caelen L, LeBoit PE. Merkel cells and sclerosing epithelial neoplasms. Am J Dermatopathol 2000; 22:311–315.

70. Thewes M, Worret WI, Engst R, et al. Stromelysin-3: a po-

tent marker for histopathologic differentiation between desmoplastic trichoepithelioma and morphealike basal cell carcinoma. Am J Dermatopathol 1998; 20:140–142.

71. Ito M, Tazawa T, Shimuzu N. Cell differentiation in human anagen hair and hair follicles studied with anti-hair keratin monoclonal antibodies. J Invest Dermatol 1986; 86:563–569.

72. Lynch MH, O'Guin M, Hardy C, et al. Acidic and basic hair/nail (hard) keratins: their colocalization in upper cortical and cuticle cells of the human hair follicle and their relationship to soft keratins. J Cell Biol 1986; 103:2593–2606.

73. Wick MR, Cooper PH, Swanson PE, et al. Microcystic adnexal carcinoma: an immunohistochemical comparison with other cutaneous appendage tumors. Arch Dermatol 1990; 126:189–194.

74. Tateyama H, Eimoto T, Tada T, et al. Malignant pilomatrixoma: an immunohistochemical study with antihair keratin antibody. Cancer 1992; 69:127–132.

75. Amaral ALMP, Nascimento A, Goellner JR. Proliferating pilar (trichilemmal) cyst: report of two cases, one with carcinomatous transformation, and one with distant metastases. Arch Pathol Lab Med 1984; 108:808–810.

76. Swanson PE, Marrogi AJ, Williams DJ, et al. Tricholemmal carcinoma: clinicopathologic study of 10 cases. J Cutan Pathol 1992; 19:100–109.

77. Dreno B, Mousset S, Stalder JF, et al. A study of intermediate filaments (cytokeratin, vimentin, neurofilament) in two cases of Merkel cell tumor. J Cutan Pathol 1985; 12:37–45.

78. Hartschuh W, Reinecke M, Weihe E, et al. VIP-immunoreactivity in the skin of various mammals: immunohistochemical, radioimmunological, and experimental evidence for a dual localization in cutaneous nerves and Merkel cells. Peptides 1984; 5:239–245.

79. Chen-Chew SB, Leung PY. Species variability in the expression of met- and leu-enkephalin-like immunoreactivity in mammalian Merkel cell dense-core granules: a light and electron microscopic immunohistochemical study. Cell Tissue Res 1992; 269:347–351.

80. Narisawa Y, Hashimoto K, Kohda H. Immunohistochemical demonstration of the expression of neurofilament proteins in Merkel cells. Acta Derm Venereol 1994; 74:441–443.

81. Gallego R, Garcia-Caballero T, Fraga M, et al. Neural cell adhesion molecule immunoreactivity in Merkel cells and Merkel cell tumors. Virchows Arch A 1995; 426:317–321.

82. Fantini F, Johansson O. Neurochemical markers in human cutaneous Merkel cells: an immunohistochemical investigation. Exp Dermatol 1995; 4:365–371.

83. Kanitakis J, Bourchany D, Faure M, et al. Merkel cells in hyperplastic and neoplastic lesions of the skin: an immunohistochemical study using an antibody to keratin 20. Dermatology 1998; 196:208–212.

84. Jensen K, Kohler S, Rouse RV. Cytokeratin staining in Merkel cell carcinoma: an immunohistochemical study of cytokeratins 5/6, 7, 17, and 20. Appl Immunohistochem Mol Morphol 2000; 8:310–315.

85. Kurokawa M, Nabeshima K, Akiyama Y, et al. CD56: a useful marker for diagnosing Merkel cell carcinoma. J Dermatol Sci 2003; 31:219–224.

86. Garcia-Caballero T, Pintos E, Gallego R, et al. MOC-31/EpCAM immunoreactivity in Merkel cells and Merkel cell carcinomas. Histopathology 2003; 43:480–484.

87. Mott RT, Smoller BR, Morgan MB. Merkel cell carcinoma: a clinicopathologic study with prognostic implications. J Cutan Pathol 2004; 31:217–223.

88. Bickle K, Glass LF, Messina JL, et al. Merkel cell carcinoma: a clinical, histopathologic, and immunohistochemical review. Semin Cutan Med Surg 2004; 23:46–53.

89. Heenan PJ, Cole JM, Spagnolo DV. Primary cutaneous neuroendocrine carcinoma (Merkel cell tumor): an adnexal epithelial neoplasm. Am J Dermatopathol 1990; 12:7–16.

90. Battifora H, Silva EG. The use of antikeratin antibodies in the immunohistochemical distinction between neuroendocrine (Merkel cell) carcinoma of the skin, lymphoma, and oat cell carcinoma. Cancer 1986; 58:1040–1046.

91. Lau SK, Luthringer DJ, Eisen RN. Thyroid transcription factor-1: a review. Appl Immunohistochem Mol Morphol 2002; 10:97–102.

92. Leech SN, Kolar AJ, Barrett PD, et al. Merkel cell carcinoma can be distinguished from metastatic small cell carcinoma using antibodies to cytokeratin 20 and thyroid transcription factor-1. J Clin Pathol 2001; 54:727–729.

93. Jacinto CM, Grant-Kels JM, Knibbs DR, et al. Malignant primitive neuroectodermal tumor presenting as a scalp nodule. Am J Dermatopathol 1991; 13:63–70.

94. Patterson JW, Maygarden SJ. Extraskeletal Ewing's sarcoma with cutaneous involvement. J Cutan Pathol 1986; 13:46–58.

95. Banerjee SS, Agbamu DA, Eyden BP, et al. Clinicopatho-

logical characteristics of peripheral primitive neuroectodermal tumor of skin and subcutaneous tissue. Histopathology 1997; 31:355–366.

96. Hasegawa SL, Davison JM, Rutten A, et al. Primary cutaneous Ewing's sarcoma: immunophenotypic and molecular cytogenetic evaluation of five cases. Am J Surg Pathol 1998; 22:310–318.

97. Chao TK, Chang YL, Sheen TS. Extraskeletal Ewing's sarcoma of the scalp. J Laryngol Otol 2000; 114:73–75.

98. Taylor GB, Chan YF. Subcutaneous primitive neuroectodermal tumor in the abdominal wall of a child: long-term survival after local excision. Pathology 2000; 32:294–298.

99. Nicholson SA, McDermott MB, Swanson PE, et al. CD99 and cytokeratin-20 in small-cell and basaloid tumors of the skin. Appl Immunohistochem Mol Morphol 2000; 8:37–41.

100. Devoe K, Weidner N. Immunohistochemistry of small round-cell tumors. Semin Diagn Pathol 2000; 17:216–224.

101. Rossi S, Orvieto E, Furlanetto A, et al. Utility of the immunohistochemical detection of FLI-1 expression in round-cell and vascular neoplasms using a monoclonal antibody. Mod Pathol 2004; 17:547–552.

102. Faure P, Chittal S, Gorguet B, et al. Immunohistochemical profile of cutaneous B-cell lymphoma on cryostat and paraffin sections. Am J Dermatopathol 1990; 12:122–133.

103. Ralfkiaer E. Immunohistological markers for the diagnosis of cutaneous lymphomas. Semin Diagn Pathol 1991; 8:62–72.

104. Rest EB, Horn TD. Immunophenotypic analysis of benign and malignant cutaneous lymphoid infiltrates. Clin Dermatol 1991; 9:261–272.

105. Hsi ED, Yegappan S. Lymphoma immunophenotyping: a new era in paraffin section immunohis-tochemistry. Adv Anat Pathol 2001; 8:218–239.

106. Chen CC, Raikow RB, Sonmez-Alpan E, et al. Classification of small B-cell lymphoid neoplasms using a paraffin section immunohistochemical panel. Appl Immunohistochem Mol Morphol 2000; 8:1–11.

107. Baldassano MF, Bailey EM, Ferry JA, et al. Cutaneous lymphoid hyperplasia and cutaneous marginal zone lymphoma: comparison of morphologic and immunophenotypic features. Am J Surg Pathol 1999; 23:88–96.

108. Schmitt IM, Manente L, DiMatteo A, et al. Lymphoblastic lymphoma of the pre-B phenotype with cutaneous presentation. Dermatology 1997; 195:289–292.

109. Dorfman DM, Kraus M, Perez-Atayde AR, et al. CD99 (p30/32-MIC2) immunoreactivity in the diagnosis of leukemia cutis. Mod Pathol 1997; 10:283–288.

110. deBoer CJ, van Krieken JH, Schuuring E, et al. Bcl-1/cyclin-D1 in malignant lymphoma. Ann Oncol 1997; 8(Suppl 2): 109–117.

111. Quintanilla-Martinez L, Zukerberg LR, Ferry JA, et al. Extramedullary tumors of lymphoid or myeloid blasts: the role of immunohistology in diagnosis and classification. Am J Clin Pathol 1995; 104:431–443.

112. Audouin J, Comperat E, LeTourneau A, et al. Myeloid sarcoma: clinical and morphologic criteria useful for diagnosis. Int J Surg Pathol 2003; 11:271–282.

113. Segal GH, Stoler MH, Fishleder AJ, et al. Reliable and cost-effective paraffin section immunohistology of lymphoproliferative disorders. Am J Surg Pathol 1991; 15: 1034–1041.

114. Cerroni L, Smolle J, Soyer HP, et al. Immunophenotyping of cutaneous lymphoid infiltrates in frozen and paraffinembedded tissue sections: a comparative study. J Am Acad Dermatol 1990; 22:405–413.

115. Fartasch M, Goerdt S, Hornstein OP. Possibilities and limits of paraffin-embedded cell markers in diagnosis of primary cutaneous histiocytosis. Hautarzt 1995; 46:144–153.

116. Nemes Z, Thomazy V. Diagnostic significance of histiocyte-related markers in malignant histiocytosis and true histiocytic lymphoma. Cancer 1988; 62:1970–1980.

117. Andrade RE, Wick MR, Frizzera G, et al. Immunophenotyping of hematopoietic malignancies in paraffin sections. Hum Pathol 1988; 19:394–402.

118. Kurtin PJ, Pinkus GS. Leukocyte common antigen – a diagnostic discriminant between hematopoietic and nonhematopoietic neoplasms in paraffin sections using monoclonal antibodies: correlation with immunologic studies and ultrastructural localization. Hum Pathol 1985; 16:353–365.

119. Falini B, Mason DY. Proteins encoded by genes involved in chromosomal alterations in lymphoma and leukemia: clinical value of their detection by immunocytochemistry. Blood 2002; 99:409–426.

120. Cerroni L, Beham-Schmid C, Kerl H. Cutaneous Hodgkin's disease: an immunohistochemical analysis. J Cutan Pathol 1995; 22:229–235.

121. Segal GH, Stoler MH, Tubbs RR. The 'CD43 only' phenotype. An aberrant, nonspecific immunophenotype requiring comprehensive analysis for lineage resolution. Am J Clin Pathol 1992; 97:861–865.
122. Goldstein NS, Ritter JH, Argenyi ZB, et al. Granulocytic sarcoma: potential diagnostic clues from immunostaining patterns seen with 'anti-lymphoid' antibodies. Int J Surg Pathol 1995; 2:199–206.
123. Kiyokawa N, Sekino T, Matsui T, et al. Diagnostic importance of CD179a/b as markers of precursor B-cell lymphoblastic lymphoma. Mod Pathol 2004; 17:423–429.
124. Torlakovic E, Torlakovic G, Nguyen PL, et al. The value of anti-pax-5 immunostaining in routinely fixed and paraffin-embedded sections: a novel pan pre-B and B-cell marker. Am J Surg Pathol 2002; 26:1343–1350.
125. Fucich LF, Freeman SF, Boh EE, et al. Atypical cutaneous lymphoid infiltrates and a role for quantitative immunohistochemistry and gene rearrangement studies. Int J Dermatol 1999; 38:749–756.
126. Yang B, Tubbs RR, Finn W, et al. Clinicopathologic reassessment of primary cutaneous B-cell lymphomas with immunophenotypic and molecular genetic characterization. Am J Surg Pathol 2000; 24:694–702.
127. Nihal M, Mikkola D, Horvath N, et al. Cutaneous lymphoid hyperplasia: a lymphoproliferative continuum with lymphomatous potential. Hum Pathol 2003; 34:617–622.
128. Gilliam AC, Wood GS. Cutaneous lymphoid hyperplasias. Semin Cutan Med Surg 2000; 19:133–141.
129. Magro CM, Crowson AN, Porcu P, et al. Automated kappa and lambda light chain mRNA expression for the assessment of B-cell clonality in cutaneous B-cell infiltrates: its utility and diagnostic application. J Cutan Pathol 2003; 30:504–511.
130. Leinweber B, Colli C, Chott A, et al. Differential diagnosis of cutaneous infiltrates of B lymphocytes with follicular growth pattern. Am J Dermatopathol 2004; 26:4–13.
131. Alaibac M, Pigozzi B, Belloni-Fortina A, et al. CD7 expression in reactive and malignant human skin T-lymphocytes. Anticancer Res 2003; 23:2707–2710.
132. Murphy M, Fullen D, Carlson JA. Low CD7 expression in benign and malignant cutaneous lymphocytic infiltrates: experience with an antibody reactive with paraffin-embedded tissue. Am J Dermatopathol 2002; 24:6–16.
133. Rijlaarsdam U, Willemze R. Cutaneous pseudo-T-cell lymphomas. Semin Diagn Pathol 1991; 8:102–108.
134. Smolle J, Tome R, Soyer HP, et al. Immunohistochemical classification of cutaneous pseudolymphomas: delineation of distinct patterns. J Cutan Pathol 1990; 17:149–159.
135. Griesser H, Feller AC, Sterry W. T-cell receptor and immunoglobulin gene rearrangements in cutaneous T-cell-rich pseudolymphomas. J Invest Dermatol 1990; 95:292–295.
136. Ritter JH, Adesokan PN, Fitzgibbon JF, et al. Paraffin section immunohistochemistry as an adjunct to morphologic analysis in the diagnosis of cutaneous lymphoid infiltrates. J Cutan Pathol 1994; 21:481–493.
137. Van Vloten WA. Cutaneous lymphoma. Basel, Switzerland: S. Karger; 1989.
138. Giannotti B, Pimpinelli N. Modern diagnosis of cutaneous lymphoma. Recent Results Cancer Res 2002; 160:303–306.
139. Cerroni L, Goteri G. Differential diagnosis between cutaneous lymphoma and pseudolymphoma. Anal Quant Cytol Histol 2003; 25:191–198.
140. Toonstra J. Actinic reticuloid. Semin Diagn Pathol 1991; 8:109–116.
141. Magro CM, Crowson AN, Kovatich AJ, et al. Drug-induced reversible lymphoid dyscrasia: a clonal lymphomatoid dermatitis of memory and activated T cells. Hum Pathol 2003; 34:119–129.
142. Burg G, Dummer R, Haeffner A, et al. From inflammation to neoplasia: mycosis fungoides evolves from reactive inflammatory conditions (lymphoid infiltrates) transforming into neoplastic plaques and tumors. Arch Dermatol 2001; 137:949–952.
143. LeBoit PE. Variants of mycosis fungoides and related cutaneous T-cell lymphomas. Semin Diagn Pathol 1991; 8:73–81.
144. Wood GS, Abel EA, Hoppe RT, et al. Leu-8 and Leu-9 antigen phenotypes: immunological criteria for the distinction of mycosis fungoides from cutaneous inflammation. J Am Acad Dermatol 1986; 14:1006–1013.
145. Bignon YJ, Souteyrand P. Genotyping of cutaneous T-cell lymphomas and pseudolymphomas. Curr Prob Dermatol 1990; 19:114–123.
146. Ceballos KM, Gascoyne RD, Martinka M, et al. Heavy multinodular cutaneous lymphoid infiltrates: clinicopathologic features and B-cell clonality. J Cutan Pathol 2002; 29:159–167.

147. Kerl H, Smolle J. Classification of cutaneous pseudolymphomas. Curr Prob Dermatol 1989; 19:167–176.
148. Hurt MA, Santa Cruz DJ. Cutaneous inflammatory pseudotumors. Am J Surg Pathol 1990; 14:764–772.
149. Toyota N, Matsuo S, Iizuka H. Immunohistochemical differential diagnosis between lymphocytoma cutis and malignant lymphoma in paraffin-embedded sections. J Dermatol 1991; 18:586–591.
150. Picker LJ, Weiss LM, Medeiros LJ, et al. Immunophenotypic criteria for the diagnosis of non-Hodgkin's lymphoma. Am J Pathol 1987; 128:181–201.
151. Ngan BY, Picker LJ, Medeiros LJ, et al. Immunophenotypic diagnosis of non-Hodgkin's lymphoma in paraffin sections: coexpression of L60 (Leu-22) and L26 antigens correlates with malignant histologic findings. Am J Clin Pathol 1989; 91:579–583.
152. Utz GL, Swerdlow SH. Distinction of follicular hyperplasia from follicular lymphoma in B5-fixed tissues: comparison of MT2 and bcl-2 antibodies. Hum Pathol 1993; 24:1155–1158.
153. Triscott JA, Ritter JH, Swanson PE, et al. Immunoreactivity for bcl-2 protein in cutaneous lymphomas and lymphoid hyperplasias. J Cutan Pathol 1995; 22:2–10.
154. Mirza I, Macpherson N, Paproski S, et al. Primary cutaneous follicular lymphoma: an assessment of clinical, histopathologic, immunophenotypic, and molecular features. J Clin Oncol 2002; 20:647–655.
155. Goodlad JR, Krajewski AS, Batstone PJ, et al. Primary cutaneous follicular lymphoma: a clinicopathologic and molecular study of 16 cases in support of a distinct entity. Am J Surg Pathol 2002; 26:733–741.
156. Lawnicki LC, Weisenburger DD, Aoun P, et al. The t(14;18) and bcl-2 expression are present in a subset of primary cutaneous follicular lymphoma: association with lower grade. Am J Clin Pathol 2002; 118:765–772.
157. Kim BK, Surti U, Pandya AG, et al. Primary and secondary cutaneous diffuse large B-cell lymphomas: a multiparameter analysis of 25 cases including fluorescence in-situ hybridization for t(14;18) translocation. Am J Surg Pathol 2003; 27:356–364.
158. Hoefnagel JJ, Vermeer MH, Jansen PM, et al. Bcl-2, Bcl-6 and CD10 expression in cutaneous B-cell lymphoma: further support for a follicle centre cell origin and differential diagnostic significance. Br J Dermatol 2003; 149:1183–1191.
159. Vergier B, Belaud-Rotureau MA, Benassy MN, et al. Neoplastic cells do not carry bcl-2-JH rearrangements detected in a subset of primary cutaneous follicle center B-cell lymphomas. Am J Surg Pathol 2004; 28:748–755.
160. Kuo TT. Cutaneous manifestations of Kikuchi's histiocytic necrotizing lymphadenitis. Am J Surg Pathol 1990; 14:872–879.
161. Spies J, Foucar K, Thompson CT, et al. The histopathology of cutaneous lesions of Kikuchi's disease (necrotizing lymphadenitis): a report of five cases. Am J Surg Pathol 1999; 23:1040–1047.
162. Lee CS, Lim HW. Cutaneous diseases in Asians. Dermatol Clin 2003; 21:669–677.
163. Yen HR, Lin PY, Chuang WY, et al. Skin manifestations of Kikuchi-Fujimoto disease: case report and review. Eur J Pediatr 2004; 163:210–213.
164. Kaudewitz P, Burg G. Lymphomatoid papulosis and Ki-1 (CD30)-positive cutaneous large cell lymphomas. Semin Diagn Pathol 1991; 8:117–124.
165. Stein H, Mason DY, Gerdes J, et al. The expression of the Hodgkin's disease-associated antigen Ki-1 in reactive and neoplastic tissue. Blood 1985; 66:848–858.
166. Cepeda LT, Pieretti M, Chapman SF, et al. CD30-positive atypical lymphoid cells in common non-neoplastic cutaneous infiltrates rich in neutrophils and eosinophils. Am J Surg Pathol 2003; 27:912–918.
167. Kuo TT. Kikuchi's disease (histiocytic necrotizing lymphadenitis): a clinicopathologic study of 79 cases with an analysis of histologic subtypes, immunohistology, and DNA ploidy. Am J Surg Pathol 1995; 19:798–809.
168. Ruzicka T, Evers J. Clinical course and therapy of Langerhans cell histiocytosis in children and adults. Hautarzt 2003; 54:148–155.
169. Singh A, Prieto VG, Czelusta A, et al. Adult Langerhans cell histiocytosis limited to the skin. Dermatology 2003; 207:157–161.
170. Aoki M, Aoki R, Akimoto M, et al. Primary cutaneous Langerhans cell histiocytosis in an adult. Am J Dermato Pathol 1998; 20: 281-284.
171. Stefanato CM, Andersen WK, Calonje E, et al. Langerhans cell histiocytosis in the elderly: a report of three cases. J Am Acad Dermatol 1998; 39:375–378.
172. Rowden G, Connelly EM, Winkelmann RK. Cutaneous his-

tiocytosis X: the presence of S100 protein and its use in diagnosis. Arch Dermatol 1983; 119:553–559.

173. Emile JF, Wechsler J, Brousse N, et al. Langerhans cell histiocytosis: definitive diagnosis with the use of monoclonal antibody O10 on routinely paraffin-embedded samples. Am J Surg Pathol 1995; 19:636–641.

174. Pinkus GS, Lones MA, Matsumura F, et al. Langerhans cell histiocytosis: immunohistochemical expression of fascin, a dendritic cell marker. Am J Clin Pathol 2002; 118:335–343.

175. Slone SP, Fleming DR, Buchino JJ. Sinus histiocytosis with massive lymphadenopathy and Langerhans cell histiocytosis express the cellular adhesion molecule CD31. Arch Pathol Lab Med 2003; 127:341–344.

176. Weiss LM, Grogan TM, Muller-Hermelink HK, et al. Follicular dendritic cell sarcoma/tumor. In: Tumors of haematopoeitic and lymphoid tissues. Washington, DC: WHO/IARC Press; 2001:286–288.

177. Favara BE, Feller AC, Pauli M, et al. Contemporary classification of histiocytic disorders: the WHO Committee on Histiocytic/Reticulum Cell Proliferations. Reclassification Working Group of the Histiocyte Society. Med Pediatr Oncol 1997; 29:157–166.

178. Shamoto M, Hosokawa S, Shinzato M, et al. Comparison of Langerhans cells and interdigitating reticulum cells. Adv Exp Med Biol 1993; 329:311–314.

179. Davaris DXG, Ling FCK, Prentice RSA. Congenital self-healing histiocytosis: report of two cases with histochemical and ultrastructural studies. Am J Dermatopathol 1991; 13: 481–487.

180. Kapila PK, Grant-Kels JM, Allred C, et al. Congenital spontaneously regressing histiocytosis: case report and review of the literature. Pediatr Dermatol 1985; 2:312–317.

181. Gianotti R, Alessi E, Caputo R. Benign cephalic histiocytosis: a distinct entity or a part of a wide spectrum of histiocytic proliferative disorders of children? A histopathological study. Am J Dermatopathol 1993; 15:315–319.

182. Pena-Penabad C, Unamuno P, Garcia-Silva J, et al. Benign cephalic histiocytosis: case report and literature review. Pediatr Dermatol 1994; 11:164–167.

183. Jih DM, Salcedo SL, Jaworsky C. Benign cephalic histiocytosis: a case report and review. J Am Acad Dermatol 2002; 47:908–913.

184. Flynn KJ, Dehner LP, Gajl-Peczalska KJ, et al. Regressing atypical histiocytosis: a cutaneous proliferation of atypical neoplastic histiocytes with unexpectedly indolent biological behavior. Cancer 1982; 49:959–970.

185. Headington JT, Roth MS, Schnitzer B. Regressing atypical histiocytosis: a review and critical appraisal. Semin Diagn Pathol 1987; 4:28–37.

186. Headington JT, Roth MS, Ginsburg D, et al. T-cell receptor gene rearrangement in regressing atypical histiocytosis. Arch Dermatol 1987; 123:1183–1187.

187. Motley RJ, Jasani B, Ford AM, et al. Regressing atypical histiocytosis, a regressing cutaneous phase of Ki-1-positive anaplastic large cell lymphoma: immunocytochemical, nucleic acid, and cytogenetic studies of a new case in view of current opinion. Cancer 1992; 70:476–483.

188. Turner ML, Gilmour HM, McLaren KM, et al. Regressing atypical histiocytosis: report of two cases with progression to high-grade T-cell non-Hodgkin's lymphoma. Hematol Pathol 1993; 7:33–47.

189. Drews R, Samel A, Kadin ME. Lymphomatoid papulosis and anaplastic large cell lymphomas of the skin. Semin Cutan Med Surg 2000; 19:109–117.

190. Stein H, Foss HD, Durkop H, et al. CD30+ anaplastic large cell lymphoma: a review of its histopathologic, genetic, and clinical features. Blood 2000; 96:3681–3695.

191. Kadin ME, Carpenter C. Systemic and primary cutaneous anaplastic large cell lymphoma. Semin Hematol 2003; 40: 244–256.

192. Liu HL, Hoppe RT, Kohler S, et al. CD30+ cutaneous lymphoproliferative disorders: the Stanford experience in lymphomatoid papulosis and primary cutaneous anaplastic large cell lymphoma. J Am Acad Dermatol 2003; 49:1049–1058.

193. Willemze R, Meijer CJ. Primary cutaneous CD30-positive lymphoproliferative disorders. Hematol Oncol Clin North Am 2003; 17:1319–1332.

194. Cerio R, Black MM. Regressing atypical histiocytosis and lymphomatoid papulosis: variants of the same disorder? Br J Dermatol 1990; 123:515–521.

195. Yashiro N, Kitajima J, Kobayashi H, et al. Primary anaplastic large-cell lymphoma of the skin: a case report suggesting that regressing atypical histiocytosis and lymphomatoid papulosis are subsets. J Am Acad Dermatol 1994; 30:358–363.

196. Camisa C, Helm TN, Sexton C, et al. Ki-1-positive anaplas-

tic large-cell lymphoma can mimic benign dermatoses. J Am Acad Dermatol 1993; 29:696–700.

197. Brown JR, Skarin AT. Clinical mimics of lymphoma. Oncologist 2004; 9:406–416.

198. Steinhoff M, Hummel M, Anagnostopoulos I, et al. Single-cell analysis of CD30+ cells in lymphomatoid papulosis demonstrates a common clonal T-cell origin. Blood 2002; 15:578–584.

199. Banerjee SS, Heald J, Harris M. Twelve cases of Ki-1-positive anaplastic large cell lymphoma of skin. J Clin Pathol 1991; 44:119–125.

200. Beljaards RC, Meijer CJ, Scheffer E. Prognostic significance of CD30 (Ki-1/Ber-H2) expression in primary cutaneous large-cell lymphoma of T-cell origin: a clinicopathologic and immunohistochemical study of 20 patients. Am J Pathol 1989; 135:1169–1178.

201. Kadin ME, Levi E, Kempf W. Progression of lymphomatoid papulosis to systemic lymphoma is associated with escape from growth inhibition by transforming growth factor-beta and CD30 ligand. Ann NY Acad Sci 2001; 94:59–68.

202. ten Berge RL, Oudejans JJ, Ossenkoppele GJ, et al. ALK-negative systemic anaplastic large-cell lymphoma: differential diagnostic and prognostic aspects – a review. J Pathol 2003; 200:4–15.

203. Bhawan J, Bacchetta C, Joris I, et al. A myofibroblastic tumor: infantile digital fibroma (recurrent digital fibrous tumor of childhood). Am J Pathol 1979; 94: 9–28.

204. Blusje LG, Bastiaens M, Chang A, et al. Infantile-type digital fibromatosis tumor in an adult. Br J Dermatol 2000; 143: 1107–1108.

205. Kanwar AJ, Kaur S, Thami GP, et al Congenital infantile digital fibromatosis. Pediatr Dermatol 2002; 19:370–371.

206. Kang SK, Chang SE, Choi JH, et al. A case of congenital infantile digital fibromatosis. Pediatr Dermatol 2002; 19:462–463.

207. Guillen DR, Cockerell CJ. Cutaneous and subcutaneous sarcomas. Clin Dermatol 2001; 19:262–268.

208. Diaz-Cascajo C, Borghi S, Weyers W, et al. Fibroblastic/myofibroblastic sarcomas of the skin: a report of five cases. J Cutan Pathol 2003; 30:128–134.

209. Hayes MM, Dietrich BE, Uys CJ. Congenital hemangiopericytomas of skin. Am J Dermatopathol 1986; 8:148–153.

210. Ferreira CM, Maceira JM, Coelho JM. Congenital hemangiopericytoma of the skin. Int J Dermatol 1997; 36: 521–523.

211. Schurch W, Seemayer TA, Lagace R, et al. The intermediate filament cytoskeleton of myofibroblasts: an immunofluorescence and ultrastructural study. Virchows Archiv A 1984; 403: 323–336.

212. Coffin CM, Neilson KA, Ingels S, et al. Congenital generalized myofibromatosis: a disseminated angiocentric myofibromatosis. Pediatr Pathol Lab Med 1995; 15:571–587.

213. Beham A, Badve S, Suster S, et al. Solitary myofibroma in adults: clinicopathological analysis of a series. Histopathology 1993; 22:335–341.

214. Mentzel T, Calonje E, Nascimento AG, et al. Infantile hemangiopericytoma versus infantile myofibromatosis: study of a series suggesting a continuous spectrum of infantile myofibroblastic lesions. Am J Surg Pathol 1994; 18:922–930.

215. Strauchen JA, Dimitriu-Bona A. Malignant fibrous histiocytoma: expression of monocyte/macrophage differentiation antigens detected with monoclonal antibodies. Am J Pathol 1986; 124:303–309.

216. Mechterscheimer G. Towards the phenotyping of soft tissue tumors by cell surface markers. Virchows Arch A 1991; 419: 7–28.

217. Mechterscheimer G, Staudter M, Majdie O. Expression of HLA-A,B,C, beta-microglobulin, HLA-DR, -DP, -DQ, and HLA-D-associated invariant chain in soft tissue tumors. Int J Cancer 1990; 46:813–823.

218. Swanson PE, Wick MR. HLA-DR (Ia-like) reactivity in tumors of bone and soft tissue: an immunohistochemical comparison of monoclonal antibodies LN3 and LK803 in routinely processed specimens. Mod Pathol 1990; 3:113–119.

219. Crocker J, Burnett D, Jones EL. Immunohistochemical demonstration of cathepsin B in the macrophages of benign and malignant lymphoid tissues. J Pathol 1984; 142:87–94.

220. Loftus B, Loh LC, Curran B, et al. MAC387: its nonspecificity as a tumor marker or marker of histiocytes. Histopathology 1991; 17:251–255.

221. Cerio R, Spaull J, Oliver GF, et al. A study of factor XIIIa and MAC387 immunolabeling in normal and pathological skin. Am J Dermatopathol 1990; 12:221–233.

222. Gray MH, Smoller BR, McNutt NS, et al. Neurofibromas and neurotized nevi are immunohisto-chemically distinct neoplasms. Am J Dermatopathol 1990; 12:234–241.

223. Nemes Z, Thomazy V. Factor XIIIa and the classic histiocytic markers in malignant fibrous histiocytoma: a comparative immunohistochemical study. Hum Pathol 1988; 19:822–829.
224. Silverman JS, Tamsen A. High-grade malignant fibrous histiocytomas have bimodal cycling populations of factor XIIIa+ dendrophages and dedifferentiated mesenchcymal cells possibly derived from CD34+ fibroblasts. Cell Vis 1998; 5:73–76.
225. Nikkels AF, Arrese-Estrada J, Pierard-Franchimont C, et al. CD68 and factor XIIIa expressions in granular-cell tumor of the skin. Dermatology 1993; 186:106–108.
226. Hirose T, Kudo E, Hasegawa T, et al. Expression of intermediate filaments in malignant fibrous histiocytomas. Hum Pathol 1989; 20:871–877.
227. Longacre TA, Smoller BR, Rouse RV. Atypical fibroxanthoma: multiple immunohistologic profiles. Am J Surg Pathol 1993; 17:1199–1209.
228. Hasegawa T, Hasegawa F, Hirose T, et al. Expression of smooth muscle markers in so-called malignant fibrous histiocytomas. J Clin Pathol 2003; 56:666–671.
229. Abenoza P, Lillemoe T. CD34 and factor XIIIa in the differential diagnosis of dermatofibroma and dermatofibrosarcoma protuberans. Am J Dermatopathol 1993; 15:429–434.
230. Altman DA, Nickoloff BJ, Fivenson DP. Differential expression of factor XIIIa and CD34 in cutaneous mesenchymal tumors. J Cutan Pathol 1993; 20:154–158.
231. Goldblum JR, Tuthill RJ. CD34 and factor XIIIa – immunoreactivity in dermatofibrosarcoma protuberans and dermatofibroma. Am J Dermatopathol 1997; 19:147–153.
232. Wick MR, Ritter JH, Lind AC, et al. The pathological distinction between 'deep penetrating' dermatofibroma and dermatofibrosarcoma protuberans. Semin Cutan Med Surg 1999; 18:91–98.
233. Weiss SW, Nickoloff BJ. CD34 is expressed by a distinctive cell population in peripheral nerve, nerve sheath tumors, and related lesions. Am J Surg Pathol 1993; 17:1039–1045.
234. Suster S, Fisher C. Immunoreactivity for the human hematopoietic progenitor cell antigen (CD34) in lipomatous tumors. Am J Surg Pathol 1997; 21:195–200.
235. Cowper SE, Kilpatrick T, Proper S, et al. Solitary fibrous tumor of the skin. Am J Dermatopathol 1999; 21:213–219.
236. Ramdial PK, Madaree A. Aggressive CD34-positive fibrous scalp lesion of childhood: extrapulmonary solitary fibrous tumor. Pediatr Devel Pathol 2001; 4:267–275.
237. Hardisson D, Cuevas-Santos J, Contreras F. Solitary fibrous tumor of the skin. J Am Acad Dermatol 2002; 46(Suppl 2):S37–S40.
238. Goldblum JR. Giant cell fibroblastoma: a report of three cases with histologic and immunohistochemical evidence of a relationship to dermatofibrosarcoma protuberans. Arch Pathol Lab Med 1996; 120:1052–1055.
239. Terrier-Lacombe MJ, Guillou L, Maire G, et al. Dermatofibrosarcoma protuberans, giant cell fibroblastoma, and hybrid lesions in children: a clinicopathologic comparative analysis of 28 cases with molecular data – a study from the French Federation of Cancer Centers Sarcoma Group. Am J Surg Pathol 2003; 27:27–39.
240. Silverman JS, Tamsen A. A cutaneous case of giant cell angiofibroma occurring with dermatofibrosarcoma protuberans and showing bimodal CD34+ fibroblastic and factor XIIIa+ histiocytic immunophenotype. J Cutan Pathol 1998; 25:265–270.
241. Sandberg AA, Bridge JA. Update on the cytogenetics and molecular genetics of bone and soft tissue tumors: dermatofibrosarcoma protuberans and giant cell fibroblastoma. Cancer Genet Cytogenet 2003; 140:1–12.
242. Billings SD, Folpe AL. Cutaneous and subcutaneous fibrohistiocytic tumors of intermediate malignancy: an update. Am J Dermatopathol 2004; 26:141–155.
243. Zelger B. It's a dermatofibroma: CD34 is irrelevant! Am J Dermatopathol 2002; 24:453–454.
244. O'Connell JX, Trotter MJ. Fibrosarcomatous dermato-fibrosarcoma protuberans with myofibroblastic differentiation: a histologically distinctive variant. Mod Pathol 1996; 9:273–278.
245. Diaz-Cascajo C. Myoid differentiation in dermatofibrosarcoma protuberans and its fibrosarcomatous variant. J Cutan Pathol 1997; 24:197–198.
246. Zamecnik M. Myoid cells in the fibrosarcomatous variant of dermatofibrosarcoma protuberans. Histopathology 2000; 36:186.
247. Morimitsu Y, Hisaoka M, Okamoto S, et al. Dermatofibrosarcoma protuberans and its fibrosarcomatous variant with areas of myoid differentiation: a report of three cases. Histopathology 1998; 32:547–551.

248. Diaz-Cascajo C, Weyers W, Borrego L, et al. Dermatofibrosarcoma protuberans with fibrosarcomatous areas: a clinicopathologic and immunohistochemical study of four cases. Am J Dermatopathol 1997; 19:562–567.

249. Mentzel T, Beham A, Katenkamp D, et al. Fibrosarcomatous (high-grade) dermatofibrosarcoma protuberans: clinicopathologic and immunohistochemical study of a series of 41 cases with emphasis on prognostic significance. Am J Surg Pathol 1998; 22:576–587.

250. Sigel JE, Bergfeld WF, Goldblum JR. A morphologic study of dermatofibrosarcoma protuberans: expansion of a histologic profile. J Cutan Pathol 2000; 27:159–163.

251. Diedhiou A, Larsimont D, Vandeweyer E, et al. Fibro-sarcomatous variant of dermatofibrosarcoma protuberans: clinicopathologic analysis of 4 cases. Ann Pathol 2001; 21:164–167.

252. Davis DA, Sanchez RL. Atrophic and plaque-like dermatofibrosarcoma protuberans. Am J Dermatopathol 1998; 20:498–501.

253. Brooks JJ. The significance of double phenotypic patterns and markers in human sarcomas: a new model of mesenchymal differentiation. Am J Pathol 1986; 125:113–123.

254. Monteagudo C, Calduch L, Navarro S, et al. CD99-immunoreactivity in atypical fibroxanthoma: a common feature of diagnostic value. Am J Clin Pathol 2002; 117:126–131.

255. Prieto VG, Reed JA, Shea CR. Immunohistochemistry of dermatofibromas and benign fibrous histiocytomas. J Cutan Pathol 1995; 22:336–341.

256. Swanson PE, Stanley MW, Scheithauer BW, et al Primary cutaneous leiomyosarcoma: a histologic and immunohistochemical study of nine cases, with ultrastructural correlation. J Cutan Pathol 1988; 15:129–141.

257. Spencer JM, Amonette RA. Tumors with smooth muscle differentiation. Dermatol Surg 1996; 22:761–768.

258. Watanabe K, Kusakabe T, Hoshi N, et al. H-caldesmon in leiomyosarcoma and tumors with smooth muscle cell-like differentiation: its specific expression in the smooth muscle cell tumor. Hum Pathol 1999; 30:392–396.

259. Schadendorf D, Haas N, Ostmeier H, et al. Primary leiomyosarcoma of the skin: a histological and immunohistochemical analysis. Acta Derm Venereol 1993; 73:143–145.

260. Jensen ML, Jensen OM, Michalski W, eet al. Intradermal and subcutaneous leiomyosarcoma: a clinicopathological and immunohistochemical study of 41 cases. J Cutan Pathol 1996; 23:458–463.

261. Altinok G, Dogan AL, Aydin SO, et al Primary leiomyosarcomas of the skin. Scand J Plast Reconstr Surg Hand Surg 2002; 36:56–59.

262. Iwata J, Fletcher CDM. Immunohistochemical detection of cytokeratin and epithelial membrane antigen in leiomyosarcoma: a systematic study of 100 cases. Pathol Int 2000; 50:7–14.

263. Dervan PA, Tobbia IN, Casey M, et al. Glomus tumors: an immunohistochemical profile of 11 cases. Histopathology 1989; 14:483–491.

264. Kaye VN, Dehner LP. Cutaneous glomus tumor: a comparative immunohistochemical study with pseudoangiomatous intradermal melanocytic nevi. Am J Dermatopathol 1991; 13: 2–6.

265. Haupt HM, Stern JB, Berlin SJ. Immunohistochemistry in the differential diagnosis of nodular hidradenoma and glomus tumor. Am J Dermatopathol 1992; 14:310–314.

266. Park JH, Oh SH, Yang MH, et al. Glomangiosarcoma of the hand: a case report and review of the literature. J Dermatol 2003; 30:827–833.

267. Mentzel T, Hugel H, Kutzner H. CD34-positive glomus tumor: clinicopathologic and immunohistochemical analysis of six cases with myxoid stromal changes. J Cutan Pathol 2002; 29:421–425.

268. Requena L, Sangueza OP. Benign neoplasms with neural differentiation: a review. Am J Dermatopathol 1995; 17:75–96.

269. George E, Swanson PE, Wick MR. Malignant peripheral nerve sheath tumors of the skin. Am J Dermatopathol 1989; 11: 213–221.

270. Demir Y, Tokyol C. Superficial malignant schwannoma of the scalp. Dermatol Surg 2003; 29:879–881.

271. Guillen DR, Cockerell CJ. Cutaneous and subcutaneous sarcomas. Clin Dermatol 2001; 19:262–268.

272. Leroy K, Dumas V, Martin-Garcia N, et al. Malignant peripheral nerve sheath tumors associated with neurofibromatosis type 1: a clinicopathologic and molecular study of 17 patients. Arch Dermatol 2001; 137:908–913.

273. Wick MR, Swanson PE, Scheithauer BW, et al. Malignant peripheral nerve sheath tumor: an immunohistochemical study of 62 cases. Am J Clin Pathol 1987; 87:425–433.

274. Swanson PE, Scheithauer BW, Wick MR. Peripheral nerve sheath neoplasms: clinicopathologic and immunochemical observations. Pathol Ann 1995; 30(Pt.2):1–82.

275. Miettinen M, Cupo W. Neural cell adhesion molecule distribution in soft tissue tumors. Hum Pathol 1993; 24:62–66.

276. Gray MH, Rosenberg AE, Dickersin GR, et al. Glial fibrillary acidic protein and keratin expression by benign and malignant peripheral nerve sheath tumors. Hum Pathol 1989; 20:1089–1096.

277. Stefansson K, Wollman RL. S100 protein in granular cell tumors (granular cell myoblastomas). Cancer 1982; 49:1834–1838.

278. LeBoit PE, Barr RJ, Burall S, et al. Primitive polypoid granular cell tumor and other cutaneous granular cell neoplasms of apparent non-neural origin. Am J Surg Pathol 1991; 15:48–58.

279. Hitchcock MG, Hurt MA, Santa Cruz DJ. Cutaneous granular cell angiosarcoma. J Cutan Pathol 1994; 21:256–262.

280. Le BH, Boyer PJ, Lewis JE, et al. Granular cell tumor: immunohistochemical assessment of inhibin-alpha, protein gene product 9.5, S100 protein, CD68, and Ki-67 proliferative index with clinical correlation. Arch Pathol Lab Med 2004; 128:771–775.

281. Fine SW, Li M. Expression of calretinin and the alpha-subunit of inhibin in granular cell tumors. Am J Clin Pathol 2003; 119:259–264.

282. Skelton HG, Williams J, Smith KJ. The clinical and histologic spectrum of cutaneous fibrous perineuriomas. Am J Dermatopathol 2001; 23:190–196.

283. Baran R, Perrin C. Subungual perineurioma: a peculiar location. Br J Dermatol 2002; 146:125–128.

284. Zamecnik M, Koys F, Gomoleak P. Atypical cellular perineurioma. Histopathology 2002; 40:296–299.

285. Baran R, Perrin C. Perineurioma: a tendon-sheath-fibroma-like variant in a distal subungual location. Acta Derm Venereol 2003; 83:60–61.

286. Mentzel T. Cutaneous perineurioma: clinical and histological findings and differential diagnosis. Pathologe 2003; 24:207–213.

287. Hewan-Lowe K, Furlong B, Mackay B. Perineurial cell differentiation in benign tumors and tumor-like proliferations of peripheral nerves. Ultrastruct Pathol 1993; 17:263–270.

288. Mentzel T, Dei Tos AP, Fletcher CDM. Perineurioma (storiform perineurial fibroma): clinicopathological analysis of four cases. Histopathology 1994; 25:261–267.

289. Giannini C, Scheithauer BW, Jenkins RB, et al. Soft tissue perineurioma: evidence for an abnormality of chromosome 22, criteria for diagnosis, and review of the literature. Am J Surg Pathol 1997; 21:164–173.

290. Fetsch JF, Miettinen M. Sclerosing perineurioma: a clinicopathologic study of 19 cases of a distinctive soft tissue lesion with a predilection for the fingers and palms of young adults. Am J Surg Pathol 1997; 21:1433–1442.

291. Hirose T, Scheithauer BW, Sano T. Perineurial malignant peripheral nerve sheath tumor (MPNST): a clinicopathologic, immunohistochemical, and ultrastructural study of seven cases. Am J Surg Pathol 1998; 22:1368–1378.

292. Zelger B, Weinlich G, Zelger B. Perineurioma: a frequently-unrecognized entity with emphasis on a plexiform variant. Adv Clin Pathol 2000; 4:25–33.

293. Burgues O, Monteagudo C, Noguera R, et al. Cutaneous sclerosing Pacinian-like perineurioma. Histopathology 2001; 39:498–502.

294. Rosenberg AS, Langee CL, Stevens GL, et al. Malignant peripheral nerve sheath tumor with perineurial differentiation: 'malignant perineurioma.' J Cutan Pathol 2002; 29:362–367.

295. Folpe AL, Billings SD, McKenney JK, et al. Expression of claudin-1, a recently described tight junction-associated protein, distinguishes soft tissue perineurioma from potential mimics. Am J Surg Pathol 2002; 26:1620–1626.

296. Laskin WB, Fetsch JF, Miettinen M. The 'neurothekeoma:' immunohistochemical analysis distinguishes the true nerve sheath myxoma from its mimics. Hum Pathol 2000; 31:1230–1241.

297. Page RN, King R, Mihm MC Jr, et al. Microophthalmia transcription factor and NKI/C3 expression in cellular neurothekeoma. Mod Pathol 2004; 17:230–234.

298. Fullen DR, Lowe L, Su LD. Antibody to S100 A6 protein is a sensitive immunohistochemical marker for neurothekeoma. J Cutan Pathol 2003; 30:118–122.

299. Misago N, Satoh T, Narisawa Y. Cellular neurothekeoma with histiocytic differentiation. J Cutan Pathol 2004; 31:568–572.

300. Calonje E, Wilson-Jones E, Smith NP, et al. Cellular neurothekeoma: an epithelioid variant of pilar leiomyoma? Morphological and immunohistochemical analysis of a series. Histopathology 1992; 20:397–404.

301. Swanson PE, Wick MR. Immunohistochemical evaluation of vascular neoplasms. Clin Dermatol 1991; 9:243–253.

302. Requena L, Sangueza OP. Cutaneous vascular proliferations: Part III: Malignant neoplasms, other cutaneous neoplasms with a significant vascular component, and disorders erroneously considered as vascular neoplasms. J Am Acad Dermatol 1998; 38:143–175.

303. Miettinen M, Holthofer H, Lehto VP, et al Ulex europaeus I lectin as a marker for tumors derived from endothelial cells. Am J Clin Pathol 1983; 79:32–36.

304. Leader M, Collins M, Patel J, et al. Staining for factor VIII-related antigen and Ulex europaeus agglutinin I (UEA-I) in 230 tumors. An assessment of their specificity for angiosarcoma and Kaposi's sarcoma. Histopathology 1986; 10:1153–1162.

305. Ramani P, Bradley NJ, Fletcher CDM. QBEND/10, a new monoclonal antibody to endothelium: assessment of its diagnostic utility in paraffin sections. Histopathology 1990; 17: 237–242.

306. Suster S, Wong TY. On the discriminatory value of anti-HPCA-1 (CD34) in the differential diagnosis of benign and malignant cutaneous vascular proliferations. Am J Dermatopathol 1994; 16:355–363.

307. DeYoung BR, Swanson PE, Argenyi ZB, et al. CD31 immunoreactivity in mesenchymal neoplasms of the skin and subcutis: report of 145 cases and review of putative immunohistological markers of endothelial differentiation. J Cutan Pathol 1995; 22:215–222.

308. Appleton MA, Attanoos RL, Jasani B. Thrombomodulin as a marker of vascular and lymphatic tumors. Histopathology 1996; 29:153–157.

309. Folpe AL, Chand EM, Goldblum JR, et al. Expression of FLI-1, a nuclear transcription factor, distinguishes vascular neoplasms from potential mimics. Am J Surg Pathol 2001; 25: 1061–1066.

310. Gray MH, Rosenberg AE, Dickersin GR, et al. Cytokeratin expression in epithelioid vascular neoplasms. Hum Pathol 1990; 21:212–217.

311. Traweek ST, Liu J, Battifora H. Keratin gene expression in non-epithelial tissues: detection with polymerase chain reaction. Am J Pathol 1993; 142:1111–1118.

312. Robin YM, Guillou L, Michels JJ, et al. Human herpesvirus-8 immunostaining: a sensitive and specific method for diagnosing Kaposi's sarcoma in paraffin-embedded sections. Am J Clin Pathol 2004; 121:330–334.

313. Cheuk W, Wong KO, Wong CS, et al. Immunostaining for human herpesvirus 8 latent nuclear antigen-1 helps distinguish Kaposi's sarcoma from its mimickers. Am J Clin Pathol 2004; 121:335–342.

314. Patel RM, Goldblum JR, His ED. Immunohistochemical detection of human herpes virus-8 latent nuclear antigen-1 is useful in the diagnosis of Kaposi's sarcoma. Mod Pathol 2004; 17:456–460.

315. O'Hara CD, Nascimento AG. Endothelial lesions of soft tissues: a review of reactive and neoplastic entities with emphasis on low-grade malignant (borderline) vascular tumors. Adv Anat Pathol 2003; 10:69–87.

316. Fletcher CDM, Beham A, Schmid C. Spindle-cell hemangioendothelioma: a clinicopathological and immunohistochemical study indicative of a non-neoplastic lesion. Histopathology 1991; 18:291–301.

317. Mentzel T, Beham A, Calonje E, et al. Epithelioid hemangioendothelioma of skin and soft tissues: clinicopathologic and immunohistochemical study of 30 cases. Am J Surg Pathol 1997; 21:363–374.

318. Mentzel T, Mazzoleni G, Dei Tos AP, et al. Kaposiform hemangioendothelioma in adults: clinicopathologic and immunohistochemical analysis of three cases. Am J Clin Pathol 1997; 108:450–455.

319. Billings SD, Folpe AL, Weiss SW. Epithelioid sarcoma-like hemangioendothelioma. Am J Surg Pathol 2003; 27:48–57.

320. Arber DA, Kandalaft PL, Mehta P, et al. Vimentin-negative epithelioid sarcoma. The value of an immunohistochemical panel that includes CD34. Am J Surg Pathol 1993; 17:302–307.

321. Manivel JC, Wick MR, Dehner LP, et al. Epithelioid sarcoma: an immunohistochemical study. Am J Clin Pathol 1987; 87: 319–326.

322. Wick MR, Manivel JC. Epithelioid sarcoma and isolated necrobiotic granuloma: a comparative immunohistochemical study. J Cutan Pathol 1986; 13:253–260.

323. Wick MR, Manivel JC. Epithelioid sarcoma and epithelioid hemangioendothelioma: an immunohistochemical and lectin-histochemical comparison. Virchows Arch A 1987; 410:309–316.

324. Chase DR, Enzinger FM, Weiss SW, et al. Keratin in epithe-

lioid sarcoma: an immunohistochemical study. Am J Surg Pathol 1984; 8:435–441.

325. Wakely P Jr. Epithelioid/granular soft tissue lesions: correlation of cytopathology and histopathology. Ann Diagn Pathol 2000; 4:316–328.

326. Humble SD, Prieto VG, Horenstein MG. Cytokeratin 7 and 20 expression in epithelioid sarcoma. J Cutan Pathol 2003; 30:242–246.

327. Laskin WB, Miettinen M. Epithelioid sarcoma: new insights based on an extended immunohistochemical analysis. Arch Pathol Lab Med 2003; 127:1161–1168.

328. Miettinen M, Fetsch JF. Distribution of keratins in normal endothelial cells and a spectrum of vascular tumors: implications in tumor diagnosis. Hum Pathol 2000; 31:1062–1067.

329. Lin L, Skacel M, Sigel JE, et al. Epithelioid sarcoma: an immunohistochemical analysis evaluating the utility of cytokeratin 5/6 in distinguishing superficial epithelioid sarcoma from spindled squamous cell carcinoma. J Cutan Pathol 2003; 30:114–117.

330. Laskin WB, Miettinen M. Epithelial-type and neural-type cadherin expression in malignant noncarcinomatous neoplasms with epithelioid features that involve the soft tissues. Arch Pathol Lab Med 2002; 126:425–431.

331. Peydro-Olaya A, Llombart-Bosch A, Carda-Batalla C, et al. Electron microscopy and other ancillary techniques in the diagnosis of small round-cell tumors. Semin Diagn Pathol 2003; 20:25–45.

332. Lloveras B, Googe PB, Goldberg DE, et al. Estrogen receptors in skin appendage tumors and extramammary Paget's disease. Mod Pathol 1991; 4:487–490.

333. Swanson PE, Mazoujian G, Mills SE, et al. Immunoreactivity for estrogen receptor protein in sweat gland tumors. Am J Surg Pathol 1991; 15:835–841.

334. Wallace ML, Longacre TA, Smoller BR. Estrogen and progesterone receptors and anti-gross cystic disease fluid protein-15 (BRST-2) fail to distinguish metastatic breast carcinoma from eccrine neoplasms. Mod Pathol 1995; 8:897–901.

335. Wick MR, Ockner DM, Mills SE, et al. Homologous carcinomas of the breasts, skin, and salivary glands: a histologic and immunohistochemical comparison of ductal mammary carcinoma, ductal sweat gland carcinoma, and salivary duct carcinoma. Am J Clin Pathol 1998; 109:75–84.

336. Busam KJ, Tan LK, Granter SR, et al. Epidermal growth factor, estrogen, and progesterone receptor expression in primary sweat gland carcinomas and primary and metastatic mammary carcinomas. Mod Pathol 1999; 12:786–793.

337. Voytek TM, Ricci A Jr, Cartun RW. Estrogen and progesterone receptors in primary eccrine carcinoma. Mod Pathol 1991; 4:582–585.

338. Baujnedcht T, Gross G, Hagedorn M. Epidermal growth factor receptors in different skin tumors. Dermatologica 1985; 171:16–20.

339. Nazini MN, Dykes RI, Marks R. Epidermal growth factor receptors in human epidermal tumors. Br J Dermatol 1990; 123:153–161.

340. Springer EA, Robinson JK. Patterns of epidermal growth factor receptors in basal cell carcinomas and squamous cell carcinomas. J Dermatol Surg Oncol 1991; 17:20–24.

341. Ellis DL, Nanney LB, King LE Jr. Increased epidermal growth factor receptors in seborrheic keratoses and acrochordons of patients with the dysplastic nevus syndrome. J Am Acad Dermatol 1990; 23:1070–1077.

342. Hasebe T, Mukai K, Yamaguchi N, et al. Prognostic value of immunohistochemical staining for proliferating cell nuclear antigen, p53, and c-erbB-2 in sebaceous gland carcinoma and sweat gland carcinomas: comparison with histopathological parameters. Mod Pathol 1994; 7:37–43.

344. Seelentag WK, Gunthert U, Saremaslani P, et al. CD44 standard and variant isoform expression in normal human skin appendages and epidermis. Histochem Cell Biol 1996; 106: 283–289.

345. Hale LP, Patel DD, Clark RE, et al. Distribution of CD44 variant isoforms in human skin: differential expression in components of benign and malignant epithelia. J Cutan Pathol 1995; 22:536–545.

346. Prieto VG, Reed JA, McNutt NS, et al. Differential expression of CD44 in malignant cutaneous epithelial neoplasms. Am J Dermatopathol 1995; 17:447–451.

347. Penneys NS, Shapiro S. CD44 expression in Merkel cell carcinoma may correlate with risk of metastasis. J Cutan Pathol 1994; 21:22–26.

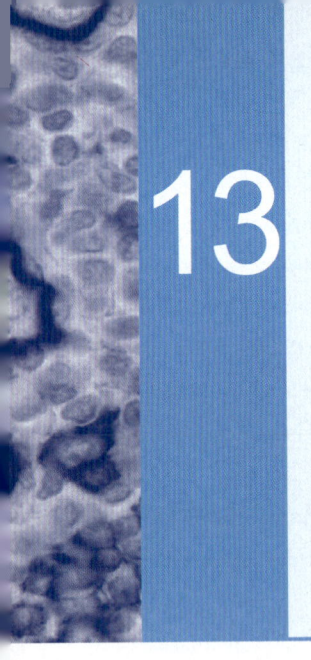

13 胃肠道、胰腺、胆管、胆囊和肝的免疫组织化学

原作者：Neal S. Goldstein and David S. Bosler
译　者：张建平，甄军晖
审校者：张廷国，孟　斌，孙妍琳，郝春燕

目　录

引言	446
抗原/抗体生物学	446
食管	447
胃	451
小肠	460
阑尾、结肠和直肠	462
肛门	471
胰腺、肝外胆管和胆囊	472
肝和胰外胆管	478

引　言

本章包括3个部分：①胃肠道；②胰胆管系统，包括肝外胆管、胆囊；③肝。本章内容包括了上述器官大量准确而实用的免疫组化研究及相关文献。免疫组化结果分析取决于标准化的方法技术，因此，无抗原修复预处理及技术落后的研究不在讨论之列。

抗原/抗体生物学

在免疫组化诊断方面，食管、胃和胰胆管腺癌低分子量和高分子量细胞角蛋白均为阳性，结肠直肠腺癌、肝细胞癌、类癌和高级别神经内分泌癌以低分子量角蛋白阳性为主[1]，食管和肛门的鳞状细胞癌则以高分子量细胞角蛋白阳性为主。

细胞角蛋白7（CK7）：CK7是一种中间丝，主要表达于胰胆管导管上皮、肾集合管的上皮细胞和近端胃肠道黏膜细胞。CK7的表达局限在腺癌的亚型和起源于非角化黏膜的鳞状细胞癌。

细胞角蛋白19（CK19）：与抗CK19抗体反应的CK19的表达见于几乎所有的正常腺上皮细胞和低级别肿瘤中。CK19表达与细胞增殖呈负相关，有丝分裂较多的高级别腺癌CK19阳性减弱[2]。

细胞角蛋白20（CK20）：CK20的免疫组化染色表达不一，在小肠，仅高分化的小肠绒毛细胞CK20阳性，大部分未成熟的基底增殖区细胞CK18阳性，结肠中仅表面上皮细胞层CK20阳性。小肠肿瘤的CK20的阳性强度及范围均高于结肠癌[3]。

CDX2：CDX2是肠道细胞增殖分化所必需的同源异型框基因[4]，在结肠直肠腺癌、某些胰胆管和胃腺癌中可能起抑癌基因的作用[5]。

MUCs：黏蛋白核多肽是胃肠道黏蛋白的主链大分子，主要形成覆盖黏膜表面的黏液-胶样层[6]。MUC1在正常的肠上皮细胞和肠道杯状细胞中表达，MUC2正常由肠道杯状细胞分泌，MUC5AC由胃小凹黏液细胞和肿瘤的杯状细胞表达，MUC6由胃窦细胞和胃底腺细胞分泌。

p53：正常的p53蛋白半衰期很短，细胞中含量很低，用免疫组化方法无法检测到。突变型p53蛋白的半衰期比正常p53蛋白长，在细胞内蓄积，能被p53抗体检测到。理论上，p53的过表达作为*p53*基因突变的标志，是免疫组化检测肿瘤(异型性)的试金石。但实际上并非如此，因为染色与基因变异间的关系并不精确[7]。

癌胚抗原（CEA）：CEA是包括胆汁糖蛋白和非特异性交叉反应抗原超家族糖蛋白的一员。多克隆和许多单克隆抗体可与CEA超家族的许多糖蛋白抗原反应[1]。新CEA单克隆抗体能与CEA糖蛋白特异抗原决定簇反应，可显著降低坏死和中性粒细胞的背景着色。

绒毛蛋白：绒毛蛋白是刷状缘微丝相关的肌动蛋白结合蛋白，与小根（rootlet）形成有关，在结肠直肠腺癌胞质中弥漫着色，刷状缘着色明显[8-11]。

肝细胞石蜡抗原1（HepPar1）：HepPar1抗体的目标抗原位于肝细胞的线粒体。在良性或恶性肝细胞或者肝样分化细胞胞质中呈粗颗粒状染色，通常膜下着色较深[12-15]。在非肝细胞性腺癌细胞中HepPar1也可阳性，但胞质均匀染色，不呈粗颗粒状。

CD117：CD117可识别胞浆Ⅲ型受体酪氨酸激酶蛋白（KIT）激动剂——跨膜c-kit蛋白，是胃肠间质瘤（GIST）的特异标志物。

hMLH1、hMSH2、hMSH6：这些抗体可识别错配修复复合体的蛋白质成分，弱阳性或阴性提示无该蛋白或为突变的蛋白。

突触素（Syn）：突触素是一种存在于细胞膜的钙通道膜糖蛋白，它的表达与CgA无关[16]。

嗜铬素A（CgA）：是一种位于神经内分泌颗粒的可溶性酸性糖蛋白[16, 17]，经过翻译后修饰可位于胃肠道及相关肿瘤不同部位[18]。CgA特异性高，但敏感性低于突触素[16]。大部分非肿瘤性神经内分泌病变和低级别神经内分泌肿瘤的CgA染色呈弥漫强阳性，染色强度取决于胞浆内神经内分泌颗粒的数目。但是有些类癌的CgA染色为弱阳性，可能与肿瘤细胞胞浆中胺的类型有关。

Leu-7（CD57）：是一种细胞膜抗原，属于CD57蛋白家族，抗CD57抗体可与神经内分泌颗粒内的一个蛋白抗原决定簇发生交叉反应[16, 17]。

食 管

Barrett 食管与胃贲门

Barrett食管的定义及与贲门的区别一直是争论的热点，在文献报道中应用免疫组化来区分这两种黏膜的意义、用途和结果分析似乎主要取决于作者所持的各自观点[19]。最近关于Barrett食管形态学的研讨会一致认为CK7、CK20、MUCs或CDX2（图13.1）免疫组化染色的诊断意义不大[20]。免疫组化在诊断Barrett食管或者区分Barrett食管和肠上皮化生的贲门黏膜方面的意义有待于进一步研究。

Barrett 食管异型增生

许多分子改变与Barrett食管肿瘤形成有关[21-37]，这些基因的改变是免疫组化辅助形态学诊断和异型增生分级的基础[21, 22, 25]。p53是唯一证实有效的分子相关抗体。随着异型增生级别的增加，p53核染色的强度和范围也有所增加，大部分Barrett食管相关腺癌均呈p53核弥漫阳性反应[28]。许多作者建议p53核阳性反应可有助于Barrett食管异型增生或癌前病变的组织学诊断[29]。但是由于p53在反应性增生和低级别异型增生中均可呈阳性，所以p53的临床应用有限[30]。Barrett食管中，p53的免疫反应呈灶性弱阳性的形态学范畴包括反应性增生、不确定的异型增生和轻度异型增生，高级别异型增生的上皮细胞核p53反应呈弥漫强阳性分布。p53在活组织检查除外出现人工挤压、组织刨平、污染、组织破碎时区分Barrett食管伴反应性增生和高级别上皮的异型增生最有帮助。

> **诊断要点：Barrett 食管**
>
> 1. 虽然免疫组化在鉴别肠上皮化生方面很有帮助，但在区分Barrett食管和贲门黏膜方面并不可靠。
> 2. p53弥漫强阳性有助于区分高级别异型增生和非异型增生的柱状上皮黏膜。

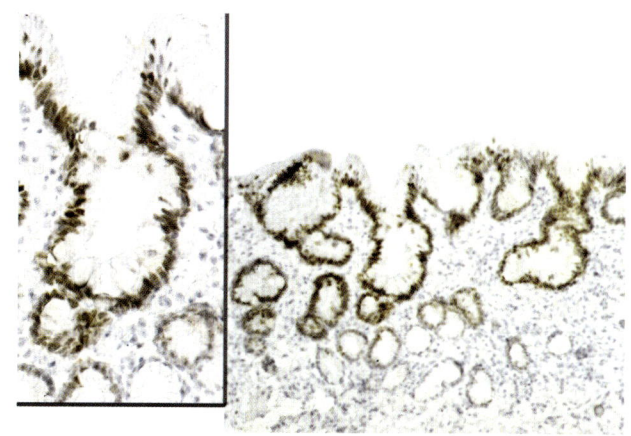

图13.1 Barrett食管的柱状黏膜肠上皮化生，肠上皮化生细胞核CDX2阳性

食管间质肿瘤

平滑肌瘤和胃肠间质瘤

食管的远端 1/3 是平滑肌瘤的好发部位，瘤组织结蛋白和肌动蛋白（平滑肌特异性HHF-35或平滑肌）染色均呈弥漫强阳性，CD34 或 CD117 呈阴性[31,32]。偶发的食管原发性胃肠间质瘤与胃原发的胃肠间质瘤免疫组化染色相似，CD34 和 CD117 均呈阳性[33,34]。

颗粒细胞瘤

食管中段和远段的颗粒细胞瘤的免疫表型和其他部位的颗粒细胞瘤相同，S-100 蛋白、CD57 和波形蛋白呈弥漫强阳性。结蛋白染色可用于区分颗粒细胞肿瘤和伴有胞浆颗粒样改变的平滑肌瘤，在颗粒细胞瘤结蛋白为阴性或个别细胞呈弱阳性，在平滑肌瘤中结蛋白呈弥漫强阳性，细胞角蛋白（大部分是细胞角蛋白 CAM5.2）上皮细胞膜抗原和单克隆CEA 均呈阴性[35,36]。

食管黑色素瘤

原发的食管恶性黑素瘤少见，与皮肤的黑素瘤相同，波形蛋白、S-100、HMB-45、melan-A(MAb A-103)和酪氨酸酶阳性（图 13.2）[37,38]。

> **诊断要点：胃肠间质瘤和颗粒细胞瘤**
>
> 1. 食管胃肠间质瘤很少见，CD117、CD34、结蛋白和肌动蛋白可区分形态学上相似的平滑肌瘤和胃肠间质瘤。
> 2. 颗粒细胞瘤S-100、CD57和波形蛋白阳性，结蛋白阴性。

食管神经内分泌肿瘤

食管类癌的免疫表型与肺的类癌相同，突触素、嗜铬素、单克隆 CEA 和 TTF-1（个人经验）呈弥漫阳性[39-41]。

原发的食管高级别神经内分泌（小细胞）癌可主要表现为鳞状细胞癌或腺癌的一部分[42,43]，突触素、嗜铬素和CD56(NCAM)阳性[16]。因为食管小细胞癌的CK19、CK20 或 34βE12 呈阴性[44,45]，所以我们认为细胞角蛋白CAM5.2 或 35βH11 最有助于食管小细胞癌诊断[44,45]，也有近一半的食管小细胞癌TTF-1呈阳性。

> **诊断要点：食管神经内分泌肿瘤**
>
> 1. 突触素和嗜铬素是免疫组化诊断食管神经内分泌肿瘤的主要依据。
> 2. 在食管小细胞癌中细胞角蛋白CAM5.2 或 35βH11 优于其他角蛋白，尤其适用于挤压的小的活组织碎片。

鳞状细胞癌

鳞状细胞癌细胞中，中分子量及高分子量的细胞角蛋白阳性，仅极少数低分子量角蛋白阳性（图 13.3），因此大部分鳞状细胞癌的细胞角蛋白抗体 CAM5.2、AE1/AE3、34βE12、CK5/6、CK14 和 CK19 呈弥漫阳性分布[46-54]。通常，细胞角蛋白 34βE12 的阳性反应和弥漫程度均强于 CK5/6（图 13.4、13.5）。抗 CK18 的抗体与大部分 CAM5.2 阳性反应对应[46]。鳞状细胞癌级别越高，CK19 染色越强，原位癌CK19也呈阳性，而正常鳞状上皮黏膜为阴性（图 13.6）。大约70%的低级别鳞状细胞癌近50%的肿瘤细胞CK19阳性，而几乎所有的高级别肿瘤CK19 呈弥漫强阳性[46]。

其他适于诊断的弥漫强阳性抗体还有p63（核染色）[55]、血栓调节素、上皮细胞膜抗原和选择性单克隆 CEA 系列抗体。

阴性抗体包括 CK7、CK20、CK35βH11、Ber-EP4、TTF-1 和 WT-1[47,48,56,57]。虽然包括CK7，但大概 15%~30% 的鳞状细胞癌偶见少数细胞和散在的细胞簇 CK7 由弱至强的阳性表达[46,49]。若以超过50% 的肿瘤细胞呈阳性为标准，鳞状细胞癌 CK7/CK20 为阴性。

TTF-1 偶尔可区分原发的肺鳞状细胞癌和食管鳞状细胞癌，虽然这两种肿瘤的 TTF-1 通常为阴性，但有时 TTF-1 在原发的肺鳞状细胞癌胞核中呈弥漫强阳性而食管鳞状细胞癌始终为阴性。TTF-1细胞核染色呈弥漫的至少中等强度阳性时才可判断为阳性，TTF-1很容易由于抗原修复和边缘效应而产生假阳性。

有时，区分低分化鳞状细胞癌和原发的食管腺癌尤为重要，此时可用CK7、CK20 和 CK5/6 系列进行鉴别[49]。鳞状细胞癌包括低分化非角化鳞状细胞癌，其 CK7-、CK20- 和 CK5+，而食管、胃和肺腺癌为CK7+、CK20+ 和 CK5/6-。

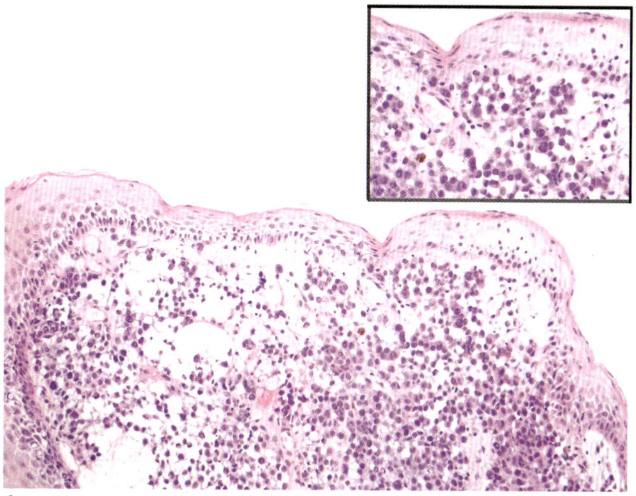

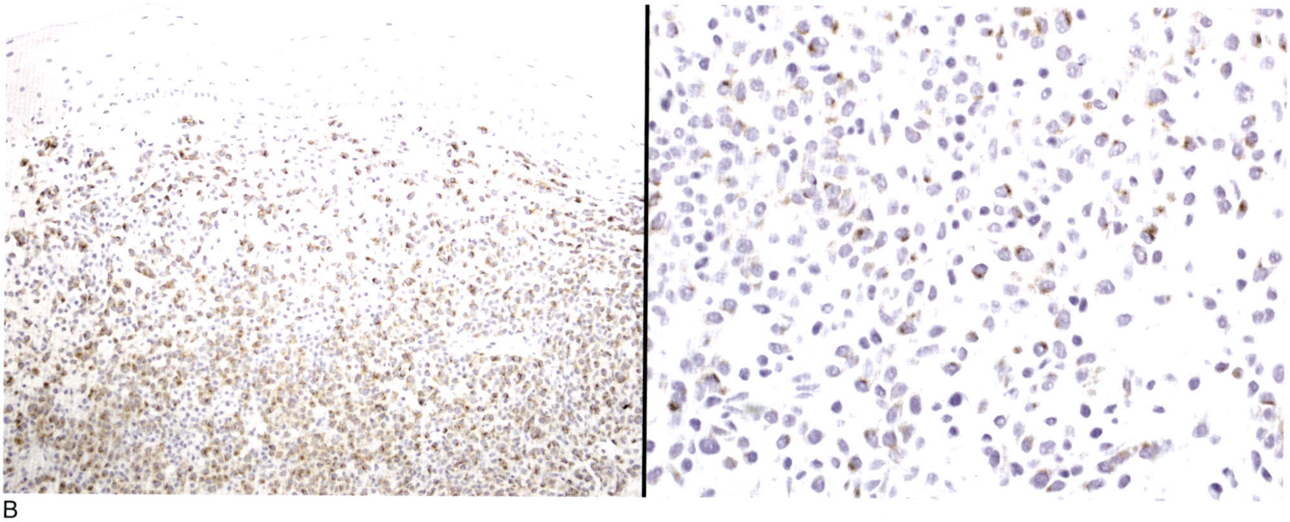

胃肠道、胰腺、胆管、胆囊和肝的免疫组织化学 13

图13.2 （A）食管黑色素瘤。在正常鳞状黏膜下方，未分化的肿瘤细胞在黏膜下散在浸润。（B）食管黑色素瘤。肿瘤细胞胞浆酪氨酸酶呈中等强度弥漫阳性，许多细胞核周点状着色，高尔基带着色更明显

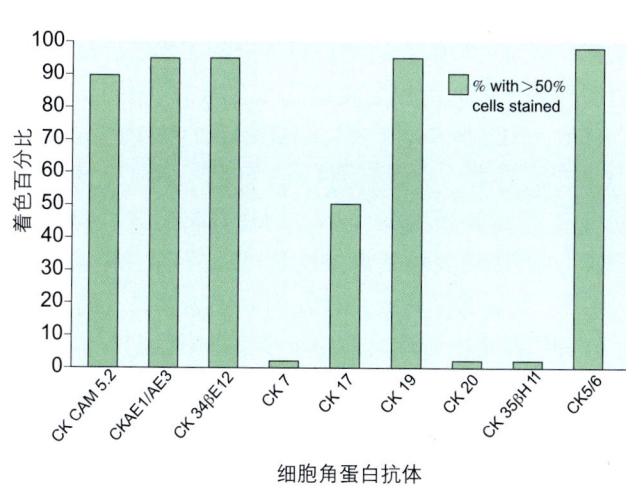

图 13.3 食管鳞状细胞癌细胞角蛋白免疫组化染色

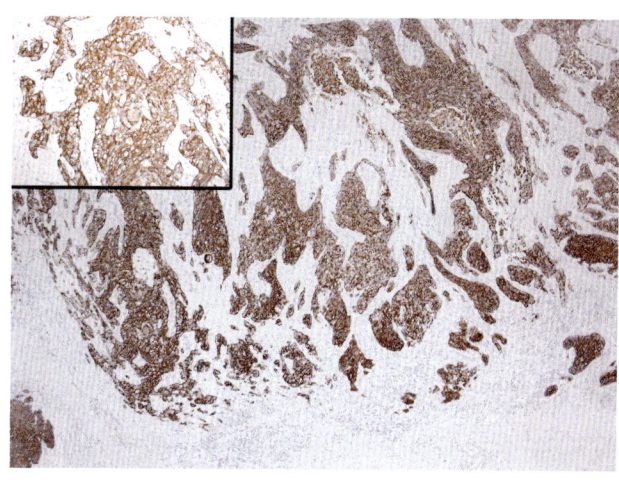

图 13.4 食管鳞状细胞癌细胞角蛋白 34βE12 呈弥漫强阳性。插图示：与周围强阳性的鳞癌细胞相对比，癌巢中央角化珠呈阴性，轮廓清晰。与图 13.5 中 CK5/6 染色结果正好相反

449

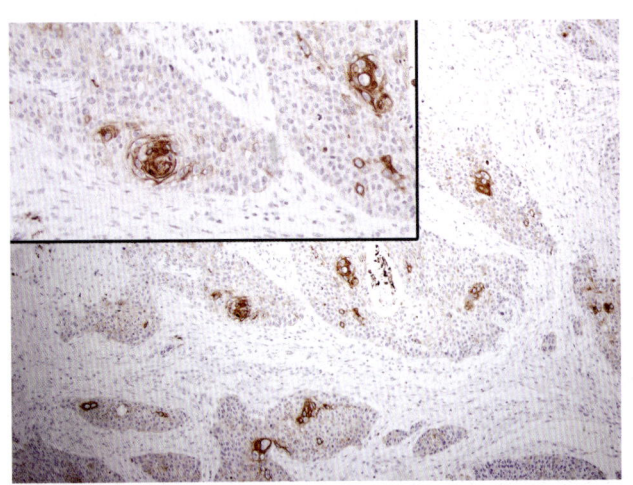

图13.5 食管鳞状细胞癌。CK5/6阳性主要局限于中央角化珠。插图示：少数散在癌细胞也呈强阳性

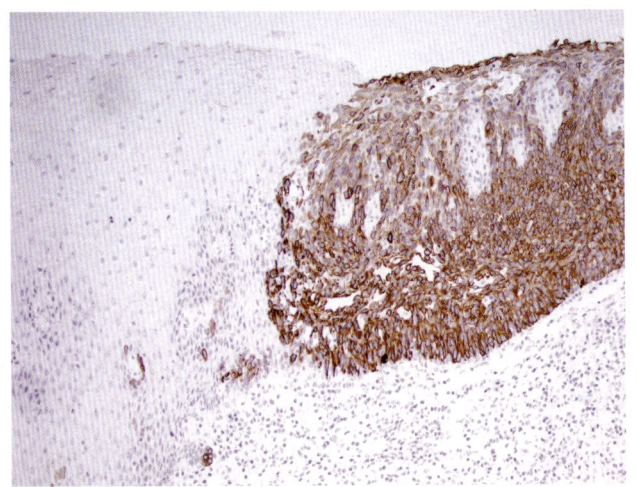

图13.6 食管正常黏膜和鳞状细胞原位癌，CK19在癌上皮呈强阳性，正常黏膜阴性

区分鳞状细胞癌和胸腺癌偶尔有重要的临床意义。CD5在原发的胸腺癌中呈弥漫强阳性，而食管鳞状细胞癌呈阴性。但必须注意的是胸腺癌中选择性CD5阳性反应主要取决于抗原修复液的pH值和抗体克隆，某些CD5抗体在食管鳞状细胞癌和胸腺癌中均呈弥漫强阳性表达[58, 59]。

某些间皮瘤在形态上和临床上均与低分化、非角化、原发食管鳞状细胞癌相似，两者calretinin和CK5/6均为阳性，只有WT-1作为诊断间皮瘤的唯一阳性标志[60]。

> **诊断要点：食管鳞状细胞癌**
>
> 1. 大多数鳞状细胞癌的CAM5.2、CK5/6和p63呈弥漫强阳性。
> 2. CK7、CK20和CEA在Ⅲ级鳞状细胞癌中或者为阴性或者呈局灶阳性，然而这些抗体在Ⅲ级腺癌中均呈弥漫阳性表达。
> 3. CD5如果检测准确，可用于区分食管鳞状细胞癌和胸腺癌。

鳞状细胞癌变型

基底细胞样（鳞状细胞）癌　基底细胞癌是低分化鳞状细胞癌在形态上和基因上的变型[61]。基底细胞样癌-经典的鳞状细胞癌或基底细胞样癌-腺癌的混合型较常见。文献报道bcl-2在基底细胞样鳞状细胞癌中为阳性，而经典的低分化鳞状细胞癌为阴性[62]。CK5/6、CK单克隆-OSCAR、CK13、CK14、CK19和p63典型地在基底细胞样(鳞状细胞)癌呈弥漫强阳性，而CK CAM5.2、35βH11和AE1/AE3通常为阴性或灶性弱阳性[63-66]。在细胞角蛋白阳性的抗体中，CK13、14和19的阳性程度最强[67, 68]。在癌巢周围假栅栏样的单层癌细胞伴典型的肌上皮分化，CK19、S-100和肌动蛋白均为阳性[63]，其结果与高级别乳腺癌相似，免疫组化肌上皮细胞分化特征性弥漫阳性[69]。

腺样囊性癌　腺样囊性癌一词是指高级别唾液腺型腺样囊性癌和伴有筛状结构的基底细胞样鳞状细胞癌。大多数报道认为食管腺样囊性癌即是基底细胞样鳞状细胞癌[63]。食管唾液腺型腺样囊性癌CAM5.2和AE1/AE3为弥漫强阳性。导管型细胞34βE12和CEA阳性，而基底样细胞S-100、肌动蛋白和波形蛋白阳性[63, 66]。

实体型基底细胞样（鳞状上皮）、假腺样囊性基底细胞样、唾液腺型腺样囊性癌和高级别神经内分泌癌在形态上相似，通常很难区分，尤其是活检的小组织碎片。此时应用免疫组化十分有益（图13.7）。CK5/6、AE1/AE3、CK7、34βE12、CK19、p63、CEA、嗜铬素、突触素或Leu7可用于鉴别上述3种病变[52, 66]。如果组织碎小，切片数量有限，p63、CK7、CK19和突触素可提供最可靠判定结果（个人经验）。虽然部分高级别神经内分泌癌核周（高尔基带）细胞角蛋白阳性，但由于其结果不稳定及其结果判断的差异而使其应用受限。CK7常是高级别神经内分泌癌的唯一阳性标志。结果判断时应注意避免将基底细胞样癌坏死碎片的突触素非特异性染色误认为真正的胞浆阳性颗粒。

> **诊断要点**：鳞状细胞癌变型
>
> 1. 基底细胞样鳞状细胞癌癌巢的中央区 CK5/6 和 p63 阳性，其周围边缘栅栏样细胞 CK19 常阳性，AE1/AE3 通常阴性或局灶弱阳性。
> 2. 大部分腺样囊性癌是基底细胞样鳞状细胞癌，真正的腺样囊性癌极其少见。
> 3. 高级别（小细胞）神经内分泌癌突触素呈弥漫阳性并且核周 CAM5.2 点状阳性，而基底细胞样癌细胞角蛋白弥漫阳性。

食管腺癌

大部分研究发现食管腺癌和贲门腺癌的免疫表型相同[70-73]，某些大样本病例比较统计研究（但并不是所有的研究）提示食管腺癌和贲门腺癌的 CK7/CK20 染色类型有显著差异[26, 74, 75]。然而，由于两组染色结果实际存在交错重叠，使得对个别肿瘤界限的判断无明显意义。

伴有梭形细胞或间叶细胞分化的癌

癌组织中梭形细胞或两三种间叶细胞成分与共存癌克隆性相关。其形态结构表现为多向去分化，并伴有细胞角蛋白表达减少。细胞角蛋白克隆 OSCAR (Signet，Dedham，MA) 和 CK5/6 的阳性程度最强且大多数为弥漫阳性。CK OSCAR 是区分肿瘤性梭形细胞和反应性肌纤维母细胞的首选抗体。CK5/6 在纺锤形、多边形及圆形的梭形细胞呈阳性，而细长梭形细胞呈阴性。CAM5.2、35βH11 和 AE1/AE3 常为阴性[77-80]，3 种抗体中 AE1/AE3 的阳性程度最强，且多弥漫分布[81]。肿瘤性梭形细胞肌动蛋白可呈阳性，但结蛋白通常为阴性，因此可与平滑肌肉瘤明显区分。也可出现真正的梭形细胞横纹肌肉瘤分化，其肌动蛋白和结蛋白均阳性[77]。

> **诊断要点**：Barrett 食管和癌
>
> 1. 多成分癌由与克隆相关的不同成分组成。
> 2. 单克隆细胞角蛋白 OSCAR 是区分肌纤维母细胞和肿瘤性梭形细胞首选的细胞角蛋白抗体。
> 3. Barrett 食管和贲门黏膜的免疫组化研究是一个活跃领域，大多数研究集中在 CK7/CK20、MUC 蛋白、绒毛蛋白、Hep (HepPar1)、DAS-1、PDX-1 和 CDX2[6, 20, 76, 82-93]。
> 4. 虽然上述所有抗体均可产生令人信服的阳性结果，但是，尤其是当涉及化生性病变时，无一抗体可表现为一致性可重复的诊断结果以确保其临床应用。

胃

非肿瘤性病变

乳糜泻（Celiac disease）

淋巴细胞性胃炎常表现为乳糜泻，偶尔为幽门螺杆菌感染。黏膜表面上皮内淋巴细胞的密度通常低于十二指肠，胃上皮内淋巴细胞为 T 淋巴细胞，CD45RO、CD3、CD7 和 CD8 呈阳性。

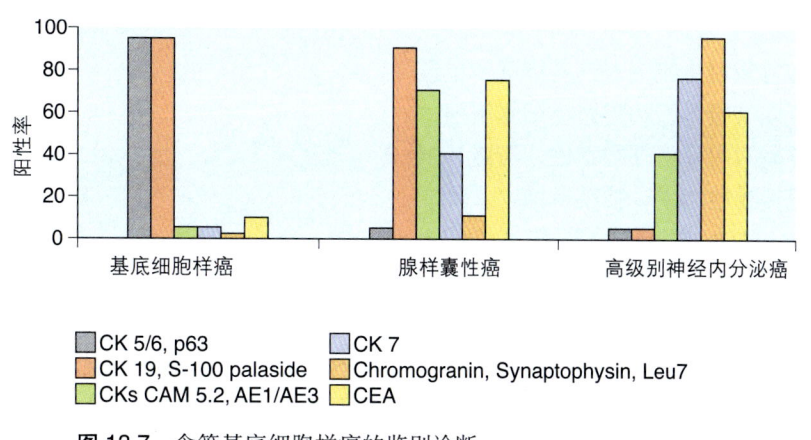

图 13.7　食管基底细胞样癌的鉴别诊断

幽门螺杆菌

质子泵抑制剂药物疗法和幽门螺杆菌根除药物疗法降低了幽门螺杆菌的密度,并且将螺旋形的幽门螺杆菌变为球形[94-96]。在改良的Giemsa染色或其他的组织化学染色中球形幽门螺杆菌很难与黏蛋白小体或细胞外碎屑区别。免疫组化是检测幽门螺杆菌可靠的、敏感的方法,尤其当幽门螺杆菌呈球形或细菌数目很少时(图13.8)[94, 96-100]。

胃底腺样息肉

胃底腺样息肉为散发性病变,与长期的质子泵抑制剂治疗有关,部分为家族性腺瘤息肉(FAP)综合征和Zollinger-Ellison综合征。这些病变的形态学区别甚微,据报道散发息肉和Zollinger-Ellison综合征相关息肉的CK7呈阳性,而β-连环蛋白在散发息肉中呈阳性,在FAP相关息肉中呈阴性[101-103]。

> **诊断要点:非肿瘤性胃部病变**
>
> 1. 对可疑的乳糜泻,可以用淋巴细胞标志物来显示上皮内淋巴细胞。
> 2. 免疫组化染色可用于其他方法难以检测的由治疗引起细菌变形的幽门螺杆菌。
> 3. CK7和β-连环蛋白的联合应用可以帮助区分FAP引起的胃底腺样息肉、Zollinger-Ellison综合征的胃底腺样息肉和散发的胃底腺样息肉。

神经内分泌细胞病变

胃底黏膜的神经内分泌细胞主要是肠嗜铬样细胞(ECL cell),而胃窦黏膜主要是产胃泌素的内分泌细胞。胃窦和胃底的神经内分泌细胞嗜铬素A和突触素均呈弥漫强阳性[16, 104, 105]。

高胃泌素血症和胃酸过少均会对这些细胞产生影响。高胃泌素血症可以诱导胃底肠嗜铬样细胞增殖,而胃酸过少可诱导胃窦的内分泌细胞增生。与这些细胞增生有关的病变包括线性增生、微结节增生、腺瘤样增生和类癌[104-111]。虽然常规苏木精-伊红染色示胃底黏膜肠嗜铬样细胞和胃窦内分泌细胞的数量正常,但免疫组化染色显示实际肠嗜铬样细胞数量更多。大多数Zollinger-Ellison综合征的病人均存在线性、微结节或腺瘤样肠嗜铬样细胞增生,尤其是在胃大弯的泌酸腺黏膜[112]。

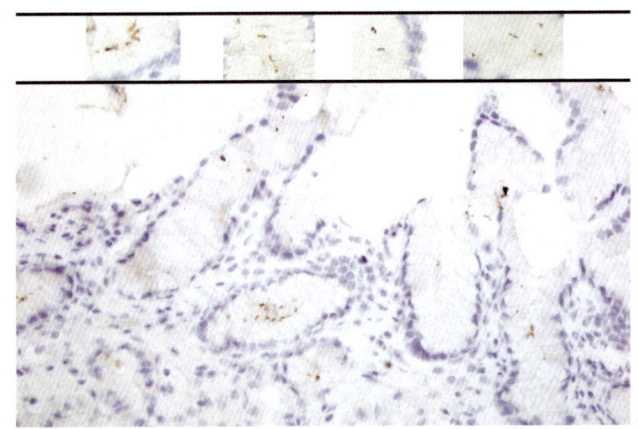

图13.8 胃窦黏膜大量幽门螺杆菌感染。大量幽门螺杆菌侵入邻近柱状黏液细胞的细胞膜之间生长。图片上方的插图示形态多样的幽门螺杆菌,包括球形的、螺旋形的、杆状的和哑铃状的细菌

人型囊泡单胺转运体(human vesicular monoamine tansporter isoform 2,VMAT-2)仅存在于肠嗜铬样细胞及其肿瘤细胞中,其作用可调节细胞囊泡内组胺的积聚,最近研发的VMAT-2抗体将成为区分胃底黏膜的肠嗜铬样细胞和胃窦的内分泌细胞类癌的实用标记。

胃类癌CDX2呈阴性,而回肠和结肠类癌CDX2呈阳性[113, 114],大约有10%胃类癌CK7呈阳性[115],而CK20均呈阴性。

> **诊断要点:神经内分泌病变**
>
> 1. 嗜铬素A和突触素能显示高胃泌素血症、胃酸过少和Zollinger-Ellison综合征中胃底和胃窦的神经内分泌细胞的增生。
> 2. 与结肠类癌相比,胃类癌CDX2为阴性。
> 3. AE1/AE3和CAM5.2在胃类癌中为阳性,有助于胃类癌与由其他神经内分泌肿瘤(如嗜铬细胞瘤和腹膜后副神经节瘤)累及胃肠道的继发病变相区别。

间质病变

胃肠间质瘤

CD117和c-kit基因 随着对胃肠间质瘤的重要分子机制c-kit原癌基因突变的认识深入,胃肠间质瘤的分类和诊断发生了根本性的变化。90%~100%的胃肠间质瘤中能检测到c-kit基因突变[116-121]。KIT蛋白是Ⅲ型酪氨酸激酶跨膜受体,促进细胞增殖和/或

抑制细胞凋亡，c-kit 基因突变导致了 KIT 蛋白结构性激活。抗 c-kit 蛋白抗体免疫组化可以检测 KIT 蛋白，称为 CD117 抗原。c-kit 激活突变及 CD117 免疫组化染色可将胃肠间质瘤从过去的平滑肌瘤、平滑肌肉瘤、胃自主神经肿瘤和一些神经鞘瘤的肿瘤中区分出来，并使这一组肿瘤统一并使其分类简化[122-125]。胃肠间质的 Cajal 间质细胞参与调节肠的能动性，CD117 呈阳性，提示胃肠间质瘤来源于 Cajal 细胞或向 Cajal 细胞分化[126, 127]。虽然 c-kit 基因突变使其 CD117 阳性，但 CD117 阳性并不一定意味着有 c-kit 基因突变。例如，大约有 25% 的 1 型神经纤维瘤病发展为 CD117 和 CD34 阳性的胃肠间质瘤[123]，但并没有 c-kit 基因突变，而是 NF-1 相关的神经纤维瘤病中常见的 NF-1（17q11.2）基因突变。

胃肠间质瘤（GISTs）CD117 染色 胃、上腹部和网膜的胃肠间质瘤中 95%～100% CD117 阳性（图 13.9）[128-132]。一些作者认为胃肠间质瘤的诊断仅限于 CD117 阳性的肿瘤[33, 119, 131, 133]。尽管这种方法简化了胃肠间质瘤的定义，但如何对待 CD117 阴性的胃肠间质瘤样肿瘤却是个问题[134]。许多 CD117 阴性并伴有典型胃肠间质瘤形态特征的肿瘤与 CD117 阳性的肿瘤具有相似的基因激活突变[123, 135, 136]。这些 CD117 阴性的胃肠间质瘤具有典型的上皮样细胞形态，发生在网膜或腹膜[123, 135-137]，此胃肠间质瘤亚型具有血小板衍生的生长因子受体突变。

胃肠间质瘤中 CD117 阳性反应部位有明显差异。近假包膜的肿瘤细胞 CD117 常为阴性或弱阳性，穿刺活组织检查中 CD117 阴性的胃肠间质瘤并不少见（个人经验），然而在手术切除的胃肠间质瘤中 CD117 阴性者少见（2%～5%）。胃肠间质瘤中 CD117 通常为细胞浆强阳性，核周高尔基带点状阳性和细胞膜阳性可同时存在，但膜阳性不出现在胞浆阴性时。

CD117 及化疗 甲磺酸伊马替尼化疗抑制正常和突变的 KIT 蛋白的酪氨酸激酶活性。已经证明这种药物对抑制大部分病人胃肠间质瘤的肿瘤生长有效[138]。无 c-kit 基因突变的胃肠间质瘤对甲磺酸伊马替尼的反应比突变的胃肠间质瘤差。文献中对甲磺酸伊马替尼疗反应的免疫组化阳性程度大小不等。尽管有些差异可能由于免疫组化技术所致，但 CD117 弱阳性仍对甲磺酸伊马替尼治疗有效。考虑到文献资料的差异及甲磺酸伊马替尼强而有益的治疗效果，胃肠间质瘤胞浆 CD117 局灶或片状弱阳性目前应认为是 CD117 阳性。

CD117 与非胃肠间质瘤病变 CD117 在非胃肠间质瘤病变中的免疫反应已有报道，CD117 阳性的腹内纤维瘤病的比例越来越高[33, 139]。同时 CD117 阳性的软组织肉瘤也较多。

其他抗体 胃肠间质瘤有不同程度的神经或平滑肌分化[31-33, 123, 126, 128-130, 142-153]。

大约 70% 的胃肠间质瘤 CD34 呈弥漫强阳性，其余 30% 的胃肠间质瘤染色呈斑片状、弱阳性或中度阳性。与伴有平滑肌分化的胃肠间质瘤相比，伴有神经分化的胃肠间质瘤 CD34 阳性的细胞数目和染色强度均较低。CD34 并不是胃肠间质瘤的特异性标志，CD34 阳性的肿瘤还包括孤立性纤维性肿瘤、胃炎性纤维性息肉和去分化脂肪肉瘤。CD99 在大部分的胃肠间质瘤中也呈弥漫强阳性。大约 25% 的胃肠间质瘤中肌特异性肌动蛋白（HHF-35）和平滑肌肌动蛋白呈强阳性，其他 50% 的胃肠间质瘤呈局部弱阳性。大部分胃肠间质瘤中结蛋白为阴性（图 13.9D）。大约近 2% 胃肠间质瘤结蛋白呈强阳性，但是近 33% 胃肠间质瘤结蛋白呈局灶弱阳性。约 50% 的肿瘤细胞胞浆和/或细胞核的 S-100 呈灶性阳性。细胞角蛋白，最常见的是 CAM5.2 和 35βH11，在胃肠间质瘤中呈斑片状阳性，偶尔呈强阳性。细胞角蛋白 AE1/AE3 常呈弱阳性，而且仅在极少数的单个细胞和小细胞簇染色。印戒细胞胃肠间质瘤的细胞角蛋白呈阴性。在胃的胃肠间质瘤中，突触素可呈弥漫强阳性，但嗜铬素呈阴性。

> **诊断要点：胃肠间质瘤**
>
> 1. CD117 表达于 c-kit 基因突变导致的 KIT 蛋白升高，是胃肠间质瘤的敏感标记。
> 2. 胃肠间质瘤 CD117 也可呈阴性，是由于肿瘤局灶变异及取材局限所致，或者是极少数（2%～5%）具有上皮样形态特征 CD117 阴性的胃肠间质瘤独特亚型。
> 3. 尽管 CD117 是诊断胃肠间质瘤免疫组化染色的主要依据，但其他抗体联合应用也可帮助确定诊断，包括 CD34、CD99、HHF-35、平滑肌肌动蛋白、S-100 和低分子量细胞角蛋白。

神经鞘瘤 胃神经鞘瘤少见，且具有许多胃肠间质瘤的形态特征[142, 144, 154, 155]，其中 S-100、CD57

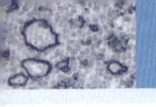

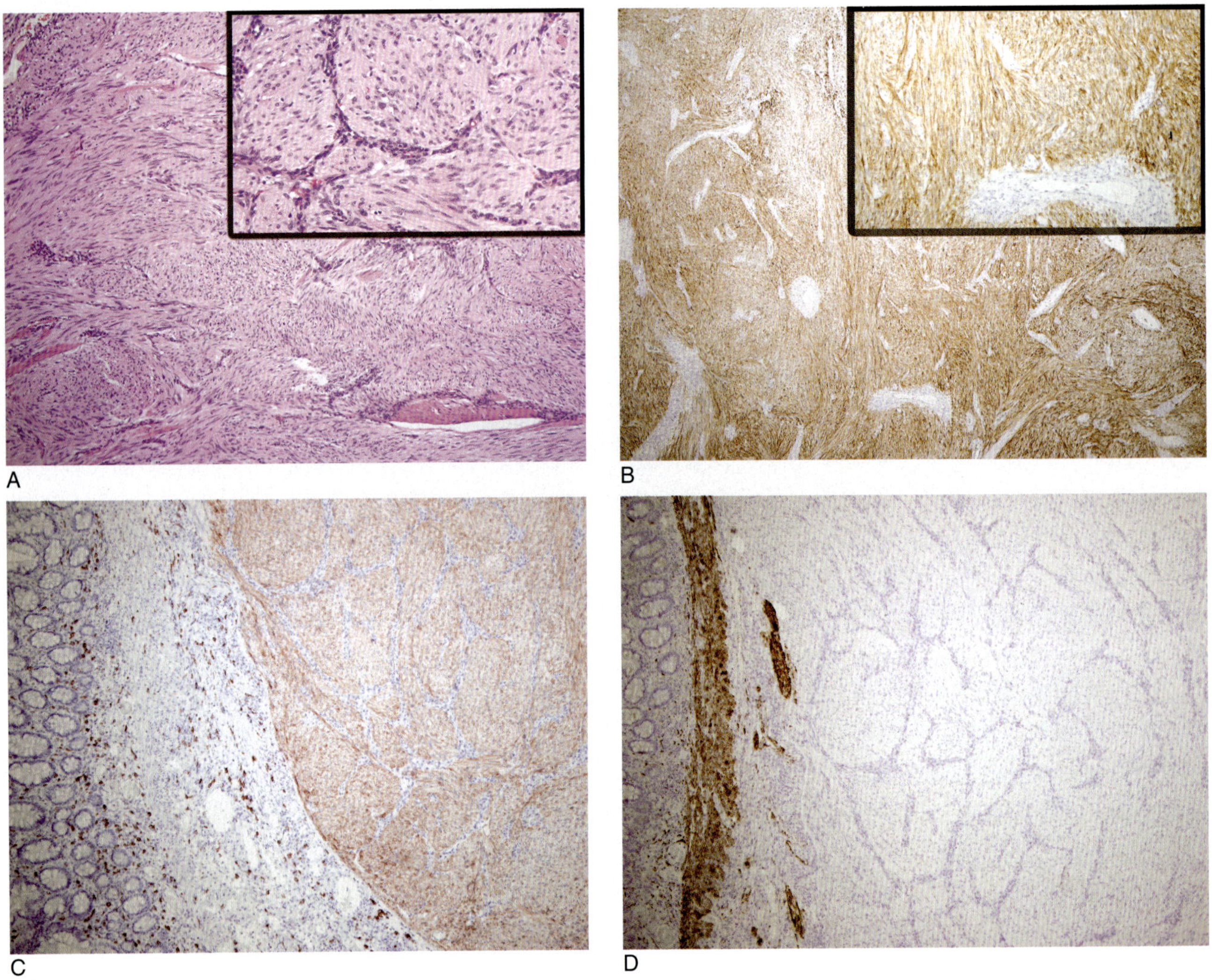

图13.9 （A）胃肠间质瘤。插图：肿瘤细胞的形态与平滑肌细胞相似；（B）胃肠间质瘤。肿瘤细胞的CD117呈弥漫强阳性。插图：血管周围的结缔组织尽管形态上与肿瘤细胞相似，但CD117呈阴性；（C）胃肠间质瘤。除了肿瘤细胞中的CD117阳性，黏膜肥大细胞的CD117也呈阳性。这些细胞提供了有效的阳性内对照；（D）胃肠间质瘤。肿瘤细胞结蛋白呈阴性，黏膜肌结蛋白呈强阳性

(Leu7)和GFAP呈弥漫强阳性，但CD117、CD34和平滑肌肌动蛋白呈阴性。

纤维瘤病 应用多聚色原体显色检测时，腹内纤维瘤病CD117呈阴性[156]。病变细胞CD34呈弱阳性斑片状分布，而且染色强度低于孤立性纤维性肿瘤。大部分纤维瘤病的平滑肌肌动蛋白和结蛋白呈阳性[31]。如果染色程序不标准，腹内纤维瘤病很容易出现CD117和CD34假阳性[139]。

孤立性纤维瘤和假瘤

孤立性纤维瘤较少发生在上腹部和肠系膜[33, 157-159]，其CD34、CD99和平滑肌肌动蛋白呈阳性，CD117阴性[33, 155, 160]。结节性纤维假瘤在这个部位很少发生，和胃肠间质瘤一样CD117呈强阳性，但形态特征与胃肠间质瘤明显不同。

间质病变的鉴别诊断

免疫组化可用于鉴别上腹部的间质肿瘤，包括胃肠间质瘤、神经鞘瘤、孤立性纤维瘤和间质纤维瘤病[33, 161]。这些病变有许多共同的形态特征，尤其是穿刺活检标本中，CD117、CD34、S-100、GFAP、CD99、β-连环蛋白和结蛋白抗体是较实用的诊断抗体组合（图13.10）。

诊断要点：间质病变的鉴别诊断

1. 免疫组化有助于区分胃肠间质瘤和许多与其形态相似的病变，包括神经鞘瘤、纤维瘤病和孤立性纤维瘤。
2. CD117、CD34、S-100、GFAP、CD99、β-连环蛋白和结蛋白为诊断这些间质病变的实用抗体组合。

胃腺癌

细胞角蛋白 见图13.11。胃腺癌中AE1/AE3和35βH11呈弥漫强阳性[48]。细胞角蛋白CAM5.2在大约2/3的胃腺癌中呈弥漫强阳性，其余1/3呈斑片状弱阳性及中度阳性[162]。CK18和19（全腺癌角蛋白）呈弥漫强阳性[53, 163-166]。

CK7：细胞中CK7的表达是胃上皮细胞和胃腺癌的重要标记。大约50%的胃腺癌中CK7呈斑片状及弥漫强阳性，30%少数细胞簇强阳性，20%呈弱阳性或阴性（图13.12）[164-170]。

CK20：大约40%的胃腺癌中CK20呈强阳性，斑片状或弥漫分布，20%呈斑片状弱阳性，40%呈阴性（图13.13）[164, 166, 167, 169, 171, 172]。

CK7/CK20联合染色：胃腺癌的CK7/CK20联合染色差别很大。不同的阳性标准使染色结果较为复杂，一般阳性标准的阳性细胞比例在1%~25%这一

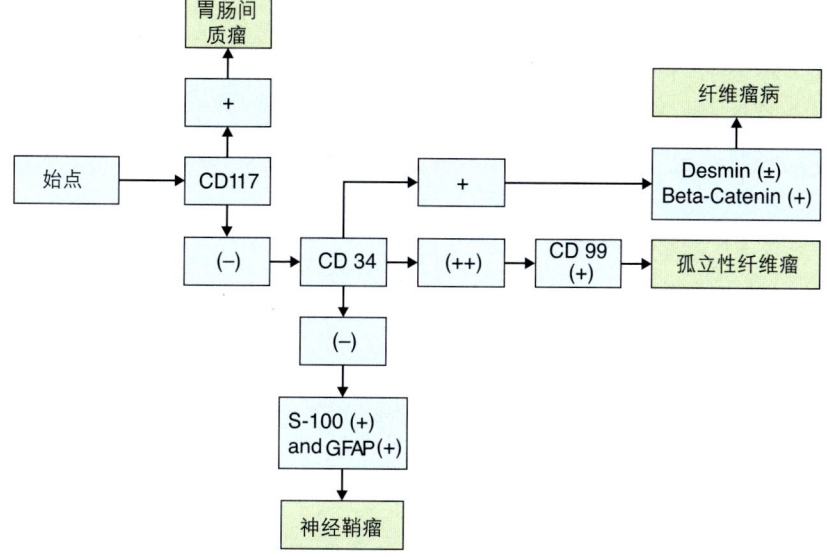

图13.10 间质肿瘤的免疫组化鉴别诊断

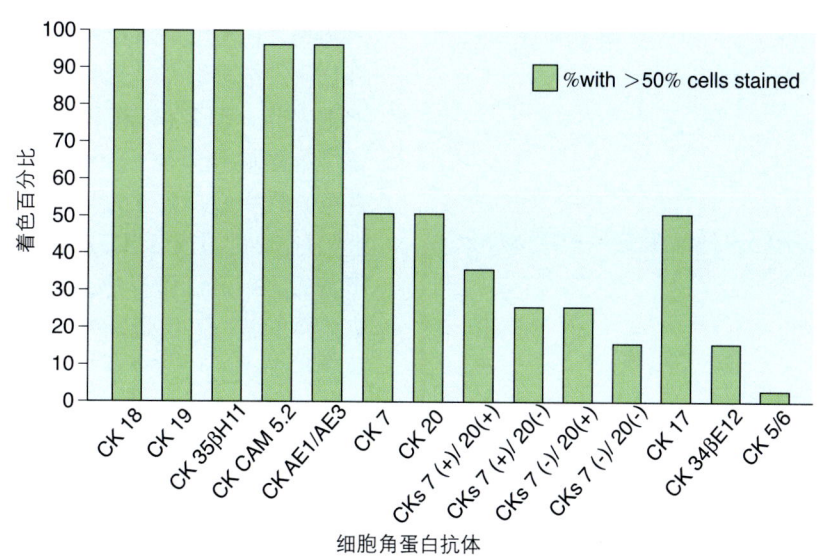

图13.11 胃腺癌中细胞角蛋白的表达

范围。CK7/CK20 染色结果有 4 种类型，每一类型均占少数，无主要类型，故应用价值有限。大约有 35% 的胃腺癌 CK7+/CK20+，25% 为 CK7-/CK20+，25% 为 CK7+/CK20-，15% 为 CK7-/CK20-[1, 164, 166, 169, 173-177]。这些百分比随染色阳性标准不同而异，差别可高达 30%。

> **诊断要点：胃腺癌角蛋白表达**
> 1. 许多细胞角蛋白在腺癌中呈弥漫强阳性。
> 2. CK7/CK20 联合染色的类型对区分胃腺癌和胃肠道的其他腺癌无使用价值。

其他的抗体　见表 13.1。

雌激素受体（ER）：对胃腺癌中 ER 阳性问题已争论多年。胃腺癌中微弱的 ER 着色最初被认为是假阳性反应，后来确认核着色是真阳性，缺乏核着色认为是假阳性。近来的研究使此问题较为明了，ER mRNA 和 ER 核受体蛋白在男性和女性腺癌中普遍存在低水平表达[178, 179]。低水平 ER 表达的免疫组化检测主要取决于抗体克隆和免疫组化操作[70, 171, 180-182]，与高敏感性兔单克隆抗体的应用有关。此类抗体在某些胃腺癌中由于操作程序原因而呈弥漫强阳性，致使其过表达而掩饰了器官部位的差异性。用标准的稀释方法和操作步骤，1D5 克隆抗体在胃腺癌中偶尔可微弱着色，着色细胞<5%，高分化腺癌的阳性程度常高于低分化腺癌[183]。

孕激素受体（PR）：某些研究显示在肠型或印戒细胞型胃腺癌中 PR 阴性[171]，但其他的研究显示 25% 的胃腺癌中 PR 呈阳性[184, 185]。与雌激素受体染色一样，有些问题也没有完全解决。

> **诊断要点：胃癌激素受体**
> ER 或 PR 在转移腺癌中呈弱阳性并不排除原发胃癌转移。

胃肿瘤的微卫星不稳定型

微卫星不稳定（MSI）是由于错配修复复合体缺失导致的一组癌的特征。微卫星高度不稳定的腺癌可表现为综合征（遗传性非息肉性结肠直肠癌，HNPCC）或散发。错配修复复合体 hMLH1、hMSH2 和 hMSH6 蛋白抗体若检测呈阴性则为微卫星不稳定。综合征病人表现为 3 种抗体中任一抗体的缺失，以 hMSH2 最常见。几乎所有微卫星高度不稳定的胃腺癌均为散发（非综合征）腺癌，表现为 hMLH1 蛋白的缺失[186, 187]。

依据细胞类型进行胃腺癌组织学类型的学者发现小凹型肿瘤通常是微卫星高度不稳定型（hMLH1 阳性减弱），完全肠化生型肿瘤通常是微卫星稳定型（MSS，hMLH1 阳性），但 p53 染色发现其抑癌基因缺失[188, 189]。

> **诊断要点：微卫星不稳定性胃癌**
> 1. 微卫星不稳定性时 hMLH1、hMSH2 或 hMSH6 蛋白表达减少。
> 2. 小凹型胃腺癌倾向于微卫星高度不稳定型，而肠化生型胃腺癌具有抑癌基因缺失。

梭形细胞分化（肉瘤样癌）

与结肠和食管癌相似，胃癌组织也有梭形细胞分化，癌细胞通常波形蛋白阳性，仅少数的细胞角蛋白阳性[190, 191]，详见食管癌章节讨论。

卵黄囊、肝样和绒毛膜癌分化

见图 13.14。

所谓卵黄囊、透明细胞或肝细胞样分化在胃组织中常见，虽然在典型的腺癌中伴卵黄囊或肝样分化很常见，但单一卵黄囊或肝样分化的肿瘤极少见。此种分化的细胞形态呈透明细胞、生殖细胞癌样，或肝细胞癌样，AFP 和/或 HepPar1 免疫组化呈单个细胞或小细胞簇强阳性[192-195]。与神经内分泌相关抗体的着色方式相似，典型的肠型腺癌和印戒细胞癌均呈局灶阳性[162-169]。仅 AFP 或 HepPar1 阳性不足以诊断为卵黄囊癌或肝细胞样癌。AFP 的表达仅与位于 13 号染色体的某一基因沉默有关，卵黄囊或肝细胞样分化与预后无关。

绒毛膜癌样分化也常见于一般类型腺癌中，其癌细胞 β-人绒毛膜促性腺激素（β-hCG）和 PLAP 阳性。β-hCG 阳性常见于一般肠型腺癌或印戒细胞癌，大约 33% 的多克隆抗体呈阳性，60% 的单克隆抗体呈阳性。

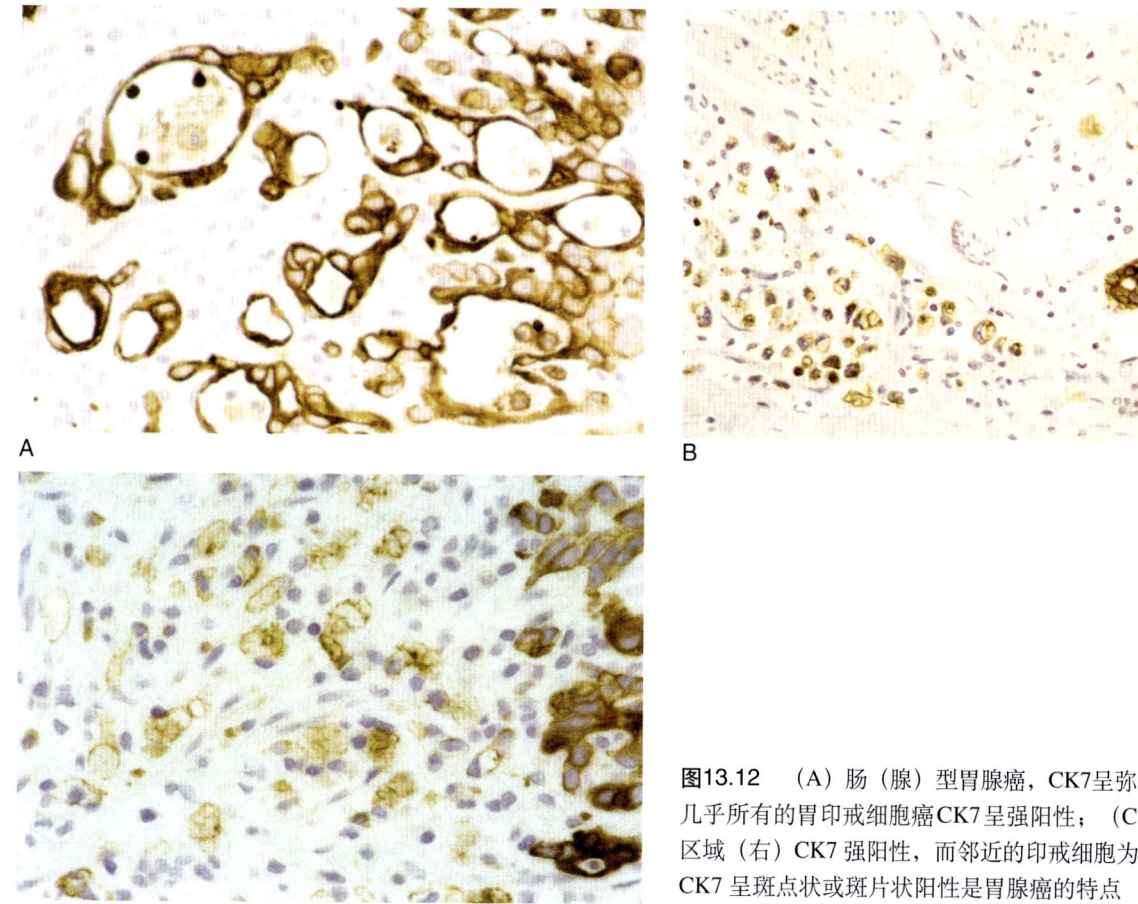

图13.12 （A）肠（腺）型胃腺癌，CK7呈弥漫强阳性；（B）几乎所有的胃印戒细胞癌CK7呈强阳性；（C）胃腺癌的腺样区域（右）CK7强阳性，而邻近的印戒细胞为阴性或弱阳性。CK7呈斑点状或斑片状阳性是胃腺癌的特点

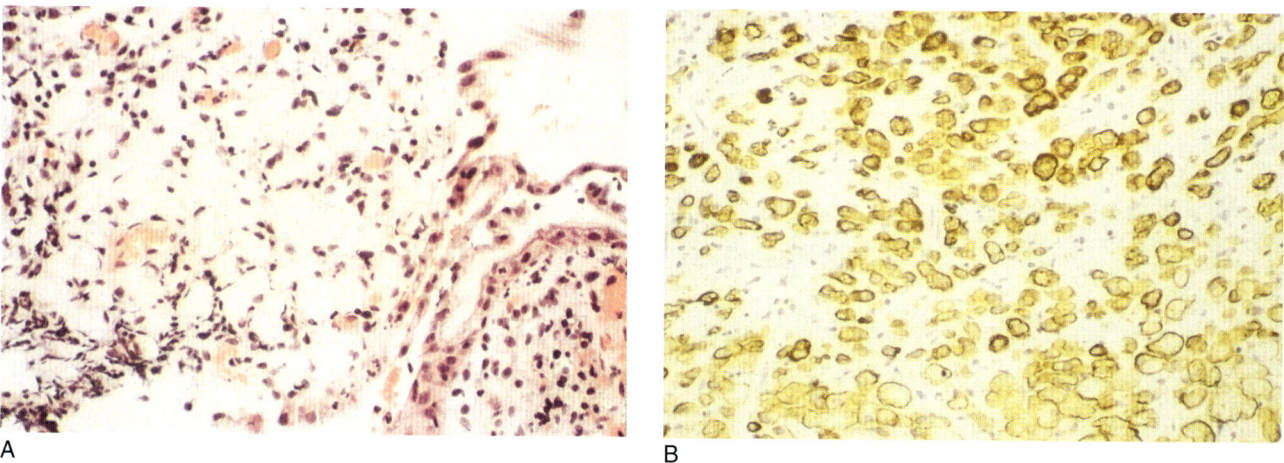

图13.13 （A）固有层内胃印戒细胞不甚明显；（B）CK20染色可见大量肿瘤性印戒细胞，而苏木精-伊红染色并不易见

伴有神经内分泌分化的胃腺癌

组织学特征无神经内分泌细胞分化的肠型或印戒细胞型胃腺癌的嗜铬素和突触素可呈阳性[16, 197, 198]。这两种抗体的任何一种均可呈弥漫阳性，且阳性程度随着方法敏感性的增加而增强[199]。胃癌突触素或嗜铬素阳性非常普遍，以至于认为胃癌预期染色结果理应阳性。嗜铬素或突触素阳性的胃腺癌如果无神经内分泌细胞分化的特征不能认为是神经内分泌肿瘤，另一种神经内分泌细胞的标记物CD56在此类肿瘤中几乎总是阴性。

表13.1 胃腺癌抗体染色

抗体	染色	注释	参考文献
CK5/6	R	转移癌可为灶性阳性	52-54
CK17	R		164-211
CK18	+		
EMA	+		411, 592
KP1 (CD68)	S	约33%的肿瘤阳性，阳性肿瘤细胞<33%	593
CA 19-9	S	约50%~70%呈胞浆或膜阳性，多数印戒细胞呈阳性	171, 329, 338, 339
CEA	+		73, 162, 594-596
Ber-EP4	+		162, 597, 598
CD99 (MIC 2)	S	阳性仅限于肠型肿瘤	599, 600
GCDFP-15	N	极少数（<1%）印戒细胞阳性	171, 203, 601, 602
CD30	N		603
Vimentin	R		330, 604
Calretinin	N		459
S-100	S	约20%肿瘤阳性，阳性细胞<25%	605
B72.3	+		162, 205, 606
CDX2	+	约70%阳性，通常呈非均质片状	113,114, 207, 292, 607
HepPar1	S	约50% 3级及印戒细胞灶性阳性	14
P504s	S	约25%肿瘤胞浆呈粗颗粒阳性	279
CA 125	S	单个细胞或小灶性阳性	164, 329, 608
TTF-1 and Surfactant-A	N		318, 609
p63	R	3级和未分化癌（鳞癌）呈片状阳性	54
Villin	S		113
α-inhibin	N		610

+，阳性；S，偶尔阳性；R，罕见阳性；N，阴性

> **诊断要点：胃癌**
>
> 1. 胃癌组织细胞形态各异，常见梭形细胞、卵黄囊/透明细胞/肝样细胞和绒毛膜癌样细胞分化。这些不同的细胞均有相应的免疫组化染色帮助证实形态学分化。
> 2. 某些抗体可区分形态学上不同分化，例如AFP、HepPar1和β-hGC，但形态上典型的腺癌细胞中也呈阳性。因此，如果没有组织学支持仅有抗体阳性尚不能证实其不同亚型分化。
> 3. 嗜铬素和突触素在典型腺癌中也可呈阳性，这种腺癌不应认为是神经内分泌癌。

鉴别诊断抗体组合

乳腺小叶癌与胃印戒细胞癌 抗体：GCDFP-15、ER、CK20、单克隆CEA、CDX2（图13.15）

胃印戒细胞癌和转移的乳腺小叶癌形态学相似，如果没有免疫组化的帮助有时二者难以鉴别[200, 201]。GCDFP-15在胃癌呈阴性，在大约50%的乳腺小叶癌中呈阳性[171, 202-205]。尽管偶尔有学者报道胃癌的ER阳性，但最近几乎所有的研究均一致认为呈阴性[70, 202]。大部分乳腺小叶癌中大多数癌细胞ER阳性[202]。胃印戒细胞癌中CDX2和CK20通常阳性，而乳腺小叶癌完全阴性(0%)[113, 173, 201, 206, 207]。同分异构的单克隆CEA在胃腺癌中呈弥漫阳性，在乳腺小叶癌中阴性。其他的相同抗原决定簇的CEA抗体在两种肿瘤中均可能为阳性。

乳腺导管腺癌和肠型胃腺癌 抗体：ER、CK17、CEA、绒毛蛋白、CDX2（图13.16）

肠型胃癌的ER阴性[70, 202]，而大约60%的乳腺导管癌ER阳性[70, 204, 208-210]。约有50%的乳腺导管癌CK17阳性，而在肠型胃腺癌中没有CK17阳性的报道[211]。CK17阳性的乳腺导管癌通常分化较差，阳性细胞常位于癌巢中央。绒毛蛋白阳性提示可能是胃原发癌，而乳腺导管癌的绒毛蛋白阴性[9,10,212]。CDX2在约70%

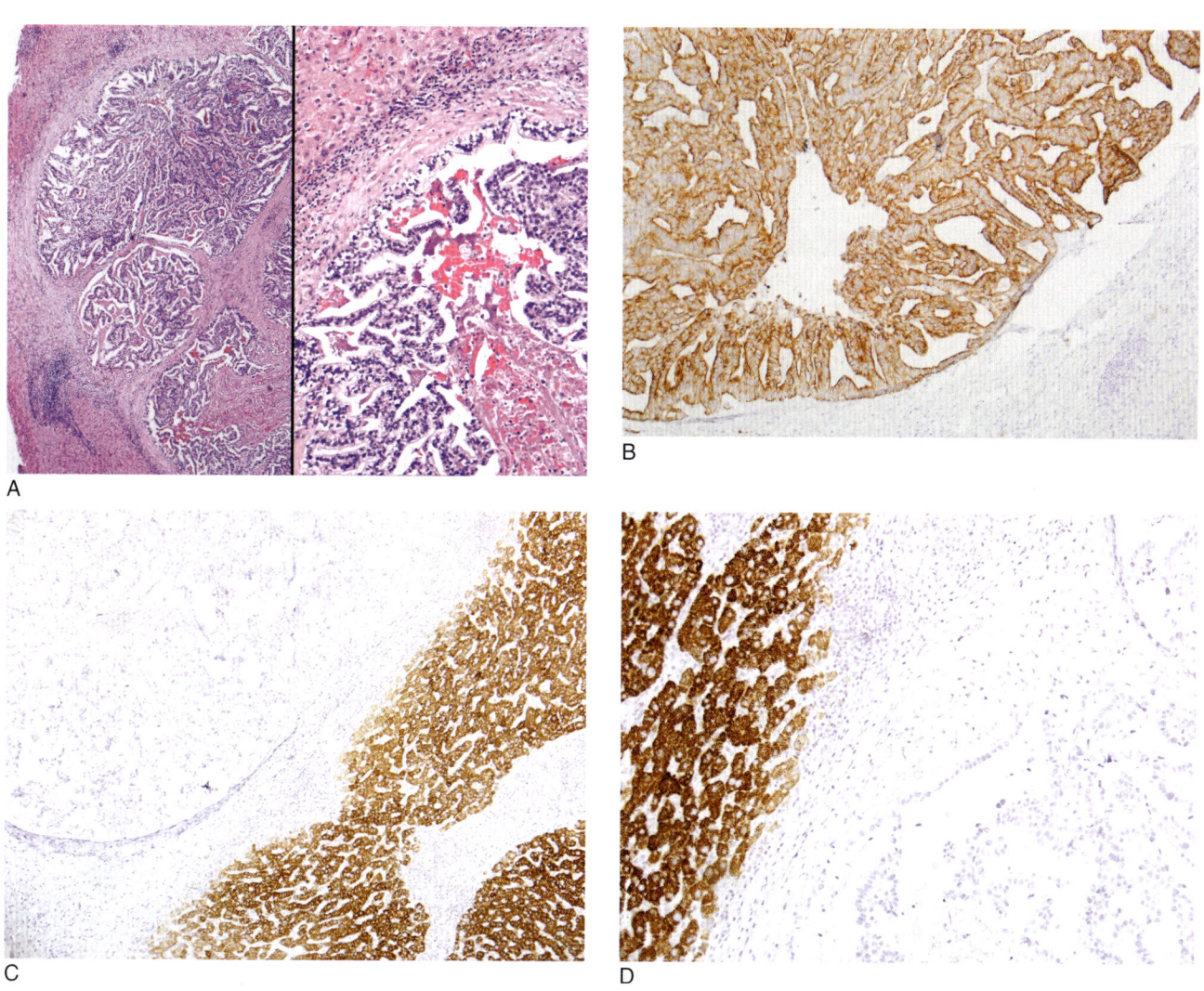

图 13.14 （A）胃/原发的卵黄囊和透明细胞腺癌肝转移；（B）AFP 免疫组化染色弥漫强阳性，容易与肝细胞癌混淆；（C）转移的胃/原发腺癌细胞核 TTF-1 阴性，良性肝细胞中 TTF-1 呈弥漫强阳性，在胞浆中呈粗颗粒分布；（D）高倍镜下良性肝细胞的 TTF-1 胞浆阳性。胃腺癌细胞核及胞浆 TTF-1 阴性，而 TTF-1 在肺腺癌细胞核常呈强阳性

的胃腺癌中阳性，在乳腺导管腺癌中阴性[113, 207]。

胰胆管腺癌与肠型胃腺癌 抗体：CK17、CA125

90% 以上的胰胆管腺癌中 CK17 呈斑片状或弥漫强阳性。大多数胰胆管腺癌中 CK17 阳性的细胞占 50% 以上，而在肠型胃腺癌中无阳性细胞（0%）[211]。50% 以上的胰胆管腺癌 CA125 呈阳性，而在胃癌中几乎全为阴性（见后述的胰胆管腺癌部分）。胃癌中 CA125 阳性的细胞不到 10%。如果癌中 CA125 阳性细胞多于 50%，强烈提示可能是胰胆管腺癌。CK7 和 CK20 在这两种癌中的染色相似，对鉴别诊断没有意义[173]。

肺腺癌与胃腺癌 抗体：CK7、CK20、TTF-1、表面活性剂 A（surfactant-A）、CDX2（表 13.2）

肺原发的印戒细胞癌形态与胃印戒细胞癌相同[213]，只有当其中一种癌的染色结果为 CK7-/CK20+ 时，CK7 和 CK20 才能鉴别二者。约有 40% 的胃腺癌 CK7-/CK20+，而肺腺癌中无此表现[167, 169, 170, 172, 173, 204, 213-216]。甲状腺转录因子-1（TTF-1）和表面活性剂 A 在大多数肺腺癌中阳性，而在胃腺癌阴性[213, 214, 217, 218]。约有 70% 的胃腺癌 CDX2 阳性，肺腺癌阴性(包括肺印戒细胞癌)[113, 207]。

高级别神经内分泌癌

高级别神经内分泌癌（也称小细胞癌）常与典型胃腺癌毗连，或为典型胃腺癌的组成部分。高级别神经内分泌癌的形态及神经内分泌免疫组化特点易于与普通腺癌区分。最好做嗜铬素和突触素的免疫组化染色，以避免将组织挤压的伴有真性神经内分泌分化的

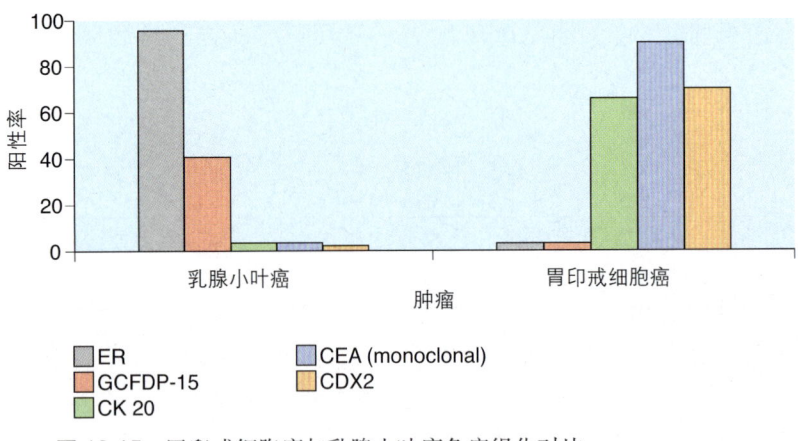

图 13.15 胃印戒细胞癌与乳腺小叶癌免疫组化对比

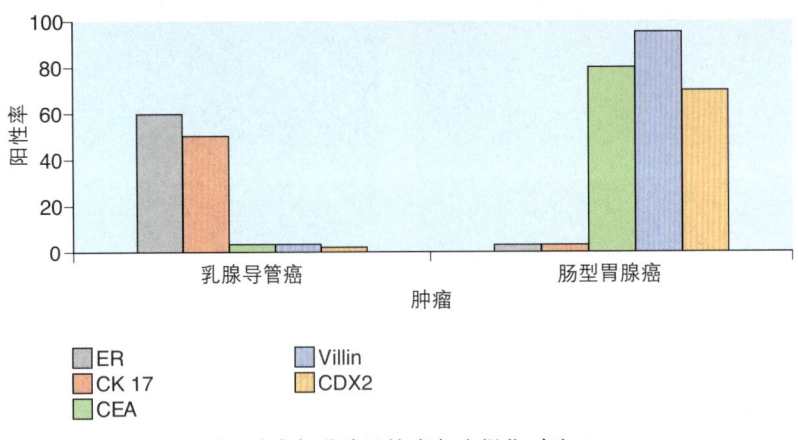

图 13.16 肠型胃腺癌与乳腺导管癌免疫组化对比

表13.2 肺腺癌与胃腺癌鉴别

抗体	胃腺癌	肺腺癌
CK7-/CK20+	S	N
CDX2	+	N
TTF-1 or Surfactant-A	N	+

+, 阳性；S, 偶尔阳性；R, 罕见阳性；N, 阴性

普通腺癌诊断为高级别神经内分泌癌。神经内分泌癌CK20阴性，少数TTF-1阳性[44, 219]。高级别神经内分泌癌CK5/6也呈阴性[52]。

核调节及细胞周期分子：研究表明 E- 钙黏素、p16 及 CDX2 是肿瘤预后较差的标志物[220, 221]。Rb 蛋白、cyclin D1、p53 和 Ki-67(MIB-1)是区分肠上皮化生和高分化腺癌的辅助检测方法。错配修复复合体(hMLH1、hMSH2 和 hMSH6) 抗体阴性是诊断遗传性非息肉结肠癌（HNPCC）的实用标记[222]。MUC1、MUC5A、MUC5B联合染色可显示胃癌细胞肠型或胃

型分化，对估计预后有一定价值[223, 226]，但对区分不同部位的腺癌没有价值[165, 227]。胃肠间质瘤 p27 和 MIB-1（Ki-67）标记指数可能预示肿瘤复发，这些标记比组织学特征更可靠，尤其是伴有不明确的组织学特征的胃肠间质瘤亚型。

小 肠

乳糜泻与上皮内淋巴细胞

乳糜泻的主要病理改变是绒毛上皮内淋巴细胞增生，大部分的上皮内淋巴细胞是活化的T细胞，包括α/β型（CD4-、CD8-/+）和δ/γ型（CD4-、CD8-）T细胞。乳糜泻中上皮内淋巴T细胞的主要免疫表型是 CD3+/CD4-/CD8-。正常的和非腹腔疾病的绒毛上皮内淋巴细胞表型混杂，包括CD3+/CD4+、CD3+/CD8+和CD3+/CD4-/CD8-T细胞。一些学者认为这些抗原对于黏膜活检组织中上皮内淋巴细胞的检测特异性较高[228, 229]。

神经内分泌病变

十二指肠内分泌细胞增生与未经治疗的腹腔疾病有关，其细胞突触素和嗜铬素阳性。

类癌

小肠类癌根据其部位分为两种：十二指肠类癌和空回肠类癌。这两种肿瘤突触素、嗜铬素、CD57和绒毛蛋白阳性[106, 230-232]。大部分十二指肠类癌胃泌素阳性，导致Zollinger-Ellison综合征；Zollinger-Ellison综合征病人最常见的类癌部位在十二指肠壶腹[106, 233-236]。靠近Oddi括约肌和Vater壶腹的类癌形态上与腺癌相似，嗜铬素和突触素阳性可将两者区分。然而此部位少数类癌嗜铬素和突触素呈阴性或弱阳性[237, 238]。在这种情况下，生长抑素抗体效果较好，因为生长抑素在小肠类癌中几乎总是呈阳性，在腺癌中为阴性。

小肠类癌CK7和TTF-1阴性，约有25%的CK20阳性，大部分小肠类癌CEA和CDX2阳性[113, 115, 231, 239]。免疫组化可以区分形态相似的肺肿瘤、胰腺肿瘤和结肠类癌的一个亚型。肝内转移类癌（低级别神经内分泌癌）与原发部位肿瘤的免疫组化鉴别诊断见图13.17。

> **诊断要点：小肠类癌**
>
> 1. 小肠类癌突触素、嗜铬素、CD57和绒毛蛋白呈特异性阳性。
> 2. 如果常规神经内分泌抗体不能确诊，生长抑素有助于区分腺癌和靠近Oddi括约肌或Vater壶腹的类癌。

小肠的胃肠间质瘤

小肠的胃肠间质瘤主要发生在十二指肠或近端空肠，少数发生在远端空肠或回肠[240]。与胃的胃肠间质瘤相似，小肠的胃肠间质瘤CD117呈弥漫强阳性[241]。与发生于胃的胃肠间质瘤相比，小肠胃肠间质瘤中CD34阳性率较低（50%），而SMA阳性率较高（39%）[114, 241]，bcl-2通常呈弥漫阳性[242]。约20%的小肠胃肠间质瘤S-100阳性，10%的CK18阳性，单一抗体阳性者不能诊断为神经鞘瘤、恶性外周神经鞘瘤或癌。

小肠腺癌和Vater壶腹腺癌

远端小肠腺癌的免疫组化表型与结肠腺癌相似，CK18和CK19均呈弥漫强阳性[165]。CK7约33%阳性，CD20约50%阳性（图13.18）[165]。抗体配套染色时，约60%为CK7-/CK20+，20%CK7+/CK20+，其余的20%为CK7-/CK20-或CK7+/CK20-[243]。小肠腺癌绒毛蛋白和CDX2也呈弥漫阳性[113]，约50%MUC1或MUC2阳性，33%的MUC5A阳性[165]。与结肠肿瘤相比，大多数小肠腺癌具有较高比例的微卫星不稳定性[244, 245]。

Vater壶腹腺癌常认为与小肠腺癌、胰管腺癌有明显差别，临床的差别更明显。几乎所有Vater壶腹腺癌CK18、CK19和CK7阳性，50%CK20阳性[165, 246]。约33%的MUC1、MUC2和MUC5A阳性[165]，33%左右的CDX2呈强阳性。临床上很难区分十二指肠腺癌和胃腺癌、Vater壶腹腺癌，它们的免疫表型也很相似。十二指肠腺癌的免疫表型及阳性率和胃腺癌、Vater壶腹腺癌、胰管腺癌及结肠腺癌几乎相同[243]。Vater壶腹腺癌和胰管腺癌的免疫表型相同[246]。

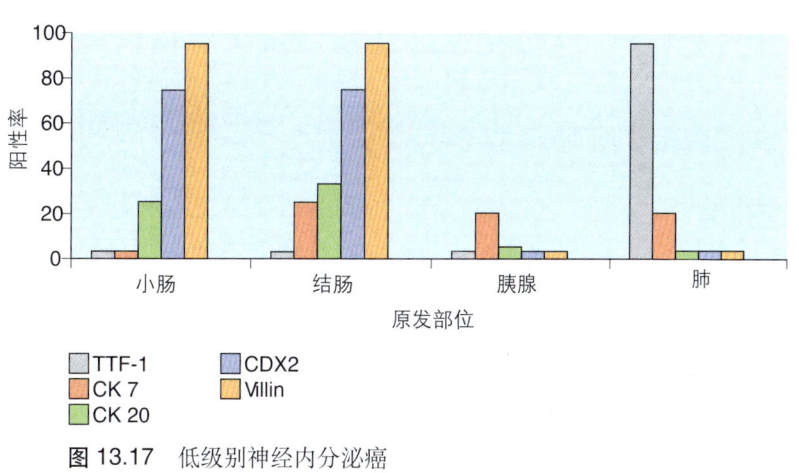

图13.17 低级别神经内分泌癌

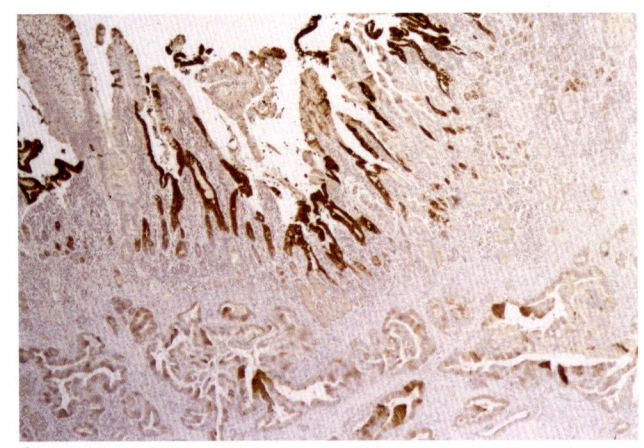

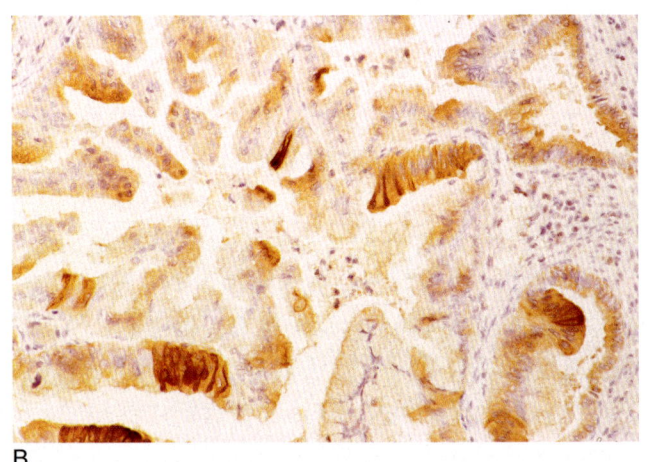

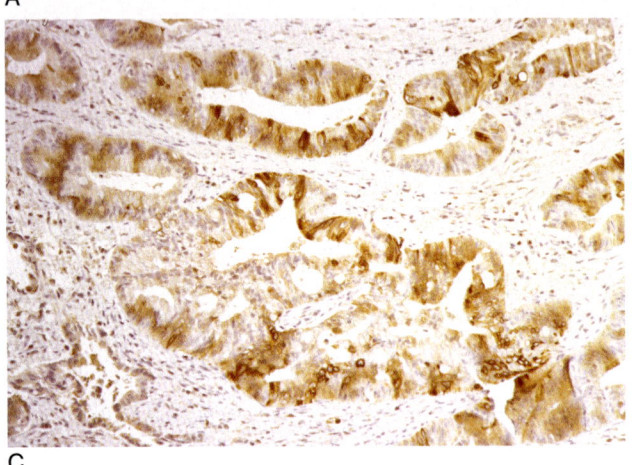

图13.18 （A）Vater壶腹原发腺癌穿透肠壁直接浸润胰腺实质。壶腹黏膜表面隐窝细胞CK20强阳性，黏膜下层浸润的腺癌阳性强度较弱；（B）高倍镜下，浸润至Vater壶腹黏膜下的腺癌中CK20呈斑片状弱阳性；（C）胰腺实质内的腺癌较黏膜下腺癌CK20弥漫阳性更强。胰胆管腺癌的免疫表型常随所浸润的周围组织而变化。因此，转移的胰胆管腺癌通常难以诊断

> **诊断要点：小肠肿瘤**
>
> 1. 小肠的胃肠间质瘤S-100或CK18可阳性，但并不能诊断为神经鞘瘤、恶性外周神经鞘瘤或癌，尤其是在典型的胃肠间质瘤中。
> 2. 大部分（60%）远端小肠腺癌呈CK7-/CK20+，与结肠腺癌相似。
> 3. 与结肠癌相比，多数小肠腺癌有微卫星不稳定性。
> 4. 虽然通常认为Vater壶腹腺癌与小肠腺癌、胰管腺癌明显不同，但这些肿瘤之间，包括结肠腺癌，它们的免疫表型却很相似，免疫组化在鉴别诊断上的作用有限。

阑尾、结肠和直肠

阑尾

类癌

典型的非杯状细胞阑尾类癌在癌巢周围常有S-100阳性的支持细胞环绕[247]。多数阑尾类癌CK20阳性，CK7阴性或局灶阳性[174, 248]。

阑尾杯状细胞类癌是类癌腺癌混合性肿瘤的一种常见类型[16, 249, 250]。这些肿瘤的形态学谱包括伴有少数杯状细胞的管状类癌、杯状细胞类癌和混合型印戒细胞/黏液腺癌-类癌。有少量混杂杯状细胞的管状类癌（类癌细胞和杯状细胞）细胞角蛋白阳性，例如角蛋白AE1/AE3阳性。与典型的阑尾类癌CEA常为阴性或仅有局灶弱阳性不同，杯状细胞类癌CEA呈强阳性。类癌细胞巢突触素和嗜铬素强阳性，黏液/杯状细胞中突触素比嗜铬素染色更强，阳性比例更大。尽管杯状细胞通常是CK7阴性和CK20阳性，但少数肿瘤细胞的CK7和CK20可同时呈阳性（图13.19～13.22）[174]。与结直肠印戒细胞腺癌和临床侵袭性结肠类癌不同，杯状细胞和典型类癌的E-钙黏素和β-连环蛋白呈强阳性[251]。腺癌/类癌混合性肿瘤的腺体成分中突触素和嗜铬素常为阴性，恶性细胞常为CK7+/CK20+，少数呈CK7-/CK20+[174]。腺瘤/类癌混合肿瘤中，每一种上皮成分都表达各自的免疫表型。

胃肠道、胰腺、胆管、胆囊和肝的免疫组织化学 | 13

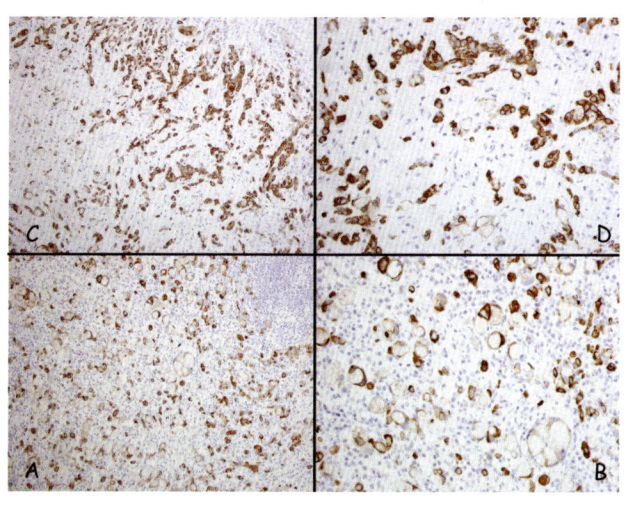

图 13.19 阑尾腺癌 CK20 阳性类型多样，此图显示 4 种类型

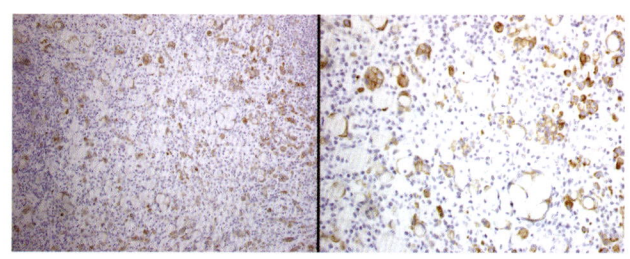

图 13.20 阑尾类腺癌的 CK7 染色通常呈不规则斑片状阳性。右图：一些黏液细胞 CK7 呈阳性，而邻近的癌巢为阴性

> **诊断要点：阑尾类癌**
>
> 1. 杯状细胞类癌 CEA 呈强阳性，与典型阑尾类癌不同。
> 2. 杯状细胞类癌和典型阑尾类癌的 E-钙黏素和 β-连环蛋白呈阳性，与结直肠印戒细胞癌和侵袭性结肠类癌不同。
> 3. 腺癌/类癌混合肿瘤的腺体成分中突触素和嗜铬素常为阴性。

腺瘤与腺癌

非黏液腺瘤和腺癌的免疫表型与结肠腺癌相同，约 25% 的 CK7 呈局灶阳性，95% 的 CK20 呈斑片状或弥漫阳性。[176, 252]

黏液增生性腺瘤、囊腺瘤、腺癌和腹腔内增生性黏液瘤细胞产生的腹膜假性黏液瘤的免疫表型与结直肠黏液腺癌不同（图 13.23）[165, 176, 252-257]。与结直肠黏液腺癌相似的是，CK8、CK13、CK18、CK19 和 CK20 均呈弥漫强阳性，约 20% 的 MUC1 呈阳性，98% 的 MUC2 呈弥漫强阳性；与结直肠腺癌不同的是，约

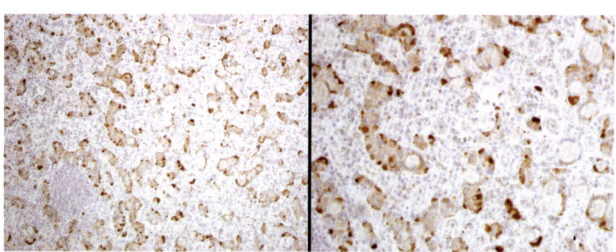

图 13.21 阑尾类腺癌中癌巢内和小管内单个神经内分泌细胞内嗜铬素阳性。右图：高倍镜显示，腺癌细胞内嗜铬素为阴性

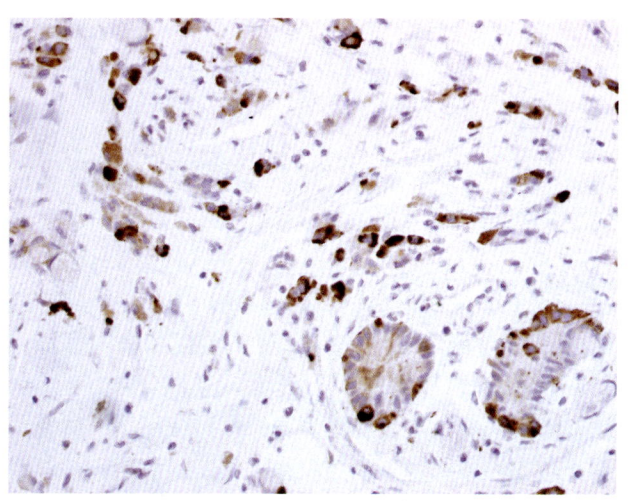

图 13.22 间质和腺癌腺体内孤立的神经内分泌细胞的突触素阳性。与嗜铬素相比，突触素阳性更强、更广泛

33% 同时表达 CK7，阳性细胞约占 25%～75%（图 13.24～13.26）。这些病变中 CK7 阳性细胞的比例明显高于典型结直肠腺癌。结直肠腺癌的阳性细胞较少，偶尔簇状细胞阳性。约 80% 的阑尾/原发黏液腺癌 MUC5A 阳性，与胃、胰腺和卵巢原发黏液腺癌及卵巢黏液交界性肿瘤（胃肠亚型）相似（图 13.23）。相反，结肠黏液腺癌的 MUC5A 阴性[165, 258]。由于抑癌基因的等位缺失导致 Dpc4（SMAD4）阴性最初认为是胰胆管腺癌独有的，但后来的研究表明许多部位的黏液腺癌，包括阑尾和结肠均由相同的机制导致 Dpc4 缺失[253]。腹膜假黏液瘤细胞还同时表达 MUC2 及部分表达 MUC5AC，这是阑尾型肿瘤上皮细胞的特征。相反，伴有局部种植的卵巢黏液肿瘤仅 MUC5AC 阳性[259]。

原发和转移的黏液腺癌的免疫组化鉴别比较困难，尤其是在卵巢[260, 261]。以作者的观点，CK7、CK20、CDX2、MUC2、MUC5A、绒毛蛋白和 β-连环蛋白的抗体组合囊括了可能的原发部位的范围，提出了最可靠的诊断依据。CK7 完全阴性且 CK20 弥漫强阳性支持结直肠腺癌，而 CK7 弥漫阳性、CK20

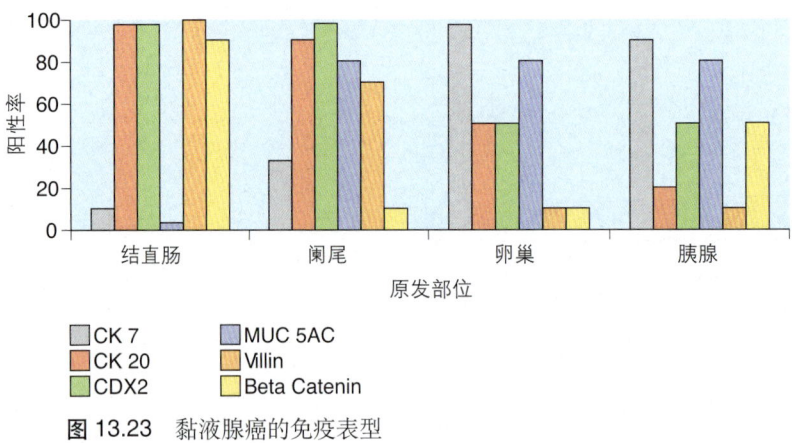

图13.23 黏液腺癌的免疫表型

完全阴性支持卵巢原发肿瘤。CK20局灶阳性既可见于阑尾也可见于卵巢的原发肿瘤，因此无诊断意义[167, 169, 172, 173, 176, 204, 215, 252, 262-267]。CDX2在细胞核的弥漫强阳性提示结直肠原发黏液腺癌。卵巢和胰腺的黏液肿瘤CDX2也呈阳性，但阳性的强度和范围都低于结肠黏液腺癌[113, 207, 268, 269]。绒毛蛋白的染色类型也可帮助鉴别诊断。阑尾和结直肠原发黏液腺癌的绒毛蛋白染色是刷状缘型，而胰腺和卵巢的黏液腺癌是胞浆阳性无刷状缘反应[111]。结肠原发黏液腺癌细胞核β-连环蛋白强阳性，而卵巢原发黏液肿瘤细胞核呈斑片状弱阳性[270]。

> **诊断要点：阑尾和结直肠的黏液肿瘤**
>
> 1. 阑尾黏液肿瘤比结直肠黏液腺癌CK7阳性反应相对较强，且MUC5A阳性，而结肠黏液肿瘤MUC5A呈阴性。
> 2. CK7、CK20、CDX2、MUC2、MUC5A、绒毛蛋白和β-连环蛋白的抗体组合有助于鉴别原发和转移的黏液腺癌。

结肠和直肠

先天性巨结肠病（Hirschsprung's disease）

直肠活检组织免疫组化染色有助于发现先天性巨结肠的神经节细胞，神经节细胞的神经特异性烯醇化酶(NSE)和组织蛋白酶D（cathepsin D）阳性[271]。围绕神经元的卫星细胞S-100强阳性，从而在神经元周围形成一可见的、阴性的空晕。抗体阳性位于无神经节区过渡带及正常有神经节肠道的黏膜下和肠肌层的神经节及神经纤维。calretinin在有神经节的肠道正常神经节和神经中为阳性，在先天性巨结肠的无神经节部位（包括无神经节部位中肥大的神经纤维）中呈阴性。

结、直肠间质肿瘤

神经鞘和神经纤维病变 胃肠道可见黏膜神经节细胞瘤和神经纤维瘤，可为孤立性病变或者是多发性内分泌肿瘤（MEN）综合征Ⅱb型和von Recklinghausen病的组成部分，大多为结肠和阑尾的偶发病变（图13.27）。免疫组化染色结果取决于神经节细胞和施万细胞成分[272]。神经节细胞中NSE、突触素和神经微丝（NF）阳性。大部分病例的梭形细胞S-100阳性，围绕神经节细胞的卫星细胞S-100也呈阳性。神经鞘瘤常累及黏膜下层和固有层，向腔内呈息肉状突出，临床上与腺瘤样息肉相似，S-100均呈弥漫强阳性，GFAP弱阳性[273]。虽然CD34阳性细胞数从少到多数量不等，但CD117一致阴性。伴大量肥大细胞的神经鞘瘤CD117常表现为阳性，但仔细观察CD117阳性仅限于肥大细胞。

结直肠的胃肠间质瘤与平滑肌肿瘤 大多数结肠的胃肠间质瘤发生在乙状结肠、直肠和肛门[151, 152, 274]。结肠的胃肠间质瘤常有平滑肌瘤的形态表现。与真性平滑肌瘤相比，大多数结肠的胃肠间质瘤（与胃原发的胃肠间质瘤相同）CD117和CD34阳性，平滑肌肌动蛋白(SMA)阴性[275]。肛门、直肠的胃肠间质瘤的结蛋白、S-100、GFAP和NF均阴性。

结肠的平滑肌瘤常起源于黏膜肌层，表现为腔内小的息肉样病变，SMA、肌特异性肌动蛋白（MSA）和结蛋白均呈弥漫强阳性，CD117、CD34和S-100阴性[31, 32, 275, 276]。远端直肠的平滑肌肉瘤的免疫组化表型与腹膜后原发肿瘤相似，CD117阴性[275]。

胃肠道、胰腺、胆管、胆囊和肝的免疫组织化学 13

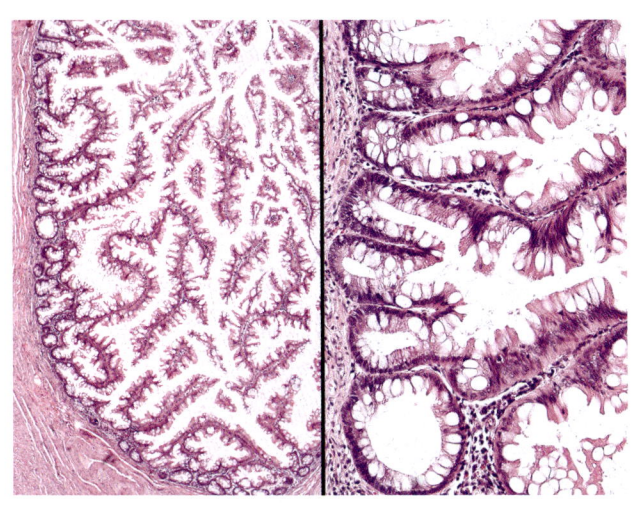

图13.24 阑尾黏液肿瘤，低级别，非浸润性。高倍镜下，肿瘤细胞在形态上与卵巢原发黏液交界肿瘤相似

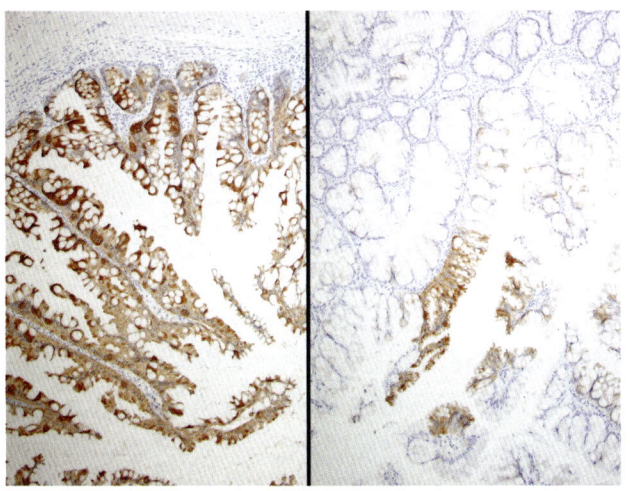

图13.25 大多数阑尾原发黏液肿瘤的CK20阳性（左），CK7阴性或局灶阳性（右）

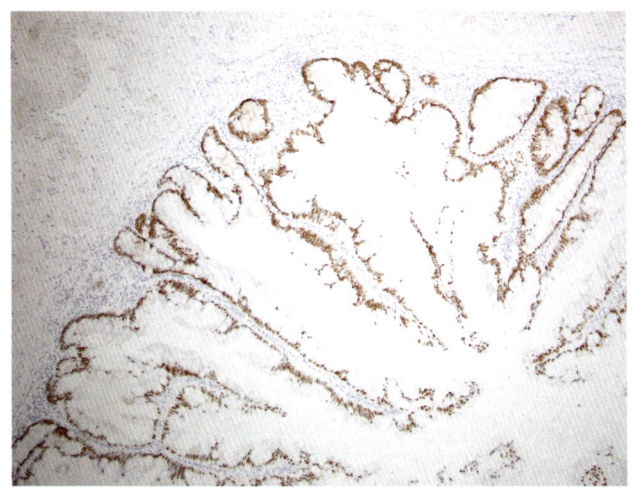

图13.26 阑尾黏液肿瘤细胞核中CDX2呈典型的强阳性

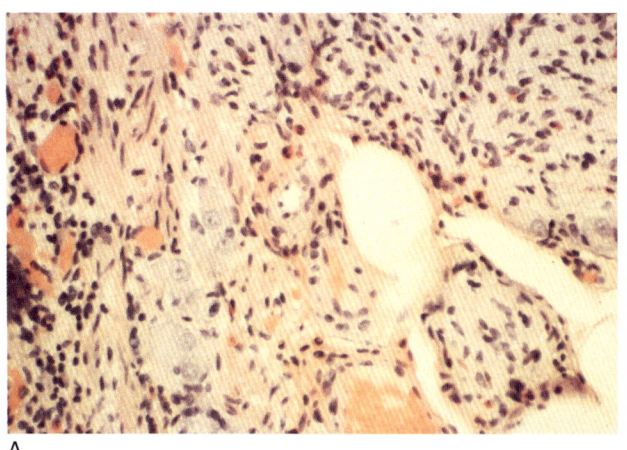

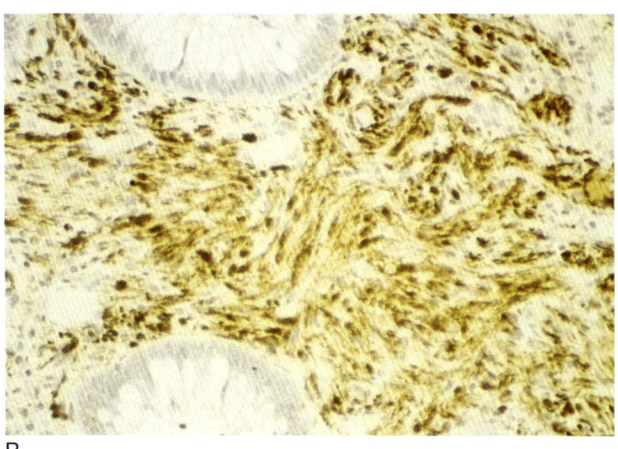

图13.27 （A）大多数单个的、小的结肠黏膜的神经节细胞瘤为偶发；（B）结肠神经节细胞瘤形态上与胃肠间质瘤相似，特别是当神经节细胞很少时。图中神经节细胞瘤间质的S-100呈强阳性，而胃肠间质瘤常为阴性

结直肠类癌 结肠类癌主要发生在两个部位，盲肠/近端右结肠和远端乙状结肠/直肠。大部分盲肠和近端右结肠类癌由肠嗜铬细胞组成，血清素、嗜铬素和突触素阳性（图13.28A）。多数右结肠类癌缺乏S-100阳性的支持细胞，与空肠和回肠类癌相同。约50%的CK20阳性，25%的CK7阳性[115]，没有特征性的CK7/20联合染色类型。细胞角蛋白AE1/AE3在个别细胞中呈斑驳状阳性（图13.28B），右结肠类癌的TTF-1一致呈阴性[239]。

乙状结肠和直肠类癌与伴有神经内分泌分化的前列腺腺癌的形态特点相似，前列腺酸性磷酸酶阳性[277,278]。与前列腺的原发腺癌不同的是，乙状结肠和直肠类癌的前列腺特异性抗原(PSA)和P504s阴性[279]。约50%~80%的直肠乙状结肠类癌嗜铬素阳性，100%的突触素阳性[106, 230, 277, 278, 280-282]，约25%的癌

465

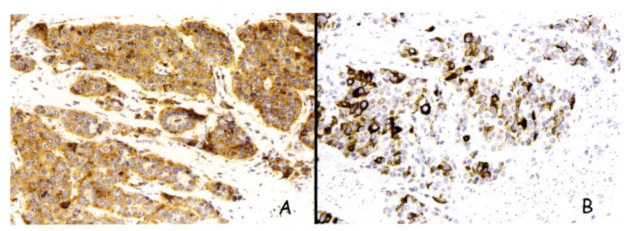

图13.28 结肠类癌的嗜铬素（左图）比AE1/AE3（右图）染色更为弥漫强阳性

胚抗原呈弱阳性[277]，约50%的直肠类癌波形蛋白阳性[108, 287]，类癌CD117阴性。回肠和阑尾类癌及其转移类癌的CDX2呈弥漫强阳性[283]。相反，原发的胃、十二指肠、胰腺和直肠的低级别神经内分泌癌的细胞核内CDX2呈斑片状弱阳性。肺、胃、胰腺、小肠和结肠低级别类癌的鉴别诊断抗体组合类型的比较见图13.17。

> **诊断要点：结直肠类癌**
> 1. 右结肠类癌由肠嗜铬细胞组成，血清素、嗜铬素和突触素阳性，免疫组化类型与空回肠类癌相同。
> 2. 直肠乙状结肠类癌与前列腺腺癌具有相同的形态特点，且前列腺酸性磷酸酶均为阳性，但前者前列腺特异性抗原和P504s阴性。

结直肠腺癌

结直肠腺癌细胞含有大多数低分子量细胞角蛋白，主要是CK8、CK18、CK19和CK20（图13.29），其中广谱AE1/AE3、CAM5.2和35βH11呈阳性，CK17局灶阳性，34βH12阴性[1, 48, 51, 211, 265, 284, 285]。

CK7：约50%的结直肠腺癌CK7阴性，40%局灶阳性（阳性细胞占5%～50%），10%弥漫（>50%）阳性[8, 52, 165, 167-170, 175, 177, 255, 262, 263, 265, 284, 286-288]。在低分化癌[174]和通过锯齿状肿瘤信号转导通道产生的微卫星不稳定性腺癌中，CK7阳性细胞的百分数和阳性强度较高[289]。

CK20：约5%的腺癌CK20阴性，3%～15%局灶阳性，85%～100%弥漫阳性（图13.30）[8, 165, 176, 171, 172, 262, 263, 265, 284-286, 290]。CK20的阳性强度并不随着肿瘤级别的增高而降低[49]，CK20阳性减弱常见于微卫星不稳定性（MSI-high）的腺癌[289]。

CK7/CK20 联合染色：结直肠腺癌主要表现为CK20弥漫强阳性，CK7完全阴性。大约20%呈CK7+/CK20+[291]。

CDX2：在几乎所有的结直肠腺癌（98%～100%）细胞的细胞核中呈弥漫强阳性[113, 114, 207, 292]，但对结直肠腺癌并无特异性。在胰胆管、胃、小肠和卵巢的黏液腺癌和子宫内膜样腺癌中也呈阳性，但是与结直肠腺癌相比，阳性程度通常较弱并且呈斑片状。

绒毛蛋白：结直肠腺癌的胞浆中弥漫阳性，伴有刷状缘着色加重（图13.31）[8-11]。其他抗体染色见表13.3。

腺癌的变型及亚型

印戒细胞腺癌 结肠印戒细胞腺癌，包括完全为印戒细胞或者是混有黏液或腺体的腺癌，与腺性结肠腺癌的免疫表型相同[164, 203]。

结直肠锯齿状腺瘤通路和微卫星不稳定表型
约15%～20%的结直肠腺癌是由于错配修复复合体功能缺失引起的，导致了微卫星不稳定性（MSI）。在非遗传性散在发生的腺癌中，hMLH1错配修复启动子基因的超甲基化导致了hMLH1蛋白表达的缺陷。hMLH1蛋白是错配修复复合体必需的组成成分。由这种分子通路导致的肿瘤多数发生在右侧，常见于老年女性病人。家族性腺癌（遗传性非息肉病结直肠癌综合征）经常有hMSH2、hMLH1和hMSH6基因的种系突变，导致其蛋白产物减少或异常[293]。错配修复复合体的hMLH1、hMSH2和hMSH6蛋白抗体阴性可用来 筛选高度微卫星不稳定性的肿瘤[294]。这种筛选可以决定哪些病人需要进一步的遗传检测。遗传性非息肉病结直肠癌综合征病人可表现为3种抗体中任何一种缺失（图13.32、13.33），肿瘤浸润最深部位的细胞核阴性是由于错配修复缺陷引起的腺癌的特点。抗体染色强度通常由弱至强呈均质分布。因此，确定有高度微卫星不稳定性肿瘤至少应有一种抗体为完全阴性。与典型的管状腺癌相比，印戒细胞腺癌和黏液腺癌常有高度微卫星不稳定性，其hMLH1、hMSH2或hMSH6抗体的免疫反应呈核阴性。

高度微卫星不稳定性腺癌中，CDX2和CK20的表达减少或缺失，CK7阳性增强[289, 295]。这些免疫表型的改变常见于直肠和伴有广泛黏液分化的肿瘤[296]。

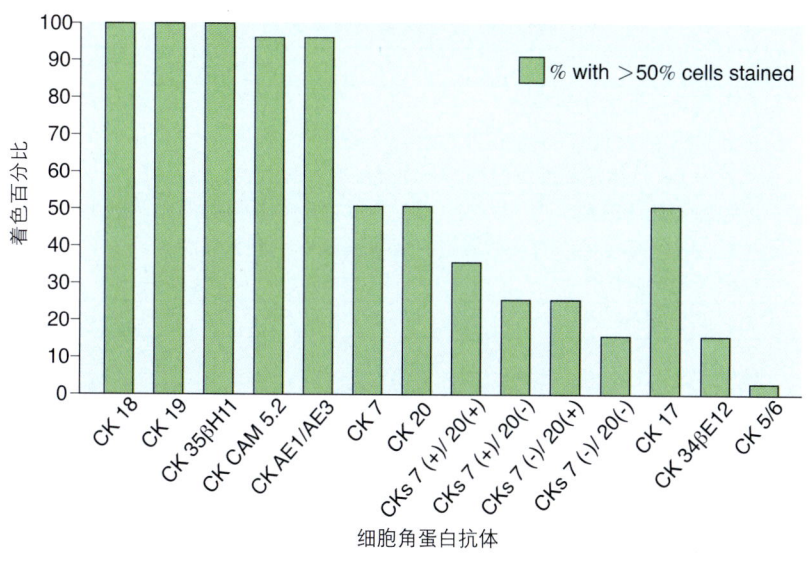

图 13.29　结直肠腺癌中细胞角蛋白的表达

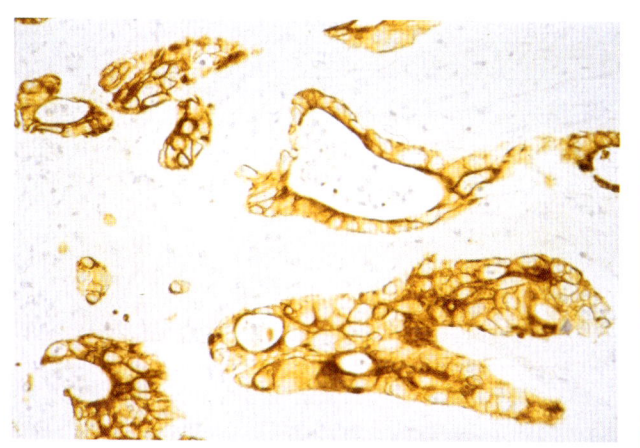

图 13.30　结直肠腺癌最常见的 CK20 阳性类型

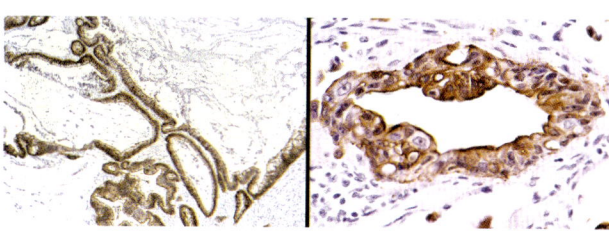

图13.31　高倍和低倍镜显示，结直肠黏液腺癌中，绒毛蛋白在胞浆呈均匀弥漫阳性，微绒毛腔和胞膜微绒毛刷状缘的着色增强。虽然非结肠腺癌的绒毛蛋白也呈阳性，但无微绒毛刷状缘结构着色

高级别神经内分泌癌

高级别神经内分泌癌常为低分化腺癌的一部分[297]，癌细胞含有大多数低分子量细胞角蛋白，大部分细胞CAM5.2、35βH11 和 CK OSCAR 阳性，呈核周点状阳性[298, 299]。常见实性非角化鳞状细胞癌的病灶，尤其是在远端结直肠癌中病灶细胞 34βE12、CK5/6 和p63 阳性。在挤压变形的组织中常保持着核周点状细胞角蛋白阳性，是有助于诊断的形态特征。AE1/AE3 仅在少部分细胞中呈弱阳性[300]。高级别（小细胞未分化）神经内分泌癌 CK20 常为阴性（图 13.34）[299]。在高级别神经内分泌癌的绝大部分细胞中突触素呈阳性（图 13.35），而嗜铬素常为阴性或弱阳性[42, 301-306]，Leu7的反应与嗜铬素相似[303, 307, 308]。轻度复染可以明显增强对这些肿瘤细胞胞浆颗粒状着色的检测。少数高级别神经内分泌癌的CD117阳性。但是，免疫反应阳性与 c-kit 近膜（外显子 11）的突变无关。

透明细胞腺癌

大部分透明细胞腺癌的免疫表型与一般的结直肠腺癌相同[309]。极少数原发的结肠癌和透明细胞癌的甲胎蛋白阳性。

未分化的肿瘤和伴有横纹肌样分化的癌

这些肿瘤的免疫组化与伴有梭形细胞分化的低分化癌相似（图 13.36）[310]。胃肠道内横纹肌样癌两个最常见的发生部位是结肠和胃，通常是典型腺癌的组成部分。

表13.3　结直肠腺癌抗体染色

抗体	染色	评论	参考文献
ER and PR	R	男女病例均呈低度受体表达 少部分腺癌敏感性鼠单克隆抗体检测呈核弱阳性，新型兔单克隆 ER 抗体使阳性细胞数和阳性强度均有所增强	70, 171, 180, 182, 204, 205, 611-614, 614-620
Synaptophysin	S	一般腺癌可灶性阳性 无神经内分泌分化形态特征的典型的结肠腺癌可呈灶性突触素及嗜铬素阳性	16, 198, 621-624
Chromogranin A	R	少见，单个细胞阳性	16, 198, 621-625
MUC 1	+		165
MUC 2	+		165
MUC 5A	N		165
CK5/6	N		52,54
CEA	+		73, 171, 205, 262, 324, 326, 327, 595,626
CA 19-9	S		171, 205, 329, 338, 339, 626
Ber-EP4	+		216, 597, 598
GCDFP-15	N		171, 204, 205, 601, 602
CD30	N		603
CA 125	R	"阳性"肿瘤呈单个细胞或小灶性阳性	205, 608
Calretinin	R		60, 459
PLAP	S	通常为细胞膜强阳性	
S-100	S	0%～25% 结肠腺癌阳性，"阳性"病例表明阳性细胞数小于 20%	212, 324, 605
B72.3	+	通常为细胞浆弥漫强阳性	205
TTF-1	N		217
Surfactant-A (PE-10)	N		312
α-inhibin	R	大的 5% 为强阳性，75% 为弱阳性	610
HepPar1	N	极少数为胞浆溶酶体假阳性	14, 196, 375, 627

+，阳性；S，有时阳性；R，极少阳性；N，阴性

诊断要点：结直肠癌

1. 结直肠腺癌呈典型的CK20、CDX2和绒毛蛋白阳性。CK7常呈局灶阳性反应，有些学者认为是阴性。
2. hMLH1、hMSH2和hMSH6可以用来筛选高度微卫星不稳定性的肿瘤。
3. 高度微卫星不稳定性的结肠腺癌可表现为CDX2 和 CK20 阳性的减弱，CK7 阳性增强。
4. 高级别神经内分泌癌常是高级别腺癌的组成部分，通常CK20 阴性、突触素阳性，此时应注意是否存在高级别鳞癌。

鉴别诊断组合

结肠腺癌与肺腺癌　抗体：CK7、CK20、表面活性剂 A、TTF-1 和 CDX2（图 13.37）

CK20 弥漫阳性是诊断结直肠腺癌的可靠依据[287]，而 CK7 的弥漫强阳性是肺腺癌的有力证据。CK20 或 CK7 任何一种抗体呈局灶阳性均无诊断意义，因为其均可见于肺或结直肠腺癌[172, 173, 215, 287]。绝大多数 1 级和 2 级非黏液肺腺癌的表面活性剂 A（PE-10）和TTF-1呈阳性，而结肠腺癌呈阴性[217,312-318]。结直肠腺癌 CDX2 阳性，而非黏液肺腺癌 CDX2 呈阴性[113, 207]。

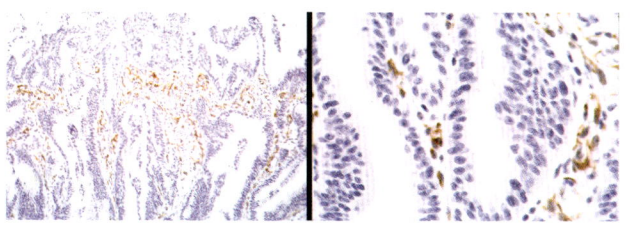

图 13.32 一位患有遗传性非息肉病结肠癌综合征的46岁病人的侵袭性乙状结肠癌的高倍和低倍图像。肿瘤细胞核hMLH2完全阴性，而周围间质的细胞核呈强阳性。只有核染色的完全缺失才能认为是错配修复酶缺陷的潜在标志

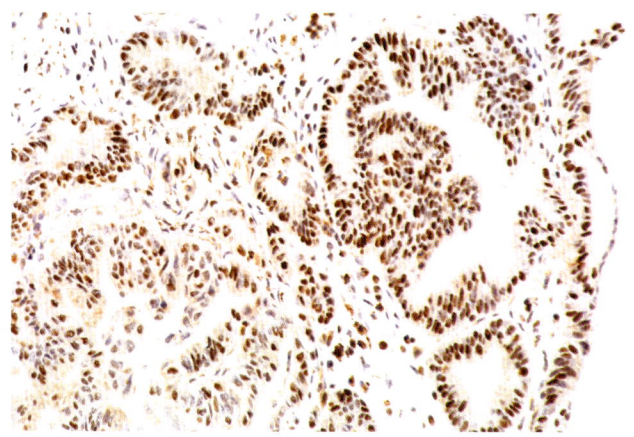

图 13.33 非综合征结直肠腺癌的hMLH1特征性核阳性图像。hMLH1和hMSH2两种抗体都呈阳性，预示着肿瘤细胞的错配修复复合体完好无损

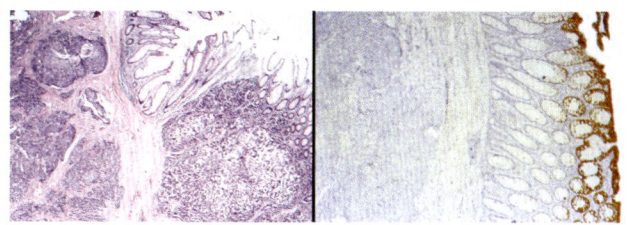

图 13.34 高级别结肠神经内分泌癌。肿瘤细胞的CK20阴性（右图）。注意仅正常黏膜的典型表面上皮阳性，隐窝上皮细胞为阴性

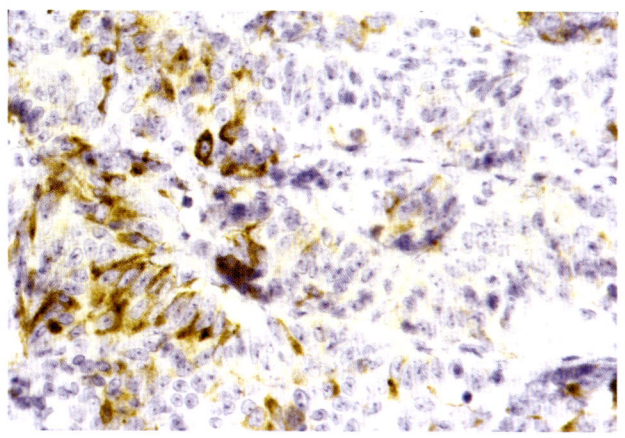

图13.35 高级别结肠神经内分泌癌的突触素呈局灶弱阳性至中度阳性

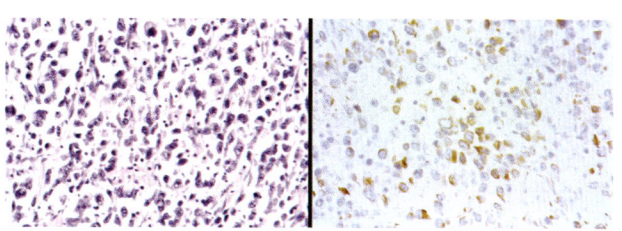

图13.36 多形性未分化结直肠腺癌。CK OSCAR（左图）是证明肿瘤细胞上皮性质的最佳角蛋白抗体

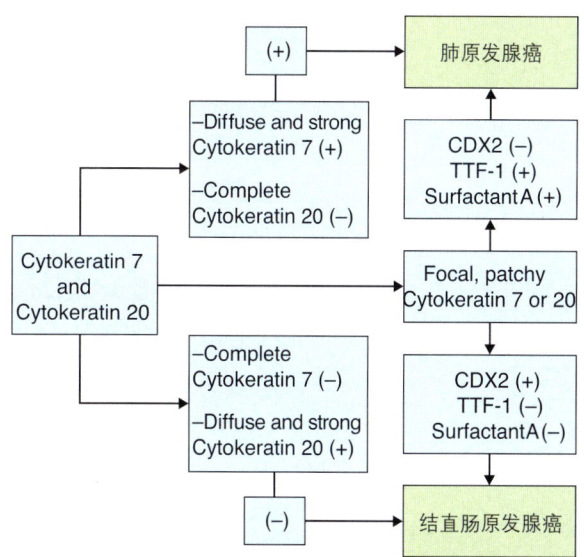

图13.37 结肠腺癌与肺腺癌的免疫组化鉴别诊断

肺原发黏液性细支气管肺泡癌和杯状细胞腺癌的免疫表型与普通的肺腺癌不同[10, 319, 320]。此型CDX2和CK20阳性，与转移的结直肠腺癌相似[321, 322]，鉴别要点是肺黏液腺癌CDX2呈中等强度，局灶阳性，而结直肠腺癌中呈弥漫强阳性。

结肠腺癌与苗勒管子宫内膜样腺癌　抗体：CK7、CK20、CEA、CA125、波形蛋白、CD56、CDX2、ER（图13.38）

CK7是有用的首选抗体，在95%以上的子宫内膜样腺癌中阳性，在极少数的结直肠腺癌中呈阳性。相反，CK20在子宫内膜样腺癌中阴性，而在结直肠腺癌中呈阳性[176, 169, 170, 172, 173, 204, 262, 264, 265, 267, 323]。另外可用来鉴别这两个部位腺癌的抗体组合包括单克隆CEA（注意，不是多克隆）[162, 205, 262, 265, 276, 323-328]、CDX2[113, 207]（113;207）、CA125[205, 262, 267, 329]、波形蛋白[263-324, 330]、CD56[331,332]和ER。

结肠腺癌和移行细胞癌 抗体：CK7、CDX2、CK5/6、p63、CK34βE12、血栓调节素（图13.39）

鉴别诊断时，CDX2是目前唯一的结肠腺癌一致阳性鉴别的抗体，因为CDX2在移行细胞癌呈完全阴性。CK7和血栓调节素的弥漫强阳性是多数移行细胞癌的特征，二者中任何一种呈阳性都是诊断移行细胞癌的有力依据[333]。许多伴有鳞状细胞分化的低分化移行细胞癌CK5/6、CK34βE12和p63阳性。

结肠腺癌与尿道上皮和脐尿管腺癌 抗体：CK7和血栓调节素

CK7和血栓调节素任一种的弥漫阳性都是诊断尿路上皮腺癌的依据[334, 335]，阴性则无诊断意义，不是结肠原发肿瘤的诊断依据。

结肠腺癌与前列腺癌 抗体：CDX2、CA19-9、CEA、CK20、PSA、P504s

CDX2和CA19-9在结直肠腺癌中阳性，而在前列腺癌中阴性。CK20和CEA弥漫强阳性时支持结直肠腺癌的诊断，二者在高级别前列腺癌中也呈局灶阳性。PSA和P504s在前列腺癌中呈阳性，在结直肠腺癌中阴性。与其他抗体相似，P504s或PSA阴性并不是非前列腺癌的诊断依据。许多高级别前列腺癌的PSA和P504s可以是阴性[172, 173, 265, 279, 336-339]。

结肠腺癌与高级别神经内分泌癌 抗体：AE1/AE3、CAM5.2、CK20、嗜铬素、CDX2（图13.40）

高级别神经内分泌癌（大细胞型）或低分化腺癌细胞通常呈实性片状生长、细胞大、胞浆较少、核染色质细腻[42, 303, 306, 340]，二者的混合性癌并不少见。仅靠形态学诊断高级别神经内分泌癌时要慎重。低分化的结直肠腺癌常有神经内分泌的表现，但突触素和嗜铬素阴性[341]。两者鉴别非常重要，因为其治疗和预后均不同。

通常利用免疫组化来区分低分化（也称未分化）的腺癌和高级别神经内分泌癌。约66%的低分化/未分化腺癌的突触素和嗜铬素呈阴性或仅有孤立的细胞阳性[16, 302, 342]，约33%的肿瘤中小的细胞簇突触素阳性，阳性细胞少于20%[340-342]，这些突触素阳性的细

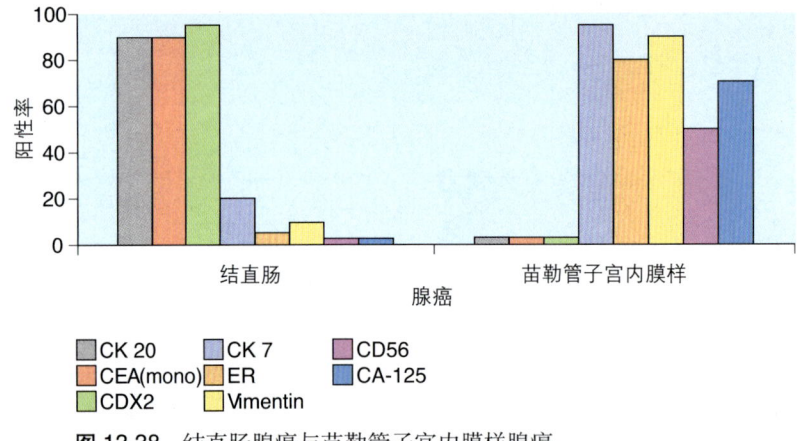

图13.38　结直肠腺癌与苗勒管子宫内膜样腺癌

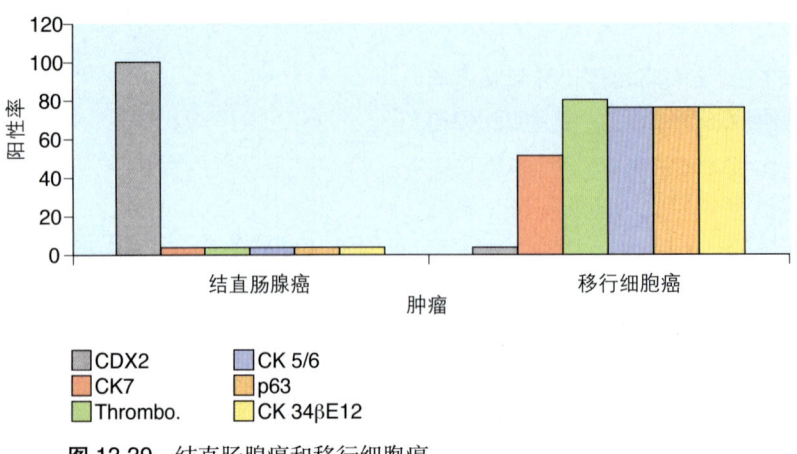

图13.39　结直肠腺癌和移行细胞癌

胃肠道、胰腺、胆管、胆囊和肝的免疫组织化学

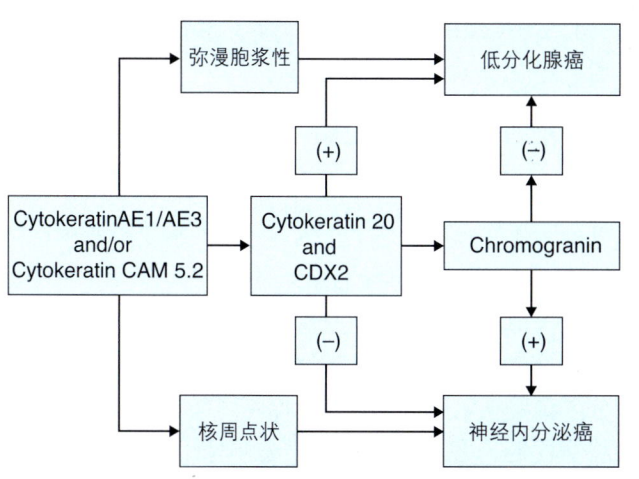

图13.40　结肠腺癌与高级别神经内分泌癌的免疫组化鉴别诊断

胞同时表达CK20，且表现为胞浆弥漫阳性，而不是像高级别神经内分泌癌呈核周点状阳性。

肛　门

鳞状细胞癌

肛门鳞状细胞癌与胃肠道其他部位的鳞状细胞癌相似（见前面的食管部分）[1, 343]。基底细胞样、梭形细胞和泄殖腔原型鳞癌与一般的鳞状细胞癌免疫组化表型相同（图 13.41、13.42）[344]。

肛门腺癌

肛门腺癌与发生于长期瘘管的黏液腺癌不同，肛门腺癌形成了仅有少量黏液蛋白的小腺体，CK7呈弥散阳性，CK20阴性[345]。

肛门Paget病

肛门Paget病上皮内的腺癌细胞的AE1/AE3和CAM5.2呈弥漫阳性[346-348]。CK7在肿瘤细胞呈弥漫阳性而在周围正常的鳞状上皮呈阴性，因而更为实用[346, 348-352]。33%～50%的Paget病中共同表达CK7和CK20[346, 348-352]。约66%的CK7+/CK20-的肛门Paget病深部无恶性病变，而90%的CK7+/CK20+的Paget病伴有深部恶性病变，原发恶性肿瘤常位于结肠、直肠或尿路上皮[346, 349, 350, 353]。大多数肛门Paget病细胞CEA和Ber-EP4阳性[346-349]，约50%的GCDFP-15阳性[346, 349, 350, 354]，34βE12和S-100阴性[349, 352]。

> **诊断要点**：肛门恶性肿瘤
>
> 1. 肛门腺癌呈CK7+/CK20-。
> 2. 肛门Paget病细胞多数是CK7+/CK20-。CK7+/CK20+的Paget病细胞通常存在深部恶性病变。

有治疗作用的抗体

表皮生长因子受体（EGFR）：EGFR是酪氨酸激酶受体。EGFR的人单克隆抗体化疗可阻断其作用活性。EGFR呈胞膜和/或胞浆阳性，在浸润最深或转移部位的阳性反应最强且弥漫分布（图 13.43）[355]。在长期储存的组织块制作的切片中，EGFR的阳性强度减弱[356]，可以通过增加抗体的浓度和抗原修复来增强阳性反应。为了确定病人是否适合EGFR抗体化疗，胞膜或胞浆阳性都应认为是阳性。两个或更多肿瘤细胞的反应即是阳性结果。正常的神经束膜表达EGFR，可以作为阳性内对照标志物。

错配修复复合体状态：hMLH1或hMSH2在腺癌细胞核呈阴性可检测错配修复复合体的缺陷，与预后较好的结肠腺癌亚型相关。

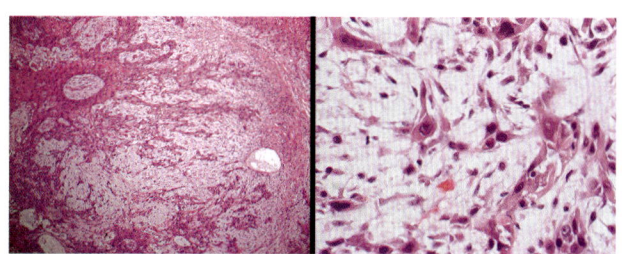

图 13.41　肛门鳞癌伴有梭形细胞（肉瘤样）分化

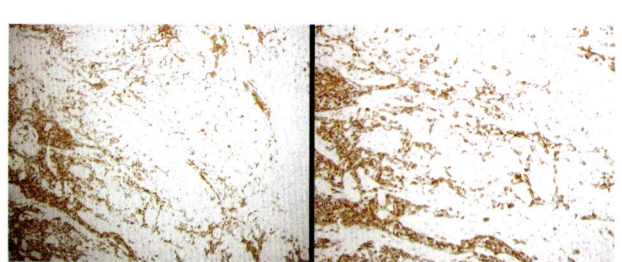

图 13.42　肿瘤的上皮和梭形细胞 CK OSCAR 均呈阳性，其他角蛋白抗体在梭形细胞癌中的阳性强度减弱。因此，OSCAR是梭形细胞和未分化癌首选的角蛋白抗体

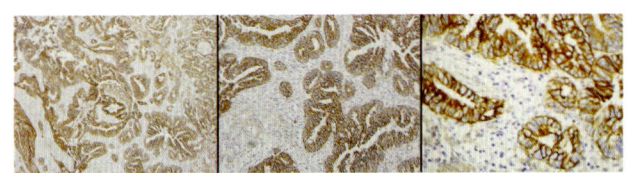

图13.43 图片显示EGFR在结直肠腺癌中较常见的阳性反应类型

胰腺、肝外胆管和胆囊

本部分对胰腺、肝外胆管系统和胆囊的免疫组化进行讨论。胆管腺癌和胰腺导管、肝外胆管以及胆囊黏液性肿瘤的免疫表型高度相似。免疫组化可用于切除标本、芯针活检标本和细针吸取标本。

正常实质细胞

在正常胰腺，腺泡、内分泌和导管细胞表达CK 8、CK18和CK20，导管细胞表达CK7和CK19。正常胰腺组织是许多抗体极好的阳性对照物，包括突触素、嗜铬素、AE1/AE3、CK7、CAM5.2、CK19、Bg8、CEA和CA19-9。

神经内分泌和内分泌细胞肿瘤

低级别胰腺内分泌肿瘤（类癌）、中级别和高级别（小细胞未分化）癌可累及Vater壶腹、胰腺、胆管系统和胆囊[237, 357-360]。根据细胞内或分泌的主要激素对内分泌细胞肿瘤进行免疫组化分类，此分类与肿瘤预后及临床行为有一定关联，但免疫组化在这方面的应用已完全被敏感的血清酶检测取代了。此外，多数胰腺内分泌肿瘤表达不止一种激素和/或激素前体，从而限制了应用免疫组化评估激素表达水平在实际诊断中的作用[361]。

低级别胰腺内分泌肿瘤

低级别胰腺内分泌肿瘤突触素、嗜铬素、蛋白基因产物9.5（PGP9.5）和CD57(Leu7)呈弥漫强阳性[16, 105-107, 230, 233, 238, 361-374]。多数低级别胰腺内分泌肿瘤的CK8、CK18和CAM5.2也呈阳性，约半数肿瘤AE1/AE3和CK19阳性。具有更高级别细胞学特征的肿瘤CK19着色常减弱。CK7和CK20常为阴性或仅极少数细胞阳性[115, 172, 371, 272]。TTF-1、CDX2和HepPar1在胰腺内分泌肿瘤中呈阴性[113, 115, 239, 375]。这些相关的阴性标记可用于小腺泡肿瘤的鉴别诊断（见下文）。肠神经内分泌肿瘤（类癌）和胰腺内分泌肿瘤免疫组化异同见图13.17。

高级别胰腺神经内分泌癌

高级别神经内分泌癌的突触素和嗜铬素的阳性强度和范围均较弱，而CD56和CD57则常呈胞膜强阳性[16, 17, 331, 332]。根据CD56的免疫反应诊断此类肿瘤时应谨慎小心，因为甲状腺滤泡癌和乳头腺癌、肝细胞癌及鳞状细胞癌也呈阳性[331]。高级别胰腺神经内分泌癌降钙素也呈阳性，因而有可能将其误认为甲状腺髓样癌，尤其是发生在肝或肺时[365, 371, 372, 376]。

> **诊断要点：** 胰腺神经内分泌肿瘤
>
> 1. 低级别神经内分泌癌的激素和激素前体免疫组化检测已被血清酶检测取代。
> 2. 高级别神经内分泌肿瘤的突触素和嗜铬素常呈弱阳性，而CD56和CD57通常为胞膜强阳性。由于CD56缺乏特异性，所以不能作为单独诊断依据。

非浸润性肿瘤

导管原位腺癌

目前认为浸润性导管腺癌是由重度非典型增生——胰腺上皮内瘤变（PanIN）进一步发展而来的[377, 387]。原位腺癌属于导管原位腺癌（PanIN-3），恶性上皮细胞局限于上皮内。PanIN-3的细胞角蛋白染色类型与浸润性导管腺癌相似（见下文）。另外，PanIN-3细胞CEA、CA19-9、CA125和CK19阳性[379, 380]，MUC1阳性而MUC2阴性[381]（图13.44）。

导管内乳头状黏液性肿瘤

导管内乳头状黏液性肿瘤（IPMNs）是一组形态特征与黏液囊性肿瘤和导管原位癌明显不同的肿瘤[381-387]。IPMNs几乎总是呈CK7弥漫阳性，CK20、CEA、CA19-9、CA125和CK19阴性[379, 380, 388, 389]。资料显示IPMNs有3种免疫学表型和形态学类型：肠型IPMNs由绒毛状腺瘤型上皮细胞组成，CDX2和MUC2阳性，MUC1阴性；胰腺型MUC1阳性，CDX2和MUC2阴性；第三型为"无表型"，由胃小凹黏液细胞组成，通常3种抗体均呈阴性。IPMNs微卫星稳定，hMLH1、hMSH2和hMSH6抗体呈弥漫阳性[390, 391]。图 13.44 强调了这 3 型非浸润性胰腺肿瘤的免疫表型不同。

黏液囊性肿瘤

黏液性囊腺瘤、黏液性交界性囊腺瘤和非浸润性黏液性囊腺癌的免疫组化相似[389]，CK7几乎均呈弥漫强阳性、CK20大部分阳性（图13.45、13.46），CA125多呈灶性阳性（图 13.47）[176, 253, 392]，CEA 和 CA19-9 弥漫强阳性[388, 392-394]，MUC5AC 和 Dpc4 也呈弥漫强阳性[253, 395]。约10%的肿瘤上皮内偶尔混有内分泌细胞，其分布类似于导管腺癌，这些内分泌细胞可通过嗜铬素或突触素阳性检测出来[396, 397]。这些非浸润性黏液性肿瘤MUC1常为阴性，MUC2在偶尔出现的杯状细胞中阳性。黏液囊性肿瘤和 IPMNs 的免疫表型区别见图 13.44。

卵巢样间质可出现在黏液囊性肿瘤的周围，这些部位的波形蛋白、平滑肌肌动蛋白和肌特异性肌动蛋白常为阳性。约20%~80%（平均33%）的肿瘤中有雌激素受体表达[396, 398, 399]。鞘膜样间质部位的α-抑制素和calretinin 阳性，呈片状分布[400]。CD34 阴性[401]。

浆液性囊腺瘤（微囊性腺瘤）

浆液性囊腺瘤内衬上皮细胞层的 AE1/AE3 和 EMA 呈弥漫强阳性[402-404]。CAM5.2 有部分作者报道呈阴性[402, 403]，部分作者报道呈弥漫阳性。囊肿内衬细胞的CEA、Ⅷ因子或嗜铬素阴性[402, 403, 405]。CA19-9可呈局灶阳性。多数肿瘤MUC1 和 MUC6 阳性[406]。

> **诊断要点**：胰腺黏液肿瘤
> 1. PanIN-3 CK 免疫组化染色与浸润性导管腺癌相似。
> 2. IPMNs 的 CK7+/CK20-、CEA、CA19-9、CA125 和 CK19 阴性。
> 3. 黏液囊性肿瘤的 CK7+/CK20+，CEA、CA19-9、MUC5AC 和 Dpc4 也均呈阳性。

浸润性肿瘤

胰胆管腺癌

胰腺导管腺癌与胆总管、胆囊导管和胆囊腺癌的免疫表型相似，在此作为一组肿瘤讨论[56, 169, 173, 291, 407, 408]。无论是否起源于非浸润性PanIN-3或导管内乳头状/黏液性肿瘤，浸润性腺癌的免疫学表型相似。一些研究发现壶腹腺癌的免疫表型与小肠腺癌相似，而不似胰胆管腺癌（见胃肠部分的相关讨论）[243]。这些部位的组织学差异已有描述。

CK：胰胆管腺癌细胞的 CK8、CK18 和 CK19、35βH11、CAM5.2 及 AE1/AE3 均为阳性[49, 243, 409-413]，CK17也呈弥漫阳性[211, 414]。鳞状分化的部位CK5/6和p63 阳性[52, 54, 415]。

CK7：导管腺癌 CK7 阳性染色形态不一，总的来说，大约90%的胰胆管腺癌呈片状或弥漫阳性（图 13.48、13.49），阳性染色通常很强[165, 168-170, 176, 177, 243, 246, 253, 290, 291, 413-416]。

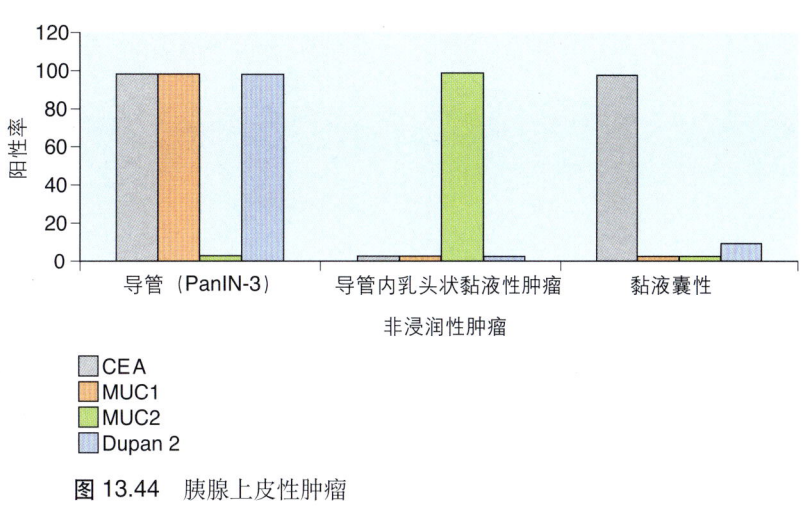

图 13.44　胰腺上皮性肿瘤

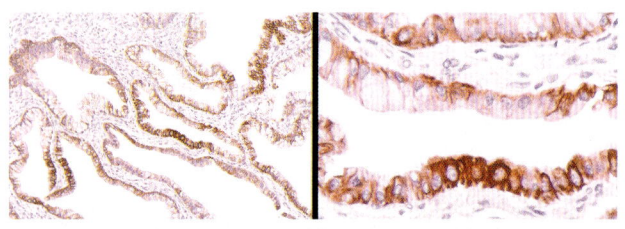

图13.45　胰腺黏液囊性肿瘤CK7呈斑驳片状阳性

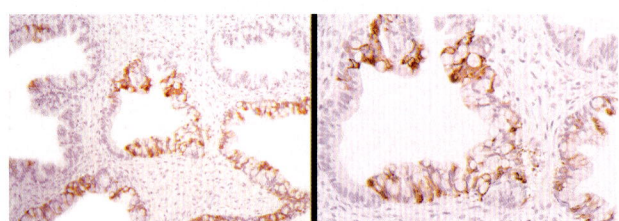

图13.46　与CK7相似，多数胰腺黏液囊性肿瘤的CK20也呈斑驳片状阳性

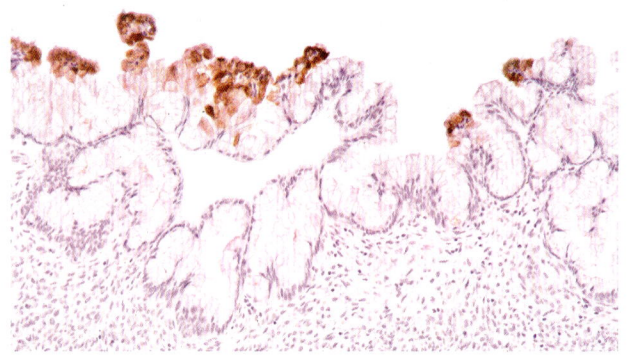

图13.47　黏液囊性肿瘤典型的CA125呈局灶阳性

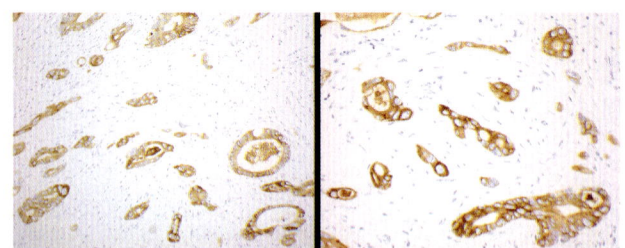

图13.48　在许多浸润性胰腺导管腺癌中可见CK7呈弥漫阳性

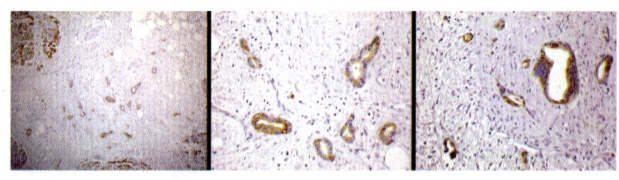

图13.49　CK7在浸润性胰腺导管腺癌中呈不同类型的局灶弱阳性，这种形式也常见于导管内肿瘤

CK20：约50%局灶或广泛阳性（图13.50），其余50%阴性。

CK7/20联合染色类型：文献报道CK7/20的染色结果各不相同。胰胆管腺癌、胃腺癌和尿路上皮癌是最常见的CK7和CK20阳性的肿瘤。胰胆管腺癌中最常见的染色类型是CK7+/CK20+（60%的肿瘤：范围25%～65%），其次是CK7+/CK20−（25%的肿瘤：范围0%～65%），CK7−/CK20−（范围：0%～35%），最后是CK7−/CK20+（范围：0%～10%）[169, 172, 173, 176, 243, 246, 253, 290, 291, 414, 416]。

CDX2：胰胆管腺癌通常呈CDX2阳性。与结肠腺癌相比，胰胆管腺癌的核染色通常较弱，呈斑片状[113, 114, 207, 292, 419]。

CEA：几乎所有的胰胆管腺癌CEA呈阳性。如果肿瘤CEA阴性，则应考虑其他诊断，如转移癌或神经内分泌癌[162, 407-409, 414, 420]。胰腺导管腺癌可有内分泌细胞成分，包括两种肿瘤类型：导管腺癌伴有散在内分泌细胞和由导管和内分泌细胞匀密混合组成的肿瘤。此混合性肿瘤中单一类型细胞的免疫学表型与其各自单纯类型肿瘤细胞相同。其他抗体的免疫反应见表13.4。

> **诊断要点：胰腺癌**
>
> 1. 胰胆管腺癌以CK7+/CK20+为主。
> 2. 胰胆管腺癌的CEA、CDX2和CA19-9呈典型阳性。
> 3. CEA阴性应考虑其他诊断的可能性。

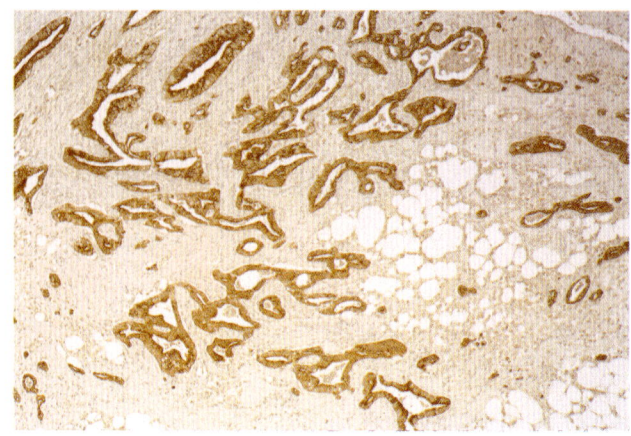

图13.50　胰腺导管腺癌的CK20呈弥漫阳性。背景着色是由于广泛的脂肪坏死和非特异性染色。生物素封闭和过氧化氢处理对减少这种背景着色作用不大

表13.4　胰胆导管腺癌抗体染色

抗体	染色	评价	参考文献
Synaptophysin	S	通常灶性弱阳性	332,628
Chromogranin	S	通常灶性阳性	332,628
CA19.9	+	通常为顶浆及膜阳性，腺腔内无定形碎片均也阳性	338,339,407,408,447,629,630
EMA	+		411,412,420,631,632
CA125	S	男性及女性胰腺癌中大约50%为腔缘胞浆阳性	329,414,633
B72.3	+	通常为顶浆及膜阳性，腺腔内无定形碎片也阳性	630,634
Calretinin	S	阳性染色与使用的抗体高度相关	60,459
AFP	N	典型的导管肿瘤阳性，透明细胞及肝样癌细胞偶尔阳性	162,635
Ber-EP4	+		162,597
ER	N		70,171,182,202,208
PR	N		171,182
PAP	N		636
PSA	N		636,637
Vimentin	N		171,330,410
α-inhibin	N		610
WT-1	N		414
P504s	R	大约10%癌阳性	279
TTF-1	N		214,217,313,548,638-640
Surfactant-A	N		313,318
MUC1	+		165,381,641　44
MUC2	N		165,381,641　44
MUC5AC	+		165,253,641
CA19-9	+		641
Dupan 2	+		641
HepPar1	N		13,14,375,627
Villin	S	大约50%阳性	113
Dpc4/ SMAD4	+		253,645-647
CD5	+		648
CD7	+		648
CK5/6	S	大约50%肿瘤阳性	649
Mesothelin	+		650

+, 通常阳性; S, 有时阳性; R, 偶尔阳性; N, 阴性

鉴别诊断与抗体组合

乳腺导管腺癌与胰胆管腺癌　抗体：CK17、ER、CK20、CDX2

CK17在大部分胰胆管腺癌中呈弥漫强阳性；相反，在多数乳腺导管腺癌中呈阴性，也有极少数的CK17阳性细胞，通常位于实性高级别癌巢的中心。CK20与CK17相似。CDX2在许多胰胆管腺癌中呈阳性，而在乳腺导管腺癌中呈阴性。胰胆管腺癌ER为阴性。

肺腺癌与胰胆管腺癌　抗体：TTF-1、表面活性剂A、CKLO、CA125、CDX2（图13.51）

TTF-1和表面活性剂载脂蛋白A（PE-10）在许多肺腺癌中呈阳性，而在胰胆管腺癌中呈阴性。在胰胆管腺癌中可能呈阳性而在肺腺癌中呈阴性的抗体包括CK20、CA125和CDX2。

苗勒管浆液性乳头状腺癌和胰胆管腺癌　抗体：WT-1、ER、CDX2、CK20、CK17（图13.52）

几乎所有的卵巢和原发的腹膜浆液性乳头状癌的WT-1和ER为阳性。在胰胆管腺癌中可能呈阳性而在浆液性乳头状腺癌中呈阴性的抗体包括CDX2、

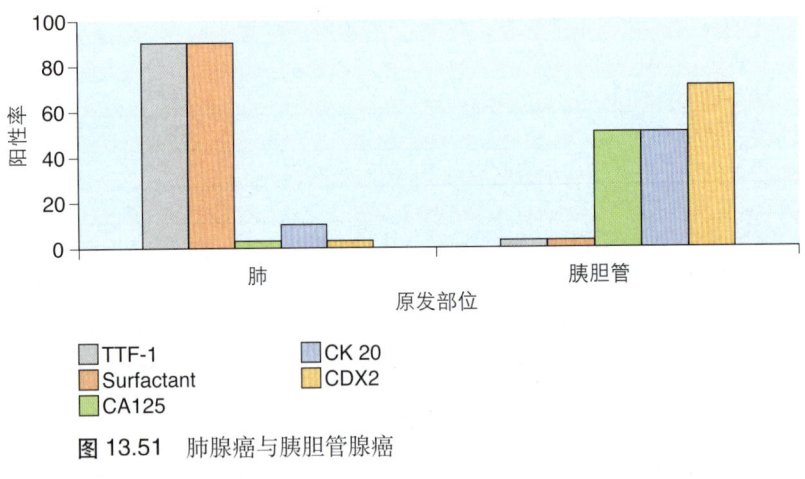

图 13.51 肺腺癌与胰胆管腺癌

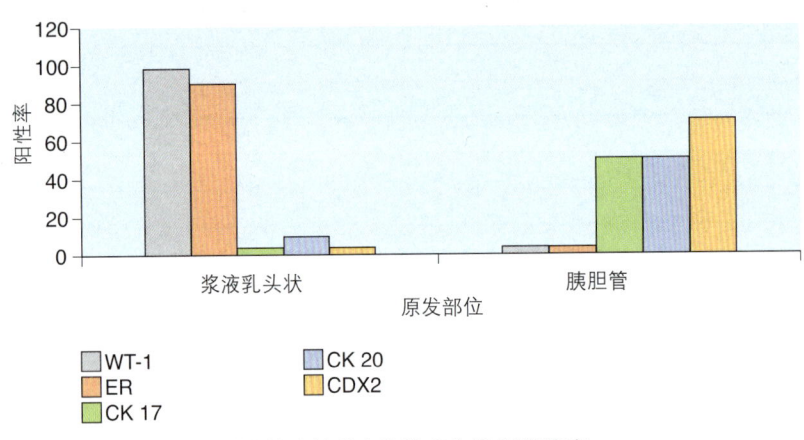

图 13.52 苗勒管浆液性乳头状腺癌和胰胆管腺癌

CK20 和 CK17。

浸润性黏液性腺癌

浸润性黏液性腺癌的CK7和CK20的阳性类型与浸润性导管腺癌相似。与导管腺癌相比，浸润性黏液性腺癌CA125和MUC1阴性，MUC2阳性[388, 396, 400, 421, 422]。浸润性黏液性腺癌微卫星稳定，因此 hMLH1、hMSH2 和 hMSH6 抗体呈弥漫阳性[423]。

未分化的、多形性和巨细胞肿瘤

未分化及多形性癌是分化较差的癌，它们常与腺癌和鳞癌混合存在，或者表现为黏液囊性肿瘤壁上的结节。在这些肿瘤细胞中阳性反应最强、分布最弥漫的抗体是单克隆广谱细胞角蛋白 OSCAR。而 AE1/AE3、CAM5.2、35βH11、CK8和CK18的阳性强度较弱，并呈斑片状[410, 424-429]，CK7和CK19通常呈局灶强阳性。如果要证实肿瘤为癌，建议使用一系列角蛋白，EMA和CEA通常呈阴性[424, 426, 430-433]。多数未分化癌（肉瘤样）和多形性癌肿瘤细胞波形蛋白呈弥漫强阳性[410, 426, 431-433]，HMB-45、MART-1或酪氨酸酶阴性。多核、分叶状多形性巨细胞出现在高级别多形性癌。

横纹肌样细胞可为一种多形性癌的亚型，或者偶见于去分化高级别神经内分泌癌[434]。横纹肌样未分化癌细胞的角蛋白 OSCAR 阳性反应最强，CAM5.2或AE1/AE3的阳性强度较弱。除了出现细胞角蛋白，作为中间丝的重要成分，波形蛋白呈典型的核周旋涡状染色[435, 436]。

破骨细胞样巨细胞最常见于高级别或未分化癌的间质成分，偶尔混有多核的多叶核巨癌细胞，也可见于黏液囊性肿瘤未分化癌的囊壁结节[425, 431, 437, 438]。这些细胞与骨巨细胞瘤中形态相似的细胞免疫表型相同[437, 439]。作为间质细胞，其CD68、CD45(LCA)、CD71、α-抗胰凝乳蛋白酶和波形蛋白阳性，EMA、细胞角蛋白或溶菌酶阴性[431, 433]。

> **诊断要点**：高级别胰腺癌
>
> 1. 建议使用一组角蛋白抗体来鉴别多形性或未分化胰腺癌的癌分化，包括CK7、CK8、CK18、CK19、AE1/AE3、OSCAR、CAM5.2和35βH11。
> 2. 横纹肌样和破骨细胞样巨细胞可出现在分化差的胰腺癌中，与其他类型肿瘤中形态相同细胞的免疫组化染色相似。

腺泡细胞癌

腺泡细胞癌形态上一般与胰腺神经内分泌肿瘤相似。大部分腺泡细胞癌的AE1/AE3、CAM5.2、CK7、CK8、CK16和CK19阳性，CK7常常是胞膜阳性，而其他的角蛋白抗体通常是胞浆弥漫阳性（图13.53、13.54）。CK AE1/AE3阳性细胞少于CAM5.2[410, 440-442]。腺泡细胞癌免疫组化淀粉酶、胰蛋白酶和α-抗胰凝乳蛋白酶阳性[390, 441, 443-446]。虽然突触素在10%~50%的肿瘤中呈阳性，但嗜铬素和CEA呈阴性[440, 444, 445, 447-449]。波形蛋白和AFP通常也呈阴性[410]。

腺泡/内分泌混合性肿瘤是由腺泡细胞和内分泌细胞紧密混合组成的。混合肿瘤的单一类型细胞的免疫学表型都与各自单纯肿瘤同类型细胞相同。

胰腺囊实性（乳头状）肿瘤

α-1-抗胰蛋白酶和波形蛋白是报道最一致的抗体，在肿瘤中呈弥漫强阳性[450, 451]。在33%~66%的肿瘤中的少数细胞细胞角蛋白 AE1/AE3 和 CK20 呈阳性。在更少的肿瘤（5%~20%）中，细胞角蛋白CAM5.2、CK7、CK8、CK18和CK19呈阳性[410, 452]。由于β-连环蛋白基因突变导致β-连环蛋白抗体在细胞核的强阳性反应，为此肿瘤的特征性表现[453]。在大部分已报道的肿瘤中，缺乏明确的神经内分泌颗粒。尽管33%~50%的肿瘤突触素呈弥漫阳性，但在报道的病例中嗜铬素阳性不到5%（图13.55）[450, 454, 455]。约20%的肿瘤雌激素受体呈弥漫阳性[450, 451]。据报道有些病例孕激素受体呈广泛阳性[456, 457]。肿瘤的EMA[450, 458]、calretinin[459]、AFP[4450]、CEA、CA19-9[440, 450, 456]或S-100[450]阴性。

微腺泡肿瘤和实性肿瘤的鉴别诊断　见表13.5。

具有实性或微腺泡结构的肿瘤包括神经内分泌癌、胰胆管腺癌、腺泡癌和囊实性（乳头状）癌[447, 460]。

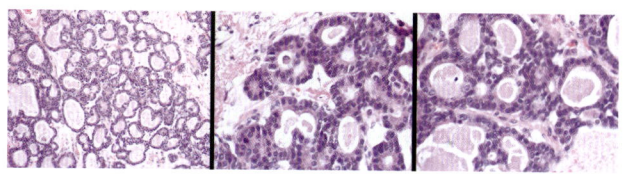

图13.53　腺泡细胞癌。此类肿瘤形态上与低级别内分泌肿瘤和一些导管腺癌相似

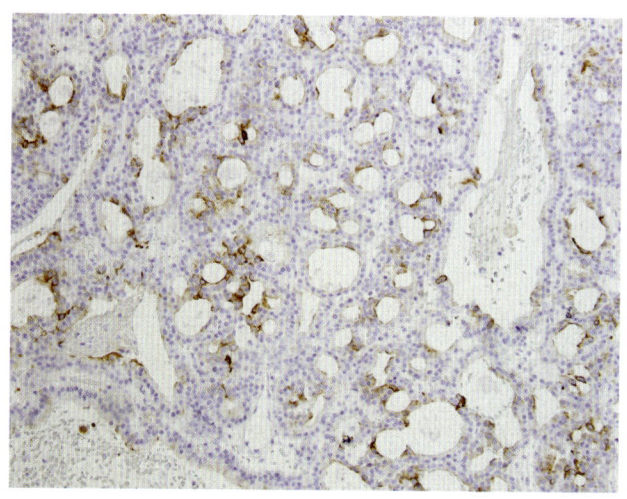

图13.54　与前面提到的肿瘤中CK7呈胞浆和/或核周点状染色不同，腺泡癌细胞的CK7呈典型的胞膜染色

与本组任何肿瘤不同，神经内分泌癌的神经内分泌抗体突触素、嗜铬素、CD56和CD57呈弥漫强阳性。虽然囊实性（乳头状）瘤偶呈突触素阳性，但嗜铬素或其他神经内分泌标志呈阴性。CK7、CEA、CA19-9、EMA、CAM5.2和CK19在导管腺癌中呈阳性，而在囊实性（乳头状）瘤中呈阴性，这对区分囊实性（乳头状）癌和胰胆管腺癌很有意义。腺泡细胞癌的脂肪酶呈阳性，可以与囊实性（乳头状）瘤鉴别，然而由于许多实验室没有这种抗体，而波形蛋白在囊实性（乳头状）瘤中呈弥漫强阳性，因此可作为鉴别诊断抗体。

> **诊断要点**：胰腺肿瘤的鉴别
>
> 1. 神经内分泌标志，突触素、嗜铬素、CD56和CD57可用于神经内分泌癌与其他肿瘤包括胰腺实性和微腺泡瘤的鉴别诊断。
> 2. CK7、CEA、CA19-9、EMA、CAM5.2和CK19在导管腺癌中呈阳性，在囊实性（乳头状）瘤中呈阴性。
> 3. 腺泡细胞癌的脂肪酶呈阳性是其特征。
> 4. 囊实性（乳头状）瘤的波形蛋白呈弥漫强阳性。

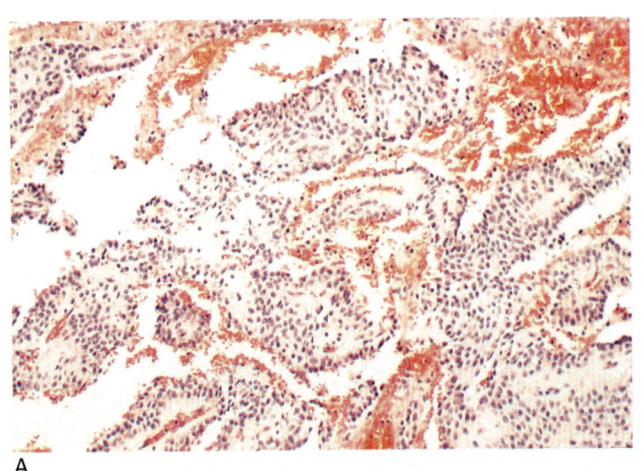
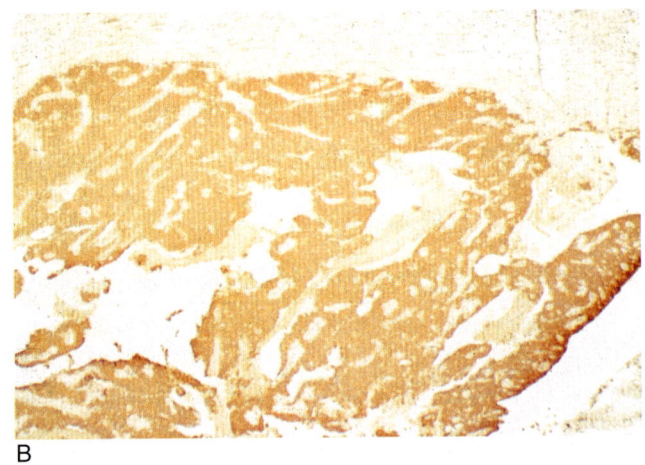

图 13.55 （A）胰腺囊实性肿瘤；（B）此类肿瘤突触素常呈弥漫阳性反应

表13.5 微腺泡癌免疫组化鉴别诊断

抗体	肿瘤			
	神经内分泌	胰胆管	腺泡	囊实性（乳头状）
Synaptophysin	+	S	N	S
Chromogranin	+	S	N	R
CD56	+	N	N	N
CD57	+	N	N	N
Alpha-1-anti-chymotrypsin	R	R	+	+
Lipase	N	N	+	N
CK7	R	+	S	R
CK19	S	+	S	R
EMA	N	+	R	N
CEA	R	+	R	N
CA 19-9	S	+	S	N
Vimentin	R	N	N	+

+，阳性；S，有时阳性；R，偶尔阳性；N，阴性

透明细胞和肝样肿瘤

透明细胞癌在胰腺、肝外导管和胆囊中已描述过[461]。这一部分肿瘤包括富含糖原的典型导管腺癌、卵黄囊样癌、肝样癌和血管周上皮样细胞瘤[409, 461-463]。用于透明细胞肿瘤鉴别诊断的抗体组分别在各自的章节中讨论。

血管周上皮样细胞瘤

血管周上皮样细胞瘤（PEComas）常由透明细胞组成，可发生在胰腺内及其周围。这些肿瘤形态上常与胰腺的内分泌肿瘤、透明细胞癌和胃肠间质瘤相似[464]。虽然细胞具有上皮样特征，但角蛋白AE1/AE3或CAM5.2、嗜铬素或脂肪酶呈阴性。与其他器官的糖瘤相同，其肌动蛋白和HMB-45呈阳性[465]，Myo-D1也呈弥漫胞浆阳性[466]。

肝和胰外胆管

正常组织结构及良性病变

肝细胞

生物素：肝细胞含有丰富的生物素，可产生强烈的非特异性着色[467-472]，抗原修复后更加明显[473]。故如果应用基于生物素的染色系统，需应用一抗前先行阻断内源性肝细胞生物素。

细胞角蛋白：胚胎肝细胞含有CK8、CK18和

CK19。妊娠第10周CK19表达消失。成熟的肝细胞只含有CK8和CK18，并呈弥漫强阳性。CAM5.2和35βH11[474-479]：CAM5.2 在门静脉周围、腺泡1区和直接围绕在终末及肝下小静脉周围的薄层肝细胞内阳性反应最强[475]。CK7、CK19、CK20和34βE12呈阴性[56, 475, 476, 478-482]。

HepPar1：HepPar1在肝细胞中呈粗颗粒状、胞浆阳性，不伴有腔缘着色增强[12, 480, 483]。

其他抗体：TTF-1呈特征性的粗颗粒状胞浆强阳性，但肝细胞核呈阴性[483]。多克隆CEA在正常肝细胞腔缘呈薄层膜着色。正常肝细胞的AFP呈阴性。

肝内胆管与胆管周围腺体

细胞角蛋白：肝内胆管上皮细胞的CK7、CK8、CK18、CK19、AE1/AE3、35βH11和34βE12呈弥漫强阳性（图13.56）[475-477, 479, 480]。CD20阴性[56]。

其他抗体：CA19-9 和 CEA 阴性[484]。

肝窦内皮细胞

正常肝的窦内皮细胞与正常动脉和静脉的内皮细胞不同，其大部分呈CD34、Ⅷ因子、CD31或Ulex阴性。

内科性疾病

慢性胆道及胆小管梗阻

慢性胆道梗阻（不考虑病因）表现为与汇管区直接相邻的实质内或汇管区周围小胆管内的立方形肝细胞样细胞增殖，称为增生的胆小管（图 13.57）[485]，是由正常存在和/或组成小管的干细胞增殖而来，连接胆管与Hering管[482, 485-487]。不管其小管形态如何，均表达胆管上皮型角蛋白或具有胆管上皮细胞和肝细胞的免疫表型特征[487-490]。

原发性胆汁性肝硬化与硬化性胆管炎

虽然这两种疾病的病理过程不同，但在穿刺活检诊断上它们有相似的问题。门脉炎症，增生挤压胆管管腔使其模糊不清，难以区分胆管和增殖的胆小管（图13.57）。两种疾病的汇管区都可有旺炽性胆小管增殖，缺乏胆管。这种情况下CK7有助于鉴别，因为CK7在胆管中呈强阳性，而在邻近肝动脉无胆管的部位呈阴性[491]。在这两种疾病中，胆管周血管丛围绕在中等及大的小叶间胆管周围，可见有损伤

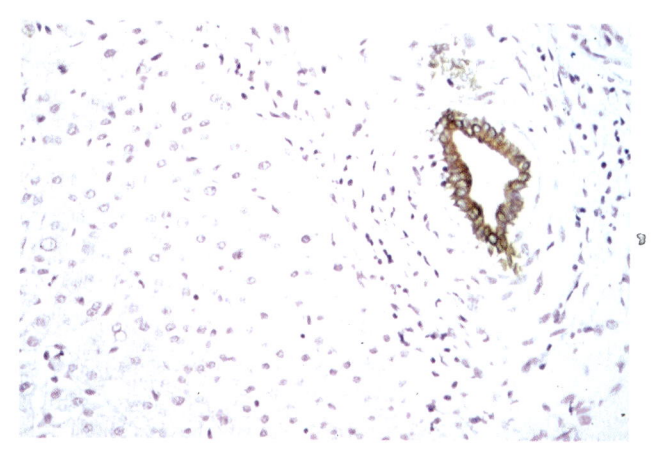

图13.56　良性病变或正常胆管的CK7呈强阳性

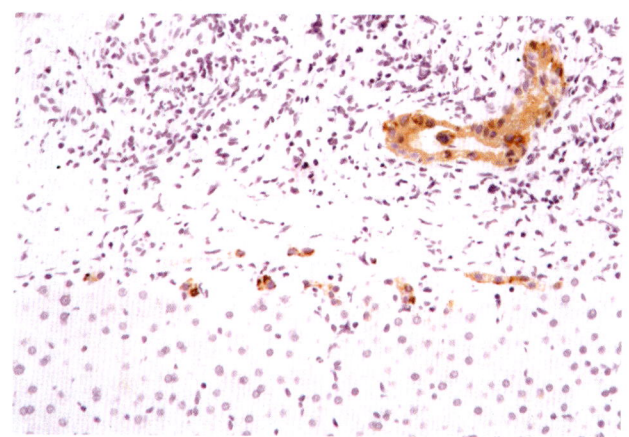

图13.57　CK7有助于确定和评价在原发性胆汁性肝硬化中胆管损伤的程度。沿汇管区周围实质分布的反应性增生的胆小管，CK7也呈阳性

或丢失。两种疾病血管损伤的类型不同，在硬化性胆管炎（PSC），同心环状的胶原将管周毛细血管与导管基底膜分离，数量通常只有轻度减少；而在原发性胆汁性肝硬化（PBC），导管周围的毛细血管的解剖部位正常，但由于围管性炎症导致毛细血管密度显著降低。用CD31或CD34显示血管的结构有助于确定这两种疾病的不同类型[492]。

肝硬化与局灶性结节性增生

肝硬化再生性结节周围的肝细胞常表达胆管型细胞角蛋白，CK7和CK19呈阳性[481]，这种阳性也见于结节状再生性增生[476]。有些作者认为肝细胞表达CK7和CK19意味着其为干细胞表型，或出现胆管和肝细胞双重分化，与在慢性胆道梗阻汇管区周围增殖细胞中的所见相同[493-497]。在这种肝细胞中免疫组化AFP呈阳性亦支持该理论[498, 499]。二者邻近纤维间隔

的窦内皮细胞与正常窦内皮相比免疫表型也发生了变化，其 CD31 和 CD34 呈阳性[500]。

灶性结节性增生 FNH 的肝硬化样结节周围的肝细胞 CK7 和 CK19 也呈阳性。一些 CK7 阳性的细胞是纤维间隔内导管结构的延续[477, 494]。与结节性再生性增生一样，FNH 病变的窦内皮细胞也呈周围毛细血管型免疫表型，CD31 和 CD34 阳性[500]。

脂肪肝与 Mallory 小体

Mallory 小体（MBs）是胞浆内聚集的异常细胞角蛋白中间丝（图 13.58）[495, 501]。大部分 Mallory 小体是由高和低分子量中间丝碎片组成，CK 34βE12、CK18、CK19 和 CAM5.2 阳性。

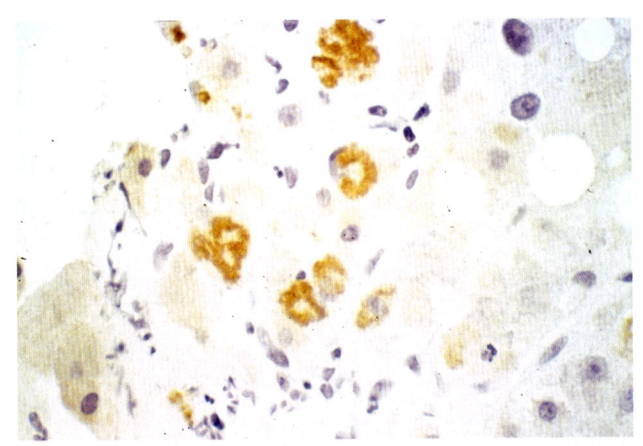

图 13.58 Mallory 小体由异常角蛋白碎片组成，典型的 AE1/AE3 阳性反应最强

> **诊断要点**：非肿瘤性肝的免疫组化
> 1. 出现在慢性胆管梗阻、FNH 结节周围和再生性结节性增生中的肝细胞样或胆管样细胞的增生，可表现为混合性免疫表型。
> 2. 在门脉致密炎症背景下，CK7 有助于鉴别胆管和活动性胆管损伤。
> 3. CD31 或 CD34 可以突出显示血管结构，有助于鉴别门系胆管周围血管丛在原发性胆汁性肝硬化和硬化性胆管炎中的不同改变。

良性肝肿瘤

肝细胞腺瘤

构成腺瘤的肝细胞与正常的、非肝硬化的肝细胞免疫组化谱相同[477]。CD34（Q Bend 10）是区分腺瘤和肝细胞癌（HCC）的辅助抗体，在腺瘤的正常肝窦内皮细胞中 CD34 呈阴性，而在 HCC 的内皮细胞中呈阳性[205]。

胆管（胆管周）错构瘤和腺瘤

这两种病变中构成胆管的细胞的免疫表型与正常胆管相同，CK7 和 CK19 呈弥漫阳性。

恶性肝肿瘤

肝母细胞瘤

肝母细胞瘤能向上皮、间质/间叶、内分泌、黑色素细胞和神经系分化[485, 487, 503]。按照形态学标准，伴有肝分化的细胞可以分类为胚胎型、胎儿型、小细胞型或间变型[485]。肝母细胞瘤对多种抗体呈阳性染色。大约 50% 的胚胎型或胎儿型癌细胞的嗜铬素呈阳性，约 75% 的 AFP 呈阳性，广谱的低分子量和高分子量 CK 阳性[504, 505]。与 HCC 不同，约 75% 的肝母细胞瘤的波形蛋白呈阳性。

一般型肝细胞癌

最初认为肝细胞癌（HCC）和胆管癌（CC）的免疫学表型分别与良性肝细胞和肝内胆管上皮相同[474, 506]。现在认识到，这两种癌常表现为异常免疫表型分化，但不能因此而改变诊断。

相关抗体 见表 13.6。

CK：HCC 细胞主要含有低分子量 CK8 和 CK18，高分子量 CK 很少[476, 477, 507, 508]。因此，CAM5.2[162, 411, 478, 509, 510]、OSCAR 和 35βH11[411, 478, 479, 481] 呈阳性，通常是胞膜和胞浆弥漫阳性[511]。

CK AE1/AE3：约 20% 的 HCC AE1/AE3 为阳性，多为弱阳性[412, 512, 513]。HCC 中 AE1/AE3 的表达状况与肿瘤级别相关。分化好者 AE1/AE3 呈斑片状阳性，而在分化差者仅有 33% 呈阳性（图 13.59）[412]。在中度分化和分化差的肿瘤中，阳性反应发生在孤立的细胞或散在簇状细胞，因而可形成不同的组织学形态，包括腺泡状结构[513]。

CK7：总体上，约 15%（范围 0%~25%）的 HCC CK7 呈阳性[173, 265, 476, 514, 515]，50% 的 HCC CK7 阴性，30% 有局灶阳性，10%~20% 的 HCC 有不到 50% 的细胞着色，0%~5% 的 HCC 阳性细胞多于 50%（图 13.60）[265, 516]。CK7 阳性程度也与 HCC 的级别有关，

表13.6　肝细胞癌抗体染色

抗体	染色	评价	参考文献
34βE12	N	偶尔细胞呈弱阳性	1,479,481
CK17	N		211
CA19-9	N		265,338,339,481,517,520
CA125	R	大约10%肝细胞癌阳性	329
Vimentin	R	大约5%肝细胞癌阳性，通常仅见于高级别（Ⅲ级）肿瘤	330,478,481,516,525,526
Calretinin	N		459
CD56	+	大多数肝细胞癌呈弱阳性	331
CD57	R	3%~15%肝细胞癌阳性	162,521
Synaptophysin	R	大约5%呈灶性阳性	511,651,652
Chromogranin	R	大约5%呈灶性阳性	651,652
Inhibin	N	如果不能很好地封闭生物素，可呈广泛假阳性	471,519,543
Melan-A (A103)	N		543
Factor XⅢa	S		480,481,521
EMA	+	高级别（Ⅲ级）肿瘤染色增强	411,412,478,520,592
Ber-EP4	S	高级别（Ⅲ级）肿瘤染色增强	162
MOC-31	N		519,522,653,654
CK5/6	N		649
ER	N		182
PR	R		182

+, 阳性; S, 有时阳性; R, 偶尔阳性; N, 阴性

分化差的 HCC 中阳性细胞数最多[477, 508, 514]。

CK20：HCC 约 20%CK20 阳性（范围：10%~30%）[172, 173, 265, 480]，呈斑片状弱阳性[56]。约 80%CK20 呈阴性，15%呈灶状阳性，5%的 HCC 阳性细胞不到 50%[265, 480]。

CK7/20 联合染色：约 75% 的 HCC 呈 CK7-/CK20-，15%呈 CK7+/CK20-，5%呈 CK7+/CK20+，没有 CK7-/CK20+ 类型[173]。

CK19：CK19染色类似CK7。约10%的HCC CK19 阳性，通常呈斑片状[265, 476, 478, 515, 517-519]。多数阳性病例仅表现为恶性肝细胞的局灶阳性[265]。少数研究报道阳性率达 30%~100%[480, 513, 514, 520]（与 CK7 相似，CK19 阳性程度与 HCC 分级相关[514, 520]）。

CEA（单克隆）：几乎所有的研究都报道在不到 5%的HCC中单克隆CEA呈阳性（范围：0%~5%），表现为明显的斑片状染色[162, 265, 412, 481, 511, 519, 521]。

CEA（多克隆）：与单克隆 CEA 相反，HCC 中多克隆CEA常为阳性，总阳性率约70%（范围：60%~95%），可为丛管状或胞浆弥漫型染色[4]。多克隆 CEA 的丛管状染色对HCC是特异性的，在其他腺癌中尚未观察到此种染色形式（见其后鉴别诊断）。总体上，约 40%~80% 的 HCC 表现为丛管状染色类型[162, 481, 509, 518-520, 522]。多克隆 CEA 的丛管状阳性与HCC的分级呈负相关，在分化好的HCC中75%呈多克隆CEA丛管状阳性，中分化HCC为70%阳性，分化差的为 25%~50% 阳性（图 13.61）[162, 412, 511, 518]。约 50% 的 HCC 为多克隆 CEA 胞浆弥漫阳性[162]。

肝细胞癌的 CD10 也呈丛管状阳性，与多克隆CEA相似。大部分非肝细胞癌为阴性，即使阳性也不表现为丛管状阳性类型[13, 519, 522, 523]。

AFP：HCC约50%AFP呈阳性，报道的阳性范围是 20%~75%[13, 162, 265, 481, 483, 509, 511, 513, 519-521, 524, 525]。阳性反应与肿瘤级别呈负相关。只有 5%~20% 的 3 级 HCC AFP 呈阳性[162, 520, 526]。

HepPar1：HCC约80%~100%HepPar1抗体呈阳性（范围：40%~100%）。通常为中到强弥漫阳性，但偶尔会出现阴性区域（图 13.62）[13-15, 193, 194, 375, 480, 483, 511, 513, 519, 522, 527]。阳性染色为胞浆内大量小囊泡[511]。阳性反应的分布与 HCC 的分级无关[480]。与 AFP 相比，HepPar1 敏感性和特异性更强。

CD34 和 CD31：虽然肝细胞（良性或恶性）的 CD34和CD31呈阴性，但这两种抗体可作为鉴别HCC 的辅助抗体，并且有助于区别 HCC 与肝细胞腺瘤、局灶性结节性增生和再生性肝硬化结节[502, 528-531]。HCC的细胞索、小梁和腺泡被环形的内皮细胞层包绕，该细胞层呈 CD34 或 CD31 阳性，即使窦状结构

不清仍可染色（图13.63）。环绕良性肝病灶的窦内皮细胞 CD34 和 CD31 呈阴性[500, 529, 531, 532]，据此认为内皮细胞可从窦内向末梢毛细血管型内皮细胞转化[532]。CD34 在围绕 HCC 的窦内皮细胞中阳性反应最强[500, 528]。邻近转移癌结节的窦内皮细胞也发生了末梢毛细血管化，与其内皮细胞表达 CD34 相符。然而，转移癌中的各个癌巢并没有环形内皮细胞层的包绕[533]。

肝细胞癌的胆管型分化

在形态不典型的 HCC 中，胆管型分化细胞角蛋白 AE1/AE3、CK7、CK19、单克隆 CEA 呈阳性，以上任何一种抗体阳性在形态不典型的 HCC 的发生率约30%。我们和其他学者均认为仅有局部阳性不能将形态不典型的 HCC 认为是 HCC-CC 混合肿瘤。我们在免疫组化上将 HCC-CC 混合肿瘤限定于伴以上抗体阳性的形态学上的 HCC-CC 混合肿瘤。同时也包括既不具有 HCC 或 CC 明确形态特征但有二者免疫表型的Ⅲ级未分化癌。

> **诊断要点**：肝细胞癌
>
> 1. HCC 主要表现为低分子量 CK8 和 CK18、CAM5.2、OSCAR 和 35βH11 阳性，仅少数 AE1/AE3 呈弱阳性。
> 2. HCC 通常呈 CK7 阴性，CK20 阴性。
> 3. 多克隆 CEA 的丛管状染色是 HCC 特异性的，阳性反应随着肿瘤级别的增高而减弱。在高级别 HCC 中，弥漫性胞浆多克隆 CEA 染色反应增强。
> 4. 对于 HCC，HepPar1 比 AFP 更具敏感性和特异性。

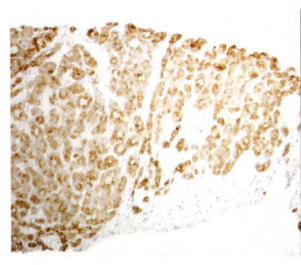
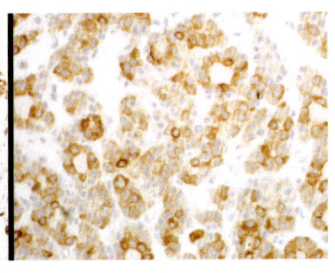

图13.59 肝细胞癌。低倍镜下（左图），肿瘤表现为AE1/AE3弥漫强阳性。然而，在高倍镜下（右图），可见许多肿瘤细胞呈阴性

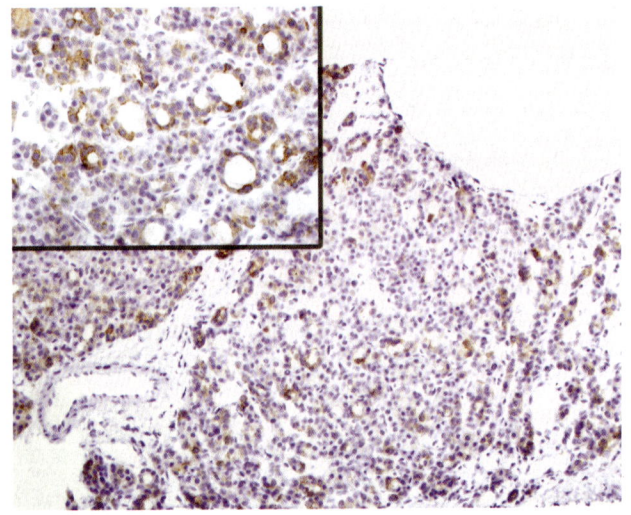

图13.60 另一个典型低级别肝细胞癌，CK7呈局灶阳性。不能因此认为是胆管分化或混合性肝癌

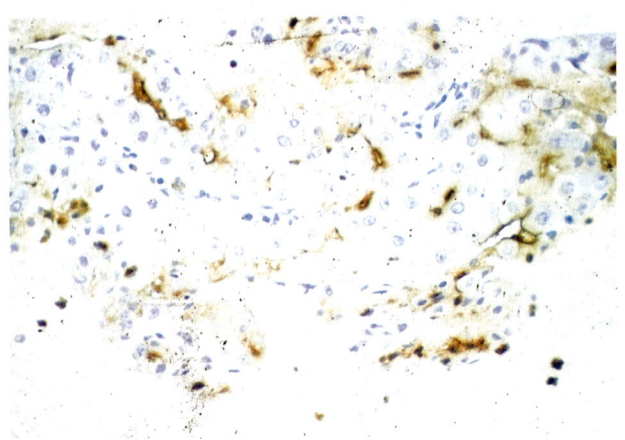

图13.61 肝细胞癌的多克隆 CEA 染色，呈丛管状阳性

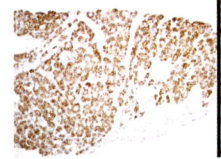
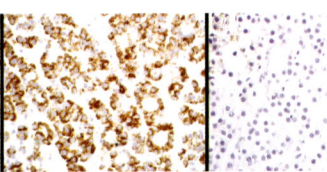

图13.62 肝细胞癌的HepPar1染色。大部分肿瘤细胞呈粗颗粒状强阳性（左图和中间图）。但在阳性细胞区之间常有灶状或片状阴性区（右图）

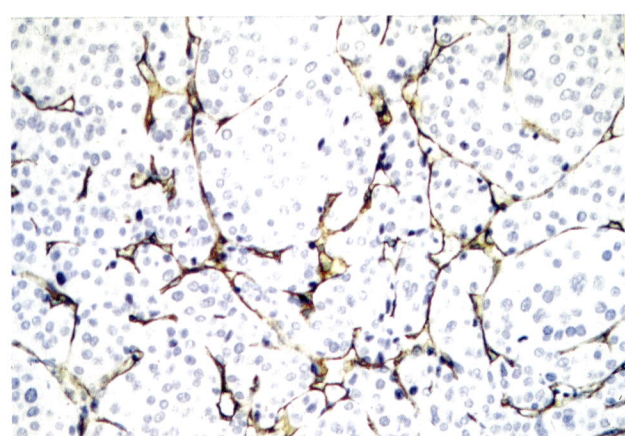

图13.63 肝细胞癌的小梁和腺泡被 CD34 阳性的环形内皮细胞层包绕。正常的肝窦内皮细胞 CD34 阴性

肝细胞癌变型

梭形细胞肝细胞癌

高级别肝细胞癌偶尔可出现梭形细胞HCC成分[516, 525]。免疫表型除梭形细胞波形蛋白阳性外，与一般型Ⅲ级上皮样HCC相似。梭形细胞HCC波形蛋白通常呈阳性，而Ⅲ级上皮样HCC为阴性。约50%的病例恶性梭形细胞呈CAM5.2和波形蛋白共表达，为该形态肿瘤的特征。与Ⅲ级上皮样HCC一样，大部分梭形细胞HCC呈HepPar1阳性，AFP阴性。梭形细胞的形态与免疫组化检测E-钙黏素丢失相关。

纤维板层肝细胞癌

纤维板层HCC与一般型HCC相似之处包括CAM5.2（CK8和18）和HepPar1呈阳性，CK19呈局灶阳性[12, 535]。与一般型HCC不同之处为纤维板层HCC的CK7[535]和A1AT[500, 502, 529, 533, 536]呈弥漫强阳性。纤维板层HCC和一般型HCC的免疫组化区别见图13.64。AFP在约20%的纤维板层型中呈阳性[536-542]。在一般型与纤维板层HCC混合性肿瘤中，AFP在纤维板层区域缺乏染色，而在一般型HCC区则有较强染色。偶尔在纤维板层HCC的胞浆中可见到嗜酸性大颗粒（透明小体），呈白蛋白抗体阳性，A1AT和AFP阴性。尽管纤维板层HCC预后较好，但其基质抗原谱与临床上侵袭性HCC相似。伴有突触素阳性的神经内分泌分化偶尔可出现于纤维板层HCC[467]。

> **诊断要点**：肝细胞癌变型
>
> 1. CAM5.2和波形蛋白共表达是梭形细胞HCC变型的特征。
> 2. 除了CK7呈弥漫阳性和A1AT呈局灶阳性以外，HCC的纤维板层型与一般型HCC的免疫表型相似。

鉴别诊断与抗体组合

肝细胞癌与肾细胞癌　抗体：HepPar1、AFP、CK7、波形蛋白

转移性肾细胞癌，尤其是由嗜酸细胞构成的，可能与HCC很难区别。低级别HCC可通过HepPar1和AFP呈阳性而与肾细胞癌区分，高级别HCC则可用HepPar1和CK7阳性与肾细胞癌区别。肾细胞癌（RCC）可通过波形蛋白阳性来确定。但依靠HepPar1鉴别诊断时应慎重，在含有大量胞浆溶酶体的肾细胞中HepPar1呈胞浆粗颗粒状阳性，与HCC细胞中真正的阳性反应相似，在这种情况下，必须检查阴性对照切片。HCC和RCC的CD10均呈阳性。

肝细胞癌与肾上腺癌　抗体：HepPar1、抑制素、melan-A（A103）、CAM5.2（图13.65）

HCC的CAM5.2和HepPar1阳性，抑制素和melan-A阴性[543]。相反，约60%的肾上腺癌抑制素和melan-A阳性，HepPar1阴性[543, 544]。肾上腺癌也表现微弱的CAM5.2染色[478]。

肝细胞癌与神经内分泌癌　抗体：AE1/AE3、CAM5.2、HepPar1、AFP、嗜铬素、突触素、CD57、CEA（单克隆）、TTF-1

有些HCC的肿瘤细胞很小，类似原发或转移的神经内分泌癌，包括低级别类癌和高级别小细胞癌。此HCC变型称为"小细胞HCC"。小细胞HCC的免疫组化表现与一般型HCC相同，AE1/AE3、CAM5.2（无核周小点）和HepPar1呈胞浆弥漫阳性，有时AFP也呈阳性。神经内分泌相关抗体，包括CD57、嗜铬素和突触素呈阴性。

肝原发性或转移性神经内分泌癌（类癌——小细胞神经内分泌癌）的突触素、嗜铬素和CD57（Leu7）阳性，HepPar1和AFP阴性[12, 16, 17, 105-107, 230, 233, 238, 332, 361-369, 521, 545-547]。高级别神经内分泌癌的AE1/AE3或CAM5.2呈典型的核周点状阳性[369, 410]。转移的肺和前肠神经内分泌癌，以及肝原发的神经内分泌肿瘤，单克隆CEA和TTF-1呈阳性，而在HCC中都呈阴性[548]。因为CD56（NCAM, Leu19）在HCC中也可能为阳性，故不能用来区别这两种肿瘤。

胆管癌

胆管癌（CC）的免疫表型与肝外胰胆管腺癌相似[476]，但也有一些细微的差别。CC中CK17和20、Dpc4/SMAD以及p53的表达少于胰胆管腺癌，而CK7的表达多于胰胆管腺癌[284, 291, 514, 549]。

细胞角蛋白：CC细胞主要含低分子量CK和少量高分子量CK，包括CK7、CK8、CK18和CK19[474, 479, 506, 507, 510, 518]。细胞角蛋白AE1/AE3、CAM5.2和35βH11通常为强阳性[162, 412, 481, 509-511]。

CK 7：几乎所有CC其CK7都呈阳性（范围：

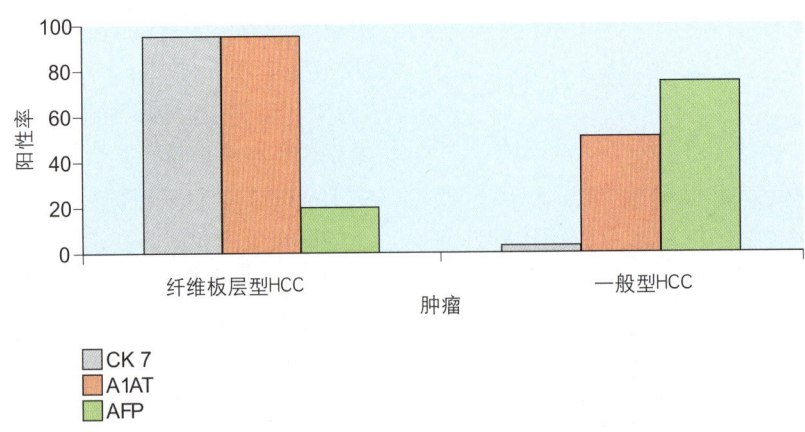

图 13.64 纤维板层型与一般型肝细胞癌

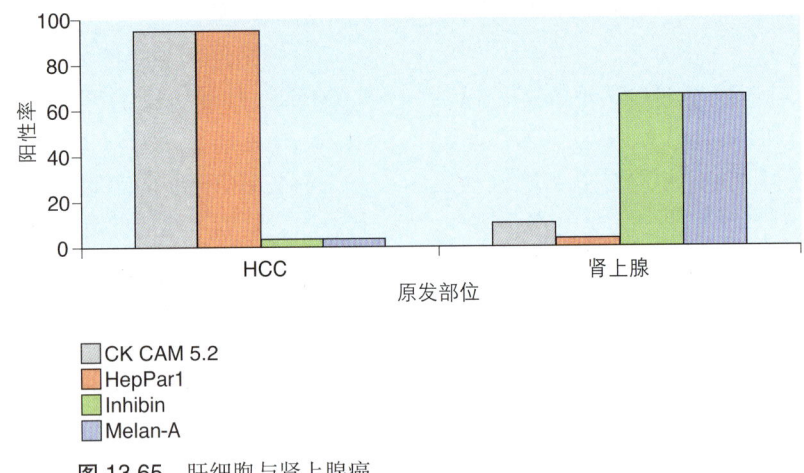

图 13.65 肝细胞与肾上腺癌

80%~100%)（图13.66）[265, 284, 416, 476, 515, 517, 550]。

CK20：约20%的CC其CK20呈阳性（范围：5%~50%)[172, 243, 265, 284, 480, 550]。

CK7/CK20联合染色：约75%的CC呈CK7+/CK20-，20%呈CK7+/CK20+，剩余的5%呈CK7-/CK20-或CK7-/CK20+[284, 416]。

CK17：50%的CC呈CK17阳性，从散在、单个细胞到弥漫阳性[211]，与其不同，几乎90%的肝外胰胆管腺癌呈阳性[211]。

CK19：约98%的CC CK19呈阳性（范围：85%~100%)[265, 284, 476, 480, 481, 511, 514, 517, 518, 520, 550]。

CEA（单克隆）：约60%~90%的CC单克隆CEA呈阳性[162, 265, 412, 481, 511, 521, 551]。

CEA（多克隆）：85%~100%的CC多克隆CEA呈弥漫强阳性[162, 412, 509, 511, 518, 520, 522, 526, 552]。

CA19-9：约90%的CC CA19-9呈阳性[265, 338, 339, 481, 484, 520, 551-554]。

MOC-31：几乎所有的CC MOC-31都呈阳性[522]。

CDX2：约75%的CC CDX2呈中等到强阳性，斑片状分布。

CC中其他抗体染色情况见表13.7。

> **诊断要点：胆管癌**
>
> 1. 胆管癌的免疫表型与胰胆管腺癌相似，主要是低分子量角蛋白阳性，CK7+/CK20-为主，以及CK19、CEA、CA19-9、CDX2和MOC-31阳性。
> 2. 鉴别胆管癌和转移性苗勒管乳头状浆液性癌比较困难，因为两者均为CK7和CA125阳性。雌激素受体在苗勒管乳头状浆液性癌中呈局灶阳性，在胆管癌中呈阴性（图13.67）。

鉴别诊断与抗体组合

肝细胞癌与胆管癌 抗体：CK7、CK19、CEA（单克隆和多克隆）、CA19-9、B72.3、MOC-31、

表 13.7　胆管癌抗体染色

抗体	染色	评价	参考文献
EMA	+		412,550,592
CD15 (Leu-M1)	+	大约 80%CC 阳性	162,521
Ber-EP4	+		162
CA125	S	大约 60%CC 弥漫强阳性	329
AFP	R		
HepPar1	R		
A1AT	R		
CA19-9	+	见上文	
Synaptophysin	N		
B72.3	+		
GCDFP-15	N		655
34βE12	+	通常单个细胞或小簇细胞阳性	
CK5/6	S	大约 20%CC 阳性	650
AFP	R	偶尔单个瘤细胞呈弱阳性	162,265,481,509,511,520,521,524,526,552
HepPar1	R	5%CC 通常弱阳性，偶尔单个黏液柱状细胞阳性	12,480,511
A1AT	R	10%CC 散在阳性，但伴有 A1AT 缺陷的 CC 呈弥漫阳性	509,517,521,552
B72.3	S	大约 50%CC 阳性	162,521

+, 阳性; S, 有时阳性; R, 偶尔阳性; N, 阴性

HepPar1、AFP（表 13.8）

鉴别 CCs 的阳性抗体包括 CK7、CK19、单克隆 CEA、CA19-9、B72.3 和 MOC-31。在 HCC 中这些抗体呈局灶弱阳性或阴性[162, 265, 339, 412, 481, 519-522, 555]。鉴别 HCC 的阳性抗体包括多克隆 CEA、HepPar1 和 AFP[12, 15, 480, 511]。多克隆 CEA 在部分到几乎所有的 HCC 中呈丛管状染色，而在几乎全部 CC 中呈胞浆弥漫阳性。

胆管癌和结肠腺癌　抗体：CK7、CK20

这两种肿瘤的 CK7 和 CK20 的染色正相反。肝内

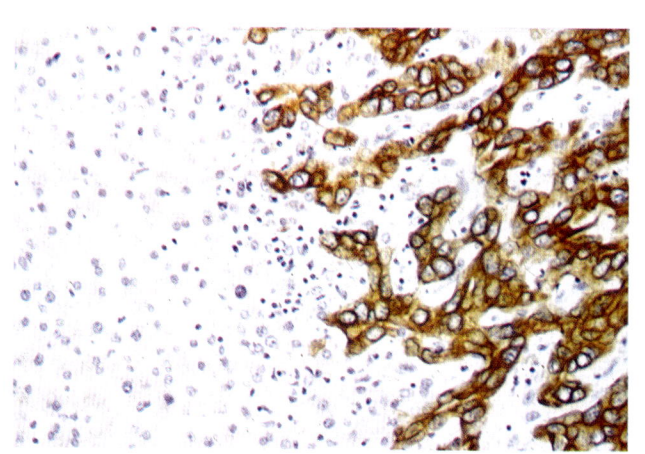

图 13.66　胆管癌细胞的 CK7 呈特征性的弥漫阳性。相邻的肝细胞呈阴性

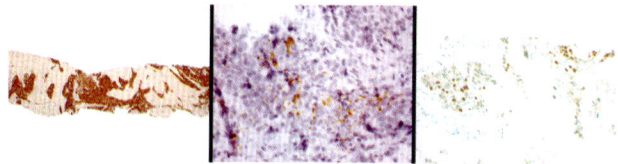

图 13.67　肝转移性苗勒管乳头状浆液性癌。肿瘤细胞呈 CK7 弥漫阳性（左），CA125 局灶阳性（中），与胆管癌免疫表型相似。与胆管癌不同的是，苗勒管乳头状浆液性癌通常有雌激素受体灶性阳性染色（右）

胆管癌通常 CK7 呈弥漫强阳性，CK20 阳性较少[265]。相反，结肠腺癌通常为 CK20 广泛阳性，CK7 很少阳性。联合染色时，约 75% 的 CC 呈 CK7+/CK20-，而约 75% 的结肠腺癌呈 CK7-/CK20+。两种肿瘤的其他阳性类型则可能有相当多的重叠[173, 204, 215, 264, 284]。

胆管癌变型

梭形细胞（肉瘤样）CC　梭形细胞（肉瘤样）CC 通常与低分化典型的 CC 混合存在。梭形细胞 CC 的 CEA 和 AFP 常呈阴性[556, 557]。可混有波形蛋白阳性的横纹肌样细胞。梭形细胞灶的低分子量角蛋白也可呈局灶阳性，包括 AE1/AE3、CAM5.2 或 35βH11 及 EMA[556, 558]。S-100 和 AFP 呈阴性[556]。用免疫组化鉴别单纯梭形细胞 CC 和单纯梭形细胞 HCC 并不可靠。

表13.8 肝细胞癌与胆管癌鉴别

抗体	肿瘤	
	HCC	CC
AE1/AE3	R~N	+
CK7	R	+
CK17	N	S
CK19	R	+
CEA（单克隆）	R	+
CEA（多克隆，丛管状）	S	N
CA19-9	N	+
B72.3	R	+
MOC-31	N	+
HepPar1	+	R
AFP	U	R

+,阳性；S,有时阳性；R,偶尔阳性；N,阴性

所幸的是，这两种肿瘤的梭形细胞类型通常都与高级别典型的（上皮样结构）HCC或CC伴随。做免疫组化时应注意选择上皮样结构区域，不要选择梭形细胞区域。

混合性肝-胆管癌 作者在免疫组化上将混合性或复合性HCC-CC限定为伴有二者免疫表型的形态学上的复合性HCC-CC或低分化癌[559, 560]，并与肿瘤的级别密切相关。一些作者将具有HCC免疫表型特征的形态上为胆管腺癌的肿瘤称为"胆管细胞癌"。在高分化的混合肿瘤中，可以根据形态学区分HCC和CC成分[561]。在分化较差的肿瘤中，CC的管状区域与呈腺泡、小梁状或实性的HCC样区域相邻[561]。由未分化癌细胞组成的、既无CC也无HCC形态特征的原发性肝癌不应归为混合性HCC-CC癌，我们认为这类肿瘤最好归类为未分化癌（见下文）。在有明确的HCC及CC区域的肿瘤中[碰撞癌（collision type carcinomas）]，无论有无过渡区，其每一种形态区域的免疫学表型均与其相应的单纯性肿瘤相同[480, 514, 521]。大部分肿瘤中，在CC的管状结构与HCC的小梁或实性结构相邻处，小管和小梁通常呈CK7和CK19阳性[514, 561]。这些细胞含有白蛋白mRNA，此为肝细胞分化特点。在小管移行区CK20和AFP也常呈阳性[480, 561]。在非典型的HCC或CC中，仅根据其具有肝和胆管分化的免疫组化双表型不足以证明为混合性HCC-CC，因为此类细胞可见于组织学上非典型的HCC、CC以及混合性HCC-CC[477]。CC中细胞角蛋白34βE12表达减少是预后好的标志。

低分化和未分化癌

有些作者将低分化或未分化的原发性肝癌分类为混合性HCC-CC。在分化差的HCC中胆管型角蛋白阳性是不足以诊断混合性HCC-CC的，原因前面已经讲过。这些肿瘤的CK7和CK19常为阳性，而CEA、CA19-9、AFP和HepPar1为阴性。

胆管囊腺瘤与囊腺癌

肝内胆管囊腺瘤和囊腺癌的细胞角蛋白反应谱与胰胆管囊腺瘤和囊腺癌相似，大部分呈斑片状CK7和CK20染色，CA125常呈灶状反应。伴随的浸润性腺癌和胆管癌相似。上皮细胞的AE1/AE3和CEA呈弥漫强阳性[562]。在50%的肿瘤中可见掺杂的、单个的嗜铬素和突触素阳性细胞。有些肿瘤在囊肿内衬上皮周围围绕着卵巢样间质，这些间质细胞的波形蛋白、SMA和结蛋白阳性，但CK、EMA、CEA、嗜铬素或突触素阴性[562-564]。在这些间质细胞中，偶尔也有雌激素和孕激素受体的表达[565, 566]。

导管内乳头状黏液瘤

导管内乳头状黏液瘤（IPMT）的形态和免疫组化与更为常见的胰腺IPMT相同[567, 568]。

肝和胆囊的原发性神经内分泌肿瘤

肝的神经内分泌癌多数是转移性的，也有极少数胆囊原发性神经内分泌癌的报道[569]。肝原发性神经内分泌癌，从低级别类癌到高级别（小细胞未分化）癌均有报道。它们的免疫表型与小肠近端的神经内分泌癌最接近[570-574]。中级别和高级别原发性肝神经内分泌癌的降钙素可能阳性。因此鉴别原发的和转移的肝神经内分泌癌时，降钙素阳性不能诊断为转移的甲状腺髓样癌。

> **诊断要点：混合性和高级别肝癌**
>
> 1. 混合性或复合性HCC-CC的诊断应限定为具有HCC和CC两种形态和免疫表型的肿瘤。
> 2. 低分化或未分化的原发性肝癌通常是CK7和CK19阳性，而CEA、CA19-9、AFP和HepPar1阴性。单独的胆管型细胞角蛋白的表达不足以诊断为混合性HCC-CC。
> 3. 肝内胆管囊腺瘤和囊腺癌的细胞角蛋白表达谱与胰胆管囊腺瘤和囊腺癌相似，AE1/AE3、CA19-9和CEA阳性。

间质病变

血管平滑肌脂肪瘤（血管周上皮样细胞肿瘤）

血管平滑肌脂肪瘤（AML）属于血管周上皮样细胞肿瘤（PEComa），偶尔会发生在肝，更常见的是由原发于肾的肿瘤转移所致[575-580]。如果肿瘤主要由平滑肌细胞组成，其形态上与HCC和转移的肾细胞癌相似。这些AML中的所谓的平滑肌细胞其结蛋白和肌动蛋白常呈弱阳性[367]，HMB-45、MART-1(melan-A)和ER呈斑片状强阳性[367, 575, 581-583]。与HCC相反，这些细胞的角蛋白呈阴性，波形蛋白阳性。

上皮样血管内皮瘤

上皮样血管内皮瘤（EHE）是中级别到高级别的恶性血管肿瘤。肿瘤细胞的形态从上皮样到树突状[584]，无论何种形态，其CD31和CD34都呈阳性[584-588]，染色呈斑片状。15%~50%的EHE细胞AE1/AE3呈阳性[584]，约30%呈CAM5.2阳性[584, 589, 590]。EHE细胞的S-100和SMA呈局灶阳性[584]，而EMA呈阴性[584, 591]。

> **诊断要点**：血管平滑肌脂肪瘤
>
> 主要由平滑肌细胞组成的肝内血管平滑肌脂肪瘤，形态上可与HCC和转移的肾细胞癌类似，可根据细胞角蛋白阴性，HMB-45、MART-1(melan-A)和ER呈斑片状阳性来区别。

参考文献

1. Gown AM. Immunohistochemical determination of primary sites of carcinomas. J Histotechnol 1999; 22:209–215.
2. Stammberger P, Baczako K. Cytokeratin 19 expression in human gastrointestinal mucosa during human prenatal development and in gastrointestinal tumours: relation to cell proliferation. Cell Tissue Res 1999; 298:377–381.
3. Zhou Q, Toivola DM, Feng N, et al. Keratin 20 helps maintain intermediate filament organization in intestinal epithelia. Mol Biol Cell 2003; 14:2959–2971.
4. Hinoi T, Lucas PC, Kuick R, et al. CDX2 regulates liver intestine-cadherin expression in normal and malignant colon epithelium and intestinal metaplasia. Gastroenterology 2002; 123:1565–1577.
5. Bonhomme C, Duluc I, Martin E, et al. The CDX2 homeobox gene has a tumour suppressor function in the distal colon in addition to a homeotic role during gut development. Gut 2003; 52:1465–1471.
6. Van Klinken BJ, Dekker J, Buller HA, et al. Biosynthesis of mucins (MUC2-6) along the longitudinal axis of the human gastrointestinal tract. Am J Physiol 1997; 273:G296–G302.
7. Ireland AP, Clark GW, DeMeester TR. Barrett's esophagus. The significance of p53 in clinical practice. Ann Surg 1997; 225:17–30.
8. Tan J, Sidhu G, Greco MA, et al. Villin, cytokeratin 7, and cytokeratin 20 expression in pulmonary adenocarcinoma with ultrastructural evidence of microvilli with rootlets. Hum Pathol 1998; 29:390–396.
9. Bacchi CE, Gown AM. Distribution and pattern of expression of villin, a gastrointestinal-associated cytoskeletal protein, in human carcinomas: A study employing paraffin-embedded tissue. Lab Invest 1991; 64:418–424.
10. Savera AT, Torres FX, Lindin MD, et al. Primary versus metastatic pulmonary adenocarcinoma: An immunohistochemical study using villin and cytokeratins 7 and 20. Appl Immunohistochem 1996; 4:86–94.
11. Nishizuka S, Chen ST, Gwadry FG, et al. Diagnostic markers that distinguish colon and ovarian adenocarcinomas: identification by genomic, proteomic, and tissue array profiling. Cancer Res 2003; 63:5243–5250.
12. Wennerberg AE, Nalesnik MA, Coleman WB. Hepatocyte paraffin 1: a monoclonal antibody that reacts with hepatocytes and can be used for differential diagnosis of hepatic tumors. Am J Pathol 1993; 143:1050–1054.
13. Chu PG, Ishizawa S, Wu E, et al. Hepatocyte antigen as a marker of hepatocellular carcinoma: an immuno-histochemical comparison to carcinoembryonic antigen, CD10, and alpha-fetoprotein. Am J Surg Pathol 2002; 26:978–988.
14. Fan Z, Montgomery K, Rouse RV. Hep par 1 antibody stain for the differential diagnosis of hepatocellular carcinoma: 676 tumors tested using tissue microarrays and conventional tissue sections. Mod Pathol 2003; 16:137–144.
15. Lamps LW, Folpe AL. The diagnostic value of hepatocyte paraffin antibody 1 in differentiating hepatocellular neoplasms from nonhepatic tumors: a review. Adv Anat Pathol 2003;

10:39-43.

16. Mertz H, Vyberg M, Paulsen SM, et al. Immunohistochemical detection of neuroendocrine markers in tumors of the lungs and gastrointestinal tract. Appl Immunohistochem 1998; 6: 175–180.

17. Capella C, Heitz PU, Hofler H, et al. Revised classification of neuroendocrine tumors of the lung, pancreas and gut. Virchows Arch 1995; 425:547–560.

18. Portela-Gomes GM, Stridsberg M. Chromogranin A in the human gastrointestinal tract: an immunocytochemical study with region-specific antibodies. J Histochem Cyto-chem 2002 50:1487–1492.

19. Kilgore SP, Ormsby AH, Gramlich TL, et al. The gastric cardia: fact or fiction? Am J Gastroenterol 2000; 95:921–924.

20. Faller G, Borchard F, Ell C, et al. Histopathological diagnosis of Barrett's mucosa and associated neoplasias: results of a consensus conference of the Working Group for Gastroenterological Pathology of the German Society for Pathology on 22 September 2001 in Erlangen. Virchows Arch 2003; 443:597–601.

21. Reid BJ, Blount PL, Rabinovitch PS. Biomarkers in Barrett's esophagus. Gastrointest Endosc Clin N Am 2003; 13:369–397.

22. Raouf AA, Evoy DA, Carton E, et al. Loss of Bcl-2 expression in Barrett's dysplasia and adenocarcinoma is associated with tumor progression and worse survival but not with response to neoadjuvant chemoradiation. Dis Esophagus 2003; 16:17–23.

23. Croft J, Parry EM, Jenkins GJ, et al. Analysis of the premalignant stages of Barrett's oesophagus through to adenocarcinoma by comparative genomic hybridization. Eur J Gastroenterol Hepatol 2002; 14:1179–1186.

24. Copelli SB, Mazzeo C, Gimenez A, et al. Molecular analysis of p53 tumor-suppressor gene and microsatellites in preneoplastic and neoplastic lesions of the colon and esophagus. Oncol Rep 2001; 8:923–929.

25. Chatelain D, Flejou JF. High-grade dysplasia and super-ficial adenocarcinoma in Barrett's esophagus: histological mapping and expression of p53, p21 and Bcl-2 oncoproteins. Virchows Arch 2003; 442:18–24.

26. Taniere P, Borghi-Scoazec G, Saurin JC, et al. Cytokeratin expression in adenocarcinomas of the esophagogastric junction: a comparative study of adenocarcinomas of the distal esophagus and of the proximal stomach. Am J Surg Pathol 2002; 26:1213–1221.

27. Weiss MM, Kuipers EJ, Hermsen MA, et al. Barrett's adenocarcinomas resemble adenocarcinomas of the gastric cardia in terms of chromosomal copy number changes, but relate to squamous cell carcinomas of the distal oesophagus with respect to the presence of high-level amplifications. J Pathol 2003; 199:157–165.

28. Symmans PJ, Linehan JM, Brito MJ, et al. p53 expression in Barrett's esophagus, dysplasia, and adenocarcinoma using antibody DO-7. J Pathol 1994; 173:221–226.

29. Cawley HM, Meltzer SJ, De Benedetti VM, et al. Anti-p53 antibodies in patients with Barrett's esophagus or esophageal carcinoma can predate cancer diagnosis. Gastroenterology 1998; 115:19–27.

30. Levine DS. Barrett's esophagus and p53. Lancet 1994; 344: 212–213.

31. Miettinen M. Gastrointestinal stromal tumors. An immunohistochemical study of cellular differentiation. Am J Clin Pathol 1988; 89:601–610.

32. Saul SH, Rast ML, Brooks JJ. The immunohistochemistry of gastrointestinal stromal tumors. Evidence supporting an origin from smooth muscle. Am J Surg Pathol 1987; 11:464–473.

33. Miettinen M, Sobin LH, Sarlomo-Rikala M. Immunohistochemical spectrum of GISTs at different sites and their differential diagnosis with a reference to CD117 (KIT). Mod Pathol 2000; 13:1134–1142.

34. Miettinen M, Sarlomo-Rikala M, Sobin LH, et al. Esophageal stromal tumors: a clinicopathologic, immunohistochemical, and molecular genetic study of 17 cases and comparison with esophageal leiomyomas and leiomyosarcomas. Am J Surg Pathol 2000; 24:211–222.

35. Fanberg-Smith JC, Meiss-Kindblom JM, Fante R, et al. Malignant granular cell tumor of soft tissue: Diagnostic criteria and clinicopathologic correlation. Am J Surg Pathol 1998; 22:779–794.

36. Goldblum JR, Rice TW, Zuccaro G, et al. Granular cell tumors of the esophagus: a clinical and pathologic study of 13 cases. Ann Thorac Surg 1996; 62:860–865.

37. Fetsch PA, Marincola FM, Filie A, et al. Melanoma-associated antigen recognized by T cells (MART-1). Cancer Cytopathol 1999; 87:37–42.

38. Lohmann CM, Hwu WJ, Iversen K, et al. Primary malignant melanoma of the oesophagus: a clinical and pathological study with emphasis on the immunophenotype of the tumours for melanocyte differentiation markers and cancer/testis antigens. Melanoma Res 2003; 13:595–601.

39. Gupta NM, Goenka MK, Atri A, et al. Carcinoid tumour of the esophagus: a rare esophageal cancer. Eur J Surg 1996; 162:841–844.

40. Schnirer II, Yao JC, Ajani JA. Carcinoid – a comprehensive review. Acta Oncol 2003; 42:672–692.

41. Salgado MC, Vasconcelos-Teixeira A, Macedo-Pinto I, et al. Small cell carcinoma of the esophagus. Hepatogastroenterology 1991; 38(Suppl 1):22–25.

42. Takubo K, Nakamura K-I, Sawabe M, et al. Primary undifferentiated small cell carcinoma of the esophagus. Hum Pathol 1999; 30:216–221.

43. Osugi H, Takemura M, Morimura K, et al. Clinicopathologic and immunohistochemical features of surgically resected small cell carcinoma of the esophagus. Oncol Rep 2002; 9: 1245–1249.

44. Cheuk W, Kwan MY, Suster S, et al. Immunostaining for thyroid transcription factor 1 and cytokeratin 20 aids the distinction of small cell carcinoma from Merkel cell carcinoma, but not pulmonary from extrapulmonary small cell carcinomas. Arch Pathol Lab Med 2001; 125:228–231.

45. Cheuk W, Chan JK. Thyroid transcription factor-1 is of limited value in practical distinction between pulmonary and extrapulmonary small cell carcinomas. Am J Surg Pathol 2001; 25:545–546.

46. Lam KY, Loke SL, Shen XC, et al. Cytokeratin expression in non-neoplastic oesophageal epithelium and squamous cell carcinoma of the oesophagus. Virchows Arch 1995; 426:345–349.

47. Suo Z, Holm R, Nesland JM. Squamous cell carcinomas: An immunohistochemical study of cytokeratins and involucrin in primary and metastatic tumors. Histopathology 1993; 23: 45–54.

48. Shah KD, Tabibzadeh SS, Gerber MA. Comparison of cytokeratin expression in primary and metastatic carcinomas. Diagnostic application in surgical pathology. Am J Clin Pathol 1987; 87:708–715.

49. Moll R. Cytokeratins as markers of differentiation in the diagnosis of epithelial tumors. Sub-Cellular Biochem 1998; 31: 205–262.

50. Clover J, Oates J, Edwards C. Anti-cytokeratin 5/6: a positive marker for epithelioid mesothelioma. Histopathology 1997; 31:140–143.

51. Ordonez NG. Value of cytokeratin 5/6 immunostaining in distinguishing epithelial mesothelioma of the pleura from lung adenocarcinoma. Am J Surg Pathol 1998; 22:1215–1221.

52. Chu PG, Weiss LM. Expression of cytokeratin 5/6 in epithelial neoplasms: an immunohistochemical study of 509 cases. Mod Pathol 2002; 15:6–10.

53. Scarpatetti M, Tsybrovskyy O, Popper HH. Cytokeratin typing as an aid in the differential diagnosis of primary versus metastatic lung carcinomas, and comparison with normal lung. Virchows Arch 2002; 440:70–76.

54. Kaufmann O, Fietze E, Mengs J, et al. Value of p63 and cytokeratin 5/6 as immunohistochemical markers for the differential diagnosis of poorly differentiated and undifferentiated carcinomas. Am J Clin Pathol 2001; 116:823–830.

55. Di Como CJ, Urist MJ, Babayan I, et al. p63 expression profiles in human normal and tumor tissues. Clin Cancer Res 2002; 8:494–501.

56. Moll R, Lowe A, Laufer J, et al. Cytokeratin 20 in human carcinomas. A new histodiagnostic marker detected by monoclonal antibodies. Am J Pathol 1992; 140:427–447.

57. Rossen K, Thomsen HK: Ber-EP4 immunoreactivity depends on the germ layer origin and maturity of the squamous epithelium. Histopathology 2001; 39:386–389.

58. Tateyama H, Eimoto T, Tada T, et al. Immunoreactivity of a new CD5 antibody with normal epithelium and malignant tumors including thymic carcinoma. Am J Clin Pathol 1999; 111:235–240.

59. Kornstein MJ, Rosai J. CD5 labeling of thymic carcinomas and other nonlymphoid neoplasms. Am J Clin Pathol 1998; 109:722–726.

60. Ordonez NG. Value of calretinin immunostaining in differentiating epithelial mesothelioma from lung adenocarcinoma. Mod Pathol 1998; 11:929–933.

61. Owonikoko T, Loberg C, Gabbert HE, et al. Comparative analysis of basaloid and typical squamous cell carcinoma of the oesophagus: a molecular biological and immuno-histochemical study. J Pathol 2001; 193:155–161.

62. Sarbia M, Bittinger F, Porschen R, et al. bcl-2 expression and prognosis in squamous-cell carcinomas of the esophagus.

Int J Cancer 1996; 69:324–328.

63. Tsang WY, Chan JKC, Lee KC, et al. Basaloid-squamous carcinoma of the upper aerodigestive tract and so-called adenoid cystic carcinoma of the esophagus: the same tumor type? Histopathology 1991; 19:35–46.

64. Banks ER, Frierson HF Jr, Mills SE, et al. Basaloid squamous cell carcinoma of the head and neck: a clinicopathologic and immunohistochemical study of 40 cases. Am J Surg Pathol 1992; 16:939–946.

65. Luna MA, El-Naggar A, Parichatikanond P, et al. Basaloid-squamous carcinoma of the upper digestive tract. Cancer 1990; 66:537–542.

66. Tsubochi H, Suzuki T, Suzuki S, et al. Immunohistochemical study of basaloid squamous cell carcinoma, adenoid cystic and mucoepidermoid carcinoma in the upper aero-digestive tract. Anticancer Res 2000; 20:1205–1211.

67. Abe K, Sasano H, Itakura Y, et al. Basaloid-squamous carcinoma of the esophagus: a clinicopathologic, DNA ploidy, and immunohistochemical study of 7 cases. Am J Surg Pathol 1996; 20:453–461.

68. Kawahara K, Makimoto K, Maekawa T, et al. An immunohistochemical examination of basaloid squamous cell carcinoma of the esophagus: report of a case. Surg Today 2001; 31 655–659.

69. Popnikolov NK, Ayala AG, Graves K, et al. Benign myoepithelial tumors of the breast have immunophenotypic characteristics similar to metaplastic matrix-producing and spindle cell carcinomas. Am J Clin Pathol 2003; 120:161–167.

70. Deamant FD, Pombo MT, Battifora H. Estrogen receptor immunohistochemistry as a predictor of site of origin in metastatic breast cancer. Appl Immunohistochem 1993; 1:188–192.

71. Driessen A, Nafteux P, Lerut T, et al. Identical cytokeratin expression pattern CK7+/CK20- in esophageal and cardiac cancer: etiopathological and clinical implications. Mod Pathol 2004; 17:49–55.

72. Gulmann C, Counihan I, Grace A, et al. Cytokeratin 7/20 and mucin expression patterns in oesophageal, cardia and distal gastric adenocarcinomas. Histopathology 2003; 43:453–461.

73. Sheahan K, O'Brien MJ, Burke B, et al. Differential reactivities of carcinoembryonic antigen (CEA) and CEA-related monoclonal and polyclonal antibodies in common epithelial malignancies. Am J Clin Pathol 1990; 94:157–164.

74. Ormsby AH, Goldblum JR, Rice TW, et al. The utility of cytokeratin subsets in distinguishing Barrett's-related oesophageal adenocarcinoma from gastric adenocarcinoma. Histopathology 2001; 38:307–311.

75. Shen B, Ormsby AH, Shen C, et al. Cytokeratin expression patterns in noncardia, intestinal metaplasia-associated gastric adenocarcinoma: implication for the evaluation of intestinal metaplasia and tumors at the esophagogastric junction. Cancer 2002; 94:820–831.

76. Flucke U, Steinborn E, Dries V, et al. Immunoreactivity of cytokeratins (CK7, CK20) and mucin peptide core antigens (MUC1, MUC2, MUC5AC) in adenocarcinomas, normal and metaplastic tissues of the distal oesophagus, oesophago-gastric junction and proximal stomach. Histo-pathology 2003; 43:127–134.

77. Guarino M, Reale D, Micoli G, eet al. Carcinosarcoma of the esophagus with rhabdomyoblastic differentiation. Histopathology 1993; 22:493–498.

78. Lauwers GY, Grant LD, Scott GV, et al. Spindle cell squamous carcinoma of the esophagus: analysis of ploidy and tumor proliferative activity in a series of 13 cases. Hum Pathol 1998; 29:863–868.

79. Ooi A, Kawahara E, Okada Y, et al. Carcinosarcoma of the esophagus. An immunohistochemical and electron microscopic study. Acta Pathol Jpn 1986; 36:151–159.

80. Rosty C, Prevot S, Tiret E, et al. Adenocarcinosarcoma in Barrett's esophagus: Report of a case. Int J Surg Pathol 1996; 4:43–48.

81. Iezzoni JC, Mills SE. Sarcomatoid carcinomas (carcinosarcomas) of the gastrointestinal tract: A review. Semin Diagn Pathol 1993; 10:176–187.

82. Piazuelo MB, Haque S, Delgado A, et al. Phenotypic differences between esophageal and gastric intestinal metaplasia. Mod Pathol 2004; 17:62–74.

83. Jovanovic I, Tzardi M, Mouzas IA, et al. Changing pattern of cytokeratin 7 and 20 expression from normal epithelium to intestinal metaplasia of the gastric mucosa and gastroesophageal junction. Histol Histopathol 2002; 17:445–454.

84. Kurtkaya-Yapicier O, Gencosmanoglu R, Avsar E, et al. The utility of cytokeratins 7 and 20 (CK7/20) immunohistochemistry in the distinction of short-segment Barrett esophagus from gastric intestinal metaplasia: Is it reliable? BMC Clin Pathol 2003; 3:5.

85. Ormsby AH, Goldblum JR, Rice TW, et al. Cytokeratin subsets can reliably distinguish Barrett's esophagus from intestinal metaplasia of the stomach. Hum Pathol 1999; 30:288–294.
86. Odze R. Cytokeratin 7/20 immunostaining: Barrett's oesophagus or gastric intestinal metaplasia? Lancet 2002; 359:1711–1713.
87. Glickman JN, Wang H, Das KM, et al. Phenotype of Barrett's esophagus and intestinal metaplasia of the distal esophagus and gastroesophageal junction: an immunohistochemical study of cytokeratins 7 and 20, Das-1 and 45 MI. Am J Surg Pathol 2001; 25:87–94.
88. Mohammed IA, Streutker CJ, Riddell RH. Utilization of cytokeratins 7 and 20 does not differentiate between Barrett's esophagus and gastric cardiac intestinal metaplasia. Mod Pathol 2002; 15:611–616.
89. Warson C, Van De Bovenkamp JH, Korteland-Van Male AM, et al. Barrett's esophagus is characterized by expression of gastric-type mucins (MUC5AC, MUC6) and TFF peptides (TFF1 and TFF2), but the risk of carcinoma development may be indicated by the intestinal-type mucin, MUC2. Hum Pathol 2002; 33:660–668.
90. Ormsby AH, Vaezi MF, Richter JE, et al. Cytokeratin immunoreactivity patterns in the diagnosis of short-segment Barrett's esophagus. Gastroenterology 2000; 119:683–690.
91. Latchford A, Eksteen B, Jankowski J. The continuing tale of cytokeratins in Barrett's mucosa: as you like it. Gut 2001; 49:746–747.
92. Chu PG, Jiang Z, Weiss LM. Hepatocyte antigen as a marker of intestinal metaplasia. Am J Surg Pathol 2003; 27:952–959.
93. Phillips RW, Frierson HF Jr, Moskaluk CA. CDX2 as a marker of epithelial intestinal differentiation in the esophagus. Am J Surg Pathol 2003; 27:1442–1447.
94. Goldstein NS. Chronic inactive gastritis and coccoid *Helicobacter pylori* in patients treated for gastroesophageal reflux disease or with *H. pylori* eradication therapy. Am J Clin Pathol 2002; 118:719–726.
95. Andersen LP, Dorland A, Karacan H, et al. Possible clinical importance of the transformation of *Helicobacter pylori* into coccoid forms. Scand J Gastroenterol 2000; 35:897–903.
96. Cao J, Li ZQ, Borch K, et al. Detection of spiral and coccoid forms of *Helicobacter pylori* using a murine monoclonal antibody. Clin Chim Acta 1997; 267:183–196.
97. Ashton-Key M, Diss TC, Isaacson PG. Detection of *Helicobacter pylori* in gastric biopsy and resection specimens. J Clin Pathol 1996; 49:107–111.
98. Jonkers D, Houben G, de Bruine A, et al. Prevalence of gastric metaplasia in the duodenal bulb and distribution of *Helicobacter pylori* in the gastric mucosa. A clinical and histopathological study in 96 consecutive patients. Ital J Gastroenterol Hepatol 1998; 30:481–483.
99. Rotimi O, Cairns A, Gray S, et al. Histological identification of *Helicobacter pylori*: comparison of staining methods. J Clin Pathol 2000; 53:756–759.
100. van der Wouden EJ, Thijs JC, van Zwet AA, et al. Reliability of biopsy-based diagnostic tests for *Helicobacter pylori* after treatment aimed at its eradication. Eur J Gastroenterol Hepatol 1999; 11:1255–1258.
101. Burt RW. Gastric fundic gland polyps. Gastroenterology 2003; 125:1462–1469.
102. Declich P, Isimbaidi G, Sironi M, et al. Sporadic fundic gland polyps: an immunohistochemical study of their antigenic profile. Pathol Res Pract 1996; 192:808–815.
103. Sekine S, Shibata T, Yamauchi Y, et al. Beta-catenin mutations in sporadic fundic gland polyps. Virchows Arch 2002; 440:381–386.
104. Muller J, Kirchner T, Muller-Hermelink HK. Gastric endocrine cell hyperplasia and carcinoid tumors in atrophic gastritis type A. Am J Surg Pathol 1987; 11:909–917.
105. Thomas RM, Baybick JH, Elsayed AM, et al. Gastric carcinoids. An immunohistochemical and clinicopathologic study of 104 patients. Cancer 1994; 73:2053–2058.
106. Al-Khafaji B, Noffsinger AE, Miller MA, et al. Immuno-histologic analysis of gastrointestinal and pulmonary carcinoid tumors. Hum Pathol 1998; 29:992–999.
107. Bordi C, Yu JY, Baggi MT, et al. Gastric carcinoids and their precursor lesions. A histologic and immunohistochemical study of 23 cases. Cancer 1991; 67:663–672.
108. Kimura N, Sasano N, Namiki TS, et al. Coexpression of cytokeratin, neurofilament, and vimentin in carcinoid tumors. Virchows Arch 1989; 415:69–77.
109. Klappenbach RS, Kurman RJ, Sinclair CF, et al. Composite carcinoma-carcinoid tumors of the gastrointestinal tract. A morphologic, histochemical, and immunocytochemical study. Am J Clin Pathol 1985; 84:137–143.
110. Ordonez NG, Mackay B, El-Naggar A, et al. Clear cell carci-

110. ...noid tumour of the stomach. Histopathology 1993; 22:190–193.
111. Reinecke P, Borchard F. Pattern of gastric endocrine cells in microcarcinoidosis – an immunohistochemical study of 14 gastric biopsies. Virchows Arch 1996; 428:237–241.
112. Peghini PL, Annibale B, Azzoni C, et al. Effect of chronic hypergastrinemia on human enterochromaffin-like cells: insights from patients with sporadic gastrinomas. Gastroenterology 2002; 123:68–85.
113. Werling RW, Yaziji H, Bacchi CE, et al. CDX2, a highly sensitive and specific marker of adenocarcinomas of intestinal origin: an immunohistochemical survey of 476 primary and metastatic carcinomas. Am J Surg Pathol 2003; 27:303–310.
114. Moskaluk CA, Zhang H, Powell SM, et al. CDX2 protein expression in normal and malignant human tissues: an immunohistochemical survey using tissue microarrays. Mod Pathol 2003; 16:913–919.
115. Cai YC, Banner B, Glickman J, et al. Cytokeratin 7 and 20 and thyroid transcription factor 1 can help distinguish pulmonary from gastrointestinal carcinoid and pancreatic endocrine tumors. Hum Pathol 2001; 32:1087–1093.
116. Taniguchi M, Nishida T, Hirota S, et al. Effect of c-kit mutation on prognosis of gastrointestinal stromal tumors. Cancer Res 1999; 59:4297–4300.
117. Kitamura Y, Hirota S, Nishida T. Molecular pathology of c-kit proto-oncogene and development of gastrointestinal stromal tumors. Ann Chir Gynaecol 1998; 87:282–286.
118. Bernet L, Zuniga A, Cano R. Characterization of GIST/GIPACT tumors by inmunohistochemistry and exon 11 analysis of c-kit by PCR. Rev Esp Enferm Dig 2003; 95:688–697.
119. Miettinen M, Lasota J. Gastrointestinal stromal tumors (GISTs): definition, occurrence, pathology, differential diagnosis and molecular genetics. Pol J Pathol 2003; 54:3–24.
120. Allander SV, Nupponen NN, Ringner M, et al. Gastro-intestinal stromal tumors with KIT mutations exhibit a remarkably homogeneous gene expression profile. Cancer Res 2001; 61:8624–8628.
121. Rubin BP, Singer S, Tsao C, et al. KIT activation is a ubiquitous feature of gastrointestinal stromal tumors. Cancer Res 2001; 61:8118–8121.
122. Miettinen M, El Rifai W, Sobin HL, et al. Evaluation of malignancy and prognosis of gastrointestinal stromal tumors: a review. Hum Pathol 2002; 33:478–483.
123. Fuller CE, Williams GT. Gastrointestinal manifestations of type 1 neurofibromatosis (von Recklinghausen's disease). Histopathology 1991; 19:1–11.
124. Antonioli DA. Gastrointestinal autonomic nerve tumors: Expanding the spectrum of gastrointestinal stromal tumors. Arch Pathol Lab Med 1989; 113:831–833.
125. Lee JR, Joshi V, Griffin JW Jr, et al. Gastrointestinal autonomic nerve tumor: immunohistochemical and molecular identity with gastrointestinal stromal tumor. Am J Surg Pathol 2001; 25:979–987.
126. Sicar K, Hewlett BR, Huizinga JD, et al. Interstitial cells of Cajal as precursors of gastrointestinal stromal tumors. Am J Surg Pathol 1999; 23:377–389.
127. Chan JK. Mesenchymal tumors of the gastrointestinal tract: a paradise for acronyms (STUMP, GIST, GANT, and now GIPACT), implication of c-kit in genesis, and yet another of the many emerging roles of the interstitial cell of Cajal in the pathogenesis of gastrointestinal diseases? Adv Anat Pathol 1999; 6:19–40.
128. Wong NA, Young R, Malcomson RD, et al. Prognostic indicators for gastrointestinal stromal tumours: a clinicopathological and immunohistochemical study of 108 resected cases of the stomach. Histopathology 2003; 43:118–126.
129. Greenson JK. Gastrointestinal stromal tumors and other mesenchymal lesions of the gut. Mod Pathol 2003; 16:366–375.
130. Tazawa K, Tsukada K, Makuuchi H, et al. An immunohistochemical and clinicopathological study of gastrointestinal stromal tumors. Pathol Int 1999; 49:786–798.
131. de Silva CM, Reid R. Gastrointestinal stromal tumors (GIST): C-kit mutations, CD117 expression, differential diagnosis and targeted cancer therapy with Imatinib. Pathol Oncol Res 2003; 9:13–19.
132. Goldblum JR. Gastrointestinal stromal tumors. A review of characteristic morphologic, immunohistochemical, and molecular genetic features. Am J Clin Pathol 2002; 117(Suppl):S49–S61.
133. Hasegawa T, Matsuno Y, Shimoda T, et al. Gastrointestinal stromal tumor: consistent CD117 immunostaining for diagnosis, and prognostic classification based on tumor size and MIB-1 grade. Hum Pathol 2002; 33:669–676.
134. Fletcher CD, Berman JJ, Corless C, et al. Diagnosis of gastrointestinal stromal tumors: A consensus approach. Hum Pathol 2002; 33:459–465.

135. Duensing A, Heinrich MC, Fletcher CD, et al. Biology of gastrointestinal stromal tumors: KIT mutations and beyond. Cancer Invest 2004; 22:106–116.
136. Duensing A, Medeiros F, McConarty B, et al. Mechanisms of oncogenic KIT signal transduction in primary gastro-intestinal stromal tumors (GISTs). Oncogene 2004; 23:3999–4006.
137. Hornick JL, Fletcher CD. The significance of KIT (CD117) in gastrointestinal stromal tumors. Int J Surg Pathol 2004; 12:93–97.
138. Singer S, Rubin BP, Lux ML, et al. Prognostic value of KIT mutation type, mitotic activity, and histologic subtype in gastrointestinal stromal tumors. J Clin Oncol 2002; 20:3898–3905.
139. Yantiss RK, Spiro IJ, Compton CC, et al. Gastrointestinal stromal tumor versus intra-abdominal fibromatosis of the bowel wall: a clinically important differential diagnosis. Am J Surg Pathol 2000; 24:947–957.
140. Hornick JL, Fletcher CD. Immunohistochemical staining for KIT (CD117) in soft tissue sarcomas is very limited in distribution. Am J Clin Pathol 2002; 117:188–193.
141. Sabah M, Leader M, Kay E. The problem with KIT: clinical implications and practical difficulties with CD117 immunostaining. Appl Immunohistochem Mol Morphol 2003; 11:56–61.
142. Suster S. Gastrointestinal stromal tumors. Semin Diagn Pathol 1996; 13:297–313.
143. Suster S, Fletcher CD. Gastrointestinal stromal tumors with prominent signet-ring cell features. Mod Pathol 1996; 9:609–613.
144. Miettinen M, Virolainen M, Maarit SR. Gastrointestinal stromal tumors – value of CD34 antigen in their identification and separation from true leiomyomas and schwannomas. Am J Surg Pathol 1995; 19:207–216.
145. Dhimes P, Lopez-Carreira M, Ortega-Serrano MP, et al. Gastrointestinal autonomic nerve tumors and their separation from other gastrointestinal stromal tumors: an ultrastructural and immunohistochemical study of seven cases. Virchows Arch 1995; 426:27–35.
146. Franquemont DW, Frierson HF Jr. Muscle differentiation and clinicopathologic features of gastrointestinal stromal tumors. Am J Surg Pathol 1992; 16:947–954.
147. Brown DC, Theaker JM, Banks PM, et al. Cytokeratin expression in smooth muscle and smooth muscle tumours. Histopathology 1987; 11:477–486.
148. Herrera GA, Cerezo L, Jones JE, et al. Gastrointestinal autonomic nerve tumors. 'Plexosarcomas'. Arch Pathol Lab Med 1989; 113:846–853.
149. Yao T, Aoyagi K, Hizawa K, et al. Gastric epithelioid stromal tumor (leiomyoma) with granular changes. Int J Surg Pathol 1996; 4:37–42.
150. Shek TW, Luk IS, Loong F, et al. Inflammatory cell-rich gastrointestinal autonomic nerve tumor: An expansion of its histologic spectrum. Am J Surg Pathol 1996; 20:325–331.
151. Tworek JA, Goldblum JR, Weiss SW, et al. Stromal tumors of the abdominal cavity: A clinicopathologic study of 20 cases. Am J Surg Pathol 1999; 23:937–345.
152. Tworek JA, Goldblum JR, Weiss SW, et al. Stromal tumors of the anorectum: a clinicopathologic study of 22 cases. Am J Surg Pathol 1999; 23:946–954.
153. Miettinen M, Monihan JM, Sarlomo-Rikala M, et al. Gastrointestinal stromal tumors/smooth muscle tumors (GISTs) primary in the omentum and mesentery: Clinicopathologic and immunohistochemical study of 26 cases. Am J Surg Pathol 1999; 23:1109–1118.
154. Prevot S, Bienvenu L, Vaillant JC, et al. Benign schwannoma of the digestive tract: A clinicopathologic and immunohistochemical study of five cases, including a case of esophageal tumor. Am J Surg Pathol 1999; 23:431–436.
155. Sarlomo-Rikala M, Kovatich AJ, Barusevicius BS, et al. CD117: A sensitive marker for gastrointestinal stromal tumors that is more specific than CD34. Mod Pathol 1998; 11: 728–734.
156. Montgomery E, Torbenson MS, Kaushal M, et al. Beta-catenin immunohistochemistry separates mesenteric fibromatosis from gastrointestinal stromal tumor and sclerosing mesenteritis. Am J Surg Pathol 2002; 26:1296–1301.
157. Young RH, Clement PB, McCaughey WT. Solitary fibrous tumors ('fibrous mesotheliomas') of the peritoneum. A report of three cases and a review of the literature. Arch Pathol Lab Med 1990; 114:493–495.
158. Fukunaga M, Naganuma H, Ushigome S, et al. Malignant solitary fibrous tumour of the peritoneum. Histopathology 1996; 28:463–466.
159. Fukunaga M, Naganuma H, Nikaido T, et al. Extrapleural solitary fibrous tumor: a report of seven cases. Mod Pathol

1997; 10:443–450.

160. Shidham VB, Chivukula M, Gupta D, et al. Immunohistochemical comparison of gastrointestinal stromal tumor and solitary fibrous tumor. Arch Pathol Lab Med 2002; 126:1189–1192.

161. Graadt van Roggen JF, van Velthuysen ML, Hogendoorn PC. The histopathological differential diagnosis of gastro-intestinal stromal tumours. J Clin Pathol 2001; 54:96–102.

162. Ma CK, Zarbo RJ, Frierson HF Jr, et al. Comparative immunohistochemical study of primary and metastatic carcinomas of the liver. Am J Clin Pathol 1993; 99:551–557.

163. McKinley M, Listrom MB, Fenoglio-Preiser C. Cytokeratin 19: A potential marker of colonic differentiation. Surg Pathol 1990; 3:107–113.

164. Goldstein NS, Long A, Kuan SF, et al. Colon signet ring cell adenocarcinoma: immunohistochemical characterization and comparison with gastric and typical colon adenocarcinomas. Appl Immunohistochem Mol Morphol 2000; 8:183–188.

165. Lee MJ, Lee HS, Kim WH, et al. Expression of mucins and cytokeratins in primary carcinomas of the digestive system. Mod Pathol 2003; 16:403–410.

166. Kim MA, Lee HS, Yang HK, et al. Cytokeratin expression profile in gastric carcinomas. Hum Pathol 2004; 35:576–581.

167. Wauters CC, Smedts F, Gerrits LG, et al. Keratins 7 and 20 as diagnostic markers of carcinomas metastatic to the ovary. Hum Pathol 1995; 26:852–855.

168. Ramaekers FC, van Niekerk CC, Poels L, et al. Use of monoclonal antibodies to keratin 7 in the differential diagnosis of adenocarcinomas. Am J Pathol 1990; 136:641–655.

169. Tot T. Adenocarcinomas metastatic to the liver: The value of cytokeratins 20 and 7 in the search for unknown primary tumors. Cancer 1999; 85:171–177.

170. Baars JH, De Ruijter JLM, Smedts F, et al. The applicability of a keratin 7 monoclonal antibody in routinely Papanicolaou-stained cytologic specimens for the differential diagnosis of carcinoma. Am J Clin Pathol 1994; 101:257–261.

171. Kaufmann OK, Deidesheimer T, Muehlenberg M, et al. Immunohistochemical differentiation of metastatic breast carcinomas from metastatic adenocarcinomas of other common primary sites. Histopathology 1996; 29:233–240.

172. Miettinen M. Keratin 20: immunohistochemical marker for gastrointestinal, urothelial, and Merkel cell carcinomas. Mod Pathol 1995; 8:384–388.

173. Wang NP, Zee S, Zarbo RJ, et al. Coordinate expression of cytokeratins 7 and 20 defines unique subsets of carcinomas. Appl Immunohistochem 1995; 3:99–107.

174. Kende AI, Carr NJ, Sobin LH. Expression of cytokeratins 7 and 20 in carcinomas of the gastrointestinal tract. Histopathology 2003; 42:137–140.

175. Park SY, Kim HS, Hong EK, et al. Expression of cytokeratins 7 and 20 in primary carcinomas of the stomach and colorectum and their value in the differential diagnosis of metastatic carcinomas to the ovary. Hum Pathol 2002; 33:1078–1085.

176. Cathro HP, Stoler MH. Expression of cytokeratins 7 and 20 in ovarian neoplasia. Am J Clin Pathol 2002; 117:944–951.

177. Chu P, Wu E, Weiss LM. Cytokeratin 7 and cytokeratin 20 expression in epithelial neoplasms: a survey of 435 cases. Mod Pathol 2000; 13:962–972.

178. Zhao XH, Gu SZ, Liu SX, et al. Expression of estrogen receptor and estrogen receptor messenger RNA in gastric carcinoma tissues. World J Gastroenterol 2003; 9:665–669.

179. Singh S, Poulsom R, Wright NA, et al. Differential expression of estrogen receptor and estrogen inducible genes in gastric mucosa and cancer. Gut 1997; 40:516–520.

180. Cameron BL, Butler JA, Rutgers J, et al. Immunohistochemical determination of the estrogen receptor content of gastrointestinal adenocarcinomas. Am Surg 1992; 58:758–760.

181. Yokozaki H, Takekura N, Takanashi A, et al. Estrogen receptors in gastric adenocarcinoma: a retrospective immunohistochemical analysis. Virchows Arch 1988; 413:297–302.

182. Nash JW, Morrison C, Frankel WL. The utility of estrogen receptor and progesterone receptor immunohistochemistry in the distinction of metastatic breast carcinoma from other tumors in the liver. Arch Pathol Lab Med 2003; 127:1591–1595.

183. Theodoropoulos GE, Lazaris AC, Panoussopoulos D, et al. Significance of estrogen receptors and cathepsin D tissue detection in gastric adenocarcinoma. J Surg Oncol 1995; 58: 176–183.

184. Sica V, Nola E, Contieri E, et al. Estradiol and progesterone receptors in malignant gastrointestinal tumors. Cancer Res 1984; 44:4670–4674.

185. Tokunaga A, Nishi K, Matsukura N, et al. Estrogen and progesterone receptors in gastric cancer. Cancer 1986; 57: 1376–1379.

186. Grogg KL, Lohse CM, Pankratz VS, et al. Lymphocyte-rich gastric cancer: associations with Epstein-Barr virus,

microsatellite instability, histology, and survival. Mod Pathol 2003; 16:641–651.
187. Jung HY, Jung KC, Shim YH, et al. Methylation of the hMLH1 promoter in multiple gastric carcinomas with microsatellite instability. Pathol Int 2001; 51:445–451.
188. Ohmura K, Tamura G, Endoh Y, et al. Microsatellite alterations in differentiated-type adenocarcinomas and precancerous lesions of the stomach with special reference to cellular phenotype. Hum Pathol 2000; 31:1031–1035.
189. Endoh Y, Tamura G, Ajioka Y, et al. Frequent hypermethylation of the hMLH1 gene promoter in differentiated-type tumors of the stomach with the gastric foveolar phenotype. Am J Pathol 2000; 157:717–722.
190. Cruz JJ, Paz JI, Cordero M, et al. Carcinosarcoma of the stomach with endocrine differentiation. A case report. Tumori 1991; 77:355–357.
191. Fukuda T, Kamishima T, Ohnishi Y, et al. Sarcomatoid carcinoma of the small intestine: histologic, immunohistochemical and ultrastructural features of three cases and its differential diagnosis. Pathol Int 1996; 46:682–688.
192. Roberts CC, Colby TV, Batts KP. Carcinoma of the stomach with hepatocyte differentiation (hepatoid adenocarcinoma). Mayo Clin Proc 1997; 72:1154–1160.
193. Terracciano LM, Glatz K, Mhawech P, et al. Hepatoid adenocarcinoma with liver metastasis mimicking hepatocellular carcinoma: an immunohistochemical and molecular study of eight cases. Am J Surg Pathol 2003; 27:1302–1312.
194. Maitra A, Murakata LA, Albores-Saavedra J. Immunoreactivity for hepatocyte paraffin 1 antibody in hepatoid adenocarcinomas of the gastrointestinal tract. Am J Clin Pathol 2001; 115:689–694.
195. Plaza JA, Vitellas K, Frankel WL. Hepatoid adeno-carcinoma of the stomach. Ann Diagn Pathol 2004; 8:137–141.
196. Villari D, Caruso R, Grosso M, et al. Hep Par 1 in gastric and bowel carcinomas: an immunohistochemical study. Pathology 2002; 34:423–426.
197. Blumenfeld W, Chandhoke DK, Sagerman P, et al. Neuroendocrine differentiation in gastric adenocarcinomas. An immunohistochemical study. Arch Pathol Lab Med 1996; 120: 478–481.
198. Park JG, Choe GY, Helman LJ, et al. Chromogranin-A expression in gastric and colon cancer tissues. Int J Cancer 1992; 51:189–194.
199. Qvigstad G, Sandvik AK, Brenna E, et al. Detection of chromogranin A in human gastric adenocarcinomas using a sensitive immunohistochemical technique. Histochem J 2000; 32:551–556.
200. Shimizu M, Matsumoto T, Hirokawa M, et al. Gastric metastasis from breast cancer: a pitfall in gastric biopsy specimens. Pathol Int 1998; 48:240–241.
201. Briest S, Horn LC, Haupt R, et al. Metastasizing signet ring cell carcinoma of the stomach mimicking bilateral inflammatory breast cancer. Gynecol Oncol 1999; 74:491–494.
202. Battifora H. Metastatic breast carcinoma to the stomach simulating linitis plastica. Appl Immunohistochem 1994; 2:225–228.
203. Raju U, Ma CK, Shaw A. Signet ring variant of lobular carcinoma of the breast: A clinicopathologic and immuno-histochemical study. Mod Pathol 1993; 6:516–520.
204. Perry A, Parisi JE, Kurtin PJ. Metastatic adenocarcinoma to the brain: an immunohistochemical approach. Hum Pathol 1997; 28:938–943.
205. Brown RW, Campagna LB, Dunn JK, et al. Immunohistochemical identification of tumor markers in metastatic adenocarcinoma. A diagnostic adjunct in the determination of primary site. Am J Clin Pathol 1997; 107:12–19.
206. Tot T. The role of cytokeratins 20 and 7 and estrogen receptor analysis in separation of metastatic lobular carcinoma of the breast and metastatic signet ring cell carcinoma of the gastrointestinal tract. APMIS 2000; 108:467–472.
207. Barbareschi M, Murer B, Colby TV, et al. CDX-2 homeobox gene expression is a reliable marker of colorectal adenocarcinoma metastases to the lungs. Am J Surg Pathol 2003; 27: 141–149.
208. Ollayos CW, Riordan GP, Rushin JM. Estrogen receptor detection in paraffin sections of adenocarcinoma of the colon, pancreas, and lung. Arch Pathol Lab Med 1994; 118:630–632.
209. Cohen C, Guarner J, DeRose PB. Mammary Paget's disease and associated carcinoma: An immunohistochemical study. Arch Pathol Lab Med 1993; 117 291–294.
210. Wallace ML, Longacre TA, Smoller BR. Estrogen and progesterone receptors and anti-gross cystic disease fluid protein 15 (BRST-2) fail to distinguish metastatic breast carcinoma from eccrine neoplasms. Mod Pathol 1995; 8:897–901.
211. Miettinen M, Nobel MP, Tuma BT, et al. Keratin 17: Immu-

nohistochemical mapping of its distribution in human epithelial tumors and its potential applications. Appl Immunohistochem 1997; 5:152–159.

212. Drier JK, Swanson PE, Cherwitz DL, et al. S100 protein immunoreactivity in poorly differentiated carcinomas: Immunohistochemical comparison with malignant mela-noma. Arch Pathol Lab Med 1987; 111:447–452.

213. Merchant SH, Amin MB, Tamboli P, et al. Primary signet-ring cell carcinoma of lung: immunohistochemical study and comparison with non-pulmonary signet-ring cell carcinomas. Am J Surg Pathol 2001; 25:1515–1519.

214. Harlamert HA, Mira J, Bejarano PA, et al. Thyroid transcription factor-1 and cytokeratins 7 and 20 in pulmonary and breast carcinoma. Acta Cytol 1998; 42:1382–1388.

215. Loy TS, Calaluce RD. Utility of cytokeratin immunostaining in separating pulmonary adenocarcinomas from colonic adenocarcinomas. Am J Clin Pathol 1994; 102:764–767.

216. Moch H, Oberholzer M, Dalquen P, et al. Diagnostic tools for differentiating between pleural mesothelioma and lung adenocarcinoma in paraffin embedded tissue. Part I. immunohistochemical findings. Virchows Arch 1993; 423:19–27.

217. Bejarano PA, Baughman RP, Biddinger PW, et al. Surfactant proteins and thyroid transcription factor-1 in pulmonary and breast carcinomas. Mod Pathol 1996; 9:445–452.

218. Di Loreto C, Puglisi F, Damante G, et al. TTF-1 protein expression in pleural malignant mesotheliomas and adenocarcinomas of the lung. Cancer Lett 1998; 124:73–78.

219. Kaufmann O, Dietel M. Expression of thyroid transcription factor-1 in pulmonary and extrapulmonary small cell carcinomas and other neuroendocrine carcinomas of various primary sites. Histopathology 2000; 36:415–420.

220. Chen HC, Chu RY, Hsu PN, et al. Loss of E-cadherin expression correlates with poor differentiation and invasion into adjacent organs in gastric adenocarcinomas. Cancer Lett 2003; 201:97–106.

221. Mizoshita T, Tsukamoto T, Nakanishi H, et al. Expression of CDX2 and the phenotype of advanced gastric cancers: relationship with prognosis. J Cancer Res Clin Oncol 2003; 129: 727–734.

222. Chiaravalli AM, Furlan D, Facco C, et al. Immunohistochemical pattern of hMSH2/hMLH1 in familial and sporadic colorectal, gastric, endometrial and ovarian carcinomas with instability in microsatellite sequences. Virchows Arch 2001; 438:39–48.

223. Wang JY, Chang CT, Hsieh JS, et al. Role of MUC1 and MUC5AC expressions as prognostic indicators in gastric carcinomas. J Surg Oncol 2003; 83:253–260.

224. Pinto-de-Sousa J, David L, Reis CA, et al. Mucins MUC1, MUC2, MUC5AC and MUC6 expression in the evaluation of differentiation and clinicobiological behaviour of gastric carcinoma. Virchows Arch 2002; 440:304–310.

225. Lee HS, Lee HK, Kim HS, et al. MUC1, MUC2, MUC5AC, and MUC6 expressions in gastric carcinomas: their roles as prognostic indicators. Cancer 2001; 92:1427–1434.

226. Gurbuz Y, Kahlke V, Kloppel G. How do gastric carcinoma classification systems relate to mucin expression patterns? An immunohistochemical analysis in a series of advanced gastric carcinomas. Virchows Arch 2002; 440:505–511.

227. Wang RQ, Fang DC. Alterations of MUC1 and MUC3 expression in gastric carcinoma: relevance to patient clinicopathological features. J Clin Pathol 2003; 56:378–384.

228. Goldstein NS. Proximal small-bowel mucosal villous intraepithelial lymphocytes. Histopathology 2004; 44:199–205.

229. Goldstein NS. Non-gluten sensitivity-related small bowel villous flattening with increased intraepithelial lymphocytes: not all that flattens is celiac sprue. Am J Clin Pathol 2004; 121:546–550.

230. Le Gall F, Vallet VS, Thomas D, et al. Immunohistochemical study of secretogranin II in 62 neuroendocrine tumors of the digestive tract and of the pancreas in comparison with other granins. Pathol Res Pract 1997; 193:179–185.

231. Burke AP, Thomas RM, Elsayed AM, et al. Carcinoids of the jejunum and ileum: an immunohistochemical and clinico-pathologic study of 167 cases. Cancer 1997; 79:1086–1093.

232. Zhang PJ, Harris KR, Alobeid B, et al. Immunoexpression of villin in neuroendocrine tumors and its diagnostic implications. Arch Pathol Lab Med 1999; 123:812–816.

233. Burke AP, Federspiel BH, Sobin LH, et al. Carcinoids of the duodenum. A histologic and immunohistochemical study of 65 tumors. Am J Surg Pathol 1989; 13:828–837.

234. De Schryver-Kecskemeti K, Clouse RE, Kraus FT. Surgical pathology of gastric and duodenal neuroendocrine tumors masquerading clinically as common polyps. Semin Diagn Pathol 1984; 1:5–12.

235. Lundqvist M, Eriksson B, Oberg K, et al. Histogenesis of a

duodenal carcinoid. Pathol Res Pract 1989; 184:217–222.

236. Stamm B, Hedinger CE, Saremaslani P. Duodenal and ampullary carcinoid tumors. A report of 12 cases with pathological characteristics, polypeptide content and relation to the MEN I syndrome and von Recklinghausen's disease (neurofibromatosis). Virchows Arch 1986; 408:475–489.

237. Pai SA, Krishnamurthy S, Soman CS. Psammomatous carcinoid tumor of the duodenum. Indian J Gastroenterol 1994; 13:26–27.

238. Makhlouf HR, Burke AP, Sobin LH. Carcinoid tumors of the ampulla of Vater: A comparison with duodenal carcinoid tumors. Cancer 1999; 85:1241–1249.

239. Oliveira AM, Tazelaar HD, Myers JL, et al. Thyroid transcription factor-1 distinguishes metastatic pulmonary from well-differentiated neuroendocrine tumors of other sites. Am J Surg Pathol 2001; 25:815–819.

240. Brainard JA, Goldblum JR. Stromal tumors of the jejunum and ileum: a clinicopathologic study of 39 cases. Am J Surg Pathol 1997; 21:407–416.

241. Miettinen M, Kopczynski J, Makhlouf HR, et al. Gastrointestinal stromal tumors, intramural leiomyomas, and leiomyosarcomas in the duodenum: a clinicopathologic, immunohistochemical, and molecular genetic study of 167 cases. Am J Surg Pathol 2003; 27:625–641.

242. Suster S, Fisher C, Moran CA: Expression of bcl-2 oncoprotein in benign and malignant spindle cell tumors of soft tissue, skin, serosal surfaces, and gastrointestinal tract. Am J Surg Pathol 1998; 22:863–872.

243. Alexander J, Krishnamurthy S, Kovacs D, et al. Cyto-keratin profile of extrahepatic pancreaticobiliary epithelia and their carcinomas. Appl Immunohistochem 1997; 5:216–222.

244. Svrcek M, Jourdan F, Sebbagh N, et al. Immunohistochemical analysis of adenocarcinoma of the small intestine: a tissue microarray study. J Clin Pathol 2003; 56:898–903.

245. Planck M, Ericson K, Piotrowska Z, et al. Microsatellite instability and expression of MLH1 and MSH2 in carcinomas of the small intestine. Cancer 2003; 97:1551–1557.

246. Goldstein NS, Bassi D. Cytokeratins 7, 17, and 20 reactivity in pancreatic and ampulla of Vater adenocarcinomas. Percentage of positivity and distribution is affected by the cut-point threshold. Am J Clin Pathol 2001; 115:695–702.

247. Moyana TN, Satkunam NA. A comparative immunohistochemical study of jejunoileal and appendiceal carcinoids. Implications for histogenesis and pathogenesis. Cancer 1992; 70:1081–1082.

248. Wilander E, Scheibenpflug L. Cytokeratin expression in small intestinal and appendiceal carcinoids. A basis for classification. Acta Oncol 1993; 32:131–134.

249. Anderson NH, Somerville JE, Johnston CF, et al. Appendiceal goblet cell carcinoids: a clinicopathological and immunohistochemical study. Histopathology 1991; 18:61–65.

250. Bak M, Asschenfeldt P. Adenocarcinoid of the vermiform appendix. A clinicopathologic study of 20 cases. Dis Colon Rectum 1988; 31:605–612.

251. Barshack I, Goldberg I, Chowers Y, et al. Different beta-catenin immunoexpression in carcinoid tumors of the appendix in comparison to other gastrointestinal carcinoid tumors. Pathol Res Pract 2002; 198:531–536.

252. Guerrieri C, Franlund B, Fristedt S, et al. Mucinous tumors of the vermiform appendix and ovary, and pseudomyxoma peritonei: histogenetic implications of cytokeratin 7 expression. Hum Pathol 1997; 28:1039–1045.

253. Ji H, Isacson C, Seidman JD, et al. Cytokeratins 7 and 20, Dpc4, and MUC5AC in the distinction of metastatic mucinous carcinomas in the ovary from primary ovarian mucinous tumors: Dpc4 assists in identifying metastatic pancreatic carcinomas. Int J Gynecol Pathol 2002; 21:391–400.

254. Ronnett BM, Shmookler BM, Diener-West M, et al. Immunohistochemical evidence supporting the appendiceal origin of pseudomyxoma peritonei in women. Int J Gynecol Pathol 1997; 16:1–9.

255. Ronnett BM, Kurman RJ, Shmookler BM, et al. The morphologic spectrum of ovarian metastases of appendiceal adenocarcinomas: a clinicopathologic and immunohistochemical analysis of tumors often misinterpreted as primary ovarian tumors or metastatic tumors from other gastrointestinal sites. Am J Surg Pathol 1997; 21:1144–1155.

256. Guerrieri C, Franlund B, Boeryd B. Expression of cytokeratin 7 in simultaneous mucinous tumors of the ovary and appendix. Mod Pathol 1995; 8:573–576.

257. Seidman JD, Elsayed AM, Sobin LH, et al. Association of mucinous tumors of the ovary and appendix. A clinicopathologic study of 25 cases. Am J Surg Pathol 1993; 17:22–34.

258. Albarracin CT, Jafri J, Montag AG, et al. Differential expression of MUC2 and MUC5AC mucin genes in primary ovarian and metastatic colonic carcinoma. Hum Pathol 2000;

31:672–677.

259. O'Connell JT, Hacker CM, Barsky SH. MUC2 is a molecular marker for pseudomyxoma peritonei. Mod Pathol 2002; 15:958–972.

260. Seidman JD, Kurman RJ, Ronnett BM. Primary and metastatic mucinous adenocarcinomas in the ovaries: incidence in routine practice with a new approach to improve intraoperative diagnosis. Am J Surg Pathol 2003; 27:985–993.

261. Lee KR, Young RH. The distinction between primary and metastatic mucinous carcinomas of the ovary: gross and histologic findings in 50 cases. Am J Surg Pathol 2003; 27:281–292.

262. Berezowski K, Stastny JF, Kornstein MJ. Cytokeratins 7 and 20 and carcinoembryonic antigen in ovarian and colonic carcinoma. Mod Pathol 1996; 9:426–429.

263. Lagendijk JH, Mullink H, Van Diest PJ, et al. Tracing the origin of adenocarcinomas with unknown primary using immunohistochemistry: differential diagnosis between colonic and ovarian carcinomas as primary sites. Hum Pathol 1998; 29:491–497.

264. Loy TS, Calaluce RD, Keeney GL. Cytokeratin immunostaining in differentiating primary ovarian carcinoma from metastatic colonic adenocarcinoma. Mod Pathol 1996; 9: 1040–1044.

265. Maeda T, Kajiyama K, Adachi E, et al. The expression of cytokeratins 7, 19, and 20 in primary and metastatic carcinomas of the liver. Mod pathol 1996; 9:901-909.

266. Ueda G, Sawada M, Ogawa H, et al. Immunohistochemical study of cytokeratin 7 for the differential diagnosis of adenocarcinomas in the ovary. Gynecol Oncol 1993; 51:219–223.

267. Young RH, Hart WR. Metastatic intestinal carcinomas simulating primary ovarian clear cell carcinoma and secretory endometrioid carcinoma: a clinicopathologic and immunohistochemical study of five cases. Am J Surg Pathol 1998; 22:805–815.

268. Fraggetta F, Pelosi G, Cafici A, et al. CDX2 immunoreactivity in primary and metastatic ovarian mucinous tumours. Virchows Arch 2003; 443:782–786.

269. Tornillo L, Moch H, Diener PA, et al. CDX-2 immunostaining in primary and secondary ovarian carcinomas. J Clin Pathol 2004; 57:641–643.

270. Chou YY, Jeng YM, Kao HL, et al. Differentiation of ovarian mucinous carcinoma and metastatic colorectal adenocarcinoma by immunostaining with beta-catenin. Histopathology 2003; 43:151–156.

271. Mackenzie JM, Dixon MF. An immunohistochemical study of the enteric neural plexi in Hirschsprung's disease. Histopathology 1987; 11:1055–1066.

272. d'Amore ES, Manivel JC, Pettinato G, et al. Intestinal ganglioneuromatosis: mucosal and transmural types. A clinicopathologic and immunohistochemical study of six cases. Hum Pathol 1991; 22:276–286.

273. Miettinen M, Shekitka KM, Sobin LH. Schwannomas in the colon and rectum: a clinicopathologic and immunohistochemical study of 20 cases. Am J Surg Pathol 2001; 25:846–855.

274. Miettinen M, Sobin LH. Gastrointestinal stromal tumors in the appendix: a clinicopathologic and immunohistochemical study of four cases. Am J Surg Pathol 2001; 25:1433–1437.

275. Miettinen M, Furlong M, Sarlomo-Rikala M, et al. Gastrointestinal stromal tumors, intramural leiomyomas, and leiomyosarcomas in the rectum and anus: a clinicopathologic, immunohistochemical, and molecular genetic study of 144 cases. Am J Surg Pathol 2001; 25:1121–1133.

276. Miettinen M, Sarlomo-Rikala M, Sobin LH. Mesenchymal tumors of muscularis mucosae of colon and rectum are benign leiomyomas that should be separated from gastrointestinal stromal tumors – a clinicopathologic and immunohistochemical study of eighty-eight cases. Mod Pathol 2001; 14: 950–956.

277. Federspiel BH, Burke AP, Sobin LH, et al. Rectal and colonic carcinoids: A clinicopathologic study of 84 cases. Cancer 1990; 65:135–140.

278. Axumi N, Traweek ST, Battifora H. Prostatic acid phosphatase in carcinoid tumors: Immunohistochemical and immunoblot studies. Am J Surg Pathol 1991; 15:785–790.

279. Jiang Z, Fanger GR, Woda BA, et al. Expression of alpha-methylacyl-CoA racemase (P504s) in various malignant neoplasms and normal tissues: a study of 761 cases. Hum Pathol 2003; 34:792–796.

280. Nash SV, Said JW. Gastroenteropancreatic neuroendocrine tumors. A histochemical and immunohistochemical study of epithelial (keratin proteins, carcinoembryonic antigen) and neuroendocrine (neuron-specific enolase, bombesin and chromogranin) markers in foregut, midgut, and hindgut tumors. Am J Clin Pathol 1986; 86:415–422.

281. Fahrenkamp AG, Wibbeke C, Winde G, et al. Immunohis-

tochemical distribution of chromogranins A and B and secretogranin II in neuroendocrine tumors of the gastrointestinal tract. Virchows Arch 1995; 426:361–367.
282. Azzoni C, Bonato M, D'Adda T, et al. Well-differentiated endocrine tumors of the middle ear and of the hindgut have immunohistochemical and ultrastructural features in common. Virchows Arch 1995; 426:411–418.
283. Barbareschi M, Roldo C, Zamboni G, et al. CDX-2 homeobox gene product expression in neuroendocrine tumors: its role as a marker of intestinal neuroendocrine tumors. Am J Surg Pathol 2004; 28:1169–1176.
284. Sasaki A, Kawano K, Aramaki M, et al. Immunohistochemical expression of cytokeratins in intrahepatic cholangiocarcinoma and metastatic adenocarcinoma of the liver. J Surg Oncol 1999; 70:103–108.
285. O'hara BJ, Paetau A, Miettinen M. Keratin subsets and monoclonal antibody HMBE-1 in chordoma: Immunohistochemical differential diagnosis between tumors simulating chordoma. Hum Pathol 1998; 29:119–126.
286. Fujisaki J, Shimoda T. Expression of cytokeratin subtypes in colorectal mucosa, adenoma, and carcinoma. Gastro-enterol Jpn 1993; 28:647–656.
287. Scarpatetti M, Tsybrovskyy O, Popper HH. Cytokeratin typing as an aid in the differential diagnosis of primary versus metastatic lung carcinomas, and comparison with normal lung. Virchows Arch 2002; 440:70–76.
288. Rubin BP, Skarin AT, Pisick E, et al. Use of cytokeratins 7 and 20 in determining the origin of metastatic carcinoma of unknown primary, with special emphasis on lung cancer. Eur J Cancer Prev 2001; 10:77–82.
289. Hinoi T, Tani M, Lucas PC, et al. Loss of CDX2 expression and microsatellite instability are prominent features of large cell minimally differentiated carcinomas of the colon. Am J Pathol 2001; 159:2239–2248.
290. Tot T. Cytokeratins 20 and 7 as biomarkers: usefulness in discriminating primary from metastatic adenocarcinoma. Eur J Cancer 2002; 38:758–763.
291. Rullier A, Le Bail B, Fawaz R, et al. Cytokeratin 7 and 20 expression in cholangiocarcinomas varies along the biliary tract but still differs from that in colorectal carcinoma metastasis. Am J Surg Pathol 2000; 24:870–876.
292. Li MK, Folpe AL. CDX-2, a new marker for adenocarcinoma of gastrointestinal origin. Adv Anat Pathol 2004; 11:101–105.
293. Wright CL, Stewart ID. Histopathology and mismatch repair status of 458 consecutive colorectal carcinomas. Am J Surg Pathol 2003; 27:1393–1406.
294. Jover R, Paya A, Alenda C, et al. Defective mismatch-repair colorectal cancer: clinicopathologic characteristics and usefulness of immunohistochemical analysis for diagnosis. Am J Clin Pathol 2004; 122:389–394.
295. McGregor DK, Wu TT, Rashid A, et al. Reduced expression of cytokeratin 20 in colorectal carcinomas with high levels of microsatellite instability. Am J Surg Pathol 2004; 28:712–718.
296. Kanazawa T, Watanabe T, Kazama S, et al. Poorly differentiated adenocarcinoma and mucinous carcinoma of the colon and rectum show higher rates of loss of heterozygosity and loss of E-cadherin expression due to methylation of promoter region. Int J Cancer 2002; 102:225–229.
297. Rossi G, Bertolini F, Sartori G, et al. Primary mixed adenocarcinoma and small cell carcinoma of the appendix: a clinicopathologic, immunohistochemical, and molecular study of a hitherto unreported tumor. Am J Surg Pathol 2004; 28: 1233–1239.
298. Sarsfield P, Anthony PP. Small cell undifferentiated ('neuroendocrine') carcinoma of the colon. Histopathology 1990; 16:357–363.
299. Chan JKC, Suster S, Wenig BM, et al. Cytokeratin 20 immunoreactivity distinguishes Merkel cell (primary cutaneous neuroendocrine) carcinomas and salivary gland small cell carcinomas from small cell carcinomas of various sites. Am J Surg Pathol 1997; 21:226–234.
300. Robey-Cafferty SS, Silva EG, Cleary KR. Anaplastic and sarcomatoid carcinoma of the small intestine: a clinicopathologic study. Hum Pathol 1988; 20:858–863.
301. Kaizaki Y, Fujii T, Kawai T, et al. Gastric neuroendocrine carcinoma associated with chronic atrophic gastritis type A. J Gastroenterol 1997; 32:643–649.
302. Burke AP, Shekitka KM, Sobin LH. Small cell carcinomas of the large intestine. Am J Clin Pathol 1991; 95:315–321.
303. Gaffey MJ, Mills SE, Lack EE. Neuroendocrine carcinoma of the colon and rectum. A clinicopathologic, ultrastructural, and immunohistochemical study of 24 cases. Am J Surg Pathol 1990; 14:1010–1023.
304. Matsui K, Jin XM, Kitagawa M, et al. Clinicopathologic features of neuroendocrine carcinomas of the stomach: Appraisal

of small cell and large cell variants. Arch Pathol Lab Med 1998; 122:1010–1017.
305. Sarker AB, Hoshida Y, Akagi S, et al. An immunohistochemical and ultrastructural study of case of small-cell neuroendocrine carcinoma in the ampullary region of the duodenum. Acta Pathol Jpn 1992; 42:529–535.
306. Saclarides TJ, Szeluga D, Staren ED. Neuroendocrine cancers of the colon and rectum: Results of a ten-year experience. Dis Colon Rectum 1994; 37:635–642.
307. Eichhorn JH, Young RH, Scully RE. Nonpulmonary small cell carcinomas of extragenital origin metastatic to the ovary. Cancer 1993; 71:177–186.
308. Zamboni G, Franzin G, Bonetti F, et al. Small-cell neuroendocrine carcinoma of the ampullary region. A clinicopathologic, immunohistochemical, and ultrastructural study of three cases. Am J Surg Pathol 1990; 14:703–713.
309. Jewell LD, Barr JR, McCaughey WTE, et al. Clear-cell epithelial neoplasms of the large intestine. Arch Pathol Lab Med 1988; 112:197–199.
310. Yang AH, Chen WYK, Chiang H. Malignant rhabdoid tumor of colon. Histopathology 1994; 24:89–91.
311. Amrikachi M, Ro JY, Ordonez NG, et al. Adenocarcinomas of the gastrointestinal tract with prominent rhabdoid features. Ann Diagn Pathol 2002; 6:357–363.
312. Nicholson AG, McCormick CJ, Shimosato Y, et al. The value of PE-10, a monoclonal antibody against pulmonary surfactant, in distinguishing primary and metastatic lung tumors. Histopathology 1995; 27:57–60.
313. Zamecnik J, Kodet R. Value of thyroid transcription factor-1 and surfactant apoprotein A in the differential diagnosis of pulmonary carcinomas: a study of 109 cases. Virchows Arch 2002; 440:353–361.
314. Moldvay J, Jackel M, Bogos K, et al. The role of TTF-1 in differentiating primary and metastatic lung adenocarcinomas. Pathol Oncol Res 2004; 10:85–88.
315. Chang YL, Lee YC, Liao WY, et al. The utility and limitation of thyroid transcription factor-1 protein in primary and metastatic pulmonary neoplasms. Lung Cancer 2004; 44:149–157.
316. Srodon M, Westra WH. Immunohistochemical staining for thyroid transcription factor-1: a helpful aid in discerning primary site of tumor origin in patients with brain metastases. Hum Pathol 2002; 33:642–645.
317. Reis-Filho JS, Carrilho C, Valenti C, et al. Is TTF1 a good immunohistochemical marker to distinguish primary from metastatic lung adenocarcinomas? Pathol Res Pract 2000; 196: 835–840.
318. Kaufmann O, Dietel M. Thyroid transcription factor-1 is the superior immunohistochemical marker for pulmonary adenocarcinomas and large cell carcinomas compared to surfactant proteins A and B. Histopathology 2000; 36:8–16.
319. Goldstein NS, Thomas M. Mucinous and nonmucinous bronchioloalveolar adenocarcinomas have distinct staining patterns with thyroid transcription factor and cytokeratin 20 antibodies. Am J Clin Pathol 2001; 116:319–325.
320. Shah RN, Badve S, Papreddy K, et al. Expression of cytokeratin 20 in mucinous bronchioloalveolar carcinoma. Hum Pathol 2002; 33:915–920.
321. Yatabe Y, Koga T, Mitsudomi T, et al. CK20 expression, CDX2 expression, K-ras mutation, and goblet cell morphology in a subset of lung adenocarcinomas. J Pathol 2004; 203: 645–652.
322. Saad RS, Cho P, Silverman JF, et al. Usefulness of CDX2 in separating mucinous bronchioloalveolar adenocarcinoma of the lung from metastatic mucinous colorectal adenocarcinoma. Am J Clin Pathol 2004; 122:421–427.
323. DeCostanzo DC, Elias JM, Chumas JC. Necrosis in 84 ovarian carcinomas: a morphologic study of primary versus metastatic colonic carcinoma with a selective immunohistochemical analysis of cytokeratin subtypes and carcinoembryonic antigen. Int J Gynecol Pathol 1997; 16:245–249.
324. Coffin CM, Swanson PE, Wick MR, et al. An immunohistochemical comparison of chordoma with renal cell carcinoma, colorectal adenocarcinoma, and myxopapillary ependymoma: A potential diagnostic dilemma in the diminutive biopsy. Mod Pathol 1993; 6:531–538.
325. Helle M, Krohn K. Immunohistochemical reactivity of monoclonal antibodies to human milk fat globule with breast carcinoma and with other normal and neoplastic tissues. Acta Pathol Microbiol Immunol Scand 1986; 94:43–51.
326. Ghoneim AHA, Brisson ML, Fuks A, et al Monoclonal anti-CEA antibodies in the discrimination between primary pulmonary adenocarcinoma and colon carcinoma metastatic to the lung. Mod Pathol 1990; 3:613–618.
327. Lash RH, Hart WR. Intestinal adenocarcinomas metastatic to the ovaries: A clinicopathologic evaluation of 22 cases.

Am J Surg Pathol 1987; 11:114–121.

328. Lagendijk JH, Mullink H, Van Diest PJ, et al. Immunohistochemical differentiation between primary adenocarcinomas of the ovary and ovarian metastases of colonic and breast origin. Comparison between a statistical and an intuitive approach. J Clin Pathol 1999; 52:283–290.

329. Loy TS, Quesenberry JT, Sharp SC. Distribution of CA 125 in adenocarcinomas. An immunohistochemical study of 481 cases. Am J Clin Pathol 1992; 98:175–179.

330. Azumi N, Battifora H. The distribution of vimentin and keratin in epithelial and nonepithelial neoplasms. Am J Clin Pathol 1987; 88:286–296.

331. Shipley WR, Hammer RD, Lennington WJ, et al. Paraffin immunohistochemical detection of CD56, a useful marker for neural cell adhesion molecule (NCAM), in normal and neoplastic fixed tissues. Appl Immunohistochem 1997; 5:87–93.

332. Kaufmann OK, George T, Dietel M. Utility of 123C3 monoclonal antibody against CD56 (NCAM) for the diagnosis of small cell carcinomas on paraffin sections. Hum Pathol 1997; 28:1373–1378.

333. Ordonez NG. Value of thrombomodulin immunostaining in the diagnosis of transitional cell carcinoma: A comparative study with carcinoembryonic antigen. Histopathology 1997; 31:517–524.

334. Wang HL, Lu DW, Yerian LM, et al. Immunohistochemical distinction between primary adenocarcinoma of the bladder and secondary colorectal adenocarcinoma. Am J Surg Pathol 2001; 25:1380–1387.

335. Tamboli P, Mohsin SK, Hailemariam S, et al. Colonic adenocarcinoma metastatic to the urinary tract versus primary tumors of the urinary tract with glandular differentiation: a report of 7 cases and investigation using a limited immunohistochemical panel. Arch Pathol Lab Med 2002; 126:1057–1063.

336. Goldstein NS. Immunophenotypic characterization of 225 prostate adenocarcinomas with intermediate or high Gleason scores. Am J Clin Pathol 2002; 117:471–477.

337. Torbenson M, Dhir R, Nangia A, et al. Prostatic carcinoma with signet ring cells: a clinicopathologic and immunohistochemical analysis of 12 cases, with review of the literature. Mod Pathol 1998; 11:552–559.

338. Gatalica D, Miettinen M. Distribution of carcinoma antigens CA 19-9 and CA 15-3: Immunohistochemical study of 400 tumors. Appl Immunohistochem 1994; 2:205–211.

339. Loy TS, Sharp SC, Andershock CJ, et al. Distribution of CA 19-9 in adenocarcinomas and transitional cell carcinomas. An immunohistochemical study of 527 cases. Am J Clin Pathol 1993; 99:726–728.

340. Grabowski P, Schonfelder J, Ahnert-Hilger G, et al. Expression of neuroendocrine markers: a signature of human undifferentiated carcinoma of the colon and rectum. Virchows Arch 2002; 441:256–263.

341. Wick MR, Weatherby RP, Weiland LH. Small cell neuroendocrine carcinoma of the colon and rectum: clinical, histologic, and ultrastructural study and immunohistochemical comparison with cloacogenic carcinoma. Hum Pathol 1987; 18:9–21.

342. Staren ED, Gould VE, Jansson DS, et al. Neuroendocrine differentiation in 'poorly differentiated' colon carcinomas. Am Surg 1990; 56 412–419.

343. Iyer PV, Leong AS. Poorly differentiated squamous cell carcinomas of the skin can express vimentin. J Cutan Pathol 1992; 19:34–39.

344. Levy R, Czernobilsky B, Geiger B. Cytokeratin polypeptide expression in a cloacogenic carcinoma and in the normal anal canal epithelium. Virchows Arch 1991; 418:447–455.

345. Hobbs CM, Lowry MA, Owen D, et al. Anal gland carcinoma. Cancer 2001; 92:2045–2049.

346. Battles OE, Page DL, Johnson JE. Cytokeratins, CEA, and mucin histochemistry in the diagnosis and characterization of extramammary Paget's disease. Am J Clin Pathol 1997; 108:6–12.

347. Helm KF, Goellner JR, Peters MS. Immunohistochemical stains in extramammary Paget's disease. Am J Dermato-pathol 1992; 14:402–407.

348. Smith KJ, Tuur S, Corvette D, et al. Cytokeratin 7 staining in mammary and extramammary Paget's disease. Mod Pathol 1997; 10:1069–1074.

349. Nowak MA, Guerriere-Kovach P, Pathan A, et al. Perianal Paget's disease: distinguishing primary and secondary lesions using immunohistochemical studies including gross cystic disease fluid protein-15 and cytokeratin 20 expression. Arch Pathol Lab Med 1998; 122:1077–1081.

350. Goldblum JR, Hart WR. Perianal Paget's disease: a histologic and immunohistochemical study of 11 cases with and

without associated rectal adenocarcinoma. Am J Surg Pathol 1998; 22:170–179.

351. Lundquist K, Kohler S, Rouse RV. Intraepidermal cytokeratin 7 expression is not restricted to Paget cells but is also seen in Toker cells and Merkel cells. Am J Surg Pathol 1999; 23: 212–219.

352. Ohnishi T, Watanabe S. The use of cytokeratins 7 and 20 in the diagnosis of primary and secondary extramammary Paget's disease. Br J Dermatol 2000; 142:243–247.

353. Ramalingam P, Hart WR, Goldblum JR. Cytokeratin subset immunostaining in rectal adenocarcinoma and normal anal glands. Arch Pathol Lab Med 2001; 125:1074–1077.

354. Ordonez NG, Awalt H, Mackay B. Mammary and extramammary Paget's disease. An immunocytochemical and ultrastructural study. Cancer 1987; 59:1173–1183.

355. Goldstein NS, Armin M. Epidermal growth factor receptor immunohistochemical reactivity in patients with American Joint Committee on Cancer Stage IV colon adenocarcinoma: implications for a standardized scoring system. Cancer 2001; 92:1331–1346.

356. Atkins D, Reiffen KA, Tegtmeier CL, et al. Immunohistochemical detection of EGFR in paraffin-embedded tumor tissues: variation in staining intensity due to choice of fixative and storage time of tissue sections. J Histochem Cytochem 2004; 52:893–901.

357. Oikawa I, Hirata K, Katsuramaki T, et al. Neuroendocrine carcinoma of the extrahepatic biliary tract with positive immunostaining for gastrin-releasing peptide: report of a case. Surg Today 1998; 28:1192–1195.

358. Moller CJ, Christgau S, Williamson MR, et al. Differential expression of neural cell adhesion molecule and cadherins in pancreatic islets, glucagonomas, and insulinomas. Mol Endocrinol 1992; 6:1332–1342.

359. Kotoulas C, Panayiotides J, Antiochos C, et al. Huge non-functioning pancreatic cystic neuroendocrine tumour: a case report. Eur J Surg Oncol 1998; 24:74–76.

360. Aronsky D, Z'graggen K, Stauffer E, et al. Primary neuroendocrine tumors of the cystic duct. Digestion 1999; 19:493–496.

361. Lam KY, Lo CY. Pancreatic endocrine tumour: a 22-year clinico-pathological experience with morphological, immunohistochemical observation and a review of the literature. Eur J Surg Oncol 1997; 23:36–42.

362. Azzoni C, Doglioni C, Viale G, et al. Involvement of BCL-2 oncoprotein in the development of enterochromaffin-like cell gastric carcinoids. Am J Surg Pathol 1996; 20:433–441.

363. Hayashi H, Nakagawa M, Kitagawa S, et al. Immunohistochemical analysis of gastrointestinal carcinoids. Gastroenterol Jpn 1993; 28:483–490.

364. Davtyan H, Nieberg R, Reber HA. Pancreatic cystic endocrine neoplasms. Pancreas 1990; 5:230–233.

365. Capella C, Riva C, Rindi G, et al. Histopathology, hormone products, and clinico-pathologic profile of endocrine tumors of the upper small intestine: A study of 44 cases. Endocr Pathol 1991; 2:92–110.

366. Gilligan CJ, Lawton GP, Tang LH, et al. Gastric carcinoid tumors: The biology and therapy of an enigmatic and controversial lesion. Am J Gastroenterol 1995; 90:338–352.

367. Rindi G, Paolotti D, LaRosa S, et al. The tumours of the endocrine pancreas. Eur J Histochem 1998; 42:63–66.

368. Chejfec G, Falkmer S, Grimelius L, et al. Synaptophysin. A new marker for pancreatic neuroendocrine tumors. Am J Surg Pathol 1987; 11:241–247.

369. Shah IA, Schlageter MO, Netto D. Immunoreactivity of neurofilament proteins in neuroendocrine neoplasms. Mod Pathol 1991; 4:215–219.

370. Rindi G, Ubiali A, Villanacci V. The phenotype of gut endocrine tumours. Dig Liver Dis 2004; 36(Suppl 1):S26–S30.

371. Erickson LA, Lloyd RV. Practical markers used in the diagnosis of endocrine tumors. Adv Anat Pathol 2004; 11:175–189.

372. Chetty R, Asa SL. Pancreatic endocrine tumors. Adv Anat Pathol 2004; 22:202–210.

373. Gurevich L, Kazantseva I, Isakov VA, et al. The analysis of immunophenotype of gastrin-producing tumors of the pancreas and gastrointestinal tract. Cancer 2003; 98:1967–1976.

374. Hoang MP, Hruban RH, Albores-Saavedra J. Clear cell endocrine pancreatic tumor mimicking renal cell carcinoma: a distinctive neoplasm of von Hippel-Lindau disease. Am J Surg Pathol 2001; 25:602–609.

375. Kakar S, Muir T, Murphy LM, et al. Immunoreactivity of Hep Par 1 in hepatic and extrahepatic tumors and its correlation with albumin in situ hybridization in hepatocellular carcinoma. Am J Clin Pathol 2003; 119:361–366.

376. O'Connor TP, Wade TP, Sunwoo YC, et al. Small cell undifferentiated carcinoma of the pancreas. Report of a patient with

tumor marker studies. Cancer 1992; 70:1514–1519.

377. Andea A, Sarkar F, Adsay VN. Clinicopathological correlates of pancreatic intraepithelial neoplasia: a comparative analysis of 82 cases with and 152 cases without pancreatic ductal adenocarcinoma. Mod Pathol 2003; 16:996–1006.

378. Takaori K, Kobashi Y, Matsusue S, et al. Clinicopathological features of pancreatic intraepithelial neoplasias and their relationship to intraductal papillary-mucinous tumors. J Hepatobiliary Pancreat Surg 2003; 10:125–136.

379. Agoff SN, Crispin DA, Bronner MP, et al. Neoplasms of the ampulla of Vater with concurrent pancreatic intraductal neoplasia: a histological and molecular study. Mod Pathol 2001; 14:139–146.

380. Moore PS, Orlandini S, Zamboni G, et al. Pancreatic tumours: molecular pathways implicated in ductal cancer are involved in ampullary but not in exocrine nonductal or endocrine tumorigenesis. Br J Cancer 2001; 84:253–262.

381. Levi E, Klimstra DS, Adsay NV, et al. MUC1 and MUC2 in pancreatic neoplasia. J Clin Pathol 2004; 57:456–462.

382. Adsay NV, Merati K, Basturk O, et al. Pathologically and biologically distinct types of epithelium in intraductal papillary mucinous neoplasms: delineation of an 'intestinal' pathway of carcinogenesis in the pancreas. Am J Surg Pathol 2004; 28:839–848.

383. Hruban RH, Takaori K, Klimstra DS, et al. An illustrated consensus on the classification of pancreatic intraepithelial neoplasia and intraductal papillary mucinous neoplasms. Am J Surg Pathol 2004; 28:977–987.

384. Abraham SC, Lee JH, Boitnott JK, et al. Microsatellite instability in intraductal papillary neoplasms of the biliary tract. Mod Pathol 2002; 15:1309–1317.

385. Abraham SC, Lee JH, Hruban RH, et al. Molecular and immunohistochemical analysis of intraductal papillary neoplasms of the biliary tract. Hum Pathol 2003; 34:902–910.

386. Suzuki Y, Atomi Y, Sugiyama M, et al. Cystic neoplasm of the pancreas: a Japanese multiinstitutional study of intraductal papillary mucinous tumor and mucinous cystic tumor. Pancreas 2004; 28:241–246.

387. Biankin AV, Kench JG, Dijkman FP, et al. Molecular pathogenesis of precursor lesions of pancreatic ductal adenocarcinoma. Pathology 2003; 35:14–24.

388. Stommer P, Gebhardt C, Schultheiss KH. Adenocarcinoma of the pancreas with a predominant intraductal component: a special variety of ductal adenocarcinoma. Pancreas 1990; 5:114–118.

389. Adsay NV, Adair CF, Heffess CS, et al. Intraductal oncocytic papillary neoplasms of the pancreas. Am J Surg Pathol 1996; 20:980–994.

390. Fabre A, Sauvanet A, Flejou JF, et al. Intraductal acinar cell carcinoma of the pancreas. Virchows Arch 2001; 438:312–315.

391. Handra-Luca A, Couvelard A, Degott C, et al. Correlation between patterns of DNA mismatch repair hMLH1 and hMSH2 protein expression and progression of dysplasia in intraductal papillary mucinous neoplasms of the pancreas. Virchows Arch 2004; 444:235–238.

392. Paal E, Thompson LD, Przygodzki RM, et al. A clinicopathologic and immunohistochemical study of 22 intraductal papillary mucinous neoplasms of the pancreas, with a review of the literature. Mod Pathol 1999; 12:518–528.

393. Nagai E, Ueki T, Chijiiwa K, et al. Intraductal papillary mucinous neoplasms of the pancreas associated with so-called 'mucinous ductal ectasia.' Histochemical and immunohistochemical analysis of 29 cases. Am J Surg Pathol 1995; 19:576–589.

394. Ohta T, Nagakawa T, Fukushima W, et al. Immunohistochemical study of carcinoembryonic antigen in mucinous cystic neoplasm of the pancreas. Eur Surg Res 1992; 24:37–44.

395. Luttges J, Feyerabend B, Buchelt T, et al. The mucin profile of noninvasive and invasive mucinous cystic neoplasms of the pancreas. Am J Surg Pathol 2002; 26:466–471.

396. Thompson LD, Becker RC, Przygodzki RM, et al. Mucinous cystic neoplasm (mucinous cystadenocarcinoma of low-grade malignant potential) of the pancreas: a clinicopathologic study of 130 cases. Am J Surg Pathol 1999; 23:1–16.

397. Terada T, Ohta T, Kitamura Y, et al. Endocrine cells in intraductal papillary-mucinous neoplasms of the pancreas. A histochemical and immunohistochemical study. Virchows Arch 1997; 431:31–36.

398. Weihing RR, Shintaku IP, Geller SA, et al. Hepatobiliary and pancreatic mucinous cystadenocarcinomas with mesenchymal stroma: analysis of estrogen receptors/progesterone receptors and expression of tumor-associated antigens. Mod Pathol 1997; 10:372–379.

399. Izumo A, Yamaguchi K, Eguchi T, et al. Mucinous cystic

tumor of the pancreas: immunohistochemical assessment of 'ovarian-type stroma.' Oncol Rep 2003; 10:515–525.

400. Zamboni G, Scarpa A, Bogina G, et al. Mucinous cystic tumors of the pancreas: clinicopathological features, prognosis, and relationship to other mucinous cystic tumors. Am J Surg Pathol 1999; 23:410–422.

401. Fukushima N, Mukai K. 'Ovarian-type' stroma of pancreatic mucinous cystic tumor expresses smooth muscle phenotype [letter]. Pathol Int 1997; 47:806–808.

402. Shorten SD, Hart WR, Petras RE. Microcystic adenomas (serous cystadenomas) of pancreas. A clinicopathologic investigation of eight cases with immunohistochemical and ultrastructural studies. Am J Surg Pathol 1986; 10:365–372.

403. Alpert LC, Truong LD, Bossart MI, et al. Microcystic adenoma (serous cystadenoma) of the pancreas. A study of 14 cases with immunohistochemical and electron-microscopic correlation. Am J Surg Pathol 1988; 12:251–263.

404. Perez-Ordonez B, Naseem A, Lieberman PH, et al. Solid serous adenoma of the pancreas. The solid variant of serous cystadenoma? Am J Surg Pathol 1996; 20:1401–1405.

405. Ishikawa T, Nakao A, Nomoto S, et al. Immunohistochemical and molecular biological studies of serous cystadenoma of the pancreas. Pancreas 1998; 16:40–44.

406. Kosmahl M, Wagner J, Peters K, et al. Serous cystic neoplasms of the pancreas: an immunohistochemical analysis revealing alpha-inhibin, neuron-specific enolase, and MUC6 as new markers. Am J Surg Pathol 2004; 28:339–346.

407. Yamaguchi K, Enjoji M, Tsuneyoshi M. Pancreatoduodenal carcinoma: a clinicopathologic study of 304 patients and immunohistochemical observation for CEA and CA19-9. J Surg Oncol 1991; 47:148–154.

408. Yamaguchi K, Enjoji M. Carcinoma of the pancreas: a clinicopathologic study of 96 cases with immunohistochemical observations. Jpn J Clin Oncol 1989; 19:14–22.

409. Luttges J, Vogel I, Menke M, et al. Clear cell carcinoma of the pancreas: an adenocarcinoma with ductal phenotype. Histopathology 1998; 32:444–448.

410. Hoorens A, Prenzel K, Lemoine NR, et al. Undifferentiated carcinoma of the pancreas: analysis of intermediate filament profile and Ki-ras mutations provides evidence of a ductal origin. J Pathol 1998; 185:53–60.

411. Thomas P, Battifora H. Keratins versus epithelial membrane antigen in tumor diagnosis: an immunohistochemical comparison of five monoclonal antibodies. Hum Pathol 1987; 18: 728–734.

412. Christensen WN, Boitnott JK, Kuhajda FP. Immunoperoxidase staining as a diagnostic aid for hepatocellular carcinoma. Mod Pathol 1989; 2:8–12.

413. Shimonishi T, Miyazaki K, Nakanuma Y. Cytokeratin profile relates to histological subtypes and intrahepatic location of intrahepatic cholangiocarcinoma and primary sites of metastatic adenocarcinoma of liver. Histopathology 2000; 37:55–63.

414. Goldstein NS, Bassi D, Uzieblo A. WT1 is an integral component of an antibody panel to distinguish pancreaticobiliary and some ovarian epithelial neoplasms. Am J Clin Pathol 2001; 116:246–252.

415. Tot T. The value of cytokeratins 20 and 7 in discriminating metastatic adenocarcinomas from pleural mesotheliomas. Cancer 2001; 92:2727–2732.

416. Duval JV, Savas L, Banner BF. Expression of cytokeratins 7 and 20 in carcinomas of the extrahepatic biliary tract, pancreas, and gallbladder. Arch Pathol Lab Med 2000; 124:1196–1200.

417. Albores-Saavedra J, Delgado R, Henson DE. Well-differentiated adenocarcinoma, gastric foveolar type, of the extrahepatic bile ducts: A previously unrecognized and distinctive morphologic variant of bile duct carcinoma. Ann Diagn Pathol 1999; 3:75–80.

418. Cabibi D, Licata A, Barresi E, et al. Expression of cytokeratin 7 and 20 in pathological conditions of the bile tract. Pathol Res Pract 2003; 199:65–70.

419. Tot T. Identifying colorectal metastases in liver biopsies: the novel CDX2 antibody is less specific than the cyto-keratin 20+/7- phenotype. Med Sci Monit 2004; 10:BR139–BR143.

420. Heyderman E, Larkin SE, O'Donnell PJ, et al. Epithelial markers in pancreatic carcinoma: immunoperoxidase localisation of DD9, CEA, EMA and CAM 5.2. J Clin Pathol 1990; 43:448–452.

421. Nishihara K, Fukuda T, Tsuneyoshi M, et al. Intraductal papillary neoplasm of the pancreas. Cancer 1993; 72:689–696.

422. Adsay V, Logani S, Sarkar F, et al. Foamy gland pattern of pancreatic ductal adenocarcinoma: a deceptively benign-appearing variant. Am J Surg Pathol 2000; 24:493–504.

423. Luttges J, Beyser K, Pust S, et al. Pancreatic mucinous noncystic (colloid) carcinomas and intraductal papillary mucinous carcinomas are usually microsatellite stable. Mod

424. Motoo Y, Kawashima A, Watanabe H, et al. Undifferentiated (anaplastic) carcinoma of the pancreas showing sarcomatous change and neoplastic cyst formation. Int J Pancreatol 1997; 21:243–248.
425. Watanabe M, Miura H, Inoue H, et al. Mixed osteoclastic/pleomorphic-type giant cell tumor of the pancreas with ductal adenocarcinoma: histochemical and immunohistochemical study with review of the literature. Pancreas 1997; 15: 201–208.
426. Marinho A, Nogueira R, Schmitt F, et al. Pancreatic mucinous cystadenocarcinoma with a mural nodule of anaplastic carcinoma. Histopathology 1995; 26:284–287.
427. Higashi M, Takao S, Sato E. Sarcomatoid carcinoma of the pancreas: a case report with immunohistochemical study. Pathol Int 1999; 49:453–456.
428. Wenig BM, Albores-Saavedra J, Buetow PC, et al. Pancreatic mucinous cystic neoplasm with sarcomatous stroma: a report of three cases. Am J Surg Pathol 1997; 21:70–80.
429. Paal E, Thompson LD, Frommelt RA, et al. A clinicopathologic and immunohistochemical study of 35 anaplastic carcinomas of the pancreas with a review of the literature. Ann Diagn Pathol 2001; 5:129–140.
430. Nishihara K, Nagai E, Izumi Y, et al. Adenosquamous carcinoma of the gallbladder: a clinicopathological, immunohistochemical and flow-cytometric study of twenty cases. Jpn J Cancer Res 1994; 85 389–399.
431. Imai Y, Morishita S, Ikeda Y, et al. Immunohistochemical and molecular analysis of giant cell carcinoma of the pancreas: a report of three cases. Pancreas 1999; 18:308–315.
432. Nishihara K, Katsumoto F, Kurokawa Y, et al. Anaplastic carcinoma showing rhabdoid features combined with mucinous cystadenocarcinoma of the pancreas. Arch Pathol Lab Med 1997; 121:1104–1107.
433. Gatteschi B, Saccomanno S, Bartoli FG, et al. Mixed pleomorphic-osteoclast-like tumor of the pancreas. Light microscopical, immunohistochemical, and molecular biological studies. Int J Pancreatol 1995; 18:169–175.
434. Perez-Montiel MD, Frankel WL, Suster S. Neuroendocrine carcinomas of the pancreas with 'rhabdoid' features. Am J Surg Pathol 2003; 27:642–649.
435. Nishihara K, Tsuneyoshi M. Undifferentiated spindle cell carcinoma of the gallbladder: a clinicopathologic, immunohistochemical, and flow cytometric study of 11 cases. Hum Pathol 1993; 24:1298–1305.
436. Al Nafussi A, O'Donnell M. Poorly differentiated adenocarcinoma with extensive rhabdoid differentiation: clinicopathological features of two cases arising in the gastrointestinal tract. Pathol Int 1999; 49:160–163.
437. Westra WH, Sturm P, Drillenburg P, et al. K-ras oncogene mutations in osteoclast-like giant cell tumors of the pancreas and liver: genetic evidence to support origin from the duct epithelium. Am J Surg Pathol 1998; 22:1247–1254.
438. Bergman S, Medeiros LJ, Radr T, et al. Giant cell tumor of the pancreas arising in the ovarian-like stroma of a mucinous cystadenocarcinoma. Int J Pancreatol 1995; 18:71–75.
439. Goldberg RD, Michelassi F, Montag AG. Osteoclast-like giant cell tumor of the pancreas: immunophenotypic similarity to giant cell tumor of bone. Hum Pathol 1991; 22:618–622.
440. Caruso RA, Inferrera A, Tuccari G, et al. Acinar cell carcinoma of the pancreas. A histologic, immunocytochemical and ultrastructural study. Histol Histopathol 1994; 9:53–58.
441. Ordonez NG. Pancreatic acinar cell carcinoma. Adv Anat Pathol 2001; 8:144–159.
442. Hartman GG, Ni H, Pickleman J. Acinar cell carcinoma of the pancreas. Arch Pathol Lab Med 2001; 125:1127–1128.
443. Kuerer H, Shim H, Pertsemlidis D, et al. Functioning pancreatic acinar cell carcinoma: immunohistochemical and ultrastructural analyses. Am J Clin Oncol 1997; 20:101–107.
444. Morohoshi T, Kanda M, Horie A, et al. Immunocytochemical markers of uncommon pancreatic tumors. Cancer 1987; 59:739–747.
445. Klimstra DS, Heffess CS, Oertel JE, et al. Acinar cell carcinoma of the pancreas. A clinicopathologic study of 28 cases. Am J Surg Pathol 1992; 16:815–837.
446. Toyota N, Takada T, Ammori BJ, et al. Acinar cell carcinoma of the pancreas showing finger-print-like zymogen granules by electron microscopy: immunohistochemical study. J Hepatobiliary Pancreat Surg 2000; 7:102–106.
447. Lonardo F, Cubilla AL, Klimstra DS. Microadenocarcinoma of the pancreas – morphologic pattern or pathologic entity? A reevaluation of the original series. Am J Surg Pathol 1996; 20:1385–1393.
448. di Sant'Agnese PA. Acinar cell carcinoma of the pancreas. Ultrastruct Pathol 1991; 15:573–577.
449. Skacel M, Ormsby AH, Petras RE, et al. Immunohistochem-

449. istry in the differential diagnosis of acinar and endocrine pancreatic neoplasms. Appl Immunohistochem Mol Morphol 2000; 8:203–209.

450. Yamaguchi K, Miyagahara T, Tsuneyoshi M, et al. Papillary cystic tumor of the pancreas: an immunohistochemical and ultrastructural study of 14 patients. Jpn J Clin Oncol 1989; 19:102–111.

451. Pettinato G, Manivel JC, Ravetto C, et al. Papillary cystic tumor of the pancreas: A clinicopathologic study of 20 cases with cytologic, immunohistochemical, ultrastructural, and flow cytometric observations and a review of the literature. Am J Clin Pathol 1992; 98:478–488.

452. Mao C, Guvendi M, Domenico DR, et al. Papillary cystic and solid tumors of the pancreas: a pancreatic embryonic tumor? Studies of three cases and cumulative review of the world's literature. Surgery 1995; 118:821–828.

453. Tanaka Y, Kato K, Notohara K, et al. Frequent beta-catenin mutation and cytoplasmic/nuclear accumulation in pancreatic solid-pseudopapillary neoplasm. Cancer Res 2001; 61: 8401–8404.

454. von Herbay A, Sieg B, Otto HF. Solid-cystic tumour of the pancreas. An endocrine neoplasm? Virchows Arch 1990; 416: 535–538.

455. Pettinato G, Di Vizio D, Manivel JC, et al. Solid-pseudopapillary tumor of the pancreas: a neoplasm with distinct and highly characteristic cytological features. Diagn Cytopathol 2002; 27:325–334.

456. Wunsch LP, Flemming P, Werner U, et al. Diagnosis and treatment of papillary cystic tumor of the pancreas in children. Eur J Pediatr Surg 1997; 7:45–47.

457. Kosmahl M, Seada LS, Janig U, et al. Solid-pseudopapillary tumor of the pancreas: its origin revisited. Virchows Arch 2000; 436 473–480.

458. Remadi S, Mac GW, Doussis-Anagnostopoulou I, et al. Papillary-cystic tumor of the pancreas. Diagn Cytopathol 1996; 15:398–402.

459. Doglioni C, Dei Tos AP, Laurino L, et al. A novel immunocytochemical marker for mesothelioma. Am J Surg Pathol 1996; 20:1037–1046.

460. Klimstra DS, Lonardo F. Microglandular carcinoma of the pancreas [letter]. Am J Clin Pathol 1997; 107:711–713.

461. Vardaman C, Albores-Saavedra J. Clear cell carcinomas of the gallbladder and extrahepatic bile ducts. Am J Surg Pathol 1995; 19:91–99.

462. Sadeghi S, Krigman H, Maluf H. Perivascular epithelioid clear cell tumor of the common bile duct. Am J Surg Pathol 2004; 28:1107–1110.

463. Yano T, Ishikura H, Wada T, et al. Hepatoid adenocarcinoma of the pancreas. Histopathology 1999; 35:90–92.

464. Ritter JH, Mills SE, Gaffey MJ, et al. Clear cell tumors of the alimentary tract and abdominal cavity. Semin Diagn Pathol 1997; 14:213–219.

465. Zamboni G, Pea M, Martignoni G, et al. Clear cell 'sugar' tumor of the pancreas. A novel member of the family of lesions characterized by the presence of perivascular epithelioid cells. Am J Surg Pathol 1996; 20:722–730.

466. Panizo-Santos A, Sola I, De Alava E, et al. Angiomyolipoma and PEComa are immunoreactive for MyoD1 in cell cytoplasmic staining pattern. Appl Immunohistochem Mol Morphol 2003; 11:156–160.

467. Wang JH, Dhillon AP, Sankey EA, et al. 'Neuroendocrine' differentiation in primary neoplasms of the liver. J Pathol 1991; 163:61–67.

468. Miller RT, Kubier P. Blocking of endogenous avidin-binding activity in immunohistochemistry: The use of egg whites. Appl Immunohistochem 1997; 5:63–66.

469. Rodriguez-Soto J, Warnke RA, Rouse RV. Endogenous avidin-binding activity in paraffin-embedded tissue revealed after microwave treatment. Appl Immunohistochem 1997; 5: 59–62.

470. Dodson A, Campbell F. Biotin inclusions: a potential pitfall in immunohistochemistry avoided. Histopathology 1999; 34: 178–179.

471. Iezzoni JC, Mills SE, Pelkey TJ, et al. Inhibin is not an immunohistochemical marker for hepatocellular carcinoma. An example of the potential pitfall in diagnostic immunohistochemistry caused by endogenous biotin. Am J Clin Pathol 1999; 111:229–234.

472. Nayler SJ, Goetsch S, Cooper K. Biotin inclusions: a potential pitfall in immunohistochemistry. Histopathology 1998; 33:87.

473. Bussolati G, Gugliotta P, Volante M, et al. Retrieved endogenous biotin: a novel marker and a potential pitfall in diagnostic immunohistochemistry [see comments]. Histopathology 1997; 31:400–407.

474. Moll R, Franke WW, Schiller DL, et al. The catalog of hu-

man cytokeratins: patterns of expression in normal epithelia, tumors and cultured cells. Cell 1982; 31:11–24.

475. Van Eyken P, Sciot R, van Damme B, et al. Keratin immunohistochemistry in normal human liver. Cytokeratin pattern of hepatocytes, bile ducts and acinar gradient. Virchows Arch A Pathol Anat Histopathol 1987; 412:63–72.

476. Fischer HP, Altmannsberger M, Weber K, et al. Keratin polypeptides in malignant epithelial liver tumors. Differential diagnostic and histogenetic aspects. Am J Pathol 1987; 127:530–537.

477. Van Eyken P, Sciot R, Desmet VJ. Immunocytochemistry of cytokeratins in primary human liver tumors. APMIS Suppl 1991; 23:77–85.

478. Gaffey MJ, Traweek ST, Mills SE, et al. Cytokeratin expression in adrenocortical neoplasia: an immunohistochemical and biochemical study with implications for the differential diagnosis of adrenocortical, hepatocellular, and renal cell carcinoma. Hum Pathol 1992; 23:144–153.

479. Lai Y-S, Thung SN, Gerber MA, et al. Expression of cytokeratins in normal and diseased livers and in primary liver carcinomas. Arch Pathol Lab Med 1989; 113:134–138.

480. Leong AS, Sormunen RT, Tsui WM, et al. Hep Par 1 and selected antibodies in the immunohistological distinction of hepatocellular carcinoma from cholangiocarcinoma, combined tumors and metastatic carcinoma. Histopathology 1998; 33:318–324.

481. Hurlimann J, Gardiol D. Immunohistochemistry in the differential diagnosis of liver carcinomas. Am J Surg Pathol 1991; 15:280–288.

482. Shah KD, Gerber MA. Development of intrahepatic bile ducts in humans. Immunohistochemical study using monoclonal cytokeratin antibodies. Arch Pathol Lab Med 1989; 113:1135–1138.

483. Wieczorek TJ, Pinkus JL, Glickman JN, et al. Comparison of thyroid transcription factor-1 and hepatocyte antigen immunohistochemical analysis in the differential diagnosis of hepatocellular carcinoma, metastatic adenocarcinoma, renal cell carcinoma, and adrenal cortical carcinoma. Am J Clin Pathol 2002; 118:911–921.

484. Nakajima T, Kondo Y. Well-differentiated cholangiocarcinoma: diagnostic significance of morphologic and immunohistochemical parameters. Am J Surg Pathol 1989. 13: 569–573.

485. Ruck P, Xiao JC, Kaiserling E. Small epithelial cells and the histogenesis of hepatoblastoma. Electron microscopic, immuno–electron microscopic, and immunohistochemical findings. Am J Pathol 1996; 148:321–329.

486. Desmet VJ, Van Eyken P, Sciot R. Cytokeratins for probing cell lineage relationships in developing liver. Hepatology 1990; 12:1249–1251.

487. Ruck P, Xiao JC, Pietsch T, et al. Hepatic stem-like cells in hepatoblastoma: expression of cytokeratin 7, albumin and oval cell associated antigens detected by OV-1 and OV-6. Histopathology 1997; 31:324–329.

488. Demetris AJ, Seaberg EC, Wennerberg AE, et al. Ductular reaction after submassive necrosis in humans. Special emphasis on analysis of ductular hepatocytes. Am J Pathol 1996; 149:439–448.

489. Halme L, Karkkainen P, Isoniemi H, et al. Carbohydrate 19-9 antigen as a marker of non-malignant hepatocytic ductular transformation in patients with acute liver failure. A comparison with alpha-fetoprotein and carcinoembryonic antigen. Scand J Gastroenterol 1999; 34:426–431.

490. Haque S, Haruna Y, Saito K, et al. Identification of bipotential progenitor cells in human liver regeneration. Lab Invest 1996; 75:699–705.

491. Rubio CA. The detection of bile ducts in liver biopsies by cytokeratin 7. In Vivo 1998; 12:183–186.

492. Washington K, Gottfried MR. Expression of p53 in adenocarcinoma of the gallbladder and bile ducts. Liver 1996; 16: 99–104.

493. Van Eyken P, Sciot R, Desmet VJ. A cytokeratin immunohistochemical study of cholestatic liver disease: evidence that hepatocytes can express 'bile duct-type' cytokeratins. Histopathology 1989; 15:125–135.

494. Van Eyken P, Sciot R, Callea F, et al. A cytokeratin-immunohistochemical study of focal nodular hyperplasia of the liver: further evidence that ductular metaplasia of hepatocytes contributes to ductular 'proliferation.' Liver 1989; 9:372–377.

495. Van Eyken P, Sciot R, Desmet VJ. A cytokeratin immunohistochemical study of alcoholic liver disease: evidence that hepatocytes can express 'bile duct-type' cytokeratins. Histopathology 1988; 13:605–617.

496. Sell S. Is there a liver stem cell? Cancer Res 1990; 50:3811–3815.

497. Gerber MA, Thung SN. Liver stem cells and development.

Lab Invest 1993; 68:253–254.

498. Theise ND, Fiel IM, Hytiroglou P, et al. Macroregenerative nodules in cirrhosis are not associated with elevated serum or stainable tissue alpha-fetoprotein. Liver 1995; 15:30–34.

499. Goldstein NS, Blue DE, Hankin RH, et al. Serum alpha-fetoprotein levels in patients with chronic hepatitis C: relationships with serum alanine amino transferase values, histologic activity index, and hepatocyte MIB-1 scores. Am J Clin Pathol 1999; 111:811–816.

500. Ruck P, Xiao JC, Kaiserling E. Immunoreactivity of sinusoids in hepatocellular carcinoma. An immunohistochemical study using lectin UEA-1 and antibodies against endothelial markers, including CD34. Arch Pathol Lab Med 1995; 119: 173–178.

501. Hazan R, Denk H, Franke WW, et al. Change of cytokeratin organization during development of Mallory bodies as revealed by a monoclonal antibody. Lab Invest 1986; 54:543–553.

502. Gottschalk-Sabag S, Ron N, Glick T. Use of CD34 and factor VIII to diagnose hepatocellular carcinoma on fine needle aspirates. Acta Cytol 1998; 42:691–696.

503. Haas JE, Muczynski KA, Krailo M, et al. Histopathology and prognosis in childhood hepatoblastoma and hepatocarcinoma. Cancer 1989; 64:1082–1095.

504. Schmidt D, Harms D, Lang W. Primary malignant hepatic tumours in childhood. Virchows Arch A Pathol Anat Histopathol 1985; 407:387–405.

505. Van Eyken P, Sciot R, Callea F, et al. The development of the intrahepatic bile ducts in man: a keratin-immunohistochemical study. Hepatology 1988; 8:1586–1595.

506. Denk H, Krepler R, Lackinger E, et al. Biochemical and immunocytochemical analysis of the intermediate filament cytoskeleton in human hepatocellular carcinomas and in hepatic neoplastic nodules of mice. Lab Invest 1982; 46:584–596.

507. Osborn M, van Lessen G, Weber K, et al. Differential diagnosis of gastrointestinal carcinomas by using monoclonal antibodies specific for individual keratin polypeptides. Lab Invest 1986; 55:497–504.

508. Van Eyken P, Sciot R, Paterson A, et al. Cytokeratin expression in hepatocellular carcinoma: an immunohistochemical study. Hum Pathol 1988; 19:562–568.

509. Johnson DE, Powers CN, Rupp G, et al. Immunocytochemical staining of fine-needle aspiration biopsies of the liver as a diagnostic tool for hepatocellular carcinoma. Mod Pathol 1992; 5:117–123.

510. Johnson DE, Herndier BG, Medeiros LJ, et al. The diagnostic utility of the keratin profiles of hepatocellular carcinoma and cholangiocarcinoma. Am J Surg Pathol 1988; 12:187–197.

511. Minervini MI, Demetris AJ, Lee RG, et al. Utilization of hepatocyte-specific antibody in the immunocytochemical evaluation of hepatocyte-specific antibody in the immunocytochemical evaluation of liver tumors. Mod Pathol 1997; 10:686–692.

512. Listrom MB, Dalton LW. Comparison of keratin monoclonal antibodies MAK-6, AE1:AE3, and CAM-5.2. Am J Clin Pathol 1987; 88:297–301.

513. Wu PC, Fang JW, Lau VK, et al. Classification of hepatocellular carcinoma according to hepatocellular and biliary differentiation markers. Clinical and biological implications. Am J Pathol 1996; 149:1167–1175.

514. D'Errico A, Baccarini P, Fiorentino M, et al. Histogenesis of primary liver carcinomas: strengths and weaknesses of cytokeratin profile and albumin mRNA detection. Hum Pathol 1996; 27:599–604.

515. Maeda T, Adachi E, Kajiyama K, et al. Combined hepatocellular and cholangiocarcinoma: Proposed criteria according to cytokeratin expression and analysis of clinicopathologic features. Hum Pathol 1995; 26:956–964.

516. Maeda T, Adachi E, Kajiyama K, et al. Spindle cell hepatocellular carcinoma. A clinicopathologic and immunohistochemical analysis of 15 cases. Cancer 1996; 77:51–57.

517. Zhou H, Fischer HP. Liver carcinoma in PiZ alpha-1-antitrypsin deficiency. Am J Surg Pathol 1998; 22:742–748.

518. Balaton AJ, Nehama-Sibony M, Gotheil C, et al. Distinction between hepatocellular carcinoma, cholangiocarcinoma, and metastatic carcinoma based on immunohistochemical staining for carcinoembryonic antigen and for cytokeratin 19 on paraffin sections. J Pathol 1988; 156:305–310.

519. Lau SK, Prakash S, Geller SA, et al. Comparative immunohistochemical profile of hepatocellular carcinoma, cholangiocarcinoma, and metastatic adenocarcinoma. Hum Pathol 2002; 33:1175–1181.

520. Tsuji M, Kashihara T, Terada N, et al. An immunohistochemical study of hepatic atypical adenomatous hyper-plasia, hepatocellular carcinoma, and cholangiocarcinoma with alpha-

fetoprotein, carcinoembryonic antigen, CA19-9, epithelial membrane antigen, and cytokeratins 18 and 19. Pathol Int 1999; 49:310–317.

521. Fucich LF, Cheles MK, Thung SN, et al. Primary vs metastatic hepatic carcinoma. An immunohistochemical study of 34 cases. Arch Pathol Lab Med 1994; 118:927–930.

522. Morrison C, Marsh W Jr, Frankel WL. A comparison of CD10 to pCEA, MOC-31, and hepatocyte for the distinction of malignant tumors in the liver. Mod Pathol 2002; 15:1279–1287.

523. Borscheri N, Roessner A, Rocken C. Canalicular immunostaining of neprilysin (CD10) as a diagnostic marker for hepatocellular carcinomas. Am J Surg Pathol 2001; 25:1297–1303.

524. McCluggage WC, Maxwell P, Patterson A, et al. Immunohistochemical staining of hepatocellular carcinoma with monoclonal antibody against inhibin. Histopathology 1997; 30:518–522.

525. Kakizoe S, Kojiro M, Nakashima K. Hepatocellular carcinoma with sarcomatous change: Clinicopathologic and immunohistochemical studies of 14 autopsy cases. Cancer 1987; 59:310–316.

526. Brumm C, Schulze C, Charels K, et al. The significance of alpha-fetoprotein and other tumour markers in differential immunocytochemistry of primary liver tumours. Histo-pathology 1989; 14:503–513.

527. Fasano M, Theise ND, Nalesnik MA, et al. Immunohistochemical evaluation of hepatoblastomas with use of the hepatocyte-specific marker, hepatocyte paraffin 1, and the polyclonal anti-carcinoembryonic antigen. Mod Pathol 1998; 11:934–938.

528. Kimura H, Nakajima T, Kagawa K, et al. Angiogenesis in hepatocellular carcinoma as evaluated by CD34 immunohistochemistry. Liver 1998; 18:14–19.

529. Ruck P, Xiao JC, Kaiserling E. QBend 10 (CD34) in the diagnosis of hepatocellular carcinoma. Histopathology 1996; 29:593–594.

530. Cui S, Hano H, Sakata A, et al. Enhanced CD34 expression of sinusoid-like vascular endothelial cells in hepatocellular carcinoma. Pathol Int 1996; 46:751–756.

531. Pitman MB, Szyfelbein WM. Significance of endothelium in the fine-needle aspiration biopsy diagnosis of hepatocellular carcinoma. Diagn Cytopathol 1995; 12:208–214.

532. Haratake J, Scheuer PJ. An immunohistochemical and ultrastructural study of the sinusoids of hepatocellular carcinoma. Cancer 1990; 65:1985–1993.

533. Terayama N, Terada T, Nakanuma Y. An immunohistochemical study of tumour vessels in metastatic liver cancers and the surrounding liver tissue. Histopathology 1996; 29:37–43.

534. Adamek HE, Spiethoff A, Kaufmann V, et al. Primary clear cell carcinoma of noncirrhotic liver: immunohistochemical discrimination of hepatocellular and cholangiocellular origin. Dig Dis Sci 1998; 43:33–38.

535. Van Eyken P, Sciot R, Brock P, et al. Abundant expression of cytokeratin 7 in fibrolamellar carcinoma of the liver. Histopathology 1990; 17:101–107.

536. Berman MA, Burnham JA, Sheahan DG. Fibrolamellar carcinoma of the liver: an immunohistochemical study of nineteen cases and a review of the literature. Hum Pathol 1988; 19:784–794.

537. McCloskey JJ, Germain-Lee EL, Perman JA, et al. Gynecomastia as a presenting sign of fibrolamellar carcinoma of the liver. Pediatrics 1988; 82:379–382.

538. Vecchio FM. Fibrolamellar carcinoma of the liver: a distinct entity within the hepatocellular tumors. A review. Appl Pathol 1988; 6:139–148.

539. Andreola S, Audisio RA, Lombardi L. A light microscopic and ultrastructural study of two cases of fibrolamellar hepatocellular carcinoma. Tumori 1986; 72:609–616.

540. Singson RC, Fraiman M, Geller SA. Hepatocellular carcinoma with fibrolamellar pattern in a patient with autoimmune cholangitis. Mt Sinai J Med 1999; 66:109–112.

541. Eckstein RP, Bambach CP, Stiel D, et al. Fibrolamellar carcinoma as a cause of bile duct obstruction. Pathology 1988; 20:326–331.

542. Mierau GW, Orsini EN Jr. Diagnosis of human tumors. Case 1: Hepatocarcinoma, fibrolamellar type. Ultrastruct Pathol 1983; 5:273–279.

543. Renshaw AA, Granter SR. A comparison of A103 and inhibin reactivity in adrenal cortical tumors: distinction from hepatocellular carcinoma and renal tumors. Mod Pathol 1998; 11:1160–1164.

544. Loy TS, Phillips RW, Linder CL. A103 immunostaining in the diagnosis of adrenal cortical tumors: an immunohistochemical study of 316 cases. Arch Pathol Lab Med 2002; 126:170–172.

545. Wiedenmann B, Waldherr R, Buhr H, et al. Identification of

gastroenteropancreatic neuroendocrine cells in normal and neoplastic human tissue with antibodies against synaptophysin, chromogranin A, secretogranin I (chromogranin B), and secretogranin II. Gastroenterology 1988; 95:1364–1374.

546. Wiedenmann B, Kuhn C, Schwechheimer K, et al. Synaptophysin identified in metastases of neuroendocrine tumors by immunocytochemistry and immunoblotting. Am J Clin Pathol 1987; 88:560–569.

547. Gould VE, Wiedenmann B, Lee I, et al. Synaptophysin expression in neuroendocrine neoplasms as determined by immunocytochemistry. Am J Pathol 1987; 126:243–257.

548. Folpe AL, Gown AM, Lamps LW, et al. Thyroid tran-scription factor-1: immunohistochemical evaluation in pulmonary neuroendocrine tumors. Mod Pathol 1999; 12:5–8.

549. Argani P, Shaukat A, Kaushal M, et al. Differing rates of loss of DPC4 expression and of p53 overexpression among carcinomas of the proximal and distal bile ducts. Cancer 2001; 91:1332–1341.

550. Tihan T, Blumgart LH, Klimstra DS. Clear cell papillary carcinoma of the liver: an unusual variant of peripheral cholangiocarcinoma [see comments]. Hum Pathol 1998; 29: 196–200.

551. Terada T, Nakanuma Y. Pathological observations of intrahepatic peribiliary glands in 1,000 consecutive autopsy livers. II. A possible source of cholangiocarcinoma. Hepatology 1990; 12:92–97.

552. Terada T, Kida T, Nakanuma Y, et al. Intrahepatic cholangiocarcinomas associated with nonbiliary cirrhosis. A clinicopathologic study. J Clin Gastroenterol 1994; 18:335–342.

553. Yamato T, Sasaki M, Hoso M, et al. Intrahepatic cholangiocarcinoma arising in congenital hepatic fibrosis: report of an autopsy case. J Hepatol 1998; 28:717–722.

554. Sasaki M, Nakanuma Y, Shimizu K, et al. Pathological and immunohistochemical findings in a case of mucinous cholangiocarcinoma. Pathol Int 1995; 45:781–786.

555. Saad RS, Luckasevic TM, Noga CM, et al. Diagnostic value of HepPar1, pCEA, CD10, and CD34 expression in separating hepatocellular carcinoma from metastatic carcinoma in fine-needle aspiration cytology. Diagn Cytopathol 2004; 30: 1–6.

556. Nakajima T, Tajima Y, Sugano I, et al. Intrahepatic cholangiocarcinoma with sarcomatous change. Clinicopathologic and immunohistochemical evaluation of seven cases. Cancer 1993; 72:1872–1877.

557. Imazu H, Ochiai M, Funabiki T. Intrahepatic sarcomatous cholangiocarcinoma. J Gastroenterol 1995; 30:677–682.

558. Honda M, Enjoji M, Sakai H, et al. Case report: intra-hepatic cholangiocarcinoma with rhabdoid transformation. J Gastroenterol Hepatol 1996; 11:771–774.

559. Kim H, Park C, Han KH, et al. Primary liver carcinoma of intermediate (hepatocyte-cholangiocyte) phenotype. J Hepatol 2004; 40:298–304.

560. Tickoo SK, Zee SY, Obiekwe S, et al. Combined hepatocellular-cholangiocarcinoma: a histopathologic, immunohistochemical, and in situ hybridization study. Am J Surg Pathol 2002; 26:989–997.

561. Taguchi J, Nakashima O, Tanaka M, et al. A clinicopathological study on combined hepatocellular and cholangiocarcinoma. J Gastroenterol Hepatol 1996; 11:758–764.

562. Devaney K, Goodman ZD, Ishak KG. Hepatobiliary cystadenoma and cystadenocarcinoma. A light microscopic and immunohistochemical study of 70 patients. Am J Surg Pathol 1994; 18:1078–1091.

563. Siren J, Karkkainen P, Luukkonen P, et al. A case report of biliary cystadenoma and cystadenocarcinoma. Hepatogastroenterology 1998; 45:83–89.

564. Yanase M, Ikeda H, Ogata I, et al. Primary smooth muscle tumor of the liver encasing hepatobiliary cystadenoma without mesenchymal stroma. Am J Surg Pathol 1999; 23:854–859.

565. Scott FR, More L, Dhillon AP. Hepatobiliary cystadenoma with mesenchymal stroma: expression of oestrogen receptors in formalin-fixed tissue. Histopathology 1995; 26:555–558.

566. Grayson W, Teare J, Myburgh JA, et al. Immunohistochemical demonstration of progesterone receptor in hepatobiliary cystadenoma with mesenchymal stroma. Histopathology 1996; 29:461–463.

567. Ishida M, Seki K, Honda K, et al. Intraductal mucinous tumors occurring simultaneously in the liver and pancreas. J Gastroenterol 2002; 37:1073–1078.

568. Nakanuma Y, Sasaki M, Ishikawa A, et al. Biliary papillary neoplasm of the liver. Histol Histopathol 2002; 17:851–861.

569. Sinkre PA, Murakata L, Rabin L, et al. Clear cell carcinoid tumor of the gallbladder: another distinctive manifestation of von Hippel-Lindau disease. Am J Surg Pathol 2001; 25:1334–1339.

570. Pilichowska M, Kimura N, Ouchi A, et al. Primary hepatic carcinoid and neuroendocrine carcinoma: clinicopathological and immunohistochemical study of five cases. Pathol Int 1999; 49:318–324.

571. Miura K, Shirasawa H. Primary carcinoid tumor of the liver. Am J Clin Pathol 1988; 89:561–564.

572. Yamamoto J, Abe Y, Nishihara K, et al. Composite glandular-neuroendocrine carcinoma of the hilar bile duct: report of a case. Surg Today 1998; 28:758–762.

573. Piatti B, Caspani B, Giudici C, et al. Fine needle aspiration biopsy of hepatocellular carcinoma resembling neuroendocrine tumor. A case report. Acta Cytol 1997; 41:583–586.

574. Ordonez NG, Mackay B. Granular cell tumor: A review of the pathology and histogenesis. Ultrastruct Pathol 1999; 23:207–222.

575. Terris B, Flejou JF, Picot R, et al. Hepatic angiomyolipoma. A report of four cases with immunohistochemical and DNA-flow cytometric studies. Arch Pathol Lab Med 1996; 120:68–72.

576. Cha I, Cartwright D, Guis M, et al. Angiomyolipoma of the liver in fine-needle aspiration biopsies: its distinction from hepatocellular carcinoma. Cancer 1999; 87:25–30.

577. Nonomura A, Mizukami Y, Kadoya M. Angiomyolipoma of the liver: a collective review. J Gastroenterol 1994; 29:95–105.

578. Adachi S, Hanada M, Kobayashi Y, et al. Heavily melanotic perivascular epithelioid clear cell tumor of the kidney. Pathol Int 2004; 54:261–265.

579. Stone CH, Lee MW, Amin MB, et al. Renal angiomyo-lipoma: further immunophenotypic characterization of an expanding morphologic spectrum. Arch Pathol Lab Med 2001; 125:751–758.

580. Folpe AL, Goodman ZD, Ishak KG, et al. Clear cell myomelanocytic tumor of the falciform ligament/ligamentum teres: a novel member of the perivascular epithelioid clear cell family of tumors with a predilection for children and young adults. Am J Surg Pathol 2000; 24:1239–1246.

581. Nonomura A, Minato H, Kurumaya H. Angiomyolipoma predominantly composed of smooth muscle cells: problems in histological diagnosis. Histopathology 1998; 33 20–27.

582. Takahashi N, Kitahara R, Hishimoto Y, et al. Malignant transformation of renal angiomyolipoma. Int J Urol 2003; 10:271–273.

583. Cho NH, Shim HS, Choi YD, eet al. Estrogen receptor is significantly associated with the epithelioid variants of renal angiomyolipoma: a clinicopathological and immunohistochemical study of 67 cases. Pathol Int 2004; 54:510–515.

584. Meis-Kindblom JM, Kindblom LG. Angiosarcoma of soft tissue: a study of 80 cases. Am J Surg Pathol 1998; 22:683–697.

585. Anthony PP, Ramani P. Endothelial markers in malignant vascular tumours of the liver: superiority of QB-END/10 over von Willebrand factor and Ulex europaeus agglutinin 1. J Clin Pathol 1991; 44:29–32.

586. Demetris AJ, Minervini MI, Raikow RB, et al. Hepatic epithelioid hemangioendothelioma: Biologic questions based on pattern of recurrence in an allograft and tumor immunophenotype. Am J Surg Pathol 1997; 21:263–270.

587. Dietze O, Davies SE, Williams R, et al. Malignant epithelioid haemangioendothelioma of the liver: a clinicopathological and histochemical study of 12 cases. Histopathology 1989; 15:225–237.

588. Eckstein RP, Ravich RB. Epithelioid hemangioendothelioma of the liver. Report of two cases histologically mimicking veno-occlusive disease. Pathology 1986; 18:459–462.

589. Hayashi Y, Inagaki K, Hirota S, et al. Epithelioid hemangioendothelioma with marked liver deformity and secondary Budd-Chiari syndrome: pathological and radiological correlation. Pathol Int 1999; 49:547–552.

590. Makhlouf HR, Ishak KG, Goodman ZD. Epithelioid hemangioendothelioma of the liver: a clinicopathologic study of 137 cases. Cancer 1999; 85:562–582.

591. Scoazec JY, Degott C, Reynes M, et al. Epithelioid hemangioendothelioma of the liver: an ultrastructural study. Hum Pathol 1989; 20:673–681.

592. Pinkus GS, Kurtin PJ. Epithelial membrane antigen – A diagnostic discriminant in surgical pathology: Immunohistochemical profile in epithelial, mesenchymal, and hematopoietic neoplasms using paraffin sections and monoclonal antibodies. Hum Pathol 1985; 16:929–940.

593. McHugh M, Miettinen M. KP1 (CD68): Its limited specificity for histiocytic tumors. Appl Immunohistochem 1994; 2:

186–190.

594. Berner A, Nesland JM. Endocrine profile in gastric carcinomas. An immunohistochemical study. Histol Histopathol 1991; 6:317–323.

595. Fowler LJ, Maygarden SJ, Novotny DB. Human alveolar macrophage-56 and carcinoembryonic antigen monoclonal antibodies in the differential diagnosis between primary ovarian and metastatic gastrointestinal carcinomas. Hum Pathol 1994; 25:666–670.

596. Bhatnagar J, Heroman W, Murphy M, et al. Immunohistochemical detection of carcinoembryonic antigen in esophageal carcinomas: a comparison with other gastrointestinal neoplasms. Anticancer Res 2002; 22:1849–1857.

597. Sheibani K, Shin SS, Kezirian J, et al. Ber-EP4 antibody as a discriminant in the differential diagnosis of malignant mesothelioma versus adenocarcinoma. Am J Surg Pathol 1991; 15:779–784.

598. Gaffey MJ, Mills SE, Swanson PE, et al. Immunoreactivity for Ber-EP4 in adenocarcinomas, adenomatoid tumors, and malignant mesotheliomas. Am J Surg Pathol 1992; 16:593–599.

599. Stevenson AJ, Chatten J, Bertoni F, et al. CD99 (p30/32^{MIC2}) neuroectodermal/Ewing's sarcoma antigen as an immunohistochemical marker: Review of more than 600 tumors and literature experience. Appl Immunohistochem 1994; 2:231–240.

600. Jung KC, Park WS, Bae YM, et al. Immunoreactivity of CD99 in stomach cancer. J Korean Med Sci 2002; 17:483–489.

601. Mazoujian G, Pinkus GS, Davis S, et al. Immunohistochemistry of a gross cystic disease fluid protein (GCDFP-15) of the breast: A marker of apocrine epithelium and breast carcinomas with apocrine features. Am J Pathol 1983; 110:105–112.

602. Wick MR, Lillemoe TJ, Copland GT, et al. Gross cystic disease fluid protein-15 as a marker for breast cancer: Immunohistochemical analysis of 690 human neoplasms and comparison with alpha-lactalbumin. Hum Pathol 1989; 20:281–287.

603. Millward C, Weidner N. CD30 (Ber-H2) expression in nonhematopoetic tumors. Appl Immunohistochem 1998; 6:164–168.

604. Ueyama T, Nagai E, Yao T, et al. Vimentin-positive gastric carcinomas with rhabdoid features. A clinicopathologic and immunohistochemical study [see comments]. Am J Surg Pathol 1993; 17:813–819.

605. Herrera GA, Turbat-Herrera EA, Lott RL. S-100 protein expression by primary and metastatic adenocarcinomas. Am J Clin Pathol 1988; 89:168–176.

606. El-Habashi A, El-Morsi B, Freeman SM, et al. Tumor oncogenic expression in malignant effusions as a possible method to enhance cytologic diagnostic sensitivity: An immunocytochemical study of 87 cases. Am J Clin Pathol 1995; 103 206–214.

607. Mizoshita T, Tsukamoto T, Inada K, et al. Immunohistochemically detectable CDX2 is present in intestinal phenotypic elements in early gastric cancers of both differentiated and undifferentiated types, with no correlation to nonneoplastic surrounding mucosa. Pathol Int 2004; 54: 392–400.

608. Koelma IA, Nap M, Rodenburg CJ, et al. The value of tumor marker CA 125 in surgical pathology. Histopathology 1987; 11:287–294.

609. Lau SK, Luthringer DJ, Eisen RN. Thyroid transcription factor-1: a review. Appl Immunohistochem Mol Morphol 2002; 10:97–102.

610. McCluggage WC, Maxwell P. Adenocarcinomas of various sites may exhibit immunoreactivity with antiinhibin antibodies. Histopathology 1999; 35:216–220.

611. Di Leo A, Messa C, Russo F, et al. Prognostic value of cytosolic estrogen receptors in human colorectal carcinoma and surrounding mucosa. Preliminary results. Dig Dis Sci 1994; 39:2038–2042.

612. Hendrickse CW, Jones CE, Donovan IA, et al. Oestrogen and progesterone receptors in colorectal cancer and human colonic cancer cell lines. Br J Surg 1993; 80:636–640.

613. Meggouh F, Lointier P, Pezet D, et al. Status of sex steroid hormone receptors in large bowel cancer. Cancer 1991; 67: 1964–1970.

614. Dawson PM, Shousha S, Blair SD, et al. Estrogen receptors in colorectal carcinoma. J Clin Pathol 1990; 43:149–151.

615. Sciascia C, Olivero G, Comandone A, et al. Estrogen receptors in colorectal adenocarcinomas and in other large bowel diseases. Int J Biol Markers 1990; 5:38–42.

616. Francavilla A, Di Leo A, Polimeno L, et al. Nuclear and cytosolic estrogen receptors in human colon carcinoma and in surrounding noncancerous colonic tissue. Gastroenterology 1987; 93:1301–1306.

617. Galandiuk S, Miseljic S, Yang A-R, et al. Expression of hormone receptors, cathepsin D, and HER-2/neu oncoprotein in normal colon and colonic disease. Arch Surg 1993; 128:637–642.

618. Singh S, Sheppard MC, Langman MJ. Sex differences in the incidence of colorectal cancer: an exploration of estrogen and progesterone receptors. Gut 1993; 34:611–615.

619. Singh S, Poulsom R, Hanby AM, et al. Expression of estrogen receptor and estrogen-inducible genes pS2 and ERD5 in large bowel mucosa and cancer. J Pathol 1998; 184:153–160.

620. Brentani MM, Liberato MH, Macedo TM, et al. Steroid receptors in Brazilian patients with large bowel cancer. Braz J Med Biol Res 1993; 26:277–284.

621. Lapertosa G, Baracchini P, Delucchi F. Prevalence and prognostic significance of endocrine cells in colorectal adenocarcinomas. Pathologica 1994; 86:170–173.

622. Syversen U, Halvorsen T, Marvik R, et al. Neuroendocrine differentiation in colorectal carcinomas. Eur J Gastroenterol Hepatol 1995; 7:667–674.

623. Jansson D, Gould VE, Gooch GT, et al. Immunohistochemical analysis of colon carcinomas applying exocrine and neuroendocrine markers. APMIS 1988; 96:1129–1139.

624. Mori M, Mimori K, Kamakura T, et al. Chromogranin positive cells in colorectal carcinoma and transitional mucosa. J Clin Pathol 1995; 48:754–758.

625. Romeo R, Pellitteri R, Mazzone V, et al. Chromogranin A expression in human colonic adenocarcinoma. Ital J Anat Embryol 2002; 107:177–183.

626. Taguchi T, Kijima H, Mitomi T, et al. Immunohistochemical study of colorectal adenocarcinomas and adenomas with antibodies against carcinoembryonic antigen (CEA), CA19-9, keratin, alpha-tubulin and secretory component (SC). Gastroenterol Jpn 1991; 26:294–302.

627. Siddiqui MT, Saboorian MH, Gokaslan ST, et al. Diagnostic utility of the HepPar1 antibody to differentiate hepatocellular carcinoma from metastatic carcinoma in fine-needle aspiration samples. Cancer 2002; 96:49–52.

628. Kamisawa T, Fukayama M, Tabata I, et al. Neuroendocrine differentiation in pancreatic duct carcinoma: special emphasis on duct-endocrine cell carcinoma of the pancreas. Pathol Res Pract 1996; 192:901–908.

629. Ohshio G, Ogawa K, Kudo H, et al. Immunohistochemical studies on the localization of cancer associated antigens DU-PAN-2 and CA19-9 in carcinomas of the digestive tract. J Gastroenterol Hepatol 1990; 5:25–31.

630. Toshkov I, Mogaki M, Kazakoff K, et al. The patterns of coexpression of tumor-associated antigens CA 19-9, TAG-72, and DU-PAN-2 in human pancreatic cancer. Int J Pancreatol 1994; 15:97–103.

631. Berho M, Blaustein A, Willis I, et al. Microglandular carcinoma of the pancreas: immunohistochemical and ultrastructural study of an unusual variant of pancreatic carcinoma that may closely resemble a neuroendocrine neoplasm. Am J Clin Pathol 1996; 105:727–732.

632. Zhu L, Kim K, Domenico DR, et al. Adenocarcinoma of duodenum and ampulla of Vater: clinicopathology study and expression of p53, c-neu, TGF-alpha, CEA, and EMA. J Surg Oncol 1996; 61:100–105.

633. Wick MR, Mills SE, Dehner LP, et al. Serous papillary carcinomas arising from the peritoneum and ovaries: A clinicopathologic and immunohistochemical comparison. Int J Gynecol Pathol 1989; 8:179–188.

634. Loy TS, Nashelsky MB. Reactivity of B72.3 with adenocarcinomas. An immunohistochemical study of 476 cases. Cancer 1993; 72:2495–2498.

635. Scheithauer W, Chott A, Knoflach P. Alpha-fetoprotein-positive adenocarcinoma of the pancreas. Int J Pancreatol 1989; 4:99–103.

636. Van Krieken JHJM. Prostate marker immunoreactivity in salivary gland neoplasms: A rare pitfall in immunohistochemistry. Am J Surg Pathol 1993; 17:410–414.

637. Papsidero LD, Croghan GA, Asirwatham J, et al. Immunohistochemical demonstration of prostate-specific antigen in metastases with the use of monoclonal antibody F5. Am J Pathol 1985; 121:451–454.

638. Bohinski RJ, Bejarano PA, Balko G, et al. Determination of lung as the primary site of cerebral metastatic adenocarcinomas using monoclonal antibody to thyroid transcription factor-1. J Neurooncol 1998; 40:227–231.

639. Khoor A, Whitsett JA, Stahlman MT, et al. Utility of surfactant protein B precursor and thyroid transcription factor 1 in differentiating adenocarcinoma of the lung from malignant mesothelioma. Hum Pathol 1999; 30:695–700.

640. Hecht JL, Pinkus JL, Weinstein LJ, et al. The value of thyroid transcription factor-1 in cytologic preparations as a marker for metastatic adenocarcinoma of lung origin. Am J

Clin Pathol 2001; 116:483–488.

641. Tajiri T, Tate G, Kunimura T, et al. Histologic and immunohistochemical comparison of intraductal tubular carcinoma, intraductal papillary-mucinous carcinoma, and ductal adenocarcinoma of the pancreas. Pancreas 2004; 29:116–122.

642. Tamada S, Goto M, Nomoto M, et al. Expression of MUC1 and MUC2 mucins in extrahepatic bile duct carcinomas: its relationship with tumor progression and prognosis. Pathol Int 2002; 52:713–723.

643. Yonezawa S, Nakamura A, Horinouchi M, et al. The expression of several types of mucin is related to the biological behavior of pancreatic neoplasms. J Hepatobiliary Pancreat Surg 2002; 9:328–341.

644. Chhieng DC, Benson E, Eltoum I, et al. MUC1 and MUC2 expression in pancreatic ductal carcinoma obtained by fine-needle aspiration. Cancer 2003; 99:365–371.

645. Wilentz RE, Su GH, Dai JL, et al. Immunohistochemical labeling for Dpc4 mirrors genetic status in pancreatic adenocarcinomas: a new marker of Dpc4 inactivation. Am J Pathol 2000; 156:37–43.

646. Tascilar M, Offerhaus GJ, Altink R, et al. Immunohistochemical labeling for the Dpc4 gene product is a specific marker for adenocarcinoma in biopsy specimens of the pancreas and bile duct. Am J Clin Pathol 2001; 116:831–837.

647. Iacobuzio-Donahue CA, Klimstra DS, Adsay NV, et al. Dpc-4 protein is expressed in virtually all human intraductal papillary mucinous neoplasms of the pancreas: comparison with conventional ductal adenocarcinomas. Am J Pathol 2000; 157: 755–761.

648. Chu PG, Arber DA, Weiss LM. Expression of T/NK-cell and plasma cell antigens in nonhematopoietic epithelioid neoplasms. An immunohistochemical study of 447 cases. Am J Clin Pathol 2003; 120:64–70.

649. Vlasoff DM, Baschinsky DY, Frankel WL. Cytokeratin 5/6 immunostaining in hepatobiliary and pancreatic neoplasms. Appl Immunohistochem Mol Morphol 2002; 10:147–151.

650. Argani P, Iacobuzio-Donahue C, Ryu B, et al. Mesothelin is overexpressed in the vast majority of ductal adenocarcinomas of the pancreas: identification of a new pancreatic cancer marker by serial analysis of gene expression (SAGE). Clin Cancer Res 2001; 7:3862–3868.

651. Zhao M, Zimmermann A. Apoptosis in hepatocellular carcinomas with neuroendocrine differentiation. Histol Histopathol 1997; 12:973–980.

652. Zhao M, Laissue JA, Zimmermann A. 'Neuroendocrine' differentiation in hepatocellular carcinomas (HCCs): immunohistochemical reactivity is related to distinct tumor cell types, but not to tumor grade. Histol Histopathol 1993; 8:617–626.

653. Proca DM, Niemann TH, Porcell AI, et al. MOC31 immunoreactivity in primary and metastatic carcinoma of the liver. Report of findings and review of other utilized markers. Appl Immunohistochem Mol Morphol 2000; 8:120–125.

654. Porcell AI, De Young BR, Proca DM, et al. Immunohistochemical analysis of hepatocellular and adenocarcinoma in the liver: MOC31 compares favorably with other putative markers. Mod Pathol 2000; 13 773–778.

655. Akasofu M, Kawahara E, Kurumaya H, et al. Immunohistochemical detection of breast specific antigens and cytokeratins in metastatic breast carcinoma in the liver. Acta Pathol Jpn 1993; 43:736–744.

14 前列腺、膀胱、睾丸和肾的免疫组织化学

原　著：David G. Bostwick, Jun Ma, Junqi Qian, Deborah Josefson and Lina Liu

译　者：连瑞虹，杨熙明

审校者：高　鹏，郝春燕，孟　斌，吴晓娟，张翠娟

目　录

引言	515
前列腺	**515**
抗原/抗体生物学	515
前列腺神经内分泌细胞	522
前列腺免疫组化	524
增殖抗原	530
细胞外基质蛋白	530
钙黏素	532
CD（分化抗原）	532
基质蛋白酶	532
生长因子及其受体	533
雄激素受体	533
微血管密度	533
治疗后前列腺癌的诊断	538
放射治疗后的免疫表型	539
前列腺良性肿瘤的免疫组化研究	540
不同类型前列腺癌的免疫组化研究	540
前列腺软组织肿瘤的免疫组化研究	542
膀　胱	**564**
抗原/抗体生物学	564
尿路上皮癌的分型	571
膀胱软组织肿瘤和梭形细胞病变	572
膀胱恶性淋巴瘤	573
睾　丸	**587**
睾丸、附属结构和外生殖器	587
抗原/抗体生物学	587
睾丸肿瘤	589
附属结构和外生殖器肿瘤	599
睾丸的良性、局部浸润和恶性软组织肿瘤	601
肾	**610**
引言	610
抗原/抗体生物学	610
儿童肾细胞肿瘤	611
成人肾肿瘤	612

引　言

本章目的在于介绍前列腺、膀胱、睾丸和肾脏组织肿瘤的诊断。前面章节已经对重要抗体在特异肿瘤诊断中的应用进行了讨论，同时还讨论了抗体组合在这些器官鉴别诊断中的应用。本章内容分为4个部分，分别对泌尿生殖系统的4个器官进行论述。

前列腺

David G. Bostwick, Jun Ma and Junqi Qian

抗原/抗体生物学

前列腺特异性抗原

前列腺特异性抗原（PSA）是一种34kD、单链、237个氨基酸的糖蛋白，几乎全部由前列腺上皮细胞产生[1]。PSA是一种丝氨酸蛋白酶，属于激肽释放酶家族，与人腺体激肽释放酶2的基因序列具有高

度同源性。它表现出糜蛋白酶样、胰蛋白酶样和酯酶样活性。在血清中，PSA 主要以与 α-1 抗糜蛋白酶形成复合物的形式存在。PSA 分泌于精液中，能够通过蛋白水解作用促使新鲜精液中的大凝胶蛋白——精液凝固蛋白 I 和 II 以及纤维连接蛋白中的凝胶液化，从而使精液呈液体状。精液中少量的 PSA 以复合物形式存在。游离的、未形成复合物形式的 PSA 只占血清 PSA 的一小部分，PSA 的相关参数如游离/总 PSA 比值可能比单独 PSA 水平更有意义[1]。PSA 的生成受到血液循环中雄激素与雄激素受体相互作用的控制[2, 3]。

在正常和增生性前列腺组织中，PSA 均匀地分布于腺上皮分泌细胞的顶部（图 14.1A）。在低分化腺癌组织中，PSA 的染色强度降低（图 14.1B）[4]。虽然在前列腺外组织和肿瘤中可见 PSA 免疫组化阳性，但是这些阳性反应部位常呈片状或较弱（表 14.1）。PSA 也是前列腺源性肿瘤的一种灵敏而特异的免疫组化标记物（图 14.2）。这对于低分化或未分化癌的鉴别诊断非常有用[4]。

除了良性前列腺组织增生（BPH）和肿瘤外，血清 PSA 在有些情况下也可能升高，包括前列腺炎、PIN、急性尿潴留、肾衰竭及涎腺炎。尽管尚存争议，但是血清 PSA 水平升高作为肿瘤早期检测的指标仍然被认为是一种减少前列腺癌死亡率的有效方法[5]。PSA 能够准确预测肿瘤的状态，而且能够比其他任何方法提前几个月检测到肿瘤的复发[6]。然而，这种方法的低特异性使其应用受到局限（47%，阈值为 4.0ng/ml）。2/3 的血清 PSA 水平 ≥ 4ng/ml 的男性其

表 14.1 在前列腺外组织和肿瘤中 PSA 的免疫组化反应

前列腺外组织
尿道及尿道周围腺体（男性和女性）
膀胱，包括膀胱黏膜和腺体
肛门，包括肛门腺体（男性）
脐尿管残留
中性粒细胞
前列腺外肿瘤
尿道及尿道周围腺体腺癌（女性）
膀胱绒毛腺癌和腺癌
发生于雄性外生殖器的乳腺外 Paget 病
涎腺多形性腺瘤（男性）
涎腺癌（男性）
乳腺癌[448]
成熟畸胎瘤
这些结果中尚有很多未经证实或还存在疑问。在这些前列腺外组织中的很多位点，免疫组化可能表现为弱阳性、散在颗粒状或阴性

活检结果为阴性。此外，在 PSA 水平为 2.5～4ng/ml 的男性中通过活检发现前列腺癌的几率达到 20%～30%。这提示，以 2.5ng/ml PSA 作为前列腺癌筛查的阈值更适当。同时，一些最新的基因检测方法，如 uPM3、GSTP1 和端粒酶对于前列腺癌检测的准确性研究也在进行当中[4, 5]。

PSA 在诊断残余肿瘤、肿瘤复发以及与治疗模式无关的治疗后肿瘤进展情况时，是一个非常灵敏而准确的指标。在根治性前列腺切除术后，如果血清 PSA 水平超过 0.2ng/ml 即可认为是肿瘤复发的生物化学指征[7, 8]。然而，在 26%～29% 的根治性前列腺切除术

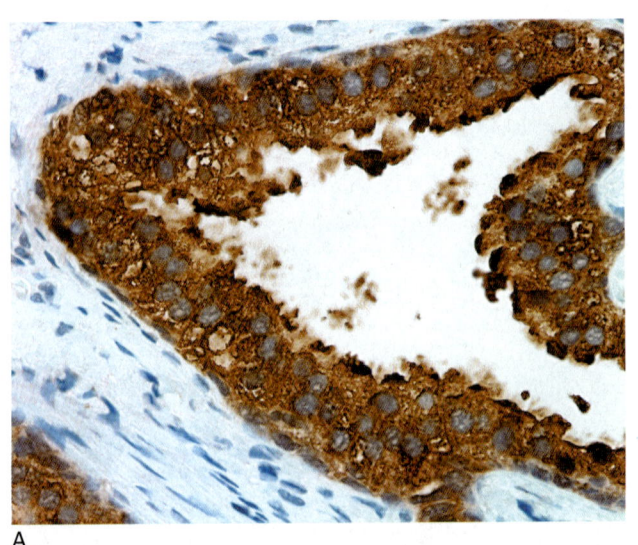

图 14.1　（A）正常前列腺上皮组织中的 PSA 抗体免疫组化。（B）在低分化前列腺腺癌细胞中 PSA 阳性强度降低

前列腺、膀胱、睾丸和肾的免疫组织化学 14

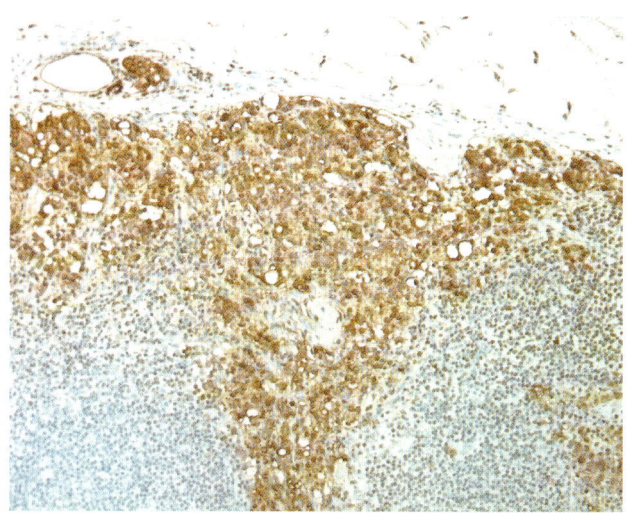

图14.2 在淋巴结内前列腺转移癌组织中PSA的免疫组化结果

表14.2 在184例前列腺癌根治性手术标本中，PSMA和PSA在良性前列腺组织及前列腺肿瘤组织中免疫组化结果对比	
	免疫组化细胞的百分比 + 标准差（范围）
PSMA	
良性	69.5+17.3(20～90)
高度 PIN	77.9+13.7(30～100)
肿瘤	80.2+13.7(30～100)
PSA	
良性	81.3+11.8(20～90)
高度 PIN	64.8+17.3(10～90)
肿瘤	74.2+16.2(10～90)

的标本中，外科手术切缘包含伴有或不伴有肿瘤的良性前列腺腺体组织。在45%的全部进行包埋的前列腺切除标本中，手术切缘只有良性腺体存在[9]。这些患者中1/3的人可以在术后血清中检测到PSA，同时这其中的一半患者PSA浓度的改变表明肿瘤有复发[10, 11]。这种PSA浓度水平的升高是以各临床实验室的检测正常范围为各自标准判定的，而不是一个绝对数值[7, 8, 12]。

前列腺酸性磷酸酶

很多年来，前列腺酸性磷酸酶（PAP）在人类的正常和增生性前列腺组织和前列腺癌组织中的免疫组织化学定位和分布一直被认为是前列腺的特异标志物[13-34]。在正常和增生的前列腺组织中，PAP均匀分布于腺体上皮分泌细胞的顶端。在肿瘤细胞以及高分化腺癌的腺体上皮细胞中阳性反应更强且更均匀，而在中度或低分化腺癌组织中阳性反应更弱且更不均匀[35, 36]。近几年，PAP表达的检测被其他组织标记物的检测所代替，包括PSA、其他人腺体激肽释放酶和PSMA[35]。

前列腺特异性膜抗原

前列腺特异性膜抗原（PSMA）是一种膜结合抗原，对于良性和恶性前列腺上皮细胞具有高度特异性[27-36]。根据使用单克隆抗体7E11.C5的研究，表明它存在于正常人的血清中，在前列腺腺癌、肿瘤临床进展期以及激素治疗无效的肿瘤患者中，其血清浓度会升高[37-39]。在对某些患者的预后进行预测时，PSMA可能比前列腺特异抗原更有优势（表14.2）[38-45]。

PSMA与转铁蛋白受体部分同源，它的细胞外结构域也具有NAALADase酶活性[46]。作者在本研究中所使用的抗体7E11.C5，能识别胞浆内结构域的头6个N-末端氨基酸。另一个PSMA的抗体是3F5.4G6，能够识别细胞外结构域部分的C-末端部分附近的8个氨基酸区域[40]。结合SPEC扫描7E11.C5抗体被成功用于检测前列腺癌的软组织及骨转移，以及术前及术后前列腺的诊断[27-30, 35, 41, 42, 47, 48]。

在每一个前列腺组织中，PSMA都在上皮细胞胞浆中呈强阳性反应[37, 39, 42]。从良性上皮组织到高级别PIN以及前列腺腺癌的发展过程中，阳性反应细胞的数量不断增加。高级别PIN表现为中度免疫组化阳性，表明这一显微镜下所见的只是一部分而非全部肿瘤的表型特征，这与其他的腺体标记物的研究相似[40]。PSMA最广泛、最强的阳性反应可见于高级别肿瘤中。在Gleason 4或5级的肿瘤中，实际上每个细胞均呈阳性反应[49]。一项研究表明：在高级别癌中免疫组化阳性的不均一性高于低级别癌[42]。但其他作者的研究结果与此相反[40]。PSMA的表达在前列腺癌组织中上调，前列腺癌组织中编码PSMA的mRNA量几乎是其重组型的100倍[45, 49]。

PSMA在前列腺组织外的表达是非常有限的，有报道主要在十二指肠黏膜、部分近端肾小管、部分结肠隐窝神经内分泌细胞、泌乳的乳腺以及涎腺和颌下腺中有表达[38, 39, 42]。有一报道在毛细血管内皮细胞中有表达[50-52]，但是作者在前列腺中未能证实该结果[40, 44]。前列腺外肿瘤的PSMA通常为阴性，包括肾细胞癌、尿道上皮癌和结肠腺癌[42]。

PSMA在肿瘤细胞中的免疫组化阳性并不能作为PSA生物化学肿瘤复发或经外科手术切除、局限于器

517

官内、边缘阴性肿瘤复发的指标[40]；这些发现与血清学研究不同，血清学研究发现PSMA浓度的升高表明外科手术失败[38, 53, 54]。

PSMA对于临床诊断与治疗非常有用。由于PSMA表达于前列腺癌的淋巴结[39,42]转移及骨髓转移灶（图14.3），故它可以用来诊断不明原发部位的转移癌。血清PSMA对疾病的预后有意义，特别是在肿瘤转移时，另外它与检测群体的肿瘤分期具有较好的相关性。此外，PSMA还可应用于反转录PCR（RT-PCR）分析当中，以检测循环系统中含有PSMA的细胞（可能为肿瘤细胞），在原发前列腺癌[47, 48]的患者中其阳性率为42%[45]和75%[55]。这种含有PSMA的细胞很明显是由于行前列腺癌根治术而进入循环系统的[49]，但是在雄激素去势治疗时这种细胞数量减少[42, 56]。抗体-放射性标记的核苷酸与PSMA结合被成功地用来明确动物和人前列腺癌的定位[41, 43, 44, 57-60]，并用来治疗裸鼠体内的人前列腺癌[35, 49]。

人腺体激肽释放酶2

人激肽释放酶家族包括3个成员：hK1、hK2和hK3（PSA）。hK2 mRNA和PSA mRNA主要位于前列腺上皮细胞中并受雄激素的调节[61-64]。此外，hK2的氨基酸与PSA具有78%的同源性，并主要表达于前列腺组织中，表明PSA可能是对诊断和监测前列腺癌有价值的临床标记物[63-65]。hK2在肿瘤组织中表达的强度和范围要大于PIN，而其在PIN中的表达要强于良性上皮中的表达。原发性Gleason 4级和5级的肿瘤中，hK2几乎在所有细胞中呈阳性反应，而在低级别癌中阳性反应强度则更加不均一[66]。与hK2截然不同，PSA和PAP的免疫组化在良性上皮组织中最强，在PIN和肿瘤组织中阳性反应较弱[66, 67]。对于hK2和PSA免疫组化呈阳性的细胞数量不能作为肿瘤复发的预测因素[68]。hK2的组织表达不受PSA和PAP的调节[69]。

α-甲基脂酰辅酶A消旋酶/P504S

α-甲基脂酰辅酶A消旋酶（AMACR，P504S，旋光酶）基因产物，也称为P504S蛋白，是一种涉及侧链脂肪酸β-氧化的酶。最近它被确定为几种人类肿瘤及其癌前病变的新的肿瘤标记物，包括前列腺癌[70-75]。初步的研究表明，消旋酶在97%~100%的前列腺癌中呈强烈而均一的阳性反应。最近的研究表明，在针吸细胞学活检组织中，消旋酶在80%~100%的微小前列腺癌组织中呈阳性反应，而在形态学较少见的前列腺癌组织中阳性反应下降且更不均一，包括萎缩、泡沫状腺体和假性增生的肿瘤组织（表14.3）。作者发现，91%的浸润性前列腺癌的消旋酶免疫组化仍然为阳性，并被另一项研究所证实[76]。此外，消旋酶阳性表达还可见于绝大多数高级别前列腺上皮内瘤变、10%~15%的非典型腺瘤样增生、少量的良性腺体，极少见于精囊腺上皮[71-77]。Jiang等人发现消旋酶用于前列腺腺癌检测的敏感性和特异性分别为97%和92%；阳性和阴性预测值均为95%。消旋酶在前列腺腺癌组织中的免疫组化强度和范围要明显高于良性前列腺组织[78]。

消旋酶、高分子量细胞角蛋白（HMWCK）和p63（基底细胞标记物）所组成的"鸡尾酒"式染色方法被越来越多地用于前列腺针吸细胞学活检组织中疑难病例的诊断[79]。仅依据基底细胞免疫组化阴性结果还不能诊断恶性肿瘤，因为有时良性腺体可能免疫组化也呈阴性，所以前列腺癌特异标记物，例如消旋酶，其免疫组化阳性结果对于恶性肿瘤的确诊很有价值。最近一项研究发现，根据消旋酶阳性表达，有10%（307例中的34例）的形态学可疑、基底细胞标记物阴性的被病理医生诊断为非典型增生的病例实际为癌，大约有50%（76例中的34例）经泌尿生殖系统专家诊断为非典型增生的病例实际诊断为癌。作者将"鸡尾酒"式免疫组化染色方法用于常规工作中，发现它对于诊断微小前列腺癌非常有用（图14.4）。目前已经具有商品化的多克隆和单克隆抗体[80]。优化"鸡尾酒"式抗体的染色条件，对于镜下染色判读来说是非常重要的[77]。尽管敏感性和特异性有局

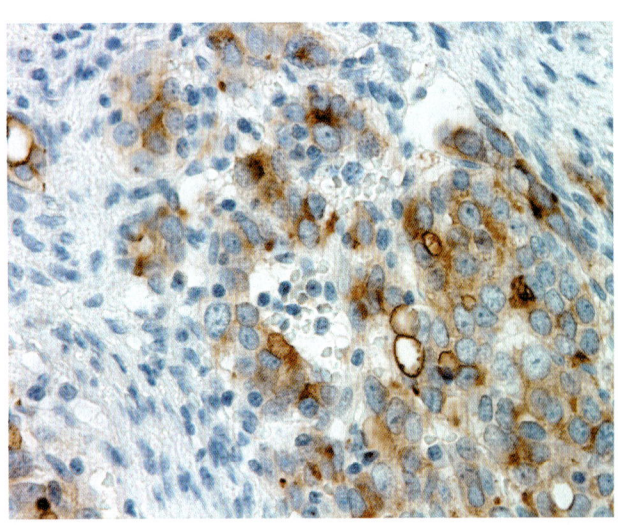

图14.3 在前列腺癌淋巴结转移组织中PSMA免疫组化阳性

前列腺、膀胱、睾丸和肾的免疫组织化学 14

表 14.3　α- 甲基脂酰辅酶 A 消旋酶（AMACR）在良性及恶性前列腺组织中的免疫组化结果

	免疫组化阳性比例（范围）	免疫组化阳性的腺体（范围）	染色强度（-,1+,2+,3+）
良性	8%(0%～10%)	4.6%(0%～24.5%)	-～1+
AAH	14%(10%～17%)	15.1%(1%～50%)	-～1+
高度 PIN	88%(80%～100%)	21.8%(2.7%～57.7%)	1+～2+
恶性肿瘤	97%(80%～100%)	35.0%(6.2%～78.2%)	2+～3+

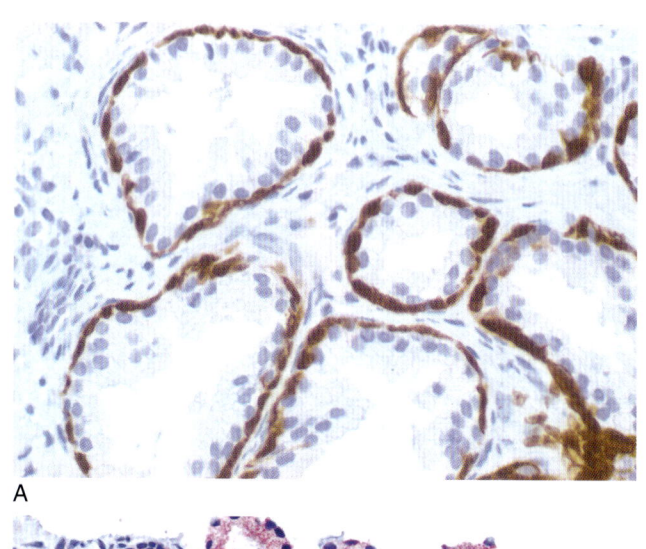

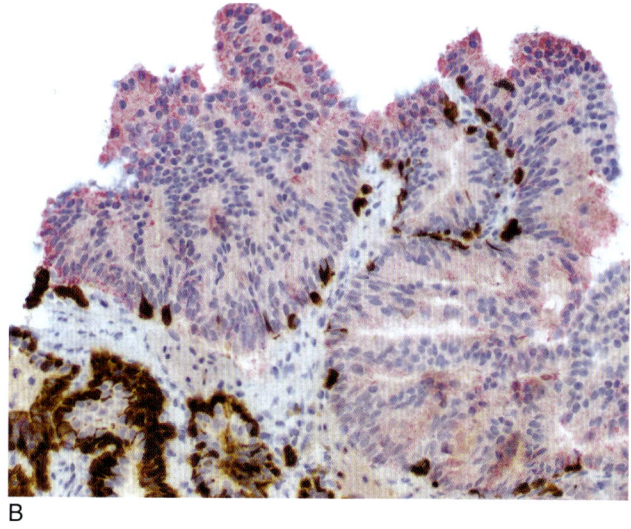

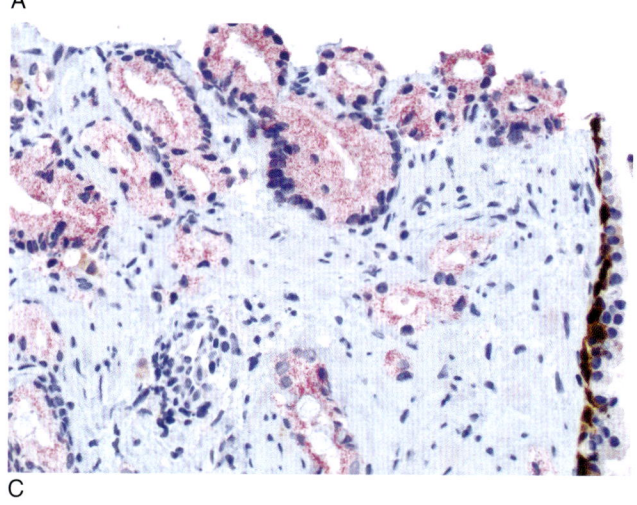

图14.4　（A）消旋酶/34βE12/p63"鸡尾酒"式染色方法在良性前列腺上皮、高度PIN（B）和肿瘤（C）组织中的免疫组化结果

限，但是消旋酶免疫组化检测还是迅速地成为一种标准的辅助诊断方法，用于前列腺活检组织学上仅根据HE染色应考虑为不典型病例而非恶性肿瘤病例的明确诊断[81]。

其他上皮诊断标记物

很多上皮标记物都被用于前列腺癌的诊断。例如，前列腺癌相关的诊断标记物-1仅表达于前列腺癌中[82]。P2x蛋白可以被用来进行前列腺癌的早期诊断。一个新的前列腺癌标记物EPCA，表达于前列腺癌患者的整个前列腺中，但是在非前列腺癌患者的前列腺中不表达。据报道，EPCA用来诊断前列腺癌患者比目前的诊断方法提前 5 年或更多[83]。Leroy 等人报道，MUC6蛋白仅表达于精囊-射精管，而在前列腺腺癌和正常前列腺组织中不表达，这表明MUC6对于精囊腺癌和前列腺腺癌的鉴别诊断有价值[84]。然而，这些抗体在前列腺癌诊断当中的应用需要进一步评价。

> **诊断要点**：前列腺抗原在诊断中的价值
>
> 1. Hk2，类似PSMA，在高级别恶性肿瘤中免疫组化更强。
> 2. PSA 和 AMACR（P504）对于前列腺癌具有高度特异性，很大程度上代替了 PAP 的应用。

角蛋白34βE12（角蛋白903；高分子量角蛋白）

实际上，所有正常前列腺基底细胞的单克隆基底细胞特异性抗角蛋白34βE12染色都呈阳性。在大多数情况下，基底细胞层能够形成完整的阳性反应条带（图14.5）。分泌细胞和基质细胞呈阴性。

这个标记物是最常用的前列腺基底细胞免疫组化标记物[85-87]，最近将这一标记物在石蜡包埋切片中的使用方法进行了优化[88]。角蛋白34βE12对福尔马林敏感，所以如果用福尔马林固定组织，就需要用酶消化或加热的方法进行预处理。用胃蛋白酶进行预消化或微波修复后，抗原的免疫组化反应强度会由于1周或更长时间的福尔马林固定而出现下降。而应用加热平台进行热诱导的抗原修复可以使结果稳定，即便是长达1个月的福尔马林固定也不会使抗原的免疫组化性下降[88]。当采用加热平台进行热诱导时，在不同的福尔马林固定时间点，抗体的免疫组化染色强度与胃蛋白酶或微波修复相比都更稳定且更强。用加热平台处理后，很少会在肿瘤细胞中见到弱阳性反应，但是用胃蛋白酶或微波修复抗原就不同。该作者的试验室研究报道认为，与单用蛋白酶消化相比，用热EDTA溶液与蛋白酶结合使用可以明显增强非肿瘤前列腺上皮基底细胞的染色强度[89]。在小叶中，非反应性良性腺泡最多见于周围腺泡，小团成簇并向外突起的腺泡离大导管或大导管末端最远[90]。更多的近端腺泡呈非连续的阳性反应区域。电子显微镜下观察可见，有时含腺腔的细胞的腺泡与基底膜相连，没有基底细胞浆进入，而其他的腺泡可见非常微弱的基底细胞胞浆的进入过程及少量成束的中间丝。

根据应用抗角蛋白34βE12（图14.6）抗体进行的研究结果，认为PIN级别的提高与基底细胞层断裂现象的增加有关。在56%的高级别PIN中可见基底细胞层的断裂，与远端腺泡相比，这种情况在与浸润性肿瘤毗邻的腺泡中更常见。断裂的数量随着PIN级别的升高而增加。早期浸润癌出现于腺体膨出的位点以及基底细胞断裂的位点与PIN相关（图14.7）[91]。PIN的筛状结构可能会被误认为是筛状腺癌，抗角蛋白抗体免疫组化方法无法进行鉴别诊断[92]。

肿瘤细胞通常不能与这种抗体发生反应，尽管其中混合有良性腺泡可能会被误认为是肿瘤组织反应阳性（图14.8）。抗角蛋白34βE12免疫组化方法可能提示在局部非典型增生的腺体中是否存在或缺乏基底细胞，这可以帮助建立良性或恶性肿瘤的诊断。作者相信，这种抗体可以被成功地应用于病理，结合光镜下所见进行结果判读；仅仅依靠免疫组化阴性（无基底细胞着色）就作出肿瘤的诊断在诊断免疫组织化学中是没有先例和不被接受的[93]。但是，最近的研究报道指出，在应用这种免疫组化标记物进行辅助诊断后，可疑病例明显减少[94]，或减少68%[85]，或从5.1%下降到1.0%[95]。对例如放射性治疗等治疗后前列腺活检组织的治疗效果评价，是抗角蛋白34βE12抗体最大的用途之一（见下文）[77,96]。

除了PIN和恶性肿瘤之外，基底细胞层的断裂或缺失还可见于炎症腺泡、非典型性腺瘤样增生（图14.9）以及萎缩后增生（图14.10），如果仅仅依靠可疑病灶的免疫组化结果进行判断，则可能会误诊为恶性肿瘤[93,97,98]。另外，Cowper腺体的基底细胞可能不会表达

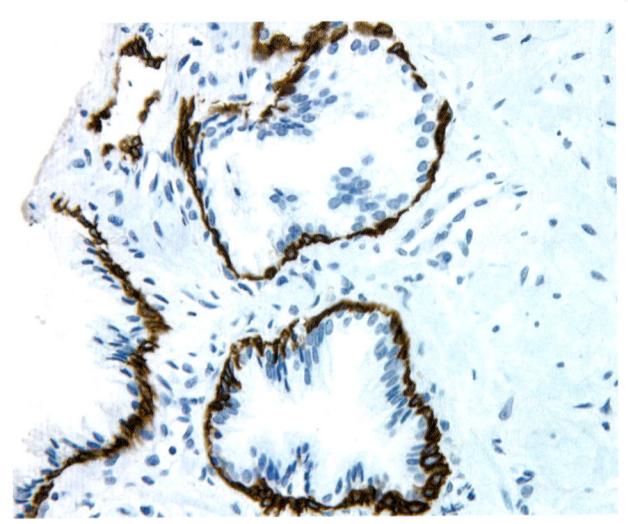

图14.5 34βE12免疫组化阳性结果显示在正常前列腺腺泡中的完整基底细胞层

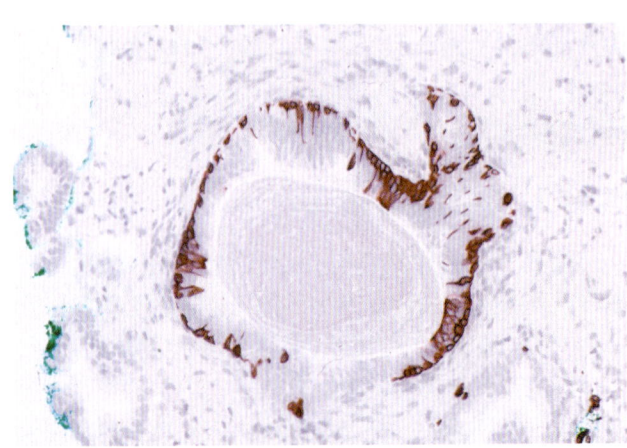

图14.6 34βE12阳性的基底细胞层在高级别PIN中出现断裂

前列腺、膀胱、睾丸和肾的免疫组织化学 14

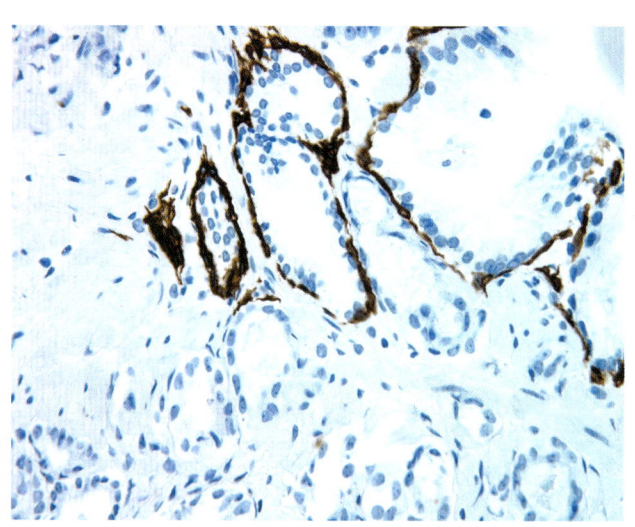

图 14.7 早期浸润癌出现于腺体膨出的位点以及基底细胞断裂的位点与 PIN 相关

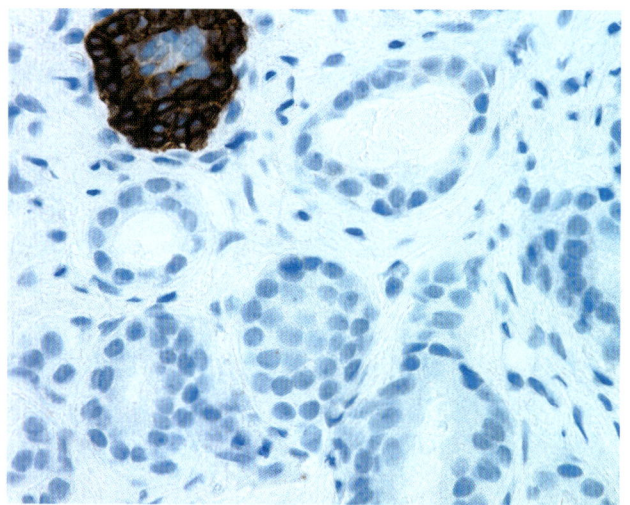

图 14.8 34βE12 免疫组化结果显示在前列腺癌腺泡中缺少基底细胞层

角蛋白 34βE12[99]，尽管对此尚存争议[100]。前列腺癌细胞表达高分子角蛋白罕见报道，包括高级别腺癌的转移灶；这些病例在表型上不具备基底细胞/腺样囊性癌的特征[101]。

基底细胞增生在组织学上与恶性肿瘤相似，故对于可疑病例推荐使用抗角蛋白 34βE12 抗体以辅助诊断[79, 102-104]。

CK5 和 CK14 mRNA 及其蛋白质在良性腺泡和 PIN 的基底细胞中表达，CK14 mRNA 在大多数 PIN 病灶中的腔面细胞中低水平表达；这样，如果 PIN 正如目前所持观点来源于基底细胞，那么 CK14 的翻译将被抑制而使得 CK14 mRNA 持续存在[105, 106]。CK8 mRNA 及其蛋白质表达于正常和异常前列腺组织的所有上皮细胞中。CK19 mRNA 及其蛋白质表达于良性腺泡的基底细胞和腔细胞中。CK16 mRNA 的表达方式与 CK19 相似，但是未检测到 CK16 蛋白质[105]。

作者们常规准备一些所有前列腺活检组织的未染色切片以备免疫组化之用，因为小的可疑病灶常常会由于组织块的重切而丢失；一项研究表明，52 个可疑病例中有 31 例被漏诊[107]。

p63

最近，一种核蛋白 p63 作为一种具有诊断价值的基底细胞标记物而被应用。据报道，p63 免疫组化染色在鉴定前列腺标本的基底细胞方面的灵敏性和特异性至少与高分子量细胞角蛋白相同（图 14.5）[108]。Shah 等人发现，p63 比 34βE12 在良性基底细胞的诊断方面

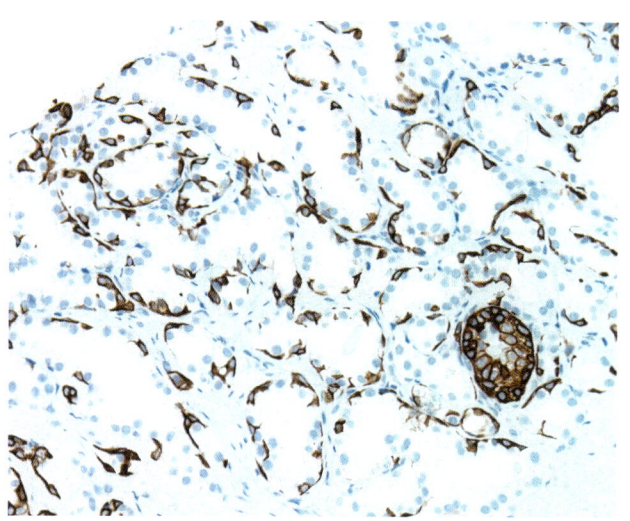

图 14.9 非典型腺瘤样增生组织中抗体 34βE12 阳性的区域提示为基底细胞

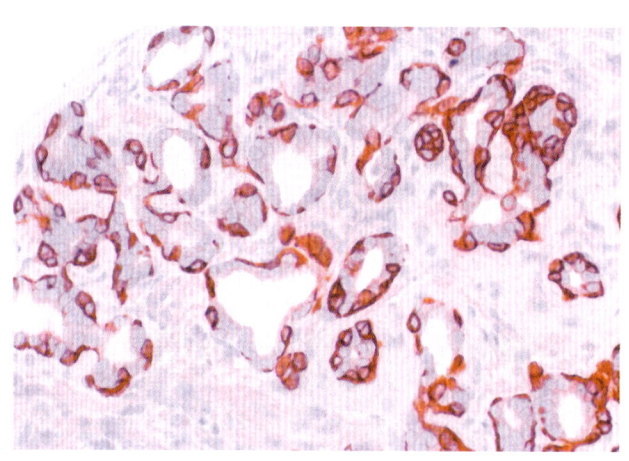

图 14.10 前列腺萎缩后增生，基底细胞 34βE12 呈阳性反应

更敏感，特别是对于 TURP 标本来说，在诊断有争议的病例时比 34βE12 更有优势[109]。Zhou 等人的研究表明，基底细胞"鸡尾酒"式（34βE12 和 p63）免疫组化染色方法能够提高基底细胞检测的灵敏性并降低染色的差异性，这使得基底细胞免疫组化结果更稳定[110]。p63 基因也在呼吸道上皮、乳腺和支气管肌上皮、人胎盘细胞滋养层细胞、淋巴结和生发层的散在细胞以及肺鳞状细胞癌中表达[111]。由消旋酶、高分子量角蛋白（HMWCK）以及 p63（基底细胞标记物）组成的三重染色方法正成为前列腺癌诊断的一种标准的联合染色方法而被应用（图 14.5）[112, 113, 114]。

其他基底细胞标记物

近来，大量的免疫组化标记物在前列腺中被确定，这其中的很多首先在上皮细胞基底层中被发现（表 14.4）。这些标记物包括细胞增殖标记物、分化标记物和遗传标记物。这些标记物中的很多被首先定位于基底细胞而非分泌细胞，表明它们在生长调节中起作用。

至少局部的基底细胞表现出对角蛋白 5、10、11、13、14、16 和 19 具有免疫反应性；这其中，只有角蛋白 19 也在分泌细胞中被发现[97, 98, 111, 115-123]。仅在分泌细胞中被发现的角蛋白包括角蛋白 7、8 和 18。最近，一种钙结合蛋白 S100A6（钙周期蛋白）被发现仅在良性腺体的基底细胞中表达，而不在恶性肿瘤细胞中表达[106, 124]。

基底细胞通常不会对前列腺特异抗原（PSA）、前列腺酸性磷酸酶（PAP）和 S-100 蛋白表现出免疫反应性，只有极少数的单个细胞嗜铬素和神经特异性烯醇化酶呈阳性反应。相反，正常分泌性腔细胞 PSA 和 PAP 总是呈阳性反应。前列腺基底细胞不总是表现出肌上皮分化[122, 125]，这与乳腺、涎腺、胰腺和其他部位的基底细胞情况相反。

> **诊断要点**：前列腺基底细胞的诊断应用
> 1. 前列腺周围出现基底细胞是良性或癌前病变的标志。
> 2. 在针吸细胞学活检组织中，角蛋白 903（K903、34βE12）与 p63 和 AMACR 配合使用，在鉴别非典型增生与浸润癌时具有很高的灵敏性和特异性。

前列腺神经内分泌细胞

神经内分泌细胞，也叫做内分泌-旁分泌细胞，是广泛分布的神经内分泌调节系统的一部分。在人前列腺中，可以根据形态学和分泌产物来鉴别神经内分泌细胞亚群（图 14.11A）[126-132]。在 LNCaP 细胞系中，可以通过药物增加细胞内 dbcAMP 水平（如 dbcAMP、福斯高林、异丙肾上腺素和肾上腺素）来诱导出旁分泌-内分泌表型。在体外研究中，撤除这些促分化试剂则导致旁分泌-内分泌分化的逆转[133]。前列腺中大多数内分泌细胞含有 5-羟色胺[134]、CgA[135-137]和其他神经内分泌细胞标记物，但呈不持续表达。前列腺中的神经内分泌细胞可能涉及生长、分化和分泌功能的调节（图 14.11B）。由于大鼠、几内亚猪、猫和狗的前列腺中缺乏 CgA 免疫组化阳性的细胞，故阻碍了以这些动物模型为基础进行人类前列腺神经内分泌细胞生理的研究[138]。

在人类，前列腺癌具有 3 种神经内分泌分化类型：①少见的小细胞神经内分泌癌（图 14.12），②少见的类癌样癌，③常见的前列腺癌伴局部神经内分泌分化。实际上，所有前列腺腺癌都至少包含一小部分神经内分泌细胞，但是还需要特殊的实验以鉴别这些细胞，如组织化学和免疫组织化学[129, 130, 136, 137, 139-144]。典型的神经内分泌分化现象包括一些在光镜下不易发现的散在细胞，但是可以通过一个或多个标记物的免疫组化方法来鉴别。前列腺癌中的神经内分泌细胞是恶性的，缺少雄激素受体表达[129, 130, 136, 145, 146]。大约 10% 的腺癌可见含有大的嗜酸性颗粒的细胞（以前叫做伴 Paneth 细胞样改变的腺癌），通常仅包括极少量的散在细胞及小的细胞簇，故可能被忽略[147, 148]。在正常上皮和腺癌组织中含有大的嗜酸性颗粒的细胞与肠道和其他部位的 Paneth 细胞在光镜下观察相似，但是它们所具有的神经内分泌分化功能（产生嗜铬素、神经特异性烯醇化酶和 5-羟色胺）以及它们缺少溶菌酶表达的特点是与 Paneth 细胞不同的[147]。良性前列腺上皮和腺癌中的神经内分泌细胞的数量实际上比含有大的嗜酸性颗粒的细胞的数量要多，这表明大多数神经内分泌细胞在 HE 染色的切片中不易被发现。

大多数神经内分泌癌病例具有典型的局部体征和前列腺腺癌的症状，尽管在这些病人中也经常出现癌旁症状。Cushing 综合征是最常见的，无一例外地与

表14.4　前列腺基底细胞分化标记物

生物标记物	功能	免疫组化结果
PCNA	细胞增殖标记物	高达 79% 的阳性细胞为基底细胞
MIB-1	细胞增殖标记物	高达 77% 的阳性细胞为基底细胞
Ki-67	细胞增殖标记物	高达 81% 的阳性细胞为基底细胞
雄激素受体	前列腺上皮细胞生长必需的核受体	强阳性；肿瘤细胞也呈阳性
前列腺特异抗原	使精液中凝胶液化的酶	极少基底细胞阳性；主要位于分泌型腔细胞中
角蛋白 8.12	角蛋白 13、16	强阳性
角蛋白 4.62	角蛋白 19	中度阳性
角蛋白 PKK1	角蛋白 7、8、17、18	中度阳性
角蛋白 312C8-1	角蛋白 14	强阳性
角蛋白 34βE12	角蛋白 5、10、11	强阳性；主要用于诊断
p63	$p53$ 基因家族成员之一	强阳性；主要用于诊断
S100A6	钙结合蛋白	强阳性
表皮生长因子受体	膜结合型 170kD 糖蛋白，调节 EGF 活性	强阳性；极少肿瘤细胞阳性
CuZn-超氧化物歧化酶	催化超氧化物阴离子残基的酶	强阳性
IV 型胶原酶	涉及细胞外基质降解的酶	强阳性；肿瘤细胞中阳性强度下降
VII 型胶原	半桥粒复合物的一部分	强阳性；肿瘤细胞阴性
整合素 α1、2、4、6 和 β1、4	细胞外基质黏附分子	强阳性；大多数肿瘤细胞阳性降低，但是 α6 和 β1 阳性强度不变
雌激素受体	激素受体	中度阳性
bcl-2	抑制凋亡的癌蛋白	强阳性；大多数肿瘤细胞也呈强阳性
c-erbB2	EGF 家族的癌蛋白	强阳性；大多数肿瘤细胞也呈强阳性
谷胱苷肽 S 转移酶基因（GSTP1）	激活亲电子性致癌物的酶	强阳性；极少肿瘤细胞阳性
C-CAM	上皮细胞黏附分子	强阳性；肿瘤细胞阴性
TGF-B	调节细胞增殖和分化的生长因子	强阳性；肿瘤细胞阴性
组织蛋白酶 B	降解基底膜的酶，可能涉及肿瘤浸润和转移	多数基底细胞阳性；肿瘤细胞也呈阳性
孕激素受体	激素受体	中度阳性

PCNA：增殖细胞核抗原
根据正文查阅参考文献

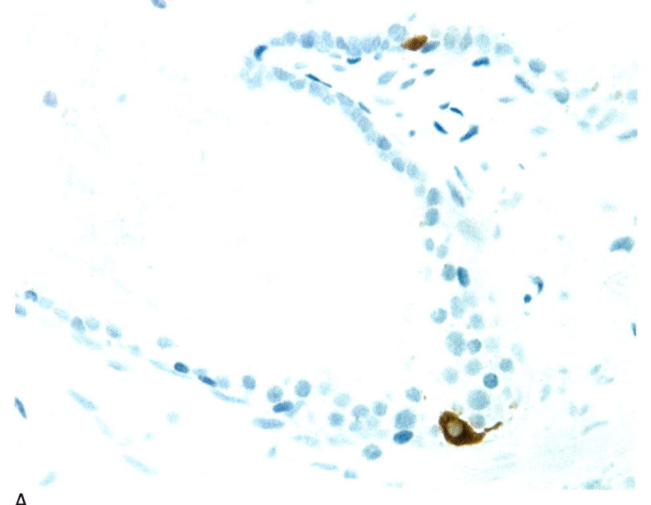

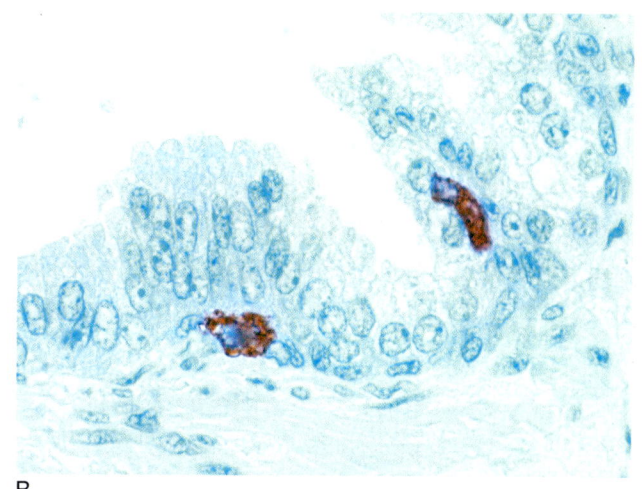

A　　　　　　　　　　　　　　　　B

图 14.11　CgA 在正常前列腺上皮（A）和高级别 PIN 细胞（B）中的免疫组化结果

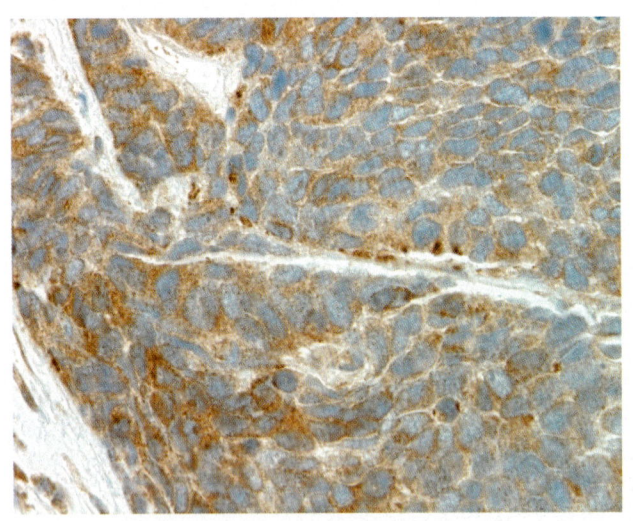

图14.12 小细胞前列腺癌中突触素的免疫组化结果

肿瘤细胞中 ACTH 免疫组化阳性反应有关[149-152]；其他临床症状包括恶性高钙血症[153]、异常抗利尿激素综合征（SIADH）和肌无力（Eaton-Lambert）综合征。小细胞癌侵袭性强，致死率高[129,148,154,155]。前列腺神经内分泌癌具有不同的组织病理学，从类癌样型（低度恶性神经内分泌癌）到小细胞未分化型（燕麦细胞）癌（高度恶性神经内分泌癌）[91,144,156,157]。这些肿瘤在形态学上与肺部及其他位点的同类型肿瘤一致。在很多病例中，至少在局部还可见到典型的腺泡型腺癌，有时还可见到过渡型。在那些拟诊断Gleason 5型神经内分泌癌的病例中，建议应用免疫组化方法进行辅助诊断。还可见混合型，包括一个同时包含小细胞癌、腺癌、典型类癌和梭形细胞癌的病例[148]。在恶性细胞中可能会检测到大量的分泌产物，包括5-羟色胺、降钙素、ACTH、人绒毛膜促性腺激素、甲状腺刺激素、铃蟾肽、降钙素-基因调节肽、双向调节因子、存活素和抑制素[158,159]。同样的细胞可能表达肽激素、PSA 和 PAP，但是单纯的小细胞癌 PSA 免疫组化通常为阴性。在福尔马林固定的前列腺组织切片中，5-羟色胺、嗜铬素和突触素是鉴别神经内分泌细胞最常用的标记物[137,160-168]。在超微结构上，前列腺小细胞癌和类癌包含不同数量的圆形、规则的膜结合神经分泌颗粒[160-166]。胞浆中的神经分泌颗粒经常清晰可见。细胞小，常伴有分散的染色质和小而不明显的核仁。

根据大多数而非全部报道，神经内分泌细胞对于良性上皮、原发前列腺腺癌和淋巴结转移病例没有明显的临床或预后价值（表14.4）[127-129,135-140,145,147,150,154,168-178]。Aprikian及同事研究发现，神经内分泌分化与病理分期或转移无关[178]。作者曾经发现，在高级别前列腺 PIN 及肿瘤中，免疫组化阳性的神经内分泌细胞的数量与各种临床及病理因素，包括分期在内，无明显关系[171,179]。Allen 等人对120名患者进行了研究，发现神经内分泌分化与患者预后没有明显的相关性[108]。相反，Weinstein 和同事对104名临床诊断为未扩散前列腺癌进行了研究，发现神经内分泌分化与患者的成活率有关，但是他们的研究仅仅局限于 Gleason 5 和 6 级的肿瘤，所以他们的结论可能受到选择偏差的影响[177]。Frierson 等人认为神经内分泌分化预示了患者的存活时间，但是这仅仅是根据一种模型分析而得出的结论[181]。Krijnen 等人报道，神经内分泌分化与早期激素治疗失败有关，这表明这些细胞是非雄激素依赖性的[146]。他们的研究结果表明，肿瘤中大量的神经内分泌细胞的出现可能提示预后不良，这可能是由于对激素生长调节不敏感造成的，但是很多研究并不支持这种观点（表14.5）[168,182]。一些作者最近报道，与良性前列腺上皮和原发性前列腺癌相比，肿瘤的淋巴结转移灶所含有的嗜铬素和5-羟色胺阳性的细胞较少，这提示神经内分泌细胞标记物表达水平的下降与肿瘤的进展有关[144]。神经内分泌细胞的表达在对行根治性前列腺切除术、伴淋巴结转移的前列腺癌患者的预后分析中无临床使用价值。

前列腺免疫组化

前列腺的免疫反应主要通过细胞免疫进行调节。在基质中含有大量的淋巴细胞，T细胞在前列腺基质和上皮内占90%以上。基质中的T细胞主要为辅助/诱导T细胞，而上皮内的T细胞主要为细胞毒性/抑制T细胞（CD4/CD8比值倒置），这种发现与以往的报道一致[143,183,184]。在上皮内部分CD4/CD8比值的倒置，表明细胞毒性/抑制T细胞可能是阻止腺腔内外源物质通过尿道逆行进入前列腺体的第一道屏障。有趣的是，淋巴细胞的数量（T细胞或B细胞，基质或上皮内的细胞）在患者的不同年龄组、不同的种族或者不同的解剖学上的带区（外周带、中心带或移行带）之间没有明显的区别[11]。这些结果表明，淋巴细胞功能和分布的调节受到了严格的调控，从出生到至少70多岁，前列腺体都会处在一个相对稳定的免疫监控之下。最近一个研究表明，肿瘤中CD4+的T淋巴细胞的浸润与肿瘤分期无关，但是与前列腺癌患者的预后不良有关[185]。

表14.5 在前列腺腺癌中，用免疫组化方法所得到的神经内分泌分化的预测值：研究结果汇总

	患者数量	不同肿瘤的患者数量	组织类型	NE标记物	肿瘤病例的阳性值(%)	NE染色结果的定量标准	肿瘤转归	多变量研究	随访时间	评价
对预后无预测作用										
Aprikian 等，1993[178]	78	31例原发肿瘤，16例转移癌，21例已烯雌酚治疗的肿瘤，10例激素不敏感性肿瘤	根治性前列腺切除术和TURP标本	CgA，NSE，5-羟色胺，降钙素，ACTH，生长激素抑制素，胃泌素释放肽，TSH	原发性未治疗肿瘤中的77%，转移癌中的56%	无阳性细胞(-)，偶尔可见NE细胞(+)，大量细胞(++)，大多数细胞(+++)	复发或转移，无激素依赖性，肿瘤进展	是，分析指标包括肿瘤分级、分期、浸润和无激素依赖性	未提供	NE细胞与肿瘤分期或转移无关
Cohen 等，1994[449]	38	临床 II、III 期	耻骨后前列腺切除术标本	CgA，NSE	CgA阳性率为29%；NSE的阳性率为24%	未见阳性细胞(-)，偶尔可见阳性细胞(+)，每个腺泡结构中1~3个阳性细胞(++)，每个腺泡结构中>3个阳性细胞(+++)	PSA试验失败，组织活检中发现复发或转移，骨扫描或X光检查阳性发现	是，肿瘤分级、分期和NE染色	4.2年（范围：4~6年）	CgA在预测肿瘤进展方面无应用价值
Bostwick 等，1994[344]	26	pT1b期1例，pT2a+b期10例，pT2c期13例，pT3a期1例，T3c期肿瘤1例，在手术前无雄激素去势治疗或放射治疗史	全标本包埋，根治性前列腺切除术标本	CgA，NSE，5-羟色胺，hCG，降钙素，ACTH，TSH，泌乳素，胰高血糖素	92%	高倍视野平均阳性细胞比率(×640)	肿瘤分级，分期	是，逐级回归，这些分析包括肿瘤分级、分期、肿瘤体积、微血管浸润	未提供	在前列腺癌中，NE的分化下调。NE的分化与各种临床和病理因素无关

续表

患者	患者数量	不同肿瘤的例数	组织类型	NE标记物	肿瘤病例的阳性值(%)	NE染色结果的定量标准	肿瘤转归	多变量研究	随访时间	评价
Noordzij等, 1995[175]	90	pT2期肿瘤22例, pT3期肿瘤66例, pT4期肿瘤2例, pN1期肿瘤5例, PN2期肿瘤2例	根治性前列腺切除术标本	CgA, 嗜铬素B	78%	未见阳性细胞(-), 少量阳性细胞, 广泛散在分布(±), 一些阳性细胞, 更有规则的分布或成形成簇状(++), 大量阳性细胞或成形成大的簇状(+++)	组织学上可见局部肿瘤复发或转移, 肿瘤导致的死亡	是, Cox回归曲线模型, 包括肿瘤分级、分期	7.2年(范围: 0.1~16.9年)	NE分化与Gleason评分、病理分期或肿瘤导致的死亡无关
Allen等, 1995[180]	120	T0期肿瘤17例, T1期肿瘤6例, T2期肿瘤17例, T3期肿瘤38例, T4期肿瘤42例	针吸细胞学活检, TURP, 根治性前列腺切除术标本	CgA, NSE	31%	阴性(只要可见阳性细胞), 阴性(无阳性细胞)	全身扩散, 肿瘤相关的存活情况	是, 相关分析因素包括分级、分期和存活率	>5年(范围未提供)	NE细胞与肿瘤分级、分期者的存活情况无关
Speights等, 1997[450]	33	高级别肿瘤23例, T1a低级别肿瘤10例, 所有病例通过TURP进行诊断; 一些接受雄激素撤退治疗的患者	TURP标本	CgA, NSE, 突触素(也包括MIB-1)	高级别肿瘤: "几乎全部"; 低级别肿瘤: 50%	每个标记物计数1000个良性和恶性肿瘤细胞	PSA实验失败(不确定), 活检证明复发, 临床治疗失败或转移, 23例高级别肿瘤中的14例扩散	是, 使用Cox回归曲线模型用来对不同的随访时间和Gleason评分进行说明	高级别肿瘤为13.4个月(范围: 1~42个月)	与低级别肿瘤相比, 在高级别肿瘤中, NE细胞的数量更多, 增殖指数(MIB-1染色)更高
McWilliams等, 1997[140]	92	T1~2期64例, T3期9例, M1期19例	TURP标本	CgA, NSE	52%	阳性(>10%的肿瘤细胞阳性), 阴性(<10%的肿瘤细胞阴性)	肿瘤相关的存活情况(33例因肿瘤死亡), 肿瘤转移(5例)	是, 分析因素包括肿瘤分级、分期、血管浸润和骨转移	9年(7~13年)	NE细胞的分化与肿瘤分级不良相关, 与肿瘤分期和肿瘤相关的存活情况

526

续表

患者	不同肿瘤的患者数量	组织类型	NE标记物	肿瘤病例的阳性值（%）	NE染色结果的定量标准	肿瘤转归	多变量研究	随访时间	评价
Pruneri 等，1998[136]	64	A期7例，B期13例，C期30例，D期14例，57例未接受激素治疗	前列腺切除术（5例），根治性前列腺切除术（28例）；TURP（31例）	CgA，嗜铬素B，分泌粒蛋白Ⅱ	86%	至少在50个肿瘤区域计数阳性细胞的数量	总体和无病存活情况	是，总体分析包括分期和分级	3.6年（范围：1.5~7.3年）	NE分化与高Gleason评分相关，但是与分期和患者存活情况无关
Casella 等，1998[173]	105	T2和更高期；根据随访信息的有效性选择患者；各种不同的治疗方法	针吸细胞学活检	CgA	25%（仅限于活检标本）	主观判断为"少"或"多"	肿瘤相关的存活情况	三组分析：偏差未提供。Gleason分析，评分和Ki-67指数，具有预测价值，但是无NE	未提供	NE分化在激素不敏感性肿瘤中更常见且更强
Tan 等，1999[451]	41	临床分期：A，6例；B，10例；C，1例；D，24例	前列腺切除术，TURP标本	CgA，NSE	53.6%	无染色（-），极少，分散单个阳性细胞（+），小簇阳性细胞（++），有时可见大的融合的阳性细胞群（+++）	全身扩散，肿瘤相关的存活情况	是，分析参数包括：肿瘤分期，分级和全身扩散	5年（范围未提供）	NE分化与高Gleason评分，分级和患者存活情况无关
Bostwick 等，2002[144]	196	行根治性前列腺切除术，淋巴结阳性	行根治性前列腺切除术的单张切片或转移的淋巴结	CgA，5-羟色胺	CgA的阳性率为98.5%；5-羟色胺阳性率为94.9%	主观判断数量增加10%，显色强度分别测定	全身扩散，肿瘤相关的存活情况和各种因素影响的存活情况	是，Cox比例危险模型包括肿瘤分级，多倍体，体积，扩散和存活情况	6.8年（范围：0.3~11年）	CgA的表达水平与肿瘤相关的或各种因素的存活情况无明显相关性。5-羟色胺的表达水平与肿瘤相关的存活情况有关，但是与各种因素的存活情况无关

续表

患者	不同肿瘤的患者数量	组织类型	NE标记物	肿瘤病例的阳性值(%)	NE染色结果的定量标准	肿瘤转归	多变量研究	随访时间	评价
患者预后的预测									
Abrahamson 等, 1989[137]	25	雄激素去势治疗之后, 用TURP检测的肿瘤(A1、A2、B1期)	TURP或前列腺摘除术标本	CgA	92%	主观判断: 阴性(0), 分离的单个细胞(±), 少量细胞(+), 中等量细胞(++), 大量细胞(+++)	在TURP标本中的肿瘤分级	否	5.5年(范围: 1~11年)	25个病例中的大多数出现了明显的肿瘤扩散, 同时NE细胞数量相应增加
Cohen 等, 1990, 1992[452,453]	90	TURP或针吸细胞学活检测的B(22)、C(20)、D(48)期肿瘤	TURP或针吸细胞学活检标本	CgA, NSE	52%	阴性(未见NE细胞), 阳性(单个细胞或成组的NE细胞)	肿瘤相关的存活情况	是, 分级和NE阳性时肿瘤扩散的指标	>4年(范围: 4~7年)	NE分化是比Gleason评分更重要的预后因素
Weinstein 等, 1996[177]	104	临床判断为局部未扩散的前列腺癌(T1~2), 行根治性前列腺切除未治疗	根治性前列腺切除术单张切片	CgA	62%	每个×100视野中NE细胞的最大数量	PSA实验失败	是, Cox比例危险模型包括Gleason评分、NE染色和肿瘤扩散	8年(范围: 7~10年)	NE分化可能是中等Gleason评分的预后指标
Krijnen 等, 1997[146]	72	雄激素去势治疗之后, 用TURP检测的肿瘤, 包括T1b期12例, T2期3例, T3期36例, T4期21例	TURP标本	CgA	55%	每1mm²的肿瘤组织中阳性细胞和阳性细胞团的数量	与扩散无关的存活情况	是, Cox比例危险模型, 分级和NE染色具有预测价值	3年(范围: 0.1~7.9年)	NE细胞数量和Gleason评分是肿瘤扩散的独立预后因素

续表

	患者数量	不同肿瘤的患者数量	组织类型	NE标记物	肿瘤病例的阳性值（%）	NE染色结果的定量标准	肿瘤转归	多变量研究	随访时间	评价
Theodorescu 等，1997[181]	71	T1～2期肿瘤，行根治性前列腺切除术而无后续治疗，直至复发	根治性前列腺切除术单张切片	CgA（也包括组织蛋白酶）	24%	主观判断：阴性（0），极少阳性肿瘤细胞（1），<1%（2），1%～10%（3），11%～25%（4），26%～50%（5），或>50%（6）；所计数的细胞数量未提供，作为结果分析，只有2～6被认为是阳性	肿瘤相关的存活情况，51%的患者复发，24%死于前列腺癌	是，Cox比例危险模型包括Gleason分级、分期、标本中肿瘤的百分率	随访时间的中位数为10.6年；53%的患者随访期在10年以上	CgA在单变量模型和只采用一个变量为研究模型的多变量研究中具有临床意义，但是在双变量模型中无意义；组织蛋白酶D在单变量或多变量研究中不能预测存活情况
Borre 等，2000[315]	221	对患者进行观察随访	诊断性活检标本	VEGF和NE标记物		半定量：弱、中等和强阳性	肿瘤相关的存活情况，57%死于前列腺癌	是，模型包括VEGF表达和微血管数量	随访时间的中位数为15年	NE分化与微血管的数量、VEGF表达情况和存活明显相关
Yu 等，2001[182]	30	临床诊断为局部的前列腺癌（T1～2）	标本类型不确定	CgA、NSE、5-羟色胺	80% 43% 77%	-，无阳性；+，<2%细胞；++，<25%细胞；+++，>25%细胞	CgA与肿瘤分级、分期、PSA和存活情况相关	否	平均随访期为3.7年	神经内分泌细胞可能成为前列腺癌后不良预后的独立标志物

NE，神经内分泌；NSE，神经特异性烯醇化酶；TURP，经尿道前列腺切除术；VEGF，血管内皮生长因子

增殖抗原

增殖细胞核抗原

增殖细胞核抗原（PCNA）标记指数在良性的、正常的前列腺上皮和局限于器官内而未扩散的肿瘤组织中是最低的，但是随着肿瘤细胞从分化良好到低分化的方向发展，PCNA的标记指数逐渐升高[186]，尽管差别较大[102, 176, 187-197]。PCNA指数与肿瘤分期的关系是非常明显的[189, 198, 199]。因此，高PCNA标记指数可能表明前列腺癌的扩散[200]、肿瘤转移[201]，可能是一种独立的预后标志物[188]。然而，PCNA还可以代表未分裂细胞的DNA损伤，这样它可能不能成为判断细胞增殖的最佳方法。

Ki-67 和 MIB-1

在前列腺癌中，在传统的Gleason分级、病理分期和DNA多倍体的预后指标的基础上，Ki-67或MIB-1的高增殖指数几乎不能对患者的预后提供更有价值的信息[202]。然而，Ki-67标记指数可能能够区分局限于器官内未扩散的肿瘤与转移癌（图14.13）[189]。因此，Ki-67/MIB-1增殖指数的升高能够反映肿瘤的进展[172, 173, 203]。这进一步可以从Ki-67的表达与表皮生长因子受体[204]、突变p53[204-206]、特殊的染色体畸变[207]以及周围神经浸润[208]的关系中看出。综上所述，这些结果提示Ki-67的表达可能是肿瘤复发、扩散[172, 173, 203]和存活情况[205, 209-212]的一个弱相关标志物。

其他角蛋白

在前列腺上皮中，根据定位、形态学、分化程度和细胞特异标志物，可以分成3种细胞类别：分泌腔细胞、基底细胞和内分泌细胞[102, 213]。腔细胞和基底细胞有特征性的角蛋白表达[214]。基底细胞表型的可塑性表明，它们含有一个干细胞亚群能够产生所有的上皮细胞[102, 215]。

根据干细胞模型，有至少3种细胞亚型，包括干细胞、扩增细胞和变行细胞。抗角蛋白抗体免疫组化至少能够鉴别出3种细胞亚群，其中之一被认为是扩增细胞[213]。这些储备干细胞亚群在前列腺癌组织中缺失。在干细胞模型中，扩增细胞被认为是前列腺上皮分化过程中变行细胞（腔细胞）的前体，所以角蛋白的表达提示这一细胞亚群可能是肿瘤转化作用的目

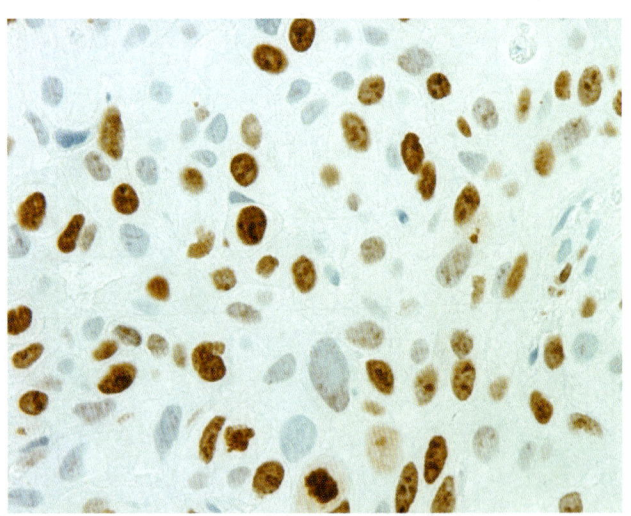

图14.13 低分化前列腺癌MIB-1免疫组化染色

标[122, 216-220]。

细胞角蛋白在正常、增生和恶性前列腺上皮细胞中表达不同[220]。前列腺癌PC3、DU145和LNCAP细胞系免疫印迹分析表明，角蛋白8和18表达，而角蛋白5、7和15不表达，这几种角蛋白只在良性前列腺组织中可见。同时标记角蛋白18和PSA，可以在50%的骨髓抽取物中检测到转移的前列腺癌细胞[221]。对细胞角蛋白8和18片段的分析，能够鉴别出高度恶性肿瘤和转移癌患者[222]。血清角蛋白18是监测治疗过程中前列腺癌细胞凋亡和坏死的潜在标记物[223]。

细胞外基质蛋白

层粘连蛋白

在正常的前列腺、BPH和分化良好的肿瘤中，层粘连蛋白以一种致密的、均一的形式定位于腺泡、血管基底膜、平滑肌和神经纤维。分化不良的肿瘤基底膜层粘连蛋白反应为阴性。然而，与许多其他的蛋白相同，高级别肿瘤的胞浆、细胞表面和分泌物质中也会出现层粘连蛋白阳性反应[156, 224-228]。

整合素

细胞黏附和迁移是肿瘤浸润的重要特征，并且部分受到整合素的调控。整合素是同源连接蛋白的大家族，它与各种不同的细胞外基质成分相互作用。这些受体蛋白与细胞外基质结合并发生反应。它

们包括2个非共价结合的跨膜糖蛋白亚基，分别叫做α和β亚基，这两个亚基在与基质蛋白的结合过程中都发挥作用。整合素结合依赖于二价阳离子。很多细胞外基质成分，包括层粘连蛋白和纤维连接蛋白，都能够识别并结合多种形式的整合素异源二聚体。在高级别前列腺癌中[229]，通过同时使用相同的免疫组化方法，可以发现E-钙黏素与β1整合素的表达是相应的。尽管整合素在人前列腺癌中的表达量明显下降，但其中的例外是α6整合素（层粘连蛋白受体），其在整个前列腺肿瘤的进展过程中持续表达[230]。前列腺癌的进展可能受到原发肿瘤细胞周围的基底细胞生化特性的影响[231]。

正常的基底细胞与半桥粒样结构形成局部黏附结构，并表现出半桥粒样相关蛋白的极性分布，包括BP180、BP230、HD1、网格蛋白、层粘连蛋白λ2、VII胶原和相应的整合素-层粘连蛋白受体α6β1和α6β4。这些蛋白的表达和分布也存在于PIN中。相反，肿瘤一律缺少半桥粒样结构、整合素α6β4、BP180、层粘连蛋白λ2和VII胶原，但是表达BP230、网格蛋白、HD1和整合素-层粘连蛋白受体α3β1和α6β1。这些结果表明，尽管在肿瘤组织中可以检测到基底细胞层，但是它的成分和细胞连接也是异常的。半桥粒蛋白和α3β1以及α6β1整合素在PIN中也存在。α6β1和层粘连蛋白在肿瘤中的反常表达可能有助于肿瘤的浸润[231, 232]。

层粘连蛋白5是一种细胞外基质蛋白，参与半桥粒的组成，半桥粒将正常的基底细胞与其下的基底膜相连。这些半桥粒复合物在前列腺癌组织中缺失，可能导致恶性细胞与附着结构的黏附性下降，这样使得恶性细胞易于浸润及向邻近组织迁移。半桥粒结构的破坏导致上皮-基质连接的稳定性下降，这使得恶性细胞容易浸润和扩散[233]。前列腺癌还具有内功素的细胞表面受体。内功素是一种存在于基底膜的糖蛋白，与层粘连蛋白形成复合物。这种异源二聚体受体等同于整合素α3β1[234]。纯化的内功素可以促进细胞的黏附和细胞的扩散。

整合素表达上的不同可能在临床应用中是有价值的。整合素的α4亚基仅仅表达于非肿瘤来源的细胞，而前列腺癌细胞表达整合素α2bβ3[235, 236]。整合素B/C表达于良性前列腺组织，但是在肿瘤组织中检测不到，这与它在体外研究中所表现出的生长抑制作用相一致[237, 238]。整合素β4在基质溶解因子作用下发生选择性断裂，可能能够解释它在肿瘤组织中的缺失[226, 239, 240]。

骨桥蛋白

骨桥蛋白是一种酸性的、可逆磷酸化的黏着糖蛋白，由骨组织和所有腺腔上皮细胞分泌，包括前列腺。在后者，它主要聚集于细胞顶端[241-244]。它是一种Ca^{2+}结合蛋白，通过-Gly-Arg-Gly-Asp-Ser-结合结构域的作用促进细胞的黏附和扩散[245]。细胞与骨桥蛋白的黏附作用部分通过细胞表面整合素[29]进行调节，整合素也是其他黏附因子的受体，包括玻璃粘连蛋白、纤维蛋白原、von Willebrand因子、凝血酶敏感素和纤维连接蛋白[246]。骨桥蛋白的表达随着肿瘤的转化而增加。最近在大鼠Dunning前列腺癌模型中的研究表明，在不同类型的细胞中，骨桥蛋白mRNA水平和肿瘤的转移潜力直接相关。在人类组织中，应用免疫组化方法证明在浸润性前列腺癌细胞中有高水平的骨桥蛋白表达。

胶原蛋白

胶原是一种重要的细胞外基质成分。目前已经鉴别出超过19种类型，由33个基因编码。I、II、III、V和XI型组成原纤维胶原，而IV、VI和XII～XIX型代表不同结构的非纤维胶原成员。除了它们在基底膜-基质的相互关系中发生作用外，XIX型胶原与血管的明显关系，提示这种胶原与其他相关的胶原类型参与了血管生成和肿瘤的发生[248, 249]。IV型胶原是基底膜的一种主要成分，组成网状结构对抗机械阻力。它同时也在上皮细胞与基底膜的黏附过程中起重要作用。IV型胶原的α链在正常前列腺、PIN和癌组织基底膜中的分布研究表明，在癌组织中α5（IV）和α2（IV）链的缺失具有特异性，而经典的α1（IV）和α2（IV）链则稳定表达。此外，VII型胶原与α5（IV）链共同存在[250]。

其他基质蛋白

在前列腺组织中所发现的其他细胞外基质成分包括纤维连接蛋白（这种物质在前列腺癌患者的组织中表达水平更高[251]）、基底膜蛋白多糖（一种多结构域的硫酸类肝素蛋白多糖）[252]和蛋白多糖（结合有糖胺聚糖的大分子物质）。tenascin是间质组织细胞外基质中的一种六面体糖蛋白成分，在胚胎发育、几乎所有器官的肿瘤形成过程，以及前列腺癌中高表达[253]。在出生后的发育过程中，tenascin优先分布于外周带[227, 254-256]。

钙黏素

钙黏素（钙黏蛋白）在钙依赖性细胞与细胞之间的黏附过程中发挥作用。3种主要的钙黏素为E-钙黏素（与多种上皮细胞有关）、N-钙黏素（神经和肌肉细胞）和P-钙黏素（胎盘细胞和表皮）。在发育过程中，所有这些类型在其他组织中都会一过性表达。在缺乏钙的情况下，钙黏素将发生构象改变，并被蛋白水解酶迅速降解。E-钙黏素聚集于成熟上皮细胞的黏着小带（zonula adherens），通过细胞间连环蛋白与肌动蛋白细胞骨架连接[257]。

钙黏素途径的功能异常与肿瘤的浸润和扩散有关[128, 229, 258-272]。E-钙黏素的表达与肿瘤级别、分期、转移、复发和存活呈负相关[229, 262, 265, 269, 273-279]。P-钙黏素在前列腺癌中不表达，可能反映了基底细胞层的缺失而非转录水平的下调。连环蛋白，特别是α-连环蛋白，在细胞黏附复合物功能异常的形成过程中也具有重要作用。前列腺腺泡、射精管和精囊腺上皮细胞表达E-钙黏素，但是不表达N-钙黏素。P-钙黏素的表达局限于基底细胞中，P-钙黏素免疫组化阳性的细胞其PSA表达阴性。前列腺癌通常P-钙黏素表达阴性，但是一些肿瘤也可见局部阳性区域，常位于PSA阴性的射精管附近。P-钙黏素和PSA在同一组织中的单一表达，表明这些蛋白涉及细胞调节的不同机制[280, 281]。

CD（分化抗原）

CD（分化抗原）蛋白是另一个跨膜糖蛋白家族，具有细胞外基质黏附功能。其中之一，CD44和它的异构体，可能与前列腺癌的恶性转移有关[277, 282-284]。CD44抑制肿瘤的转移而不影响原发肿瘤的生长。在前列腺癌出现转移的临床进展过程中，CD44表达阴性[285-287]。针对CD44（基底细胞）和CD57（分泌细胞）在不同细胞上的表达，利用相应抗体，采用流式细胞技术对上皮细胞亚群进行分离[52]。当前列腺组织被胶原酶溶解为分散的单个细胞后，CD57阳性细胞中PSA的表达消失。当CD57阳性细胞与间质细胞重新组合后，PSA的表达又出现。两种细胞都表达一种新的前列腺标记物——CD38[288]。在BPH和肿瘤组织中，CD38的表达完全缺失。

基质蛋白酶

细胞外基质的局部降解是组织更新、细胞穿过基底膜移行和肿瘤转移的需要。这种降解通过蛋白酶的作用完成。蛋白水解酶包括两种主要类型，即金属蛋白酶如胶原酶和基质溶解因子，以及丝氨酸蛋白酶如激肽释放酶和尿激酶型纤溶酶原激活因子（uPA）。uPA能够将纤溶酶原转化为纤溶酶，进而在细胞移行和组织更新的过程中使细胞周围的蛋白水解。uPA由肿瘤细胞和间质细胞作为一种无活性的酶原形式（pro-uPA）分泌[289]。有活性的uPA将纤溶酶原转化为纤溶酶，反过来降解肿瘤间质的成分如纤维素、纤维连接蛋白、蛋白多糖和层粘连蛋白；它也可能激活Ⅳ型胶原酶前体，使得Ⅳ型胶原降解，Ⅳ型胶原是基底膜的主要组成部分。与良性组织相比，原发性肿瘤和转移瘤中uPA的浓度升高[290-294]。在良性组织中，Ⅳ型胶原酶的表达最少，但是在所有Gleason级别的肿瘤和PIN组织中则呈强表达[295-296]。

在肿瘤细胞的产生和浸润过程中，可能会出现蛋白水解级联反应[291]。蛋白酶如金属蛋白酶（MMP）的作用常由于蛋白酶抑制因子如组织蛋白酶抑制因子（TIMP）的存在而局限于特定的区域。MMP的活性在肿瘤组织中比在BPH中要高。Pro-MMP-9的分子量为92kD，只在肿瘤细胞中表达，特别是在那些具有扩散和转移现象的肿瘤组织中[297, 298]。这些蛋白酶的很多异构体和它们的抑制因子都在前列腺中存在。TIMP-1、TIMP-2、MMP-2和MMP-9的表达水平被认为是前列腺癌预后的独立判断指标。

基质溶解因子（MAT）是MMP家族的另一成员，涉及组织的更新过程。它表达于BPH和肿瘤的上皮组织中，这与绝大多数MMP相反，后者是由间质产生的[299]。

组织蛋白酶B是一种溶酶体半胱氨酸蛋白酶，参与细胞外基质蛋白的降解和许多实体肿瘤中肿瘤细胞从一个生物区室向另一个生物区室的转移，包括前列腺癌。Sinha等人报道，CB/stefin A（半胱氨酸蛋白酶抑制剂）的比值可以用来预测前列腺癌的侵袭性。高比值的组织蛋白酶B和stefin A与骨盆淋巴结转移有关[300-302]。

透明质酸（HA）是一种糖胺聚糖，能促进肿瘤的转移。CD44糖蛋白是HA的细胞表面受体，CD44v6异构体与肿瘤转移有关。HYAL-1型透明质酸酶（HAase）表达于肿瘤细胞中，像其他的HAase一样，将HA降解为血管源性物质。Ekici等人报道，HA、HYAL-1及结合的HA-HYAL-1的免疫组化结果对于预测肿瘤的进展分别具有96%、84%和84%的敏感性。特异性分别为61%（HA）、80.5%（HYAL-1）和87.8%（HA-HYAL-1），与前列腺癌的其他预测指标无关[303,304]。

生长因子及其受体

前列腺癌的进展伴随着生长因子及其受体表达的改变。肿瘤转化过程的一个特征是肿瘤细胞中生长因子、受体、癌基因和肿瘤抑制基因的表达出现多种同时发生的改变。因此，出现于肿瘤细胞中的多种改变可能是相互作用的和/或由一个或更多共同的转化过程所诱导。

雄激素受体

雄激素受体（AR）的基因突变存在于未经激素治疗的前列腺癌组织和激素不敏感性肿瘤中[212,305]。突变型AR经雌激素和弱雄激素激活后，可能使肿瘤细胞中的AR被肾上腺雄激素或外源性雌激素激活，从而对睾丸雄激素撤退治疗不产生反应[306]。由于前列腺癌组织中含有比正常组织更低水平的5α-还原酶和DHT，所以这种突变可能会使肿瘤即便是在无雄激素撤退时仍然具有生长优势[307]。还有人认为，在不依赖于雄激素的前列腺癌的发展过程中，HER-2家族与雄激素受体在功能上具有协同作用[308]。

微血管密度

微血管密度（MVD）有望成为前列腺癌患者治疗后的预后评价指标。与肿瘤细胞相关的因子不同，微血管密度是一种宿主间质因子，它在肿瘤组织中具有明显的、局限的不均一性。在很多研究报道中指出了它对于病理分期的预测值，但是并非所有研究都持此观点。另外，最近的研究表明，微血管密度可能是肿瘤复发和患者存活的预测因素。抑制血管生成可能是一种有效的化学预防的手段，特别是对那些有前列腺癌高危因素的男性。最近提出了分析前列腺癌和其他肿瘤中微血管密度的标准[309-311]。用CD34免疫组化方法判断前列腺癌中的微血管密度比用CD31更准确[312,313]。

在前列腺肿瘤的发生过程中，血管的形成被分为两个阶段。血管形成前阶段可能持续数年；在此期间，上皮细胞生长有限，可能形成高级别前列腺上皮内瘤变（PIN）和小的、局灶性的浸润癌。血管形成阶段形成与新的血管出现时，此时肿瘤中的血管加速形成，促进了肿瘤的生长并可能导致临床扩散。血管生成的"开关"可能部分受到组织因子及其诱导血管内皮生长因子（VEGF，一种促血管生成因子）的能力和抑制凝血酶敏感素2（一种抗血管生成因子）的能力的调节。前列腺癌表达高水平的组织因子，这种表达与微血管密度和血清PSA相关[314]。另外，VEGF的表达与微血管密度、肿瘤分期以及采用保守治疗的患者的存活情况相关[315]。

在前列腺肿瘤的中心区，微血管密度比肿瘤的外周区高（图14.14A），但是有一定的变异系数（分别为106/mm^{2}和50/mm^2）[316-318]。通过对最大密度区域（称之为"热点"）的研究，发现由于取材方式的不同，通过病理活检以及取相应的根治性前列腺癌切除术后的组织标本所得到的微血管密度的结果也不同[316,317]，但是这种观点受到经验的否定[319,320]。最佳的微血管密度的计算方法是通过计算机分析程序，在减去腺腔空间后所得到的微血管密度数值。这种计算方法可能比人工计算单位面积的血管总数更精确[319]。最近一种新的方法被用来从三维视角观察和分析前列腺中的微血管，这种方法需要制成一系列的前列腺标本切片[321]。这种方法包括常规组织处理、电脑将数字化的一系列组织切片重新构建成三维结构，然后计算几何参数和MVD。在一个给定的体积中的血管总长度称为"血管长度密度"，在鉴别良性前列腺组织和肿瘤方面比微血管密度更好。结果表明，与肿瘤相关的微血管和良性组织中的微血管相比，在定位、大小以及曲度方面更均匀。

关于良性前列腺疾病和结节性增生病变中微血管密度的资料是有限的。在一项研究中，MVD在增生性结节中的平均值是99/mm^2[322]，与肿瘤的数值相似（图14.14B），明显高于正常移行带的数值（70/mm^2）[323]。血管密度在小间质结节中也升高。超过1mm^{3}的增生结节可能包括一个类似于肿瘤的"血管生成开关"[324]，使得微血管密度的升高与肿瘤细胞增生同步。将肿瘤组织与同一标本中的良性组织进行对比可能是不适当的，因为那些包含有肿瘤组织的标本其良性区域中的血管密度也增加[323]，尽管大多数研究否认这种可能性[319]。

高级别前列腺PIN作为浸润癌的最常见的癌前病变[319]，实际上总是伴随有间质小毛细血管的增生。高级别PIN中的MVD比邻近的良性前列腺组织中的MVD更高[316,317]，毛细血管更短，间隔更宽，有更多的开放腔隙及弯曲的外部轮廓，并且环绕有更多的内皮细胞[325]。PIN中的MVD数值介于良性上皮和肿瘤之间，进一步证明了PIN是前列腺癌的癌前病变。

微血管密度分析有望成为前列腺癌病理分期和患者预后的评价指标[303]。与前列腺癌有关的微血管比良性前列腺组织或增生前列腺组织中的微血管更短，并具有更多弯曲的血管[325,326]。众多的证据表明，血管密度的分析在前列腺癌患者的治疗中具有重要的作用[327]。多项研究对微血管密度与肿瘤分期的关系进行了探讨（表14.6）[316,320,322,326,328-341]。可能是由于评价方法简单而且组织来源丰富，大多数研究将前列腺切除术标本的MVD值与病理分期进行了对比。测定两个同时进行针吸细胞学活检组织中的MVD值，并将这一数值与前列腺切除标本的病理分期相联系[342]。其他的研究是将用放射治疗[343]或主要用保守治疗[330]的患者经尿道前列腺切除的标本的MVD值与临床分期进行比较；然而，与病理分期相比，临床分期可能会非常不准确，所以在解释这些结果时应该谨慎[171]。很多针对前列腺切除术的标本的研究发现MVD与病理分期有关[322,338,344]。然而，在一项研究中发现，只有在低级别肿瘤中可以看到pT2期和pT3期肿瘤的MVD值有重要的区别，而在另一项研究中则结果刚好相反。Silberman等人认为MVD与肿瘤分期无关[345]，但是只对Gleason 6分和7分的患者进行了有限的研究；之后，令人惊讶的是，作者将这一研究结果与另一个采用不同选择标准的研究结果进行了合并。Barth等人发现MVD和分期无明显相关[326]。肿瘤活检组织中的MVD值与相应的前列腺切除标本的MVD值呈正相关，是前列腺外扩散的一个独立的预测指标[338,346]。优化的微血管密度与Gleason评分和血清PSA浓度合并使用时，这些方法对肿瘤分期的预测价值明显升高。微血管浸润也和分期、分级和其他参数有关[329]，尽管其他的报道否认这些结果。大量的证据证明了MVD与肿瘤分期之间的关系，尽管不同的方法之间以及不同的病例组织间存在一定的差异[340,341,347]。

通常认为，MVD不是最佳的前列腺癌复发的预测指标（表14.7）[174,311,315,320,321,330,331,337,339,348-354]。在一些研究中，选择那些采用外科手术治疗或外照射治疗的患者[331]，微血管密度[332,335,337]和微血管浸润[335]预示生物化学方法（PSA）的失败。然而，在那些用放射性治疗的患者中，对MVD的分析结果并未得出其与分级无关的结论[331]。当大多数患者仅采用激素姑息疗法治疗时，MVD并未预测出肿瘤进展与分级无关[330]。在行根治性前列腺切除术的患者中，对于pT2期和Gleason 6分和7分的病例的分析认为MVD与生物化学方法的失败无关[353]。这些作者发现pT3期的患者也具有相似的结果[350]。其他的研究结果认为，MVD[330,354]或微血管浸润[356]具有预测肿瘤相关性存活情况的价值，但是无独立的预测价值（表14.7）。这种预测价值在单变量分析中被分级[330,356]或分期[354]的

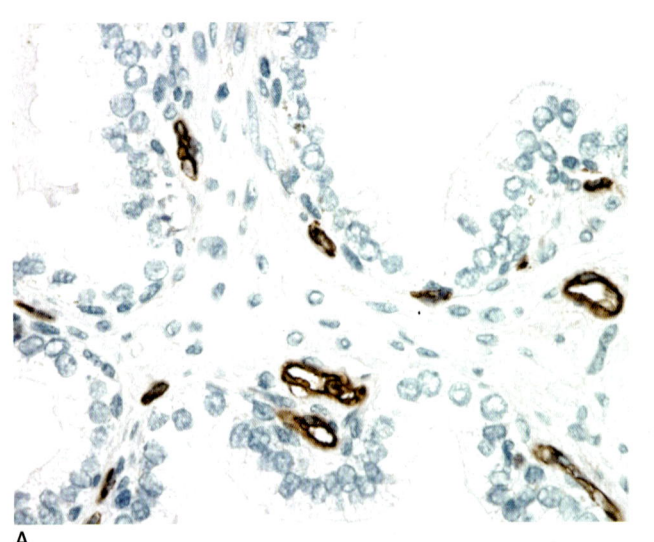

A

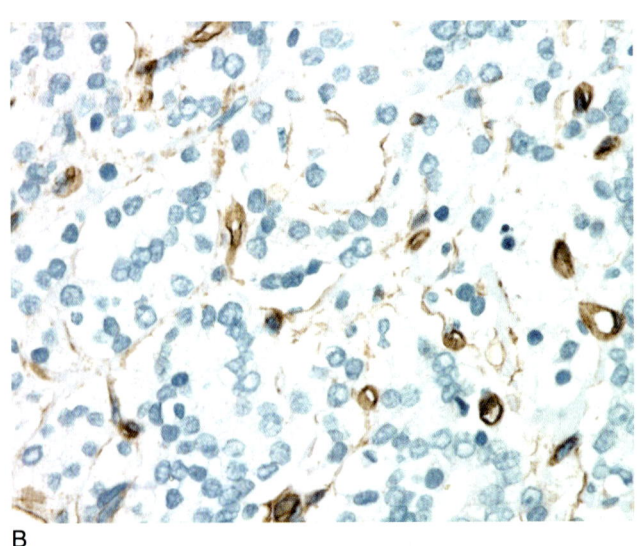

B

图14.14 在良性前列腺病灶（A）和癌性病灶（B）中标记CD34抗体的微血管

表14.6 微血管密度或微血管浸润与前列腺癌分期的关系

第一作者/年份	病例特点	患者数量	抗体或染色	定量测定指标	结 果
Wakui, 1992[333]	行TURP、前列腺切除术或尸检,包括43例骨髓转移和58例无骨髓转移病例	101	波形蛋白	DIA	对于pT2、pT3期,低级别肿瘤中的MVD值比中、高级别肿瘤中的MVD值低;对于pT4期,各级别间无差异
Bigler, 1993[323]	行前列腺切除术,未扩散或转移癌	15	F Ⅷ	DIA;毛细血管面积与肿瘤面积比值	在高级别肿瘤中比值高2倍,但是在中、低级别肿瘤中则无此情况
Fregene, 1993[332]	行前列腺切除术,伴或不伴LN转移	34	F Ⅷ	立体学	MVD:T2期和T3期没有区别,但在LN转移的患者中升高。对照组包括34例良性活检标本
Weidner, 1993[335]	行前列腺切除术,包括29例转移癌和45例非转移癌,或者术后PSA水平升高	74	F Ⅷ	立体学,热点	在转移癌中(77)MVD值比非转移癌(39)的MVD值高;通过多变量分析,MVD值在预测肿瘤转移方面优于Gleason评分
Hall, 1994[331]	TUR诊断为pT1~2期,用外照射治疗	25	F Ⅷ	立体学,热点	伴有EPE的患者的MVD值比那些不伴EPE的患者高。在放射治疗后出现扩散的患者比那些没有扩散的患者的MVD值高(在200倍视野下,96对46);此结果没有独立于肿瘤分级进行分析
Brawer, 1994[316]	行前列腺切除术,伴(9)和不伴(19)边缘阳性,或LN(4)或骨(5)转移	37	F Ⅷ	DIA	在预测分期方面,MVD值优于Gleason评分。在包含边缘阳性和LN或骨转移的患者的MVD值比边缘阴性的患者高
Vesalainen, 1994[330]	TUR诊断为pT1~2期。在大多数病例中,保守治疗或随访11年;2例行前列腺切除术,1例放射治疗,2例雌激素治疗,23例睾丸切除术	88	Ⅳ型胶原	热点,血管表面密度DIA(mm^2/mm^3组织)	不同分期中,血管表面密度不同
Salomao, 1995[329]	行前列腺切除术;pT2期和pT3期	210	HE染色	N/A	53%的标本出现MV浸润,与分期、分级、体积和边缘状态有关

续表

第一作者/年份	病例特点	患者数量	抗体或染色	定量测定指标	结果
Barth, 1996[326]	行前列腺切除术；pT2~4 期；级别为低、中和高度	41	F Ⅷ	血管表面密度 DIA（mm²/mm³ 组织）	微血管数量随着分期和分级的提高而提高，但是 MVD 值下降。正常组织作为对照（未指明来源）
Bostwick, 1996[346]	对 115 例 pT2 期和 71 例 pT3 期行前列腺切除术的病例进行定量研究	186	F Ⅷ	DIA；优化的微血管密度减去该组织的腺腔空间	MVD 能够独立预测 EPE
Silberman, 1997[337]	行前列腺切除术，只有 6 级和 7 级；pT2 期（31%），pT3 期（69%）	109	CD31	立体学，热点	MVD 与分期无关，但与 EPE 有关
Rogatsch, 1997[338]	行前列腺切除术，对 pT2 和 pT3 期将活检标本与前列腺切除术标本进行对比	36	CD31	立体学，热点	MVD 与分期有关；活检标本与前列腺切除术标本呈正相关
Rubin, 1999[347]	对临床诊断为未扩散肿瘤行根治性前列腺切除术	87	CD31	热点	MVD 值与 Gleason 评分、分期、手术边缘情况、精囊腺浸润或 PSA 无关

TUR：经尿道切除术；FⅧ：Ⅷ因子相关抗原；热点（见前文）；DIA，计算机辅助的数字影像学分析；LN，淋巴结；MV，微血管；MVD，微血管密度；EPE，前列腺外扩张；分级指 Gleason 分级

表14.7 微血管密度或微血管浸润分析与前列腺癌复发、扩散和存活情况的关系

第一作者/年份	病例特点	患者数量	抗体	定量测定指标	结果
Bahnson, 1989[356]	行根治性前列腺切除术	55		微血管浸润	微血管浸润的患者肿瘤临床扩散的可能性要高 4 倍
Hall, 1994[331]	经 TUR 诊断的 pT1~2，用外照射治疗	25	F Ⅷ	立体学，热点	与无 EPE 的患者相比，伴有 EPE 的患者的 MVD 值更高。在放射治疗后出现扩散的患者具有更高的 MVD 值（在200倍视野下，97 对 46）
Vesalainen, 1994[330]	pT1~2。在大多数病例中，保守治疗和随访时间为 11 年	88	Ⅳ型胶原 11 年	热点。血管表面密度 DIA（mm²/mm³ 组织）	血管表面密度不是临床肿瘤扩散的独立预测因子，还依赖于分级
McNeal, 1996[335]	>0.5cm³ 的肿瘤行前列腺切除术	357	CD34		在 7% 的 <4cc 的肿瘤和 24% 的 >4cc 的肿瘤中出现 MV 浸润。MV 浸润与肿瘤分级和体积一同成为 PSA 失败（升高至>0.07ng/ml）的独立预测因子

续表

第一作者/年份	病例特点	患者数量	抗体或染色	定量测定指标	结 果
Silberman, 1997[337]	行前列腺切除术；只有5~7级；pT2期（75%）和pT3（25%）	87	CD31	热点	MVD是肿瘤扩散的独立预测指标（43例扩散，29例未扩散）
Gettman, 1998[353]	pT2期肿瘤患者用根治性前列腺切除术；只有6级或以上的病例	148	FⅧ	DIA；优化的微血管密度减去相应组织中的腺腔空间	在这组选择队列中，MVD不是临床复发和/或生化指标再次出现异常的有意义的单变量或多变量预测指标
Gettman, 1999[350]	pT3期肿瘤患者行根治性前列腺切除术	211	FⅧ	DIA；优化的微血管密度减去相应组织中的腺腔空间	在这组选择队列中，MVD不是临床复发和/或生化指标再次出现异常的有意义的多变量预测指标
De la Taille, 2000[312]	行根治性前列腺切除术	102	CD31与CD34		MVD与CD34共同成为生化指标失败的多变量预测因子
Bahnson, 1989[356]	局部肿瘤，pT2~pT3期	55	HE染色	N/A	38%的标本出现MV浸润；扩散和死亡的危险性增加4倍；但是在多变量研究中，这一变量依赖于分级
Vesalainen, 1994[330]	pT1~2期。在大多数病例中，保守治疗和随访时间为11年	88	Ⅳ型胶原	热点。血管表面密度的DIA（mm²/mm³组织）	MVD对存活情况无独立的预测价值；依赖于分级
Lissbrant, 1997[354]	通过TURP检测肿瘤；大多数患者采用保守治疗	98	FⅧ	热点	MVD可以预测存活情况（56%死亡）。因为出现转移灶，所以无独立预测价值
Borre, 2000[315]	保守治疗的患者；随访时间中位数为15年	221	Ⅷ因子和血管内皮生长因子（VEGF）	半定量计数	MVD和VEGF的表达相互关联，与分期和肿瘤特异性存活率也相关；然而，VEGF在多变量分析中，对于肿瘤未扩散的患者的存活率无预测价值
Erbersdobler, 2002[341]	根治性前列腺切除术标本	75	CD34	热点	外周带区肿瘤的MVD比移行带区高
Grossfeld, 2002[340]	从85名病理分期为T3期的患者中得到的根治性前列腺切除术标本	85	CD34	热点	病理分期为T3期的前列腺肿瘤患者行根治性前列腺切除术后，其MVD值与预后之间无明显相关性

TUR：经尿道切除术；FⅧ：Ⅷ因子相关抗原；热点（见前文）；DIA，计算机辅助的数字影像学分析；LN，淋巴结；MV，微血管；MVD，微血管密度；EPE，前列腺外扩张；分级指Gleason分级

结果所否定。

治疗后前列腺癌的诊断

PSA、PAP 和角蛋白 34βE12

PSA、PAP 和基底细胞特异的角蛋白 34βE12 的免疫组化在治疗后肿瘤的鉴别中被使用。PSA和PAP在治疗后的肿瘤细胞中持续存在，角蛋白 34βE12 为阴性，这表明肿瘤组织缺乏基底细胞层（图14.15）[179]。

神经内分泌标记物

雄激素撤退治疗之后，各种神经内分泌分化标记物的表达无变化，如嗜铬素、烯醇化酶、β-hCG和5-羟色胺[91, 136, 357]。

增殖细胞核抗原

在雄激素撤退治疗后，PCNA的免疫组化反应强度下降，表明雄激素能够调节参与细胞增殖周期性蛋白的表达[179, 358, 359]。

雄激素和雌激素受体

雄激素受体在雄激素敏感和雄激素不敏感的前列腺组织的细胞中都存在，这表明雄激素不敏感性的形成不可能是缺乏雄激素受体表达的结果。通过免疫组化方法研究，发现这些受体广泛分布于正常前列腺的分泌细胞、BPH、高级别PIN[360-366]以及局部和转移性前列腺癌[203, 367-370]组织中。在采用雄激素撤退治疗之后，具有雄激素受体的肿瘤细胞的比例并不能预测发生肿瘤扩散的时间，尽管在那些对治疗反应比较差的肿瘤中的免疫组化阳性反应更加不均一。在受体蛋白发生氨基酸替代的标本中免疫反应更强[179]。

根据免疫组织化学的研究，在正常的前列腺间质细胞中雌激素受体呈低水平表达，但是在经过雄激素撤退治疗后，特别是在围绕前列腺腺泡的区域雌激素受体表达升高[371-379]。肿瘤细胞无反应[91]。

黏糖蛋白 A-80

Gould 及其同事发现，高分子量黏糖蛋白 A-80 免疫组化在肿瘤性前列腺上皮组织中呈特异的强表达，在雄激素撤退治疗后，实际上每个细胞都呈阳性表达[380]。令人感兴趣的是，胶体池和血管外皮细胞瘤样区域也有阳性表达，表明这些区域的一部分是破裂的恶性腺泡的残迹。这一标记物的出色的稳定性和它对异型增生及恶性上皮细胞的良好的特异性使它的常规使用价值增加，但是目前还没有商品化的黏糖蛋白 A-80。

微血管密度

针对临床诊断为局部前列腺癌的病例，经过雄激素撤退治疗后，根据免疫组化研究结果，发现微血管的平均值比未经治疗的肿瘤中的值要低[381, 382]。

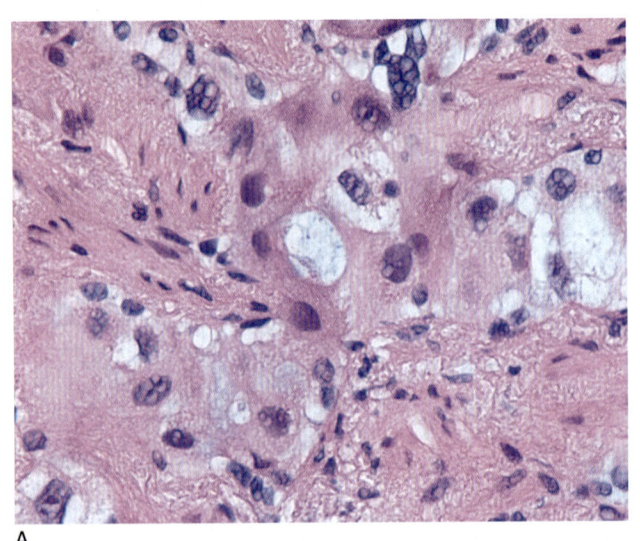
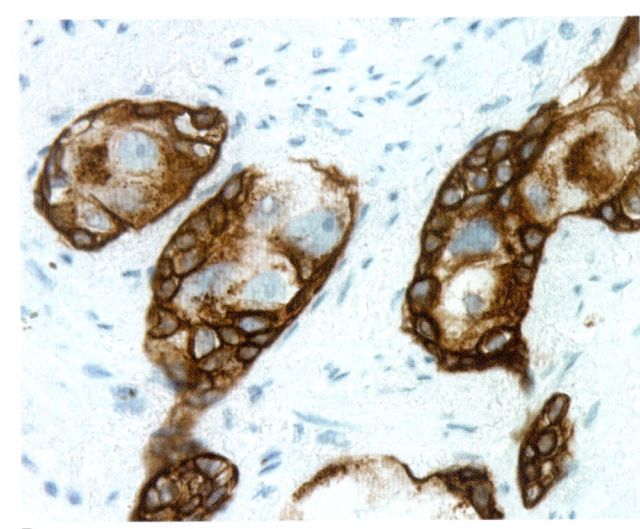

图 14.15 （A）良性前列腺组织伴随放射性改变；（B）免疫组化显示基底细胞阳性

放射治疗后的免疫表型

除了出于治疗目的而采用放射治疗（RT）外，原发部位肿瘤的生物学特征还不十分清楚。尽管局部持续存在或复发的肿瘤可能与预后不良有关，但是同时使用治疗后PSA监测、经直肠超声引导的前列腺活检和早期治疗，使得有机会在肿瘤早期和更易治疗的阶段发现局部持续存在的肿瘤。不同的生物标记物在前列腺癌中的预后价值以往已经被研究过，但是与放射治疗后持续存在的肿瘤有关的发现几乎没有。

PAP、PSA 和角蛋白 34βE12

没有权威的方法能够监测放射性治疗后肿瘤的改变。PAP表达通常持续存在[383]，表明能够产生蛋白质的肿瘤细胞可能具有细胞分裂和转移的特性。PSA和角蛋白34βE12的表达也在放射治疗后持续存在[384]，常有助于对治疗后的腺癌和其他相似疾病的鉴别诊断。大多数报告指出，如果前列腺肿瘤不能够在外放射治疗12个月后从组织学的水平上消失，那么它可能是具有生物学活性的[67, 385-388]。

p53 和增殖标记物

在放射性治疗后，大部分肿瘤可见p53在核内的表达升高（图14.16），p53蛋白的过表达与前列腺癌细胞的增生有关。p53在核内的积聚也与放射治疗后的预后不良有关，还可能在放射治疗后肿瘤复发时表达增高[384, 389-400]。p53突变会使得其对DNA-损伤试剂的敏感性下降，p53功能的缺失可能与放射治疗的不敏感有关[384, 389-400]。

Prendergast 等人对 18 名前列腺癌治疗后局部复发的肿瘤进行了研究，发现72%的肿瘤p53核阳性；在5名治疗前做过活检的患者中，所有人的p53均为核阳性[397]。免疫组化结果与单链构象多态性和DNA测序分析结果有关[397]。这种发现表明p53的改变可能在治疗前已经存在，可能可以作为治疗前肿瘤复发的标记物。PCNA在治疗后前列腺活检组织中免疫组化持续阳性，表明其与局部肿瘤的复发有关[9]。在那些放射治疗后行前列腺切除术的患者中，大多数（96%）从组织学上观察其前列腺癌处于明显的增殖状态，MIB-1免疫组化阳性[10, 399]。与作者研究机构中那些未经放射性治疗而行前列腺切除术的患者的组织标本（平均2.7%，未发表）相比，平均Ki-67标记指

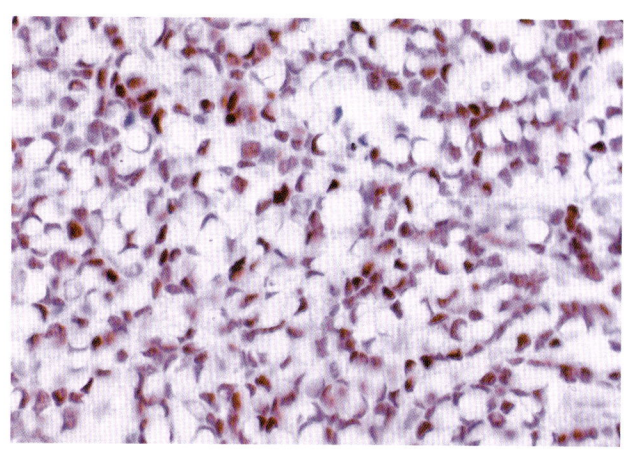

图14.16　在分化不良的前列腺癌细胞中 p53 免疫组化结果

数在复发性前列腺癌中升高（7.0%）。细胞增殖率较高的患者p53蛋白的过表达也增加，这表明这些肿瘤具有生物活性。

作者的研究方案中不包括对下述两个问题的研究，即肿瘤的生物学特性是否随着时间的变化而改变（即时间依赖性的肿瘤"克隆进化"），或者是否肿瘤的复发是由于本身是具有侵袭潜能的肿瘤[9]。实际上，p53蛋白的免疫组化在那些治疗后肿瘤复发的患者治疗前的组织标本中也可呈阳性表达。另外p53蛋白异常表达与患者的不良预后之间的关系，可能也表明这些患者在采用放射治疗之前已经具有较恶性的肿瘤类型。

最近的研究表明，Ki-67是肿瘤远处转移和男性前列腺癌患者经放射治疗合并雄激素撤退治疗后的肿瘤死亡率的有力的预测指标[157]。Hintz等人描述了两种在用激素治疗的过程中出现 Ki-67 表达波动的情况：第一种类型是在用醋酸亮丙瑞林治疗起效后，Ki-67 的表达下降，而后在撤掉醋酸亮丙瑞林后，Ki-67 的表达又反弹至基础水平的120%以下；第二种类型也是在使用醋酸亮丙瑞林之初出现 Ki-67 的表达下降，但随后出现反弹至120%以上。第二种类型与第一种类型相比，与PSA监测更高的失败率有关。Ki-67-SI 可能对于采取不同治疗方案（包括度他雄胺的使用）的患者的分层有帮助[401, 402]。

糖蛋白 A-80

除了组织结构和细胞学的改变外，糖蛋白A-80在放射性治疗后的前列腺组织中稳定而持久的表达[403]。所有的病例都可以在肿瘤细胞的胞浆和恶性腺泡的腔内物质中观察到 A-80 的稳定表达，并常为强阳性。

免疫组化的弥漫程度和反应强度与肿瘤大小和级别无关。强阳性通常可见于陈旧扭曲变形的腺泡、透明细胞、单个肿瘤细胞中，胶体池中只有很少或没有可辨认的肿瘤细胞。在53%的病例中存在PIN，其中79%A-80强阳性；萎缩或高度增生的腺泡虽然存在一定程度的异型性，但免疫组化通常为阴性[403]。

前列腺良性肿瘤的免疫组化研究

硬化性腺病

硬化性腺病发现于20年前，当时诊断为腺瘤样或假腺瘤样肿瘤，表现为在致密的梭形细胞的间质中，小腺泡局限性增生。在我们对诊断为前列腺癌的经尿道切除的标本进行研究时发现，硬化性腺病占到10%[404]。硬化性腺病是在良性前列腺增生经尿道切除术的标本中偶然发现的，存在于不到2%的标本中；几乎没有病例与血清PSA浓度的升高有关。硬化性腺病通常呈单一、微小瘤体的生长模式，但是可能会呈多灶性及弥漫性分布。腺泡结构完整，从小至中等大小，但是可能形成微小的细胞巢或细胞团伴有腺腔发育不良。这些围绕腺泡的细胞有一些表现出透明至嗜伊红特点的胞浆，经常可见明显的细胞边缘。这些基底细胞层可能局部突起和增生，特别是在由于多细胞的间质结构存在而形成很厚的边缘的腺泡中。在某些区域，腺泡与周围高度增生的、富含成纤维细胞的间质融合而使基底物质稀疏。通常不存在明显的上皮细胞或间质细胞的异型性，但是在一些病例中也可能会出现明显的细胞异型性（Bostwick，未发表）。根据间质中明显的成纤维细胞的增生来鉴别硬化性腺病与腺癌，后者很少见到成纤维细胞增生。硬化性腺病细胞具有良性特征，上皮细胞和间质细胞无突出的核增大。在硬化性腺病中，偶尔可见透明样腺泡周围间质，具有完整的细胞层[405]，常与结节性增生有关，具有S-100蛋白的免疫表型，肌动蛋白免疫组化阳性（图14.17），超微结构研究显示肌上皮分化[406-410]。

不同类型前列腺癌的免疫组化研究

不同组织类型的腺癌的生物学行为可能与典型的腺泡腺癌不同，正确的临床治疗方案的选择依赖于快速诊断及与其他部位肿瘤的鉴别诊断。生长于前列腺的罕见肿瘤也使其组织发生学成为新的课题。在本节，重点讲述那些具有突出的免疫表型的不同类型的腺癌；读者可以参考专门的泌尿外科病理学书籍作为补充资料，以了解这些罕见肿瘤的临床行为和其他病理学特征。

导管癌（具有子宫内膜样特征的腺癌、乳头状腺癌、子宫内膜样腺癌）

导管癌占到前列腺腺癌总数的0.8%。在前列腺尿道部分和大的尿道周围前列腺导管中，肿瘤呈息肉状或乳头状生长。大多数作者将这种肿瘤称做伴有子宫内膜样特征的腺癌或单纯导管癌。"子宫内膜"一词不应该用于前列腺。

在就医时，大多数患者的肿瘤仍局限于前列腺或尿道组织中，并且至少77%的病例同时合并浸润性

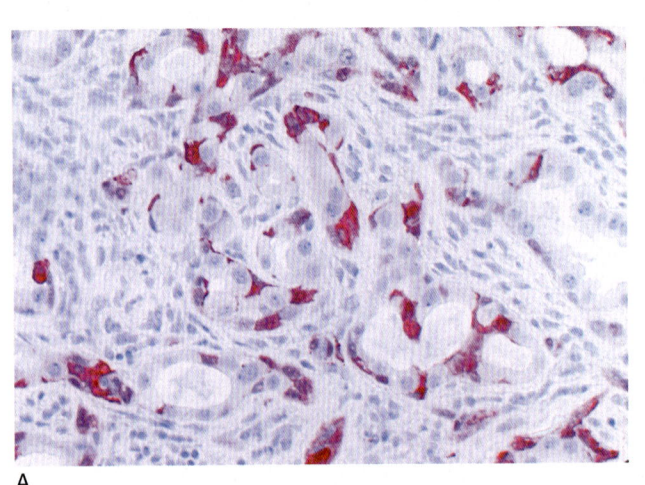

A

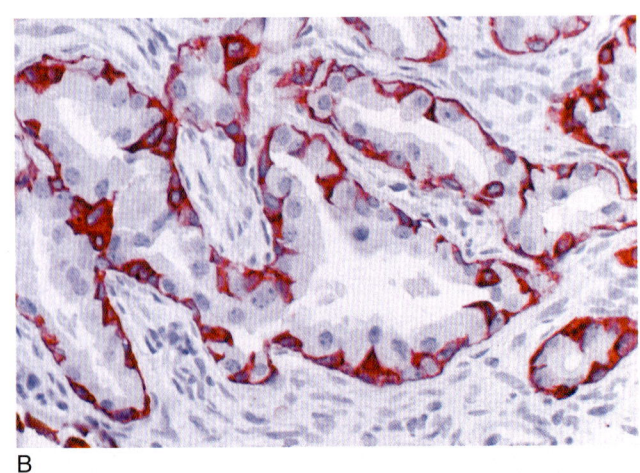

B

图14.17 （A）硬化性腺病，基底细胞中S-100蛋白免疫组化强阳性表达。（B）硬化性腺病，基底细胞中平滑肌细胞肌动蛋白免疫组化强阳性表达

腺泡性前列腺腺癌。导管癌的预后与典型的腺泡性腺癌的预后相同，但是也有研究报道不同的结果。血清PSA浓度在确诊时可能是正常的，除非患者出现了骨转移。

导管癌通常位于大尿道周围的前列腺导管和精阜中，由被复层柱状上皮包绕的乳头状结构或腺泡结构形成的瘤体所构成。可见两种结构类型：乳头状和筛状。这两种类型在大约一半的病例中同时存在，两种类型都可见核异型性并常可见有丝分裂象。PAP和PSA免疫组化在导管癌中呈稳定的强表达；CEA免疫组化偶尔在局部也会出现阳性结果[411-414]。

导管癌的鉴别诊断包括前列腺尿路上皮癌、大腺体Gleason 3级腺泡腺癌、异位的前列腺组织、良性息肉、肾源性肿瘤转移、乳头状增生性尿道炎、内翻型乳头（状）瘤和严重的黏膜皱褶。在导管癌中通常可以见到腺泡分化的表现，这可以与尿路上皮癌进行鉴别；在疑难病例或较小的标本中，PSA和PAP免疫组化方法常可以鉴别诊断（导管癌呈阳性，尿路上皮癌呈阴性）。在毗邻的尿道黏膜中出现尿路上皮的异型性增生是尿路上皮癌的有力证据，但并不能确诊。

黏液癌（胶样癌）

单纯的前列腺黏液癌很少见，尽管典型的腺泡样腺癌常可于局部产生黏液，特别在高剂量雌激素治疗后[176,415-417]。这种肿瘤对内分泌治疗或放射性治疗的反应可能不会太好，而且具有高度的侵袭性[418]。

在至少1/3的前列腺癌病例中可见局灶性的黏液腺分化，但是黏液癌的诊断需要至少25%的肿瘤含有细胞外黏液池。黏液癌组织中可见肿瘤细胞巢和细胞团漂浮在黏液当中，与乳腺黏液癌相似。目前已知有3种类型的黏液癌：腺泡状黏液癌伴腺腔扩张、筛状癌伴腺腔扩张以及胶样癌伴含有细胞团的黏液湖。腺癌还有其他的组织类型，包括筛状和粉刺状癌。胶状微结节在产生黏液的肿瘤中是伴随现象，可能由细胞外酸性黏蛋白组成[419]。

黏液癌组织中，PAS、阿辛蓝和黏蛋白胭脂红的免疫组化结果与其他的前列腺黏蛋白相似，但是作者在实际工作中很少使用这些抗体。大多数研究发现，良性腺泡产生中性黏蛋白，而恶性腺泡产生酸性黏蛋白，良性腺泡很少产生酸性黏蛋白。酸性黏蛋白可见于非典型性腺瘤样增生、黏液样化生、前列腺上皮内瘤变、硬化性腺病和基底细胞异常增生。黏液癌细胞中包含有PSA和PAP，但是通常不产生CEA。鉴别诊断包括直肠、尿道膀胱或Cowper腺体的黏液癌。这些鉴别诊断非常重要，因为其治疗和预后是非常不同的。PSA和PAP免疫组化在前列腺黏液癌中至少呈局灶性阳性反应，则可明确肿瘤的前列腺来源。最近的研究表明，黏液癌组织中消旋酶（P504）通常为阳性[420]。

印戒细胞癌

前列腺印戒细胞癌非常少见[416,421-427]。除了所有的印戒细胞癌均为高度恶性之外，其临床表现与典型的腺泡样腺癌相似。该肿瘤预后不佳。

印戒细胞癌的诊断条件是25%或者更多的肿瘤细胞为印戒细胞，也有些作者认为应该有50%以上为印戒细胞。在很多情况下，印戒细胞是Gleason 5型肿瘤的一种细胞成分。肿瘤细胞的胞核被透明胞浆取代现象明显。印戒细胞在2.5%的腺泡样腺癌中存在，但是这一数量不足以诊断为印戒细胞癌[424]。黏蛋白、类脂、PSA、PAP和CEA的组织化学和免疫组织化学结果是不同的，印戒细胞可能是由胞浆、黏蛋白颗粒和脂肪空泡形成的。

前列腺印戒细胞癌的鉴别诊断包括，来源于其他部位的相似肿瘤，特别是肠道和胃来源的肿瘤。前列腺来源的肿瘤应该与锁骨上淋巴结转移性印戒细胞癌鉴别，后者黏蛋白免疫组化阴性；PSA和PAP免疫组化在鉴别诊断上也有用途。一些人为造成的假象有时也会与印戒细胞癌相似，它常发生在淋巴瘤、良性淋巴细胞和挖空状平滑肌细胞中，常导致诊断困难。在这些病例中，可疑细胞的PSA和PAP免疫组化染色为阴性，而CD45（白细胞共同抗原）和平滑肌肌动蛋白免疫组化分别在炎性细胞和平滑肌细胞中呈阳性表达[427]。

肉瘤样癌（癌肉瘤、化生性癌）

肉瘤样癌被很多人认为与癌肉瘤为同义词[150,428-431]。将这些肿瘤定义为肉瘤样癌的作者认为它是一种上皮样肿瘤，但表现出梭形细胞（间充质细胞）分化；定义为癌肉瘤的作者认为它是一种腺癌，但混合有异源性的恶性软组织成分。无论如何定义，这些肿瘤都是罕见的。

患者一般为老年男性，表现出尿道排尿不畅症状，与典型的腺癌相似。血清PSA浓度可能在诊断时仍为正常水平。大约一半的患者之前有典型腺泡状腺癌经放射性治疗或雄激素撤退治疗的病史。对该病有不同的治疗方法，但都不能有效改善预后不佳的结局。

从病理学上讲，区分肉瘤样癌与癌肉瘤是困难的，并且无临床意义。然而，转移灶可能包含癌和/或肉瘤成分，所以认真寻找原发病灶对于鉴别肿瘤的某一成分是有用的。合并存在的腺癌几乎总是高级别的（Gleason 9 或 10）。根据 Dundore 等人的研究，骨肉瘤是最常见的软组织成分，伴有或不伴有软骨组织分化及平滑肌肉瘤[428]。在上皮成分中，角蛋白、PSA 和 PAP 免疫组化胞浆阳性，与典型的前列腺腺癌相似。在软组织成分中，波形蛋白免疫组化结果常为阳性，结蛋白、肌动蛋白和 S-100 蛋白的免疫组化结果常有不同。超微结构研究发现，肉瘤组织中的肿瘤细胞偶尔也可见桥粒和纤丝样结构，提示可能表达细胞角蛋白。

该病的鉴别诊断包括肉瘤，尽管用免疫组化染色和电镜观察可以鉴别，但这种鉴别诊断可能比较困难并且在临床上也不重要。由于角蛋白在一些平滑肌肉瘤中也可呈阳性表达，所以根据这种结果诊断为上皮来源分化并不充分[432]。

腺样囊性癌/基底细胞癌

腺样囊性癌/基底细胞癌是由浸润在间质中的不同大小的基底细胞团所组成（图14.18A）。由于所报道的病例数少而且随访期有限，所以腺样囊性癌/基底细胞癌的恶性潜能情况并不十分清楚，但是一些病例出现了前列腺外组织的恶性浸润和远处转移。目前，腺样基底细胞作为一种具有潜在侵袭特征的肿物常采用烧灼法治疗[103, 104, 433, 434]。

腺样囊性癌/基底细胞癌具有两种结构类型：腺样囊性结构和基底细胞样结构[103, 104, 433]。腺样囊性结构由不规则、成团的基底细胞簇组成，其间含有圆形的透明小孔，其内大多含有黏液样物质，类似于涎腺腺样囊性癌。基底细胞样结构由不同大小的圆形基底细胞样细胞团组成，周围有明显的栅栏样结构。这些结构类型经常是同时存在的，尽管也有单一结构类型的肿瘤存在[434]。

两种结构类型在组织学上都与基底细胞增生和基底细胞腺瘤相似，但是肿瘤常侵及前列腺的大片组织，并且很少或无组织界限，且常可浸润周围神经[103, 104, 433]。腺样囊性癌/基底细胞癌的角蛋白 34βE12 免疫组化结果常可变；可能存在腔细胞阳性（图14.18B）或周围基底细胞阳性（图14.18C）。该肿瘤的 p63 和角蛋白 7 及 34βE12 的免疫组化呈阳性表达，但是角蛋白 20 呈阴性表达[434]。极少散在的细胞 PSA 和 PAP 免疫组化反应呈阳性，但是这些细胞可能是偶尔混入的分泌腺腔细胞的残迹；其他的细胞可能表现出嗜铬素阳性。无定形的腔内物质对所有的免疫抗体反应均为阴性[434]。

前列腺软组织肿瘤的免疫组化研究

前列腺的软组织肿瘤与其他器官来源的相应的软组织肿瘤的免疫表型相似。少见的肿瘤如术后梭形细胞结节、炎性假瘤和横纹肌肉瘤是膀胱中最常见的肿瘤，将在下一节中对它们进行介绍。在本节中，我们重点介绍前列腺软组织肿瘤的共同的或显著的免疫表型。

平滑肌肉瘤

平滑肌肉瘤常为一巨大的肿瘤，占据了前列腺和前列腺周围组织。它是成年人中最常见的肉瘤，占到所有前列腺肉瘤的26%。患者年龄从40岁到71岁不等（平均59岁），也有少量研究报道在年轻人中也有发生[428, 435]。尽管对于前列腺的平滑肌瘤与低级别的平滑肌肉瘤的鉴别标准还不十分明确，但是可能与其他器官中的相应肿瘤的鉴别相似，包括细胞构成、细胞间变程度、核分裂象及坏死的数量、血管浸润和肿瘤大小。

平滑肌特异性的肌动蛋白和波形蛋白通常在肿瘤细胞中表现为胞浆强阳性，而结蛋白则为弱阳性。大多数肿瘤细胞的细胞角蛋白（AE1/AE3）和 S-100 阴性，但是也有例外，特别在那些具有上皮样特点的细胞中，角蛋白免疫组化可能为阳性[171]。

肿瘤的局部复发和远处转移常见，预后不佳。确诊后的平均存活期不足 3 年（范围 0.2～6.5 年），大多数患者死于肿瘤复发[171]。极少有长期存活者的报道。尽管资料有限，但根治性手术切除仍被认为是最佳的治疗方法[171]。

叶状肿瘤（叶状囊肉瘤）

前列腺叶状肿瘤是一种少见的病变，它应该被看做是一种肿瘤而非异型性增生，因为在一些病例中常可见早期复发、浸润性生长和具有向前列腺外扩散的潜能[436-443]。多次复发后出现的去分化现象也进一步证明了该肿瘤具有侵袭性生长的特性[443]。尽

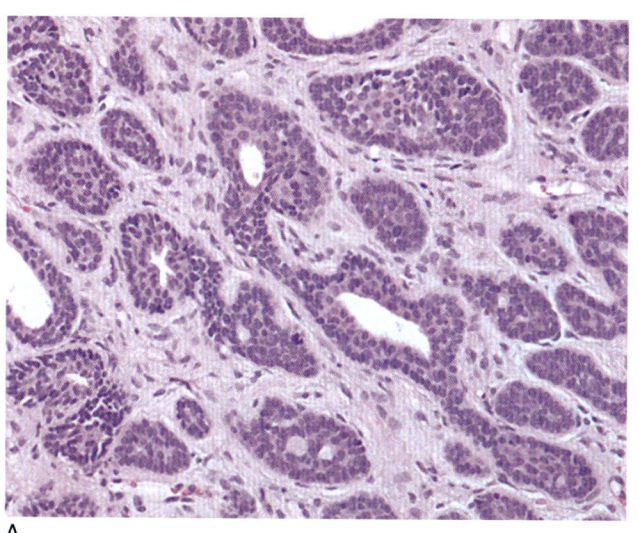
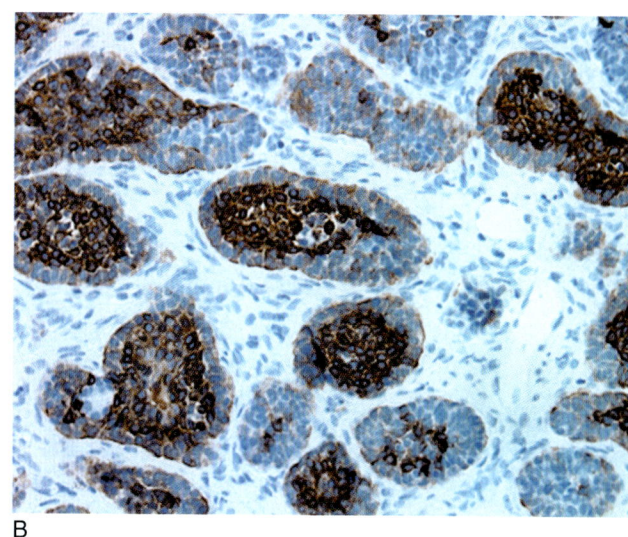
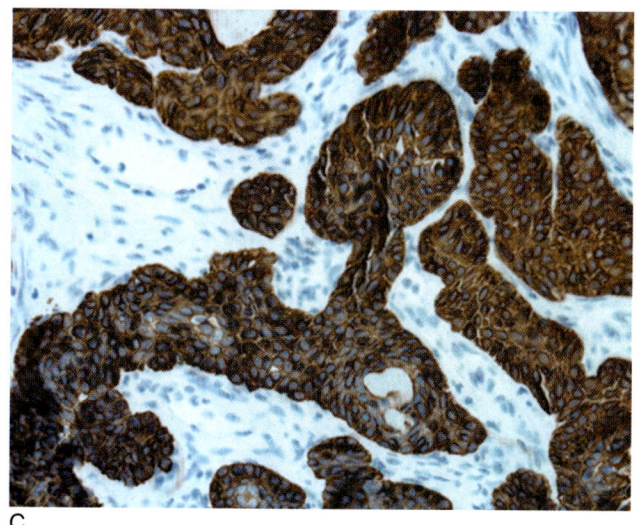

图 14.18 腺样囊性癌/基底细胞癌是由浸润在间质中的不同大小的基底细胞团所组成（A）。囊性癌/基底细胞癌的角蛋白 34βE12 免疫组化结果常可变；可有腔细胞阳性（B）和周围基底细胞阳性（C）

管在一些报道中强调肿瘤具有良性的临床过程[444]，但是文献中越来越多的证据证明一些患者会出现局部复发[443]。

前列腺叶状肿瘤患者的典型症状是尿道梗阻、血尿和排尿困难。患者可能会出现严重的尿道梗阻。这种症状的出现年龄经常比典型的前列腺增生的出现年龄要早。大多数肿瘤的大小从 4cm 到 25cm，有一研究报道肿瘤达 58cm，重 11.2kg[445]。在经尿道前列腺切除过程中，泌尿外科医生可能会看到海绵状或囊状结构的病变前列腺[159]。

前列腺叶状肿瘤具有一系列组织学特征，与乳腺组织的相应肿瘤相似（图 14.19）。该肿瘤可以分为低级别、中级别和高级别 3 组，但是即便是低级别肿瘤也可能复发[443]。高级别前列腺叶状肿瘤的间质/上皮比值高，间质细胞丰富，生长活跃，细胞异型性明显，核分裂活性增高。随着时间的推移，低级别肿瘤的肉瘤成分可能会增加，尤其在多年后经过多次复发之后

会出现这种情况[443]。有报道一个叶状肿瘤的病例组织中伴有局部分化良好的腺癌组织[445]。

免疫组织化学研究表明，在大多数间质细胞中，波形蛋白和肌动蛋白的免疫组化呈胞浆强阳性反应；在腔上皮细胞中，PSA、PAP 和角蛋白 AE1/AE3 呈胞浆强阳性反应；在基底上皮细胞中，高分子量角蛋白 34βE12 呈强阳性反应；结蛋白和 S-100 蛋白为阴性反应（表 14.8）。

这种肿瘤的组织发生学还不清楚[446]，但是认为不应该来源于苗勒管，原因如下：①在成年人前列腺组织中无苗勒管痕迹，在生命的早期阶段，前列腺囊中的苗勒上皮被泌尿生殖窦取代；② PSA 和 PAP 在成年人前列腺囊上皮中呈阳性反应，表明该组织具有内胚层（前列腺样）特征；以及③ PSA 在前列腺叶状肿瘤上皮中呈阳性反应。

叶状肿瘤肯定具有侵袭潜能，所以应采用个性化的治疗方案以期将肿瘤完全切除。低级别肿瘤可能会

被采取保守治疗，但是会发现复发后的肿瘤恶性级别升高，故需要将肿瘤完全切除[443]。很少情况下，伴有明显恶性间质成分的肿瘤会导致肺、骨骼和腹壁出现肉瘤转移。淋巴结转移尚未见到[159]。

叶状肿瘤的鉴别诊断包括间质增生伴胞核异常、巨大多腔性前列腺囊腺瘤、异常增生伴囊性腺泡以及囊肿如苗勒管囊肿和先天性及获得性精囊腺囊肿（表14.9）。叶状肿瘤也可能来源于精囊腺，作为一种前列腺上精囊后肿物，但是这种肿瘤可以与前列腺来源的肿瘤相鉴别，因为该肿瘤上皮的PSA和PAP免疫组化结果为阴性。间质增生伴细胞核异型性实际上是一种细胞损伤状态，表现为在邻近增生的腺泡或在结节性增生的间质组织细胞中出现大、深染、退行性变的细胞核。前列腺的巨大多腔性囊腺瘤是一种实体肿瘤，其中包含有由前列腺上皮包绕的囊性结构，而前列腺上皮又由致密的纤维性间质所环绕。前列腺囊性腺瘤由向内生长的乳头状上皮组织和少量的间质组织所构成。结节状增生通常在增生的结节组织中含有小的囊性腺泡，有时可能存在小的不常见的纤维腺瘤样组织，易被误诊为叶状肿瘤。苗勒管囊肿（主要在中部）和精囊腺囊肿（主要在侧部）通常是单腔性，并缺乏前列腺上皮被膜以及叶状肿瘤的间质细胞形态特征。前列腺原发性肉瘤如平滑肌肉瘤也需要进行鉴别诊断，但是这种肿瘤主要是梭形细胞呈单相、致密的增生，而缺少叶状肿瘤的上皮成分。当存在明显的恶性梭形细胞成分时，还需要考虑肉瘤样癌，但是在这种肿瘤增生的梭形细胞中，存在恶性上皮成分或上皮分化的特征，以此鉴别[159, 447]。

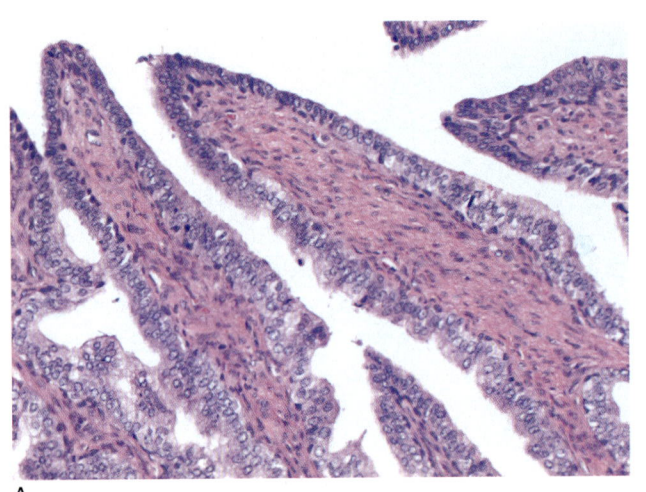
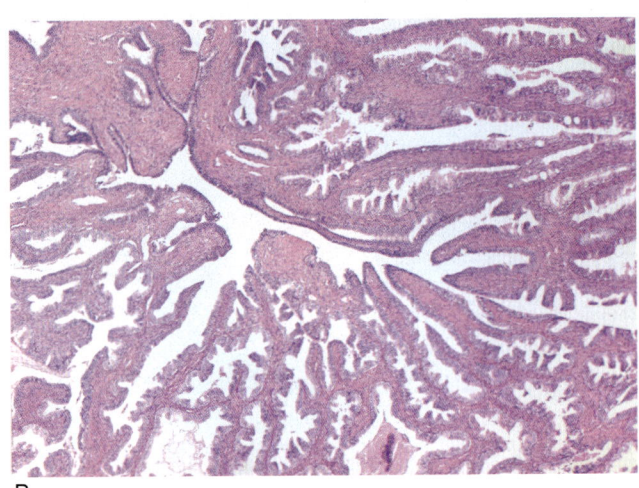

图14.19 叶状肿瘤。低级别前列腺叶状肿瘤，伴有上皮环绕的间质组织向腺腔内凸出，形成叶片样（×200）（A）；低级别前列腺叶状肿瘤，间质/上皮比值降低，细胞中等异型性，无核分裂象（×400）（B）

表14.8 前列腺叶状肿瘤：7个病例中的免疫组化结果*

病例号	PSA	PAP	角蛋白 AE1/AE3	角蛋白 34βE12	S-100 蛋白	嗜铬素	5-羟色胺	雌激素受体	孕激素受体	雄激素受体	波形蛋白	结蛋白	肌动蛋白
1	++	+++	++	+	-	-	-	-	-	++	++	-	+++
2†	++	+++	+++	+++	-	-	-	-	-	-	+++	+++	+++
3	+++	+++	++	-	-	-	-	-	-	-	+++	-	++
4	+++	+++	+	+	-	-	-	-	-	+++	+++	-	+
5	+++	+++	+++	++	-	-	-	-	-	-	+++	-	+
6	++	++	++	+	-	-	-	-	-	-	+	-	+
7	+++	+++	++	+++	-	-	-	NT	NT	NT	+++	-	+

* 未提供7号病例的免疫组化染色的切片
- 至 +++ 的判断是根据阳性细胞的数量（+ ≤ 25%；++ = 25% ~ 50%；+++ ≥ 50%）

†除了病例2，其余病例均使用单一抗体同批实验以避免内部差异
NT：未检测

表14.9 前列腺或精囊腺的叶状肿瘤：鉴别诊断

特　征	叶状肿瘤	间质增生伴异型性（平滑肌瘤样型）*	间质增生伴异型性（浸润型）*	平滑肌肉瘤**
临床特征				
患者平均年龄（范围）		68岁（57~80）	69岁（59~80）	61岁（41~78）
症　状	尿道梗阻症状，血尿或伴随症状	尿道梗阻症状，或伴随症状	尿道梗阻症状，或伴随症状	尿道梗阻症状，会阴部疼痛
膀胱镜/肉眼观察		间质结节	间质结节	肿瘤直径3~21cm（平均9cm）
血清PSA	正常范围	正常范围	正常范围	正常范围
结　构	双相型，包括变形的囊性扩张或裂缝样上皮腺体，经常可见叶状凸起，合并凝集的间质	实性的、局限的、扩张的间质结节，伴有丰富的平滑肌组织和异型的间质细胞	Ⅲ期增生性间质结节伴弥漫性的异型细胞和典型增生腺泡周围的均一浸润；基质中细胞减少、松散，伴有大而扩张的血管	巨大结节样肿瘤，含有梭形细胞
细胞学	良性上皮；异型间质细胞数量不等，伴挖空细胞核和多核性；出现核分裂象和坏死，表明肿瘤的恶性级别升高	异型巨大间质细胞，伴挖空的细胞核，常可见多核现象；无核分裂象或坏死	异型巨大间质细胞，伴挖空的细胞核，常可见多核现象；无核分裂象或坏死	梭形或上皮样肿瘤细胞，伴多形性、核分裂象，常见坏死
免疫组织化学				
波形蛋白	通常+++	+	+++	++
结蛋白	通常-；很少+++	+++	通常+	通常-；很少+
肌动蛋白	+	+++	+	通常-；很少+
雌激素受体	-	-	-	NT
孕激素受体	通常-；很少+	通常++	通常+++	NT
雄激素受体	通常-；很少++	+++	+++	NT
角蛋白AE1/AE3	++（上皮）	-	-	通常-（在27%的病例中呈+）
角蛋白34βE12	++（上皮）	-	-	NT
PSA	+++	-	-	-
PAP	+++	-	-	-
S-100蛋白	-	-	-	-
随　诊	常复发，间质过度生长的出现表明具有明显的恶性潜能	良性；非常少见实体肿瘤复发	良性；非常少见实体肿瘤复发	恶性；存活期平均为22个月（3~72个月）

* 资料来自Wang和Bostwick，1997
** 资料来自Cheville等，1996
PSA，前列腺特异抗原；PAP，前列腺酸性磷酸酶；NT，未检测

参考文献

1. Akdas A, Cevik I, Tarcan T, et al. The role of free prostate-specific antigen in the diagnosis of prostate cancer. Br J Urol 1997; 79:920.
2. Rocchi P, Muracciole X, Fina F, et al. Molecular analysis integrating different pathways associated with androgen-independent progression in LuCaP 23.1 xenograft. Oncogene 2004; 23:9111–9119.
3. Kim J, Coetzee GA. Prostate specific antigen gene regulation by androgen receptor. J Cell Biochem 2004; 93:233.
4. Bostwick DG. Prostate-specific antigen. Current role in diagnostic pathology of prostate cancer. Am J Clin Pathol 1994; 102:S31.
5. Ablin RJ. A retrospective and prospective overview of prostate-specific antigen. J Cancer Res Clin Oncol 1997; 123:583.
6. Brawer MK, Benson MC, Bostwick DG, et al. Prostatespecific antigen and other serum markers: current concepts from the World Health Organization Second International Consultation on Prostate Cancer. Semin Urol Oncol 1999; 17:206.
7. Ishibashi M. [Progress in standardization of total PSA immunoassays]. Rinsho Byori 2004; 52:618.
8. Hernandez J, Thompson IM. Prostate-specific antigen: a review of the validation of the most commonly used cancer biomarker. Cancer 2004; 101:894.
9. Cheng L, Darson MF, Bergstralh EJ, et al. Correlation of margin status and extraprostatic extension with progression of prostate carcinoma. Cancer 1999; 86:1775.
10. Cheng L, Leibovich BC., Bergstralh EJ, et al. p53 alteration in regional lymph node metastases from prostate carcinoma: a marker for progression? Cancer 1999; 85:2455.
11. Montironi R, Mazzucchelli R, Algaba F, et al. Prostatespecific antigen as a marker of prostate disease. Virchows Arch 2000; 436:297.
12. Roehl KA, Han M, Ramos CG, et al. Cancer progression and survival rates following anatomical radical retropubic prostatectomy in 3,478 consecutive patients: long-term results. J Urol 2004; 172:910.
13. Shevchuk MM, Romas NA, Ng PY, et al. Acid phosphatase localization in prostatic carcinoma. A comparison of monoclonal antibody to heteroantisera. Cancer 1983; 52:1642.
14. Lippert MC, Bensimon H, Javadpour N. Immunoperoxidase staining of acid phosphatase in human prostatic tissue. J Urol 1982; 128:1114.
15. Ordonez NG, Ayala AG, von Eschenbach AC, et al. Immunoperoxidase localization of prostatic acid phosphatase in prostatic carcinoma with sarcomatoid changes. Urology 1982; 19:210.
16. Nadji M, Morales AR. Immunohistochemistry of prostatic acid phosphatase. Ann NY Acad Sci 1982; 390:133.
17. Jobsis AC, De Vries GP, Meijer AE, et al. The immunohistochemical detection of prostatic acid phosphatase: its possibilities and limitations in tumour histochemistry. Histochem J 1981; 13:961.
18. Ablin RJ. Immunohistological localization of prostatic acid phosphatase. Allergol Immunopathol (Madr) 1979; 7:361.
19. Epstein JI, Eggleston JC. Immunohistochemical localization of prostate-specific acid phosphatase and prostate-specific antigen in stage A2 adenocarcinoma of the prostate: prognostic implications. Hum Pathol 1984; 15:853.
20. Pollen JJ, Dreilinger A. Immunohistochemical identification of prostatic acid phosphatase and prostate specific antigen in female periurethral glands. Urology 1984; 23:303.
21. Broghamer WL Jr, Richardson ME, Faurest S, et al. Prostatic acid phosphatase immunoperoxidase staining of cytologically positive effusions associated with adenocarcinomas of the prostate and neoplasms of undetermined origin. Acta Cytol 1985; 29:274.
22. Song GX, Lin CT, Wu JY, et al. Immunoelectron microscopic demonstration of prostatic acid phosphatase in human hyperplastic prostate. Prostate 1985; 7:63.
23. Mori K, Wakasugi C. Immunocytochemical demonstration of prostatic acid phosphatase: different secretion kinetics between normal, hyperplastic and neoplastic prostates. J Urol 1985; 133:877.
24. Raynor RH, Hazra TA, Moncure CW, et al. Biochemical nature of the prostate-associated antigen identified by the monoclonal antibody, KR-P8. Prostate 1986; 9:21.
25. Keillor JS, Aterman K. The response of poorly differentiated prostatic tumors to staining for prostate specific antigen and prostatic acid phosphatase: a comparative study. J Urol 1987; 137:894.
26. van Dieijen-Visser MP, Delaere KP, Gijzen AH, et al. A comparative study on the diagnostic value of prostatic acid phosphatase (PAP) and prostatic specific antigen (PSA) in patients

with carcinoma of the prostate gland. Clin Chim Acta 1988; 174:131.

27. Ersev A, Ersev D, Turkeri L, et al. The relation of prostatic acid phosphatase and prostate specific antigen with tumour grade in prostatic adenocarcinoma: an immunohistochemical study. Prog Clin Biol Res 1990; 357:129.

28. Sakai H, Shiraishi K, Minami Y, et al. Immunohistochemical prostatic acid phosphatase level as a prognostic factor of prostatic carcinoma. Prostate 1991; 19:265.

29. Garde SV, Sheth AR, Porter AT, et al. A comparative study on expression of prostatic inhibin peptide, prostate acid phosphatase and prostate specific antigen in androgen independent human and rat prostate carcinoma cell lines. Cancer Lett 1993; 70:159.

30. Grob BM, Schellhammer PF, Brassil DN, et al. Changes in immunohistochemical staining of PSA, PAP, and TURP-27 following irradiation therapy for clinically localized prostate cancer. Urology 1994; 44:525.

31. De Marzo AM, Bradshaw C, Sauvageot J, et al. CD44 and CD44v6 downregulation in clinical prostatic carcinoma: relation to Gleason grade and cytoarchitecture. Prostate 1998; 34:162.

32. Bettencourt MC, Bauer JJ, Sesterhenn IA, et al. CD34 immunohistochemical assessment of angiogenesis as a prognostic marker for prostate cancer recurrence after radical prostatectomy. J Urol 1998; 160:459.

33. Sinha AA, Quast BJ, Wilson MJ, et al. Codistribution of procathepsin B and mature cathepsin B forms in human prostate tumors detected by confocal and immunofluorescence microscopy. Anat Rec 1998; 252:281.

34. Perlman EJ, Epstein JI, Long PP, et al. Cytogenetic and ploidy analysis of prostatic adenocarcinoma. Mod Pathol 1993; 6:348.

35. Goldstein NS. Immunophenotypic characterization of 225 prostate adenocarcinomas with intermediate or high Gleason scores. Am J Clin Pathol 2002; 117:471.

36. Varma M, Berney DM, Jasani B, et al. Technical variations in prostatic immunohistochemistry: need for standardisation and stringent quality assurance in PSA and PSAP immunostaining. J Clin Pathol 2004; 57:687.

37. Lopes AD, Davis WL, Rosenstraus MJ, et al. Immunohistochemical and pharmacokinetic characterization of the site-specific immunoconjugate CYT-356 derived from antiprostate monoclonal antibody 7E11-C5. Cancer Res 1990; 50:6423.

38. Murphy GP, Elgamal AA, Su SL, et al. Current evaluation of the tissue localization and diagnostic utility of prostate specific membrane antigen. Cancer 1998; 83:2259.

39. Troyer JK, Beckett ML, Wright GL Jr. Detection and characterization of the prostate-specific membrane antigen (PSMA) in tissue extracts and body fluids. Int J Cancer 1995; 62:552.

40. Sweat SD, Pacelli A, Murphy GP, et al. Prostate-specific membrane antigen expression is greatest in prostate adenocarcinoma and lymph node metastases. Urology 1998; 52:637.

41. Seckin B, Anthony CT, Murphy B, et al. Can prostatespecific antigen be used as a valid end point to determine the efficacy of chemotherapy for advanced prostate cancer? World J Urol 1996; 14:S26.

42. Zaviacic M, Ruzickova M, Blazekova J, et al. Immunohistochemical distribution of rabbit polyclonal antiurinary protein 1 antibody in the female (Skene's gland) and male prostate: new marker for neuroendocrine cells? Acta Histochem 1997; 99:267.

43. Gregorakis AK, Holmes EH, Murphy GP. Prostate-specific membrane antigen: current and future utility. Semin Urol Oncol 1998; 16:2.

44. Elgamal AA, Holmes EH, Su SL, et al. Prostate-specific membrane antigen (PSMA): current benefits and future value. Semin Surg Oncol 2000; 18:10.

45. Chang SS. Monoclonal antibodies and prostate-specific membrane antigen. Curr Opin Investig Drugs 2004; 5:611.

46. Brooks JD, Bova GS, Ewing CM, et al. An uncertain role for p53 gene alterations in human prostate cancers. Cancer Res 1996; 56:3814.

47. Hessels D, Verhaegh GW, Schalken JA, et al. Applicability of biomarkers in the early diagnosis of prostate cancer. Expert Rev Mol Diagn 2004; 4:513.

48. Ghosh A, Heston WD. Tumor target prostate specific membrane antigen (PSMA) and its regulation in prostate cancer. J Cell Biochem 2004; 91:528.

49. Marchal C, Redondo M, Padilla M, et al. Expression of prostate specific membrane antigen (PSMA) in prostatic adenocarcinoma and prostatic intraepithelial neoplasia. Histol Histopathol 2004; 19:715.

50. Chang SS, O'Keefe DS, Bacich DJ, et al. Prostate-specific

membrane antigen is produced in tumor-associated neovasculature. Clin Cancer Res 1999; 5:2674.

51. Reimer CL, Borras AM, Kurdistani SK, et al. Altered regulation of cyclin G in human breast cancer and its specific localization at replication foci in response to DNA damage in p53+/+ cells. J Biol Chem 1999; 274:11022.

52. Nevalainen MT, Valve EM, Ahonen T, et al. Androgen-dependent expression of prolactin in rat prostate epithelium in vivo and in organ culture. Faseb J 1997; 11:1297.

53. Ross JS, Sheehan CE, Fisher HA, et al. Correlation of primary tumor prostate-specific membrane antigen expression with disease recurrence in prostate cancer. Clin Cancer Res 2003; 9:6357.

54. Schmidt B, Anastasiadis AG, Seifert HH, et al. Detection of circulating prostate cells during radical prostatectomy by standardized PSMA RT-PCR: association with positive lymph nodes and high malignant grade. Anticancer Res 2003; 23:3991.

55. Israeli RS, Powell CT, Corr JG, et al. Expression of the prostate-specific membrane antigen. Cancer Res 1994; 54:1807.

56. Mottaz AE, Markwalder R, Fey MF, et al. Abnormal p53 expression is rare in clinically localized human prostate cancer: comparison between immunohistochemical and molecular detection of p53 mutations. Prostate 1997; 31:209.

57. Troyer JK, Beckett ML, Wright GL Jr. Location of prostate-specific membrane antigen in the LNCaP prostate carcinoma cell line. Prostate 1997; 30:232.

58. Gong MC, Chang SS, Sadelain M, et al. Prostate-specific membrane antigen (PSMA)-specific monoclonal antibodies in the treatment of prostate and other cancers [In Process Citation]. Cancer Metastasis Rev 1999; 18:483.

59. Salgaller ML, Lodge PA, McLean JG, et al. Report of immune monitoring of prostate cancer patients undergoing T-cell therapy using dendritic cells pulsed with HLA-A2-specific peptides from prostate-specific membrane antigen (PSMA). Prostate 1998; 35:144.

60. Zhang WM, Finne P, Leinonen J, et al. Characterization and immunological determination of the complex between prostate-specific antigen and alpha2-macroglobulin. Clin Chem 1998; 44:2471.

61. Partin AW, Catalona WJ, Finlay JA, et al. Use of human glandular kallikrein 2 for the detection of prostate cancer: preliminary analysis. Urology 1999; 54:839.

62. Tremblay RR, Deperthes D, Tetu B, et al. Immunohistochemical study suggesting a complementary role of kallikreins hK2 and hK3 (prostate-specific antigen) in the functional analysis of human prostate tumors. Am J Pathol 1997; 150:455.

63. Darson MF, Pacelli A, Roche P, et al. Human glandular kallikrein 2 (hK2) expression in prostatic intraepithelial neoplasia and adenocarcinoma: a novel prostate cancer marker. Urology 1997; 49:857.

64. Darson MF, Pacelli A, Roche P, et al. Human glandular kallikrein 2 expression in prostate adenocarcinoma and lymph node metastases. Urology 1999; 53:939.

65. Steuber T, Niemela P, Haese A, et al. Association of free prostate-specific antigen subfractions and human glandular kallikrein 2 with volume of benign and malignant prostatic tissue. Prostate 2005; 63:13–18.

66. Haese A, Graefen M, Steuber T, et al. Total and Gleason grade 4/5 cancer volumes are major contributors of human kallikrein 2, whereas free prostate specific antigen is largely contributed by benign gland volume in serum from patients with prostate cancer or benign prostatic biopsies. J Urol 2003; 170:2269.

67. Civantos F. Difficulties in interpreting specimens after neoadjuvant hormonal therapy and radiation with illustration of neuroendocrine differentiation. Mol Urol 2000; 4:117.

68. Vaisanen V, Eriksson S, Ivaska KK, et al. Development of sensitive immunoassays for free and total human glandular kallikrein 2. Clin Chem 2004; 50:1607.

69. Fuessel S, Sickert D, Meye A, et al. Multiple tumor marker analyses (PSA, hK2, PSCA, trp-p8) in primary prostate cancers using quantitative RT-PCR. Int J Oncol 2003; 23:221.

70. Evans AJ. Alpha-methylacyl-CoA racemase (P504S): overview and potential uses in diagnostic pathology as applied to prostate needle biopsies. J Clin Pathol 2003; 56:892.

71. Jiang Z, Woda BA, Rock KL, et al. P504S: a new molecular marker for the detection of prostate carcinoma. Am J Surg Pathol 2001; 25:1397.

72. Jiang Z, Fanger GR, Woda BA, et al. Expression of alpha-methylacyl-CoA racemase (P504s) in various malignant neoplasms and normal tissues: a study of 761 cases. Hum Pathol 2003; 34:792.

73. Jiang Z, Wu CL, Woda BA, et al. P504S/alpha-methylacyl-CoA racemase: a useful marker for diagnosis of small foci of prostatic carcinoma on needle biopsy. Am J Surg Pathol 2002;

26:1169.

74. Wu CL, Yang XJ, Tretiakova M, et al. Analysis of alpha-methylacyl-CoA racemase (P504S) expression in high-grade prostatic intraepithelial neoplasia. Hum Pathol 2004; 35:1008.

75. Magi-Galluzzi C, Luo J, Isaacs WB, et al. Alpha-methylacyl-CoA racemase: a variably sensitive immunohistochemical marker for the diagnosis of small prostate cancer foci on needle biopsy. Am J Surg Pathol 2003; 27:1128.

76. Yang XJ, Laven B, Tretiakova M, et al. Detection of alpha-methylacyl-coenzyme A racemase in postradiation prostatic adenocarcinoma. Urology 2003; 62:282.

77. Yang XJ, Wu CL, Woda BA, et al. Expression of alpha-methylacyl-CoA racemase (P504S) in atypical adenomatous hyperplasia of the prostate. Am J Surg Pathol 2002; 26:921.

78. Jiang Z, Wu CL, Woda BA, et al. Alpha-methylacyl-CoA racemase: a multi-institutional study of a new prostate cancer marker. Histopathology 2004; 45:218.

79. Zhou M, Aydin H, Kanane H, et al. How often does alpha-methylacyl-CoA-racemase contribute to resolving an atypical diagnosis on prostate needle biopsy beyond that provided by basal cell markers? Am J Surg Pathol 2004; 28:239.

80. Sanderson SO, Sebo TJ, Murphy LM, et al. An analysis of the p63/alpha-methylacyl coenzyme A racemase immunohistochemical cocktail stain in prostate needle biopsy specimens and tissue microarrays. Am J Clin Pathol 2004; 121:220.

81. Tacha DE, Miller RT. Use of p63/P504S monoclonal antibody cocktail in immunohistochemical staining of prostate tissue. Appl Immunohistochem Mol Morphol 2004; 12:75.

82. Ohkia A, Hu Y, Wang M, et al. Evidence for prostate cancer-associated diagnostic marker-1: immunohistochemistry and in situ hybridization studies. Clin Cancer Res 2004; 10:2452.

83. Dhir R, Vietmeier B, Arlotti J, et al. Early identification of individuals with prostate cancer in negative biopsies. J Urol 2004; 171:1419.

84. Leroy X, Ballereau C, Villers A, et al. MUC6 is a marker of seminal vesicle-ejaculatory duct epithelium and is useful for the differential diagnosis with prostate adenocarcinoma. Am J Surg Pathol 2003; 27:519.

85. Novis DA, Zarbo RJ, Valenstein PA. Diagnostic uncertainty expressed in prostate needle biopsies. A College of American Pathologists Q-probes Study of 15,753 prostate needle biopsies in 332 institutions. Arch Pathol Lab Med 1999; 123:687.

86. Wojno KJ, Epstein JI. The utility of basal cell-specific anti-cytokeratin antibody (34 beta E12) in the diagnosis of prostate cancer. A review of 228 cases. Am J Surg Pathol 1995; 19:251.

87. Kahane H, Sharp JW, Shuman GB, et al. Utilization of high molecular weight cytokeratin on prostate needle biopsies in an independent laboratory. Urology 1995; 45:981.

88. Varma M, Linden MD, Amin MB. Effect of formalin fixation and epitope retrieval techniques on antibody 34betaE12 immunostaining of prostatic tissues [see comments]. Mod Pathol 1999; 12:472.

89. Iczkowski KA, Cheng L, Crawford BG, et al. Steam heat with an EDTA buffer and protease digestion optimizes immunohistochemical expression of basal cell-specific antikeratin 34betaE12 to discriminate cancer in prostatic epithelium. Mod Pathol 1999; 12:1.

90. Goldstein NS, Underhill J, Roszka J, et al. Cytokeratin 34 beta E-12 immunoreactivity in benign prostatic acini. Quantitation, pattern assessment, and electron microscopic study. Am J Clin Pathol 1999; 112:69.

91. Bostwick DG, Qian J, Maihle NJ. Amphiregulin expression in prostatic intraepithelial neoplasia and adenocarcinoma: a study of 93 cases. Prostate 2004; 58:164.

92. Amin MB, Schultz DS, Zarbo RJ. Analysis of cribriform morphology in prostatic neoplasia using antibody to high-molecular-weight cytokeratins. Arch Pathol Lab Med 1994; 118:260.

93. Ramnani DM, Bostwick DG. Basal cell-specific anti-keratin antibody 34betaE12: optimizing its use in distinguishing benign prostate and cancer [editorial; comment]. Mod Pathol 1999; 12:443.

94. Cohen RJ, McNeal JE, Edgar SG, et al. Characterization of cytoplasmic secretory granules (PSG) in prostatic epithelium and their transformation-induced loss in dysplasia and adenocarcinoma. Hum Pathol 1998; 29:1488.

95. Freibauer C. Diagnosis of prostate carcinoma on biopsy specimens improved by basal-cell-specific anti-cytokeratin antibody (34 beta E12). Wien Klin Wochenschr 1998; 110:608.

96. Brawer MK, Nagle RB, Pitts W, et al. Keratin immunoreactivity as an aid to the diagnosis of persistent adenocarcinoma in irradiated human prostates. Cancer 1989; 63:454.

97. Bostwick DG, Brawer MK. Prostatic intra-epithelial neoplasia and early invasion in prostate cancer. Cancer 1987; 59:788.

98. Hedrick L, Epstein JI. Use of keratin 903 as an adjunct in the diagnosis of prostate carcinoma. Am J Surg Pathol 1989; 13: 389.

99. Saboorian MH, Huffman H, Ashfaq R, et al. Distinguishing Cowper's glands from neoplastic and pseudoneoplastic lesions of prostate: immunohistochemical and ultrastructural studies. Am J Surg Pathol 1997; 21:1069.

100. Cina SJ, Epstein JI. Adenocarcinoma of the prostate with atrophic features. Am J Surg Pathol 1997; 21:289.

101. Kim YW, Park YK, Park JH, et al. Adenosquamous carcinoma of the prostate. Yonsei Med J 1999; 40:396.

102. Bonkhoff H, Stein U, Remberger K. The proliferative function of basal cells in the normal and hyperplastic human prostate. Prostate 1994; 24:114.

103. Epstein JI, Armas OA. Atypical basal cell hyperplasia of the prostate. Am J Surg Pathol 1992; 16:1205.

104. Devaraj LT, Bostwick DG. Atypical basal cell hyperplasia of the prostate. Immunophenotypic profile and proposed classification of basal cell proliferations. Am J Surg Pathol 1993; 17:645.

105. Yang Y, Hao J, Liu X, et al. Differential expression of cytokeratin mRNA and protein in normal prostate, prostatic intraepithelial neoplasia, and invasive carcinoma. Am J Pathol 1997; 150:693.

106. Abrahams NA, Bostwick DG, Ormsby AH, et al. Distinguishing atrophy and high-grade prostatic intraepithelial neoplasia from prostatic adenocarcinoma with and without previous adjuvant hormone therapy with the aid of cytokeratin 5/6. Am J Clin Pathol 2003; 120:368.

107. Zijlmans HJ, Bonnet J, Burton J, et al. Detection of cell and tissue surface antigens using up-converting phosphors: a new reporter technology. Anal Biochem 1999; 267:30.

108. Weinstein MH, Signoretti S, Loda M. Diagnostic utility of immunohistochemical staining for p63, a sensitive marker of prostatic basal cells. Mod Pathol 2002; 15:1302.

109. Shah RB, Zhou M, LeBlanc M, et al. Comparison of the basal cell-specific markers, 34betaE12 and p63, in the diagnosis of prostate cancer. Am J Surg Pathol 2002; 26:1161.

110. Zhou M, Shah R, Shen R, et al. Basal cell cocktail (34betaE12 + p63) improves the detection of prostate basal cells. Am J Surg Pathol 2003; 27:365.

111. Reis-Filho JS, Simpson PT, Martins A, et al. Distribution of p63, cytokeratins 5/6 and cytokeratin 14 in 51 normal and 400 neoplastic human tissue samples using TARP-4 multi-tumor tissue microarray. Virchows Arch 2003; 443:122.

112. Signoretti S, Waltregny D, Dilks J, et al. p63 is a prostate basal cell marker and is required for prostate development. Am J Pathol 2000; 157:1769.

113. Yang A, Kaghad M, Wang Y, et al. p63, a p53 homolog at 3q27-29, encodes multiple products with transactivating, death-inducing, and dominant-negative activities. Mol Cell 1998; 2:305.

114. Parsons JK, Gage WR, Nelson WG, et al. p63 protein expression is rare in prostate adenocarcinoma: implications for cancer diagnosis and carcinogenesis. Urology 2001; 58:619.

115. Kitajima K, Tokes ZA. Immunohistochemical localization of keratin in human prostate. Prostate 1986; 9:183.

116. Purnell DM, Heatfield BM, Anthony RL, et al. Immunohistochemistry of the cytoskeleton of human prostatic epithelium. Evidence for disturbed organization in neoplasia. Am J Pathol 1987; 126:384.

117. Dhom G, Seitz G, Wernert N. Histology and immunohistochemistry studies in prostate cancer. Am J Clin Oncol 1988; 11:S37.

118. Wernert N, Luchtrath H, Seeliger H, et al. Papillary carcinoma of the prostate, location, morphology, and immunohistochemistry: the histogenesis and entity of so-called endometrioid carcinoma. Prostate 1987; 10:123.

119. Guinan P, Shaw M, Targonski P, et al. Evaluation of cytokeratin markers to differentiate between benign and malignant prostatic tissue. J Surg Oncol 1989; 42:175.

120. Nagle RB, Ahmann FR, McDaniel KM, et al. Cytokeratin characterization of human prostatic carcinoma and its derived cell lines. Cancer 1987; Res 47:281.

121. O'Malley FP, Grignon DJ, Shum DT. Usefulness of immunoperoxidase staining with high-molecular-weight cytokeratin in the differential diagnosis of small-acinar lesions of the prostate gland. Virchows Arch A Pathol Anat Histopathol 1990; 417:191.

122. Srigley JR, Dardick I, Hartwick RW, et al. Basal epithelial cells of human prostate gland are not myoepithelial cells. A comparative immunohistochemical and ultrastructural study with the human salivary gland. Am J Pathol 1990; 136:957.

123. Shah IA, Schlageter MO, Stinnett P, et al. Cytokeratin immunohistochemistry as a diagnostic tool for distinguishing malignant from benign epithelial lesions of the prostate [see

comments]. Mod Pathol 1991; 4:220.

124. Rehman I, Cross SS, Azzouzi AR, et al. S100A6 (calcyclin) is a prostate basal cell marker absent in prostate cancer and its precursors. Br J Cancer 2004; 91:739.

125. Howat AJ, Mills PM, Lyons TJ, et al. Absence of S-100 protein in prostatic glands. Histopathology 1988; 13:468.

126. Mahapokai W, Xue Y, van Garderen E, et al. Cell kinetics and differentiation after hormonal-induced prostatic hyperplasia in the dog. Prostate 2000; 44:40.

127. Mucci NR, Akdas G, Manely S, et al. Neuroendocrine expression in metastatic prostate cancer: evaluation of high throughput tissue microarrays to detect heterogeneous protein expression. Hum Pathol 2000; 31:406.

128. Aaltomaa S, Lipponen P, Ala-Opas M, et al. Alpha-catenin expression has prognostic value in local and locally advanced prostate cancer. Br J Cancer 1999; 80:477.

129. Helpap B, Kollermann J. Atypical acinar proliferations of the prostate. Pathol Res Pract 1999; 195:795.

130. Bonkhoff H, Stein U, Welter C, et al. Differential expression of the pS2 protein in the human prostate and prostate cancer: association with premalignant changes and neuroendocrine differentiation. Hum Pathol 1995; 26:824.

131. Buchholz NP, Moch H, Feichter GE, et al. Clinical and pathological features of highly malignant prostatic carcinomas with metastases to the penis. Urol Int 1994; 53:135.

132. Kamiya N, Akakura K, Suzuki H, et al. Pretreatment serum level of neuron specific enolase (NSE) as a prognostic factor in metastatic prostate cancer patients treated with endocrine therapy. Eur Urol 2003; 44:309.

133. Djakiew D, Delsite R, Pflug B, et al. Regulation of growth by a nerve growth factor-like protein which modulates paracrine interactions between a neoplastic epithelial cell line and stromal cells of the human prostate. Cancer Res 1991; 51:3304.

134. di Sant'Agnese PA, de Mesy Jensen KL, Churukian CJ, et al. Human prostatic endocrine-paracrine (APUD) cells. Distributional analysis with a comparison of serotonin and neuron-specific enolase immunoreactivity and silver stains. Arch Pathol Lab Med 1985; 109:607.

135. McCormick DL, Rao KV. Chemoprevention of hormone-dependent prostate cancer in the Wistar-Unilever rat. Eur Urol 1999; 35:464.

136. Pruneri G, Galli S, Rossi RS, et al. Chromogranin A and B and secretogranin II in prostatic adenocarcinomas: neuroendocrine expression in patients untreated and treated with androgen deprivation therapy. Prostate 1998; 34:113.

137. Abrahamsson PA, Falkmer S, Falt K, et al. The course of neuroendocrine differentiation in prostatic carcinomas. An immunohistochemical study testing chromogranin A as an 'endocrine marker.' Pathol Res Pract 1989; 185:373.

138. Angelsen A, Mecsei R, Sandvik AK, et al. Neuroendocrine cells in the prostate of the rat, guinea pig, cat, and dog. Prostate 1997; 33:18.

139. Falkmer S, Askensten U, Grimelius L, et al. Cytochemical markers and DNA content of neuroendocrine cells in carcinoma of the prostate gland during tumour progression. Acta Histochem Suppl 1990; 38:127.

140. McWilliam LJ, Manson C, George NJ. Neuroendocrine differentiation and prognosis in prostatic adenocarcinoma. Br J Urol 1997; 80:287.

141. Xue Y, Smedts F, Umbas R, et al. Changes in keratin expression during the development of benign prostatic hyperplasia. Eur Urol 1997; 32:332.

142. Guy L, Begin LR, Al-Othman K, et al. Neuroendocrine cells of the verumontanum: a comparative immunohistochemical study. Br J Urol 1998; 82:738.

143. Bostwick DG, Alexander EE, Singh R, et al. Antioxidant enzyme expression and reactive oxygen species damage in prostatic intraepithelial neoplasia and cancer. Cancer 2000; 89:123.

144. Bostwick DG, Qian J, Pacelli A, et al. Neuroendocrine expression in node positive prostate cancer: correlation with systemic progression and patient survival. J Urol 2002; 168:1204.

145. Chen SF, Xu Y, Ip MP. Electrochemical enzyme immunoassay for serum prostate-specific antigen at low concentrations. Clin Chem 1997; 43:1459.

146. Krijnen JL, Janssen PJ, Ruizeveld de Winter JA, et al. Do neuroendocrine cells in human prostate cancer express androgen receptor? Histochemistry 1993; 100:393.

147. Adlakha H, Bostwick DG. Paneth cell-like change in prostatic adenocarcinoma represents neuroendocrine differentiation: report of 30 cases [see comments]. Hum Pathol 1994; 25:135.

148. Weaver MG, Abdul-Karim FW, Srigley JR. Paneth cell-like change and small cell carcinoma of the prostate. Two divergent forms of prostatic neuroendocrine differentiation. Am J

Surg Pathol 1992; 16:1013.

149. Fjellestad-Paulsen A, Abrahamsson PA, Bjartell A, et al. Carcinoma of the prostate with Cushing's syndrome. A case report with histochemical and chemical demonstration of immunoreactive corticotropin-releasing hormone in plasma and tumoral tissue. Acta Endocrinol (Copenh) 1988; 119:506.

150. Frkovic-Grazio S, Kraljic I, Trnski D, et al. Immunohistochemical staining and serotest markers during development of a sarcomatoid and small cell prostate tumor. Anticancer Res 1994; 14:2151.

151. Hagood PG, Johnson FE, Bedrossian CW, et al. Small cell carcinoma of the prostate. Cancer 1991; 67:1046.

152. Watanabe K, Hoshi N, Hiraki H, et al. Neoplastic endocrine cells in prostatic carcinoma: a case report with immunocytochemical and electron microscopic findings. Fukushima J Med Sci 1995; 41:51.

153. Iwamura M, Abrahamsson PA, Schoen S, et al. Immunoreactive parathyroid hormone-related protein is present in human seminal plasma and is of prostate origin. J Androl 1994; 15:410.

154. Oesterling JE, Hauzeur CG, Farrow GM. Small cell anaplastic carcinoma of the prostate: a clinical, pathological and immunohistological study of 27 patients. J Urol 1992; 147:804.

155. Schron DS, Gipson T, Mendelsohn G. The histogenesis of small cell carcinoma of the prostate. An immunohistochemical study. Cancer 1984; 53:2478.

156. Yu HM, Frank DE, Zhang J, et al. Basal prostate epithelial cells stimulate the migration of prostate cancer cells. Mol Carcinog 2004; 41:85.

157. Pollack A, Cowen D, Troncoso P, et al. Molecular markers of outcome after radiotherapy in patients with prostate carcinoma: Ki-67, bcl-2, bax, and bcl-x. Cancer 2003; 97:1630.

158. Xing N, Qian J, Bostwick D, et al. Neuroendocrine cells in human prostate over-express the anti-apoptosis protein survivin. Prostate 2001; 48:7.

159. Bostwick DG, Hossain D, Qian J, et al. Phyllodes tumor of the prostate: long-term followup study of 23 cases. J Urol 2004; 172:894.

160. di Sant'Agnese PA. Neuroendocrine differentiation in prostatic adenocarcinoma does not represent true Paneth cell differentiation [editorial; comment]. Hum Pathol 1994; 25:115.

161. di Sant'Agnese PA. Neuroendocrine differentiation in human prostatic carcinoma. Hum Pathol 1992; 23:287.

162. di Sant'Agnese PA. Neuroendocrine differentiation in carcinoma of the prostate. Diagnostic, prognostic, and therapeutic implications. Cancer 1992; 70:254.

163. di Sant'Agnese PA, Cockett AT. Neuroendocrine differentiation in prostatic malignancy. Cancer 1996; 78:357.

164. Di Sant'Agnese PA, Cockett AT. The prostatic endocrine-paracrine (neuroendocrine) regulatory system and neuroendocrine differentiation in prostatic carcinoma: a review and future directions in basic research [see comments]. J Urol 1994; 152:1927.

165. di Sant'Agnese PA. Neuroendocrine differentiation in prostatic carcinoma: an update. Prostate Suppl 1998; 8:74.

166. di Sant'Agnese PA. Neuroendocrine cells of the prostate and neuroendocrine differentiation in prostatic carcinoma: a review of morphologic aspects. Urology 1998; 51:121.

167. Bostwick DG, Myers RP, Oesterling JE. Staging of prostate cancer. Semin Surg Oncol 1994; 10:60.

168. Dizeyi N, Bjartell A, Nilsson E, et al. Expression of serotonin receptors and role of serotonin in human prostate cancer tissue and cell lines. Prostate 2004; 59:328.

169. Abrahamsson PA, Cockett AT, di Sant'Agnese PA. Prognostic significance of neuroendocrine differentiation in clinically localized prostatic carcinoma. Prostate Suppl 1998; 8:37.

170. Berner A, Waere H, Nesland JM, et al. DNA ploidy, serum prostate specific antigen, histological grade and immunohistochemistry as predictive parameters of lymph node metastases in T1-T3/M0 prostatic adenocarcinoma. Br J Urol 1995; 75:26.

171. Cheville JC, Dundore PA, Nascimento AG, et al. Leiomyosarcoma of the prostate. Report of 23 cases. Cancer 1995; 76:1422.

172. Bubendorf L, Sauter G, Moch H, et al. Ki67 labelling index: an independent predictor of progression in prostate cancer treated by radical prostatectomy. J Pathol 1996; 178:437.

173. Casella R, Bubendorf L, Sauter G, et al. Focal neuroendocrine differentiation lacks prognostic significance in prostate core needle biopsies. J Urol 1998; 160:406.

174. Krupski T, Petroni GR, Frierson HF Jr, et al. Microvessel density, p53, retinoblastoma, and chromogranin A immunohistochemistry as predictors of disease-specific survival following radical prostatectomy for carcinoma of the prostate. Urology 2000; 55:743.

175. Noordzij MA, van der Kwast TH, van Steenbrugge GJ, et al. Determination of Ki-67 defined growth fraction by monoclonal antibody MIB-1 in formalin-fixed, paraffin-embedded prostatic cancer tissues. Prostate 1995; 27:154.

176. van de Voorde W, Baldewijns M, Lauweryns J. Florid basal cell hyperplasia of the prostate. Histopathology 1994; 24:341.

177. Weinstein MH, Partin AW, Veltri RW, et al. Neuroendocrine differentiation in prostate cancer: enhanced prediction of progression after radical prostatectomy. Hum Pathol 1996; 27:683.

178. Aprikian AG, Cordon-Cardo C, Fair WR, et al. Characterization of neuroendocrine differentiation in human benign prostate and prostatic adenocarcinoma. Cancer 1993; 71:3952.

179. Bostwick DG, Qian J, Civantos F, et al. Does finasteride alter the pathology of the prostate and cancer grading? Clin Prostate Cancer 2004; 2:228.

180. Allen SM. An enzyme linked immunosorbent assay (ELISA) for detection of seminal fluid using a monoclonal antibody to prostatic acid phosphatase. J Immunoassay 1995; 16:297.

181. Theodorescu D, Broder SR, Boyd JC, et al. Cathepsin D and chromogranin A as predictors of long term disease specific survival after radical prostatectomy for localized carcinoma of the prostate. Cancer 1997; 80:2109.

182. Yu DS, Hsieh DS, Chen HI, et al. The expression of neuropeptides in hyperplastic and malignant prostate tissue and its possible clinical implications. J Urol 2001; 166:871.

183. el-Demiry MI, Hargreave TB, Busuttil A, et al. Lymphocyte sub-populations in the male genital tract. Br J Urol 1985; 57:769.

184. Theyer G, Kramer G, Assmann I, et al. Phenotypic characterization of infiltrating leukocytes in benign prostatic hyperplasia. Lab Invest 1992; 66:96.

185. McArdle PA, Canna K, McMillan DC, et al. The relationship between T-lymphocyte subset infiltration and survival in patients with prostate cancer. Br J Cancer 2004; 91:541.

186. Nemoto R, Kawamura H, Miyakawa I, et al. Immunohistochemical detection of proliferating cell nuclear antigen (PCNA)/cyclin in human prostate adenocarcinoma. J Urol 1993; 149:165.

187. Accetta PA, Gardner WA Jr. Adenosquamous carcinoma of prostate. Urology 1983; 22:73.

188. Botticelli AR, Casali AM, Botticelli L, et al. Immunohistochemical detection of cell-cycle associated markers on paraffin embedded and formalin fixed needle biopsies of prostate cancer: correlation of p120 protein expression with AgNOR, PCNA/cyclin, Ki-67/MIB1 proliferation-scores and Gleason gradings. Eur J Histochem 1998; 42:41.

189. Cher ML, Chew K, Rosenau W, et al. Cellular proliferation in prostatic adenocarcinoma as assessed by bromodeoxyuridine uptake and Ki-67 and PCNA expression. Prostate 1995; 26:87.

190. Helpap B. Cell kinetic studies on prostatic intraepithelial neoplasia (PIN) and atypical adenomatous hyperplasia (AAH) of the prostate. Pathol Res Pract 1995; 191:904.

191. Hepburn PJ, Glynne-Jones E, Goddard L, et al. Cell proliferation in prostatic carcinoma: comparative analysis of Ki-67, MIB-1 and PCNA. Histochem J 1995; 27:196.

192. Igawa M, Urakami S, Shiina H, et al. Association of nm23 protein levels in human prostates with proliferating cell nuclear antigen expression at autopsy. Eur Urol 1996; 30:383.

193. Ljung G, Egevad L, Norberg M, et al. Assessment of proliferation indicators in residual prostatic adenocarcinoma cells after radical external beam radiotherapy. Prostate 1996; 29:303.

194. Montironi R, Galluzzi CM, Diamanti L, et al. Proliferating cell nuclear antigen (PCNA) in prostatic invasive adenocarcinoma. Is the proliferation state in the marginal zone of the tumour higher than in the central part? Anticancer Res 1993; 13:129.

195. Naito S, Sakamoto N, Kotoh S, et al. Proliferating cell nuclear antigen in needle biopsy specimens of prostatic carcinoma. Eur Urol 1994; 26:164.

196. Sakr WA, Sarkar FH, Sreepathi P, et al. Measurement of cellular proliferation in human prostate by AgNOR, PCNA, and SPF. Prostate 1993; 22:147.

197. Visakorpi T, Kallioniemi OP, Koivula T, et al. Expression of epidermal growth factor receptor and ERBB2 (HER-2/Neu) oncoprotein in prostatic carcinomas. Mod Pathol 1992; 5:643.

198. Limas C, Frizelle SP. Proliferative activity in benign and neoplastic prostatic epithelium. J Pathol 1994; 174:201.

199. Carroll PR, Waldman FM, Rosenau W, et al. Cell proliferation in prostatic adenocarcinoma: in vitro measurement by 5-bromodeoxyuridine incorporation and proliferating cell nuclear antigen expression. J Urol 1993; 149:403.

200. Idikio HA. Expression of proliferating cell nuclear antigen

in node-negative human prostate cancer. Anticancer Res 1996; 16:2607.
201. Minardi D, Galosi AB, Giannulis I, et al. Comparison of proliferating cell nuclear antigen immunostaining in lymph node metastases and primary prostate adenocarcinoma after neoadjuvant androgen deprivation therapy. Scand J Urol Nephrol 2004; 38:19.
202. Coetzee LJ, Layfield LJ, Hars V, et al. Proliferative index determination in prostatic carcinoma tissue: is there any additional prognostic value greater than that of Gleason score, ploidy and pathological stage? [see comments]. J Urol 1997; 157:214.
203. Sadi MV, Barrack ER. Androgen receptors and growth fraction in metastatic prostate cancer as predictors of time to tumour progression after hormonal therapy. Cancer Surv 1991; 11:195.
204. Glynne-Jones E, Goddard L, Harper ME. Comparative analysis of mRNA and protein expression for epidermal growth factor receptor and ligands relative to the proliferative index in human prostate tissue. Hum Pathol 1996; 27:688.
205. Moul JW. Angiogenesis, p53, bcl-2 and Ki-67 in the progression of prostate cancer after radical prostatectomy. Eur Urol 1999; 35:399.
206. Thompson SJ, Mellon K, Charlton RG, et al. P53 and Ki-67 immunoreactivity in human prostate cancer and benign hyperplasia. Br J Urol 1992; 69:609.
207. Henke RP, Kruger E, Ayhan N, et al. Numerical chromosomal aberrations in prostate cancer: correlation with morphology and cell kinetics. Virchows Arch A Pathol Anat Histopathol 1993; 422:61.
208. Aaltomaa S, Lipponen P, Vesalainen S, et al. Value of Ki-67 immunolabelling as a prognostic factor in prostate cancer. Eur Urol 1997; 32:410.
209. Moul JW, Maygarden SJ, Ware JL, et al. Cathepsin D and epidermal growth factor receptor immunohistochemistry does not predict recurrence of prostate cancer in patients undergoing radical prostatectomy. J Urol 1996; 155:982.
210. Bettencourt MC, Bauer JJ, Sesterhenn IA, et al. Ki-67 expression is a prognostic marker of prostate cancer recurrence after radical prostatectomy [see comments]. J Urol 1996; 156:1064.
211. Mashal RD, Lester S, Corless C, et al. Expression of cell cycle-regulated proteins in prostate cancer. Cancer Res 1996; 56:4159.
212. Li R, Heydon K, Hammond ME, et al. Ki-67 staining index predicts distant metastasis and survival in locally advanced prostate cancer treated with radiotherapy: an analysis of patients in radiation therapy oncology group protocol 86-10. Clin Cancer Res 2004; 10:4118.
213. Verhagen AP, Aalders TW, Ramaekers FC, et al. Differential expression of keratins in the basal and luminal compartments of rat prostatic epithelium during degeneration and regeneration. Prostate 1988; 13:25.
214. Soeffing WJ, Timms BG. Localization of androgen receptor and cell-specific cytokeratins in basal cells of rat ventral prostate. J Androl 1995; 16:197.
215. Deshmukh N, Scotson J, Dodson AR, et al. Differential expression of acidic and basic fibroblast growth factors in benign prostatic hyperplasia identified by immunohistochemistry. Br J Urol 1997; 80:869.
216. Foster BA, Gingrich JR, Kwon ED, et al. Characterization of prostatic epithelial cell lines derived from transgenic adenocarcinoma of the mouse prostate (TRAMP) model. Cancer Res 1997; 57:3325.
217. Robinson EJ, Neal DE, Collins AT. Basal cells are progenitors of luminal cells in primary cultures of differentiating human prostatic epithelium. Prostate 1998; 37:149.
218. Wang X, Hsieh JT. Androgen repression of cytokeratin gene expression during rat prostate differentiation: evidence for an epithelial stem cell-associated marker. Chin Med Sci J 1994; 9:237.
219. Verhagen AP, Ramaekers FC, Aalders TW, et al. Colocalization of basal and luminal cell-type cytokeratins in human prostate cancer. Cancer Res 1992; 52:6182.
220. Sherwood ER, Theyer G, Steiner G, et al. Differential expression of specific cytokeratin polypeptides in the basal and luminal epithelia of the human prostate. Prostate 1991; 18:303.
221. Oberneder R, Riesenberg R, Kriegmair M, et al. Immunocytochemical detection and phenotypic characterization of micrometastatic tumour cells in bone marrow of patients with prostate cancer. Urol Res 1994; 22:3.
222. De Marzo AM, Marchi VL, Epstein JI, et al. Proliferative inflammatory atrophy of the prostate: implications for prostatic carcinogenesis. Am J Pathol 1999; 155:1985.
223. Linder S, Havelka AM, Ueno T, et al. Determining tumor

apoptosis and necrosis in patient serum using cytokeratin 18 as a biomarker. Cancer Lett 2004; 214:1.
224. Fuchs ME, Brawer MK, Rennels MA, et al. The relationship of basement membrane to histologic grade of human prostatic carcinoma. Mod Pathol 1989; 2:105.
225. Sinha AA, Gleason DF, Wilson MJ, et al. Immunohistochemical localization of laminin in the basement membranes of normal, hyperplastic, and neoplastic human prostate. Prostate 1989; 15:299.
226. Nagle RB, Knox JD, Wolf C, et al. Adhesion molecules, extracellular matrix, and proteases in prostate carcinoma. J Cell Biochem Suppl 1994; 19:232.
227. Xue Y, Li J, Latijnhouwers MA, et al. Expression of periglandular tenascin-C and basement membrane laminin in normal prostate, benign prostatic hyperplasia and prostate carcinoma. Br J Urol 1998; 81:844.
228. Nagakawa O, Akashi T, Hayakawa Y, et al. Differential expression of integrin subunits in DU-145/AR prostate cancer cells. Oncol Rep 2004; 12:837.
229. Murant SJ, Handley J, Stower M, et al. Co-ordinated changes in expression of cell adhesion molecules in prostate cancer. Eur J Cancer 1997; 33:263.
230. Rabinovitz I, Nagle RB, Cress AE. Integrin alpha 6 expression in human prostate carcinoma cells is associated with a migratory and invasive phenotype in vitro and in vivo. Clin Exp Metastasis 1995; 13:481.
231. Nagle RB, Hao J, Knox JD, et al. Expression of hemidesmosomal and extracellular matrix proteins by normal and malignant human prostate tissue. Am J Pathol 1995; 146:1498.
232. Knox JD, Mack CF, Powell WC, et al. Prostate tumor cell invasion: a comparison of orthotopic and ectopic models. Invasion Metastasis 1993; 13:325.
233. Hao J, Yang Y, McDaniel KM, et al. Differential expression of laminin 5 (alpha 3 beta 3 gamma 2) by human malignant and normal prostate. Am J Pathol 1996; 149:1341.
234. Dedhar S, Saulnier R, Nagle R, et al. Specific alterations in the expression of alpha 3 beta 1 and alpha 6 beta 4 integrins in highly invasive and metastatic variants of human prostate carcinoma cells selected by in vitro invasion through reconstituted basement membrane. Clin Exp Metastasis 1993; 11:391.
235. Trikha M, Raso E, Cai Y, et al. Role of alphaII(b)beta3 integrin in prostate cancer metastasis. Prostate 1998; 35:185.
236. Moro L, Greco M, Ditonno P, et al. Transcriptional regulation of the beta1C integrin splice variant in human prostate adenocarcinoma. Int J Oncol 2003; 23:1601.
237. Fornaro M, Manzotti M, Tallini G, et al. Beta1C integrin in epithelial cells correlates with a nonproliferative phenotype: forced expression of beta1C inhibits prostate epithelial cell proliferation. Am J Pathol 1998; 153:1079.
238. Fornaro M, Tallini G, Bofetiado CJ, et al. Down-regulation of beta 1C integrin, an inhibitor of cell proliferation, in prostate carcinoma. Am J Pathol 1996; 149:765.
239. von Bredow DC, Nagle RB, Bowden GT, et al. Cleavage of beta 4 integrin by matrilysin. Exp Cell Res 1997; 236:341.
240. Tantivejkul K, Kalikin LM, Pienta KJ. Dynamic process of prostate cancer metastasis to bone. J Cell Biochem 2004; 91:706.
241. Tozawa K, Yamada Y, Kawai N, et al. Osteopontin expression in prostate cancer and benign prostatic hyperplasia. Urol Int 1999; 62:155.
242. Thalmann GN, Sikes RA, Devoll RE, et al. Osteopontin: possible role in prostate cancer progression. Clin Cancer Res 1999; 5:2271.
243. Devoll RE, Pinero GJ, Appelbaum ER, et al. Improved immunohistochemical staining of osteopontin (OPN) in paraffin-embedded archival bone specimens following antigen retrieval: anti-human OPN antibody recognizes multiple molecular forms. Calcif Tissue Int 1997; 60:380.
244. Brown LF, Papadopoulos-Sergiou A, Berse B, et al. Osteopontin expression and distribution in human carcinomas. Am J Pathol 1994; 145:610.
245. Oldberg A, Antonsson P, Hedbom E, et al. Structure and function of extracellular matrix proteoglycans. Biochem Soc Trans 1990; 18:789.
246. Angelucci A, Festuccia C, Gravina GL, et al. Osteopontin enhances the cell proliferation induced by the epidermal growth factor in human prostate cancer cells. Prostate 2004; 59:157.
247. Coppola D, Szabo M, Boulware D, et al. Correlation of osteopontin protein expression and pathological stage across a wide variety of tumor histologies. Clin Cancer Res 2004; 10:184.
248. Myers JC, Li D, Bageris A, et al. Biochemical and immunohistochemical characterization of human type XIX defines a

249. Petrioli R, Rossi S, Caniggia M, et al. Analysis of biochemical bone markers as prognostic factors for survival in patients with hormone-resistant prostate cancer and bone metastases. Urology 2004; 63:321.

250. Dehan P, Waltregny D, Beschin A, et al. Loss of type IV collagen alpha 5 and alpha 6 chains in human invasive prostate carcinomas. Am J Pathol 1997; 151:1097.

251. Suer S, Sonmez H, Karaaslan I, et al. Tissue sialic acid and fibronectin levels in human prostatic cancer. Cancer Lett 1996; 99:135.

252. Murdoch AD, Liu B, Schwarting R, et al. Widespread expression of perlecan proteoglycan in basement membranes and extracellular matrices of human tissues as detected by a novel monoclonal antibody against domain III and by in situ hybridization. J Histochem Cytochem 1994; 42:239.

253. Schenk S, Muser J, Vollmer G, et al. Tenascin-C in serum: a questionable tumor marker. Int J Cancer 1995; 61:443.

254. Shiraishi T, Kato H, Komada S, et al. Tenascin expression and postnatal development of the human prostate. Int J Dev Biol 1994; 38:391.

255. Ibrahim SN, Lightner VA, Ventimiglia JB, et al. Tenascin expression in prostatic hyperplasia, intraepithelial neoplasia, and carcinoma. Hum Pathol 1993; 24:982.

256. Xue Y, Smedts F, Latijnhouwers MA, et al. Tenascin-C expression in prostatic intraepithelial neoplasia (PIN): a marker of progression? Anticancer Res 1998; 18:2679.

257. Koksal IT, Ozcan F, Kilicaslan I, et al. Expression of E-cadherin in prostate cancer in formalin-fixed, paraffin-embedded tissues: correlation with pathological features. Pathology 2002; 34:233.

258. Bryden AA, Freemont AJ, Clarke NW, et al. Paradoxical expression of E-cadherin in prostatic bone metastases. Br J Urol Int 1999; 84:1032.

259. Brewster SF, Oxley JD, Trivella M, et al. Preoperative p53, bcl-2, CD44 and E-cadherin immunohistochemistry as predictors of biochemical relapse after radical prostatectomy. J Urol 1999; 161:1238.

260. Bussemakers MJ, van Moorselaar RJ, Giroldi LA, et al. Decreased expression of E-cadherin in the progression of rat prostatic cancer. Cancer Res 1992; 52:2916.

261. Cheng L, Nagabhushan M, Pretlow TP, et al. Expression of E-cadherin in primary and metastatic prostate cancer. Am J Pathol 1996; 148:1375.

262. De Marzo AM, Knudsen B, Chan-Tack K, et al. E-cadherin expression as a marker of tumor aggressiveness in routinely processed radical prostatectomy specimens. Urology 1999; 53:707.

263. Giroldi LA, Bringuier PP, Schalken JA. Defective E-cadherin function in urological cancers: clinical implications and molecular mechanisms. Invasion Metastasis 1994; 14:71.

264. Jarrard DF, Paul R, van Bokhoven A, et al. P-Cadherin is a basal cell-specific epithelial marker that is not expressed in prostate cancer. Clin Cancer Res 1997; 3:2121.

265. Kuczyk M, Serth J, Machtens S, et al. Expression of Ecadherin in primary prostate cancer: correlation with clinical features. Br J Urol 1998; 81:406.

266. Morita N, Uemura H, Tsumatani K, et al. E-cadherin and alpha-, beta- and gamma-catenin expression in prostate cancers: correlation with tumour invasion. Br J Cancer 1999; 79:1879.

267. Pan Y, Matsuyama H, Wang N, et al. Chromosome 16q24 deletion and decreased E-cadherin expression: possible association with metastatic potential in prostate cancer. Prostate 1998; 36:31.

268. Rembrink K, Otto T, Goepel M, et al. E-cadherin: expression of the epithelial cell-cell-adhesion molecule in prostatic carcinoma and normal prostate. Investig Urol 1994; 5:24.

269. Ross JS, Figge HL, Bui HX, et al. E-cadherin expression in prostatic carcinoma biopsies: correlation with tumor grade, DNA content, pathologic stage, and clinical outcome. Mod Pathol 1994; 7:835.

270. Ruijter E, van de Kaa C, Aalders T, et al. Heterogeneous expression of E-cadherin and p53 in prostate cancer: clinical implications. BIOMED-II Markers for Prostate Cancer Study Group. Mod Pathol 1998; 11:276.

271. Umbas R, Schalken JA, Aalders TW, et al. Expression of the cellular adhesion molecule E-cadherin is reduced or absent in high-grade prostate cancer. Cancer Res 1992; 52:5104.

272. Umbas R, Isaacs WB, Bringuier PP, et al. Relation between aberrant alpha-catenin expression and loss of E-cadherin function in prostate cancer. Int J Cancer 1997; 74:374.

273. Schalken J. Molecular diagnostics and therapy of prostate cancer: new avenues. Eur Urol 1998; 34:3.

274. Rennie PS, Nelson CC. Epigenetic mechanisms for progres-

sion of prostate cancer. Cancer Metastasis Rev 1998; 17:401.

275. Richmond PJ, Karayiannakis AJ, Nagafuchi A, et al. Aberrant E-cadherin and alpha-catenin expression in prostate cancer: correlation with patient survival. Cancer Res 1997; 57:3189.

276. Otto T, Rembrink K, Goepel M, et al. E-cadherin: a marker for differentiation and invasiveness in prostatic carcinoma. Urol Res 1993; 21:359.

277. Cohen MB, Griebling TL, Ahaghotu CA, et al. Cellular adhesion molecules in urologic malignancies. Am J Clin Pathol 1997; 107:56.

278. Schalken JA. New perspectives in the treatment of prostate cancer. Eur Urol 1997; 31:20.

279. Patriarca C, Petrella D, Campo B, et al. Elevated E-cadherin and alpha/beta-catenin expression after androgen deprivation therapy in prostate adenocarcinoma. Pathol Res Pract 2003; 199:659.

280. Soler AP, Harner GD, Knudsen KA, et al. Expression of P-cadherin identifies prostate-specific-antigen-negative cells in epithelial tissues of male sexual accessory organs and in prostatic carcinomas. Implications for prostate cancer biology. Am J Pathol 1997; 151:471.

281. Jonsson BA, Adami HO, Hagglund M, et al. 160C/A polymorphism in the E-cadherin gene promoter and risk of hereditary, familial and sporadic prostate cancer. Int J Cancer 2004; 109:348.

282. Bourrguignon LY, Iida N, Welsh CF, et al. Involvement of CD44 and its variant isoforms in membrane–cytoskeleton interaction, cell adhesion and tumor metastasis. J Neurooncol 1995; 26:201.

283. Furuya Y, Isaacs JT. Proliferation-dependent vs. independent programmed cell death of prostatic cancer cells involves distinct gene regulation. Prostate 1994; 25:301.

284. Woodson K, Hayes R, Wideroff L, et al. Hypermethylation of GSTP1, CD44, and E-cadherin genes in prostate cancer among US blacks and whites. Prostate 2003; 55:199.

285. Kauffman EC, Robinson VL, Stadler WM, et al. Metastasis suppression: the evolving role of metastasis suppressor genes for regulating cancer cell growth at the secondary site. J Urol 2003; 169:1122.

286. Vis AN, van Rhijn BW, Noordzij MA, et al. Value of tissue markers p27(kip1), MIB-1, and CD44s for the pre-operative prediction of tumour features in screen-detected prostate cancer. J Pathol 2002; 197:148.

287. Ekici S, Ayhan A, Kendi S, et al. Determination of prognosis in patients with prostate cancer treated with radical prostatectomy: prognostic value of CD44v6 score. J Urol 2002; 167:2037.

288. Kramer G, Steiner G, Fodinger D, et al. High expression of a CD38-like molecule in normal prostatic epithelium and its differential loss in benign and malignant disease. J Urol 1995; 154:1636.

289. Al-Ejeh F, Croucher D, Ranson M. Kinetic analysis of plasminogen activator inhibitor type-2: urokinase complex formation and subsequent internalisation by carcinoma cell lines. Exp Cell Res 2004; 297:259.

290. Schmitt M, Janicke F, Moniwa N, et al. Tumor-associated urokinase-type plasminogen activator: biological and clinical significance. Biol Chem Hoppe Seyler 1992; 373:611.

291. Frenette G, Tremblay RR, Lazure C, et al. Prostatic kallikrein hK2, but not prostate-specific antigen (hK3), activates single-chain urokinase-type plasminogen activator. Int J Cancer 1997; 71:897.

292. Reese JH, McNeal JE, Redwine EA, et al. Tissue type plasminogen activator as a marker for functional zones, within the human prostate gland. Prostate 1988; 12:47.

293. Lyon PB, See WA, Xu Y, et al. Diversity and modulation of plasminogen activator activity in human prostate carcinoma cell lines. Prostate 1995; 27:179.

294. Van Veldhuizen PJ, Sadasivan R, Cherian R, et al. Urokinase-type plasminogen activator expression in human prostate carcinomas. Am J Med Sci 1996; 312:8.

295. Stearns ME, Wang M, Stearns M. IL-10 blocks collagen IV invasion by 'invasion stimulating factor' activated PC-3 ML cells: upregulation of TIMP-1 expression. Oncol Res 1995; 7:157.

296. Forbes K, Gillette K, Kelley LA, et al. Increased levels of urokinase plasminogen activator receptor in prostate cancer cells derived from repeated metastasis. World J Urol 2004; 22:67.

297. Hamdy FC, Fadlon EJ, Cottam D, et al. Matrix metalloproteinase 9 expression in primary human prostatic adenocarcinoma and benign prostatic hyperplasia. Br J Cancer 1994; 69:177.

298. Still K, Robson CN, Autzen P, et al. Localization and quantification of mRNA for matrix metalloproteinase-2 (MMP-2) and tissue inhibitor of matrix metalloproteinase-2 (TIMP-2)

298. in human benign and malignant prostatic tissue. Prostate 2000; 42:18.

299. Mohler JL, Chen Y, Hamil K, et al. Androgen and glucocorticoid receptors in the stroma and epithelium of prostatic hyperplasia and carcinoma. Clin Cancer Res 1996; 2:889.

300. Sinha AA, Quast BJ, Wilson MJ, et al. Prediction of pelvic lymph node metastasis by the ratio of cathepsin B to stefin A in patients with prostate carcinoma. Cancer 2002; 94:3141.

301. Sinha AA, Quast BJ, Wilson MJ, et al. Ratio of cathepsin B to stefin A identifies heterogeneity within Gleason histologic scores for human prostate cancer. Prostate 2001; 48:274.

302. Sinha AA, Jamuar MP, Wilson MJ, et al. Plasma membrane association of cathepsin B in human prostate cancer: biochemical and immunogold electron microscopic analysis. Prostate 2001; 49:172.

303. Ekici S, Cerwinka WH, Duncan R, et al. Comparison of the prognostic potential of hyaluronic acid, hyaluronidase (HYAL-1), CD44v6 and microvessel density for prostate cancer. Int J Cancer 2004; 112:121.

304. Alam TN, O'Hare MJ, Laczko I, et al. Differential expression of CD44 during human prostate epithelial cell differentiation. J Histochem Cytochem 2004; 52:1083.

305. Olapade-Olaopa EO, Muronda CA, MacKay EH, et al. Androgen receptor protein expression in prostatic tissues in black and Caucasian men. Prostate 2004; 59:460.

306. Mizokami A, Koh E, Fujita H, et al. The adrenal androgen androstenediol is present in prostate cancer tissue after androgen deprivation therapy and activates mutated androgen receptor. Cancer Res 2004; 64:765.

307. Mohler JL, Gregory CW, Ford OH. 3rd, et al. The androgen axis in recurrent prostate cancer. Clin Cancer Res 2004; 10: 440.

308. Di Lorenzo G, Autorino R, De Laurentiis M, et al. HER-2/neu receptor in prostate cancer development and progression to androgen independence. Tumori 2004; 90:163.

309. Siegal JA, Yu E, Brawer MK. Topography of neovascularity in human prostate carcinoma. Cancer 1995; 75:2545.

310. Weidner N. Intratumoral vascularity as a prognostic factor in cancers of the urogenital tract. Eur J Cancer 1996; 32A:2506.

311. Bostwick DG, Grignon DJ, Hammond ME, et al. Prognostic factors in prostate cancer. College of American Pathologists Consensus Statement 1999. Arch Pathol Lab Med 2000; 124: 995.

312. Burchardt M, Burchardt T, Chen MW, et al. Vascular endothelial growth factor-A expression in the rat ventral prostate gland and the early effects of castration. Prostate 2000; 43: 184.

313. Trojan L, Thomas D, Friedrich D, et al. Expression of different vascular endothelial markers in prostate cancer and BPH tissue: an immunohistochemical and clinical evaluation. Anticancer Res 2004; 24:1651.

314. Abdulkadir SA, Carvalhal GF, Kaleem Z, et al. Tissue factor expression and angiogenesis in human prostate carcinoma [see comments]. Hum Pathol 2000; 31:443.

315. Borre M, Nerstrom B, Overgaard J. Association between immunohistochemical expression of vascular endothelial growth factor (VEGF), VEGF-expressing neuroendocrine-differentiated tumor cells, and outcome in prostate cancer patients subjected to watchful waiting [In Process Citation]. Clin Cancer Res 2000; 6:1882.

316. Brawer MK, Deering RE, Brown M, et al. Predictors of pathologic stage in prostatic carcinoma. The role of neovascularity. Cancer 1994; 73 678.

317. Brawer MK. Quantitative microvessel density. A staging and prognostic marker for human prostatic carcinoma. Cancer 1996; 78:345.

318. Eberhard A, Kahlert S, Goede V, et al. Heterogeneity of angiogenesis and blood vessel maturation in human tumors: implications for antiangiogenic tumor therapies. Cancer Res 2000; 60:1388.

319. Gould VE, Doljanskaia V, Gooch G, et al. Immunolocalization of glycoprotein A-80 in prostatic carcinoma and prostatic intraepithelial neoplasia. Hum Pathol 1996; 27:547.

320. Yorukoglu K, Sagol O, Ozkara E, et al. Comparison of microvascularization in diagnostic needle biopsies and radical prostatectomies in prostate carcinoma. Eur Urol 1999; 35: 109.

321. Shiraishi T, Watanabe M, Muneyuki T, et al. A clinicopathological study of p53, p21 (WAF1/CIP1) and cyclin D1 expression in human prostate cancers. Urol Int 1998; 61:90.

322. Deering RE, Bigler SA, Brown M, et al. Microvascularity in benign prostatic hyperplasia. Prostate 1995; 26:111.

323. Bigler SA, Deering RE, Brawer MK. Comparison of microscopic vascularity in benign and malignant prostate tissue. Hum Pathol 1993; 24:220.

324. Folkman J, Watson K, Ingber D. et al. Induction of angio-

genesis during the transition from hyperplasia to neoplasia. Nature 1989; 339:58.

325. Montironi R, Diamanti L, Thompson D, et al. Analysis of the capillary architecture in the precursors of prostate cancer: recent findings and new concepts. Eur Urol 1996; 30:191.

326. Barth PJ, Weingartner K, Kohler HH, et al. Assessment of the vascularization in prostatic carcinoma: a morphometric investigation. Hum Pathol 1996; 27:1306.

327. Offersen BV, Borre M, Overgaard J. Quantification of angiogenesis as a prognostic marker in human carcinomas: a critical evaluation of histopathological methods for estimation of vascular density. Eur J Cancer 2003; 39:881.

328. Volavsek M, Masera A, Ovcak Z. Tumor neoangiogenesis in rebiopsied patients with prostatic carcinoma. Acta Med Croatica 1999; 53:73.

329. Salomao DR, Graham SD, Bostwick DG. Microvascular invasion in prostate cancer correlates with pathologic stage. Arch Pathol Lab Med 1995; 119:1050.

330. Vesalainen S, Lipponen P, Talja M, et al. Tumor vascularity and basement membrane structure as prognostic factors in T1-2MO prostatic adenocarcinoma. Anticancer Res 1994; 14:709.

331. Hall MC, Troncoso P, Pollack A, et al. Significance of tumor angiogenesis in clinically localized prostate carcinoma treated with external beam radiotherapy. Urology 1994; 44:869.

332. Fregene TA, Khanuja PS, Noto AC, et al. Tumor-associated angiogenesis in prostate cancer. Anticancer Res 1993; 13:2377.

333. Wakui S, Furusato M, Itoh T, et al. Tumour angiogenesis in prostatic carcinoma with and without bone marrow metastasis: a morphometric study. J Pathol 1992; 168:257.

334. Furusato M, Wakui S, Sasaki H, et al. Tumour angiogenesis in latent prostatic carcinoma. Br J Cancer 1994; 70:1244.

335. Weidner N, Carroll PR, Flax J, et al. Tumor angiogenesis correlates with metastasis in invasive prostate carcinoma. Am J Pathol 1993; 143:401.

336. Bostwick DG, Wheeler TM, Blute M, et al. Optimized microvessel density analysis improves prediction of cancer stage from prostate needle biopsies. Urology 1996; 48:47.

337. Silberman MA, Partin AW, Veltri RW, et al. Tumor angiogenesis correlates with progression after radical prostatectomy but not with pathologic stage in Gleason sum 5 to 7 adenocarcinoma of the prostate. Cancer 1997; 79:772.

338. Rogatsch H, Hittmair A, Reissigl A, et al. Microvessel density in core biopsies of prostatic adenocarcinoma: a stage predictor? J Pathol 1997; 182:205.

339. Rubin MA, Buyyounouski M, Bagiella E, et al. Microvessel density in prostate cancer: lack of correlation with tumor grade, pathologic stage, and clinical outcome. Urology 1999; 53:542.

340. Grossfeld GD, Carroll PR, Lindeman N, et al. Thrombospondin-1 expression in patients with pathologic stage T3 prostate cancer undergoing radical prostatectomy: association with p53 alterations, tumor angiogenesis, and tumor progression. Urology 2002; 59:97.

341. Erbersdobler A, Fritz H, Schnoger S, et al. Tumour grade, proliferation, apoptosis, microvessel density, p53, and bcl-2 in prostate cancers: differences between tumours located in the transition zone and in the peripheral zone. Eur Urol 2002; 41:40.

342. Offersen BV, Borre M, Overgaard J. Immunohistochemical determination of tumor angiogenesis measured by the maximal microvessel density in human prostate cancer. APMIS 1998; 106:463.

343. Tilley WD, Lim-Tio SS, Horsfall DJ, et al. Detection of discrete androgen receptor epitopes in prostate cancer by immunostaining: measurement by color video image analysis. Cancer Res 1994; 54:4096.

344. Bostwick DG, Dousa MK, Crawford BG, et al. Neuroendocrine differentiation in prostatic intraepithelial neoplasia and adenocarcinoma. Am J Surg Pathol 1994; 18:1240.

345. Cina SJ, Silberman MA, Kahane H, et al. Diagnosis of Cowper's glands on prostate needle biopsy. Am J Surg Pathol 1997; 21:550.

346. Bostwick DG. Progression of prostatic intraepithelial neoplasia to early invasive adenocarcinoma. Eur Urol 1996; 30:145.

347. Shabisgh A, Tanji N, D'Agati V, et al. Early effects of castration on the vascular system of the rat ventral prostate gland. Endocrinology 1999; 140:1920.

348. de la Taille A, Katz AE, Bagiella E, et al. Microvessel density as a predictor of PSA recurrence after radical prostatectomy. A comparison of CD34 and CD31. Am J Clin Pathol 2000; 113:555.

349. Strohmeyer D, Rossing C, Strauss F, et al. Tumor angiogenesis is associated with progression after radical prostatectomy

in pT2/pT3 prostate cancer. Prostate 2000; 42:26.

350. Gettman MT, Pacelli A, Slezak J, et al. Role of microvessel density in predicting recurrence in pathologic stage T3 prostatic adenocarcinoma. Urology 1999; 54:479.

351. Cetinkaya M, Gunce S, Ulusoy E, et al. Relationship between prostate specific antigen density, microvessel density and prostatic volume in benign prostatic hyperplasia and advanced prostatic carcinoma. Int Urol Nephrol 1998; 30:581.

352. Borre M, Offersen BV, Nerstrom B, et al. Microvessel density predicts survival in prostate cancer patients subjected to watchful waiting. Br J Cancer 1998; 78:940.

353. Gettman MT, Bergstralh EJ, Blute M, et al. Prediction of patient outcome in pathologic stage T2 adenocarcinoma of the prostate: lack of significance for microvessel density analysis. Urology 1998; 51:79.

354. Lissbrant IF, Stattin P, Damber JE, et al. Vascular density is a predictor of cancer-specific survival in prostatic carcinoma. Prostate 1997; 33:38.

355. McNeal JE, Yemoto CE. Significance of demonstrable vascular space invasion for the progression of prostatic adenocarcinoma. Am J Surg Pathol 1996; 20:1351.

356. Bahnson RR, Dresner SM, Gooding W, et al. Incidence and prognostic significance of lymphatic and vascular invasion in radical prostatectomy specimens. Prostate 1989; 15:149.

357. Berruti A, Dogliotti L, Mosca A, et al. Circulating neuroendocrine markers in patients with prostate carcinoma. Cancer 2000; 88:2590.

358. Bostwick DG, Aquilina JW. Prostatic intraepithelial neoplasia (PIN) and other prostatic lesions as risk factors and surrogate endpoints for cancer chemoprevention trials. J Cell Biochem Suppl 1996; 25:156.

359. Polito M, Muzzonigro G, Minardi D, et al. Effects of neoadjuvant androgen deprivation therapy on prostatic cancer. Eur Urol 1996; 30:26.

360. van der Kwast TH, Labrie F, Tetu B. Persistence of high-grade prostatic intra-epithelial neoplasia under combined androgen blockade therapy. Hum Pathol 1999; 30:1503.

361. Tsuji M, Kanda K, Murakami Y, et al. Biologic markers in prostatic intraepithelial neoplasia: immunohistochemical and cytogenetic analyses. J Med Invest 1999; 46:35.

362. Harper ME, Glynne-Jones E, Goddard L, et al. Expression of androgen receptor and growth factors in premalignant lesions of the prostate. J Pathol 1998; 186:169.

363. Magi-Galluzzi C, Xu X, Hlatky L, et al. Heterogeneity of androgen receptor content in advanced prostate cancer. Mod Pathol 1997; 10:839.

364. Lyne JC, Melhem MF, Finley GG, et al. Tissue expression of neu differentiation factor/heregulin and its receptor complex in prostate cancer and its biologic effects on prostate cancer cells in vitro. Cancer J Sci Am 1997; 3:21.

365. Leav I, McNeal JE, Kwan PW, et al. Androgen receptor expression in prostatic dysplasia (prostatic intraepithelial neoplasia) in the human prostate: an immunohistochemical and in situ hybridization study. Prostate 1996; 29:137.

366. Van der Kwast TH, Tetu B, Fradet Y, et al. Androgen receptor modulation in benign human prostatic tissue and prostatic adenocarcinoma during neoadjuvant endocrine combination therapy. Prostate 1996; 28:227.

367. Takeda H, Akakura K, Masai M, et al. Androgen receptor content of prostate carcinoma cells estimated by immunohistochemistry is related to prognosis of patients with stage D2 prostate carcinoma. Cancer 1996; 77:934.

368. Hobisch A, Culig Z, Radmayr C, et al. Androgen receptor status of lymph node metastases from prostate cancer. Prostate 1996; 28:129.

369. Hobisch A, Culig Z, Radmayr C, et al. Distant metastases from prostatic carcinoma express androgen receptor protein. Cancer Res 1995; 55:3068.

370. Loda M, Fogt F, French FS, et al. Androgen receptor immunohistochemistry on paraffin-embedded tissue. Mod Pathol 1994; 7:388.

371. Hiramatsu M, Maehara I, Orikasa S, et al. Immunolocalization of oestrogen and progesterone receptors in prostatic hyperplasia and carcinoma. Histopathology 1996; 28:163.

372. Ehara H, Koji T, Deguchi T, et al. Expression of estrogen receptor in diseased human prostate assessed by non-radioactive in situ hybridization and immunohistochemistry. Prostate 1995; 27:304.

373. Bodker A, Balslev E, Juul BR, et al. Estrogen receptors in the human male bladder, prostatic urethra, and prostate. An immunohistochemical and biochemical study. Scand J Urol Nephrol 1995; 29:161.

374. Kirschenbaum A, Ren M, Erenburg I, et al. Estrogen receptor messenger RNA expression in human benign prostatic hyperplasia: detection, localization, and modulation with a long-acting gonadotropin-releasing hormone agonist. J Androl

1994; 15:528.

375. Konishi N, Nakaoka S, Tsuzuki T, et al. Expression of nm23-H1 and nm23-H2 proteins in prostate carcinoma. Jpn J Cancer Res 1993; 84:1050.

376. Brolin J, Lowhagen T, Skoog L. Immunocytochemical detection of the androgen receptor in fine needle aspirates from benign and malignant human prostate. Cytopathology 1992; 3:351.

377. Schulze H, Claus S. Histological localization of estrogen receptors in normal and diseased human prostates by immunocytochemistry. Prostate 1990; 16:331.

378. Mobbs BG, Johnson IE. Changes in tumor characteristics during progression of the R3327 HI experimental prostatic carcinoma. Prostate 1990; 16:127.

379. Seitz G, Wernert N. Immunohistochemical estrogen receptor demonstration in the prostate and prostate cancer. Pathol Res Pract 1987; 182:792.

380. Gould VE, Doljanskaia V, Gooch GT, et al. Stability of the glycoprotein A-80 in prostatic carcinoma subsequent to androgen deprivation therapy. Am J Surg Pathol 1997; 21:319.

381. Matsushima H, Goto T, Hosaka Y, et al. Correlation between proliferation, apoptosis, and angiogenesis in prostate carcinoma and their relation to androgen ablation. Cancer 1999; 85:1822.

382. Andriole GL, Humphrey P, Ray P, et al. Effect of the dual 5alpha-reductase inhibitor dutasteride on markers of tumor regression in prostate cancer. J Urol 2004; 172:915.

383. Ljung G, Norberg M, Holmberg L, et al. Characterization of residual tumor cells following radical radiation therapy for prostatic adenocarcinoma; immunohistochemical expression of prostate-specific antigen, prostatic acid phosphatase, and cytokeratin 8. Prostate 1997; 31:91.

384. Ljung G, Egevad L, Norberg M, et al. Expression of p21 and mutant p53 gene products in residual prostatic tumor cells after radical radiotherapy. Prostate 1997; 32:99.

385. Bostwick DG, Egbert BM, Fajardo LF. Radiation injury of the normal and neoplastic prostate. Am J Surg Pathol 1982; 6:541.

386. Cheng L, Sebo TJ, Slezak J, et al. Predictors of survival for prostate carcinoma patients treated with salvage radical prostatectomy after radiation therapy. Cancer, 1998; 83:2164.

387. Cheng L, Cheville JC, Pisansky T, M. et al. Prevalence and distribution of prostatic intraepithelial neoplasia in salvage radical prostatectomy specimens after radiation therapy. Am J Surg Pathol 1999; 23:803.

388. Cheng L, Cheville JC, Bostwick DG. Diagnosis of prostate cancer in needle biopsies after radiation therapy. Am J Surg Pathol 1999; 23:1173.

389. Larson TR, Bostwick DG, Corica A. Temperature-correlated histopathologic changes following microwave thermoablation of obstructive tissue in patients with benign prostatic hyperplasia. Urology 1996; 47:463.

390. Scherr DS, Vaughan ED Jr, Wei J, et al. BCL-2 and p53 expression in clinically localized prostate cancer predicts response to external beam radiotherapy [published erratum appears in J Urol 1999 Aug;162(2):503]. J Urol 1999; 162:12.

391. Rakozy C, Grignon DJ, Li Y, et al. p53 gene alterations in prostate cancer after radiation failure and their association with clinical outcome: a molecular and immunohistochemical analysis. Pathol Res Pract 1999; 195:129.

392. Cheng L, Sebo TJ, Cheville JC, et al. p53 protein overexpression is associated with increased cell proliferation in patients with locally recurrent prostate carcinoma after radiation therapy. Cancer 1999; 85:1293.

393. Rakozy C, Grignon DJ, Sarkar FH, et al. Expression of bcl-2, p53, and p21 in benign and malignant prostatic tissue before and after radiation therapy. Mod Pathol 11:892. 1998;

394. Kyprianou N, Rock S. Radiation-induced apoptosis of human prostate cancer cells is independent of mutant p53 overexpression. Anticancer Res 1998; 18:897.

395. Huang A, Gandour-Edwards R, Rosenthal SA, et al. p53 and bcl-2 immunohistochemical alterations in prostate cancer treated with radiation therapy. Urology 1998; 51:346.

396. Grignon DJ, Caplan R, Sarkar FH,. et al. p53 status and prognosis of locally advanced prostatic adenocarcinoma: a study based on RTOG 8610. J Natl Cancer Inst 1997; 89:158.

397. Prendergast NJ, Atkins MR, Schatte EC, et al. p53 immunohistochemical and genetic alterations are associated at high incidence with post-irradiated locally persistent prostate carcinoma. J Urol 1996; 155:1685.

398. Stattin P, Damber JE, Modig H, et al. Pretreatment p53 immunoreactivity does not infer radioresistance in prostate cancer patients. Int J Radiat Oncol Biol Phys 1996; 35:885.

399. Grossfeld GD, Olumi AF, Connolly JA, et al. Locally recurrent prostate tumors following either radiation therapy or radical prostatectomy have changes in Ki-67 labeling index, p53

and bcl-2 immunorea-ctivity. J Urol 1998; 159:1437.
400. Kim HE, Han SJ, Kasza T, et al. Platelet-derived growth factor (PDGF)-signaling mediates radiation-induced apoptosis in human prostate cancer cells with loss of p53 function. Int J Radiat Oncol Biol Phys 1997; 39:731.
401. Hintz BL, Koo C, Murphy JF. Pattern of proliferative index (Ki-67) after anti-androgen manipulation reflects the ability of irradiation to control prostate cancer. Am J Clin Oncol 2004; 27:85.
402. Li R, Wheeler T, Dai H, et al. High level of androgen receptor is associated with aggressive clinicopathologic features and decreased biochemical recurrence-free survival in prostate: cancer patients treated with radical prostatectomy. Am J Surg Pathol 2004; 28:928.
403. Magi-Galluzzi C, Nagy S, Bostwick DG, et al. Demonstrability of the glycoprotein A-80 in postradiation prostatic carcinoma. Hum Pathol 1999; 30:1474.
404. Bostwick DG, Ramnani D, Cheng L. Treatment changes in prostatic hyperplasia and cancer, including androgen deprivation therapy and radiotherapy. Urol Clin North Am 1999; 26:465.
405. Luque RJ, Lopez-Beltran A, Perez-Seoane C, et al. Sclerosing adenosis of the prostate. Histologic features in needle biopsy specimens. Arch Pathol Lab Med 2003; 127:e14.
406. Collina G, Botticelli AR, Martinelli AM, et al. Sclerosing adenosis of the prostate. Report of three cases with electronmicroscopy and immunohistochemical study. Histopathology 1992; 20:505.
407. Grignon DJ, Ro JY, Srigley JR, et al. Sclerosing adenosis of the prostate gland. A lesion showing myoepithelial differentiation. Am J Surg Pathol 1992; 16:383.
408. Jones EC, Clement PB, Young RH. Sclerosing adenosis of the prostate gland. A clinicopathological and immunohistochemical study of 11 cases. Am J Surg Pathol 1991; 15:1171.
409. Sakamoto N, Tsuneyoshi M, Enjoji M. Sclerosing adenosis of the prostate. Histopathologic and immunohistochemical analysis. Am J Surg Pathol 1991; 15:660.
410. Young RH, Clement PB. Sclerosing adenosis of the prostate. Arch Pathol Lab Med 1987; 111:363.
411. Oxley JD, Abbott CD, Gillatt DA, et al. Ductal carcinomas of the prostate: a clinicopathological and immunohistochemical study. Br J Urol 1998; 81:109.
412. Grizzle WE, Myers RB, Arnold MM, et al. Evaluation of biomarkers in breast and prostate cancer. J Cell Biochem Suppl 1994; 19:259.
413. Millar EK, Sharma NK, Lessells AM. Ductal (endometrioid) adenocarcinoma of the prostate: a clinicopathological study of 16 cases. Histopathology 1996; 29:11.
414. Bock BJ, Bostwick DG. Does prostatic ductal adenocarcinoma exist? Am J Surg Pathol 1999; 23:781.
415. McNeal JE, Alroy J, Villers A, et al. Mucinous differentiation in prostatic adenocarcinoma. Hum Pathol 1991; 22:979.
416. Uchijima Y, Ito H, Takahashi M, et al. Prostate mucinous adenocarcinoma with signet ring cell. Urology 1990; 36:267.
417. Ro JY, Grignon DJ, Ayala AG, et al. Mucinous adenocarcinoma of the prostate: histochemical and immunohistochemical studies. Hum Pathol 1990; 21:593.
418. Legrier ME, de Pinieux G, Boye K, et al. Mucinous differentiation features associated with hormonal escape in a human prostate cancer xenograft. Br J Cancer 2004; 90:720.
419. Arangelovich V, Tretiakova M, SenGupta E, et al. Pathogenesis and significance of collagenous micronodules of the prostate. Appl Immunohistochem Mol Morphol 2003; 11:15.
420. Beach R, Gown AM, De Peralta-Venturina MN, et al. P504S immunohistochemical detection in 405 prostatic specimens including 376 18-gauge needle biopsies. Am J Surg Pathol 2002; 26:1588.
421. Dodson MK, Cliby WA, Pettavel PP, et al. Female urethral adenocarcinoma: evidence for more than one tissue of origin? Gynecol Oncol 1995; 59:352.
422. Skodras G, Wang J, Kragel PJ. Primary prostatic signet-ring cell carcinoma. Urology 1993; 42:338.
423. Segawa T, Kakehi Y. Primary signet ring cell adenocarcinoma of the prostate: a case report and literature review. Hinyokika Kiyo 1993; 39:565.
424. Guerin D, Hasan N, Keen CE. Signet ring cell differentiation in adenocarcinoma of the prostate: a study of five cases. Histopathology 1993; 22:367.
425. Ben-Izhak O, Lichtig C. Signet-ring cell carcinoma of the prostate mimicking primary gastric carcinoma. J Clin Pathol 1992; 45:452.
426. Ro JY, Grignon DJ, Ayala AG, et al. Blue nevus and melanosis of the prostate. Electron-microscopic and immunohistochemical studies. Am J Clin Pathol 1988; 90:530.
427. Torbenson M, Dhir R, Nangia A, et al. Prostatic carcinoma

with signet ring cells: a clinicopathologic and immunohistochemical analysis of 12 cases, with review of the literature. Mod Pathol 1998; 11:552.

428. Dundore PA, Cheville JC, Nascimento AG, et al. Carcinosarcoma of the prostate. Report of 21 cases. Cancer 1995; 76: 1035.

429. Lindboe CF, Mjones J. Carcinosarcoma of prostate. Immunohistochemical and ultrastructural observations. Urology 1992; 40:376.

430. Delahunt B, Eble JN, Nacey JN, et al. Sarcomatoid carcinoma of the prostate: progression from adenocarcinoma is associated with p53 over-expression. Anticancer Res 1999; 19:4279.

431. Ro JY, el-Naggar AK, Amin MB, et al. Pseudosarcomatous fibromyxoid tumor of the urinary bladder and prostate: immunohistochemical, ultrastructural, and DNA flow cytometric analyses of nine cases. Hum Pathol 1993; 24:1203.

432. Renshaw AA, Granter SR. Metastatic, sarcomatoid, and PSA- and PAP-negative prostatic carcinoma: diagnosis by fine-needle aspiration. Diagn Cytopathol 2000; 23:199.

433. Grignon DJ, Ro JY, Ordonez NG, et al. Basal cell hyperplasia, adenoid basal cell tumor, and adenoid cystic carcinoma of the prostate gland: an immunohistochemical study. Hum Pathol 1988; 19:1425.

434. Iczkowski KA, Ferguson KL, Grier DD, et al. Adenoid cystic/basal cell carcinoma of the prostate: clinicopathologic findings in 19 cases. Am J Surg Pathol 2003; 27:1523.

435. Nazeer T, Barada JH, Fisher HA, et al. Prostatic carcinosarcoma: case report and review of literature. J Urol 1991; 146:1370.

436. Kim HS, Lee JH, Nam JH, et al. Malignant phyllodes tumor of the prostate. Pathol Int 1999; 49:1105.

437. Umekita Y, Yoshida H. Immunohistochemical study of hormone receptor and hormone-regulated protein expression in phyllodes tumour: comparison with fibroadenoma. Virchows Arch 1998; 433:311.

438. Cacic M, Petrovic D, Tentor D, et al. Cystosarcoma phyllodes of the prostate. Scand J Urol Nephrol 1996; 30:501.

439. Lopez-Beltran A, Gaeta JF, Huben R, et al. Malignant phyllodes tumor of prostate. Urology 1990; 35:164.

440. Ito H, Ito M, Mitsuhata N, et al. Phyllodes tumor of the prostate: a case report. Jpn J Clin Oncol 1989; 19:299.

441. Manivel C, Shenoy BV, Wick MR, et al. Cystosarcoma phyllodes of the prostate. A pathologic and immunohistochemical study. Arch Pathol Lab Med 1986; 110:534.

442. Yokota T, Yamashita Y, Okuzono Y, et al. Malignant cystosarcoma phyllodes of prostate. Acta Pathol Jpn 1984; 34: 663.

443. Bostwick D, Qian J, Ramnani D. et al. Prostatic phyllodes tumor. Long term follow-up study of 23 cases. J Urol 2004; 172:894.

444. Reese J H, Lombard CM, Krone K, et al. Phyllodes type of atypical prostatic hyperplasia: a report of 3 new cases. J Urol 1987; 138:623.

445. Kerley SW, Pierce P, Thomas J. Giant cystosarcoma phyllodes of the prostate associated with adenocarcinoma. Arch Pathol Lab Med 1992; 116:195.

446. McCarthy RP, Zhang S, Bostwick DG, et al. Molecular genetic evidence for different clonal origins of epithelial and stromal components of phyllodes tumor of the prostate. Am J Pathol 2004; 165:1395.

447. Bhat DM, Poflee SV, Kotwal MN. et al. Giant cystosarcoma phyllodes tumor of prostate: Case report of a rare entity. Indian J Cancer 2004; 41:129.

448. Alanen KA, Kuopio T, Collan YU, et al. Immunohistochemical labelling for prostate-specific antigen in breast carcinomas. Breast Cancer Res Treat 1999; 56:169.

449. Cohen RJ, Haffejee Z, Steele GS, et al. Advanced prostate cancer with normal serum prostate-specific antigen values. Arch Pathol Lab Med 1994; 118:1123.

450. Speights VO Jr, Cohen MK, Riggs MW, et al. Neuroendocrine stains and proliferative indices of prostatic adenocarcinomas in transurethral resection samples. Br J Urol 1997; 80: 281.

451. Tan MO, Karaoglan U, Celik B, et al. Prostate cancer and neuroendocrine differentiation. Int Urol Nephrol 1999; 31: 75.

452. Cohen RJ, Glezerson G, Haffejee Z. Prostate-specific antigen and prostate-specific acid phosphatase in neuroendocrine cells of prostate cancer. Arch Pathol Lab Med 1992; 116:65.

453. Cohen RJ, Glezerson G, Haffejee Z, et al. Prostatic carcinoma: histological and immunohistological factors affecting prognosis. Br J Urol 1990; 66:405.

膀 胱

David G. Bostwick and Junqi Qian

抗原/抗体生物学

尿路上皮癌（urothelial carcinoma）的形态学，特别是当肿瘤呈低分化或在转移灶中时，往往不是很清楚，并且常与其他低分化非尿路上皮癌的图像重叠。但是一些生物标记物能够帮助判断肿瘤的尿路上皮来源。

细胞角蛋白7和20

细胞角蛋白7（CK7）广泛存在于上皮组织中，包括肺、宫颈、乳腺、胆管、肾集合管、尿路上皮和间皮组织。然而，在肠道上皮、肝细胞、肾近端和远端肾小管以及鳞状上皮中则很少阳性。抗CK7抗体的主要用途在于鉴别非胃肠道来源的腺癌。相反，细胞角蛋白20（CK20）存在于人类消化道上皮、胃小凹细胞、尿路上皮伞细胞和表皮Merkel细胞中。CK20相对局限的组织分布在不明来源的肿瘤的鉴别诊断中是有意义的，特别是当与CK7联合使用时。

大多数尿路上皮癌病例中两种角蛋白均为强阳性（图14.20～14.21）[1-8]。相反，肝细胞癌、前列腺腺癌、肾细胞癌、鳞状细胞癌和神经内分泌肿瘤中CK7和CK20通常均为阴性。CK7-/CK20+的免疫表型在结直肠腺癌的诊断上高度特异，而CK7+/CK20-常可见于绝大多数来源于其他部位的肿瘤，包括卵巢、子宫内膜、乳腺、肺和恶性间皮瘤（表14.10）[9]。

其他器官特异性的生物学标记物的使用进一步提高了CK7和CK20的鉴别诊断价值。例如，Basssily等对59名前列腺腺癌标本和28例尿路上皮癌标本中的CK7和CK20以及前列腺特异抗原（PSA）的表达进行了研究[10]。对于前列腺腺癌，5例只有CK7阳性，5例只有CK20局灶性阳性，1例二者均为阳性，48例二者均为阴性；PSA则除了1例低分化前列腺癌以外，其余均为阳性。对于尿路上皮肿瘤，6例只有CK7阳性，1例CK20阳性，17例二者均为阳性，4例二者均阴性；所有尿路上皮癌的PSA均阴性。他

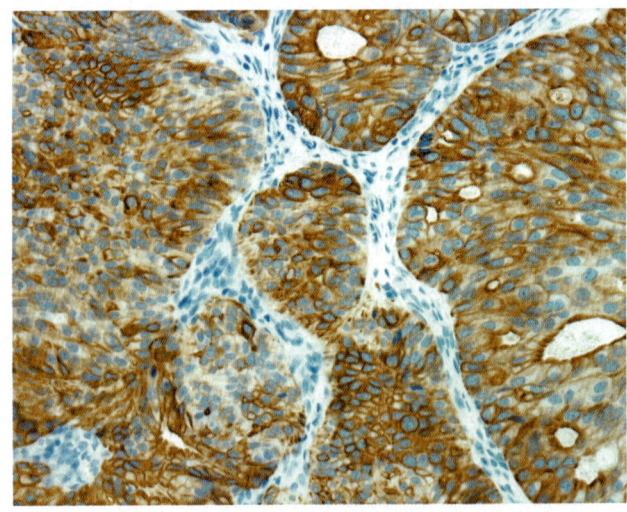

图14.20　尿路上皮癌细胞中细胞角蛋白7的免疫组化结果

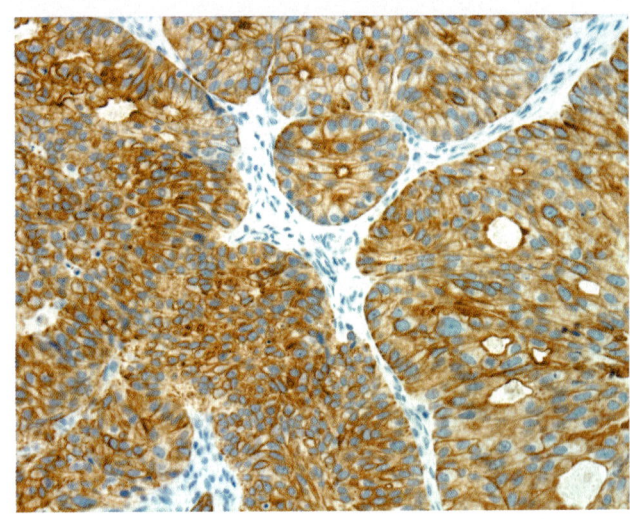

图14.21　尿路上皮癌细胞中细胞角蛋白20的免疫组化结果

们总结得出，PSA对于将前列腺癌与尿路上皮癌进行鉴别是有价值的，但是CK7和CK20在两种组织中均为阳性，则有助于尿路上皮癌的诊断。然而，如果只有一个标记物阳性或两者均为阴性，那么这些标记物在两种肿瘤的鉴别诊断上的用途就很有限。Ormsby等人对癌胚抗原125（CA125）、CK7和CK20在原发性精囊腺癌与其他来源肿瘤在鉴别诊断上的应用价值进行了研究[11]。他们发现，精囊腺癌只有一种免疫表型：CK7阳性、CK20阴性、CA125阳性、PSA和PAP阴性；这种组合的结果，再与组织形态学特征相结合，就可以将精囊腺癌与其他肿瘤相鉴别，包括前列腺腺癌（CA125阴性、PSA/PAP阳性）、膀胱尿路上皮癌（CK20阳性、CA125阴性）、直肠腺癌（CA125阴性、CK7阴性、CK20阳性）、膀

表14.10　角蛋白7和20在尿路上皮癌鉴别诊断中的应用

CK7+/CK20+	CK7-/CK20-	CK7+/CK20-	CK7-/CK20+
尿路上皮癌	肝细胞癌	乳腺癌	结直肠腺癌
胰腺癌	肾细胞癌	肺非小细胞癌	
卵巢黏液癌	前列腺腺癌	原发性精囊腺癌	
	鳞状细胞癌	卵巢浆液性癌	
	神经内分泌癌	间皮瘤	
		子宫内膜腺癌	

胱腺癌（CA125阴性）[12]。膀胱尿路上皮癌和卵巢移行细胞癌在免疫表型上有很大区别；卵巢癌很少表达CEA并从不表达CK20或凝血酶敏感素（thrombospondin），这与膀胱癌相反[13, 14]。Cheng等人报道，非典型性肾源性化生的组织，高分子量角蛋白、细胞角蛋白7和EMA均为阳性表达，但是细胞角蛋白20和CEA常为阴性[15]。

CK20的表达主要局限于良性和反应性尿路上皮的表层伞细胞及少量的中间层细胞中，甚至在有严重炎性反应时也会出现。然而，在细胞异型增生和原位癌时，这些细胞表达的局限性通常会完全丧失，至少在组织局部是这样的，研究发现，36例中有31例的CK20在整个尿路上皮全层表达阳性[3]。这样，CK20的异常表达与形态学特点相结合有助于诊断细胞异型增生，还可能在鉴别反应性增生时具有很大的应用价值，因为反应性增生的诊断是最困难的。CK20的异常表达还能够预测尿路上皮异常增生患者的复发，尽管这一观点还需要进一步证明[2]。最近，有报道CK20和34βE12抗原是膀胱癌复发的有力的预测标记物[16]。

> **诊断要点**：常见盆腔肿瘤
> 1. 绝大多数前列腺癌为CK7-/CK20-、CA125-。
> 2. 绝大多数尿路上皮癌为CK7+/CK20+、CA125-。
> 3. 精囊腺癌为CK7+/CK20-、CA125+。
> 4. 绝大多数结直肠癌为CK20+/CK7-、CA125-。

高分子量细胞角蛋白抗体克隆34βE12

单克隆抗体克隆34βE12对于高分子量角蛋白（HMWCK）1、5、10和14是特异的，其Moll分类分别相当于68、58、56.5和50kD。据报道，HMWCK抗体克隆34βE12对于高级别浸润性尿路上皮癌来说是非常敏感的生物学标记物，特别是当用于微波加热修复时。然而，也有相反的结果被报道[18]。在有鳞状上皮分化的肿瘤组织中，对34βE12的免疫组化结果的解释要慎重。如果在"常见"的高级别癌中HMWCK的免疫组化反应为弥漫性阳性反应，则提示为尿路上皮癌而非前列腺癌，如果HMWCK的阳性反应局限于鳞状上皮分化区则不能除外前列腺癌。

Uroplakin

Uroplakin（UP）是尿路上皮特异性跨膜蛋白，只在尿路上皮中存在，对于尿路上皮癌来说是一个非常好的特异性肿瘤标记物[19, 20]。通过对基因组5′端区域的克隆研究，并与染色体3q片段相比较发现，该蛋白的基因长31kb，具有8个外显子，其中包括1个非编码外显子1。采用免疫组织化学方法，Kageyama等人对行根治性膀胱切除术的尿路上皮癌的患者标本和尸检标本中UPⅠa的表达进行了研究[21]。在63例膀胱切除术的患者中有61例的原发病变部位（96.8%）为阳性（10%或以上的阳性肿瘤细胞）。根据病理学分级，在中度至分化良好的尿路上皮癌患者中，18例中有17例（94.4%）为高表达（50%或以上的阳性肿瘤细胞），而在分化不良的肿瘤细胞中，45例中有36例（80.0%）为高表达。对于肿瘤浸润组织，22例表层浸润中有20例（90.9%）为高表达，41例肌层浸润中有33例（80.5%）为高表达。在转移癌中，18例中有13例为阳性反应（72.2%）[21, 22]。在将uroplakin抗体应用于FNA细胞涂片时，使用95%的乙醇固定细胞，这样能够提高转移性尿路上皮癌对抗体的敏感性，而同时又可以保持其对于石蜡包埋组织的特异性[23]。

由于使用单一的生物学标记物具有局限性，故采用一组标记物组合来确定肿瘤的尿路上皮来源。Parker等人[18]使用的一组标记物组合包括uroplakin Ⅲ

（UROⅢ）抗体、血栓调节蛋白（THR）抗体、高分子量细胞角蛋白（HMWCK）抗体和细胞角蛋白20（CK20）抗体，广泛应用于112种尿路上皮肿瘤的诊断，他们发现这一方法在所有尿路上皮肿瘤中的总阳性率如下：UROⅢ，64/112（57.1%）；THR，77/112（68.8%）；HMWCK，88/110（80%）；CK20，53/110（48.2%）（表14.11）。4种标记物的表达随着肿瘤的分级和分期的不同而不同。所有小细胞癌中，这4种标记物的表达均为阴性。在形态学上，不同肿瘤的亚型与常见的尿路上皮癌的免疫组化结果相似。组织芯片分析表明，在非尿路上皮肿瘤的组织中UROⅢ的表达阴性。THR在少数非尿路上皮组织中的表达为阳性[37例非小细胞肺癌中10例表达阳性（27%），36例淋巴瘤中2例表达阳性（5.6%）]。HMWCK在43.8%的非小细胞性肺癌中表达，在其他的非尿路上皮细胞肿瘤中则为阴性。根据以前的研究结果，UROⅢ在肿瘤中的表达实质上已经确定了肿瘤的尿路上皮来源；然而，UROⅢ在一半以上的尿路上皮肿瘤中仅呈弱阳性表达。THR、HMWCK和CK20的共表达有力地证明了肿瘤的尿路上皮来源。3种非UROⅢ标记物（THR、HMWCK、CK20）中的2种共表达阳性表明肿瘤来源于尿路上皮，但是需要临床病理学作参考[18]。

> **诊断要点：尿路上皮癌**
>
> 血栓调节蛋白、HMWCK和CK20的共表达提示尿路上皮癌可能性极大。

表14.11 在不同级别和分期的非小细胞尿路上皮肿瘤中的免疫组化结果

	UROⅢ	THR	HMWCK	CK20
LMP (n=14)	12 (86%)	12 (86%)	13 (93%)*	6 (43%)
LG (n=16)	12 (75%)	16 (100%)	10 (63%)	8 (50%)
HG (n=16)	13 (81%)	12 (75%)	11 (69%)a	
INV (n=36)	14 (39%)	22 (61%)	30 (88%)a (n=34)	17 (50%) (n=34)
MET (n=25)	13 (52%)	15 (60%)	24 (96%)a	10 (40%)

* 主要在基底细胞中
a 整个肿瘤均为阳性反应
资料来自：Parker. Am J Surg Pathol 2003; 27:1-10

Ki-67（MIB-1）

采用冰冻组织标本中阳性细胞的计数方法判断Ki-67和MIB-1的表达，再参考肿瘤的分级和分期，通常可以预测尿路上皮癌的复发（图14.22）[24-42]。MIB-1的表达与p53的表达、肿瘤侵袭性和患者预后密切相关[43-47]。

增殖细胞核抗原（细胞周期蛋白）

增殖细胞核抗原（PCNA）在膀胱癌中的标记指数从5%到92%，是基因组不稳定[48]、癌复发[49-51]、放射治疗反应[52]和存活情况的预测因子[32, 53-55]。相反，一些报道认为PCNA不能预测临床预后[38, 56]。二倍体尿路上皮细胞癌的PCNA标记指数在30%以下的肿瘤不会复发，而非整倍体的肿瘤的PCNA的标记指数在30%以上的通常会复发[57]。PCNA的表达与膀胱癌细胞的核形态测定结果有关[58]。

癌基因、肿瘤抑制基因和致突变基因

几种癌基因和肿瘤抑制基因在尿路上皮癌的形成过程中发挥了重要的作用（表14.12）。最可能发挥作用的因子包括p53、视网膜母细胞瘤、Her-2/neu和ras家族基因。

p53基因

p53，一个53kD的DNA结合磷酸蛋白，是一种肿瘤抑制基因蛋白。p53基因位于17号染色体（17p13.1）的短臂。这一转录因子调节细胞的生长和抑制细胞进入S期。p53的突变或功能失活在很多人类肿瘤中是

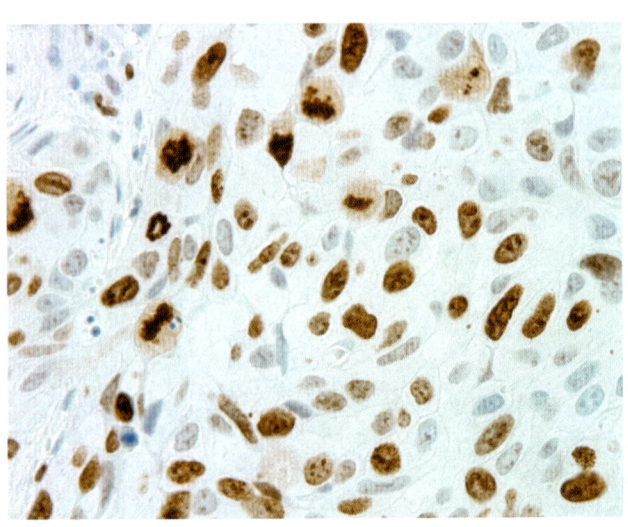

图14.22 尿路上皮癌细胞中的MIB-1免疫组化染色

共同存在的现象，反映了正常生长调节作用的缺失[59]。突变导致细胞半衰期延长，并使得p53蛋白在肿瘤细胞核中积聚到一定的水平，用免疫组化方法可以检测得到[60]。p53蛋白的过表达与各种肿瘤的不良预后有关[61,62]。

大多数p53抗体在用于脱蜡的福尔马林固定的组织切片免疫组化时，需要抗原修复过程。免疫组化结果可能是不相同的，因为固定不同、组织预处理不同以及抗体结合位点不同[63]。免疫组化的结果依赖于p53错义突变而导致的p53蛋白在细胞内的积聚量。发生这一现象的原因不清楚，目前的研究表明，免疫组化并不总是能检测到p53的突变。野生型p53蛋白可能在p53激活的环境中积累，包括低氧和DNA损伤。而且，不是所有的p53错义突变都会导致p53蛋白的积累，所以有可能造成免疫组化的假阴性结果。最终，由于位点和突变程度的不同，可能会有不同程度的p53失活。虽然如此，但是免疫组化结果与p53突变之间还是有很明显的正相关关系[64]。良性尿路上皮很少阳性，而在18%～78%的癌组织中可以看到p53的表达[65-69]。不同的分界点用来确定阳性和阴性结果，最常见的标准为0%[70,71]、10%[33,69,72,73]和20%[43,61,62,66,67,74,75]。免疫组化结果的不均一性反映了肿瘤内部组织来源的异源性。尿沉积细胞可能被用来对p53突变进行基因分析[76,77]。

在尿路上皮癌中，核p53蛋白免疫组化结果与肿瘤的高级别（图14.23）[33,78-82]、高分期[33,79-81,83,84]、血管浸润[79]、肿瘤复发与侵袭[61,62,72,78]、存活情况[40,61,62,67,85-89]以及p53突变包括17p缺失和17多倍体[33,37,43,67,74,75,82,90-93]有关。免疫组化结果可能对患者的预后有独立的预测价值[37,43,61,62,67,71,75,85,86,93-98]，但是也有不同观点[33,65,70,80,99-101]。T1期膀胱癌中p53免疫组化阳性细胞数高于20%的肿瘤比低于20%的肿瘤有更高的扩散几率（分别为每年21%和3%的扩散率）[86]。相似的，原位癌中p53免疫组化阳性细胞数高于20%的肿瘤比低于20%的肿瘤有更高的扩散几率（分别为每年86%和16%的扩散率）[85]。这些结果均被其他作者的研究所证实[67,72,102,103]。相反，最近一项包括p53和bcl-2在内的研究表明，只有肿瘤的分级和分期才是患者存活的预测因子[33]。无论肿瘤级别如何，p53的存在都无法预测T1期患者行经尿道切除术后对bacillus Galmette-Guerin治疗的临床反应[44,45,104,105]。

p53的预测价值当与其他因子结合使用时可能会

表14.12	尿路上皮癌的选择标记物
Propietary 商品化标记物	
BTA™	
NMP22	
Immunocyt™	
增殖标记物	
增殖细胞核抗原（PCNA）	
Ki-67	
MIB-1	
癌抗原、肿瘤抑制抗原和致突变基因	
p53	
视网膜母细胞瘤基因（Rb）	
Her-2/neu	
ras	
bcl-2	
生长因子和受体	
表皮生长因子受体（EGFR）	
酸性成纤维细胞生长因子	
碱性成纤维细胞生长因子	
细胞黏附标记物	
E-钙黏素	
整合素	
细胞周期蛋白D1	
CD44	
F和G肌动蛋白	
端粒酶血管生成标记物	
微血管密度	
血管内皮生长因子	
其他标记物	
自分泌动力因子	
腔上皮抗原（LEA135）	
雄激素受体	
尿激酶型纤溶酶原激活因子	
FHIT基因	
细胞角蛋白20	
T138	
透明质酸	

增加。p53的免疫组化结果与DNA的非整倍体现象密切相关，当均为阳性时，预示浸润癌患者的预后不良[48]；相反，另一研究结果认为p53表达与DNA非整倍体的存在无关[100]。

在尿路上皮癌中，p53的改变可能会导致细胞对损伤DNA的化疗药物的敏感性增加，包括阿霉素和顺铂[106,107]。在p53突变的患者中，辅助化疗方法的采用会使肿瘤复发的风险下降3倍，并使中位随访期为9年的患者的存活期增加2.6倍[106,107]。无p53基因

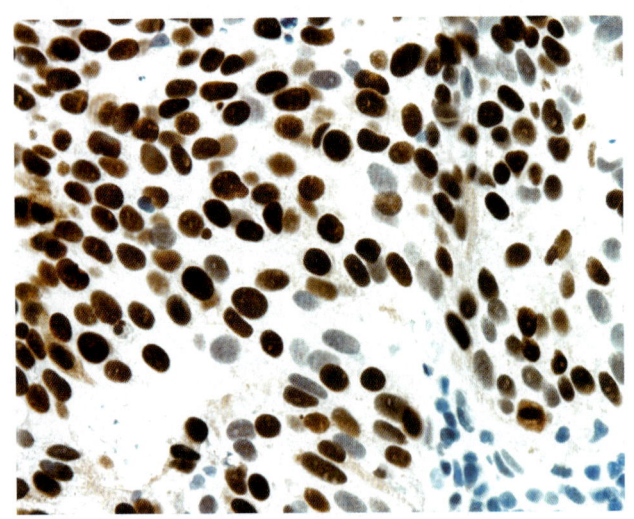

图 14.23 尿路上皮细胞癌中的 p53 的免疫组化结果

突变的患者采用化疗未见存活期延长。这些结果表明,具有肿瘤扩散和死亡高风险的患者(那些具有 p53 基因突变的患者)可能是辅助化疗的最大受益者,那么 p53 蛋白的检测可以鉴别出这样的患者[108, 109]。

野生型 p53 可以导致细胞凋亡,而突变的 p53 蛋白则抑制细胞凋亡,这与 bcl-2 相似。这样,一个非常有趣的发现是,bcl-2 在低级别和低分期的尿路上皮癌中更常表达,而突变的 p53 在高级别和高分期的肿瘤中更常表达。一种可能的解释是,突变型 p53 蛋白延长了带有基因缺陷的细胞的存活期,使得它们更加不稳定而在临床上更具侵袭性;相反,bcl-2 可能只是在早期延长细胞的存活期,使得它们开始获得基因缺陷[16, 33]。

p53 蛋白可以被病毒蛋白产物灭活,如人乳头瘤病毒(HPV)16 分泌的 E6 蛋白。HPV 偶尔可在乳头状非浸润和浸润癌中被检测到,HPV 的存在与更高级别和分期的肿瘤有关[110-114]。HPV 阳性的肿瘤患者标本中很少出现 p53 突变,这表明该肿瘤另一种不同的病原学途径[115]。而且,p53 能够激活原癌基因核抗原 MDM2[116, 117]。这种蛋白在 67% 的未浸润和早期浸润膀胱癌的病例中表达升高,但是只有在 27% 的侵犯肌层的肿瘤中表达。p16 基因位于 9 号染色体,可以在高达 60% 的与血吸虫病相关的鳞状细胞癌的病例中出现表达异常,但是只有 18% 的尿路上皮癌出现表达异常[118-120]。此外,p16 和 p53 的异常是相互排斥的,这表明二者在膀胱癌的发病机制上存在互补的作用[119, 121]。同时检测 p53 和 nm23-H-1,发现其与患者的预后不佳有明显的关系[122]。

p53 诱导 p53 依赖性基因。这类基因当中的一个原型是 Cip-1(WAF-1),编码一个 21kD 的蛋白,能够抑制启动细胞周期 G1 期的细胞周期蛋白依赖性激酶。p53 基因的突变使得其激活 Cip-1 的功能丧失,随之丧失了抑制细胞周期蛋白依赖性激酶和抑制 G1 期启动的功能[83]。p53 蛋白依赖性细胞周期蛋白依赖性激酶抑制因子的发现将这个基因与细胞周期调节的酶作用机制联系起来。p53 基因的突变通常为错义突变,主要集中在一段基因产物的特定区域,在氨基酸 130 至 290 之间,所涉及的氨基酸残基包括 117~142、171~181、239~258 和 270~286 区域。这些区域在种属间是高度保守的,对于维持正常的 p53 功能是必要的。围绕密码子 280 和 285 的区域是 p53 基因突变的热点区域[123-125]。

p53 基因杂合性缺失出现在人类多种肿瘤中。因此,当 p53 正常的等位基因缺失或失活时,p53 成为人类肿瘤发生的最可能的促进因素。在杂合性状态下的转化激活可能是突变型和野生型 p53 形成寡聚复合物的结果。在经突变 p53 基因转化的细胞中,发生改变的蛋白复合物存在于胞浆中。

突变的 p53 基因能够与 ras 基因相互作用,在内源性野生型 p53 蛋白存在的情况下转化原代培养的成纤维细胞[64]。在一些肿瘤中,第 17 号染色体基因的缺失常与其他的染色体异常同时存在,表明 p53 突变是肿瘤发生过程中的晚期事件。反映染色体不稳定性的肿瘤细胞非整倍体现象,可能在 p53 基因突变的肿瘤细胞的选择中发挥作用。这一过程可能导致剩余的野生型等位基因的丢失,并导致正常的 p53 蛋白生长控制功能的失活[59]。

大约 65% 的原位癌病例可见 p53 基因突变[117, 126],相比于非典型增生和异常增生 28%~33% 的比例要高得多[68, 69]。这种高突变频率与浸润性尿路上皮癌相似,可以在基因水平上解释为原位癌具有向浸润癌进展的潜能[117]。此外,p53 基因突变的种系遗传也可见于有肿瘤倾向的家族,包括那些 Li-Fraumeni 综合征患者。在 18 例浸润性膀胱癌的患者中有 11 例出现 p53 基因突变,最常见的基因突变是单碱基损伤替换。11 例患者中的 7 例出现错义突变,3 例出现无意义突变。在尿沉积细胞[127]中也可检测到 p53 突变,这可能是肿瘤扩散的预测指标[76, 128-134]。在对 23 名患者中的 25 例膀胱癌标本所进行的研究中发现,在侵犯肌层组织中 p53 基因的突变率要明显高于无肌层侵犯的肿瘤(分别为 58% 和 8%)。根据一项研究所示,高级别膀胱癌中，36%的病例出现不同的p53基因突变[64]。这些分子生物学研究证实了 p53 蛋白免疫组化在膀胱癌组织中的表达结果。在尿路上皮癌和其他人类肿瘤中Cip-1和MTS-1基因突变的检测结果表明，p53蛋白调节途径中不同基因的改变可能导致相似的生物学功能。

> **诊断要点**：尿路上皮癌中的 p53 蛋白
> p53+ 的尿路上皮癌的患者对化疗的反应更好。

视网膜母细胞瘤基因

视网膜母细胞瘤（Rb）基因位于染色体 13q14 上，编码一种105kD蛋白，调节所有成年人细胞的基因转录。正常的基因产物抑制调节细胞周期的基因表达。细胞周期蛋白和细胞周期蛋白依赖性激酶能够通过磷酸化过程使Rb基因失活。pRb能够被HPV16中相应的开放阅读框架编码的蛋白E6所灭活，而无需Rb基因的突变[110]。MTS-1 基因编码 p16 蛋白，它是Rb的上游调节因子，能够保持Rb蛋白处于激活状态或者低磷酸化状态。一些研究表明，p16的缺失与Rb蛋白的失活有关，也许可以解释某些研究中Rb缺失或过表达的患者预后相同的情况[135]。

pRb 在所有人类组织中都表达。Rb 基因的突变失活和pRb 表达的减少可见于视网膜母细胞瘤和其他肿瘤中。在人类肿瘤中，Rb 基因的两种主要的改变类型是基因缺失或突变。主要的基因大片段的缺失会导致基因产物正常功能的缺如[136]。基因突变，包括能改变基因功能的核苷酸替代，可以使转录起始位点、剪切位点、密码子终止位点发生改变，并出现氨基酸替代以及其他使转录不稳定的改变，使基因产物长度变短或使信使 RNA 发生修饰。这些变化会导致Rb 蛋白功能的缺失[137, 138]。在膀胱癌中，Rb 的变化表现为点突变而非大片段的缺失。Rb 基因是在高级别侵犯肌层的膀胱癌的进展和扩散过程中起主要作用的基因之一[24, 72, 101, 135, 139-149]。Rb 功能的缺失可见于 30% 的高级别乳头状和非乳头状尿路上皮癌。Rb 功能的缺失与 Rb 基因杂合性的缺失，以及高级别和侵犯肌层组织有关。

pRb表达的增加与pRb超磷酸化有关，而pRb超磷酸化反过来又与p16的表达和/或细胞周期蛋白D1的表达增加有关。最近的研究发现表明，p53、p21

和pRb基因表达的改变在促进膀胱癌的进展过程中具有协同作用[150]。pRb的表达改变与尿路上皮癌患者的存活期缩短有关[72, 138]。良性尿路上皮黏膜和非浸润性尿路上皮癌的大多数细胞都可见pRb免疫组化反应阳性[151]。pRb的免疫组化检测是预测肿瘤进展的一个有用指标，但并未常规使用[78, 140, 152-155]。

Her-2/neu；p185（c-erbB2）

在尿路上皮癌中，Her-2/neu的免疫组化阳性部位通常在细胞膜（图14.24）[156]，尽管有时胞浆也会有阳性信号[157]。阳性细胞呈弥漫性分布，而不是分布于表层或基底细胞中。在正常和感染的尿路上皮中，Her-2/neu 蛋白的表达频率从 2% 到 65% 不等，并在 19% 的异常增生病例和64%的原位癌中表达[158]。免疫组化反应的强度与尿路上皮癌的分期[159, 160]、复发[161]和患者存活情况有关[162, 163]，尽管也有一些报道认为 Her-2/neu 的免疫组化结果与预后无关[164]。

在正常和异常增生的活检组织中，都可以观察到单纯的表皮细胞 Her-2/neu 阳性。然而，弥漫性的阳性反应和p53的过表达都与异常增生的进展有关。用荧光原位杂交方法进行分析表明，在原位癌（CIS）中可见 Her-2/neu 基因的扩增和 p53 的缺失，同时在所有 6 例 CIS 组织中，都可见 17 号染色体的拷贝数呈明显的不均一性。这些结果表明了在膀胱原位癌中，基因组具有明显的不稳定性，表明erbB-2和p53基因都发生了改变[165]。

bcl-2

在大约一半的尿路上皮癌病例中，bcl-2 的免疫组化阳性反应可见于良性和异常增生的尿路上皮中，

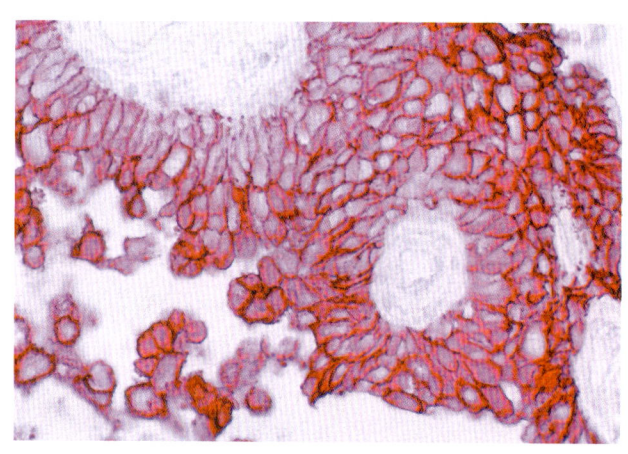

图 14.24 Her-2/neu 在尿路上皮癌中的免疫组化染色

但是在原位癌中则呈阴性反应[33, 166]。在高分期和高级别肿瘤中，bcl-2 表达下降[33, 37, 54, 94, 102, 167-182]。bcl-2 的表达有望成为经放射性治疗后的肿瘤患者对辅助化疗反应的标记物[25, 144, 183, 184]。

细胞黏附标记物

E- 钙黏素

正常人尿路上皮的 E- 钙黏素免疫组化呈均一阳性，在细胞边缘呈膜阳性[185, 186]。腔膜附近的表皮细胞呈阴性反应，与基膜相连的部分细胞也呈阴性反应。21% 的低级别肿瘤和 76% 的浸润癌组织 E- 钙黏素的表达异常[178]。E- 钙黏素的表达与肿瘤分期的关系表明，它在肿瘤的浸润过程中起作用[188]。E-钙黏素的表达与存活率又有明显的关系；相反，正常E-钙黏素阳性反应的出现预示着患者即便为高分期肿瘤，其预后也良好[185, 186, 188-197]。E-钙黏素的血清浓度与肿瘤分级、肿瘤数量、肿瘤复发和转移有关，但是与肿瘤组织切片中的免疫组化结果无关[199, 200]。

整合素

正常的上皮细胞不表达 α1、α4 和 α5 整合素亚单位，但是在细胞膜中可以表达α2和α3，且在基底细胞中比在腔细胞中表达更强[193, 201-203]。α2β1 的表达逐渐下降，而在某种程度上，从Ta和T1期肿瘤到T2~3期肿瘤的发展过程中，α3β1 的表达在增加[203]。在正常的尿路上皮中，α6β1整合素与VII型胶原共同定位于基底细胞和固有膜的交界处[203]。在对 57 名患者的研究中发现，整合素家族中的这一成员如果在尿路上皮癌中的表达低，则患者的预后较强阳性表达或阴性表达的患者要好[201]。在 83% 的非浸润性膀胱癌中，整合素的表达在上基底部和基底部细胞中，而 VII 型胶原仍存在于半桥粒锚定复合物中。这一结果表明，在低级别肿瘤中，锚定复合物是正常的或仅轻度改变，而在83%的浸润性肿瘤中，整合素、VII 型胶原或二者的缺失则表明细胞的异常状态[203]。

细胞周期蛋白 D1

良性及异常增生的尿路上皮，包括内翻性乳头状瘤，并不表达细胞周期蛋白D1[204]。对细胞周期蛋白D1在尿路上皮癌中免疫组化的研究则得到了相反的结论。一项研究表明，Ta期和T1期乳头状尿路上皮癌呈细胞核细胞周期蛋白D1 阳性，但是在浸润癌和非乳头状癌中则为阴性，其反应强度随着肿瘤级别的升高而下降[204]。细胞周期蛋白D1的表达与PCNA及p53的表达呈负相关，这表明细胞周期蛋白D1在细胞增殖的负调控中发挥作用以促进肿瘤的分化。相反，其他的研究发现细胞周期蛋白D1的表达与肿瘤的分级和分期无关，尽管细胞周期蛋白D1免疫组化阳性的肿瘤比细胞周期蛋白D1阴性的肿瘤复发快[205, 206]。在 81% 非肌层浸润的癌组织和 38% 肌层浸润的癌组织中发现细胞周期蛋白D1mRNA的过表达[207, 208]。通过对比研究，大约 10%～15% 的膀胱癌有 11q13 区的扩增[207]。越来越多的结果表明，细胞周期蛋白D1基因的改变可能是尿路上皮癌发生过程中的一个早期事件[205, 209, 210]。一项研究表明，细胞周期蛋白D1和细胞周期蛋白D3的过表达与T1和T3期膀胱癌患者的存活情况有关[45, 211]。

CD44

正常的尿路上皮表达 CD44，但是在早期非浸润性乳头状尿路上皮癌中表达最高，并随着浸润的发生而表达下降[186, 212-222]。尿样中脱落的癌细胞中可检测到CD44蛋白异构体和mRNA片段[212, 215]。可溶性CD44蛋白在血清中可以检测到，与健康对照组相比，膀胱癌患者的血清中 CD44 蛋白水平更低[223]。CD44v6的免疫组化反应可以将膀胱小细胞癌（阴性）与低分化的尿路上皮细胞癌（通常为阳性）相鉴别[224]。

微血管密度

微血管密度增加是尿路上皮癌淋巴结转移、复发和存活情况[128, 226-231]的预测因子[225]，是独立的预后预测因子[226, 227, 232]。

血管内皮生长因子

血管内皮细胞生长因子（VEGF）和基本的成纤维细胞生长因子是膀胱癌细胞血管生成的主要诱导因子[223-237]。肿瘤组织中的VEGF mRNA和蛋白水平比良性尿路上皮组织高[236]，VEGF 的表达增高预示预后不良[238-241]，并且与高级别膀胱癌有关[242]。凝血酶敏感素-1作为VEGF的一个抑制因子，在血管的生成过程中发挥重要作用；它的低表达与从抗血管生成到血管生成的转化有关，这一现象发生于尿路上皮癌的早期[233]。

表皮生长因子受体

表皮生长因子受体（EGFR）在很多上皮肿瘤中

过表达，包括膀胱癌[243]。检测EGFR可能在对膀胱癌的治疗措施的选择上具有临床意义[244, 245]。

其他生物学标记物

对其他的生物学标记物的研究和评价比较有限。自分泌动力因子（AMF-R或gp78）在良性尿路上皮中不表达，而其在尿路上皮癌中的表达则是患者经外科手术治疗后的独立预后预测因子[246]。表面糖蛋白腔上皮抗原（LEA135）的免疫组化结果分析表明，其表达水平在高级别和高分期的肿瘤中降低[247]。雄激素受体作为甾体激素核受体超家族成员之一，在绝大多数尿路上皮癌中表达[248]，但是在良性尿路上皮中则为阴性。尿激酶型纤溶酶原激活因子是一种丝氨酸蛋白酶，其表达是淋巴结阴性、肌层浸润的膀胱癌患者独立的预后预测指标，但是对于上尿路道肿瘤来说则并非如此[250-254]。脆弱三联组氨酸（FHIT）基因位于3p14.2染色体上，在大多数原发性尿路上皮癌中都呈异常表达[255]。细胞角蛋白20在尿路上皮肿瘤细胞中表达，但是在正常上皮中不表达，从膀胱癌患者的尿液中提取的mRNA的分析表明其敏感性为91%，特异性为67%[256]。肿瘤进展标记物T138可以检测表面抗原，再参考肿瘤分期，可以成为肿瘤转移的独立预测指标[257]。糖胺聚糖透明质酸能够促进细胞的迁移和黏附，用酶联免疫吸附方法检测其在尿液中的水平，发现尿路上皮癌的患者体内升高3～5倍[258-262]。

尿路上皮癌的分型

有几种不同类型的尿路上皮癌，包括混合分化型（表14.13）。识别这些不同变型的肿瘤可能在预后判断上有价值。3种具有独特的或意想不到的免疫表型的变型如下；关于其他类型，读者可以通过其他泌尿系统病理学专业书籍来了解[263]。

嵌套型尿路上皮癌

嵌套型尿路上皮癌的特征是，具有小的融合细胞团和发育不良的小管，轻度异型的肿瘤细胞浸入膀胱的固有膜和/或固有肌膜。除了不太明显的组织形态学的改变外，该病变据报道具有一定的侵袭行为。Lin等报道，通过免疫组化分析发现嵌套型尿路上皮癌与常见的高危型尿路上皮癌具有某些共同特征，如p27表达的缺失和高增殖指数。常见的和嵌套型尿路上皮癌中，p53、bcl-2或EGFR的免疫组化常为阴性反应[264]。

小细胞癌（高级别神经内分泌癌）

包含部分或全部小细胞未分化癌的尿路上皮癌是很少见的，治疗（如放射性治疗）后，这种肿瘤发生的可能性增加，这与前列腺小细胞癌相似。其他部位的小细胞癌的免疫组化结果是比较典型的，说明其具有临床侵袭过程（表14.14）[216, 265-268]。

27例小细胞癌中，有25例C44v6免疫组化结果阴性，2例为阳性细胞少于10%的弱阳性；相反，所有中度或低分化尿路上皮癌的病例都表现为有50%～100%的阳性细胞的中等强度的阳性反应。CD44v6免疫组化能够鉴别低分化的尿路上皮癌与小细胞癌，而且还可以检测出混合型小细胞尿路上皮分化[216]。

膀胱小细胞癌具有大量的基因组改变（平均：每个肿瘤11.3个）[269]。基因缺失最常见于10q（10个有缺失基因的肿瘤中7个发生于此区域）、4q、5q（每10个里有5个发生于此区域）和13q（4/10）。这些区域可能含有与这一特殊肿瘤类型相关的肿瘤抑制基因。获得DNA序列的区域主要集中在8q（5/10）、5p、6p和10q（4/10）。高水平的基因扩增可见于1p22-32、3q26.3、8q24和12q4-21区域。这些基因座可能是与小细胞膀胱癌有关的癌基因的准确定位位点。对一个既含有小细胞癌又含有尿路上皮癌的肿瘤进行分析的结果显示，小细胞癌能够通过基因的改变而从尿路上皮癌发展而来[269]。

表14.13　尿路上皮癌的变型
嵌套型
微乳头状型
微囊型
淋巴上皮瘤样
淋巴瘤样或浆细胞瘤样
内翻型乳头瘤样
尿路上皮癌伴合体滋养层巨细胞分化
巨细胞型
透明细胞型（糖原丰富）
肉瘤样型
混合分化型
癌伴肿瘤相关性间质反应
小细胞癌（高级别神经内分泌癌）

尿路上皮癌伴合体滋养层巨细胞

巨细胞可见于12%的尿路上皮癌中，有时会产生一定量的β-人绒毛膜促性腺激素（β-hCG），表明其具备合体滋养层细胞分化特征[270]。hCG反应细胞的数量与肿瘤的级别呈负相关[271]。hCG分泌入血清可能与对放射治疗反应较差有关[272]。最主要的鉴别诊断是绒毛膜癌；大多数但不是所有的以往报道为原发性膀胱绒毛膜癌的病例，实际上是尿路上皮癌伴合体滋养层细胞分化。

表14.14 膀胱小细胞癌的免疫组化结果

抗体	阳性病例
神经特异性烯醇化酶（NSE）	90%
神经丝（neurofilament）	84%
人乳脂球蛋白	67%
上皮细胞膜抗原（EMA）	63%
角蛋白 AE1/AE3；CAM5.2	61%
癌胚抗原（CEA）	50%
突触素	46%
LeuM1	43%
嗜铬素	41%
5-羟色胺	38%
Leu7	35%
S-100蛋白	34%
5-羟色胺	31%
舒血管肠肽	17%
波形蛋白	17%
促肾上腺皮质激素（ACTH）	9%

膀胱软组织肿瘤和梭形细胞病变

膀胱软组织肿瘤的免疫组化反应与身体其他部位的相应软组织肿瘤相似。最常见的类型为成年型肉瘤、平滑肌肉瘤，可能会误诊为肉瘤样（梭形细胞）癌，本书其他部分所描述的常规免疫组化方法对于临床鉴别诊断经常是有用的（表14.15）。

两种非常类似于恶性肿瘤的肿瘤，即手术后梭形细胞瘤和炎性肌纤维母细胞瘤，具有特征性的免疫组化结果，可以用来将它们与肉瘤和肉瘤样癌相鉴别。

术后梭形细胞结节

术后梭形细胞结节（PSCN）是一种在下泌尿生殖道内不常见的病变，通常在术后3个月之内形成。它看上去像一个易碎的赘生物，包含有交叉排列的梭形细胞，细胞经常出现大量的有丝分裂象，但是无异型性[273-278]。可能会出现反应性非典型性，但是细胞并不表现出明显异常。PSCN与平滑肌肉瘤有明显的相似性，但是还要与其他的肉瘤如Kaposi肉瘤相鉴别。PSCN容易与中度或高度平滑肌肉瘤相区别，因为其缺少细胞异型性，所以与低级别平滑肌肉瘤相鉴别是最困难的[279]。两者都侵及固有肌层，并且两者都可能表现出黏液样变，尽管广泛而明显的黏液样改变有助于平滑肌肉瘤的诊断。临床病史在鉴别诊断中是非常重要的，PSCN中常存在特征性的细小血管网。

免疫组化在PSCN的诊断中有价值。这种肿瘤样的增生使得80%的病例表现出细胞角蛋白阳性，而在膀胱的平滑肌肉瘤组织中则不常见。

炎性假瘤（假肉瘤样肌纤维母细胞瘤、炎性肌纤维母细胞瘤；假肉瘤性纤维肌样瘤）

所有年龄组都可能出现炎性假瘤，平均年龄为30岁；女性居多。小儿患者可能会被误诊为横纹肌瘤，在成年患者中可能被误诊为平滑肌肉瘤或肉瘤样癌[265,280-286]。一些病例出现于泌尿道感染之后，但是大多数没有明显的病因。炎性假瘤由富含酸性黏多糖间质中增生的肌纤维母细胞、纤维母细胞和内皮细胞组成，表明其为活性肉芽组织，与结节性筋膜炎相似[265]。肿瘤细胞无间变或核深染现象，完全可以排除中级别或高级别肉瘤。肿瘤组织侵入固有肌层常见，不应被认为是恶性行为的表现。肉瘤样癌有时局部组织结构可能类似于炎性假瘤，尤其在标本较小或取材较局限时应谨慎判断。还有些类型包括组织编状结构或因组织透明样变化而产生的硬化性结构。梭形细胞中波形蛋白（10/10）[287]和肌肉特异性肌动蛋白（10/10）的免疫组化均为阳性。少数病例平滑肌特异性肌动蛋白（3/8）、CK（2/10）、结蛋白（2/9）和EMA（2/8）的免疫组化结果阳性[265]。在一些病例中，至少可见到局灶性的角蛋白异常表达[265,286]。采用流式细胞技术对DNA含量进行测定可以得到二倍体矩形图（6/6）[265]。

良性软组织肿瘤

神经节细胞瘤（嗜铬细胞瘤）是一种罕见但是非常重要的肿瘤，可能发生于膀胱壁的正常神经节组织[288-294]。它可发生于任何年龄段，男、女发生率相同。极少病例与神经纤维瘤病[259]、肠道类癌[291]、长

表14.15　膀胱软组织肿瘤的免疫组化比较

	术后梭形细胞结节	炎性假瘤*	梭形细胞癌	平滑肌肉瘤	横纹肌肉瘤
角蛋白	+	-（偶有+）	+	-	-
EMA	-	-	+	-	-
波形蛋白	+	+	+	+	+
结蛋白	+	-	-	+	+
MSA	+	-	-	+	+

EMA，上皮细胞膜抗原；MSA，肌肉特异性肌动蛋白
* 炎性肌纤维母细胞瘤

期透析[296]有关。该病通常采用尿或血清中的儿茶酚胺及其代谢产物的测定以确诊。神经节瘤通常局限于壁内，常见于膀胱三角区、前壁和顶部。外被黏膜层可能是完整的或形成溃疡。

显微镜下，膀胱神经节瘤的组织结构与发生于其他部位的该肿瘤是相同的，由排列整齐的独立的细胞团（zellballen）组成，细胞团之间被明显的窦状隙血管网隔开（图14.25）。对这些肿瘤行为进行预测的病理标记物目前还不清楚[297]。生长于其他部位与肿瘤浸润行为有关的特征包括有丝分裂象、坏死和血管浸润，这些特征在膀胱肿瘤的研究中已经使用。从免疫组织化学方法看，最有用的特征是肿瘤的角蛋白、上皮细胞膜抗原和癌胚抗原的免疫组化为阴性，而神经内分泌标记物常为阳性，包括神经特异性烯醇化酶、嗜铬素（图14.26）、突触素、5-羟色胺、促生长素抑制素和其他因子。肿瘤支持细胞的S-100蛋白免疫组化阳性（图14.27）[288-294, 298-300]。

孤立性纤维瘤

这种肿瘤曾经被诊断为局限性纤维间皮瘤，很少发生于膀胱壁[301-303]。免疫组化方法在鉴别单个纤维瘤与其他膀胱软组织肿瘤是有用的[304]，该肿瘤CK34、bcl-2免疫组化常为阳性，而角蛋白和S-100蛋白常为阴性。少数细胞可能表现出肌动蛋白和肌肉特异性肌动蛋白阳性，但是不常见。

颗粒细胞瘤

膀胱颗粒细胞瘤很少见，均发生于成年人。认为这种肿瘤是神经内源性（施万细胞）的，S-100蛋白免疫组化阳性，与其他部位的颗粒细胞瘤类似[305-307]。

膀胱恶性淋巴瘤

原发性膀胱恶性淋巴瘤很少见，已报道的病例不足100例，只相当于淋巴结外淋巴瘤的0.2%[308-314]。大多数为个例报道，组织学分类有明显不同，只有少量报道对淋巴瘤的表型进行了免疫学研究[310, 315]。

显微镜下观察，可见弥漫分布的淋巴细胞位于或侵入正常结构中，但并不取代正常组织结构。常可见淋巴上皮病变。最常见的淋巴瘤类型是MALT淋巴瘤（黏膜相关性淋巴组织型），可见弥漫性分布大淋巴细胞淋巴瘤和小淋巴细胞淋巴瘤[310]。很少有淋巴瘤病变与腺癌和尿路上皮癌同时发生。

用免疫组化方法研究，发现几乎所有的膀胱淋巴瘤都是B细胞来源的淋巴瘤，并呈单克隆性。最常见的原发性淋巴瘤是低级别MALT型淋巴瘤[310]。原发性霍奇金病和免疫母细胞型肉瘤是极其少见的。主要的鉴别诊断包括慢性弥漫性膀胱炎、小细胞癌、淋巴上皮样癌（图14.28）和淋巴瘤样癌。膀胱淋巴瘤的总存活情况为：1年存活率为68%~73%，5年存活率为27%~64%[310]。

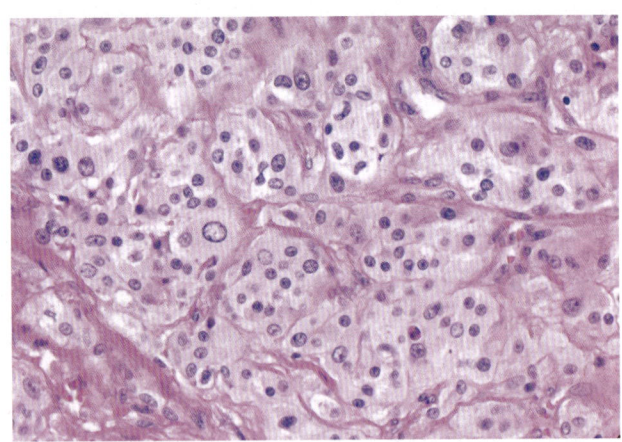

图14.25 膀胱神经节瘤,由排列整齐的独立的细胞团(zellballen)组成,细胞团之间被明显的窦状隙血管网隔开

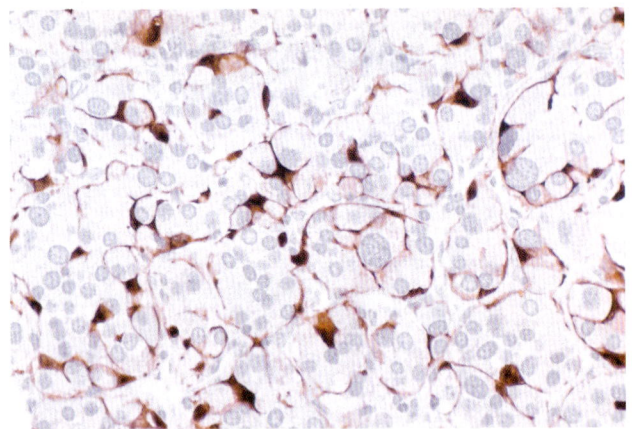

图14.27 膀胱神经节瘤。肿瘤细胞中S-100蛋白的免疫组化结果

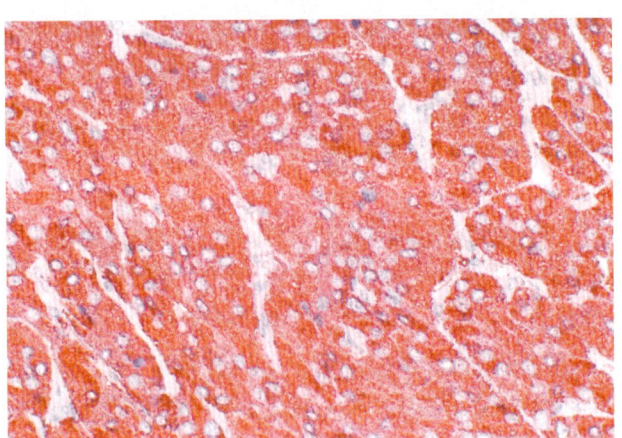

图14.26 膀胱神经节瘤。肿瘤细胞中嗜铬素的免疫组化结果

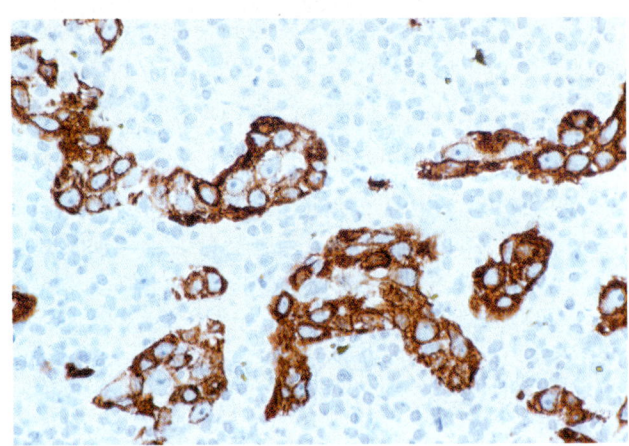

图14.28 淋巴上皮瘤样尿路上皮癌细胞中AE1/AE3的免疫组化结果

参考文献

1. Wang N, Bacchi C, Gown A. Coordinate expression of cytokeratins 7 and 20 define unique subsets of carcinomas. Appl Immunohistochem 1995; 3:88.
2. Harnden P, Mahmood N, Southgate J. Expression of cytokeratin 20 redefines urothelial papillomas of the bladder. Lancet 1999; 353:974.
3. Harnden P, Eardley I, Joyce AD, et al. Cytokeratin 20 as an objective marker of urothelial dysplasia. Br J Urol 1996; 78: 870.
4. Harnden P, Allam A, Joyce AD, et al. Cytokeratin 20 expression by non-invasive transitional cell carcinomas: potential for distinguishing recurrent from non-recurrent disease. Histopathology 1995; 27:169.
5. Baars JH, De Ruijter JL, Smedts F, et al. The applicability of a keratin 7 monoclonal antibody in routinely Papanicolaou-stained cytologic specimens for the differential diagnosis of carcinomas [see comments]. Am J Clin Pathol 1994; 101: 257.
6. Mortimer G, Jones DN, Assaf H, et al. Patterns of cytokeratin expression by neoplastic and non-neoplastic epithelium. Ir J Med Sci 1993; 162:77.
7. Vojtesek B, Staskova Z, Nenutil R. et al. A panel of monoclonal antibodies to keratin no. 7: characterization and value in tumor diagnosis. Neoplasma 1990; 37:333.
8. Reedy EA, Heatfield BM, Trump BF, et al. Correlation of cytokeratin patterns with histopathology during neoplastic progression in the rat urinary bladder. Pathobiology 1990; 58:15.
9. Gown A. Immunohistochemical detection of primary sites of carcinomas. J Histotechnol 1999; 22:7.

10. Bassily NH, Vallorosi CJ, Akdas G, et al. Coordinate expression of cytokeratins 7 and 20 in prostate adenocarcinoma and bladder urothelial carcinoma. Am J Clin Pathol 2000; 113: 383.

11. Ormsby AH, Haskell R, Jones D, et al. Primary seminal vesicle carcinoma: an immunohistochemical analysis of four cases. Mod Pathol 2000; 13:46.

12. Wang HL, Lu DW, Yerian LM, et al. Immunohistochemical distinction between primary adenocarcinoma of the bladder and secondary colorectal adenocarcinoma. Am J Surg Pathol 2001; 25:1380.

13. Ordonez NG. Transitional cell carcinomas of the ovary and bladder are immunophenotypically different. Histopathology 2000; 36:433.

14. Soslow RA, Rouse RV, Hendrickson MR, et al. Transitional cell neoplasms of the ovary and urinary bladder: a comparative immunohistochemical analysis. Int J Gynecol Pathol 1996; 15:257.

15. Cheng L, Cheville JC, Sebo TJ, et al. Atypical nephrogenic metaplasia of the urinary tract: a precursor lesion? Cancer 2000; 88:853.

16. Ramos Soler D, Navarro Fos S, Villamon Fort R, et al. [Comparative study of P 53, Bcl-2, and C-erbB-2 expression in low-grade papillary bladder tumors.]. Presented at the Arch Esp Urol, Apr, 2003.

17. Varma M, Morgan M, Amin MB, et al. High molecular weight cytokeratin antibody (clone 34betaE12): a sensitive marker for differentiation of high-grade invasive urothelial carcinoma from prostate cancer. Histopathology 2003; 42:167.

18. Parker DC, Folpe AL, Bell J, et al. Potential utility of uroplakin III, thrombomodulin, high molecular weight cytokeratin, and cytokeratin 20 in noninvasive, invasive, and metastatic urothelial (transitional cell) carcinomas. Am J Surg Pathol 2003; 27:1.

19. Yuasa T, Yoshiki T, Isono T, et al. Molecular cloning and expression of uroplakins in transitional cell carcinoma. Adv Exp Med Biol 2003; 539:33.

20. Olsburgh J, Harnden P, Weeks R, et al. Uroplakin gene expression in normal human tissues and locally advanced bladder cancer. J Pathol 2003; 199:41.

21. Kageyama S, Yoshiki T, Isono T, et al. High expression of human uroplakin Ia in urinary bladder transitional cell carcinoma. Jpn J Cancer Res 2002; 93:523.

22. Mhawech P, Uchida T, Pelte MF. Immunohistochemical profile of high-grade urothelial bladder carcinoma and prostate adenocarcinoma. Hum Pathol 2002; 33:1136.

23. Xu X, Sun TT, Gupta PK, et al. Uroplakin as a marker for typing metastatic transitional cell carcinoma on fine-needle aspiration specimens. Cancer 2001; 93:216.

24. Korkolopoulou P, Christodoulou P, Konstantinidou AE, et al. Cell cycle regulators in bladder cancer: a multivariate survival study with emphasis on p27Kip1. Hum Pathol 2000; 31:751.

25. Rodel C, Grabenbauer GG, Rodel F, et al. Apoptosis, p53, bcl-2, and Ki-67 in invasive bladder carcinoma: possible predictors for response to radiochemotherapy and successful bladder preservation. Int J Radiat Oncol Biol Phys 2000; 46:1213.

26. Zlotta AR, Schulman CC. Biological markers in superficial bladder tumors and their prognostic significance. Urol Clin North Am 2000; 27:179.

27. Pfister C, Lacombe L, Vezina MC, et al. Prognostic value of the proliferative index determined by Ki-67 immunostaining in superficial bladder tumors. Hum Pathol 1999; 30:1350.

28. Zlotta AR, Noel JC, Fayt I, et al. Correlation and prognostic significance of p53, p21WAF1/CIP1 and Ki-67 expression in patients with superficial bladder tumors treated with bacillus Calmette-Guerin intravesicle therapy [see comments]. J Urol 1999; 161:792.

29. Osen I, Fossa SD, Majak B, et al. Prognostic factors in muscle-invasive bladder cancer treated with radiotherapy: an immunohistochemical study. Br J Urol 1998; 81:862.

30. Lianes P, Charytonowicz E, Cordon-Cardo C, et al. Biomarker study of primary nonmetastatic versus metastatic invasive bladder cancer. National Cancer Institute Bladder Tumor Marker Network. Clin Cancer Res 1998; 4:1267.

31. Pfister C, Buzelin F, Casse C, et al. Comparative analysis of MiB1 and p53 expression in human bladder tumors and their correlation with cancer progression. Eur Urol 1998; 33:278.

32. Korkolopoulou P, Christodoulou P, Kapralos P, et al. The role of p53, MDM2 and c-erb B-2 oncoproteins, epidermal growth factor receptor and proliferation markers in the prognosis of urinary bladder cancer. Pathol Res Pract 1997; 193:767.

33. Nakopoulou L, Vourlakou C, Zervas A, et al. The prevalence of bcl-2, p53, and Ki-67 immunoreactivity in transitional cell

bladder carcinomas and their clinicopathologic correlates. Hum Pathol 1998; 29:146.

34. Leonardi E, Cristofori A, Reich A, et al. Bivariate analysis DNA/cytokeratin 7 and flow cytometric measurement of MIB-1 in superficial transitional carcinoma of the bladder (TCC). Methodological aspects and prognostic implications. Eur J Histochem 1997; 41:133.

35. Siu LL, Banerjee D, Khurana RJ, et al. The prognostic role of p53, metallothionein, P-glycoprotein, and MIB-1 in muscle-invasive urothelial transitional cell carcinoma. Clin Cancer Res 1998; 4:559.

36. Lee E, Park I, Lee C. Prognostic markers of intravesicle bacillus Calmette-Guerin therapy for multiple, high-grade, stage T1 bladder cancers. Int J Urol 1997; 4:552.

37. Vollmer RT, Humphrey PA, Swanson PE, et al. Invasion of the bladder by transitional cell carcinoma: its relation to histologic grade and expression of p53, MIB-1, c-erb B-2, epidermal growth factor receptor, and bcl-2. Cancer 82:715. 1998;

38. Vorreuther R, Hake R, Borchmann P, et al. Expression of immunohistochemical markers (PCNA, Ki-67, 486p and p53) on paraffin sections and their relation to the recurrence rate of superficial bladder tumors. Urol Int 1997; 59:88.

39. Popov Z, Hoznek A, Colombel M, et al. The prognostic value of p53 nuclear overexpression and MIB-1 as a proliferative marker in transitional cell carcinoma of the bladder. Cancer 1997; 80:1472.

40. Tsuji M, Kojima K, Murakami Y, et al. Prognostic value of Ki-67 antigen and p53 protein in urinary bladder cancer: immunohistochemical analysis of radical cystectomy specimens. Br J Urol 1997; 79:367.

41. Hake R, Vorreuther R, Borchmann P, et al. [Monoclonal antibodies (MIB 1, PC 10, 486p and p53) as prognostic factors for recurrent urothelial carcinoma of the urinary bladder]. Verh Dtsch Ges Pathol 1993; 77:236.

42. Pich A, Chiusa L, Comino A, et al. Cell proliferation indices, morphometry and DNA flow cytometry provide objective criteria for distinguishing low and high grade bladder carcinomas. Virchows Arch 1994; 424:143.

43. Liukkonen T, Rajala P, Raitanen M, et al. Prognostic value of MIB-1 score, p53, EGFr, mitotic index and papillary status in primary superficial (stage pTa/T1) bladder cancer: a prospective comparative study. The Finnbladder Group. Eur Urol 1999; 36:393.

44. Feil G, Krause FS, Zumbraegel A, et al. Ki67, p53, nm23, and DNA cytometry in bladder cancer: potential markers for detection of recurrence? Adv Exp Med Biol 2003; 539:99.

45. Lopez-Beltran A, Luque RJ, Alvarez-Kindelan J, et al. Prognostic factors in stage T1 grade 3 bladder cancer survival: the role of G1-S modulators (p53, p21Waf1, p27kip1, cyclin D1, and cyclin D3) and proliferation index Ki67-MIB1). Eur Urol 2004; 45:606.

46. Bol MG, Baak JP, van Diermen B, et al. Proliferation markers and DNA content analysis in urinary bladder TaT1 urothelial cell carcinomas: identification of subgroups with low and high stage progression risks. J Clin Pathol 2003; 56: 447.

47. Molinie V, Longchampt E, Ouazana D, et al. [Bladder tumors and molecular markers. Current status and perspectives]. Ann Pathol 2003; 23:306.

48. Shiina H, Igawa M, Yagi H, et al. Relationship of genetic instability with immunoreactivities for p53 protein and proliferating cell nuclear antigen in transitional cell carcinoma of the bladder. Eur Urol 1996; 30:80.

49. Blasco-Olaetxea E, Belloso L, Garcia-Tamayo J. Superficial bladder cancer: study of the proliferative nuclear fraction as a prognostic factor. Eur J Cancer 1996; 32A:444.

50. Chen G, Lin MS, Li RC. Expression and prognostic value of proliferating cell nuclear antigen in transitional cell carcinoma of the urinary bladder. Urol Res 1997; 25:25.

51. Iizumi T, Iiyama T, Tanaka W, et al. Immunohistochemical studies of proliferating cell nuclear antigen and cathepsin D in transitional cell carcinoma of the urinary bladder. Urol Int 1997; 59:81.

52. Ogura K, Habuchi T, Yamada H, et al. Immunohistochemical analysis of p53 and proliferating cell nuclear antigen (PCNA) in bladder cancer: positive immunostaining and radiosensitivity. Int J Urol 1995; 2:302.

53. Shiina H, Igawa M, Nagami H, et al. Immunohistochemical analysis of proliferating cell nuclear antigen, p53 protein and nm23 protein, and nuclear DNA content in transitional cell carcinoma of the bladder. Cancer 1996; 78:1762.

54. Plastiras D, Moutzouris G, Barbatis C, et al. Can p53 nuclear over-expression, bcl-2 accumulation and PCNA status be of prognostic significance in high-risk superficial and invasive bladder tumours? Eur J Surg Oncol 1999; 25:61.

55. Lipponen PK, Eskelinen MJ. Cell proliferation of transitional cell bladder tumours determined by PCNA/cyclin immunostaining and its prognostic value. Br J Cancer 1992; 66:171.
56. Skopelitou A, Hadjiyannakis M, Dimopoulos D, et al. p53 and c-jun expression in urinary bladder transitional cell carcinoma: correlation with proliferating cell nuclear antigen (PCNA) histological grade and clinical stage. Eur Urol 1997; 31:464.
57. Pantazopoulos, Ioakim-Liossi A, Karakitsos P, et al. DNA content and proliferation activity in superficial transitional cell carcinoma of the bladder. Anticancer Res 1997; 17:781.
58. Ogura K, Fukuzawa S, Habuchi T, et al. Correlation of nuclear morphometry and immunostaining for p53 and proliferating cell nuclear antigen in transitional cell carcinoma of the bladder. Int J Urol 1997; 4:561.
59. Dalbagni G, Cordon-Cardo C, Reuter V, et al. Tumor suppressor gene alterations in bladder carcinoma. Translational correlates to clinical practice. Surg Oncol Clin N Am 1995; 4:231.
60. Underwood MA, Reeves J, Smith G, et al. Overexpression of p53 protein and its significance for recurrent progressive bladder tumours. Br J Urol 1996; 77:659.
61. Cordon-Cardo C, Sheinfeld J, Dalbagni, G. Genetic studies and molecular markers of bladder cancer. Semin Surg Oncol 1997; 13:319.
62. Cordon-Cardo C, Reuter VE. Alterations of tumor suppressor genes in bladder cancer. Semin Diagn Pathol 1997; 14:123.
63. McShane LM, Aamodt R, Cordon-Cardo C, et al. Reproducibility of p53 immunohistochemistry in bladder tumors. National Cancer Institute, Bladder Tumor Marker Network [In Process Citation]. Clin Cancer Res 2000; 6:1854.
64. Cordon-Cardo C, Dalbagni G, Saez GT, et al. p53 mutations in human bladder cancer: genotypic versus phenotypic patterns. Int J Cancer 1994; 56:347.
65. Burkhard FC., Markwalder R, Thalmann GN, et al. Immunohistochemical determination of p3 overexpression. An easy and readily available method to identify progression in superficial bladder cancer? Urol Res 1997; 25:S31.
66. Caliskan M, Turkeri LN, Mansuroglu B, et al. Nuclear accumulation of mutant p53 protein: a possible predictor of failure of intravesicle therapy in bladder cancer. Br J Urol 1997; 79:373.
67. Esrig D, Elmajian D, Groshen S. et al. Accumulation of nuclear p53 and tumor progression in bladder cancer [see comments]. N Engl J Med 1994; 331:1259.
68. Sinik Z, Alkibay T, Ataoglu O, et al. Nuclear p53 overexpression in bladder, prostate, and renal carcinomas. Int J Urol 1997; 4:546.
69. Sinik Z, Alkibay T, Ataoglu O, et al. Correlation of nuclear p53 over-expression with clinical and histopathological features of transitional cell bladder cancer. Int Urol Nephrol 1997; 29:25.
70. Vatne V, Maartmann-Moe H, Hoestmark J. The prognostic value of p53 in superficially infiltrating transitional cell carcinoma. Scand J Urol Nephrol 1995; 29:491.
71. Casetta G, Gontero P, Russo R, et al. p53 expression compared with other prognostic factors in OMS grade-I stage-Ta transitional cell carcinoma of the bladder. Eur Urol 1997; 32:229.
72. Grossman HB, Liebert M, Antelo M, et al. p53 and RB expression predict progression in T1 bladder cancer. Clin Cancer Res 1998; 4:829.
73. Gardiner RA, Walsh MD, Allen V, et al. Immunohistological expression of p53 in primary pT1 transitional cell bladder cancer in relation to tumour progression. Br J Urol 1994; 73:526.
74. Liukkonen TJ, Lipponen PK, Helle M, et al. Immunoreactivity of bcl-2, p53 and EGFr is associated with tumor stage, grade and cell proliferation in superficial bladder cancer. Finnbladder III Group. Urol Res 1997; 25:1.
75. Raitanen MP, Tammela TL, Kallioinen M, et al. P53 accumulation, deoxyribonucleic acid ploidy and progression of bladder cancer. J Urol 1997; 157:1250.
76. Friedrich MG, Erbersdobler A, Schwaibold H, et al. Detection of loss of heterozygosity in the p53 tumor-suppressor gene with PCR in the urine of patients with bladder cancer. J Urol 2000; 163:1039.
77. Rodriguez-Alonso A, Pita-Fernandez S, Gonzalez-Carrero J, et al. p53 and ki67 expression as prognostic factors for cancer-related survival in stage T1 transitional cell bladder carcinoma. Eur Urol 2002; 41:182.
78. Lipponen PK, Liukkonen TJ. Reduced expression of retinoblastoma (Rb) gene protein is related to cell proliferation and prognosis in transitional-cell bladder cancer. J Cancer Res

Clin Oncol 1995; 121:44.

79. Dalbagni G, Presti JC Jr, Reuter VE, et al. Molecular genetic alterations of chromosome 17 and p53 nuclear overexpression in human bladder cancer. Diagn Mol Pathol 1993; 2:4.

80. Inagaki T, Ebisuno S, Uekado Y, et al. PCNA and p53 in urinary bladder cancer: correlation with histological findings and prognosis. Int J Urol 1997; 4:172.

81. Miyamoto H, Kubota Y, Shuin T, et al. Analyses of p53 gene mutations in primary human bladder cancer. Oncol Res 1993; 5:245.

82. Oyasu R, Nan L, Szumel RC, et al. p53 gene mutations in human urothelial carcinomas: analysis by immunohistochemistry and single-strand conformation polymorphism. Mod Pathol 1995; 8:170.

83. Miyamoto H, Shuin T, Ikeda I, et al. Loss of heterozygosity at the p53, RB, DCC and APC tumor suppressor gene loci in human bladder cancer. J Urol 1996; 155:1444.

84. Nakopoulou L, Constantinides C, Papandropoulos J, et al. Evaluation of overexpression of p53 tumor suppressor protein in superficial and invasive transitional cell bladder cancer: comparison with DNA ploidy. Urology 1995; 46:334.

85. Sarkis AS, Dalbagni G, Cordon-Cardo C, et al. Association of P53 nuclear overexpression and tumor progression in carcinoma in situ of the bladder. J Urol 1994; 152:388.

86. Sarkis AS, Dalbagni G, Cordon-Cardo C, et al. Nuclear overexpression of p53 protein in transitional cell bladder carcinoma: a marker for disease progression. J Natl Cancer Inst 1993; 85:53.

87. Llopis J, Alcaraz A, Ribal MJ, et al. p53 expression predicts progression and poor survival in T1 bladder tumours [In Process Citation]. Eur Urol 2000; 37:644.

88. Gao JP, Uchida T, Wang C, et al. Relationship between p53 gene mutation and protein expression: clinical significance in transitional cell carcinoma of the bladder. Int J Oncol 2000; 16:469.

89. Uchida T, Wada C, Ishida H, et al. p53 mutations and prognosis in bladder tumors. J Urol 1995; 153:1097.

90. Mayr B, Reifinger M, Alton K, et al. Novel p53 tumour suppressor mutations in cases of spindle cell sarcoma, pleomorphic sarcoma and fibrosarcoma in cats. Vet Res Commun 1998; 22:249.

91. Okamoto M, Hattori K, Fujimoto K, et al. Antisense RNA-mediated reduction of p53 induces malignant phenotype in nontumorigenic rat urothelial cells. Carcinogenesis 1998; 19:73.

92. Fujimoto K, Yamada Y, Okajima E, et al. Frequent association of p53 gene mutation in invasive bladder cancer. Cancer Res 1992; 52:1393.

93. Spruck CH 3rd, Ohneseit PF, Gonzalez-Zulueta M, et al. Two molecular pathways to transitional cell carcinoma of the bladder. Cancer Res 1994; 54:784.

94. Tzai TS, Chow NH, Lin JS, et al. The expression of p53 and bcl-2 in superficial bladder transitional cell carcinoma and its role in the outcome of postoperative intravesicle chemotherapy. Anticancer Res 1998; 18:4717.

95. Aprikian AG, Sarkis AS, Reuter VE, et al. Biological markers of prognosis in transitional cell carcinoma of the bladder: current concepts. Semin Urol 1993; 11:137.

96. Cordon-Cardo C, Dalbagni G, Sarkis AS, et al. Genetic alterations associated with bladder cancer. Important Adv Oncol 1994; 71–73.

97. Sarkis AS, Bajorin DF, Reuter VE, et al. Prognostic value of p53 nuclear overexpression in patients with invasive bladder cancer treated with neoadjuvant MVAC. J Clin Oncol 1995; 13:1384.

98. Esrig D, Spruck CH, Nichols PW, et al. p53 nuclear protein accumulation correlates with mutations in the p53 gene, tumor grade, and stage in bladder cancer. Am J Pathol 1993; 143:1389.

99. Lipponen PK. Over-expression of p53 nuclear oncoprotein in transitional-cell bladder cancer and its prognostic value. Int J Cancer 1993; 53:365.

100. al-Abadi H, Nagel R, Neuhaus P. Immunohistochemical detection of p53 protein in transitional cell carcinoma of the bladder in correlation to DNA ploidy and pathohistological stage and grade. Cancer Detect Prev 1998; 22:43.

101. Niehans GA, Kratzke RA, Froberg MK, et al. G1 checkpoint protein and p53 abnormalities occur in most invasive transitional cell carcinomas of the urinary bladder. Br J Cancer 1999; 80:1175.

102. Glick SH, Howell LP, White RW. Relationship of p53 and bcl-2 to prognosis in muscle-invasive transitional cell carcinoma of the bladder. J Urol 1996; 155:1754.

103. Watanabe R, Tomita Y, Nishiyama T, et al. Correlation of p53 protein expression in human urothelial transitional cell cancers with malignant potential and patient survival. Int J

Urol 1994; 1:43.

104. Lebret T, Becette V, Barbagelatta M, et al. Correlation between p53 overexpression and response to bacillus Calmette-Guerin therapy in a high risk select population of patients with T1G3 bladder cancer. J Urol 1998; 159:788.

105. Pages F, Flam TA, Vieillefond A, et al. p53 status does not predict initial clinical response to bacillus Calmette-Guerin intravesicle therapy in T1 bladder tumors. J Urol 1998; 159: 1079.

106. Cote RJ, Esrig D, Groshen S, et al. p53 and treatment of bladder cancer [letter; comment]. Nature 1997; 385:123.

107. Grossfeld GD, Ginsberg DA, Stein JP, et al. Thrombospondin-1 expression in bladder cancer: association with p53 alterations, tumor angiogenesis, and tumor progression. J Natl Cancer Inst 1997; 89:219.

108. Garcia del Muro X, Condom E, Vigues F, et al. p53 and p21 expression levels predict organ preservation and survival in invasive bladder carcinoma treated with a combined-modality approach. Cancer 2004; 100:1859-1867.

109. Tzai TS, Tsai YS, Chow NH. The prevalence and clinicopathologic correlate of p16INK4a, retinoblastoma and p53 immunoreactivity in locally advanced urinary bladder cancer. Urol Oncol 2004; 22:112.

110. Lopez-Beltran A, Escudero AL. Human papillomavirus and bladder cancer. Biomed Pharmacother 1997; 51:252.

111. Lopez-Beltran A, Escudero AL, Carrasco-Aznar JC, et al. Human papillomavirus infection and transitional cell carcinoma of the bladder. Immunohistochemistry and in situ hybridization. Pathol Res Pract 1996; 192:154.

112. Lopez-Beltran A, Escudero AL, Vicioso L, et al. Human papillomavirus DNA as a factor determining the survival of bladder cancer patients. Br J Cancer 1996; 73:124.

113. Lopez-Beltran A, Munoz E. Transitional cell carcinoma of the bladder: low incidence of human papillomavirus DNA detected by the polymerase chain reaction and in situ hybridization. Histopathology 1995; 26:565.

114. Khaled HM, Bahnassi AA, Zekri AR, et al. Correlation between p53 mutations and HPV in bilharzial bladder cancer. Urol Oncol 2003; 21:334.

115. Simoneau M, LaRue H, Fradet Y. Low frequency of human papillomavirus infection in initial papillary bladder tumors. Urol Res 1999; 27:180.

116. Lianes P, Orlow I, Zhang ZF, et al. Altered patterns of MDM2 and TP53 expression in human bladder cancer [see comments]. J Natl Cancer Inst 1994; 86:1325.

117. Schmitz-Drager BJ, Kushima M, Goebell P, et al. p53 and MDM2 in the development and progression of bladder cancer. Eur Urol 1997; 32:487.

118. Warren W, Biggs PJ, el-Baz M, et al. Mutations in the p53 gene in schistosomal bladder cancer: a study of 92 tumours from Egyptian patients and a comparison between mutational spectra from schistosomal and non-schistosomal urothelial tumours. Carcinogenesis 1995; 16:1181.

119. Orlow I, Lacombe L, Hannon GJ, et al. Deletion of the p16 and p15 genes in human bladder tumors [see comments]. J Natl Cancer Inst 1995; 87:1524.

120. Gonzalez-Zulueta M, Bender CM, Yang AS, et al. Methylation of the 5' CpG island of the p16/CDKN2 tumor suppressor gene in normal and transformed human tissues correlates with gene silencing. Cancer Res 1995; 55:4531.

121. Orlow I, LaRue H, Osman I, et al. Deletions of the INK4A gene in superficial bladder tumors. Association with recurrence. Am J Pathol 1999; 155:105.

122. Nakopoulou LL, Constandinides CA, Tzonou A, et al. Immunohistochemical evaluation of nm23-H1 gene product in transitional cell carcinoma of the bladder. Histopathology 1996; 28:429.

123. Xu X, Stower MJ, Reid IN, et al. A hot spot for p53 mutation in transitional cell carcinoma of the bladder: clues to the etiology of bladder cancer. Cancer Epidemiol Biomarkers Prev 1997; 6:611.

124. Ahrendt SA, Decker PA, Doffek K, et al. Microsatellite instability at selected tetranucleotide repeats is associated with p53 mutations in non-small cell lung cancer. Cancer Res 2000; 60:2488.

125. Xu X, Stower MJ, Reid IN, et al. Molecular screening of multifocal transitional cell carcinoma of the bladder using p53 mutations as biomarkers. Clin Cancer Res 1996; 2:1795.

126. Spruck CH 3rd, Gonzalez-Zulueta M, Shibata A, et al. p16 gene in uncultured tumours [letter] [see comments]. Nature 1994; 370:183.

127. Sidransky D, Von Eschenbach A, Tsai YC, et al. Identification of p53 gene mutations in bladder cancers and urine samples. Science 1991; 252:706.

128. Krupski T, Moskaluk C, Boyd JC, et al. A prospective pilot evaluation of urinary and immunohistochemical markers as

predictors of clinical stage of urothelial carcinoma of the bladder. Br J Urol 2000; 85:1027.

129. Brown FM. Urine cytology. Is it still the gold standard for screening? Urol Clin North Am 2000; 27:25.

130. Righi E, Rossi G, Ferrari G, et al. Does p53 immunostaining improve diagnostic accuracy in urine cytology? Diagn Cytopathol 1997; 17:436.

131. Sugano K, Tsutsumi M, Nakashima Y, et al. Diagnosis of bladder cancer by analysis of the allelic loss of the p53 gene in urine samples using blunt-end single-strand conformation polymorphism. Int J Cancer 1997; 74:403.

132. Mao L. Genetic alterations as clonal markers for bladder cancer detection in urine. J Cell Biochem Suppl 1996; 25:191.

133. Walther PJ. 'Wildcatting' for breakthroughs in urothelial cancer detection and management – a frustrating business [editorial; comment]. J Urol 1995; 154:1348.

134. Hruban RH, van der Riet P, Erozan YS, et al. Brief report: molecular biology and the early detection of carcinoma of the bladder – the case of Hubert H. Humphrey [see comments]. N Engl J Med 1994; 330:1276.

135. Benedict WF, Lerner SP, Zhou J, et al. Level of retinoblastoma protein expression correlates with p16 (MTS-1/INK4A/CDKN2) status in bladder cancer. Oncogene 1999; 18:1197.

136. Ishikawa J, Xu HJ, Hu SX, et al. Inactivation of the retinoblastoma gene in human bladder and renal cell carcinomas. Cancer Res 1991; 51:5736.

137. Miyamoto H, Shuin T, Torigoe S, et al. Retinoblastoma gene mutations in primary human bladder cancer. Br J Cancer 1995; 71:831.

138. Kubota Y, Miyamoto H, Noguchi S, et al. The loss of retinoblastoma gene in association with c-myc and transforming growth factor-beta 1 gene expression in human bladder cancer [see comments]. J Urol 1995; 154:371.

139. Diaz-Cano SJ, Blanes A, Rubio J, et al. Molecular evolution and intratumor heterogeneity by topographic compartments in muscle-invasive transitional cell carcinoma of the urinary bladder. Lab Invest 2000; 80:279.

140. Cordon-Cardo C. Molecular alterations in bladder cancer. Cancer Surv 1998; 32:115.

141. de Vere White RW, Stapp E. Predicting prognosis in patients with superficial bladder cancer. Oncology (Huntingt) 1998; 12:1717.

142. Ow K, Delprado W, Fisher R, et al. Relationship between expression of the KAI1 metastasis suppressor and other markers of advanced bladder cancer. J Pathol 2000; 191:39.

143. Wada T, Louhelainen J, Hemminki K, et al. Bladder cancer: allelic deletions at and around the retinoblastoma tumor suppressor gene in relation to stage and grade. Clin Cancer Res 2000; 6:610.

144. Pollack A, Wu CS, Czerniak B, et al. Abnormal bcl-2 and pRb expression are independent correlates of radiation response in muscle-invasive bladder cancer. Clin Cancer Res 1997; 3:1823.

145. Adshead JM, Kessling AM, Ogden CW. Genetic initiation, progression and prognostic markers in transitional cell carcinoma of the bladder: a summary of the structural and transcriptional changes, and the role of developmental genes. Br J Urol 1998; 82:503.

146. Orntoft TF, Wolf H. Molecular alterations in bladder cancer [editorial]. Urol Res 1998; 26:223.

147. Jahnson S, Karlsson MG. Predictive value of p53 and pRb immunostaining in locally advanced bladder cancer treated with cystectomy. J Urol 1998; 160:1291.

148. Pollack A, Czerniak B, Zagars GK, et al. Retinoblastoma protein expression and radiation response in muscleinvasive bladder cancer. Int J Radiat Oncol Biol Phys 1997; 39:687.

149. Cordon-Cardo C, Zhang ZF, Dalbagni G, et al. Cooperative effects of p53 and pRB alterations in primary superficial bladder tumors. Cancer Res 1997; 57:1217.

150. Cordon-Cardo C. p53 and RB: simple interesting correlates or tumor markers of critical predictive nature? J Clin Oncol 2004; 22:975.

151. Goodrich DW, Chen Y, Scully P, et al. Expression of the retinoblastoma gene product in bladder carcinoma cells associates with a low frequency of tumor formation. Cancer Res 1992; 52:1968.

152. Wright C, Thomas D, Mellon K, et al. Expression of retinoblastoma gene product and p53 protein in bladder carcinoma: correlation with Ki67 index. Br J Urol 1995; 75:173.

153. Geradts J, Hu SX, Lincoln CE, et al. Aberrant RB gene expression in routinely processed, archival tumor tissues determined by three different anti-RB antibodies. Int J Cancer 1994; 58:161.

154. Sanchez Zalabardo D, Rosell Costa D, Fernandez Montero JM, et al. [Prognostic value of P53, Ki67, and Rb protein in infiltrating bladder tumors]. Actas Urol Esp 2002; 26:98.

155. Chatterjee SJ, George B, Goebell PJ, et al. Hyperphosphorylation of pRb: a mechanism for RB tumour suppressor pathway inactivation in bladder cancer. J Pathol 2004; 203:762.

156. Gorgoulis VG, Barbatis C, Poulias I, et al. Molecular and immunohistochemical evaluation of epidermal growth factor receptor and c-erb-B-2 gene product in transitional cell carcinomas of the urinary bladder: a study in Greek patients. Mod Pathol 1995; 8:758.

157. Tetu B, Allard P, Fradet Y, et al. Prognostic significance of nuclear DNA content and S-phase fraction by flow cytometry in primary papillary superficial bladder cancer. Hum Pathol 1996; 27:922.

158. Underwood M, Bartlett J, Reeves J, et al. C-erbB-2 gene amplification: a molecular marker in recurrent bladder tumors? Cancer Res 1995; 55:2422.

159. Coogan CL, Estrada CR, Kapur S, et al. HER-2/neu protein overexpression and gene amplification in human transitional cell carcinoma of the bladder. Urology 2004; 63:786.

160. de Pinieux G, Colin D, Vincent-Salomon A, et al. Confrontation of immunohistochemistry and fluorescent in situ hybridization for the assessment of HER-2/neu (c-erbB-2) status in urothelial carcinoma. Virchows Arch 2004; 444:415.

161. Mellon JK, Lunec J, Wright C, et al. C-erbB-2 in bladder cancer: molecular biology, correlation with epidermal growth factor receptors and prognostic value [see comments]. J Urol 1996; 155:321.

162. Lonn U, Lonn S, Friberg S., et al. Prognostic value of amplification of c-erb-B2 in bladder carcinoma. Clin Cancer Res 1995; 1:1189.

163. Miyamoto H, Kubota Y, Noguchi S, et al. C-ERBB-2 gene amplification as a prognostic marker in human bladder cancer. Urology 2000; 55:679.

164. Moch H, Sauter G, Mihatsch MJ, et al. p53 but not erbB-2 expression is associated with rapid tumor proliferation in urinary bladder cancer. Hum Pathol 1994; 25:1346.

165. Wagner U, Sauter G, Moch H, et al. Patterns of p53, erbB-2, and EGF-r expression in premalignant lesions of the urinary bladder. Hum Pathol 1995; 26:970.

166. Li B, Kanamaru H, Noriki S, et al. Reciprocal expression of bcl-2 and p53 oncoproteins in urothelial dysplasia and carcinoma of the urinary bladder. Urol Res 1998; 26:235.

167. Kelly JD, Williamson KE, Irvine AE, et al. Apoptosis and its clinical significance for bladder cancer therapy. Br J Urol Int 1999; 83:1.

168. Miyake H, Hara I, Yamanaka K, et al. Overexpression of bcl-2 enhances metastatic potential of human bladder cancer cells. Br J Cancer 1999; 79:1651.

169. Kong G, Shin KY, Oh YH, et al. Bcl-2 and p53 expressions in invasive bladder cancers. Acta Oncol 1998; 37:715.

170. Wu TT, Chen JH, Lee YH, et al. The role of bcl-2, p53, and Ki-67 index in predicting tumor recurrence for low grade superficial transitional cell bladder carcinoma. J Urol 2000; 163:758.

171. Gazzaniga P, Gradilone A, Vercillo R, et al. Bcl-2/bax mRNA expression ratio as prognostic factor in low-grade urinary bladder cancer. Int J Cancer 1996; 69:100.

172. Keegan PE, Lunec J, Neal DE. p53 and p53-regulated genes in bladder cancer [see comments]. Br J Urol 1998; 82:710.

173. Atug F, Turkeri L, Ozyurek M, et al. Bcl-2 and p53 overexpression as associated risk factors in transitional cell carcinoma of the bladder. Int Urol Nephrol 1998; 30:455.

174. Ye D, Li H, Qian S, et al. bcl-2/bax expression and p53 gene status in human bladder cancer: relationship to early recurrence with intravesicle chemotherapy after resection. J Urol 1998; 160:2025.

175. Okamura T, Akita H, Kawai N, et al. Immunohistochemical evaluation of p53, proliferating cell nuclear antigen (PCNA) and bcl-2 expression during bacillus Calmette-Guerin (BCG) intravesicle instillation therapy for superficial bladder cancers. Urol Res 1998; 26:161.

176. Eissa S, Seada LS. Quantitation of bcl-2 protein in bladder cancer tissue by enzyme immunoassay: comparison with Western blot and immunohistochemistry. Clin Chem 1998; 44:1423.

177. Bilim VN, Tomita Y, Kawasaki T, et al. Variable bcl-2 phenotype in benign and malignant lesions of urothelium [see comments]. Cancer Lett 1998; 128:87.

178. Gazzaniga P, Gradilone A, Silvestri I, et al. Variable levels of bcl-2, bcl-x and bax mRNA in bladder cancer progression. Oncol Rep 1998; 5:901.

179. Kirsh EJ, Baunoch DA, Stadler WM. Expression of bcl-2 and bcl-X in bladder cancer. J Urol 1998; 159:1348.

180. Shiina H, Igawa M, Urakami S, et al. Immunohistochemical analysis of bcl-2 expression in transitional cell carcinoma of the bladder. J Clin Pathol 1996; 49:395.

181. Lipponen PK, Aaltomaa S, Eskelinen M. Expression of the apoptosis suppressing bcl-2 protein in transitional cell bladder tumours. Histopathology 1996; 28:135.

182. King ED, Matteson J, Jacobs SC, et al. Incidence of apoptosis, cell proliferation and bcl-2 expression in transitional cell carcinoma of the bladder: association with tumor progression [see comments]. J Urol 1996; 155:316.

183. Cooke PW, James ND, Ganesan R, et al. Bcl-2 expression identifies patients with advanced bladder cancer treated by radiotherapy who benefit from neoadjuvant chemotherapy. Br J Urol Int 2000; 85:829.

184. Matsumoto H, Wada T, Fukunaga K, et al., eds. Bax to Bcl-2 ratio and Ki-67 index are useful predictors of neoadjuvant chemoradiation therapy in bladder cancer. Jpn J Clin Oncol 2004; 34:124–130.

185. Ross JS, del Rosario AD, Figge HL, et al. E-cadherin expression in papillary transitional cell carcinoma of the urinary bladder. Hum Pathol 1995; 26:940.

186. Ross JS, del Rosario AD, Bui HX, et al. Expression of the CD44 cell adhesion molecule in urinary bladder transitional cell carcinoma. Mod Pathol 1996; 9:854.

187. Lipponen PK, Eskelinen MJ. Reduced expression of Ecadherin is related to invasive disease and frequent recurrence in bladder cancer. J Cancer Res Clin Oncol 1995; 121:303.

188. Wakatsuki S, Watanabe R, Saito K, et al. Loss of human E-cadherin (ECD) correlated with invasiveness of transitional cell cancer in the renal pelvis, ureter and urinary bladder. Cancer Lett 1996; 103:11.

189. Popov Z, Gil-Diez de Medina S, Lefrere-Belda MA, et al. Low E-cadherin expression in bladder cancer at the transcriptional and protein level provides prognostic information. Br J Cancer 2000; 83:209.

190. Garcia del Muro X, Torregrosa A, Munoz J, et al. Prognostic value of the expression of E-cadherin and beta-catenin in bladder cancer. Eur J Cancer 2000; 36:357.

191. Syrigos KN, Karayiannakis A, Syrigou EI, et al. Abnormal expression of p120 correlates with poor survival in patients with bladder cancer. Eur J Cancer 1998; 34:2037.

192. Mialhe A, Louis J, Montlevier S, et al. Expression of Ecadherin and alpha-, beta- and gamma-catenins in human bladder carcinomas: are they good prognostic factors? Invasion Metastasis 1997; 17:124.

193. Mialhe A, Louis J, Pasquier D, et al. Expression of three cell adhesion molecules in bladder carcinomas: correlation with pathological features [published erratum appears in Anal Cell Pathol 1997; 14(2):1225–1227]. Anal Cell Pathol 1997; 13:125.

194. Shimazui T, Schalken JA, Giroldi LA, et al. Prognostic value of cadherin-associated molecules (alpha-, beta-, and gamma-catenins and p120cas) in bladder tumors. Cancer Res 1996; 56:4154.

195. Fujisawa M, Miyazaki J, Takechi Y. et al. The significance of E-cadherin in transitional-cell carcinoma of the human urinary bladder. World J Urol 1996; 14:S12.

196. Giroldi LA, Bringuier PP, Schalken JA. Defective Ecadherin function in urological cancers: clinical implications and molecular mechanisms. Invasion Metastasis 1994; 14:71.

197. Ross JS, Cheung C, Sheehan C, et al. E-cadherin cell-adhesion molecule expression as a diagnostic adjunct in urothelial cytology. Diagn Cytopathol 1996; 14:310.

198. Matsumoto K, Shariat SF, Casella R, et al. Preoperative plasma soluble E-cadherin predicts metastases to lymph nodes and prognosis in patients undergoing radical cystectomy. J Urol 2003; 170:2248–2252.

199. Griffiths TR, Brotherick I, Bishop RI, et al. Cell adhesion molecules in bladder cancer: soluble serum E-cadherin correlates with predictors of recurrence. Br J Cancer 1996; 74:579.

200. Byrne RR, Shariat SF, Brown R, et al. E-cadherin immunostaining of bladder transitional cell carcinoma, carcinoma in situ and lymph node metastases with long-term followup. J Urol 2001; 165:1473.

201. Grossman HB, Lee C, Bromberg J, et al. Expression of the alpha6beta4 integrin provides prognostic information in bladder cancer. Oncol Rep 2000; 7:13.

202. Wilson CB, Leopard J, Cheresh DA, et al. Extracellular matrix and integrin composition of the normal bladder wall. World J Urol 1996; 14:S30.

203. Liebert M, Washington R, Wedemeyer G, et al. Loss of co-localization of alpha 6 beta 4 integrin and collagen VII in bladder cancer. Am J Pathol 1994; 144:787.

204. Lee CC, Yamamoto S, Morimura K, et al. Significance of cyclin D1 overexpression in transitional cell carcinomas of the urinary bladder and its correlation with histopathologic features. Cancer 1997; 79:780.

205. Shin KY, Kong G, Kim WS, et al. Overexpression of cyclin D1 correlates with early recurrence in superficial bladder cancers. Br J Cancer 1997; 75:1788.
206. Wagner U, Suess K, Luginbuhl T, et al. Cyclin D1 overexpression lacks prognostic significance in superficial urinary bladder cancer. J Pathol 1999; 188:44.
207. Bringuier PP, Tamimi Y, Schuuring E, et al. Expression of cyclin D1 and EMS1 in bladder tumours; relationship with chromosome 11q13 amplification. Oncogene 1996; 12:1747.
208. Suwa Y, Takano Y, Iki M, et al. Cyclin D1 protein overexpression is related to tumor differentiation, but not to tumor progression or proliferative activity, in transitional cell carcinoma of the bladder. J Urol 1998; 160:897.
209. Takaba K, Saeki K, Suzuki K, et al. Significant overexpression of metallothionein and cyclin D1 and apoptosis in the early process of rat urinary bladder carcinogenesis induced by treatment with N-butyl-N-(4-hydroxybutyl)nitrosamine or sodium L-ascorbate. Carcinogenesis 2000; 21:691.
210. Rabbani F, Cordon-Cardo C. Mutation of cell cycle regulators and their impact on superficial bladder cancer. Urol Clin North Am 2000; 27:83.
211. Sgambato A, Migaldi M, Faraglia B, et al. Cyclin D1 expression in papillary superficial bladder cancer: its association with other cell cycle-associated proteins, cell proliferation and clinical outcome. Int J Cancer 2002; 97:671.
212. Woodman AC, Goodison S, Drake M, et al. Noninvasive diagnosis of bladder carcinoma by enzyme-linked immunosorbent assay detection of CD44 isoforms in exfoliated urothelia [In Process Citation]. Clin Cancer Res 2000; 6:2381.
213. Miyake H, Hara I, Arakawa S, et al. Utility of competitive reverse transcription-polymerase chain reaction analysis of specific CD44 variant RNA for detecting upper urinary tract transitional-cell carcinoma. Mol Urol 1999; 3:365.
214. Lipponen P, Aaltoma S, Kosma VM, et al. Expression of CD44 standard and variant-v6 proteins in transitional cell bladder tumours and their relation to prognosis during a long-term follow-up. J Pathol 1998; 186:157.
215. Miyake H, Hara I, Gohji K, et al. Urinary cytology and competitive reverse transcriptase-polymerase chain reaction analysis of a specific CD44 variant to detect and monitor bladder cancer [see comments]. J Urol 1998; 160:2004.
216. Iczkowski KA, Shanks JH, Bostwick DG. Loss of CD44 variant 6 expression differentiates small cell carcinoma of urinary bladder from urothelial (transitional cell) carcinoma. Histopathology 1998; 32:322.
217. Muller M, Heicappell R, Habermann F, et al. Expression of CD44V2 in transitional cell carcinoma of the urinary bladder and in urine. Urol Res 1997; 25:187.
218. Naot D, Sionov RV, Ish-Shalom D. CD44: structure, function, and association with the malignant process. Adv Cancer Res 1997; 71:241.
219. Sugino T, Gorham H, Yoshida K, et al. Progressive loss of CD44 gene expression in invasive bladder cancer. Am J Pathol 1996; 149:873.
220. Takada S, Namiki M, Matsumiya K. et al. Expression of CD44 splice variants in human transitional cell carcinoma. Eur Urol 1996; 29:370.
221. Kan M, Furukawa A, Aki M, et al. Expression of CD44 splice variants in bladder cancer. Int J Urol 1995; 2:295.
222. Matsumura Y, Sugiyama M, Matsumura S, et al. Unusual retention of introns in CD44 gene transcripts in bladder cancer provides new diagnostic and clinical oncological opportunities. J Pathol 1995; 177:11.
223. Lein M, Jung K, Weiss S, et al. Soluble CD44 variants in the serum of patients with urological malignancies. Oncology 1997; 54:226.
224. Gadalla HA, Kamel NA, Badary FA, et al. Expression of CD44 protein in bilharzial and non-bilharzial bladder cancers. Br J Urol Int 2004; 93:151.
225. Jaeger TM, Weidner N, Chew K, et al. Tumor angiogenesis correlates with lymph node metastases in invasive bladder cancer. J Urol 1995; 154:69.
226. Dickinson AJ, Fox SB, Persad RA, et al. Quantification of angiogenesis as an independent predictor of prognosis in invasive bladder carcinomas. Br J Urol 1994; 74:762.
227. Bochner BH, Cote RJ, Weidner N, et al. Angiogenesis in bladder cancer: relationship between microvessel density and tumor prognosis. J Natl Cancer Inst 1995; 87:1603.
228. Hawke CK, Delahunt B, Davidson PJ. Microvessel density as a prognostic marker for transitional cell carcinoma of the bladder. Br J Urol 1998; 81:585.
229. Dinney CP, Babkowski RC, Antelo M, et al. Relationship among cystectomy, microvessel density and prognosis in stage T1 transitional cell carcinoma of the bladder. J Urol 1998; 160:1285.

230. Ozer E, Mungan MU, Tuna B, et al. Prognostic significance of angiogenesis and immunoreactivity of cathepsin D and type IV collagen in high-grade stage T1 primary bladder cancer. Urology 1999; 54:50.

231. Chaudhary R, Bromley M, Clarke NW, et al. Prognostic relevance of micro-vessel density in cancer of the urinary bladder. Anticancer Res 1999; 19:3479.

232. Goddard JC, Sutton CD, Furness PN, et al. Microvessel density at presentation predicts subsequent muscle invasion in superficial bladder cancer. Clin Cancer Res 2003; 9:2583.

233. Campbell SC, Volpert OV, Ivanovich M, et al. Molecular mediators of angiogenesis in bladder cancer. Cancer Res 1998; 58:1298.

234. Crew JP. Vascular endothelial growth factor: an important angiogenic mediator in bladder cancer. Eur Urol 1999; 35:2.

235. Sato K, Sasaki R, Ogura Y, et al. Expression of vascular endothelial growth factor gene and its receptor (flt-1) gene in urinary bladder cancer. Tohoku J Exp Med 1998; 185:173.

236. Brown LF, Berse B, Jackman RW, et al. Increased expression of vascular permeability factor (vascular endothelial growth factor) and its receptors in kidney and bladder carcinomas. Am J Pathol 1993; 143:1255.

237. Chow NH, Liu HS, Chan SH, et al. Expression of vascular endothelial growth factor in primary superficial bladder cancer. Anticancer Res 1999; 19:4593.

238. Jones A, Crew J. Vascular endothelial growth factor and its correlation with superficial bladder cancer recurrence rates and stage progression. Urol Clin North Am 2000; 27:191.

239. Crew JP, O'Brien T, Bicknell R, et al. Urinary vascular endothelial growth factor and its correlation with bladder cancer recurrence rates [see comments]. J Urol 1999; 161:799.

240. Droller MJ. Vascular endothelial growth factor is a predictor of relapse and stage progression in superficial bladder cancer. J Urol 1998; 160:1932.

241. Crew JP, O'Brien T, Bradburn M, et al. Vascular endothelial growth factor is a predictor of relapse and stage progression in superficial bladder cancer. Cancer Res 1997; 57:5281.

242. Yang CC, Chu KC, Yeh WM. The expression of vascular endothelial growth factor in transitional cell carcinoma of urinary bladder is correlated with cancer progression. Urol Oncol 2004; 22:1.

243. Colquhoun AJ, Mellon JK. Epidermal growth factor receptor and bladder cancer. Postgrad Med J 2002; 78:584.

244. Qu XJ, Yang JL, Russell PJ, et al. Changes in epidermal growth factor receptor expression in human bladder cancer cell lines following interferon-alpha treatment. J Urol 2004; 172:733.

245. Penault-Llorca F, Durando X, Bay JO. [Prognostic value of epidermal growth factor receptor]. Bull Cancer 2003; 90:S192.

246. Otto T, Bex A, Schmidt U, et al. Improved prognosis assessment for patients with bladder carcinoma. Am J Pathol 1997; 150:1919.

247. Jones HL, Delahunt B, Bethwaite PB, et al. Luminal epithelial antigen (LEA.135) expression correlates with tumor progression for transitional carcinoma of the bladder. Anticancer Res 1997; 17:685.

248. Zhuang YH, Blauer M, Tammela T, et al. Immunodetection of androgen receptor in human urinary bladder cancer. Histopathology 1997; 30:556.

249. Shariat SF, Casella R, Monoski MA, et al. The addition of urinary urokinase-type plasminogen activator to urinary nuclear matrix protein 22 and cytology improves the detection of bladder cancer. J Urol 2003; 170:2244.

250. Hasui Y, Osada Y. Urokinase-type plasminogen activator and its receptor in bladder cancer [editorial; comment] [see comments]. J Natl Cancer Inst 1997; 89:678.

251. Hasui Y, Marutsuka K, Asada Y, et al. Prognostic value of urokinase-type plasminogen activator in patients with superficial bladder cancer. Urology 1996; 47:34.

252. Hasui Y, Marutsuka K, Nishi S, et al. The content of urokinase-type plasminogen activator and tumor recurrence in superficial bladder cancer. J Urol 1994; 151:16.

253. Schmitt M, Janicke F, Moniwa N, et al. Tumor-associated urokinase-type plasminogen activator: biological and clinical significance. Biol Chem Hoppe Seyler 1992; 373:611.

254. Hasui Y, Suzumiya J, Marutsuka K, et al. Comparative study of plasminogen activators in cancers and normal mucosae of human urinary bladder. Cancer Res 1989; 49:1067.

255. Baffa R, Gomella LG, Vecchione A, et al. Loss of FHIT expression in transitional cell carcinoma of the urinary bladder. Am J Pathol 2000; 156:419.

256. Klein A, Zemer R, Buchumensky V, et al. Expression of cytokeratin 20 in urinary cytology of patients with bladder carcinoma [see comments]. Cancer 1998; 82:349.

257. Ravery V, Colombel M, Popov Z, et al. Prognostic value of epidermal growth factor-receptor, T138 and T43 expression

in bladder cancer. Br J Cancer 1995; 71:196.

258. Lokeshwar VB, Obek C, Pham HT, et al. Urinary hyaluronic acid and hyaluronidase: markers for bladder cancer detection and evaluation of grade. J Urol 2000; 163:348.

259. Lokeshwar VB, Block NL. HA-HAase urine test. A sensitive and specific method for detecting bladder cancer and evaluating its grade. Urol Clin North Am 2000; 27:53.

260. Lokeshwar VB, Soloway MS, Block NL. Secretion of bladder tumor-derived hyaluronidase activity by invasive bladder tumor cells. Cancer Lett 1998; 131:21.

261. Pham HT, Block NL, Lokeshwar VB. Tumor-derived hyaluronidase: a diagnostic urine marker for high-grade bladder cancer [published erratum appears in Cancer Res 1997; 57:1622]. Cancer Res 1997; 57:778.

262. Lokeshwar VB, Obek C, Soloway MS, et al. Tumor-associated hyaluronic acid: a new sensitive and specific urine marker for bladder cancer [published erratum appears in Cancer Res 1998; 58:3191]. Cancer Res 1997; 57:773.

263. Bostwick D, Lopez-Beltran A. Bladder biopsy interpretation. Glen Allen, VA: United Pathologists Press; 1999.

264. Lin O, Cardillo M, Dalbagni G, et al. Nested variant of urothelial carcinoma: a clinicopathologic and immunohistochemical study of 12 cases. Mod Pathol 2003; 16:1289.

265. Jones EC, Clement PB, Young RH. Inflammatory pseudotumor of the urinary bladder. A clinicopathological, immunohistochemical, ultrastructural, and flow cytometric study of 13 cases [see comments]. Am J Surg Pathol 1993; 17:264.

266. Yamaguchi T, Imamura Y, Shimamoto T, et al. Small cell carcinoma of the bladder. Two cases diagnosed by urinary cytology. Acta Cytol 2000; 44:403.

267. Eusebi V, Damiani S, Pasquinelli G, et al.: Small cell neuroendocrine carcinoma with skeletal muscle differentiation: report of three cases. Am J Surg Pathol 2000; 24:223.

268. Ali SZ, Reuter VE, Zakowski MF. Small cell neuroendocrine carcinoma of the urinary bladder. A clinicopathologic study with emphasis on cytologic features. Cancer 1997; 79:356.

269. Terracciano L, Richter J, Tornillo L, et al. Chromosomal imbalances in small cell carcinomas of the urinary bladder. J Pathol 1999; 189:230.

270. Grammatico D, Grignon DJ, Eberwein P, et al. Transitional cell carcinoma of the renal pelvis with choriocarcinomatous differentiation. Immunohistochemical and immunoelectron microscopic assessment of human chorionic gonadotropin production by transitional cell carcinoma of the urinary bladder. Cancer 1993; 71:1835.

271. Yamase HT, Wurzel RS, Nieh PT, et al. Immunohistochemical demonstration of human chorionic gonadotropin in tumors of the urinary bladder. Ann Clin Lab Sci 1985; 15:414.

272. Martin JE, Jenkins BJ, Zuk RJ, et al. Human chorionic gonadotrophin expression and histological findings as predictors of response to radiotherapy in carcinoma of the bladder. Virchows Arch A Pathol Anat Histopathol 1989; 414:273.

273. Biyani CS, Sharma N, Nicol A, et al. Postoperative spindle cell nodule of the bladder: a diagnostic problem. Urol Int 1996; 56:119.

274. Allen PW, Allen LJ. Perce the permissive pathologist: a cautionary tale of one who misdiagnosed a pseudosarcoma, killed the patient and was found out. Aust NZ J Surg 1994; 64:273.

275. Lo JW, Fung CH, Yonan T, et al. Postoperative spindle-cell nodule of urinary bladder with unusual intracytoplasmic inclusions. Diagn Cytopathol 1992; 8:171.

276. Young RH. Spindle cell lesions of the urinary bladder. Histol Histopathol 1990; 5:505.

277. Vekemans K, Vanneste A, Van Oyen P, et al. Postoperative spindle cell nodule of bladder. Urology 1990; 35:342.

278. Huang WL, Ro JY, Grignon DJ, et al. Postoperative spindle cell nodule of the prostate and bladder. J Urol 1990; 143:824.

279. Rehmani JA, Khan MA, Mehmood A, et al. Pseudotumor of urinary bladder. J Coll Physicians Surg Pak 2004; 14:53.

280. Lopez-Beltran A, Lopez-Ruiz, J, Vicioso L. Inflammatory pseudotumor of the urinary bladder. A clinicopathological analysis of two cases. Urol Int 1995; 55:173.

281. Wanibuchi H, Iwata H, Washida H, et al. A case report of inflammatory pseudotumor of the urinary bladder. Osaka City Med J 1995; 41:31.

282. Foschini MP, Scarpellini F, Rinaldi P, et al. [Inflammatory pseudotumor of the urinary bladder. Study of 4 cases and review of the literature]. Pathologica 1995; 87:653.

283. Jones EC, Young RH. Myxoid and sclerosing sarcomatoid transitional cell carcinoma of the urinary bladder: a clinicopathologic and immunohistochemical study of 25 cases. Mod Pathol 1997; 10:908.

284. Horn LC, Reuter S, Biesold M. Inflammatory pseudotumor of the ureter and the urinary bladder. Pathol Res Pract 1997; 193:607.

285. Coffin CM, Humphrey PA, Dehner LP. Extrapulmonary inflammatory myofibroblastic tumor: a clinical and pathological survey. Semin Diagn Pathol 1998; 15:85.

286. Sonobe H, Okada Y, Sudo S, et al. Inflammatory pseudotumor of the urinary bladder with aberrant expression of cytokeratin. Report of a case with cytologic, immunocytochemical and cytogenetic findings. Acta Cytol 1999; 43:257.

287. Perez Garcia FJ, Pinto Blazquez J, Gutierrez Garcia R, et al. [Inflammatory prostatic pseudotumor (fibromyxoid pseudosarcomatous tumor)]. Arch Esp Urol 2004; 57:657.

288. Moyana TN, Kontozoglou T. Urinary bladder paragangliomas. An immunohistochemical study. Arch Pathol Lab Med 1988; 112:70.

289. Salo JO, Miettinen M, Makinen J, et al. Pheochromocytoma of the urinary bladder. Report of 2 cases with ultrastructural and immunohistochemical analyses. Eur Urol 1989; 16:237.

290. Grignon DJ, Ro JY, Mackay B, et al. Paraganglioma of the urinary bladder: immunohistochemical, ultrastructural, and DNA flow cytometric studies. Hum Pathol 1991; 22:1162.

291. Lam KY, Chan AC. Paraganglioma of the urinary bladder: an immunohistochemical study and report of an unusual association with intestinal carcinoid. Aust NZ J Surg 1993; 63:740.

292. Shono T, Sakai H, Minami Y, et al. Paraganglioma of the urinary bladder: A case report and review of the Japanese literature. Urol Int 1999; 62:102.

293. Kato H, Suzuki M, Mukai M, et al. Clinicopathological study of pheochromocytoma of the urinary bladder: immunohistochemical, flow cytometric and ultrastructural findings with review of the literature. Pathol Int 1999; 49:1093.

294. Cheng L, Leibovich BC, Cheville JC, et al. Paraganglioma of the urinary bladder: can biologic potential be predicted? Cancer 2000; 88:844.

295. Burton EM, Schellhammer PF, Weaver DL, et al. Paraganglioma of urinary bladder in patient with neurofibromatosis. Urology 1986; 27:550.

296. Misawa T, Shibasaki T, Toshima R, et al. A case of pheochromocytoma of the urinary bladder in a long-term hemodialysis patient. Nephron 1993; 64:443.

297. Zhou M, Epstein JI, Young RH. Paraganglioma of the urinary bladder: a lesion that may be misdiagnosed as urothelial carcinoma in transurethral resection specimens. Am J Surg Pathol 2004; 28:4.

298. Nesi G, Vezzosi V, Amorosi A, et al. Paraganglioma of the urinary bladder. Urol Int 1996; 56:250.

299. Honma K. Paraganglia of the urinary bladder. An autopsy study. Zentralbl Pathol 1994; 139:465.

300. Hacker GW, Bishop AE, Terenghi G, et al. Multiple peptide production and presence of general neuroendocrine markers detected in 12 cases of human phaeochromocytoma and in mammalian adrenal glands. Virchows Arch A Pathol Anat Histopathol 1988; 412:399.

301. Mentzel T, Bainbridge TC, Katenkamp D. Solitary fibrous tumour: clinicopathological, immunohisto-chemical, and ultrastructural analysis of 12 cases arising in soft tissues, nasal cavity and nasopharynx, urinary bladder and prostate. Virchows Arch 1997; 430:445.

302. Bainbridge TC, Singh RR, Mentzel T, et al. Solitary fibrous tumor of urinary bladder: report of two cases. Hum Pathol 1997; 28:1204.

303. Westra WH, Grenko RT, Epstein J. Solitary fibrous tumor of the lower urogenital tract: a report of five cases involving the seminal vesicles, urinary bladder, and prostate. Hum Pathol 2000; 31:63.

304. Kim SH, Cha KB, Choi YD, et al. Solitary fibrous tumor of the urinary bladder. Yonsei Med J 2004; 45:573.

305. Park SH, Kim TJ, Chi JG. Congenital granular cell tumor with systemic involvement. Immunohistochemical and ultrastructural study. Arch Pathol Lab Med 1991; 115:934.

306. Kontani K, Okaneya T, Takezaki T. Recurrent granular cell tumour of the bladder in a patient with von Recklinghausen's disease. Br J Urol Int 1999; 84:871.

307. Fletcher MS, Aker M, Hill JT, et al. Granular cell myoblastoma of the bladder. Br J Urol 1985; 57:109.

308. Ando K, Matsuno Y, Kanai Y, et al. Primary low-grade lymphoma of mucosa-associated lymphoid tissue of the urinary bladder: a case report with special reference to the use of ancillary diagnostic studies. Jpn J Clin Oncol 1999; 29:636.

309. Yuille FA, Angus B, Roberts JT, et al. Low grade MALT lymphoma of the urinary bladder. Clin Oncol 1998; 10:265.

310. Kempton CL, Kurtin PJ, Inwards DJ, et al. Malignant lymphoma of the bladder: evidence from 36 cases that low-grade lymphoma of the MALT-type is the most common primary bladder lymphoma. Am J Surg Pathol 1997; 21:1324.

311. Fernandez Acenero MJ, Martin Rodilla C, Lopez Garcia-

Asenjo J, et al. Primary malignant lymphoma of the bladder. Report of three cases. Pathol Res Pract 1996; 192:160.

312. Ohsawa M, Aozasa K, Horiuchi K, et al. Malignant lymphoma of bladder. Report of three cases and review of the literature. Cancer 1993; 72:1969.

313. Pawade J, Banerjee SS, Harris M, et al. Lymphomas of mucosa-associated lymphoid tissue arising in the urinary bladder. Histopathology 1993; 23:147.

314. Siegel RJ, Napoli VM. Malignant lymphoma of the urinary bladder. A case with signet-ring cells simulating urachal adenocarcinoma. Arch Pathol Lab Med 1991; 115:635.

315. Koike H, Morita T, Tamura Y. [Primary malignant lymphoma of the urinary bladder: a case report]. Nippon Hinyokika Gakkai Zasshi 2004; 95:75.

睾 丸

Deborah Josefson, Junqi Qian and David G. Bostwick

睾丸、附属结构和外生殖器

睾丸肿瘤非常少见，大约占男性恶性肿瘤的1%；然而，在15至44岁的男性中，它是最常见的肿瘤[1]。在美国，白种男性中睾丸癌目前的发生率是每100 000个人中6例[2]。绝大多数睾丸肿瘤是生殖细胞瘤。在过去20年间，研究人员对睾丸癌发病机制的研究取得了巨大的进展。小管内生殖细胞瘤被认为是大多数生殖细胞肿瘤的前体[3-7]。虽然显微镜下的形态学观察仍然是诊断睾丸癌的主要依据，但是免疫组化、细胞遗传学、DNA扩增的研究和其他分子生物学技术的应用已经成为睾丸癌诊断的重要补充手段。性索间质肿瘤大约占睾丸肿瘤的4%。近年来对它的分类取得了较大的进展，在已经建立的肿瘤命名的基础上，又描述了几种新增加的形态学上的分型。

在下文中，首先对在睾丸病理学中有特殊意义的免疫组化标记物进行讨论，然后讨论睾丸、附属结构和外生殖器肿瘤的免疫组化标记物。其他的免疫组化标记物如CK、间充质细胞标记物，这些也可能在该位置的肿瘤的诊断中发挥作用的标记物将在本文的其他部分论述。

抗原/抗体生物学

胎盘样碱性磷酸酶

人类碱性磷酸酶活性来自3种主要的同工酶，它们由肝组织、骨组织和胎盘组织产生。这3种同工酶蛋白质由来自同一祖先基因的多基因座基因编码[8]。胎盘来源的碱性磷酸酶是一种膜结合的120kD的酶，正常情况下由合体滋养层细胞合成，在怀孕第12周时释放入母体血循环[9]。但是，它同时也可以被许多肿瘤组织合成，所以是一种肿瘤标记物[10]。在生理状态下，该酶参与细胞运输、细胞增殖和细胞分化，以及代谢和基因转录的调节[11]。

胎盘样碱性磷酸酶（placental-like alkaline phosphatase，PLAP）并不是仅见于生殖细胞肿瘤，通过生化方法在血清中以及通过免疫组化方法在多种肿瘤患者组织内都可以检测到这种酶，这些肿瘤包括胃肠道、妇科生殖系统、血液、肺、乳腺和泌尿系统肿瘤[12, 13]。实际上，肿瘤相关的PLAP首先是在一名小细胞肺癌的患者的血清中被发现的，以患者的名字命名为Regan同工酶[14]。一项研究表明，在生殖细胞肿瘤中，98%的精原细胞瘤、98%的小管内生殖细胞瘤、97%的胚胎癌和85%的卵黄囊瘤的PLAP免疫组化结果阳性[12]。在大多数性腺胚细胞瘤（gonadoblastomas）的生殖细胞成分中，PLAP免疫组化也为阳性。在其他生殖细胞肿瘤如绒毛膜癌和畸胎瘤中，PLAP的免疫组化结果是不同的，在大约一半的病例中呈阳性。另有报道，在卵巢的生殖细胞肿瘤中，PLAP也可阳性[15]。正常的睾丸组织只含有痕量的PLAP，在大多数病例中不能用免疫组化方法检测得到。在无小管内生殖细胞肿瘤的情况下，从不育症男性及性腺异常和隐睾患者活检中很少检测到PLAP免疫组化阳性[12]。

PLAP的免疫反应定位主要在细胞膜，有时也会在胞浆。PLAP阳性反应的分布和强度在不同的肿瘤之间以及在同一肿瘤的不同部位有所区别（表14.16）。从免疫组化方法学的角度看，这种情况是由于肿瘤细胞酶含量的不均一性以及酶本身的不均一性所造成的[13]。

α-胎球蛋白

α-胎球蛋白（AFP）在很多物理化学性质上与清蛋白相似，是一种主要的胎儿血清蛋白，正常情况下由胎儿卵黄囊、胎儿和再生的肝组织和胎儿消化道上皮产生。AFP在非精原细胞瘤型生殖细胞瘤患者中的含量上升75%，用免疫组化方法可以在肿瘤组织中检测得到[16]。单纯类型的精原细胞瘤不产生AFP[17]。睾丸肿瘤患者伴血清AFP水平升高应该按照非精原细胞瘤型生殖细胞瘤来治疗，即便是AFP不能在肿瘤组织中用免疫组化方法检测到[18]。AFP还是肝细胞癌诊断和治疗最有用的标记物（表14.17）。

绒毛膜促性腺激素

人绒毛膜促性腺激素（hCG）是第一个被发现的孕期特异性蛋白，它是一种37kD的糖蛋白，包含一个α和一个β亚基。α亚基与几个其他激素相应的亚基相同，包括甲状腺刺激素、黄体生成激素和卵泡刺激素。β亚基具有器官特异性。β-hCG由良性及恶性绒毛膜组织中的合体滋养层细胞合成，并经尿液排泄。在排卵后第8天首先出现在母体血清中，在怀孕后第8周血清浓度达到峰值，随后迅速下降并在以后的孕期中维持在低水平[19]。

作为有活性的滋养层组织的标记物，β-hCG的血清检测在妊娠滋养层疾病和睾丸肿瘤的诊断、分期、治疗监控和患者随访中都起着重要的作用[17, 20]。血清β-hCG在大多数绒癌和10%的精原细胞肿瘤的患者体内升高。当结合AFP进行检测时，有50%~90%的非精原细胞瘤型生殖细胞瘤患者的β-hCG水平升高[21]。β-hCG定位于精原细胞瘤、胚胎癌、卵黄囊瘤的合体滋养层巨细胞中，以及定位于绒毛膜癌的合体滋养层细胞中（表14.18）。

人胎盘催乳素

人胎盘催乳素（HPL）之前亦被称做人绒毛膜生长促乳素，是一种22kD的蛋白质，与生长激素部分同源[22]。HPL首先在妊娠第5周的母体血清中被检测到，在第34周时达到峰值并维持在平台期。用免疫组化方法在绒毛膜癌的合体滋养层细胞中可以检测到HPL。据报道，在睾丸中存在一种少见的滋养层细胞肿瘤变型，与子宫胎盘的滋养层细胞肿瘤相似[23]。它只含有中间滋养层细胞，这种细胞中，人胎盘催乳素呈弥漫阳性，β-hCG呈局灶性阳性（表14.19）。

抑制素

抑制素是一种32kD的二聚体糖蛋白，包含一个α和一个β亚基[24]。它主要由卵巢颗粒细胞和睾丸支持（Sertoli）细胞产生，少量由Leydig细胞产生[25]。它能够抑制卵泡刺激素从垂体的释放，从而抑制卵泡的生成[26]。抑制素被证明是卵巢性索-间质肿瘤的一种敏感的免疫组化标记物，特别是对颗粒细胞瘤[27-31]。

抑制素在发生于睾丸的性索-间质肿瘤中也表达[32-34]。在一项研究中发现，抑制素在16例Leydig细胞瘤中的15例呈阳性反应，在6例睾丸性索-间质瘤伴不同程度Sertoli或颗粒细胞分化的肿瘤中有4例呈阳性，在3例未分化型性索-间质肿瘤中有2例为阳性[33]。绝大多数阳性病例呈弥漫性、强胞浆着色。在所有病例中，非肿瘤型Leydig和支持细胞也呈抗抑制素抗体阳性反应，尽管阳性强度比肿瘤型Leydig和支持细胞要弱。在本研究中，精原细胞瘤、黑色素瘤、淋巴瘤、恶性畸胎瘤未分化型或转移性癌组织中抑制素免疫组化均为阴性反应[33]。

在另一个研究中，11例支持细胞肿瘤中有10例、所有的支持细胞腺瘤和所有的良性及恶性Leydig细胞肿瘤中抑制素A都呈阳性反应。在这项研究中，6例精原细胞瘤、1例胚胎癌和3例混合型生殖细胞瘤中抑制素免疫组化均为阴性反应[32]。合体滋养层细胞的抗抑制素抗体呈阳性反应[35, 36]。这使得对含有

表14.16　在生殖细胞中PLAP的免疫组化结果

肿　瘤	阳性病例数
精原细胞瘤	98%
小管内生殖细胞瘤	98%
胚胎癌	97%
卵黄囊瘤	85%
性腺胚细胞瘤（生殖细胞成分）	大多数
绒毛膜癌	不同
畸胎瘤	不同

表14.17　α-胎球蛋白（AFP）

在非精原细胞瘤型生殖细胞瘤（NSGCT）中上升75%
单纯类型的精原细胞瘤不产生

表14.18　人绒毛膜促性腺激素（hCG）

在50%~90%的非精原细胞瘤型生殖细胞瘤的患者中水平升高
定位于精原细胞瘤、胚胎癌、卵黄囊肿瘤和绒毛膜癌中的合体滋养层巨细胞

表14.19　人胎盘催乳素（hPL）

在绒毛膜癌的合体滋养层细胞中呈阳性表达
在一种含有中间滋养层细胞的滋养层肿瘤变型中呈弥漫性阳性分布

合体滋养层细胞的精原细胞瘤的诊断出现困难，因为抑制素在局部呈阳性反应。目前认为，抑制素是葡萄胎中间滋养层细胞和合体滋养层细胞、胎盘部位滋养层细胞肿瘤和绒毛膜癌的一个有价值的免疫组化标记物（表 14.20）[36-38]。

表 14.20 抑制素

在发生于睾丸的性索-间质细胞瘤中为阳性：支持细胞肿瘤、Leydig 细胞肿瘤、颗粒细胞瘤阳性
在中间滋养层和合体滋养层细胞中呈阳性
在精原细胞瘤、黑色素瘤、淋巴瘤、恶性畸胎瘤未分化型或转移癌中呈阴性

睾丸肿瘤

生殖细胞肿瘤

小管内生殖细胞新生物

小管内生殖细胞新生物未分化型（IGCNU）是大多数生殖细胞肿瘤的前体病变，但除外精母细胞性精原细胞瘤和小儿生殖细胞肿瘤（图 14.29）。Skakkebaek 和他的同事最早对它在浸润性生殖细胞肿瘤中的作用进行了仔细的观察[3-7]。IGCNU 可见于隐睾症、寡精性不育症、睾丸发育不良和生殖细胞瘤患者对侧睾丸的活检组织中。活检诊断为 IGCNU 的患者中，大约有 50% 在 5 年中发展为浸润性生殖细胞肿瘤[39]。在小儿和青春期前的生殖细胞肿瘤活检组织中很少见 IGCNU，这表明这些肿瘤的病因学与此不同。在没有肿瘤浸润症状的情况下，IGCNU 呈无症状状态，而只是在上述疾病的高危患者的活检组织中经显微镜观察而发现。

IGCNU 所累及的输精管很少有生精过程，管腔直径也常由于管周基膜的增厚而变小。肿瘤细胞主要位于基底层，含有增大、深染的细胞核伴一个或更多的核仁，胞浆透明并含有 PAS 阳性物质（糖蛋白），胞浆界限清楚[40]。PLAP 是一种非常灵敏而特异的 IGCNU 标记物。在 85%～98% 的患者中 PLAP 表现为胞膜阳性（图14.30），而正常的生殖细胞和支持细胞通常为阴性[41-44]。很少情况下，转移至睾丸的肿瘤可能会累及输精管而看上去与 IGCNU 难以区别。PLAP 有助于将这些肿瘤与 IGCNU 进行鉴别。另一有前景的方法是将 PLAP 与 RNA 结合序列（RBM）蛋白同时进行免疫组化双染，PLAP 检测 IGCNU，RBM 检测正常生殖细胞，这样就可以将二者进行鉴别。RBM 由 Y 染色体编码，仅持续表达于分化型男性生殖细胞中；肿瘤生殖细胞不表达 RBM。这样对于疑难病例，双染可以被用来提高 IGCNU 检测的敏感性。

在 IGCNU 中，AFP、β-hCG、癌胚抗原和人胎盘催乳素免疫反应通常为阴性[45-47]。Jacobsen 和他的同事发现，83% 的 IGCNU 病例中铁蛋白免疫组化为阳性[48]。他们还发现，在 189 例睾丸切除术的标本中，有 94% 的标本在邻近浸润性精原细胞瘤或非精原细

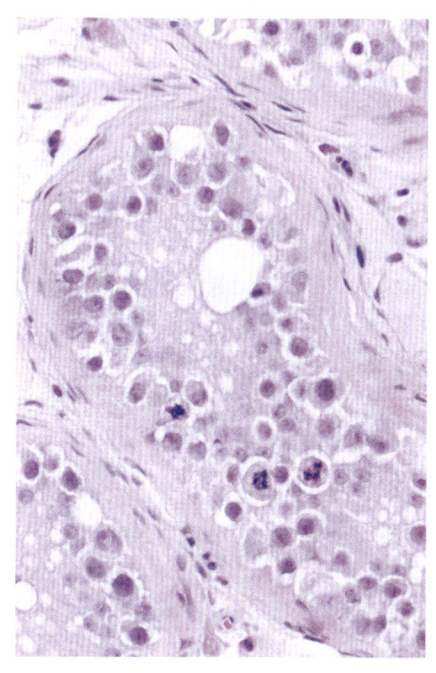

图 14.29　小管内生殖细胞瘤，未分化型（IGCNU）

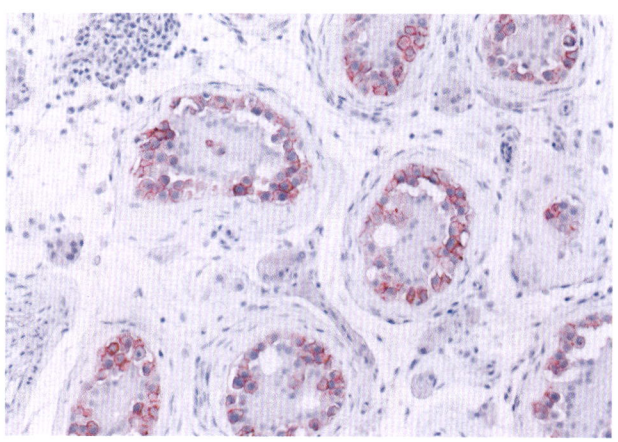

图 14.30　小管内生殖细胞瘤。肿瘤细胞表现出 PLAP 免疫组化呈膜阳性反应

胞瘤型生殖细胞肿瘤的 IGCNU 组织中，铁蛋白免疫组化呈阳性反应[49]。然而，还未见其他研究者重复得出这些研究结果[50]。

弱三联组氨酸（*FHIT*）基因表达阴性的检测对于鉴别 IGCNU 与良性病变可能也是有价值的，但是这种方法还未得到广泛的应用。FHIT 被认为是一种肿瘤抑制基因，位于染色体 3p14.2，该基因的突变与肺、宫颈、乳腺、肾和食管癌有关。高达41%的睾丸生殖细胞肿瘤也出现*FHIT*基因座的突变。FHIT通过改变细胞周期动力学和诱导细胞凋亡而发挥作用。在一项研究中发现，FHIT 表达于生殖细胞、支持细胞和 Leydig 细胞中，但是在所有 42 例 IGCNU 样本中都为阴性反应[51]。

神经特异性烯醇化酶（NSE）是一种神经内分泌分化标记物，在 IGCNU 和浸润性生殖细胞肿瘤中常为阳性[52]。在与成熟畸胎瘤邻近的 IGCNU 组织中，用免疫组化方法可以检测到肿瘤抑制基因蛋白产物 p53 的过表达[53,54]。在一小样本量的研究中，一种相对比较新的标记物分期特异性胚胎抗原（SSEA-4）被发现在 IGCNU 以及良性精原细胞和不同的生殖细胞肿瘤包括精原细胞瘤、非精原细胞瘤、胚胎癌和卵黄囊肿瘤组织中呈阳性[55]。但是这一检测结果在诊断中的应用尚存疑问。很多其他抗原也在 IGCNU 中呈阳性反应，包括 TRA-1-60、*c-kit* 原癌基因蛋白产物（Kit）、胰岛素样生长因子 1、M2A、43-9F、谷胱甘肽-S-转移酶 π、鞘糖脂 Gb3 和 CD143（一种血管紧张素转换酶）[56-63]。在浸润性生殖细胞肿瘤中，这些标记物呈不同程度的反应，但是关于它们如何辅助外科病理学的诊断目前尚无定论。

典型精原细胞瘤 精原细胞瘤是最常见的一种生殖细胞肿瘤，占所有生殖细胞肿瘤的27%~56%[64,65]。在诊断时的平均年龄大约为 40 岁，大多数患者临床表现为睾丸肿物。血清 β-hCG 在 5%~40% 的单纯局限性的肿瘤患者的体内升高，在 13%~61% 的转移癌患者体内升高[66]。血清 AFP 正常。肉眼观察，该肿瘤是一种质软、红褐色、弥漫性或多结节的肿物，可能还含有小的局灶性坏死或出血。肿瘤细胞中含有大量的透明胞浆、胞膜明显、核呈圆形囊状、核仁明显。将肿瘤细胞分隔成团的纤维组织中含有淋巴浆细胞浸润。

免疫组化结果对鉴别精原细胞瘤与其他相似的良性或恶性肿瘤方面是有价值的。PLAP 是精原细胞的一种敏感的标记物，90%~100% 的病例呈胞浆膜阳性[67-69]。PLAP 对于精原细胞瘤来说并不是特异的，在其他的生殖细胞肿瘤或癌中也可呈阳性[68]。PLAP 的免疫组化在鉴别精原细胞瘤伴过度增生的肉芽肿样反应（PLAP+）与原发性肉芽肿样睾丸炎（PLAP-）时很有用。管状精原细胞瘤是精原细胞瘤的一种组织类型，类似于支持细胞瘤，PLAP 阳性；而支持细胞瘤则与其他的性索-间质肿瘤相同，PLAP 阴性。

很少的精原细胞瘤与血清 β-hCG 水平升高有关。这样的病例通常表现为局部成簇的合体滋养层巨细胞 β-hCG 免疫组化阳性[69-72]。在一些精原细胞瘤中，并不能检测到像合体滋养层那样的β-hCG阳性细胞，它们可能为中间滋养层细胞。AFP是卵黄囊肿瘤的标记物，在精原细胞瘤中不表达。CD30 在大多数精原细胞瘤中呈阴性反应，在胚胎癌中通常呈阳性反应[73-75]。这表明，CD30在少数精原细胞瘤中的表达可能反映了它们向胚胎癌转化的初级阶段[74]。精原细胞瘤中抑制素免疫组化常为阴性，而抑制素是睾丸性索-间质肿瘤的一个灵敏而特异的标志物[76]。

通过对OCT4免疫组化的检测也可以确定精原细胞瘤。OCT4 也被称做 OCT3、OTF3 和 POU5F1，是一种由位于染色体 6p21.3 的一个基因编码的转录调节因子。OCT4在胚胎干细胞和生殖细胞中具有多向潜能，认为其可以通过对下游基因的转录调节而协助细胞正常的生长发育[77]。最近的研究表明，OCT4 是精原细胞瘤和胚胎癌的一种灵敏而特异的标记物[78]。在一个对 91 例原发睾丸肿瘤的分析中发现，51 例典型精原细胞瘤中，100% 的病例 OCT4 免疫组化均为

诊断要点：小管内生殖细胞肿瘤

1. PLAP+（85%~98%的病例，特异性标记物）。
2. 铁蛋白 +（83% 的病例）。
3. NSE+。
4. SSEA-4+。
5. AFP-。
6. β-hCG-。
7. 癌胚抗原 -。
8. 人胎盘催乳素。
9. FHIT-。
10. RBM-。

阳性。54例胚胎癌病例中有53例该抗体也为阳性。该抗体着色部位为核阳性，有极少的背景着色，两种肿瘤阳性均为+++。相反，有5例精原细胞瘤被证明OCT4呈阴性反应，与22例非生殖细胞肿瘤相同，包括Leydig细胞肿瘤、支持细胞肿瘤、性索-间质细胞瘤、颗粒细胞瘤和腺瘤样肿瘤。此外，所有的卵黄囊肿瘤、绒毛膜癌和畸胎瘤均为阴性[4]。OCT4与PLAP配合使用可能在疑难病例的鉴别诊断上有一定的作用。这一指标是否得到认可还不确定，因为PLAP是精原细胞的一个非常灵敏和有价值的标记物。

另一个有同等价值的精原细胞瘤标记物是c-kit。c-kit是一种跨膜糖蛋白和酪氨酸激酶，参与细胞的信号转导作用。c-kit与血小板源性生长因子受体、单细胞克隆刺激因子受体具有同源性。c-kit传输的信号对于生殖细胞、造血干细胞、黑色素细胞、肥大细胞和Cajal间质细胞的发育和存活都非常重要，Cajal是胃肠道蠕动功能的起搏点。在最近的一项研究中，38例精原细胞瘤中有31例抗c-kit免疫组化阳性（82%）。非精原细胞瘤型生殖细胞肿瘤则为阴性。这一研究还对睾丸肿瘤进行了突变研究，并提出了针对Kit突变的一种治疗精原细胞瘤的思路，方式类似于用Gleevac®治疗胃肠道间质瘤和慢性髓性白血病。目前正在进行特异Kit激酶抑制剂靶向治疗普遍存在Kit突变的精原细胞瘤的研究[79]。

约40%的精原细胞瘤CK表达可能为阳性，尽管在文献中这一阳性率为0%~73%之间[69,80-83]。阳性反应通常较弱，可见于单个细胞或小簇细胞。极少有病例呈CK弥漫性阳性表达。混合其中的合体滋养层细胞可能表现出CK AE1/AE3强阳性。CK8和18在精原细胞瘤中呈阳性[84,85]；CK19通常为阴性，但在胚胎癌中常弥漫表达[86,87]。少数精原细胞瘤组织也表达CK4和17[88]。EMA不表达[69]。在精原细胞瘤中还不同程度地表达结蛋白、波形蛋白、神经丝蛋白、NSE、铁蛋白、LDH、Leu7和α-1-抗胰蛋白酶，但是均无诊断价值[49,69,80,88-90]。

根据已发表的研究报告，精原细胞中p53免疫组化结果差异很大，从阴性到在90%的病例中过表达不等[91]。原发于纵隔的精原细胞瘤的K-ras和p53免疫组化结果（阳性率更低）与睾丸精原细胞瘤有所不同。睾丸和纵隔来源的精原细胞瘤其他标记物的免疫组化检测结果有一些明显的不同。纵隔精原细胞瘤中80%的病例CAM5.2呈点状强阳性，而在睾丸精原细胞瘤中这一比例只有20%[92]。

总之，在精原细胞瘤中，PLAP和c-kit表现为胞浆膜阳性，OCT4为核阳性。EMA、CK、β-hCG、AFP、CD30和抑制素通常为阴性或弱阳性。典型的精原细胞瘤与高有丝分裂指数的精原细胞瘤没有明显区别，除了后者PCNA表达增高以外（以前称做"间变性精原细胞瘤"）[93]。

PLAP是精原细胞瘤的一个灵敏的生物标记物，90%~100%的病例呈胞浆膜阳性。PLAP的免疫组化在鉴别精原细胞瘤伴过度增生的肉芽肿样反应（PLAP+）与原发性肉芽肿样睾丸炎（PLAP-）时很有用。管状精原细胞瘤是精原细胞瘤的一种组织类型，类似于支持细胞肿瘤，PLAP阳性；而支持细胞瘤则PLAP阴性，与其他性索-间质肿瘤相同。OCT4和c-kit免疫组化结果也能够比较稳定地鉴别出精原细胞瘤的细胞，可能能够与PLAP配合使用或代替

> **诊断要点**：典型精原细胞瘤
>
> 1. PLAP+（90%~100%的病例，灵敏，非特异）。
> 2. OCT4+（95%）。
> 3. c-kit+（>80%）。
> 4. CK AE1/AE3+。
> 5. CK8+、18+。
> 6. CK19-。
> 7. AFP-。
> 8. β-hCG 结果不同。
> 9. 抑制素 -。
> 10. EMA-。
> 11. CD30-/+。

PLAP成为鉴别诊断的有价值的方法。

精母细胞性精原细胞瘤

精母细胞性精原细胞瘤是一种不常见的睾丸肿瘤，常为无痛性肿瘤。这种肿瘤大约占睾丸精原细胞瘤的5%[94]。与典型的精原细胞瘤相比，其组织发生、临床表现、形态学特征和生物学行为都有所不同。它常发生于中老年人，诊断时的平均年龄为54岁（25~87岁），在青春期前儿童和青少年均尚未见报道[95]。这种肿瘤不发生于隐睾、睾丸外位点或与其他生殖细胞肿瘤有关。除了极少病例发生肉瘤样转化以外，其生物学行为通常为良性[96]。在显微镜下观察，它包含

3种细胞类型：丰富的中等大小细胞、散在的小淋巴样细胞和大细胞。精母细胞性精原细胞瘤的鉴别诊断包括恶性淋巴瘤、典型精原细胞瘤和实体性胚胎癌。

目前还没有发现非常有价值的精母细胞性精原细胞瘤的生物标记物，它的诊断主要依据常规显微镜下观察；然而，免疫组化结果在疑难病例的鉴别诊断中还是有价值的。在这些病例中，肿瘤组织常呈不典型的形态学特征，使得该肿瘤与其他生殖细胞肿瘤相似。目前可能对诊断精母细胞性精原细胞瘤有帮助的标记物包括Chk2、MAGE-A4和p19ink4d。Chk2和p19ink4d是调节蛋白，它的功能是调节生殖母细胞向精原细胞的转化以及从有丝分裂象向减数分裂象的转化。MAGE-A4参与DNA的损伤修复。在最近的一项针对25例精母细胞性精原细胞瘤的研究中发现，100%的MAGE-A4免疫组化结果阳性，94%的病例Chk2阳性。而在这组精母细胞性精原细胞瘤病例中，p53和NSE的阳性率分别为83.3%和88%。在此研究中，p19均为阴性，这表明精母细胞性精原细胞瘤来源于减数分裂前期[97]。

这些结果非常复杂，而Chk2和MAG-A4可能被证明具有诊断价值，但是它们还没有作为肿瘤标记物被广泛地认可或应用。

在一些精母细胞性精原细胞瘤中，淋巴细胞的浸润现象可能与典型精原细胞瘤相似。在一些病例中，微囊性结构的存在可能提示卵黄囊肿瘤。据报道，精母细胞性精原细胞瘤间变型与呈实性增长的胚胎癌形似[98]。精母细胞性精原细胞瘤中AFP、β-hCG、CD30、CEA、人胎盘催乳素、NSE、S-100蛋白、LCA、结蛋白、波形蛋白和肌动蛋白的免疫组化结果为阴性。在少数病例的散在细胞中，PLAP免疫组化呈胞浆和胞膜阳性[99]。EMA和CK AE1/AE3免疫组化呈阴性，而低分子量CK（CAM5.2、CK18）在大约40%的病例中可能呈包涵体样阳性，与Merkel细胞癌着色模式相似[100]。一项研究表明，4例间变性精母细胞性精原细胞瘤中有2例为p53免疫组化过表达[98]。而在另一项研究中表明，25例精母细胞性精原细胞瘤中有20例（80%）的p53为强表达[97]。

40%的精母细胞性精原细胞瘤的病例中可见c-kit原癌基因蛋白产物的表达呈阳性。在这项研究中，所有的典型的精原细胞瘤的c-kit均为阳性[101]。在另一个小样本量的研究中，精母细胞性精原细胞瘤中c-kit阳性可见于所有7个病例[102]。

胚胎癌

单纯的胚胎癌占睾丸生殖细胞肿瘤的不到5%，经常是以混合生殖细胞肿瘤中的一个成分存在（大约45%的病例）[64, 65]。好发于年轻人，诊断时平均年龄30岁。大多数患者的临床症状为睾丸肿物；极少数病例以远处转移作为首发症状。在显微镜下观察，胚胎癌由多角形细胞组成，胞浆丰富，边界不清楚，具有增大的空泡状细胞核，核仁突出，核分裂象易见。细胞排列成片状、腺体状、乳头状或管状。原始的间充质组织可能与肿瘤细胞有关，而不是未成熟畸胎瘤的表现。

绝大多数胚胎癌的细胞角蛋白AE1/AE3和CAM5.2，以及CK8、18和19为免疫组化阳性反应。一些病例CK4和17免疫组化也为阳性反应[67-69, 103, 104]。EMA、CEA和波形蛋白通常为阴性。86%~97%的胚胎癌病例中，PLAP免疫组化为阳性[67, 69]。胚胎癌中PLAP的免疫组化结果在胞浆和胞膜中都为阳性，但比在精原细胞瘤中阳性更强且更局限。OCT4有望成为胚胎癌的一种新的肿瘤标记物，在最近一项研究中发现，它在90%以上的病例中呈阳性反应。然而，它对于胚胎癌来说是非特异性的，所有的精原细胞瘤的OCT4的监测均为阳性[78, 105]。80%以上的胚胎癌CD30（Ki-1、Ber-H2）免疫组化均阳性[73-75]。CD30免疫组化很少在其他生殖细胞肿瘤中呈阳性反应，所以在鉴别转移部位的体细胞来源的肿瘤与胚胎癌时是很有实用价值的。当对睾丸外部位的低分化肿瘤进行诊断时，PLAP、panCK和CD30免疫组化阳性，而EMA免疫组化阴性有助于胚胎癌与体细胞癌的鉴别诊断。

AFP和β-hCG可能分别在33%和21%的病例的散在肿瘤细胞中呈免疫组化阳性反应[69]。对于AFP在胚胎癌中的阳性反应，有很多不同的解释：少数肿瘤细胞为真阳性，阳性细胞其实为混合在其中的卵黄囊成分，以及提示早期向卵黄囊肿瘤转化[106]。

关于胚胎癌，还有很多其他的免疫组化标记物被报道，但是应用于日常工作的意义不大。铁蛋白、单克隆抗体43-9F、LDH-1、p53、α-1-抗胰蛋白酶、Leu7、波形蛋白和人胎盘催乳素都可能在胚胎癌中呈阳性反应[69, 89, 107-109]。

> **诊断要点**：胚胎癌
>
> 1. PLAP+（86%~97%的病例；灵敏，非特异）。
> 2. panCK+。
> 3. OCT4+。
> 4. CD30+。
> 5. EMA-。

卵黄囊肿瘤

卵黄囊肿瘤是最常见的小儿睾丸肿瘤，占全部青春期前生殖细胞瘤的80%[110]。在成人中，单纯的卵黄囊肿瘤大约占睾丸生殖细胞瘤的1.5%，但是可以作为大约40%的混合型生殖细胞瘤中的一个成分[111, 112]。卵黄囊肿瘤成分是以单纯形式还是以混合形式（作为混合型生殖细胞瘤中的一个成分）出现与血清中AFP水平的升高有很大的关系[113, 114]。肉眼观察，该肿瘤呈红褐色，均一、分叶状，可见光亮的黏液性表面提示微囊状区域。常可见局部坏死和出血。不同的组织学类型可以与其他生殖细胞肿瘤或睾丸外的恶性肿瘤相似。微囊状（网状）是最常见的类型。

不同的研究报道中，有55%~100%的卵黄囊肿瘤病例的AFP免疫组化结果阳性[45, 69, 115]。阳性部位通常在胞浆，在很多病例中也可能是弱阳性或局灶性阳性。肝细胞样类型可能表现为AFP强阳性反应。胞浆和细胞外的嗜酸性玻璃样小体是卵黄囊肿瘤的一个有特征性的组织学特征，这一结构对于AFP、α-1-抗胰蛋白酶、白蛋白和转铁蛋白的免疫组化结果各不相同[64, 116]。CK在大多数病例中为强阳性[69, 81]。EMA阴性有助于鉴别卵黄囊肿瘤与睾丸外的体细胞瘤[69]。PLAP在一半以上的病例中为阳性[43, 69, 117]。梭形细胞成分表现为波形蛋白免疫组化阳性[81]。在少量病例中，肠道腺体可能表现为CEA阳性[118, 119]。α-1-抗胰蛋白酶免疫组化据报道在大约50%的病例中为阳性[45, 69]。层粘连蛋白、NSE、Leu7、p53和CD34在某些病例中也可呈阳性反应[69, 107, 118, 120]。在一项研究中，12个卵黄囊肿瘤中有7个呈局部抗CD34抗体免疫组化阳性反应。其中5个表现为局部强阳性，其余2个表现为小的成簇或单个的肿瘤细胞中弱阳性。CD34阳性反应主要见于实性或网状卵黄囊肿瘤成分中。在卵黄囊肿瘤中，CD34为局部阳性并且阳性表现不同，但是有助于该肿瘤与其他生殖细胞瘤的鉴别诊断，因为精原细胞瘤、胚胎癌和绒毛膜癌的CD34为阴性[121]。与胚胎癌不同，CD30不表达[73, 75]。另外还有鉴别小儿卵黄囊肿瘤的两种标记物为转录因子GATA4和GATA6，并且经初步证明是有临床应用价值的[122]。

> **诊断要点**：卵黄囊肿瘤
>
> 1. PLAP+（>50%的病例）。
> 2. AFP+（55%~100%的病例）。
> 3. CK+（大多数病例）。
> 4. α-1-抗胰蛋白酶+（>50%的病例）。
> 5. CD34+/-。
> 6. CD30-。
> 7. EMA-。

绒毛膜癌

单纯绒毛膜癌非常少见，大约占睾丸生殖细胞肿瘤的0.3%。睾丸绒毛膜癌通常作为混合型生殖细胞瘤的一个成分存在，大约占到病例数的8%~10%[123]。它是一种具有高度侵袭性的肿瘤，往往在刚发现时即为远处转移。与肿瘤相关的血清β-hCG水平的明显升高在大约10%的患者中可能导致男子乳腺发育。绒毛膜癌有导致出血的倾向，患者可能出现内出血症状，被称做绒毛膜癌综合征。肿瘤的浸润倾向来自于它的组成性合体滋养层细胞和细胞滋养层细胞成分的特性，它的正常功能是促进胎盘植入。肉眼观察，肿瘤呈海绵状，通常有出血或坏死区域。在显微镜下观察，大多数病例具有典型的双相表现，包括合体滋养层细胞紧密的包绕和覆盖于细胞滋养层细胞之上（图14.31）。

很多病例的正确诊断可能会因为广泛的出血、坏死表现而被影响。小的局灶性的肿瘤可能存在于坏死区的外围。β-hCG免疫组化常可以在坏死灶处鉴别出合体滋养层细胞。在所有病例中，合体滋养层细胞的β-hCG免疫组化均为强阳性（图14.32）；细胞滋养层细胞为阴性或弱阳性[45, 69, 124]。人胎盘催乳素和妊娠特异性β-1-糖蛋白（SP-1）在合体滋养层细胞与中间细胞滋养层细胞中也可呈阳性[124]。CK在细胞及合体滋养层细胞中都为强阳性表达[69, 125]。在相当高比例的病例中，EMA在合体滋养层细胞中的免疫组化常为阳性，而在精原细胞瘤、胚胎癌和卵黄囊肿瘤中则通常为阴性[69]。

大约一半的病例表现为 PLAP 免疫组化阳性[69]。CEA 在合体滋养层和细胞滋养层细胞中均为阳性表达[126]。抑制素是性索-间质肿瘤的一个标记物，在合体滋养层中为强阳性。上皮生长因子受体（EGFR）主要表达于绒毛膜癌的合体滋养层细胞中，为膜强阳性[127]。

少数绒毛膜癌病例含有大量的细胞滋养层成分，而只含有极少量的合体滋养层细胞成分，被称为单相绒毛膜癌[23]。这种肿瘤可能容易与精原细胞瘤或实性卵黄囊肿瘤混淆。免疫组化方法有助于鉴别诊断。在一篇关于单相绒毛膜癌的病例报道中，细胞滋养层细胞和少数合体滋养层细胞的 β-hCG 免疫组化结果均为弥漫分布的阳性信号。人胎盘免疫组化的阳性结果仅在后者的细胞中出现。据报道，另一种少见的滋养层细胞肿瘤也在睾丸中被发现，它与子宫胎盘部位的滋养层细胞肿瘤相似[23]。它只含有中间滋养细胞层，人胎盘催乳素弥漫性阳性，β-hCG 呈局部阳性反应。对滋养细胞层的标记物进行了研究，如 leptins、氨基肽酶、同源盒基因产物，以及 c-ras、c-erbB-2、nm23 和 p53 基因产物。但是，这些标记物只在胎盘来源的绒毛膜癌组织中进行了检测，在睾丸来源的肿瘤组织中未进行检测。这些标记物是否表达于睾丸来源的绒毛膜癌组织中尚需进一步验证。细胞表面氨基肽酶如 dipeptidyl peptidase Ⅳ 和羧肽酶-M，能够在异位滋养层细胞中检测到，故可能涉及绒毛迁移。同源盒基因在胚胎发育过程中是非常重要的，因为它们参与了器官分化和组织形成。有可能在滋养层细胞中检测到它们的表达。leptins可能类似于生长因子，可以促进滋养层细胞生长，所以这样的细胞可能具有leptin细胞表面受体[128-132]。在睾丸来源的绒毛膜癌中检测这些标记物在将来可能被证明是有应用价值的。在研究中，基因表达谱被用来对胎盘来源的绒毛膜癌进行分析[133]。

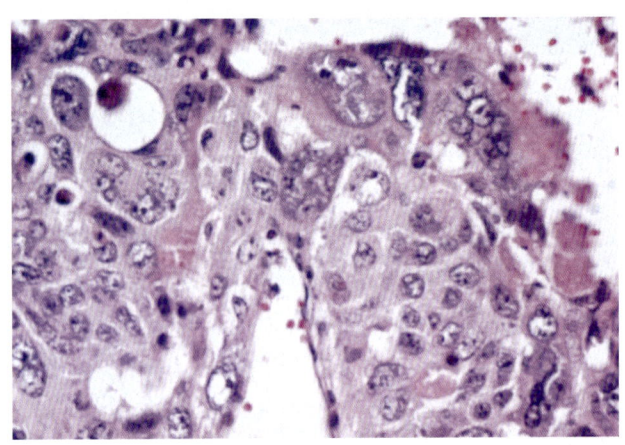

图14.31 绒毛膜癌。合体滋养层细胞与覆盖的细胞滋养层细胞紧密相关

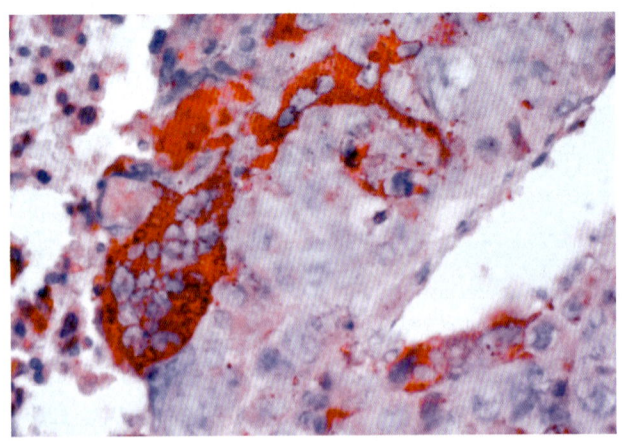

图14.32 绒毛膜癌。合体滋养层细胞中β-hCG免疫组化为强阳性

> **诊断要点：绒毛膜癌**
>
> 1. 合体滋养层细胞。
> 2. 细胞滋养层细胞。
> 3. β-hCG+（100%）。
> 4. CK+。
> 5. CEA+。
> 6. EMA+。
> 7. PLAP+（85%~98%的病例，特异）。
> 8. 抑制素-。
> 9. 妊娠特异β-1-糖蛋白+。
> 10. EGFR+。
> 11. β-hCG 少见阳性或为弱阳性。
> 12. CK+。
> 13. CEA+。

畸胎瘤

畸胎瘤在儿童中是第二常见的生殖细胞肿瘤，占全部病例的14%~20%[134-136]。在儿童中，诊断时的平均年龄为20个月，临床症状常为睾丸无痛性或痛性胀大。单纯的畸胎瘤在成年人中不常见，只占睾丸生殖细胞肿瘤的2%~3%。然而，所有生殖细胞肿瘤中的一半都含有畸胎瘤成分[111,137]。小儿成熟畸胎瘤的生物学行为是良性的，成人畸胎瘤则具有侵袭倾向，形成的转移灶可能含有非畸胎瘤性的生殖细胞成分[138-140]。肉眼观察所见与显微镜下观察所见是不同的，这依赖于组织本身所表现出的情况。

在这些肿瘤的诊断中，免疫组化方法的应用是有限的。各种标记物的免疫组化结果是肿瘤产生的组织成分的反映。具有肝样分化和腺体分化结构的细胞，具有消化道或肠型上皮结构，可能AFP免疫组化为阳性[45, 64]。在19%～36%的畸胎瘤中，AFP免疫组化结果为阳性[64, 118]。还有数量不等的病例中，其腺体成分表现为α-1-抗胰蛋白酶、CEA、铁蛋白和PLAP的免疫组化结果为阳性[118]。肌动蛋白、波形蛋白和结蛋白在周围的间质组织中常为阳性。在有肉瘤样改变的畸胎瘤中，这些标记物对于肉瘤的分型有帮助。在那些青春期前因畸胎瘤行睾丸切除术的患者中，未发现小管内生殖细胞肿瘤。与青春期前成熟畸胎瘤邻近的非典型生殖细胞中未见PLAP免疫组化阳性反应，表明这些细胞只是肿瘤前体细胞而非IGCNU[141]。

虽然免疫组化方法在诊断中无使用价值，但是它可能可以作为一种肿瘤的预后预测因子。最近的研究报告发现，Her-2/neu基因在一组生殖细胞肿瘤中呈过表达，而且与肿瘤的分期和进展有关。在这个研究中，畸胎瘤和绒毛膜样成分与生殖细胞肿瘤中的其他组织成分相比，Her-2/neu蛋白的表达更高（$P=0.0095$）。如果有研究进一步证明这一结果，那么抗Her-2/neu抗体如herceptin可能会被证明在治疗绒毛膜癌和畸胎瘤中有临床价值[142, 143]。

混合型生殖细胞肿瘤

混合型生殖细胞肿瘤包括不止一种生殖细胞肿瘤，占所有生殖细胞肿瘤的30%～60%[65, 111, 144, 145]。最常见的类型是胚胎癌伴一种或更多种的精原细胞瘤、畸胎瘤、卵黄囊肿瘤或绒毛膜癌的组织成分。实际上迄今为止，所有可能的组合都已被报道过。根据规定，精原细胞瘤中只含有合体滋养层细胞的肿瘤不能被称做混合型生殖细胞肿瘤。混合型生殖细胞肿瘤的临床特征与非精原细胞型生殖细胞肿瘤相似。AFP和β-hCG水平常升高，反映了其中的组成成分。

混合型生殖细胞肿瘤的诊断通常可以直接诊断，而很少需要免疫组化的帮助。在一些病例中，AFP的免疫组化阳性可能有助于诊断卵黄囊肿瘤微小病灶的存在，这种病灶在常规光镜下观察时经常被忽视。

性索-间质肿瘤

性索-间质肿瘤大约占所有睾丸肿瘤的5%[32]。在青春期前男性中，这种肿瘤的比例更高些。这是一种分化良好的肿瘤，类似于非肿瘤性Leydig细胞、支持细胞或间质细胞。性索-间质肿瘤可能有多种组织类型，经常与生殖细胞肿瘤或起源于该位置的其他肿瘤相混淆。在鉴别这些疑难病例方面，免疫组化方法常无明显价值。

间质（Leydig）细胞瘤

Leydig细胞瘤是最常见的性索-间质肿瘤中的一种类型，大约占睾丸肿瘤的3%[40, 146]。几乎所有的Leydig细胞肿瘤病例都是单侧发生的。双侧发生的概率只有3%。尽管儿童和成年人都可发生，但超过55%的病例发生于30岁以上的男性[40]。发生于儿童的肿瘤通常小而不可触及，由于雄激素分泌异常可出现同性性早熟。成年人则表现为睾丸肿物、男子乳腺发育、性欲或体力下降以及有时伴不育症。通常情况下，肿瘤包被完整，呈黄色或黄褐色，常可见坏死和出血灶。该肿瘤肿瘤细胞体积大、多边形、胞浆丰富、嗜酸性、胞浆界限不清（图14.33）。细胞核呈圆形、空泡状，含点状核仁。在大约30%的病例中可见Reinke类晶体，在20%的病例中可见脂色素沉积。

Leydig细胞瘤具有典型的组织学特征，但是它也可能与很多来源于睾丸的良性和恶性肿瘤相混淆，包括隐睾症中Leydig细胞增生、来源于肾上腺性征综合征的睾丸"肿瘤"、软化斑、恶性淋巴瘤、浆细胞瘤、精原细胞瘤和转移癌。抑制素的免疫组化被证明在鉴别Leydig细胞肿瘤与其他很多相似肿瘤方面具有很大的应用价值[30-34]。在一项研究中，发现抑制素的免疫组化在所有良性和恶性Leydig细胞瘤中都呈阳性反应[32]。以10例睾丸生殖细胞肿瘤作为对照，抑制素为阴性反应。另一项研究表明，16例Leydig细胞肿瘤中有15例的抑制素免疫组化为阳性[33]。在阳性病例中，免疫组化反应通常为强反应，并且弥漫分布、胞浆阳性（图14.34）。非肿瘤性支持细胞和Leydig细胞的抑制素反应也为阳性，但阳性强度比肿瘤细胞低。没有一例精原细胞瘤（共8例）、恶性黑色素瘤、睾丸淋巴瘤、恶性畸胎瘤未分化型和睾丸转移癌的抑制素呈阳性反应[33]。精原细胞瘤伴合体滋养层巨细胞的肿瘤可能表现为局灶性抑制素阳性，因为后者抑制

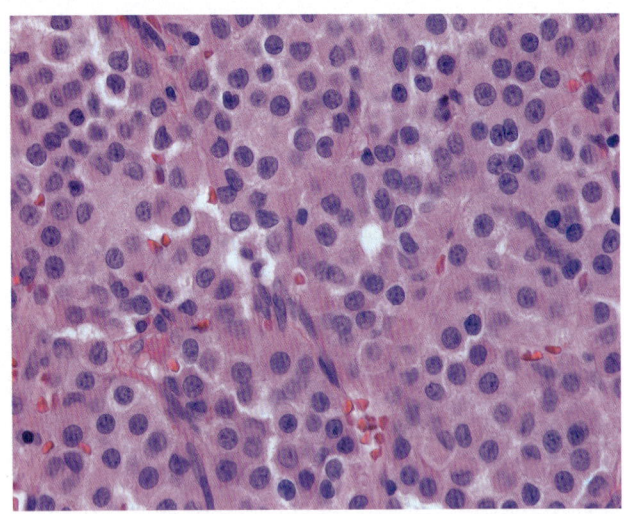

图14.33 Leydig细胞瘤。大的多边形细胞伴丰富的嗜酸性胞浆，胞浆边界不清

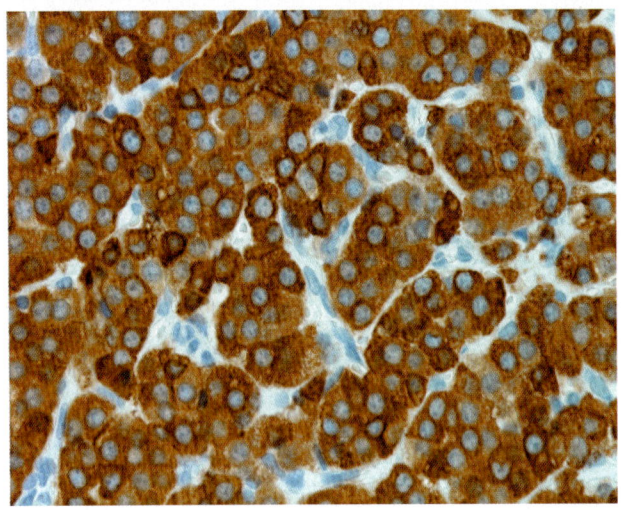

图14.34 Leydig细胞瘤。抑制素在肿瘤细胞中通常呈弥漫胞浆强阳性染色

素免疫组化可为阳性[35, 36]。

Leydig细胞瘤PLAP免疫组化为阴性，这使得这一肿瘤可以与精原细胞瘤进行鉴别。在Leydig细胞瘤中，许多抗体的免疫组化反应可以为阳性，包括CAM5.2、波形蛋白、S-100蛋白、结蛋白和EMA[33]。这些结果与卵巢脂质细胞瘤的免疫组化结果相似，包括Leydig细胞瘤[147]。CK免疫组化结果通常为弱阳性和局部阳性。一组免疫组化结果分析，包括抑制素和波形蛋白阳性，EMA和不同的CK阴性，支持了Leydig细胞瘤的诊断，而非转移癌。S-100蛋白有时在Leydig细胞瘤中呈阳性反应，因此在与恶性黑色素瘤进行鉴别诊断时是没有帮助的，但是这一鉴别诊断很少考虑。Leydig细胞瘤中HMB-45阴性。

一些研究者发现，Leydig细胞瘤表达激素敏感性的脂肪酶受体[148, 149]。这很容易理解，因为Leydig细胞是能够产生甾体激素的，甾体的生成需要胆固醇和脂肪。而有趣的是，脂肪酶受体的免疫组化结果并不具有诊断价值。

CD99是一种跨膜糖蛋白，由Mic-2基因编码，用于诊断Leydig细胞瘤，因为它在几乎所有的正常Leydig细胞和支持细胞中都呈阳性。它也在正常的颗粒细胞中表达。但是，有几项研究证实，它的价值不如抑制素[150-152]。最近一项研究表明Leydig细胞TSPY抗体也为阳性，它是一种睾丸特异的Y染色体编码的蛋白[153]。在Leydig细胞瘤中检测到这种标记物可能是有价值的。

据报道，有一种少见的含有微囊状结构的Leydig细胞瘤与卵黄囊肿瘤相似[154]。通过免疫组化，该研究中所有4个病例的波形蛋白免疫组化均为弥漫阳性；3个病例中的2个为抑制素阳性，1个为CAM5.2局灶性阳性。所有病例的PLAP和AFP均为阴性。测定增殖活性的MIB-1标记指数与Leydig细胞瘤的转移行为有关[155]。

一组正常的Leydig细胞被认为是分散的神经内分泌系统的一部分，其Syn和CgA免疫组化为阳性[156]。S-100在非肿瘤性和肿瘤性Leydig细胞中都为阳性，结果同前。在一项研究中，26例Leydig细胞瘤中有24例CgA阳性，但是7例恶性Leydig细胞瘤中只有3例为阳性[32]。恶性细胞的免疫组化阳性结果常为局灶性，并且强度较弱。33例Leydig细胞瘤中有23例Syn免疫组化结果为阳性。

> **诊断要点**：Leydig 细胞瘤
>
> 1. 抑制素和波形蛋白阳性。
> 2. CD99 阳性（50%~60%）。
> 3. EMA 阴性。
> 4. CK 免疫组化结果有差别。

支持（Sertoli）细胞瘤

支持细胞瘤占睾丸肿瘤的不到1%[157]。该肿瘤被分为3种类型：支持细胞瘤（未分类，NOS）、硬化型、大细胞钙化型支持细胞瘤。支持细胞瘤（NOS）是最常见的类型，临床表现通常为睾丸肿物。发病的平均年龄在迄今为止规模最大的关于支持细胞瘤的研究报告中为46岁[157]。60个病例中只有2个在20岁以下。硬化型支持细胞瘤是一种非常少见的类型，其特征是：在致密的硬化性间质组织中含有索状、片状和实性管状的支持细胞[158]。大细胞钙化型支持细胞瘤偶尔可见，或者并发于遗传性内分泌紊乱的患者，如Carney和Peutz-Jeghers综合征或雄激素不敏感性综合征。

抑制素A是一种支持细胞分化的灵敏的标记物[32, 33]。在一项研究中，11例支持细胞瘤中有10例（91%）和所有支持细胞腺瘤伴隐睾症的患者中抑制素免疫组化结果为阳性[32]。在这些病例中非肿瘤性支持细胞比肿瘤细胞的阳性强度更高。另报道有一例支持细胞瘤伴有不均一性肉瘤样成分[159]。在这一少见的双相恶性睾丸肿瘤中，上皮细胞成分中抑制素和波形蛋白弥漫分布的免疫组化强阳性表明了支持细胞的分化。CK AE1/AE3和CAM5.2呈局部阳性反应，EMA、单克隆和多克隆性CEA、S-100蛋白、CA19-9和PLAP在上皮成分中呈阴性。

支持细胞瘤包括大细胞钙化型的波形蛋白、CK、S-100、Syn、嗜铬素和NSE的免疫组化反应均阳性[160-163]。支持细胞瘤中细胞CK免疫组化阳性信号通常比Leydig细胞肿瘤要强。PLAP在支持细胞瘤中呈阴性反应。管型精原细胞瘤通常在结构上与支持细胞瘤相似，可以用PLAP免疫组化阳性结果和抑制素、CK免疫组化阴性结果将二者鉴别出来。

CD99在诊断支持细胞瘤时是有价值的指标。在最近一项小样本量的研究中，20例支持细胞瘤中有12例CD99呈阳性反应（60%）[150]。

> **诊断要点：支持细胞瘤**
>
> 1. 抑制素A是敏感的标记物。
> 2. CK阳性。
> 3. PLAP阴性。
> 4. 波形蛋白阳性。
> 5. S-100、Syn、CgA和NSE阳性。
> 6. CD99阳性（60%）。

颗粒细胞瘤，幼年型

幼稚型颗粒细胞瘤是一种不常见的睾丸肿瘤，经常见于新生儿和2岁以内的幼儿[164-166]。在组织学上，这些少见的肿瘤内含不规则的囊泡，被覆单层或多层颗粒细胞。未见Call-Exner小体和核沟结构，与成年型不同。肿瘤细胞表现出上皮/间充质双重分化，低分子量CK（8、18和19）以及平滑肌肌动蛋白、结蛋白和波形蛋白的免疫组化呈阳性[165, 166]。最近一项研究表明CD99免疫组化结果也为阳性；但是，标本数量（n=5 幼稚型颗粒细胞瘤；CD99在其中的3个标本中为阳性）不具有统计学意义。但是，由于CD99可以标记正常的颗粒细胞，所以可以推论大量的幼稚型颗粒细胞瘤可以表达这种标记物[167]。

颗粒细胞瘤，成年型

成年型颗粒细胞瘤也是非常少见的，常见临床表现为睾丸肿物，有时伴有男子乳腺发育[168, 169]。在显微镜下观察，它们的特征与卵巢颗粒细胞瘤相同，内含片状的肿瘤细胞伴纵向的核沟。由于该肿瘤少见，所以寻找到一个可靠的和具有统计学意义的免疫组化方法进行诊断很困难。关于这一肿瘤的免疫组化结果数据非常少。一般说来，这些肿瘤波形蛋白和抑制素为阳性，但是CK和EMA常为阴性[29, 33, 169, 170]。S-100蛋白和平滑肌肌动蛋白在少数病例中呈阳性[33, 171]。几个小规模研究中发现CD99免疫组化呈阳性。此外，在一些小规模的研究中，抗苗勒激素受体在这些肿瘤中也为阳性[172]。性索-间质肿瘤（未分类）的免疫组化结果与颗粒细胞瘤的结果相似，即平滑肌肌动蛋白和S-100蛋白阳性[171]。

> **诊断要点：颗粒细胞瘤，成年型**
>
> 1. 波形蛋白+。
> 2. 抑制素+。
> 3. CD99+。
> 4. CK-。
> 5. S-100结果有差别。
> 6. 肌动蛋白结果有差别。

纤维瘤-卵泡膜细胞瘤

纤维瘤-卵泡膜细胞瘤很少发生于睾丸间质组织[173, 174]，它们与来源卵巢的相应肿瘤无明显区别。在日常工作中，很少使用免疫组化方法对该肿瘤进行诊断。在这些肿瘤中，波形蛋白免疫组化结果为强阳性，肌动蛋白和结蛋白免疫组化结果为局灶性阳性[174]。在一项研究中发现，CK、S-100蛋白和CD34为阴性。少数睾丸性索-间质肿瘤的病例中梭形细胞成分占优势。这些肿瘤的免疫组化结果与颗粒细胞瘤的结果相似，包括S-100蛋白阳性和平滑肌肌动蛋白阳性[171]。对卵巢肿瘤的免疫组化研究表明，11例卵泡膜细胞瘤中的10例和11例纤维瘤中的3例抑制素免疫组化结果为阳性[175]。

混合型性索-间质和生殖细胞肿瘤

性腺母细胞瘤 性腺母细胞瘤是一种独特的睾丸肿瘤，它含有巢状生殖细胞群，肿瘤细胞类似于支持细胞或颗粒细胞[176-178]。该肿瘤来源于遗传缺陷的性腺和未下降的睾丸，与生殖细胞肿瘤的形成相关。少数病例发生于正常性腺。80%的病例表型为女性，20%的病例表型为男性。大多数病例为XY或XO/XY嵌合体核型[179]。性腺母细胞瘤通常为良性，但是为发展为其他生殖细胞肿瘤的标志，因此被认为是该肿瘤的前体病变。高达50%的性腺母细胞瘤伴有局灶性的恶性生殖细胞肿瘤。

一项免疫组化研究表明，所有ITGCN的标记物，包括PLAP、抗M2A抗体、43-0F和TRA-1-60都为阳性[176]。然而，生殖细胞群通常是异源性的，因此会导致肿瘤免疫组化结果的不同。在这些肿瘤中，支持样细胞与CK和波形蛋白抗体发生反应。围绕细胞团的玻璃样物质的层粘连蛋白免疫组化反应阳性[177]。有一项研究表明，所研究的2个病例的Wilms肿瘤基因（WT-1）、苗勒抑制物质（MIS）、抑制素和p53的免疫组化均为阳性[178]。抑制素在性索-间质肿瘤中为阳性，在生殖细胞肿瘤中为阴性；MIS在两种细胞成分中均为阳性；WT-1只在性索区域为阳性；p53在生殖细胞中为阳性。在一个小样本量的研究中，发现性腺母细胞瘤中E-钙黏素为阴性，而β-连环蛋白为阳性[31, 180]。

最近发现一种因子有望成为性腺母细胞瘤的新标记物：睾丸特异性蛋白，由Y染色体编码（TSPY），由位于Y染色体短臂上的一个串联重复序列基因家族调控。在正常情况下，它在早期精原细胞的发育过程中发挥作用，被认为主要是在精原细胞的增殖过程中发挥功能。性腺母细胞瘤能够被抗TSPY的抗体所标记出来[181]。另外，最近有报道，成性腺细胞瘤同时还表达生殖细胞系标记物VASA。

> **诊断要点：性腺母细胞瘤**
> 1. 性腺母细胞瘤细胞对于所有ITGCN标记物都为阳性反应。
> 2. TSPY抗体可能是性腺母细胞瘤的一个新的、灵敏的和相对特异的标记物。
> 3. 然而，生殖细胞群通常是异源性的。

造血细胞肿瘤、转移瘤和其他少见的睾丸肿瘤

苗勒乳头状浆液性肿瘤 据报道，在睾丸组织中发现有一些卵巢型上皮肿瘤存在，包括低度恶性的浆液性乳头状囊性瘤、浆液性乳头状癌、黏液性囊腺瘤、Brenner肿瘤、子宫内膜样腺癌、黏液性囊腺癌和透明细胞腺癌[182-186]。低度恶性的浆液性乳头状囊性瘤是这组肿瘤中最常见的，从形态学上与卵巢来源的肿瘤不易区分。有报道，在1个病例中LeuM1、CA125、ER、PR、CK7免疫组化为阳性，CK20免疫组化为弱阳性[182]。CEA为阴性。在同一个报道中发现，所有9个卵巢乳头状浆液性瘤病例都表达CK7、CA125和ER，9例中的8例表达PR，9例中的5例表达LeuM1，9例中的2例弱表达CK20。另一项关于睾丸旁乳头状浆液性癌的研究中发现，CK AE1/AE3、S-100蛋白、EMA、Ber-EP4、LeuM1、B72.3、CEA和PLAP的免疫组化为阳性[183]。

原发性类癌肿瘤 原发性类癌肿瘤是一种罕见的无痛性肿瘤，有转移潜能[187, 188]。其组织学及免疫组化特征与那些来源于肺、胃肠道和其他部位的相应肿瘤相同。在这些肿瘤中，CgA、5-羟色胺、NSE、CK、胃泌素、P物质和血管活性肠肽呈免疫组化阳性[178]。大约25%的睾丸类癌的发生与畸胎瘤相关[187, 189]。在睾丸类癌中，类癌综合征未见报道。

> **诊断要点：原发性类癌**
>
> 在睾丸的原发性类癌中，CgA、5-羟色胺、NSE、CK、胃泌素、P物质和血管活性肠肽呈免疫组化阳性。

淋巴瘤 睾丸淋巴瘤大约占所有睾丸肿瘤的5%，老年患者占到一半以上[190, 191]。在鉴别老年患者的睾丸肿瘤时应该考虑淋巴瘤，以及精母细胞性精原细胞瘤和转移癌。绝大多数睾丸肿瘤病例为B细胞淋

巴瘤，但是也可见T细胞淋巴瘤以及T/NK细胞淋巴瘤[192-194]。在大多数病例中，睾丸淋巴瘤与典型的精原细胞瘤、精母细胞性精原细胞瘤和胚胎癌的区别通常是明显的。淋巴瘤呈明显的间质浸润生长型。在少数病例中，肿瘤细胞浸润曲精小管，从而表现为管内生长型。相反，在一些精原细胞肿瘤病例中，肿瘤周围的淋巴细胞表现为明显的管间生长型。在疑难病例中，LCA和B、T细胞标记物的阳性反应有助于对将淋巴瘤与原发性生殖细胞肿瘤相鉴别。淋巴瘤中，PLAP和CK为阴性。

间变型大细胞淋巴瘤（ALCL）与胚胎癌的鉴别可能会特别困难。ALCL可能表现为管内生长型伴坏死，与胚胎癌相似[191]。CD45、CD3、CD45RO、CD43阳性，以及B细胞标记物、PLAP和CK阴性有助于正确诊断。

> **诊断要点：淋巴瘤**
>
> 1. 淋巴瘤：LCA+、B 或 T 细胞标记物 +、PLAP 和 CK-。
> 2. ALCL：CD45+、CD3+、CD45RO+、CD43+、B 细胞标记物 -、PLAP-、CK-。

浆细胞瘤 睾丸浆细胞瘤的发生率大约是每1000个睾丸肿瘤中有1例[195]。大多数睾丸浆细胞瘤表现为来源于另一位置的转移癌，或者是系统性浆细胞恶液质的一个征象[196]。由于这种肿瘤很少见，大多数病例一开始常被认为是精原细胞瘤、精原母细胞性精原细胞瘤或淋巴瘤。从免疫组化结果来看，大多数浆细胞瘤表达单型细胞浆免疫球蛋白（通常为IgG或IgA型），并常缺乏B细胞标记物，如CD20。很多病例不表达CD45[197]。UCHL-1（CD45RO）在浆细胞瘤常为阳性。EMA的表达可能要与上皮性肿瘤鉴别，但是CK通常为阴性。PLAP 在睾丸浆细胞瘤中常为阴性。

> **诊断要点：浆细胞瘤**
>
> 1. 单型细胞浆免疫球蛋白表达阳性（通常为 IgG 或 IgA 型）。
> 2. CD45RO 常表达阳性。
> 3. B 细胞标记物阴性。
> 4. EMA 可能为阳性，CK 通常阴性。
> 5. PLAP 阴性。

白血病 继发性睾丸损害在急性白血病中是非常常见的。大约5%的急性淋巴母细胞性白血病的男性儿童会出现睾丸损害，这种损害或者为白血病首发症状，或者发生于疾病的过程中，或者成为第一个复发位置[198]。在尸检中，64%的急性白血病患者和22%的慢性白血病患者都发现有睾丸浸润[199]。粒细胞性肉瘤在睾丸中也有报道，这会使诊断变得困难，因为在鉴别诊断时经常不会考虑到它[200-202]。大多数病例一开始被误诊为恶性淋巴瘤或浆细胞瘤。在一些病例中，嗜酸性颗粒在嗜酸性髓细胞中的出现提示诊断正确。在粒细胞性肉瘤中，氯醋酸酯酶染色阳性，并且溶菌酶、髓过氧化物酶和LCA的免疫组化为阳性。B、T细胞标记物和CK常为阴性[200]。

转移癌 睾丸可能很少有转移癌发生[203-205]。这些病例常造成误诊，因为睾丸肿物常为转移癌的第一个临床表现。最常见的原发性肿瘤来自前列腺和肺[203]。在前列腺癌睾丸切除术的标本中，有6%存在癌转移位点[206]。其他的原发性肿瘤/部位包括：黑色素瘤、结肠、肾、胃、胰腺、膀胱、输尿管、胆管、涎腺和甲状腺。神经母细胞瘤、类癌、视网膜母细胞瘤和间皮瘤也可转移至睾丸。肿瘤的形态依赖于原发部位，可能与原发的生殖细胞瘤相似。老年人、双侧性或多病灶、相关的临床病史（如果存在）、间质生长型和淋巴血管浸润表现都支持原发性生殖细胞肿瘤转移癌的诊断。在疑难病例中，一个基本的免疫组化组合包括：CK、EMA、PLAP、PSA、LCA和HMB-45，对于诊断应该是有价值的。根据初步研究结果，其他的标记物如抑制素、CD30和B、T细胞抗原可能也是有价值的。据报道，尚有少数前列腺腺癌转移到附睾，与腺瘤样肿瘤类似[207]。前列腺酸性磷酸酶和前列腺特异性抗原可以帮助正确诊断。

附属结构和外生殖器肿瘤

腺瘤样瘤

腺瘤样瘤是睾丸附属结构中最常见的良性肿瘤，占睾丸旁肿瘤的60%[40]。在典型的病例中，该肿瘤含有圆形、椭圆形或砂粒样管状物，由立方形或扁平形细胞围绕。然而，这种间皮肿瘤能够表现出各种不同的组织学类型，能够与性索-间质肿瘤、印戒细胞腺癌、恶性间皮瘤和卵黄囊肿瘤相似。腺瘤样肿瘤中，CK、EMA和波形蛋白为均一阳性[208, 209]。血栓调节素可能为阳性，其他的间皮细胞标记物如 HBME-1 和 OC125 也可为阳性。这些抗体在腺瘤样肿瘤中的显色部位在胞膜[210]。一种间皮细胞的新的标记物 D2-40 尚未在腺瘤样肿瘤中检测到。

据报道，CEA、Ber-EP4、B72.3、LeuM1、Ⅷ因子相关抗原、CD34 和 OCT4 在肿瘤中为阴性。由于血管标记物免疫组化常为阴性，所以易与组织细胞样血管瘤相鉴别，组织细胞样血管瘤是来源于该部位的一种罕见相似肿瘤[40,211]。组织细胞样血管瘤中波形蛋白、Ⅷ因子相关抗原和 Ulex europaeus I 凝集素为阳性，但是 CK 和 EMA 为阴性。根据肉眼和显微镜下观察，大多数腺瘤样瘤与恶性间皮瘤的鉴别是可以完成的。肿瘤大、边界不清、镜下呈双相表现的肿瘤，更有可能是恶性间皮瘤。细胞异型性和明显的乳头状成分也支持间皮瘤的诊断。一些腺瘤样瘤表现为实性生长型伴明显的嗜酸性胞浆并缺少空泡，与性索-间质肿瘤相似。有些特征支持后者的诊断，包括大量的脂褐素沉积、泡沫状胞浆、Reinke 类晶体、抑制素免疫组化强阳性，以及 CK 阴性或弱阳性。腺瘤样瘤中，抗抑制素抗体的免疫组化结果尚不清楚。

> **诊断要点：腺瘤样瘤**
>
> 1. CK、EMA、波形蛋白均一阳性反应。
> 2. 间皮标记物血栓调节素、HBME-1 和 OC125 阳性。
> 3. CEA、Ber-EP4、B72.3、LeuM1、Ⅷ因子相关抗原和 CD34 阴性。
> 4. 血管标记物阴性。

乳腺外 Paget 病

乳腺外 Paget 病可能来源于真皮内顶浆分泌细胞，可以认为是表皮内腺癌具有皮肤浸润潜能[40]。很多病例继发于具有泌尿生殖系统或结肠直肠潜在恶性的类 Paget 病[212-214]。在组织学上，该肿瘤含有大的空泡状细胞，表皮基底细胞的胞浆为淡嗜伊红色。主要的鉴别诊断包括黑色素瘤、原位鳞状细胞癌。肿瘤细胞的 CK、EMA 和 CEA 免疫组化阳性，S-100 蛋白和 HMB-45 为阴性[214]。空泡状胞浆也可以被黏蛋白胭脂红和阿辛蓝染色。

最近的研究表明，受体结合癌抗原或 RCAS1 可能是乳腺外 Paget 病的一种有诊断价值的标记物。在一项研究中，63 例乳腺外 Paget 病病例中的 59 例（93.7%）呈阳性[215-217]。

间皮瘤

鞘膜恶性间皮瘤是一种非常少见的肿瘤，临床表现常为鞘膜积液或睾丸旁肿物[218-220]。发病的平均年龄为 53.5 岁。组织学特征与那些来源于胸膜和腹腔的相应肿瘤相似。在一项研究中，全部 8 个肿瘤都表现为 CK 阳性，5 例病例中的 4 例为 EMA 和波形蛋白阳性[218]。所有检测的肿瘤中，CEA、B72.3、LeuM1 和 Ber-EP4 均为阴性。

calretinin 是一种钙结合蛋白，被认为是间皮分化的特异标志物，据不同的研究报道，这种标记物的阳性率在 87.5%～92%[221-223]。阳性部位为胞浆和胞核，伴或不伴膜阳性，形成一种具有特征性的"煎蛋"样表现[221]。反应性间皮细胞和其他良性的间皮细胞增殖时也可为阳性。腺瘤样瘤与恶性间皮瘤的免疫组化结果分析无明显区别[219]。二者的鉴别诊断主要依靠肉眼观察和显微镜下形态学观察。血栓调节素、CK5/6 和 CD44H 在间皮瘤与转移性腺癌的鉴别诊断中很有价值，特别是当肿瘤侵犯胸膜时[222]。

一种新的间皮瘤标记物最近被报道，认为它很有应用前景。D2-40 是近期被认可并进行商品化销售的单克隆抗体，最近一篇报道指出，53 例恶性间皮瘤中有 51 例（96%）该标记物为阳性。同一研究还指出，它的敏感性相当于 calretinin，超过 CK5/6 和 WT-1。令人感兴趣的是，D2-40 最初被研究用来检测表达于胎儿睾丸生殖母细胞表面的唾液糖蛋白，从而对生殖细胞瘤进行检测。它还可以标记淋巴管内皮[224]。

结缔组织增生型小圆细胞瘤

结缔组织增生型小圆细胞瘤（DSRCT）是一种高度恶性的肿瘤，首先由 Gerald 和 Rosai 于 1989 年报道。该肿瘤主要发生于十几岁的年轻人，男性居多（男女比例为 >5:1）。肿瘤最常发生于腹腔，出现腹部疼痛、膨胀和腹水。

DSRCT 也可发生于睾丸旁组织[225, 226]。在这一区域，它的典型表现为年轻男性出现阴囊肿物。典型 DSRCT 患者的平均年龄为 28 岁。肉眼和显微镜下观察发现，肿瘤可能侵及睾丸旁软组织、被囊和附睾。肿瘤的组成为均一的小细胞形成的细胞巢和细胞岛，由结缔组织间质分隔成多个结节。肿瘤的免疫组化结果分析表现出多系分化的特点,包括上皮、间充质和神经元的特征。肿瘤细胞中,CK、波形蛋白、结蛋白和NSE为阳性,HBA-71为阴性反应。DSRCT属于肿瘤中的Ewing肉瘤(ES)家族,肿瘤的形态学和免疫组化特征与原始神经外胚层肿瘤或PNET相似。PNET和ES的特征性免疫组化结果为CD99阳性,CD99也称作O13。

许多研究表明,WT-1是用于鉴别DSRCT和PNET的可靠指标。WT-1在DSRCT呈阳性,而在PNET呈阴性。然而,横纹肌肉瘤WT-1亦呈阳性。

其他需要与DSRCT进行鉴别诊断的肿瘤还有胚胎性横纹肌肉瘤、恶性淋巴瘤和视网膜原基瘤,这些肿瘤也都含有"小圆蓝细胞"。胚胎性横纹肌肉瘤具有黏液样间质,常见于非常年轻的人。横纹肌母细胞瘤常具有深染的、丰富的嗜伊红胞浆和纵行横纹,如果出现这种形态特征,则有助于横纹肌母细胞瘤的诊断。肌细胞生成素是早期肌肉分化的标记物,用来鉴别横纹肌母细胞瘤与DSRCT。

恶性淋巴瘤组织中无DSRCT肿瘤中那样的肿瘤细胞巢和细胞簇。这种肿瘤还缺少硬化型间质和DSRCT的免疫组化特征。在疑难病例的诊断中,用RT-PCR对石蜡切片组织进行分析,如判断有ES/WT-1嵌合基因的存在则可最终确诊为DSRCT,因为DSRCT具有特征性的融合基因t(11;22)(p13;q12),该融合基因是由于染色体易位造成的。

最近一项研究发现,DSRCT中结缔组织生长因子CCN2过表达,认为这种因子可能具有促进这些肿瘤的结缔组织增生的作用。用免疫组织化学方法和原位杂交方法,研究者发现,CCN2 mRNA和蛋白质共同定位于肿瘤本身和间质成纤维细胞及血管内皮细胞附近[228]。这一结果的诊断用途还不清楚。

视网膜原基瘤

这一少见的肿瘤有多种命名,包括黑色素神经外胚瘤和黑色素错构瘤[229-231]。典型的患者发病年龄不足1岁,常因疾病累及上颌骨而发现。少数病例累及附睾[231]。有一例黑色素神经外胚瘤的病例报道,该肿瘤为未成熟睾丸畸胎瘤的主要成分[232]。组织学上,它由两种细胞组成:大的柱状细胞或立方形上皮样细胞,具有泡状细胞核和突出的核仁,以及一群小的神经母细胞样的细胞,具有少量的胞浆和深染的细胞核。这种肿瘤表现出多表型的分化,具有上皮和神经标记物的表达,产生黑色素,偶尔产生神经胶质以及表达横纹肌母细胞瘤的标记物[230]。两种细胞群对NSE、Syn和HMB-45的免疫组化均为阳性[230]。S-100蛋白的表达可见于大的细胞中。在一些病例中,还可见EMA、GFAP、结蛋白和Leu7的表达。绝大多数大细胞表达CK和波形蛋白。这一肿瘤的生物学行为通常为良性的。视网膜原基瘤有时与DSRCT相似,而后者常预后不佳。两种肿瘤的鉴别主要是根据两种细胞类型的不同以及前者产生黑色素这一特征。在疑难病例的鉴别诊断中,特别是当黑色素沉着、两种细胞类型不易区分以及间质硬化时,HMB-45和S-100免疫组化结果将支持视网膜原基瘤的诊断。

睾丸的良性、局部浸润和恶性软组织肿瘤

实际上,在睾丸旁组织中,可以看到全部类型的间充质肿瘤[40]。在少数病例中,睾丸实质本身可能被累及。在这一区域中已经被报道过的良性或局部浸润的软组织肿瘤包括平滑肌瘤、脂肪瘤、脂肪肉瘤、横纹肌瘤、纤维瘤(除外性索-间质来源的肿瘤)、毛细血管瘤、海绵状血管瘤、组织细胞样血管瘤、血管肌纤维瘤和浸润性血管黏液瘤[40,233-235]。在成人中,发生于该区域的最常见的肉瘤为脂肪肉瘤[236],在儿童中则为横纹肌肉瘤[237,238]。另外,平滑肌肉瘤、恶性纤维组织细胞瘤、横纹肌样肿瘤和纤维瘤病也有报道。这些软组织肿瘤的组织学和免疫组织化学特征将在本书的其他章节进行介绍。

参考文献

1. Brown LM, Pottern LM, Hoover RN, et al. Testicular cancer in the United States: trends in incidence and mortality. Int J Epidemiol 1986; 15:164–170.

2. Muir C, Waterhouse J, Mack T, et al. Cancer incidence in five continents, Vol 5. Lyon, France: International Agency for Research on Cancer; 1987.

3. Skakkebaek NE. Possible carcinoma-in-situ of the undescended testis. Lancet 1972; 2:516–517.

4. Skakkebaek NE. Carcinoma-in-situ of the testis: frequency and relationship to invasive germ cell tumors in infertile men. Histopathology 1978; 2:157–170.

5. Berthelsen JG, Skakkebaek NE. Value of testicular biopsy in

diagnosing carcinoma in situ of testis. Scand J Urol Nephrol 1981; 15:165–168.

6. Muller J, Skakkebaek NE. Abnormal germ cells in maldescended testes: a study of cell density, nuclear size and deoxyribonucleic acid content in testicular biopsies from 50 boys. J Urol 1984; 131:730–733.

7. Skakkebaek NE, Berthelsen JG, Giwercman A, et al. Carcinoma-in-situ of the testis: possible origin from gonocytes and precursor of all types of germ cell tumours except spermatocytoma. Int J Androl 1987; 10:19–28.

8. Fishman WH. Oncotrophoblast gene expression: Placental alkaline phosphatase. Adv Cancer Res 1987; 48:1.

9. Fishman WH, Bardawil WA, Habib HG, et al. The placental isoenzyme of alkaline phosphatase in sera of normal pregnancy. Am J Clin Pathol 1972; 57:65.

10. Fishman WH, Inglis NI, Stolbach LL, et al. A serum alkaline phosphatase isoenzyme of human neoplastic cell origin. Cancer Res 1968; 28:150–154.

11. Benham F, Cotell DC, Franks LM, et al. Alkaline phosphatase activity in human bladder tumor cell lines. J Histochem Cytochem 1977; 25:266–274.

12. Manivel JC, Jessurun J, Wick MR, et al. Placental alkaline phosphatase immunoreactivity in testicular germ-cell neoplasms. Am J Surg Pathol 1987; 11:21–29.

13. Koshida K, Wahren B. Placental-like alkaline phosphatase in seminoma. Urol Res 1990; 18:87–92.

14. Fishman WH, Inglis NR, Stolbach LL, et al. A serum alkaline phosphatase isoenzyme of human neoplastic cell origin. Cancer Res 1968; 28:150.

15. Aguirre P, Scully RE, Dayal Y, et al. Placental-like alkaline phosphatase in germ cell tumors of the ovary and testis [Abstract]. Lab Invest 1986; 54:2A.

16. Javadpour N. The role of biologic tumor markers in testicular cancer. Cancer 1980; 45:1755–1761.

17. Bosl GJ, Chaganti RSK. The use of tumor markers in germ cell malignancies. In: Tumor markers in adult solid malignancies. Hem Oncol Clin N Am 1994; 8:573–587.

18. Grossman BH. Tumor markers in urology. Semin Urol 1985; 3:10–17.

19. Wilson RB, Albert A, Randall M. Quantitative studies on the production, destruction and elimination of chorionic gonadotrophin in normal pregnancy. Am J Obstet Gynecol 1949; 58:960–967.

20. Horne CHW, Rankin R, Bremner RD. Pregnancy-specific proteins as markers for gestational trophoblastic disease. Int J Gynecol Pathol 1984; 3:27–39.

21. Hussa RO. Human chorionic gonadotropin, a clinical marker: Review of its biosynthesis. Ligand Rev 1981; 3:1.

22. Sherwood LM, Handwerger S, McLauren WD, et al. Comparison of the structure and function of HPL and human GH. In: Pecile A, Muller EE, eds. Second international symposium on growth hormone. Amsterdam: Excerpta Medica; 1971:8–9.

23. Ulbright TM, Young RH, Scully RE. Trophoblastic tumors of the testis other than classic choriocarcinoma: 'monophasic' choriocarcinoma and placental site trophoblastic tumor: a report of two cases. Am J Surg Pathol 1997; 21:282–288.

24. McCluggage WG, Shanks JH, Whiteside C, et al. Immunohistochemical study of testicular sex cord-stromal tumors, including staining with anti-inhibin antibody. Am J Surg Pathol 1998; 22:615–619.

25. Roberts V, Meunier H, Sanchenko PE, et al. Differential production and regulation of inhibin subunits in rat testicular cell types. Endocrinology 1989; 125:2350–2359.

26. McLachlan RI, Robertson DM, Burger HG, et al. Circulating immunoreactive inhibin levels during the normal menstrual cycle. J Clin Endocrinol Metab 1987; 65:954–961.

27. Arora DS, Cooke IE, Ganesan TS, et al. Immunohistochemical expression of inhibin/activin subunits in epithelial and granulosa cell tumors of the ovary. J Pathol 1997; 181:413–418.

28. Flemming P, Wellmann A, Maschek H, et al. Monoclonal antibodies against inhibin represent key markers of adult granulosa tumors of the ovary even in their metastases. Am J Surg Pathol 1995; 19:927–933.

29. McCluggage WG, Maxwell P, Sloan JM. Immunohistochemical staining of ovarian granulosa cell tumors with monoclonal antibody against inhibin. Hum Pathol 1997; 28:1034–1038.

30. Rishi M, Howard L, Bratthauer GL, et al. Use of monoclonal antibody against inhibin as a marker for sex cord-stromal tumors of the ovary. Am J Surg Pathol 1997; 21:583–589.

31. Stewart CJR, Jeffers MD, Kennedy A. Diagnostic value of inhibin immunoreactivity in ovarian gonadal stromal tumors and their histological mimics. Histopathology 1997; 31:67–74.

32. Iczkowski KA, Bostwick DG, Roche PC, et al. Inhibin A is a

sensitive and specific marker for testicular sex cord-stromal tumors. Mod Pathol 1998; 11:774–779.

33. McCluggage WG, Shanks JH, Whiteside C, et al. Immunohistochemical study of testicular sex cord-stromal tumors, including staining with anti-inhibin antibody. Am J Surg Pathol 1998; 22:615–619.

34. Amin MB, Young RH, Scully RE. Immunohistochemical profile of Sertoli and Leydig cell tumors of the testis [Abstract]. Mod Pathol 1998; 11:78A.

35. McCluggage WB, Ashe P, McBride H, et al. Localization of the cellular expression of inhibin in trophoblastic tissue. Histopathology 1998; 32:252–256.

36. Pelkey TJ, Frierson HF Jr, Mills SE, et al. Detection of the alpha-subunit of inhibin in trophoblastic neoplasia. Hum Pathol 1999; 30:26–31.

37. Minami S, Yamoto M, Nakano R. Immunohistochemical localization of inhibin/activin subunits in human placenta. Obstet Gynecol 1992; 80:410–414.

38. Minami S, Yamoto M, Nakano R. Immunohistochemical localization of inhibin/activin subunits in hydatidiform mole and invasive mole. Obstet Gynecol 1993; 82:414–418.

39. Skakkebaek NE, Berthelsen JG, Muller J. Carcinoma-in-situ of the undescended testis. Urol Clin North Am 1982; 9:377.

40. Ulbright TM, Amin MB, Young RH. Tumors of the testis, adnexa, spermatic cord, and scrotum. AFIP Fascicle 1999; 41–58.

41. Beckstead JH. Alkaline phosphatase histochemistry in human germ cell neoplasms. Am J Surg Pathol 1983; 7:341–349.

42. Jacobsen GK, Norgaard-Pedersen B. Placental alkaline phosphatase in testicular germ cell tumors and carcinomain-situ of the testis: an immunohistochemical study. Acta Pathol Microbiol Immunol Scand [A] 1984; 92:323–329.

43. Manivel JC, Jessurun J, Wick MR, et al. Placental alkaline phosphatase immunoreactivity in testicular germ cell tumors. Am J Surg Pathol 1987; 11:21–29.

44. Burke AP, Mostofi FK. Intratubular malignant germ cells in testicular biopsies: clinical course and identification by staining for placental alkaline phosphatase. Mod Pathol 1988; 1: 475–479.

45. Jacobsen GK, Jacobsen M. Alpha-fetoprotein (AFP) and human chorionic gonadotropin (HCG) in testicular germ cell tumors: a prospective immunohistochemical study. Acta Pathol Microbiol Scand 1983; 91:165–176.

46. Jacobsen GK, Jacobsen M, Claussen PP, et al. Immunohistochemical demonstration of tumor-associated antigens in carcinoma-in-situ of the testis. Int J Androl 1981; 4(suppl): 203.

47. Sigg C, Hedinger C. Atypical germ cells of the testis: comparative, ultrastructural and histochemical investigations. Virchows Arch (A) 1984; 402:439.

48. Jacobsen GK, Jacobsen M, Praetorius C. Ferritin as a possible marker protein of carcinoma-in-situ of the testis. Lancet 1980; 2:533–534.

49. Jacobsen GK, Jacobsen M. Ferritin in testicular germ cell tumors. An immunohistochemical study. Acta Pathol Microbiol Immunol Scand [A] 1983; 91(3):177–181.

50. Coffin CM, Ewing S, Dehner LP. Frequency of the intratubular germ cell neoplasia with invasive testicular germ cell tumors. Histologic and immunocytochemical features. Arch Pathol Lab Med 1985; 109:555–559.

51. Eyzaguirre E, Gatalica Z. Loss of FHIT expression in testicular germ cell tumors and intratubular germ cell neoplasia. Mod Pathol 2002; 15:1068.

52. Kang JL, Meyts E, Skakkebaek NE. Immunoreactive neuron-specific enolase is expressed in testicular carcinoma-in-situ. J Pathol 1996; 178:161–165.

53. Kuczyk MA, Serth J, Bokemeyer C, et al. Overexpression of the p53 oncoprotein in carcinoma-in-situ of the testis. Pathol Res Pract 1994; 190: 993–998.

54. Kuczyk MA, Serth J, Bokemeyer C, et al. Alterations in the p53 tumor suppressor gene in carcinoma-in-situ of the testis. Cancer 1996; 78:1958–1966.

55. Tokuyama S, Saito S, Takahashi T, et al. Immunostaining of stage-specific embryonic antigen-4 in intratubular germ cell neoplasia unclassified and in testicular germ-cell tumors. Oncol Rep 2003; 10:1097.

56. Giwercman A, Andrews PW, Jorgensen N, et al. Immunohistochemical expression of embryonal marker TRA-1-60 in carcinoma-in-situ and germ cell tumors of the testis. Cancer 1993; 72:1308–1314.

57. Giwercman A, Lindenberg S, Kimber SJ, et al. Monoclonal antibody 43-9-F as a sensitive immunohistochemical marker of carcinoma-in-situ of human testis. Cancer 1990; 65:1135–1142.

58. Rajpert-De Meyts E, Kvist M, Skakkebaek NE. Heterogene-

ity of expression of immunohistochemical tumor markers in testicular carcinoma-in-situ: pathogenetic relevance. Virchows Arch 1996; 428:133–139.

59. Drescher B, Lauke H, Hartmann M, et al. Immunohistochemical pattern of insulin-like growth factor (IGF) I, IGF II and IGF-binding proteins 1 to 6 in carcinoma-in-situ of the testis. Mol Pathol 1997; 50:298–303.

60. Giwercam A, Cantell L, Marks A. Placental-like alkaline phosphatase as a marker of carcinoma-in-situ of the testis. Comparison with monoclonal antibodies M2A and 43-9F. APMIS 1991; 99: 586–594.

61. Jorgensen N, Giwercam A, Muller J, et al. Immunohistochemical markers of carcinoma-in-situ of the testis are also expressed in normal infantile germ cells. Histopathology 1993; 22:373–378.

62. Klys HS, Whillis D, Howard G, et al. Glutathione-S-transferase expression in the human testis and testicular germ cell neoplasia. Br J Cancer 1992; 66:589–593.

63. Kang JL, Rajpert-De Meyts E, Wiels J, et al. Expression of the glycolipid globotriaosylceramide (Gb3) in testicular carcinoma-in-situ. Virch Arch 1995; 426:369–374.

64. Mostofi FK, Sesterhenn IA. Pathology of germ cell tumors of testes. Prog Clin Biol Res 1985; 203:1–34.

65. Mostofi FK, Spaander P, Grigor K, et al. Consensus on pathological classifications of testicular tumors. Prog Clin Biol Res 1990; 357:267.

66. Rustin GJS, Vogelzand NJ, Sleijfer DT, et al. Consensus statement on circulating tumor markers and staging patients with germ cell tumors. Prog Clin Biol Res 1990; 357:277.

67. Manivel JC, Jesserun J, Wick MR, et al. Placental alkaline phosphatase immunoreactivity in testicular germ cell neoplasms. Am J Surg Pathol 1987; 11:21–29.

68. Wick MR, Swanson PE, Manivel JC. Placental alkaline-like phosphatase reactivity in human tumors. Hum Pathol 1987; 18:946–954.

69. Niehans GA, Manival JC, Copland GT, et al. Immunohistochemistry of germ cell and trophoblastic neoplasms. Cancer 1988; 62:1113–1123.

70. Bosman FT, Giard RW, Kruseman AC, et al. Human chorionic gonadotropin and alpha-fetoprotein in testicular germ cell tumors: a retrospective immunohistochemical study. Histopathology 1980; 4:673–684.

71. Jacobsen GK, Jacobsen M. Alpha-fetoprotein (AFP) and human chorionic gonadotropin in testicular germ cell tumors. A prospective immunohistochemical study. Acta Pathol Microbiol Scant [A] 1983; 91:165–176.

72. von Hochstetter AR, Sigg C, Saremaslani P, et al. The significance of giant cells in human testicular seminomas. A clinicopathological study. Virchows Arch [A] 1985; 407:309–322.

73. Ferreiro JA. Ber-H2 expression in testicular germ cell tumors. Hum Pathol 1994; 25:522–524.

74. Hittmair A, Rogatsch H, Hobisch A, et al. CD30 expression in seminoma. Hum Pathol 1996; 27:1166–1171.

75. Pallesen G, Hamilton-Dutoit SJ. Ki-1 (CD30) antigen is regularly expressed in tumor cells of embryonal carcinoma. Am J Pathol 1988; 133:446–450.

76. Iczkowski KA, Bostwick DG, Roche PC, et al. Inhibin A is a sensitive and specific marker for testicular sex cord-stromal tumors. Mod Pathol 1998; 11:774.

77. Looijenga LH, Stoop H, de Leeuw HP, et al. POU5F1 (OCT3/4) identifies cells with pluripotent potential in human germ cell tumors. Cancer Res 2003; 63:2244.

78. Jones TD, Ulbright TM, Eble JN, et al. OCT4 staining in testicular tumors: a sensitive and specific marker for seminoma and embryonal carcinoma. Am J Surg Pathol 2004; 28: 935.

79. Heinrich MC, Blanke CD, Druker BJ, et al. Inhibition of KIT tyrosine kinase activity: a novel molecular approach to the treatment of KIT-positive malignancies. J Clin Oncol 2002; 20:1692.

80. Eglen DE, Ulbright TM. The differential diagnosis of cytokeratin, alpha-fetoprotein, and alpha-1-antitrypsin immunoperoxidase reactions. Am J Surg Pathol 1987; 88:328.

81. Miettinen M, Virtanen I, Talerman A. Intermediate filament proteins in human testis and testicular germ cell tumors. Am J Surg Pathol 1985; 120:402.

82. Rao S, Iczkowski KA, Cheville JC. Cytokeratin expression in seminoma and embryonal carcinoma of the testis [Abstract] Mod Pathol 1998; 11:92A.

83. Cheville JC, Rao S, Iczkowski KA, et al. Cytokeratin expression in seminoma of the human testis. Am J Clin Pathol 2000; 113:583–588.

84. Moll F, Franke WW, Schiller DR, et al. The catalog of human cytokeratins: patterns of expression in normal epithelia, tumors, and cultured cells. Cell 1982; 31:11–14.

85. Ramaekers F, Feitz W, Moesker O, et al. Antibodies to

cytokeratin and vimentin in testicular tumor diagnosis. Virchows Arch [A] 1985; 408:127–142.

86. Denk H, Moll R, Weybora W, et al. Intermediate filaments and desmosomal plaque proteins in testicular seminomas and non-seminomatous germ cell tumors as revealed by immunohistochemistry. Virchows Arch [A] 1987; 410:295–307.

87. Bartkova J, Rejthar A, Bartek J, et al. Differentiation patterns in testicular germ cell tumors as revealed by a panel of monoclonal antibodies. Tumor Biol 1987; 49:196–202.

88. Fogel M, Lifschitz-Mercer B, Moll R, et al. Heterogeneity of intermediate filament expression in human testicular seminomas. Differentiation 1990; 45:242–249.

89. Murakami SS, Said JW. Immunohistochemical localization of lactate dehydrogenase isoenzyme 1 in the germ cell tumors of the testis. Am J Clin Pathol 1984; 81:293–296.

90. Pauls K, Fink L, Franke FE. Angiotensin-converting enzyme (CD143) in neoplastic germ cells. Lab Invest 1999; 79:1425.

91. Przygodzki RM, Moran CA, Suster S, et al. Primary mediastinal and testicular seminomas: a comparison of K-ras-2 gene sequence and p53 immunoperoxidase analysis of 26 cases. Hum Pathol 1996; 27:975–979.

92. Suster S, Moran, Dominguez-Malagon H, et al. Germ cell tumors of the mediastinum and testis: a comparative immunohistochemical study of 120 cases. Hum Pathol 1998; 29:737–742.

93. Suzuki T, Sasano H, Aoki H, et al. Immunohistochemical comparison between anaplastic seminoma and typical seminoma. Acta Pathol Jpn 1993; 43:751–757.

94. Talerman A. Spermatocytic seminoma: A clinicopathologic study of 22 cases. Cancer 1980; 45:2169–2176.

95. Eble JN. Spermatocytic seminoma. Hum Pathol 1994; 25:1035–1042.

96. Burke AP, Mostofi FK. Spermatocytic seminoma, a clinicopathologic study of 79 cases. J Urol Pathol 1993; 1:21–32.

97. Rajpert-De Meyts E, Jacobsen GK, Bartkova J, et al.: The immunohistochemical expression pattern of Chk2, p53, p19INK4d, MAGE-A4 and other selected antigens provides new evidence for the premeiotic origin of spermatocytic seminoma. Histopathology 2003; 42:217.

98. Albores-Saavedra J, Huffman H, Alvarado-Cabrero I, et al. Anaplastic variant of spermatocytic seminoma. Hum Pathol 1996; 27:650–655.

99. Dekker I, Rozeboom T, Delemarre J, et al. Placental-like alkaline phosphatase and DNA flow cytometry in spermatocytic seminoma. Cancer 1992; 69:993–996.

100. Cummings OW, Ulbright TM, Eble JN, et al. Spermatocytic seminoma: An immunohistochemical study. Hum Pathol 1994; 25:54–59.

101. Kraggerud SM, Berner A, Bryne M, et al. Spermatocytic seminoma as compared to classical seminoma: an immunohistochemical and DNA flow cytometric study. APMIS 1999; 107:297–302.

102. Decaussin M, Borda A, Bouvier R, et al. [Spermatocytic seminoma. A clinicopathological and immunohistochemical study of 7 cases]. Ann Pathol 2004; 24:161.

103. Battifora H, Sheibani K, Tubbs RR, et al. Antikeratin antibodies in tumor diagnosis: distinction between seminoma and embryonal carcinoma. Cancer 1984; 54:843–848.

104. Lifschitz-Mercer B, Fogel M, Moll R, et al. Intermediate filament protein profiles of human testicular non-seminomatous germ cell tumors: correlation of cytokeratin synthesis to cell differentiation. Differentiation 1991; 48:191–198.

105. Cheng L. Establishing a germ cell origin for metastatic tumors using OCT4 immunohistochemistry. Cancer 2004; 101:2006–2010.

106. Stiller D, Bahn H, Pressler H. Immunohistochemical demonstration of alpha-fetoprotein in testicular germ cell tumors. Acta Histochem Suppl 1986; 33:225–231.

107. Bartkova J, Bartek J, Lukas J, et al. p53 protein alterations in human testicular cancer including preinvasive intratubular germ cell neoplasia. Int J Cancer 1991; 49:196–202.

108. Visfeldt J, Giwercman A, Skakkebaek NE. Monoclonal antibody 43-9F: an immunohistochemical marker of embryonal carcinoma of the testis. APMIS 1992; 100:63–70.

109. Ulbright TM, Orazi A, de Riese W, et al. The correlation of p53 protein expression with proliferative activity and occult metastases in clinical stage I non-seminomatous germ cell tumors of the testis. Mod Pathol 1994; 7:64–68.

110. Brown NJ. Yolk-sac tumour ('orchioblastoma') and other testicular tumours of childhood. In: Pugh RC, ed. Pathology of the testis. Oxford: Blackwell Scientific; 1976:356–370.

111. von Hochstetter AR, Hedinger CE. The differential diagnosis of testicular germ cell tumors in theory and in practice: a critical analysis of two major systems of classification and review of 389 cases. Virchows Arch [A] 1982; 396:247.

112. Talerman A. Endodermal sinus (yolk sac) tumor elements in testicular germ cell tumors in adults: comparison of prospective and retrospective studies. Cancer 1980; 46:1213.

113. Talerman A, Haije WG, Baggerman L. Histological patterns in germ cell tumors associated with raised serum alpha fetoprotein (AFP). Scant J Immunol Suppl 1978; 8:97.

114. Talerman A, Haije WG, Baggerman L. Serum alpha fetoprotein (AFP) in patients with germ cell tumors of the gonads and extragonadal sites. Correlation between endodermal sinus (yolk sac) tumor and raised serum AFP. Cancer 1980; 46:380.

115. Mostofi FK, Sesterhenn IA, Davis CJ Jr. Immunopathology of germ cell tumors of the testis. Semin Diagn Pathol 1987; 4:320–341.

116. Wold LE, Kramer SA, Farrow GM. Testicular yolk sac and embryonal carcinomas in pediatric patients: comparative immunohistochemical and clinicopathologic study. Am J Clin Pathol 1984; 81:427.

117. Burke AP, Mostofi FK. Placental alkaline phosphatase immunohistochemistry of intratubular malignant germ cells and associated testicular germ cell tumors. Hum Pathol 1988; 19: 663–670.

118. Jacobsen GK, Jacobsen M, Clausen PP. Distribution of tumor-associated antigens in the various histologic components of germ cell tumors of the testis. Am J Surg Pathol 1981; 5: 257–266.

119. Ulbright TM, Roth LM, Brodhecker CA. Yolk sac differentiation in germ cell tumors: a morphologic study of 50 cases with emphasis on hepatic, enteric and parietal yolk sac features. Am J Surg Pathol 1986; 10:151–164.

120. Visfeldt J, Jorgensen N, Muller J, et al. Testicular germ cell tumors of childhood in Denmark, 1943–1989: incidence and evaluation of histology using immunohistochemical techniques. J Pathol 1994; 174:39–47.

121. Hamazaki S, Okada S. Expression of CD34 antigen in testicular mixed germ cell tumor. Pathol Int 2003; 53:853.

122. Siltanen S, Heikkila P, Bielinska M, et al. Transcription factor GATA-6 is expressed in malignant endoderm of pediatric yolk sac tumors and in teratomas. Pediatr Res 2003; 54:542.

123. Ulbright TM, Amin MB, Young RH. Tumors of the testis, adnexa, spermatic cord, and scrotum. Atlas of tumor pathology, 3rd Series, Fascicle 25. Washington, DC: Armed Forces Institute of Pathology; 1999.

124. Manivel JC, Niehans G, Wick MR, et al. Intermediate trophoblast in germ cell neoplasms. Am J Surg Pathol 1987; 11: 693–701.

125. Clark RK, Damjanov I. Intermediate filaments of human trophoblast and choriocarcinoma cell lines. Virchows Arch [A] 1985; 407:203–208.

126. Lind HM, Haghighi P. Carcinoembryonic antigen staining in choriocarcinoma. Am J Clin Pathol 1986; 86:538–540.

127. Hechelhammer L, Storkel S, Odermatt B, et al. Epidermal growth factor receptor is a marker for syncytiotrophoblastic cells in testicular germ cell tumors. Virchows Arch 2003; 443: 28.

128. Zhao J, Kunz TH, Tumba N, et al. Comparative analysis of expression and secretion of placental leptin in mammals. Am J Physiol Regul Integr Comp Physiol 2003; 285:R438.

129. Bifulco G, Trencia A, Caruso M, et al. Leptin induces mitogenic effect on human choriocarcinoma cell line (JAr) via MAP kinase activation in a glucose-dependent fashion. Placenta 2003; 24:385.

130. Cauzac M, Czuba D, Girard J, et al. Transduction of leptin growth signals in placental cells is independent of JAKSTAT activation. Placenta 2003; 24:378.

131. Challier J, Galtier M, Bintein T, et al. Placental leptin receptor isoforms in normal and pathological pregnancies. Placenta 2003; 24:92.

132. Masuzaki H, Ogawa Y, Sagawa N, et al. Nonadipose tissue production of leptin: leptin as a novel placenta-derived hormone in humans. Nat Med 1997; 3:1029.

133. Cui JQ, Shi YF, Zhou HJ, et al. The changes of gene expression profiles in hydatidiform mole and choriocarcinoma with hyperplasia of trophoblasts. Int J Gynecol Cancer 2004; 14: 984.

134. Brosman SA. Testicular tumors in prepubertal children. Urology 1979; 13:581–588.

135. Grady RW, Ross JH, Kay R. Epidemiological features of testicular teratomas in prepubertal population. J Urol 1997; 158: 1191–1192.

136. Kay R. Prepubertal testicular tumor registry. J Urol 1993; 150:671–674.

137. Barsky SH. Germ cell tumors of the testis. In: Javadpour N, Barsky SH, eds. Surgical pathology of urologic diseases. Baltimore: William & Wilkins; 1987:224–246.

138. Leibovitch I, Foster RS, Ulbright TM, et al. Adult primary

138. pure teratoma of the testis. The Indiana Experience. Cancer 1995; 75:2244–2250.
139. Simmonds PD, Lee AH, Theaker JM, et al. Primary pureteratoma of the testis. J Urol 1996; 155:939–942.
140. Stevens MJ, Normal AR, Fisher C, et al. Prognosis of testicular teratoma differentiated. Br J Urol 1994; 73:701–706.
141. Jorgensen N, Muller J, Giwercman, et al. DNA content and expression of tumour markers in germ cells adjacent to germ cell tumours in childhood: probably a different origin for infantile and adolescent germ cell tumors. J Pathol 1995; 176: 269–278.
142. Mandoky L, Geczi L, Bodrogi I, et al. Clinical relevance of HER-2/neu expression in germ-cell testicular tumors. Anticancer Res 2004; 24:2219.
143. Mandoky L, Geczi L, Bodrogi I, et al. Expression of HER-2/neu in testicular tumors. Anticancer Res 2003; 23:3447.
144. Mostofi FK. Testicular tumors: Epidemiologic, etiologic and pathologic features. Cancer 1973; 32:1186.
145. Mostofi FK, Sesterhenn IA, Davis DJ. Developments in histopathology of testicular germ cell tumors. Semin Urol 1988; 6:171.
146. Kim I, Young RH, Scully RE. Leydig cell tumors of the testis: A clinicopathologic study of 40 cases and review of the literature. Am J Surg Pathol 1985; 9:177.
147. Seidman JD, Abbondanzo SL, Bratthauer GL. Lipid cell (steroid cell) tumor of the ovary: immunophenotype with analysis of potential pitfall due to endogenous biotin-like activity. Int J Gynecol Pathol 1995; 14:331–338.
148. Arenas MI, Lobo MV, Caso E, et al. Normal and pathological human testes express hormone-sensitive lipase and the lipid receptors CLA-1/SR-BI and CD36. Hum Pathol 2004; 35:34.
149. Johnson WJ, Jang SY, Bernard DW. Hormone sensitive lipase mRNA in both monocyte and macrophage forms of the human THP-1 cell line. Comp Biochem Physiol B Biochem Mol Biol 2000; 126:543.
150. Comperat E, Tissier F, Boye K. et al. Non-Leydig sex-cord tumors of the testis. The place of immunohistochemistry in diagnosis and prognosis. A study of twenty cases. Virchows Arch 2004; 444:567.
151. Gordon MD, Corless C, Renshaw AA, et al. CD99, keratin, and vimentin staining of sex cord-stromal tumors, normal ovary, and testis. Mod Pathol 1998; 11:769.
152. Verajakorva E, Laato M, Pollanen P. CD99 and CD106 (VCAM-1) in human testis. Asian J Androl 2002; 4:243.
153. Honecker F, Stoop H, de Krijger RR, et al. Pathobiological implications of the expression of markers of testicular carcinoma in situ by fetal germ cells. J Pathol 2004; 203:849.
154. Billings SD, Roth LM, Ulbright TM. Microcystic Leydig cell tumors mimicking yolk sac tumor: a report of four cases. Am J Surg Pathol 1999; 23:546–551.
155. Cheville JC, Sebo TJ, Lager DG, et al. Leydig cell tumor of the testis: a clinicopathologic, DNA content, and MIB-1 comparison of nonmetastasizing and metastasizing tumors. Am J Surg Pathol 1998; 22:1361–1367.
156. Middendorff R, Davidoff MS, Mayer H, et al. Neuroendocrine characteristics of human Leydig cell tumors. Andrologia 1995; 27:351–355.
157. Young RH, Koelliker DD, Scully RE. Sertoli cell tumors of the testis, not otherwise specified. A clinicopathologic analysis of 60 cases. Am J Surg Pathol 1998; 22:709–721.
158. Zukerberg LR, Young RH, Scully RE. Sclerosing Sertoli cell tumor of the testis: a report of 10 cases. Am J Surg Pathol 1991; 15:829–834.
159. Gilcrease MZ, Delgado R, Albores-Saavedra J. Testicular Sertoli cell tumor with a heterologous sarcomatous component: immunohistochemical assessment of Sertoli cell differentiation. Arch Pathol Lab Med 1998; 122:907–911.
160. Cano-Valdez AM, Chanona-Vilchis J, Dominguez-Malagon H. Large cell calcifying Sertoli cell tumor of the testis: a clinicopathological, immunohistochemical, and ultrastructural study of two cases. Ultrastruct Pathol 1999; 23:259–265.
161. Plata C, Algaba F, Andujar M, et al. Large cell calcifying Sertoli cell tumor of the testis. Histopathology 1995; 26:255–259.
162. Kratzer SS, Ulbright TM, Talerman A, et al. Large cell calcifying Sertoli cell tumor of the testis: contrasting features of six malignant and six benign tumors and a review of the literature. Am J Surg Pathol 1997; 21:1271–1280.
163. Bufo P, Pennella A, Serio G, et al. Malignant large cell calcifying Sertoli cell tumor of the testis. Report of a case in an elderly man and review of the literature. Pathologica 1999; 91:107–114.
164. Lawrence WD, Young RH, Scully RE; Juvenile granulosa cell tumor of the infantile testis: A report of 14 cases. Am J Surg Pathol 1985; 9:87.

165. Groisman GM, Dische MR, Fine EM, et al. Juvenile granulosa cell tumor of the testis: a comparative immunohistochemical study with normal infantile gonads. Pediatr Pathol 1993; 13:389–400.

166. Perez-Atayde AR, Joste N, Mulhern H. Juvenile granulosa cell tumor of the infantile testis. Evidence of a dual epithelial-smooth muscle differentiation. Am J Surg Pathol 1996; 20:72–79.

167. Kommoss F, Oliva E, Bittinger F, et al. Inhibin-alpha CD99, HEA125, PLAP, and chromogranin immunoreactivity in testicular neoplasms and the androgen insensitivity syndrome. Hum Pathol 2000; 31:1055.

168. Talerman A. Pure granulosa cell tumor of the testis: Report of a case and review of the literature. Appl Pathol 1985; 3:117.

169. Jiminez-Quintero LP, Ro JY, Zavala-Pompa A, et al. Granulosa cell tumor of the adult testis: a clinicopathologic study of seven cases and a review of the literature. Hum Pathol 1993; 24:1120–1125.

170. Morgan DR, Brame KG. Granulosa cell tumor of the testis displaying immunoreactivity for inhibin. Br J Urol Int 1999; 83:731–732.

171. Renshaw AA, Gordon M, Corless CL. Immunohistochemistry of unclassified sex cord-stromal tumors of the testis with a predominance of spindle cells. Mod Pathol 1997; 10:693–700.

172. Matias-Guiu X, Pons C, Prat J. Mullerian inhibiting substance, alpha-inhibin, and CD99 expression in sex cord-stromal tumors and endometrioid ovarian carcinomas resembling sex cord-stromal tumors. Hum Pathol 1998; 29:840.

173. Nistal M, Martinez-Garcia C, Paniagua R. Testicular fibroma. J Urol 1992; 147:1617–1619.

174. Jones MA, Young RH, Scully RE. Benign fibromatous tumors of the testis and paratesticular region: A report of 9 cases with a proposed classification of fibromatous tumors and tumor-like lesions. Am J Surg Pathol 1997; 21:296–305.

175. Kommoss F, Oliva E, Bhan AK, et al. Inhibin expression in ovarian tumors and tumor-like lesions: an immunohistochemical study. Mod Pathol 1998; 11:656–664.

176. Jorgensen N, Muller J, Jaubert F, et al. Heterogeneity of gonadoblastoma germ cells: similarities with immature germ cells, spermatogonia and testicular carcinoma in situ cells. Histopathology 1997; 30:177–186.

177. Roth LM, Eglen DE. Gonadoblastoma: Immunohistochemical and ultrastructural observations. Int J Gynecol Pathol 1989; 8:72–81.

178. Hussong J, Crussi FG, Chou PM. Gonadoblastoma: immunohistochemical localization of Mullerian-inhibiting substance, inhibin, WT-1, and p53. Mod Pathol 1997; 10:1101–1105.

179. Gravholt CH, Fedder J, Naeraa RW, et al. Occurrence of gonadoblastoma in females with Turner syndrome and Y chromosome material: a population study. J Clin Endocrinol Metab 2000; 85:3199.

180. Honecker F, Kersemaekers AM, Molier M, et al. Involvement of E-cadherin and beta-catenin in germ cell tumours and in normal male fetal germ cell development. J Pathol 2004; 204:167.

181. Zeeman AM, Stoop H, Boter M, et al. VASA is a specific marker for both normal and malignant human germ cells. Lab Invest 2002; 82:159.

182. Carano KS, Soslow RA. Immunophenotypic analysis of ovarian and testicular Mullerian papillary serous tumors. Mod Pathol 1997; 10:414–420.

183. Jones MA, Young RH, Srigley JR, et al. Paratesticular serous papillary carcinoma. A report of six cases. Am J Surg Pathol 1995; 19:1359–1365.

184. Caccamo D, Social M, Truchet C. Malignant Brenner tumor of the testis and epididymis. Arch Pathol Lab Med 1991; 115:524–527.

185. Elbadawi A, Batchvarov MM, Linke CA. Intratesticular papillary mucinous cystadeno-carcinoma. Urology 1970; 26:853–865.

186. Young RH, Scully RE. Testicular and paratesticular tumors and tumor-like lesions of ovarian common epithelium and mullerian types. A report of 4 cases and review of the literature. Am J Clin Pathol 1986; 86:146–152.

187. Zavala-Pompa A, Ro JY, el-Naggar A, et al. Primary carcinoid tumor of testis. Immunohistochemical, ultrastructural, and DNA flow cytometric study of three cases with a review of the literature. Cancer 1993; 72:1726–1732.

188. Kim HJ, Cho MY, Park YN, et al. Primary carcinoid tumor of the testis: immunohistochemical, ultrastructural and DNA flow cytometric study of two cases. J Korean Med Sci 1999; 14:57–62.

189. Miliauskas JR. Carcinoid tumor occurring in a mature tes-

ticular teratoma. Pathology 1991; 23:72–74.
190. Ferry JA, Harris NL, Young RH, et al. Malignant lymphoma of the testis, epididymis, and spermatic cord: a clinicopathological study of 69 cases with immunophenotypic analysis. Am J Surg Pathol 1994; 18:376–390.
191. Ferry JA, Ulbright TM, Young RH. Anaplastic large cell lymphoma of the testis: a lesion that may be confused with embryonal carcinoma. J Urol Pathol 1996; 5:139–147.
192. Akhtar M, Al-Dayel F, Siegrist K, et al. Neutrophil-rich Ki-1-positive anaplastic large cell lymphoma presenting as a testicular mass. Mod Pathol 1996; 9:812–815.
193. Hsueh C, Gonzalez-Crussi F, Murphy SB. Testicular angiocentric lymphoma of post-thymic T-cell type in a child with T-cell acute lymphoblastic leukemia in remission. Cancer 1993; 72:1801–1805.
194. Guler G, Altinok G, Uner AH, et al. CD56+ lymphoma presenting as a testicular tumor. Leuk Lymphoma 1999; 36:207–211.
195. Levin HS, Mostofi FK. Symptomatic plasmacytoma of the testis. Cancer 1970; 25:1193–1203.
196. Chica G, Johnson DE, Ayala AG. Plasmacytoma of testis presenting as primary testicular tumor. Urology 1978; 11:90–92.
197. Ferry JA, Young RH, Scully RE. Testicular and epididymal plasmacytoma: a report of 7 cases, including three that were the initial manifestation of plasma cell myeloma. Am J Surg Pathol 1997; 21:590–598.
198. Gutjahr P, Humpl T. Testicular lymphoblastic leukemia/lymphoma. World J Urol 1995; 13:230–232.
199. Givler RL. Testicular involvement in leukemia and lymphoma. Cancer 1969; 23:1290–1295.
200. Ferry JA, Srigley JR, Young RH. Granulocytic sarcoma of the testis: a report of two cases of a neoplasm prone to misinterpretation. Mod Pathol 1997; 10:320–325.
201. Economopoulos T, Alexopoulos C, Anagnostou D, et al. Primary granulocytic sarcoma of the testis. Leukemia 1994; 8:199–200.
202. Neiman RS, Barcos M, Berard C, et al. Granulocytic sarcoma: a clinicopathologic study of 61 biopsies cases. Cancer 1981; 48:1426–1437.
203. Pater SR, Richardson RL, Kvols L. Metastatic cancer to the testes: a report of 20 cases and review of the literature. J Urol 1989; 142:1003–1005.
204. Haupt HM, Mann RB, Trump DL, et al. Metastatic carcinoma involving the testis. Clinical and pathologic distinction from primary testicular neoplasms. Cancer 1984; 54:709–714.
205. Meacham RB, Mata JA, Espada R, et al. Testicular metastasis as the first manifestation of colon carcinoma. J Urol 1988; 140:621–622.
206. Johansson JE, Lannes P. Metastases to the spermatic cord, epididymis and testicles from carcinoma of the prostate – five cases. Scand J Urol Nephrol 1983; 17:249–251.
207. Rizk CC, Scholes J, Chen SK, et al. Epididymal metastasis from prostatic adenocarcinoma mimicking adenomatoid tumor. Urology 1990; 36:526–530.
208. Detassis C, Pusiol T, Piscioli F, et al. Adenomatoid tumor of the epididymis: immunohistochemical study of 8 cases. Urol Int 1986; 41:232–234.
209. Delahunt B, Eble JN, King D, et al. Immunohistochemical evidence for mesothelial origin of paratesticular adenomatoid tumor. Histopathology 2000; 36:109–115.
210. Delahunt B, Eble JN, King D, et al. Immunohistochemical evidence for mesothelial origin of paratesticular adenomatoid tumour. Histopathology 2000; 36:109.
211. Banks ER, Mills SE. Histiocytoid (epithelioid) hemangioma of the testis. The so-called vascular variant of 'adenomatoid tumor.' Am J Surg Pathol 1990; 14:584–589.
212. Hoch WH. Adenocarcinoma of the scrotum (extramammary Paget's disease): case report and review of the literature. J Urol 1984; 132:137–139.
213. Koh KB, Nazarina AR. Paget's disease of the scrotum: report of a case with underlying carcinoma of the prostate. Br J Dermatol 1995; 133:306–307.
214. Ordonez NG, Awalt H, Mackay B. Mammary and extramammary Paget's disease: an immunocytochemical and ultrastructural study. Cancer 1987; 59:1173–1183.
215. Enjoji M, Noguchi K, Watanabe H, et al. A novel tumour marker RCAS1 in a case of extramammary Paget's disease. Clin Exp Dermatol 2003; 28:211.
216. Akashi T, Oimomi H, Nishiyama K, et al. Expression and diagnostic evaluation of the human tumor-associated antigen RCAS1 in pancreatic cancer. Pancreas 2003; 26:49.
217. Takahashi H, Iizuka H, Nakashima M, et al. RCAS1 antigen is highly expressed in extramammary Paget's disease and in advanced stage squamous cell carcinoma of the skin. J Dermatol Sci 2001; 26:140.

218. Jones MA, Young RH, Scully RE. Malignant mesothelioma of the tunica vaginalis. A clinicopathologic analysis of 11 cases with review of the literature. Am J Surg Pathol 1995; 19:815–825.

219. Moch H, Ohnacker H, Epper R, et al. A new case of malignant mesothelioma of the tunica vaginalis testis. Immunohistochemistry in comparison with an adenomatoid tumor of the testis. Pathol Res Pract 1994; 190:400–404.

220. Kamiya M, Eimoto T. Malignant mesothelioma of the tunica vaginalis. Pathol Res Pract 1990; 186:680–684.

221. Chhieng DC, Yee H, Schaefer D, et al. Calretinin staining pattern aids in the differentiation of mesothelioma from adenocarcinoma in serous effusions. Cancer 2000; 90:194–200.

222. Cury PM, Butcher DN, Fisher C, et al. Value of the mesothelium-associated antibodies thrombomodulin, cytokeratin 5/6, calretinin, and CD44H in distinguishing epithelioid pleural mesothelioma from adenocarcinoma metastatic to the pleura. Mod Pathol 2000; 13:107–112.

223. Doglioni C, Dei Tos AP, Laurino L, et al. Calretinin: a novel immunocytochemical marker for mesothelioma: Am J Surg Pathol 1996; 20:1037–1046.

224. Chu AY, Litzky LA, Pasha TL, et al. Utility of D2-40, a novel mesothelial marker, in the diagnosis of malignant mesothelioma. Mod Pathol 2005; 18:105–110.

225. Cummings OW, Ulbright TM, Young RH, et al. Desmoplastic small round cell tumors of the paratesticular region. A report of six cases. Am J Surg Pathol 1997; 21:219–225.

226. Kawano N, Inayama Y, Nagashima Y, et al. Desmoplastic small round-cell tumor of the paratesticular region: report of an adult case with demonstration of EWS and WT1 gene fusion using paraffin-embedded tissue. Mod Pathol 1999; 12:729–734.

227. Carpentieri DF, Nichols K, Chou PM, et al. The expression of WT1 in the differentiation of rhabdomyosarcoma from other pediatric small round blue cell tumors. Mod Pathol 2002; 15:1080.

228. Rachfal AW, Luquette MH, Brigstock DR. Expression of connective tissue growth factor (CCN2) in desmoplastic small round cell tumour. J Clin Pathol 2004; 57:422.

229. Johnson RE, Scheithauer BW, Dahlin DC. Melanotic neuroectodermal tumor of infancy. A review of seven cases. Cancer 1983; 52:661–666.

230. Pettinato G, Manivel JC, d'Amore ES, et al. Melanotic neuroectodermal tumor of infancy: a reexamination of histogenetic problem based on immunohistochemical, ultrastructural, and flow cytometric study of 10 cases. Am J Surg Pathol 1991; 15:233–245.

231. Jurincic-Winkler C, Metz KA, Klippel KF. Melanotic neuroectodermal tumor of infancy (MNTI) in the epididymis. A case report with immunohistological studies and special consideration of malignant features. Zentrabl Pathol 1994; 140:181–185.

232. Anagnostaki L, Krag JG, Horn T, et al. Melanotic neuroectodermal as a predominant component of an immature testicular teratoma. Case report with immunohistochemical investigations. APMIS 1992; 100:809–816.

233. Lioe TF, Biggart JD. Tumors of the spermatic cord and paratesticular tissue. A clinicopathological study. Br J Urol 1993; 71:600233. Urologic Surg Path 606.

234. Srigley JR, Hartwick RW. Tumors and cysts of the paratesticular region. Pathol Annul 1990; 25:51–108.

235. Schwartz SL, Swierzewski SJ III, Sondak VK, et al. Liposarcoma of the spermatic cord: report of 6 cases and review of the literature. J Urol 1995; 153:154–157.

236. Leuschner I, Newton WA Jr, Schmidt D, et al. Spindle cell variants of embryonal rhabdomyosarcoma in the paratesticular region. A report of the Intergroup Rhabdomyosarcoma Study. Am J Surg Pathol 1993; 17:221–230.

237. Loughlin KR, Retik AB, Weinstein JT, et al. Genitourinary rhabdomyosarcoma in children. Cancer 1989; 63:1600–1606.

肾

Lina Liu, Junqi Qian and David G. Bostwick

引 言

肾有很多不同类型的良性和恶性肿瘤，对于病理医生来说，其中很多肿瘤诊断起来比较困难。肾最常见的肿瘤是儿童 Wilms 瘤和成人肾细胞癌。本节将详述这些肿瘤在诊断中常遇到的难点问题。

抗原/抗体生物学

用于肾肿瘤诊断的大多数抗体在本章的其他部分

已经进行了介绍。本节主要对一些针对特殊肿瘤诊断有价值的其他抗体进行介绍。

儿童肾细胞肿瘤

肾母细胞（Wilms）瘤

Wilms瘤在儿童肾肿瘤中占到80%以上。Wilms瘤通常巨大，直径一般在5cm以上[1-3]。肿瘤切面的典型表现为实性、质软、灰色或粉红色，类似于脑组织。显微镜下观察，典型的Wilms瘤由胚基、上皮和间质组成。胚基通常有3种排列方式：螺旋型、结节型和弥漫型。上皮成分主要由内衬原始柱状或立方形细胞的小管或囊组成。在Wilms瘤的间质中可看到各种类型的软组织[1-3]。

Wilms瘤的胚基成分表现出胚胎组织和早期上皮分化的免疫组化特征，表明胚基细胞具有分化成管状上皮细胞和间质细胞的功能[4-9]。未分化的胚基细胞只含有中间丝波形蛋白，而有一定分化程度的胚基细胞则含有波形蛋白和CK；间质细胞则表达波形蛋白。神经特异性烯醇化酶（NSE）在胚基中也为阳性表达（表14.21）[4, 7, 9-11]。而且，在胚基和管状结构之间上皮抗原表达的逐渐增加也反映了胚基细胞向管状结构的过渡[7, 9, 12]。Wilms瘤的鉴别诊断总结于表14.21[9, 12-15]。

肾透明细胞肉瘤

透明细胞肉瘤（儿童骨转移肾肿瘤）是一种高度恶性的肿瘤，诊断时的平均年龄为36个月（2个月到14岁）。男女比例为2∶1。典型的大体特征包括瘤体巨大、黏液样结构、有坏死灶和明显的囊状结构。目前已发现9种主要的组织学类型，包括经典型、黏液型、硬化型、细胞型、上皮型、栅栏型、梭形细胞型、席纹状型和间变型；实际上，所有的肿瘤都包含多种类型的组织学特征。在这种肿瘤中，波形蛋白持续表达阳性，而CK和MIC2表达常为阴性（表14.21）[16-20]。α-1-抗胰凝乳蛋白酶表达阳性[21, 22]。

肾横纹肌样瘤

横纹肌样瘤是小儿恶性程度最高的肾肿瘤，常发生广泛转移，患者通常在诊断后12个月内死亡[1-3]。镜下观察，肿瘤呈灰黄色或淡褐色，边界明显，易切除。在组织学上，横纹肌样瘤由弥漫且分布均一的中

表14.21 Wilms瘤、透明细胞肉瘤和横纹肌样瘤免疫组化表型特征

肿瘤	免疫组化标记物	鉴别诊断
Wilms瘤（胚基）	波形蛋白+ NSE+ CK+	神经母细胞瘤： 　波形蛋白- 　神经丝+ 　Syn+，NSE+ Ewing肉瘤： 　MIC2（HBA71）+ 横纹肌肉瘤： 　结蛋白+ 淋巴瘤：LCA+
透明细胞肉瘤	CK- 波形蛋白+（大多数） α-1-抗胰凝乳蛋白酶+ EMA- MSA- 结蛋白-	Wilms瘤： 　波形蛋白+ 　NSE+ 　CK+ 横纹肌样瘤： 　CK（S） 　波形蛋白+ 　EMA+
横纹肌样瘤	CK（S） 波形蛋白+ EMA+ S-100蛋白（S） 肌动蛋白- 结蛋白（S） 肌红蛋白-	Wilms瘤： 　波形蛋白+ 　NSE+，CK+ 透明细胞肉瘤： 　CK- 　波形蛋白（S） 　EMA-

+，几乎总为阳性；S，有时阳性；R，很少阳性

等或大多边形细胞组成，胞浆丰富呈嗜酸性，胞核圆形，核膜增厚，核仁增大[1-3]。免疫组化显示波形蛋白阳性，在一些病例中，也可见到低分子量角蛋白（CAM5.2）、上皮细胞膜抗原（EMA）、神经特异性烯醇化酶（NSE）、S-100蛋白和结蛋白呈阳性[24-28]。鉴别诊断总结于表14.21[24-28]。

中胚叶肾瘤

尽管中胚叶肾瘤只占到原发性小儿肾肿瘤的不足3%，但是在3个月以内的婴儿当中，它仍然是最常见的肾肿瘤[1-3]。该肿瘤无包膜，切面与平滑肌瘤相似。典型的组织学变化包括呈中度增殖的、稠密的、交错排列的梭形细胞，伴伸长的细胞核，常浸润肾及周围组织。年龄稍大的儿童可见细胞性亚型，具有更丰富的细胞以及中度的细胞异型性[1-3]。中胚叶肾瘤波形蛋白阳性（表14.22）[29-32]。

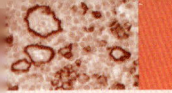

表14.22	良性肾肿瘤和肿瘤样结构
肿瘤或肿瘤样病变	免疫组化表达谱
多房性囊肿	CK+
	EMA+
中胚叶肾瘤	波形蛋白+
	结蛋白（S）
	肌特异性肌动蛋白(S)
	CK-
	结蛋白-
嗜酸细胞瘤	细胞角蛋白 AE1/AE3+
	低分子量角蛋白+
	碳酸酐酶+
	带3阴离子交换蛋白+
	CD117+（大多数）
	波形蛋白+
血管平滑肌脂肪瘤	HMB-45+（在平滑肌）
	肌特异性肌动蛋白+
	结蛋白+
	波形蛋白+
	CK-
	CD117（S）
	S-100蛋白-
后肾腺瘤	CK+
	波形蛋白+
	平滑肌肌动蛋白（S）
	CEA-, S-100-, NSE-,
	嗜铬素-, 神经丝-,
	EMA-
肾盂囊性错构瘤	CK+
	EMA+
	平滑肌肌动蛋白
肾小球旁细胞瘤	肾素+
	平滑肌肌动蛋白+
	肌特异性肌动蛋白+
	波形蛋白+
	CD34+
	CK-, NSE-, 结蛋白-,
	S-100蛋白-

+，几乎总为阳性；S，有时阳性；R，很少阳性

成人肾肿瘤

良性上皮性肿瘤

乳头状腺瘤

乳头状腺瘤比较小，直径小于0.5cm，通常位于皮质浅层。该肿瘤由带有少量胞浆的小细胞组成，呈乳头

状或管状结构[1-3]。如果胞浆有较多的透明胞浆，则无论肿瘤大小都应考虑为透明细胞癌。从细胞遗传学上讲，乳头状腺瘤表现为7、17号染色体三体或17号染色体四体。关于这种肿瘤的免疫组化研究比较有限[33, 34]。

肾嗜酸细胞腺瘤

肾嗜酸细胞腺瘤是一种肾皮质的良性肿瘤，30年以前曾被称做"颗粒型"肾细胞癌。肾嗜酸细胞腺瘤肉眼观察最具特征的是肿瘤呈红褐至褐色，与典型的透明细胞癌的明黄色不同[35-37]。显微镜下观察，嗜酸细胞腺瘤的基本特征是，肿瘤细胞形态均一，胞浆呈嗜酸性粗颗粒状（图14.35）。细胞核呈圆形、空泡状，位于细胞中央。局部细胞由于多倍体化而导致细胞核出现多形性，并且双核细胞增多，细胞核互相重叠，具有鉴别诊断价值[1-3]。细胞遗传学特征包括：肿瘤为异源性，伴有一致性的Y染色体和1号染色体与着丝粒相关部分的缺失，以及少量病例出现染色体互换易位 t (5; 11) (q35; q13)[33, 34]。

免疫组化观察，嗜酸细胞腺瘤细胞角蛋白 AE1/AE3（图14.36）和低分子量角蛋白阳性，但是波形蛋白阴性（表14.23)[35, 36, 38-44]。大约70%的嗜酸细胞腺瘤（图14.37）和80%的嫌色性肾细胞癌表达 c-kit (CD117)，而其他类型的肾细胞癌则为阴性[45, 46]。嗜酸细胞腺瘤的CK7为阴性，该标记物可用来鉴别嫌色性肾细胞癌（RCC）[40]。据报道，带3蛋白（band 3 protein）仅在嗜酸细胞腺瘤中呈阳性，但是在其他类型的肾上皮性肿瘤中则为阴性。当Hale胶体铁染色结果不确定或意义不明确或为阴性时，CK7和带3蛋白可被用来进行鉴别诊断[47]。嗜酸细胞腺瘤的RCC抗体也呈阴性，但是CD10在一些病例中可以为阳性[35]。早先有报道认为Ron原癌基因产物可以作为肾嗜酸细胞腺瘤的表型标记物[48]，但是现在有一些相反的报道，根据另一项研究和作者的经验，这一标记物在鉴别诊断中的应用价值还需要进一步研究（图14.38、14.39）。

> **诊断要点**：肾嗜酸细胞腺瘤
> 1. 波形蛋白-。
> 2. 细胞角蛋白 AE1/AE3+。
> 3. 碳酸酐酶+。
> 4. CD117+（大多数）。
> 5. CK7-。
> 6. RCC 抗体-。

前列腺、膀胱、睾丸和肾的免疫组织化学 14

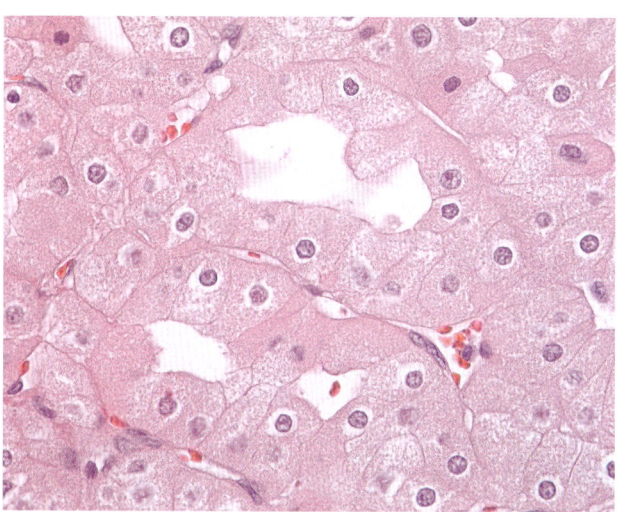

图14.35 肾嗜酸细胞腺瘤具有形态均一的肿瘤细胞，胞浆呈嗜酸性粗颗粒状

其他的良性肾肿瘤和肿瘤样病变

表14.22总结了良性肾肿瘤和肿瘤样病变的免疫组化结果[52]。例如，肾盂囊性错构瘤表现为CK、EMA和平滑肌肌动蛋白（SMA）阳性[68]。肾小球旁细胞瘤通常表现为肾素、肌动蛋白和CD34阳性（图14.40）[69-76]。血管平滑肌脂肪瘤中的平滑肌呈HMB-45阳性[77-81]。c-kit在血管平滑肌脂肪瘤中的表达情况目前还有争议。一项研究表明，在全部21例血管平滑肌脂肪瘤病例（6例为肾来源，15例为肝来源）中，c-kit均为阳性反应[82]，而在另一项研究中所有23例肾血管平滑肌脂肪瘤则都为阴性[45]。

肾细胞癌

肾细胞癌（RCC）是泌尿生殖系统第三常见肿瘤。在美国，据估计2004年将有35 710例新增确诊肾

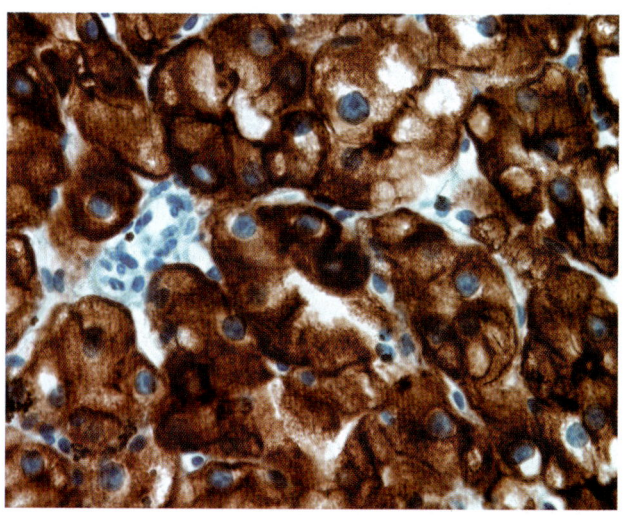

图14.36 嗜酸细胞腺瘤角蛋白AE1/AE3的免疫组化结果

表14.23	肾嗜酸细胞腺瘤免疫组化结果
免疫组化	
波形蛋白 -	PAS-
CK AE1/3+	低分子量 CK+
碳酸酐酶 +	带3阴离子交换蛋白 +
CD117+（大多数）	Hale胶体铁染色 -
CK7-	CD10（S）
RCC 抗体 -	
鉴别诊断	
嫌色性肾细胞癌：Hale胶体铁染色+，CK7+，带3蛋白	
透明细胞肾细胞癌：波形蛋白+，带3蛋白-，CD10+，RCC抗体+，CD117-	

+，几乎总为阳性；S，有时阳性；R，很少阳性

后肾腺瘤

后肾腺瘤是一种最近才报道的肾腺瘤[50-62]。该肿瘤含有双倍体DNA[63,64]，最近的研究表明该肿瘤具有 *met* 癌基因突变[33,34]。对该肿瘤的免疫组化特征还不十分清楚（表14.24）[57,61,62]。几项研究表明，后肾腺瘤由不成熟的肾上皮细胞组成。例如，Nonomura等人研究报道，大多数肿瘤细胞的S-100蛋白阳性，有时α-1-抗胰蛋白酶和波形蛋白也为阳性[65,66]，CK、溶菌酶和Leu7为明显的胞膜阳性，只有乳头状或大的管状结构中的肿瘤细胞呈EMA阳性，LeuM1和HMB-45肿瘤细胞为阴性。Tsuji报道后肾腺瘤的波形蛋白为阳性[67]。

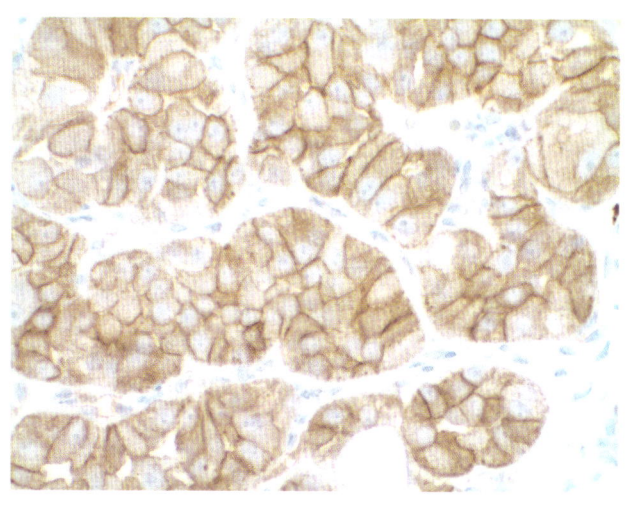

图14.37 肾嗜酸细胞腺瘤细胞中CD117免疫组化结果

613

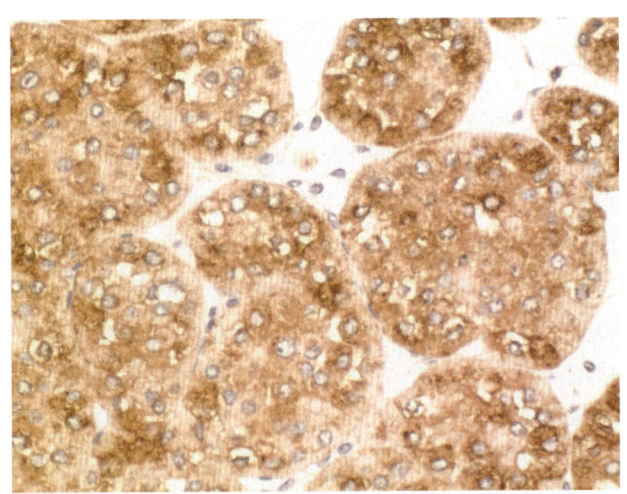

图 14.38　肾嗜酸细胞腺瘤细胞中的 Ron 免疫组化结果

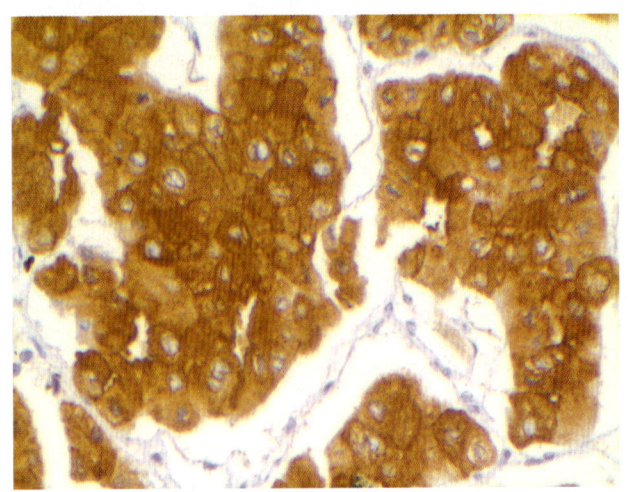

图 14.39　肾嫌色细胞癌细胞中的 Ron 免疫组化结果

表14.24　后肾腺瘤免疫组化结果	
免疫组化	
CK+	波形蛋白 +
Leu7+	S-100 蛋白（S）
EMA（S）	CEA-
SMA（S）	结蛋白 -
糖原（PAS）-	油红 O-
HMB-45-	NSE-
嗜铬素 -	神经丝 -
鉴别诊断	
成人 Wilms 瘤：波形蛋白 +，NSE+，CK+	
肾腺瘤：EMA+	
乳头状肾细胞癌：CK7+，7 和 17 号染色体三体	
类癌：神经内分泌标记物阳性	

+，几乎总为阳性；S，有时阳性；R，很少阳性

癌病例，将导致大约 12 480 例死亡。其中男性病例是女性病例的 2～3 倍，未见明显的种族差异。发病高峰为五六十岁的人群，35 岁以下患者少见[83]。表 14.25 总结了肾上皮性肿瘤的现代分类[84]。

透明细胞肾细胞癌

最常见的肾细胞癌类型是透明细胞肾细胞癌[1-3]，大约占总病例的 80%。其特征为多结节性和多彩性瘤性肿块，切面以黄色为主，兼有灰色和白色病灶。镜下观察，胞浆呈透明及空白状（图 14.41）[1-3]，虽然前述的颗粒型 RCC 也包括在透明细胞类肿瘤中，但是那些肿瘤的胞浆是嗜酸性的。透明细胞 RCC 的 3 号染色体有部分或全部丢失，或位于染色体 3p 臂上的基因突变，导致一个或更多的肿瘤抑制基因的丢失。VHL 基因位于染色体 3p25-26，这一区域在透明细胞

肾细胞癌中经常缺失[33, 34]。

大多数但非全部肾肿瘤能够根据形态学和免疫组化结果进行鉴别；然而，在透明细胞肾细胞癌与嫌色细胞癌之间，以及这些肿瘤中的颗粒性/嗜酸性变型与肾嗜酸细胞腺瘤之间都存在形态学上的相似性[1-3]。只有有限的免疫组化标记物有助于这些肿瘤的鉴别诊断，但都不具有确定性。表 14.26 总结了透明细胞 RCC 的免疫组化结果[20, 35, 39, 41, 85-92]。

> **诊断要点：透明细胞癌**
>
> 1. 高分子量 CK-。
> 2. 癌胚抗原（CEA）-。
> 3. S-100 蛋白 -。
> 4. 带 3 蛋白 -。
> 5. 抑制素（inhibin）-。
> 6. 黏蛋白（mucin）-。
> 7. 油红 O（脂质）+，Hale 胶体铁染色 -。
> 8. 低分子量角蛋白 +。
> 9. 上皮细胞膜抗原（EMA）+。
> 10. 波形蛋白 +。
> 11. 碳酸酐酶（G250）+。
> 12. CD10+。
> 13. RCC 抗体 +。

细胞角蛋白、上皮细胞膜抗原和波形蛋白　一组包括 CK、EMA 和波形蛋白在内的抗体组合可能有助于 RCC 的鉴别诊断[20, 35, 39, 41, 85-92]。透明细胞 RCC 的

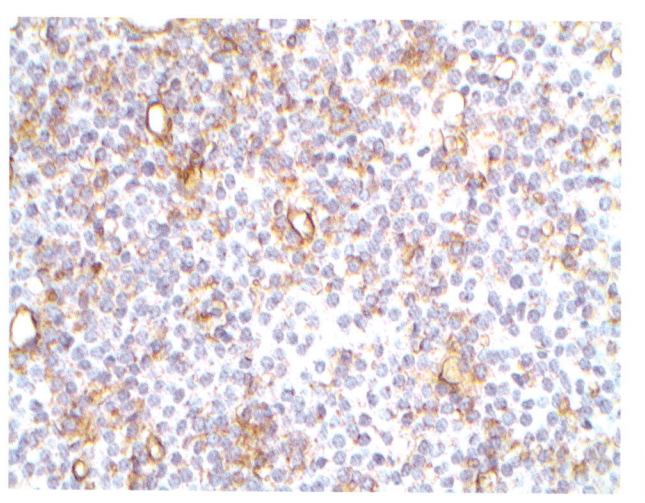

图 14.40　肾小球旁细胞瘤 CD34 免疫组化结果

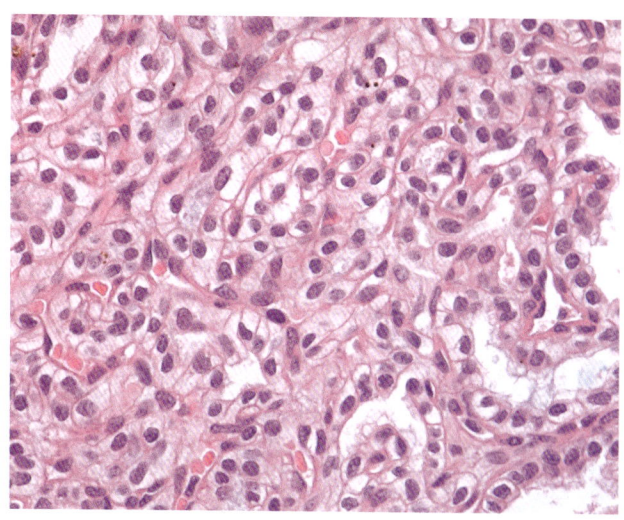

图 14.41　透明细胞肾细胞癌

表 14.25　肾上皮性肿瘤的分类（WHO，2004）
良性上皮性肿瘤
乳头状腺瘤
嗜酸细胞腺瘤
后肾腺瘤
肾细胞癌
透明细胞肾细胞癌
多房性囊性肾细胞癌
乳头状肾细胞癌
嫌色性肾细胞癌
Bellini 集合管癌
肾髓质癌
Xp11 易位性癌
神经母细胞瘤相关性肾癌
黏液管状和梭形细胞癌
肾细胞癌，未分类型

低分子量（LMW）角蛋白（CAM5.2）、CK18、AE1/AE3、EMA（图 14.42）和波形蛋白通常为阳性（图 14.43）；但是 CK7、CK20、高分子量（HMW）角蛋白（34βE12、CK19）[41, 93, 94]、CEA[95]、S-100 蛋白[20, 96]、HMB-45[95] 和抑制素[97, 98] 为阴性。

在不同的研究中，这些标记物的阳性率不同。例如，Medeiros 等人发现，55 例肾细胞癌病例中有 48 例表达角蛋白。CAM5.2 阳性率为 84%，AE1 阳性率为 67%，AE1 阳性的肿瘤中有 2 例 CAM5.2 阴性的肿瘤，EMA 的阳性率为 64%，包括 3 例 CAM5.2 阴性的肿瘤。波形蛋白阳性率为 47%，S-100 蛋白阳性病例只有 1 例[90, 100]。

当诊断转移性肾细胞癌、尿路上皮癌或其他肿瘤有困难时，免疫组化结果可以帮助鉴别诊断。尿路上皮癌表达所有的 CK 和癌胚抗原，但是其波形蛋白为阴性。神经节细胞瘤嗜铬素阳性，并且支持细胞 S-100 蛋白呈散在阳性。转移性黑色素瘤的 S-100 蛋白和 HMB-45 阳性[20, 95, 98, 101, 102]。

RCC 抗体和 CD10　　RCC 抗体与一个表达于肾近曲小管上皮细胞的 200kD 的糖蛋白结合。Yoshida 等人[103] 报道，这一抗体在 93% 的原发性肾细胞癌和 84% 的转移性肾细胞癌中呈阳性，但是不能够对肿瘤亚型进行区分。CD10（急性淋巴细胞白血病抗原，CALLA）表达于肾小管上皮细胞的刷状缘。Avery 等人用 RCC 抗体和 CD10 对常见的肾肿瘤进行鉴别诊断[35]，他们发现 85% 的透明细胞癌的细胞膜表面 RCC 抗体阳性，94% 的病例 CD10 阳性。几乎所有的乳头状癌病例（14 例中有 13 例）也表现为 RCC 和 CD10 强阳性。相反，19 例嫌色细胞癌两种标记物均为表面膜染色阴性。嗜酸细胞腺瘤的 RCC 也为阴性（9 例全为阴性），但 CD10 在一些病例中为阳性（9 例中有 3 例阳性）。这些结果表明，RCC 和 CD10 表面膜阳性可用于证实疑似透明细胞或乳头状肾癌的诊断，而嫌色细胞癌两种标记物应为阴性。RCC 阴性也有助于嗜酸细胞腺瘤的诊断。此外，CK7 有助于鉴别嗜酸细胞腺瘤（CK7-）和嫌色细胞癌（CK7+）[35, 36, 38-40, 85, 103-107]。应用包括波形蛋白、EMA、CEA、RCC、CD10 和 CK7 在内的抗体组合有助于肾细胞肿瘤的鉴别诊断。

透明细胞癌的其他诊断标记物　　最近，cDNA 微阵列分析和免疫组化研究表明，谷胱甘肽转移酶 -α（GST-α）在区分肾细胞癌亚型中有应用价值。GST-α 在透明细胞亚型中呈高表达（90%），但在其他亚型中不表达或仅偶尔表达[108]。

表14.26 透明细胞肾细胞癌免疫组化结果

免疫组化	
低分子量角蛋白 +	高分子量角蛋白 -
EMA+	CEA-
波形蛋白 +	S-100 蛋白 -
碳酸酐酶（G250）+	带 3 蛋白 -
CD10+	抑制素 -
RCC 抗体 +	黏蛋白 -
谷胱甘肽 S-转移酶 α (GST-α)+	油红 O（脂质）-
胎盘碱性磷酸酶（PLAP）+	Hale 胶体铁染色 -
PAS/糖原 +	

鉴别诊断标记物
肾上腺皮质癌
抑制素 +
EMA-
CK-
CD10+
肾盂尿路上皮癌
CEA+
高分子量角蛋白 +
CK7+
CK20+
CK19+
波形蛋白 -
乳头状肾细胞癌
碳酸酐酶（G250）-
α-甲基-CoA-乙酰基消旋酶 +
嫌色性肾细胞癌
Hale 胶体铁染色（酸性黏多糖）+
CK7+
波形蛋白 -
细小白蛋白（parvalbumin）+
碳酸酐酶 II +
CD117+
脂质和糖原（PAS 染色）-
嗜酸细胞腺瘤
带 3 蛋白 +
波形蛋白-
CD117+
黑色素瘤
S-100+
HMB-45+
CK-
EMA-

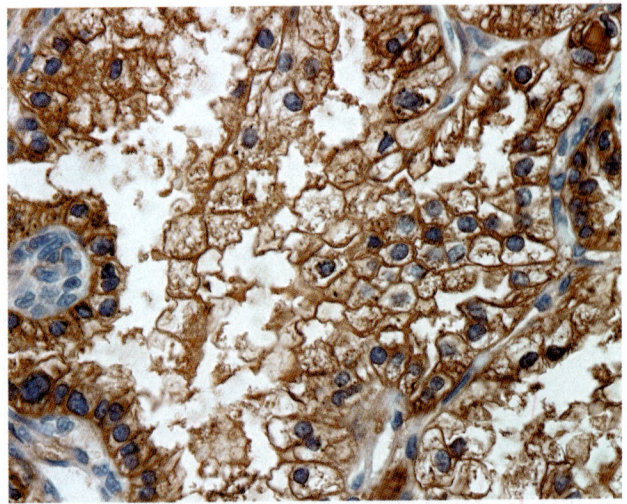

图 14.42 透明细胞肾细胞癌中 EMA 免疫组化结果

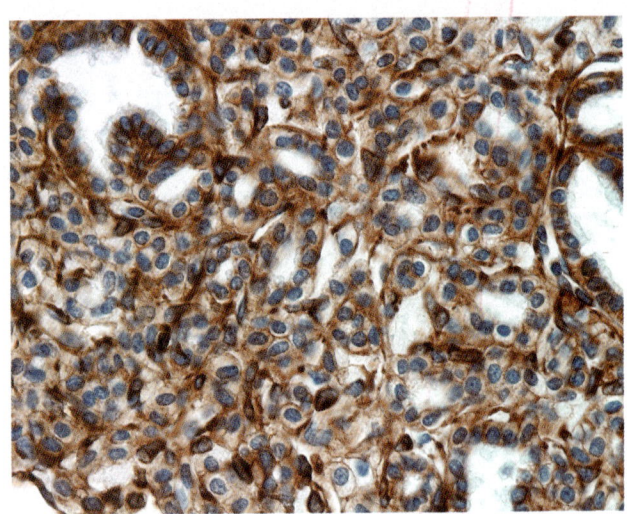

图 14.43 透明细胞肾细胞癌中波形蛋白免疫组化结果

钙黏素（cadherin）在肾细胞癌中的应用尚存争议。Taki 等人报道，E-钙黏素在透明细胞亚型中为阴性，但在嫌色细胞癌和嗜酸细胞腺瘤中为阳性[42]。

Fisher 等人报道，E-钙黏素的表达与肿瘤进展有关[109]。

G250 是一种识别碳酸酐酶IX（CA IX）的抗体[110,111]。正常情况下，肾上皮细胞内的碳酸酐酶被 pVHL 基因所抑制。在透明细胞癌中，VHL 功能的缺失导致CA IX 抗原表达并与G250抗体发生反应[110,111]。碳酸酐酶IX抗原在透明细胞癌中表达，但是在正常的肾细胞和乳头状癌中为阴性。然而，G250 对于肾细胞癌来说并不是特异的，它也在正常的消化道黏膜和胆管上皮中着色[110,111]。

抗 α-抑制素是一种肽激素抗体，据报道有助于肾上腺皮质癌（抑制素+）与透明细胞肾细胞癌（抑制素-）的鉴别诊断[112]。FHIT 基因位于人染色体 3p14.2，在许多恶性肿瘤中该基因缺失，包括透明细胞肾癌，导致 FHIT 蛋白的表达缺失[113-115]。其他标记物如 CD44 和 IL-6 据报道在透明细胞癌中也呈阳性表达[90, 91, 109, 116, 117]。

乳头状肾细胞癌

乳头状肾细胞癌是肾癌第二常见亚型，具有明显的大体特征、组织学特征和细胞遗传学特征[118-120]。肉眼观察，可见典型的球状轮廓和点状结构[1-3, 121]。在显微镜下观察，复杂的乳头状结构为其特征性结构，间质常伴有泡沫状巨噬细胞浸润。乳头状癌可分为2种亚型：1型，乳头状结构由单层的含有少量淡染胞浆的细胞覆盖（图14.44）；2型，乳头状结构由假复层上皮细胞覆盖，细胞内含有大量嗜酸性胞浆（图14.45）。1型肿瘤的 Fuhrman 核分级常较低，比2型肿瘤的预后更好[120]。细胞遗传学特征包括染色体 3q、7、8、12、16、17 和 20 三体，并有 Y 染色体丢失[122-124]。

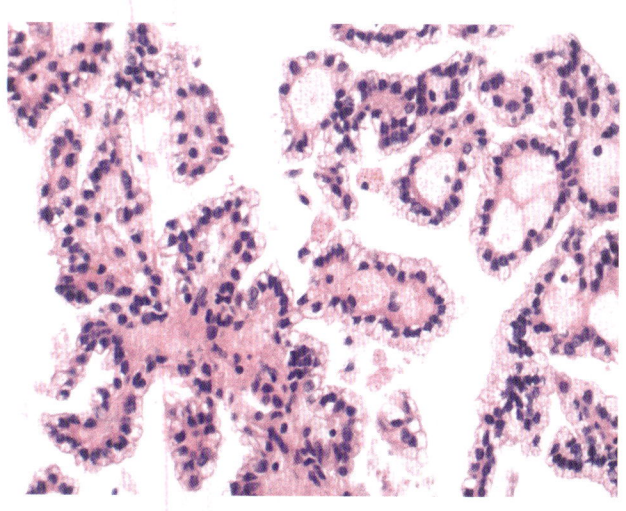

图14.44 1型乳头状RCC，乳头状结构由含有少量胞浆的小细胞覆盖，细胞核呈小椭圆形，核仁不明显

对乳头状癌的免疫组化研究比较有限（表14.27）[113, 118, 119, 125, 126]。Renshaw 等人对 36 个病例用不同的角蛋白抗体和CEA抗体进行了研究，发现100%（全部36例）的病例AE1/AE3阳性（图14.46），92%（36例中33例）的病例胼胝角蛋白（callus keratins）阳性（图14.47）；只有3%（36例中的1例）角蛋白34βE12阳性，11%（36例中的4例）CEA 为弱阳性[119, 126]。α-甲基-CoA-消旋酶（AMACR）是乳头状肾细胞癌的另一个标记物（图14.48），对于鉴别肾细胞癌亚型和鉴别不明来源的转移性乳头状癌有应用价值[108, 127]。此外，MUC1（EMA）有助于鉴别1型和2型乳头状癌，该标记物在1型表达，而在2型中很少表达（图14.49）[128, 129]。

> **诊断要点：** 乳头状肾细胞癌
>
> 1. 细胞角蛋白 AE1/AE3+。
> 2. 波形蛋白+。
> 3. 消旋酶+。

嫌色性肾细胞癌

嫌色性肾细胞癌是由特征性的大多边形细胞组成，胞浆透明或呈轻微网状，胞膜明显（图14.50）[1-3]。另一个具有诊断价值的特征是，常规染料胞浆染色不

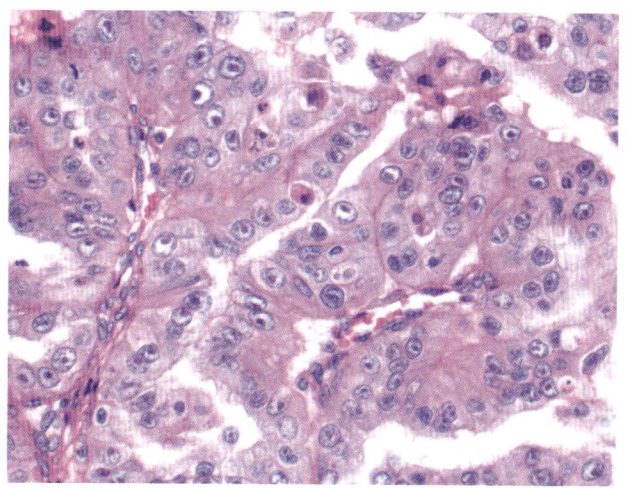

图14.45 2型乳头状RCC，乳头状结构由富含嗜酸性胞浆的大细胞覆盖，呈假复层上皮样结构，细胞核为大球形，核仁明显

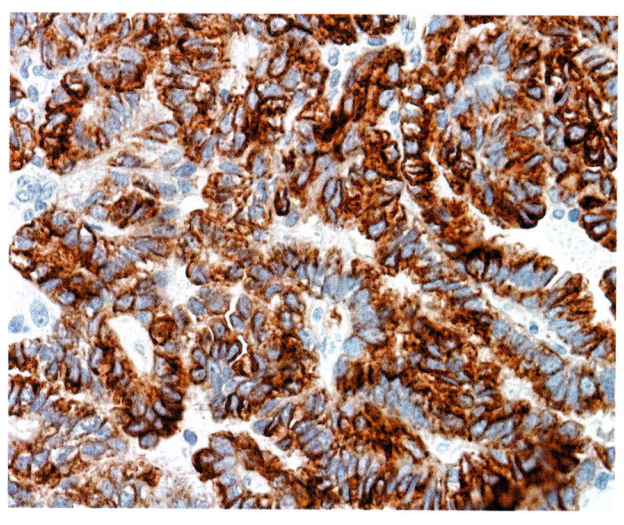

图14.46 乳头状肾细胞癌细胞角蛋白AE1/AE3免疫组化结果

617

表14.27 乳头状肾细胞癌免疫组化结果	
免疫组化	
细胞角蛋白 AE1/3+	低分子量角蛋白（CK7）+
波形蛋白 +	高分子量角蛋白 -
消旋酶 +	Ulex europaeus 凝集素 -
黏蛋白 -	碳酸酐酶（G250）-
糖原 +	MUC1：1 型癌 +
鉴别诊断	
集合管癌 　　黏蛋白+，高分子量 CK+	
后肾腺瘤 　　紧密排列的肾小管，内衬细胞胞核均匀，胞浆稀少；伴有纤维血管轴心的乳头结构少见，EMA-	

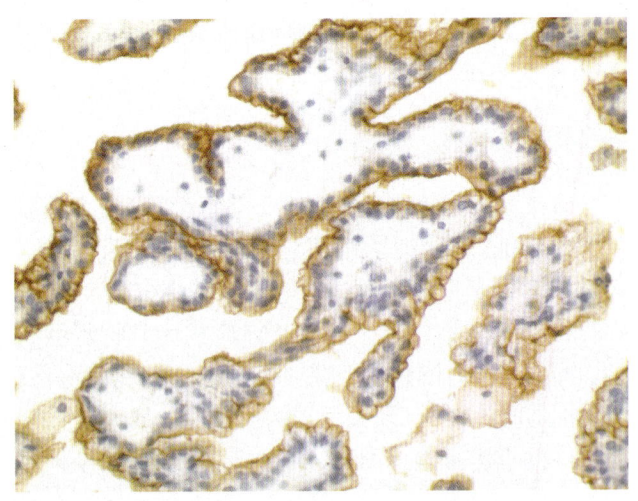

图 14.49　1 型乳头状肾细胞癌 EMA 免疫组化结果

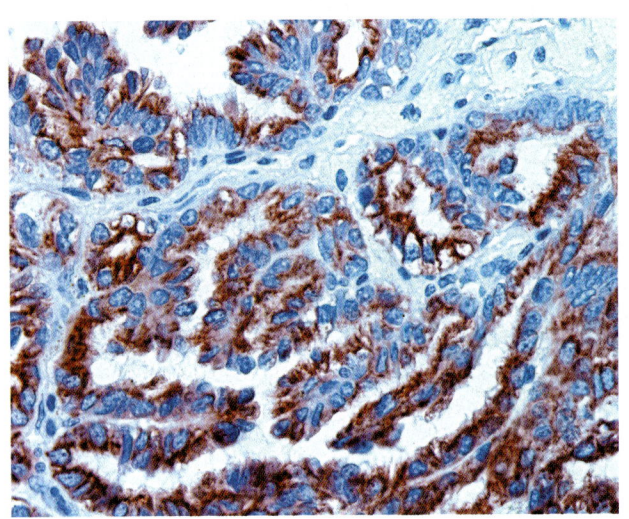

图14.47　乳头状肾细胞癌细胞角蛋白（CAM5.2）免疫组化结果

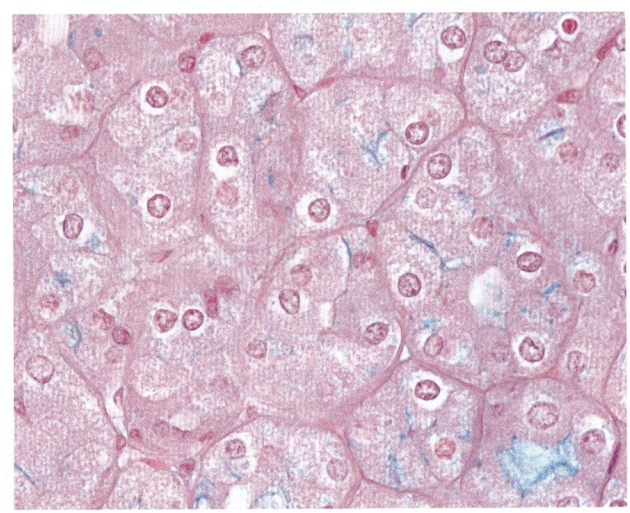

图14.50　嫌色性肾细胞癌，表现为大的多边形细胞，胞浆透明或呈轻微网状，细胞膜明显

明显，但是 Hale 胶体铁染色胞浆广泛着色[1-3]。细胞遗传学特征为大片段的染色体（即1、2、6、10、13、17 和 21）丢失。这些结果已经被荧光原位杂交和比较基因组杂交分析所证实[33, 34]。

尽管超微结构和免疫组化研究显示，这些肿瘤细胞所表现出来的几个特征与那些集合管的插入细胞相似，但是大样本量的免疫组化抗体组合研究不多（表 14.28）[43, 101, 107, 125, 130-132]。Taki 等人将 21 例嫌色性细胞癌病例的免疫组化结果与透明细胞癌和肾嗜酸细胞腺瘤进行了对比[42]，发现嫌色细胞癌 EMA 阳性（图 14.51），而波形蛋白为阴性。细胞角蛋白在 3 种肾肿瘤中没有显示恒定的免疫反应性。所有的嫌色细胞癌和肾嗜酸细胞腺瘤的 E- 钙黏素都为阳性，但 N- 钙黏素则为阴性，而所有透明细胞癌的 E- 钙黏素都

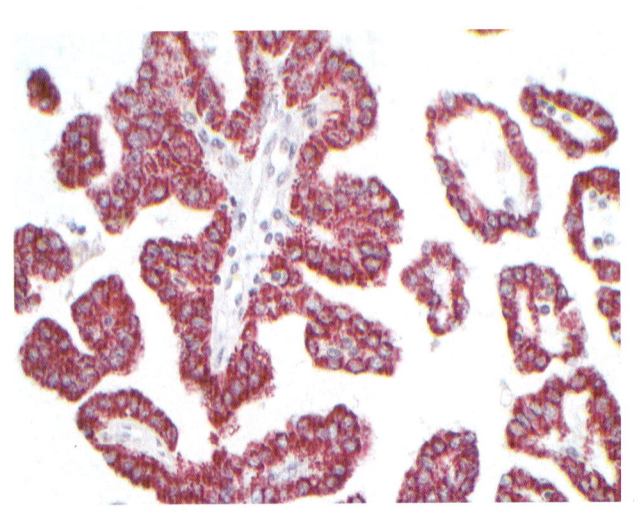

图 14.48　乳头状肾细胞癌消旋酶（P504S）免疫组化结果

表14.28 嫌色性肾细胞癌免疫组化结果	
免疫组化	
Hale 胶体铁染色 +	波形蛋白 -
低分子量角蛋白 +	CD10-
高分子量角蛋白 (S)	RCC 抗体 -
角蛋白 AE1/3+	碳酸酐酶Ⅱ +
E- 钙黏素 +	N- 钙黏素 -
EMA+	带 3 蛋白 -
微小白蛋白 +	CD117+
脂质和糖原 (PAS)-	阿辛蓝 -
CK7+	
鉴别诊断	
嗜酸细胞腺瘤	
CK7-，Hale 胶体铁染色 -，带 3 蛋白 +	
肾透明细胞癌	
波形蛋白 +,Hale 胶体铁染色 -,RCC 抗体 +,CD10+,CD117-	

> **诊断要点：嫌色性肾细胞癌**
> 1. 波形蛋白 -。
> 2. CK7+。
> 3. CD10-。
> 4. RCC 抗体 -。
> 5. 碳酸酐酶Ⅱ+。
> 6. N- 钙黏素 -。
> 7. CD117+。
> 8. Hale 胶体铁染色 +。

肾集合管癌

肾集合管癌（CDC）是一种少见的、独特的肾肿瘤，可能发生于肾髓质集合管[1-3]。实际上该肿瘤形态上总是表现为中级别或高级别，提示预后不良。以前所报道的低级别集合管癌最近被重新分类为黏液管状和梭形细胞癌（见下文）。

典型的集合管癌位于肾髓质中央，并扩展到肾皮质。组织学类型包括乳头状型、管状型、实体型和肉瘤样型（图14.53）。典型的可见明显的间质结缔组织增生、血管淋巴管侵入和急性炎症，还可见胞浆内黏蛋白成分[1-3]。细胞遗传学特征包括染色体8p和染色体 13 的缺失，还可见[1, 6, 14, 15]和 22 号染色体呈单体性[33, 34]。

典型的免疫组化表达谱包括，广谱角蛋白（AE1/AE3）、低分子量（CAM5.2）和高分子量角蛋白（CK19和34βE12）（图14.54）、EMA、波形蛋白（图14.55）和 Ulex europaeus 凝集素（UEA-1）阳性；CEA 的免

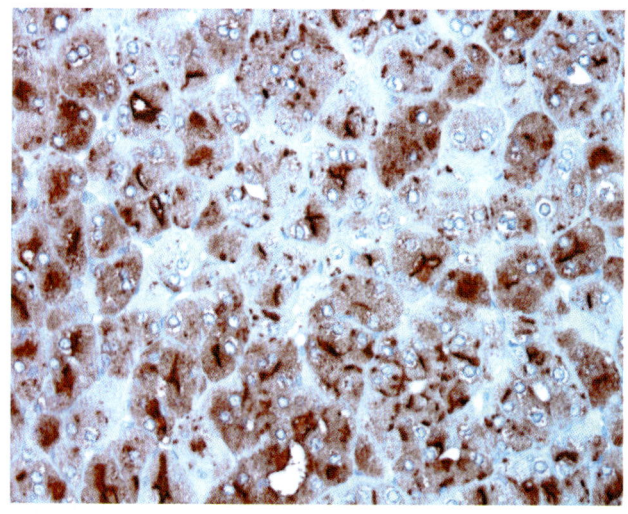

图 14.51 嫌色性肾细胞癌 EMA 的免疫组化结果

为阴性，但58% 的病例 N- 钙黏素为阳性。其他研究发现，微小白蛋白（parvalbumin）在嫌色性细胞癌中稳定表达。E-钙黏素、微小白蛋白、波形蛋白抗体组合，再配合 Hale 胶体铁染色，被认为在嫌色细胞癌与透明细胞癌的鉴别诊断中有应用价值[42, 133, 134]。据报道，碳酸酐酶Ⅱ+和桩蛋白（paxillin）在所有的嫌色细胞癌和嗜酸细胞腺瘤中均为阳性，但只有少数其他几种肾癌亚型为阳性[108, 135]。Leroy 等人报道，当Hale胶体铁染色结果不确定时，CK7在鉴别肾嗜酸细胞腺瘤（CK7-）和嫌色细胞癌（CK7+）（图 14.52）时有价值[40]。

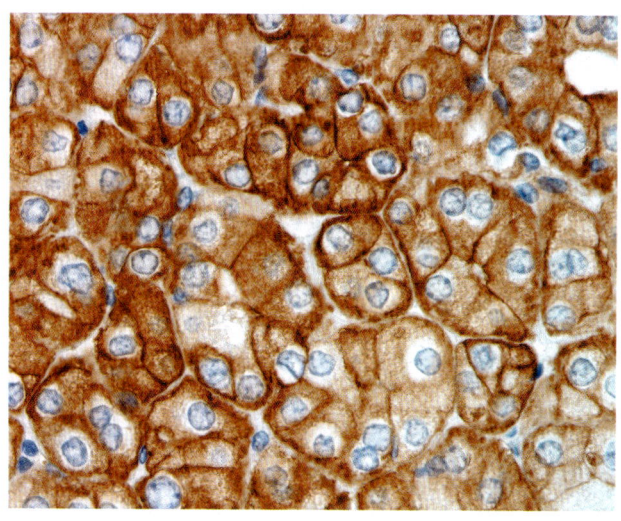

图 14.52 嫌色性肾细胞癌 CK7 的免疫组化结果

疫染色在 CDC 中不一致（表 14.29）。组织化学和免疫组织化学检测在集合管癌的诊断中常常是必需的。该肿瘤预后不佳，大多数患者在发现后 2 年内发生转移或死亡[120, 121, 136, 137]。

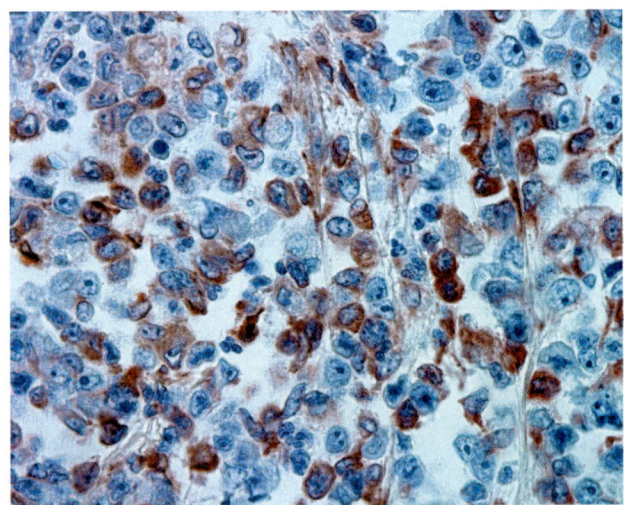

图 14.55　集合管癌波形蛋白免疫组化结果

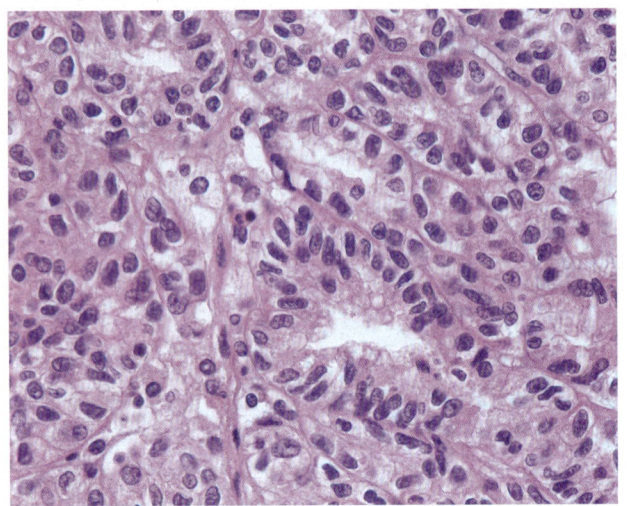

图 14.53　集合管癌，管状型

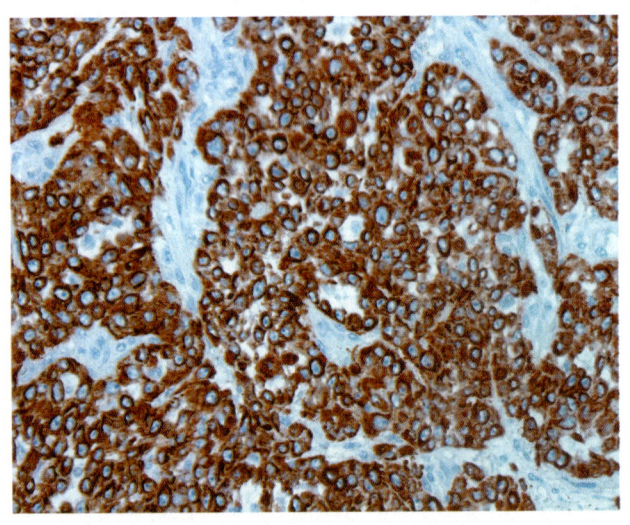

图 14.54　集合管癌高分子量角蛋白（34βE12）免疫组化结果

黏液管状和梭形细胞癌

　　黏液管状和梭形细胞癌是肾细胞癌家族中新近认识的肿瘤类型，具有独特的形态学、免疫组化和细胞遗传学特征[138-143]，是一类少见的肿瘤，女性多见（女：男为 2 : 1）。肉眼观察，肿瘤边界清楚，呈灰色或淡棕色。显微镜下观察，肿瘤由均一的立方形细胞构成，胞浆呈嗜酸性，局部形成空泡，细胞核呈低级别。肿瘤细胞常形成相互连接的小管，在泡状黏液样

表14.29　集合管癌免疫组化结果	
免疫组化	
黏蛋白 +	波形蛋白 +
EMA+	花生凝集素 +
低分子量角蛋白 +	UEA-1+
高分子量角蛋白 +	CEA 灶状 +
CK13-	LeuM1-
鉴别诊断	
乳头状肾细胞癌	
Ulex europaeus 凝集素 -	
高分子量角蛋白 -	
透明细胞肾细胞癌	
Ulex europaeus 凝集素 -	
高分子量角蛋白 -	
肾盂尿路上皮癌	
波形蛋白 -，CK13+，CK19+	

间质中可见呈索状生长的小区域和梭形细胞。

　　肿瘤显示多个一致性的染色体缺失（1、4、6、8、9、13、14、15、22）。免疫组化结果和遗传学发现表明，肿瘤来源于集合管上皮[141]，而超微结构分析表明，肿瘤有向 Henle 环或远曲小管分化的倾向[140]。临床预后较佳，可复发，但尚未发现远处转移或致死。

　　针对该肿瘤只有有限的免疫组化数据（表 14.30）。黏液管状和梭形细胞癌典型的免疫组化结果为，高分子量 CK、EMA 和花生凝集素（PNA）阳性，但是低分子量 CK 为弱阳性或阴性。大多数病例的波形蛋白为阳性。

表14.30 黏液管状和梭形细胞癌免疫组化结果

免疫组化	
高分子量角蛋白+	PAS-
低分子量角蛋白（CAM5.2，19和20）弱阳性或阴性	CEA-
	RCC-
CK7+	绒毛素-
EMA+	SMA-
波形蛋白+	结蛋白-
花生凝集素（PNA）+	S-100-
黏蛋白：Hale胶体铁染色+，阿辛蓝+	HMB-45-
	CD15-
	Ulex europaeus凝集素（UEA）-
	Tamm-Hosrsfall蛋白（THP）-
鉴别诊断	
肾细胞癌伴肉瘤样分化　梭形多形性细胞，核仁明显，分裂象常见　高分子量CK-	
经典型集合管癌　浸润性生长，多形性细胞，明显的核异型性，促结缔组织增生，UEA阳性或阴性	
后肾腺瘤　典型的小腺泡成分，缺少间质成分，缺少梭形细胞成分，EMA-	
血管平滑肌脂肪瘤　HMB-45+	
其他的平滑肌肿瘤　SMA+，结蛋白+	

参考文献

1. Bostwick DG, Murphy GP. Diagnosis and prognosis of renal cell carcinoma: highlights from an international consensus workshop. Semin Urol Oncol 1998; 16:46.

2. Bostwick DG, Eble JN. Diagnosis and classification of renal cell carcinoma. Urol Clin North Am 1999; 26:627.

3. Storkel S, Eble JN, Adlakha K,. et al. Classification of renal cell carcinoma: Workgroup No. 1. Union Internationale Contre le Cancer (UICC) and the American Joint Committee on Cancer (AJCC). Cancer 1997; 80:987.

4. Nagao T, Sugano I, Ishida Y, et al. Cystic partially differentiated nephroblastoma in an adult: an immunohistochemical, lectin histochemical and ultrastructural study. Histopathology 1999; 35:65.

5. Froberg K, Brown RE, Gaylord H, et al. Intra-abdominal desmoplastic small round cell tumor: immunohistochemical evidence for up-regulation of autocrine and paracrine growth factors. Ann Clin Lab Sci 1999; 29:78.

6. Eble JN, Bonsib SM. Extensively cystic renal neoplasms: cystic nephroma, cystic partially differentiated nephroblastoma, multilocular cystic renal cell carcinoma, and cystic hamartoma of renal pelvis. Semin Diagn Pathol 1998; 15:2.

7. Folpe AL, Patterson K, Gown AM. Antibodies to desmin identify the blastemal component of nephroblastoma. Mod Pathol 1997; 10:895.

8. Ellison DA, Silverman JF, Strausbauch PH, et al. Role of immunocytochemistry, electron microscopy, and DNA analysis in fine-needle aspiration biopsy diagnosis of Wilms' tumor. Diagn Cytopathol 1996; 14:101.

9. Leuschner I, Harms D, Schmidt D. Renal cell carcinoma in children: histology, immunohistochemistry, and follow-up of 10 cases. Med Pediatr Oncol 1991; 19:33.

10. Juszkiewicz, P. [Immunohistochemical evaluation of the percentage of proliferating neoplastic cells of Wilms' tumor in children by means of the MIB-1 monoclonal antibody]. Ann Acad Med Stetin 1997; 43:113.

11. Tarnowski BI, Hazen-Martin DJ, Garvin AJ, et al. Characterization of a monoclonal antibody recognizing the blastemal element of Wilms' tumors and fetal kidneys. Pediatr Pathol 1994; 14:849.

12. Domagala W, Chosia M, Bedner E, et al. Immunocytochemistry in fine needle aspirates of small cell-, round-, blue-cell malignant tumors of childhood (neuroblastoma, nephroblastoma, lymphoma, Ewing's sarcoma, rhabdomyosarcoma). Patol Pol 1991; 42:79.

13. Ohshio G, Ogawa K, Kudo H, et al. Immunohistochemical distribution of CA19-9 in normal and tumor tissues of the kidney. Urol Int 1990; 45:1.

14. Schmidt D, Harms D, Pilon VA. Small-cell pediatric tumors: histology, immunohistochemistry, and electron microscopy. Clin Lab Med 1987; 7:63.

15. Takagi M, Takakuwa T, Ushigome S, et al. Sarcomatous variants of Wilms' tumor. Immunohistochemical and ultrastructural comparison with classical Wilms' tumor. Cancer 1987; 59:963.

16. Argani P, Perlman EJ, Breslow NE, et al. Clear cell sarcoma

of the kidney: a review of 351 cases from the National Wilms' Tumor Study Group Pathology Center. Am J Surg Pathol 2000; 24:4.

17. Choi YJ, Jung WH, Jung SH, et al. Clear cell sarcoma of the kidney – immunohistochemical study and flow cytometric DNA analysis of 7 cases. Yonsei Med J 1994; 35:336.

18. Oda H, Shiga J, Machinami R. Clear cell sarcoma of kidney. Two cases in adults. Cancer 1993; 71:2286.

19. Ogawa K, Nakashima Y, Yamabe H, et al. Clear cell sarcoma of the kidney. An immunohistochemical study. Acta Pathol Jpn 1986; 36:681.

20. Amin MB, de Peralta-Venturina MN, Ro JY, et al. Clear cell sarcoma of kidney in an adolescent and in young adults: a report of four cases with ultrastructural, immunohistochemical, and DNA flow cytometric analysis. Am J Surg Pathol 1999; 23:1455.

21. Altmannsberger M, Osborn M, Schafer H, et al. Distinction of nephroblastomas from other childhood tumors using antibodies to intermediate filaments. Virchows Arch B Cell Pathol Incl Mol Pathol 1984; 45:113.

22. Fleming S, Gibson AA. Proteinase inhibitors in the kidney and its tumours. Histopathology 1986; 10:1303.

23. Weeks DA, Beckwith JB, Mierau GW, et al. Rhabdoid tumor of kidney. A report of 111 cases from the National Wilms' Tumor Study Pathology Center. Am J Surg Pathol 1989; 13:439.

24. Hirose M, Yamada T, Toyosaka A, et al. Rhabdoid tumor of the kidney: a report of two cases with respective tumor markers and a specific chromosomal abnormality, del(11p13). Med Pediatr Oncol 1996; 27:174.

25. Kaiserling E, Ruck P, Handgretinger R, et al. Immunohistochemical and cytogenetic findings in malignant rhabdoid tumor. Gen Diagn Pathol 1996; 141:327.

26. Liu Y, Li P, Liu S. [Malignant rhabdoid tumor of kidney: a clinicopathologic and immunohistochemical study of 15 patients]. Chung Hua Ping Li Hsueh Tsa Chih 1995; 24:72.

27. Ueyama T, Nagai E, Yao T, et al. Vimentin-positive gastric carcinomas with rhabdoid features. A clinicopathologic and immunohistochemical study [see comments]. Am J Surg Pathol 1993; 17:813.

28. Fischer HP, Thomsen H, Altmannsberger M,. et al. Malignant rhabdoid tumour of the kidney expressing neurofilament proteins. Immunohistochemical findings and histogenetic aspects. Pathol Res Pract 1989; 184:541.

29. Bisceglia M, Carosi I, Vairo M, et al. Congenital mesoblastic nephroma: report of a case with review of the most significant literature. Pathol Res Pract 2000; 196:199.

30. Siracusano S, Bosincu L, Onida A, et al. Congenital mesoblastic nephroma (CMN) with an unusual immunohistochemical feature. Arch Esp Urol 1999; 52:299.

31. Nadasdy T, Roth J, Johnson DL, et al. Congenital mesoblastic nephroma: an immunohistochemical and lectin study. Hum Pathol 1993; 24:413.

32. Boccon-Gibod L, Ben Lagha N. [Atypical congenital mesoblastic nephroma (atypical Bolande's tumor)]. Arch Anat Cytol Pathol 1992; 40:333.

33. Storkel S. [Epithelial tumors of the kidney. Pathological subtyping and cytogenetic correlation]. Urologe A 1999; 38:425.

34. van den Berg E, Dijkhuizen T, Oosterhuis JW, et al. Cytogenetic classification of renal cell cancer. Cancer Genet Cytogenet 1997; 95:103.

35. Avery AK, Beckstead J, Renshaw AA, et al. Use of antibodies to RCC and CD10 in the differential diagnosis of renal neoplasms. Am J Surg Pathol 2000; 24:203.

36. Cohen C, McCue PA, Derose PB. Histogenesis of renal cell carcinoma and renal oncocytoma. An immunohistochemical study. Cancer 1988; 62:1946.

37. Eble JN, Hull MT. Morphologic features of renal oncocytoma: a light and electron microscopic study. Hum Pathol 1984; 15:1054.

38. Beham A, Ratschek M, Zatloukal K, et al. Distribution of cytokeratins, vimentin and desmoplakins in normal renal tissue, renal cell carcinomas and oncocytoma as revealed by immunofluorescence microscopy. Virchows Arch A Pathol Anat Histopathol 1992; 421:209.

39. Bonsib SM, Bromley C, Lager DJ. Renal oncocytoma: diagnostic utility of cytokeratin-containing globular filamentous bodies. Mod Pathol 1991; 4:16.

40. Leroy X, Moukassa D, Copin MC, et al. Utility of cytokeratin 7 for distinguishing chromophobe renal cell carcinoma from renal oncocytoma. Eur Urol 2000; 37:484.

41. Markovic-Lipkovski J, Brasanac D, Todorovic V, et al. Immunomorphological characteristics of renal cell carcinoma. Histol Histopathol 1995; 10:651.

42. Taki A, Nakatani Y, Misugi K, et al. Chromophobe renal cell

carcinoma: an immunohistochemical study of 21 Japanese cases. Mod Pathol 1999; 12:310.
43. Storkel S, Steart PV, Drenckhahn D, et al. The human chromophobe cell renal carcinoma: its probable relation to intercalated cells of the collecting duct. Virchows Arch B Cell Pathol Incl Mol Pathol 1989; 56:237.
44. van den Berg E, van der Hout AH, Oosterhuis JW, et al. Cytogenetic analysis of epithelial renal-cell tumors: relationship with a new histopathological classification. Int J Cancer 1993; 55:223.
45. Pan CC, Chen PC, Chiang H. Overexpression of KIT (CD117) in chromophobe renal cell carcinoma and renal oncocytoma. Am J Clin Pathol 2004; 121:878.
46. Petit A, Castillo M, Santos M, et al. KIT expression in chromophobe renal cell carcinoma: comparative immunohistochemical analysis of KIT expression in different renal cell neoplasms. Am J Surg Pathol 2004; 28:676.
47. Bonsib SM, Bromley C. Immunocytochemical analysis of band 3 protein in renal cell carcinoma, nephroblastoma, and oncocytoma. Arch Pathol Lab Med 1994; 118:702.
48. Rampino T, Gregorini M, Soccio G, et al. The Ron proto-oncogene product is a phenotypic marker of renal oncocytoma. Am J Surg Pathol 2003; 27:779.
49. Patton KT, Tretiakova MS, Yao JL, et al. Expression of RON proto-oncogene in renal oncocytoma and chromophobe renal cell carcinoma. Am J Surg Pathol 2004; 28:1045.
50. Keshani de Silva V, Tobias V, Kainer G, et al. Metanephric adenoma with embryonal hyperplasia of Bowman's capsular epithelium: previously unreported association [In Process Citation]. Pediatr Dev Pathol 2000; 3:472.
51. Renshaw AA, Freyer DR, Hammers YA. Metastatic metanephric adenoma in a child. Am J Surg Pathol 2000; 24:570.
52. Tamboli P, Ro JY, Amin MB, et al. Benign tumors and tumor-like lesions of the adult kidney. Part II: Benign mesenchymal and mixed neoplasms, and tumor-like lesions. Adv Anat Pathol 2000; 7:47.
53. Birgisson H, Einarsson GV, Steinarsdottir M, et al. Metanephric adenoma. Scand J Urol Nephrol 1999; 33:340.
54. Monge Mirallas JM, Asensio Lahoz A, Martinez Bretones F, et al. [Metanephric adenoma of the kidney and chronic myeloproliferative syndrome. An unusual association]. Actas Urol Esp 1999; 23:359.
55. Patankar T, Punekar S, Madiwale C, et al. Metanephric adenoma in a solitary kidney. Br J Radiol 1999; 72:80.
56. Imamoto T, Furuya Y, Ueda T, et al. Metanephric adenoma of the kidney. Int J Urol 1999; 6:200.
57. Martin L, Justrabo E, Michel F, et al. Metanephric adenoma of the kidney. A clinicopathologic, immunohistochemical and electron microscopic study of two cases. Ann Pathol 1998; 18:120.
58. Grignon DJ, Eble JN. Papillary and metanephric adenomas of the kidney. Semin Diagn Pathol 1998; 15:41.
59. Granter SR, Fletcher JA, Renshaw AA. Cytologic and cytogenetic analysis of metanephric adenoma of the kidney: a report of two cases. Am J Clin Pathol 1997; 108:544.
60. Renshaw AA, Maurici D, Fletcher JA. Cytologic and fluorescence in situ hybridization (FISH) examination of metanephric adenoma. Diagn Cytopathol 1997; 16:107.
61. Ban S, Yoshii S, Tsuruta A, et al. Metanephric adenoma of the kidney: ultrastructural, immunohistochemical and lectin histochemical studies. Pathol Int 1996; 46:661.
62. Gatalica Z, Grujic S, Kovatich A, et al. Metanephric adenoma: histology, immunophenotype, cytogenetics, ultrastructure. Mod Pathol 1996; 9:329.
63. Brown JA, Anderl KL, Borell TJ, et al. Simultaneous chromosome 7 and 17 gain and sex chromosome loss provide evidence that renal metanephric adenoma is related to papillary renal cell carcinoma. J Urol 1997; 158:370.
64. Brown JA, Sebo TJ, Segura JW. Metaphase analysis of metanephric adenoma reveals chromosome Y loss with chromosome 7 and 17 gain. Urology 1996; 48:473.
65. Nonomura A, Mizukami Y, Hasegawa T, et al. Metanephric adenoma of the kidney: an electron microscopic and immunohistochemical study with quantitative DNA measurement by image analysis. Ultrastruct Pathol 1995; 19:481.
66. Nonomura A, Mizukami Y, Hasegawa T, et al. Metanephric adenoma of the kidney. Pathol Int 1995; 45:160.
67. Tsuji M, Murakami Y, Kanayama H, et al. A case of renal metanephric adenoma: histologic, immunohistochemical and cytogenetic analyses. Int J Urol 1999; 6:203.
68. Mensch LS, Trainer TD, Plante MK. Cystic hamartoma of the renal pelvis: a rare pathologic entity. Mod Pathol 1999; 12:417.
69. Kuroda N, Moriki T, Komatsu F, et al. Adult-onset giant juxtaglomerular cell tumor of the kidney. Pathol Int 2000; 50:249.
70. Hashimoto Y, Nakazawa H, Okuda H, et al. [A juxtaglom-

erular cell tumor. Analysis of immunohistochemistry, electron microscopy and in situ hybridization]. Nippon Hinyokika Gakkai Zasshi 1998; 89:907.

71. Hayami S, Sasagawa I, Suzuki H, et al. Juxtaglomerular cell tumor without hypertension. Scand J Urol Nephrol 1998; 32: 231.

72. Caregaro L, Menon F, Gatta A, et al. Juxtaglomerular cell tumor of the kidney. Clin Exp Hypertens 1994; 16:41.

73. Kodet R, Taylor M, Vachalova H, et al. Juxtaglomerular cell tumor. An immunohistochemical, electron-microscopic, and in situ hybridization study. Am J Surg Pathol 1994; 18:837.

74. Lopez GAJA, Blanco Gonzalez J, Ortega Medina L, et al. Juxtaglomerular cell tumor of the kidney. Morphological, immunohistochemical and ultrastructural studies of a new case. Pathol Res Pract 1991; 187:354.

75. Lindop GB, Stewart JA, Downie TT. The immunocytochemical demonstration of renin in a juxtaglomerular cell tumour by light and electron microscopy. Histopathology 1983; 7: 421.

76. Martin SA, Mynderse LA, Lager DJ, et al. Juxtaglomerular cell tumor: a clinicopathologic study of four cases and review of the literature. Am J Clin Pathol 2001; 116:854.

77. L'Hostis H, Deminiere C, Ferriere JM, et al. Renal angiomyolipoma: a clinicopathologic, immuno-histochemical, and follow-up study of 46 cases. Am J Surg Pathol 1999; 23:1011.

78. Watanabe K, Suzuki T. Mucocutaneous angiomyolipoma. A report of 2 cases arising in the nasal cavity. Arch Pathol Lab Med 1999; 123:789.

79. Jungbluth AA, Busam KJ, Gerald WL, et al. A103: An anti-melan-A monoclonal antibody for the detection of malignant melanoma in paraffin-embedded tissues [see comments]. Am J Surg Pathol 1998; 22:595.

80. Gupta RK, Nowitz M, Wakefield SJ. Fine-needle aspiration cytology of renal angiomyolipoma: report of a case with immunocytochemical and electron microscopic findings. Diagn Cytopathol 1998; 18:297.

81. Gyure KA, Prayson RA. Subependymal giant cell astrocytoma: a clinicopathologic study with HMB45 and MIB-1 immunohistochemical analysis. Mod Pathol 1997; 10: 313.

82. Makhlouf HR, Remotti HE, Ishak KG. Expression of KIT (CD117) in angiomyolipoma. Am J Surg Pathol 2002; 26: 493.

83. Greenlee RT, Murray T, Bolden S, et al. Cancer statistics, 2000. CA Cancer J Clin 2000; 50:7.

84. Eble JN, Epstein JI, Sesterhenn IA, eds. World Health Organization Classification of Tumours. Pathology and Genetics of Tumours of the Urinary System and Male Genital Organs. Lyon: IARC Press; 2004.

85. Beham A, Ratschek M, Zatloukal K, et al. [Immunohistochemical analysis of 42 renal cell carcinomas and one oncocytoma with mono- and polyclonal antibodies against vimentin and cytokeratin]. Verh Dtsch Ges Pathol 1989; 73: 392.

86. Bonsib SM, Bray C. Cytokeratin-containing globular filamentous bodies in renal oncocytoma. Ultrastruct Pathol 1991; 15: 521.

87. Chu P, Arber DA. Paraffin-section detection of CD10 in 505 nonhematopoietic neoplasms. Frequent expression in renal cell carcinoma and endometrial stromal sarcoma. Am J Clin Pathol 2000; 113:374.

88. Coffin CM, Swanson PE, Wick MR, et al. An immunohistochemical comparison of chordoma with renal cell carcinoma, colorectal adenocarcinoma, and myxopapillary ependymoma: a potential diagnostic dilemma in the diminutive biopsy. Mod Pathol 1993; 6:531.

89. Gerharz CD, Moll R, Storkel S, et al. Ultrastructural appearance and cytoskeletal architecture of the clear, chromophilic, and chromophobe types of human renal cell carcinoma in vitro. Am J Pathol 1993; 142:851.

90. Gilcrease MZ, Guzman-Paz M, Niehans G, et al. Correlation of CD44S expression in renal clear cell carcinomas with subsequent tumor progression or recurrence [see comments]. Cancer 1999; 86:2320.

91. Heider KH, Ratschek M, Zatloukal K, et al. Expression of CD44 isoforms in human renal cell carcinomas. Virchows Arch 1996; 428:267.

92. Jin TX, Kakehi Y, Moroi S, et al. [E-cadherin expression and histopathological features in renal cell carcinomas]. Hinyokika Kiyo 1995; 41:653.

93. Waldherr R, Schwechheimer K. Co-expression of cytokeratin and vimentin intermediate-sized filaments in renal cell carcinomas. Comparative study of the intermediate-sized filament distribution in renal cell carcinomas and normal human kidney. Virchows Arch A Pathol Anat Histopathol 1985; 408:

94. Martin de las Mulas J, Espinosa de los Monteros A, Carrasco L, et al. Immunohistochemical distribution pattern of intermediate filament proteins in 50 feline neoplasms. Vet Pathol 1995; 32:692.
95. Sim SJ, Ro JY, Ordonez NG, et al.: Metastatic renal cell carcinoma to the bladder: a clinicopathologic and immunohistochemical study. Mod Pathol 1999; 12:351.
96. Banner BF, Burnham JA, Bahnson RR, et al. Immunophenotypic markers in renal cell carcinoma. Mod Pathol 1990; 3:129.
97. Gaffey MJ, Mills SE, Askin FB et al. Clear cell tumor of the lung. A clinicopathologic, immuno-histochemical, and ultrastructural study of eight cases [see comments]. Am J Surg Pathol 1990; 14:248.
98. Amo-Takyi BK, Handt S, Gunawan B, et al. A cytogenetic approach to the differential diagnosis of metastatic clear cell renal carcinoma. Histopathology 1998; 32:436.
99. Medeiros LJ, Gelb AB, Weiss LM. Low-grade renal cell carcinoma. A clinicopathologic study of 53 cases. Am J Surg Pathol 1987; 11:633.
100. Medeiros LJ, Michie SA, Johnson DE, et al. An immunoperoxidase study of renal cell carcinomas: correlation with nuclear grade, cell type, and histologic pattern. Hum Pathol 1988; 19:980.
101. Akhtar M, Kardar H, Linjawi T, et al. Chromophobe cell carcinoma of the kidney. A clinicopathologic study of 21 cases. Am J Surg Pathol 1995; 19:1245.
102. Kletscher BA, Qian J, Bostwick DG, et al. Prospective analysis of the incidence of ipsilateral adrenal metastasis in localized renal cell carcinoma. J Urol 1996; 155:1844.
103. Yoshida K, Moriguchi H, Sumi S, et al. Alterations of asparagine-linked sugar chains of N-acetyl beta-Dhexosaminidase during human renal oncogenesis: a preliminary study using serial lectin affinity chromatography. J Chromatogr B Biomed Sci Appl 1999; 723:75.
104. Yoshida K, Hosoya Y, Sumi S, et al. Studies of the expression of epidermal growth factor receptor in human renal cell carcinoma: a comparison of immunohistochemical method versus ligand binding assay. Oncology 1997; 54:220.
105. Yoshida SO, Imam A. Monoclonal antibody to a proximal nephrogenic renal antigen: immunohistochemical analysis of formalin-fixed, paraffin-embedded human renal cell carcinomas. Cancer Res 1989; 49:1802.
106. Yoshida K, Sumi S, Honda M, et al. Serial lectin affinity chromatography demonstrates altered asparagine-linked sugar chain structures of gamma-glutamyltransferase in human renal cell carcinoma. J Chromatogr B Biomed Appl 1995; 672:45.
107. Cochand-Priollet B, Molinie V, Bougaran J, et al. Renal chromophobe cell carcinoma and oncocytoma. A comparative morphologic, histochemical, and immunohistochemical study of 124 cases. Arch Pathol Lab Med 1997; 121:1081.
108. Takahashi M, Yang XJ, Sugimura J, et al. Molecular subclassification of kidney tumors and the discovery of new diagnostic markers. Oncogene 2003; 22:6810.
109. Fischer C, Georg C, Kraus S, et al. CD44s, E-cadherin and PCNA as markers for progression in renal cell carcinoma. Anticancer Res 1999; 19:1513.
110. Oosterwijk E, Bander NH, Divgi CR., et al. Antibody localization in human renal cell carcinoma: a phase I study of monoclonal antibody G250. J Clin Oncol 1993; 11:738.
111. Uemura H, Nakagawa Y, Yoshida K, et al. MN/CA IX/G250 as a potential target for immunotherapy of renal cell carcinomas. Br J Cancer 1999; 81:741.
112. Renshaw AA, Granter SR. A comparison of A103 and inhibin reactivity in adrenal cortical tumors: distinction from hepatocellular carcinoma and renal tumors. Mod Pathol 1998; 11:1160.
113. Eyzaguirre EJ, Miettinen M, Norris BA, et al. Different immunohistochemical patterns of FHIT protein expression in renal neoplasms. Mod Pathol 1999; 12:979.
114. Hadaczek P, Siprashvili Z, Markiewski M, et al. Absence or reduction of FHIT expression in most clear cell renal carcinomas. Cancer Res 1998; 58:2946.
115. Hadaczek P, Kovatich A, Gronwald J, et al. Loss or reduction of FHIT expression in renal neoplasias: correlation with histogenic class. Hum Pathol 1999; 30:1276.
116. Fujita J, Takenawa J, Kaneko Y, et al. [Anti-interleukin-6 (IL-6) therapy of IL-6-producing renal cell carcinoma]. Hinyokika Kiyo 1992; 38:1333.
117. Li N, Tsuji M, Kanda K, et al. Analysis of CD44 isoform v10 expression and its prognostic value in renal cell carcinoma. Br J Urol Int 2000; 85:514.
118. Amin MB, Corless CL, Renshaw AA, et al. Papillary (chromophil) renal cell carcinoma: histomorphologic char-

acteristics and evaluation of conventional pathologic prognostic parameters in 62 cases [see comments]. Am J Surg Pathol 1997; 21:621.

119. Renshaw AA, Corless CL. Papillary renal cell carcinoma. Histology and immunohistochemistry. Am J Surg Pathol 1995; 19:842.

120. Delahunt B, Eble JN. Papillary renal cell carcinoma: a clinicopathologic and immunohistochemical study of 105 tumors. Mod Pathol 1997; 10:537.

121. Srigley JR, Eble JN. Collecting duct carcinoma of kidney. Semin Diagn Pathol 1998; 15:54.

122. Corless C., Aburatani H, Fletcher JA, et al. Papillary renal cell carcinoma: quantitation of chromosomes 7 and 17 by FISH, analysis of chromosome 3p for LOH, and DNA ploidy. Diagn Mol Pathol 1996; 5:53.

123. Kattar MM, Grignon DJ, Wallis T, et al. Clinicopathologic and interphase cytogenetic analysis of papillary (chromophilic) renal cell carcinoma. Mod Pathol 1997; 10: 1143.

124. Henke RP, Erbersdobler A. Numerical chromosomal aberrations in papillary renal cortical tumors: relationship with histopathologic features. Virchows Arch 2002; 440:604.

125. Mai KT, Burns BF. Chromophobe cell carcinoma and renal cell neoplasms with mucin-like changes. Acta Histochem 2000; 102:103.

126. Renshaw AA, Zhang H, Corless CL, et al. Solid variants of papillary (chromophil) renal cell carcinoma: clinicopathologic and genetic features. Am J Surg Pathol 1997; 21:1203.

127. Tretiakova MS, Sahoo S, Takahashi M, et al. Expression of alpha-methylacyl-CoA racemase in papillary renal cell carcinoma. Am J Surg Pathol 2004; 28:69.

128. Leroy X, Zini L, Leteurtre E, et al. Morphologic subtyping of papillary renal cell carcinoma: correlation with prognosis and differential expression of MUC1 between the two subtypes. Mod Pathol 2002; 15:1126.

129. Langner C, Ratschek M, Rehak P, et al. Expression of MUC1 (EMA) and E-cadherin in renal cell carcinoma: a systematic immunohistochemical analysis of 188 cases. Mod Pathol 2004; 17:180.

130. Wechsel HW, Petri E, Feil G, et al. Renal cell carcinoma: immunohistological investigation of expression of the integrin alpha v beta 3. Anticancer Res 1999; 19:1529.

131. Morell-Quadreny L, Gregori-Romero M, Llombart-Bosch A. Chromophobe renal cell carcinoma. Pathologic, ultrastructural, immunohistochemical, cytofluorometric and cytogenetic findings. Pathol Res Pract 1996; 192:1275.

132. Weiss LM, Gaffey MJ, Warhol MJ, et al. Immunocytochemical characterization of a monoclonal antibody directed against mitochondria reactive in paraffinembedded sections. Mod Pathol 1991; 4:596.

133. Martignoni G, Pea M, Chilosi M, et al. Parvalbumin is constantly expressed in chromophobe renal carcinoma. Mod Pathol 2001; 14:760.

134. Young AN, de Oliveira Salles PG, Lim SD, et al. Beta defensin-1, parvalbumin, and vimentin: a panel of diagnostic immunohistochemical markers for renal tumors derived from gene expression profiling studies using cDNA microarrays. Am J Surg Pathol 2003; 27:199.

135. Kuroda N, Guo L, Toi M, et al. Paxillin: application of immunohistochemistry to the diagnosis of chromophobe renal cell carcinoma and oncocytoma. Appl Immunohistochem Mol Morphol 2001; 9:315.

136. MacLennan GT, Farrow GM, Bostwick DG. Low-grade collecting duct carcinoma of the kidney: report of 13 cases of low-grade mucinous tubulocystic renal carcinoma of possible collecting duct origin. Urology 1997; 50:679.

137. Tickoo SK, Amin MB, Linden MD, et al. The MIB-1 tumor proliferation index in adult renal epithelial tumors with granular cytoplasm: biologic implications and differential diagnostic potential. Mod Pathol 1998; 11:1115.

138. Eble JN. Mucinous tubular and spindle cell carcinoma and post-neuroblastoma carcinoma: newly recognised entities in the renal cell carcinoma family. Pathology 2003; 35:499.

139. Hes O, Hora M, Perez-Montiel DM, et al. Spindle and cuboidal renal cell carcinoma, a tumour having frequent association with nephrolithiasis: report of 11 cases including a case with hybrid conventional renal cell carcinoma/spindle and cuboidal renal cell carcinoma components. Histopathology 2002; 41:549.

140. Parwani AV, Husain AN, Epstein JI, et al. Low-grade myxoid renal epithelial neoplasms with distal nephron differentiation. Hum Pathol 2001; 32:506.

141. Rakozy C, Schmahl GE, Bogner S, et al. Low-grade tubular-mucinous renal neoplasms: morphologic, immunohistochemical, and genetic features. Mod Pathol 2002; 15:1162.

142. Renshaw AA. Subclassification of renal cell neoplasms: an

update for the practising pathologist. Histopathology 2002; 41:283.

143. Weber A, Srigley J, Moch H. [Mucinous spindle cell carcinoma of the kidney. A molecular analysis]. Pathologe 2003; 24:453.

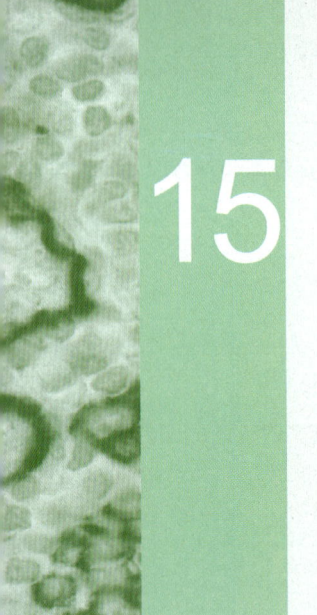

15 小儿肿瘤的免疫组织化学

原作者：Cheryl M. Coffin and Deborah Belchis

译　者：李　丽

审校者：年　坤，郝春燕

目　录

引言　　　　　　　　　　　　　　　　628
抗原／抗体生物学　　　　　　　　　　628
肿瘤　　　　　　　　　　　　　　　　629
小结　　　　　　　　　　　　　　　　645

引　言

　　小儿与青少年实体瘤包含多种诊断上较困难的肿瘤，就基本形态来讲，这些肿瘤为小圆细胞肿瘤和梭形细胞肿瘤。免疫组织化学和分子学诊断技术极大地推动了这些肿瘤的分类[1-4]。辅助诊断技术在病理诊断、复发瘤与转移瘤的评价以及部分病例的预后分级中愈来愈显示出其重要性。肿瘤科、外科、放射科、放疗科（放射肿瘤科）、医学遗传学和病理科等多学科之间的密切交流与沟通应当予以重视。此外，辅助检查应当与光镜所见结合起来，并且足量取材非常关键。免疫组织化学技术是一种非常有用的诊断工具，但同时在诊断某些特殊病例时也存在陷阱[5,6]。组织固定不良、坏死、局灶阳性表达、在小组织标本（如芯针组织活检）中出现的人为改变以及其他技术因素均可影响免疫组化的结果。一些技术，如应用于白血病、淋巴瘤[7]的流式细胞术、电镜技术[8-12]和分子学检测[13,14]对支持诊断和预后评估是必要的。因此，肿瘤标本的取材和组织处理规范化可给病理诊断提供重要指导[15-20]。

　　本章主要讨论小儿和青少年实体瘤的诊断和免疫组织化学表现，包括神经母细胞瘤及相关的神经母细胞性肿瘤、横纹肌肉瘤、Ewing 肉瘤／原始神经外胚层肿瘤、促结缔组织增生性小圆细胞肿瘤、恶性横纹肌样瘤、Wilms 瘤和骨肉瘤。很多病例光镜检查结合临床与影像学表现即可诊断。另外有些肿瘤以圆形细胞或梭形细胞为主，要视不同的临床、影像以及形态学表现进行鉴别诊断。例如，婴儿肾上腺肿块伴血清与尿儿茶酚胺水平升高，光镜下神经纤维背景上可见神经母细胞，伴钙化和纤维血管间隔，即可诊断为神经母细胞瘤。但是原始横纹肌肉瘤则需要免疫组织化学甚至分子学检查才能作出诊断。至于何时进行特殊检查要根据肿瘤的复杂程度及病理医师的经验。往往首次开出的一组免疫组化指标是诊断和支持诊断的第一步，如果结果与镜下所见不一致，可再使用一组范围稍广的指标。不管何种病例，采用一组指标，而不是依靠单一指标是一条重要的诊断原则。

抗原／抗体生物学

　　多种不同的抗体可用于小儿实体瘤的免疫组织化学分析。一些常用抗体将在其他章节有介绍，本章主要介绍对于上述肿瘤有特殊重要性的抗体，如生肌转录调节蛋白、CD99、FLI-1 蛋白、WT-1 蛋白和 hSNF5/INI-1 蛋白。

　　生肌调节蛋白　成肌素（myf-4）、Myo-D1、myf-5 和 mrf-4-herculin/myf-6 组成生肌转录调节蛋白的一个家族，参与骨骼肌分化，其表达早于结蛋白及肌动蛋白等结构蛋白。成肌素和 Myo-D1 在横纹肌肉瘤表达阳性，即便在那些分化较差、缺乏明确的横纹肌母细胞分化形态学特征（如有横纹的带状细胞）的病例中也有表达。大量研究证实了 Myo-D1 是横纹肌肉瘤特异性标记物[21-27]，这与肌特异性肌动蛋白与结蛋白不同，后两者可表达于包括骨骼肌、平滑肌以及纤维母-肌纤维母源性肿瘤在内的多种肿瘤。Myo-D1 胞浆着色可见于非肌源性肿瘤，如神经母细胞瘤，因此观察 Myo-D1 着色情况时细胞核着色这一点非常重要。有骨骼肌分化的肿瘤如 Wilms 瘤、外胚层间叶瘤和有多向分化的恶性外周神经鞘瘤可表达生肌转录调节蛋白[28]，非肿瘤性骨骼肌细胞成肌素可呈细胞核阳性表达[26]，有研究显示横纹肌肉瘤不同亚型成肌素着色模式不同[29]。

CD99（p30/32，mic2） 该组抗体用来检测一种跨膜糖蛋白，是位于 Xp22.32 pter 和 Yq11 pter 的拟常染色体区 mic2 基因的表达产物[30]。采用 O13、12E7、HBA-71 在内的一系列抗体可以检测到 CD99 在 85%~95% 的 ES/PTEN 病例中呈细胞膜强阳性表达[31-33]，若 CD99 阴性，应采取进一步检查，如增加免疫组化指标、电镜或分子学检测以支持 ES/PNET 诊断，并排除其他小圆细胞肿瘤。CD99 在急性淋巴母细胞白血病/淋巴母细胞淋巴瘤、急性髓性白血病、粒细胞肉瘤、间叶性软骨肉瘤、滑膜肉瘤、血管肿瘤以及其他一些恶性肿瘤中也有表达[34-39]。有人认为抗原修复可提高 CD99 在多种肿瘤中的表达。尤其临床表现不典型时，鉴别 ES/PNET 与急性淋巴母细胞白血病/淋巴母细胞淋巴瘤应提高警惕，因为二者免疫组化有重叠[34, 40]。CD99 对于鉴别 ES/PNET 和神经母细胞瘤尤其有用[41]。多种肿瘤均能表达 CD99，提示鉴别诊断小圆细胞肿瘤时应采用一组免疫组化指标。

FLI-1 ES/PNET 存在 t(11;12)(q24;q12) 易位，导致 EWS-FLI-1/1 基因融合，因此 FLI-1 蛋白过度表达[42]。接近 70% 的 ES/PNET 病例可观察到 FLI-1 细胞核表达，但同时 90% 的淋巴母细胞淋巴瘤和血管肿瘤亦可见 FLI-1 表达[43, 44]。若能考虑到淋巴母细胞淋巴瘤与血管肿瘤均表达 FLI-1，该抗体作为诊断 ES/PNET 的指标之一还是有用的。

WT-1 作为针对 WT 基因 (WT-1) C-末端表达蛋白产物的抗体，可用于诊断促结缔组织增生性小圆细胞肿瘤。抗 C-末端 WT-1 抗体在促结缔组织增生性小圆细胞肿瘤中呈细胞核强阳性[45-47]，Wilms 瘤和横纹肌肉瘤也有 WT-1 细胞核表达[36, 46, 47]。作者曾观察到少数其他小圆细胞肿瘤病例，包括 ES/PNET，WT-1 表达阳性，因此进一步评价该抗体是必要的。

hSNF5/INI-1 非典型畸胎瘤/横纹肌样瘤频繁出现 hSNF5/INI-1 基因缺失和突变伴 INI-1 蛋白表达降低或缺失。INI-1 抗体可以用于检测 INI-1 缺失，表现为免疫组化呈阴性，而功能性 INI-1 在正常组织和其他肿瘤组织中呈阳性。近期研究发现中枢神经系统的非典型畸胎瘤/横纹肌样瘤，INI-1 细胞核表达阴性[48]。尚无中枢神经系统以外恶性横纹肌样瘤的相关研究。

肿 瘤

神经母细胞瘤和神经母细胞性肿瘤

肾上腺和交感神经系统的神经母细胞性肿瘤来源于神经嵴的迁移性神经外胚层肿瘤，包括神经母细胞瘤、节细胞神经母细胞瘤和节细胞神经瘤[49]。根据神经母细胞的分化程度和 schwannian 间质发育情况对神经母细胞性肿瘤进行分类。现在使用的名词由国际神经母细胞瘤病理协会命名，包括神经母细胞瘤、节细胞神经母细胞瘤（混合型、schwannian 间质丰富型）、节细胞神经瘤、节细胞神经母细胞瘤结节型（包括混合型、schwannian 间质丰富型、间质为主型和间质消减型）[20, 50]。神经母细胞性肿瘤是 2 岁以内儿童最常见的颅外恶性实体瘤，常见于 10 岁以下的青少年。最常见的发病部位为肾上腺，其次是腹部、胸部、颈部和骨盆等有交感神经节的部位。根据 schwannian 间质的多少、分化程度、坏死和出血情况大体所见有所不同。

典型的神经母细胞瘤为富于细胞的神经母细胞性肿瘤，在神经纤维背景上由"小蓝细胞"组成，"小蓝细胞"呈不同程度菊形团排列，可见纤维血管间质、不同分化阶段的神经母细胞，伴或不伴明显的神经节细胞（图 15.1）[20, 50]，无显著的 schwannian 间质。神经节神经母细胞瘤有两种亚型：混合型与结节型。混合型神经节神经母细胞瘤 schwannian 间质内可见局灶与神经母细胞瘤相似的神经母细胞成分，但间质成分占肿瘤的 50% 以上。结节型则相反，有单个或多个肉眼可见的神经母细胞结节，可见显著的混合型神经节神经母细胞瘤和节细胞神经瘤图像。节细胞神经瘤主要由 schwannian 间质构成，以及散在分布的成熟节细胞，伴或不伴稀疏的不同分化阶段的神经母细胞和不成熟节细胞成分。

尽管神经母细胞瘤具有神经元特征分化，但免疫组化并无特殊性。神经母细胞对一系列神经元标记物阳性表达，如神经特异性烯醇化酶（图 15.2）、CD57、

CD56、PGP9.5（蛋白基因产物9.5）、GD2（人神经母细胞瘤细胞膜上的一种神经节苷脂）、NB84（神经母细胞瘤细胞系的一种抗体）、突触素（图15.3）、嗜铬素和神经丝蛋白[20, 50-55]。其中部分标记物敏感性很强，但缺乏特异性，如神经特异性烯醇化酶、CD57、CD56和PGP9.5。反之，特异性较高的标记物如突触素、嗜铬素与神经丝蛋白，敏感性则较低。内分泌标记物偶为阳性，尤其是分泌型腹泻相关血管活性肠肽在神经母细胞瘤呈阳性表达。schwannian间质S-100阳性表达，尤其分化好的神经母细胞瘤间质S-100阳性更显著[56]。神经母细胞瘤分化越高，神经元标记物阳性越强，阳性率也越高，但不能据此判断预后[57]。在神经母细胞瘤呈阴性的标记物包括结蛋白、肌源性标记物（如成肌素、Myo-D1等）、波形蛋白、白细胞共同抗原及CD99，能帮助与其他"小蓝细胞"恶性肿瘤进行鉴别。白细胞共同抗原或CD45可用于将神经母细胞瘤活检小组织标本、治疗后标本及疑难病例[52]与慢性炎症区分开来。神经元标记物还能用于检测骨髓转移[58]。90%以上的神经母细胞瘤病例ALK-1阳性，这容易成为与间变性大细胞淋巴瘤及部分横纹肌肉瘤鉴别的陷阱[59]。

目前已经发现了一系列神经母细胞瘤分子遗传学异常，但无一有诊断特异性[60, 61]。1号染色体短臂缺失或重排是最常见的染色体异常[4, 60, 61]，N-myc是一种非常重要的评估预后的分子标记物，N-myc扩增提示预后不良[62, 63]。

用于预后评估的标记物有多种，细胞增殖相关抗原如Ki-67和REPP86，在侵袭性强及预后不良的神经母细胞瘤表达较强，而在生存期较长的肿瘤中则常表达缺如[64-66]。细胞表面糖蛋白CD44在组织分化好的

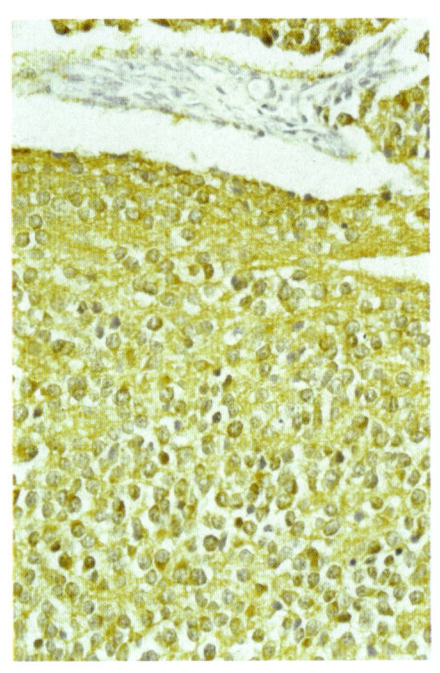

图15.2 神经特异性烯醇化酶在神经母细胞瘤呈胞浆弥漫阳性（免疫过氧化物酶染色，×400）

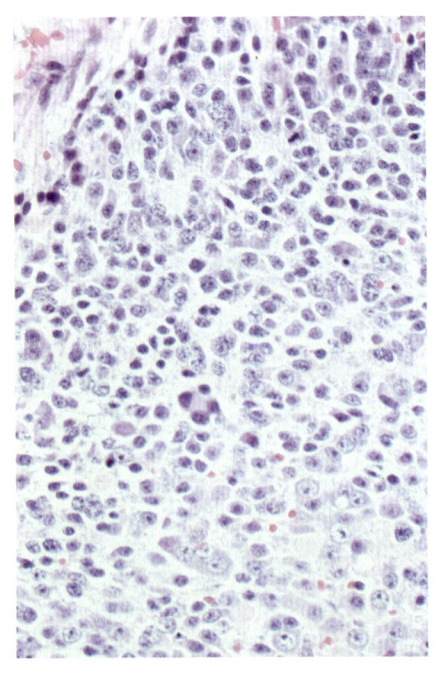

图15.1 有分化的神经母细胞瘤主要由小圆蓝细胞组成，可见少量大细胞，细胞核空泡状，胞质丰富而红染（HE染色，×200）

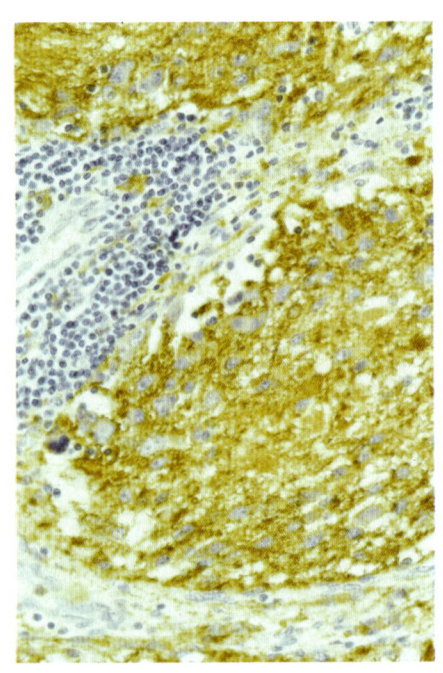

图15.3 突触素在神经母细胞瘤呈胞浆强阳性（免疫过氧化物酶染色，×400）

神经母细胞瘤呈阳性,阴性多见于分化差的病例[67-69]。c-kit对于预后的意义目前还有争议[70, 71]。凋亡标记物bcl-2与bax蛋白的表达与化疗反应性相关,可能会成为有用的评价预后的标记物[72]。基质金属蛋白酶及其特异性组织抑制剂有望用于预后评估[73]。TRK-A高表达伴或不伴有TRK-C表达与组织分化好和预后好相关。分化差和预后不好的肿瘤则表达TRK-B及其配体BDNF[49, 60, 61, 74-78]。

无明显节细胞或schwannian分化的低分化或未分化神经母细胞瘤与其他"小蓝细胞"肿瘤非常难区分,尤其是ES/PNET、白血病/淋巴瘤、横纹肌肉瘤及恶性横纹肌样瘤。合理使用肌源性标记物与淋巴造血组织标记物有助于识别横纹肌肉瘤、白血病和淋巴瘤。神经母细胞瘤通常波形蛋白、CD99阴性,据此可与ES/PNET鉴别[51]。恶性横纹肌样瘤除表达其他间叶标记物外,还表达波形蛋白、角蛋白与上皮细胞膜抗原,据此,可与神经母细胞瘤区分开来[79]。

> **诊断要点:** 神经母细胞瘤与神经母细胞性肿瘤
>
> 1. 神经母细胞性肿瘤表达神经元标记物,包括神经特异性烯醇化酶、Leu7、PGP9.5、突触素、嗜铬素等,但敏感性与特异性各异。
> 2. 神经母细胞性肿瘤通常呈波形蛋白、结蛋白、特异性肌源性抗原(如成肌素、Myo-D1)、角蛋白以及CD99阴性。
> 3. 在分化性神经母细胞瘤、节细胞神经母细胞瘤、节细胞瘤的schwannian间质呈S-100阳性表达。
> 4. TRK-A阳性提示神经母细胞瘤预后良好,而N-myc扩增则预后不佳。
> 5. 其他标记物如CD44和增殖相关抗原将来对预后分级会有帮助。

横纹肌肉瘤

横纹肌肉瘤(RMS)是儿童最常见的软组织肉瘤,占儿童实体瘤的5%~10%、软组织肉瘤的一半左右。这种原始的恶性肿瘤有胚胎性骨骼肌的形态与生物学特征[80, 81]。儿童和青少年RMS组织学亚型由RMS国际分类定义[80, 82-84]。在最近的方案中,WHO修正了此分类并且纳入多形性横纹肌肉瘤,该型主要见于成人。尽管各型横纹肌肉瘤均有骨骼肌分化特征,该瘤却通常发生于无骨骼肌分布的部位。临床上横纹肌肉瘤有两个发病高峰,一半以上的病例发生于10岁以内,另一发病高峰则见于青年。绝大多数胚胎性横纹肌肉瘤发生于5岁以下儿童,腺泡状横纹肌肉瘤则可见于任何年龄。胚胎性横纹肌肉瘤最常见部位为头、颈、泌尿生殖道,而腺泡状横纹肌肉瘤则好发于肢体末端[85]。大部分横纹肌肉瘤形成边界不清的肿块,鱼肉状,灰白或灰黑色,但某些类型有其特征性的大体表现,梭形细胞横纹肌肉瘤形成坚实的纤维性包块,切面漩涡状,似平滑肌肿瘤,葡萄状横纹肌肉瘤则形成息肉状外观,可见成串的广基或有蒂的结节,表面被覆上皮[85]。

儿童和青少年横纹肌肉瘤的WHO组织学分类,其主要亚型有葡萄状、梭形细胞、胚胎性(非特指)和腺泡状横纹肌肉瘤。非特指胚胎性横纹肌肉瘤约占横纹肌肉瘤的49%,细胞形态多样,可表现为从原始间叶细胞到高分化肿瘤性横纹肌细胞各种不同分化阶段的细胞,分化较好的细胞包括横纹肌母细胞、带状细胞、肌管等(图15.4),分化较差的细胞呈纺锤状或星芒状,胞浆少,细胞核和胞浆均不成熟。胚胎性横纹肌肉瘤这种原始的图像给病理鉴别诊断造成很大困难。葡萄状胚胎性横纹肌肉瘤约占横纹肌肉瘤的6%,特点是上皮下可见致密的多层肿瘤细胞,分化不一,显示不同程度的肌源性特征。梭形细胞胚胎性横纹肌肉瘤约占3%,包含细长的梭形细胞,排列成纺锤状、漩涡状或车辐状,肿瘤细胞间有多少不等的胶原纤维,这种图像与平滑肌肉瘤相似。葡萄状和梭形细胞胚胎性横纹肌肉瘤均为组织学形态/预后较好的亚型,而非特指胚胎性横纹肌肉瘤次之,腺泡状横纹肌肉瘤约占31%,属于组织学形态/预后不良的亚型。典型的腺泡状横纹肌肉瘤肿瘤细胞被网络状的纤维间隔分隔,肿瘤细胞沿纤维间隔排列,肿瘤细胞圆形,偶见多核细胞,胞浆有肌源性特征,散布于腺泡内(图15.5)。各型腺泡状横纹肌肉瘤的共同特征为细胞呈圆形,大小不一,横纹肌母细胞和带状细胞分化不明显,核圆或椭圆,核膜清晰,染色质粗糙,核仁不清或多个核仁。其微腺泡亚型和实体亚型,以及某些有灶性腺泡结构的胚胎性横纹肌肉瘤病例,在诊断时有一定难度。尽管横纹肌肉瘤国际分类尚未采用"间变"一词,但间变性均可见于胚胎性横纹肌肉瘤和腺泡状横纹肌肉瘤,并进一步归入组织学形态/预后不良的一类[83, 85-87]。

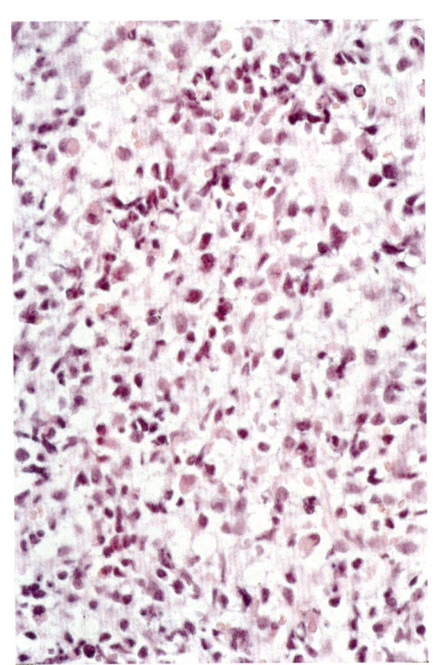

图 15.4 胚胎性横纹肌肉瘤由小圆细胞、多角形细胞、梭形细胞组成，胞浆嗜酸红染，多少不等，染色质浓染（HE染色，×200）

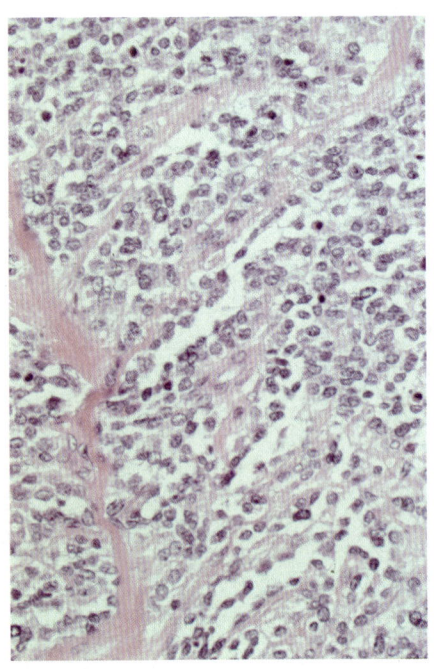

图 15.5 腺泡状横纹肌肉瘤小圆肿瘤细胞沿纤维血管间隔排列，中央为散在单个肿瘤细胞（HE 染色，×200）

图15.6列出了横纹肌肉瘤的免疫表型特点[21-26, 88, 89]。典型的阳性免疫标记物有波形蛋白、成肌素、Myo-D1、肌特异性肌动蛋白和结蛋白。早期免疫组织化学研究着重于肌动蛋白、肌凝蛋白、肌酸激酶、α-actinin、肌球蛋白和原肌球蛋白[90, 91]。其中只有肌球蛋白是骨骼肌分化的特异性标记物。尽管肌球蛋白特异性高，但只在不到一半的横纹肌肉瘤中呈阳性[92-95]。结蛋白（图15.7、15.8）和肌特异性肌动蛋白（图15.9、15.10）是敏感性非常强的标记物，但特异性不够，平滑肌细胞和肌纤维母细胞增生均可呈阳性[94-100]。对于横纹肌肉瘤，结蛋白多克隆抗体较单克隆抗体敏感性更强，胎儿重链肌凝蛋白在相当比例的病例呈阳性，但由于其缺乏特异性[100]，很少使用。横纹肌肉瘤分化程度影响免疫组化的结果，高分化横纹肌肉瘤 肌球蛋白、肌特异性肌动蛋白和结蛋白阳性率高。同时还取决于组织的固定方式，福尔马林固定切片、乙醇固定切片或冰冻切片的免疫组化反应性也有所不同[94]。

在一些疑似横纹肌肉瘤的病例应用生肌转录调节

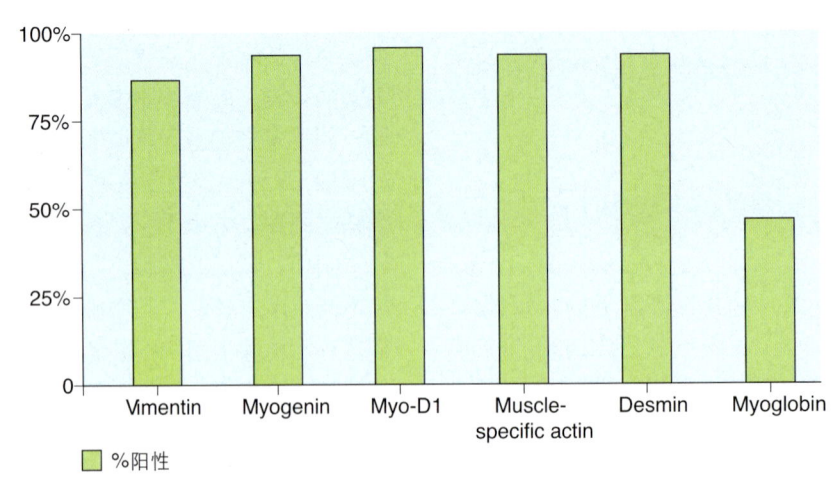

图 15.6 横纹肌肉瘤的免疫组化谱

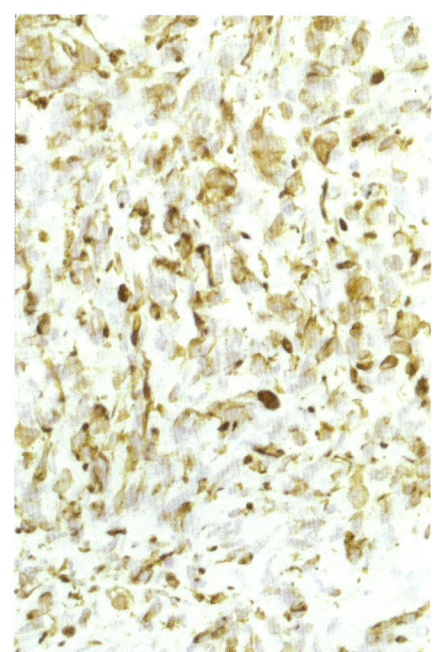

图15.7 胚胎性横纹肌肉瘤 结蛋白呈胞浆阳性，细长形的带状细胞尤为明显（免疫过氧化物酶染色，×200）

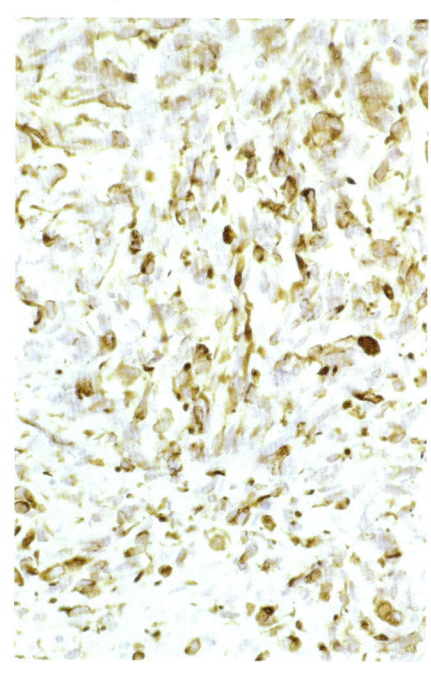

图15.9 胚胎性横纹肌肉瘤的梭形细胞和横纹肌母细胞显示肌特异性肌动蛋白呈胞浆阳性（免疫过氧化物酶染色，×400）

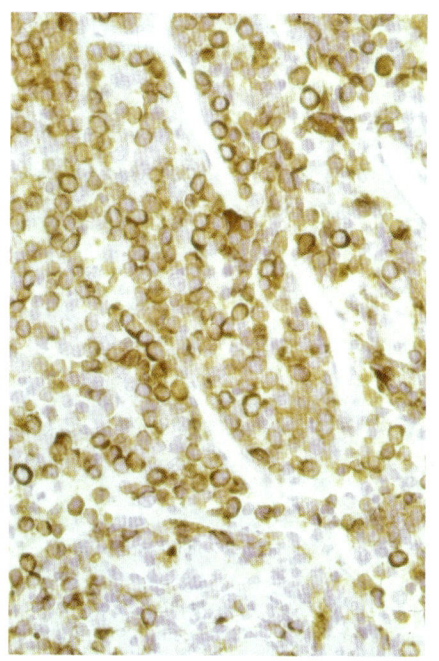

图15.8 腺泡状横纹肌肉瘤 结蛋白呈胞浆强阳性（免疫过氧化物酶染色，×400）

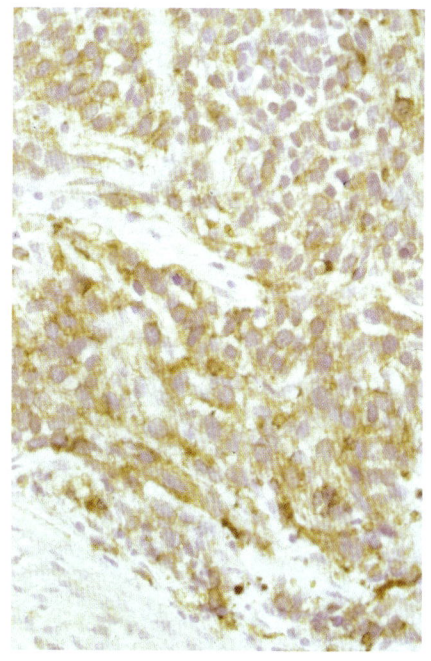

图15.10 腺泡状横纹肌肉瘤肌特异性肌动蛋白呈弥漫胞浆阳性（免疫过氧化物酶染色，×400）

蛋白成肌素（也称myf-4）和Myo-D1可以很好地确定有无骨骼肌分化。成肌素和Myo-D1是在横纹肌分化早期表达的生肌转录调节蛋白，在横纹肌肉瘤呈细胞核着色，为其特异而敏感的标记物[21-23, 25-27]。这两种生肌转录调节蛋白较肌球蛋白更敏感，较结蛋白和肌特异性肌动蛋白更特异。成肌素在腺泡状横纹肌肉瘤显示细胞核弥漫强阳性（图15.11），但在胚胎性横纹肌肉瘤阳性强度和分布则不一致（图15.12）[21, 23, 25, 26]。Myo-D1在横纹肌肉瘤主要呈细胞核阳性（图15.13），但在横纹肌母细胞及其他类型肿瘤细胞则胞浆也可着色[24]。从实际应用来讲，成肌素要优于Myo-D1，因为Myo-D1背景强，并且有胞浆着

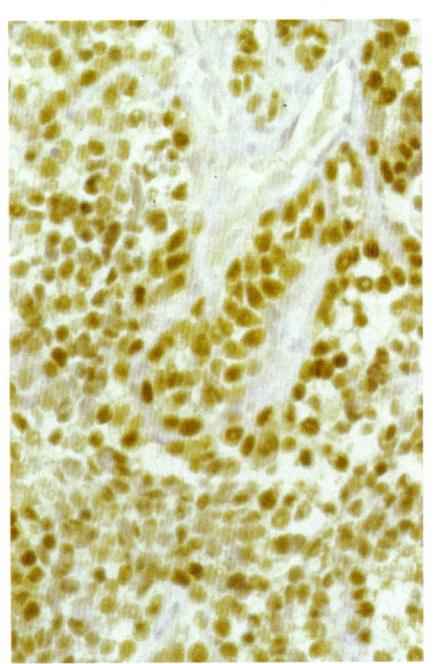

图15.11 腺泡状横纹肌肉瘤 成肌素呈胞核阳性，显示出腺泡状结构（免疫过氧化物酶染色，×400）

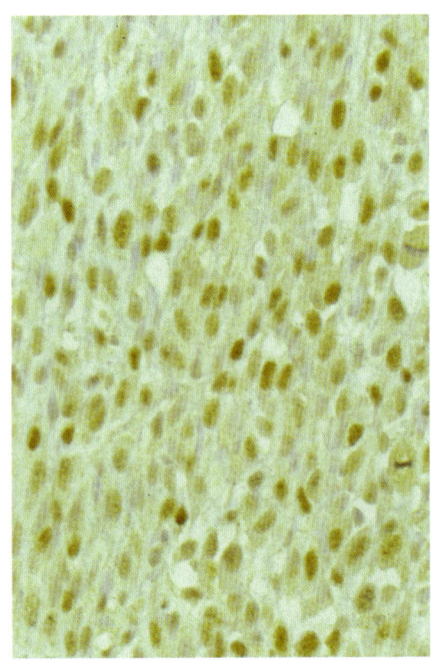

图15.13 Myo-D1 在横纹肌肉瘤呈胞核阳性，但因胞浆背景太强而不易辨认（免疫过氧化物酶染色，×400）

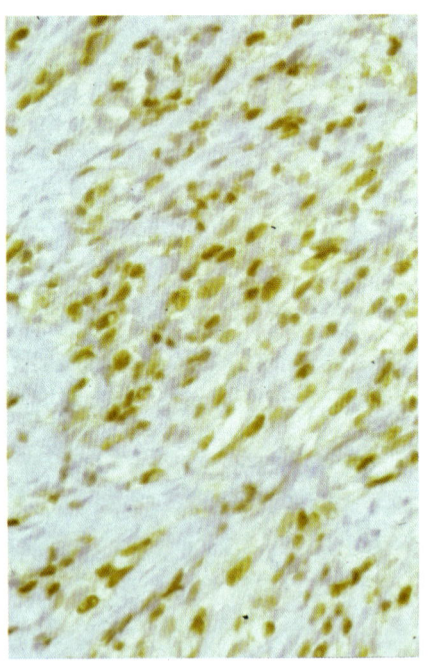

图15.12 胚胎性横纹肌肉瘤 成肌素胞核阳性程度不一（免疫过氧化物酶染色，×400）

色[21, 26]。然而，应注意横纹肌肉瘤各亚型免疫组化着色的多样性，有时会导致小标本出现假阴性。成肌素和Myo-D1均能用RT-PCR检出，但对于横纹肌肉瘤，成肌素比 Myo-D1 更特异[101]。

还有其他一些免疫组化指标在横纹肌肉瘤也呈阳性，如果不能将组织学与免疫组化结果结合分析，容易导致错误诊断。少数横纹肌肉瘤病例可观察到CD99、平滑肌肌动蛋白、ALK-1、CK、68kD神经丝蛋白以及S-100阳性[21, 23, 94, 102-104]。大部分的横纹肌肉瘤呈胎盘碱性磷酸酶阳性和WT-1胞浆阳性，但二者并无特异性[105, 106]。WT-1 在横纹肌肉瘤为胞浆着色，而在 Wilms 瘤则为胞核着色。

采用一组免疫组化指标对诊断横纹肌肉瘤最有帮助，可用成肌素、Myo-D1、肌特异性肌动蛋白和结蛋白来检测肿瘤的骨骼肌表型[7, 26, 89]。肌特异性肌动蛋白与结蛋白阳性亦见于平滑肌肿瘤、纤维瘤病、Wilms瘤、外胚层间质瘤、ES/PNET、恶性横纹肌样瘤、骨化性肌炎、恶性纤维组织细胞瘤及肝胚胎性肉瘤，但在神经母细胞瘤和视网膜母细胞瘤通常为阴性[94, 96, 97]。尽管成肌素和Myo-D1为骨骼肌分化特异抗原，但在有横纹肌或横纹肌母细胞特点的肿瘤如横纹肌性Wilms瘤、外胚层间质瘤、多向分化的恶性外周神经鞘瘤以及胚胎性、萎缩及再生的横纹肌均可对这些标记物有反应[21, 25, 26]。成肌素和Myo-D1通常在神经母细胞瘤、ES/PNET、纤维母-肌纤维母肿瘤、平滑肌肿瘤、腺泡状软组织肉瘤、滑膜肉瘤、恶性横纹肌样瘤、DSRCT、嗅神经母细胞瘤、造血组织肿瘤和癌呈阴性[21, 23, 25, 26]。

近年来，细胞遗传学与分子遗传学研究在横纹肌肉瘤及其各亚型的评价中占据重要地位[13, 14, 83-85, 87]。

大部分的腺泡状横纹肌肉瘤存在与PAX相关的两种易位中的一种。其中t（2;13）(q35;q14)易位较常见，其嵌合产物为PAX 3-FKHR，t（1;13）(p36;q14)易位少见，其嵌合产物为PAX 7-FKHR。少数腺泡状横纹肌肉瘤不显示上述任何一种易位。常规细胞遗传学方法、RT-PCR或荧光原位杂交（FISH）均可检测到易位。胚胎性横纹肌肉瘤显示多种细胞遗传学异常，包括11p15.5杂合性缺失及11q上可能存在肿瘤相关位点，但至今尚未发现特征性的遗传学异常。

横纹肌肉瘤的预后相关标记物有p53和增殖抗原，免疫组化检测PCNA或MIB-1（Ki-67）显示的高增殖指数与生存率低、复发率高、肿瘤进展快相关[107,108]。p53过度表达与MIB-1高表达、预后差相关[109,110]。间变性横纹肌肉瘤同样呈p53阳性[87]。

> **诊断要点：横纹肌肉瘤**
>
> 1. 根据横纹肌肉瘤国际分类，横纹肌肉瘤分为胚胎性、腺泡状、梭形细胞和葡萄状等亚型，很多病例仅靠光镜即可诊断。
> 2. 横纹肌肉瘤免疫组化标记物包括生肌转录调节蛋白，成肌素与Myo-D1、肌特异性肌动蛋白、结蛋白和肌球蛋白。
> 3. 成肌素和Myo-D1是横纹肌肉瘤特异性和敏感性最高的指标，但不同亚型着色分布与着色模式不同。
> 4. 对于疑难病例，RT-PCR或FISH检测染色体易位可能对于腺泡状横纹肌肉瘤的诊断有帮助，但尚未发现胚胎性横纹肌肉瘤存在特异的遗传学异常。
> 5. CK、CD99及其他一些标记物在横纹肌肉瘤中的异常表达易导致误诊。

Ewing肉瘤/原始神经外胚层肿瘤

Ewing肉瘤/原始神经外胚层肿瘤（ES/PNET）是一种原始小圆细胞肉瘤，伴不同程度神经外胚层分化[111]。过去根据光镜、电镜及免疫组化显示的神经外胚层分化特征，ES与PNET的诊断是分开的，但是近年认识到二者有共同的分子遗传学异常、临床过程和预后，属同一实体。ES与PNET作为同一概念已经收入当前的WHO骨与软组织分类中[111]。

ES/PNET是儿童第二常见的骨与软组织肉瘤，骨较常见，骨外ES/PNET占到15%[112]，男性多见。骨的ES/PNET多起源于长骨、骨盆和肋骨[111]，亦可作为播散性肿瘤，发生在体表或深部软组织而无明显的原发灶，或发生于内脏器官如肾[112-116]。ES/PNET可见于任何年龄，发病年龄不是诊断的考虑因素，发病高峰为10～20岁，大多数病人就诊时不超过20岁。肿瘤常呈有坏死、出血的灰白或灰黑色肿块，极少数病例与周围神经有关联[111]。

ES/PNET组织学图像，由小而一致的圆细胞到大而不规则的细胞组成，甚至呈梭形细胞（图15.14）。小圆肿瘤细胞核圆，染色质细腻，胞浆稀少，细胞界限不清，大肿瘤细胞核轮廓不整，形成假菊形团或巢状排列。地图状坏死常见，坏死区内可见残存的细胞团，围绕在血管周围。超微结构显示从未分化间叶细胞到神经分化的特点。肿瘤细胞通常含有中间丝、细胞连接（包括桥粒），还可见丰富的糖原、电子致密颗粒和神经小管[8,117,118]。

图15.15列举了ES/PNET的各种免疫标记物[40,119-121]。典型的免疫表型为波形蛋白、CD99（O13、HBA-71、mic-2）阳性，神经特异性烯醇化酶、CD57、突触素、CK不同程度阳性。极少数病例对结蛋白和神经胶质酸性蛋白（glial fibrillary acidic protein, GFAP）呈阳性，白细胞共同抗原和肌动蛋白通常阴性[30,52,120]。神经标记物表达情况与预后没有关系[119]。

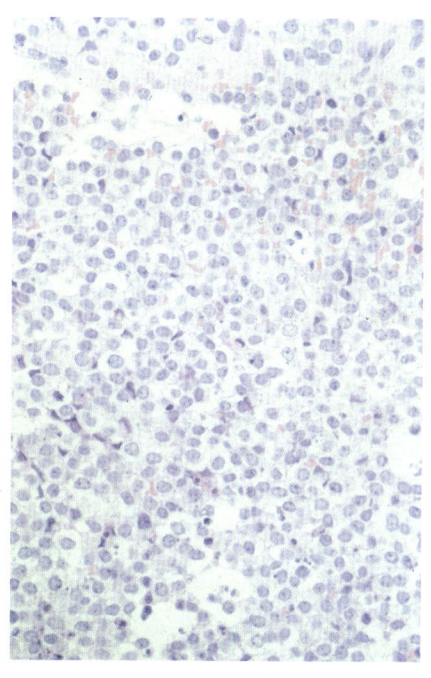

图15.14 ES/PNET肿瘤细胞紧密排列成片状，细胞小到中等大小，圆，边界不清，胞浆少且透明，核圆或椭圆，染色质细（HE染色，×200）

CD99一般呈细胞膜阳性（图15.16），最初被看做ES/PNET高度特异性标记物，但目前认为尽管其敏感性高达84%～100%，特异性却有限[32, 33, 41, 122]。CD99是一种细胞表面抗原，但与EWS基因的易位无关。其他CD99阳性与ES/PNET相似的肿瘤包括横纹肌肉瘤、神经胶质肿瘤、神经内分泌肿瘤、部分癌、淋巴母细胞淋巴瘤、Wilms瘤、子宫肉瘤、肾透明细胞肉瘤、畸胎瘤、骨肉瘤和间叶性软骨肉瘤[32, 33, 39, 123]。所幸Wilms瘤的胚基成分CD99为阴性。鉴别ES/PNET与淋巴母细胞淋巴瘤非常困难，因为二者CD99均为细胞膜浆着色[32, 124]。结合TdT、CD43、CD34、CD10、CD79a免疫组化染色结果和基因重排分析可将淋巴母细胞淋巴瘤与ES/PNET区分开来[40, 124]。波形蛋白在大部分ES/PNET呈阳性，而在淋巴母细胞淋巴瘤只有不到25%的阳性率。神经特异性烯醇化酶不是鉴别二者的可靠指标（图15.17）。

ES/PNET可有位于染色体22q12上的*EWS*基因与其他基因的易位，其中位于11q24上的*FLI-1*基因最常见，EWS/FLI-1包括几种融合转录亚型[125-129]。常规细胞遗传学、FISH和RT-PCR可检测到这些基因异常[13, 14]。*EWS*和*FLI-1*基因易位导致的FLI-1蛋白过度表达可见于71%～100%的ES/PNET病例[43, 44]，仅

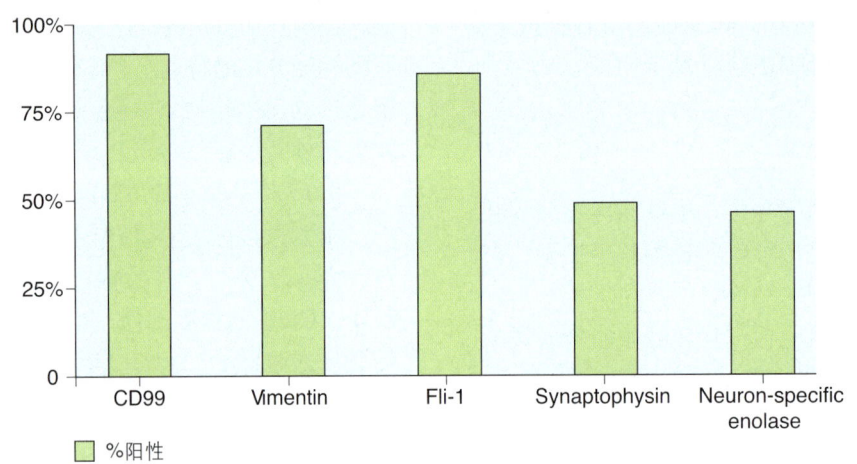

图15.15　ES/PNET的免疫组化谱

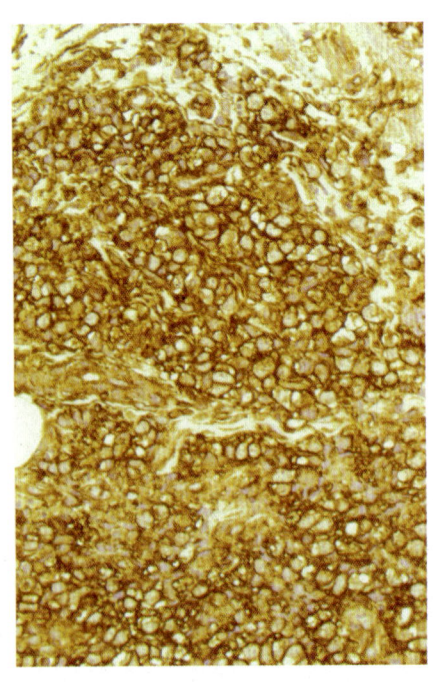

图15.16　CD99（O13）在ES/PNET呈胞膜和胞浆着色（免疫过氧化物酶染色，×400）

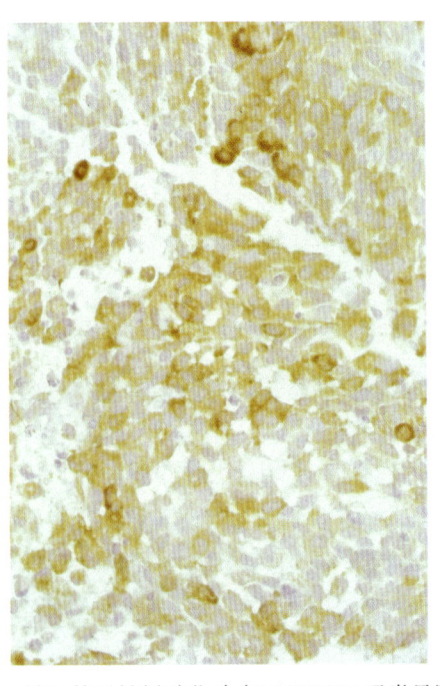

图15.17　神经特异性烯醇化酶在ES/PNET通常呈阳性，但也可见于其他多种肿瘤（免疫过氧化物酶染色，×400）

细胞核着色才视作阳性（图15.18）。但其他一些与ES/PNET难以鉴别的肿瘤免疫组化也呈现FLI-1阳性，如近90%的淋巴母细胞淋巴瘤、DSRCT、恶性黑色素瘤、Merkel细胞癌、滑膜肉瘤、部分癌及血管肿瘤（如血管瘤、血管肉瘤、上皮样血管内皮瘤、血管球瘤、Kaposi肉瘤）。尽管有文献报道在横纹肌肉瘤未观察到FLI-1阳性，但笔者曾观察到多例横纹肌肉瘤尤其是腺泡状横纹肌肉瘤呈FLI-1阳性。当组织学形态典型时，根据光镜下以及免疫组化CD99和FLI-1阳性，而淋巴母细胞、上皮及肌源性标记物阴性时可诊断ES/PNET[130]。有人主张把RT-PCR作为明确ES/PNET诊断的一种常规手段[123]，但是现在证明除非是不常见的ES/PNET组织学亚型如上皮样、梭形细胞或结蛋白阳性肿瘤，否则不需要遗传学检测。

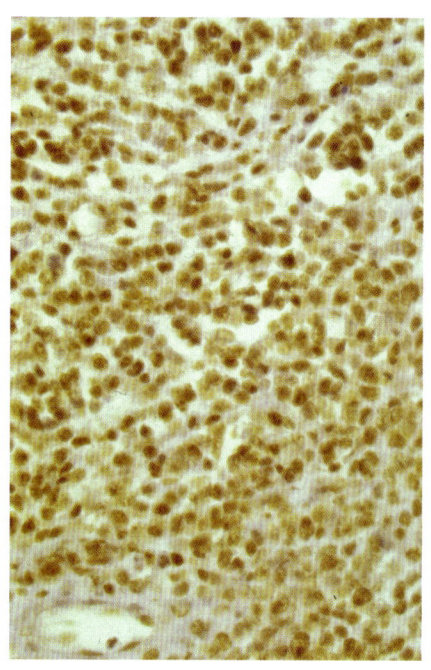

图15.18　FLI-1在ES/PNET呈细胞核着色，但也可见于其他小圆细胞肿瘤，尤其是淋巴母细胞淋巴瘤（免疫过氧化物酶染色，×400）

诊断要点： Ewing肉瘤／原始神经外胚层肿瘤

1. 组织学上，ES/PNET从原始小圆细胞肿瘤至肿瘤主要由圆细胞组成，并形成小叶状或形成假菊形团。
2. 免疫组化特点为：波形蛋白、CD99、FLI-1阳性，神经标记物阳性程度不一。
3. ES/PNET存在涉及*EWS*基因的一系列细胞遗传学异常，最常见的是发生于染色体11和22的易位。
4. FLI-1表达仅见于存在染色体22上的*EWS*基因与染色体11上的*FLI-1*基因易位的病例。
5. 利用免疫组化可将ES/PNET与横纹肌肉瘤及其他相似的"小蓝细胞"肿瘤鉴别开来，CD99、FLI-1均不够特异，需要一组免疫组化指标帮助鉴别诊断。
6. CD99在淋巴瘤/白血病呈强阳性容易造成一个严重的诊断陷阱，不过使用一组免疫组化指标可以避免诊断错误。
7. 细胞遗传学和分子遗传学检测在疑难病例的鉴别诊断中有帮助。

促结缔组织增生性小圆细胞肿瘤

促结缔组织增生性小圆细胞肿瘤（DSRCT）是一种主要见于儿童和青年的多形性恶性肿瘤，侵袭性强，男性多见，发病年龄涵盖婴幼儿到50岁之内的成年人[138-140]。典型的DSRCT为腹膜广泛播散的结节，也可见于胸腔、睾丸旁区、头颈部、中枢神经系统和肢体末端[141-144]。肉眼，肿瘤为巨大的多结节肿块，表面凸起，光滑[145,146]。

典型的组织学形态表现为小圆肿瘤细胞呈巢状排列，被致密的胶原纤维或纤维黏液样间质分隔[145]，肿瘤细胞可为小圆细胞、棒状细胞或透明细胞，可见中央坏死及囊性变（图15.19）[145]。组织结构多样，可形成菊形团，可见局灶上皮分化，间质富于血管，核分裂多见。电镜下见胞浆内中间丝多少不一，即某些DSRCT光镜下所见到的横纹[11]。

DSRCT可同时表达上皮性标记物与间叶性抗原。波形蛋白、CK、上皮细胞膜抗原、结蛋白、神经特异性烯醇化酶和WT-1阳性有一定特异性。图15.20是来自7组研究报告的DSRCT免疫组化表达情况[36,45-47,139,145,147]。几乎所有病例均表达波形蛋白（图15.21），约90%的病例同时表达角蛋白（图15.22）和上皮细胞膜抗原（图15.23）。有人发现细胞角蛋白CAM5.2比细胞角蛋白AE1/AE3敏感[36]，而另外有人报道二者阳性率相似[47]。结蛋白（图15.24）为胞浆弥漫或点灶状着色。使用抗C-末端WT-1抗体，近90%的病例呈细胞核阳性（图15.25）。只有不到30%的DSRCT表达CD99，并且缺乏ES/PNET的细胞膜阳性模式。神经特异性烯醇化酶在79%的DSRCT病例中有表达，但是其他神经标记物如突触素、嗜铬素、神经丝蛋白、胶质酸性蛋白及S-100为阴性或很少表达[36, 46, 47, 139, 145, 147]。此外，即便有也只有极少数DSRCT对平滑肌肌动蛋白、肌特异性肌动蛋白或肌球蛋白和成肌素呈阳性反应，Myo-D1阴性。CD57、CD15、CA125、Ber-EP4、MOC-31、胎盘碱性磷酸酶和Her-2阳性易误导诊断[36, 147]。曾有calretinin和c-kit阳性的散发病例[36]。

尽管免疫组化对于明确DSRCT的诊断非常有用，但仍可能难以与其他组织学多样的小细胞肿瘤鉴别，如极少数ES/PNET、Wilms瘤、恶性横纹肌样瘤和滑膜肉瘤。尽管与DSRCT一样对结蛋白、肌球蛋白、肌特异性肌动蛋白呈阳性，但横纹肌肉瘤的特点是成肌素和Myo-D1阳性。如果不能识别胚基为主型Wilms瘤的上皮成分，鉴别诊断将比较困难，不过分子或细胞遗传学检测有助于其与DSRCT的鉴别。滑膜肉瘤较DSRCT有不同的组织学图像，免疫组化bcl-2强阳性，此外，尚存在X染色体与染色体18易位。恶性横纹肌样瘤也是一种形态多样的小细胞恶性肿瘤，WT-1阴性，无EWS/WT-1融合，但有与INI-1有关的遗传学异常。在遇到疑难或临床表现不典型的病例时，采用FISH或RT-PCR技术检测t（11;22）（p13;q12）易位和EWS-WT-1基因重排以支持DSRCT的诊断。由上述易位引起的WT-1过度表达可通过抗C-末端WT-1抗体检测，表现为细胞核着色[45, 46, 149]。

最近曾通过免疫组化发现DSRCT病例自分泌生长因子和旁分泌生长因子如转化生长因子β-1、血小板源性生长因子受体α、血小板源性生长因子-AB链、胰岛素样生长因子2和结缔组织生长因子表达上升[155, 156]。尚未发现这些结果有诊断、治疗和预后意义。

> **诊断要点：促结缔组织增生性小圆细胞肿瘤**
>
> 1. 波形蛋白、CK、上皮细胞膜抗原、结蛋白和WT-1共同表达支持DSRCT的诊断。
> 2. 分子学或细胞遗传学检测发现EWS-WT-1基因融合支持DSRCT的诊断。
> 3. WT-1阳性和缺乏CD99细胞膜阳性着色模式有助于DSRCT与ES/PTEN的鉴别。
> 4. 生肌调节蛋白、成肌素和Myo-D1阴性有助于DSRCT与横纹肌肉瘤鉴别，二者结蛋白、肌球蛋白和肌动蛋白均为阳性。
> 5. WT-1阳性和EWS-WT-1基因融合能鉴别DSRCT与恶性横纹肌样瘤，后者也是一种组织学多样的小细胞恶性肿瘤。

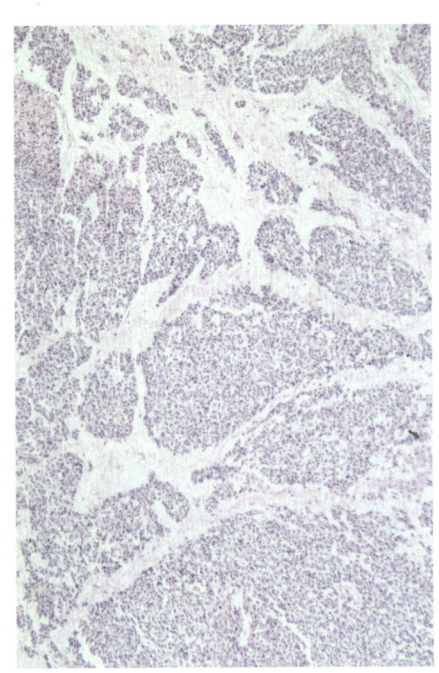

图15.19　DSRCT肿瘤细胞圆形或多边形，被纤维组织分隔成巢状（HE染色，×100）

恶性横纹肌样瘤

恶性横纹肌样瘤是发生于婴幼儿和儿童的一种有高度侵袭性、有广泛转移倾向的恶性肿瘤[157-159]。最早描述见于肾[159-161]和中枢神经系统[162, 163]，目前知道也可见于其他脏器、肾外软组织及先天性散发病例，有累及中枢神经系统及其他部位的家族性病例的报道[79, 158, 164, 165]。大多数肿瘤发生于儿童，且无性别差别，真正的恶性横纹肌样瘤成人罕见。这些原始肿瘤形态多样，因肿瘤细胞呈横纹肌细胞样外观而得名。肉眼肿瘤为灰白或灰褐色肿块，柔软，有灶性出血和坏死。

组织学上，恶性横纹肌样瘤肿瘤细胞密集，呈巢状或条索状排列，细胞核圆或椭圆，空泡状，中央为嗜酸性大核仁，胞浆丰富，嗜酸，偏心性（图15.26）。组织学图像多样常见，部分肿瘤只有少量典型的横纹肌样细胞或呈现原始"小蓝细胞"特点，黏液样背景，细胞排列松散，肿瘤细胞条索之间为多量胶原沉积，并散在非肿瘤性破骨细胞样巨细胞，极少数肿瘤有局灶上皮分化，核分裂多见。电镜下发现胞浆内中间丝呈漩涡状，即光镜下见到的典型横纹肌样细胞内的嗜酸性颗粒。

免疫组化作为辅助方法对于恶性横纹肌样瘤诊断意义不大，因为很多肿瘤都有横纹肌样外观。图15.27显示了从4组研究中挑选出来的恶性横纹肌样

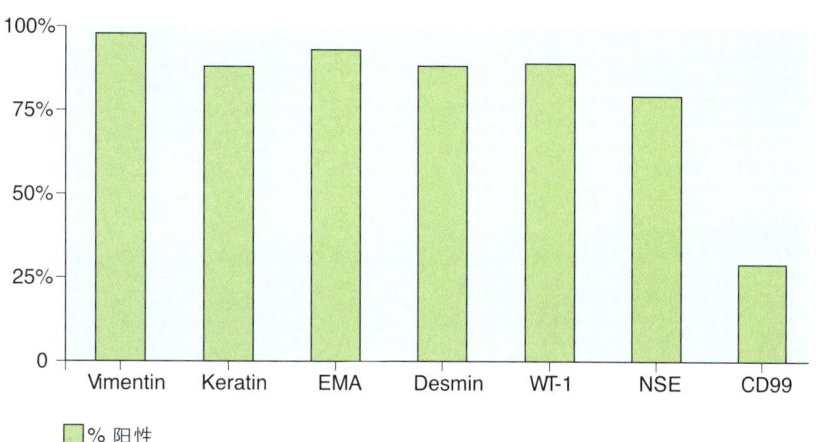

图 15.20 DSRCT 的免疫组化谱

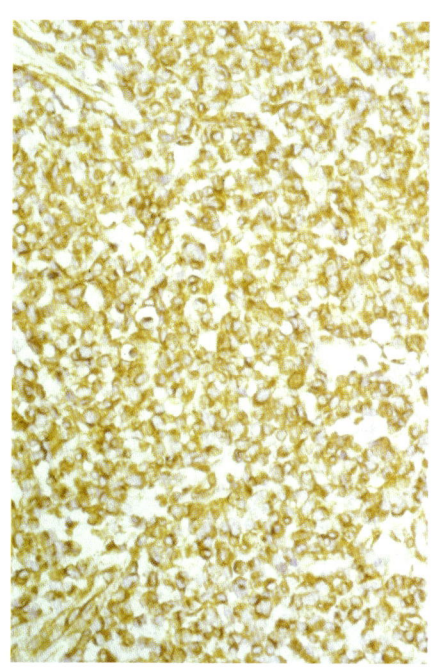

图 15.21 波形蛋白在 DSRCT 呈弥漫胞浆阳性（免疫过氧化物酶染色，×400）

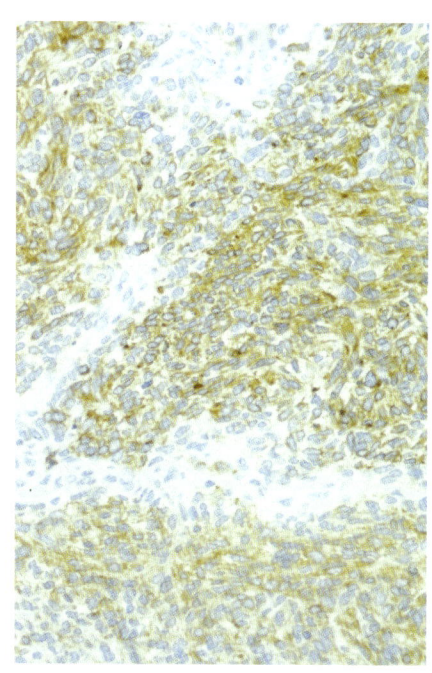

图 15.22 CK 在 DSRCT 呈胞浆阳性（免疫过氧化物酶染色，×200）

瘤最常用的免疫组化指标[79, 158, 164, 165]。该肿瘤是一种形态多样的肿瘤，可同时表达波形蛋白（图 15.28），至少一种上皮标记物如 CK（图 15.29）或上皮细胞膜抗原（图15.30），神经外胚层标记物如神经特异性烯醇化酶、突触素（图15.31），或 CD99、间叶组织标记物如肌特异性肌动蛋白（图15.32）和 S-100[79, 158, 164, 165]。其他标记物如平滑肌肌动蛋白、癌胚抗原、胶质酸性蛋白和神经丝蛋白也可能呈阳性[162, 165]。而成肌素、肌球蛋白、HMB-45、嗜铬素和 CD34 通常为阴性[165]。横纹肌样嗜酸性胞浆内包涵体包括波形蛋白和CK8在内的细胞骨架蛋白。该肿瘤存在人CK基因突变[167]。

染色体 22q11 异常是恶性横纹肌样瘤的特点[79, 164, 165]。其细胞遗传学异常包括 22 染色体单体、22q11 缺失、22q11.2 易位、INI-1（hSNF5）基因突变或杂合性缺失[157, 170-172]。FISH 是一种检测染色体缺失非常有用的方法[173]。近来，中枢神经系统恶性横纹肌样瘤免疫组化分析显示 INI-1 蛋白阴性（图 15.33），与 hSNF-5/INI-1 基因突变和缺失密切相关[48]。

最近的研究表明中枢神经系统恶性横纹肌样瘤表达胰岛素样生长因子2、胰岛素样生长因子1型受体和组织蛋白酶 D[174]，而不表达 β-连环素[175]。

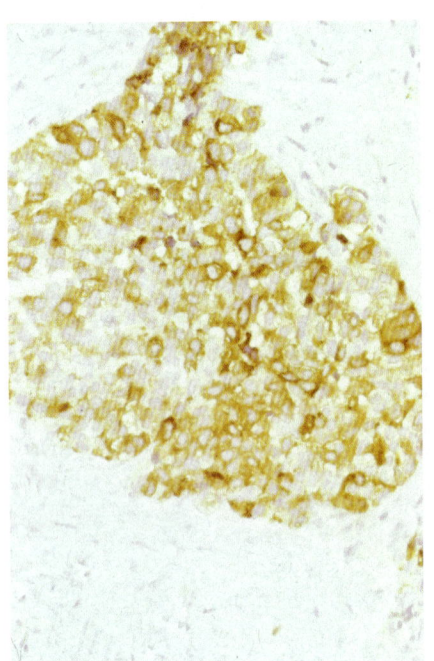

图 15.23 上皮细胞膜抗原在 DSRCT 呈胞浆和胞膜阳性（免疫过氧化物酶染色，×400）

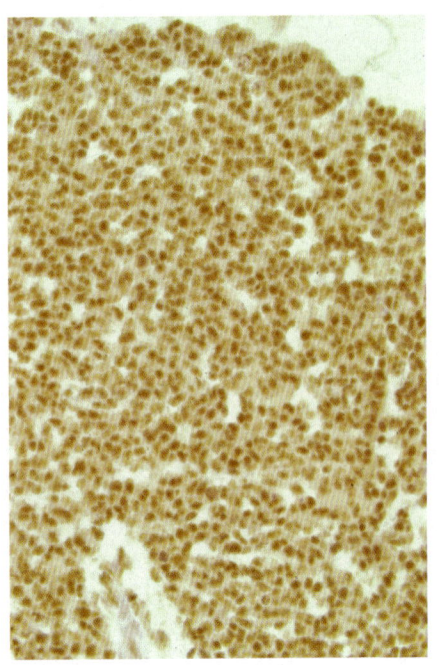

图 15.25 采用抗 C-末端 WT-1 抗体，DSRCT 肿瘤细胞呈弥漫核着色（免疫过氧化物酶染色，×400）

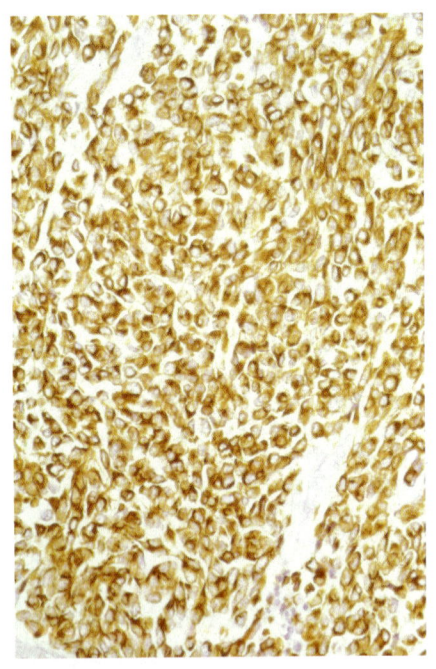

图 15.24 结蛋白在 DSRCT 呈弥漫胞浆强阳性（免疫过氧化物酶染色，×400）

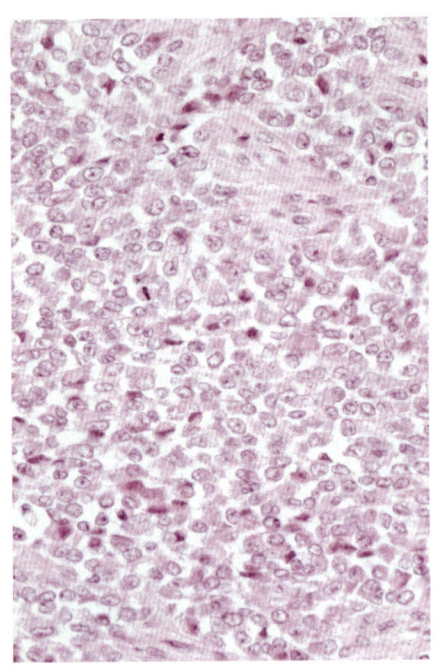

图 15.26 恶性横纹肌样瘤由成片的圆形肿瘤细胞构成，细胞核呈空泡状，核仁明显，胞浆嗜酸，多少不等，胞浆内偶见大的嗜酸性小体（HE 染色，×200）

免疫组化多样性给恶性横纹肌样瘤鉴别诊断带来困难，尤其是与 DSRCT、横纹肌肉瘤、脉络丛癌和上皮样肉瘤鉴别。与其他相似肿瘤比较，恶性横纹肌样瘤无 INI-1 蛋白表达，并且应用横纹肌分化的标记物如成肌素和 Myo-D1 对于鉴别诊断非常有帮助。对于有疑问的病例，细胞遗传学和分子遗传学分析可作为辅助诊断手段。

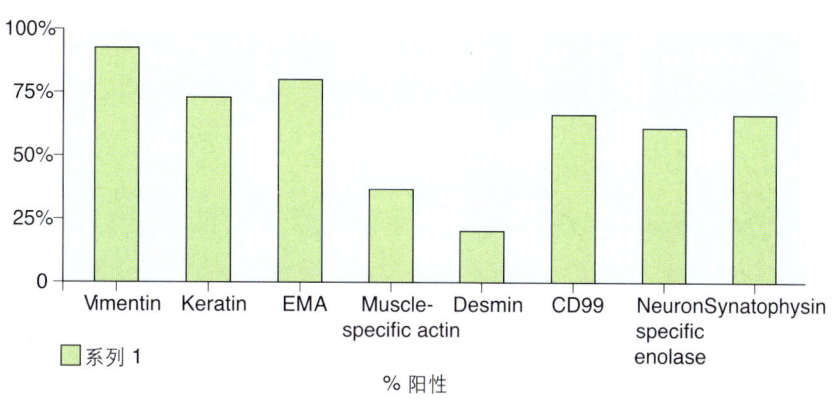

图 15.27 恶性横纹肌样瘤的免疫组化谱

诊断要点：恶性横纹肌样瘤

1. 恶性横纹肌样瘤是一种有高度侵袭性、形态多样、有广泛转移或播散倾向的恶性肿瘤。
2. 恶性横纹肌样瘤中的横纹肌样肿瘤细胞比例多少不一，组织学图像多样，可与ES/PNET、髓母细胞瘤、横纹肌肉瘤、DSRCT、上皮样肉瘤和其他一些原始恶性肿瘤形态相似。
3. 恶性横纹肌样瘤显示波形蛋白弥漫阳性，至少一种上皮标记物局灶阳性，间叶和神经外胚层标记物阳性程度不一。
4. INI-1蛋白表达阴性支持恶性横纹肌样瘤诊断，可帮助与其他无 *INI-1* 突变或缺失、INI-1阳性肿瘤进行鉴别诊断。
5. 若分子遗传学检测证实染色体 22q11 异常则支持恶性横纹肌样瘤的诊断。

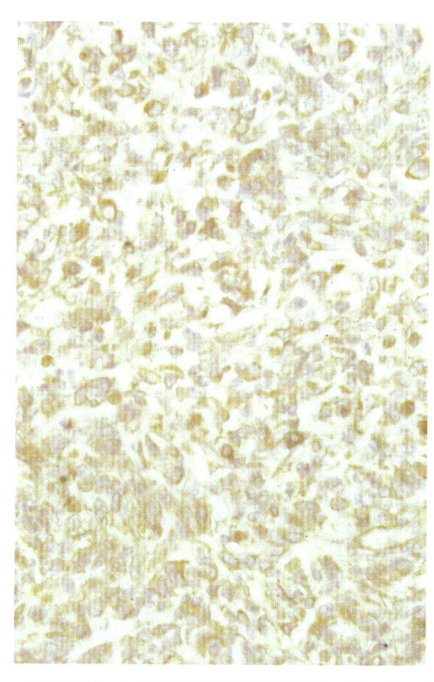

图15.28 波形蛋白在恶性横纹肌样瘤呈胞浆阳性（免疫过氧化物酶染色，×400）

Wilms 瘤

Wilms 瘤即肾母细胞瘤，是儿童最常见的肾肿瘤。98% 的病例发生于 10 岁以前，无性别差异，来源于肾胚基细胞，组织学可重复肾发生各阶段的图像，并可有不同分化方向[176]。大多数 Wilms 瘤为单源性，7% 为多源性，5% 为双源性。肿瘤为边界非常清楚的圆形实性肿物，质软，切面灰白或灰褐色。

典型的 Wilms 瘤包含 3 种成分，即肾胚基成分、上皮成分、间质成分（图 15.34）。3 种成分所占比例各异，亦可见双相分化或单相分化。胚基细胞小，圆或椭圆，排列紧密，呈弥漫结节状或蜿蜒条索状。上皮成分可排列成原始管样结构，呈菊形团样外观，或形成明显的管状或乳头状结构。异源上皮成分包括黏液上皮和鳞状上皮。间质分化包括纤维组织、平滑肌、骨骼肌、脂肪组织、软骨、骨和神经组织（包括神经节细胞、神经纤维和神经胶质细胞）[176, 177]。北美国家 Wilms 瘤研究组织和欧洲 SIOP 标准共同规范了 Wilms 瘤的病理学评估标准[16, 19, 178]。5% 的 Wilms 瘤肿瘤细胞核有间变，特征为多极性，多核，核显著增大，染色质密集。胚基成分容易给诊断带来困难，因为其图像与其他小圆细胞相似。蓝染的胚基细胞一致聚集成片，细胞之间黏附性降低。需与淋巴瘤、ES/PNET、神经母细胞瘤、DSRCT 和横纹肌肉瘤鉴别。

Wilms 瘤无特别的免疫表型。胚基成分对波形蛋白通常呈阳性，结蛋白也多为阳性（图 15.35）[176, 179]。

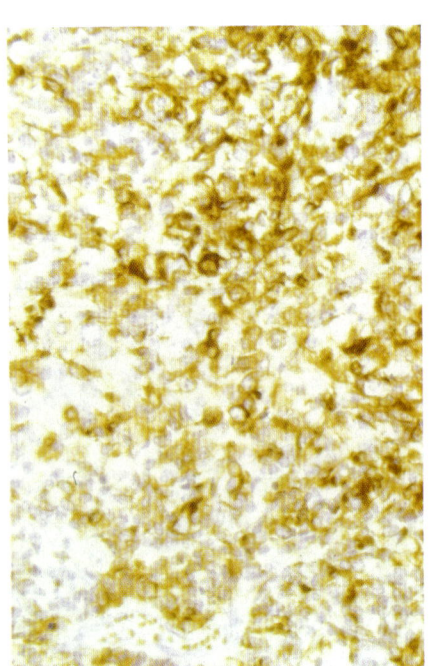

图15.29 恶性横纹肌样瘤显示细胞角蛋白CAM5.2程度不等的胞浆阳性（免疫过氧化物酶染色，×400）

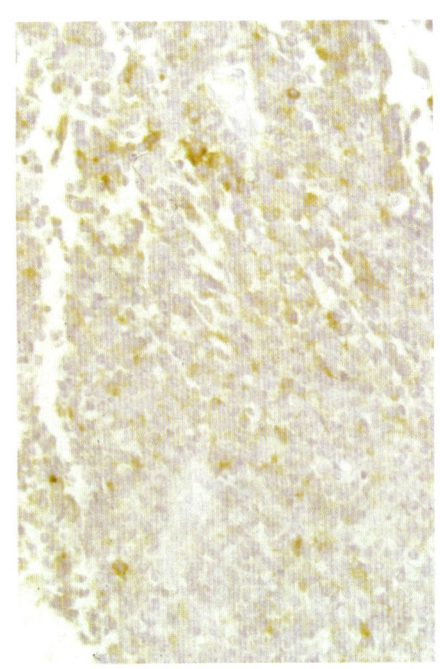

图15.31 突触素在恶性横纹肌样瘤呈胞浆弱阳性，着色较淡（免疫过氧化物酶染色，×400）

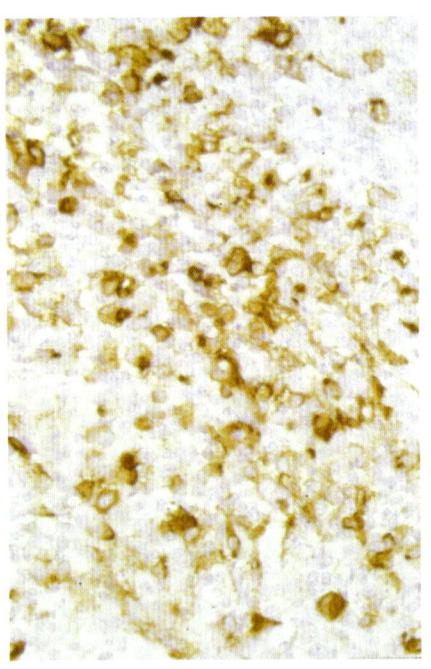

图15.30 上皮细胞膜抗原在恶性横纹肌样瘤呈局灶胞浆强阳性（免疫过氧化物酶染色，×400）

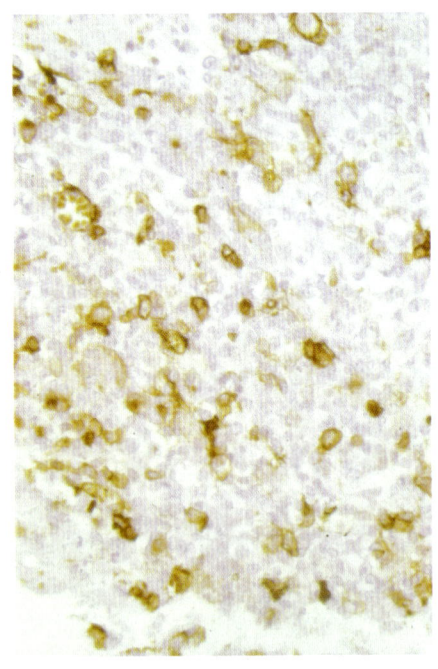

图15.32 肌特异性肌动蛋白在恶性横纹肌样瘤呈局灶胞浆阳性（免疫过氧化物酶染色，×400）

其他肌肉标记物如成肌素和Myo-D1在胚基成分为阴性表达，在骨骼肌分化区则为阳性。WT-1在胚基成分为阳性，在早期上皮分化区为局灶阳性，细胞核着色（图15.36）[180]。一些上皮分化较成熟的区域如肾小管通常CK（图15.37）、CD56、CD57阳性。胚基

组织对神经特异性烯醇化酶和CK也可有局灶阳性，但CD99阴性[176]。Wilms瘤的神经分化区神经特异性烯醇化酶、突触素、嗜铬素为阳性，但胶质酸性蛋白和S-100蛋白表达情况则差别较大[177,181]。CD99阴性有助于把胚基成分为主的Wilms瘤与ES/PNET区分

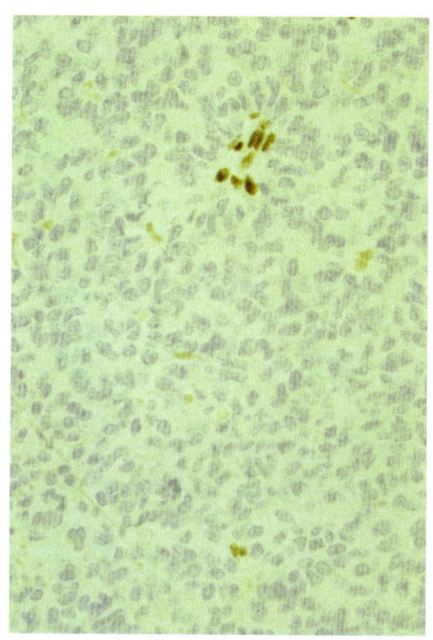

图 15.33 中枢神经系统恶性横纹肌样瘤显示 INI-1 蛋白阴性表达，与 hSNF5/INI-1 基因缺失和突变有关（免疫过氧化物酶染色，×400）

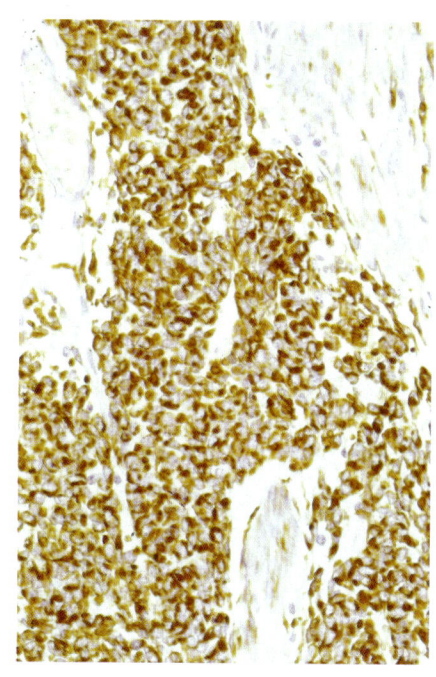

图 15.35 结蛋白在 Wilms 瘤胚基区呈胞浆强阳性（免疫过氧化物酶染色，×400）

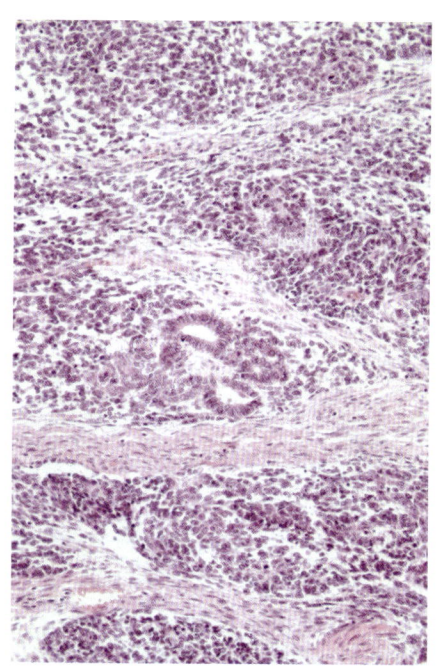

图 15.34 典型的 Wilms 瘤组织学图像包含3种成分，小管状上皮分化成分、片状排列的圆形原始胚基细胞和纤维间质（HE 染色，×200）

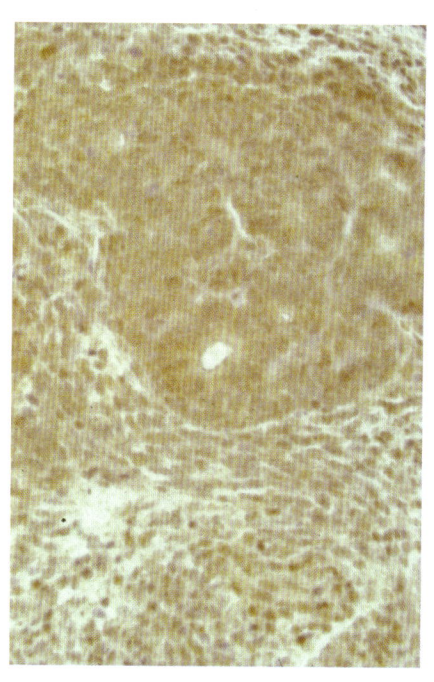

图 15.36 WT-1 在 Wilms 瘤胚基区和原始上皮区呈胞核阳性（免疫过氧化物酶染色，×400）

开来。总之，正确诊断 Wilms 瘤最重要的依据是临床上幼儿肾肿块的病史和组织学出现胚基、上皮和间质3种成分。

评估 Wilms 瘤预后的重要免疫组化指标包括 p53、CD44、生长因子、增殖相关抗原、血管源性标记物以及凋亡标记物。p53 突变见于 73%～100% 的间变性 Wilms 瘤（图 15.38、15.39）[182]。但有研究表明 p53 阳性与肿瘤进展和复发相关，尽管还存在争议[183,184]。同时认为 bcl-2 表达增加导致的凋亡失控亦影响预后[187]。CD44 在胚基成分表达与临床分期、肿瘤进展速

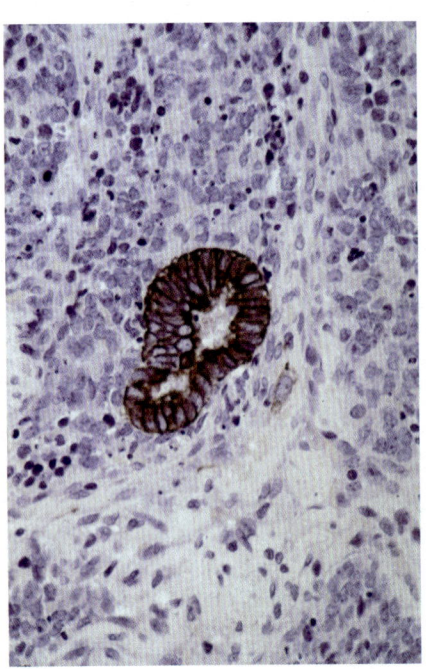

图 15.37　CK 在 Wilms 瘤管状上皮分化区呈阳性（免疫过氧化物酶染色，×400）

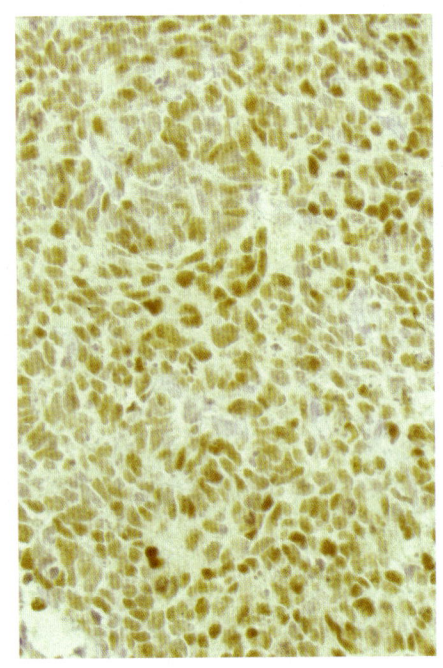

图 15.39　间变性 Wilms 瘤显示 p53 呈胞核阳性，这与 p53 突变有关（免疫过氧化物酶染色，×400）

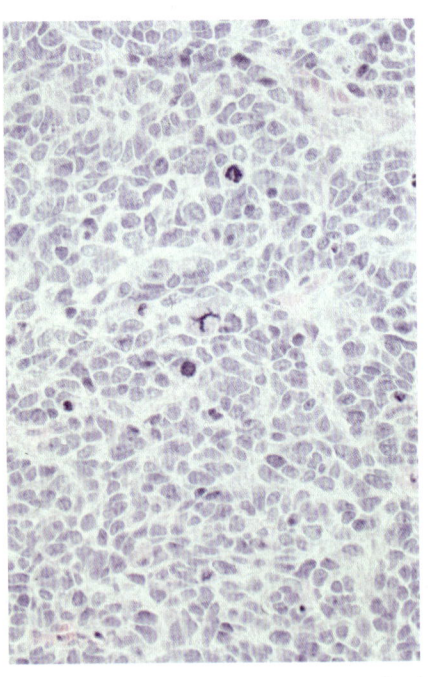

图15.38　间变性Wilms瘤特点为细胞核大，染色质浓染，可见病理性核分裂象（HE染色，×400）

> **诊断要点：Wilms 瘤**
>
> 1. 诊断 Wilms 瘤通常要将典型的组织学图像与临床资料如发病年龄和部位结合起来。
> 2. 胚基成分为主的 Wilms 瘤易于与其他相似的"小蓝细胞"肿瘤混淆，尤其是在活检小组织中。
> 3. 肌源性标记物如成肌素和 Myo-D1 在胚基成分为主型 Wilms 瘤不表达，因此在结蛋白阳性、胚基成分为主型 Wilms 瘤可作为一个有用的鉴别诊断工具。CD99同样为一个有用的鉴别诊断指标，在胚基成分为主的 Wilms 瘤表达阴性，而在 ES/PNET 阳性。
> 4. 与 Wilms 瘤鉴别困难的肾肿瘤有肾原发性 ES/PNET、小细胞滑膜肉瘤、白血病/淋巴瘤和转移的腺泡状横纹肌肉瘤。

骨肉瘤

　　骨肉瘤是最常见的骨原发恶性肿瘤，常见类型为高级别骨肉瘤，可见成骨现象。尽管骨肉瘤是一种好发于青年的恶性肿瘤，发病高峰为 10～20 岁，60% 的患者于 25 岁前发病，但也有 30% 病例为 40 岁以上的患者，男性发病率高于女性，尤其是青年患者。最常见的部位为四肢长骨干骺端或骨干，肿块体积大，鱼肉状，

度和死亡时间相关[188]。转化生长因子α和表皮生长因子受体通过促进增生和转化可使肿瘤进展加快。PCNA高表达提示肿瘤处于进展期和预后差。血管内皮生长因子及其受体 FLI-1 阳性提示预后差[189]。

有时质地较硬，含数量不等的钙化灶、骨和软骨。

光镜下，肿瘤由多形性肿瘤细胞构成，细胞呈梭形、圆形或椭圆形，上皮样、浆细胞样、透明细胞、多核细胞，通常出现一种以上的细胞形态。诊断骨肉瘤必须查见类骨组织，还可见多少不等的骨形成、软骨及纤维组织。传统的骨肉瘤组织学亚型包括骨母细胞性、软骨母细胞性、纤维母细胞性[190]。电镜同样发现多种细胞类型，具有骨母细胞、破骨细胞、软骨母细胞及纤维母细胞的特征[191]。

骨肉瘤没有特别的免疫组化表型，在不同比例的病例中可表达不同类型的抗原，如骨钙素、CK、上皮细胞膜抗原、结蛋白、平滑肌肌动蛋白、Ⅳ型胶原蛋白、S-100、XIII因子等[192, 193]。免疫组化对于与骨肉瘤相似肿瘤的鉴别有帮助，如肉瘤样癌，其他肉瘤如滑膜肉瘤、淋巴瘤和恶性黑色素瘤。CD99阳性容易造成误诊，尤其是以小圆细胞为主的骨肉瘤。

对多种有预后和生物学意义的免疫组化指标进行了研究。尽管有关Her-2/ERB B2胞浆着色与胞核着色的遗传学基础和意义尚存在争议[194-196]，但目前认为Her-2/ERB B2阳性预示患者预后差及肺转移几率增高[197-200]。其他与预后差相关的标记物有ephrin[201]、细胞色素P450 CYP 3A4/5[202]、p-糖蛋白过度表达[197, 203, 204]、p53[197, 105, 206]、增殖抗原如Ki-67和PCNA[38, 205, 206]。

也有数据表明生存素（survivin）呈细胞核阳性提示预后好。曾有人观察到成骨蛋白7和8高表达，β-连环素细胞浆和细胞核着色，但这些抗原对于预后的意义尚不明了[208, 209]。

> **诊断要点：骨肉瘤**
>
> 1. 骨肉瘤是一种免疫组化多样性的肿瘤，缺乏特异的标记物。
> 2. 成骨现象是诊断骨肉瘤的关键特征。
> 3. 在与骨转移瘤或肉瘤样癌、ES/PNET、滑膜肉瘤、恶性黑色素瘤及其他恶性肿瘤鉴别时，若骨肉瘤表达CK、上皮细胞膜抗原、CD99和S-100，容易造成诊断误区。

小 结

总的来说，应用特异性高和敏感性高的免疫组化指标可帮助病理医师更准确地对小儿肿瘤进行分类，尤其是小圆细胞肿瘤和梭形细胞肿瘤（表15.1）。临床针对性治疗要求更精确的病理诊断。免疫组化只是病理医师用来对儿童和青少年实体瘤进行分类的方法之一，某些病例还可采用细胞遗传学和分子学检测、

表15.1　部分小儿肿瘤主要病理学和免疫组化特征

诊断	组织学	免疫表型
神经母细胞瘤	小圆细胞成片状或巢状排列，核分裂、核碎裂、神经纤维、菊形团、纤维血管间质以及schwannian间质多少不等	NSE、突触素、嗜铬素、神经丝、CD57、CD56、PGP9.5
横纹肌肉瘤	腺泡状：可见腺泡状或实性结构，小圆细胞呈不同程度的横纹肌母细胞分化，可见横纹肌母巨细胞和透明细胞 胚胎性：黏液样背景上可见原始梭形、星芒状、圆形、多角形细胞，多少不等的横纹肌母细胞、带状细胞、多核细胞和肌管形成	腺泡状：成肌素、Myo-D1、结蛋白、肌特异性肌动蛋白 胚胎性：成肌素、Myo-D1、肌特异性肌动蛋白
ES/PNET	小圆细胞片状排列，核圆、染色质细腻、胞浆少，菊形团多少不等，核仁明显，可见梭形细胞和坏死	波形蛋白、CD99、突触素、FLI-1
DSRCT	小圆细胞巢状排列，间质纤维化明显，中央有坏死，多少不等的囊性变和上皮分化	多形性：CK、上皮细胞膜抗原、波形蛋白、结蛋白、WT-1（C-末端）、CD99
恶性横纹肌样瘤	多边形或小圆细胞呈片状或管状，核大、空泡状，中央为显著大核仁，胞浆偏心、丰富，可见玻璃样嗜酸性球状包涵体，核分裂多见	多形性：波形蛋白、CK、上皮细胞膜抗原、CD99阳性不等、突触素、S-100蛋白、肌特异性肌动蛋白、INI-1阴性
Wilms瘤	胚基、上皮、间质3种成分，胚基细胞小、圆或椭圆，结节状或蜿蜒状排列，上皮成分形成原始菊形团样结构或管状、乳头状结构，间质包括纤维、骨骼肌、脂肪、软骨、骨及神经	胚基：波形蛋白、结蛋白 上皮：CK 间质：视分化不同而各异
骨肉瘤	肿瘤多形性、间变、细胞异型性明显，有类骨及骨组织形成	多样，无特异性免疫表型

流式细胞学及电镜技术。实用、方便、费用低廉使得免疫组化成为儿童外科病理的一种重要的诊断工具，同时病理医师必须对着色模式、敏感性、特异性以及常见的诊断误区有清楚的认识。

参考文献

1. Ordonez NG. Application of immunocytochemistry in the diagnosis of soft tissue sarcomas: a review and update. Adv Anat Pathol 1998; 5(2):67–85.
2. Parham DM. Immunohistochemistry of childhood sarcomas: old and new markers. Mod Pathol 1993; 6(2):133–138.
3. Coindre JM. Immunohistochemistry in the diagnosis of soft tissue tumours. Histopathology 2003; 43(1):1–16.
4. Meis-Kindblom JM, Stenman G, Kindblom LG. Differential diagnosis of small round cell tumors. Semin Diagn Pathol 1996; 13(3):213–241.
5. Leong AS. Pitfalls in diagnostic immunohistology. Adv Anat Pathol 2004; 11(2):86–93.
6. Sebire NJ, Ramsay AD, Levitt G, et al. Aberrant immunohistochemical expression in nonrhabdomyosarcoma soft tissue sarcomas of infancy: retrospective review of clinical material. Pediatr Dev Pathol 2002; 5(6):579–586.
7. Zutter MM, Hess JL. Guidelines for the diagnosis of leukemia or lymphoma in children. Am J Clin Pathol 1998; 109(4 Suppl 1):S9–S22.
8. Mierau GW, Berry PJ, Orsini EN. Small round cell neoplasms: can electron microscopy and immunohistochemical studies accurately classify them? Ultrastruct Pathol 1985; 9(1–2):99–111.
9. Mierau GW, Berry PJ, Malott RL, et al. Appraisal of the comparative utility of immunohistochemistry and electron microscopy in the diagnosis of childhood round cell tumors. Ultrastruct Pathol 1996; 20(6):507–517.
10. Mierau GW, Weeks DA, Hicks MJ. Role of electron microscopy and other special techniques in the diagno-sis of childhood round cell tumors. Hum Pathol 1998; 29(12):1347–1355.
11. Peydro-Olaya A, Llombart-Bosch A, Carda-Batalla C, et al. Electron microscopy and other ancillary techniques in the diagnosis of small round cell tumors. Semin Diagn Pathol 2003; 20(1):25–45.
12. Brahmi U, Srinivasan R, Komal HS, et al. Comparative analysis of electron microscopy and immunocytochemistry in the cytologic diagnosis of malignant small round cell tumors. Acta Cytol 2003; 47(3):443–449.
13. Kushner BH, LaQuaglia MP, Cheung NK, et al. Clinically critical impact of molecular genetic studies in pediatric solid tumors. Med Pediatr Oncol 1999; 33(6):530–535.
14. McManus AP, Gusterson BA, Pinkerton CR, et al. The molecular pathology of small round-cell tumours – relevance to diagnosis, prognosis, and classification. J Pathol 1996; 178(2):116–121.
15. Askin FB, Perlman EJ. Neuroblastoma and peripheral neuroectodermal tumors. Am J Clin Pathol 1998; 109(4 Suppl 1):S23–S30.
16. Qualman SJ, Bowen J, Amin MB, et al. Protocol for the examination of specimens from patients with Wilms tumor (nephroblastoma) or other renal tumors of childhood. Arch Pathol Lab Med 2003; 127(10):1280–1289.
17. Qualman SJ, Bowen J, Parham DM, et al. Protocol for the examination of specimens from patients (children and young adults) with rhabdomyosarcoma. Arch Pathol Lab Med 2003; 127(10):1290–1297.
18. Coffin CM, Dehner LP. Pathologic evaluation of pediatric soft tissue tumors. Am J Clin Pathol 1998; 109(4 Suppl 1):S38–S52.
19. Boccon-Gibod LA. Pathological evaluation of renal tumors in children: International Society of Pediatric Oncology approach. Pediatr Dev Pathol 1998; 1(3):243–248.
20. Shimada H, Ambros IM, Dehner LP, et al. Terminology and morphologic criteria of neuroblastic tumors: recommendations by the International Neuroblastoma Pathology Committee. Cancer 1999; 86(2):349–363.
21. Wang NP, Marx J, McNutt MA, et al. Expression of myogenic regulatory proteins (myogenin and MyoD1) in small blue round cell tumors of childhood. Am J Pathol 1995; 147(6):1799–1810.
22. Dias P, Parham DM, Shapiro DN, et al. Myogenic regulatory protein (MyoD1) expression in childhood solid tumors: diagnostic utility in rhabdomyosarcoma. Am J Pathol 1990; 137(6):1283–1291.
23. Cui S, Hano H, Harada T, et al. Evaluation of new monoclonal anti-MyoD1 and anti-myogenin antibodies for the diagnosis of rhabdomyosarcoma. Pathol Int 1999; 49(1):62-68.
24. Engel ME, Mouton SC, Emms M. Paediatric rhabdomyosarcoma: MyoD1 demonstration in routinely pro-

cessed tissue sections using wet heat pretreatment (pressure cooking) for antigen retrieval. J Clin Pathol 1997; 50(1):37–39.

25. Kumar S, Perlman E, Harris CA, et al. Myogenin is a specific marker for rhabdomyosarcoma: an immunohistochemical study in paraffin-embedded tissues. Mod Pathol 2000; 13(9):988–993.

26. Cessna MH, Zhou H, Perkins SL, et al. Are myogenin and myoD1 expression specific for rhabdomyosarcoma? A study of 150 cases, with emphasis on spindle cell mimics. Am J Surg Pathol 2001; 25(9):1150–1157.

27. Sebire NJ, Malone M. Myogenin and MyoD1 expression in paediatric rhabdomyosarcomas. J Clin Pathol 2003; 56(6): 412–416.

28. Dias P, Parham DM, Shapiro DN, et al. Monoclonal antibodies to the myogenic regulatory protein MyoD1: epitope mapping and diagnostic utility. Cancer Res 1992; 52(23):6431–6439.

29. Dias P, Chen B, Dilday B, et al. Strong immunostaining for myogenin in rhabdomyosarcoma is significantly associated with tumors of the alveolar subclass. Am J Pathol 2000; 156(2):399–408.

30. Stevenson AJ, Chatten J, Bertoni F, et al. (p30/32^{MIC2}) neuroectodermal/Ewing's sarcoma antigen as an immunohistochemical marker: Review of more than 600 tumors and the literature experience. Appl Immunohistochem 1994; 2:231–240.

31. Perlman EJ, Dickman PS, Askin FB, et al. Ewing's sarcoma – routine diagnostic utilization of MIC2 analysis: a Pediatric Oncology Group/Children's Cancer Group Intergroup Study. Hum Pathol 1994; 25(3):304–307.

32. Weidner N, Tjoe J. Immunohistochemical profile of monoclonal antibody O13: antibody that recognizes glycoprotein p30/32MIC2 and is useful in diagnosing Ewing's sarcoma and peripheral neuroepithelioma. Am J Surg Pathol 1994; 18(5):486–494.

33. Ambros IM, Ambros PF, Strehl S, et al. MIC2 is a specific marker for Ewing's sarcoma and peripheral primitive neuroectodermal tumors. Evidence for a common histogenesis of Ewing's sarcoma and peripheral primitive neuroectodermal tumors from MIC2 expression and specific chromosome aberration. Cancer 1991; 67(7):1886–1893.

34. Ramani P, Rampling D, Link M. Immunocytochemical study of 12E7 in small round-cell tumours of childhood: an assessment of its sensitivity and specificity. Histopathology 1993; 23(6):557–561.

35. Riopel M, Dickman PS, Link MP, et al. MIC2 analysis in pediatric lymphomas and leukemias. Hum Pathol 1994; 25(4):396–399.

36. Zhang PJ, Goldblum JR, Pawel BR, et al. Immunophenotype of desmoplastic small round cell tumors as detected in cases with EWS-WT1 gene fusion product. Mod Pathol 2003; 16(3):229–235.

37. Granter SR, Renshaw AA, Fletcher CD, et al. CD99 reactivity in mesenchymal chondrosarcoma. Hum Pathol 1996; 27(12):1273–1276.

38. Folpe AL, Schmidt RA, Chapman D, et al. Poorly differentiated synovial sarcoma: immunohistochemical distinction from primitive neuroectodermal tumors and high-grade malignant peripheral nerve sheath tumors. Am J Surg Pathol 1998; 22(6):673–682.

39. Fellinger EJ, Garin-Chesa P, Triche TJ, et al. Immunohistochemical analysis of Ewing's sarcoma cell surface antigen p30/32MIC2. Am J Pathol 1991; 139(2):317–325.

40. Ozdemirli M, Fanburg-Smith JC, Hartmann DP, et al. Differentiating lymphoblastic lymphoma and Ewing's sarcoma: lymphocyte markers and gene rearrangement. Mod Pathol 2001; 14(11):1175–1182.

41. Pappo AS, Douglass EC, Meyer WH, et al. Use of HBA 71 and anti-beta 2-microglobulin to distinguish peripheral neuroepithelioma from neuroblastoma. Hum Pathol 1993; 24(8):880–885.

42. Nilsson G, Wang M, Wejde J, et al. Detection of EWS/FLI-1 by immunostaining. An adjunctive tool in diagnosis of Ewing's sarcoma and primitive neuroectodermal tumor on cytological samples and paraffin-embedded archival material. Sarcoma 1999; 3:25–32.

43. Folpe AL, Hill CE, Parham DM, et al. Immunohistochemical detection of FLI-1 protein expression: a study of 132 round cell tumors with emphasis on CD99-positive mimics of Ewing's sarcoma/primitive neuroectodermal tumor. Am J Surg Pathol 2000; 24(12):1657–1662.

44. Rossi S, Orvieto E, Furlanetto A, et al. Utility of the immunohistochemical detection of FLI-1 expression in round cell and vascular neoplasm using a monoclonal antibody. Mod Pathol 2004; 17(5):547–552.

45. Hill DA, Pfeifer JD, Marley EF, et al. WT1 staining reliably differentiates desmoplastic small round cell tumor from Ewing sarcoma/primitive neuroectodermal tumor. An immunohistochemical and molecular diagnostic study. Am J Clin Pathol 2000; 114(3):345–353.

46. Barnoud R, Sabourin JC, Pasquier D, et al. Immunohistochemical expression of WT1 by desmoplastic small round cell tumor: a comparative study with other small round cell tumors. Am J Surg Pathol 2000; 24(6):830–836.

47. Lae ME, Roche PC, Jin L, et al. Desmoplastic small round cell tumor: a clinicopathologic, immunohistochemical, and molecular study of 32 tumors. Am J Surg Pathol 2002; 26(7): 823–835.

48. Judkins AR, Mauger J, et al. Immunohistochemical analysis of hSNF5/INI1 in pediatric CNS neoplasms. Am J Surg Pathol 2004; 28(5):644–650.

49. Schwab M, Shimada H, Joshi V, et al. Neuroblastic tumors of adrenal gland and sympathetic nervous system. In: Kleihues P, Cavenee WK, eds. World Health Organization classification of tumors. tumors of the nervous system. Lyon, France: IARC Press; 2000.

50. Shimada H, Ambros IM, Dehner LP, et al. The International Neuroblastoma Pathology Classification (the Shimada system). Cancer 1999; 86(2):364–372.

51. Miettinen M, Chatten J, Paetau A, et al. Monoclonal antibody NB84 in the differential diagnosis of neuroblastoma and other small round cell tumors. Am J Surg Pathol 1998; 22(3): 327–332.

52. Parham DM. Neuroectodermal and neuroendocrine tumors principally seen in children. Am J Clin Pathol 2001; 115 (Suppl):S113–S128.

53. Wick MR. Immunohistology of neuroendocrine and neuroectodermal tumors. Semin Diagn Pathol 2000; 17(3):194–203.

54. Joshi VV. Peripheral neuroblastic tumors: pathologic classification based on recommendations of International Neuroblastoma Pathology Committee (modification of Shimada classification). Pediatr Dev Pathol 2000; 3(2):184–199.

55. Carter RL, al-Sams SZ, Corbett RP, et al. A comparative study of immunohistochemical staining for neuron-specific enolase, protein gene product 9.5 and S-100 protein in neuroblastoma, Ewing's sarcoma and other round cell tumours in children. Histopathology 1990; 16(5):461–467.

56. Shimada H, Aoyama C, Chiba T, et al. Prognostic subgroups for undifferentiated neuroblastoma: immunohistochemical study with anti-S-100 protein antibody. Hum Pathol 1985; 16(5):471–476.

57. Brook FB, Raafat F, Eldeeb BB, et al. Histologic and immunohistochemical investigation of neuroblastomas and correlation with prognosis. Hum Pathol 1988; 19(8):879–888.

58. Moss TJ, Reynolds CP, Sather HN, et al. Prognostic value of immunocytologic detection of bone marrow metastases in neuroblastoma. N Engl J Med 1991; 324(4):219–226.

59. Lamant L, Pulford K, Bischof D, et al. Expression of the ALK tyrosine kinase gene in neuroblastoma. Am J Pathol 2000; 156(5):1711–1721.

60. Brodeur GM, Maris JM, Yamashiro DJ, et al. Biology and genetics of human neuroblastomas. J Pediatr Hematol Oncol 1997; 19(2):93–101.

61. Brodeur GM, Nakagawara A, Yamashiro DJ, et al. Expression of TrkA, TrkB and TrkC in human neuroblastomas. J Neurooncol 1997; 31(1–2):49–55.

62. Brodeur GM. Molecular pathology of human neuroblastomas. Semin Diagn Pathol 1994; 11(2):118–125.

63. Brodeur GM. Molecular basis for heterogeneity in human neuroblastomas. Eur J Cancer 1995; 31A(4):505–510.

64. Mejia C, Navarro S, Pellin A, et al. Prognostic significance of cell proliferation in human neuroblastoma: comparison with other prognostic factors. Oncol Rep 2003; 10(1):243–247.

65. Krams M, Hero B, Berthold F, et al. Proliferation marker KI-S5 discriminates between favorable and adverse prognosis in advanced stages of neuroblastoma with and without MYCN amplification. Cancer 2002; 94(3):854–861.

66. Krams M, Heidebrecht HJ, Hero B, et al. Repp86 expression and outcome in patients with neuroblastoma. J Clin Oncol 2003; 21(9):1810–1818.

67. Munchar MJ, Sharifah NA, Jamal R, et al. CD44s expression correlated with the International Neuroblastoma Pathology Classification (Shimada system) for neuroblastic tumours. Pathology 2003; 35(2):125–129.

68. Comito MA, Savell VH, Cohen MB. CD44 expression in neuroblastoma and related tumors. J Pediatr Hematol Oncol 1997; 19(4):292–296.

69. Combaret V, Gross N, Lasset C, et al. Clinical relevance of CD44 cell-surface expression and N-myc gene amplification in a multicentric analysis of 121 pediatric neuroblastomas. J

Clin Oncol 1996; 14(1):25–34.

70. Krams M, Parwaresch R, Sipos B, et al. Expression of the c-kit receptor characterizes a subset of neuroblastomas with favorable prognosis. Oncogene 2004; 23(2):588–595.

71. Vitali R, Cesi V, Nicotra MR, et al. c-Kit is preferentially expressed in MYCN-amplified neuroblastoma and its effect on cell proliferation is inhibited in vitro by STI-571. Int J Cancer 2003; 106(2):147–152.

72. Gallo G, Giarnieri E, Bosco S, et al. Aberrant bcl-2 and bax protein expression related to chemotherapy response in neuroblastoma. Anticancer Res 2003; 23(1B):777–784.

73. Ara T, Fukuzawa M, Kusafuka T, et al. Immunohistochemical expression of MMP-2, MMP-9, and TIMP-2 in neuroblastoma: association with tumor progression and clinical outcome. J Pediatr Surg 1998; 33(8):1272–1278.

74. Nakagawara A, Arima-Nakagawara M, Scavarda NJ, et al. Association between high levels of expression of the TRK gene and favorable outcome in human neuroblastoma. N Engl J Med 1993; 328(12):847–854.

75. Nakagawara A, Liu XG, Ikegaki N, et al. Cloning and chromosomal localization of the human TRK-B tyrosine kinase receptor gene (NTRK2). Genomics 1995; 25(2):538–546.

76. Kramer K, Gerald W, LeSauteur L, et al. Prognostic value of TrkA protein detection by monoclonal antibody 5C3 in neuroblastoma. Clin Cancer Res 1996; 2(8):1361–1367.

77. Kramer K, Gerald W, LeSauteur L, et al. Monoclonal antibody to human Trk-A: diagnostic and therapeutic potential in neuroblastoma. Eur J Cancer 1997; 33(12):2090–2091.

78. Tanaka T, Hiyama E, Sugimoto T, et al. trk A gene expression in neuroblastoma. The clinical significance of an immunohistochemical study. Cancer 1995; 76(6):1086–1095.

79. White FV, Dehner LP, Belchis DA, et al. Congenital disseminated malignant rhabdoid tumor: a distinct clinicopathologic entity demonstrating abnormalities of chromosome 22q11. Am J Surg Pathol 1999; 23(3):249–256.

80. Asmar L, Gehan EA, Newton WA, et al. Agreement among and within groups of pathologists in the classification of rhabdomyosarcoma and related childhood sarcomas. Report of an international study of four pathology classifications. Cancer 1994; 74(9):2579–2588.

81. Miller RW, Young JL Jr, Novakovic B. Childhood cancer. Cancer 1995; 75(1 Suppl):395–405.

82. Newton WA Jr, Gehan EA, Webber BL, et al. Classification of rhabdomyosarcomas and related sarcomas. Pathologic aspects and proposal for a new classification – an Intergroup Rhabdomyosarcoma Study. Cancer 1995; 76(6):1073–85.

83. Qualman SJ, Coffin CM, Newton WA, et al. Intergroup Rhabdomyosarcoma Study: update for pathologists. Pediatr Dev Pathol 1998; 1(6):550–561.

84. Coffin CM. The new international rhabdomyosarcoma classification, its progenitors, and considerations beyond morphology. Adv Anatomic Pathol 1997; 4:1–16.

85. Parham D, Barr FG. Pathology and genetics of tumors of soft tissue and bone. In: Fletcher CD, Unni KK, Mertens F, eds. World Health Organization classification of tumours. Lyon, France: IARC Press; 2002:146–152.

86. Kodet R, Newton WA Jr, Hamoudi AB, et al. Childhood rhabdomyosarcoma with anaplastic (pleomorphic) features. A report of the Intergroup Rhabdomyosarcoma Study. Am J Surg Pathol 1993; 17(5):443–453.

87. Parham DM. Pathologic classification of rhabdomyosarcomas and correlations with molecular studies. Mod Pathol 2001; 14(5):506–514.

88. Kodet R. Rhabdomyosarcoma in childhood. An immunohistological analysis with myoglobin, desmin and vimentin. Pathol Res Pract 1989; 185(2):207–213.

89. Coffin CM, Rulon J, Smith L, et al. Pathologic features of rhabdomyosarcoma before and after treatment: a clinicopathologic and immunohistochemical analysis. Mod Pathol 1997; 10(12):1175–1187.

90. Tsokos M. The role of immunocytochemistry in the diagnosis of rhabdomyosarcoma. Arch Pathol Lab Med 1986; 110(9):776–778.

91. Scupham R, Gilbert EF, Wilde J, et al. Immunohistochemical studies of rhabdomyosarcoma. Arch Pathol Lab Med 1986; 110(9):818–821.

92. Brooks JJ. Immunohistochemistry of soft tissue tumors. Myoglobin as a tumor marker for rhabdomyosarcoma. Cancer 1982; 50(9):1757–1763.

93. Leader M, Patel J, Collins M, et al. Myoglobin: an evaluation of its role as a marker of rhabdomyosarcomas. Br J Cancer 1989; 59(1):106–109.

94. Parham DM, Webber B, Holt H, et al. Immunohistochemical study of childhood rhabdomyosarcomas and related neoplasms. Results of an Intergroup Rhabdomyosarcoma study project. Cancer 1991; 67(12):3072–3080.

95. Carter RL, McCarthy KP, Machin LG, et al. Expression of desmin and myoglobin in rhabdomyosarcomas and in developing skeletal muscle. Histopathology 1989; 15(6):585–595.

96. Schmidt RA, Cone R, Haas JE, et al. Diagnosis of rhabdomyosarcomas with HHF35, a monoclonal antibody directed against muscle actins. Am J Pathol 1988; 131(1):19–28.

97. Azumi N, Ben-Ezra J, Battifora H. Immunophenotypic diagnosis of leiomyosarcomas and rhabdomyosarcomas with monoclonal antibodies to muscle-specific actin and desmin in formalin-fixed tissue. Mod Pathol 1988; 1(6):469–474.

98. Dodd S, Malone M, McCulloch W. Rhabdomyosarcoma in children: a histological and immunohistochemical study of 59 cases. J Pathol 1989; 158(1):13–18.

99. Dias P, Kumar P, Marsden HB, et al. Evaluation of desmin as a diagnostic and prognostic marker of childhood rhabdomyosarcomas and embryonal sarcomas. Br J Cancer 1987; 56(3):361–365.

100. Eusebi V, Ceccarelli C, Gorza L, et al. Immunocytochemistry of rhabdomyosarcoma. The use of four different markers. Am J Surg Pathol 1986; 10(4):293–299.

101. Michelagnoli MP, Burchill SA, Cullinane C, et al. Myogenin – a more specific target for RT-PCR detection of rhabdomyosarcoma than MyoD1. Med Pediatr Oncol 2003; 40(1):1–8.

102. Cessna MH, Zhou H, Sanger WG, et al. Expression of ALK1 and p80 in inflammatory myofibroblastic tumor and its mesenchymal mimics: a study of 135 cases. Mod Pathol 2002; 15(9):931–938.

103. Miettinen M, Rapola J. Immunohistochemical spectrum of rhabdomyosarcoma and rhabdomyosarcoma-like tumors. Expression of cytokeratin and the 68 kD neurofilament protein. Am J Surg Pathol 1989; 13(2):120–132.

104. Coindre JM, de Mascarel A, Trojani M, et al. Immunohistochemical study of rhabdomyosarcoma. Unexpected staining with S100 protein and cytokeratin. J Pathol 1988; 155(2):127–132.

105. Goldsmith JD, Pawel B, Goldblum JR, et al. Detection and diagnostic utilization of placental alkaline phosphatase in muscular tissue and tumors with myogenic differentiation. Am J Surg Pathol 2002; 26(12):1627–1633.

106. Carpentieri DF, Nichols K, Chou PM, et al. The expression of WT1 in the differentiation of rhabdomyosarcoma from other pediatric small round blue cell tumors. Mod Pathol 2002; 15(10):1080–1086.

107. Tokuc G, Dogan O, Ayan I, et al. Prognostic value of proliferating cell nuclear antigen immunostaining in pediatric rhabdomyosarcomas. Acta Paediatr Jpn 1998; 40(6):573–579.

108. San Miguel-Fraile P, Carrillo-Gijon R, Rodriguez-Peralto JL, et al. Prognostic significance of DNA ploidy and proliferative index (MIB-1 index) in childhood rhabdomyosarcoma. Am J Clin Pathol 2004; 121(3):358–365.

109. Ayan I, Dogan O, Kebudi R, et al. Immunohistochemical detection of p53 protein in rhabdomyosarcoma: association with clinicopathological features and outcome. J Pediatr Hematol Oncol 1997; 19(1):48–53.

110. Takahashi Y, Oda Y, Kawaguchi K, et al. Altered expression and molecular abnormalities of cell-cycle-regulatory proteins in rhabdomyosarcoma. Mod Pathol 2004; 17(6):660–669.

111. Ushigome S, Machinami R, Sorensen PH. Ewing sarcoma/primitive neuroectodermal tumour (PNET). In: Fletcher CD, Unni KK, Mertens F, eds. Pathology and genetics of tumors of soft tissue and bone. World Health Organization classification of tumours. Lyon, France: IARC Press; 2002:298–300.

112. Coffin CM, Dehner LP. Peripheral neurogenic tumors of the soft tissues in children and adolescents: a clinicopathologic study of 139 cases. Pediatr Pathol 1989; 9(4):387–407.

113. de Alava E, Gerald WL. Molecular biology of the Ewing's sarcoma/primitive neuroectodermal tumor family. J Clin Oncol 2000; 18(1):204–213.

114. Hasegawa SL, Davison JM, Rutten A, et al. Primary cutaneous Ewing's sarcoma: immunophenotypic and molecular cytogenetic evaluation of five cases. Am J Surg Pathol 1998; 22(3):310–318.

115. Marley EF, Liapis H, Humphrey PA, et al. Primitive neuroectodermal tumor of the kidney – another enigma: a pathologic, immunohistochemical, and molecular diagnostic study. Am J Surg Pathol 1997; 21(3):354–359.

116. Lawlor ER, Mathers JA, Bainbridge T, et al. Peripheral primitive neuroectodermal tumors in adults: documentation by molecular analysis. J Clin Oncol 1998; 16(3):1150–1157.

117. Moll R, Lee I, Gould VE, et al. Immunocytochemical analysis of Ewing's tumors. Patterns of expression of intermediate filaments and desmosomal proteins indicate cell type heterogeneity and pluripotential differentiation. Am J Pathol 1987; 127(2):288–304.

118. Llombart-Bosch A, Lacombe MJ, Peydro-Olaya A, et al. Malignant peripheral neuroectodermal tumours of bone other

than Askin's neoplasm: characterization of 14 new cases with immunohistochemistry and electron micro-scopy. Virchows Arch A Pathol Anat Histopathol 1988; 412(5):421–430.
119. Shanfeld RL, Edelman J, Willis JE, et al. Immunohistochemical analysis of neural markers in peripheral primitive neuroectodermal tumors (pPNET) without light microscopic evidence of neural differentiation. Appl Immunohistochem 1997; 5(2):78–86.
120. Fellinger EJ, Garin-Chesa P, Glasser DB, et al. Comparison of cell surface antigen HBA71 (p30/32MIC2), neuron-specific enolase, and vimentin in the immunohistochemical analysis of Ewing's sarcoma of bone. Am J Surg Pathol 1992; 16(8):746–755.
121. Gu M, Antonescu CR, Guiter G, et al. Cytokeratin immunoreactivity in Ewing's sarcoma: prevalence in 50 cases confirmed by molecular diagnostic studies. Am J Surg Pathol 2000; 24(3):410–416.
122. Hamilton G, Fellinger EJ, Schratter I, et al. Characteriza-tion of a human endocrine tissue and tumor-associated Ewing's sarcoma antigen. Cancer Res 1988; 48(21):6127–6131.
123. Scotlandi K, Serra M, Manara MC, et al. Immunostaining of the p30/32MIC2 antigen and molecular detection of EWS rearrangements for the diagnosis of Ewing's sarcoma and peripheral neuroectodermal tumor. Hum Pathol 1996; 27(4):408–416.
124. Lucas DR, Bentley G, Dan ME, et al. Ewing sarcoma vs lymphoblastic lymphoma. A comparative immunohistochemical study. Am J Clin Pathol 2001; 115(1):11–17.
125. Kumar S, Pack S, Kumar D, et al. Detection of EWS-FLI-1 fusion in Ewing's sarcoma/peripheral primitive neuroectodermal tumor by fluorescence in situ hybridization using formalin-fixed paraffin-embedded tissue. Hum Pathol 1999; 30(3):324–330.
126. Fritsch MK, Bridge JA, Schuster AE, et al. Performance characteristics of a reverse transcriptase-polymerase chain reaction assay for the detection of tumor-specific fusion transcripts from archival tissue. Pediatr Dev Pathol 2003; 6(1):43–53.
127. Dagher R, Pham TA, Sorbara L, et al. Molecular confirmation of Ewing sarcoma. J Pediatr Hematol Oncol 2001; 23(4):221–224.
128. Sandberg AA, Bridge JA. Updates on cytogenetics and molecular genetics of bone and soft tissue tumors: Ewing sarcoma and peripheral primitive neuroectodermal tu-mors. Cancer Genet Cytogenet 2000; 123(1):1–26.
129. Delattre O, Zucman J, Melot T, et al. The Ewing family of tumors – a subgroup of small-round-cell tumors defined by specific chimeric transcripts. N Engl J Med 1994; 331(5):294–299.
130. Folpe AL, Goldblum JR, Rubin BP, et al. When can Ewing sarcoma/primitive neuroectodermal tumor (ES/PNET) be diagnosed without genetic confirmation? A study of 62 proven cases. Mod Pathol 2004; 17(Suppl 1):13A.
131. Amir G, Issakov J, Meller I, et al. Expression of p53 gene product and cell proliferation marker Ki-67 in Ewing's sarcoma: correlation with clinical outcome. Hum Pathol 2002; 33(2):170–174.
132. de Alava E, Antonescu CR, Panizo A, et al. Prognostic impact of p53 status in Ewing sarcoma. Cancer 2000; 89(4):783–792.
133. Maitra A, Roberts H, Weinberg AG, et al. Aberrant expression of tumor suppressor proteins in the Ewing family of tumors. Arch Pathol Lab Med 2001; 125(9):1207–1212.
134. Smithey BE, Pappo AS, Hill DA. C-kit expression in pediatric solid tumors: a comparative immunohistochemical study. Am J Surg Pathol 2002; 26(4):486–492.
135. Daugaard S, Kamby C, Sunde LM, et al. Ewing's sarcoma. A retrospective study of histological and immunohistochemical factors and their relation to prog-nosis. Virchows Arch A Pathol Anat Histopathol 1989; 414(3):243–251.
136. Parham DM, Hijazi Y, Steinberg SM, et al. Neuroectodermal differentiation in Ewing's sarcoma family of tumors does not predict tumor behavior. Hum Pathol 1999; 30(8):911–918.
137. Pinto A, Grant LH, Hayes FA, et al. Immunohistochemical expression of neuron-specific enolase and Leu 7 in Ewing's sarcoma of bone. Cancer 1989; 64(6):1266–1273.
138. Ordonez NG, Zirkin R, Bloom RE. Malignant small-cell epithelial tumor of the peritoneum coexpressing mesenchymal-type intermediate filaments. Am J Surg Pathol 1989; 13(5):413–421.
139. Gerald WL, Miller HK, Battifora H, et al. Intra-abdominal desmoplastic small round-cell tumor. Report of 19 cases of a distinctive type of high-grade polyphenotypic malignancy affecting young individuals. Am J Surg Pathol 1991; 15(6):499–513.
140. Gonzalez-Crussi F, Crawford SE, Sun CC. Intra-abdominal

desmoplastic small-cell tumors with divergent differentiation. Observations on three cases of childhood. Am J Surg Pathol 1990; 14(7):633–642.

141. Kawano N, Inayama Y, Nagashima Y, et al. Desmoplastic small round-cell tumor of the paratesticular region: report of an adult case with demonstration of EWS and WT1 gene fusion using paraffin-embedded tissue. Mod Pathol 1999; 12(7):729–734.

142. Parkash V, Gerald WL, Parma A, et al. Desmoplastic small round cell tumor of the pleura. Am J Surg Pathol 1995; 19(6):659–665.

143. Tison V, Cerasoli S, Morigi F, et al. Intracranial desmoplastic small-cell tumor. Report of a case. Am J Surg Pathol 1996; 20(1):112–117.

144. Backer A, Mount SL, Zarka MA, et al. Desmoplastic small round cell tumour of unknown primary origin with lymph node and lung metastases: histological, cytological, ultrastructural, cytogenetic and molecular findings. Virchows Arch 1998; 432(2):135–141.

145. Gerald WL, Ladanyi M, de Alava E, et al. Clinical, pathologic, and molecular spectrum of tumors associated with t(11;22)(p13;q12): desmoplastic small round-cell tumor and its variants. J Clin Oncol 1998; 16(9):3028–3036.

146. Ordonez NG. Desmoplastic small round cell tumor: I: a histopathologic study of 39 cases with emphasis on unusual histological patterns. Am J Surg Pathol 1998; 22(11):1303–1313.

147. Ordonez NG. Desmoplastic small round cell tumor: II: an ultrastructural and immunohistochemical study with emphasis on new immunohistochemical markers. Am J Surg Pathol 1998; 22(11):1314–1327.

148. Antonescu CR, Gerald WL, Magid MS, et al. Molecular variants of the EWS-WT1 gene fusion in desmoplastic small round cell tumor. Diagn Mol Pathol 1998; 7(1):24–28.

149. Barnoud R, Delattre O, Peoc'h M, et al. Desmoplastic small round cell tumor: RT-PCR analysis and immunohistochemical detection of the Wilms, tumor gene WT1. Pathol Res Pract 1998; 194(10):693–700.

150. de Alava E, Ladanyi M, Rosai J, et al. Detection of chimeric transcripts in desmoplastic small round cell tumor and related developmental tumors by reverse transcriptase polymerase chain reaction. A specific diagnostic assay. Am J Pathol 1995; 147(6):1584–1591.

151. Gerald WL, Rosai J, Ladanyi M. Characterization of the genomic breakpoint and chimeric transcripts in the EWS-WT1 gene fusion of desmoplastic small round cell tumor. Proc Natl Acad Sci USA 1995; 92(4):1028–1032.

152. Ladanyi M, Gerald W. Fusion of the EWS and WT1 genes in the desmoplastic small round cell tumor. Cancer Res 1994; 54(11):2837–2840.

153. Ladanyi M. The emerging molecular genetics of sarcoma translocations. Diagn Mol Pathol 1995; 4(3):162–173.

154. Leuschner I, Radig K, Harms D. Desmoplastic small round cell tumor. Semin Diagn Pathol 1996; 13(3):204–212.

155. Froberg K, Brown RE, Gaylord H, et al. Intra-abdominal desmoplastic small round cell tumor: immunohistochemical evidence for up-regulation of autocrine and paracrine growth factors. Ann Clin Lab Sci 1998; 28(6):386–393.

156. Rachfal AW, Luquette MH, Brigstock DR. Expression of connective tissue growth factor (CCN2) in desmoplastic small round cell tumour. J Clin Pathol 2004; 57(4):422–425.

157. Schofield D. Extrarenal rhabdoid tumour. In: Fletcher CDM, Unni KK, eds. Pathology and genetics of tumors of soft tissue and bone. World Health Organization classification of tumours. Lyon, France: IARC Press; 2002:219–220.

158. Kodet R, Newton WA Jr, Sachs N, et al. Rhabdoid tumors of soft tissues: a clinicopathologic study of 26 cases enrolled on the Intergroup Rhabdomyosarcoma Study. Hum Pathol 1991; 22(7):674–684.

159. Tsuneyoshi M, Daimaru Y, Hashimoto H, et al. Malignant soft tissue neoplasms with the histologic features of renal rhabdoid tumors: an ultrastructural and immunohistochemical study. Hum Pathol 1985; 16(12):1235–1242.

160. Beckwith JB, Palmer NF. Histopathology and prognosis of Wilms' tumors: results from the First National Wilms' Tumor Study. Cancer 1978; 41(5):1937–1948.

161. Tsokos M, Kouraklis G, Chandra RS, et al. Malignant rhabdoid tumor of the kidney and soft tissues. Evidence for a diverse morphological and immunocytochemical phenotype. Arch Pathol Lab Med 1989; 113(2):115–120.

162. Rorke LB, Packer RJ, Biegel JA. Central nervous system atypical teratoid/rhabdoid tumors of infancy and childhood: definition of an entity. J Neurosurg 1996; 85(1):56–65.

163. Burger PC, Yu IT, Tihan T, et al. Atypical teratoid/rhabdoid tumor of the central nervous system: a highly malignant tumor of infancy and childhood frequently mistaken for medulloblastoma: a Pediatric Oncology Group study. Am J

Surg Pathol 1998; 22(9):1083–1092.
164. Parham DM, Weeks DA, Beckwith JB. The clinicopathologic spectrum of putative extrarenal rhabdoid tumors. An analysis of 42 cases studied with immunohistochemistry or electron microscopy. Am J Surg Pathol 1994; 18(10):1010–1029.
165. Fanburg-Smith JC, Hengge M, Hengge UR, et al. Extrarenal rhabdoid tumors of soft tissue: a clinicopathologic and immunohistochemical study of 18 cases. Ann Diagn Pathol 1998; 2(6):351–362.
166. Gessi M, Giangaspero F, Pietsch T. Atypical teratoid/rhabdoid tumors and choroid plexus tumors: when genetics 'surprise' pathology. Brain Pathol 2003; 13(3):409–414.
167. Shiratsuchi H, Saito T, Sakamoto A, et al. Mutation analysis of human cytokeratin 8 gene in malignant rhabdoid tumor: a possible association with intracytoplasmic inclusion body formation. Mod Pathol 2002; 15(2):146–153.
168. Biegel JA, Burk CD, Parmiter AH, et al. Molecular analysis of a partial deletion of 22q in a central nervous system rhabdoid tumor. Genes Chromosomes Cancer 1992; 5(2):104–108.
169. Schofield DE, Beckwith JB, Sklar J. Loss of heterozygosity at chromosome regions 22q11-12 and 11p15.5 in renal rhabdoid tumors. Genes Chromosomes Cancer 1996; 15(1):10–17.
170. Uno K, Takita J, Yokomori K, et al. Aberrations of the hSNF5/INI1 gene are restricted to malignant rhabdoid tumors or atypical teratoid/rhabdoid tumors in pediatric solid tumors. Genes Chromosomes Cancer 2002; 34(1):33–41.
171. Sevenet N, Lellouch-Tubiana A, Schofield D, et al. Spectrum of hSNF5/INI1 somatic mutations in human cancer and genotype–phenotype correlations. Hum Mol Genet 1999; 8(13):2359–2368.
172. Sevenet N, Sheridan E, Amram D, et al. Constitutional mutations of the hSNF5/INI1 gene predispose to a variety of cancers. Am J Hum Genet 1999; 65(5):1342–1348.
173. Bruch LA, Hill DA, Cai DX, et al. A role for fluorescence in situ hybridization detection of chromosome 22q dosage in distinguishing atypical teratoid/rhabdoid tumors from medulloblastoma/central primitive neuroectodermal tu-mors. Hum Pathol 2001; 32(2):156–162.
174. Ogino S, Cohen ML, Abdul-Karim FW. Atypical teratoid/rhabdoid tumor of the CNS: cytopathology and immunohistochemistry of insulin-like growth factor-II, insulin-like growth factor receptor type 1, cathepsin D, and Ki-67. Mod Pathol 1999; 12(4):379–385.
175. Saito T, Oda Y, Itakura E, et al. Expression of intercellular adhesion molecules in epithelioid sarcoma and malignant rhabdoid tumor. Pathol Int 2001; 51(7):532–542.
176. Perlman E, Grosfeld JL, Togashi K, et al. Pathology and genetics of tumors of the urinary system and male genital organs. In: Eble JN, Sauter G, Epstein JI, Sesterhenn IA, eds. World Health Organization classification of tumors. Lyon, France: IARC Press; 2004:48–52.
177. Hussong JW, Perkins SL, Huff V, et al. Familial Wilms' tumor with neural elements: characterization by histology, immunohistochemistry, and genetic analysis. Pediatr Dev Pathol 2000; 3(6):561–567.
178. Vujanic GM, Sandstedt B, Harms D, et al. Revised International Society of Paediatric Oncology (SIOP) working classification of renal tumors of childhood. Med Pediatr Oncol 2002; 38(2):79–82.
179. Folpe AL, Patterson K, Gown AM. Antibodies to desmin identify the blastemal component of nephroblastoma. Mod Pathol 1997; 10(9):895–900.
180. Muir TE, Cheville JC, Lager DJ. Metanephric adenoma, nephrogenic rests, and Wilms' tumor: a histologic and immunophenotypic comparison. Am J Surg Pathol 2001; 25(10):1290–1296.
181. Magee F, Mah RG, Taylor GP, et al. Neural differentiation in Wilms' tumor. Hum Pathol 1987; 18(1):33–37.
182. el Bahtimi R, Hazen-Martin DJ, Re GG, et al. Immunophenotype, mRNA expression, and gene structure of p53 in Wilms' tumors. Mod Pathol 1996; 9(3):238–244.
183. Sredni ST, de Camargo B, Lopes LF, et al. Immunohistochemical detection of p53 protein expression as a prognostic indicator in Wilms' tumor. Med Pediatr Oncol 2001; 37(5):455–458.
184. D'Angelo MF, Kausik SJ, Sebo TJ, et al. p53 immuno-positivity in histologically favorable Wilms' tumor is not related to stage at presentation or to biological aggression. J Urol 2003; 169(5):1815–1817.
185. Ghanem MA, Van der Kwast TH, Den Hollander JC, et al. The prognostic significance of apoptosis-associated proteins BCL-2, BAX and BCL-X in clinical nephroblastoma. Br J Cancer 2001; 85(10):1557–1563.
186. Ghanem MA, Van Steenbrugge GJ, Van Der Kwast TH, et al.

Expression and prognostic value of CD44 isoforms in nephroblastoma (Wilms' tumor). J Urol 2002; 168(2):681–686.

187. Ghanem MA, Van Der Kwast TH, Den Hollander JC, et al. Expression and prognostic value of epidermal growth factor receptor, transforming growth factor-alpha, and c-erb B-2 in nephroblastoma. Cancer 2001; 92(12):3120–3129.

188. Skotnicka-Klonowicz G, Kobos J, Los E, et al. Prognostic value of proliferating cell nuclear antigen in Wilms' tumour in children. Eur J Surg Oncol 2002; 28(1):67–71.

189. Ghanem MA, van Steenbrugge GJ, Sudaryo MK, et al. Expression and prognostic relevance of vascular endo-thelial growth factor (VEGF) and its receptor (FLT-1) in nephroblastoma. J Clin Pathol 2003; 56(2):107–113.

190. Raymond AK, Ayala AG, Knuutila S. Conventional osteosarcoma. In: World Health Organization Classification of Tumors. Pathology and Genetics, Tumors of Soft Tissue and Bones. Fletcher CDM, Unni KK, Mertens F (eds). IARC Press, Lyons. 2002:264–270.

191. Ferguson RJ, Yunis EJ. The ultrastructure of human osteosarcoma: a study of nine cases. Clin Orthop 1978; 131: 234–246.

192. Okada K, Hasegawa T, Yokoyama R, et al. Osteosarcoma with cytokeratin expression: a clinicopathological study of six cases with an emphasis on differential diagnosis from metastatic cancer. J Clin Pathol 2003; 56(10):742–746.

193. Hasegawa T, Hirose T, Kudo E, et al. Immunophenotypic heterogeneity in osteosarcomas. Hum Pathol 1991; 22(6):583–590.

194. Kilpatrick SE, Geisinger KR, King TS, et al. Clinicopathologic analysis of HER-2/neu immunoexpression among various histologic subtypes and grades of osteosarcoma. Mod Pathol 2001; 14(12):1277–1283.

195. Akatsuka T, Wada T, Kokai Y, et al. ErbB2 expression is correlated with increased survival of patients with osteosarcoma. Cancer 2002; 94(5):1397–1404.

196. Tsai JY, Aviv H, Benevenia J, et al. HER-2/neu and p53 in osteosarcoma: an immunohistochemical and fluorescence in situ hybridization analysis. Cancer Invest 2004; 22(1):16–24.

197. Ferrari S, Bertoni F, Zanella L, et al. Evaluation of P-glycoprotein, HER-2/ErbB-2, p53, and bcl-2 in primary tumor and metachronous lung metastases in patients with high-grade osteosarcoma. Cancer 2004; 100(9):1936–1942.

198. Gorlick R, Huvos AG, Heller G, et al. Expression of HER2/erbB-2 correlates with survival in osteosarcoma. J Clin Oncol 1999; 17(9):2781–2788.

199. Onda M, Matsuda S, Higaki S, et al. ErbB-2 expression is correlated with poor prognosis for patients with osteosarcoma. Cancer 1996; 77(1):71–78.

200. Zhou H, Randall RL, Brothman AR, et al. Her-2/neu expression in osteosarcoma increases risk of lung metastasis and can be associated with gene amplification. J Pediatr Hematol Oncol 2003; 25(1):27–32.

201. Varelias A, Koblar SA, Cowled PA, et al. Human osteo-sarcoma expresses specific ephrin profiles: implications for tumorigenicity and prognosis. Cancer 2002; 95(4):862–869.

202. Dhaini HR, Thomas DG, Giordano TJ, et al. Cytochrome P450 CYP3A4/5 expression as a biomarker of outcome in osteosarcoma. J Clin Oncol 2003; 21(13):2481–2485.

203. Serra M, Scotlandi K, Reverter-Branchat G, et al. Value of P-glycoprotein and clinicopathologic factors as the basis for new treatment strategies in high-grade osteosarcoma of the extremities. J Clin Oncol 2003; 21(3):536–542.

204. Pakos EE, Ioannidis JP. The association of P-glycoprotein with response to chemotherapy and clinical outcome in patients with osteosarcoma. A meta-analysis. Cancer 2003; 98 (3):581–589.

205. Nakashima H, Nishida Y, Sugiura H, et al. Telomerase, p53 and PCNA activity in osteosarcoma. Eur J Surg Oncol 2003; 29(7):564–567.

206. Junior AT, de Abreu Alves F, Pinto CA, et al. Clinicopathological and immunohistochemical analysis of twenty-five head and neck osteosarcomas. Oral Oncol 2003; 39(5):521–530.

207. Trieb K, Lehner R, Stulnig T, et al. Survivin expression in human osteosarcoma is a marker for survival. Eur J Surg Oncol 2003; 29(4):379–782.

208. Haydon RC, Deyrup A, Ishikawa A, et al. Cytoplasmic and/or nuclear accumulation of the beta-catenin protein is a frequent event in human osteosarcoma. Int J Cancer 2002; 102 (4):338–342.

209. Sulzbacher I, Birner P, Trieb K, et al. The expression of bone morphogenetic proteins in osteosarcoma and its relevance as a prognostic parameter. J Clin Pathol 2002; 55(5):381–385.

16 女性生殖系统的免疫组织化学

原作者：Robert A. Soslow, Christina Isacson and Charles Zaloudek

译　者：杨　斌，张　询

审校者：张庆慧，张廷国，刘志艳

目　录

引言	655
外阴、阴道和宫颈	655
子宫体	666
妊娠滋养层细胞疾病	676
卵巢	677

引　言

本章主要论述免疫组化在妇科病理诊断中的应用。自本书第一版发行以来，为提高妇科病理诊断的准确性，大量新抗体被用于研究和临床工作。如用于外阴和宫颈鳞状上皮瘤变的p16、用于子宫内膜腺癌的β-钙黏素以及用于鉴别子宫内膜间质肿瘤与其他相似组织学病变的CD10等。

本章分为4节：①外阴、阴道和宫颈，②子宫体，③妊娠滋养层细胞疾病，④卵巢、输卵管与腹膜。每节的第一部分简述在诊断中最有价值的相关抗体，以及这些抗体的属性及应用，请参照表16.1列注的常用抗体及属性。每节的第二部分则讨论免疫组化如何解决疑难妇科病变的诊断及鉴别诊断。

需要强调的是，在使用这些抗体并评价其意义时，必须与常规HE切片和临床病理密切结合。

外阴、阴道和宫颈

外阴、阴道和宫颈最常见的诊断问题是上皮性病变，免疫组化检测能改进对前期病变（如湿疣、鳞状上皮内病变）认识的准确性以及分类，有助于对发生于这些部位的各种类型恶性肿瘤诊断的准确性和分类。

抗原/抗体生物学特性：外阴、阴道和宫颈

细胞角蛋白

细胞角蛋白常被用于评价外阴、阴道、宫颈的复层鳞状上皮病变，包括AE1/AE3（pan-CK）、CAM5.2（低分子量角蛋白）、CK7和CK20。正常的复层鳞状上皮均表达AE1/AE3，而不表达低分子量的角蛋白（如CAM5.2）。尽管癌前病变 [外阴上皮内瘤变（VIN）、阴道上皮内瘤变（VAIN）、宫颈上皮内瘤变（CIN）] 以及鳞癌可有低分子量角蛋白表达，然而因低分子量角蛋白在异型增生的表达不具特异性，因此诊断价值不大[7, 8]。CK7和CK20在鳞状上皮通常不表达。宫颈管腺体表达CK7，但不表达CK20，相似于上生殖道（子宫内膜、输卵管及卵巢）[1]。CK7及CK20表达对外阴Paget病的鉴别诊断以及累及下生殖道的非生殖源性肿瘤（如结肠及泌尿系肿瘤）的确有重要价值。

细胞增殖标志物

细胞增殖标志物，诸如细胞增殖核抗原（PCNA）和Ki-67抗原，已被病理医生用于识别和分类肿瘤及其他疾病的客观指标。Ki-67抗原是一类非组蛋白的核蛋白，它表达于除G_0期外的其他所有细胞周期。MIB-1是由重组Ki-67抗原诱发的单克隆抗

表16.1 妇科病理诊断抗体

抗体	克隆	公司	稀释度	修复	对照	阳性部位
34βE12	34βE12	DAKO	1:50	微波30分钟	腮腺	细胞浆
AE1/AE3	AE1、AE3	B-M	1:8000	胰蛋白酶10分钟	结肠	细胞浆
AFP	C3	BioGenex	1:300	不修复	胎肝	细胞浆
B72.3	B72.3	BioGenex	1:100	微波10分钟	肺癌	细胞膜
Ber-EP4	Ber-EP4	DAKO	1:200	胰蛋白酶10分钟	乳腺	细胞膜
BRST-2	GCDFP-15	Signet	1:50	不修复	乳腺癌	细胞浆
Beta-catenin	14	Becton-Dickinson	1:200	微波30分钟	结肠癌	细胞核
c-kit	多克隆	DAKO	1:1000	微波	GIST	细胞浆
CD10	56C6	Novocastra	1:40 ON	微波	肾	胞膜和胞浆
CD15	MMA	Becton-Dickinson	1:150	压力锅	霍奇金病	细胞膜
CD30	Ber-H2	DAKO	1:25	微波15分钟	霍奇金病	细胞浆
CD34	QBend10	Immunotech	1:2000	微波30分钟	扁桃体	细胞浆
CD44	A308	NeoMarkers	1:100	微波10分钟	扁桃体	细胞膜
CD44v6	VFF7	Bender Med	1:20	微波10分钟	结肠	细胞膜
CD45	ZB11+PD7/26	DAKO	1:100	微波	扁桃体	细胞膜
CD56	123C3	Zymed	1:100	微波30分钟	小细胞癌	细胞浆
CD99	O13	Signet	1:200	压力锅	胸腺	细胞膜
CD117	多克隆	DAKO	1:25	微波	精原细胞瘤	细胞膜
CEA	B01-94-11M	BioGenex	1:1000	不修复	结肠	细胞浆/膜
CK7	OV-TL12/30	DAKO	1:100	微波10分钟	乳腺	细胞浆
CK20	KS20.8	DAKO	1:1000	微波20分钟	结肠	细胞浆
Caldesmon	h-CD	DAKO	1:100	水浴40分钟	平滑肌	细胞浆
Calretinin	多克隆	BioGenex	1:100	微波20分钟	间皮瘤	细胞浆/核
CDX2	CDX2-88	BioGenex	1:25 ON	微波	结肠	核
Chromogranin	LK2H10	BioGenex	1:400	不修复	胰腺	细胞浆
Desmin	D33	DAKO	1:300	微波10分钟	结肠	细胞浆
EMA	E29	DAKO	1:200	压力锅	扁桃体	细胞浆/膜
ER	1D5	DAKO	1:25	压力锅	乳腺	核
HCG	多克隆	DAKO	1:1000	不修复	胎盘	细胞浆
HMB-45	HMB-45	Enzo	1:50	不修复	黑色素瘤	细胞浆
HPL	多克隆	BioGenex	1:200	不修复	胎盘	细胞浆
Inhibin	R1	Serotec	1:20	压力锅	卵巢	细胞浆
Melan-A	A103	DAKO	1:400	微波20分钟	黑色素瘤	细胞浆
MIB-1	7B11	Zymed	1:50	压力锅	乳腺癌	核
MOC-31	MOC-31	DAKO	1:40	微波	结肠癌	细胞膜
p16	E6H4	DAKO	1:400	微波30分钟	横纹肌肉瘤	细胞浆/核
p53	1801	BioGenex	1:150	压力锅	卵巢癌	核
p63	4A4	DAKO	1:800	微波30分钟	胰腺癌	核
PLAP	多克隆	DAKO	1:500	不修复	胎盘	细胞浆
PR	PR88	BioGenex	1:50	压力锅	乳腺癌	核
PTEN(phospho)	多克隆	Cell Signaling	1:200	微波	子宫内膜癌	细胞浆
S-100	多克隆	DAKO	1:4000	不修复	皮肤	细胞浆/核
SMA	1A4	DAKO	1:400	不修复	结肠癌	细胞浆
Synaptophysin	Sy 38	DAKO	1:100	不修复	脑组织	细胞浆
Vimentin	V9	DAKO	1:100	微波10分钟	结肠癌	细胞浆
WT-1	6F-H2	DAKO	1:25	微波	Wilms瘤	细胞核

体[9]。MIB-1和多克隆Ki-67抗体（DAKO，Carpenteria，CA）皆能识别固定组织中Ki-67抗原。由于Ki-67抗原会在离开细胞周期后迅速被裂解，而PCNA则持续存在，所以Ki-67抗体作为细胞增殖标志物优于PCNA[10]。

应用MIB-1免疫组化分析时，不能只报阳性或阴性，其Ki-67阳性细胞的百分比及分布更有意义。正常情况下Ki-67阳性细胞仅限于皮肤及黏膜鳞状上皮的基层及旁基层。上皮内瘤变时MIB-1阳性细胞在数目及分布位置上皆随病变程度而增加[11, 12]。Ki-67阳性表达也可见于良性病变及组织修复反应。后者多伴有正常鳞状上皮组织成熟分化的丧失[13]。应用细胞增殖标志物为病变诊断及特定情况下的质控提供较为客观的方法。Ki-67不仅仅是阴性或阳性，更重要的是阳性细胞的百分数及特异性的分布。经用抗原暴露法（如组织经微波处理）之后，Ki-67的核染色更明显和清晰，因而更易识别。此外切片中的上皮细胞或淋巴细胞可作为阳性对照，偶尔少量的正常宫颈管上皮细胞也能被Ki-67标记[14]。

p63

p63是抑癌基因*p53*的同源家族，与胚胎发育有关，可表达于有鳞状细胞的器官，也见于非肿瘤性鳞状化生的宫颈管上皮细胞核、上皮内瘤变和浸润性鳞癌。不表达于腺癌或神经内分泌肿瘤。因此p63抗体可用于区别低分化鳞癌与腺癌，或用于小细胞神经内分泌癌与低分化鳞癌（尤其是基底细胞样或小细胞的变型）的鉴别。

p16

p16是细胞周期调控成分。在人乳头状病毒HPV（肿瘤蛋白产物E6和E7）相关的肿瘤细胞内呈细胞核及细胞浆着色。因此是检测HPV的替代标记物。异常的MIB-1标记与p16过表达可确定高危型的HPV病变，如浸润性宫颈鳞癌/高级别上皮内瘤变（HSIL）、腺癌/原位腺癌（AIS）以及一组低度鳞状上皮病变。p16阴性和MIB-1表达属于低危型HPV病变（一组LSIL病变和所有的湿疣）的特征。需要指出的是p16表达在宫颈管腺癌是普遍而弥漫的，但在宫颈内膜腺癌仅呈斑片状着色或完全阴性。因此p16染色有助于宫颈管腺癌与宫颈内膜癌的鉴别诊断。

神经内分泌标志物

神经内分泌标志物嗜铬素和突触素可用于宫颈神经内分泌肿瘤的鉴别诊断，包括类癌、大细胞性神经内分泌肿瘤和小细胞癌[31]。单个或孤立的神经内分泌细胞可见于子宫颈恶性腺瘤（adenoma malignum）[32]、腺癌、鳞癌[33]及子宫内膜腺癌[34]。神经细胞黏附分子NCAM和CD56在自然杀伤细胞（NK）和NK细胞肿瘤的表达早为人知，目前NCAM和CD56也被作为一种辅助性的神经内分泌标志物[35, 36]。

鉴别诊断

原发性Paget病与继发性Paget病、表浅播散型黑色素瘤和Paget样的外阴上皮内瘤变

Paget病是一种鳞状上皮内腺癌，其特征是在表皮或部分皮肤附属器内可见空泡状核的胞浆丰富淡染的大Paget细胞（图16.1A）。免疫组化可协助乳腺外Paget病与表浅扩散型黑色素瘤和Paget样外阴上皮内瘤变（VIN）的鉴别诊断。免疫组化也可用于识别盆腔内的恶性肿瘤在表皮的扩散（继发性Paget病）。一组有助于鉴别诊断乳腺外Paget病的免疫组化抗体包括：角蛋白（AE1/AE3、CK7/CK20）、CEA、GCDFP和S-100（表16.2）。

CK7弥漫而均匀一致地表达于Paget细胞的胞浆，但在鳞状上皮细胞不表达（图16.1B）[37, 38]。CK7可用于鉴别Paget细胞是否存在于手术切缘，以及判断早期间质浸润。但是CK7也可标记与Paget细胞相似的上皮内Toker细胞[39]。有报道称Paget样VIN的肿瘤性鳞状细胞CK7也呈强阳性[40]，因此要准确区分Paget病与Paget样VIN，需用高分子量角蛋白，后者在Paget样VIN呈阳性。但低分子量角蛋白如CK8（通常用CAM5.2）、CEA和GCDFP，在典型Paget病呈阳性，在VIN则阴性。所以尽管CK7阳性细胞是Paget病的敏感标志物，但它并不具有特异性。CK20也应包括在这一组诊断抗体之列，尤其当考虑到其他内脏肿瘤有可能继发性累及表皮时。原发性Paget病CK20阴性（图16.1C），CK20阳性可见于直肠癌、移行细胞癌和极少数原发性乳腺外Paget病的转移灶[37, 41, 42]。

当疑有Paget病时，下述抗体作用不大：广谱细胞角蛋白、CEA和GCDFP或BRST-2。由于AE1/AE3

可同时标记鳞状上皮和Paget细胞，故其应用价值有限。CEA单抗可在多数Paget病表达（图16.1D），但表达程度可能较弱[37]。尽管GCDFP对Paget病不像CK7那样敏感，却也是有用的标志物（图16.1E）。GCDFP常常表达于原发性外阴Paget病，而少见于与内脏恶性肿瘤有关的继发性病变[37, 43]。若病变CK20+/ GCDFP- 则应考虑结肠/泌尿道癌，特别须注意，上皮内病变同时表达CK7+/CK20+ 极为罕见。非肿瘤性Toker细胞为CK7+/CK20-，非肿瘤性Merkel细胞为CK7-/CK20+，而Merkel细胞癌在上皮内扩散时为CK7-/CK20+。

几乎所有的黑色素瘤都表达S-100，尽管偶尔Paget细胞也呈S-100阳性，而Paget病时一般S-100阴性（图16.1F）。若此组抗体中有任何一种阳性，HMB-45应被视为黑色素瘤的诊断性抗体。与黑色素细胞有关的抗体还包括MART-1/A103、小眼转录因子和酪氨酸酶[43]。它们的应用与HMB-45相似。如果角蛋白和黑色素标记物均为阴性，应考虑有Paget样特征的皮肤T细胞淋巴瘤[43]。

> **诊断要点：外阴原发性Paget病**
> 1. Paget细胞CK7弥漫强阳性。
> 2. Paget细胞典型的为CEA+/GCDFP+。
> 3. 若GCDFP-/CK20+ 应考虑继发性Paget病。
> 4. 鲍温样VIN的非典型鳞状细胞和上皮内的Toker细胞均表达CK7。
> 5. 树突状细胞S-100阳性，而Paget细胞通常S-100阴性。

尖锐湿疣、鳞状上皮乳头状瘤和纤维上皮性息肉

细胞增殖标志物可作为检测HPV相关病变的辅助手段。然而正如免疫组化方法检测HPV一样，它缺乏敏感性[44]。常见外阴外生性病变的鉴别诊断包括尖锐湿疣、纤维上皮性息肉和鳞状上皮乳头状瘤。尽管挖空细胞样病变（koilocytosis）是HPV相关病变的特征性改变，这一现象却不多见于外阴湿疣。湿疣的诊断主要依赖一些非特征性变化，诸如乳头状瘤样病变、表皮增厚、过度角化和单个细胞异常角化。MIB-1和Ki-67在正常外阴皮肤及黏膜的表达局限于旁基层，其在外阴上皮内瘤变和湿疣的表达可上延至表皮上2/3层[12, 45]。研究表明，MIB-1阳性表达与HPV原位杂交所测的分布相似（图16.2A~C），皆位于所有尖锐湿疣的上2/3上皮层。相反，MIB-1阳性细胞在全部10例鳞状上皮乳头状瘤（图16.2D~F）和12/14例纤维上皮性息肉（图16.2G~I）仅限于基层及旁基层细胞。因此对模棱两可的湿疣，MIB-1染色有助于校正HPV DNA阴性时的过诊断和HPV DNA阳性时的低诊断。

分化型的VIN3与鳞状上皮增生

湿疣、基底细胞样和鲍温样VIN3（普通型VIN3）均是与HPV相关的病变。分化型的VIN3（differentiated VIN），也称单纯型VIN3（simplex VIN），通常并非源于HPV感染[47, 47]。分化型的VIN3常与鳞状上皮增生和/或硬化性苔藓有关。与分化型VIN3有关的浸润癌是高分化和角化型，反之源于普通型VIN3的浸润癌为基底细胞样和非角化型。病变本身呈棘皮症样、过度角化和角化不全。分化型VIN3表层有含核的角化细胞（parakeratosis）。除基底细胞外，几乎整个表层增厚（图16.3A、B）。成熟的角化细胞有嗜酸性胞浆、核大、染色质松解且核仁明显[49, 50]。可见宽、厚、圆形的基底层轮廓和分支网状的边缘以及奇异的基底角化。Ki-67可标记其增生活性，基底层阳性但外底层阴性（与湿疣和基底细胞样VIN3相反）。增殖指数在鳞状上皮增生和硬化性苔藓不显著，后者与分化型VIN3相似，建议此时使用p53作为辅助诊断[48]。p53在大约75%的分化型VIN3的基底层和外底层呈弥漫强阳性表达（图16.3C），而在鳞状上皮增生和硬化性苔藓中局灶性弱表达或不表达[48]。要注意的是，限于基底鳞状细胞呈斑块状着色的p53偶尔也见于正常皮肤、一定数量增生的鳞状上皮、硬化性苔藓和脂溢性角化病[51]。分化型VIN3被认为是高度鳞状上皮病变，可能比普通型VIN3更易发生浸润性癌。低度分化型VIN目前认识不足，相反普通型VIN组织学与宫颈鳞状上皮内病变相似，两者免疫表型也相似，将于下一部分讨论。

外阴、阴道、宫颈鳞状上皮和腺上皮内病变

研究了Ki-67（MIB-1）在宫颈肿瘤中的表达[11, 14, 52-56]，证实在高度鳞状上皮内病变（HSIL）中，包括外阴和阴道的VAIN 2级和3级，Ki-67的表达弥漫均一地分布于病变的全层；尽管在低度鳞状上皮内病变（LSIL）中的阳性细胞百分数较低，但仍能在表层

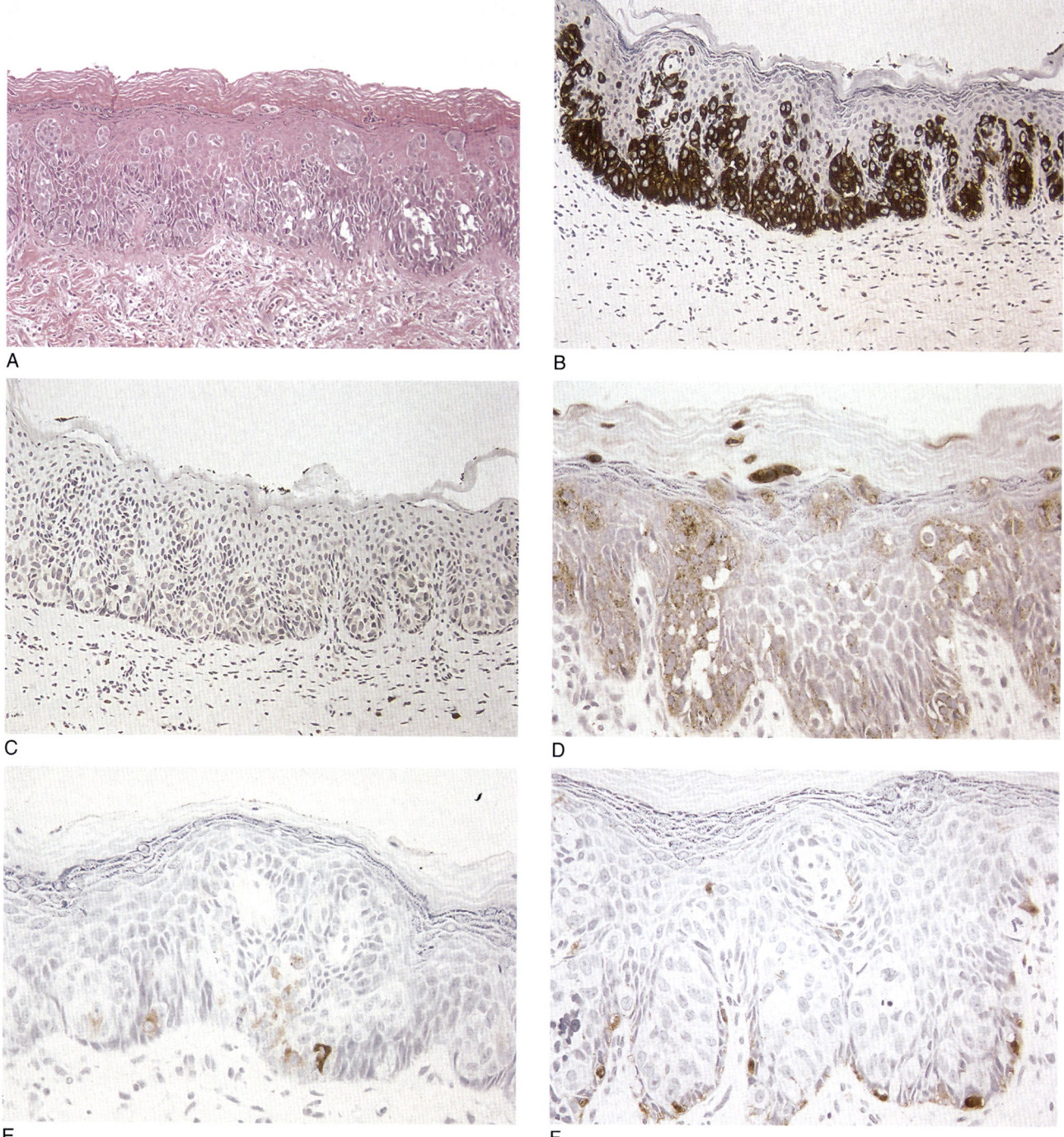

图 16.1 乳腺外Paget病的免疫组化谱。(A) HE染色;(B) CK7在病变细胞中呈强阳性表达;(C) CK20阴性表达;(D) CEA显示胞浆中呈颗粒状中度阳性;(E) GCDFP呈局部弱阳性;(F) S-100显示树突状细胞阳性,病变细胞未着色

上皮见到阳性细胞。HPV相关病变的细胞增生主要归于由HPV肿瘤蛋白,特别是早期蛋白E6和E7诱导的细胞分裂增加。

尽管组织学特点仍被视为诊断上皮内病变的最重要的工具,但当诊断特征不是一目了然时,Ki-67可起一定的作用(表16.3)。正常宫颈黏膜中Ki-67表达限于旁基层细胞并呈均匀一致的线状染色带(图16.4A、B)。应注意到,正常黏膜基底细胞本身并不着色。鳞状上皮化生时,尽管旁基层细胞和局灶基底层细胞可着色(图16.4E、F),但与正常鳞状上皮黏膜相比没有显著区别[11, 52],包括炎症区域[54]。SIL病变时,不仅旁基层细胞与基底层细胞着色数目增加,Ki-67

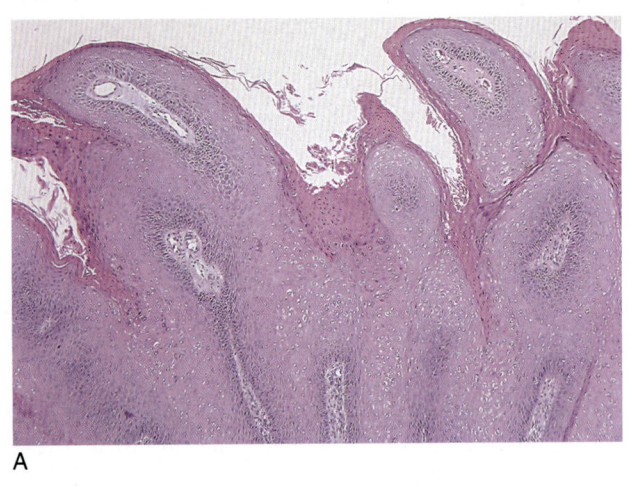
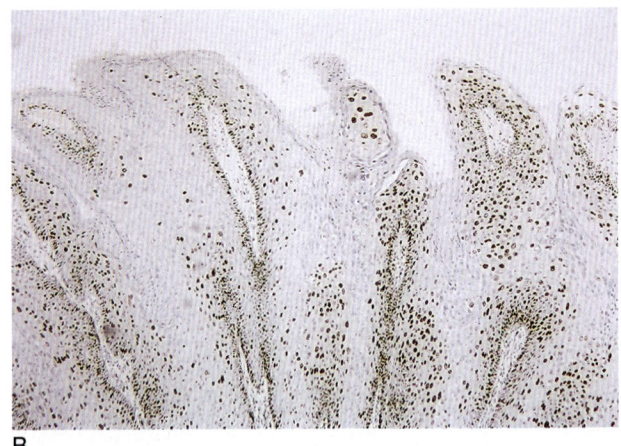
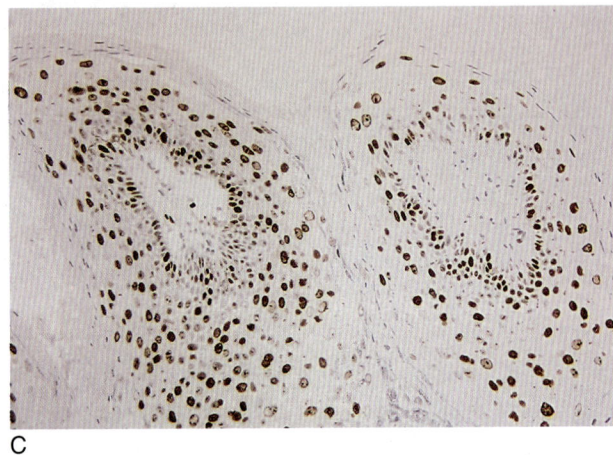
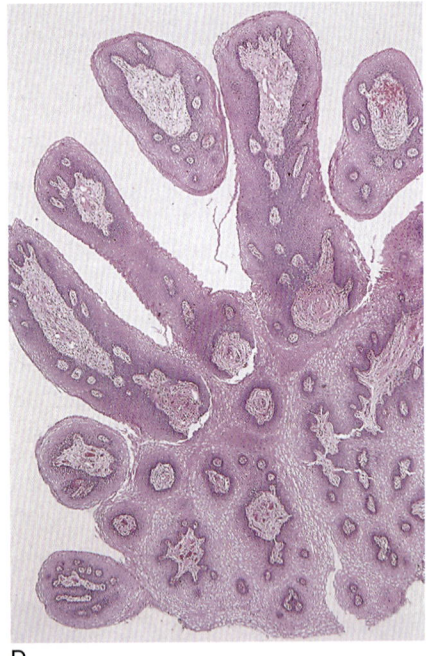
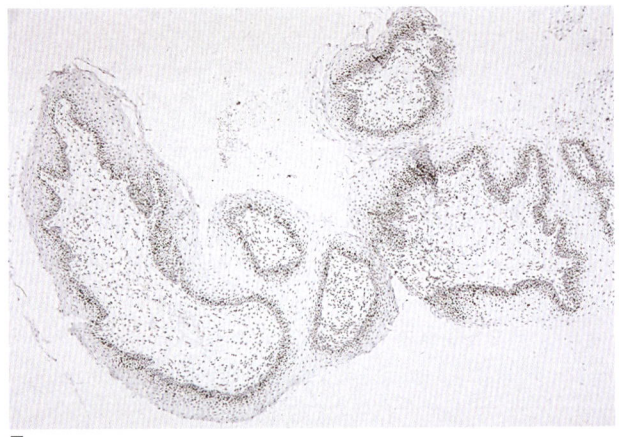
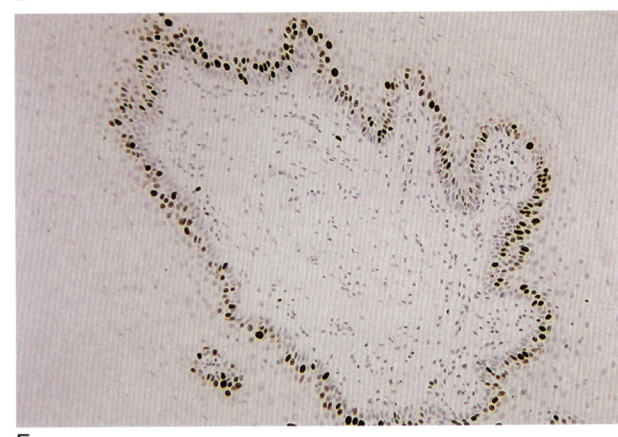

图16.2 常见外阴外生性病变的 Ki-67 免疫组化染色。(A~C) 尖锐湿疣：除基底细胞层着色以外，上皮全层均显示Ki-67阳性；(D~F)，鳞状细胞乳头状瘤

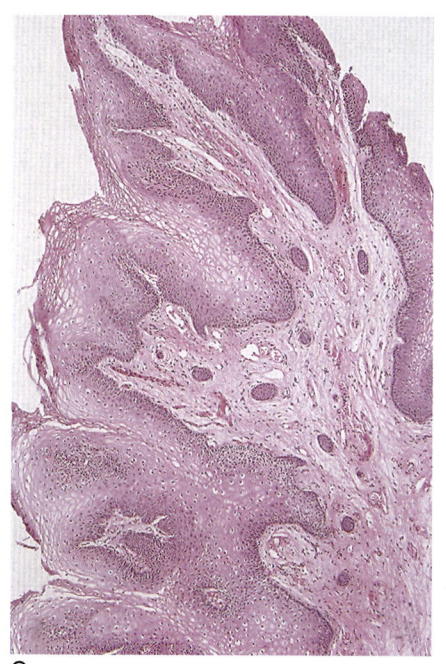

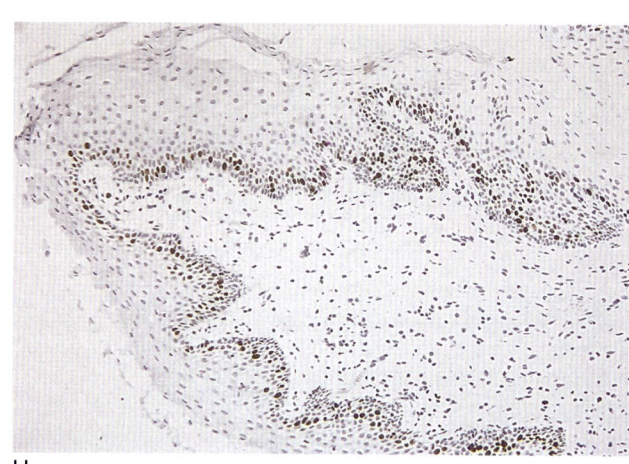

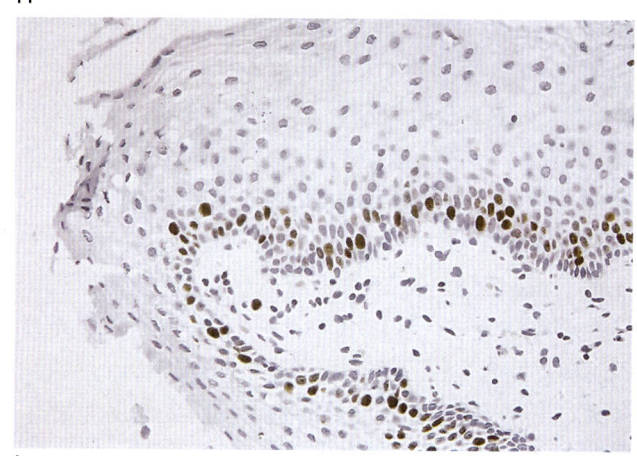

图 16.2 续 （G～I）纤维上皮性息肉，类似于正常皮肤或鳞状上皮黏膜，仅显示外底层细胞线状着色，表层及中层上皮 Ki-67 阴性

表 16.2 外阴 Paget 样病变

疾病类型	AE1/AE3	CK7	CK20	CEA	GCDFP	S-100	LCA
Paget 病	S	+	S	S	S	R	N
继发性 Paget 病	+	+	S	+	N	N	N
Paget 样外阴上皮内瘤变	+	N	N	N	N	N	N
表浅播散型黑色素瘤	N	N	N	N	N	+	N
淋巴瘤	N	N	N	N	N	N	+

N，阴性；+，阳性；S，有时阳性；R，极少阳性

阳性细胞也扩延至中间层细胞（LSIL，图16.4G、H）或表层全部细胞（HSIL，图16.4I、J）。Ki-67通常也能使上皮内淋巴细胞着色，因此可有假阳性。

萎缩由于缺乏成熟性，可形如HSIL病变。但其典型的组织学为良性核形态且缺乏核分裂象。Ki-67阴性也可用于确认萎缩（图16.4C、D）[53,55]。非典型不成熟鳞状化生（AIM）可酷似HSIL，尽管与正常相比，Ki-67指数在AIM较为增加，但其表达与正常宫颈、LSIL和HSIL有很大的重叠性。因此，提示AIM是一组异质性病变[13]。

MIB-1的表达也可用于腺体肿瘤性病变（如原位腺癌和腺癌）与宫颈炎、微腺体增生和输卵管子宫内膜样化生的鉴别诊断（表16.3）[56,57]。在肿瘤性腺体增加的MIB-1阳性细胞百分数和分布很像HSIL和鳞癌。

HPV感染与p16表达的关系已用于诊断。因此可用p16和MIB-1表达一道来区别宫颈肿瘤和如下相似病变（表16.3）：HSIL与萎缩、HSIL与非典型反应和再生、HSIL与非典型不成熟化生、宫颈原位腺癌与反应性腺体不典型增生。多项研究已验证了这一

表16.3 宫颈鳞状上皮和腺上皮病变

疾病类型	MIB-1	p16
低级别鳞状上皮上皮内瘤变	+*	S
高级别鳞状上皮上皮内瘤变	+*	+
反应性鳞状上皮或腺上皮非典型性	N	N
非典型不成熟化生	S	N
原位腺癌	+	+
管状化生	N	S

* 鳞状上皮旁基层表达
N，阴性；+，阳性；S，有时阳性

工作[20-28, 30]。本表格缺乏包括LSIL的鉴别诊断，是因为只有少部分的LSIL与人类乳头状瘤病毒的E6、E7有关。p16在LSIL的表达率是60%～80%，而HSIL接近100%（图16.4 K）[22, 24, 28]，因此，如果病变形态和其他免疫组化结果支持诊断，即使p16阴性也不能排除LSIL。另外LSIL和HSIL表达p16的情况也不同，p16阳性的LSIL中含有的免疫反应细胞较少，染色强度也较弱。在LSIL中，p16标记严格限于下1/3的鳞状上皮，全层均匀标记则更多见于HSIL。尽管如此，作者在使用p16区分鳞状上皮病变程度上仍有顾虑。一些研究显示绝大多数p16标记胞浆，偶尔胞核[22]；而另一些学者则明确表示应该核强阳性[24, 28]。我们认为胞浆明显着色且核着色，限于HSIL/重度异型。不同结论可能源于不同克隆抗体和/或方法。

p16在宫颈管腺体的表达已有研究定论（图16.5），这是因为几乎所有常见的宫颈管腺癌与高危型HPV感染有关。注意下列宫颈腺癌亚型可能与HPV感染无关：恶性腺瘤（或微偏腺癌）、中肾腺癌，以及浆液和透明细胞腺癌[58, 59]。据我们所知，对这些特殊类型肿瘤，尚无p16表达的大量研究。另一个重要的陷阱是p16在输卵管子化生和输卵管子宫内膜化生的表达，p16偶尔也见于良性子宫内膜成分中。因此，作者推荐对所有病例应联合使用Ki-67和p16，尽管子宫内膜和输卵管化生可弱表达p16，MIB-1指数却非常低。

由于Ki-67和p16能客观提高诊断率，因此，质量评价和质量保证也是重要的。本书已记载了数个研究结果[24, 29, 46, 60]。

有一点应引起注意：尽管已发表的资料明确支持p16作为中等和高危型HPV感染的代言者，但仍有几个实验室资料提示p16应用方面的困难，甚至认为是有缺陷的。显然有必要增加用于任何抗体的最优

化的实验数据方面的研究工作。

免疫组化也可应用于宫颈涂片和液基细胞学[61, 62]。最近研究显示，用空气干燥涂片，0.3%过氧化氢阻断，和在磷酸缓冲液中的抗生物素-生物素过氧化物酶法给予最佳Ki-6标记效果[61]。最近也有将p16免疫组化用于细胞学的报道[63-66]，而这些结果提示p16能作为传统筛查方法的辅助诊断。但由于在子宫内膜组织、输卵管子宫内膜化生和输卵管型别中偶尔有p16表达，由此造成的假阳性令人关注。

> **诊断要点**：鳞状上皮内病变／腺上皮内病变
>
> 1. Ki-67在鳞状上皮病变旁基层细胞核的表达，无论伴/或不伴有p16表达，均支持LSIL。
> 2. Ki-67表达增加伴p16表达支持HSIL。
> 3. Ki-67和p16在腺体病变弥漫表达支持宫颈管腺癌，而仅表达其中一种抗体则排除腺癌诊断。

恶性腺瘤、高分化腺癌和良性腺体病变

有时鉴别宫颈的良性与恶性腺病变常较为困难，尤其当恶性病变为高分化如恶性腺瘤时。有人提出使用CEA、Ki-67和p53免疫组化有助于鉴别诊断。许多研究证实，CEA细胞浆的表达见于多数宫颈腺癌，而正常宫颈腺上皮为阴性[32, 67-69]。但是，因为CEA在恶性腺瘤时的表达可局灶性或弥散性，所以CEA在肿瘤的活检标本或刮除术时可能为阴性反应[32]。CEA与Ki-67和p53结合已成为一组有用的鉴别诊断抗体[69]。与形态学上酷似的正常宫颈和良性腺体增生，如隧道样腺簇增生（tunnel clusters）和微腺管增生相比，高增殖指数或CEA阳性，或两者均阳性，则限定于腺癌和恶性腺瘤以及原位腺癌（AIS）。此外，p53过表达（腺体核着色达10%），除去鲜红微腺体过度增生（florid microglandular hyperplasia）外，仅见于肿瘤性腺体。许多恶性腺瘤p53呈阴性，有趣的是，恶性腺瘤能显示胃肠道分化的不同级别和类型特点[59]。

宫颈管腺癌与子宫内膜腺癌

宫颈管与子宫体腺癌在形态学上有重叠（图16.6A），区分宫颈腺癌和子宫内膜腺癌大多可根据组织学不同的癌前病变，如原位腺癌（AIS）和核复杂性异常增生加以鉴别。也可凭肿瘤在宫颈或子宫体的分布优势而区分。宫颈腺癌100%表达CEA而仅有50%的

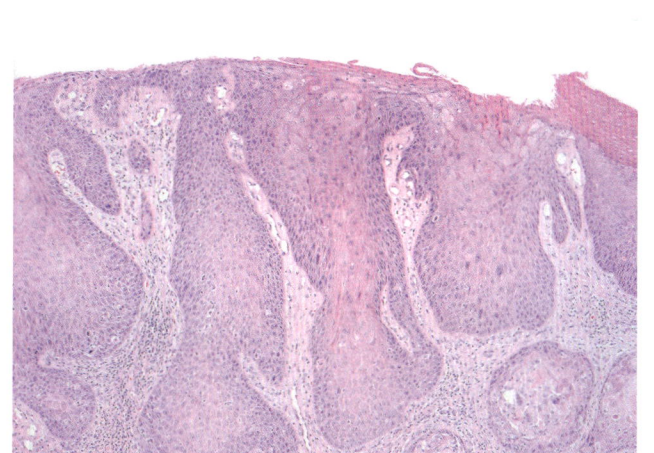
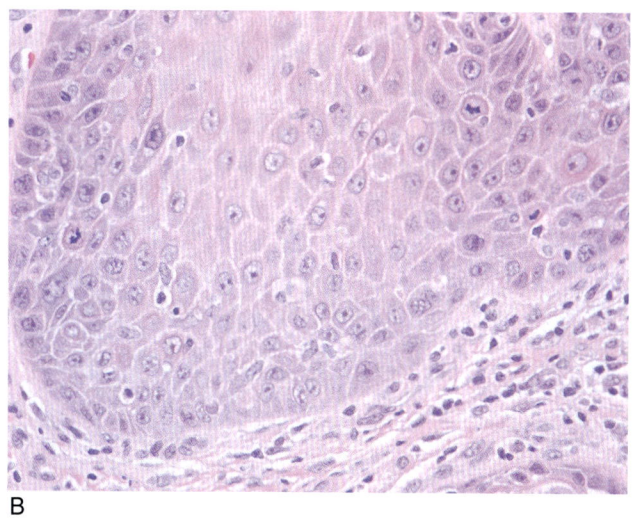

图16.3 分化型（单纯型）VIN3。（A）一个红润的分化型VIN3向下浸润的例子，角化型鳞状细胞癌；（B）高倍镜显示分化型VIN3的胞浆特点；（C）p53蛋白在分化型VIN3基底层和外底层的过表达，能区别鳞状上皮增生（p53阴性）

子宫体腺癌表达CEA，由于表达重叠性太大，因此CEA在个案病例诊断时缺乏临床应用价值[70-72]。CEA在子宫内膜腺癌的表达呈腺腔弱阳性，而在宫颈腺癌为瘤细胞胞浆和腺腔呈强阳性（图16.6B）。波形蛋白染色更有临床价值（表16.4），因为波形蛋白与低分子量细胞角蛋白同时表达见于多数子宫内膜腺癌，但很少见于宫颈腺癌（图16.6C）[73, 74]。目前，人们运用包括雌激素受体（ER）、孕激素受体（PR）和p16的一组抗体来鉴别宫颈和子宫体腺癌[29, 30, 75]。如子宫体分化型内膜样腺癌常有ER/PR表达（见下文"子宫体"），而与高危型HPV感染有关的宫颈腺癌常有p16过表达。因此1级和2级子宫体内膜样腺癌（FIGO1、2）应表达ER/PR和波形蛋白，而大多数宫颈腺癌ER/PR阴性（图16.6D），但CEA和p16阳性（图16.6E）。关于p16在区别宫颈和子宫内膜癌的特异性仍存有争议。但在鉴别子宫内膜的浆液性癌时p16免疫组化有重要意义。

所以当出现宫颈或子宫内膜来源不明的腺癌时，我们提倡应密切与临床联系。

表16.4 子宫颈腺癌和子宫内膜腺癌*

	CEA**	Vimentin	ER/PR	p16
子宫颈	+	N	N	+
子宫内膜*	N	+	+	S

* 子宫内膜样型
** 细胞浆
N，阴性；+，阳性；S，有时阳性

> **诊断要点**：子宫内膜的内膜样癌和宫颈内膜癌
>
> 1. 多数典型的宫颈管腺癌表达CEA和p16。
> 2. 多数典型的内膜样子宫体腺癌表达波形蛋白和ER/PR。

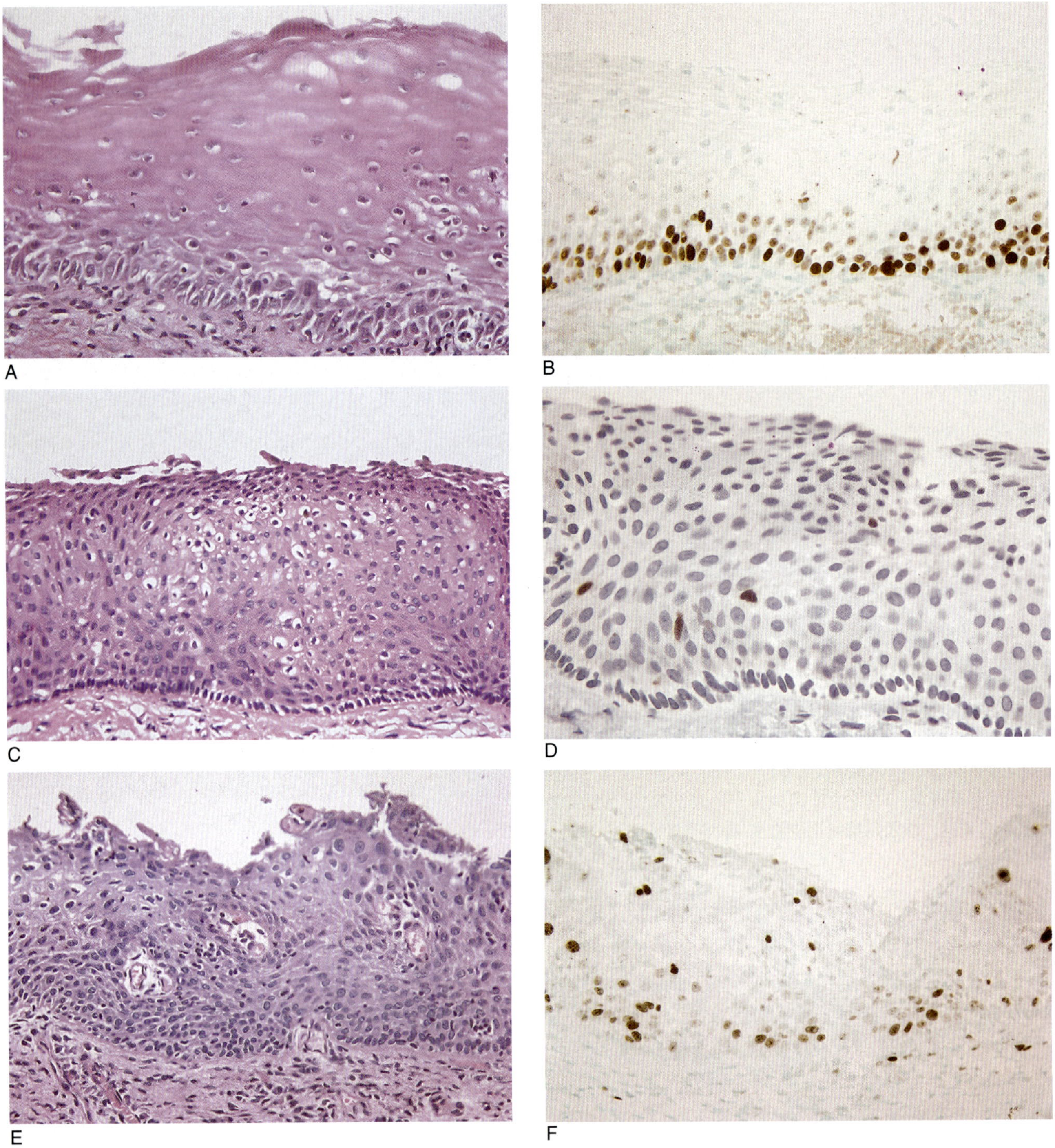

图 16.4　Ki-67 在正常宫颈染色（A 和 B）、绝经后萎缩的上皮（C 和 D）和炎性鳞状化生（E 和 F）

微腺体增生和黏液性子宫内膜腺癌

这两类病变在组织学上有明显的相似性[76, 77]，年轻患者近期服用激素会出现有核下空泡特点的微腺体增生（MGH）。黏液性子宫内膜癌（MEA）见于老年患者，腺体可有鳞状上皮化生，至少中度细胞异型，有核分裂象，出现间质泡沫细胞，因不表达 CEA 而表达 ER/PR 区别于宫颈管腺癌。MGH 通常 CEA 阴性，ER/PR 阳性，因此这些抗体对子宫内膜腺癌诊断作用不大。一组更有用的免疫标记物包括波形蛋白和 MIB-1。波形蛋白在大多数子宫内膜腺癌和 MEA 中表达，增殖指数接近 10%，相反 MGH 不表达波形蛋白，通常仅偶尔核表达 MIB-1（＜1%）。

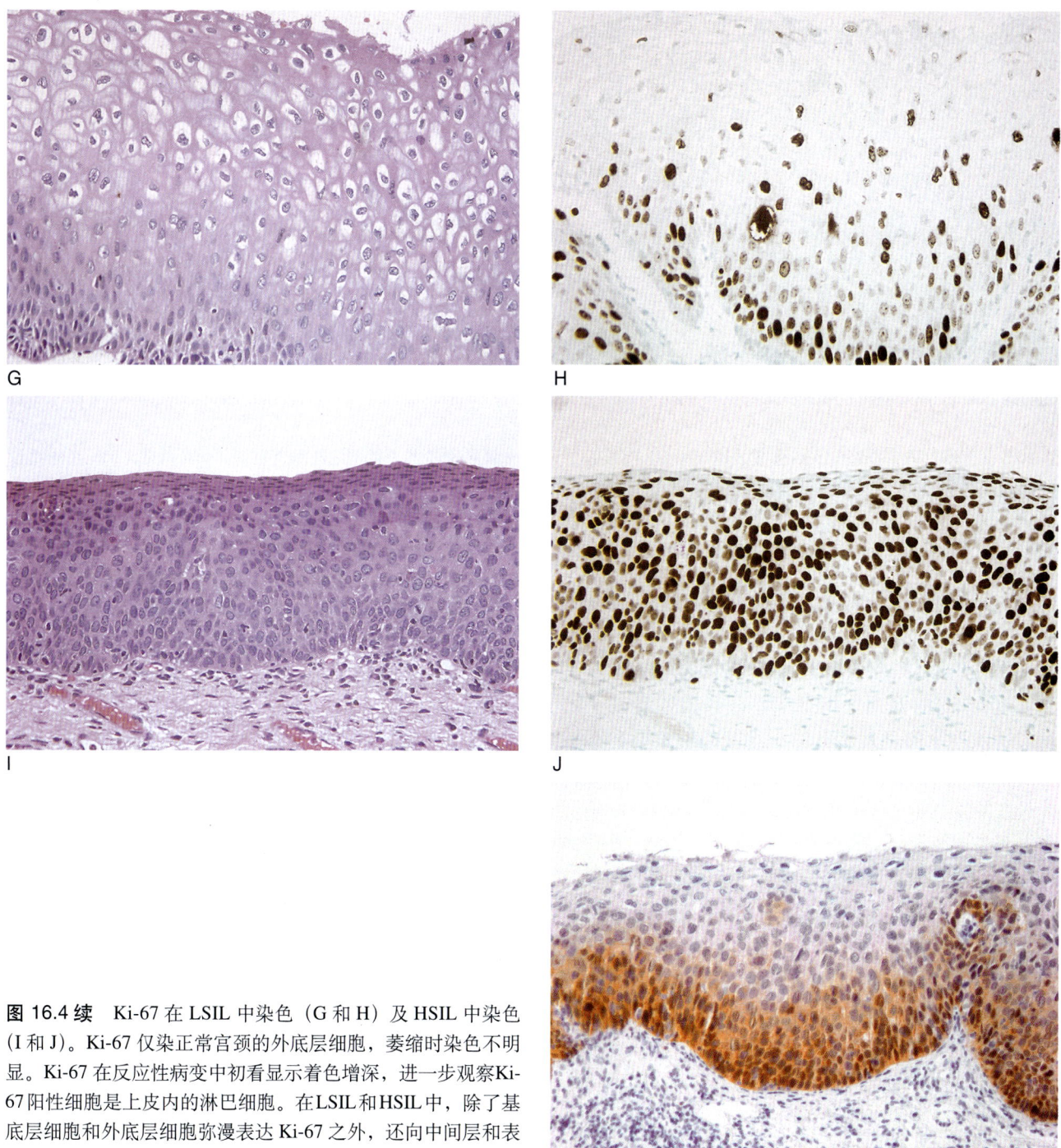

图 16.4 续　Ki-67 在 LSIL 中染色（G 和 H）及 HSIL 中染色（I 和 J）。Ki-67 仅染正常宫颈的外底层细胞，萎缩时染色不明显。Ki-67 在反应性病变中初看显示着色增深，进一步观察Ki-67 阳性细胞是上皮内的淋巴细胞。在 LSIL 和 HSIL 中，除了基底层细胞和外底层细胞弥漫表达 Ki-67 之外，还向中间层和表层扩展，LSIL 显示表层细胞斑块状着色，而 HSIL 则全层弥漫表达。（K）在 HSIL 中 p16 呈强阳性核浆表达

Arias-Stella 反应和透明细胞癌

　　Arias-Stella（A-S）反应非常像透明细胞癌。MIB-1 和 p53 有助于鉴别诊断[78]。一项研究显示，27 例 A-S 反应的病例中只有 3 例细胞核 MIB-1 阳性＞5%，这 3 例核标记在 5% 和 25% 之间。与其相比，11 例透明细胞癌中有 9 例核标记＞5%，其中有 6 例＞25%。

尽管透明细胞癌一般比 A-S 反应增殖指数更高，但也有重叠。p53结果相似，多数 A-S 反应是阴性，偶尔 p53＞25%。透明细胞癌更倾向显示 p53 核阳性，11 例中有 7 例核阳性＞25%。有趣的是，不到 5% 的透明细胞癌显示＞75% 的阳性细胞，这一特点进一步提示 p53 基因突变和浆液癌密切相关（参考 "浆液癌与子宫内膜样癌"）。

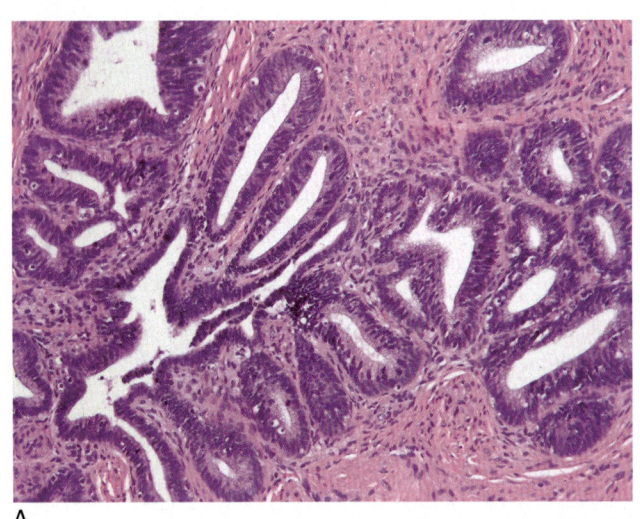 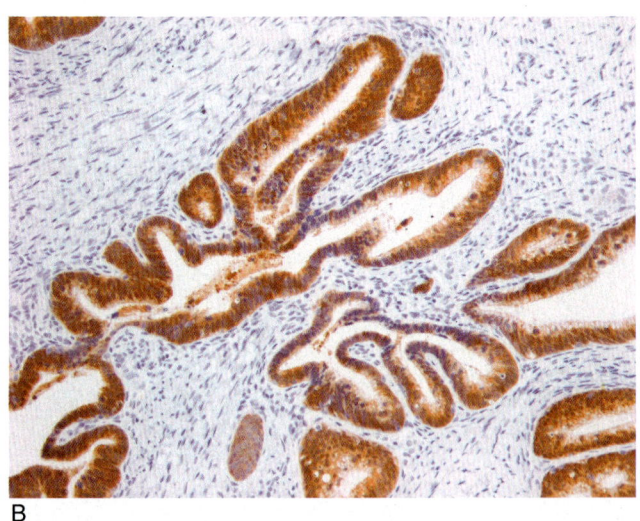

图 16.5 宫颈内膜原位癌，p16 弥漫表达（A，B）与反应性宫颈内膜病变和大多数增生性病变对照，p16 阴性，p16 在输卵管化生和子宫内膜斑块状着色是一种重要陷阱

大细胞神经内分泌癌、小细胞癌、鳞状细胞癌与淋巴瘤

为了与其他低分化癌鉴别，大细胞性神经内分泌肿瘤的神经内分泌特性应由免疫组化证实（表16-5）[31]。这些肿瘤可表达嗜铬素和突触素或两者同时表达[79]。由于近60%的宫颈小细胞癌不表达嗜铬素或突触素，所以当全部呈现所有的小细胞癌组织形态特征时，免疫组化染色并不为诊断所必需。但如果一肿瘤具有大多数而非全部小细胞癌的组织学特征时，免疫组化证实神经内分泌特性是有帮助的。假如一肿瘤的形态学呈临界图像且仅表达细胞角蛋白而不表达神经内分泌标记物时，此肿瘤有可能是小细胞鳞状上皮癌而非真正小细胞癌[45]。由于小细胞癌常需与淋巴瘤鉴别诊断，所以也应包括使用白细胞共同抗原（LCA）。

CD56作为一种神经内分泌分化标记物。研究表明，只有50%~70%的肺小细胞癌表达突触素和嗜铬素，而CD56抗体表达几乎达到100%[35]。在宫颈小细胞神经内分泌癌的临床病理研究中，21例中观察到15例有CD56表达，21例中有16例表达嗜铬素，21例中有19例表达突触素[36]。CD56特异性好，肺癌在缺乏神经内分泌分化时很少表达CD56。CD56被作为鉴别宫颈小细胞癌和基底细胞样/小细胞鳞癌重要的抗体。标记鳞状上皮的高分子量角蛋白（CK5/6或34βE12）和p63可作为优选抗体，尤其是嗜铬素和突触素阴性或不明确时[16, 17]。CD56表达而CK5/6或p63阴性，支持神经内分泌肿瘤，如小细胞癌，反之支持鳞癌。由于上述病变均与高危型HPV感染有关，p16的免疫组化一般无意义[81]。

子宫体

子宫体可发生各种类型上皮性和间叶来源的肿瘤，并常引起一些诊断问题，免疫组化有助于鉴别子宫内膜腺癌的组织类型以及浆液性癌的癌前病变、子宫内膜上皮内癌。间叶肿瘤也可引起诊断问题，免疫组化尤其能区别子宫内膜间质肿瘤和平滑肌肿瘤。

抗原/抗体生物学特性：子宫体肿瘤

上皮标记物（角蛋白和EMA）

一般来讲，为了证实肿瘤源于上皮组织，表达细胞角蛋白（AE1/AE3和CAM5.2）足以证实。但细胞角蛋白在子宫体的表达不仅仅限于上皮细胞。子宫内膜间质细胞和平滑肌细胞皆可局部性地表达角蛋白，尽管染色较弱[82-84]。典型的例子是恶性混合性苗勒管肿瘤（MMMT），其肿瘤细胞除表达间质标记物外，

表16.5 小细胞宫颈癌

疾病类型	Chromogranin**	CD56	高分子量 CK	LCA
神经内分泌癌*	+	+	N	N
鳞状细胞癌	N	N	+	N
淋巴瘤	N	S	N	+

* 包括小细胞癌
** 和/或突触素
N，阴性；+，阳性；S，有时阳性；hMW CK，高分子量CK（也可用p63）；LCA，淋巴细胞共同抗原

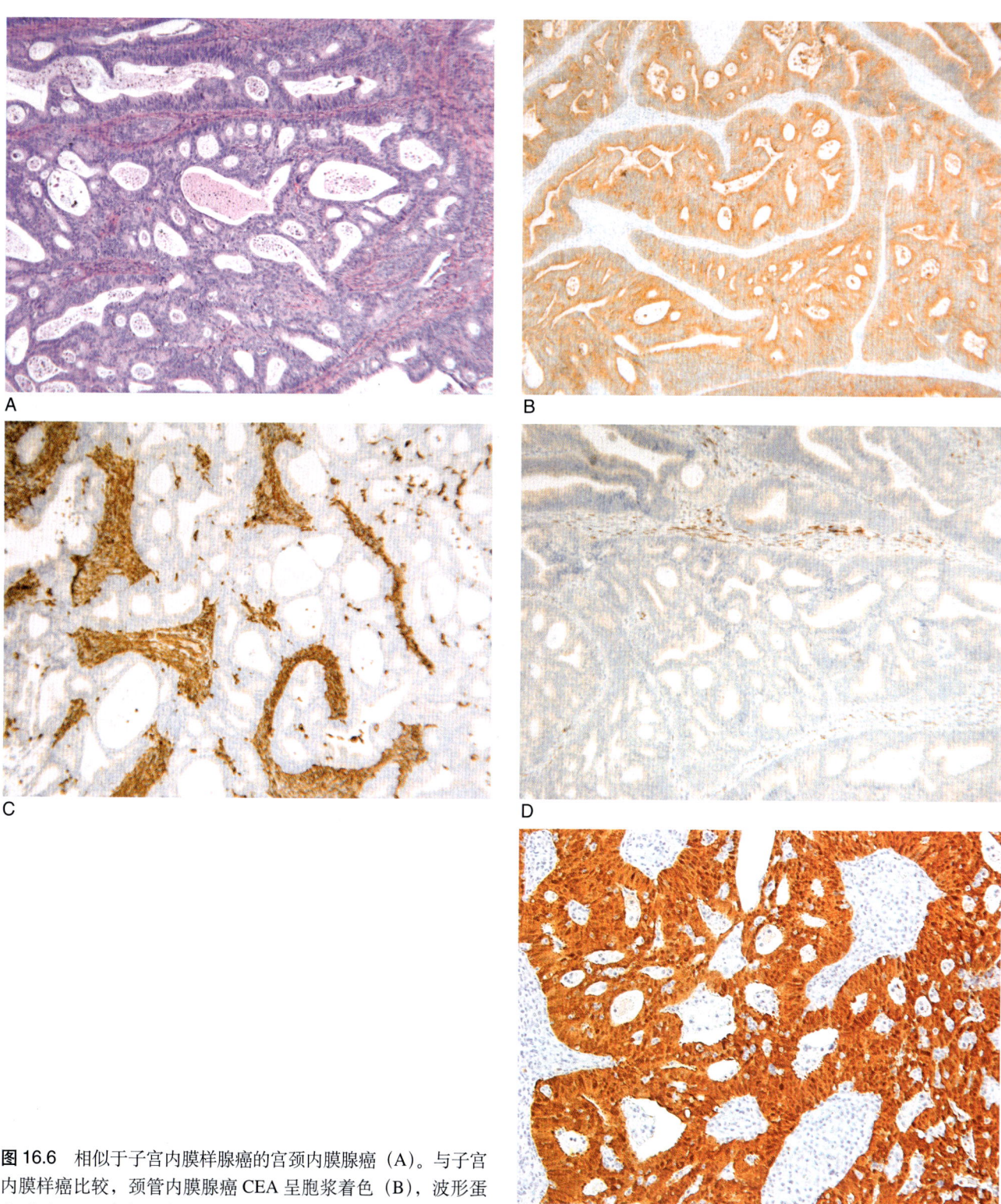

图16.6 相似于子宫内膜样腺癌的宫颈内膜腺癌（A）。与子宫内膜样癌比较，颈管内膜腺癌 CEA 呈胞浆着色（B），波形蛋白（C）、ER（D）阴性。p16 的表达在宫颈内膜腺癌占优（E）

也表达角蛋白和其他上皮标记物，如上皮细胞膜抗原（EMA）和CK7。

波形蛋白

波形蛋白是中间丝的一种，可见于正常增殖期内膜上皮细胞和多数子宫内膜癌[70,74]。正如前述，波形蛋白与低分子量角蛋白的共同表达有助于鉴别子宫内膜癌与子宫颈腺癌（前文已讨论）。

p53

大多数（80%）子宫浆液癌及其癌前病变子宫内膜上皮内癌（EIC）有p53的过表达[85-87]。最常用的抗p53蛋白的抗体可分为突变型和野生型，只有突变型 *p53* 基因导致弥漫和强的过表达。由于 *p53* 基因突变而出现异常p53蛋白，使得我们可通过免疫组化手段评价p53。因 *p53* 基因突变使其蛋白降解减少，故出现瘤细胞核着色，这种着色方式是显著的，即大于75%的瘤细胞强着色，与邻近未受累的萎缩子宫内膜形成明显对比。复杂性非典型增生和1级子宫内膜样腺癌罕见p53表达，即使有，也呈微弱和灶状[88-91]。随着肿瘤的级别增加，p53表达增强，一些3级的子宫内膜样腺癌呈强阳性[88-90, 92]。

β-钙黏素、PTEN、ER/PR

最近发现一些与p53相呼应的标记物，包括与子宫内膜样分化有关的抗体：ER/PR、β-钙黏素和PTEN[90-104]。众所周知，ER和PR在正常子宫组织、良性肿瘤和恶性肿瘤中皆表达。ER和PR在子宫内膜样腺癌中呈中等强度表达，在透明细胞癌中不表达或偶尔弱表达[88, 93, 104]。而在低分化子宫内膜样癌、浆液癌和透明细胞癌一样呈弱表达[94-96]。

β-钙黏素与细胞粘连有关，作为Wnt信号转导通路的成分之一，当其他因子突变或失稳定时易位到核内。核内β-钙黏素表达也可出现在50%的子宫内膜样腺癌中[97, 98, 104-106]，但在浆液癌罕见[98, 104]。*PTEN* 是抑癌基因，其与40%~75%的子宫内膜样腺癌的发病有关。与p53比较，在绝大多数p53突变的病例中，PENT表达上调，PTEN突变则免疫组化阴性（正常组织阳性）。PTEN丢失在浆液癌报道非常少见[98-104]。

肌性标记物

肌动蛋白（MSA和SMSA）、结蛋白、h-钙调素结合蛋白用于鉴别平滑肌细胞。正常子宫内膜间质细胞表达波形蛋白和肌动蛋白，但不表达角蛋白和EMA[83]。一些作者发现，结蛋白可见于正常间质细胞和内膜间质细胞肿瘤。但也有研究报告结蛋白可作为可靠的标记物用于平滑肌与内膜间质细胞的鉴别[84, 107, 108]。抑制素是一种激素肽类，正常时见于卵巢的卵泡颗粒层细胞。已证实子宫间质细胞肿瘤的性索样成分表达抑制素[109]。有时平滑肌也表达角蛋白，但是即使高表达角蛋白的平滑肌肿瘤，尤其是上皮样平滑肌肿瘤也同时表达肌性分化标记物，因此鉴别诊断并不困难[110]。有报道子宫间质细胞肿瘤可染色角蛋白，但上皮细胞膜抗原EMA一般不表达[82-84, 107]。抗结蛋白抗体可用于标记癌肉瘤中横纹肌样成分，但是，由于免疫表型的重叠性，在缺乏恶性异源性成分（heterologous elements）时，免疫组化在鉴别癌肉瘤与低分化癌时几乎没有任何价值[111]。h-钙调素结合蛋白是较MSA、SMA和结蛋白更具特异性的平滑肌分化标记物，能更好地识别子宫内膜间质肿瘤和这些肿瘤的平滑肌分化[112, 113]。这样，h-钙调素结合蛋白及其他肌源性标记物在部分有平滑肌分化的子宫内膜间质肿瘤中表达就不足为奇了。平滑肌肿瘤中证实有抗垂体催产素受体的抗体，但子宫内膜间质肿瘤中没有发现[114]。

CD10 和 WT-1

CD10被认为是急性淋巴母细胞淋巴病抗原，目前用于识别肿瘤性和非肿瘤性子宫内膜间质细胞[115-117]。它具有划分两类肿瘤的潜能：即腺肌症（adenomyosis）和浸润性子宫内膜癌、子宫内膜间质肿瘤与平滑肌肿瘤。然而使用CD10也存在复杂性，包括可着染浸润癌周围的子宫肌细胞，偶尔也可着染平滑肌肿瘤。CD10在伴有异质性分化的子宫内膜间质肿瘤可为阴性。WT-1是Wilms瘤的抑癌基因产物，可表达于子宫内膜间质和内膜间质肿瘤，但也表达于平滑肌肿瘤，因此无法鉴别这两类肿瘤[118, 119]。

鉴别诊断

浸润性子宫内膜样癌和累及腺肌症的子宫内膜样癌

CD10有助于区别浸润性子宫内膜癌和累及腺肌症的腺癌。由于CD10表达于内膜间质，而不表达于子宫肌层平滑肌，从理论上，位于子宫肌层的腺癌表达CD10将支持累及腺肌症的浸润癌[120, 121]。遗憾的是，在这一假设中至少有两个问题。事实上，许多浸润性腺癌被周边表达CD10的组织所围绕，而这种组织形态学表现类似于腺肌症的内膜间质[120, 121]。另一种不太常见的情况是化生间质。偶尔在子宫内膜癌中出现内膜间质，此支持子宫内膜癌经过了平滑肌或纤维母细胞化生，这种间质与内膜息肉类似。此化生的间质只局灶或弱表达CD10，所以，CD10阴性并不能完全除外子宫内膜间质和腺肌症。

子宫内膜上皮内癌与子宫内膜增生，包括化生

p53 抑癌基因正常用于证实子宫浆液癌及其癌前病变子宫内膜上皮内癌（EIC）。p53 的过表达体现为弥漫性强染色。这一染色特点可用于鉴别表浅子宫浆液癌或 EIC 与类似良性病变[85, 87]。子宫刮除术和子宫全切标本中常常见到细胞高度不典型性的表浅内膜病变（图16.7A）。若没有子宫肌层浸润，鉴别诊断应包括 EIC、表浅子宫浆液癌及内膜表层化生性改变，诸如嗜酸性变、输卵管化生和退变性改变（图 16.7D）。EIC 可能与肿瘤性内膜增生混淆，如复杂性不典型增生和子宫内膜癌 FIGO 1级。结合使用 Ki-67 和 p53 有助于鉴别诊断。辅加 Ki-67 可标示浆液癌（包括 EIC）中的不典型增生细胞（图 16.7B、C），而反应性或化生性病变则不表达 Ki-67 和 p53（图 16.7E、F）。

子宫浆液癌与子宫内膜样癌

子宫内膜样癌与浆液癌是子宫内膜癌中最主要的两个组织学类型。两者有着不同的临床表现和生物学行为。免疫组化不但用于显示其不同的生物途径，也用于鉴别诊断（表16.6）。区别的重要意义在于子宫浆液癌有较子宫内膜样癌更恶性的生物行为和导致不成比例的临床死亡[122, 123]。浆液癌（USC）有别于内膜样癌（UEC），因为大于80%的浆液癌为 p53 强阳性（图 16.8A～F）。相反，p53 阳性细胞仅见于 20% 的子宫内膜样癌[89]。p53 在高分化（1级）和中分化（2级）的内膜样癌呈阴性或弱阳性。同样在非典型复杂增生为阴性。分子生物学已证实 90% 的浆液癌有 *p53* 基因突变[86]，而仅 10%～20% 的子宫内膜样癌 *p53* 基因突变，后者多为高级别癌[86]。在评价 p53 免疫染色方面应特别注意，首要考虑的是许多病理学家认为的大于75%的细胞着色是否就是 p53 过表达，而斑块状和/或局灶以及和/或弱 p53 表达则不可靠。当腺体结构占优势时，浆液癌可被误认为内膜样癌。

虽然 p53 免疫组化对评价子宫内膜肿瘤有重要性，但有时也存在困难。有15%的浆液癌不表达 p53[89]。而 FIGO3 级的子宫内膜样腺癌可以表达 p53（图 16.8 G、H），因此 p53+ 本身意义不大。我们认为当鉴别 3 级 FIGO 子宫内膜癌时，不应推荐 p53。而对于高分化的子宫内膜样腺癌，诸如乳头结构和腺管形成但有高度级别的核时，p53 则有助于鉴别诊断（图 16.9A）。

最近增加一些有用的标记物，如 MIB-1、ER/PR、β- 钙黏素和 PTEN。当考虑浆液癌时，MIB-1 较为有用，尤其是当瘤细胞不表达 p53 时。MIB-1 弥漫而强着色（大于75%的细胞）支持浆液癌。当然若 p53 弥漫强阳性，MIB-1 也弥漫着色绝对支持浆液癌。ER/PR 在 FIGO1 级、2 级子宫内膜癌呈阳性（图 16.9B），但在浆液癌、透明细胞癌和 FIGO3 级子宫内膜癌中弱阳性或不表达[88, 93-96, 104]。ER、PR 可作为一组抗体的一部分来区别子宫内膜样癌和浆液癌。

大约 35%～50% 的子宫内膜样癌 β- 钙黏素核着色（图16.9C），与仅细胞膜着色的子宫内膜样癌和浆液癌形成对比。β-钙黏素在几乎所有的子宫内膜样癌（不考虑亚型）呈细胞膜强染色，但只有核的强着色才有助于诊断。这种现象说明有子宫内膜分化[97, 98, 104-106]。因此膜着色而核不着色无意义。可能核着色仅限于鳞状分化的区域，通常是灶状分布。所以仔细阅读切片非常重要。

与 p53 比较，PTEN 在大多数 *p53* 基因突变的病例中表达上调，PTEN 突变则不着色（与正常组织对比），PTEN 通常不在子宫内膜样癌中表达（图16.9D），浆液癌也只有少数表达[99-104]，为了避免 PTEN 免疫组化中的假阳性，建议使用于一组免疫组化抗体。因基因突变 PTEN 在子宫内膜样癌可不着色，故应建立明确的内对照。子宫内膜样癌由于 PTEN 遗传学变化可致组织不着色，而其周围的内膜间质和子宫肌层即可作为合适的内对照。评价 PTEN 阴性及其意义具有挑战性，尤其是当 PTEN 遗传改变，与其相关的免疫组化研究还未得到肯定证实时。只要表明 PTEN 着色很少即可，因为很可能存在 PTEN 遗传学改变；作者曾提出以 10% 着色作为界线来区别 PTEN 阴性（小于10%）和 PTEN 阳性（大于10%），以鉴别 UEC/USC[104]，但这一提案尚未得到证实。

诊断要点：子宫内膜样癌和浆液性乳头状癌

1. 最好使用一组抗体而不是只用 p53 进行 UEC/USC 的鉴别诊断。
2. 大多数研究中使用一组抗体包括 p53、ER/PR 和 MIB-1 是有意义的。
3. 大约有10%的疑难病例免疫组化不能提供结论性的信息。
4. 密切联系传统形态学特征和临床资料非常关键。

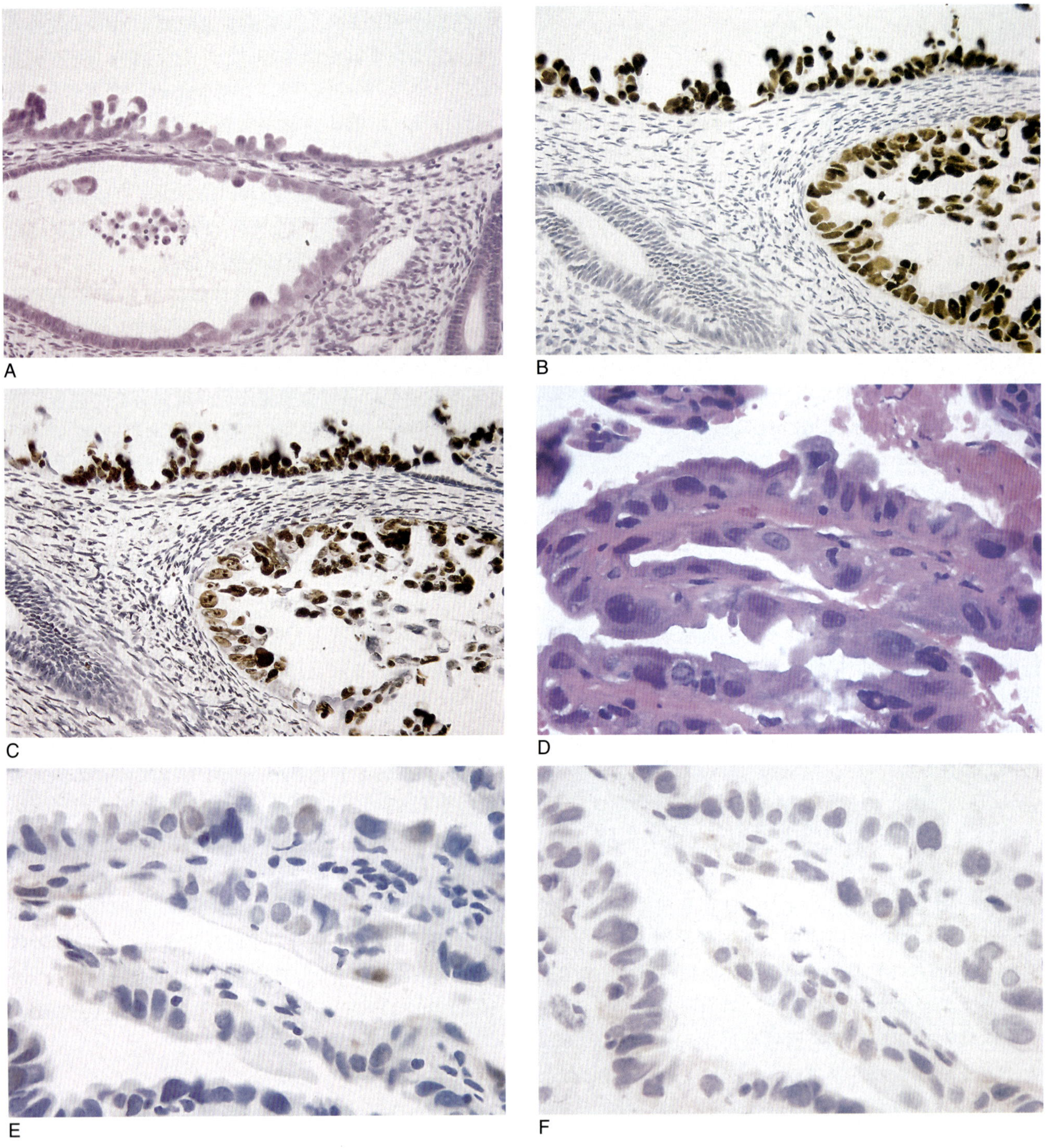

图 16.7 p53 和 Ki-67 在子宫内膜表层化生及退行性变与子宫内膜表面浆液性癌及子宫内膜上皮内癌（EIC）的比较。EIC（A~C）与化生及退行性变对照（D~F），p53（B 和 E）和 Ki-67（C 和 F）在 EIC 呈均匀一致的核强染

表 16-6 子宫浆液性癌和子宫内膜样癌比较

病变类型	p53*	ER/PR	MIB-1	PTEN	β-catenin
浆液性	S	S	高	保持	正常
子宫内膜样	R	S	低	有时消失	正常或异常**

* 只有 75% 以上的细胞着色时算作阳性
** 单纯核着色视为异常
S，有时阳性；R，很少阳性

子宫内膜间质肿瘤与平滑肌肿瘤

诊断子宫间叶组织肿瘤最常见的困惑是鉴别子宫内膜间质肿瘤与子宫平滑肌瘤（图 16.10A）。富于细胞型子宫肌瘤很容易被误诊为子宫内膜间质结节[84]。从免疫组化角度，子宫内膜间质肿瘤、平滑肌瘤和平滑肌肉瘤之间有许多重叠性反应[82,83]。平滑肌肌动蛋

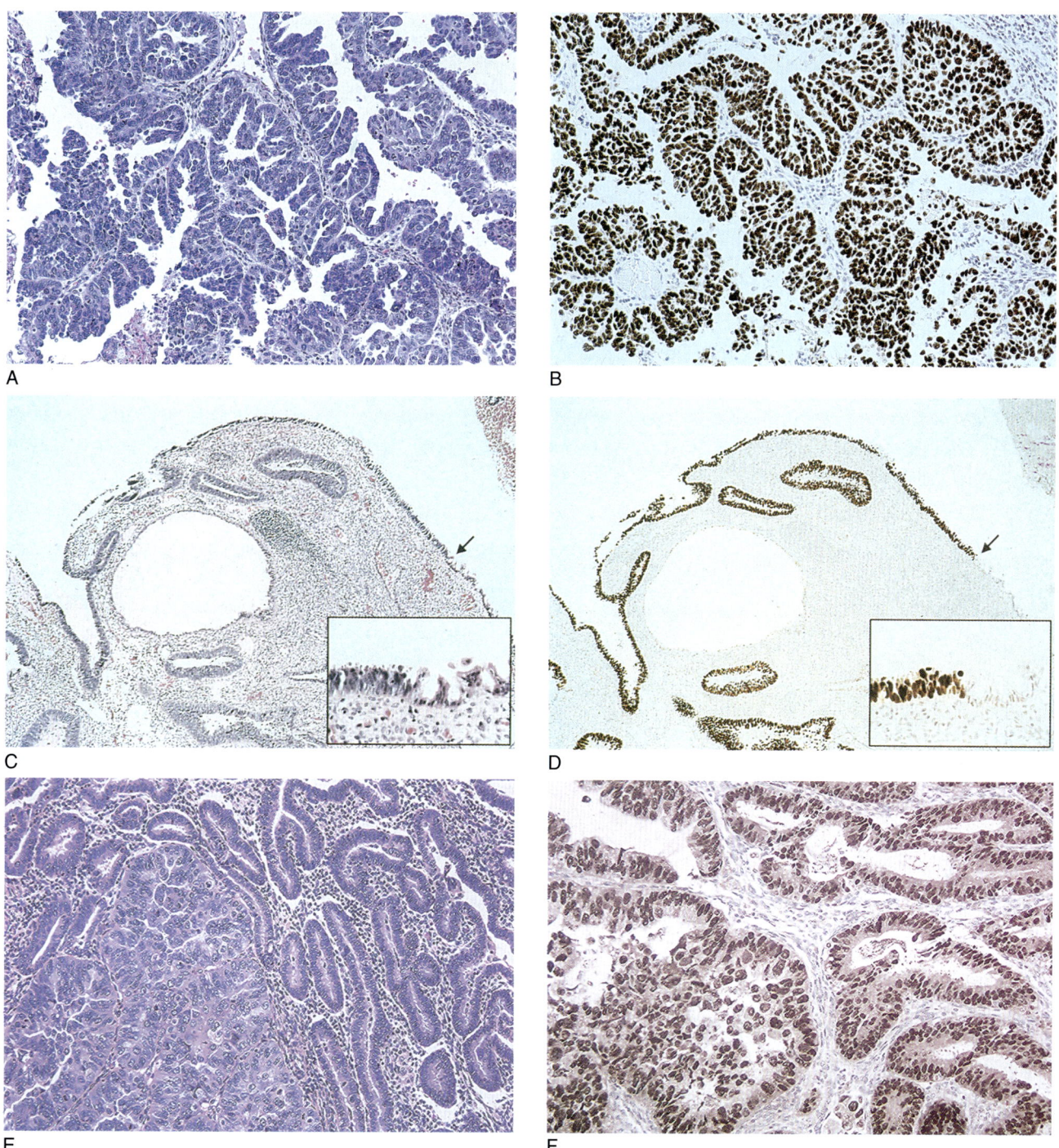

图 16.8 p53 在子宫浆液癌（USC）与子宫内膜样癌（UEC）的免疫组化比较。USC 显示 p53 弥漫及强阳性的核染色（A 和 B），类似染色可见于 USC 的癌前病变 EIC（C 和 D）。腺体结构在 USC 并非不常见（E），p53 在 USC 腺体的强阳性表达（F）则有助于与单纯性增生伴不典型增生和子宫内膜样腺癌的鉴别诊断。

白（SMA）可见于间质细胞和平滑肌细胞，然而间质细胞缺乏结蛋白表达。h-钙调素结合蛋白是一种肌动蛋白和原肌球蛋白的结合蛋白。它可用于子宫体平滑肌肿瘤的鉴别[112, 113]。两篇研究发现 h- 钙调素结合蛋白与结蛋白相比对平滑肌分化细胞更具特异性，可用于平滑肌瘤与子宫内膜间质肿瘤的鉴别。后者不表达 h- 钙调素结合蛋白（图 16.10B）。CD10 可作为 h- 钙调素结合蛋白的补充，它作为平滑肌细胞的对应物，能更完美地表达子宫内膜间质细胞（图 16.10C）。而 CD10 对子宫内膜间质分化并非完全特异；目前研究

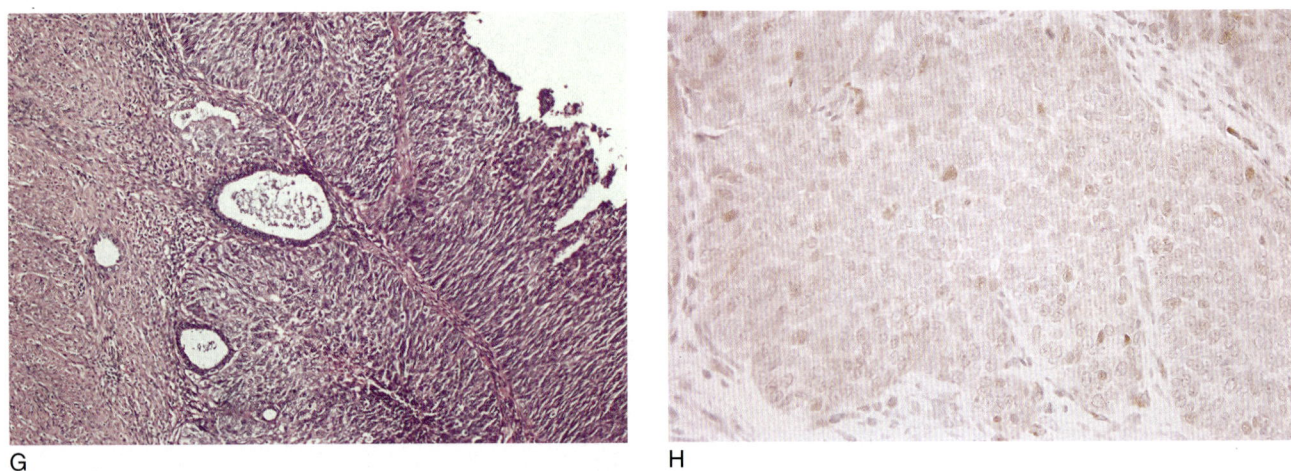

G

H

图 16.8 续 尽管 p53 在低度子宫内膜样癌极少表达，但在高度恶性的子宫内膜样癌（G）可明显过表达（H）。p53 在 FIGO 高度恶性的子宫内膜样癌（3级）的表达与USC相比，通常后者p53表达更弥漫、更强染（A~D 摘自Tashiro H, Isacson C, Levine R, et al. Am J Pathol,1997; 150:177-185）

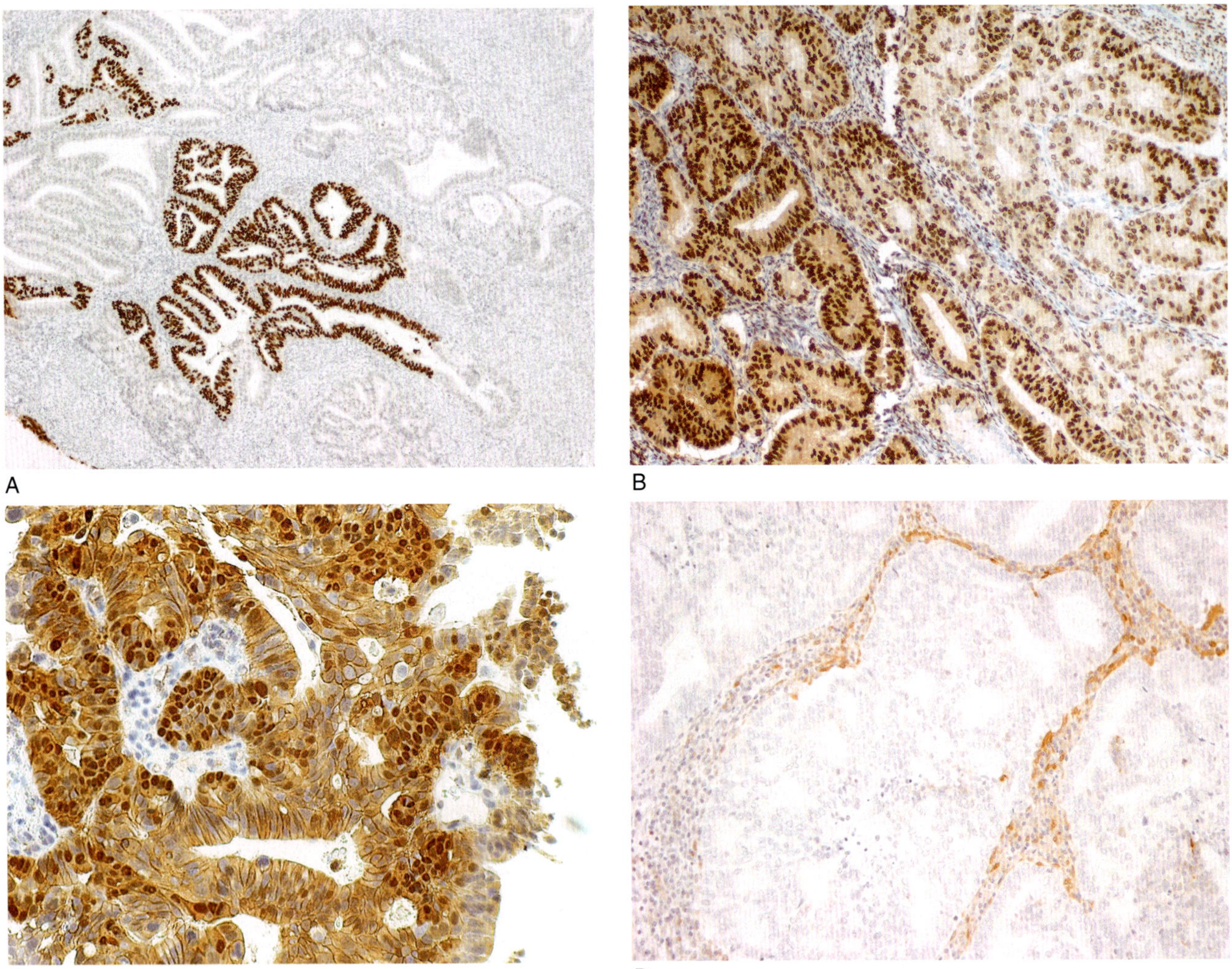

A

B

C

D

图 16.9 子宫内膜样癌（UEC）与子宫内膜浆液性癌（USC）的免疫组化指标比较。USC 特异性表达 p53（A），UEC 当有腺体结构时，表达ER（B）通常至少局灶核、浆着色β-钙黏素（C），PTEN阴性（D）（A~D摘自Darvishian F, Hummer AJ, Thaler H, et al. Am J Surg Pathol 2004; 28:1568-1578）

发现CD10也可见于平滑肌肿瘤[116]。子宫内膜间质肿瘤几乎都表达ER/PR（图16.10D）。与子宫内膜组织学相似的孤立性纤维性肿瘤，既可表达PR，也可表达CD10（图16.10E）。WT-1表达也曾在子宫内膜间质肿瘤和平滑肌肿瘤中描述（表16.7）[119]。

表16-7 内膜间质肿瘤				
病变类型	SMA	Desmin	h-caldesmon	CD10
内膜间质	S	R	N	+*
平滑肌	+	+	+	S

N，阴性；+，阳性；S，有时阳性；R，很少阳性
* 有些内膜间质变型CD10并不呈弥漫阳性

子宫内膜间质肿瘤有几种变型。如子宫内膜间质结节、低度恶性子宫间质肉瘤，由于出现平滑肌的分化被称之为混合型的子宫内膜间质/平滑肌瘤和间质肌瘤（图16.11A）[107, 124]。纤维黏液样变[108, 124]、性索分化，如"类似卵巢性索间质肿瘤的子宫肿瘤"[125]，甚至出现子宫内膜样腺体或上皮样细胞的变型[126]。对理解这些肿瘤免疫表型的关键是变异或化生成分，因其常失去内膜间质的表型，而获取相应化生成分的表型[124]。因此子宫内膜间质结节的平滑肌变型可表达肌源性标记物（图16.11B），而CD10常阴性[116, 124]。低度恶性内膜间质肉瘤的子宫内膜腺体，即上皮变型，可表达上皮性标记物，如EMA，一般不表达CD10。同样，内膜间质结节成分中的性索间质成分，即性索变型，可表达抑制素而CD10阴性[109]。存在混合类型进一步说明其复杂性，如一些伴性索特点的间质肿瘤可同时表达肌性标记物和角蛋白[116]。

> **诊断要点：子宫间质肿瘤**
>
> 1. 典型的子宫内膜间质肿瘤CD10阳性而结蛋白和h-钙调素结合蛋白阴性。
> 2. 对混合性子宫内膜间质的变型，重点检测近似于增殖期子宫内膜间质的成分。
> 3. 表达CD10，但无h-钙调素结合蛋白和/或结蛋白表达的区域，支持内膜间质成分。

子宫内膜间质肉瘤和伴有血管周细胞瘤样结构的软组织肿瘤

子宫内膜间质肉瘤继原发瘤十余年后转移（尤其到肺），也可作为原发肿瘤出现在子宫外（特别是卵巢和腹膜后）。假定观察到许多子宫内膜间质肿瘤具有血管周细胞瘤样结构，应考虑与下列肿瘤鉴别：单相分化的滑膜肉瘤、孤立性纤维性肿瘤和血管周细胞瘤。最近详细公布了一组关于上述病变免疫组化的鉴别表（表16.8）[127]。几乎所有子宫内膜间质肉瘤包括变型和子宫外肿瘤，都至少局灶性表达ER/PR和CD10（图16.10A~D）。有趣的是，超过50%的肿瘤表达SMA[83, 84, 116, 127]，几乎1/4肿瘤表达AE1/AE3[82, 127]。除去子宫内膜间质肿瘤内的腺体成分之外，EMA为阴性[83, 127]。CD10在几乎所有的内膜间质肉瘤中都表达。弥漫强阳性膜着色只见于近50%的非变型肿瘤，而变型肿瘤较少。在这些肿瘤中CD10着色方式是斑块状的胞浆和膜着色。与内膜间质肉瘤相似的上述着色方式见于50%的血管周细胞瘤和60%以上的孤立性纤维性肿瘤（图16.10E）[127]。而CD34表达几乎普遍出现在血管周细胞瘤和孤立性纤维肿瘤。但内膜间质肉瘤不表达[116, 127]。因此应建立CD10、ER和CD34的一组抗体，即使只有CD10局灶阳性，但所有间质肉瘤都表达ER，几乎没有一例表达CD34。相反孤立性纤维性肿瘤和血管周细胞肿瘤都表达CD34，不表达ER。我们不推荐使用PR，原因是PR既能表达于间质肉瘤又能表达于近50%的孤立性纤维性肿瘤和血管周细胞肿瘤[127]。

良性和恶性平滑肌肿瘤

鉴别平滑肌瘤与平滑肌肉瘤是妇科病理常遇到的难题之一。众所周知，形态学标准异常重要，但这些形态学标准常常缺乏。遗憾的是免疫组化并不能提供太多的帮助。研究ER/PR、p53、bcl-2和MIB-1在平滑肌瘤的表达皆有所报道[128-131]。子宫平滑肌肉瘤的p53和MIB-1的阳性较平滑肌瘤高，而ER/PR和bcl-2的表达较低。由于这一组抗体在平滑肌瘤、不典型

表16.8 内膜间质肿瘤和周细胞瘤的比较					
病变类型	CD10	ER	PR	CD34	AE1/AE3
内膜间质肉瘤	+	+	+	N	S
孤立性纤维性肿瘤/血管周细胞瘤	S	N	S	+	N
单相性滑膜肉瘤	N	N	N	N	S

N，阴性；+，阳性；S，有时阳性

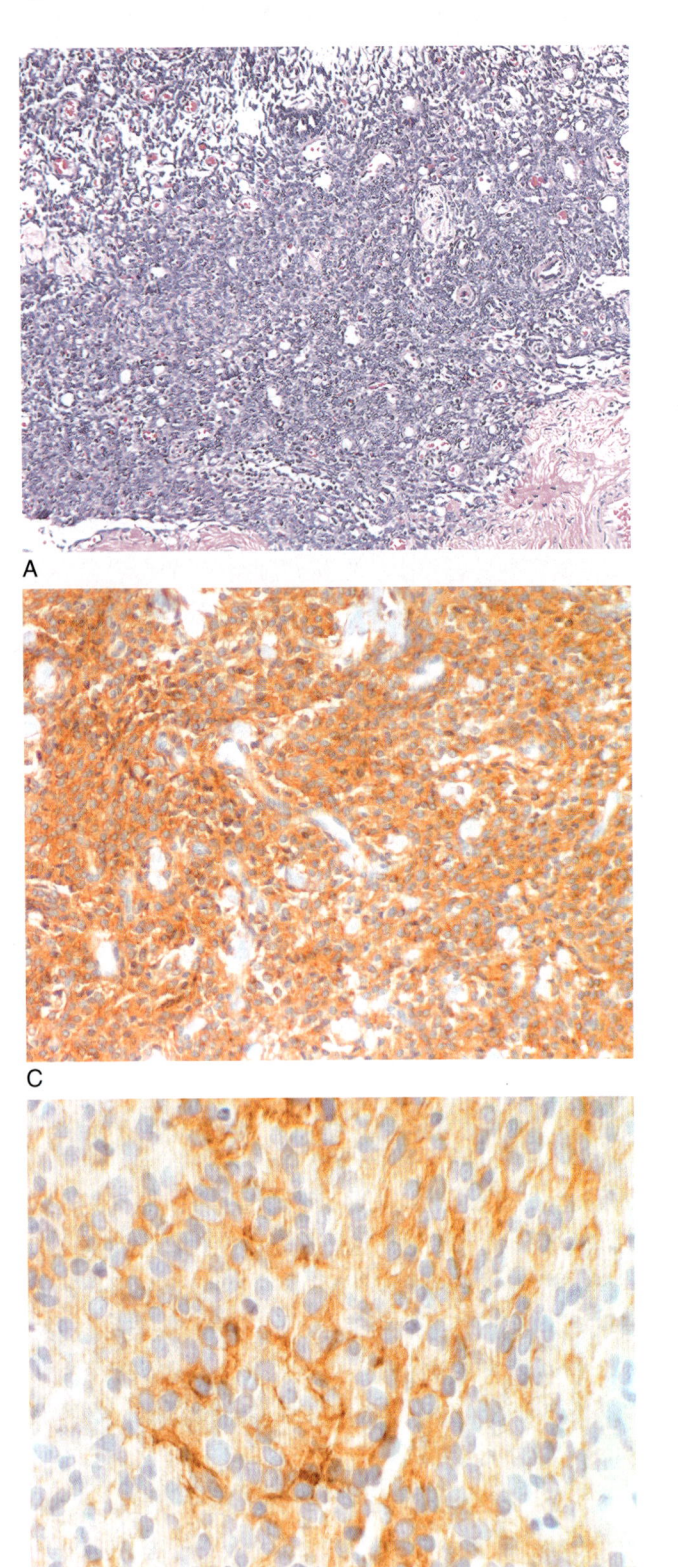

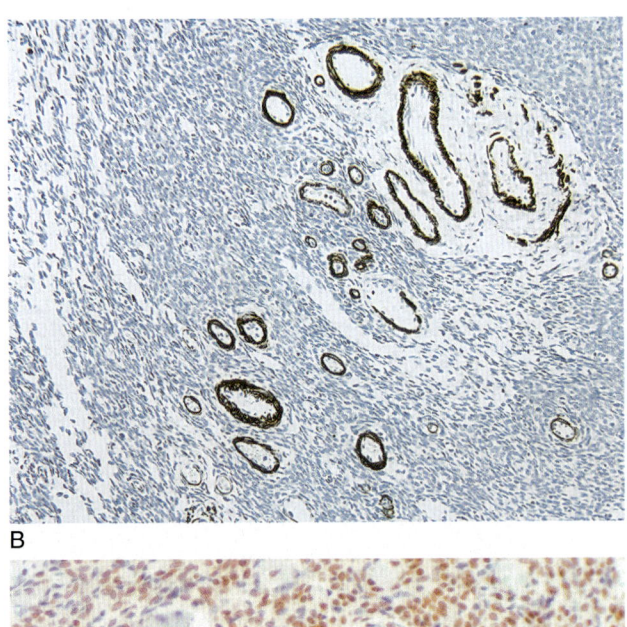

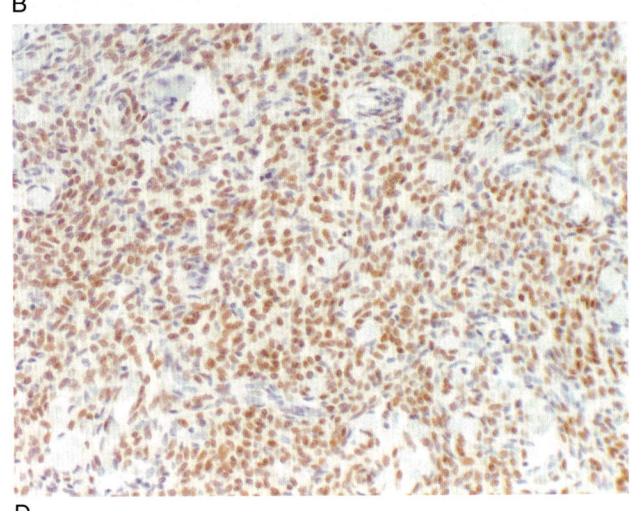

图16.10 子宫内膜间质肿瘤。子宫内膜间质肿瘤（增生结节和肉瘤）以及细胞性平滑肌瘤在形态学上有明显相似之处。尽管结蛋白的表达通常能将这些肿瘤区别开来，新近推出的h-钙调素结合蛋白抗体似乎对于平滑肌分化更有特异性。A组合显示h-钙调素结合蛋白在子宫内膜间质肿瘤呈阴性表达（B）。子宫内膜间质肿瘤常表达CD10（C）和ER（D）以及PR。几种组织学近似于转移的子宫内膜间质肉瘤，如孤立性纤维性肿瘤也能表达PR和CD10（E），虽然许多子宫内膜间质肿瘤弥漫强表达CD10，但也可呈斑块状，这种着色方式能在孤立性纤维性肿瘤和血管周细胞瘤见到，两肿瘤均有鹿角状血管图像（C~E摘自 Bhargava R, Shia J, Hummer A, et al. Mod Pathol, 2005;18:40-47）

平滑肌瘤和平滑肌肉瘤的表达较广，缺乏定量性区分指标，所以临床应用有限。MIB-1弥漫表达也不是诊断平滑肌肉瘤的常规标准之一作为孤立变量，ER/PR、p53和MIB-1对评价平滑肌肉瘤预后有意义[131]。在多个变量中肿瘤的分期仍是最重要的预后因素。

应特别注意上皮样平滑肌肿瘤，其组织形态可使人想起其他的几类肿瘤，诸如原发和转移癌、黑色素瘤、滋养层细胞肿瘤和子宫内膜间质肿瘤，以及有性索分化的肿瘤。要注意不便单独使用角蛋白来鉴别癌和上皮样平滑肌肿瘤。尽管子宫上皮样平滑肌瘤的免

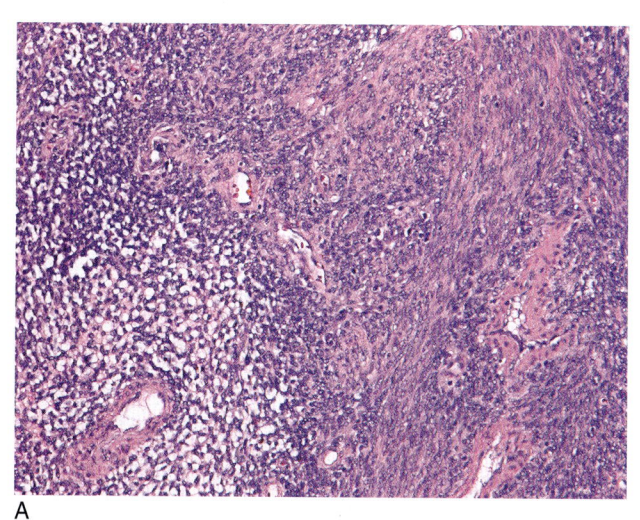 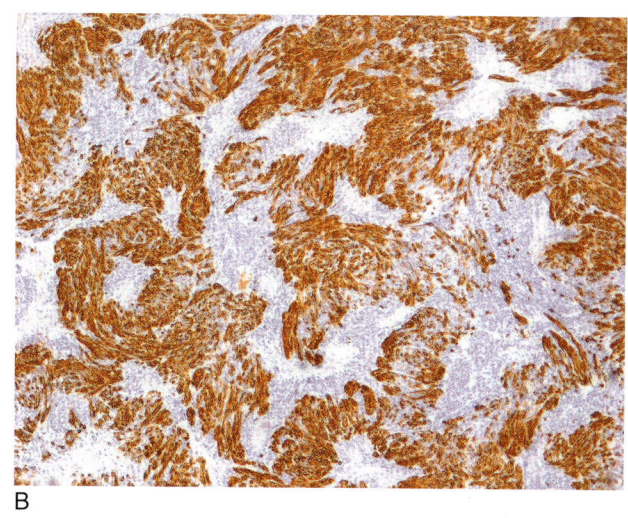

图 16.11 伴平滑肌分化的子宫内膜间质肿瘤。相似于子宫内膜间质的区域（A，左侧）与相似平滑肌的区域对比（A，右侧）。CD10标记子宫内膜间质细胞，而肌源性标记，如h-钙调素结合蛋白标记平滑肌分化的区域（B），当典型子宫内膜间质出现时，一般诊断子宫内膜间质肿瘤。由于分化的多样性，如有平滑肌分化，诊断不应轻易放弃

疫表型资料非常有限，许多病理学家的经验是上皮样平滑肌瘤至少能局灶表达角蛋白[110, 116]。而角蛋白在真正的癌呈强阳性和弥漫性表达（包括几种角蛋白的亚型）。由于许多子宫上皮样平滑肌瘤并不弥漫表达结蛋白和h-钙调素结合蛋白，因此如果单独评价结蛋白一种抗体而不是一组抗体，有可能出现主观性错误[116]。我们提倡使用一种以上的肌源性抗体进行鉴别，基于这一原因，免疫组化应包括CAM5.2、AE1/AE3、结蛋白、h-钙调素结合蛋白和SMA。

血管周上皮样细胞肿瘤（PEComas）最近在子宫曾有报道[132]，其组织学特点与上皮样平滑肌瘤有重叠，特别是当出现透明胞浆时。PEComas与结节性硬化伴增生性血管肌脂肪瘤和血管平滑肌瘤病有关，由特化的或混合的肌细胞组成，可表达肌性标记物和与黑色素分化相关的抗体，即HMB-45和melan-A[132, 133]。8例子宫PEComas病人中，有一人患结节硬化综合征[132]，但是子宫PEComas和结节硬化的相关性仍需阐明。因此，子宫PEComas和常见的子宫上皮样平滑肌肿瘤是否有重要的临床区别尚不清楚。

子宫内膜未分化癌和未分化肉瘤、癌肉瘤

癌肉瘤（MMMT）的诊断定义较明确，即分别有癌与肉瘤成分。假如在HE切片中不能区别这两种成分，癌肉瘤的诊断通常困难或无法证实。换句话讲，对于形态上是未分化的肿瘤可有未分化癌、原发或转移黑色素瘤、淋巴瘤/白血病，以及未分化子宫肉瘤。可通过角蛋白、S-100、LCA、CD34、肌源性抗体来

区别。我们不主张用CD10，因为当肿瘤属于高度异型时（高度不分化时），CD10无法标记子宫内膜间质。角蛋白弥漫而强表达支持癌，弥漫肌源性标记而无角蛋白表达时支持伴有肌源性表达的肉瘤。在很多病例中，尽管使用一组免疫标记物鉴别未分化肿瘤的类型，包括癌和肉瘤，但免疫组化结果往往令人迷惑——上皮或者间叶抗体都被标记或者互补。如果某一区域的瘤组织界限明确地表达角蛋白，而其他区域明确表达间叶抗体，则认为是癌肉瘤，如果肿瘤原发于子宫，上皮和间叶区域不明确，且免疫组化标记不清晰，我们认为应诊断"未分化的恶性肿瘤"，与相关的妇科医师进行一次讨论是有价值的，如有关免疫组化的工作范围、手术计划和辅助治疗。仔细充分检查子宫切除标本，比花时间对活检标本进行免疫检测来了解肿瘤来源更有必要。如有可能，在切除子宫之前需除外转移性肿瘤和淋巴瘤/白血病。

c-kit（CD117）

由于发现瘤组织中存在大量有意义的c-kit使胃肠道间叶瘤和慢性髓性白血病得到了一个良好的辅助治疗药物，即格列卫（Gleevec）®。多项研究发现子宫平滑肌和内膜间质肿瘤不表达c-kit或极少表达[116, 134, 135]。另外有人证实c-kit在平滑肌瘤和癌肉瘤中有表达[135-137]。需要注意的是，最近一项研究发现，c-kit免疫组化可在平滑肌肉瘤和癌肉瘤表达，但却没有c-kit基因的突变[137]。因此我们认为用c-kit抗体确定子宫平滑肌肿瘤和子宫内膜间质肿瘤是否用Gleevec治疗是无

意义的,我们之所以推荐c-kit与CD34一道分析是因为鉴别既包括了妇科平滑肌肿瘤又包括胃肠道间质肿瘤[116]。

预后因子

尽管分期和分级仍是子宫内膜癌最重要的预后指标,但近来更多采用免疫组化来预测预后,p53过表达与预后有关,目前一些研究认为p53过表达是子宫内膜癌预后不良的因素[138-141]。

妊娠滋养层细胞疾病

子宫可发生不同的滋养层病变。有些是非肿瘤性良性增生性病变,如胎盘部位结节。葡萄胎通常是一种临床良性演变过程,但能复发或进展为妊娠滋养层细胞疾病。恶性滋养层细胞肿瘤包括绒毛膜癌、胎盘部位滋养层细胞肿瘤(PSTT)和上皮样滋养层细胞肿瘤(ETT)。由于各种滋养层细胞具有明确的免疫表型,因此通过免疫组化手段有助于滋养层细胞病变的诊断。

抗原/抗体生物学特性: 妊娠滋养层细胞疾病

滋养层细胞,无论细胞滋养层细胞、中间滋养层细胞或合体滋养层细胞皆弥漫性地强烈表达细胞角蛋白(AE1/AE3)[142]。抑制素、CD10和CK18也作为良好的广谱滋养层细胞的标记物,合体滋养层细胞和一些中间滋养层细胞可强表达hCG。人胎盘催乳素(hPL)可标记植入型的中间滋养层细胞[143]和合体滋养层细胞。胎盘碱性磷酸酶(PLAP)标记与hPL相似[144],但此处标记的中间滋养层细胞具有绒毛膜的特点[143, 145]。其他关于中间滋养层细胞的标记物也曾有报道,Mel-Cam(又称CD146)是涉及细胞与细胞之间反应的免疫球蛋白基因家族细胞膜糖蛋白[146]。抗此蛋白的抗体显示对中间滋养层细胞的特异性,其染色程度从滋养层细胞的基底到顶端逐渐加深[146]。

近期关于p63鉴别不同类型的滋养层细胞的详细报道提供了有说服力的一组抗体:hPL、hCG、p63、Ki-67,甚至包括CK18在鉴别诊断[147]中的作用(图16.12)。首先,滋养层病变弥漫表达CK18。大量合体

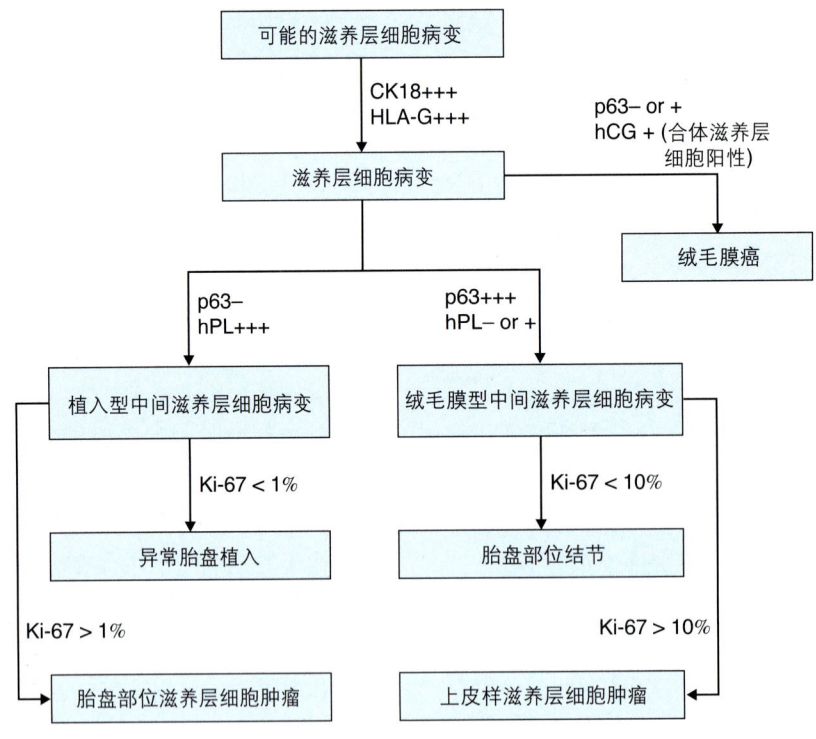

图16.12 用来鉴别诊断滋养层细胞病变的一组抗体的免疫组化运算法则。首先进行CK18和HLA-G染色,如果这两个抗体均呈弥漫阳性,那么该病变为滋养层细胞病变。如果p63在细胞滋养层细胞中呈阳性,hCG在合体细胞滋养层细胞中呈阳性,那么该病变为绒毛膜细胞癌。如果p63呈阴性,而hPL弥漫阳性,那么该病变为异常胎盘植入或为PSTT。这两个病变可通过Ki-67染色进行鉴别。如果p63弥漫阳性,hPL仅为局灶阳性,该病变为PSN或ETT。这两个病变也可通过Ki-67染色进行鉴别(+++,弥漫阳性;+,局灶阳性;-,阴性)(摘自Shih IeM, Kurman RJ. Am J Surg Pathol 2004; 28: 1177-1183)

滋养层细胞表达hCG，密切与细胞滋养层细胞混合有助于绒癌诊断。对于多数合体滋养层细胞有hPL表达，但p63阴性的病变，属于不全植入型中间滋养层细胞的病变（异常胎盘植入与胎盘部位滋养细胞肿瘤）；p63表达与变化不定的hPL有助于绒毛膜中间滋养层细胞病变的诊断（胎盘部位结节与上皮样滋养层细胞肿瘤）。Ki-67指数小于1%时，更支持异常胎盘植入反应，而不是PSTT，Ki-67指数不到10%时，更支持胎盘部位结节，而不是ETT。

滋养层细胞病变有：葡萄胎（部分、完全和侵袭性）、绒癌、胎盘部位滋养层细胞肿瘤、上皮样滋养层细胞肿瘤、异常胎盘植入和胎盘部位结节。免疫组化对葡萄胎诊断的作用甚微，尽管p57的出现有助于诊断，将在下文讨论[148-151]。

鉴别诊断

早期完全性葡萄胎、部分胎块和水肿性流产

鉴别完全性葡萄胎与其相似病变的形态标准是肯定的，特别对于来自于第二个3个月孕体（胚体）的组织。因为绒毛体积增大和滋养层细胞增生没有后期妊娠明显，在第一个3个月期早期发现异常妊娠往往很困难。通过使用p57蛋白（一种母系转录基因产物）免疫组化，对葡萄胎组织的形态学、流式细胞学和细胞遗传学的研究是有辅助价值的。完全性葡萄胎、部分性葡萄胎和非葡萄胎的流产组织中的中间层滋养细胞表达p57蛋白，完全性葡萄胎中的细胞滋养层细胞和绒毛间质细胞不表达p57[148-151]。

胎盘部位结节、鳞状上皮内病变和鳞状上皮癌

胎盘部位结节由中间滋养层细胞构成，形成结节样和玻璃样间质成分。在刮宫术标本中，它常被误为鳞状上皮内病变或浸润性角化型鳞状细胞癌。使用一组抗体诸如抑制素、Ki-67和CK18。CK18和抑制素表达滋养层细胞病变，一般不表达鳞状上皮肿瘤。Ki-67指数在HSIL和鳞癌的阳性率为60%以上[11]，而胎盘部位结节的阳性率低于10%～15%[152]。

胎盘部位滋养层细胞肿瘤与胎盘部位结节

细胞角蛋白及hPL的染色可见于胎盘部位滋养层细胞肿瘤，也可见于胎盘部位结节内的正常中间滋养层细胞。Ki-67指数（阳性细胞百分数）在胎盘部位结节几乎为零，而在胎盘部位滋养层细胞肿瘤则为14%（±7%）[153]，Ki-67指数在异常胎盘植入较低。另一种方法是使用p63来鉴别胎盘部位结节和胎盘部位滋养层细胞肿瘤。p63在胎盘部位结节的中间滋养层细胞表达，但在胎盘部位滋养层细胞肿瘤中不表达[147]。

滋养层细胞与蜕膜

广谱细胞角蛋白主要表达于滋养层细胞，但一般不表达于蜕膜细胞[142]。当确认宫腔妊娠的子宫刮除术标本中的中间滋养层细胞时，可使用hPL、抑制素或Mel-CAM免疫组化染色[146,154]。

绒毛膜癌、胎盘部位滋养层细胞肿瘤与低分化肿瘤

绒毛膜癌是一含双相细胞成分的肿瘤，由合体滋养层细胞与单核细胞组成，单核细胞可为中间层细胞或细胞滋养层细胞。有时绒毛膜癌可酷似低分化癌。鉴别诊断还包括胎盘部位滋养层细胞肿瘤。特别是有多核巨细胞出现时，应有一组免疫组化染色，包括hCG、CK18、hPL和抑制素。绒癌因含有大量合体滋养层细胞，所以可表达hCG。表达hCG的细胞与单核细胞关系密切，相反胎盘部位滋养层细胞肿瘤在片状排列的中间滋养层细胞中，有大量随意分布的合体滋养层细胞。滋养层细胞肿瘤弥漫表达CK18，但鳞状上皮则阴性。一般来说，抑制素是判断滋养层细胞的良好标记物，它在酷似滋养层细胞肿瘤的鳞癌中不表达；hPL也表达于大多数滋养层细胞肿瘤。此外，Ki-67也有助于鉴别诊断，胎盘部位滋养层细胞肿瘤的Ki-67阳性指数较低（14%±7%），而绒毛膜癌和其他癌症的Ki-67阳性指数常常在60%以上[11,153]。

免疫组化不能区别妊娠性绒癌和生殖细胞绒癌，也不能将妊娠性绒癌从含滋养叶成分的非生殖细胞癌中区分出来，后者可以在宫颈鳞癌、膀胱移行细胞癌中见到[155,156]。偶尔在癌组织中见到合体滋养层细胞表达hCG也不奇怪。

卵 巢

卵巢原发性肿瘤可分为四大类：上皮性肿瘤、性索-间质肿瘤、生殖细胞肿瘤及其他类型肿瘤。后者包括多种原发和转移性肿瘤，如间叶肿瘤、淋巴瘤和白血病以及转移性上皮性肿瘤。输卵管的肿瘤主要是上皮性的，与卵巢相应肿瘤相似。卵巢和输卵管肿瘤的详细分类见《WHO乳腺与女性生殖系统肿瘤病理学与遗传学》分册[157]。通常借助常规HE切片即能

正确诊断卵巢和输卵管肿瘤。然而卵巢肿瘤每一主要类型都有独特的免疫组化特征，因此免疫组织化学也常用于确定诊断。卵巢肿瘤相对不常见，因而病理学家对此常显经验不足。免疫组织化学染色可用于提示或支持某一诊断。它对低分化肿瘤的分类意义重大，而且也是诊断和分类某些转移性或其他部位肿瘤累及卵巢的必要手段。

抗原／抗体生物学特性：卵巢和输卵管

相对少量的抗体即可满足大多数卵巢和输卵管肿瘤的诊断。这些核心性抗体的特性见下文。有时其他辅助抗体对诊断也有帮助，在下文相应部分讨论。

细胞角蛋白

角蛋白是形成上皮细胞骨架的中间丝蛋白。它们存在于所有上皮细胞中，所以细胞角蛋白有助于筛查肿瘤是否为上皮源性。Moll等根据人体细胞角蛋白分子量和等电点的不同将其分类[158]。已有20种上皮性角蛋白多肽被确定。其中一些抗体具有特异的组织分布，这可用于肿瘤的鉴别诊断。那些能识别许多不同细胞角蛋白的广谱抗体最适用于筛查，如联合使用AE1/AE3和CAM5.2。

细胞角蛋白7 细胞角蛋白7（CK7）是Ⅱ型碱性低分子量角蛋白，见于许多器官的单层上皮，包括女性生殖道的所有上皮[1,158]。卵巢和输卵管上皮性肿瘤均表现为CK7胞浆和／或胞膜阳性[159-161]。女性生殖道肿瘤的这种特征性着色方式常与其他角蛋白如CK20联合使用，来鉴别女性生殖道的原发腺癌和转移性腺癌[162,163]。由于某些原发卵巢肿瘤CK7阴性而且一定数量的卵巢转移性癌CK7阳性[164]，因此需要一组免疫染色来评价此类肿瘤。

细胞角蛋白20 细胞角蛋白20（CK20）是Ⅰ型酸性低分子量细胞角蛋白，最初描述于1992年[165]。见于正常胃组织、肠道组织、尿路上皮和Merkel细胞。CK20表达于大肠和小肠大多数腺癌、卵巢黏液性肿瘤以及Merkel细胞癌，也常见于尿路上皮癌和胃、胰腺及胆管的腺癌[163,166]。CK20是鉴别卵巢原发黏液性肿瘤和卵巢各种转移性肿瘤的有用指标[167-169]，多数原发的非黏液性上皮性肿瘤CK20阴性。

抗腺癌的抗体

那些在腺癌阳性而间皮细胞阴性的抗体被集成一组用于鉴别腺癌和间皮细胞瘤。这些抗体包括CD15、BerEP4、单克隆癌胚抗原（mCEA）和MOC-31。CD15（LeuM1）主要应用于血液病理学，因为它表达于中性粒细胞、组织细胞、免疫母细胞和经典型R-S细胞，但它也表达于各种腺癌。据报道，约1/3～2/3卵巢浆液性癌和更多的子宫内膜样癌以及透明细胞腺癌呈阳性着色[170,171]。着色可为颗粒状胞浆／胞膜。BerEP4为直接针对上皮细胞糖蛋白的单克隆抗体，几乎所有卵巢和腹膜的浆液性癌均显示胞膜弥漫强阳性[170-172]。单克隆CEA除了在卵巢黏液性腺癌中表现为典型阳性外，在卵巢其他肿瘤中罕见阳性[170,172-179]。子宫内膜样腺癌的鳞状上皮分化区域也显示CEA阳性。多克隆CEA特异性似乎不如单克隆CEA，其在卵巢癌着色比例略高。B72.3是针对肿瘤相关糖蛋白（TAG-72）的一种单克隆抗体。它常阳性表达于卵巢癌，表现为胞浆颗粒状着色[170,172,181]。这种着色很难解释，因为常有黏蛋白和其他分泌物的着色背景。MOC-31是直接针对糖蛋白的一种单克隆抗体，多数卵巢癌表现胞膜强阳性[170]。所有上述抗体在间皮瘤均阴性或罕见阳性。通常BerEP4、MOC-31和B72.3在检测卵巢表面上皮性肿瘤方面比LeuM1和CEA更敏感，因此可与间皮瘤阳性标记物calretinin和CK5/6联合使用，来鉴别卵巢肿瘤和间皮瘤。

CA125

CA125是被单克隆抗体OC125识别的一种高分子量糖蛋白，它具有细胞内、跨膜和细胞外结构域[182-184]。OC125与M11的结合位点位于细胞外结构域[182]。CA125常表达于卵巢原发性非黏液性上皮性癌，但也可表达于多种其他女性生殖道癌，包括宫颈癌、子宫内膜癌、输卵管癌以及某些非女性生殖道肿瘤包括胰腺癌、乳腺癌、结肠癌、肺癌和甲状腺癌[185-187]。正常子宫内膜CA125阳性，因此可作为阳性对照[188]。间皮瘤CA125也可阳性[181]。评估CA125（OC125）的表达意义有限，因为女性生殖道表面上皮增生、生殖道外的转移癌和间皮增生都可表达CA125[185,189]。

抑制素

抑制素是一种32kD的二价糖蛋白激素，参与垂体-性腺轴反馈系统的调节[190-193]。卵巢分泌的抑制素由一个α亚单位与两个β亚单位之一相连而成。抑制素A是由一个α亚单位与一个β-A亚单位相连；抑制素B则是一个β亚单位与一个β亚单位相连。该单克隆抗体通常经免疫组织化学识别抑制素A。抑制素是卵巢性索-间质肿瘤敏感而且相对特异的标志物，它在妇科肿瘤中的主要用途就是鉴别这类肿瘤[194-199]。伴随癌的黄素化间质细胞可表达抑制素[194, 196, 200]，这会导致误认为是癌表达抑制素。一般来说抑制素在癌中表达并不常见，若有，其强而弥漫表达也是例外[194, 196, 200-202]。肾上腺皮质肿瘤也常表达抑制素[203-208]。

calretinin

calretinin为一种29kD的钙结合蛋白，最初发现于中枢神经系统[209]。它与S-100蛋白同属于EF-hand蛋白家族[210, 211]。后来的研究表明calretinin存在于良性间皮细胞和间皮瘤，现今已广泛用做间皮瘤的标记物。它着色部位在胞浆和胞核，核着色是间皮瘤必需的特异表现。calretinin也见于肥大细胞、施万细胞瘤、颗粒细胞瘤、肾上腺皮质肿瘤和卵巢的性索-间质肿瘤，后者对于妇科病理学家而言尤为有趣。与抑制素相比，calretinin具有更广范围的性索-间质肿瘤谱，而且在这些肿瘤中它也更敏感但特异性稍差[199, 212-214]。它通常与抑制素及其他抗体组成一组来使用。

WT-1

WT-1即Wilms瘤基因，位于11p13。它在泌尿生殖道的发育中起作用，并被认为具有抑癌功能[215]。Wilms瘤基因产物为位于细胞核的一种DNA结合蛋白。核阳性着色见于Wilms瘤[216]、促纤维增生性小圆细胞肿瘤[217-219]和间皮瘤[220, 221]。WT-1表达于卵巢表面上皮、包涵囊肿和正常输卵管上皮[222]；也表达于卵巢、输卵管和腹膜浆液性癌[221]，但在子宫内膜浆液性癌中的表达有限。WT-1单克隆或多克隆抗体均可获得。浆液性癌着色敏感性高，某些研究中报道90%以上病例为核阳性[220, 223]。其他报道表达WT-1的卵巢肿瘤有移行细胞癌、高血钙型小细胞癌和某些性索-间质肿瘤[199, 224, 225]。

胎盘碱性磷酸酶

胎盘碱性磷酸酶（PLAP）是恶性生殖细胞肿瘤的标记物，尤其对无性细胞瘤和胚胎性癌。然而，其阳性着色也可见于某些上皮性肿瘤，特别是浆液性癌[226, 227]。PLAP是无性细胞瘤和含有相关细胞的肿瘤的有用标记物，如性腺母细胞瘤。尽管无性细胞瘤通常表达PLAP，但表达也并不能证明该肿瘤就是无性细胞瘤，因为非无性细胞性生殖细胞肿瘤和某些癌也表达PLAP。

CD117

CD117蛋白为c-kit基因表达的跨膜蛋白，具有酪氨酸激酶生长因子受体活性。它存在于各种正常人体组织的细胞类型中，包括乳腺上皮、生殖细胞、黑色素细胞、不成熟髓细胞和肥大细胞[230, 231]。CD117阳性着色见于许多肿瘤，但强阳性表达主要见于肥大细胞疾病和胃肠道间质瘤，而且是其首选标记物[230, 232-234]。少数卵巢浆液性癌CD117呈强阳性[230]。在卵巢病理学中，CD117是无性细胞瘤最有用的标记物，几乎所有病例均表现为胞膜弥漫强阳性[231, 235]。胚胎性癌不表达CD117，而对无性细胞瘤而言，比PLAP更具特异性。转移性恶性黑色素瘤偶尔与无性细胞瘤相似，值得注意的是黑色素瘤偶尔也表达CD117，但通常表现为胞浆着色。

甲胎蛋白

甲胎蛋白（AFP）为一种胎儿肿瘤糖蛋白，表达卵黄囊瘤及其变型，包括肝样和子宫内膜样卵黄囊瘤[236-241]。其他常表达AFP阳性的卵巢肿瘤有罕见的肝样腺癌[242-244]、转移性肝细胞癌[243, 245]以及伴有异源性肝细胞分化的Sertoli-Leydig细胞肿瘤[246-248]。在卵巢生殖细胞肿瘤中，AFP表达几乎全部限于卵黄囊瘤[238, 249]，尽管胚胎性癌和畸胎瘤中的肝组织/肠道组织也可局灶阳性[250-254]。有罕见报道AFP阳性的卵黄囊瘤起源于体细胞性（somatic）腺癌如子宫内膜样腺癌[255, 256]。然而多数情况下，结合相应的形态学特征，卵巢肿瘤AFP阳性提示为生殖细胞源性卵黄囊瘤。

人绒毛膜促性腺激素

人绒毛膜促性腺激素（hCG）是由合体滋养层细胞分泌的糖蛋白激素，由二硫键将一个α链与一个β链相连而成。α链与卵泡刺激素（FSH）、黄体生成激素（LH）和促甲状腺激素相似。β链是该激素独特的免疫组织化学抗体位点。在生殖细胞肿瘤，hCG表达限于合体滋养层细胞和部分中间滋养层细胞。含有合体滋养层细胞的原发卵巢肿瘤（包括绒毛膜癌和一些无性细胞瘤和胚胎性癌）均表达hCG[245, 257-259]。极少数低分化癌表现为绒癌样分化，而且这些肿瘤中的合体滋养层细胞表达hCG[260]。此外，偶有报道某些缺乏合体滋养层细胞的癌也表达 hCG[261, 262]。

S-100 蛋白

S-100 蛋白是小酸性 EF-hand 钙结合蛋白的多基因家族，最初发现于脑提取物[263-265]。恶性黑色素瘤几乎总是 S-100 蛋白强阳性，因此，S-100 蛋白染色是筛查卵巢原发或转移性恶性黑色素瘤的实用方法[266]。S-100蛋白也可见于许多其他肿瘤血浆中，包括一些癌[267, 268]、外周神经鞘瘤和含有肌上皮细胞的肿瘤以及肿瘤中的树突状细胞。对诊断不明的病例可通过HMB-45或melan-A（A103）阳性来肯定恶性黑色素瘤的诊断[269-271]。对于恶性黑色素瘤，HMB-45 和 melan-A 比 S-100 更具特异性，但其敏感性稍差[272]。HMB-45 也表达于淋巴-血管平滑肌瘤病和血管平滑肌瘤[273-279]，而melan-A可表达于黄素化细胞、Leydig细胞和异位肾上腺组织[202, 280]。

CD45

CD45，也称白细胞共同抗原（LCA），为酪氨酸磷酸酶跨膜蛋白家族。它表达于除了红系和巨核细胞之外的所有造血细胞。商业化单克隆抗体能有效地标记良性或恶性淋巴样细胞，因而可用于筛查肿瘤以判定其是否可能为造血系统肿瘤[281]。LCA 通常为膜着色。浆细胞肿瘤呈弱阳性或根本不着色，而在髓细胞白血病中着色形式多样。如果某肿瘤被怀疑为淋巴造血系统肿瘤，应采用其他多种标记来进一步确定，这将在淋巴瘤一章详细讨论（见第 4 章和第 5 章）。

神经内分泌分化

神经内分泌分化标记物有助于诊断原发或转移性神经内分泌癌和原始神经外胚层肿瘤，以及确定原发性和继发性类癌。有关这类抗体的讨论详见内分泌肿瘤一章（见第 9 章）。嗜铬素和突触素是常用的最特异的神经内分泌分化的标记物。NSE 和 CD56（神经细胞黏附分子，NCAM）用于筛查时特异性稍差，但敏感性较好。

上皮性肿瘤

上皮性肿瘤占卵巢所有肿瘤的 60%，大约占所有恶性肿瘤的95%。多数输卵管肿瘤是上皮性的。角蛋白有助于鉴别上皮性肿瘤。广谱角蛋白如 AE1/AE3 可用来确定肿瘤的上皮性质。低至中度级别上皮性癌容易诊断，而卵巢癌通常分化差，有些不易诊断为癌。角蛋白和EMA阳性提示癌。在卵巢癌评价中，特异性抗角蛋白抗体已具有独立的意义。CK7免疫染色是女性生殖道（包括卵巢和输卵管）上皮性肿瘤的特征。卵巢和输卵管原发性上皮性肿瘤几乎100%CK7 阳性（图 16.13A）[159-162,169]，因此 CK7 阴性提示可能为转移癌。CK20也有助于评价卵巢和输卵管肿瘤。除了肠型黏液性肿瘤外，其他原发上皮性肿瘤 CK20 通常为阴性（图 16.13B）。因此，CK7-/CK20+ 免疫表型提示卵巢转移性肿瘤，尤其可能来

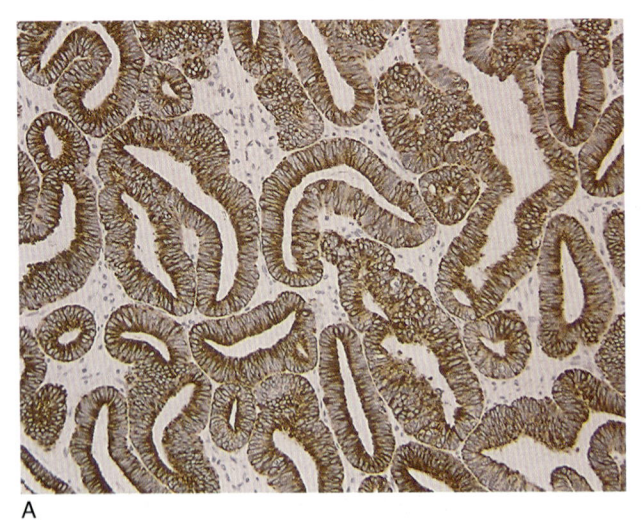

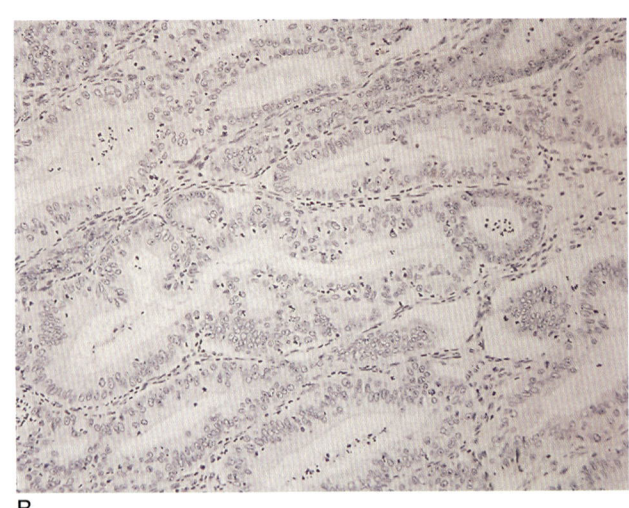

图 16.13 细胞角蛋白亚型在原发性上皮性肿瘤中的染色。（A）正如此例子宫内膜样腺癌，CK7 在原发性上皮性肿瘤中通常为弥漫强阳性；（B）除黏液性肿瘤外，原发性上皮性肿瘤CK20 阴性

女性生殖系统的免疫组织化学

自肠道或阑尾。

浆液性肿瘤

正如其他卵巢原发上皮性肿瘤一样，浆液性肿瘤表现为 CK7+/CK20-（表 16.9）[159, 161]。在交界性浆液性肿瘤中，角蛋白染色可明确显示微小浸润灶[282]。浆液性癌细胞膜可表现为 CA125 强阳性（图 16.14）[283]。近 50% 浆液性癌可表达 ER/PR[284]。30%~50% 浆液性癌呈细胞核 p53 强阳性[223, 284, 285]。有时借助此染色可显示卵巢表面和输卵管内的原位癌。良性和交界性浆液性肿瘤包括微乳头性交界性肿瘤 p53 为阴性。Wilms 瘤基因产物 WT-1 胞核阳性着色通常见于卵巢、输卵管和腹膜浆液性癌，尽管染色范围和强度各有不同（图 16.15）[178, 220, 223, 286, 287]，阳性染色也见于交界性浆液性肿瘤[287]。子宫内膜浆液性癌 WT-1 阴性[288]或仅局灶弱阳性[223]，因此 WT-1 阴性而 p53 强阳性提示转移性浆液性癌很可能来自子宫内膜而非卵巢。卵巢性索-间质肿瘤也呈 WT-1 核阳性[199]。

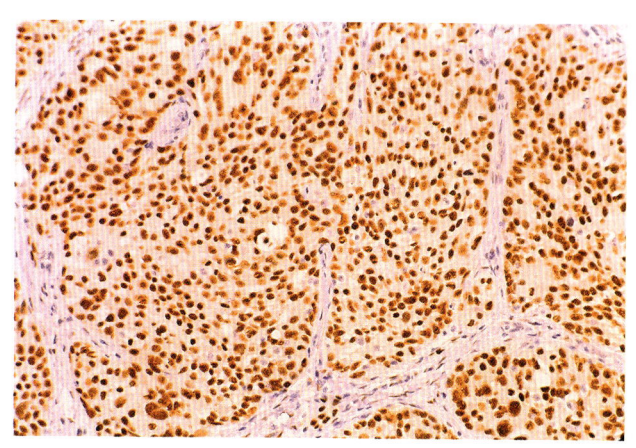

图 16.15　浆液性癌 WT-1 阳性表达。这里显示绝大多数瘤细胞核着色，是卵巢浆液性癌的一个特征

黏液性肿瘤

免疫组织化学在卵巢黏液性肿瘤的诊断和分类中起着重要作用。卵巢原发黏液性肿瘤有两类。肠型细胞型最常见，但少部分黏液性肿瘤具有宫颈内膜样或浆黏液（seromucinous）表型。此两类黏液性肿瘤具有不同的免疫表型，可借此区分这两类肿瘤。细胞角蛋白或上皮细胞膜抗原可有助于确定微小浸润灶。

肠型黏液性肿瘤 CK7 弥漫强阳性表达（图 16.16A）[169]。大多数也表达 CK20[162]。在卵巢原发黏液性肿瘤中，CK20 倾向为斑片状着色而且着色范围和强度不同（图 16.16B）。有些病理学家提倡采用较高的阳性结果阈值（亦即，>25% 或 >50% 肿瘤细胞着色），以提高结果评判的重复性；这种方案若被采纳，那么仅 40%~50% 卵巢黏液性癌将被认为是 CK20 阳性[161, 178]。CK7 强阳性结合 CK20 不同程度阳性或阴性，可明确区别原发黏液性肿瘤和转移性结直肠癌，因为后者 CK7 阴性而 CK20 弥漫强阳性（表 16.10）[159, 161-163, 283]。然而重要的是要记住偶有原发和转移性肿瘤细胞角蛋白可异常表达。尤其直肠腺癌 CK7 可阳性而偶尔卵巢原发黏液性肿瘤 CK7 阴性[289]。单克隆和多克隆 CEA 显示腺腔内黏液（luminal mucin）、细胞顶部边缘（apical cell border）和肿瘤细胞胞浆着色[178, 290]。在大多数病例中，免疫染色可明显着色绒毛处的肿瘤细胞顶部边缘[291]。在柱状细胞肿瘤中嗜铬素和突触素散在表达位于基底部的内分泌细胞。黏液性肿瘤的上皮抑制素阴性，但囊壁周围间质细胞常因部分或全部黄素化故强表达抑制素。肠型黏液性肿瘤雌激素和孕激素受体常为阴性。

几种新的免疫染色可能有助于评价卵巢黏液性肿

表16.9　卵巢常见上皮性肿瘤免疫表型				
	CK7	CK20	WT-1	Vimentin
浆液性	+	N	+	S
黏液性*	+	+	N	N
内膜样	+	N	N	+
透明细胞性	+	N	N	N
移行细胞性	+	N	+	N

*肠型黏液样肿瘤
N，阴性；+，阳性；S，有时阳性

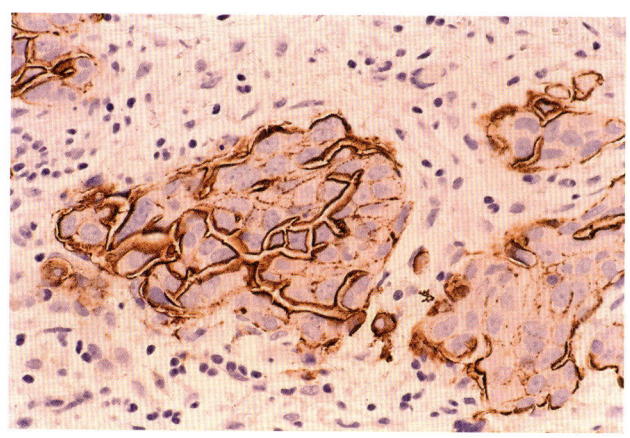

图 16.14　许多非黏液性卵巢上皮性肿瘤，尤其浆液性肿瘤可表达 CA125。这是微小浆液性癌，发现于有卵巢癌家族史的一位妇女，显示典型的胞膜着色

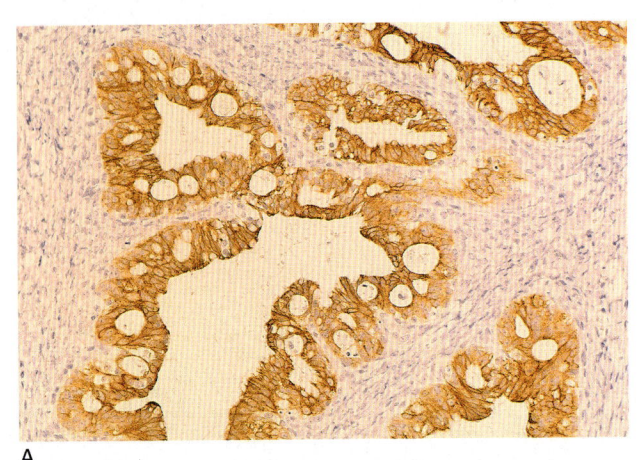
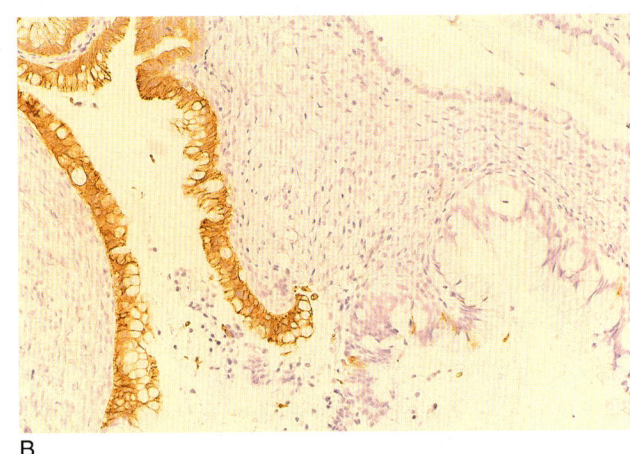

图 16.16 原发肠型黏液性肿瘤的细胞角蛋白亚型。(A) 正如其他原发上皮性肿瘤，肠型黏液性肿瘤通常强阳性表达CK7；(B) 与原发上皮肿瘤不同，肠型黏液性肿瘤通常为CK20阳性。CK20染色倾向于斑片状（如图）而且可不如转移性结直肠腺癌强。后者为典型的 CK7-/CK20+

瘤。黏蛋白基因产物 MUC5A 以及胰腺癌抑癌基因产物 DPC4 通常在卵巢黏液性癌中阳性[169]，而CK17为阴性[178]。卵巢黏液性肿瘤 DPC4 失表达而CK17阳性提示可能来自胰腺癌转移。Cdx基因编码同源核转录因子，涉及肠上皮细胞的增殖和分化。CDX2核弥漫强阳性着色见于正常肠上皮、大多数结直肠腺癌和其卵巢转移灶[291-293]。卵巢肿瘤的染色结果报道有争议，有人报道多数黏液性卵巢腺癌为阳性着色[291,294]，而其他人报道为阴性或仅局灶、弱阳性[164,295]。非黏液性卵巢肿瘤CDX2阴性。利用CDX2来鉴别卵巢原发性黏液性癌和转移性结直肠黏液性癌有待进一步评价。

累及卵巢的黏液性肿瘤可发生腹膜假黏液瘤。卵巢肿瘤外观从良性囊腺瘤到腺癌变化多样，尽管大多数类似于肠型交界性黏液性肿瘤。临床病理学和分子研究表明多数情况下腹膜假黏液瘤为继发于胃肠道尤其是阑尾的肿瘤，而卵巢肿瘤为转移性肿瘤的继发受累。免疫组织化学染色倾向支持这一观点，因为多数肿瘤缺乏 CK7 而肠黏蛋白 MUC2 却阳性[296,297]。

黏液性肿瘤囊壁偶尔可见到附壁结节（mural nodules）。黏液性肿瘤可为良性、交界性或癌。已描述有 3 种附壁结节：间变性癌[298]、肉瘤[299]和肉瘤样反应性梭形细胞结节[300]。间变性癌明显恶性，常弥漫性强表达细胞角蛋白，且常伴有波形蛋白表达[301,302]。肉瘤性附壁结节为恶性梭形或上皮样细胞，表达波形蛋白但不表达细胞角蛋白[303]。肉瘤样结节形态变化多样，但通常细胞异型性和分裂活性不如恶性结节。良性增生结节，除表达波形蛋白之外，通常呈弱、局灶性细胞角蛋白表达[304,305]。

浆黏液性肿瘤与肠型黏液性肿瘤免疫表型不同。其 CK7 阳性（图 16.17A）。与肠型黏液性肿瘤比较，无论阳性结果阈值多大，它们皆倾向于CK20阴性（图 16.17B）。肠型黏液性肿瘤CEA 阳性，而除了交界性浆黏液性肿瘤中的嗜酸性分化细胞 CEA 强阳性表达外，浆黏液性肿瘤倾向于 CEA 阴性[290]。浆黏液性肿瘤常表现为胞核 ER/PR 及胞浆波形蛋白阳性[306]。

子宫内膜样癌

子宫内膜样癌 CK7 阳性而 CK20 阴性或至多局灶性弱阳性（图 16.13）[293]。转移性结直肠癌通常与子宫内膜样癌相似；CK7 弥漫强阳性表达而CK20阴性可用于鉴别子宫内膜样癌和转移结直肠腺癌（表16.10）[159]。CDX2 在子宫内膜样癌为斑片状表达，而弥漫强阳性表达则提示为转移性结直肠腺癌[293]。最后，子宫内膜样癌无CEA的胞浆着色，尽管在鳞状分化区域可有局灶阳性[73]。大多数子宫内膜样癌显示核周或胞浆底部波形蛋白着色[73]。某些子宫内膜样癌的生长方式与性

表16.10 原发和转移性腺癌						
	CK7	CK20	CDX2	DPC4	CK17	mCEA
原发黏液性	+	+	S	+	N	+
原发内膜样	+	N	N	+	N	N
转移性结直肠	N	+	+	+	N	+
转移性前列腺	S	S	N	N (50%)	+	+

N, 阴性；+, 阳性；S, 有时阳性

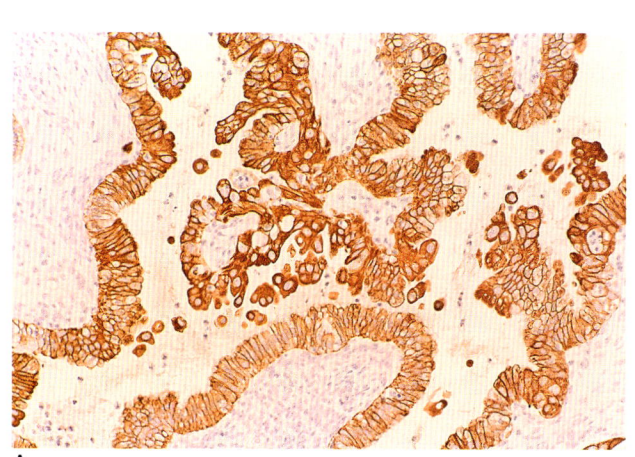 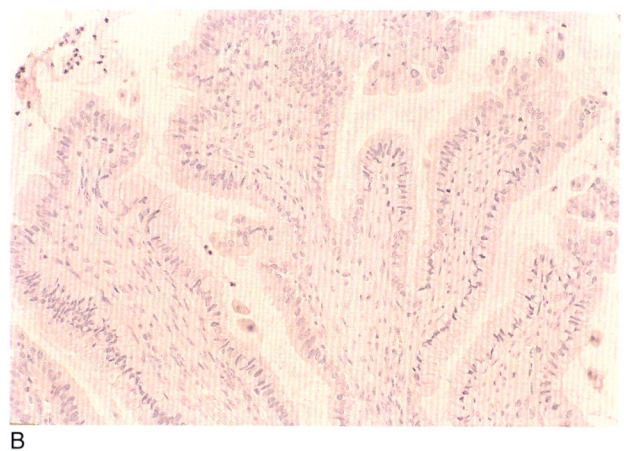

图 16.17 原发宫颈型黏液性肿瘤（浆黏液性肿瘤）的细胞角蛋白亚型。此型黏液性肿瘤具有典型的"苗勒"免疫表型。（A）宫颈型黏液性肿瘤显示 CK7 弥漫强阳性；（B）与肠型黏液性肿瘤不同的是，宫颈型黏液性肿瘤 CK20 阴性

索 - 间质肿瘤如 Sertoli 细胞瘤、Sertoli-Leydig 细胞瘤或颗粒细胞瘤相似。其中，Sertoli 样变型子宫内膜样癌最常见。免疫组织化学染色有助于鉴别这些子宫内膜癌变型与性索-间质肿瘤，因为子宫内膜样癌EMA阳性（图16.18），雌、孕激素受体阳性，而抑制素或 calretinin 阴性（表 16.11）[307]。相反，性索 - 间质肿瘤细胞角蛋白可阳性，而 EMA 阴性，而且呈抑制素胞浆着色、calretinin 胞浆和胞膜着色[201]。

癌肉瘤、腺肉瘤和子宫内膜样间质肉瘤分类如同卵巢子宫内膜样肿瘤[157]。这些肿瘤的准确诊断需要确认上皮性成分或正确确认各种间叶细胞类型。在癌肉瘤和腺肉瘤，细胞角蛋白或 EMA 免疫组织化学检测可帮助病理学家识别间叶性肿瘤中的上皮成分[308, 309]。结蛋白和成肌素可有助于确认横纹肌母细胞的存在，软骨样成分通常S-100 阳性。子宫内膜样间质肉瘤CD10 显著阳性[115]，而易于引起混淆的性索 - 间质肿瘤则抑制素和calretinin 典型阳性。含有局灶上皮样或性索样分化的子宫内膜样间质肉瘤会出现特殊的诊断问题，因为这些成分可表达抑制素或calretinin[310]。除了CD10 弥漫着色外，子宫内膜样间质肉瘤倾向于强阳性表达 ER/PR。

透明细胞癌

正如卵巢其他原发上皮性肿瘤一样，透明细胞癌显示出典型的免疫反应方式。肿瘤细胞呈细胞角蛋白、CK7（图 16.19A）、高分子量角蛋白和上皮膜抗原阳性[311, 312]。它们也表达 CD15（图 16.19B），但通常不表达CK20[311]。ER/PR结果各有不同。一组研究检测ER和PR常有表达[313]，而其他研究则发现ER和

PR 阳性不常见于透明细胞癌[312]。这种不一致的原因尚不清楚，尽管所研究的肿瘤级别或所选技术的不同是最可能的原因。有报道p53呈核弥漫阳性[311]，但也有相反的报道[314, 315]。作者的经验是 p53 若有着色的话，其分布通常不规律并且比浆液性癌弱，后者核染

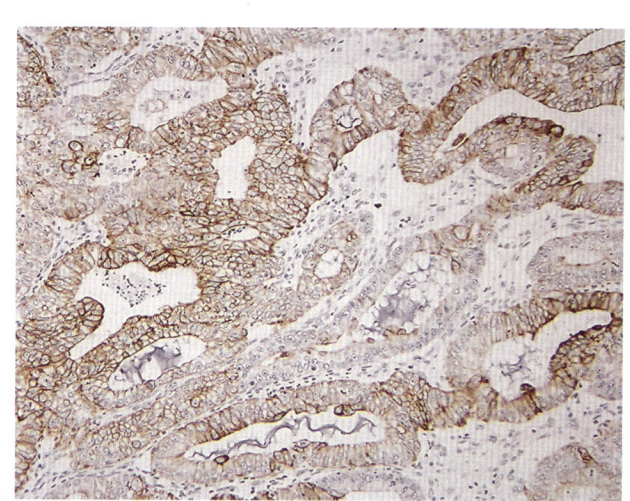

图 16.18 子宫内膜样癌，包括"Sertoli样"变型，显示EMA弥漫强阳性，如本图所示。Sertoli 细胞和 Sertoli-Leydig 细胞肿瘤 EMA 阴性

表16.11 子宫内膜癌与性索间质肿瘤的比较				
	CK	EMA	Inhibin	Calretinin
子宫内膜癌	+	+	N	N
颗粒细胞瘤	S	N	+	+
Sertoli-Leydig 细胞瘤	+	N	+	+
Sertoli 细胞瘤	+	N	+	+

N，阴性；+，阳性；S，有时阳性

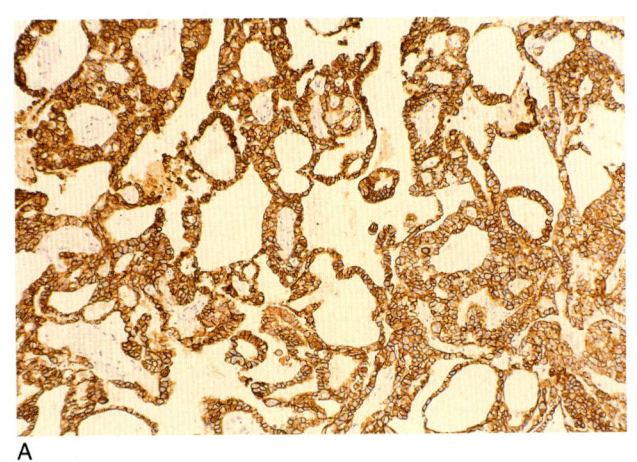
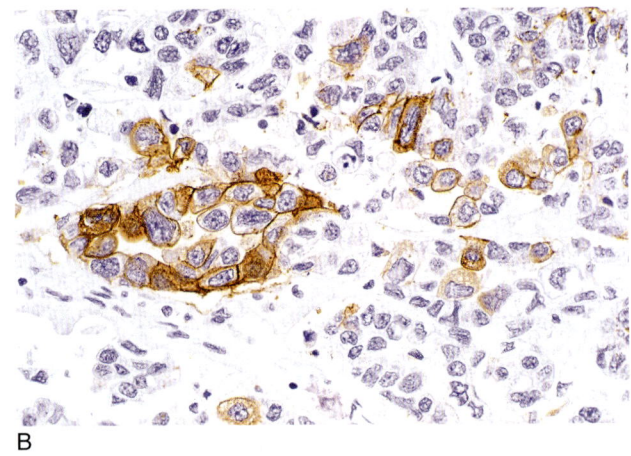

图16.19 透明细胞癌。(A) 透明细胞癌CK7弥漫强阳性;(B) 虽然CD15首先应用于血液病理学,但它能染某些腺癌包括透明细胞癌,如本图示。卵黄囊瘤是重要的鉴别诊断,其CK7和CD15为阴性

色倾向于强而弥漫。这可用于透明细胞癌和浆液性癌鉴别有困难的情况下,p53和WT-1胞核弥漫强阳性支持浆液性癌的诊断。透明细胞癌腺体间的基质或乳头内常含有淀粉样嗜酸性透明物质。这种物质不见于其他类型上皮性肿瘤,因其层粘连蛋白和Ⅳ型胶原阳性而被认为是基底膜物质[316, 317]。

过去透明细胞癌和卵黄囊瘤被认为是同一类型肿瘤("中肾瘤")。在某些病例中,卵黄囊瘤仍存在鉴别诊断问题,因为这些肿瘤的组织学表现有一定程度的重叠。知晓患者年龄、临床情况以及血清甲胎蛋白(AFP)水平有助于鉴别诊断。透明细胞癌通常AFP阴性而卵黄囊瘤通常至少局灶阳性(表16.12)[171]。另一方面,透明细胞癌CD15和EMA强阳性,而卵黄囊瘤为阴性或弱阳性[240]。据报道CK7在卵巢的卵黄囊瘤中为阴性[171],但作者观察到约1/3睾丸卵黄囊瘤CK7阳性,也有其他作者报道卵巢卵黄囊瘤有CK7表达[241]。然而,透明细胞癌几乎总是CK7阳性,因此CK7不表达有助于卵黄囊瘤的诊断。

肾细胞癌透明细胞变型可与卵巢原发透明细胞癌相似。原发透明细胞癌CK7阳性,而转移性肾透明细胞癌很少CK7阳性[312]。鉴别诊断的其他有用指标是CD10[318],它在卵巢原发透明细胞癌为阴性,而在转移性肾透明细胞癌为阳性而且常为胞膜浓染。在透明细胞癌中很可能阳性的其他指标包括高分子量角蛋白、CA125、ER/PR[313]。另一方面,肾细胞癌抗原阳性染色有助于转移性肾细胞癌的诊断[312]。最有用的组合包括CK7、CD10和肾细胞癌抗原[312]。CK7弥漫强阳性染色、CD10和肾细胞癌抗原阴性有助于诊断卵巢原发透明细胞癌。

Brenner瘤和移行细胞肿瘤

新近研究表明Brenner瘤上皮和尿路上皮具有相似的免疫表型,表明Brenner瘤的移行细胞样上皮代表真正的尿路上皮化生。所有作者均报道Brenner瘤为CK7阳性并且多数为CEA阳性[224, 319-321]。虽然并非所有作者观察到同样的染色模式,多数最近的报道表明Brenner瘤染色似尿路上皮,即CK7、尿激酶Ⅲ(uroplakin Ⅲ)[322]和血栓调节素(thrombomodulin)(图16.20)阳性,以及某些报道中CK20阳性[320, 323]。一些作者未能检测到CK20和血栓调节素这些尿路上

表16.12 透明细胞癌与Yolk Sac肿瘤的比较

	CK	CK7	EMA	CD15	AFP
透明细胞癌	+	+	+	+	N
Yolk Sac肿瘤	+	N	N	N	+

N, 阴性;+, 阳性

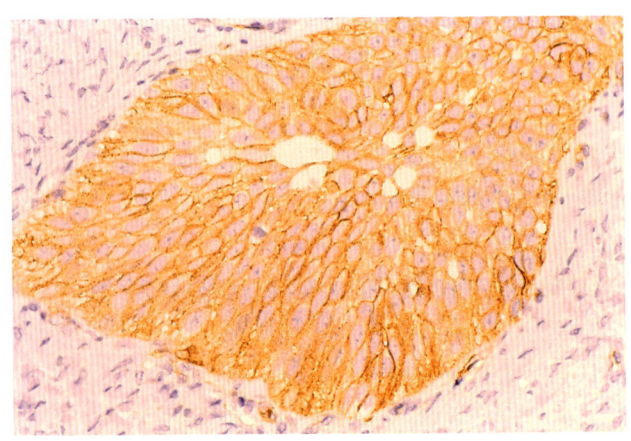

图16.20 Brenner瘤的上皮样成分CK7阳性。也有报道尿路上皮分化标志物如尿激酶着色,本图示血栓调节素为胞浆和胞膜阳性

女性生殖系统的免疫组织化学 16

皮的免疫标记物[319, 321]。良性Brenner瘤较交界性和恶性Brenner瘤更常表达尿路上皮标记[224]。卵巢移行细胞癌具有与其他表面上皮癌尤其是浆液性癌相同的免疫组织化学特征，而且其免疫表型不同于尿路上皮型移行细胞癌。卵巢移行细胞癌表达 CK7 和 CA125，罕见表达尿路上皮标记物如CK13、CK20、尿激酶Ⅲ或血栓调节素，但常表达 WT-1[224, 321, 324, 325]。如同卵巢其他非黏液型上皮性肿瘤一样，移行细胞癌表达间皮素（mesothelin），而尿路上皮型移行细胞癌则不然[326]。免疫染色组合包括CK7、CK20、血栓调节素、WT-1，以及如果可能的话，尿激酶Ⅲ，它们有助于鉴别卵巢原发移行细胞癌和来自膀胱的转移性移行细胞癌。然而，以作者实验室经验而言，尿激酶Ⅲ缺乏敏感性，因此在诊断工作中不再使用。

其他上皮性肿瘤

原发未分化/低分化癌的免疫表型尚未很好定义。作者的经验是高级别癌能表达常见的上皮性标记物如细胞角蛋白和EMA。它们有助于鉴别低分化癌和癌肉瘤以及各种低分化非上皮性肿瘤，如淋巴瘤。有两类小细胞癌发生于卵巢。神经内分泌性小细胞癌可单独发生于卵巢，而更多见的是与某种更普通的原发上皮性肿瘤如黏液性或子宫内膜样癌混合存在。肺小细胞癌可转移至卵巢。神经内分泌性小细胞癌表达常见的神经内分泌标记物，如NSE（图16.21）和CD56。某些病例表达突触素和/或嗜铬素。这些肿瘤有时显示有限的细胞角蛋白表达，可表现为胞浆点状染色或边缘染色模式，高度提示为小细胞癌。肺外小细胞癌可表达甲状腺转录因子（TTF-1），因此TTF-1阳性并不一定表明卵巢的小细胞癌是来自肺癌转移。

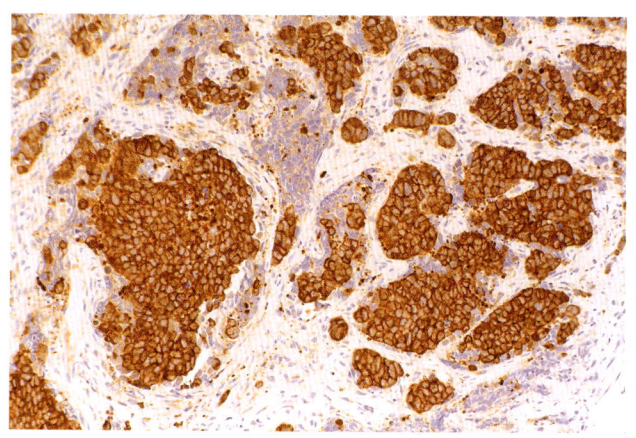

图16.21 神经内分泌性小细胞癌。此肿瘤发生于子宫内膜样腺癌。肿瘤细胞 NSE 强阳性

第二型小细胞癌是高血钙型小细胞癌，常发生于卵巢。这是主要发生于年轻女性卵巢的一种高度恶性肿瘤。约2/3患者具有高钙血症。此瘤的本质有争议，但最近研究表明它最好归类为上皮性肿瘤。免疫组织化学染色表明其上皮性表型，因为多数肿瘤显示EMA和细胞角蛋白阳性[225, 327-329]。最近一项研究表明相当一部分病例 WT-1、CD10 和 p53 染色阳性[225]。其他染色为非特异性，但常阳性的有波形蛋白、NSE、嗜铬素和CD99[327, 329]。偶有肿瘤着染甲状旁腺激素相关蛋白或甲状旁腺激素[328]，但是伴随于小细胞癌的高钙血症的原因尚待阐明。抑制素阴性、calretinin常弱阳性以及EMA阳性有助于鉴别小细胞癌和幼年性颗粒细胞瘤，也表明小细胞癌并非性索-间质肿瘤[197, 214, 225, 327]。

其他需要与卵巢小细胞癌鉴别诊断的原发性和转移性小圆细胞肿瘤包括：淋巴瘤、黑色素瘤[226, 330]、促纤维增生性小圆细胞肿瘤[331-334]、Ewing肉瘤/原始神经外胚层肿瘤（ES/PNET）[335]以及原发和转移性小圆细胞肉瘤，包括胚胎性和腺泡状横纹肌肉瘤[336-338]。用于鉴别这些肿瘤的抗体包括CD45和相关的淋巴瘤标记物（图16.22），S-100、HMB-45和相关恶性黑色素瘤标记，细胞角蛋白、结蛋白、WT-1、NSE用于促纤维增生性小圆细胞肿瘤（图16.23），用于ES/PNET的CD99和FLI-1，以及用于横纹肌肉瘤的结蛋白和成肌素。

> **诊断要点：卵巢上皮性肿瘤**
>
> 1. 卵巢所有常见的原发上皮性肿瘤均表达 CK7。
> 2. 如果上皮性肿瘤CK7阴性，考虑为转移癌或前面讨论过的罕见原发性上皮性肿瘤。
> 3. 浆液性癌和移行细胞癌通常 WT-1 阳性。
> 4. 许多原发性卵巢肿瘤为 CK20 阴性。例外的是肠型黏液性卵巢肿瘤，其CK20和CK7均阳性。

卵巢性索-间质肿瘤

源自卵巢性索或卵巢间叶组织的肿瘤占所有卵巢肿瘤的5%～12%[339, 340]。纤维-卵泡膜肿瘤的良性肿瘤相对常见。其他性索-间质肿瘤和间叶肿瘤罕见。最常见的恶性性索-间质肿瘤是颗粒细胞瘤，占所有卵巢恶性肿瘤的1%～2%[340, 341]。有两型颗粒细胞瘤：成年型，主要发生于绝经后妇女；幼年型，主要发生

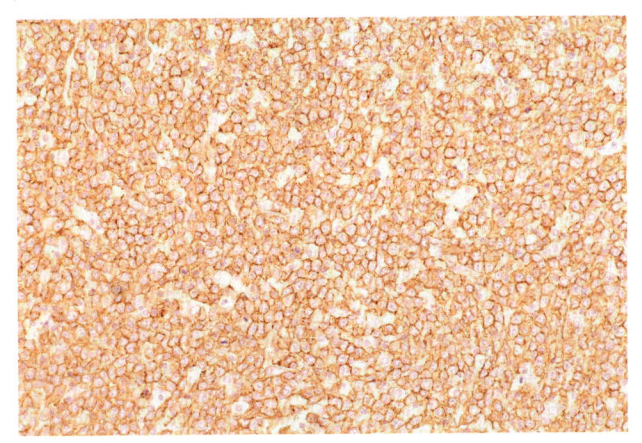

图 16.22 卵巢淋巴瘤。这种弥漫浸润性肿瘤证实为大B细胞性淋巴瘤。CD20免疫染色显示瘤细胞膜强阳性

肿瘤中为阳性；CD99在很多性索-间质肿瘤中阳性；而EMA在性索-间质肿瘤中总是阴性，在鉴别诊断中它能排除许多类型的癌。抑制素是最特异的性索-间质肿瘤标记物[190, 194, 195, 197, 198, 200, 201, 327, 342, 343]。Calretinin更为敏感，能着染更多肿瘤和肿瘤类型，但其特异性稍差，因为它还在间皮瘤和约20%的上皮性肿瘤中表达[213, 214, 342]。与抑制素相比，calretinin在肿瘤细胞中着色更强、更弥漫。抑制素着色倾向于斑片状且强度不一。

纤维瘤、卵泡膜瘤及其相关肿瘤

纤维瘤是良性间质肿瘤，为梭形纤维母细胞伴丰富的胶原纤维。纤维瘤很少采用免疫组化；因为HE切片表现通常可以确诊。纤维瘤和相关肿瘤如富于细胞的纤维瘤和纤维肉瘤仅偶见抑制素着色，但多数为calretinin阳性[197, 199, 214]。

于儿童。其他易于引起诊断问题，需要免疫组织化学来解决的性索-间质肿瘤包括Sertoli-Leydig细胞瘤、Sertoli细胞瘤、具有环形小管的性索肿瘤、Leydig细胞瘤以及未分类的类固醇细胞肿瘤。

数种抗体已被证明非常有助于诊断性索-间质瘤。它们是抑制素和calretinin，在大多数性索-间质

卵泡膜瘤为良性梭形细胞肿瘤，与纤维瘤不同的是它常有激素活性，通常分泌雌激素；另外肿瘤细胞形态也有不同，它倾向于肥胖、胞浆透明或空泡状；

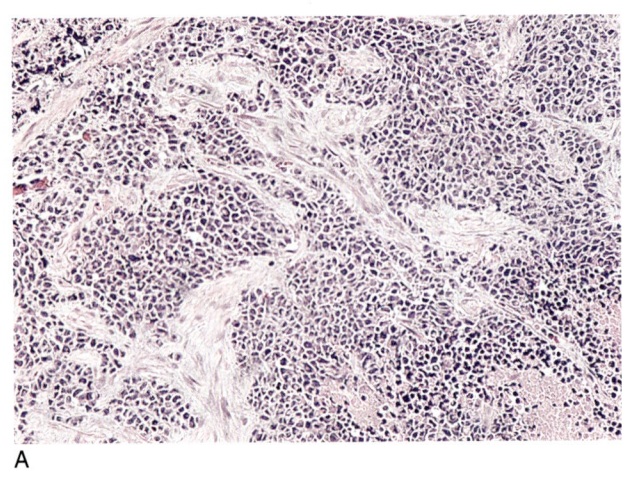

A

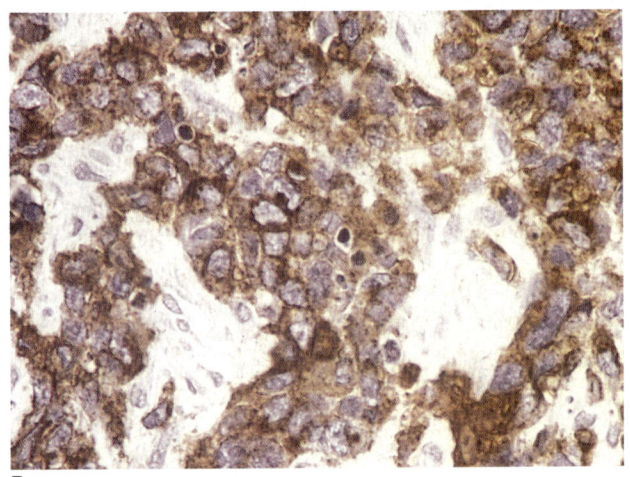

B

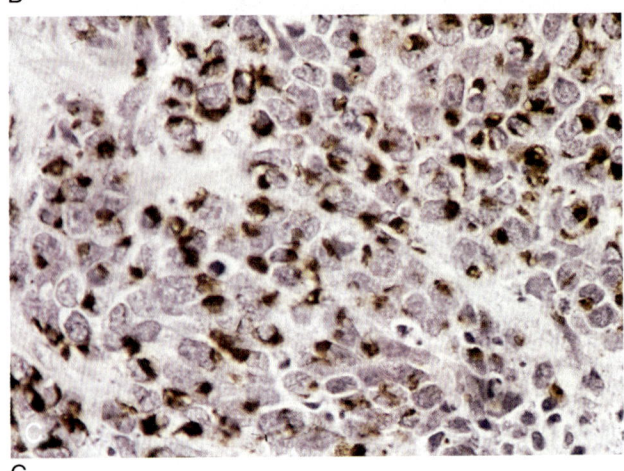

C

图 16.23 促纤维增生性小圆细胞性肿瘤累及卵巢。（A）肿瘤细胞巢状生长，在癌巢间为增生的纤维间质；（B）肿瘤细胞显示细胞膜上细胞角蛋白强阳性，并倾向于着染EMA和NSE（图片未显示）；（C）核周结蛋白点状着色是DSRCT的特点（获Anjali Saqi，MD授权）

女性生殖系统的免疫组织化学　16

其背景间质胶原比纤维瘤少。卵泡膜瘤通常抑制素和calretinin均阳性[195-197, 199, 214]。抑制素强阳性支持卵泡膜瘤而非纤维瘤的诊断。肌源性标志物如平滑肌肌动蛋白（SMA）也通常为阳性[344]。

卵巢硬化性间质瘤为良性无激素活性肿瘤[345, 346]。组织学表现呈多样性，细胞丰富的梭形细胞区与细胞稀少的纤维化区交替存在。散在分布分支状扩张的血管呈"血管周细胞瘤样"。邻近血管的肿瘤细胞通常呈多角形和模糊不清肌样。肿瘤细胞波形蛋白阳性并常表达 SMA，SMA 染色集中于肿瘤脉管周围的肥胖细胞[347-349]。50%以上的硬化性间质瘤均阳性表达抑制素和calretinin[197, 214, 347]。数位作者已将所观察到的这些肿瘤的高血管密度与血管内皮生长因子（VEGF）关联起来[346, 350]。血管标志物如CD31和CD34染色能确定这些明显的分支状血管。

颗粒细胞瘤

卵巢颗粒细胞瘤分两型。成年型最常见。它是一种潜在低度恶性的惰性肿瘤；可扩散至卵巢外、复发以及导致死亡[351, 352]。复发倾向于晚期，某些病例复发可见于首次治疗20余年后[353]。镜下，肿瘤细胞小而一致，核深染，胞浆稀少。核分裂度相当低。该肿瘤因瘤细胞的特征性排列而易于辨认，包括岛屿状、微滤泡、梁状和弥漫性。抑制素和 calretinin 免疫组化染色有助于作出颗粒细胞瘤的诊断（表16.13）[195, 197, 199, 200, 213, 214, 327, 354]。抑制素和calretinin均为典型强阳性，calretinin着色弥漫而抑制素弥漫或斑片状（图16.24A）[194]。这些染色并不特异，因为其他类型性索-间质肿瘤也呈阳性而且偶尔癌也呈弱阳性。在

表16.13　颗粒细胞瘤的鉴别诊断

	I	CR	CK	EMA	LCA	CD99	CGR/SYN
颗粒细胞瘤	+	+	S	N	N	+	N
癌	N	N	+	+	N	N	N
类癌	N	N	+	+	N	N	+
淋巴瘤	N	N	N	N	+	S	N
小细胞癌	N	S	S	S	N	S	S

I，抑制素；CR，calretinin；CK，细胞角蛋白；EMA，上皮细胞膜抗原；LCA，白细胞共同抗原；CGR，嗜铬素；SYN，突触素
N，阴性；+，阳性；S，有时阳性

30%~60% 肿瘤中，低分子量角蛋白为阳性，通常呈斑片状（图16.24B）[355-358]，但颗粒细胞瘤 EMA 阴性[355]。其他常见阳性的指标有SMA、S-100和CD99[201, 353, 358, 359]。

经常误认为颗粒细胞瘤的肿瘤是卵巢原发或转移性低分化癌。癌表现出颗粒细胞瘤所不具有的特征如极性（bilaterality）、高级别核以及高核分裂指数。此外，免疫组化有助于建立正确的诊断，因为癌通常强而弥漫地表达角蛋白和 EMA。它们通常着染 CK7 或 CK20 等角蛋白亚型，并且抑制素和calretinin 为阴性。类癌也类似颗粒细胞瘤，尤其当它们呈岛屿状、微腺样或弥漫时。正确诊断的线索包括其他畸胎瘤成分和肿瘤细胞具有粗的、块状的核染色质以及颗粒性胞浆。它们的免疫表型与颗粒细胞瘤不同，类癌倾向于强而弥漫性表达角蛋白而抑制素和calretinin 为阴性，表达神经内分泌标志物如突触素和嗜铬素。

卵巢第二种类型颗粒细胞瘤为幼年型颗粒细胞瘤[360, 361]。它主要发生于儿童和年轻女性，但也可见于任何年龄包括绝经后妇女[362]。幼年型颗粒细胞瘤局

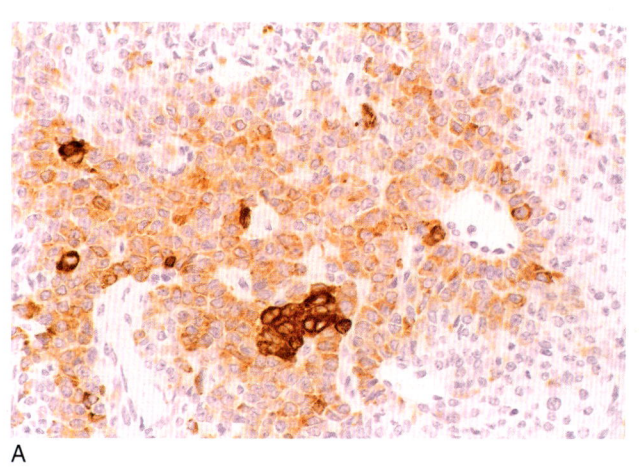
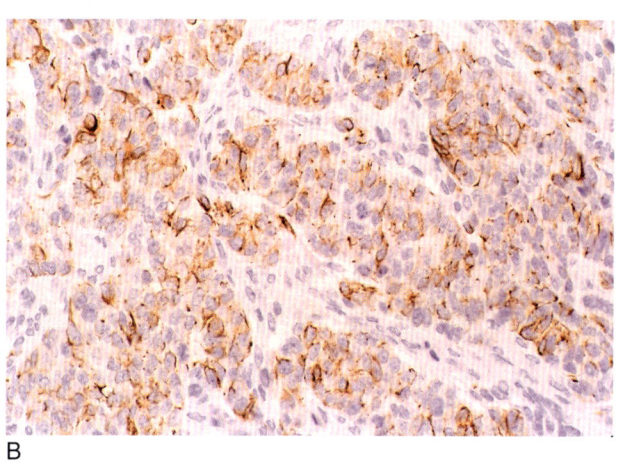

图16.24　成人型颗粒细胞瘤。（A）颗粒细胞瘤抑制素阳性，但强度及分布不均。如图示，有些细胞胞浆强阳性，而有些细胞弱阳性或阴性；（B）颗粒细胞瘤细胞角蛋白的表达，为斑片状中等强度胞浆着色，但许多颗粒细胞瘤细胞角蛋白阴性

限于卵巢内时预后相当好,但其组织学表现惊人。肿瘤细胞大、核异型、核仁显著。胞浆丰富并常黄素化。核分裂象常见。肿瘤细胞呈大滤泡样或弥漫排列。其免疫表型与成年型颗粒细胞瘤一样。肿瘤细胞着染抑制素和calretinin[196, 197, 201],而且常CD99胞膜强阳性(图16.25)[201]。细胞角蛋白表达见于某些肿瘤,但EMA为阴性。免疫组化有助于鉴别幼年型颗粒细胞瘤和高血钙型小细胞癌(表16.13)。幼年型颗粒细胞瘤为抑制素阳性而小细胞癌抑制素阴性[197, 327]。小细胞癌细胞角蛋白着色强而且约50%表达EMA,而幼年型颗粒细胞瘤EMA阴性[327]。calretinin染色可见于小细胞癌,但通常比幼年型颗粒细胞瘤染色弱[225]。文献中报道小细胞癌表达CD99的结果有争议,有些作者报道为阴性而其他作者报道约半数病例为阳性[225, 327]。尽管小细胞癌可为CD99阴性,但几乎所有幼年型颗粒细胞瘤均为CD99阳性。

Sertoli-Leydig 细胞瘤

Sertoli-Leydig细胞瘤主要发生于年轻女性而且约半数有男性化(virilizing)[363]。高分化型的Sertoli细胞排列成良好的小管,纤维性间质中含有簇状排列的多角形Leydig细胞[364, 365],没有不成熟的间质和Sertoli细胞。更常见的中间型和低分化Sertoli-Leydig细胞瘤含有不同程度不成熟的Sertoli细胞,呈小梁状、巢状,或衬覆圆形或网状小管[364, 366-368]。间质富于细胞且不成熟,在多数肿瘤中可见单个或成簇的Leydig细胞。许多患者肿瘤局限于卵巢并具有很好的预后。因为难于辨认不同细胞类型,而且由于其他类型肿瘤特别是子宫内膜样癌的Sertoli样变型具有与Sertoli-Leydig细胞瘤某些共同的组织学特征,免疫组化染色在Sertoli-Leydig细胞瘤诊断中显得很重要。Sertoli细胞表达细胞角蛋白,突出了小管并勾勒出不成熟Sertoli细胞条索、巢状和片状结构,Sertoli细胞不表达EMA(图16.26)[201, 369, 370]。间质细胞和Leydig细胞CK和EMA阴性。抑制素和calretinin在Sertoli-Leydig细胞瘤中通常阳性,尽管呈斑片状着色但在Sertoli-Leydig细胞表达最强[190, 194-197, 214, 327, 342, 371]。虽然罕见子宫内膜样癌弱阳性表达抑制素,但多数为阴性,因此抑制素和EMA联合使用有助于鉴别Sertoli-Leydig细胞瘤和子宫内膜样癌的Sertoli样变型(表16.11)[307, 308, 370, 372, 373]。Sertoli细胞倾向于CD99胞膜强阳性[295]。Sertoli细胞还表现为WT-1胞核强表达,这也见于与Sertoli-Leydig细胞瘤鉴别的各种腺癌[341]。约

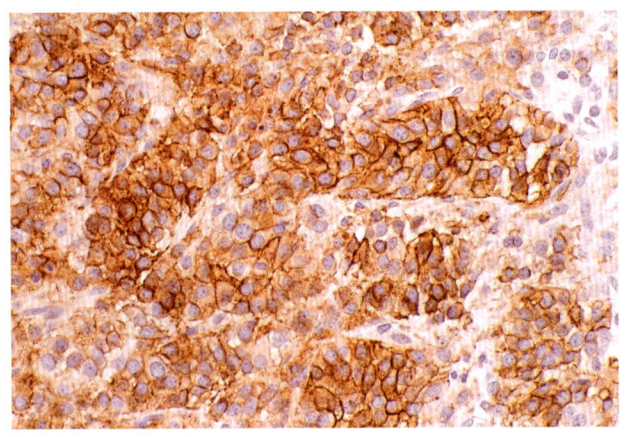

图16.25 幼年型颗粒细胞瘤。几乎所有瘤细胞胞膜强表达CD99

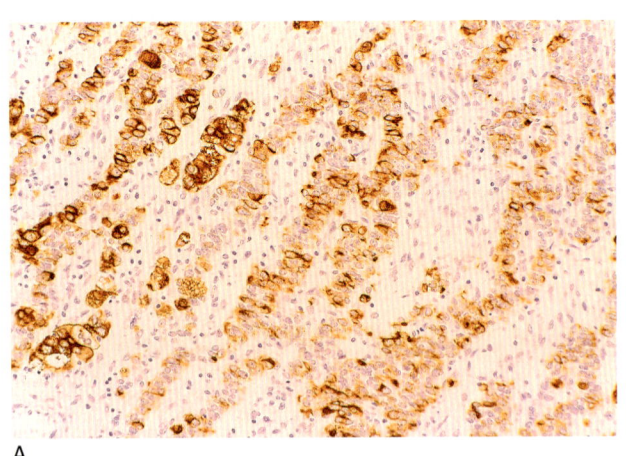

A

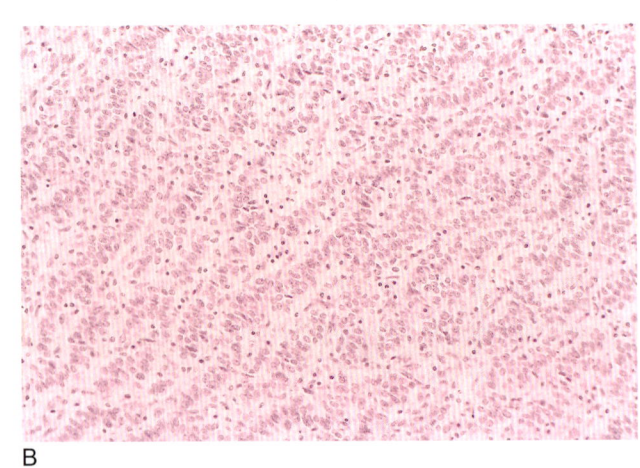

B

图16.26 Sertoli-Leydig细胞瘤。Sertoli细胞的条索和小管不易辨认。(A)细胞角蛋白有助于诊断,呈条索和小管状排列的Sertoli细胞特异性的胞浆着色,如图所示;(B)Sertoli细胞Sertoli细胞索及小管EMA阴性,与子宫内膜样癌Sertoli样变型形成对比,其角蛋白和EMA均阳性(已在图16.18描述)

20%Sertoli-Leydig细胞瘤存在异源性成分，免疫染色有助于它们的识别和归类。胃肠型上皮是最常见的异源性成分[347]，呈细胞角蛋白和EMA阳性但抑制素阴性。嗜铬素、血清素以及各种肽类如皮质激素、生长抑素和降钙素免疫染色常见于异源性肠上皮[375]。Sertoli-Leydig细胞瘤罕见地表现局灶性异源性肝样分化，可分泌甲胎蛋白（图16.27）[246, 248]。肝样细胞着染低分子量细胞角蛋白（CK8/18）、抗肝细胞抗体和甲胎蛋白，但不表达抑制素。异源性类癌分化是嗜铬素和/或突触素阳性。局灶异源性横纹肌母细胞（rhabdomyoblastic）分化是预后差的表现，通常结蛋白和成肌素阳性[376]。

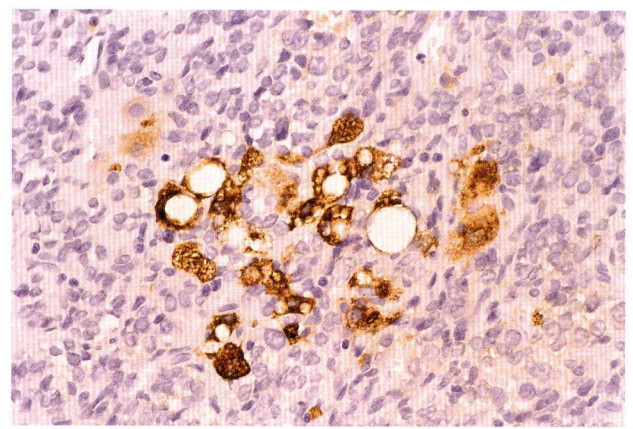

图16.27　Sertoli-Leydig细胞瘤。显示局灶异源性肝样分化，这种肝样细胞胞浆强表达AFP，也表达抗肝细胞抗体

Sertoli 细胞瘤

Sertoli细胞瘤为罕见的良性肿瘤，其中Sertoli细胞排列成小管或小梁状[377]。它们缺乏原始间质和Sertoli-Leydig细胞瘤的Leydig细胞。嗜酸性和富于脂质的变型已被描述[378]。免疫组织化学有助于确定诊断并鉴别Sertoli细胞瘤和Sertoli型子宫内膜样癌以及转移性癌。Sertoli细胞瘤呈波形蛋白和细胞角蛋白强阳性，不表达EMA。但抑制素和calretinin阳性，多数也表达CD99[214]。Sertoli型子宫内膜样癌不仅表达细胞角蛋白也表达EMA，但抑制素和calretinin常阴性[307, 369, 370, 372, 373]。

伴有环形小管的性索肿瘤（SCTAT）

SCTAT为一种未分类性索-间质肿瘤，可有两种临床情况。约1/3的SCTAT患者伴有Peutz-Jeghers综合征和小的，常是镜下的微小肿瘤，后者通常多灶并发生于双侧。2/3 SCTAT患者不伴有Peutz-Jeghers综合征。它们为较大的具有激素活性、可复发或转移的单侧肿瘤。不管临床情况如何，肿瘤由核位于基底部的柱状细胞组成，围绕着嗜酸性透明物轴心的柱状细胞排列成紧密的环形小管。SCTAT具有与其他性索-间质肿瘤相似的免疫表型：波形蛋白、细胞角蛋白、抑制素和calretinin阳性[196, 197, 199, 379]，但上皮细胞膜抗原阴性。超微结构显示嗜酸性轴心和间质的透明物质为基底膜物质。至少某些病例层粘连蛋白和Ⅳ型胶原阳性。

Leydig 细胞瘤

Leydig细胞瘤为良性卵巢肿瘤，常分泌大量的睾酮，因此在肿瘤尚小的情况下即引起症状。它们由多角形Leydig细胞组成，具有泡状核，常有显著核仁和丰富的嗜酸性或淡染的空泡状胞浆。胞浆特征性地含有嗜酸性透明小球或棒状包涵体。后者即为著名的Reinke结晶，它们的存在是Leydig细胞瘤的诊断依据。大多数Leydig细胞瘤发生于卵巢门（hilum），因此有时称为门细胞瘤。非门部Leydig细胞瘤和间质Leydig细胞瘤常难以诊断，因为Reinke结晶的存在为诊断所需要，但这仅见于约50%病例。免疫组织化学染色通常不是Leydig细胞瘤诊断所必需，对Leydig细胞瘤与其他性索-间质肿瘤及瘤样病变的鉴别没有帮助意义（如黄素化卵泡膜瘤、未分类的Steroid细胞瘤以及妊娠黄体瘤）。Leydig细胞抑制素、calretinin和melan-A阳性，而角蛋白和上皮细胞膜抗原常阴性[371]。

类固醇细胞瘤

类固醇细胞肿瘤倾向为大的单侧性肿瘤。多数有激素活性并分泌睾酮或其他激素。显微镜下，它们由具有丰富胞浆的大多角形细胞构成。有些细胞具有透明、空泡状胞浆，类似于肾上腺皮质细胞。除缺乏Reinke结晶之外，其他细胞具有致密的嗜酸性胞浆，类似Leydig细胞。同一种类固醇细胞瘤中可存在两种类型的细胞，但以某种细胞类型为主。细胞大、核异型性显著以及核分裂指数高与恶性行为相关。类固醇细胞肿瘤特征性着染抑制素、calretinin和melan-A[194,197,342,380]。calretinin染色比抑制素和melan-A强而弥漫[342]。多数肿瘤波形蛋白阳性，而且40%～50%表达细胞角蛋白[381]。上皮细胞膜抗原为阴性。某些肿瘤可表达S-100或HMB-45，尽管比较弱且局灶性，但MART-1阴性[342]。

> **诊断要点：性索-间质肿瘤**
>
> 1. 性索-间质肿瘤 CK 可阳性或阴性。
> 2. 性索-间质肿瘤 EMA 阴性。EMA 阳性着色提示原发或转移性上皮性肿瘤（形态与性索-间质肿瘤相似）。
> 3. 抑制素是性索-间质肿瘤相对特异的指标。
> 4. 在性索-间质肿瘤 calretinin 更为敏感，但特异性不如抑制素。

生殖细胞肿瘤

生殖细胞肿瘤可被分为三大类。第一类包括常见良性囊性畸胎瘤，在实际操作中占生殖细胞肿瘤的绝大部分，另外较少见的是实性成熟型畸胎瘤。这些肿瘤大体和镜下比较特异，含有皮肤和皮肤附属器，以及来源于其他胚层的良性组织。神经胶质组织常很明显。单纯良性畸胎瘤的诊断很少需要免疫组织化学。第二类包括良性囊性畸胎瘤的变型，以某一胚层分化为主或单胚层畸胎瘤。这类肿瘤包括卵巢甲状腺肿、类癌和来源于良性囊性畸胎瘤的恶性肿瘤如癌和恶性黑色素瘤。免疫组化有助于这类肿瘤的诊断。第三类由恶性生殖细胞肿瘤构成：无性细胞瘤、卵黄囊瘤、胚胎性癌、绒毛膜癌、多胚瘤以及包含两种或两种以上单纯成分的混合性生殖细胞瘤。这些罕见肿瘤常发生于年轻患者。治疗采取保守手术，结合术后化疗。准确诊断为正确治疗所必需，因而常采用免疫组织化学来辅助诊断。最常用于恶性生殖细胞肿瘤诊断的抗体包括CD117、PLAP、AFP、CD30、hCG、广谱角蛋白如 AE1/AE3 以及 EMA，详见下述。

无性细胞瘤

无性细胞瘤常显示PLAP和CD117（c-kit）胞膜强阳性（图 16.28）[228]。CD117 尤其能鉴别其他肿瘤，如胚胎性癌、卵黄囊瘤不显示CD117胞膜阳性，而CD117胞膜阳性着色为无性细胞瘤特征性表现（表 16.14）[171]。最近，无性细胞瘤，像睾丸的精原细胞瘤和胚胎性癌，表达核转录因子 OCT4 胞核强阳性[382]。其他类

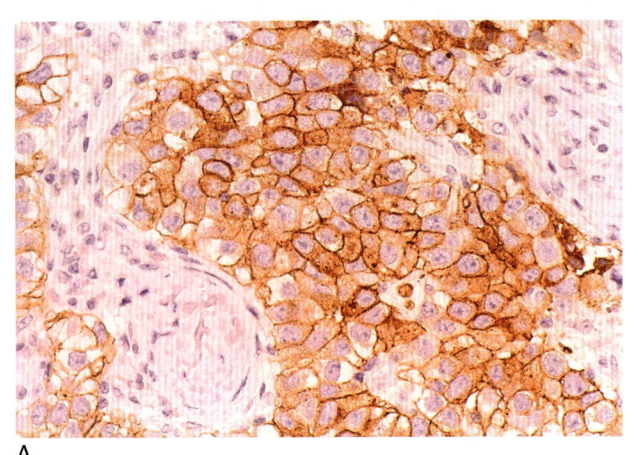
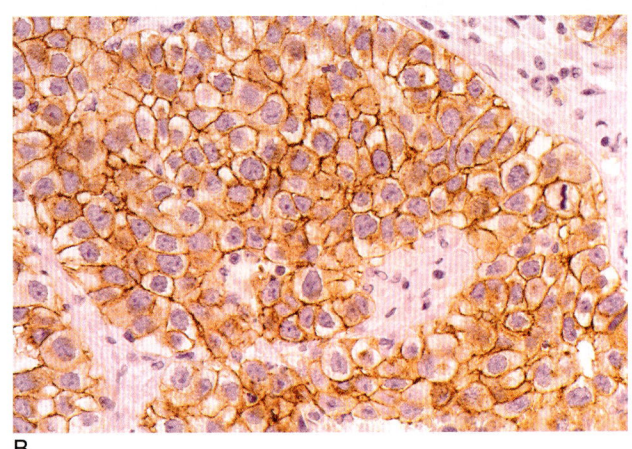

图 16.28 无性细胞瘤显示：(A) PLAP 胞膜和胞浆强阳性，(B) CD117（c-kit）胞膜强阳性

表16.14 无性细胞瘤的鉴别诊断

	PLAP	CD117	OCT4	CK	CD30	S-100	LCA	MPO
无性细胞瘤	+	+	+	N	N	N	N	N
胚胎性癌	+	N	+	+	+	N	N	N
卵黄囊瘤	+	N	N	+	N	N	N	N
淋巴瘤	N	N	N	N	N	N	+	N
粒细胞肉瘤	N	+	N	N	N	N	+	+
恶性黑色素瘤	N	N	N	N	N	+	N	N

PLAP：胎盘碱性磷酸酶；CD117 (c-kit)：膜阳性；CK：细胞角蛋白，少数无性细胞瘤呈弱阳性，AE1/AE3 在胚胎性癌呈膜阳性，在卵黄囊肿瘤呈胞浆阳性；LCA：白细胞共同抗原；MPO：髓过氧化物酶
N，阴性；+，阳性

型生殖细胞瘤如卵黄囊瘤和绒毛膜癌，不表达OCT4，正如大多数其他生殖细胞肿瘤一样。最重要的例外是透明细胞癌，少数病例中显示局灶阳性（<10%肿瘤细胞）[382]。无性细胞瘤可显示CK斑片状阳性，但不像其他生殖细胞肿瘤和上皮性肿瘤呈弥漫强阳性[228]。EMA、CD30、S-100蛋白、淋巴标记物和神经内分泌标记物均为阴性。约5%无性细胞瘤含有合体滋养层巨细胞（STGC），显示hCG胞浆强阳性（图16.29)[259]。

卵黄囊瘤

卵黄囊瘤为不常见的恶性生殖细胞肿瘤，其组织学具有多种复杂形态。免疫组织化学染色可有助于诊断。最有用的染色是甲胎蛋白，它是卵黄囊瘤特异性标记物（图16.30)[236]。甲胎蛋白染色不易掌握，而且弥漫强阳性并不见于每一例肿瘤。甲胎蛋白常表现为斑片状着色，当只有小灶卵黄囊瘤时常不表达AFP。然而75%以上的卵黄囊瘤AFP呈胞浆阳性。卵黄囊瘤中常可见腺腔内分泌物及透明小体，两者也表达AFP。AFP的阳性表达特别有助于一些罕见的变型卵黄囊瘤的诊断，例如子宫内膜样型和腺样型卵巢囊瘤[175,178]。肝样型卵黄囊瘤AFP阳性，也表达抗肝细胞抗体，呈胞浆阳性[243]。虽然该染色结果有助于这种罕见变型卵黄囊瘤的诊断，但是不能区分肝样型卵黄囊瘤和卵巢肝样癌及转移性肝细胞癌，因为后两者AFP也为阳性。卵黄囊瘤表达广谱CK，AE1/AE3胞浆呈弥漫阳性（图16.31），这与胚胎性癌的胞膜阳性不同，据此可进行鉴别诊断（表16.15）。卵黄囊瘤EMA、CD15通常阴性[240,249]，有报道CK7也为阴性[171]。胎盘碱性磷酸酶（PLAP）常阳性，由于其他类型的生

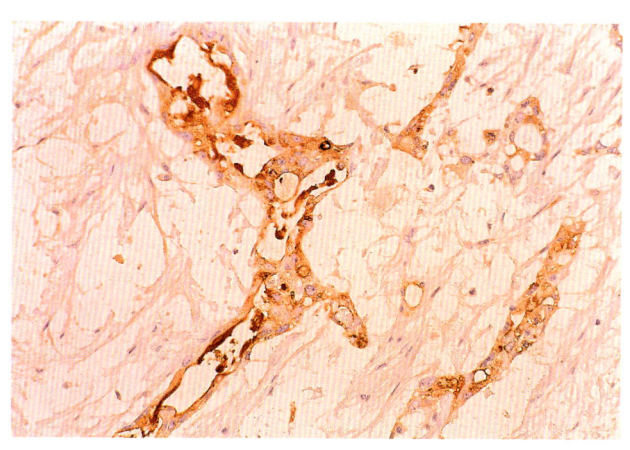

图16.30 卵黄囊瘤。显示AFP染色阳性，特征性的弱至中等强度、斑片状阳性。AFP弥漫强阳性较少见

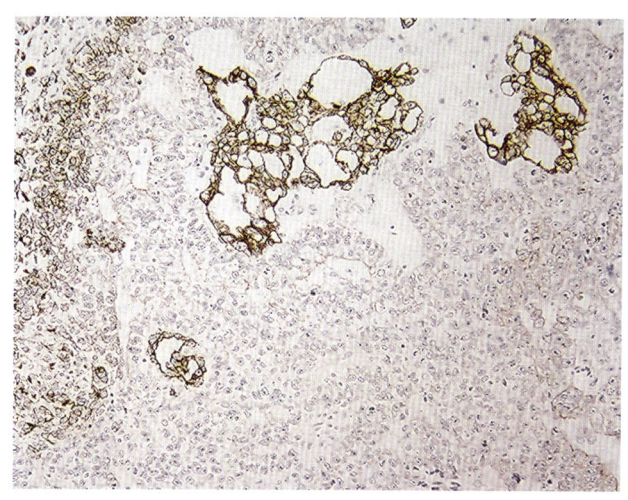

图16.31 混合性生殖细胞肿瘤。用AE1/AE3染色勾勒出肿瘤的不同成分。卵黄囊瘤区（上）显示胞浆角蛋白强阳性。周围无性细胞瘤成分角蛋白阴性

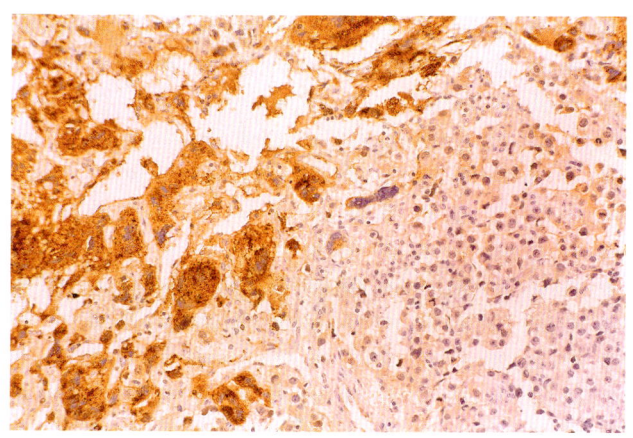

图16.29 无性细胞瘤。患者血清β-hCG升高，肿瘤含有许多合体滋养层巨细胞。图示hCG胞浆弥漫强阳性（左），而无性细胞瘤细胞为hCG阴性（右）

表16.15 细胞角蛋白AE1/AE3在生殖细胞肿瘤中的染色模式

	胞膜着色	胞浆着色
无性细胞瘤	N	通常为N，有时候呈点状弱阳性或胞浆边缘染色
胚胎性癌	+	N
卵黄囊瘤	N	+
胚胎性癌或无性细胞瘤中的绒癌和STGC	N	+

N，阴性；+，阳性；S，有时阳性

殖细胞肿瘤和一些上皮性肿瘤也为阳性，因此PLAP缺乏特异性[249]。卵黄囊瘤细胞外的透明样物质层粘连蛋白阳性。免疫组化染色显示，卵黄囊瘤中除了偶尔出现的合体滋养层巨细胞hCG呈胞浆阳性之外，其他肿瘤细胞则为阴性。

胚胎性癌

胚胎性癌在睾丸是一种相对常见的生殖细胞肿瘤，但却罕见于卵巢。免疫组化胚胎性癌通常PLAP阳性，CD30染色胞膜呈强阳性（图16.32）。胚胎性癌CD117阴性，CK阳性（AE1/AE显示特征性的膜阳性），EMA阴性。胚胎性癌CK和CD30弥漫阳性而CD117阴性，这一特点可与无性细胞瘤鉴别。在睾丸中仅有胚胎性癌和精原细胞瘤这两种肿瘤显示核转录因子OCT4胞核阳性[383]。卵巢无性细胞瘤也能显示这一抗体[382]，而在卵巢的胚胎性癌尚未检测，但基于睾丸中的这种研究结果，预计其为阳性。OCT4阳性不能鉴别胚胎性癌和无性细胞瘤，但能与其他类型的生殖细胞肿瘤和分化差的表面上皮来源的癌进行鉴别，因后者通常会与胚胎性癌混淆。胚胎性癌中常见合体滋养层巨细胞，这种细胞hCG阳性。在一些胚胎性癌中还注意到AFP呈斑片状阳性，这种着色方式尚不清楚：是细胞着色还是向卵黄囊瘤早期功能分化，还是一种难以辨认的卵黄囊成分。

绒毛膜癌

卵巢中单纯的绒毛膜癌罕见，常为混合性生殖细胞肿瘤的一部分。它以细胞滋养层细胞、中间滋养层细胞和合体滋养层细胞混合构成为特征。合体滋养层巨细胞hCG染色胞浆阳性，而细胞滋养层细胞、中间滋养层细胞阴性。由于血清中hCG可能引起强背景染色，因此有些难以解释hCG的染色结果。抑制素也可以作为合体滋养层细胞的一种标记物，其具有背景染色弱的优点[384-387]。值得注意的是，滋养层细胞CD10也为阳性[388]。所有的滋养层细胞CK阳性，但EMA阴性。具有丰富胞浆的合体滋养层细胞显示CK弥漫强阳性，因此即使在低倍镜下也容易识别。绒毛膜癌多为混合性生殖细胞肿瘤的一部分或者以单纯形式出现，罕见卵巢癌伴有绒毛膜癌分化的报道[260]。

畸胎瘤

免疫组织化学对评估成熟型和未成熟型畸胎瘤的作用不大。畸胎瘤可能含有丰富的神经胶质，这可以通过GFAP加以证实。细胞增殖指数标记物Ki-67（MIB-1）偶尔能够为区分成熟型和未成熟型畸胎瘤提供一些帮助。例如，成熟型畸胎瘤中的室管膜样型菊形团结构常显示较低的细胞增殖指数，而在未成熟型畸胎瘤中的神经管常显示较高的细胞增殖指数。未成熟型畸胎瘤患者血清AFP水平增高。对这些病例进行AFP免疫组织化学染色，阳性部位位于内胚层的腺样小囊、未成熟的肠上皮和肝细胞[250, 389]。

免疫组织化学对诊断单胚层畸胎瘤起了很大的作用。例如卵巢的甲状腺肿，它具有大囊腔而少有滤泡[390]，异常的生长方式，或由胞浆透明或嗜酸的细胞混合而成[391]，或与甲状腺腺瘤或甲状腺癌形态相似[392]。这需要依据瘤细胞胞浆和胶质表达甲状腺球蛋白，或瘤细胞胞核TTF-1（甲状腺转录因子）阳性进行诊断[390, 391]（图16.33）。发生在卵巢不同类型的类癌，可能

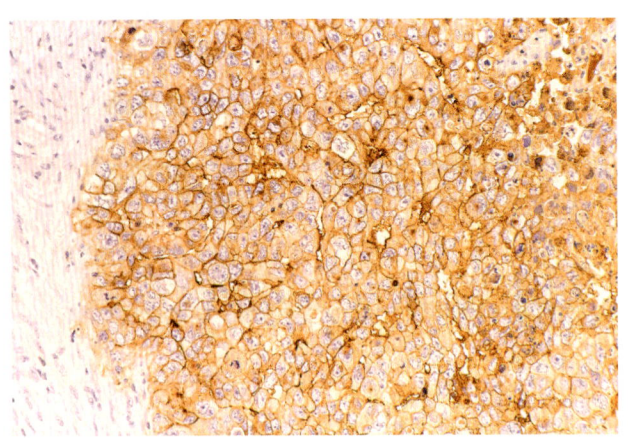

图16.32　胚胎性癌。CD30染色显示瘤细胞胞膜强阳性是胚胎性癌的特征。AE1/AE3染色，胚胎性癌同样显示为膜阳性，这与卵黄囊瘤的胞浆阳性不同（见图16.31）

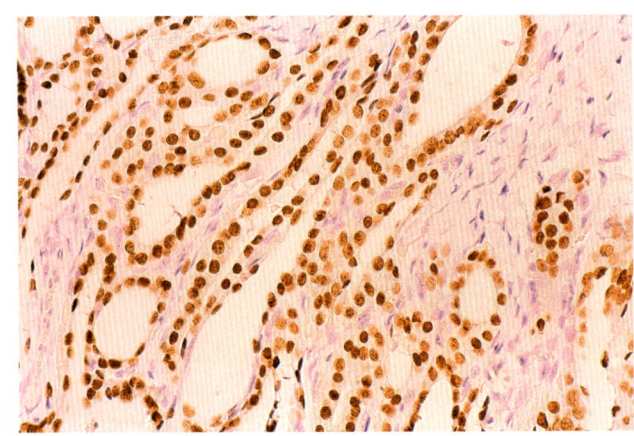

图16.33　卵巢甲状腺肿是一种单胚层畸胎瘤，以甲状腺组织为主要成分。甲状腺细胞显示细胞核TTF-1强阳性，如图所示。肿瘤细胞胞浆和胶质甲状腺球蛋白染色阳性

与其他畸胎瘤成分相关或无关。卵巢中类癌的类型包括岛状型、梁状型、甲状腺肿和黏液型类癌。类癌可以与其他卵巢肿瘤相似，因此免疫组化有助于对其作出正确的诊断。岛状型和梁状型类癌与性索-间质肿瘤相似，例如颗粒细胞瘤、Sertoli细胞瘤或者Sertoli-Leydig细胞瘤，但在类癌中CK呈弥漫强阳性，神经内分泌标记物嗜铬素和突触素阳性，抑制素和calretinin阴性，据此可作出正确的诊断（图16.34）。类癌也可表达多种肽类激素，如血清素[393]。甲状腺肿类癌局部显示甲状腺分化，可能会与富于细胞的卵巢甲状腺或恶性卵巢甲状腺肿混淆。在这种肿瘤中，向甲状腺分化的区域甲状腺球蛋白阳性，类癌的区域嗜铬素和突触素阳性，故能帮助诊断[394-396]。一些甲状腺肿类癌降钙素阳性。大多数甲状腺肿类癌具有有趣的特性，虽然它们不表达PSA[394,395]，但却表达PSAP。此外，那些伴有严重便秘综合征的甲状腺肿类癌患者YY蛋白阳性[397]。黏液型类癌往往嗜铬素、突触素和/或血清素阳性，免疫表型可以帮助其与不同类型的原发或转移性黏液性肿瘤进行鉴别[398]。

性腺母细胞瘤

性腺母细胞瘤由原始生殖细胞和性索细胞混合而成，典型结构是瘤细胞以玻璃样透明物为核心环绕排列。在一些性腺母细胞瘤病例中出现侵袭性恶性生殖细胞肿瘤，通常是精原细胞瘤。能显示生殖细胞的免疫组织化学染色有PLAP、CD117、OCT4，性索细胞波形蛋白、CK和抑制素阳性[197,343,382,399,400]。与肿瘤细胞互相混合的玻璃样透明物质层粘连蛋白阳性，说明它是一种基底膜样物质。

> **诊断要点：生殖细胞瘤**
>
> 1. 恶性生殖细胞肿瘤常表达PLAP。
> 2. CD117是无性细胞瘤的特异标记物，胚胎性癌表达CD30，卵黄囊瘤表达AFP。
> 3. AE1/AE3在很多恶性生殖细胞肿瘤中表达，着色方式有助于肿瘤分类（上面已讨论）。
> 4. 一种新标记物OCT4只在无性细胞瘤和胚胎性癌表达。

转移性肿瘤

卵巢的转移性肿瘤常见，常为上皮来源的肿瘤，占卵巢恶性肿瘤的10%。虽然各种类型、各个部位的肿瘤都有可能转移至卵巢，但是最常见的卵巢转移性肿瘤的原发部位为消化道，尤其是大肠、胃和阑尾；乳腺；女性生殖道，包括子宫内膜和宫颈；还有胰腺[401]。鉴别原发于卵巢表面的上皮性肿瘤和生殖道外的上皮性肿瘤可能比较困难，特别是在外科医生和/或病理科医生不了解病史的情况下。尽管形态学线索是有用的，但是许多病例的组织病理学形态却让人困惑，对于这些病例，免疫组织化学就格外有价值。免疫组织化学最有助于判定非生殖系统的转移性肿瘤，而对鉴别卵巢原发性肿瘤与生殖系统其他部位原发性肿瘤转移至卵巢，例如原发于子宫内膜的肿瘤，就十分困难，免疫组织化学染色对鉴别没有帮助。

在常见的上皮性肿瘤中，浆液性肿瘤通常容易判定是原发性肿瘤，形态极少会与转移性肿瘤相似。另一方面，转移性腺癌的形态常常与黏液性和子宫内膜样肿瘤相似。最近报道有77%的卵巢黏液癌是转移来的[402]。原发性卵巢黏液性和子宫内膜样肿瘤常为单侧发生，并且原发性黏液性肿瘤的直径多大于10cm[402]。小的黏液型肿瘤（直径<10cm）或双侧发生的黏液性或子宫内膜样性肿瘤，应该判断它们是否为转移性肿瘤。这一原则不仅适用于明显的侵袭性肿瘤（癌），而且适用于交界性肿瘤。来自阑尾、结肠、胰腺和膀胱的转移性黏液性腺癌，其形态有时与交界性黏液性和子宫内膜样肿瘤有明显的交叉。应该用抗体CK7和CK20来判断肿瘤是否来自于上述这些部位

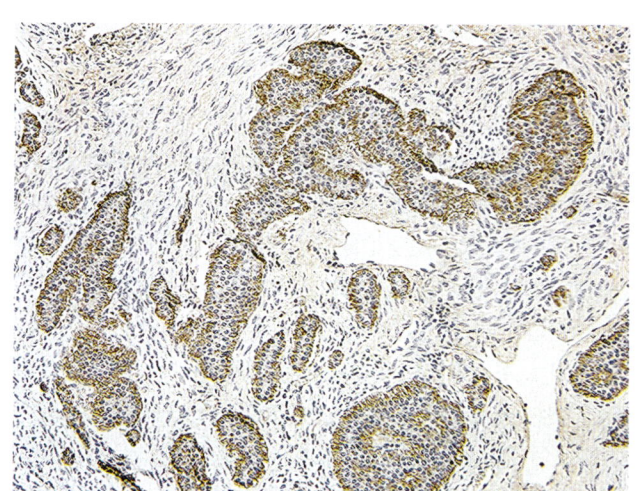

图16.34 卵巢类癌可以和其他组织一起作为畸胎瘤的一部分；它们也可以原发于卵巢，而与其他畸胎瘤组织无关，在这些病例中它们被视作单胚层畸胎瘤；也可以由阑尾、小肠或其他部位转移而来。不论其来源，类癌对嗜铬素、突触素呈胞浆阳性染色

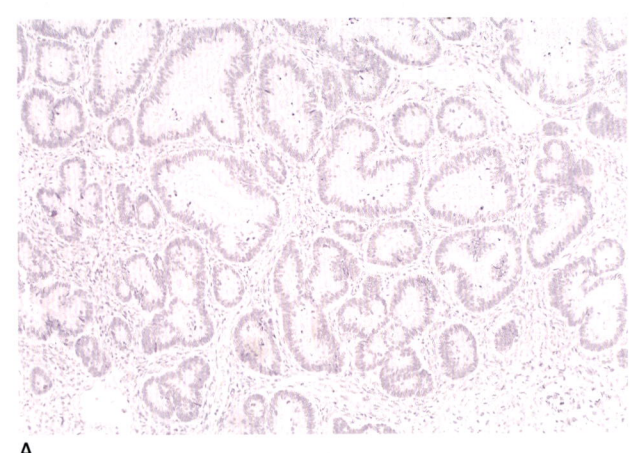
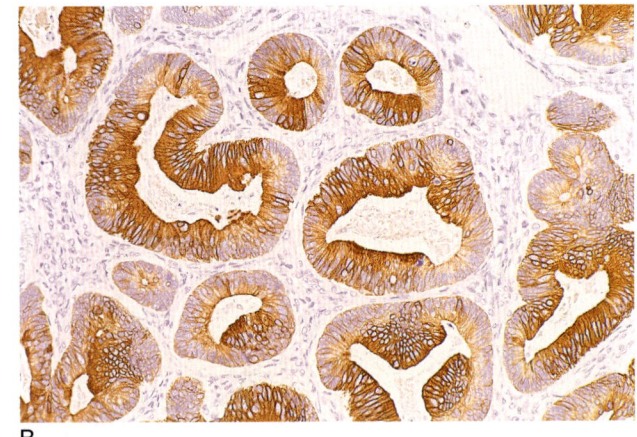

图 16.35 结直肠腺癌是最常转移到卵巢的肿瘤。转移性结直肠腺癌特征性的 CK7 阴性（A），但是 CK20 弥漫强阳性（B）

（表 16.10）。虽然会有例外，但是原发性卵巢癌几乎总是CK7弥漫强阳性，转移性结直肠癌CK7常完全阴性（图16.35A）或仅有小灶阳性。直肠和阑尾来源的肿瘤有时可能表达CK7[169,403]。转移性结直肠肿瘤常呈弥漫强阳性表达CK20（图16.35B）。子宫内膜样癌极少CK20阳性。卵巢原发性黏液性癌CK20阳性，但是其阳性表达较转移性结直肠癌明显弱并且局限。因此，CK7+/CK20- 和 CK7+/CK20+ 支持卵巢原发，CK7-/CK20+ 强烈支持转移[168,404]。新抗体可有一定的作用，包括CDX2，为一种核转录因子，对结肠肿瘤的判定有效（图16.36）；DPC4（Smad4）为一种核因子，50%的胰腺癌失表达。关于这些抗体的使用在黏液性肿瘤的部分中已有详细讨论。来自于胃的转移性腺癌多为双侧性，虽然在一些肿瘤可以出现腺样结构，但是多为印戒细胞（Krukenberg瘤）或低分化形态。卵巢肿瘤中出现印戒细胞表明这种肿瘤可能是转移性的，胃是最有可能的原发部位。转移性胃癌多为CK7阳性（一项研究中阳性率为56%），实际上部分病例（33%）CK20也为阳性[404]。因此，要作出正确的诊断，形态学比免疫组织化学更重要。

来自于胰腺、胆道，甚至是消化道的转移性肿瘤偶尔也可能与透明细胞癌相似[405]；这些肿瘤也可以通过CK7、CK20和DPC4的表达来鉴别。胰腺癌CK7和CK20的表达是不稳定的，有些病例会和卵巢原发性黏液癌重叠。原发性卵巢癌尚未明确DPC4的缺失，因此如果能用充分的病例来证实这个结果，将是很有意义的。转移性肾透明细胞癌和卵巢原发性透明细胞癌也很相似，但是两者的鉴别很少会有困难，因为肾肿瘤通常不会转移到卵巢。转移性肾透明细胞癌CK7阴性，但 CD10 胞膜强阳性。原发性透明细胞癌 CK7+/CD10-。最后，当移行细胞肿瘤无良性Brenner瘤的成分时，与转移性的尿路上皮癌的鉴别十分重要。原发性卵巢移行细胞癌 CK7 阳性。但转移性尿路上皮癌CK7也阳性，而CK20、血栓调节素、尿激酶也常会阳性，后面这些结果能区别原发性卵巢移行细胞癌。

其他转移到卵巢的原发性肿瘤，包括乳腺、肺、甲状腺的肿瘤，免疫组织化学有助于它们的鉴别。乳腺癌的鉴别很少存在困难，因为患者通常知道自己有乳腺肿瘤的病史[406,407]，并且转移性乳腺癌的形态学特点能与大多数卵巢癌鉴别。乳腺癌和卵巢癌的免疫组织化学结果有很大的重叠。两者CK7均阳性，CK20均阴性，可能都表达ER和PR。一些乳腺癌表达GCDFP-15，这一染色有助于乳腺癌和卵巢癌的鉴别[160,408]。作者实践中发现和其他文献报道[409]，GCDFP-15 缺乏敏感性，因此它还没有被证实是转移性乳腺癌的有效抗体。WT-1在浆液性卵巢癌中的表达较在转移性乳腺癌中的表达更为普遍。甲状腺转录因子（TTF-1）是一种

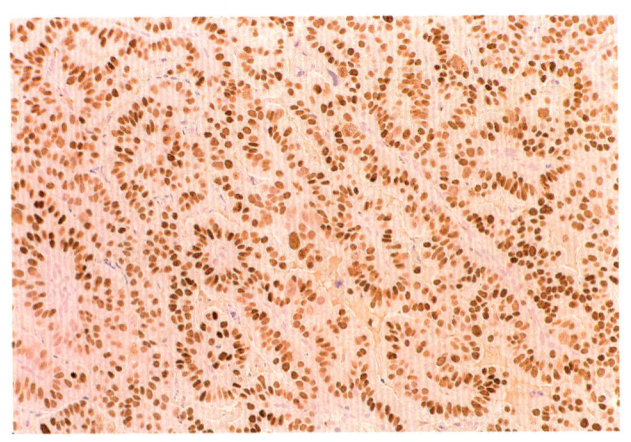

图 16.36 来自于阑尾的转移性腺癌转录因子CDX2染色胞核弥漫强阳性，CDX2 是一种新的结肠腺癌标记物

核转录因子，特异性地表达于甲状腺和肺肿瘤。甲状腺肿瘤偶有转移到卵巢，依据肿瘤的组织学类型，能够通过 TTF-1 和甲状腺球蛋白或降钙素的表达被证实[410]。肺腺癌和肺小细胞癌对 TTF-1 的表达比率高，这种标记物有助于区别肺癌来源的卵巢转移性肿瘤[410]。但是肺外小细胞癌 TTF-1 也会阳性[411-413]，所以 TTF-1 阳性并不能够表明卵巢转移性小细胞癌来自肺；临床病理联系对判定肿瘤原发部位是必不可少的[414]。

事实上任何类型的肿瘤，包括软组织肿瘤和造血系统肿瘤，例如淋巴瘤和白血病，都能累及卵巢，它们可以是原发的也可以是远处转移来的。它们中的大多数具有特异的免疫组织化学特性，能够支持诊断，这在本书的其他章节有详细描述。

> **诊断要点：卵巢转移性肿瘤**
>
> 1. 5%～10% 的卵巢恶性肿瘤是转移性的。
> 2. 结直肠腺癌是最常见的转移癌，与卵巢子宫内膜样癌相似。
> 3. CK7/CK20 对鉴别卵巢转移癌最有用。
> 4. 除黏液癌 CK7+/CK20+ 之外，原发卵巢癌通常为 CK7+/CK20-。
> 5. 转移瘤通常但并不总是 CK7 阴性。
> 6. 转移性结直肠癌通常但并不总是 CK20+。
> 7. CDX2 有助于识别转移性肠道来源的癌，尽管目前尚不清楚为何原发性黏液癌表达 CDX2。
> 8. 有助于识别转移癌的其他抗体，前面已详述。

间皮瘤

浆液性肿瘤不仅可以起源于卵巢内的包涵上皮，也可以起源于卵巢和腹膜表面，因此，临床甚至病理上间皮瘤的发生是可能的。然而女性发生腹膜间皮瘤不常见，并极少局限于卵巢[415-417]。蜕膜样变间皮瘤好发于腹膜，有些病例是年轻女性；免疫表型与普通间皮瘤一致[418-420]。腹膜间皮瘤与浆液性癌的鉴别可以依靠常规光镜观察，但是浆液性癌与胸膜间皮瘤的鉴别经常要借助于免疫组织化学染色的帮助。目前可使用一组免疫组化来鉴别（表16.16）[170,172]，包括间皮瘤阳性而浆液性癌阴性的抗体，例如calretinin、CK5/6和血栓调节素；及浆液性癌阳性而间皮瘤阴性的抗体，例如BerEP4、MOC-31和B72.3（图16.37）。值得注意的是，一些对胸膜间皮瘤有价值的抗体却对腹膜间皮瘤的鉴别作用较小。CD15 仅在一小部分浆液性癌中表达，癌胚抗原在浆液性癌中罕见表达，WT-1在间皮瘤和浆液性癌中都特征性表达，因此这些抗体没有加入上述免疫组化组。

表16.16　腹膜间皮瘤和浆液性癌

	CR	CK5/6	TM	BerEP4	MOC-31	B72.3	WT-1
间皮瘤	+	+	+	N	N	N	+
浆液性癌	N	N	N	+	+	+	+

CR：calretinin；CK5/6：细胞角蛋白5/6；TM：血栓调节素
N，阴性；+，阳性

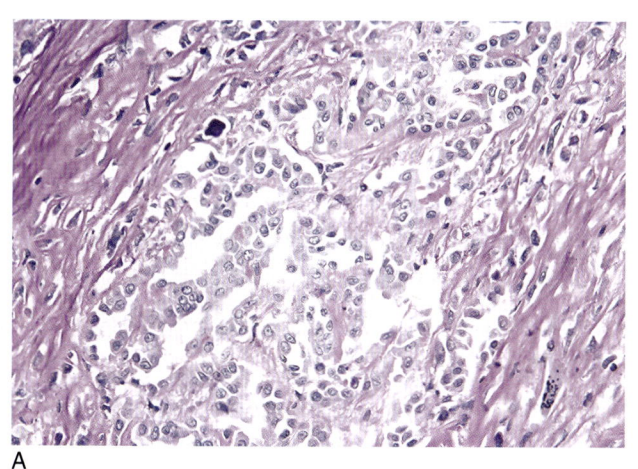
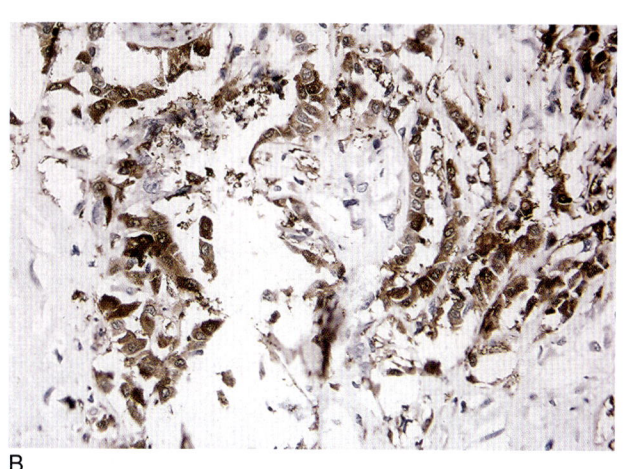

图16.37 间皮瘤。（A）管状的生长方式、立方形的肿瘤细胞，依据这些特点可以区分间皮瘤和浆液性癌，但在一些病例中两者的组织学结构会有重叠。（B）间皮瘤显示胞浆和胞核calretinin强阳性，如图所示；CK5/6染色胞浆阳性。浆液性癌这两种抗体均为阴性

输卵管和阔韧带

输卵管和阔韧带的肿瘤较卵巢肿瘤少见。多数发生于输卵管,其中上皮性肿瘤是最常见的。良性和交界性肿瘤罕见,多数输卵管肿瘤为癌。同一类型的癌发生于卵巢也可发生于输卵管。某些类型在卵巢相对常见,例如透明细胞癌和黏液性癌,在输卵管很少发生。最常见的输卵管癌的组织学类型是浆液性癌,子宫内膜样癌居第二位,再次是移行细胞癌和未分化癌。输卵管癌的免疫组织化学特征与卵巢肿瘤相似,已如前所述。在一个大的病例资料中,不同类型的癌所占的比例分别为:浆液性癌50%、子宫内膜样癌25%、移行细胞癌11%、未分化癌8%、混合型4%、透明细胞癌2%[421]。其他研究报道浆液性癌所占比例更高[422-424]。

有两种类型的肿瘤好发于输卵管和阔韧带,但罕见于卵巢,它们是腺瘤样瘤和午非管来源的女性附件肿瘤(FATWO)。

腺瘤样瘤

腺瘤样瘤是输卵管最常见的良性肿瘤[425],虽然也认为其起源于间皮下的间叶细胞,但是常认为其起源于间皮[426-428]。腺瘤样瘤体积小,直径常为1~2cm。镜下,嗜酸胞浆、立方形的细胞排列呈索状或小管状,或由扁平细胞被覆的腺样囊性裂隙。一些肿瘤细胞有明显的胞浆内空泡,这种细胞有时会与印戒细胞混淆。上皮样成分可能会出现浸润性生长,需要与腺癌进行鉴别。依据腺瘤样瘤的大体界限、温和的细胞形态、缺乏核分裂象这些特点能将其区别于恶性肿瘤。免疫组织化学研究表明腺瘤样瘤起源于间皮,CK、calretinin、CK5/6和WT-1阳性[429,430]。上皮性肿瘤的标记物,例如BerEP4、CEA和B72.3常为阴性,或多为弱阳性和局灶阳性[431]。在一项子宫腺瘤样瘤的研究中BerEP4多数为阳性[432],这与其他间皮瘤的报道和通常的经验有所不同。

女性午非源性(wolffian)的附件肿瘤

女性午非源性的附件肿瘤(FATWO)是源于阔韧带的明确肿瘤,与输卵管系膜相连,罕见于卵巢[433-435]。它可能源自中肾管残余,后者常见于该部位。大多数午非源性的附件肿瘤见于中年女性并且为良性。罕见的恶性肿瘤表现为核分裂活性或细胞异型性增强、高度增生的梭形细胞或淋巴脉管浸润或不可预料的转移。

FATWO为实性的直径2~20cm的肿瘤。它由单一多角形或梭形上皮样细胞组成,呈弥漫、梁状、管状、网状或微囊状排列。核均一深染,缺乏核分裂象和细胞异型性。主要的鉴别诊断是输卵管子宫内膜样癌变型[436,437]和性索-间质肿瘤如颗粒细胞瘤或Sertoli细胞瘤。其免疫表型与卵巢网相似,与上皮性肿瘤和性索-间质肿瘤有重叠[438]。FATWO为细胞角蛋白阳性,但多数为EMA阴性[438-440]。抑制素和calretinin常阳性[197,438]。FATWO为CD10阳性,显示胞浆着色,这有助于该肿瘤与其他肿瘤相鉴别[318]。

> **诊断要点:** 输卵管和阔韧带肿瘤
>
> 1. 输卵管和输卵管旁组织的上皮性肿瘤与卵巢肿瘤相似,且具有相似的免疫表型特征。
> 2. 没有用于鉴别原发性卵巢肿瘤和输卵管肿瘤的标记物。
> 3. 细胞角蛋白和calretinin染色有助于鉴别腺瘤样瘤。
> 4. FATWO免疫表型与上皮性和性索-间质肿瘤有重叠,但CD10胞浆阳性着色可有助于鉴别。

卵巢和输卵管肿瘤的临床和常规病理学检查具有预后意义。病理分期是最重要的预后因素。肿瘤分级和肿瘤类型也较重要,如上所述的免疫组织化学有助于卵巢肿瘤的准确分级和分类。在卵巢和输卵管癌中,尚未发现能为大众所接受的具有独立预后意义的免疫组织化学染色。

参考文献

1. Moll R, Levy R, Czernobilsky B, et al. Cytokeratins of normal epithelia and some neoplasms of the female genital tract. Lab Invest 1983; 49:599–610.
2. Puts JJ, Moesker O, Aldeweireldt J, et al. Application of antibodies to intermediate filament proteins in simple and complex tumors of the female genital tract. Int J Gynecol Pathol 1987; 6:257–274.
3. Bobrow LG, Makin CA, Law S, et al. Expression of low molecular weight cytokeratin proteins in cervical neoplasia. J Pathol 1986; 148:135–140.
4. Raju GC. Expression of the cytokeratin marker CAM5.2 in cervical neoplasia. Histopathology 1988; 12:437–443.

5. Esquius J, Brisigotti M, Matias-Guiu X, et al. Keratin expression in normal vulva, non-neoplastic epithelial disorders, vulvar intraepithelial neoplasia, and invasive squamous cell carcinoma. Int J Gynecol Pathol 1991; 10:341–355.

6. Smedts F, Ramaekers F, Leube RE, et al. Expression of keratins 1, 6, 15, 16, and 20 in normal cervical epithelium, squamous metaplasia, cervical intraepithelial neoplasia, and cervical carcinoma. Am J Pathol 1993; 142:403–412.

7. Malecha MJ, Miettinen M. Patterns of keratin subsets in normal and abnormal uterine cervical tissues. An immunohistochemical study. Int J Gynecol Pathol 1992; 11:24–29.

8. Gernow A, Nielsen B, Holund B, et al. Immunohistochemical study of possible changes in keratin expression during neoplastic transformation of the uterine mucosa. Virchows Arch A Pathol Anat Histopathol 1990; 416:287–293.

9. Cattoretti G, Becker MH, Key G, et al. Monoclonal antibodies against recombinant parts of the Ki-67 antigen (MIB 1 and MIB 3) detect proliferating cells in microwave-processed formalin-fixed paraffin sections. J Pathol 1992; 168:357–363.

10. Bravo R, Donald-Bravo H. Changes in the nuclear distribution of cyclin (PCNA) but not its synthesis depend on DNA replication. EMBO J 1985; 4:655–661.

11. Isacson C, Kessis TD, Hedrick L, et al. Both cell proliferation and apoptosis increase with lesion grade in cervical neoplasia but do not correlate with human papillomavirus type. Cancer Res 1996; 56:669–674.

12. van Hoeven KH, Kovatich AJ. Immunohistochemical staining for proliferating cell nuclear antigen, BCL2, and Ki-67 in vulvar tissues. Int J Gynecol Pathol 1996; 15:10–16.

13. Geng L, Connolly DC, Isacson C, et al. Atypical immature metaplasia (AIM) of the cervix: Is it related to high-grade squamous intraepithelial lesion (HSIL)? Hum Pathol 1999; 30:345–351.

14. Resnick M, Lester S, Tate JE, et al. Viral and histopathologic correlates of MN and MIB-1 expression in cervical intra-epithelial neoplasia. Hum Pathol 1996; 27:234–239.

15. Ince TA, Cviko AP, Quade BJ, et al. p63 coordinates anogenital modeling and epithelial cell differentiation in the developing female urogenital tract. Am J Pathol 2002; 161:1111–1117.

16. Quade BJ, Yang A, Wang Y, et al. Expression of the p53 homologue p63 in early cervical neoplasia. Gynecol Oncol 2001; 80:24–29.

17. Wang TY, Chen BF, Yang YC, et al. Histologic and immunophenotypic classification of cervical carcinomas by expression of the p53 homologue p63: A study of 250 cases. Hum Pathol 2001; 32:479–486.

18. Wang BY, Gil J, Kaufman D, et al. p63 in pulmonary epithelium, pulmonary squamous neoplasms, and other pulmonary tumors. Hum Pathol 2002; 33:921–926.

19. Wu M, Wang B, Gil J, et al. p63 and TTF-1 immunostaining. A useful marker panel for distinguishing small cell carcinoma of lung from poorly differentiated squamous cell carcinoma of lung. Am J Clin Pathol 2003; 119:696–702.

20. Amortegui AJ, Meyer MP, Elborne VL, et al. p53, retinoblastoma gene product, and cyclin protein expression in human papillomavirus virus DNA-positive cervical intraepithelial neoplasia and invasive cancer. Mod Pathol 1995; 8:907–912.

21. Xiong Y, Kuppuswamy D, Li Y, et al. Alteration of cell cycle kinase complexes in human papillomavirus E6- and E7-expressing fibroblasts precedes neoplastic transformation. J Virol 1996; 70:999–1008.

22. Keating JT, Cviko A, Riethdorf S, et al. Ki-67, cyclin E, and p16INK4 are complimentary surrogate biomarkers for human papilloma virus-related cervical neoplasia. Am J Surg Pathol 2001; 25:884–891.

23. Ishikawa M, Fujii T, Masumoto N, et al. Correlation of p16INK4A overexpression with human papillomavirus infection in cervical adenocarcinomas. Int J Gynecol Pathol 2003; 22:378–385.

24. Agoff SN, Lin P, Morihara J, et al. p16(INK4a) expression correlates with degree of cervical neoplasia: a comparison with Ki-67 expression and detection of high-risk HPV types. Mod Pathol 2003; 16:665–673.

25. Negri G, Egarter-Vigl E, Kasal A, et al. p16INK4a is a useful marker for the diagnosis of adenocarcinoma of the cervix uteri and its precursors: an immunohistochemical study with immunocytochemical correlations. Am J Surg Pathol 2003; 27:187–193.

26. Klaes R, Benner A, Friedrich T, et al. p16INK4a immunohistochemistry improves interobserver agreement in the diagnosis of cervical intraepithelial neoplasia. Am J Surg Pathol 2002; 26:1389–1399.

27. Riethdorf L, Riethdorf S, Lee KR, et al. Human papillomaviruses, expression of p16INK4A, and early endo-cer-

vical glandular neoplasia. Hum Pathol 2002; 33:899–904.

28. Tringler B, Gup CJ, Singh M, et al. Evaluation of p16INK4a and pRb expression in cervical squamous and glandular neoplasia. Hum Pathol 2004; 35:689–696.

29. Ansari-Lari MA, Staebler A, Zaino RJ, et al. Distinction of endocervical and endometrial adenocarcinomas: immunohistochemical p16 expression correlated with human papillomavirus (HPV) DNA detection. Am J Surg Pathol 2004; 28:160–167.

30. McCluggage WG, Jenkins D. p16 immunoreactivity may assist in the distinction between endometrial and endo-cervical adenocarcinoma. Int J Gynecol Pathol 2003; 22:231–235.

31. Albores-Saavedra J, Gersell D, Gilks CB, et al. Terminology of endocrine tumors of the uterine cervix: results of a workshop sponsored by the College of American Pathologists and the National Cancer Institute. Arch Pathol Lab Med 1997; 121:34–39.

32. Gilks CB, Young RH, Aguirre P, et al. Adenoma malignum (minimal deviation adenocarcinoma) of the uterine cervix: a clinicopathological and immunohistochemical analysis of 26 cases. Am J Surg Pathol 1989; 13:717–730.

33. Savargaonkar PR, Hale RJ, Mutton A, et al. Neuroendocrine differentiation in cervical carcinoma. J Clin Pathol 1996; 49:139–141.

34. Aguirre P, Scully RE, Wolfe HJ, et al. Endometrial carcinoma with argyrophil cells: a histochemical and immunohistochemical analysis. Hum Pathol 1984; 15:210–217.

35. Chu PG, Arber DA, Weiss LM. Expression of T/NK-cell and plasma cell antigens in nonhematopoietic epithelioid neoplasms. An immunohistochemical study of 447 cases. Am J Clin Pathol 2003; 120:64–70.

36. Viswanathan AN, Deavers MT, Jhingran A, et al. Small cell neuroendocrine carcinoma of the cervix: outcome and patterns of recurrence. Gynecol Oncol 2004; 93:27–33.

37. Battles OE, Page DL, Johnson JE. Cytokeratins, CEA, and mucin histochemistry in the diagnosis and characterization of extramammary Paget's disease. Am J Clin Pathol 1997; 108:6–12.

38. Smith KJ, Tuur S, Corvette D, et al. Cytokeratin 7 staining in mammary and extramammary Paget's disease. Mod Pathol 1997; 10:1069–1074.

39. Lundquist K, Kohler S, Rouse RV. Intraepidermal cytokeratin 7 expression is not restricted to Paget cells but is also seen in Toker cells and Merkel cells. Am J Surg Pathol 1999; 23:212–219.

40. Raju RR, Goldblum JR, Hart WR. Pagetoid squamous cell carcinoma in situ (pagetoid Bowen's disease) of the external genitalia. Int J Gynecol Pathol 2003; 22:127–135.

41. Goldblum JR, Hart WR. Vulvar Paget's disease: A clinicopathologic and immunohistochemical study of 19 cases. Am J Surg Pathol 1997; 21:1178–1187.

42. Goldblum JR, Hart WR. Perianal Paget's disease – A histologic and immunohistochemical study of 11 cases with and without associated rectal adenocarcinoma. Am J Surg Pathol 1998; 22:170–179.

43. Kohler S, Rouse RV, Smoller BR. The differential diagnosis of pagetoid cells in the epidermis. Mod Pathol 1998; 11:79–92.

44. Kadish AS, Burk RD, Kress Y, et al. Human papillomaviruses of different types in precancerous lesions of the uterine cervix: histologic, immunocytochemical and ultrastructural studies. Hum Pathol 1986; 17:384–392.

45. Scurry J, Beshay V, Cohen C, et al. Ki-67 expression in lichen sclerosus of vulva in patients with and without associated squamous cell carcinoma. Histopathology 1998; 32:399–404.

46. Pirog EC, Chen YT, Isacson C. MIB-1 immunostaining is a beneficial adjunct test for accurate diagnosis of vulvar condyloma acuminatum. Am J Surg Pathol 2000; 24:1393–1399.

47. Haefner HK, Tate JE, McLachlin CM, et al. Vulvar intraepithelial neoplasia: Age, morphological phenotype, papillomavirus DNA, and coexisting invasive carcinoma. Hum Pathol 1995; 26:147–154.

48. Yang B, Hart WR. Vulvar intraepithelial neoplasia of the simplex (differentiated) type – A clinicopathologic study including analysis of HPV and p53 expression. Am J Surg Pathol 2000; 24:429–441.

49. Abell MR. Intraepithelial carcinomas of epidermis and squamous mucosa of vulva and perineum. Surg Clin North Am 1965; 45:1179–1198.

50. Gosling JR, Abell MR, Drolette BM, et al. Infiltrative squamous cell (epidermoid) carcinoma of vulva. Cancer 1961; 14:330–343.

51. Santos M, Montagut C, Mellado B, et al. Immunohistochemical staining for p16 and p53 in premalignant and malignant epithelial lesions of the vulva. Int J Gynecol Pathol 2004; 23:

206–214.

52. Al-Saleh W, Delvenne P, Greimers R, et al. Assessment of Ki-67 antigen immunostaining in squamous intraepithelial lesions of the uterine cervix: Correlation with the histologic grade and human papillomavirus type. Am J Clin Pathol 1995; 104:154–160.

53. McCluggage WG, Buhidma M, Tang L, et al. Monoclonal antibody MIB1 in the assessment of cervical squamous intraepithelial lesions. Int J Gynecol Pathol 1996; 15:131–136.

54. Mittal K, Palazzo J. Cervical condylomas show higher proliferation than do inflamed or metaplastic cervical squamous epithelium. Mod Pathol 1998; 11:780–783.

55. Mittal K, Mesia A, Demopoulos RI. MIB-1 expression is useful in distinguishing dysplasia from atrophy in elderly women. Int J Gynecol Pathol 1999; 18:122–124.

56. McCluggage WG, Maxwell P, McBride HA, et al. Monoclonal antibodies Ki-67 and MIB1 in the distinction of tuboendometrial metaplasia from endocervical adeno-carcinoma and adenocarcinoma in situ in formalin-fixed material. Int J Gynecol Pathol 1995; 14:209–216.

57. van Hoeven KH, Ramondetta L, Kovatich AJ, et al. Quantitative image analysis of MIB-1 reactivity in inflammatory, hyperplastic, and neoplastic endocervical lesions. Int J Gynecol Pathol 1997; 16:15–21.

58. Pirog EC, Kleter B, Olgac S, et al. Prevalence of human papillomavirus DNA in different histological subtypes of cervical adenocarcinoma. Am J Pathol 2000; 157:1055–1062.

59. Mikami Y, Kiyokawa T, Hata S, et al. Gastrointestinal immunophenotype in adenocarcinomas of the uterine cervix and related glandular lesions: a possible link between lobular endocervical glandular hyperplasia/pyloric gland metaplasia and 'adenoma malignum'. Mod Pathol 2004; 17:962–972.

60. Pirog EC, Baergen RN, Soslow RA, et al. Diagnostic accuracy of cervical low-grade squamous intraepithelial lesions is improved with MIB-1 immunostaining. Am J Surg Pathol 2002; 26:70–75.

61. van Hoeven KH, Kovatich AJ, Oliver RE, et al. Protocol for immunocytochemical detection of SIL in cervical smears using MIB-1 antibody to Ki-67 [corrected]. Mod Pathol 1996; 9:407–412.

62. Dabbs DJ, Abendroth CS, Grenko RT, et al. Immunocytochemistry on the Thinprep processor. Diagn Cytopathol 1997; 17:388–392.

63. Saqi A, Pasha TL, McGrath CM, et al. Overexpression of p16INK4A in liquid-based specimens (SurePath) as marker of cervical dysplasia and neoplasia. Diagn Cytopathol 2002; 27:365–370.

64. Nieh S, Chen SF, Chu TY, et al. Expression of p16 INK4A in Papanicolaou smears containing atypical squamous cells of undetermined significance from the uterine cervix. Gynecol Oncol 2003; 91:201–208.

65. Yoshida T, Fukuda T, Sano T, et al. Usefulness of liquid-based cytology specimens for the immunocytochemical study of p16 expression and human papillomavirus testing: a comparative study using simultaneously sampled histology materials. Cancer 2004; 102:100–108.

66. Nieh S, Chen SF, Chu TY, et al. Expression of p16INK4A in Pap smears containing atypical glandular cells from the uterine cervix. Acta Cytol 2004; 48:173–180.

67. Speers WC, Picaso LG, Silverberg SG. Immunohistochemical localization of carcinoembryonic antigen in microglandular hyperplasia and adenocarcinoma of the endocervix. Am J Clin Pathol 1983; 79:105–107.

68. Michael H, Grawe L, Kraus FT. Minimal deviation endocervical adenocarcinoma: clinical and histologic features, immunohistochemical staining for carcinoembryonic antigen, and differentiation from confusing benign lesions. Int J Gynecol Pathol 1984; 3:261–276.

69. Cina SJ, Richardson MS, Austin RM, et al. Immunohistochemical staining for Ki-67 antigen, carcinoembryonic antigen, and p53 in the differential diagnosis of glandular lesions of the cervix. Mod Pathol 1997; 10:176–180.

70. Dabbs DJ, Geisinger KR, Norris HT. Intermediate filaments in endometrial and endocervical carcinomas. The diagnostic utility of vimentin patterns. Am J Surg Pathol 1986; 10:568–576.

71. Kudo R, Sasano H, Koizumi M, et al. Immunohistochemical comparison of new monoclonal antibody 1C5 and carcinoembryonic antigen in the differential diagnosis of adenocarcinoma of the uterine cervix. Int J Gynecol Pathol 1990; 9:325–336.

72. Maes G, Fleuren GJ, Bara J, et al. The distribution of mucins, carcinoembryonic antigen, and mucus-associated antigens in endocervical and endometrial adenocarcinomas. Int J Gynecol Pathol 1988; 7:112–122.

73. Dabbs DJ, Sturtz K, Zaino RJ. The immunohistochemical discrimination of endometrioid adenocarcinomas. Hum Pathol 1996; 27:172–177.

74. Dabbs DJ, Gesinger KR, Norris HT. Intermediate filaments in endometrial and endocervical adenocarcinomas. The diagnostic utility of vimentin patterns. Am J Surg Pathol 1986; 10:568–576.

75. Staebler A, Sherman ME, Zaino RJ, et al. Hormone receptor immunohistochemistry and human papillomavirus in situ hybridization are useful for distinguishing endocervical and endometrial adenocarcinomas. Am J Surg Pathol 2002; 26: 998–1006.

76. Qiu W, Mittal K. Comparison of morphologic and immunohistochemical features of cervical microglandular hyperplasia with low-grade mucinous adenocarcinoma of the endometrium. Int J Gynecol Pathol 2003; 22:261–265.

77. Zaloudek C, Hayashi GM, Ryan IP, et al. Microglandular adenocarcinoma of the endometrium: a form of mucinous adenocarcinoma that may be confused with microglandular hyperplasia of the cervix. Int J Gynecol Pathol 1997; 16:52–59.

78. Vang R, Barner R, Wheeler DT, et al. Immunohistochemical staining for Ki-67 and p53 helps distinguish endo-metrial Arias-Stella reaction from high-grade carcinoma, including clear cell carcinoma. Int J Gynecol Pathol 2004; 23:223–233.

79. Gilks CB, Young RH, Gersell DJ, et al. Large cell neuroendocrine carcinoma of the uterine cervix: a clinicopathologic study of 12 cases. Am J Surg Pathol 1997; 21:905–914.

80. Ambros RA, Park JS, Shah KV, et al. Evaluation of histologic, morphometric, and immunohistochemical criteria in the differential diagnosis of small cell carcinomas of the cervix with particular reference to human papillomavirus types 16 and 18. Mod Pathol 1991; 4:586–593.

81. Masumoto N, Fujii T, Ishikawa M, et al. P16 overexpression and human papillomavirus infection in small cell carcinoma of the uterine cervix. Hum Pathol 2003; 34:778–783.

82. Farhood AI, Abrams J. Immunohistochemistry of endometrial stromal sarcoma. Hum Pathol 1991; 22:224–230.

83. Franquemont DW, Frierson HF Jr, Mills SE. An immunohistochemical study of normal endometrial stroma and endometrial stromal neoplasms. Evidence for smooth muscle differentiation. Am J Surg Pathol 1991; 15:861–870.

84. Oliva E, Young RH, Clement PB, et al. Cellular benign mesenchymal tumors of the uterus: A comparative morphologic and immunohistochemical analysis of 33 highly cellular leiomyomas and six endometrial stromal nodules, two frequently confused tumors. Am J Surg Pathol 1995; 19:757–768.

85. Sherman ME, Bur ME, Kurman RJ. p53 in endometrial cancer and its putative precursors: Evidence for diverse pathways of tumorigenesis. Hum Pathol 1995; 26:1268–1274.

86. Tashiro H, Isacson C, Levine R, et al. p53 gene mutations are common in uterine serous carcinoma and occur early in their pathogenesis. Am J Pathol 1997; 150:177–185.

87. Zheng W, Khurana R, Farahmand S, et al. p53 immuno-staining as a significant adjunct diagnostic method for uterine surface carcinoma: precursor of uterine papillary serous carcinoma. Am J Surg Pathol 1998; 22:1463–1473.

88. Lax SF, Pizer ES, Ronnett BM, et al. Comparison of estrogen and progesterone receptor, Ki-67, and p53 immuno-reactivity in uterine endometrioid carcinoma and endometrioid carcinoma with squamous, mucinous, secretory, and ciliated cell differentiation. Hum Pathol 1998; 29:924–931.

89. Lax SF, Kendall B, Tashiro H, et al. The frequency of p53, K-ras mutations, and microsatellite instability differs in uterine endometrioid and serous carcinoma – Evidence of distinct molecular genetic pathways. Cancer 2000; 88:814–824.

90. Kohler MF, Nishii H, Humphrey PA, et al. Mutation of the p53 tumor-suppressor gene is not a feature of endometrial hyperplasias. Am J Obstet Gynecol 1993; 169:690–694.

91. Yu CC, Wilkinson N, Brito MJ, et al. Patterns of immunohistochemical staining for proliferating cell nuclear antigen and p53 in benign and neoplastic human endometrium. Histopathology 1993; 23:367–371.

92. Soslow RA, Shen PU, Chung MH, et al. Distinctive p53 and mdm2 immunohistochemical expression profiles suggest different pathogenetic pathways in poorly differentiated endometrial carcinoma. Int J Gynecol Pathol 1998; 17:129–134.

93. Lax SF, Pizer ES, Ronnett BM, et al. Clear cell carcinoma of the endometrium is characterized by a distinctive profile of p53, Ki-67, estrogen, and progesterone receptor expression. Hum Pathol 1998; 29:551–558.

94. Soslow RA, Shen PU, Chung MH, et al. Cyclin D1 expression in high-grade endometrial carcinomas – association with histologic subtype. Int J Gynecol Pathol 2000; 19:329–334.

95. Chambers JT, Carcangiu ML, Voynick IM, et al. Immuno-

histochemical evaluation of estrogen and progesterone receptor content in 183 patients with endometrial carcinoma. Part II: Correlation between biochemical and immunohistochemical methods and survival. Am J Clin Pathol 1990; 94:255–260.

96. Carcangiu ML, Chambers JT, Voynick IM, et al. Immunohistochemical evaluation of estrogen and progesterone receptor content in 183 patients with endometrial carcinoma. Part I: Clinical and histologic correlations. Am J Clin Pathol 1990; 94:247–254.

97. Nei H, Saito T, Yamasaki H, et al. Nuclear localization of beta-catenin in normal and carcinogenic endometrium. Mol Carcinog 1999; 25:207–218.

98. Schlosshauer PW, Ellenson LH, Soslow RA. Beta-catenin and E-cadherin expression patterns in high-grade endometrial carcinoma are associated with histological subtype. Mod Pathol 2002; 15:1032–1037.

99. Obata K, Morland SJ, Watson RH, et al. Frequent PTEN/MMAC mutations in endometrioid but not serous or mucinous epithelial ovarian tumors. Cancer Res 1998; 58:2095–2097.

100. Risinger JI, Hayes AK, Berchuck A, et al. PTEN/MMAC1 mutations in endometrial cancers. Cancer Res 1997; 57:4736–4738.

101. Simpkins SB, Peiffer-Schneider S, Mutch DG, et al. PTEN mutations in endometrial cancers with 10q LOH: additional evidence for the involvement of multiple tumor suppressors. Gynecol Oncol 1998; 71:391–395.

102. Tashiro H, Blazes MS, Wu R, et al. Mutations in PTEN are frequent in endometrial carcinoma but rare in other common gynecological malignancies. Cancer Res 1997; 57:3935–3940.

103. Yokoyama Y, Wan X, Shinohara A, et al. Expression of PTEN and PTEN pseudogene in endometrial carcinoma. Int J Mol Med 2000; 6:47–50.

104. Darvishian F, Hummer AJ, Thaler HT, et al. Serous endometrial cancers that mimic endometrioid adenocarcinomas: a clinicopathologic and immunohistochemical study of a group of problematic cases. Am J Surg Pathol 2004; 28:1568–1578.

105. Fukuchi T, Sakamoto M, Tsuda H, et al. Beta-catenin mutation in carcinoma of the uterine endometrium. Cancer Res 1998; 58:3526–3528.

106. Saegusa M, Hamano M, Kuwata T, et al. Up-regulation and nuclear localization of beta-catenin in endometrial carcinoma in response to progesterone therapy. Cancer Sci 2003; 94:103–111.

107. Oliva E, Clement PB, Young RH, et al. Mixed endometrial stromal and smooth muscle tumors of the uterus – A clinicopathologic study of 15 cases. Am J Surg Pathol 1998; 22:997–1005.

108. Oliva E, Young RH, Clement PB, et al. Myxoid and fibrous endometrial stromal tumors of the uterus: a report of 10 cases. Int J Gynecol Pathol 1999; 18:310–319.

109. Baker RJ, Hildebrandt RH, Rouse RV, et al. Inhibin and CD99 (MIC2) expression in uterine stromal neoplasms with sex-cord-like elements. Hum Pathol 1999; 30:671–679.

110. Rizeq MN, Van de Rijn M, Hendrickson MR, et al. A comparative immunohistochemical study of uterine smooth muscle neoplasms with emphasis on the epithelioid variant. Hum Pathol 1994; 25:671–677.

111. Meis JM, Lawrence WD. The immunohistochemical profile of malignant mixed mullerian tumor. Overlap with endometrial adenocarcinoma. Am J Clin Pathol 1990; 94:1–7.

112. Nucci MR, O'Connell JT, Huettner PC, et al. h-Caldesmon expression effectively distinguishes endometrial stromal tumors from uterine smooth muscle tumors. Am J Surg Pathol 2001; 25:455–463.

113. Rush DS, Tan JY, Baergen RN, et al. h-caldesmon, a novel smooth muscle-specific antibody, distinguishes between cellular leiomyoma and endometrial stromal sarcoma. Am J Surg Pathol 2001; 25:253–258.

114. Loddenkemper C, Mechsner S, Foss HD, et al. Use of oxytocin receptor expression in distinguishing between uterine smooth muscle tumors and endometrial stromal sarcoma. Am J Surg Pathol 2003; 27:1458–1462.

115. Chu PG, Arber DA, Weiss LM, et al. Utility of CD10 in distinguishing between endometrial stromal sarcoma and uterine smooth muscle tumors: an immunohistochemical comparison of 34 cases. Mod Pathol 2001; 14:465–471.

116. Oliva E, Young RH, Amin MB, et al. An immunohistochemical analysis of endometrial stromal and smooth muscle tumors of the uterus – A study of 54 cases emphasizing the importance of using a panel because of overlap in immunoreactivity for individual antibodies. Am J Surg Pathol 2002; 26:403–412.

117. McCluggage WG, Sumathi VP, Maxwell P. CD10 is a sensi-

tive and diagnostically useful immunohistochemical marker of normal endometrial stroma and of endometrial stromal neoplasms. Histopathology 2001; 39:273–278.

118. Agoff SN, Grieco VS, Garcia R, et al. Immunohistochemical distinction of endometrial stromal sarcoma and cellular leiomyoma. Appl Immunohistochem Mol Morphol 2001; 9: 164–169.

119. Sumathi VP, Al-Hussaini M, Connolly LE, et al. Endometrial stromal neoplasms are immunoreactive with WT-1 antibody. Int J Gynecol Pathol 2004; 23:241–247.

120. Srodon M, Klein WM, Kurman RJ. CD10 immunostaining does not distinguish endometrial carcinoma invading myometrium from carcinoma involving adenomyosis. Am J Surg Pathol 2003; 27:786–789.

121. Nascimento AF, Hirsch MS, Cviko A, et al. The role of CD10 staining in distinguishing invasive endometrial adeno-carcinoma from adenocarcinoma involving adenomyosis. Mod Pathol 2003; 16:22–27.

122. Carcangiu ML, Chambers JT. Uterine papillary serous carcinoma: a study on 108 cases with emphasis on the prognostic significance of associated endometrioid carcinoma, absence of invasion, and concomitant ovarian carcinoma. Gynecol Oncol 1992; 47:298–305.

123. Sherman ME, Bitterman P, Rosenshein NB, et al. Uterine serous carcinoma: A morphologically diverse neoplasm with unifying clinicopathologic features. Am J Surg Pathol 1992; 16:600–610.

124. Yilmaz A, Rush DS, Soslow RA. Endometrial stromal sarcomas with unusual histologic features: a report of 24 primary and metastatic tumors emphasizing fibroblastic and smooth muscle differentiation. Am J Surg Pathol 2002; 26:1142–1150.

125. Clement PB, Scully RE. Uterine tumors resembling ovarian sex-cord tumors. A clinicopathologic analysis of 14 cases. Am J Clin Pathol 1976; 66:512–525.

126. Clement PB, Scully RE. Endometrial stromal sarcomas of the uterus with extensive glandular differentiation: a report of three cases that caused problems in differential diagnosis. Int J Gynecol Pathol 1992; 11:163–173.

127. Bhargava R, Shia J, Hummer AJ, et al. Distinction of endometrial stromal sarcomas from 'hemangiopericytomatous' tumors using a panel of immunohistochemical stains. Mod Pathol 2005;18:40–47.

128. Zhai YL, Kobayashi Y, Mori A, et al. Expression of steroid receptors, Ki-67, and p53 in uterine leiomyosarcomas. Int J Gynecol Pathol 1999; 18:20–28.

129. Nordal RR, Kristensen GB, Stenwig AE, et al. Immuno-histochemical analysis of p53 protein in uterine sarcomas. Gynecol Oncol 1998; 70:45–48.

130. Blom R, Guerrieri C, Stal O, et al. Leiomyosarcoma of the uterus: A clinicopathologic, DNA flow cytometric, p53, and mdm-2 analysis of 49 cases. Gynecol Oncol 1998; 68:54–61.

131. Leitao MM, Soslow RA, Nonaka D, et al. Tissue microarray immunohistochemical expression of estrogen, progesterone, and androgen receptors in uterine leiomyomata and leiomyosarcoma. Cancer 2004; 101:1455–1462.

132. Vang R, Kempson RL. Perivascular epithelioid cell tumor ('PEComa') of the uterus: a subset of HMB-45-positive epithelioid mesenchymal neoplasms with an uncertain relationship to pure smooth muscle tumors. Am J Surg Pathol 2002; 26:1–13.

133. Silva EG, Deavers MT, Bodurka DC, et al. Uterine epithelioid leiomyosarcomas with clear cells: reactivity with HMB-45 and the concept of PEComa. Am J Surg Pathol 2004; 28: 244–249.

134. Klein WM, Kurman RJ. Lack of expression of c-kit protein (CD117) in mesenchymal tumors of the uterus and ovary. Int J Gynecol Pathol 2003; 22:181–184.

135. Winter WE III, Seidman JD, Krivak TC, et al. Clinicopathological analysis of c-kit expression in carcinosarcomas and leiomyosarcomas of the uterine corpus. Gynecol Oncol 2003; 91:3–8.

136. Wang L, Felix JC, Lee JL, et al. The proto-oncogene c-kit is expressed in leiomyosarcomas of the uterus. Gynecol Oncol 2003; 90:402–406.

137. Rushing RS, Shajahan S, Chendil D, et al. Uterine sarcomas express KIT protein but lack mutation(s) in exon 11 or 17 of c-KIT. Gynecol Oncol 2003; 91:9–14.

138. Ito K, Watanabe K, Nasim S, et al. Prognostic significance of p53 overexpression in endometrial cancer. Cancer Res 1994; 54:4667–4670.

139. Sung CJ, Zheng Y, Quddus MR, et al. p53 as a significant prognostic marker in endometrial carcinoma. Int J Gynecol Cancer 2000; 10:119–127.

140. Alkushi A, Lim P, Coldman A, et al. Interpretation of p53 immunoreactivity in endometrial carcinoma: establishing a clinically relevant cut-off level. Int J Gynecol Pathol 2004;

23:129–137.

141. Dupont J, Wang X, Marshall DS, et al. Wilms' tumor gene (WT1) and p53 expression in endometrial carcinomas: a study of 130 cases using a tissue microarray. Gynecol Oncol 2004; 94:449–455.

142. Daya D, Sabet L. The use of cytokeratin as a sensitive and reliable marker for trophoblastic tissue. Am J Clin Pathol 1991; 95:137–141.

143. Kurman RJ, Young RH, Norris HJ, et al. Immunocytochemical localization of placental lactogen and chorionic gonadotropin in the normal placenta and trophoblastic tumors, with emphasis on intermediate trophoblast and the placental site trophoblastic tumor. Int J Gynecol Pathol 1984; 3:101–121.

144. Huettner PC, Gersell DJ. Placental site nodule: a clinicopathologic study of 38 cases. Int J Gynecol Pathol 1994; 13:191–198.

145. Yeh IT, O'Connor DM, Kurman RJ. Vacuolated cytotrophoblast: a subpopulation of trophoblast in the chorion laeve. Placenta 1989; 10:429–438.

146. Shih IM, Kurman RJ. Expression of melanoma cell adhesion molecule in intermediate trophoblast. Lab Invest 1996; 75: 377–388.

147. Shih IM, Kurman RJ. p63 expression is useful in the distinction of epithelioid trophoblastic and placental site trophoblastic tumors by profiling trophoblastic subpopulations. Am J Surg Pathol 2004; 28:1177–1183.

148. Fukunaga M. Immunohistochemical characterization of p57 (KIP2) expression in early hydatidiform moles. Hum Pathol 2002; 33:1188–1192.

149. Fisher RA, Hodges MD, Rees HC, et al. The mater-nally transcribed gene p57 (KIP2) (CDNK1C) is abnor-mally expressed in both androgenetic and biparental complete hydatidiform moles. Hum Mol Genet 2002; 11:3267–3272.

150. Genest DR, Dorfman DM, Castrillon DH. Ploidy and imprinting in hydatidiform moles. Complementary use of flow cytometry and immunohistochemistry of the imprinted gene product p57KIP2 to assist molar classification. J Reprod Med 2002; 47:342–346.

151. Castrillon DH, Sun DQ, Weremowicz S, et al. Discrimination of complete hydatidiform mole from its mimics by immunohistochemistry of the paternally imprinted gene product p57KIP2. Am J Surg Pathol 2001; 25:1225–1230.

152. Shih IM, Seidman JD, Kurman RJ. Placental site nodule and characterization of distinctive types of intermediate trophoblast. Hum Pathol 1999; 30:687–694.

153. Shih IM, Kurman RJ. Ki-67 labeling index in the differential diagnosis of exaggerated placental site, placental site trophoblastic tumor, and choriocarcinoma: A double immunohistochemical staining technique using Ki-67 and Mel-CAM antibodies. Hum Pathol 1998; 29:27–33.

154. Angel E, Davis JR, Nagle RB. Immunohistochemical demonstration of placental hormones in the diagnosis of uterine versus ectopic pregnancy. Am J Clin Pathol 1985; 84:705–709.

155. Hameed A, Miller DS, Muller CY, et al. Frequent expression of beta-human chorionic gonadotropin (beta-hCG) in squamous cell carcinoma of the cervix. Int J Gynecol Pathol 1999; 18:381–386.

156. Bacchi CE, Coelho KI, Goldberg J. Expression of beta-human chorionic gonadotropin (beta-hCG) in non-trophoblastic elements of transitional cell carcinoma of the bladder: possible relationship with the prognosis. Rev Paul Med 1993; 111:412–416.

157. Tavassoli FA. Pathology and genetics of tumours of the breast and female genital organs. Lyon: IARC Press; 2003.

158. Moll R, Franke WW, Schiller DL, et al. The catalog of human cytokeratins: patterns of expression in normal epithelia, tumors and cultured cells. Cell 1982; 31:11–24.

159. Berezowski K, Stastny JF, Kornstein MJ. Cytokeratins 7 and 20 and carcinoembryonic antigen in ovarian and colonic carcinoma. Mod Pathol 1996; 9:426–429.

160. Lagendijk JH, Mullink H, Van Diest PJ, et al. Immunohistochemical differentiation between primary adenocarcinomas of the ovary and ovarian metastases of colonic and breast origin. Comparison between a statistical and an intuitive approach. J Clin Pathol 1999; 52:283–290.

161. Cathro HP, Stoler MH. Expression of cytokeratins 7 and 20 in ovarian neoplasia. Am J Clin Pathol 2002; 117:944–951.

162. Wang NP, Zee S, Zarbo RJ, et al. Coordinate expression of cytokeratins 7 and 20 defines unique subsets of carcinomas. Appl Immunohistochem 1995; 3:99–107.

163. Chu P, Wu E, Weiss LM. Cytokeratin 7 and cytokeratin 20 expression in epithelial neoplasms: a survey of 435 cases. Mod Pathol 2000; 13:962–972.

164. Raspollini MR, Amunni G, Villanucci A, et al. Utility of CDX-2 in distinguishing between primary and secondary (intestinal)

164. ...mucinous ovarian carcinoma: an immunohistochemical comparison of 43 cases. Appl Immunohistochem Mol Morphol 2004; 12:127–131.

165. Moll R, Lowe A, Laufer J, et al. Cytokeratin 20 in human carcinomas. A new histodiagnostic marker detected by monoclonal antibodies. Am J Pathol 1992; 140:427–447.

166. Miettinen M. Keratin 20: immunohistochemical marker for gastrointestinal, urothelial, and Merkel cell carcinomas. Mod Pathol 1995; 8:384–388.

167. Wauters CCAP, Smedts F, Gerrits LGM, et al. Keratins 7 and 20 as diagnostic markers of carcinomas metastatic to the ovary. Hum Pathol 1995; 26:852–855.

168. Loy TS, Calaluce RD, Keeney GL. Cytokeratin immunostaining in differentiating primary ovarian carcinoma from metastatic colonic adenocarcinoma. Mod Pathol 1996; 9:1040–1044.

169. Ji H, Isacson C, Seidman JD, et al. Cytokeratins 7 and 20, Dpc4, and MUC5AC in the distinction of metastatic mucinous carcinomas in the ovary from primary ovarian mucinous tumors: Dpc4 assists in identifying metastatic pancreatic carcinomas. Int J Gynecol Pathol 2002; 21:391–400.

170. Ordonez NG. Role of immunohistochemistry in distinguishing epithelial peritoneal mesotheliomas from peritoneal and ovarian serous carcinomas. Am J Surg Pathol 1998; 22:1203–1214.

171. Ramalingam P, Malpica A, Silva EG, et al. The use of cytokeratin 7 and EMA in differentiating ovarian yolk sac tumors from endometrioid and clear cell carcinomas. Am J Surg Pathol 2004; 28:1499–1505.

172. Attanoos RL, Webb R, Dojcinov SD, et al. Value of mesothelial and epithelial antibodies in distinguishing diffuse peritoneal mesothelioma in females from serous papillary carcinoma of the ovary and peritoneum. Histopathology 2002; 40:237–244.

173. Charpin C, Bhan AK, Zurawski VRJ, et al. Carcinoembryonic antigen (CEA) and carbohydrate determinant 19-9 (CA 19-9) localization in 121 primary and metastatic ovarian tumors: an immunohistochemical study with the use of monoclonal antibodies. Int J Gynecol Pathol 1982; 1:231–245.

174. Brown RW, Campagna LB, Dunn JK, et al. Immunohistochemical identification of tumor markers in metastatic adenocarcinoma. A diagnostic adjunct in the determination of primary site. Am J Clin Pathol 1997; 107:12–19.

175. Lagendijk JH, Mullink H, Van Diest PJ, et al. Tracing the origin of adenocarcinomas with unknown primary using immunohistochemistry: Differential diagnosis between colonic and ovarian carcinomas as primary sites. Hum Pathol 1998; 29:491–497.

176. Ulfig N. Calcium-binding proteins in the human developing brain. Adv Anat Embryol Cell Biol 2002; 165:III–IX; 1–92.

177. Chou YY, Jeng YM, Kao HL, et al. Differentiation of ovarian mucinous carcinoma and metastatic colorectal adenocarcinoma by immunostaining with beta-catenin. Histopathology 2003; 43:151–156.

178. Goldstein NS, Bassi D, Uzieblo A. WT1 is an integral component of an antibody panel to distinguish pancreatico-biliary and some ovarian epithelial neoplasms. Am J Clin Pathol 2001; 116:246–252.

179. Multhaupt HA, Arenas-Elliott CP, Warhol MJ. Comparison of glycoprotein expression between ovarian and colon adenocarcinomas. Arch Pathol Lab Med 1999; 123:909–916.

180. Thor A, Gorstein F, Ohuchi N, et al. Tumor-associated glycoprotein (TAG-72) in ovarian carcinomas defined by monoclonal antibody B72.3. J Natl Cancer Inst 1986; 76:995–1006.

181. Bollinger DJ, Wick MR, Dehner LP, et al. Peritoneal malignant mesothelioma versus serous papillary adenocarcinoma. A histochemical and immunohistochemical comparison. Am J Surg Pathol 1989; 13:659–670.

182. O'Brien TJ, Beard JB, Underwood LJ, et al. The CA 125 gene: An extracellular superstructure dominated by repeat sequences. Tumor Biol 2001; 22:348–366.

183. O'Brien TJ, Beard JB, Underwood LJ, et al. The CA 125 gene: A newly discovered extension of the glycosylated N-terminal domain doubles the size of this extracellular superstructure. Tumor Biol 2002; 23:154–169.

184. Bast RC Jr, Xu FJ, Yu YH, et al. CA 125: the past and the future. Int J Biol Markers 1998; 13:179–187.

185. Loy TS, Quesenberry JT, Sharp SC. Distribution of CA 125 in adenocarcinomas: An immunohistochemical study of 481 cases. Am J Clin Pathol 1992; 98:175–179.

186. Koelma IA, Nap M, Rodenburg CJ, et al. The value of tumour marker CA 125 in surgical pathology. Histopathology 1987; 11:287–294.

187. Keen CE, Szakacs S, Okon E, et al. CA 125 and thyro-globulin staining in papillary carcinomas of thyroid and ovarian origin is not completely specific for site of origin. Histopa-

thology 1999; 34:113–117.
188. Nap M, Vitali A, Nustad K, et al. Immunohistochemical characterization of 22 monoclonal antibodies against the CA 125 antigen: 2nd report from the ISOBM TD-1 workshop. Tumor Biol 1996; 17:325–331.
189. Leake J, Woolas RP, Daniel J, et al. Immunocytochemical and serological expression of CA 125: A clinicopathological study of 40 malignant ovarian epithelial tumours. Histopathology 1994; 24:57–64.
190. Zheng W, Senturk BZ, Parkash V. Inhibin immunohistochemical staining: a practical approach for the surgical pathologist in the diagnoses of ovarian sex cord-stromal tumors. Adv Anat Pathol 2003; 10:27–38.
191. Rivier C, Meunier H, Roberts V, et al. Inhibin: role and secretion in the rat. Recent Prog Horm Res 1990; 46:231–257.
192. Vale W, Rivier C, Hsueh A, et al. Chemical and biological characterization of the inhibin family of protein hormones. Recent Prog Horm Res 1988; 44:1–34.
193. Welt CK. The physiology and pathophysiology of inhibin, activin and follistatin in female reproduction. Curr Opin Obstet Gynecol 2002; 14:317–323.
194. Rishi M, Howard LN, Bratthauer GL, et al. Use of monoclonal antibody against human inhibin as a marker for sex cord-stromal tumors of the ovary. Am J Surg Pathol 1997; 21:583–589.
195. Costa MJ, Ames PF, Walls J, et al. Inhibin immunohistochemistry applied to ovarian neoplasms: A novel, effective, diagnostic tool. Hum Pathol 1997; 28:1247–1254.
196. Hildebrandt RH, Rouse RV, Longacre TA. Value of inhibin in the identification of granulosa cell tumors of the ovary. Hum Pathol 1997; 28:1387–1395.
197. Kommoss F, Oliva E, Bhan AK, et al. Inhibin expression in ovarian tumors and tumor-like lesions: an immunohistochemical study. Mod Pathol 1998; 11:656–664.
198. McCluggage WG. Value of inhibin staining in gynecological pathology. Int J Gynecol Pathol 2001; 20:79–85.
199. Deavers MT, Malpica A, Liu J, et al. Ovarian sex cord-stromal tumors: an immunohistochemical study including a comparison of calretinin and inhibin. Mod Pathol 2003; 16:584–590.
200. Pelkey TJ, Frierson HFJ, Mills SE, et al. The diagnostic utility of inhibin staining in ovarian neoplasms. Int J Gynecol Pathol 1998; 17:97–105.
201. Matias-Guiu X, Pons C, Prat J. Mullerian inhibiting substance, alpha-inhibin, and CD99 expression in sex cord-stromal tumors and endometrioid ovarian carcinomas resembling sex cord-stromal tumors. Hum Pathol 1998; 29:840–845.
202. Yao DX, Soslow RA, Hedvat CV, et al. Melan-A (A103) and inhibin expression in ovarian neoplasms. Appl Immunohistochem Mol Morphol 2003; 11:244–249.
203. McCluggage WG, Burton J, Maxwell P, et al. Immunohistochemical staining of normal, hyperplastic, and neoplastic adrenal cortex with a monoclonal antibody against alpha inhibin. J Clin Pathol 1998; 51:114–116.
204. Pelkey TJ, Frierson HFJ, Mills SE, et al. The alpha subunit of inhibin in adrenal cortical neoplasia. Mod Pathol 1998; 11:516–524.
205. Chivite A, MatiasGuiu X, Pons C, et al. Inhibin A expression in adrenal neoplasms – A new immunohistochemical marker for adrenocortical tumors. Appl Immunohistochem Mol Morphol 1998; 6:42–49.
206. Cho EY, Ahn GH. Immunoexpression of inhibin alpha-subunit in adrenal neoplasms. Appl Immunohistochem Mol Morphol 2001; 9:222–228.
207. Jorda M, De MB, Nadji M. Calretinin and inhibin are useful in separating adrenocortical neoplasms from pheochromocytomas. Appl Immunohistochem Mol Morphol 2002; 10:67–70.
208. Zhang PJ, Genega EM, Tomaszewski JE, et al. The role of calretinin, inhibin, melan-A, BCL-2, and C-kit in differentiating adrenal cortical and medullary tumors: an immunohistochemical study. Mod Pathol 2003; 16:591–597.
209. Rogers JH. Calretinin: a gene for a novel calcium-binding protein expressed principally in neurons. J Cell Biol 1987; 105:1343–1353.
210. Tos AP, Doglioni C. Calretinin: a novel tool for diagnostic immunohistochemistry. Adv Anat Pathol 1998; 5:61–66.
211. Rogers J, Khan M, Ellis J. Calretinin and other CaBPs in the nervous system. Adv Exp Med Biol 1990; 269:195–203.
212. Cao QJ, Jones JG, Li M. Expression of calretinin in human ovary, testis, and ovarian sex cord-stromal tumors. Int J Gynecol Pathol 2001; 20:346–352.
213. McCluggage WG, Maxwell P. Immunohistochemical staining for calretinin is useful in the diagnosis of ovarian sex cord-stromal tumours. Histopathology 2001; 38:403–408.
214. Movahedi-Lankarani S, Kurman RJ. Calretinin, a more sen-

215. Lee SB, Haber DA. Wilms tumor and the WT1 gene. Exp Cell Res 2001; 264:74–99.
216. Mrir TE, Cheville X, Layer DJ. Metanephric adenoma, nephrogeric rests, and Wilms' tumor – A histologic and immunophenotypic comparison. Am J Surg Pathol 2001; 25: 1290–1296.
217. Ordonez NG. Desmoplastic small round cell tumor II: An ultrastructural and immunohistochemical study with emphasis on new immunohistochemical markers. Am J Surg Pathol 1998; 22:1314–1327.
218. Hill DA, Pfeifer JD, Marley EF, et al. WT1 staining reliably differentiates desmoplastic small round cell tumor from Ewing sarcoma/primitive neuroectodermal tumor – An immunohistochemical and molecular diagnostic study. Am J Clin Pathol 2000; 114:345–353.
219. Lae ME, Roche PC, Jin L, et al. Desmoplastic small round cell tumor – A clinicopathologic, immunohistochemical, and molecular study of 32 tumors. Am J Surg Pathol 2002; 26: 823–835.
220. Hwang H, Quenneville L, Yaziji H, et al. Wilms tumor gene product: sensitive and contextually specific marker of serous carcinomas of ovarian surface epithelial origin. Appl Immunohistochem Mol Morphol 2004; 12:122–126.
221. Ordonez NG. Value of thyroid transcription factor-1, E-cadherin, BG8, WT1, and CD44S immunostaining in distinguishing epithelial pleural mesothelioma from pulmonary and nonpulmonary adenocarcinoma. Am J Surg Pathol 2000; 24: 598–606.
222. Shimizu M, Toki T, Takagi Y, et al. Immunohistochemical detection of the Wilms' tumor gene (WT1) in epithelial ovarian tumors. Int J Gynecol Pathol 2000; 19:158–163.
223. Acs G, Pasha T, Zhang PJ. WT1 is differentially expressed in serous, endometrioid, clear cell, and mucinous car-cinomas of the peritoneum, fallopian tube, ovary, and endometrium. Int J Gynecol Pathol 2004; 23:110–118.
224. Logani S, Oliva E, Amin MB, et al. Immunoprofile of ovarian tumors with putative transitional cell (urothelial) differentiation using novel urothelial markers: histogenetic and diagnostic implications. Am J Surg Pathol 2003; 27:1434–1441.
225. McCluggage WG, Oliva E, Connolly LE, et al. An immunohistochemical analysis of ovarian small cell carcinoma of hypercalcemic type. Int J Gynecol Pathol 2004; 23:330–336.
226. Nakopoulou L, Stefanaki K, Janinis J, et al. Immunotochemical expression of placental alkaline phosphatase and vimentin in epithelial ovarian neoplasms. Acta Oncol 1995; 34:511–515.
227. Nouwen EJ, Hendrix PG, Dauwe S, et al. Tumor markers in the human ovary and its neoplasms. A comparative immunohistochemical study. Am J Pathol 1987; 126:230–242.
228. Lifschitz-Mercer B, Walt H, Kushnir I, et al. Differentiation potential of ovarian dysgerminoma: An immunohistochemical study of 15 cases. Hum Pathol 1995; 26:62–66.
229. Hustin J, Gillerot Y, Collette J, et al. Placental alkaline phosphatase in developing normal and abnormal gonads and in germ-cell tumours. Virchows Arch A Pathol Anat Histopathol 1990; 417:67–72.
230. Arber DA, Tamayo R, Weiss LM. Paraffin section detection of the c-kit gene product (CD117) in human tissues: Value in the diagnosis of mast cell disorders. Hum Pathol 1998; 29: 498–504.
231. Gibson PC, Cooper K. CD117 (KIT): a diverse protein with selective applications in surgical pathology. Adv Anat Pathol 2002; 9:65–69.
232. Sarlomo-Rikala M, Kovatich AJ, Barusevicius A, et al. CD117: a sensitive marker for gastrointestinal stromal tumors that is more specific than CD34. Mod Pathol 1998; 11:728–734.
233. Miettinen M, Sarlomo-Rikala M, Lasota J. Gastrointestinal stromal tumors: Recent advances in understanding of their biology. Hum Pathol 1999; 30:1213–1220.
234. Lee JR, Joshi V, Griffin JW Jr, et al. Gastrointestinal autonomic nerve tumor – Immunohistochemical and molecular identity with gastrointestinal stromal tumor. Am J Surg Pathol 2001; 25:979–987.
235. Leroy X, Augusto D, Leteurtre E, et al. CD30 and CD117 (c-kit) used in combination are useful for distinguishing embryonal carcinoma from seminoma. J Histochem Cytochem 2002; 50:283–285.
236. Harms D, Janig U. Germ cell tumours of childhood. Report of 170 cases including 59 pure and partial yolk-sac tumours. Virchows Arch [A] 1986; 409:223–239.
237. Clement PB, Young RH, Scully RE. Endometrioid-like vari-

ant of ovarian yolk sac tumor. A clinicopathological analysis of eight cases. Am J Surg Pathol 1987; 11:767–778.

238. Kurman RJ, Norris HJ. Endodermal sinus tumor of the ovary. A clinical and pathologic analysis of 71 cases. Cancer 1976; 38:2404–2419.

239. Prat J, Bhan AK, Dickersin GR, et al. Hepatoid yolk sac tumor of the ovary (endodermal sinus tumor with hepatoid differentiation): a light microscopic, ultrastructural and immunohistochemical study of seven cases. Cancer 1982; 50:2355–2368.

240. Zirker TA, Silva EG, Morris M, et al. Immunohistochemical differentiation of clear-cell carcinoma of the female genital tract and endodermal sinus tumor with the use of alpha-fetoprotein and Leu-M1. Am J Clin Pathol 1989; 91:511–514.

241. Devouassoux-Shisheboran M, Schammel DP, Tavassoli FA. Ovarian hepatoid yolk sac tumours: morphological, immunohistochemical and ultrastructural features. Histopathology 1999; 34:462–469.

242. Ishikura H, Scully RE. Hepatoid carcinoma of the ovary. A newly described tumor. Cancer 1987; 60:2775–2784.

243. Pitman MB, Triratanachat S, Young RH, et al. Hepatocyte paraffin 1 antibody does not distinguish primary ovarian tumors with hepatoid differentiation from metastatic hepatocellular carcinoma. Int J Gynecol Pathol 2004; 23:58–64.

244. Tochigi N, Kishimoto T, Supriatna Y, et al. Hepatoid carcinoma of the ovary: a report of three cases admixed with a common surface epithelial carcinoma. Int J Gynecol Pathol 2003; 22:266–271.

245. Young RH, Gersell DJ, Clement PB, et al. Hepatocellular carcinoma metastatic to the ovary: A report of three cases discovered during life with discussion of the differential diagnosis of hepatoid tumors of the ovary. Hum Pathol 1992; 23:574–580.

246. Gagnon S, Tëtu B, Silva EG, et al. Frequency of alpha-fetoprotein production by Sertoli-Leydig cell tumors of the ovary: an immunohistochemical study of eight cases. Mod Pathol 1989; 2:63–67.

247. Hammad A, Jasnosz KM, Olson PR. Expression of alpha-fetoprotein by ovarian Sertoli-Leydig cell tumors – Case report and review of the literature. Arch Pathol Lab Med 1995; 119:1075–1079.

248. Mooney EE, Nogales FF, Tavassoli FA. Hepatocytic differentiation in retiform Sertoli-Leydig cell tumors: distinguishing a heterologous element from Leydig cells. Hum Pathol 1999; 30:611–617.

249. Niehans GA, Manivel JC, Copland GT, et al. Immuno-histochemistry of germ cell and trophoblastic neoplasms. Cancer 1988; 62:1113–1123.

250. Perrone T, Steeper TA, Dehner LP. Alpha-fetoprotein localization in pure ovarian teratoma. An immunohistochemical study of 12 cases. Am J Clin Pathol 1987; 88:713–717.

251. Kurman RJ, Norris HJ. Embryonal carcinoma of the ovary: a clinicopathologic entity distinct from endodermal sinus tumor resembling embryonal carcinoma of the adult testis. Cancer 1976; 38:2420–2433.

252. Ueda G, Abe Y, Yoshida M, et al. Embryonal carcinoma of the ovary: a six-year survival. Int J Gynaecol Obstet 1990; 31:287–292.

253. Nakashima N, Fukatsu T, Nagasaka T, et al. The frequency and histology of hepatic tissue in germ cell tumors. Am J Surg Pathol 1987; 11:682–692.

254. Furumoto M. Cellular localization of AFP, hCG and its free subunits, and SP1 in embryonal carcinoma of the testis and ovary. Pathol Res Pract 1981; 173:12–21.

255. Nogales FF, Bergeron C, Carvia RE, et al. Ovarian endometrioid tumors with yolk sac tumor component; an unusual form of ovarian neoplasm – Analysis of six cases. Am J Surg Pathol 1996; 20:1056–1066.

256. Lopez JM, Malpica A, Deavers MT, et al. Ovarian yolk sac tumor associated with endometrioid carcinoma and mucinous cystadenoma of the ovary. Ann Diagn Pathol 2003; 7:300–305.

257. Kurman RJ, Scardino PT, McIntire KR, et al. Cellular localization of alpha-fetoprotein and human chorionic gonadotropin in germ cell tumors of the testis using an indirect immunoperoxidase technique. Cancer 1977; 40:2136–2151.

258. Hustin J, Reuter AM, Franchimont P. Immunohistochemical localization of hCG and its subunits in testicular germ cell tumours. Virchows Arch A Pathol Anat Histopathol 1985; 406:333–338.

259. Zaloudek CJ, Tavassoli FA, Norris HJ. Dysgerminoma with syncytiotrophoblastic giant cells: a histologically and clinically distinctive subtype of dysgerminoma. Am J Surg Pathol 1981; 5:361–367.

260. Oliva E, Andrada E, Pezzica E, et al. Ovarian carcinomas with choriocarcinomatous differentiation. Cancer 1993; 72:

2441–2446.

261. Matias-Guiu X, Prat J. Ovarian tumors with functioning stroma. An immunohistochemical study of 100 cases with human chorionic gonadotropin monoclonal and polyclonal antibodies. Cancer 1990; 65:2001–2005.

262. Mohabeer J, Buckley CH, Fox H. An immunohistochemical study of the incidence and significance of human chorionic gonadotrophin synthesis by epithelial ovarian neoplasms. Gynecol Oncol 1983; 16:78–84.

263. Donato R. S100: a multigenic family of calcium-modulated proteins of the EF-hand type with intracellular and extracellular functional roles. Int J Biochem Cell Biol 2001; 33:637–668.

264. Donato R. Intracellular and extracellular roles of S100 proteins. Microsc Res Tech 2003; 60:540–551.

265. Heizmann CW, Fritz G, Schafer BW. S100 proteins: structure, functions and pathology. Front Biosci 2002; 7:d1356–d1368.

266. Gupta D, Deavers MT, Silva EG, et al. Malignant melanoma involving the ovary: a clinicopathologic and immunohistochemical study of 23 cases. Am J Surg Pathol 2004; 28:771–780.

267. Drier JK, Swanson PE, Cherwitz DL, et al. S100 protein immunoreactivity in poorly differentiated carcinomas. Immunohistochemical comparison with malignant melanoma. Arch Pathol Lab Med 1987; 111:447–452.

268. Herrera GA, Turbat-Herrera EA, Lott RL. S-100 protein expression by primary and metastatic adenocarcinomas. Am J Clin Pathol 1988; 89:168–176.

269. Jungbluth AA, Busam KJ, Gerald WL, et al. A103 – An anti-Melan-A monoclonal antibody for the detection of malignant melanoma in paraffin-embedded tissues. Am J Surg Pathol 1998; 22:595–602.

270. Bacchi CE, Bonetti F, Pea M, et al. HMB-45: A review. Appl Immunohistochem 1996; 4:73–85.

271. Gown AM, Vogel AM, Hoak D, et al. Monoclonal anti-bodies specific for melanocytic tumors distinguish subpopulations of melanocytes. Am J Pathol 1986; 123:195–203.

272. Wick MR, Swanson PE, Rocamora A. Recognition of malignant melanoma by monoclonal antibody HMB-45. An immunohistochemical study of 200 paraffin-embedded cutaneous tumors. J Cutan Pathol 1988; 15:201–207.

273. Hoon V, Thung SN, Kaneko M, et al. HMB-45 reactivity in renal angiomyolipoma and lymphangioleiomyomatosis. Arch Pathol Lab Med 1994; 118:732–734.

274. Gyure KA, Hart WR, Kennedy AW. Lymphangiomyomatosis of the uterus associated with tuberous sclerosis and malignant neoplasia of the female genital tract: a report of two cases. Int J Gynecol Pathol 1995; 14:344–351.

275. Longacre TA, Hendrickson MR, Kapp DS, et al. Lymphangioleiomyomatosis of the uterus simulating high-stage endometrial stromal sarcoma. Gynecol Oncol 1996; 63:404–410.

276. Anderson AE, Yang X, Young RH. Epithelioid angiomyolipoma of the ovary: a case report and literature review. Int J Gynecol Pathol 2002; 21:69–73.

277. Makhlouf HR, Ishak KG, Shekar R, et al. Melanoma markers in angiomyolipoma of the liver and kidney – A comparative study. Arch Pathol Lab Med 2002; 126:49–55.

278. Stone CH, Lee MW, Amin MB, et al. Renal angiomyolipoma – Further immunophenotypic characterization of an expanding morphologic spectrum. Arch Pathol Lab Med 2001; 125:751–758.

279. Matsui K, Tatsuguchi A, Valencia J, et al. Extrapulmonary lymphangioleiomyomatosis (LAM): Clinicopathologic features in 22 cases. Hum Pathol 2000; 31:1242–1248.

280. Busam KJ, Iversen K, Coplan KA, et al. Immunoreactivity for A103, an antibody to Melan-A (MART-1), in adreno-cortical and other steroid tumors. Am J Surg Pathol 1998; 22:57–63.

281. Weiss LM, Chang KL. CD 45: a review. Appl Immunohistochem 1993; 1:166–181.

282. Hanselaar AGJM, Vooijs GP, Mayall B, et al. Epithelial markers to detect occult microinvasion in serous ovarian tumors. Int J Gynecol Pathol 1993; 12:20–27.

283. Multhaupt HAB, Arenas-Elliott CP, Warhol MJ. Comparison of glycoprotein expression between ovarian and colon adenocarcinomas. Arch Pathol Lab Med 1999; 123:909–916.

284. Halperin R, Zehavi S, Hadas E, et al. Immunohistochemical comparison of primary peritoneal and primary ovarian serous papillary carcinoma. Int J Gynecol Pathol 2001; 20:341–345.

285. Geisler JP, Geisler HE, Wiemann MC, et al. Quantification of p53 in epithelial ovarian cancer. Gynecol Oncol 1997; 66:435–438.

286. Hashi A, Yuminamochi T, Murata S, et al. Wilms tumor gene immunoreactivity in primary serous carcinomas of the fallo-

pian tube, ovary, endometrium, and peritoneum. Int J Gynecol Pathol 2003; 22:374–377.

287. Al Hussaini M, Stockman A, Foster H, et al. WT-1 assists in distinguishing ovarian from uterine serous carcinoma and in distinguishing between serous and endometrioid ovarian carcinoma. Histopathology 2004; 44:109–115.

288. Goldstein NS, Uzieblo A. WT1 immunoreactivity in uterine papillary serous carcinomas is different from ovarian serous carcinomas. Am J Clin Pathol 2002; 117:541–545.

289. Zhang PJ, Shah M, Spiegel GW, et al. Cytokeratin 7 immunoreactivity in rectal adenocarcinomas. Appl Immunohistochem Mol Morphol 2003; 11:306–310.

290. Rutgers JL, Bell DA. Immunohistochemical characterization of ovarian borderline tumors of intestinal and mullerian types. Mod Pathol 1992; 5:367–371.

291. Werling RW, Yaziji H, Bacchi CE, et al. CDX2, a highly sensitive and specific marker of adenocarcinomas of intestinal origin: an immunohistochemical survey of 476 primary and metastatic carcinomas. Am J Surg Pathol 2003; 27:303–310.

292. Moskaluk CA, Zhang H, Powell SM, et al. Cdx2 protein expression in normal and malignant human tissues: an immunohistochemical survey using tissue microarrays. Mod Pathol 2003; 16:913–919.

293. Groisman GM, Meir A, Sabo E. The value of Cdx2 immunostaining in differentiating primary ovarian carcinomas from colonic carcinomas metastatic to the ovaries. Int J Gynecol Pathol 2004; 23:52–57.

294. Fraggetta F, Pelosi G, Cafici A, et al. CDX2 immuno-reactivity in primary and metastatic ovarian mucinous tumours. Virchows Arch 2003; 443:782–786.

295. Tornillo L, Moch H, Diener PA, et al. CDX-2 immunostaining in primary and secondary ovarian carcinomas. J Clin Pathol 2004; 57:641–643.

296. Ronnett BM, Shmookler BM, Diener-West M, et al. Immunohistochemical evidence supporting the appendiceal origin of pseudomyxoma peritonei in women. Int J Gynecol Pathol 1997; 16:1–9.

297. O'Connell JT, Tomlinson JS, Roberts AA, et al. Pseudomyxoma peritonei is a disease of MUC2-expressing goblet cells. Am J Pathol 2002; 161:551–564.

298. Prat J, Young RH, Scully RE. Ovarian mucinous tumors with foci of anaplastic carcinoma. Cancer 1982; 50:300–304.

299. Prat J, Scully RE. Sarcomas in ovarian mucinous tumors. A report of two cases. Cancer 1979; 44:1327–1331.

300. Prat J, Scully RE. Ovarian mucinous tumors with sarcoma-like mural nodules. A report of seven cases. Cancer 1979; 44:1332–1344.

301. Nichols GE, Mills SE, Ulbright TM, et al. Spindle cell mural nodules in cystic ovarian mucinous tumors: A clinicopathologic and immunohistochemical study of five cases. Am J Surg Pathol 1991; 15:1055–1062.

302. Chan YF, Ho HC, Yau SM, et al. Ovarian mucinous tumor with mural nodules of anaplastic carcinoma. Gynecol Oncol 1989; 35:112–119.

303. Baergen RN, Rutgers JL. Mural nodules in common epithelial tumors of the ovary. Int J Gynecol Pathol 1994; 13:62–71.

304. Matias-Guiu X, Aranda I, Prat J. Immunohistochemical study of sarcoma-like mural nodules in a mucinous cyst-adenocarcinoma of the ovary. Virchows Arch A Pathol Anat Histopathol 1991; 419:89–92.

305. Bague S, Rodriguez IM, Prat J. Sarcoma-like mural nodules in mucinous cystic tumors of the ovary revisited – A clinicopathologic analysis of 10 additional cases. Am J Surg Pathol 2002; 26:1467–1476.

306. Lee KR, Nucci MR. Ovarian mucinous and mixed epithelial carcinomas of mullerian (endocervical-like) type: A clinicopathologic analysis of four cases of an uncommon variant associated with endometriosis. Int J Gynecol Pathol 2003; 22:42–51.

307. Ordi J, Schammel DP, Rasekh L, et al. Sertoliform endometrioid carcinomas of the ovary: a clinicopathologic and immunohistochemical study of 13 cases. Mod Pathol 1999; 12:933–940.

308. Dellers EA, Valente PT, Edmonds PR, et al. Extrauterine mixed mesodermal tumors: an immunohistochemical study. Arch Pathol Lab Med 1991; 115:918–920.

309. De Brito PA, Silverberg SG, Orenstein JM. Carcinosarcoma (malignant mixed müllerian (mesodermal) tumor) of the female genital tract: Immunohistochemical and ultrastructural analysis of 28 cases. Hum Pathol 1993; 24:132–142.

310. Chang KL, Crabtree GS, Lim-Tan SK, et al. Primary extrauterine endometrial stromal neoplasms: a clinicopathologic study of 20 cases and a review of the literature. Int J Gynecol Pathol 1993; 12:282–296.

311. Vang R, Whitaker BP, Farhood AI, et al. Immunohistochemi-

cal analysis of clear cell carcinoma of the gynecologic tract. Int J Gynecol Pathol 2001; 20:252–259.

312. Cameron RI, Ashe P, O'Rourke DM, et al. A panel of immunohistochemical stains assists in the distinction between ovarian and renal clear cell carcinoma. Int J Gynecol Pathol 2003; 22:272–276.

313. Nolan LP, Heatley MK. The value of immunocytochemistry in distinguishing between clear cell carcinoma of the kidney and ovary. Int J Gynecol Pathol 2001; 20:155–159.

314. Ho ES, Lai CR, Hsieh YT, et al. p53 mutation is infrequent in clear cell carcinoma of the ovary. Gynecol Oncol 2001; 80:189–193.

315. Shimizu M, Nikaido T, Toki T, et al. Clear cell carcinoma has an expression pattern of cell cycle regulatory molecules that is unique among ovarian adenocarcinomas. Cancer 1999; 85:669–677.

316. Kwon TJ, Ro JY, Tornos C, et al. Reduplicated basal lamina in clear-cell carcinoma of the ovary: An immunohistochemical and electron microscopic study. Ultrastruct Pathol 1996; 20:529–536.

317. Mikami Y, Hata S, Melamed J, et al. Basement membrane material in ovarian clear cell carcinoma: correlation with growth pattern and nuclear grade. Int J Gynecol Pathol 1999; 18:52–57.

318. Ordi J, Romagosa C, Tavassoli FA, et al. CD10 expression in epithelial tissues and tumors of the gynecologic tract: a useful marker in the diagnosis of mesonephric, trophoblastic, and clear cell tumors. Am J Surg Pathol 2003; 27:178–186.

319. Ordonez NG, Mackay B. Brenner tumor of the ovary: A comparative immunohistochemical and ultrastructural study with transitional cell carcinoma of the bladder. Ultrastruct Pathol 2000; 24:157–167.

320. Riedel I, Czernobilsky B, Lifschitz-Mercer B, et al. Brenner tumors but not transitional cell carcinomas of the ovary show urothelial differentiation: immunohistochemical staining of urothelial markers, including cytokeratins and uroplakins. Virchows Arch Int J Pathol 2001; 438:181–191.

321. Soslow RA, Rouse RV, Hendrickson MR, et al. Transitional cell neoplasms of the ovary and urinary bladder: a comparative immunohistochemical analysis. Int J Gynecol Pathol 1996; 15:257–265.

322. Kaufmann O, Volmerig J, Dietel M. Uroplakin III is a highly specific and moderately sensitive immunohistochemical marker for primary and metastatic urothelial carcinomas. Am J Clin Pathol 2000; 113:683–687.

323. Ogawa K, Johansson SL, Cohen SM. Immunohistochemical analysis of uroplakins, urothelial specific proteins, in ovarian Brenner tumors, normal tissues, and benign and neoplastic lesions of the female genital tract. Am J Pathol 1999; 155:1047–1050.

324. Ordonez NG. Transitional cell carcinomas of the ovary and bladder are immunophenotypically different. Histopathology 2000; 36:433–438.

325. Riedel I, Czernobilsky B, Lifschitz-Mercer B, et al. Brenner tumors but not transitional cell carcinomas of the ovary show urothelial differentiation: immunohistochemical staining of urothelial markers, including cytokeratins and uroplakins. Virchows Arch 2001; 438:181–191.

326. Ordonez NG. Application of mesothelin immunostaining in tumor diagnosis. Am J Surg Pathol 2003; 27:1418–1428.

327. Riopel MA, Perlman EJ, Seidman JD, et al. Inhibin and epithelial membrane antigen immunohistochemistry assist in the diagnosis of sex cord-stromal tumors and provide clues to the histogenesis of hypercalcemic small cell carcinomas. Int J Gynecol Pathol 1998; 17:46–53.

328. Young RH, Oliva E, Scully RE. Small cell carcinoma of the ovary, hypercalcemic type: A clinicopathological analysis of 150 cases. Am J Surg Pathol 1994; 18:1102–1116.

329. Aguirre P, Thor AD, Scully RE. Ovarian small cell carcinoma. Histogenetic considerations based on immunohistochemical and other findings. Am J Clin Pathol 1989; 92:140–149.

330. Young RH, Scully RE. Malignant melanoma metastatic to the ovary: A clinicopathologic analysis of 20 cases. Am J Surg Pathol 1991; 15:849–860.

331. Parker LP, Duong JL, Wharton JT, et al. Desmoplastic small round cell tumor: report of a case presenting as a primary ovarian neoplasm. Eur J Gynaecol Oncol 2002; 23:199–202.

332. Slomovitz BM, Girotra M, Aledo A, et al. Desmoplastic small round cell tumor with primary ovarian involvement: case report and review. Gynecol Oncol 2000; 79:124–128.

333. Young RH, Eichhorn JH, Dickersin GR, et al. Ovarian involvement by the intra-abdominal desmoplastic small round cell tumor with divergent differentiation: A report of three cases. Hum Pathol 1992; 23:454–464.

334. Zaloudek C, Miller TR, Stern JL. Desmoplastic small cell tumor of the ovary: a unique polyphenotypic tumor with an

unfavorable prognosis. Int J Gynecol Pathol 1995; 14:260–265.
335. Kawauchi S, Fukuda T, Miyamoto S, et al. Peripheral primitive neuroectodermal tumor of the ovary confirmed by CD99 immunostaining, karyotypic analysis, and RT-PCR for EWS/FLI-1 chimeric mRNA. Am J Surg Pathol 1998; 22:1417–1422.
336. Young RH, Scully RE. Alveolar rhabdomyosarcoma metastatic to the ovary. A report of two cases and a discussion of the differential diagnosis of small cell malignant tumors of the ovary. Cancer 1989; 64:899–904.
337. Nielsen GP, Oliva E, Young RH, et al. Primary ovarian rhabdomyosarcoma: a report of 13 cases. Int J Gynecol Pathol 1998; 17:113–119.
338. Paler RJ, Felix JC. Desmin, myoglobin, and muscle-specific actin immunohistochemical staining in a case of embryonal rhabdomyosarcoma of the ovary. Appl Immunohistochem Mol Morphol 1999; 7:237–241.
339. Katsube Y, Berg JW, Silverberg SG. Epidemiologic pathology of ovarian tumors: a histopathologic review of primary ovarian neoplasms diagnosed in the Denver Standard Metropolitan Statistical Area, 1 July–31 December 1969 and 1 July–31 December 1979. Int J Gynecol Pathol 1982; 1:3–16.
340. Koonings PP, Campbell K, Mishell DR Jr, et al. Relative frequency of primary ovarian neoplasms: a 10-year review. Obstet Gynecol 1989; 74:921–926.
341. Stage AH, Grafton WD. Thecomas and granulosa-theca cell tumors of the ovary: an analysis of 51 tumors. Obstet Gynecol 1977; 50:21–27.
342. Deavers MT, Malpica A, Ordonez NG, et al. Ovarian steroid cell tumors: an immunohistochemical study including a comparison of calretinin with inhibin. Int J Gynecol Pathol 2003; 22:162–167.
343. Stewart CJR, Jeffers MD, Kennedy A. Diagnostic value of inhibin immunoreactivity in ovarian gonadal stromal tumours and their histological mimics. Histopathology 1997; 31:67–74.
344. Tiltman AJ, Haffajee Z. Sclerosing stromal tumors, thecomas, and fibromas of the ovary: an immunohistochemical profile. Int J Gynecol Pathol 1999; 18:254–258.
345. Chalvardjian A, Scully RE. Sclerosing stromal tumors of the ovary. Cancer 1973; 31:664–670.
346. Kawauchi S, Tsuji T, Kaku T, et al. Sclerosing stromal tumor of the ovary. A clinicopathologic, immunohistochemical, ultrastructural, and cytogenetic analysis with special reference to its vasculature. Am J Surg Pathol 1998; 22:83–92.
347. Sabah M, Leader M, Kay E. The problem with KIT: clinical implications and practical difficulties with CD117 immunostaining. Appl Immunohistochem Mol Morphol 2003; 11:56–61.
348. Saitoh A, Tsutsumi Y, Osamura RY, et al. Sclerosing stromal tumor of the ovary. Immunohistochemical and electron microscopic demonstration of smooth-muscle differentiation. Arch Pathol Lab Med 1989; 113:372–376.
349. Shaw JA, Dabbs DJ, Geisinger KR. Sclerosing stromal tumor of the ovary: An ultrastructural and immunohistochemical analysis with histogenetic considerations. Ultrastruct Pathol 1992; 16:363–377.
350. Ishioka S, Sagae S, Saito T, et al. A case of a sclerosing stromal ovarian tumor that expresses VEGF. J Obstet Gynaecol Res 2000; 26:35–38.
351. Fox H. Pathologic prognostic factors in early stage adult-type granulosa cell tumors of the ovary. Int J Gynecol Cancer 2003; 13:1–4.
352. Schumer ST, Cannistra SA. Granulosa cell tumor of the ovary. J Clin Oncol 2003; 21:1180–1189.
353. Hines JF, Khalifa MA, Moore JL, et al. Recurrent granulosa cell tumor of the ovary 37 years after initial diagnosis: a case report and review of the literature. Gynecol Oncol 1996; 60:484–488.
354. Shah VI, Freites NO, Maxwell P, et al. Inhibin is more specific than calretinin as an immunohistochemical marker for differentiating sarcomatoid granulosa cell tumour of the ovary from other spindle cell neoplasms. J Clin Pathol 2003; 56:221–224.
355. Costa MJ, DeRose PB, Roth LM, et al. Immunohistochemical phenotype of ovarian granulosa cell tumors: Absence of epithelial membrane antigen has diagnostic value. Hum Pathol 1994; 25:60–66.
356. Gitsch G, Kohlberger P, Steiner A, et al. Expression of cytokeratins in granulosa cell tumors and ovarian carcinomas. Arch Gynecol Obstet 1992; 251:193–197.
357. Otis CN, Powell JL, Barbuto D, et al. Intermediate filamentous proteins in adult granulosa cell tumors: An immunohistochemical study of 25 cases. Am J Surg Pathol 1992; 16:962–968.

358. Choi YL, Kim HS, Ahn G. Immunoexpression of inhibin alpha subunit, inhibin/activin betaA subunit and CD99 in ovarian tumors. Arch Pathol Lab Med 2000; 124:563–569.

359. Gordon MD, Corless C, Renshaw AA, et al. CD99, keratin, and vimentin staining of sex cord-stromal tumors, normal ovary, and testis. Mod Pathol 1998; 11:769–773.

360. Young RH, Dickersin GR, Scully RE. Juvenile granulosa cell tumor of the ovary. A clinicopathological analysis of 125 cases. Am J Surg Pathol 1984; 8:575–596.

361. Zaloudek CJ, Norris HJ. Granulosa tumors of the ovary in children: a clinical and pathologic study of 32 cases. Am J Surg Pathol 1982; 6:503–512.

362. Rakheja D, Sharma S. Pathologic quiz case – Cystic and solid ovarian tumor in a 43-year-old woman – Pathologic diagnosis: Cystic juvenile-type granulosa cell tumor of the ovary in an adult. Arch Pathol Lab Med 2002; 126:1123–1124.

363. Young RH. Sertoli-Leydig cell tumors of the ovary: review with emphasis on historical aspects and unusual forms. Int J Gynecol Pathol 1993; 12:141–147.

364. Zaloudek C, Norris HJ. Sertoli-Leydig tumors of the ovary. A clinicopathologic study of 64 intermediate and poorly differentiated neoplasms. Am J Surg Pathol 1984; 8:405–418.

365. Young RH, Scully RE. Well-differentiated ovarian Sertoli-Leydig cell tumors: a clinicopathological analysis of 23 tumors. Int J Gynecol Pathol 1984; 3:277–290.

366. Young RH, Scully RE. Ovarian Sertoli-Leydig cell tumors. A clinicopathological analysis of 207 cases. Am J Surg Pathol 1985; 9:543–569.

367. Young RH, Scully RE. Ovarian Sertoli-Leydig cell tumors with a retiform pattern – A problem in diagnosis: a report of 25 cases. Am J Surg Pathol 1983; 7:755–771.

368. Mooney EE, Nogales FF, Bergeron C, et al. Retiform Sertoli-Leydig cell tumours: clinical, morphological and immunohistochemical findings. Histopathology 2002; 41:110–117.

369. Aguirre P, Thor AD, Scully RE. Ovarian endometrioid carcinomas resembling sex cord-stromal tumors. An immunohistochemical study. Int J Gynecol Pathol 1989; 8:364–373.

370. Guerrieri C, Franlund B, Malmstrom H, et al. Ovarian endometrioid carcinomas simulating sex cord-stromal tumors: a study using inhibin and cytokeratin 7. Int J Gynecol Pathol 1998; 17:266–271.

371. Cao QJ, Jones JG, Li M. Expression of calretinin in human ovary, testis, and ovarian sex cord-stromal tumors. Int J Gynecol Pathol 2001; 20:346–352.

372. Roth LM, Liban E, Czernobilsky B. Ovarian endometrioid tumors mimicking Sertoli and Sertoli-Leydig cell tumors: Sertoliform variant of endometrioid carcinoma. Cancer 1982; 50:1322–1331.

373. Young RH, Prat J, Scully RE. Ovarian endometrioid carcinomas resembling sex cord-stromal tumors. A clinicopathologic analysis of 13 cases. Am J Surg Pathol 1982; 6:513–522.

374. Young RH, Prat J, Scully RE. Ovarian Sertoli-Leydig cell tumors with heterologous elements. I. Gastrointestinal epithelium and carcinoid: A clinicopathologic analysis of 36 cases. Cancer 1982; 50:2448–2456.

375. Aguirre P, Scully RE, DeLellis RA. Ovarian heterologous Sertoli-Leydig cell tumors with gastrointestinal-type epithelium. An immunohistochemical analysis. Arch Pathol Lab Med 1986; 110:528–533.

376. Prat J, Young RH, Scully RE. Ovarian Sertoli-Leydig cell tumors with heterologous elements. II. Cartilage and skeletal muscle. A clinicopathologic analysis of twelve cases. Cancer 1982; 50:2465–2475.

377. Young RH, Scully RE. Ovarian Sertoli cell tumors. A report of 10 cases. Int J Gynecol Pathol 1984; 2:349–363.

378. Ferry JA, Young RH, Engel G, et al. Oxyphilic Sertoli cell tumor of the ovary: a report of three cases, two in patients with the Peutz-Jeghers syndrome. Int J Gynecol Pathol 1994; 13:259–266.

379. Benjamin E, Law S, Bobrow LG. Intermediate filaments cytokeratin and vimentin in ovarian sex cord-stromal tumours with correlative studies in adult and fetal ovaries. J Pathol 1987; 152:253–263.

380. Stewart GJR, Nandini CL, Richmond JA. Value of A103 (melan-A) immunostaining in the differential diagnosis of ovarian sex cord-stromal tumours. J Clin Pathol 2000; 53:206–211.

381. Seidman JD, Abbondanzo SL, Bratthauer GL. Lipid cell (steroid cell) tumor of the ovary: immunophenotype with analysis of potential pitfall due to endogenous biotin-like activity. Int J Gynecol Pathol 1995; 14:331–338.

382. Cheng L, Thomas A, Roth LM, et al. OCT4: A novel biomarker for dysgerminoma of the ovary. Am J Surg Pathol 2004; 28:1341–1346.

383. Jones TD, Ulbright TM, Eble JN, et al. OCT4 staining in testicular tumors: a sensitive and specific marker for semi-

noma and embryonal carcinoma. Am J Surg Pathol 2004; 28: 935–940.
384. Kommoss F, Schmidt D, Coerdt W, et al. Immunohistochemical expression analysis of inhibin-alpha and -beta subunits in partial and complete moles, trophoblastic tumors, and endometrial decidua. Int J Gynecol Pathol 2001; 20:380–385.
385. McCluggage WG, Ashe P, McBride H, et al. Localization of the cellular expression of inhibin in trophoblastic tissue. Histopathology 1998; 32:252–256.
386. Pelkey TJ, Frierson HFJ, Mills SE, et al. Detection of the alpha-subunit of inhibin in trophoblastic neoplasia. Hum Pathol 1999; 30:26–31.
387. Shih IM, Kurman RJ. Immunohistochemical localization of inhibin-alpha in the placenta and gestational trophoblastic lesions. Int J Gynecol Pathol 1999; 18:144–150.
388. Oliva E, Musulen E, Prat J, et al. Transitional cell carcinoma of the renal pelvis with symptomatic ovarian metastases. Int J Surg Pathol 1995; 2:231–236.
389. Nogales FF, Avila IR, Concha A, et al. Immature endo-dermal teratoma of the ovary: Embryologic correla-tions and immunohistochemistry. Hum Pathol 1993; 24:364–370.
390. Szyfelbein WM, Young RH, Scully RE. Cystic struma ovarii: A frequently unrecognized tumor: A report of 20 cases. Am J Surg Pathol 1994; 18:785–788.
391. Szyfelbein WM, Young RH, Scully RE. Struma ovarii simulating ovarian tumors of other types. A report of 30 cases. Am J Surg Pathol 1995; 19:21–29.
392. Devaney K, Snyder R, Norris HJ, et al. Proliferative and histologically malignant struma ovarii: a clinicopathologic study of 54 cases. Int J Gynecol Pathol 1993; 12:333–343.
393. Sporrong B, Falkmer S, Robboy SJ, et al. Neurohormonal peptides in ovarian carcinoids: an immunohistochemical study of 81 primary carcinoids and of intraovarian metastases from six mid-gut carcinoids. Cancer 1982; 49:68–74.
394. Sidhu J, Sánchez RL. Prostatic acid phosphatase in strumal carcinoids of the ovary: An immunohistochemical study. Cancer 1993; 72:1673–1678.
395. Stagno PA, Petras RE, Hart WR. Strumal carcinoids of the ovary. An immunohistologic and ultrastructural study. Arch Pathol Lab Med 1987; 111:440–446.
396. Snyder RR, Tavassoli FA. Ovarian strumal carcinoid: immunohistochemical, ultrastructural, and clinicopathologic analysis. Int J Gynecol Pathol 1986; 5:187–201.
397. Matsuda K, Maehama T, Kanazawa K. Strumal carcinoid tumor of the ovary: a case exhibiting severe constipation associated with PYY. Gynecol Oncol 2002; 87:143–145.
398. Baker PM, Oliva E, Young RH, et al. Ovarian mucinous carcinoids including some with a carcinomatous component ——A report of 17 cases. Am J Surg Pathol 2001; 25:557–568.
399. Hussong J, Crussi FG, Chou PM. Gonadoblastoma: immunohistochemical localization of Mullerian-inhibiting substance, inhibin, WT-1, and p53. Mod Pathol 1997; 10: 1101–1105.
400. Roth LM, Eglen DE. Gonadoblastoma. Immunohistochemical and ultrastructural observations. Int J Gynecol Pathol 1989; 8:72–81.
401. Moore RG, Chung M, Granai CO, et al. Incidence of metastasis to the ovaries from nongenital tract primary tumors. Gynecol Oncol 2004; 93:87–91.
402. Seidman JD, Kurman RJ, Ronnett BM. Primary and metastatic mucinous adenocarcinomas in the ovaries: incidence in routine practice with a new approach to improve intra-operative diagnosis. Am J Surg Pathol 2003; 27:985–993.
403. Ronnett BM, Kurman RJ, Shmookler BM, et al. The morphologic spectrum of ovarian metastases of appendiceal adenocarcinomas – A clinicopathologic and immunohistochemical analysis of tumors often misinterpreted as primary ovarian tumors or metastatic tumors from other gastrointestinal sites. Am J Surg Pathol 1997; 21:1144–1155.
404. Park SY, Kim HS, Hong EK, et al. Expression of cytokeratins 7 and 20 in primary carcinomas of the stomach and colorectum and their value in the differential diagnosis of metastatic carcinomas to the ovary. Hum Pathol 2002; 33:1078–1085.
405. Young RH, Hart WR. Metastatic intestinal carcinomas simulating primary ovarian clear cell carcinoma and secretory endometrioid carcinoma – A clinicopathologic and immunohistochemical study of five cases. Am J Surg Pathol 1998; 22:805–815.
406. Gagnon Y, Tëtu B. Ovarian metastases of breast carcinoma. A clinicopathologic study of 59 cases. Cancer 1989; 64:892–898.
407. Young RH, Carey RW, Robboy SJ. Breast carcinoma masquerading as primary ovarian neoplasm. Cancer 1981; 48: 210–212.
408. Monteagudo C, Merino MJ, LaPorte N, et al. Value of gross cystic disease fluid protein-15 in distinguishing metastatic

breast carcinomas among poorly differentiated neoplasms involving the ovary. Hum Pathol 1991; 22:368–372.

409. Brown RW, Campagna LB, Dunn JK, et al. Immunohistochemical identification of tumor markers in metastatic adenocarcinoma – A diagnostic adjunct in the determination of primary site. Am J Clin Pathol 1997; 107:12–19.

410. Lau SK, Luthringer DJ, Eisen RN. Thyroid transcription factor-1: a review. Appl Immunohistochem Mol Morphol 2002; 10:97–102.

411. Agoff SN, Lamps LW, Philip AT, et al. Thyroid transcription factor-1 is expressed in extrapulmonary small cell carcinomas but not in other extrapulmonary neuroendocrine tumors. Mod Pathol 2000; 13:238–242.

412. Kaufmann O, Dietel M. Expression of thyroid transcription factor-1 in pulmonary and extrapulmonary small cell carcinomas and other neuroendocrine carcinomas of various primary sites. Histopathology 2000; 36:415–420.

413. Ordonez NG. Value of thyroid transcription factor-1 immunostaining in distinguishing small cell lung carcinomas from other small cell carcinomas. Am J Surg Pathol 2000; 24:1217–1223.

414. Cheuk W, Kwan MY, Suster S, et al. Immunostaining for thyroid transcription factor 1 and cytokeratin 20 aids the distinction of small cell carcinoma from Merkel cell carcinoma, but not pulmonary from extrapulmonary small cell carcinomas. Arch Pathol Lab Med 2001; 125:228–231.

415. Goldblum J, Hart WR. Localized and diffuse mesotheliomas of the genital tract and peritoneum in women – A clinicopathologic study of nineteen true mesothelial neoplasms, other than adenomatoid tumors, multicystic mesotheliomas, and localized fibrous tumors. Am J Surg Pathol 1995; 19:1124–1137.

416. Clement PB, Young RH, Scully RE. Malignant mesotheliomas presenting as ovarian masses – A report of nine cases, including two primary ovarian mesotheliomas. Am J Surg Pathol 1996; 20:1067–1080.

417. Kerrigan SAJ, Turnnir RT, Clement PB, et al. Diffuse malignant epithelial mesotheliomas of the peritoneum in women – A clinicopathologic study of 25 patients. Cancer 2002; 94:378–385.

418. Nascimento AG, Keeney GL, Fletcher CDM. Deciduoid peritoneal mesothelioma: An unusual phenotype affecting young females. Am J Surg Pathol 1994; 18:439–445.

419. Orosz Z, Nagy P, Szentirmay Z, et al. Epithelial mesothelioma with deciduoid features. Virchows Arch 1999; 434:263–266.

420. Shanks JH, Harris M, Banerjee SS, et al. Mesotheliomas with deciduoid morphology – A morphologic spectrum and a variant not confined to young females. Am J Surg Pathol 2000; 24:285–294.

421. Alvarado-Cabrero I, Young RH, Vamvakas EC, et al. Carcinoma of the fallopian tube: a clinicopathological study of 105 cases with observations on staging and prognostic factors. Gynecol Oncol 1999; 72:367–379.

422. Baekelandt M, Nesbakken AJ, Kristensen GB, et al. Carcinoma of the fallopian tube – Clinicopathologic study of 151 patients treated at the Norwegian Radium Hospital. Cancer 2000; 89:2076–2084.

423. Piura B, Rabinovich A. Primary carcinoma of the fallopian tube: study of 11 cases. Eur J Obstet Gynecol Reprod Biol 2000; 91:169–175.

424. di Re E, Grosso G, Raspagliesi F, et al. Fallopian tube cancer: incidence and role of lymphatic spread. Gynecol Oncol 1996; 62:199–202.

425. Youngs LA, Taylor HB. Adenomatoid tumors of the uterus and fallopian tube. Am J Clin Pathol 1967; 48:537–545.

426. Stephenson TJ, Mills PM. Adenomatoid tumours: an immunohistochemical and ultrastructural appraisal of their histogenesis. J Pathol 1986; 148:327–335.

427. Salazar H, Kanbour A, Burgess F. Ultrastructure and observations on the histogenesis of mesotheliomas, 'adenomatoid tumors,' of the female genital tract. Cancer 1972; 29:141–152.

428. Mai KT, Yazdi HM, Perkins DG, et al. Adenomatoid tumor of the genital tract: evidence of mesenchymal cell origin. Pathol Res Pract 1999; 195:605–610.

429. Nogales FF, Isaac MA, Hardisson D, et al. Adenomatoid tumors of the uterus: an analysis of 60 cases. Int J Gynecol Pathol 2002; 21:34–40.

430. Schwartz EJ, Longacre TA. Adenomatoid tumors of the female and male genital tracts express WT1. Int J Gynecol Pathol 2004; 23:123–128.

431. Delahunt B, Eble JN, King D, et al. Immunohistochemical evidence for mesothelial origin of paratesticular adenomatoid tumour. Histopathology 2000; 36:109–115.

432. Otis CN. Uterine adenomatoid tumors: immunohistochemi-

cal characteristics with emphasis on Ber-EP4 immunoreactivity and distinction from adenocarcinoma. Int J Gynecol Pathol 1996; 15:146–151.
433. Kariminejad MH, Scully RE. Female adnexal tumor of probable wolffian origin: a distinctive pathologic entity. Cancer 1973; 31:671–677.
434. Young RH, Scully RE. Ovarian tumors of probable wolffian origin: a report of 11 cases. Am J Surg Pathol 1983; 7:125–136.
435. Tavassoli FA, Andrade R, Merino M. Retiform wolffian adenoma. In: Fenoglio-Preiser CM, Wolffe M, Rilke F, eds. Progress in surgical pathology, vol. XI. New York: Field and Wood Medical Publishers; 1990.
436. Daya D, Young RH, Scully RE. Endometrioid carcinoma of the fallopian tube resembling an adnexal tumor of pro-bable wolffian origin: a report of six cases. Int J Gynecol Pathol 1992; 11:122–130.
437. Karpuz V, Berger SD, Burkhardt K, et al. A case of endometrioid carcinoma of the fallopian tube mimicking an adnexal tumor of probable wolffian origin. APMIS 1999; 107:550–554.
438. Devouassoux-Shisheboran M, Silver SA, Tavassoli FA. Wolffian adnexal tumor, so-called female adnexal tumor of probable wolffian origin (FATWO): immunohistochemical evidence in support of a wolffian origin. Hum Pathol 1999; 30:856–863.
439. Rahilly MA, Williams ARW, Krausz T, et al. Female adnexal tumour of probable wolffian origin: A clinicopathological and immunohistochemical study of three cases. Histopathology 1995; 26:69–74.
440. Tiltman AJ, Allard U. Female adnexal tumours of probable wolffian origin: an immunohistochemical study comparing tumours, mesonephric remnants and paramesonephric derivatives. Histopathology 2001; 38:237–242.

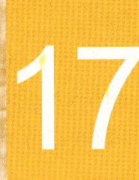

17 乳腺组织的免疫组织化学

原作者：David J. Dabbs
译　者：张庆慧
审校者：李劲松，吴晓娟

目　录

引言	716
抗原/抗体生物学	716
导管上皮增生性病变和原位癌	729
乳腺 Paget 病	731
腋窝淋巴结微转移癌	731
导管癌和小叶癌	736
小叶癌变型和以前的小叶癌变型	737
乳腺癌的全身转移	743
乳腺癌免疫组化预后因子	744

引　言

在外科病理实验室中，诊断性免疫组化方法最常用于乳腺活检标本，这主要是因为乳腺标本数量大而且常常诊断困难。免疫组化方法除了用于乳腺活检标本的病理诊断外，还经常用于对患者预后的评估。此外，转移性乳腺癌的诊断仍是当前的一个难题。

本章主要讨论以下几方面的问题：乳腺癌的间质浸润、导管癌与小叶癌的鉴别诊断、非典型增生性病变、患者预后/预测指标、免疫组化在转移性乳腺癌诊断方面的作用以及前哨淋巴结活检标本的分析。此外，还涉及免疫组化在某些乳腺特殊性病变中的应用。有关间叶性肿瘤的内容在第 3 章讲述。

抗原/抗体生物学

免疫组化在诊断间质浸润中的应用

肌上皮细胞

乳腺上皮性病变不但是外科病理学家最常面临的病变，而且也是乳腺良恶性病变鉴别诊断中最受关注的问题。需要鉴别的病变主要包括：非肿瘤性增生与恶性肿瘤（硬化性腺病与浸润性癌）、原位癌与浸润性癌（小叶性或导管性）、假浸润性良性病变（腺病、放射性瘢痕、硬化性乳头状瘤）与浸润性恶性病变等[1,2]。此外，在很多情况下免疫组化还有助于鉴别非典型性导管上皮增生（ADEH）、乳头状病变及微浸润性癌等。

在上述的所有病理诊断问题中，病变部位肌上皮细胞（myoepithelial cell，MEC）与上皮细胞之间的关系是鉴别原位癌与浸润性癌以及假浸润性病变与浸润性癌的关键（微腺型腺病除外）。微腺型腺病是一种腺泡增生呈不规则分布的良性乳腺腺病。肌上皮细胞位于基底膜的上方，包绕在导管-小叶上皮细胞的周围。肌上皮细胞的存在一直被认为是区分非浸润性肿瘤与浸润性肿瘤的重要依据[3-8]。在正常乳腺的导管和腺泡周围通常都可以看到肌上皮细胞，但是当导管或腺泡扩张，其内充满增生的细胞或被挤压时，致使肌上皮细胞难以辨认。特异性和敏感性更高的针对肌上皮细胞胞浆成分的抗体 calponin、平滑肌肌球蛋白重链抗体（smooth muscle myosin heavy chain，SMMHC）以及细胞核标记物 p63 已经取代了过去使用的 S-100、高分子量角蛋白以及平滑肌肌动蛋白抗体。

S-100抗体标记肌上皮细胞的敏感性和特异性均较差，而且结果不稳定[9-13]。此外，近年来使用的maspin和CD10，由于也可以标记其他不同类型的上皮，包括终末导管小叶单位的上皮细胞以及肿瘤细胞，其应用也在逐渐减少[14-18]。

在"鸡尾酒"式的细胞角蛋白混合抗体中，CK14和CK17除了可以标记肌上皮细胞外[19]，还可以标记腺上皮细胞，因为肌上皮细胞与腺上皮细胞紧密相邻，所以很难将这两类细胞区分开来。平滑肌肌动蛋白（SMA）抗体除了可以与肌上皮细胞反应外，还可以与间质中肌纤维母细胞反应[20-24]，因此特异性较差。由于该抗体与肌纤维母细胞有交叉反应，所以很难识别和确认肌上皮细胞，尤其在导管原位癌（DCIS），因为导管原位癌可有导管周围间质的纤维组织增生。

Nayar和Bose等发现，尽管SMA（DAKO, Carpinteria, CA）和肌特异性肌动蛋白HHF-35抗体（Enzo, Farmingdale, NY）可以标记绝大多数乳腺良性病变中的肌上皮细胞，但是它们也可以与间质中肌纤维母细胞发生交叉反应，SMA尤为明显。在大约36%的病例中见到一些导管上皮细胞也被HHF-35抗体标记，这可能与实验方法有关[13, 25]。Wang和他的同事们对各种乳腺良恶性病变中calponin和SMMHC的标记情况进行了调查总结[26]。

SMMHC是平滑肌细胞特有的结构成分，分子量200kD，它位于粗细肌丝收缩结构内，呈六边形排列[27]。calponin是一种分子量34kD的多肽，它可以调节平滑肌收缩单位中肌纤凝蛋白ATP酶的活性，是平滑肌细胞特有的成分[28, 29]。Wang和他的同事在对70例乳腺癌和各种良性硬化性病变以及乳头状病变的分析中发现：①在良性病变中，肌上皮细胞总是表达calponin和SMMHC；②与平滑肌肌动蛋白抗体1A4相比，calponin和SMMHC几乎不与纤维组织中的肌纤维母细胞发生反应，因此，后两种抗体在鉴别乳腺良恶性病变时更有意义[26]。

根据作者的经验，calponin和SMMHC都是非常好的抗体，但与SMMHC相比，calponin在一定程度上可与间质肌纤维母细胞发生反应（图17.1～17.6）。在乳腺良性增生性病变或硬化性病变中，肌上皮细胞

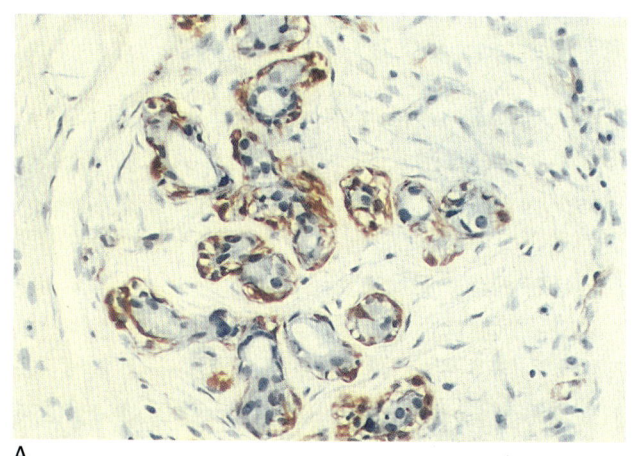

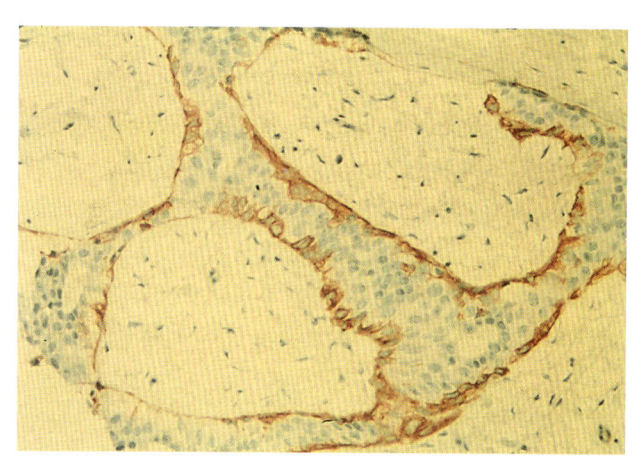

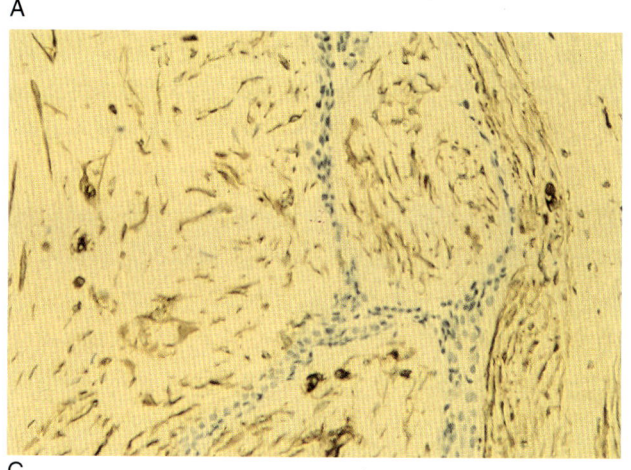

图17.1　（A）SMMHC免疫组化示乳腺小叶中的肌上皮细胞阳性。（B）SMMHC免疫组化示纤维腺瘤中的肌上皮细胞阳性。（C）波形蛋白免疫组化示纤维腺瘤中的间质细胞阳性

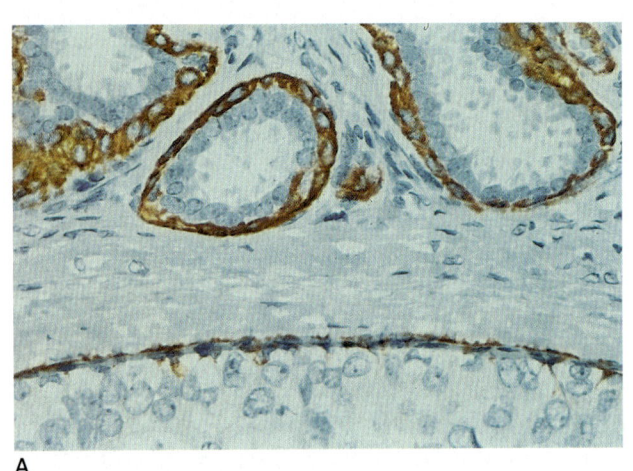
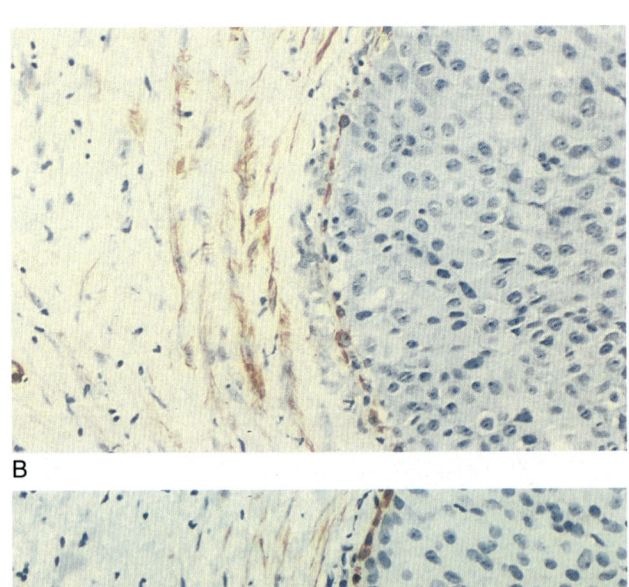
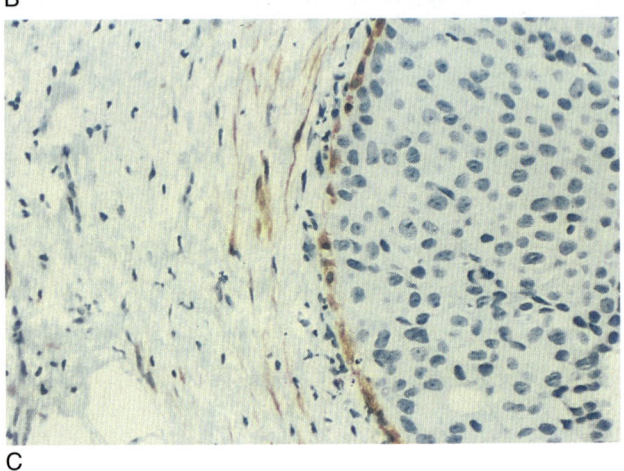

图17.2 （A）比较SMMHC在正常导管（位于图的上方）和原位癌扩张导管（位于图的下方）的染色情况。（B和C）分别显示calponin及平滑肌肌动蛋白使原位癌周围增生的间质细胞着色

SMMHC阳性，间质肌纤维母细胞阴性或仅有极少数细胞阳性。根据作者的经验，对难以诊断的乳腺活检标本，联合使用SMMHC和p63是识别肌上皮细胞的最佳选择，尤其是对诊断性穿刺活检的标本。在穿刺活检标本中原位癌和浸润癌的鉴别是非常重要的，因为许多浸润癌患者通常都要进行前哨淋巴结活检（SNLB）。

近年来，肿瘤抑制基因p53家族成员p63已被用于在多个器官中识别肌上皮细胞、基底细胞（前列腺）和肌上皮分化细胞（乳腺化生性癌和涎腺肿瘤），以及作为鳞状细胞分化的标记物[30-32]。p63用于间质浸润诊断的优势在于它只存在于细胞核中，并且不会与肌纤维母细胞发生反应，因此是显示乳腺肌上皮细胞最为特异的抗体。有人将SMMHC和p63联合使用，进行双重标记[30]。值得注意的是，大约有5%的DCIS病例无论用何种抗体标记均无肌上皮细胞的阳性表达（其肌上皮细胞均为阴性）。在这种情况下，对组织切片严格的观察评估是作出正确诊断的关键（表17.1）。

某些病例中，约5%~10%的肿瘤细胞有p63免疫反应。一般情况下，细胞核级别越高，核染色越强（图17.7）。p63仅在细胞核着色，肌上皮细胞的胞浆不着色，因此在阳性的细胞核之间有明显的"空隙"。在瘤细胞巢周围出现的任何细胞核阳性细胞都可能被认为是肌上皮细胞。但必须注意要除外在肿瘤性小导管周围核阳性的肿瘤细胞。

在穿刺活检标本中难以作出诊断的病变包括：伴有明显的导管周围纤维组织增生或大量淋巴细胞浸润时鉴别原位癌与浸润癌、小叶样生长的圆形瘤细胞团（在病理学家的眼内，浸润是"全或无"）、浸润性筛状癌、硬化性腺病（SA）（伴有或不伴有原位癌成分）、小叶癌化、伴有间质弹力纤维和纤维结缔组织增生的放射性瘢痕、小管癌（TC）和囊内乳头状癌（IPC）（图17.8~17.12）。作者[33]和其他一些学者认为，对于难以诊断的病变，识别肌上皮细胞的最佳抗体包括SMMHC和p63[34]。对于乳腺穿刺活检标本，在低级别病变而且有小叶样结构时，或伴有大量淋巴细胞浸润，或有小叶癌化，或由于在细胞周围有明显的反应性纤维组织增生而与不规则的间质浸润相似时，SMMHC和p63可以准确地将浸润癌和原位癌区分开来[34]。

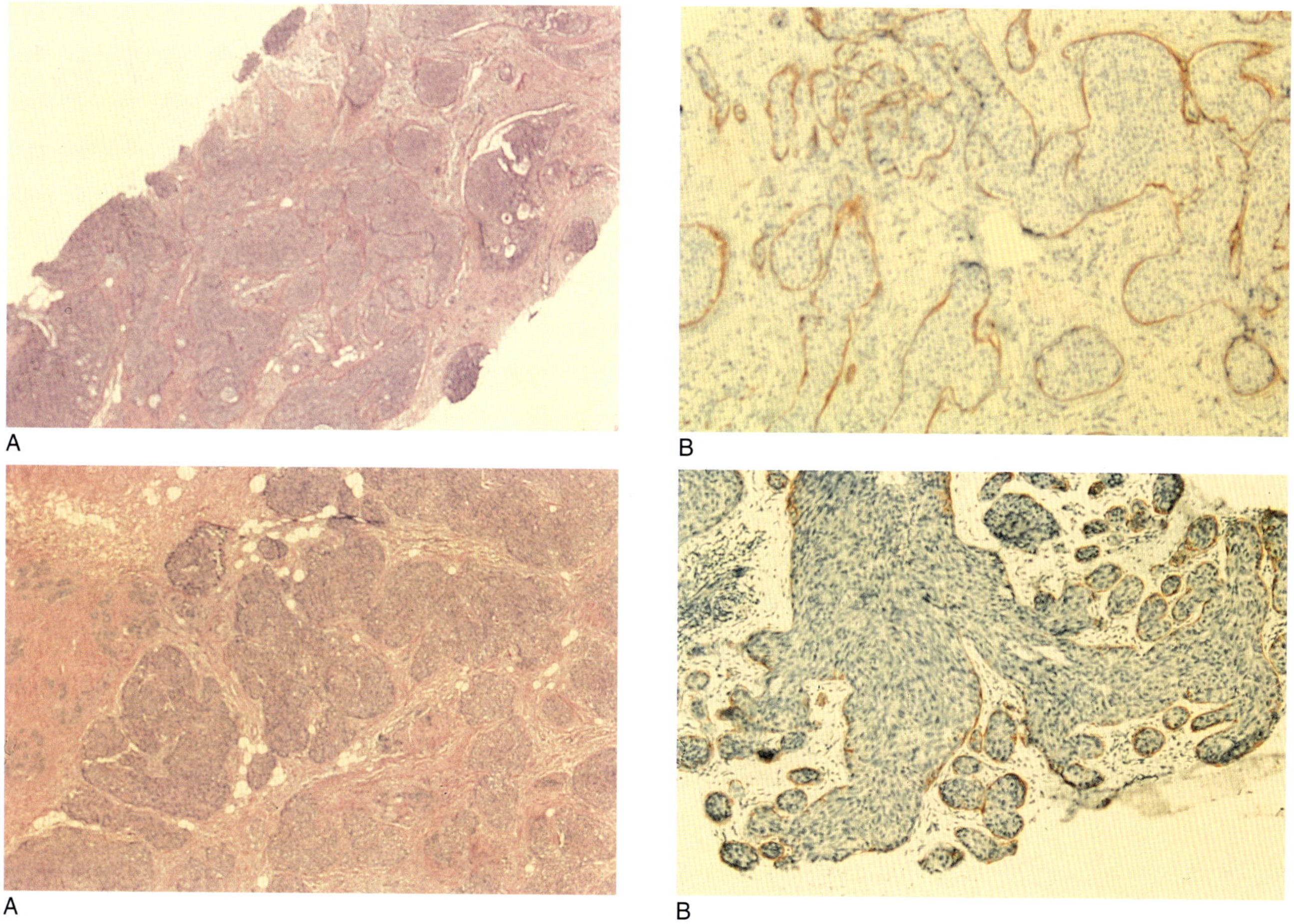

图 17.3 和图 17.4　（A）诊断有疑问的乳腺穿刺活检标本：原位癌还是浸润性癌？（B）上述两个病例，经 SMMHC 染色后，清楚地显示肌上皮细胞沿舌状的瘤细胞索边缘排列，表明这两个标本都是原位癌

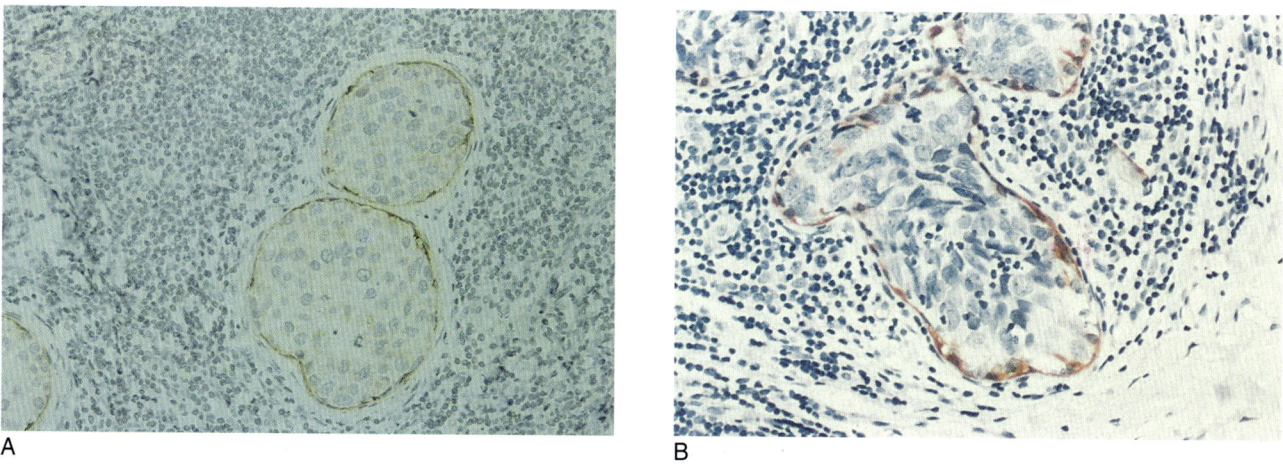

图 17.5　（A 和 B）这两例原位癌都伴有大量淋巴细胞浸润，但是经过 SMMHC 染色，可以清晰地显示肌上皮细胞

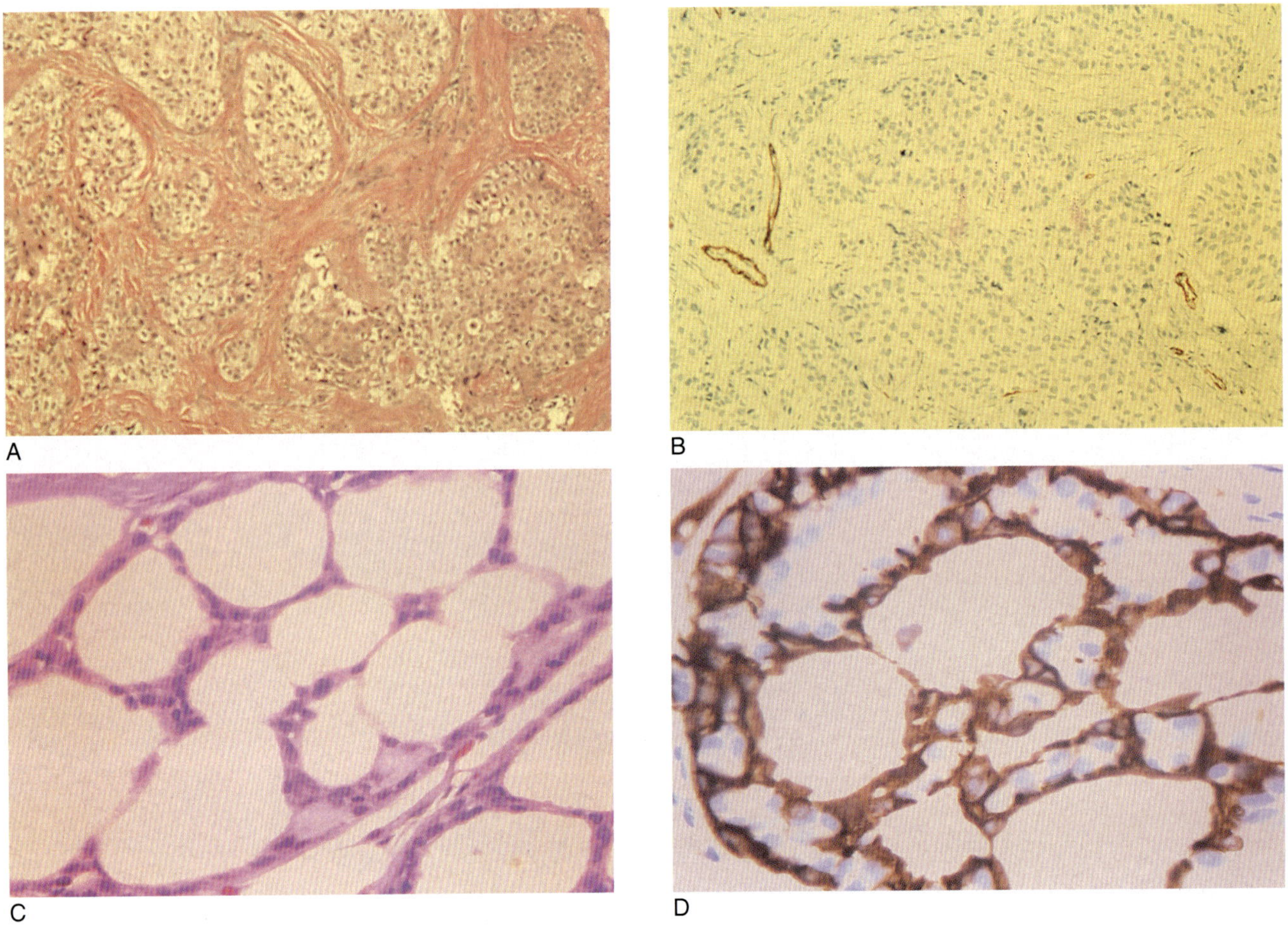

图17.6 （A）空心针穿刺活检为浸润性乳腺癌，可见（B）SMMHC染色阴性，血管可以作为阳性内对照。（C）腺样囊性癌的组织学切片，（D）经SMMHC染色，显示出肌上皮细胞与上皮细胞的关系

表17.1 乳腺组织中用于标记肌上皮细胞的抗体

抗体	阳性部位	MEC	肌纤维母细胞	微血管系统	癌
S-100	胞浆	弱阳性	不定	阴性	不定
SMA	胞浆	强阳性	中等阳性	强阳性	罕见阳性
Calponin	胞浆	强阳性	弱至中等阳性	强阳性	罕见阳性
SMMHC	胞浆	强阳性	很少阳性	强阳性	阴性
p63	胞核	强阳性	阴性	阴性	少数核阳性

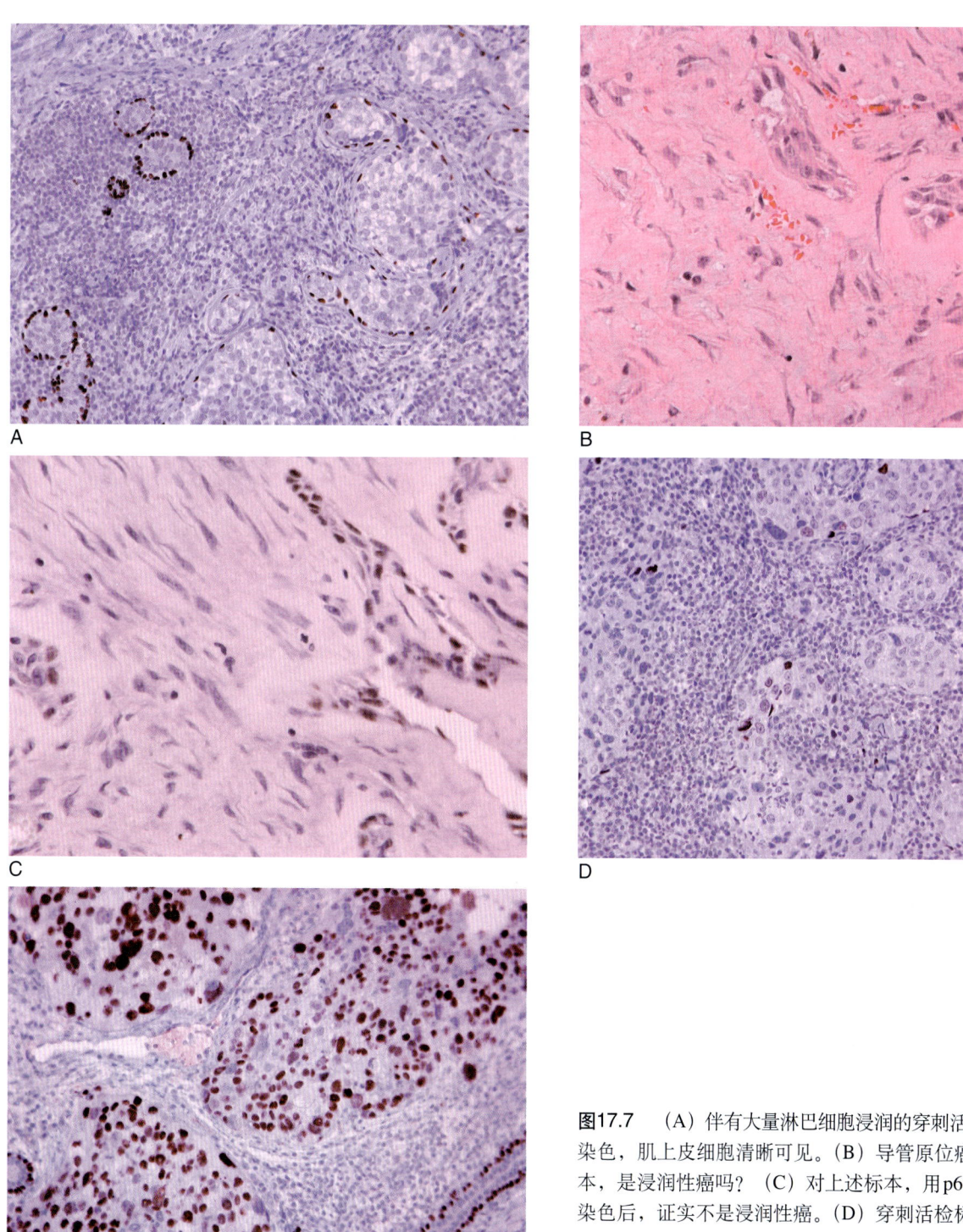

图17.7 （A）伴有大量淋巴细胞浸润的穿刺活检标本，经p63染色，肌上皮细胞清晰可见。（B）导管原位癌的手术切除标本，是浸润性癌吗？（C）对上述标本，用p63进行免疫组化染色后，证实不是浸润性癌。（D）穿刺活检标本，用p63进行免疫组化染色，极少数的肿瘤细胞呈阳性。（E）少数情况下，穿刺活检标本中的绝大多数肿瘤细胞可呈p63阳性

A B

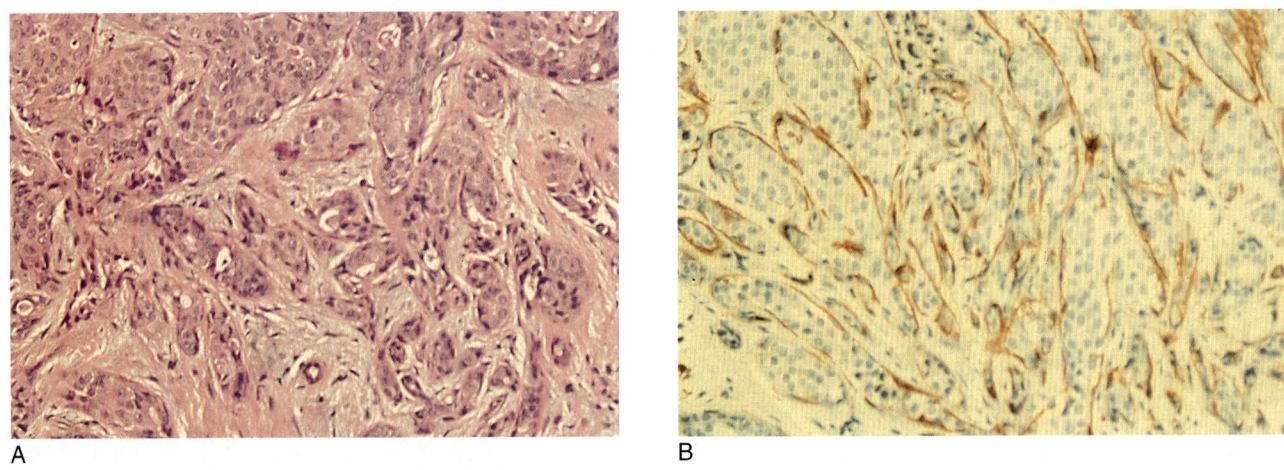

图 17.8 （A）硬化性腺病有时形态学上与癌难以区分，（B）但是经 SMMHC 染色后，可以看到细胞巢周围包绕着肌上皮细胞

A B C D

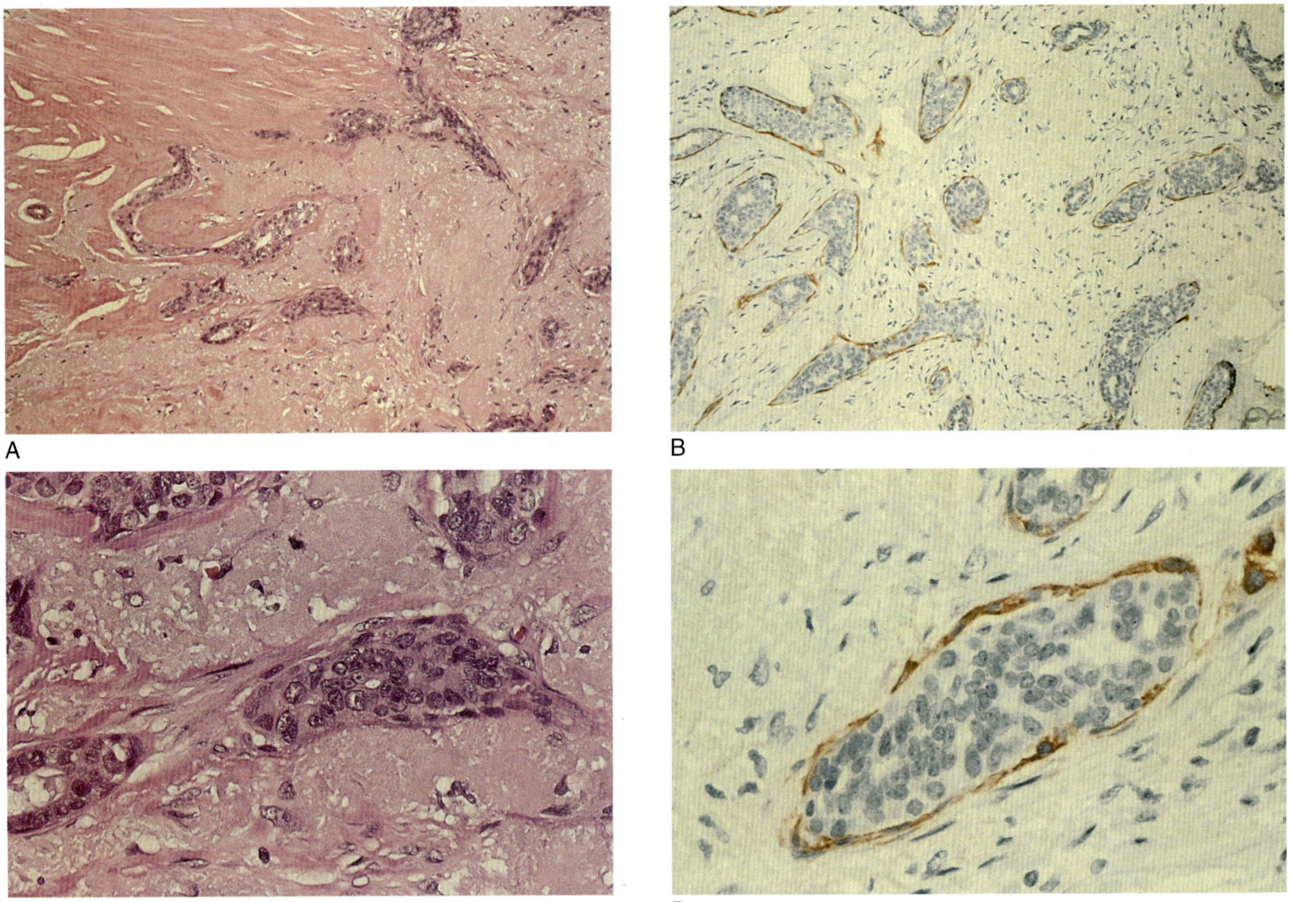

图17.9 （A，C）这是一例放射性瘢痕伴有明显的弹力纤维化，看起来很像癌，（B，D）经SMMHC染色后，肌上皮细胞呈强阳性，提示这是良性病变

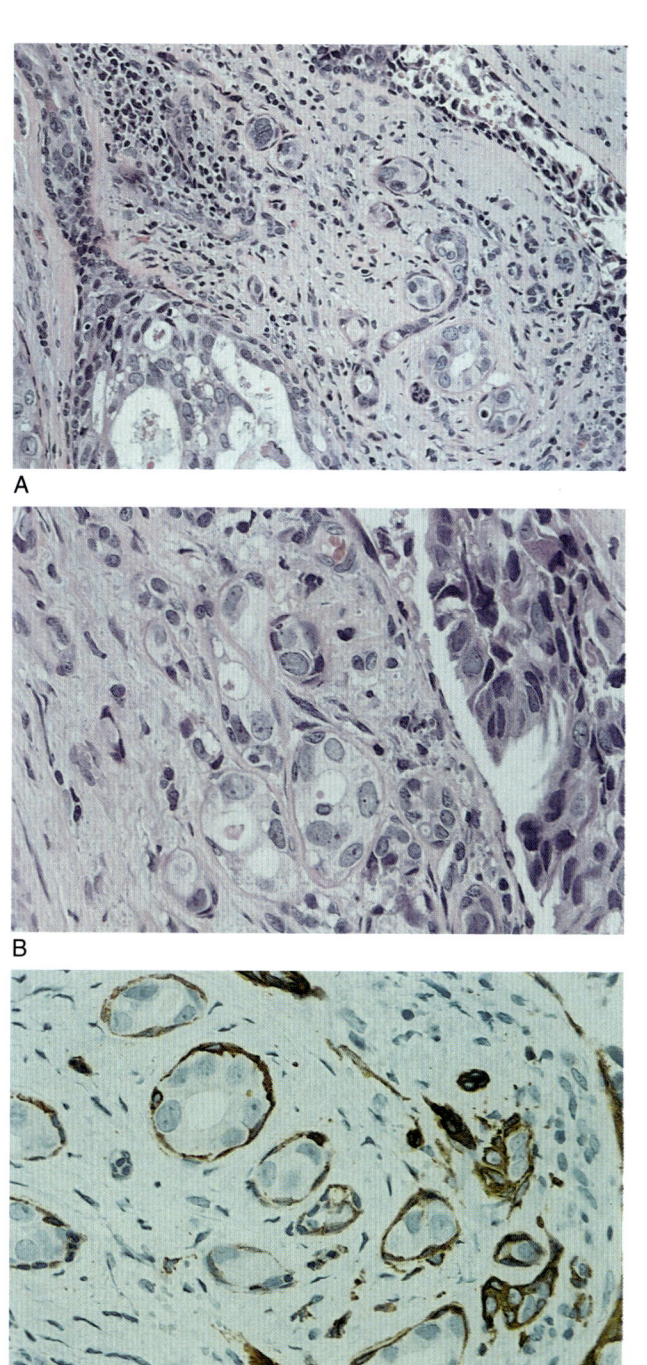
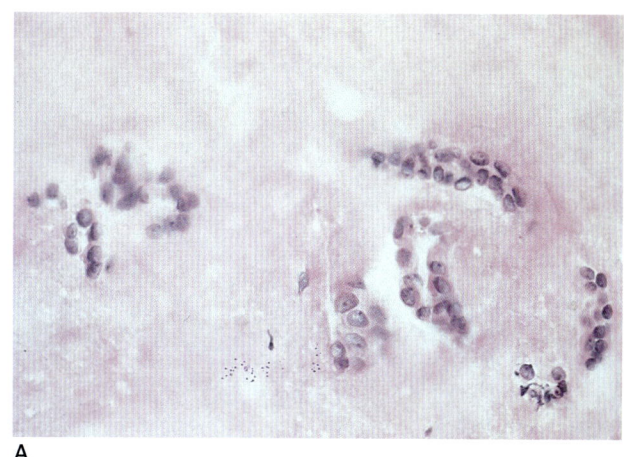
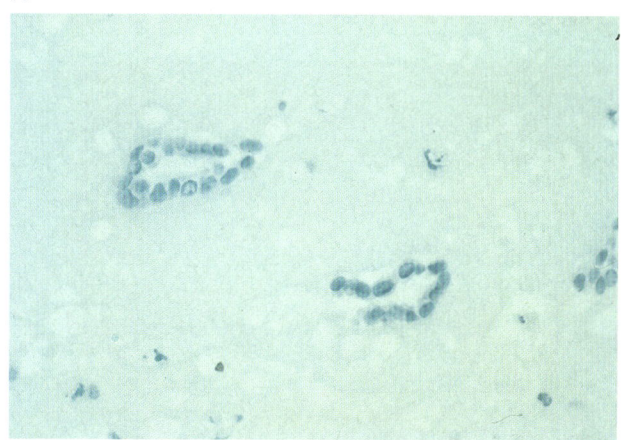
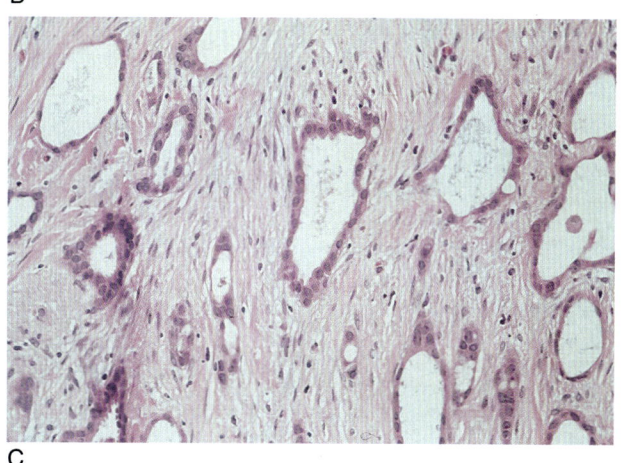

图17.10 （A，B）硬化性腺病中有原位癌形态学上看起来总是很可怕，但诊断是肯定的，（C）但是经SMMHC染色证实存在肌上皮细胞，即可作出上述诊断

图17.11 （A）乳腺穿刺细胞涂片显示异常的小管样结构，（B）SMMHC染色阴性，与小管癌相一致，（C）这一诊断在切除的组织标本中得到了证实

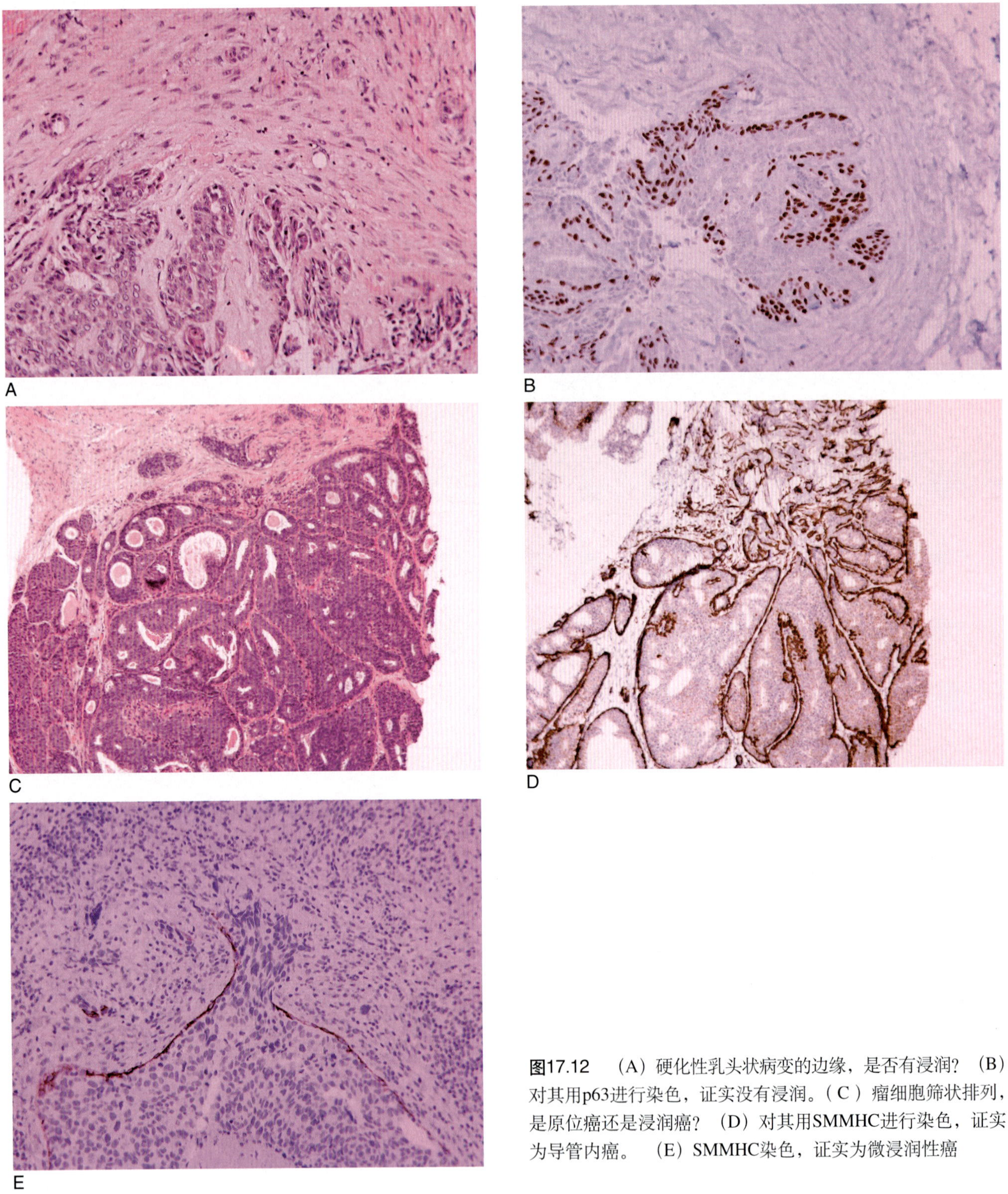

图17.12 （A）硬化性乳头状病变的边缘，是否有浸润？（B）对其用p63进行染色，证实没有浸润。（C）瘤细胞筛状排列，是原位癌还是浸润癌？（D）对其用SMMHC进行染色，证实为导管内癌。（E）SMMHC染色，证实为微浸润性癌

用于标记肌上皮细胞的抗体，如 calponin 和 SMMHC，其显著的缺点是这些抗体均可使肿瘤细胞巢周围的微血管着色。用SMMHC染色后，可见肿瘤细胞巢周围绕以一周阳性细胞，看起来很像是肌上皮细胞（图17.13），但p63染色阴性。经高倍视野观察，可以发现这些 SMMHC 阳性细胞是围绕在肿瘤细胞巢周围的微血管或淋巴管（图 17.14）[35]。

对肌上皮细胞进行免疫组化染色，有助于将3种主要的乳腺良性病变：硬化性腺病、微腺型腺病、管状腺病与小管癌相鉴别（表 17.2）。但更重要的是要对这些病变进行仔细的形态学观察[36]。

除了微腺型腺病以外，经免疫组化染色所有乳腺腺病均可见到肌上皮细胞。微腺型腺病是目前已知的唯一不含有肌上皮细胞的良性病变[37]。Lee和他的同事所描述的管状腺病与微腺型腺病和癌都很相似，管状腺病与微腺型腺病的主要区别在于有肌上皮细胞[38]。微腺型腺病S-100免疫组化染色阳性，而硬化性腺病和小管癌 S-100 阴性。

在乳腺腺病[39,40]内有大汗腺样化生或原位癌病变是不罕见的[37]。如上所述，肌上皮细胞的存在是排除浸润性癌的重要依据。

肌上皮细胞的存在也是乳腺乳头状瘤的显著特点。对于某些难以诊断的病例[41]，做肌上皮细胞免疫组化染色有助于区分导管内乳头状瘤和乳头状癌，因为真正的乳头状癌缺乏肌上皮细胞，因而不会与肌上皮细胞抗体发生反应[12,42]。在一些乳头状瘤的标本中，可以出现"不典型乳头状瘤"的区域，在这些区域内可见导管上皮不典型增生，这种不典型增生比乳头状瘤上皮的生长更加旺盛[43]。经过氧化物酶免疫组化染色[44,45]发现这些不典型增生区域缺乏肌上皮细胞，经K903和CK5/6染色，非典型乳头状瘤和导管内乳头状癌失去了高分子量角蛋白的表达（见下文）。

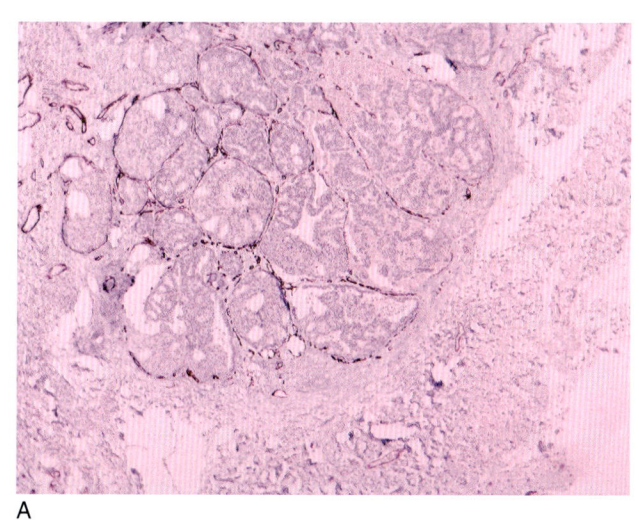

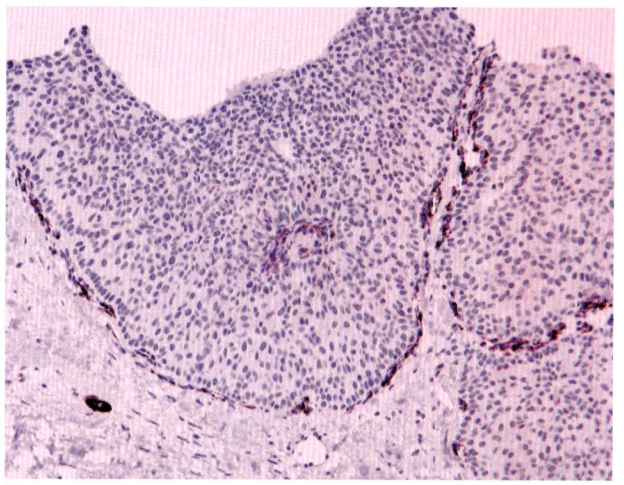

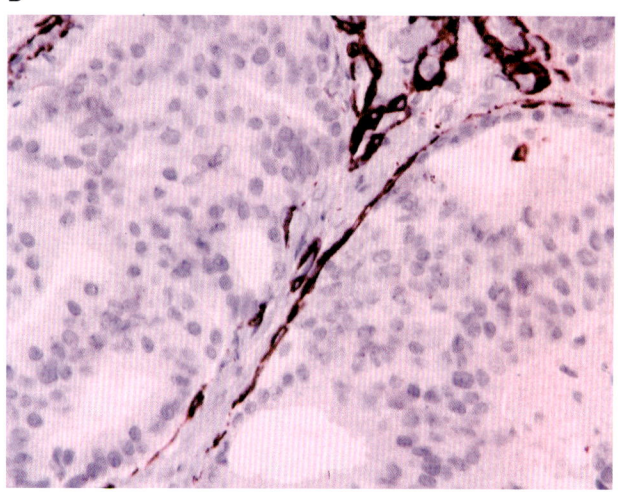

图17.13 （A，B）SMMHC染色低倍镜下观察到癌巢周围有MEC。（C）仔细观察揭示SMMHC阳性的是包绕在癌巢周围的非连续性的血管（注意管腔）

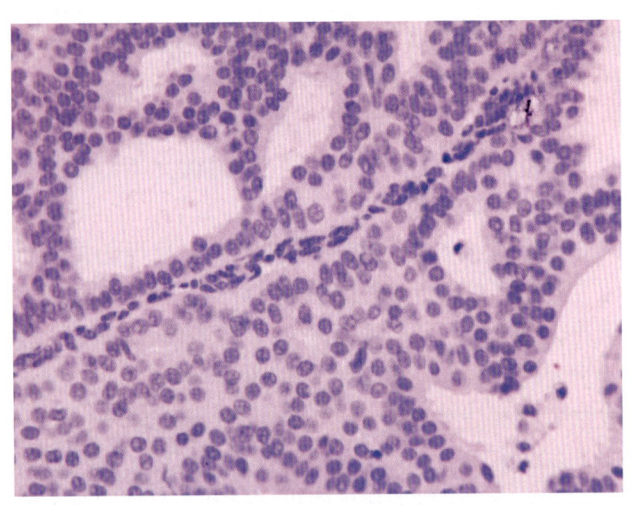

图 17.14 示无 p63 阳性染色，表明图 17.13 没有肌上皮细胞

Ⅳ型胶原是基底膜的组成成分，包绕正常与增生的良性细胞[46]，但其对鉴别浸润性癌似乎意义不大[24,47]。在大多数良性病变中都可检测到Ⅳ型胶原，但是在某些情况下，尤其是在导管原位癌和放射状瘢痕，Ⅳ型胶原的染色常不连续，结果不稳定。在绝大多数情况下，Ⅳ型胶原不连续并不意味着有微浸润。

在腺样囊性癌中（adenoid cystic carcinoma, ACC）肌上皮细胞与肿瘤性增生的上皮细胞均为肿瘤成分（图17.6C和D）。在腺样囊性癌中，肌上皮细胞可见于假筛状结构的筛孔内，而在筛状型的DCIS中，肌上皮细胞只出现在导管的外周。在腺肌上皮瘤中，肌上皮细胞的增生没有固定的形式，多数是作为间质中的细胞，或者与增生的上皮细胞混合存在。

肌上皮细胞肿瘤与原发性肉瘤

肌上皮细胞分化占优势的乳腺肿瘤包括腺肌上皮瘤、肌上皮瘤、肉瘤样癌（化生性癌）和肌上皮细胞癌（myoepithelial cell carcinoma，MECC）[48-51]。虽然大多数腺肌上皮瘤是良性的，但偶尔也可表现为像癌或肌上皮细胞癌那样侵袭性生长[52-55]。这些肿瘤的肌上皮成分免疫标记特征为细胞浆角蛋白 K903、CK5/6 强阳性，细胞核 p63 强阳性（图 17.15）。通常肿瘤细胞 S-100 蛋白阳性表达（90%），也可以表达肌组织的标记物，如calponin（86%）、肌特异性肌动蛋白、结蛋白（14%）和α-平滑肌肌动蛋白（36%）[49,51]。偶尔细胞也会表达 GFAP（46%）[49,51]。与肉瘤样癌

表17.2 小管癌、微腺型腺病、管状腺病和硬化性腺病的鉴别诊断

	组织学	肌上皮细胞	S-100 蛋白	Ⅳ型胶原
小管癌	弥漫性浸润，脂肪浸润 泪滴状开放小管 顶浆突起 间质纤维组织增生	无	无	无
微腺型腺病	弥漫性无结构的排列模式 圆形、开放的小管 无脂肪浸润 无间质纤维组织增生	无	有	有
管状腺病	模糊的小叶状排列模式 伸长的、狭窄的分支状小管 腔内分泌物 可能有脂肪浸润 间质硬化 大汗腺样改变或伴有原位癌成分	有	无	无
硬化性腺病	小叶状排列 常被挤压，没有腺腔 间质硬化 大汗腺样改变或伴有原位癌成分	有	无	无

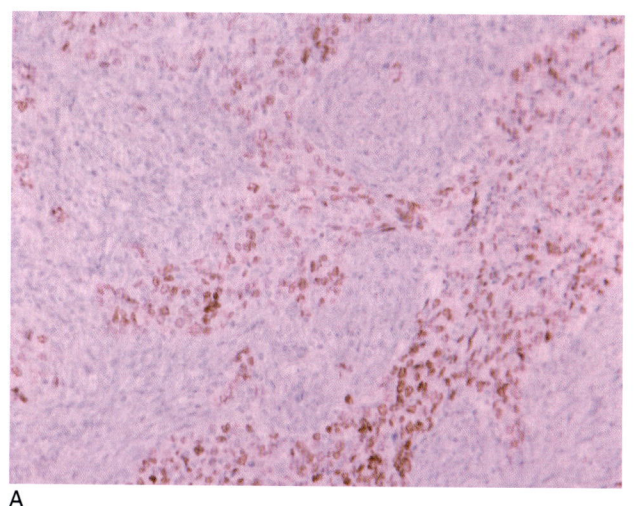 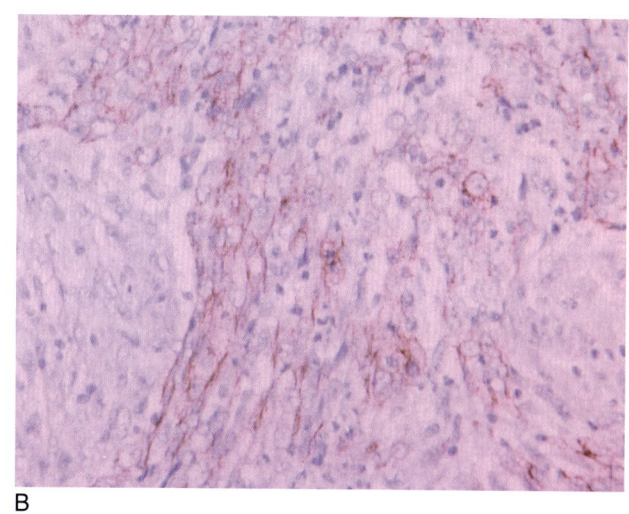

图 17.15 （A）乳腺肉瘤样癌（化生性癌）CK5/6 阳性；（B）肉瘤样癌 p63 通常阳性

不同，平滑肌标记物和 GFAP 表达更支持为单纯性肌上皮分化，而这些标记物在绝大多数肉瘤样癌呈阴性表达[56-59]。平滑肌肌动蛋白的表达是非特异的，不能作为肌上皮细胞分化的肯定性标志物。恶性肌上皮肿瘤也可有不同的异源性组织分化[48]。

肌上皮肿瘤需要与罕见的乳腺原发性梭形细胞肉瘤相鉴别，后者包括纤维肉瘤（波形蛋白阳性）、平滑肌肉瘤和横纹肌肉瘤（肌组织标记物阳性）、滑膜肉瘤（CK7 和 CK19 阳性）[60]、恶性外周神经鞘瘤（S-100 和波形蛋白阳性）和恶性纤维组织细胞瘤（波形蛋白阳性）。虽然这些肿瘤光镜下都有各自的组织学特征，但免疫组化染色有助于鉴别诊断（表 17.3）。

对于罕见的乳腺肌纤维母细胞瘤，可以通过免疫组化染色与肌上皮肿瘤相鉴别。肌纤维母细胞瘤不表达角蛋白、S-100 蛋白和 SMMHC，可以表达 CD34（图 17.16）[64]。

乳腺肉瘤样癌（癌肉瘤、梭形细胞癌、乳腺化生性癌）的免疫表型非常类似于肌上皮细胞，细胞浆内既有低分子量角蛋白 CAM5.2 的弱阳性表达，又有高分子量角蛋白 K903（34βE12）、CK5/6 以及波形蛋白的强阳性表达，而且细胞核 p63（90%）阳性。但是，绝大多数病例没有 GFAP 和平滑肌肌球蛋白重链的表达。由于乳腺化生性癌中常有鳞状上皮分化，从而使上述肿瘤的鉴别诊断变得更加复杂。免疫组化染色肌源性标记物阳性表明是单纯性肌上皮性肿瘤，而不是化生性癌。肉瘤样癌免疫组化标记谱在很大程度上与肌上皮肿瘤一致，所以一些研究者认为肌上皮细胞是化生性癌的前体细胞[59, 65-68]。Leibel[66]最近发表的文章提出，新发现的肌上皮细胞标记物 CD29 和 14-3-3 sigma 也可以出现在化生性癌中，进一步提供了这些肿瘤具有肌上皮细胞性质的证据。乳腺化生性癌中肌上皮细胞分化将为发生在其他器官的肉瘤样癌提供统一的概念。

表 17.3　乳腺肌上皮肿瘤和梭形细胞肉瘤的比较

	CK5/6	K903	p63	GFAP	S-100 蛋白	HHF-35
肌上皮癌	+	S	S	S	+	+
肉瘤样癌	+	+	+	N	N	S
纤维肉瘤	N	N	N	N	N	N
肌源性肉瘤	N	N	R~N	N	N	+
恶性外周神经鞘瘤	N	N	N	N	S	N
滑膜肉瘤	N	N	N	N	R~N	N
恶性纤维组织细胞瘤	N	N	N	N	N	N

+，总是阳性；S，有时阳性；R，很少阳性；N，阴性
GFAP，胶质纤维酸性蛋白

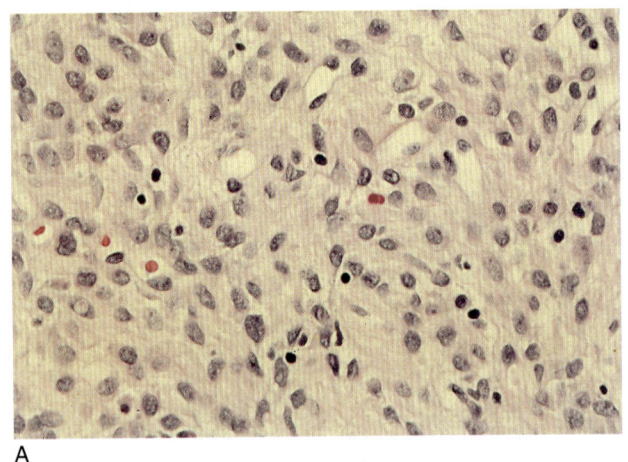
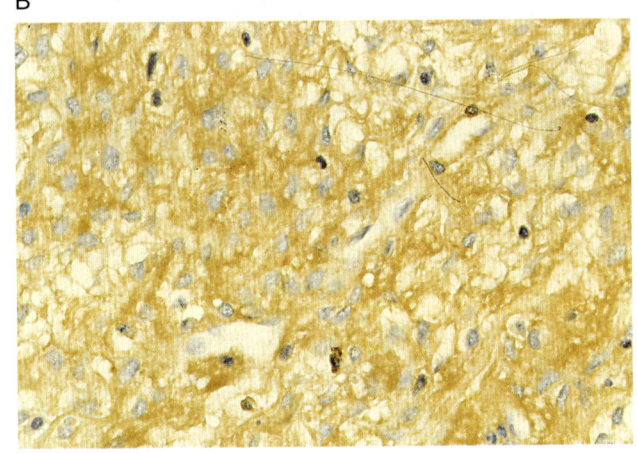

图 17.16 乳腺肌纤维母细胞瘤（A）显示结蛋白阳性（B），肌特异性肌动蛋白（HHF-35）阳性（C）

> **诊断要点：肌上皮肿瘤**
>
> 1. 腺肌上皮瘤是双相性肿瘤，一方面与导管内乳头状瘤相似，另一方面又表现出肌上皮瘤纯梭形细胞的特性。
> 2. 肌上皮分化的免疫组化染色包括 CK5/6、K903、肌特异性肌动蛋白（HHF-35）、GFAP 和 p63。
> 3. 必须仔细地进行组织形态学观察，以鉴别乳腺化生性癌（肉瘤样癌）、肌上皮癌和间叶性肿瘤，如纤维瘤病、平滑肌肉瘤和恶性纤维组织细胞瘤。
> 4. 肉瘤样癌通常有上皮分化，如鳞状上皮成分或原位癌的成分，与单纯性肌上皮肿瘤相比，肉瘤样癌缺乏肌源性标记物表达，但其 K903、CK5/6 染色阳性，p63 也几乎都是阳性表达。
> 5. 单纯性肌上皮肿瘤（肌上皮瘤或肌上皮癌）只有 27% 的病例 p63 染色阳性，27%~36% 的病例 GFAP 阳性，而 S-100 总是阳性。

乳腺微浸润性癌

乳腺微浸润性癌这一概念是指由导管内癌进展而来的早期微小浸润癌，多数是由高级别导管内癌（粉刺型）发展而来[69,70]。乳腺微浸润性癌的早期超微结构研究显示瘤细胞穿过基底膜间隙和间断的肌上皮细胞，但这些改变与光镜水平的浸润并不一致[71]。事实上，多年来有关微浸润癌有着多种概念，至今尚未达成明确一致的定义[69,70,72-77]。

Rosen 提出将微浸润癌这一概念用于单个浸润灶最大直径不超过 1.0mm 的病变[78]。这个定义的关键是，浸润灶是由伴有间质-淋巴细胞反应的不规则浸润巢或单个浸润细胞组成（图17.17）。只有具有这种形态学特征，肌上皮细胞抗体在判断有疑问的浸润灶时才有意义。当导管原位癌累及小叶时，在切片中由于切面不同，有必要做肌上皮细胞免疫染色。

诊断要点：肌上皮细胞抗体在间质浸润中的应用

1. 乳腺增生和硬化性病变周围有肌上皮细胞是良性或非浸润性病变的表现。
2. 肌上皮细胞在乳腺乳头状瘤中呈均匀分布，在细胞过度生长的导管不典型性增生和癌中逐渐消失。
3. SMMHC 和 p63 抗体是显示肌上皮细胞最好的标记物，尤其是在结缔组织增生的硬化性病变中。
4. 导管内癌很少有肌上皮细胞缺失，尤其是用 SMMHC 和 p63 抗体标记时。
5. 肌上皮细胞抗体对诊断乳腺微浸润癌起决定性作用，尤其是对不超过1mm的病灶，外形不规则，有间质反应，有单一的浸润细胞，或以上3种病变并存时。
6. 浸润性癌：SMMHC 和 p63 阴性。
7. 腺病/良性增生/硬化性病变：SMMHC 和 p63 阳性。
8. 微腺型腺病：SMMHC 阴性，S-100 阳性。
9. 注意：血管壁 SMMHC 染色可以阳性，与 p63 联合应用可以避免误判。

导管上皮增生性病变和原位癌

乳腺增生病变和原位癌中细胞角蛋白的表达有所不同[21, 79-82]。34βE12抗体可以识别CK1、CK5、CK10和CK14，这些角蛋白主要存在于导管来源的上皮细胞和鳞状上皮。正常乳腺的肌上皮细胞和腔缘细胞表达34βE12，普通型增生的导管上皮也表达，但非典型增生导管上皮的表达程度明显降低，而81%~100%导管原位癌没有34βE12表达（图17.18、17.19），但个别细胞可以阳性[79, 80, 82]。

CAM5.2 标记在大多数 DCIS 中呈现均匀一致的阳性，反应出从高分子量角蛋白到单纯性角蛋白8和18表达的变化。34βE12 在 DCIS 和 ADH 中的免疫组化染色特点相似，所以无助于这两者之间的鉴别[82]，但是有助于鉴别组织形态学上难以区别的导管上皮旺炽性增生与 DCIS。由于 D5.16B4 克隆抗体 CK5/6 在 DCIS 中几乎完全不表达，所以对 DCIS 的形态学诊断更为特异[83]。

乳头状增生性病变的诊断尤其困难。好在乳头状增生性病变细胞角蛋白的免疫组化表达与导管增生性病变相同，细胞角蛋白的免疫组化可以对导管内乳头状癌，包括结节性实性变型，与导管上皮旺炽性增生进行鉴别[84]。相反，80%~100% 小叶原位癌（lobular carcinoma in situ，LCIS）34βE12呈核周阳性染色，而 DCIS 很少阳性，但两者 CK5/6 染色均为阴性（表 17.4）。

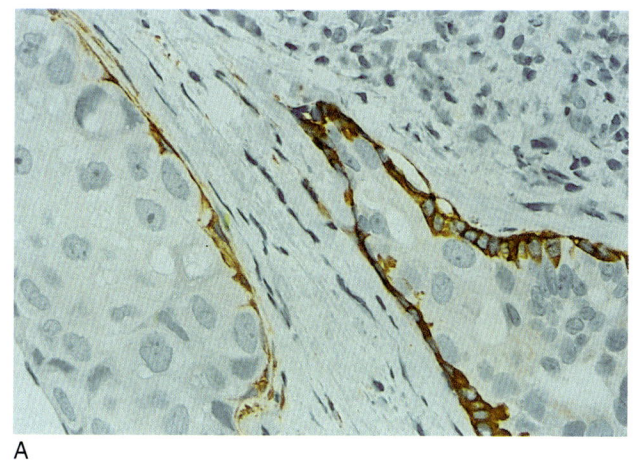
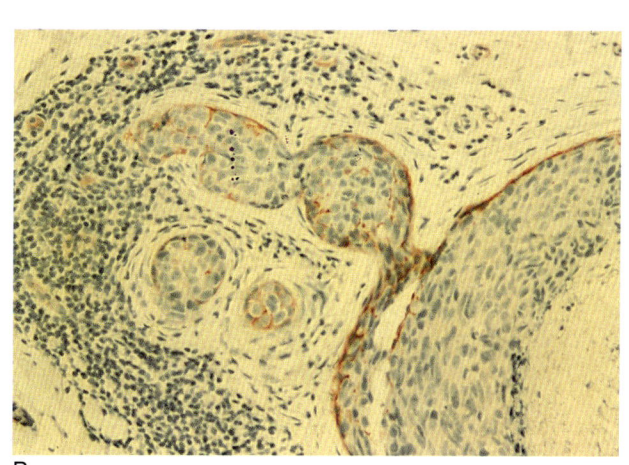

A　　　　　　　　　　　　　　　B

图17.17 （A，B）浸润性不规则病灶的鉴别诊断；SMMHC染色示肌上皮细胞阳性，排除了浸润癌

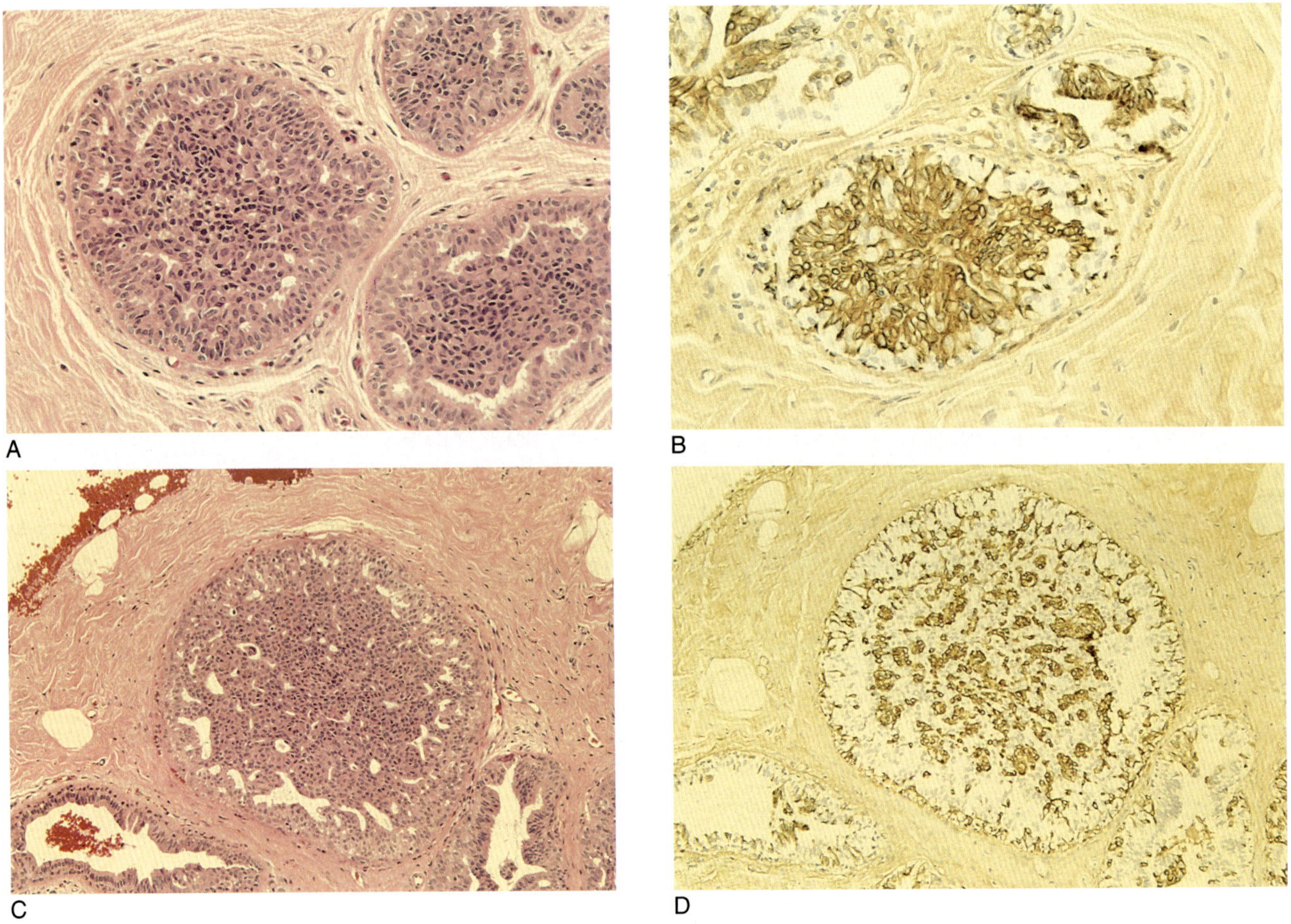

图 17.18　旺炽性导管上皮增生的病例（A，C）示典型的角蛋白 903（34βE12）强阳性表达（B，D）

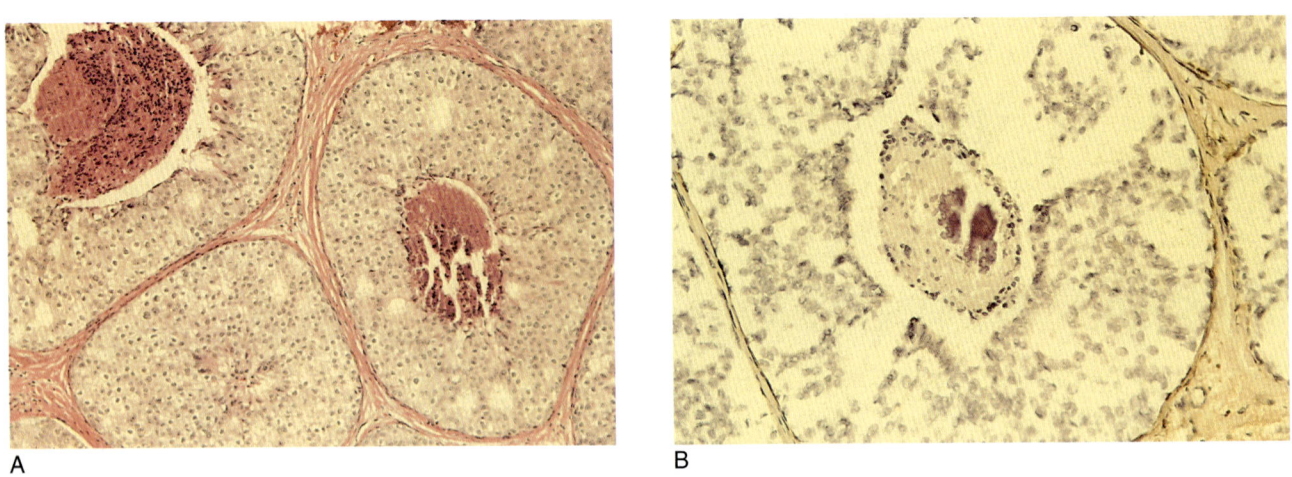

图 17.19　导管原位癌（A）角蛋白 903（34βE12）通常为阴性（B）

表17.4　乳腺上皮增生中高分子量角蛋白的表达

细胞角蛋白	DEH	ADEH	DCIS	LCIS
34βE12	4+	1+	Rare	3~4+
CK5/6	4+	1+	Neg	Neg

DEH：导管上皮增生，ADEH：不典型性导管上皮增生，DCIS：导管原位癌，LCIS：小叶原位癌
半定量范围，0~4+；Rare，很少阳性；Neg，阴性

诊断要点：增生性病变和原位癌中角蛋白的表达

1. 乳腺导管旺炽性增生中34βE12和CK5/6呈强阳性表达，有助于导管旺炽性增生和乳头状瘤与ADH/DCIS的鉴别。
2. 与34βE12抗体相比，CK5/6在DCIS中几乎或完全不表达。
3. 结合显微镜下组织形态学，34βE12或CK5/6可以帮助鉴别DCIS和旺炽性增生，而且对鉴别乳头状瘤和导管内乳头状癌也有帮助。

乳腺 Paget 病

Paget病可以发生在乳腺或者乳腺外器官。乳腺Paget病几乎总是提示存在乳腺组织内癌，可以是原位癌或浸润性癌[85-87]，而乳腺外Paget病则有可能是转移癌的征兆。

乳腺Paget病表现为乳头表皮内CK7阳性的恶性瘤细胞浸润。肿瘤细胞散在或成簇地浸润于表皮内，细胞体积大，胞浆丰富，印戒样，有时黏蛋白阳性（图17.20A~D）。表皮角质形成细胞CK7阴性。多数Paget病例CK7阳性，乳腺组织特异性的大囊肿病液体蛋白-15（gross cystic disease fluid protein-15，GCDFP-15）阳性，多克隆癌胚抗原（polyclonal carcinoembryonic antigen，pCEA）阳性，偶有病例可能CK7阴性。Paget细胞也可以通过检测雌激素受体[88]和HER/neu癌基因蛋白而加以确定[89]。

Toker细胞CK7阳性，这种细胞也可见于正常乳头的皮肤中，与Paget细胞相比，Toker细胞没有那么醒目，细胞学无异型性[90]，一般不会引起诊断困难。基于免疫表型相似，有人认为上皮内Paget细胞可能起源于Toker细胞[91]。在乳头的旺炽性乳头状瘤的患者也可以在表皮中发现一些CK7阳性细胞，在诊断乳头的Paget病时要注意此类陷阱[87,92]。另外，乳头导管的表皮内区也可以有CK7阳性细胞，应注意与Paget病相鉴别（图17.20E）[93]。

由于恶性黑色素瘤不表达任何类型的角蛋白，而且HMB-45或melan-A阳性，所以容易鉴别，实际上，乳头的恶性黑色素瘤是非常少见的。

乳腺的Paget样鳞状细胞癌（即Bowen病）很少见，应与Paget病相鉴别。Bowen病肿瘤细胞CK7阴性，K903阳性，p16阳性，而Paget病这些抗体的染色结果恰恰相反（图17.21）[94]。

偶尔在大导管中可以见到假Paget病。上皮内有大的组织细胞浸润，形成类似于Paget病的图像。这些大细胞CK7阴性而CD68强阳性（图17.22）。

诊断要点：乳腺 Paget 病

1. CK7+、GCDFP-15+、pCEA+。
2. 陷阱：在旺炽性增生的乳头导管内乳状瘤的表皮内有CK7+细胞。
3. Paget样Bowen病CK7-、p16+。

腋窝淋巴结微转移癌

历史上，对乳腺癌患者局部肿块切除或乳房切除的同时进行腋窝淋巴结清扫的目的是为临床分期和决定是否需要辅助化学治疗提供信息。尽管切除腋窝受累的淋巴结能更有效地控制局部复发，但完全腋窝淋巴结切除术（complete axillary lymph node dissection，CALND）也许并不能改变整个疾病的进程，而且这种手术还会引起上肢活动受限、疼痛和慢性淋巴水肿等。

前哨淋巴结（sentinel lymph node，SLN）这一概念是Cabanas[95]在研究阴茎癌时提出来的。最早的有关前哨淋巴结转移（sentinel lymph node metastasis，SLNM）的研究是针对黑色素瘤病人，目的是防止大范围淋巴结的切除对病人造成运动障碍。通过对黑色素瘤病人前哨淋巴结的研究发现，淋巴结的转移进程有其规律性，即转移细胞首先转移至前哨淋巴结，然后再进一步转移至远处淋巴结[96]。现在，同样的理论也被用于乳腺癌病人。在计划手术切除之前可以采用注射放射性同位素和蓝色染料的方式寻找前哨淋巴

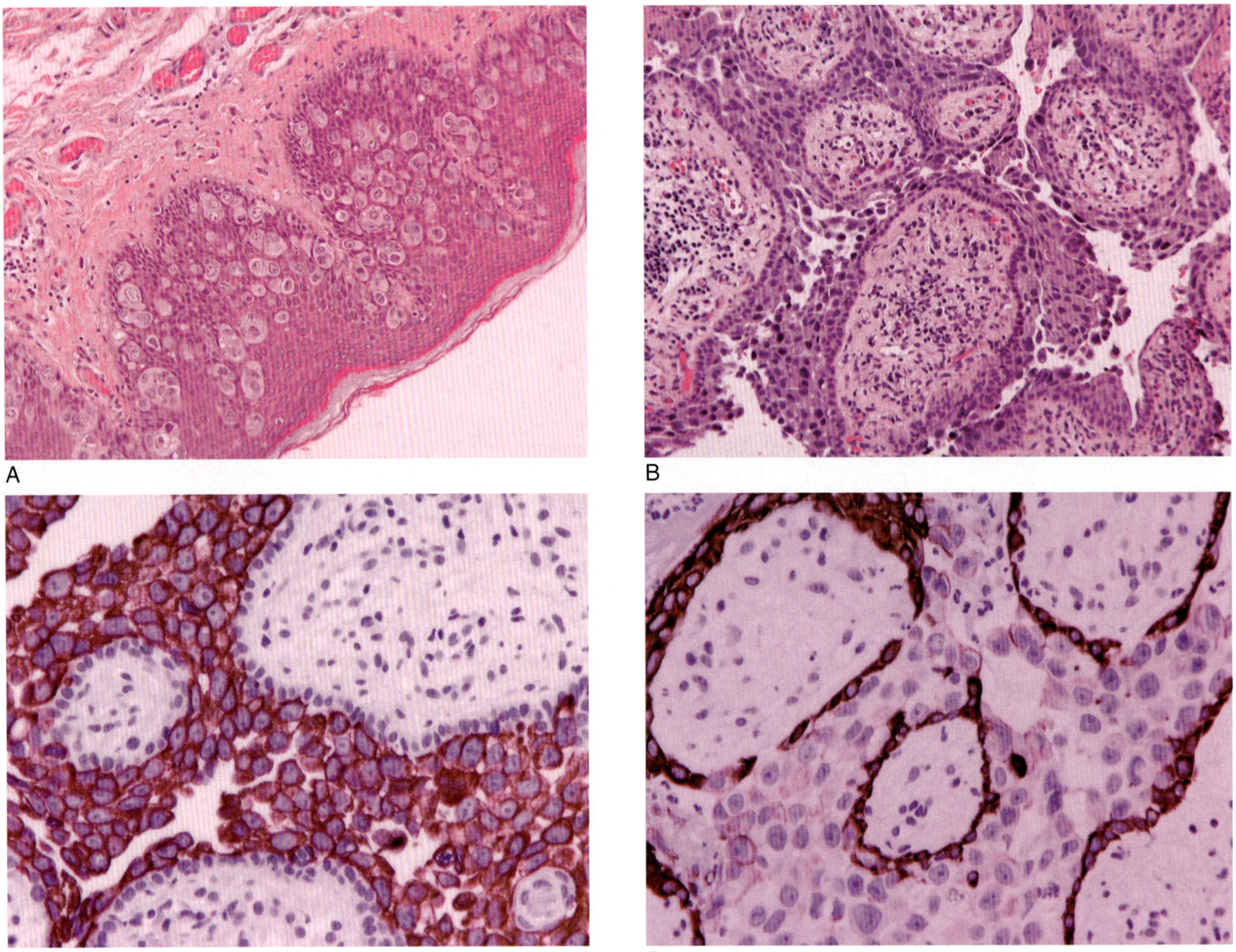

A B C D

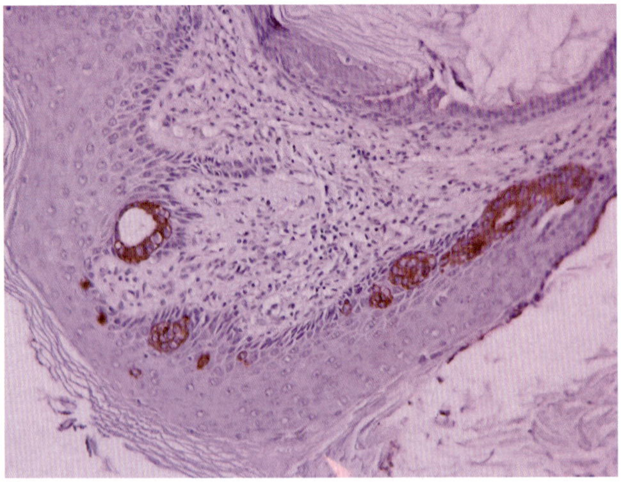

E

图17.20 （A）经典的乳头Paget病，表皮中散在肿瘤细胞；（B）乳头Paget病呈假乳头状图像；（C）Paget病肿瘤细胞CK7染色阳性，角质形成细胞阴性；（D）Paget 细胞 K903 阴性，而角质形成细胞阳性；（E）乳头腺瘤的细胞可以累及表皮并且 CK7 染色阳性，应注意与 Paget 病相鉴别

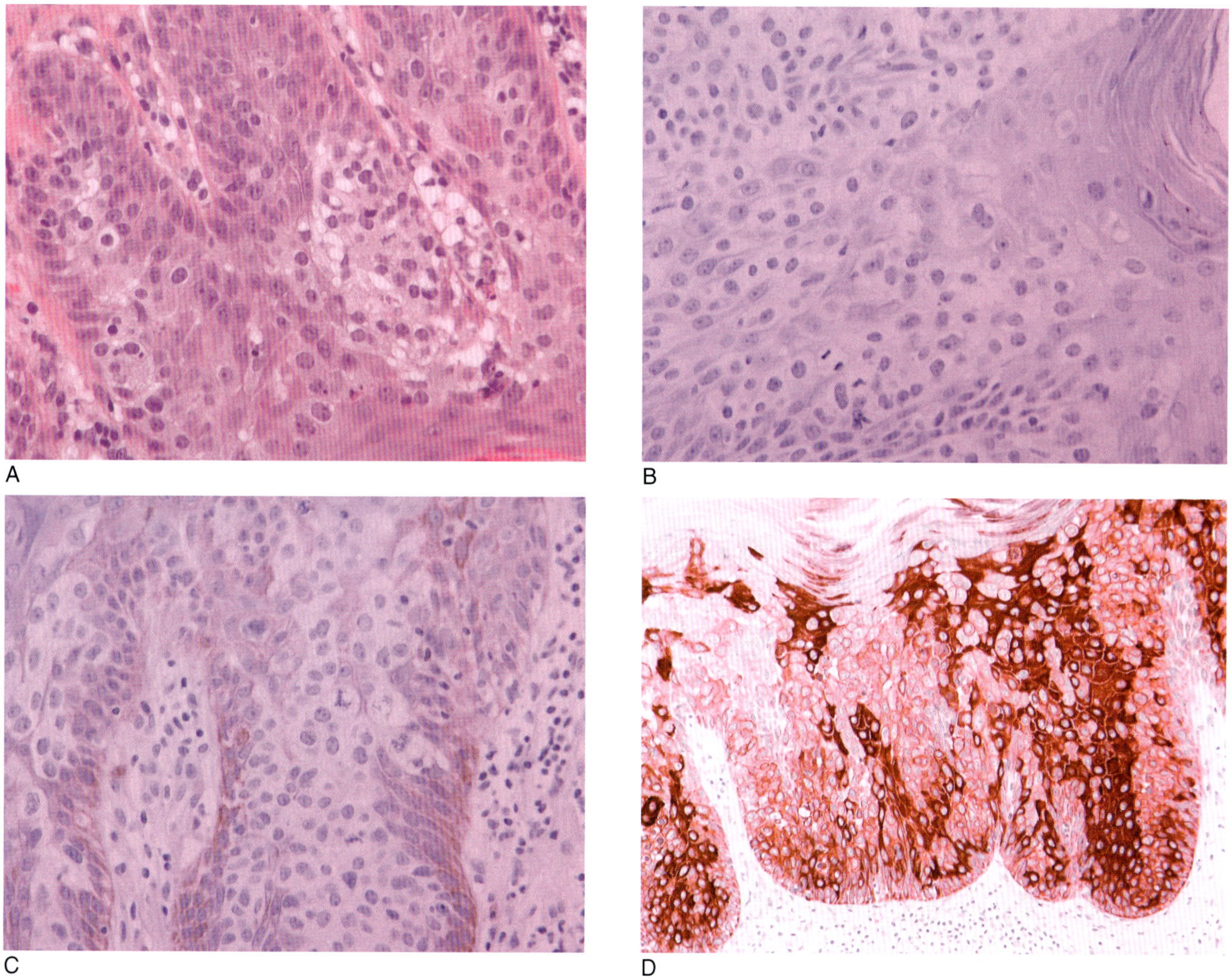

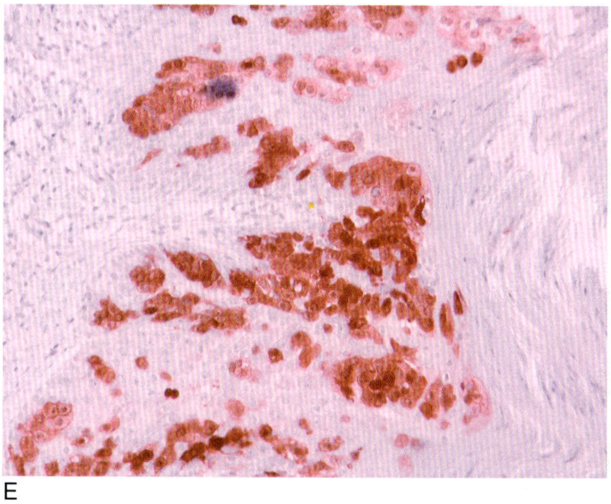

图17.21 （A）乳头皮肤中聚集着非典型淡染的细胞，病人有乳腺癌病史；（B）乳腺Paget样Bowen病，淡染的细胞CK7阴性；（C）表皮内淡染的细胞K903也阴性；（D）与角质形成细胞相比较，非典型细胞显示CK5/6着色；（E）Paget样细胞p16强阳性，确诊为Bowen病

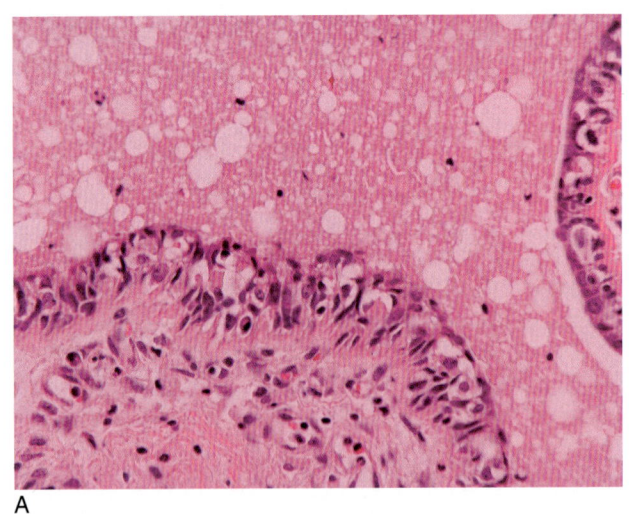
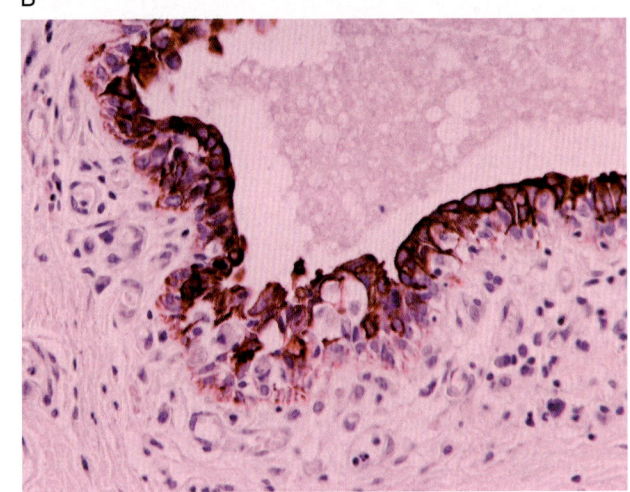

图 17.22 （A）导管扩张症伴假 Paget 病的大导管，（B）镶嵌于导管上皮中的大而透亮的细胞CD68阳性，（C）CK7阴性

结。通过可视性染料与手术中放射性同位素扫描相结合确定前哨淋巴结，将其摘取送检进行病理学检查。目前认为：如果是前哨淋巴结阴性的病人，腋窝清扫是没有必要的，但如果是前哨淋巴结阳性的病人，腋窝清扫术可以减少将来局部复发的可能性。鉴于存在以下几个实质性的问题，在这一方面仍存有争议：

1. 腋窝淋巴结微转移癌（MM）的自然进程是什么？

2. 前哨淋巴结微转移癌是临床出现腋窝局部复发的必然途径吗？

3. 前哨淋巴结微转移癌是辅助性化疗的指征吗？

4. 对切除的前哨淋巴结应该如何进行病理检查？

5. 前哨淋巴结微转移癌会对总生存率有影响吗？

6. 对某一特定患者，微转移癌能作为判断生物学行为的预测参数吗？

7. 能否识别出前哨淋巴结内"良性输送"（benign transport）的上皮成分？

这些问题对于乳腺癌病人的治疗都是非常关键和有意义的。美国癌症联合委员会（AJCC）将淋巴结微转移癌定义为瘤细胞簇不超过 2mm。最近十多年随访结果的研究认为，与淋巴结阴性患者相比，微转移癌患者无瘤生存率和总生存率有所降低，虽然差别很小但有统计学意义[97]，但尚不能作为独立的预后因素[98]。综合转移灶的大小、肿瘤的大小和其他因素一起或许能对病人将来复发的危险性作出预测。正在进行的临床试验将最终决定与病人预后有关的淋巴结转移灶的大小到底是多少。

在多数医疗机构，局部肿块切除术和乳房切除术加前哨淋巴结活检已经成为常规方法。绝大多数前哨淋巴结转移都是在被送检的前3个前哨淋巴结内发现的[99]。

对临床病理学家来说，对前哨淋巴结进行恰当的检查和分类是非常重要的，但这一方面也存在某些争议。

当前对淋巴结的标准取材[100]是肉眼下间隔2mm连续切开，两张切片做苏木精-伊红（HE）染色，一张切片做角蛋白的免疫组化染色。虽然大多数实验室都是采用这种方法，但是对整个前哨淋巴结进行大量切片的方法已经证明可以大大提高微转移癌的检出率，46%的T1期病人有前哨淋巴结微转移癌[101, 102]。Dowlatshahi等采用这种方法[102]，即垂直于前哨淋巴结的长轴间隔2mm将其切开，做一张HE染色切片，然后再每隔0.25mm对其余组织块进行切片并全部做HE染色和角蛋白免疫组织化学染色。他们认为对淋巴结在0.25mm的水平上进行检查是可行的，并且能够检测出所有的0.25mm的微转移灶[103]。

当前，尚无一致的最恰当的前哨淋巴结检测方法。最经济的方案还要等待临床试验的结果而定[104]。初步的数据显示，前哨淋巴结微转移灶并没有改变病人的预后，但毕竟随访时间太短，不足以用来下决定性的结论[105]。某些病理学术团体认为，在有关"仅有细胞角蛋白阳性的淋巴结微转移灶是否有意义"的实验数据出来之前，并不需要将角蛋白作为临床的常规检测指标。

当对前哨淋巴结进行细胞角蛋白免疫组化染色时，应该采用联合的细胞角蛋白抗体，如AE1/AE3的联合应用；不要用CAM5.2，因为它可以显示淋巴结中的树突状细胞[103]。其他角蛋白的联合应用也是可以的[106]。微转移灶瘤细胞簇的直径小于2mm，聚集在淋巴结或被膜下的淋巴窦内（图17.23），这需要和淋巴结内散在于间质内的树突状细胞相鉴别，因为这些树突状细胞角蛋白也呈阳性染色[107, 108]。确定淋巴结微转移的部位（被膜下淋巴窦和淋巴结实质内淋巴窦）是否有临床意义，仍需对大量病人进行研究。

Carter等[109]描述腋窝淋巴结被膜下淋巴窦内可以出现乳腺上皮细胞的聚集，并认为这是在乳腺活检之后"机械性运输"的结果。也有观点认为空芯针活检本身或注射同位素/染料后的乳房按摩会导致细胞机械性地移位到前哨淋巴结[110, 111]。孤立的角蛋白阳性细胞可以被输送到前哨淋巴结，但真正良性运输的主要组织学特点是CK阳性细胞与变形的红细胞、含铁血黄素还有巨噬细胞一起被输送到前哨淋巴结（图17.24）。Diaz[112]就曾在一名单纯DCIS的病人的皮肤真皮淋巴管和前哨淋巴结中发现过良性的上皮组织。这为"良性机械性运输"的概念提供了形态学的证据。

孤立的角蛋白阳性细胞的报道也不尽相同。在作者的单位，我们通过显微分级装置可以精确测量到0.25mm的瘤细胞聚集灶。也有人报道过更小的聚集灶以及病灶的数量和每个病灶中有多少个细胞。

> **诊断要点：前哨淋巴结微转移病变**
>
> 1. 间隔2mm将淋巴结连续切开，进行HE染色和AE1/AE3联合染色。
> 2. 在许多医疗机构中，前哨淋巴结检查已被作为常规方法。
> 3. 当送检多个前哨淋巴结时，97%的前哨淋巴结微转移灶会在前3个前哨淋巴结中发现。
> 4. "良性输送"的标志是角蛋白阳性细胞与变形的红细胞、含铁血黄素及巨噬细胞混合存在。

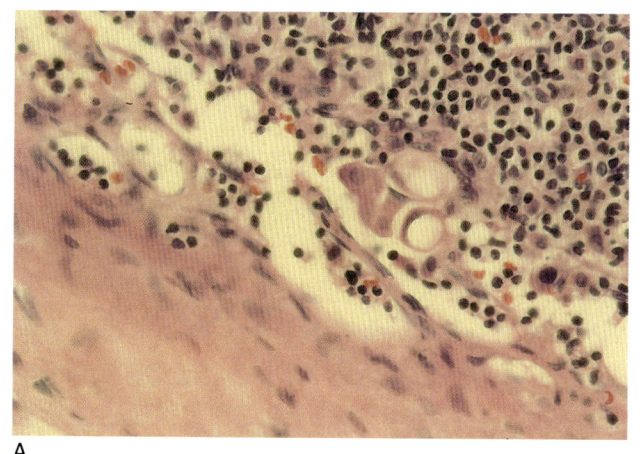
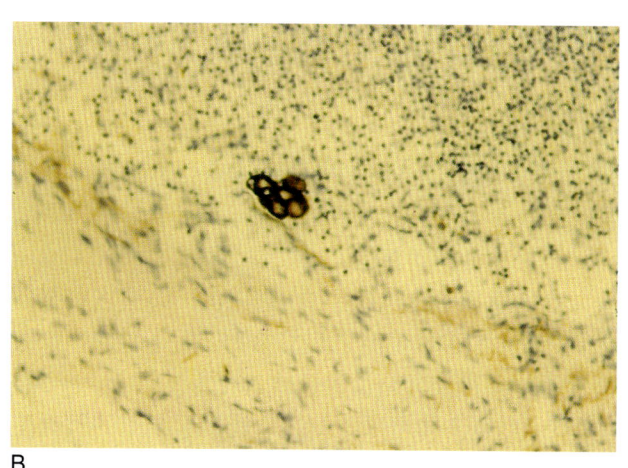

图17.23 （A）淋巴结被膜下窦内异型的瘤细胞 （B）角蛋白染色阳性，与光镜下微转移癌相一致

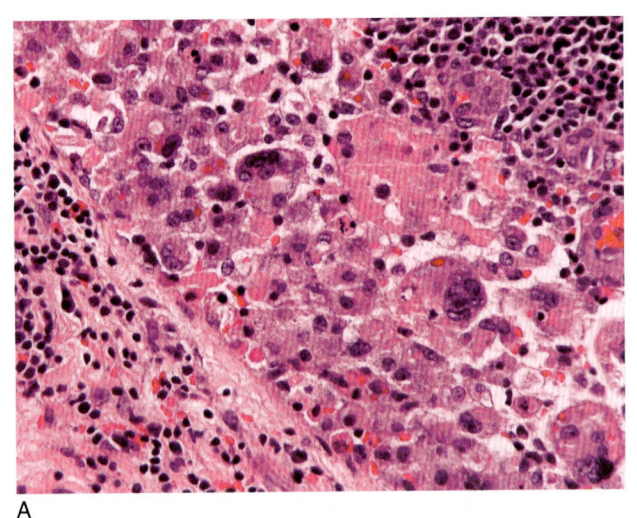
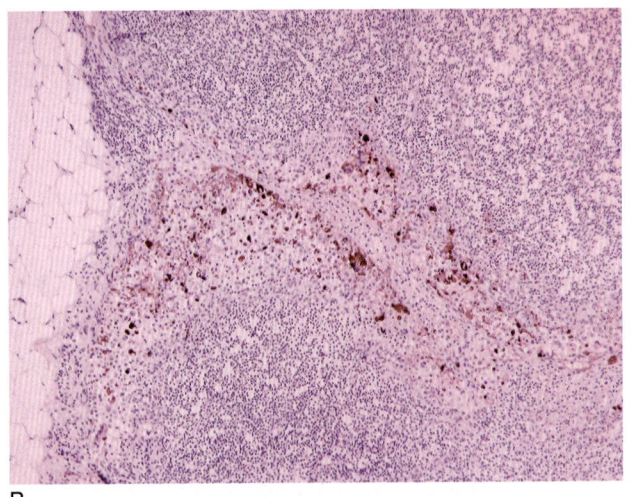
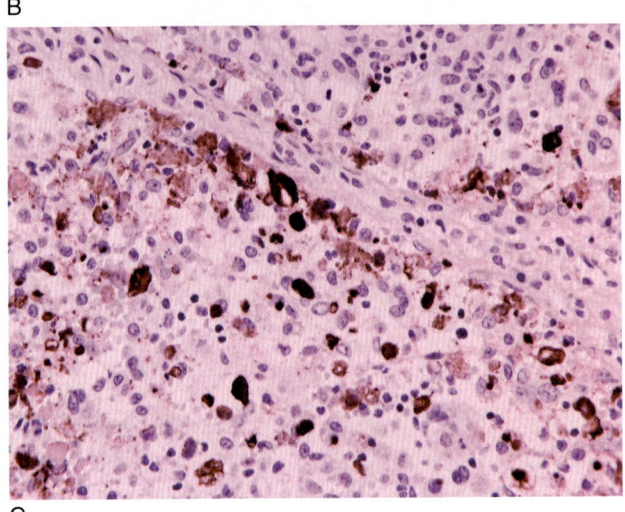

图 17.24 （A）前哨淋巴结淋巴窦中的巨细胞、巨噬细胞、破碎的红细胞和上皮细胞。（B）低倍镜下在图 A 淋巴窦内的角蛋白阳性细胞，（C）高倍镜下显示角蛋白阳性细胞与破碎的巨噬细胞和变性的红细胞共存

导管癌和小叶癌

E-钙黏素

　　E-钙黏素（ECAD）是钙依赖性跨膜蛋白，对细胞与细胞之间的黏附起重要作用，使细胞彼此黏附在一起。某些研究认为肿瘤抑制基因ECAD的缺失会降低细胞间的黏附性[113-115]，促进肿瘤转移而降低生存率[116-126]。细胞膜强而清晰的免疫着色方式可以证实导管上皮细胞之间存在 ECAD。

　　ECAD 的编码基因 *CDH1* 是定位于 16q22.1 的一个较大的基因。ECAD蛋白由胞浆区、跨膜区和胞外区构成。ECAD在细胞之间的黏附作用还要依赖于细胞膜下胞浆内连环蛋白复合体（分为 α、β、γ 3种亚型），此复合体可以将 ECAD 连接于细胞的肌动蛋白骨架上。连环蛋白或ECAD基因表达异常会导致各种病理性的 ECAD 免疫组化染色。

　　某些学者[115, 120, 127, 128]的早期研究显示在导管癌中存在钙黏素，而小叶癌中则缺乏钙黏素[129]。用ECAD染色来区分导管癌和小叶癌在一定程度上尚存在争议，但也有人认为这种方法很有效。

　　*CDH1*基因表现为特征性的双等位基因突变，该基因的异常表达必须是两个基因均有突变。小叶肿瘤普遍存在 16.22.1 的杂合性缺失，但这一点在导管肿瘤中同样也很常见。但是在LCIS中，*CDH1*基因（第二个等位基因）也会因为移码插入、缺失及无意义突变而失活，最终产生截短的 ECAD 蛋白[130-138]。在多数情况下，免疫组化染色截短的ECAD蛋白位于胞外区，结果无论是小叶原位癌还是浸润性小叶癌，都缺乏细胞膜清晰的ECAD免疫组化着色。ECAD等位基因突变是小叶肿瘤形成过程中的早期事件，表现为细胞膜的染色缺失，而ECAD等位基因突变在导管癌中是极罕见的。导致 *CDH1* 异常突变包括杂合性缺失（占80%）和高度甲基化（占20%）。突变产生截短的ECAD产物不能使相邻的细胞黏合在一起，失去黏附

性的细胞在组织学上呈弥散性分布，ECAD免疫组化染色完全丧失（例如经典的浸润性小叶癌）（图17.25）。某些研究表明细胞的这种弥散性分布模式与疾病的进一步扩散和进展有关。免疫组织学上ECAD的染色类型依赖于ECAD突变发生的部位。膜染色的缺失可能伴有胞浆的颗粒性染色（图17.26A~C），表明胞浆内存在截短蛋白的可溶性部分。近端的截短突变导致ECAD与连环蛋白复合体结合不稳定，表达截短的ECAD蛋白，表现为灶性或点状的细胞膜免疫染色（图17.26D,E）。小叶原位癌细胞有ECAD灶性细胞膜染色的病人同侧乳腺发生DCIS的危险性增加[139]。连环蛋白复合体的突变也可以导致ECAD的功能丧失和细胞膜染色缺失[140, 141]。作为LOH的结果，*CDH1*基因缺失也可见于导管癌，但这不是早期事件，与通常发生于小叶肿瘤的点突变无关。膜染色强度减弱或灶性膜染色也可见于高级别导管癌，所以只有细胞膜染色完全缺失才能被视为小叶肿瘤。

免疫组化和分子生物学的方法不仅有助于诊断，在某种程度上还要求诊断者从一种崭新的视角去看待已熟识的形态学。图17.27就很好地说明了这一点。所有的以"单行线状"方式浸润伴有低级别核的浸润性乳腺癌不一定都是小叶癌，因为浸润性导管癌也有这种浸润方式。

从形态学上估计是导管癌还是小叶癌存有争议，而且也有其局限性。经典型浸润性小叶癌（infiltrating lobular carcinoma，ILC）由均匀一致的小细胞构成，胞浆淡染，有浆细胞样的特点，生长方式完全是非黏附性的。大体上乳腺组织（或X线照片）相对正常，镜下形态学却可以是广泛弥散浸润的经典型小叶癌。这些肿瘤细胞ECAD阴性，并伴有全身性转移的特点[142]。浸润性导管癌（invasive ductal carcinoma，IDC）也可以表现出小叶癌的一些生长模式，例如肿瘤细胞的单行线状排列，靶环状排列，局部失去黏附性。虽然这种模式有一定的迷惑性，但是很容易由ECAD免疫组化染色来鉴别。对于形态学上介于小叶型和导管型之间的乳腺癌类型，绝大多数都可以通过ECAD染色来确定其类型，有一小部分是属于小叶-导管混合型癌，也可以通过ECAD来明确[143-145]。要注意肌上皮细胞ECAD染色也阳性，这可能会导致误将LCIS诊断为DCIS（图17.25）。

有人认为鉴别LCIS/ILC和DCIS/IDC有重要的治疗意义[115]。是否有必要通过空芯针活检鉴别出LCIS/ILC和IDIS/IDC仍存在争议。LCIS被视为危险因子，并不像DCIS那样属于癌前病变，但是对于这一理论的关注度和争议也越来越多。

通过一个小样本的回顾性调查研究[146-161]，也包括作者本人所做的工作提示：在空芯针活检诊断为LCIS中与诊断为非典型性导管上皮增生者的切除活检标本中浸润癌的发生率是相近似的。

最近Elsheikh对33个病人作了回顾性和前瞻性研究，通过空芯针活检诊断为LCIS的病人做肿块切除，术后发现有31%是浸润性癌，局部切除术后有25%为浸润癌或DCIS[162]。Page[163]提供的数据表明在活检发现LCIS患者的同侧乳腺发生乳腺癌的危险性增加了3倍。此外，在同一张切片上LCIS与ILC并存也是很常见的。在LCIS中出现的分子异常也可在邻近的ILC中观察到[164]。但这些信息还是有限的，须有更多的研究结果加以证实。

在某些研究中心，标准的程序是先穿刺活检诊断ILC（需要ECAD染色）后，再获得MRI信息。其理论依据是外科医生认为浸润性小叶癌很难确定肿瘤边缘，这样做将有助选择适合于乳房重造的患者。

单从形态学来鉴别浸润性导管癌（IDC）和浸润性小叶癌（ILC）以及LCIS和DCIS的可重复性还不尽理想。ILC和IDC、LCIS和DCIS之间可能有本质上的不同，单凭这一点，也应该做ECAD免疫组化染色，以助于将这些病变正确分类。

小叶癌变型和以前的小叶癌变型

多形性小叶癌

多形性小叶癌于1980年由Bassler[165]首先描述，后经Weidner[166]和Eusebi[167]进一步详述。从遗传学、免疫组化和临床特征方面，人们已充分认识到多形性小叶癌是一种特殊的临床病理类型[133, 168-171]。在组织学上该肿瘤显示3级核，不论原位癌还是浸润癌均为缺乏黏附性的方式生长（图17.28）。原位癌往往是由于在乳腺X线片上有钙化而发现。穿刺活检为原位癌，细胞为缺乏黏附性的3级核伴有粉刺样坏死和钙化。

激素受体往往呈弱阳性或阴性，细胞增殖率高，HER-2过度表达[172]，ECAD阴性[173]。比较基因组分析已证实，多形性小叶癌与导管癌的遗传谱不同[133, 174]。该类型的癌具有很强的侵袭特性，因此需要将其完全切除。

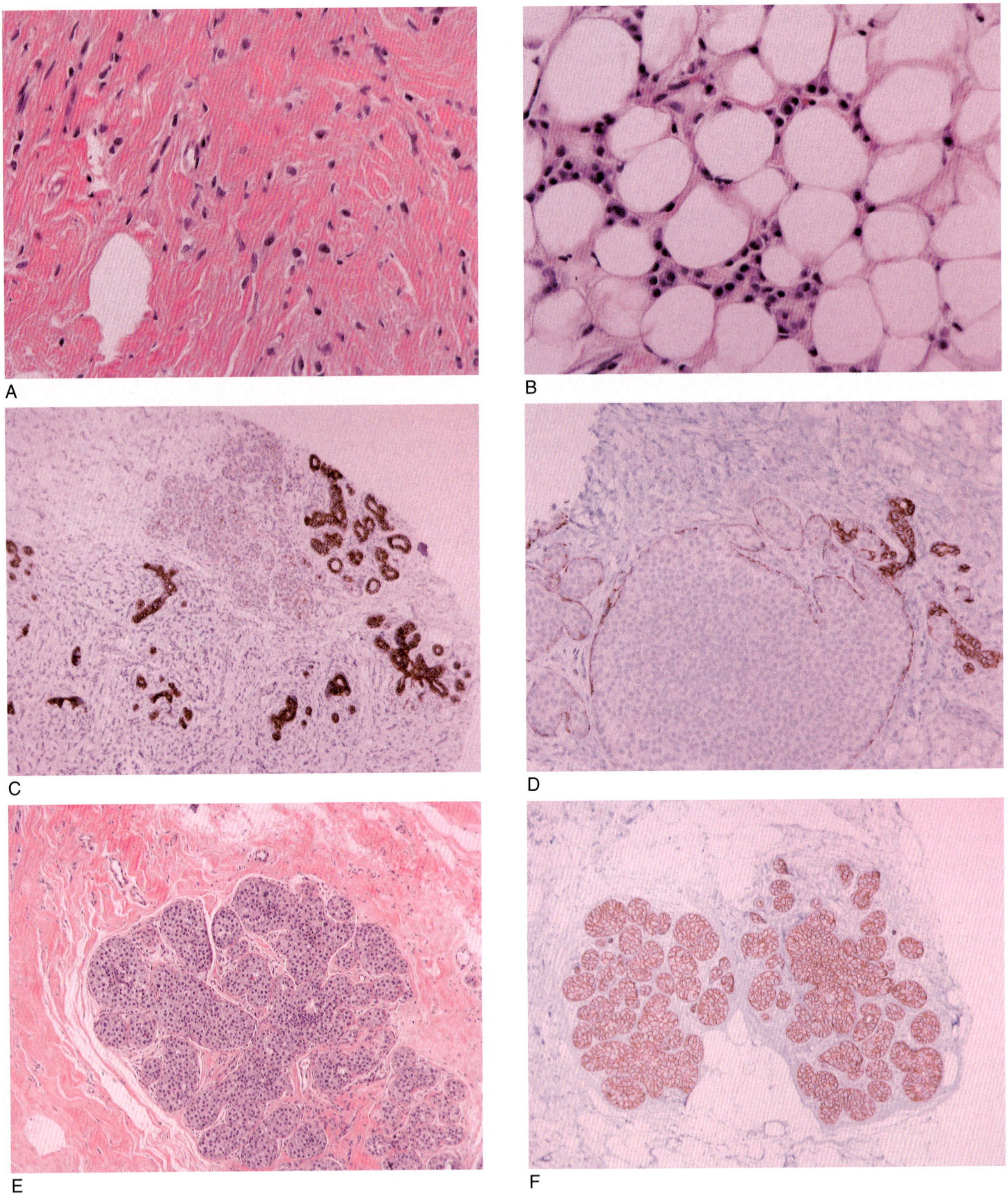

图17.25 （A,B）经典型小叶癌，肿瘤细胞体积小、淡染，呈弥漫散在分布，这是肿瘤缺乏ECAD表达、细胞无黏附性的特征。（C）肿瘤细胞ECAD阴性，正常导管小叶单位呈阳性。注意在LCIS区域免疫着色的细胞——肌上皮细胞ECAD染色阳性。（D）为高倍镜。（E）尽管提示为LCIS，但这种形态结构不能确定细胞类型。（F）ECAD表达阳性，提示为DCIS累及小叶

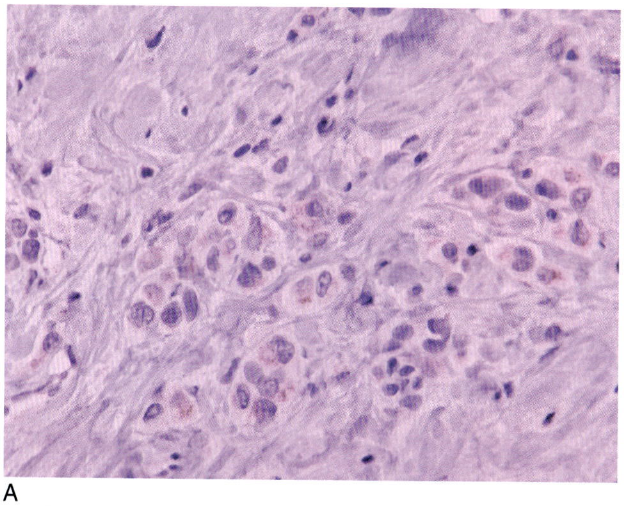

乳腺组织的免疫组织化学 17

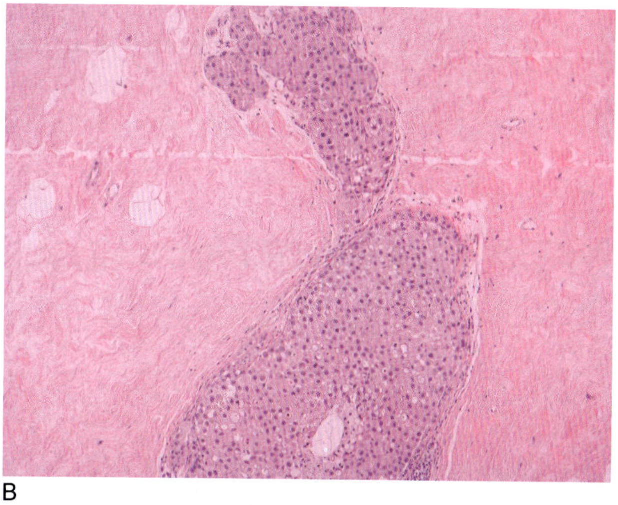

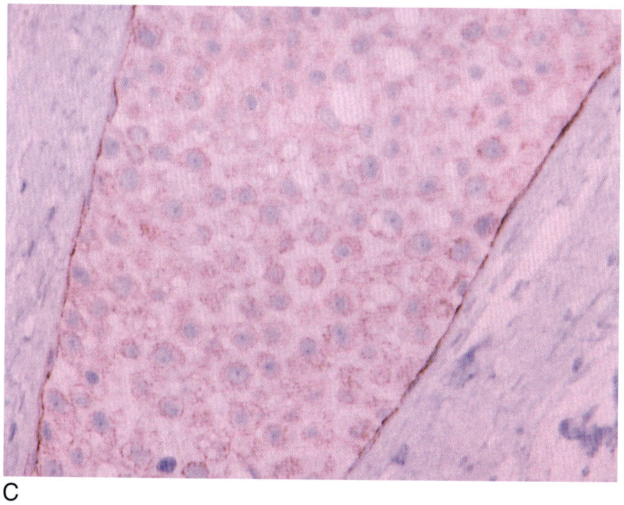

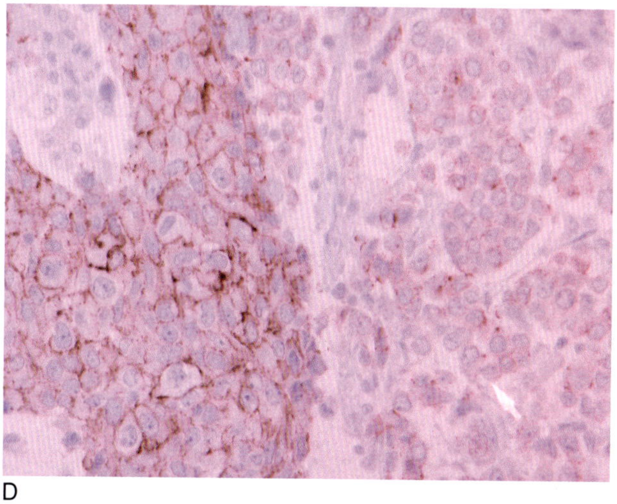

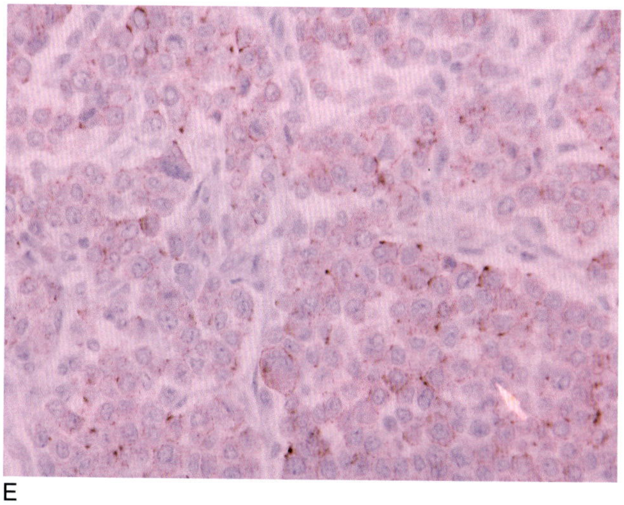

图17.26 （A）浸润性小叶癌，细胞浆ECAD着色。（B）具有大汗腺特征的导管内肿瘤，是导管性还是小叶性？（C）为（B）的ECAD染色，显示胞浆着色，提示为LCIS。（D）高级别导管癌，图片左侧显示ECAD完整胞膜着色，而右侧过渡为局灶性点状着色，细胞失去黏附性，这是ECAD分子近端发生突变的特征。（E）高倍镜视野显示ECAD局灶性点状着色

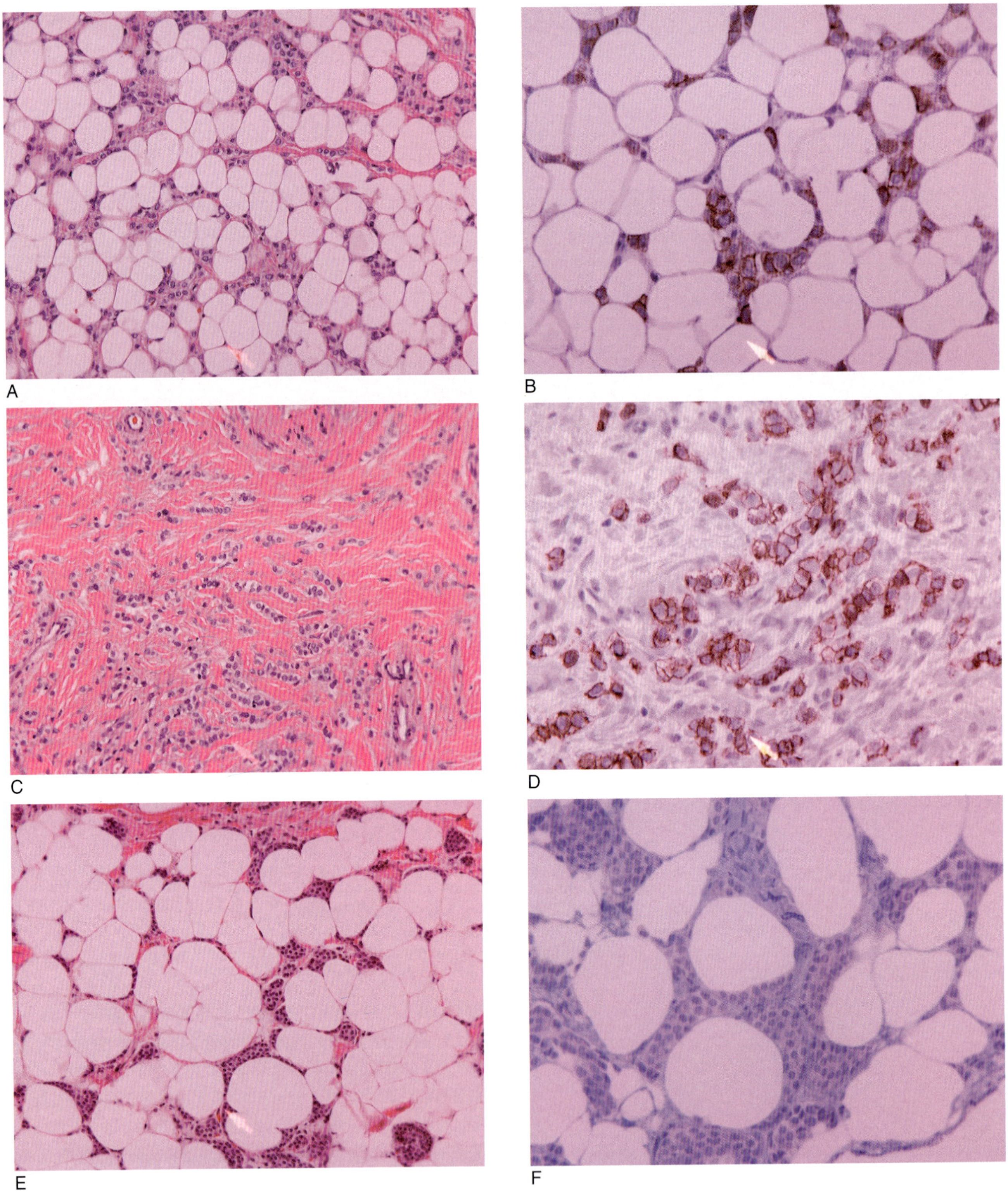

图17.27 （A）癌细胞在脂肪组织内浸润，类似小叶癌，（B）但ECAD+。（C）低级别核和细胞单行线状排列类似小叶癌，（D）但细胞膜ECAD+，提示为导管癌。（E）与（A）相比，脂肪组织内为典型的小而淡染的小叶癌细胞，（F）并且ECAD阴性

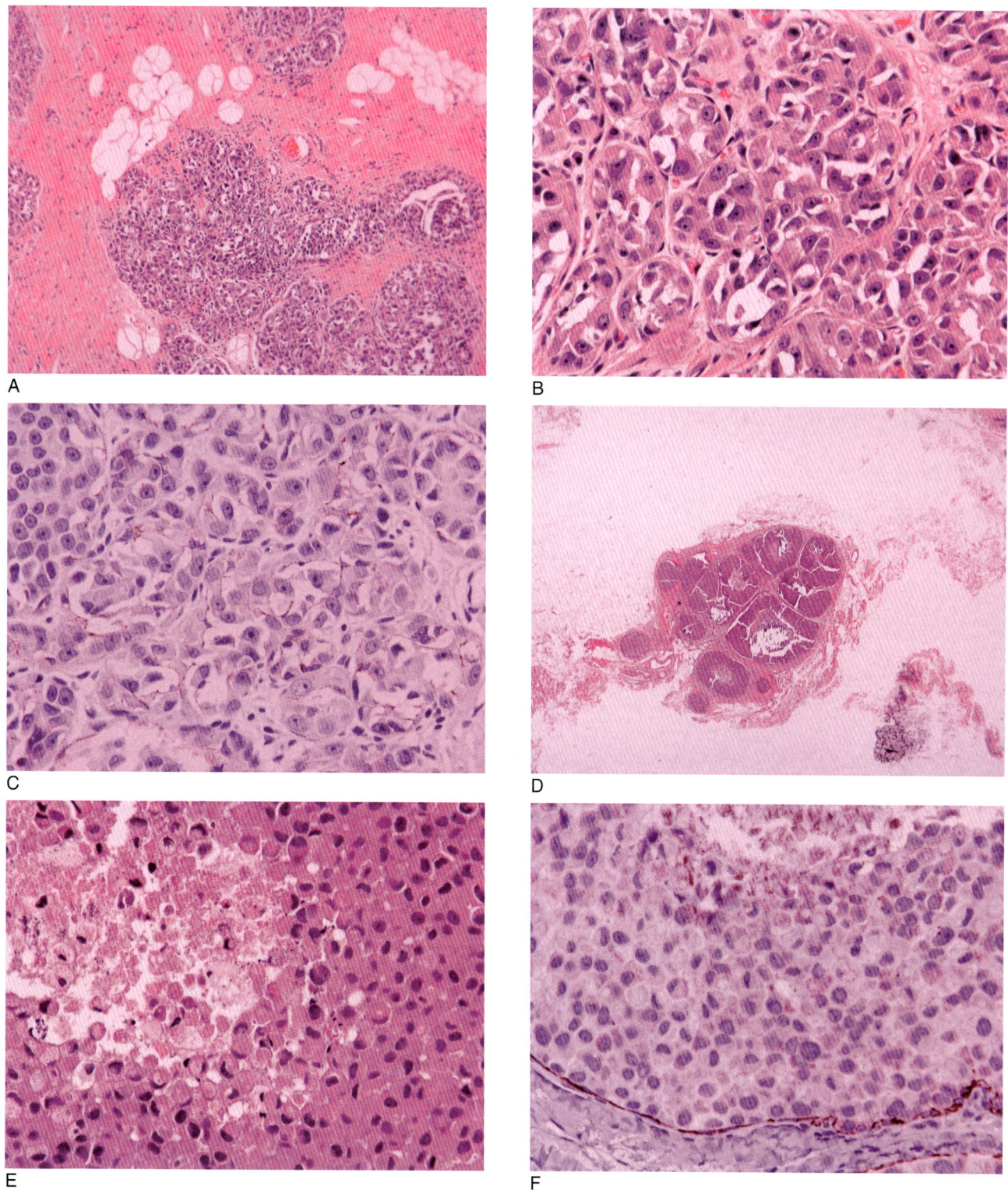

图 17.28 （A）低倍镜下多形性 LCIS 的小叶癌排列结构。（B）显示 3 级核和突出的核仁。（C）多形性 LCIS 为 ECAD 阴性。（D）低倍镜下多形性 LCIS 伴有粉刺样坏死和钙化，类似 DCIS。（E）注意多形性 LCIS 细胞无黏附性和浆细胞样的特征。（F）LCIS 中 ECAD 阴性，肌上皮细胞阳性

腺管型小叶癌

1977年首先由Fisher描述，是一种有小管状结构，瘤细胞单行排列的具有小叶癌生长方式的小叶癌，其预后介于纯小管癌和浸润性小叶癌之间[175,176]。此病变因细胞小和具有ILC单行排列以及靶心性浸润的特征，已经被列为ILC的一种变型。

Wheeler和Esposito最近的研究证明小管和小叶样细胞成分ECAD染色呈均匀一致的膜阳性（图17.29）[35,177]，并发现在这些病变中，有时以单纯的LCIS和混合性LCIS/DCIS为主。小而圆的腺管与浸润性小叶样结构混合存在，ECAD为阳性，表明该类型属于导管癌的范畴。

组织细胞样癌

1983年Filotico[178]描述了一例具有组织细胞样特征的小叶样癌。随后的报道根据其典型的浸润方式推测这是小叶癌的一种变型。最近才有这种罕见变型的免疫组化研究报道。Gupta[179]报道了最多的一组病例研究结果，发现11例中有8例没有ECAD的表达，11例中有8例伴有LCIS成分。3例有ECAD的表达，他认为这种组织细胞样形态尚缺乏特异性的临床表现，因此不足以把组织细胞样癌作为一种特殊的类型。

髓样癌

髓样癌的典型特征是高级别合体样肿瘤细胞中有大量淋巴细胞浸润。若干研究结果证实肿瘤细胞HLA-DR的过表达为髓样癌所特有[180,181]。与非典型性髓样癌和非特殊性浸润性导管癌相比，HLA-DR过表达可能有助于髓样癌的诊断。髓样癌应通过大体标本而不是通过穿刺活检标本作出最终诊断。

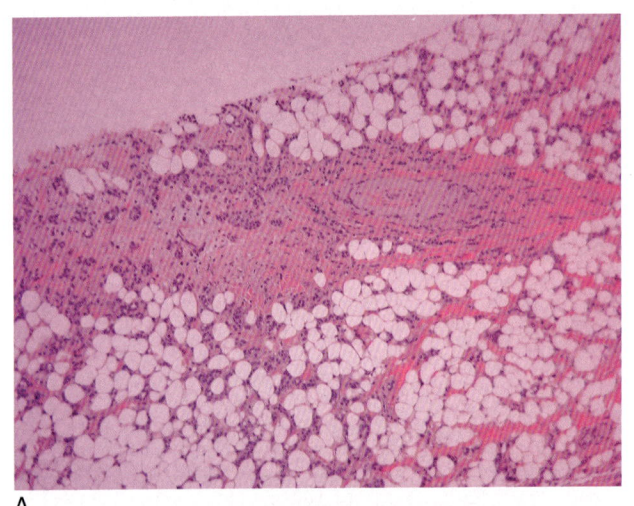

A

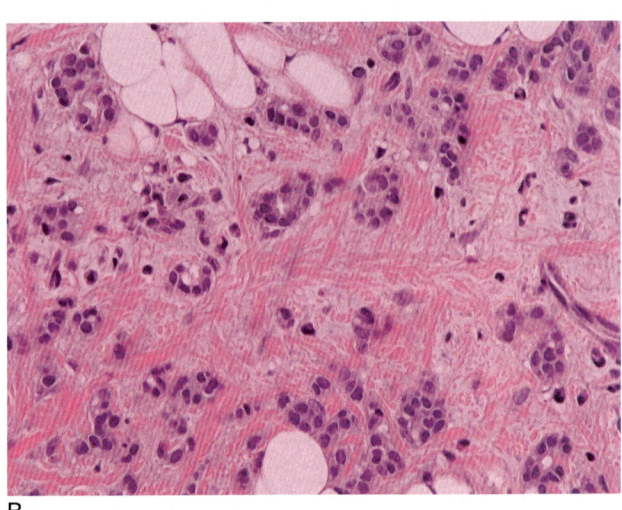

B

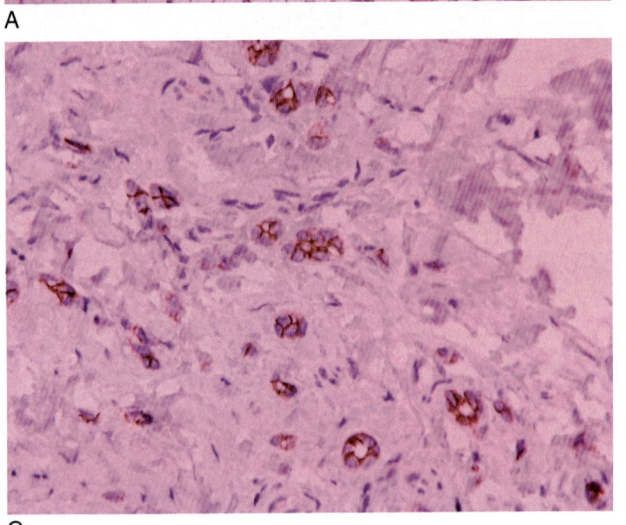

C

图17.29 （A）浸润性小管型小叶癌（TLC）与小叶癌相似，（B）小管散布于类似小叶癌的肿瘤成分中，（C）小管和单个的肿瘤细胞ECAD阳性

乳腺癌的全身转移

大囊肿病液体蛋白

由 Pearlman 等[182]和 Haagensen 等[183]首先描述，由 Murphy 与合作者[184]发现的催乳素诱导蛋白与大囊肿病液体蛋白-15（GCDGP-15）的氨基酸序列相同，并发现在乳腺囊肿液内和任何具有大汗腺特征的细胞内含有大量的催乳素诱导蛋白[167, 185, 186]。除乳腺外，GCDGP-15 还存在于其他具有大汗腺特征的细胞中，如涎腺的腺泡、大汗腺、汗腺、皮肤的 Paget 病、外阴和前列腺组织等[187-191]。

与乳腺癌形态表现相同的癌，如皮肤附属器癌和涎腺癌，其 GCDFP-15 免疫染色与乳腺癌有重叠[192]。除了这些肿瘤有免疫反应外，其他大多数肿瘤 GCDFP-15 免疫组化染色阴性[193]。乳腺癌累及皮肤（或者局部复发）可能很难与皮肤附属器肿瘤相鉴别[193]。Wick 及其同事们对形态学相似的乳腺、涎腺和皮肤附属器肿瘤研究结果发现，汗腺癌很少表达 GCDFP-15，乳腺癌极少表达 CEA，涎腺导管癌大多数缺乏雌激素受体表达[192]。

GCDFP-15 对乳腺癌的预测性价值和特异性均为 99%[187]。研究报道单克隆抗体 D6（Cambridge Research Laboratories, Cambridge, MA）的敏感性高达 74%[187]，但是其他实验室的研究报道为接近 50%[194]。

由于 GCDFP 抗体对确定为乳腺癌具有高度特异性，因此常将此抗体用于某些临床病人的筛选，结果证明该方法经常使原发部位不明的转移灶，或有乳腺癌病史而肺部出现新肿块的患者得以明确诊断。其他研究也证实了 GCDFP-15 抗体在鉴别肺内乳腺癌转移灶方面的实用性和特异性[195, 196]。

File 等应用细胞学标本检测 GCDFP-15 发现，56.5% 的复发性或转移性乳腺癌免疫染色为阳性，并观察到 GCDFP-15 必须要在福尔马林或 Bouin 固定液固定的切片中检测，酒精固定可以使抗体与 GCDFP-15 的免疫反应丧失[197]。

乳球蛋白 A

乳球蛋白基因是子宫球蛋白家族成员之一，编码一种与乳腺上皮细胞相关的糖蛋白。多数乳球蛋白研究是基于 RT-PCR 方法，尤其是对血液、骨髓和淋巴结做定量检测[198, 199]。应用 RT-PCR 检测显示，绝经后乳腺癌患者乳球蛋白的表达与肿瘤低级别、雌激素受体阳性相关[200, 201]。与 GCDFP-15 类似，乳球蛋白为胞浆着色。至编写本书时才有两篇有关的免疫组化研究论文发表。

运用组织芯片技术及乳球蛋白多克隆抗体检测，Han 发现乳球蛋白 A 对乳腺癌的敏感性可以高达 84%[202]。其他癌仅 15% 的病例染色阳性，总体敏感性与 GCDFP-15 相当。Ciampa[203, 204]的研究证实乳腺癌胸腔积液的细胞涂片敏感性为 55%。如果缺乏高度敏感性/高度特异性的乳腺癌抗体，可以采用乳球蛋白联合其他抗体来确定乳腺癌。

癌胚抗原

癌胚抗原（CEA）是一种分子量为 180kD 的糖蛋白，其中糖占 50%[205]。有多种针对不同 CEA 抗原决定簇的抗体。多克隆抗体通常与组织非特异性交叉反应抗原及胆汁糖蛋白 I 发生交叉反应[206, 207]。除了肺、结直肠癌以外，CEA 抗体 CD66e 系列还能与乳腺导管癌发生弥漫性强阳性反应。CEA 的特异性很差，不能用于转移性乳腺癌的诊断，必须要采用一组抗体以排除其他肿瘤。

细胞角蛋白

绝大多数乳腺导管癌和小叶癌表达 CK7，但有极少数细胞表达 CK20[208]。细胞角蛋白在乳腺癌与其他癌鉴别方面的作用不大，因为大多数的癌 CK7 阳性。但是，如果某个癌 CK20 弥漫性强阳性则是排除乳腺癌的有利证据，因为绝大多数具有这种表型的癌来自于胃肠道[209]。

最初认为乳腺髓样癌不表达 CK19，因此把 CK19 作为区别髓样癌和低分化导管癌的一个指标[210]。随后的研究表明两者对 CK19 染色有较大的重叠。Jensen 及 Dalal 等的研究结论是髓样癌和低分化导管癌均表达 CK19[145, 211]。Tot[204]的研究认为髓样癌和不典型髓样癌均可表达多种不同的角蛋白。

Lehr 及其同事[145]描述了 CK8 在乳腺癌中的应用。通过检测 CAM5.2，可以鉴别导管癌和小叶癌。在导管癌，CK8 染色特点是集中于细胞浆周围，使细胞表现为"墓碑样"排列。小叶癌则倾向于在核周胞浆着色，与毗邻肿瘤细胞形成"一袋大理石石子"的图像。

雌激素受体

一般认为雌激素/孕激素受体（ER/PR）可能仅存在于激素反应性组织，如乳腺。但自20世纪90年代末以来，有关这方面的文献报道一直存在争议。虽然某些研究者的结论为 ER/PR 只发现于乳腺癌、卵巢癌、子宫内膜癌的某些亚型中[196, 212, 213]，但其他研究者在肺、胃和甲状腺肿瘤也检测到了性激素受体的表达，多数表达 ER，少数表达 PR[214-218]。Vargas 等[214]用 IHC 证实雌激素相关蛋白 p29 在 98% 的非小细胞性肺癌中表达，说明雌激素轴在这一组恶性病变中可能起着较为重要的作用。同一组肿瘤使用市售的抗体 ER1D5（DAKO, Carpenteria, CA）染色则均为阴性。此组患者男女之间的生存率不同，提示受某些性别特异性 p29 相关因子的影响。

其他研究者也得出相同的结论，即对于原发部位不明的肿瘤 ER 的特异性很低。

> **诊断要点：转移性乳腺癌**
>
> 1. GCDFP-15 对确定为乳腺癌的特异性为 99%，敏感性为 55%。
> 2. 乳球蛋白 A 敏感性为 80%，但当前对其特异性尚无定论。
> 3. GCDFP-15 免疫组化染色与涎腺癌和皮肤附属器癌有交叉反应。
> 4. ER/PR 对转移性乳腺癌无特异性，但在某些鉴别诊断方面可能有一定的作用。

乳腺癌免疫组化预后因子

用于乳腺癌形态学诊断的石蜡包埋组织，同样也可以用于其他多种抗体检测。这些检测不仅可以更清楚地认识乳腺癌的生物学特性，而且还可以作为开发新的检测方法的突破口，这些新的检测结果将对患者的治疗有指导作用。

估计乳腺癌预后价值的病理学指标包括：
1. 肿瘤大小；
2. 淋巴结状况；
3. 肿瘤组织学类型；
4. 核的分级；
5. 有丝分裂活性；

6. 雌激素和孕激素受体。

这些已经纳入病理学家外科病理报告的参数指标早已被全面深入地研究，并证实其对病人的临床病程和治疗反应有重要的预测作用。绝大多数参数已作为 Scarff-Bloom-Richardson 或 Nottingham 指数并已被验证[219]。通过临床应用和长期随访已确立了 ER、PR 配体结合检测的地位，建立了阳性结果的分界点。

在前面提及的所有因素中，ER/PR 的免疫组化检测仍然有争议，因为关于究竟什么是 ER/PR 免疫组化的阳性标准至今尚未统一[220]。同样的原则也适用于表 17.5 中列出的令人眼花缭乱的 "新" 的免疫组化预后指标。大部分关于预后指标的研究都有其局限性，如未标准化，来自于小样本数据，或者是非随机临床试验采用的治疗方法不一致，或者没有可靠的随访结果等。以上所有这些指标均可检测，实际上，只要是有要求，这些指标在任何实验室都可以做。在作者实验室，许多临床医生或病人要求做这些指标，这些人都是受了当前媒体宣传的影响。作者实验室最近对所有新诊断的乳腺癌病人都做 HER-2 和 ER/PR 免疫组织化学检测。Ravdin[221] 曾提出："HER-2 检测是否适用于全部新发的乳腺癌病人？"他的答案是否定的，像其他检测一样，这项检测应该只应用于将根据此检测结果进行治疗的病人。

最近发表的某些数据提示[222, 223]，HER-2/neu 阳性病人用阿霉素化疗的效果更好一些，因此，这些病人可以将阿霉素作为一线治疗方案。

在本节中，我们讨论了一些直接、快速可能对治疗方案有提示的常规 IHC 检测指标。基于对病人预后结果的分析，表 17.5 中某些预后因素也许有一天会被

表 17.5 其他尚待确定的免疫组化预后指标
p53
Nm23
EGFR
Cathepsin D
MIB-1
微血管密度
PS2
p-糖蛋白
bcl-2
纤维母细胞生长因子
转化生长因子β
胰岛素生长因子
间质金属蛋白酶
表皮生长因子受体

加入到"高通量"预后/治疗的决策流程中去。

空芯针穿刺活检和细针针吸细胞学方法（FNA）是诊断乳腺癌最常用的方法。所有的诊断和预后检测指标（SMMHC、SMA、ER、PR、MIB-1、p53、HER-2/neu等）都可在局部活检的小组织上进行，并可获得可靠的结果[34, 224-231]。在用空芯针活检标本检测的所有指标中，只有黄体酮检测得出了假阴性的结果，原因是应用免疫过氧化物酶染色的组织存在异质性[230]。

区域淋巴管浸润的检测：D2-40

区域淋巴管是否受累是判断是否有淋巴结转移的重要提示因素。众所周知，在石蜡包埋乳腺组织中，镜下难以辨识淋巴管，如人工造成的标本收缩，导管内上皮细胞脱落，以及人为造成的细胞异位等都可造成活检标本的诊断困难。最近有一种抗体D2-40，对多种组织中的淋巴管有高度的敏感性和特异性[232-234]。在乳腺组织中，D2-40可使淋巴管内皮细胞的胞膜呈清晰、强阳性反应。淋巴管伴随血管束成为一种理想的内对照。在乳腺组织内可以确定淋巴管，免疫染色为清晰浓染的细胞膜着色（图17.30）。在肌上皮细胞和反应性的间质肌纤维母细胞中D2-40呈模糊着色。不像CD31、D2-40与乳腺的血管内皮细胞不发生反应。D2-40还可以用于其他细胞和组织的免疫染色，包括血管肉瘤、卡波西肉瘤、Cajal细胞、胃肠间质瘤、间皮瘤、卵巢浆液性癌、精原细胞瘤及淋巴结的滤泡树突状细胞等[233, 234]。

激素受体

现已认识到阻断雌激素对部分乳腺癌患者有治疗作用[235]，乳腺癌患者临床治疗反应与雌激素受体的表达有关[236]。

激素与ER/PR结合后，在细胞核中发挥其生物效应。通过免疫组化染色，在正常乳腺腺泡中可显示两种受体蛋白。因此，正常乳腺腺泡可作为检测过程中的内对照。正常乳腺上皮细胞核ER染色呈异质性并随月经周期而变化[237]。雌激素的作用之一即为诱导PR产生，而且在同一种细胞中两种激素受体的联合表达反映了细胞内ER/PR轴的精确调节作用。在乳腺癌中，大部分PR阳性的肿瘤ER也阳性，只有小于5%的PR阳性肿瘤为ER阴性[238, 239]。PR阳性病人比PR阴性病人的无病生存率要高得多[240-245]。

从20世纪90年代初期，采用免疫组化检测ER/PR的方法就取代了葡聚糖活性碳包裹法（DCC）。DCC法作为应用了多年的金标准，有着明显的不足，即：①肿瘤取材的误差；②过分依赖于获取组织的时间，肿瘤血运中断后要立即取材，需在手术室内完成操作；③正常组织的污染；④分析误差。

IHC法的优点在于：①有确切的肿瘤组织学证据；②能对肿瘤细胞核ER/PR的异质性准确评价；③通过直视和半定量法，或将两者结合可快速评估ER/PR的水平；④短期内得到实验结果；⑤价格便宜；⑥需要的组织量小。

第一代IHC抗体仅在冰冻的肿瘤标本中获得良好效果。H222（Abbot实验室，Abbot Park，IL）抗体在冰冻标本中获得非常好的效果。后来研究出用于福尔马林固定石蜡包埋组织的抗体，需强调，要想获得最佳结果，福尔马林固定的时间不能太长（<24小时）。长时间的固定可使免疫活性减退[246]，要特别注意肿瘤切片中的阳性内对照[247, 248]。

Frigo及其同事对H222抗体进行了细致的研究，他发现使用标记链卵白素法时，采用不同的固定液所得的结果并不比用福尔马林固定的标本效果好[249]。Battifora等对DCC法和IHC法进行了对比分析，通过对166名患者6年的随访研究，结论为：当使用H222抗体免疫组化法与把分界点定为20fmol/mg的DCC法比较时，两者的一致率达94%[250]。随后的研究证实使用H222抗体得到的结果与冰冻切片所得的结果类似[246, 251-257]。第二代ER抗体（ER1D5，DAKO，Carpinteria，CA）的面世以及新的抗原修复方法的使用[258-260]，使DCC法已被弃用[261]。

早期对ICA和DCC法检测ER一致性的研究结果表明：从H222表达、总体生存率、无病生存率方面来讲，它们均具有较好的相关性[262]，有高敏感性和特异性[263-267]。对IHC法的结果定量标准尚有一定的争议。概括大量的文献报道，某些作者将ER阳性标准定为大于或等于5%细胞核染色，而其他作者认为最少也应该有10%的细胞核染色，还有少数人信赖"H评分"，即包括阳性细胞核的百分比和核着色的强度。

Pertschuk等及Taylor等提出将最低的阳性标准定为细胞核染色的百分比为10%时重复性好，并且与临床结果相一致[265, 268, 269]。Ferno等也发现10%的核染色率与临床反应紧密相关，而核染色的强度没有什么实际价值[270]。Schultz等和Remmele等就可视性免

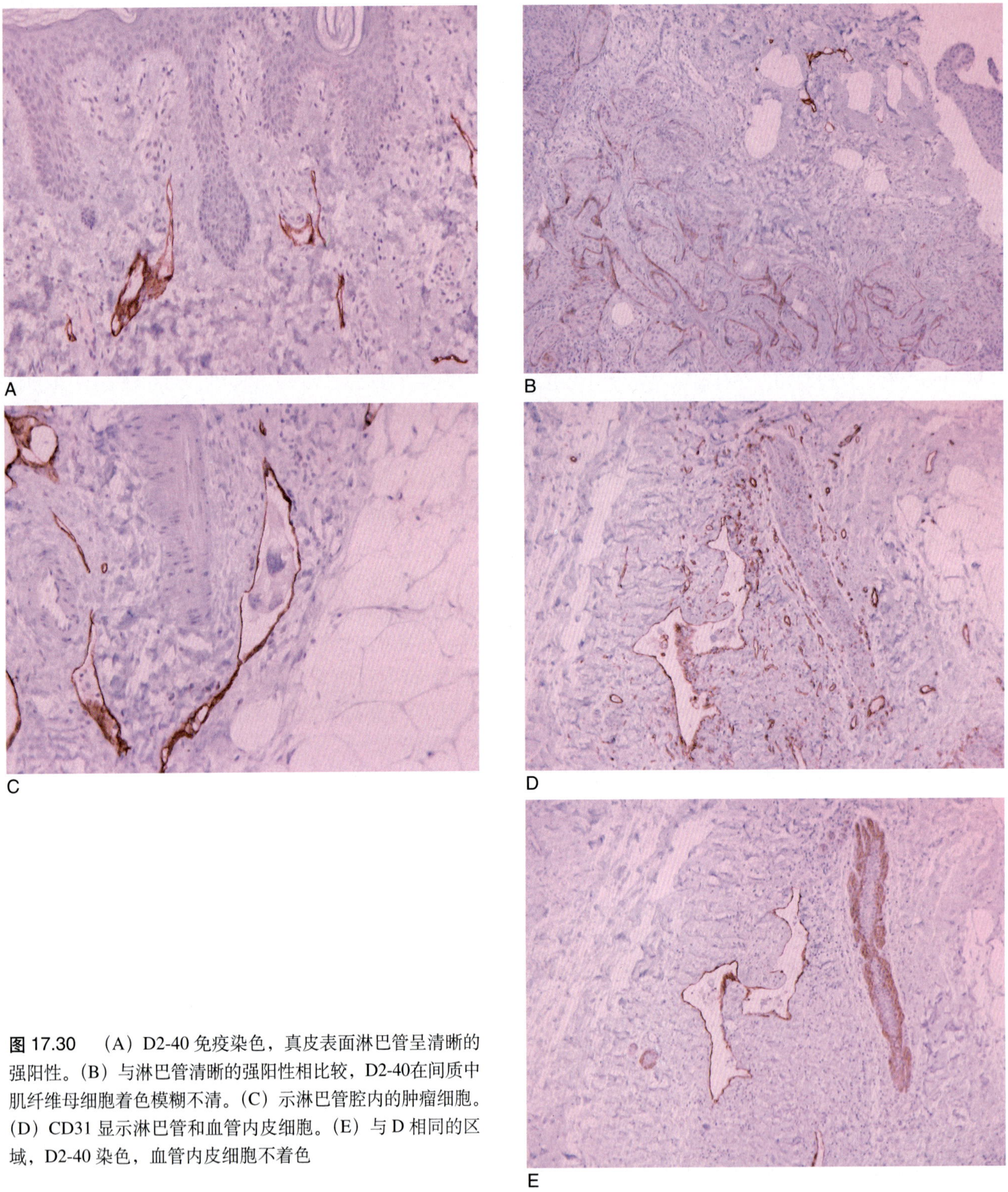

图 17.30 （A）D2-40 免疫染色，真皮表面淋巴管呈清晰的强阳性。（B）与淋巴管清晰的强阳性相比较，D2-40在间质中肌纤维母细胞着色模糊不清。（C）示淋巴管腔内的肿瘤细胞。（D）CD31 显示淋巴管和血管内皮细胞。（E）与 D 相同的区域，D2-40 染色，血管内皮细胞不着色

疫组化评分与图像分析结果进行对比，两组报告的结论为：图像定量分析并不比方便、简单、快速的可视性半定量效果好[271, 272]。

有关这方面研究的一篇综述中，Barnes等将染色强度、阳性细胞百分数以及染色的异质性程度赋予一个数值，将其作为预测内分泌治疗反应的指标。这些研究者根据DCC法相关的内分泌治疗反应的结果确定他们的分界点，其敏感性为71%，特异性为62%[273]。

Clark及其同事提出即使病人ER/PR阳性细胞百分比只有1%也对内分泌辅助治疗有效[274]。

关于ER/PR的IHC评分的可重复性研究很少，Van Diest及其同事观察到在两极（0和强阳性）时的可重复性好，而中间部分的评分很难一致，总体一致率为61%[275]。

已有报道证明福尔马林固定、石蜡包埋的组织的IHC测量法与DCC之间有较高的符合率[276, 277]。

IHC法的定量结果与生化法结果非常相似，且对预后有预测作用[278, 282]。很少有研究验证是否ER的出现即预示着对内分泌治疗有反应，即使在已作过的这方面研究中，其病人数目也很少[283]。Veronese和他的同事们在一项应用ER1D5抗体的研究中发现，65名使用他莫昔芬治疗的患者，ER免疫组化染色对治疗反应有预测作用，而且可以作为无病生存率和总体生存率的指标[284]。Barnes等及Goulding等证实，不管使用何种免疫组化评分方法，应用IHC法检测ER比DCC法要好，而且与病人的预后密切相关[285, 286]。

Harvey[287]用阳性细胞占1%作为阳性标准，选取了1982个病例，把IHC法检测ER（克隆6F11，Ventana医疗系统，Tuscon，AZ）与配体结合分析法（LBA）进行了对比，结果发现两者具有高度一致性，而且可以很好地预测临床预后。在这项研究中所应用的ER/PR评分方法被称为"Allred评分"，这种半定量的方法效果好而且简单。该评分法是将阳性细胞百分数与免疫染色强度联合起来评分（图17.31）。

Elledge，运用同样方法研究发现[288]，在转移性乳腺癌患者中用IHC法测ER可以更好地预测病人对他莫昔芬的治疗反应。作者最近发表的研究结果[289]，即对参加NSABP-B-09试验的409例淋巴结阳性患者免疫组化检测ER结果进行研究，比较在不同观察者之间的差异，对可视性半定量以及图像分析定量的数据与葡聚糖包裹活性碳法（DCC）的数据进行了对比。

结论是：任何一种测量方法均对预后有帮助，因为简便，可视性半定量法是最常用的方法，观察者间的一致性很好。

NSABP-B-29治疗方案结果证实了ER定量的重要性，肿瘤中ER高表达的患者不能从附加的化疗中获益。

Mohsin[290]是第一个通过IHC证实PR作用的人，他应用PR 1294克隆株以1%作为阳性标准，采用Allred评分系统，证实PR在预测患者无病生存率和总体生存率方面比LBA法效果好。

以前大量的关于IHC法检测ER阳性标准问题的争论，现在可以告一段落了，因为在2000年11月1日至11月3日的会议上，NIH（National Institutes of Health）乳腺癌辅助治疗方案组一致同意：免疫组化染色只要有细胞核ER阳性表达，都应对病人进行抗雌激素治疗。

可以在微小组织上对ER、PR进行IHC法检测是一个显著的优点，IHC可用于细针吸取细胞学检查（FNA）确定为癌的患者[280]，一些研究证明FNA标本与DCC法检测ER/PR有着高敏感性、专一性和一致性[226, 291]。用IHC法测ER、PR也可应用于细胞涂片，使用PreservCyt固定液（Cytyc，Boxborough，MA），染色效果良好[292, 293]。

Rosen第一个描述了肿瘤的组织病理学与ER、PR表达之间的关系[294]。ER阳性的肿瘤一般包括小叶癌、小管癌、黏液癌和乳头状癌，以及低核级别的导管癌[238, 239, 295]。

IHC法检测孕激素受体细胞核染色的异质性比检测雌激素受体大[296]，甚至可能会出现假阴性结果，尤其在空芯针活检或细针吸取细胞学检查时[230]。在作者的研究机构，空芯针活检的检测结果基本类似。因此，如果空芯针活检标本ER、PR为阴性的话，需要在乳腺肿块切除后的标本上再重复一次检测。

使用抗体1A6检测PR的敏感性、特异性及一致性的研究与ER的研究结果相似[297-300]。

另一种类型ER（ER-β）的发现开辟了ER生物学研究的新领域[301-303]。Choi[304]应用组织芯片法研究了ER-β的分布，结果证实，与ER-α相比，ER-β与预后不良的指标，如HER-2、p53、cathepsin D和Ki-67的表达密切相关，而与组织学分级、肿瘤大小或分期无关。Fuqua[305]发现ER-β与非整倍体及ER-α假阳性有关。Stefanou[306]通过一个小样本的研究得出结

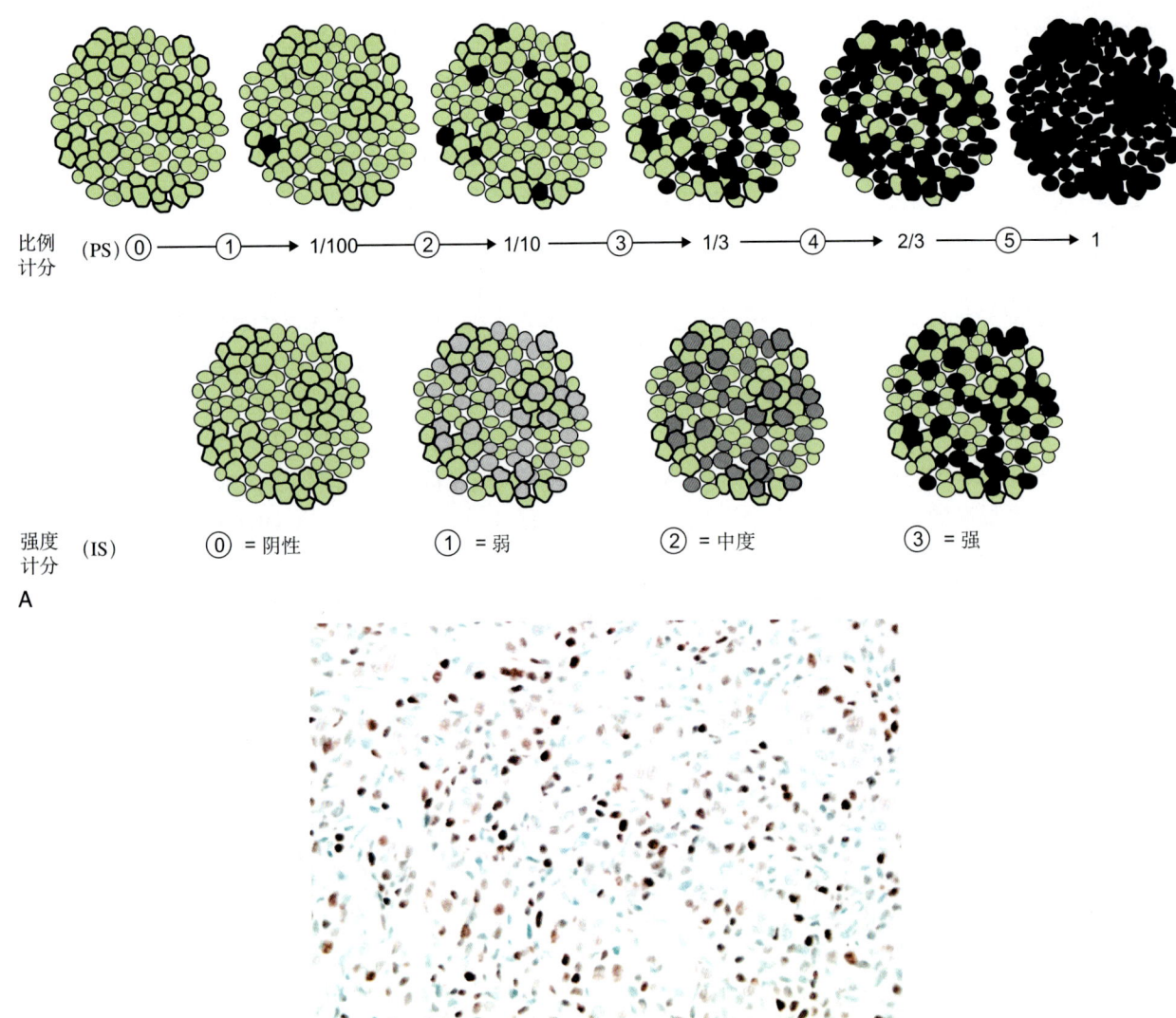

图 17.31 （A,B）一种将雌激素受体和孕激素受体细胞核染色强度和阳性百分数相结合的半定量的方法，把百分数评分（PS）与强度评分（IS）相加即得到 0 到 8 之间的总分（引自 Harvey，et al.1999）

论，即 ER-α、ER-β 的表达互不相关且与肿瘤大小、分级或淋巴结是否受累也无关。Hopp[307]得出了相似的结果并证实在接受他莫昔芬治疗的ER-β高表达的患者无病生存率和总体生存率高。ER-β 及其在确定临床方案中的作用尚需要进一步的研究。

HER-2/neu 肿瘤蛋白

HER-2/neu蛋白分子量为185kD，属于酪氨酸激酶受体家族，与表皮生长因子受体有50%的同源性，包括膜外区、跨膜区以及膜内区[308-310]。它是位于染色体 17q12-21.32 上的 *cerb-B2* 基因表达产物[311, 312]。其胞浆区具有促磷酸化和转录启动的作用，免疫组化抗

> **诊断要点：激素受体**
>
> 1. 在空芯针活检或 FNA 时 ER/PR 假阴性结果增加。故在空芯针活检时，如果ER/PR 阴性则有必要在切除的活检标本上重复 ER/PR 检测。
> 2. 最具有权威性的研究显示 1% 的细胞阳性即可认为 ER 或 PR 阳性。这与 2000 年 12 月 NIH 作出的任何程度的细胞核 ER 免疫染色均定为 ER 阳性的论述密切相关。
> 3. 激素受体的半定量检测在临床上非常有用。
> 4. 可视性半定量法检测激素受体与图像分析的效果相同。

体所结合的抗原决定簇即来源于这一区域。HER-2 受体的激活性配体至今未明。

从开始有报道提示 HER-2 扩增与临床预后不良相关后[313]，至少有涉及 15 000 名患者的 48 个与预后有关的 HER-2 基因研究课题[314]。在淋巴结阴性患者中，HER-2/neu 过度表达与预后的关系不明显[315, 316]，某些研究结果显示两者之间无明显关系[317-326]。最初，这方面研究结果是矛盾和有争议的，也许是因为应用的抗体不同，或对存档标本没有进行抗原热修复，或患者接受了辅助化疗的干扰[327]。淋巴结阳性患者的研究结果似乎很明确，通过大量的研究显示 HER-2/neu 过表达的患者预后不良[223, 314, 318, 320, 321, 323, 326, 328-337]。

当前，临床上对乳腺癌病人进行 HER-2/neu 检测的作用有两个：①用于阿霉素化疗效果的预测，②确定哪些患者适合用赫赛汀（trastuzumab）治疗。

Mass 及其同事[223]根据 HER-2 过表达情况，对 1527 名妇女的化疗反应进行研究，结论为 HER-2 阳性患者使用大剂量的阿霉素、环磷酰胺和氟尿嘧啶化疗的效果明显好于 HER-2 阴性患者。

Paik 及其同事利用国家乳腺癌外科辅助化疗计划（NSABP）项目的资料，用包括 CB11 单克隆抗体（Ventana, Tucson, AZ）和多克隆兔抗体检测存档的石蜡标本，结论为 HER-2 检测结果 2+ 的病人用阿霉素治疗效果好[222]。

1998 年，临床试验证明了赫赛汀作为一种单克隆抗体可以有效地阻断 HER-2 受体，将其与化疗联合应用时效果肯定，患者肿瘤明显缩小[338, 339]。

对部分患者，赫赛汀可作为一线辅助治疗药物。Vogel[340]报道了单独将赫赛汀作为转移患者一线药物的试验结果，有效率和临床受益率分别为 35% 和 48%。但只有 HER-2/neu 过表达的肿瘤才有效。Slamon 及其同事[341]报道采用一线化疗药物和赫赛汀治疗，患者总体生存率提高了 25%。

自 20 世纪 90 年代初以来由于对所采用的不同抗体进行了广泛研究，免疫组化测定 HER-2 的阳性标准（癌基因蛋白过表达）也在不断改进[327]。最近，免疫荧光原位杂交法（FISH）已成为检测 HER-2 的金标准，因为其在检测基因扩增方面有着明显的优势。这些检测方法的优缺点列于表 17.6。IHC 和 FISH 均适用于冰冻及福尔马林固定的组织以及细胞学涂片[342, 343]。FISH 和 IHC 两者的符合率超过 90%。

Lottner 在石蜡包埋组织中同时检测了 HER-2/neu 的基因扩增和蛋白过表达，结果发现两种方法的一致率为 97.7%，对胞浆染色要忽略不计[345]，仅观察膜阳性染色时两者的一致性最好[344]。实验中心和地方实验室检测的符合率在 92%~94% 之间[346, 347]。结果判断采用美国食品药品管理局（FDA）批准的 HercepTest Kit（DAKO, Carpinteria, CA）的评分方法，阳性结果 3+ 者为弥漫的网格状膜染色（"chicken wire"）（图 17.32）；2+ 为至少有 10% 的肿瘤细胞显示完整的膜染色，但染色较弱；少于 10% 的细胞染色并且细胞膜染色不完整都认为是阴性。利用自动细胞成像系统（ACIS）（Clarient, Irvine, CA）进行图像分析，可明显提高 HER-2 检测的可重复性和准确性[348, 349]。

IHC 检测为 2+ 时，建议再做 FISH，大约有 20% 的肿瘤可能有扩增[350]。其他情况下，如 ER/PR 阴性的肿瘤，IHC 法 HER-2 为 0 或者 1+ 时，FISH 检测有不到 3% 的肿瘤有 HER-2 扩增[350]。HER-2/neu 免疫组化着色模式通常是一致的，在同一肿瘤组织内没有明显的不同[348]。这样，乳腺空芯针活检 HER-2 的检测结果几乎就可以代表整个肿瘤的结果，与乳腺肿块切除标本染色结果的相关性很好。为了避免活检过程中过诊断（假阳性）发生，要忽略空心针活检中人工假象造成的边缘效应。

作者利用 DAKO（多克隆）、Zymed（TAB250 和多克隆）和 Ventana（CB11 单克隆）抗-P185 抗体检测了 87 例存档的乳腺癌病例，其染色结果显示，所有的抗体在敏感性和专一性上均有可比性。DAKO 抗体阳性率比其他抗体高 19%~26%。本研究的阳性率

表 17.6　HER-2/neu 免疫组化与原位杂交的优缺点对比

免疫组化	FISH	色素原位杂交
福尔马林固定或冰冻组织，酒精固定的细胞学标本	同前 需要专门的训练人员操作和分析	同前
便宜	当前很贵 可自动化	比 FISH 便宜 可自动化
光学显微镜	荧光显微镜	光学显微镜

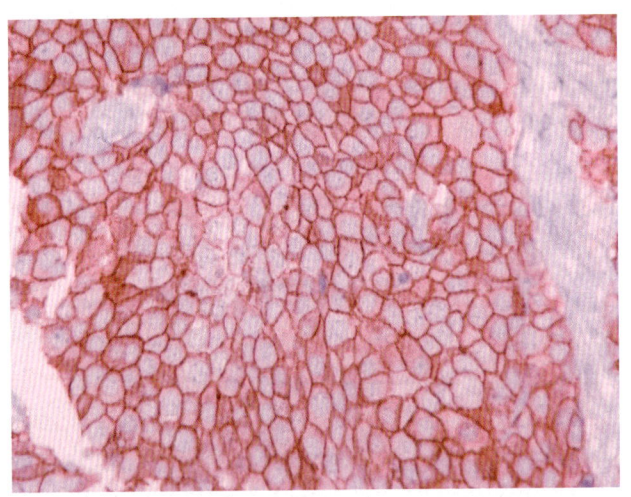

图17.32 典型的 HER-2/neu 阳性为网格状细胞膜的强染色（"chicken-wire"）（获 Dr. DC Allred 授权）

并未达到Roche和Ingle描述的60%那么高[351]。Jacobs及其同事发现用IHC检测HER-2时，各实验室间的一致性很好，这两个实验室使用的是同样的一抗，但是染色方法和评分标准不同[352]。Press报道IHC、FISH两者之间一致性也较高[353]。

IHC 检测 HER-2 的质量控制应该包括阳性病例百分比的统计和 IHC 阳性病例 FISH 扩增的百分比。实验室定期对这些相关指标进行评估对保证报告质量是至关重要的。严格按照用10%的中性福尔马林缓冲液固定，固定时间6~12小时，设立组织对照/细胞株

HER-2/neu 诊断要点

1. 根据产品说明书操作，认真地对染色结果加以解释，对获得可靠结果是十分必要的。质量控制应该包括阳性、阴性及FISH扩增病例的百分比。
2. HER-2过表达者预后不良，对阿霉素或单克隆抗体治疗方法反应好，ER阳性病人反应稍差。
3. DAKO、Ventana、Zymed公司单克隆、多克隆抗体的 IHC 结果有可比性。
4. FISH是检测基因扩增，IHC是检测过表达的基因产物。
5. FISH 和 IHC 均适用于石蜡包埋标本和针吸标本。
6. 当 IHC 检测 HER-2 为 2+ 时，或 ER/PR 阴性 HER-2 评分为 0 或 1+ 时主张再应用 FISH 检测。

对照[354]，改善观察者间报告的一致性或采用图像分析等[341,355,356]。

色素原位杂交（CISH）在HER-2/neu扩增检测方面有取代FISH的可能性[84,357]，该方法采用与HER-2基因及17号中心粒结合的探针进行原位杂交。病理学家通过光学显微镜观察得出报告。CISH和FISH之间的相关性非常好[358-361]。CISH检测HER-2/neu的实验室全自动化即将实现。使用多参数荧光法可以同时检测蛋白、多倍体、非整倍体和基因扩增[344]。

表皮生长因子受体

某些研究提出表皮生长因子受体的表达与乳腺癌恶性程度高的类型相关[362]。统计结果显示，EFGR的表达与ER阴性、肿瘤抗内分泌治疗和HER-2/neu过表达相关[363-366]。目前，用 IHC 检测 EGFR 并不是常规的临床检验项目。关于他莫昔芬与雌激素抵抗、芳香化酶抑制剂和EGFR/HER-2/neu抑制剂关系的临床研究试验正在进行中。

前列腺特异性抗原

大约 30%~40% 的女性乳腺癌中存在前列腺特异性抗原（PSA）[367-370]，在男性乳腺癌中也有报道[243,371,372]。乳腺癌 PSA 免疫活性的重要性在于要与转移的前列腺癌相鉴别[373]，尤其是对有乳腺肿块的男性患者。乳腺癌CK7和多克隆CEA为弥漫性强阳性，而前列腺癌两种抗体的染色均为阴性。可以根据这一特点将前列腺癌与男性乳腺癌区别开来，Gupta描述的两位患者其血清 PSA 均无升高[373]。

纤维上皮性肿瘤

对空芯针穿刺乳腺标本区分纤维腺瘤（FA）和分叶状肿瘤（PT）的金标准仍是形态学。目前还没有能准确区别这两种肿瘤的免疫染色方法[374]。

Komenaka[374]的一项形态学研究指出，PT的阴性预测值为93%，阳性预测值为83%。c-kit 表达与 Ki-67标记指数一样，随着肿瘤侵袭性形态学表现的增强而增强，而 PDGFRA 几乎不表达[375]，没有发现与c-kit 表达相关的分子变化。

Tse研究了纤维上皮性肿瘤 CD10 表达的情况，发现在 33 名 FA 患者中有 1 例、102 名良性 PT 患者中有 6 例、51 名交界性 PT 患者中有 16 例、28 名恶性 PT 患者中有 14 例的间质成分中有 CD10 表达[376]。但这些结果没有用在空芯针活检的标本。

参考文献

1. Joshi MG, Lee AKC, Pederson CA, et al. The role of immunocytochemical markers in the differential diagnosis of proliferative and neoplastic lesions of the breast. Mod Pathol 1996; 9:57–62.
2. Rudland PS, Leinster SJ, Winstanley J, et al. Immunocytochemical identification of cell types in benign and malignant breast diseases: Variations in cell markers accompany the malignant state. J Histochem Cytochem 1993; 41:543–553.
3. Gusterson B, Warburton MJ, Mitchell D, et al. Distribution of myoepithelial cells and basement membrane proteins in the normal breast and in benign and malignant breast diseases. Cancer Res 1982; 42:4763–4770.
4. Bussolati G, Botta G, Gugliotta P. Actin-rich (myoepithelial cells) in ductal carcinoma in situ of the breast. Virchows Arch B 1980; 34:251–259.
5. Bussolati G. Actin-rich (myoepithelial) cells in lobular carcinoma in situ of the breast. Virchows Arch B 1980; 32:165–176.
6. Bussolati G, Botto-Micca FB, Eusebi V, et al. Myoepithelial cells in lobular carcinoma in situ of the breast. Ultrastruct Pathol 1981; 2:219–230.
7. Ahmed A. The myoepithelium in human breast carcinoma. J Pathol 1974; 113:129–135.
8. Gould VE, Jao W, Battifora H. Ultrastructural analysis in the differential diagnosis of breast tumors: The significance of myoepithelial cells, basal lamina, intracytoplasmic lumina and secretory granules. Pathol Res Pract 1980; 167:45–70.
9. Hijazi YM, Lessard JL, Weiss MA, et al. Use of anti-actin and S-100 protein antibodies in differentiating benign and malignant sclerosing breast lesions. Surg Pathol 1989; 2:125–135.
10. Dwarakanath S, Lee AK, Dellilis RA, et al. S-100 protein positivity in breast carcinomas: A potential pitfall in diagnostic immunohistochemistry. Hum Pathol 1987; 18:1144–1148.
11. Raju U, Lee MW, Zarbo RJ, et al. Papillary neoplasia of the breast: Immunohistochemically defined myoepithelial cells in the diagnosis of benign and malignant papillary breast neoplasms. Mod Pathol 1989; 2:569–576.
12. Nagle R, Bocker W, Davis JR, et al. Characterization of breast carcinomas by two monoclonal antibodies distinguishing myoepithelial from luminal epithelial cells. J Histochem Cytochem 1986; 34:869–881.
13. Jarasch E, Nagle RB, Kaufman M, et al. Differential diagnosis of benign epithelial proliferations and carcinomas of the breast using antibodies to cytokeratins. Hum Pathol 1988; 19:276–289.
14. Lele SM, Graves K, Gatalica Z. Immunohistochemical detection of maspin is a useful adjunct in distinguishing radial sclerosing lesion from tubular carcinoma of the breast. Appl Immunohistochem Mol Morphol 2000; 8(1):32–36.
15. Mohsin SK, et al. Maspin expression in invasive breast cancer: association with other prognostic factors. J Pathol 2003; 199(4):432–435.
16. Umekita Y, Yoshida H. Expression of maspin is up-regulated during the progression of mammary ductal carcinoma. Histopathology 2003; 42(6):541–545.
17. Navarro R de L, Martins MT, Araujo VC de. Maspin expression in normal and neoplastic salivary gland. J Oral Pathol Med 2004; 33(7):435–440.
18. Acs G, et al. Differential expression of E-cadherin in lobular and ductal neoplasms of the breast and its biologic and diagnostic implications. Am J Clin Pathol 2001; 115(1):85–98.
19. Bocker W, Bier B, Freytag G, et al. An immunohistochemical study of the breast using antibodies to basal and luminal keratins, alpha-smooth muscle actin, vimentin, collagen IV and laminin. Part II. Virchows Arch A Pathol Anat Histopathol 1992; 421:323–330.
20. Gottlieb C, Raju U, Greenwald KA. Myoepithelial cells in the differential diagnosis of complex benign and malignant breast lesions: An immunohistochemical study. Mod Pathol 1990; 3:135–140.
21. Gugliotta P, Sapino A, Macri L, et al. Specific demonstration of myoepithelial cells by anti-alpha smooth muscle actin antibody. J Histochem Cytochem 1993; 36:659–663.
22. Raymond WA, Leong AS. Assessment of invasion in breast lesions using antibodies to basement membrane components and myoepithelial cells. Pathology 1991; 23:291–297.
23. Bose S, DeRosa CM, Ozzello L. Immunostaining of type IV collagen and smooth muscle actin as an aid in the diagnosis of breast lesions. Breast J 1999; 5:194–201.
24. Wang N, Wan BC, Skelly M, et al. Antibodies to novel myoepithelium-associated proteins distinguish benign lesions and carcinoma in situ from invasive carcinoma of the breast.

Appl Immunohistochem 1997; 5:141–151.

25. Titus MA. Myosins. Curr Opin Cell Biol 1993; 5:77–81.

26. Winder SJ, Walsh MP. Calponin: Thin fiiament-linked regulation of smooth muscle contraction. Cell Signal 1993; 5:677–686.

27. Gimoa M, Herzog M, Vancekerckhove J, et al. Smooth muscle specific expression of calponin. FEBS Lett 1990; 274:159–162.

28. Dabbs DJ, Pickeral J, Tung MY, et al. Predicting invasion in stereotactic core biopsies of breast: Qualitative differences of antibodies that detect myoepithelial cells. Mod Pathol, in press.

29. Someren A, Sewell CW. Differential diagnosis in pathology: breast disorders. New York: Igaku-Shoin; 1997.

30. Werling RW, et al. Immunohistochemical distinction of invasive from noninvasive breast lesions: a comparative study of p63 versus calponin and smooth muscle myosin heavy chain. Am J Surg Pathol 2003; 27(1):82–90.

31. Barbareschi M, et al. p63, a p53 homologue, is a selective nuclear marker of myoepithelial cells of the human breast. Am J Surg Pathol 2001; 25(8):1054–1060.

32. Kaufmann O, et al. Value of p63 and cytokeratin 5/6 as immunohistochemical markers for the differential diagnosis of poorly differentiated and undifferentiated carcinomas. Am J Clin Pathol 2001; 116(6):823–830.

33. Duan X, Dabbs D. Smooth muscle myosin heavy chain and p63 for diagnosis of difficult lesions on core biopsies of the breast. Mod Pathol 2004; 17:22A.

34. Eusebi V, Foschini MP, Betts CM, et al. Microglandular adenosis, apocrine adenosis, and tubular carcinoma of the breast: An immunohistochemical comparison. Am J Surg Pathol 1993; 17:99–109.

35. Wheeler DT, et al. Tubulolobular carcinoma of the breast: an analysis of 27 cases of a tumor with a hybrid morphology and immunoprofile. Am J Surg Pathol 2004. 28(12):1587–1593.

36. Lee KC, Chan JK, Gwi E. Tubular adenosis of the breast: A distinct benign lesion mimicking invasive carcinoma. Am J Surg Pathol 1996; 20:46–54.

37. Eusebi V, Collina G, Bussolati G. Carcinoma in situ in sclerosing adenosis of the breast: An immunohistochemical study. Semin Diagn Pathol 1989; 6:146–152.

38. Rasbridge S. Carcinoma in situ involving sclerosing adenosis: A mimic of invasive breast carcinoma. Histopathology 1995; 27:269–273.

39. Papotti M, Gugliotta P, Eusebi V, et al. Immunohistochemical analysis of benign and malignant papillary lesions of the breast. Am J Surg Pathol 1983; 7:451–461.

40. Purcell C, Norris HJ. Intraductal proliferations of the breast: A review of histologic criteria for atypical ductal hyperplasia and ductal carcinoma in situ, including apocrine and papillary lesions. Ann Diagn Pathol 1998; 2:135–145.

41. McKinney CD, Fechner RE. Papillomas of the breast: A histologic spectrum including atypical hyperplasia and duct carcinoma in situ. Pathol Annu 1995; 30:137–178.

42. Raju U, Vertes D. Breast papillomas with atypical ductal hyperplasia. Hum Pathol 1996; 27:1231–1238.

43. Barsky S, Siegal GP, Jannota F, et al. Loss of basement membrane components by invasive tumors but not their benign counterparts. Lab Invest 1983; 49:140–147.

44. Chomette G, Auriol M, Tranbaloc P, et al. Stromal changes in early invasive breast carcinoma: An immunohistochemical, histoenzymological and ultrastructural study. Pathol Res Pract 1990; 186:70–79.

45. Hill CB, Yeh IT. Myoepithelial cell staining patterns of papillary breast lesions: from intraductal papillomas to invasive papillary carcinomas. Am J Clin Pathol 2005; 123(1):36–44.

46. Simpson R, Cope N, Skalova A, et al. Malignant adenomyoepithelioma of the breast with mixed osteogenic, spindle cell and carcinomatous differentiation. Am J Surg Pathol 1998; 22:631–636.

47. Maiorano E, Ricco R, Virgintino D, et al. Infiltrating myoepithelioma of the breast. Appl Immunohistochem 1994; 2: 130–136.

48. Foschini M, Eusebi V. Carcinomas of the breast showing myoepithelial cell differentiation: A review of the literature. Virchows Arch 1998; 432:303–310.

49. Chen PC, Chen CK, Nicastri AD, et al. Myoepithelial carcinoma of the breast with distant metastasis and accompanied by adenomyoepitheliomas. Histopathology 1994; 24:543–548.

50. Young RH. Adenomyoepithelioma of the breast: A report of three cases and review of the literature. Am J Clin Pathol 1988; 89:308–314.

51. Thorner PS, Kahn HJ, Baumal R, et al. Malignant myoepithelioma of the breast: An immunohistochemical study by

light and electron microscopy. Cancer Res 1986; 57:745–750.
52. Tavassoli F., Myoepithelial lesions of the breast: Myoepitheliosis, adenomyoepithelioma and myoepithelial carcinoma. Am J Surg Pathol 1991; 15:554–568.
53. Schurch W, Potvin C, Seemayer TA. Malignant myoepithelioma (myoepithelial carcinoma) of the breast: An ultrastructural and immunohistochemical study. Ultrastruct Pathol 1985; 8:1–11.
54. Smith TA, Machen K, Fisher C, et al. Usefulness of cytokeratin subsets for distinguishing monophasic synovial sarcoma from malignant peripheral nerve sheath tumors. Am J Clin Pathol 1999; 112:641–648.
55. Deligeorgi-Politi H, Kontozoglou T, Joseph M, et al. Myofibroblastoma of the breast: Cytologic, histologic, immunohistochemical and ultrastructural findings in two cases with differing cellularity. Breast J 1997; 3:365–371.
56. Hornick JL, Fletcher CD. Cutaneous myoepithelioma: a clinicopathologic and immunohistochemical study of 14 cases. Hum Pathol 2004; 35(1):14–24.
57. Hornick JL, Fletcher CD. Myoepithelial tumors of soft tissue: a clinicopathologic and immunohistochemical study of 101 cases with evaluation of prognostic parameters. Am J Surg Pathol 2003; 27(9):1183–1196.
58. Koker MM, Kleer CG. p63 expression in breast cancer: a highly sensitive and specific marker of metaplastic carcinoma. Am J Surg Pathol 2004; 28(11):1506–1512.
59. Lacroix-Triki M, et al. Value of cytokeratin 5/6 immuno-staining using D5/16 B4 antibody in the spectrum of proliferative intraepithelial lesions of the breast. A comparative study with 34betaE12 antibody. Virchows Arch 2003; 442(6):548–554.
60. Julien M, Trojani M, Coindre JM. Myofibroblastoma of the breast: Report of 8 cases. Ann Pathol 1994; 14:143–147.
61. Wargotz ES, Weiss SW, Norris HJ. Myofibroblastoma of the breast: Sixteen cases of a distinctive benign mesenchymal tumor. Am J Surg Pathol 1987; 11:493–502.
62. Damiani S, Miettinin M, Peterse JL, et al. Solitary fibrous tumor (myofibroblastoma) of the breast. Virchows Arch 1994; 425:89–92.
63. Schwartz GF, Patchefsky AS, Finkelstein, SD, et al. Nonpalpable in situ ductal carcinoma of the breast: Predictors of multicentricity and microinvasion and implications for treatment. Arch Surg 1989; 124:29–32.
64. Patchefsky AS, Schwartz GF, Finkelstein SD, et al. Heterogeneity of intraductal carcinoma of the breast. Cancer Res 1989; 63:731–741.
65. Dunne B, et al. An immunohistochemical study of metaplastic spindle cell carcinoma, phyllodes tumor and fibromatosis of the breast. Hum Pathol 2003; 34(10):1009–1015.
66. Leibl S, et al. Metaplastic breast carcinomas: are they of myoepithelial differentiation?: immunohistochemical profile of the sarcomatoid subtype using novel myoepithelial markers. Am J Surg Pathol 2005; 29(3):347–353.
67. Popnikolov NK, et al. Benign myoepithelial tumors of the breast have immunophenotypic characteristics similar to metaplastic matrix-producing and spindle cell carcinomas. Am J Clin Pathol 2003; 120(2):161–167.
68. Reis-Filho JS, et al. Novel and classic myoepithelial/stem cell markers in metaplastic carcinomas of the breast. Appl Immunohistochem Mol Morphol 2003; 11(1):1–8.
69. Tamimi SO, Ahmed A. Stromal changes in early invasive and non-invasive breast carcinoma: An ultrastructural study. J Pathol 1986; 150:43–49.
70. Silverstein MJ, Waisman JR, Gamagami P, et al. Intraductal carcinoma of the breast (208 cases): Clinical factors influencing treatment choice. Cancer 1990; 66:102–108.
71. Schuh ME, Nemoto T, Penetrante RB, et al. Intraductal carcinoma: Analysis of presentation, pathologic findings and outcome of disease. Arch Surg 1986; 121:1303–1307.
72. Wong JH, Kopald KH, Morton DL. The impact of microinvasion on axillary node metastases and survival in patients with intraductal breast cancer. Arch Surg 1990 125:1298–1302.
73. Solin LJ, Fowble BL, Yeh I-T, et al. Microinvasive ductal carcinoma of the breast treated with breast conserving surgery and definitive radiation. Int J Radiat Oncol Biol Phys 1992; 23:961–968.
74. Rosner D, Lane WW, Penetrante R. Duct carcinoma in situ with microinvasion: A curable entity using surgery alone without need for adjuvant therapy. Cancer 1991; 67:1498–1503.
75. Force PW. Standardized management of breast cancer specimens. Am J Clin Pathol 1973; 60:789–798.
76. Rosen PP. Intraductal carcinoma. In: Breast pathology. Philadelphia: Lippincott-Raven; 1997:264–265.
77. Prasad ML, Hyjek E, Giri DD, et al. Double immunolabeling with cytokeratin and smooth-muscle actin in confirming early invasive carcinoma of breast. Am J Surg Pathol 1999; 23:

176–181.

78. Masood S, Sim SJ, Lu L. Immunohistochemical differentiation of atypical hyperplasia vs. carcinoma in situ. Cancer Detect Prev 1992; 16:225–235.
79. Soini Y, Miettinin M. Immunohistochemical evaluation of the cytoarchitecture of benign and malignant breast lesions. APMIS 1993; 100:901–907.
80. Monifar F, Man YG, Lininger RA, et al. Use of keratin 34bE12 as an adjunct in the diagnosis of mammary intraepithelial neoplasia-ductal type-benign and malignant intraductal proliferations. Am J Surg Pathol 1999; 23:1048–1058.
81. Ashikari R, Park K, Huvos A, et al. Paget's disease of the breast. Cancer 1970; 26:680–685.
82. Kister SJ, Haagensen CD. Paget's disease of the breast. Am J Surg Pathol 1977; 119:606–609.
83. Stefanou D, et al. p63 expression in benign and malignant breast lesions. Histol Histopathol 2004; 19(2):465–471.
84. Rabban JT, Lerwill MF. Cytokeratin 5/6 distinguishes solid papillary ductal carcinoma in situ form florid usual ductal hyperplasia. Mod Pathol 2005; 18(Suppl 1):47A.
85. Salvadori B, Fariselli G, Saccozzi R. Analysis of 100 cases of Paget's disease of the breast. Tumori 1976; 62:529–536.
86. Lundquist K, Kohler S, Rouse RV. Intraepidermal cytokeratin 7 expression is not restricted to Paget cells but is also seen in Toker cells and Merkel cells. Am J Surg Pathol 1999; 23:212–219.
87. Zeng Z, Melamed J, Symmans P, et al. Benign proliferative nipple duct lesions frequently contain CAM5.2 and anti-cytokeratin 7 immunoreactive cells in the overlying epidermis. Am J Surg Pathol 1999; 23:1349–1355.
88. Cabanas RM. An approach for the treatment of penile carcinoma. Cancer 1977; 39:456–466.
89. Reintgen D, Cruse CW, Wells K, et al. The orderly progression of melanoma lymph node metastasis. Ann Surg 1994; 220:759–767.
90. Tani E, Skoog L. Immunocytochemical detection of estrogen receptors in mammary Paget cells. Acta Cytol 1988; 23:825–828.
91. Marucci G, et al. Toker cells are probably precursors of Paget cell carcinoma: a morphological and ultrastructural description. Virchows Arch 2002; 441(2):117–123.
92. Meissner K, Riviere A, Haupt G, et al. Study of neu-protein expression in mammary Paget's disease with and without underlying breast carcinoma and in extramammary Paget's disease. Am J Clin Pathol 1990; 137:1305–1309.
93. Yao DX, et al. Intraepidermal cytokeratin 7 immunoreactive cells in the non-neoplastic nipple may represent inter-epithelial extension of lactiferous duct cells. Histopathology 2002; 40(3):230–236.
94. Salama ME, et al. p16INK4a expression in actinic keratosis and Bowen's disease. Br J Dermatol 2003; 149(5):1006–1012.
95. Steinhoff MM. Axillary node micrometastases: Detection and biologic significance. Breast J 1999; 5:325–329.
96. Mansi JL, Gogas H, Bliss JM, et al. Outcome of primary breast cancer patients with micrometastases: A long-term follow-up study. Lancet 1999; 354:197–202.
97. Nasser IA, Lee AK, Bosari S, et al. Occult axillary lymph node metastases in 'node negative' breast carcinoma. Hum Pathol 1993; 24:950–957.
98. Bass SS, Lyman GH, McCann CR, et al. Lymphatic mapping and sentinel lymph node biopsy. Breast J 1999; 5:288–295.
99. Dabbs DJ, Johnson R. The optimal number of sentinel lymph nodes for focused pathologic examination. Breast J 2004; 10(3):186–189.
100. Dowlatshahi K, Fan M, Bloom KJ, et al. Occult metastases in the sentinel lymph nodes of patients with early stage breast carcinoma. Cancer 1999; 86:990–996.
101. Meyer J. Sentinel lymph node biopsy: Strategies for pathologic examination of the specimen. J Surg Oncol 1998; 69:212–218.
102. Roberts SA, Pasha TL, Zhang PJ. Undesirable cytokeratin immunoreactivity of native nonepithelial cells in sentinel lymph nodes from patients with breast carcinoma. Arch Pathol Lab Med 2000; 124:1310–1313.
103. Czerniecki BJ, Scheff AM, Callans LS, et al. Immunohistochemistry with pancytokeratins improves sensitivity of sentinel lymph node biopsy in patients with breast carcinoma. Cancer 1999; 85:1098–1103.
104. Krag DN, et al. NSABP-32: Phase III, randomized trial comparing axillary resection with sentinel lymph node dissection: a description of the trial. Ann Surg Oncol 2004; 11(3 Suppl):208S–210S.
105. Chagpar A, et al. Clinical outcome of patients with lymph node-negative breast carcinoma who have sentinel lymph node micrometastases detected by immunohistochemistry.

Cancer 2005; 241:1005–1012; discussion 1012–1015.
106. Doglioni C, Dell'Orto P, Zanetti G, et al. Cytokeratin immunoreactive cells of lymph nodes and spleen in normal and pathologic conditions. Virchow's Arch A Pathol Anat Histopathol 1990; 416:479–490.
107. Iuzzolino P, Bontempini L, Doglioni C, et al. Keratin immunoreactivity in extrafollicular reticular cells of the lymph node. Am J Clin Pathol 1989; 91:239–240.
108. Carter BA, Jensen RA, Simpson JF, et al. Benign transport of breast epithelium into axillary lymph nodes after biopsy. Am J Clin Pathol 2000; 113:259–265.
109. Pearlman WH, Giueriguian JD, Sawyer ME, et al. A specific progesterone binding component of human breast fluid. J Biol Chem 1973; 248:5736–5741.
110. Diaz NM, et al. Modes of benign mechanical transport of breast epithelial cells to axillary lymph nodes. Adv Anat Pathol 2005; 12(1):7–9.
111. Diaz NM, et al. Benign mechanical transport of breast epithelial cells to sentinel lymph nodes. Am J Surg Pathol 2004; 28(12):1641–1645.
112. Diaz NM, Mayes JR, Vrcel V. Breast epithelial cells in dermal angiolymphatic spaces: A manifestation of benign mechanical transport. Hum Pathol 2005; 36(3):310–313.
113. Wong AS, Gumbiner BM. Adhesion-independent mechanism for suppression of tumor cell invasion by E-cadherin. J Cell Biol 2003; 161(6):1191–1203.
114. Berx G, et al. E-cadherin is a tumour/invasion suppressor gene mutated in human lobular breast cancers. Embo J 1995; 14(24):6107–6115.
115. Acs G, Lawton TJ, Rebbeck TR, et al. Differential expression of E-cadherin in lobular and ductal neoplasms of the breast and its biologic and diagnostic implications. Am J Clin Pathol 2001; 115:85–98.
116. Behrens J, et al. The role of E-cadherin and scatter factor in tumor invasion and cell motility. EXS 1991; 59:109–126.
117. Shiozaki H, et al. Expression of immunoreactive E-cadherin adhesion molecules in human cancers. Am J Pathol 1991; 139(1):17–23.
118. Gamallo C, et al. Correlation of E-cadherin expression with differentiation of grade and histological type in breast carcinoma. Am J Pathol 1993; 142(4):987–993.
119. Guriec N, et al. E-cadherin mRNA expression in breast carcinomas correlates with overall and disease-free survival. Invasion Metastasis 1996; 16(1):19–26.
120. Siitonen S, Kononen JT, Helin HJ, et al. Reduced E-cadherin expression is associated with invasiveness and unfavorable prognosis in breast cancer. Am J Clin Pathol 1996; 105:394–402.
121. Charpin C, et al. Reduced E-cadherin immunohistochemical expression in node-negative breast carcinomas correlates with 10-year survival. Am J Clin Pathol 1998; 109(4):431–438.
122. Yoshida R, et al. The loss of E-cadherin, alpha- and beta-catenin expression is associated with metastasis and poor prognosis in invasive breast cancer. Int J Oncol 2001; 18(3):513–520.
123. Madhavan M, et al. Cadherins as predictive markers of nodal metastasis in breast cancer. Mod Pathol 2001; 14(5):423–427.
124. Parker C, et al. E-cadherin as a prognostic indicator in primary breast cancer. Br J Cancer 2001; 85(12):1958–1963.
125. Kowalski PJ, Rubin MA, Kleer CG. E-cadherin expression in primary carcinomas of the breast and its distant metastases. Breast Cancer Res 2003; 5(6):R217–R222.
126. Brinck U, et al. Diffuse growth pattern affects E-cadherin expression in invasive breast cancer. Anticancer Res 2004; 24(4):2237–2242.
127. Moll R MM, Frixen UH, et al. Differential loss of E-cadherin expression in infiltrating ductal and lobular carcinomas. Am J Pathol 1993; 143:1731–1742.
128. Rasbridge SA, Gillett CE, Sampson SA, et al. Epithelial (E-) and placental (P-) cadherin cell adhesion molecule expression in breast carcinoma. J Pathol 1993; 169:245–250.
129. Mastracci TL, et al. E-cadherin alterations in atypical lobular hyperplasia and lobular carcinoma in situ of the breast. Mod Pathol 2005; 18:741–751.
130. Kanai Y, et al. Point mutation of the E-cadherin gene in invasive lobular carcinoma of the breast. Jpn J Cancer Res 1994; 85(10):1035–1039.
131. Graff JR, et al. E-cadherin expression is silenced by DNA hypermethylation in human breast and prostate carcinomas. Cancer Res 1995; 55(22):5195–5199.
132. Berx G, et al. E-cadherin is inactivated in a majority of invasive human lobular breast cancers by truncation mutations throughout its extracellular domain. Oncogene 1996; 13(9):1919–1925.
133. Nishizaki T. et al. Genetic alterations in lobular breast cancer by comparative genomic hybridization. Int J Cancer 1997;

74(5):513–517.

134. Etzell JE, et al. Loss of chromosome 16q in lobular carcinoma in situ. Hum Pathol 2001; 32(3):292–296.

135. Droufakou S, et al. Multiple ways of silencing E-cadherin gene expression in lobular carcinoma of the breast. Int J Cancer 2001; 92(3):404–408.

136. Sarrio D, et al. Epigenetic and genetic alterations of APC and CDH1 genes in lobular breast cancer: relationships with abnormal E-cadherin and catenin expression and microsatellite instability. Int J Cancer 2003; 106(2):208–215.

137. Cheng CW, et al. Mechanisms of inactivation of E-cadherin in breast carcinoma: modification of the two-hit hypothesis of tumor suppressor gene. Oncogene 2001; 20(29):3814–3823.

138. Sarrio D, et al. Cytoplasmic localization of p120ctn and E-cadherin loss characterize lobular breast carcinoma from pre-invasive to metastatic lesions. Oncogene 2004; 23(19):3272–3283.

139. Goldstein NS, Kestin LL, Vicini FA. Clinicopathologic implications of E-cadherin reactivity in patients with lobular carcinoma in situ of the breast. Cancer 2001; 92(4):738–747.

140. De Leeuw WJ, et al. Simultaneous loss of E-cadherin and catenins in invasive lobular breast cancer and lobular carcinoma in situ. J Pathol 1997; 183(4):404–411.

141. Gonzalez MA, et al. An immunohistochemical examination of the expression of E-cadherin, alpha- and beta/gamma-catenins, and alpha2- and beta1-integrins in invasive breast cancer. J Pathol 1999; 187(5):523–529.

142. Goldstein NS. Does the level of E-cadherin expression correlate with the primary breast carcinoma infiltration pattern and type of systemic metastases? Am J Clin Pathol 2002; 118(3):425–434.

143. Jacobs TW, et al. Carcinomas in situ of the breast with indeterminate features: role of E-cadherin staining in categorization. Am J Surg Pathol 2001; 25(2):229–236.

144. Goldstein NS, et al. E-cadherin reactivity of 95 noninvasive ductal and lobular lesions of the breast. Implications for the interpretation of problematic lesions. Am J Clin Pathol 2001; 115(4):534–542.

145. Lehr H, Folpe A, Yaziji H, et al. Cytokeratin 8 immuno-staining pattern and E-cadherin expression distinguish lobular from ductal breast carcinoma. Am J Clin Pathol 2000; 114:190–196.

146. Middleton LP, et al. Lobular carcinoma in situ diagnosed by core needle biopsy: when should it be excised? Mod Pathol 2003; 16(2):120–129.

147. O'Driscoll D, et al. Lobular carcinoma in situ on core biopsy – what is the clinical significance? Clin Radiol 2001; 56(3): 216–220.

148. Liberman L, et al. Lobular carcinoma in situ at percutaneous breast biopsy: surgical biopsy findings. AJR Am J Roentgenol 1999; 173(2):291–299.

149. Shin SJ, Rosen PP. Excisional biopsy should be performed if lobular carcinoma in situ is seen on needle core biopsy. Arch Pathol Lab Med 2002; 126(6):697–701.

150. Renshaw AA, et al. Lobular neoplasia in breast core needle biopsy specimens is not associated with an increased risk of ductal carcinoma in situ or invasive carcinoma. Am J Clin Pathol 2002; 117(5):197–799.

151. Bauer VP, et al. The management of lobular neoplasia identified on percutaneous core breast biopsy. Breast J 2003; 9(1):4–9.

152. Dmytrasz K, et al. The significance of atypical lobular hyperplasia at percutaneous breast biopsy. Breast J 2003; 9(1): 10–12.

153. Berg WA, Mrose HE, Ioffe OB. Atypical lobular hyperplasia or lobular carcinoma in situ at core-needle breast biopsy. Radiology 2001; 218(2):503–509.

154. Philpotts LE, et al. Uncommon high-risk lesions of the breast diagnosed at stereotactic core-needle biopsy: clinical importance. Radiology 2000; 216(3):831–837.

155. Lee AH, et al. Excision biopsy findings of patients with breast needle core biopsies reported as suspicious of malignancy (B4) or lesion of uncertain malignant potential (B3). Histopathology 2003; 42(4):331–336.

156. Zhang RR. Atypical lobular hyperplasia or lobular carcinoma in situ on large core needle biopsy of the breast: is surgical excision necessary? Am J Clin Pathol 2001; 116:610.

157. Pacelli A, Amrami KK. Outcome of atypical lobular hyperplasia and lobular carcinoma in situ diagnosed by core needle biopsy; clinical and surgical follow-up of 30 cases. Am J Clin Pathol 2001; 116:591A.

158. Elsheikh TM. Is follow-up surgical excision indicated when breast core needle biopsies show lobular hyperplasia or lobular carcinoma in situ? A correlative study of 22 patients. Mod Pathol 2001; 14:25A.

159. Clark B, Dabbs DJ. The quantitative significance of lobular neoplasia and atypical ductal hyperplasia in breast needle core biopsy. Mod Pathol 2005; 18 (1):30A.
160. Sapino A, et al. Mammographically detected in situ lobular carcinomas of the breast. Virchows Arch 2000; 436(5):421–430.
161. Arpino G, et al. Lobular neoplasia on core-needle biopsy – clinical significance. Cancer 2004; 101(2):242–250.
162. Elsheikh TM, Silverman JF. Follow-up surgical excision is indicated when breast core needle biopsies show atypical lobular hyperplasia or lobular carcinoma in situ: a correlative study of 33 patients with review of the literature. Am J Surg Pathol 2005; 29(4):534–543.
163. Page DL, et al. Atypical lobular hyperplasia as a unilateral predictor of breast cancer risk: a retrospective cohort study. Lancet 2003; 361(9352):125–129.
164. Vos CB, et al. E-cadherin inactivation in lobular carcinoma in situ of the breast: an early event in tumorigenesis. Br J Cancer 1997; 76(9):1131–1133.
165. Bassler R, Kronsbein H. Disseminated lobular carcinoma – a predominantly pleomorphic lobular carcinoma of the whole breast. Pathol Res Pract 1980; 166(4):456–470.
166. Weidner N, Semple JP. Pleomorphic variant of invasive lobular carcinoma of the breast. Hum Pathol 1992; 23(10):1167–1171.
167. Eusebi V, Magalhaes F, Azzopardi JG, et al. Pleomorphic lobular carcinoma of the breast: An aggressive tumor showing apocrine differentiation. Hum Pathol 1992; 23:655–662.
168. Bentz JS, Yassa N, Clayton F. Pleomorphic lobular carcinoma of the breast: clinicopathologic features of 12 cases. Mod Pathol 1998; 11(9):814–822.
169. Radhi JM. Immunohistochemical analysis of pleomorphic lobular carcinoma: higher expression of p53 and chromogranin and lower expression of ER and PgR. Histopathology 2000; 36(2):156–160.
170. Middleton LP, Palacios D, Bryant B, et al. Pleomorphic lobular carcinoma: morphology, immunohistochemistry, and molecular analysis. Am J Surg Pathol 2000; 24(12):1650–1656.
171. Frolik D, Caduff R, Varga Z. Pleomorphic lobular carcinoma of the breast: its cell kinetics, expression of oncogenes and tumour suppressor genes compared with invasive ductal carcinomas and classical infiltrating lobular carcinomas. Histopathology 2001; 39(5):503–513.
172. Sneige N, et al. Clinical, histopathologic, and biologic features of pleomorphic lobular (ductal-lobular) carcinoma in situ of the breast: a report of 24 cases. Mod Pathol 2002; 15(10):1044–1050.
173. Palacios J, et al. Frequent E-cadherin gene inactivation by loss of heterozygosity in pleomorphic lobular carcinoma of the breast. Mod Pathol 2003; 16(7):674–678.
174. Chen Y, Fitzgibbons P, Jacobs T, et al. Pleomorphic apocrine lobular carcinoma in situ. Phenotypic and genetic study of a distinct variant of lobular carcinoma. Mod Pathol 2005; 18(1):29A.
175. Fisher ER, et al. Tubulolobular invasive breast cancer: a variant of lobular invasive cancer. Hum Pathol 1977; 8(6):679–683.
176. Green I, et al. A comparative study of pure tubular and tubulolobular carcinoma of the breast. Am J Surg Pathol 1997; 21(6):653–657.
177. Esposito N, Chivukula M, Dabbs DJ. Tubulolobular carcinoma: A morphologic and immunophenotypic study of 11 cases. Mod Pathol 2001; 18 (1):33A.
178. Filotico M, et al. Histiocytoid carcinoma of the breast. A problem of differential diagnosis for the pathologist. Report of a case. Pathologica 1983; 75(1037):429–433.
179. Gupta D, et al. E-cadherin immunohistochemical analysis of histiocytoid carcinoma of the breast. Ann Diagn Pathol 2002; 6(3):141–147.
180. Lazzaro B, et al. Antigenic characterization of medullary carcinoma of the breast: HLA-DR expression in lymph node positive cases. Appl Immunohistochem Mol Morphol 2001; 9(3):234–241.
181. Feinmesser M, et al. HLA-DR and beta 2 microglobulin expression in medullary and atypical medullary carcinoma of the breast: histopathologically similar but biologically distinct entities. J Clin Pathol 2000; 53(4):286–291.
182. Haagensen DEJ, Mazoujian G, Holder WDJ, et al. Evaluation of a breast cyst fluid protein detectable in the plasma of breast carcinoma patients. Ann Surg 1977; 185:279–285.
183. Murphy LC, Lee-Wing M, Goldenberg GJ, et al. Expression of the gene encoding a prolactin-inducible protein by human breast cancers in vivo. Cancer Res 1987; 47:4160–4164.
184. Losi L, Lorenzini R, Eusebi V, et al. Apocrine differentiation in invasive carcinoma of the breast: Comparison of mono-

clonal and polyclonal gross cystic disease fluid protein-15 antibodies with prolactin-inducible protein mRNA expression. Appl Immunohistochem 1995; 3:91–98.
185. Mazoujian G, Parish TH, Haagensen DEJ, et al. Immunoperoxidase localization of GCDFP-15 with mouse monoclonal antibodies versus rabbit antiserum. J Histochem Cytochem 1988; 36:377–382.
186. Wick MR, Lillemoe TJ, Copland GT, et al. Gross cystic disease fluid protein-15 as a marker for breast cancer: Immunohistochemical analysis of 690 human neoplasms and comparison with alpha-lactalbumin. Hum Pathol 1989; 20:281–287.
187. Viacava P, Naccarato AG, Bevilacqua GS. Spectrum of GCDFP-15 expression in human fetal and adult normal tissues. Virchows Arch 1998; 432:255–260.
188. Mazoujian G, Margolis R. Immunohistochemistry of gross cystic disease fluid protein (GCDFP-15) in 65 benign sweat gland tumors of the skin. Am J Dermatopathol 1988; 10:28–35.
189. Mazoujian G, Pinkus GS, David S, et al. Immunohistochemistry of a breast gross cystic disease fluid protein (GCDFP-15): A marker of apocrine epithelium and breast carcinomas with apocrine features. Am J Pathol 1983; 110:105–112.
190. Swanson PE, Pettinato G, Lillemoe TJ, et al. Gross cystic disease fluid protein-15 in salivary gland tumors. Arch Pathol Lab Med 1991; 115:158–163.
191. Wick M, Ockner DM, Mills SE, et al. Homologous carcinomas of the breasts, skin and salivary glands: A histologic and immunohistochemical comparison of ductal mammary carcinoma, ductal sweat gland carcinoma and salivary duct carcinoma. Am J Clin Pathol 1998; 109:75–84.
192. Ormsby AH, Snow JL, Su WPD, et al. Diagnostic immunohistochemistry of cutaneous metastatic breast carcinoma: A statistical analysis of the utility of gross cystic disease fluid protein-15 and estrogen receptor protein. J Am Acad Dermatol 1995; 32:711–716.
193. Mazoujian G, Bodian C, Haagensen DEJ, et al. Expression of GCDFP-15 in breast carcinomas: Relationship to pathologic and clinical factors. Cancer 1989; 63:156–161.
194. Kaufman O, Deidesheimer T, Muehlenberg M, et al. Immunohistochemical differentiation of metastatic breast carcinomas from metastatic adenocarcinomas of other common sites. Histopathology 1996; 29:233–240.
195. Raab SS, Berg SC, Swanson PE, et al. Adenocarcinoma in the lung in patients with breast cancer: A prospective analysis of the discriminatory value of immunohistology. Am J Clin Pathol 1993; 100:27–35.
196. Fiel MI, Cernaianu G, Burstein DE, et al. Value of GCDFP-15 (BRST-2) as a specific immunocytochemical marker for breast carcinoma in cytologic specimens. Acta Cytol 1996; 40:637–641.
197. Pritchard D, Todd CW, Egan ML. Chemistry of carcinoembryonic antigen. Methods Cancer Res 1978; 14:55–85.
198. Benoy IH, et al. Real-time RT-PCR correlates with immunocytochemistry for the detection of disseminated epithelial cells in bone marrow aspirates of patients with breast cancer. Br J Cancer 2004; 91(10):1813–1820.
199. Watson MA, et al. Mammaglobin expression in primary, metastatic, and occult breast cancer. Cancer Res 1999; 59(13):3028–3031.
200. Span PN, et al. Mammaglobin is associated with low-grade, steroid receptor-positive breast tumors from postmenopausal patients, and has independent prognostic value for relapse-free survival time. J Clin Oncol 2004; 22(4):691–698.
201. Nunez-Villar MJ, et al. Elevated mammaglobin (h-MAM) expression in breast cancer is associated with clinical and biological features defining a less aggressive tumour phenotype. Breast Cancer Res 2003; 5(3):R65–R70.
202. Han JH, et al. Mammaglobin expression in lymph nodes is an important marker of metastatic breast carcinoma. Arch Pathol Lab Med 2003; 127(10):1330–1334.
203. Ciampa A, et al. Mammaglobin and CRxA-01 in pleural effusion cytology: potential utility of distinguishing metastatic breast carcinomas from other cytokeratin 7-positive/cytokeratin 20-negative carcinomas. Cancer 2004; 102(6):368–372.
204. Tot T. The cytokeratin profile of medullary carcinoma of the breast. Histopathology 2000; 37(2):175–181.
205. Svenberg T. Carcinoembryonic antigen-like substances of human bile: Isolation and partial characterization. Int J Cancer 1976; 17:588–596.
206. Nach-J Pusztaszeri G. Demonstration of a partial identity between CEA and a normal glycoprotein. Immunochemistry 1972; 9:1031–1033.
207. Pavelic ZP, Pavelic L, Pavelic K, et al. Utility of anti-carcinoembryonic antigen monoclonal antibodies for differ-

208. entiating ovarian adenocarcinomas from gastrointestinal metastases to the ovary. Gynecol Oncol 1991; 40:112–117.
208. Moll R, Lowe A, Laufer J, et al. Cytokeratin 20 in human carcinomas: A new histodiagnostic marker detected by monoclonal antibodies. Am J Pathol 1992; 140:427–447.
209. Larsimont D, Lespagnard L, Degeyten M, et al. Medullary carcinoma of the breast: A tumor lacking keratin 19. Histopathology 1994; 24:549–552.
210. Dalal P, Shousha S. Keratin 19 in paraffin sections of medullary carcinoma and other benign and malignant breast lesions. Mod Pathol 1995; 8:413–416.
211. Jensen ML, Kiaer H, Melsen F. Medullary carcinoma versus poorly differentiated ductal carcinoma: An immunohistochemical study with keratin 19 and estrogen receptor staining. Histopathology 1996; 29:241–245.
212. Bacchi CE, Garcia RL, Gown AM. Immunolocalization of estrogen and progesterone receptors in neuroendocrine tumors of the lung, skin, gastrointestinal and female genital tracts. Appl Immunohistochem 1997; 5:17–22.
213. Deamant FT, Pombo MT, Battifora H. Estrogen receptor immunohistochemistry as a predictor of site of origin in metastatic breast cancer. Appl Immunohistochem 1993; 1:188–192.
214. Vargas SO, Leslie KO, Vacek PM, et al. Estrogen receptor related protein 29 in primary non-small cell carcinoma: Pathologic and prognostic correlations. Cancer 1998; 82:1495–1500.
215. Beattie CW, Hansen NW, Thomas PA. Steroid receptors in human lung cancer. Cancer Res 1985; 45:4206–4214.
216. Kaiser U, Hofmann J, Schilli M, et al. Steroid hormone receptors in cell lines and tumor biopsies of human lung cancer. Int J Cancer 1996; 67:357–364.
217. Su JM, Shu HK, Chang H, et al. Expression of estrogen and progesterone receptors in non-small cell lung cancer: Immunohistochemical study. Anticancer Res 1996; 16:3803–3806.
218. Cagle PT, Mody DR, Schwartz MR. Estrogen and progesterone receptors in bronchogenic carcinoma. Cancer Res 1990; 50:6632–6635.
219. Genestie C, Zafrani B, Asselain B. Comparison of the prognostic value of Scarff-Bloom-Richardson and Nottingham histological grades in a series of 825 cases of breast cancer: Major importance of the mitotic count as a component of both grading systems. Anticancer Res 1998; 18:571–576.
220. Allred C, Harvey JM, Berado M, et al. Prognostic and predictive factors in breast cancer by immunohistochemical analysis. Mod Pathol 1999; 11:155–168.
221. Ravdin PM. Should HER-2 status be routinely measured for all breast cancer patients? Semin Oncol 1999; 26:117–123.
222. Paik S, Bryant J, Park C, et al. ErbB-2 and response to doxorubicin in patients with axillary lymph node-positive, hormone receptor negative breast cancer. J Natl Cancer Inst 1998; 90:1361–1370.
223. Muss HB, Thor AD, Berry DA, et al. C-erbB-2 expression and response to adjuvant therapy in women with node-positive early breast cancer. N Engl J Med 1994; 330:1260–1266.
224. Masood S. Estrogen and progesterone receptors in cytology. Diagn Cytopathol 1992; 8:475–491.
225. Masood S, Dee S, Goldstein JD. Immunocytochemical analysis of progesterone receptors in breast cancer. Am J Clin Pathol 1991; 96:59–63.
226. Marrazzo A, Taormina P, Leonardi P, et al. Immunocytochemical determination of estrogen and progesterone receptors on 219 fine-needle aspirates of breast cancer: A prospective study. Anticancer Res 1995; 15:521–526.
227. Keshgegian AA, Inverso K, Kline TS. Determination of estrogen receptor by monoclonal antireceptor antibody in aspiration biopsy cytology from breast carcinoma. Am J Clin Pathol 1988; 89:24–29.
228. Keunen-Boumeester V, Van der Kwast TH, Van Laarhoven HA, et al. Ki-67 staining in histological subtypes of breast carcinoma and fine needle aspiration smears. J Clin Pathol 1989; 134:733.
229. Jacobs TW, Sisiopikou KP, Prioleau JE, et al. Do prognostic marker studies on core needle biopsy specimens of breast carcinoma accurately reflect the marker status of the tumor? Mod Pathol 1998; 11:259–264.
230. Zidan A, Christie Brown JS, Peston D, et al. Estrogen and progesterone receptor assessment in core biopsy specimens of breast carcinoma. J Clin Pathol 1997; 50:27–29.
231. Puglisi F, Scalone PF, Bazzocchi M, et al. Image guided core breast biopsy: A suitable method for preoperative biological characterization of small (pT1) breast carcinomas. Cancer Lett 1998; 133:223–229.
232. Kaiserling E. [Immunohistochemical identification of lymph vessels with D2-40 in diagnostic pathology]. Pathologe 2004; 25(5):362–374.

233. Kahn HJ, Bailey D, Marks A. Monoclonal antibody D2-40, a new marker of lymphatic endothelium, reacts with Kaposi's sarcoma and a subset of angiosarcomas. Mod Pathol 2002; 15(4):434–440.

234. Chu AY, et al. Utility of D2-40, a novel mesothelial marker, in the diagnosis of malignant mesothelioma. Mod Pathol 2005; 18(1):105–110.

235. Beatson GT. On the treatment of inoperable cases of carcinoma of the mamma: Suggestions for a new method of treatment, with illustrative cases. Lancet 1896; 2:104–107.

236. McGuire W, Carbone P, Vollmer E. Estrogen receptors in human breast cancer. New York: Raven Press; 1975.

237. Jacquemier JD, Hassoun J, Torrente M, et al. Distribution of estrogen and progesterone receptors in healthy tissue adjacent to breast lesions at various stages – immunohistochemical study of 107 cases. Breast Cancer Res Treat 1990; 15: 109–117.

238. Reiner A, Reiner G, Spona J, et al. Histopathologic characterization of human breast cancer in correlation with estrogen receptor status: A comparison of immunocytochemical and biochemical analysis. Cancer 1988; 64:1149–1154.

239. Lesser ML, Rosen PP, Seine RT, et al. Estrogen and progesterone receptors in breast carcinoma: Correlations with epidemiology and pathology. Cancer 1981; 48:299–309.

240. Clark GM, McGuire WL. Steroid receptors and other prognostic factors in primary breast cancer. Semin Oncol 1988; 15:20–25.

241. Castagnetta L, Traina A, Carruba G, et al. The prognosis of breast cancer patients in relation to the estrogen receptor status of both primary disease and involved nodes. Br J Cancer 1992; 66:167–170.

242. Brdar B, Graf D, Padovan R, et al. Estrogen and progesterone receptors as prognostic factors in breast cancer. Tumori 1988; 74:45–52.

243. Crowe JP, Hubay CA, Pearson OH, et al. Estrogen receptor status as a prognostic indicator for stage I breast cancer patients. Breast Cancer Res Treat 1982; 2:171–176.

244. Clark GM, McGuire WL, Hubay CA, et al. Progesterone receptors as a prognostic factor in stage II breast cancer. N Engl J Med 1983; 309:1343–1347.

245. Pichon MF, Pallud C, Hacene K, et al. Prognostic value of progesterone receptor after long-term follow-up in primary breast cancer. Eur J Cancer 1992; 28:1676–1680.

246. Shintaku A, Said JW. Detection of estrogen receptors in routinely processed formalin-fixed paraffin sections of breast carcinoma: Use of DNAase pretreatment to enhance sensitivity of the reaction. Am J Clin Pathol 1987; 87:161–167.

247. Esteban JM, Battifora H, Warsi Z, et al. Quantification of estrogen receptors on paraffin embedded tumors by image analysis. Mod Pathol 1991; 4:53–57.

248. Cohen C, Unger ER, Sgoutas D, et al. Automated immunohistochemical estrogen receptor in fixed embedded breast carcinoma. Am J Clin Pathol 1991; 95:335–339.

249. Frigo B, Scopsi L, Faber M, et al. Application of an estrogen receptor-immunocytochemical assay primary monoclonal antibody to paraffin-embedded human breast tumor tissue: Personal experience and review of the literature. Appl Immunohistochem 1993; 1:136–142.

250. Battifora H, Mehta P, Ahn C, et al. Estrogen receptor immunohistochemical assay in paraffin-embedded tissue: A better gold standard? Appl Immunohistochem 1993; 1:39–45.

251. Styliandu A, Papadimitriou CS. Immunohistochemical demonstration of estrogen receptors on routine paraffin sections of breast carcinomas: A comparison with frozen sections and an enzyme immunoassay. Oncology (Basel) 1992; 49:15–21.

252. Katz RL, Patel S, Sneige N, et al. Comparison of immunocytochemical and biochemical assays for estrogen receptor in fine needle aspirates and histologic sections from breast carcinomas. Breast Cancer Res Treat 1990; 15:191–203.

253. Cowen PN, Teasdale J, Jackson P, et al. Estrogen receptor in breast cancer: Prognostic studies using a new immunohistochemical assay. Histopathology 1990; 17:319–325.

254. Cheng L, Binder SW, Fu YS. Methods in laboratory investigation: Demonstration of estrogen receptors by monoclonal antibody in formalin-fixed breast tumors. Lab Invest 1988; 58:346–353.

255. Giri DD, Dangerfield VJM, Lonsdale R, et al. Immunohistology of estrogen receptor content of adjacent cryostat sections of breast carcinoma by radioligand binding and enzyme assay. J Clin Pathol 1987; 40:734–740.

256. Jackson P, Teasdale J, Cowen PN, et al. Development and validation of a sensitive immunohistochemical estrogen receptor assay for use on archival breast cancer tissue. Histochemistry 1989; 92:149–152.

257. Graham DM, Jin L, Lloyd RV. Detection of estrogen receptor in paraffin-embedded sections of breast carcinoma by

immunohistochemistry and in situ hybridization. Am J Surg Pathol 1991; 15:475–485.
258. Leong A-Y, Milios J. Comparison of antibodies to estrogen and progesterone receptors and the influence of microwave antigen retrieval. Appl Immunohistochem 1993; 1:282–288.
259. Kell DL, Kamel O, Rouse RV. Immunohistochemical analysis of breast carcinoma estrogen and progesterone receptors in paraffin-embedded tissue: Correlation of clones ER1D5 and 1A6 with a cytosol based hormone receptor assay. Appl Immunohistochem 1993; 1:275–281.
260. Cattoretti G, Pileri S, Parravicini C, et al. Antigen unmasking on formalin-fixed, paraffin-embedded tissue sections. J Pathol 1993; 171:83–98.
261. Battifora H. Immunocytochemistry of hormone receptors in routinely processed tissue: The new gold standard [Editorial]. Appl Immunohistochem 1994; 2:143–145.
262. Mauri FA, Veronese S, Frigo B, et al. ER1D5 and H222 (ER-ICA) antibodies to human estrogen receptor protein in breast carcinomas: Results of a multicentric compara-tive study. Appl Immunohistochem 1994; 2:157–163.
263. DeSombre ER, Thorpe SM, Rose C, et al. Prognostic usefulness of estrogen receptor immunocytochemical assays for human breast cancer. Cancer Res 1986; 46:4256s–4264s.
264. Kinsel LB, Szabo E, Greene GL, et al. Immunocytochemical analysis of estrogen receptors as a predictor of prognosis in breast cancer patients: Comparison with quantitative biochemical methods. Cancer Res 1989; 49:1052–1056.
265. Pertschuk LP, Kim DS, Nayer K, et al. Immunocytochemical estrogen and progestin receptor assays in breast cancer with monoclonal antibodies: Histopathologic, demographic and biochemical correlations and relationship to endocrine response and survival. Cancer 1990; 66:1663–1670.
266. Pertschuk LP, Eisenberg KB, Carter AC, et al. Immunohistologic localization of estrogen receptors in breast cancer with monoclonal antibodies. Cancer 1985; 55:1513–1518.
267. McGuire WL, DeLaGarza M. Improved sensitivity in the measurement of estrogen receptors in human breast cancer. J Clin Endocrinol Metab 1973; 37:986–989.
268. Taylor C. Paraffin section immunocytochemistry for estrogen receptor: The time has come. Cancer 1996; 77:2419–2422.
269. Pertschuk L, Feldman J, Eisenberg K, et al. Immunohistochemical detection of progesterone receptor in breast cancer with monoclonal antibody: Relation to biochemical assay, disease-free survival, and clinical endocrine response. Cancer 1988; 62:342–349.
270. Ferno M, Andersson C, Fallenius G, et al. Estrogen receptor analysis of paraffin sections and cytosol samples of primary breast cancer in relation to outcome after adjuvant tamoxifen treatment. The South Sweden Breast Cancer Group. Acta Oncol 1996; 35:17–22.
271. Remmele W, Schicketanz KH. Immunohistochemical determination of estrogen and progesterone receptor content in human breast cancer: Computer-assisted image analysis. Pathol Res Pract 1993; 189:862–866.
272. Schultz D, Katz RL, Patel S, et al. Comparison of visual and CAS-200 quantitation of immunocytochemical staining in breast carcinoma samples. Anal Quant Cytol Histol 1992; 14:35–40.
273. Barnes DM, Millis RR, Beex LVAM, et al. Increased use of immunohistochemistry for estrogen receptor measurement in mammary carcinoma: The need for quality assurance. Eur J Cancer 1998; 34:1677–1682.
274. Clark GM, Harvey JM, Osborne CK, et al. Estrogen receptor status determined by immunohistochemistry is superior to biochemical ligand-binding (LB) assay for evaluating breast cancer patients. Proc Am Soc Clin Oncol 1997; 16:29A.
275. van Diest PJ, Weger DR, Lindholm J, et al. Reproducibility of subjective immunoscoring of steroid receptors in breast cancer. Anal Quant Cytol Histol 1996; 18:351–354.
276. Wilbur DC, Willis J, Mooney RA, et al. Estrogen and progesterone detection in archival formalin-fixed, paraffin-embedded tissue from breast carcinoma: A comparison in immunohistochemistry with the dextran-coated charcoal assay. Mod Pathol 1992; 5:79–84.
277. Tesch M, Shawwa A, Henderson R. Immunohistochemical determination of estrogen and progesterone receptor status in breast cancer. Am J Clin Pathol 1993; 99:8–12.
278. McClelland RA, Finlay P, Walker KJ, et al. Automated quantitation of immunohistochemical localized estrogen receptors in human breast cancer. Cancer Res 1990; 50:3545–3550.
279. Esteban JM, Kandalaft PI, Mehta P. Improvement of the quantification of estrogen and progesterone receptors in paraffin-embedded tumors by image analysis. Am J Clin Pathol 1993; 99:32–38.
280. Charpin C, Andrac L, Habib M-C, et al. Immunodetection in

fine-needle aspirates and multiparametric (SAMBA) image analysis: Receptors (monoclonal antiestrogen and antiprogesterone) and growth fraction (monoclonal Ki-67) evaluation in breast carcinomas. Cancer 1989; 63:863–872.

281. Layfield L, Saria EA, Conlon DH, et al. Estrogen and progesterone receptor status determined by the Ventana ES 320 automated immunohistochemical stainer and the CAS 200 image analyzer in 236 early-stage breast carcinomas: Prognostic significance. J Surg Oncol 1996; 61:177–184.

282. de Mascarel I., Soubeyran G, MacGrogan J, et al. Immunohistochemical analysis of estrogen receptors in 938 breast carcinomas. Appl Immunohistochem 1995; 3:222–231.

283. Pertschuk LP, Feldman JG, Kim YD, et al. Estrogen receptor immunocytochemistry in paraffin-embedded tissues with ER1D5 predicts breast cancer endocrine response more accurately than H222Sp gamma in frozen sections or cytosol-based ligand-binding assays. Cancer 1996; 77:2514–2519.

284. Veronese SM, Barbareschi M, Morelli L. Predictive value of ER1D5 antibody immunostaining in breast cancer: A paraffinbased retrospective study of 257 cases. Appl Immunohistochem 1995; 3:85–90.

285. Barnes DM, Harris WH, Smith P, et al. Immunohistochemical determination of estrogen receptor: Comparison of different methods of assessment of staining and correlation with clinical outcome of breast cancer patients. Br J Cancer 1996; 74:1445-1451.

286. Goulding H, Pinder S, Cannon P, et al. A new immunohistochemical antibody for the assessment of estrogen receptor status on routine formalin-fixed tissue samples. Hum Pathol 1995; 26:291–294.

287. Harvey JM, Clark GM, Osborne CK, et al. Estrogen receptor status by immunohistochemistry is superior to the ligand-binding assay for predicting response to adjuvant endocrine therapy in breast cancer. J Clinical Oncology 1999; 17(5): 1474–1481.

288. Elledge RM, et al. Estrogen receptor (ER) and progesterone receptor (PgR), by ligand-binding assay compared with ER, PgR and pS2, by immunohistochemistry in predicting response to tamoxifen in metastatic breast cancer: a Southwest Oncology Group Study. Int J Cancer 2000; 89(2):111–117.

289. Fisher ER, et al. Solving the dilemma of the immunohistochemical and other methods used for scoring estrogen receptor and progesterone receptor in patients with invasive breast carcinoma. Cancer 2005; 103(1):164–173.

290. Mohsin SK, et al. Progesterone receptor by immunohistochemistry and clinical outcome in breast cancer: a validation study. Mod Pathol 2004; 17(12):1545–1554.

291. Marcot I, Migeon C, Parache RM, et al. A comparative study of hormone receptors in breast cancer with quantitative immunocytochemistry and biochemistry. Bull Cancer 1997; 84: 613–618.

292. Tabbarra SO, Sidaway MK, Frost A, et al. The stability of estrogen and progesterone receptor expression on breast carcinoma cells stored as PreservCyt suspensions and as ThinPrep slides. Cancer 1998; 84:355–360.

293. Leung SW, Bedard YC. Estrogen and progesterone receptor contents in ThinPrep processed fine needle aspirates of breast. Am J Clin Pathol 1999; 112:50–56.

294. Rosen PP, Menendez-Botet CJ, Nisselbaum JS, et al. Pathological review of breast lesions analyzed for estrogen receptor protein. Cancer 1975; 35:3187–3194.

295. Nadji M, et al. Immunohistochemistry of estrogen and progesterone receptors reconsidered: experience with 5,993 breast cancers. Am J Clin Pathol 2005; 123(1):21–27.

296. Layfield L, Saria E, Mooney EE, et al. Tissue heterogeneity of immunohistochemically detected estrogen receptor: Implications for image analysis quantification. Am J Clin Pathol 1998; 110:758–764.

297. MacGrogan G, Soubeyran I, DeMascarel I, et al. Immunohistochemical detection of progesterone receptors in breast invasive ductal carcinomas: A correlative study of 942 cases. Appl Immunohistochem 1996; 4:219–227.

298. Gibney EM, Lawson D, DeRose PB, et al. Image cytometric progesterone quantitation: Comparison with visual semiquantitation and cytosolic assay. Appl Immunohistochem 1998; 6:62–68.

299. Elias JM, Margiotta M, Sexton TR, et al. Immunohistochemical detection of sex steroid receptors in breast carcinoma using routine paraffin sections: Comparison with frozen sections and enzyme immunoassay. J Cell Biochem Suppl 1994; 19:126–133.

300. Soomo S, Shousa S, Sinnet HD. Estrogen and progesterone receptors in screen-detected carcinoma: An immunohistological study using paraffin sections. Histopathology 1992; 21: 543–547.

301. Pennsi E. Differing roles found for estrogen's two receptors.

Science 1997; 277:1439.

302. Kuiper GGJM, Enmark E, Pelto-Huikko M, et al. Cloning of a novel receptor expressed in rat prostate and ovary. Proc Natl Acad Sci USA 1996; 93:5925–5930.

303. Paech K, Webb P, Kuiper GGJM, et al. Differential ligand activation of estrogen receptor alpha and ER beta at AP1 sites. Science 1997; 277:1508–1510.

304. Choi Y, Pinto M. Estrogen receptor beta in breast cancer: associations between ERbeta, hormonal receptors, and other prognostic biomarkers. Appl Immunohistochem Mol Morphol 2005; 13(1):19–24.

305. Fuqua SA, et al. Estrogen receptor beta protein in human breast cancer: correlation with clinical tumor parameters. Cancer Res 2003; 63(10):2434–2439.

306. Stefanou D, et al. Estrogen receptor beta (ERbeta) expression in breast carcinomas is not correlated with estrogen receptor alpha (ERalpha) and prognosis: the Greek experience. Eur J Gynaecol Oncol 2004; 25(4):457–461.

307. Hopp TA, et al. Low levels of estrogen receptor beta protein predict resistance to tamoxifen therapy in breast cancer. Clin Cancer Res 2004; 10(22):7490–7499.

308. Bargmann C, Hung MC, Weinber RA. The neu oncogene encodes an epidermal growth factor receptor-related protein. Nature 1986; 319:226–230.

309. Schecter A, Stern DF, Vaidyanathan L, et al. The neu oncogene: An erb-B-related gene encoding an 185,000 Mr tumor antigen. Nature 1984; 312:513–516.

310. King CR, Kraus MH, Aaronson SA. Amplification of a novel V-erbB-related gene in a human mammary carcinoma. Science 1985; 229:974–976.

311. Popescu NC, King CR, Kraus MH. Location of the human erbB-2 gene on normal and rearranged chromosomes 17 to bands q12-21.32. Genomics 1989; 4:362–366.

312. Shih C, Padhy LC, Murray M, et al. Transforming genes of carcinomas and neuroblastomas introduced into mouse fibroblasts. Nature 1981; 290:261–264.

313. Slamon DJ, Clark GM, Wong SG, et al. Human breast cancer: Correlation of relapse and survival with amplification of Her-2/neu oncogene. Science 1987; 235:177–182.

314. Hanna W, Kahn H.J, Trudeau M. Evaluation of Her-2/neu (erbB-2) status in breast cancer: From bench to bedside. Mod Pathol 1999; 12:827–834.

315. Clark G. Should selection of adjuvant chemotherapy for patients with breast cancer be based on erb-2 status? J Natl Cancer Inst 1998; 90:1320–1321.

316. Andrulis IL, Bull SB, Blackstein ME, et al. Neu/erbB-2 amplification identifies a poor prognosis group of women with node-negative breast cancer. J Clin Oncol 1998; 16:1340–1349.

317. Bianchi S, Paglierani M, Zampi G, et al. Prognostic significance of cerbB-2 expression in node negative breast cancer. Br J Cancer 1993; 67:625–629.

318. Borg A, Tandon AK, Sigurdsson H, et al. HER-2/neu amplification predicts poor survival in node positive breast cancer. Cancer Res 1990; 50:4332–4337.

319. Clark GM, McGuire WL. Follow-up study of HER-2/neu amplification in primary breast cancer. Cancer Res 1991; 51: 944–948.

320. Lovekin C, Ellis IO, Locker A, et al. C-erb-2 oncoprotein expression in primary and advanced breast cancer. Br J Cancer 1991; 63:439–443.

321. McCann AH, Dervan PA, O'Reagan M, et al. Prognostic significance of c-erbB-2 and estrogen receptor status in human breast cancer. Cancer Res 1991; 51:3296–3303.

322. Noguchi M, Koyasaki N, Ohta N, et al. C-erbB-2 oncoprotein expression versus internal mammary lymph node metastases as additional prognostic factors in patients with axillary lymph node positive breast cancer. Cancer 1992; 69:2953–2960.

323. O'Reilly SM, Barnes DM, Camplejohn RS, et al. The relationship between c-erbB-2 expression, S-phase fraction, and prognosis in breast cancer. Br J Cancer 1991; 63:444–446.

324. Paterson MC, Dietrich KD, Kanylik J, et al. Correlation between c-erbB-2 amplification and risk of recurrent disease in lymph node negative breast cancer. Cancer Res 1991; 54: 556–567.

325. Rosen PP, Lesser ML, Arroyo CD, et al. Immunohistochemical detection of HER-2/neu in patients with axillary lymph node-negative breast carcinoma. Cancer 1995; 75:1320–1326.

326. Toikkanen S, Helin H, Isola J, et al. Prognostic significance of HER-2 oncoprotein expression in breast cancer: A 20-year follow-up. J Clin Oncol 1992; 10:1044–1048.

327. Pres MF, Hung G, Godolphin GW, et al. Sensitivity of HER-2/neu antibodies in archival tissue samples: Potential source of error in immunohistochemical studies of oncogene expression. Cancer Res,1994; 54:2771–2777.

328. Anbazhagan R, Gelber RD, Bettelheim R, et al. Association

of c-erbB-2 expression and S phase fraction in the prognosis of node-positive breast cancer. Ann Oncol 1991; 2:47–53.

329. Borresen AL, Ottestad L, Gaustad A, et al. Amplification and protein overexpression of the neu/HER-2/c-erbB-2 proto-oncogene in human breast carcinomas: Relationship to loss of gene sequences on chromosome 17, family history and prognosis. Br J Cancer 1990; 62:585–590.

330. Gusterson BA, Gelber RD, Goldhirsch A, et al. Prognostic importance of c-erbB-2 expression in breast cancer. J Clin Oncol 1992; 10:1049–1056.

331. Marks JR, Humphrey PA, Wu K, et al. Overexpression of p53 and Her-2/neu proteins as prognostic markers in early-stage breast cancer. Ann Surg 1994; 219:332–341.

332. Quenel N, Wafflart J, Bonichon F, et al. The prognostic value of c-erbB-2 in primary breast carcinomas: A study of 942 cases. Breast Cancer Res Treat 1995; 35:283–291.

333. Rilke F, Colnaghi MI, Cascinelli N, et al. Prognostic significance of Her-2/neu expression in breast cancer and its relationship to other prognostic factors. Int J Cancer 1991; 49:44–49.

334. Winstanley J, Cooke T, Murray GD, et al. The long-term prognostic significance of c-erbB-2 in primary breast cancer. Br J Cancer 1991; 63:447–450.

335. Schonborn I, Zschiesche W, Spitzer E, et al. C-erbB-2 overexpression in primary breast cancer: Independent prognostic factor in patients at high risk. Breast Cancer Res Treat 1994; 29:287–295.

336. Tetu B, Brisson J. Prognostic significance of HER-2/neu oncoprotein expression in node-positive breast cancer: The influence of the pattern of immunostaining and adjuvant therapy. Cancer 1994; 73:2359–2365.

337. Kallioniemmi OP, Holli K, Visakorpi T, et al. Association of c-erbB-2 protein overexpression with high rate of cell proliferation, increased risk of visceral metastasis, and poor long-term survival in breast cancer. Int J Cancer 1991; 49:650–655.

338. Slamon D, Leyland-Jones B, Shak S, et al. Addition of Herceptin (humanized anti-Her-2 antibody) to first-line chemotherapy for (Her-2+/MBC) markedly increases anticancer activity: A randomized, multinational controlled phase III trial. Proc ASCO 1998; 17:98a.

339. Pegram MD, Lipton A, Hayes DF, et al. Phase II study of receptor-enhanced chemosensitivity using recombinant humanized anti-p185 Her-2/neu monoclonal antibody plus cisplatin in patients with Her-2/neu-overexpressing metastatic breast cancer refractory to chemotherapy treatment. J Clin Oncol 1998; 16:2659–2671.

340. Vogel CL, et al. Efficacy and safety of trastuzumab as a single agent in first-line treatment of HER2-overexpressing metastatic breast cancer. J Clin Oncol 2002; 20(3):719–726.

341. Slamon D, et al. Use of chemotherapy plus a monoclonal antibody against HER2 for metastatic breast cancer that overexpresses HER2. New Engl J Med 2001; 344:783–792.

342. Persons DL, Borrelli KA, Hsu PH. Quantitation of Her-2/neu and c-myc gene amplification in breast carcinoma using fluorescence in situ hybridization. Mod Pathol 1997; 10:720–727.

343. Mezzelani A, Alasio L, Bartoli C, et al. C-erbB2/neu gene and chromosome 17 analysis in breast cancer by FISH on archival cytological fine needle aspirates. Br J Cancer 1999; 80:519–525.

344. Lottner C, et al. Simultaneous detection of HER2/neu gene amplification and protein overexpression in paraffin-embedded breast cancer. J Pathol 2005; 205(5):577–584.

345. Pauletti G, Godolphin W, Press M, et al. Detection and quantification of HER-2/neu gene amplification in human breast cancer archival material using fluorescence in situ hybridization. Oncogene 1996; 13:63–72.

346. Paik S, et al. Real world performance of HER2 testing national surgical adjuvant breast and bowel project experience. J Natl Cancer Inst 2002; 94:852–854.

347. Roche P, et al. Concordance between local and central laboratory HER2 testing in the breast intergroup trial N9831. J Natl Cancer Inst 2002; 94:855–857.

348. Andersson J, et al. HER-2/neu (c-erbB-2) evaluation in primary breast carcinoma by fluorescence in situ hybridization and immunohistochemistry with special focus on intratumor heterogeneity and comparison of invasive and in situ components. Appl Immunohistochem Mol Morphol 2004; 12(1):14–20.

349. Wang S, et al. Assessment of HER-2/neu status in breast cancer. Automated Cellular Imaging System (ACIS)-assisted quantitation of immunohistochemical assay achieves high accuracy in comparison with fluorescence in situ hybridization assay as the standard. Am J Clin Pathol 2001; 116(4):495–503.

350. Owens MA, Horten BC, Da Silva MM. HER2 amplification ratios by fluorescence in situ hybridization and correlation with immunohistochemistry in a cohort of 6556 breast cancer tissues. Clin Breast Cancer 2004; 5(1):63–69.
351. Roche PC, Ingle JN. Increased HER2 with U.S. Food and Drug Administration-approved antibody. J Clin Oncol 1999; 17:434.
352. Jacobs TW, Gown AM, Yazdii H, et al. Her-2/neu protein expression in breast cancer evaluated by immunohistochemistry. Am J Clin Pathol 2000; 113:251–258.
353. Press MF, et al. Evaluation of HER-2/neu gene amplification and overexpression: comparison of frequently used assay methods in a molecularly characterized cohort of breast cancer specimens. J Clin Oncol 2002; 20(14):3095–3105.
354. Rhodes A, et al. The use of cell line standards to reduce HER-2/neu assay variation in multiple European cancer centers and the potential of automated image analysis to provide for more accurate cut points for predicting clinical response to trastuzumab. Am J Clin Pathol 2004; 122(1):51–60.
355. Zarbo RJ, Hammond ME. Conference summary, Strategic Science symposium. Her-2/neu testing of breast cancer patients in clinical practice. Arch Pathol Lab Med 2003; 127(5):549–553.
356. Cell Markers and Cytogenetics Committees College of American Pathologists. Clinical laboratory assays for HER-2/neu amplification and overexpression quality assurance, standardization, and proficiency testing. Arch Pathol Lab Med 2002; 126:803–808.
357. Ross JS, et al. HER-2/neu testing in breast cancer. Am J Clin Pathol 2003; 120 Suppl:S53–S71.
358. Hauser-Kronberger C, Dandachi N. Comparison of chromogenic in situ hybridization with other methodologies for HER2 status assessment in breast cancer. J Mol Histol 2004; 35(6):647–653.
359. Wixom CR, Albers EA, Weidner N. Her2 amplification: correlation of chromogenic in situ hybridization with immunohistochemistry and fluorescence in situ hybridization. Appl Immunohistochem Mol Morphol 2004; 12(3):248–251.
360. Madrid MA, Lo RW. Chromogenic in situ hybridization (CISH): a novel alternative in screening archival breast cancer tissue samples for HER-2/neu status. Breast Cancer Res 2004; 6(5):R593–R600.
361. Arnould L, et al. Agreement between chromogenic in situ hybridisation (CISH) and FISH in the determination of HER2 status in breast cancer. Br J Cancer 2003; 88(10):1587–1591.
362. Dabbs DJ. Correlations of morphology, proliferation indices, and oncogene activation in ductal breast carcinoma: nuclear grade, S-phase, proliferating cell nuclear antigen, p53, epidermal growth factor receptor, and c-erb-B-2. Mod Pathol 1995; 8(6):637–642.
363. Nicholson RI, et al. Relationship between EGF-R, c-erbB-2 protein expression and Ki67 immunostaining in breast cancer and hormone sensitivity. Eur J Cancer 1993; 29A(7):1018–1823.
364. Nicholson RI, et al. Epidermal growth factor receptor expression in breast cancer: association with response to endocrine therapy. Breast Cancer Res Treat 1994; 29(1):117–125.
365. Sharma AK, et al. Dual immunocytochemical analysis of oestrogen and epidermal growth factor receptors in human breast cancer. Br J Cancer 1994; 69(6):1032–1037.
366. Klijn JG, et al. The prognostic value of epidermal growth factor receptor (EGF-R) in primary breast cancer: results of a 10-year follow-up study. Breast Cancer Res Treat 1994; 29(1):73–83.
367. Diamandis EP, Yu H, Lopez-Otin C. Prostate specific antigen – a new constituent of breast fluid. Breast Cancer Res Treat 1996; 38:259–264.
368. Melegos DN, Diamandis EP. Diagnostic value of molecular forms of prostate specific antigen for female breast cancer. Clin Biochem 1996; 29:193–200.
369. Yu H, Diamandis EP, Sutherland DJ. Immunoreactive prostate specific antigen levels in female and male breast tumors and its association with steroid hormone receptors and patient age. Clin Biochem 1994; 27:75–79.
370. Yu H, Diamandis EP, Levesque M, et al. Prostate specific antigen in breast cancer, benign breast disease and normal breast tissue. Breast Cancer Res Treat 1996; 40:171–178.
371. Kidwai N, et al. Expression of androgen receptor and prostate-specific antigen in male breast carcinoma. Breast Cancer Res 2004; 6(1):R18–R23.
372. Carder PJ, et al. Expression of prostate specific antigen in male breast cancer. J Clin Pathol 2005; 58(1):69–71.
373. Gupta RK. Immunoreactivity of prostate specific antigen in male breast carcinomas: Two examples of a diagnostic pitfall in discriminating a primary breast cancer from metastatic prostate carcinoma. Diagn Cytopathol 1999; 21:167–169.

374. Komenaka IK, El-Tamer M, Pile-Spellman E, et al. Core needle biopsy as a diagnostic tool to differentiate phyllodes tumor from fibroadenoma. Arch Surg 2003; 138(9):987–990.

375. Carvalho S, et al. c-KIT and PDGFRA in breast phyllodes tumours: overexpression without mutations? J Clin Pathol 2004; 57(10):1075–1079.

376. Tse GM, et al. Stromal CD10 expression in mammary fibroadenomas and phyllodes tumours. J Clin Pathol 2005; 58(2):185–189.

18 神经系统的免疫组织化学

原作者：Paul E. McKeever
译　者：孙妍琳，郭成浩
审校者：周庚寅，张庆慧，刘志艳，张翠娟，孟　斌

目　录

引言	767
病变临床与影像学展望	768
非肿瘤脑部病变	769
肿瘤	778
囊肿	818
痴呆	820
脱髓鞘疾病	822
癫痫	823
诊断中的陷阱	824

引　言

本章主要讨论神经系统疾病的诊断性免疫组化。表18.2、18.13为总结性的内容。示意图18.1和18.2为流程图，直方图显示各病理类型的简要特点。如疑为某一特异性疾病，可以直接在表格中查寻，各个表格列出了特异性疾病的结构、免疫组化及局部解剖部位，因而能够通过表格或示意图流程查找特异性疾病。正文和图片则对这些疾病特征加以阐述[1-3]。

可以从不同的流程图和表格中寻找未知疾病的特征以帮助诊断。例如，一个肿块，本章在专门的表格中总结了肿块的鉴别诊断特征，如下所示：

1. 纤维性细胞：表18.5，图18.8~18.10。
2. 上皮样细胞：表18.6，图18.1、18.19、18.34。
3. 一种以上的细胞：表18.7，图18.29。
4. 间变性小细胞：表18.8，图18.36~18.40。
5. 合体细胞：表18.9，图18.42。

以上特征是基于细胞学和组织学的样本[3,4]。

示意图18.1主要是对透明细胞病变免疫组化的鉴别诊断。示意图18.2是对上皮样肿瘤免疫组化的鉴别诊断。

表18.1以字母顺序列出了神经系统疾病鉴别诊断的免疫组化。免疫组化应当设立对照。笔者本人的经验倾向于选择的标本要符合以下3个条件：标本内有感兴趣的病变，组织内有对所用的免疫染色呈阳性反应和阴性反应的区域，以此作为标准的组织内对照[1,5]。例如，一个染胶质纤维酸性蛋白（GFAP）的标本，在同一个组织块中应该包含神经胶质增生区（阳性对照）和血管（阴性对照）。这比用其他组织块作对照要好，其他组织块有可能不是采用同样的固定或处理方法。

个别肿瘤不能被它们正常应该表达的标记物所染色，而正常和反应性组织则保留它们预期的免疫表型[5,6]。因此，阳性免疫染色结果远比阴性结果有意义。在本章中重点阐述阳性染色的特征。

如果某个病变不能立即确诊，可以用正文、示意图流程和表格中描述的一组免疫组化染色来进行鉴别诊断。下面的例子讲述了这一方法在实际病例中的应用。

图18.1显示一中年妇女腰骶部肿瘤，HE切片显示肿瘤细胞中主要为上皮样细胞和少量的透明细胞，大部分细胞核圆形、椭圆形，染色质细（图18.1 A，表18.6）。免疫组化染色显示上皮细胞膜抗原（EMA）灶性阳性（图18.1B）。示意图18.1和18.2显示癌、脊索瘤、颅咽管瘤、垂体腺瘤和脑膜瘤EMA(+)。该肿瘤细胞角蛋白（CK）CAM5.2阴性（图18.1C），因而不符合癌、脊索瘤或颅咽管瘤的免疫组化表型。肿瘤CgA阴性（图18.1D），即无垂体腺瘤激素表达（另

表18.1 神经组织特异性免疫组化染色

抗体/来源/稀释倍数*	主要类型和组织成分	抗原修复
A6（CD45RO）/Zymed/1:50*	T淋巴细胞	枸橼酸缓冲液（pH6.0）Mw15 min
CgA/Dr. Lloyd/1:160	垂体腺瘤、副神经节瘤、神经内分泌肿瘤	枸橼酸缓冲液（pH6.0）Mw15 min
IV型胶原/DAKO/1:8	纤维化、脓肿、肉瘤、畸胎瘤、纤维性囊肿和血管壁、硬脑膜	ventana 蛋白酶1，16 min
CAM5.2 CK/BD/1:10	癌、颅咽管瘤、脊索瘤、上皮	ventana 蛋白酶2，16 min
EMA/DAKO/1:50	癌、脑膜瘤、颅咽管瘤、脊索瘤、上皮	枸橼酸缓冲液（pH6.0）Mw15 min
GFAP/DAKO/1:6400	神经胶质增生、胶质瘤、CNS实质	ventana 蛋白酶2，16 min
HV抗原/DAKO/1:1000	单纯疱疹性脑炎、CMV、带状疱疹	无
JCV/SV40 病毒抗原/Lee Biomolecular/1:500	PML	无
KP-1（CD68）/DAKO/1:1600	巨噬细胞	枸橼酸缓冲液（pH6.0）Mw15 min
L26（CD20）/DAKO/1:500	B淋巴细胞、B细胞淋巴瘤	枸橼酸缓冲液（pH6.0）Mw15 min
MIB-1/Immunotech/1:25	增生的细胞	枸橼酸缓冲液（pH6.0）Mw15 min
NF/DAKO/1:50	节细胞肿瘤、神经纤维瘤、PNET、Alzheimer病、CNS实质	枸橼酸缓冲液（pH6.0）Mw15 min
Prealbumin/DAKO/1:500	脉络丛肿瘤	无
S-100 蛋白/DAKO/1:500	胶质瘤、PNET、黑色素瘤、神经鞘瘤、神经纤维瘤、神经元和软骨样肿瘤、脊索瘤、CNS、PNS	无
Syn/BioGenex/1:600	神经元和松果体肿瘤、PNET、髓母细胞瘤	枸橼酸缓冲液（pH6.0）Mw10 min
Toxoplasma/ BioGenex/ 纯液	弓形虫病	无
Vimentin/DAKO/1:800	多种细胞，大量存在于脑膜瘤	枸橼酸缓冲液（pH6.0）Mw15 min

* 密歇根医学院病理系免疫过氧化物酶实验室专家和工作人员给予了精心指导和帮助，改自 McKeever PE. New methods of brain tumor analysis. In: Mena H, ed. Dr. Kenneth M. Earle Memorial Neuropathology Review. Washington, DC: Armed Forces Institute of Pathology; Feb 24, 2000
CMV，巨细胞病毒；CNS，中枢神经系统；EMA，上皮细胞膜抗原；GFAP，胶质纤维酸性蛋白；HV，疱疹病毒；NF，神经微丝；PML，进行性多灶性白质脑病；PNET，原始神经外胚层肿瘤；PNS，周围神经系统；Mw，从冷的缓冲液开始微波指定的时间
（表格改自McKeever PE, Blaivas M. The brain, spinal cord, and meninges. In: Sternberg SS, ed. Diagnostic Surgical Pathology. 2nd edn. New York: Raven Press; 1994:409-492）

外，GFAP、Syn和HMB-45也阴性）。表18.6总结了对含有上皮样细胞肿瘤的鉴别诊断，证实该肿瘤的免疫组化表型为脑膜瘤，并且注明了一般的特征和常见的位置。该例肿瘤中极少旋涡结构，累及脊髓膜，与正文中脑膜瘤的描述相比较，细胞为上皮样的并有局灶的合体细胞。透明细胞不是主要的，没有透明细胞变型中的胞浆内糖原，这一肿瘤应诊断为具有明显上皮样细胞的脑膜上皮细胞型脑膜瘤[1,3]。

非肿瘤性疾病的脑部活检的诊断常需要免疫组化与微生物培养、聚合酶链反应（PCR）、Western blot或电镜（EM）等研究技术相结合[7,8]。以上工作可由专业中心检测以达到明确诊断[9-12]。

病变临床与影像学展望

脑、脊髓、脑膜的主要病变，如单发性和多发性肿块、囊肿、血管畸形和脓肿等，临床上主要通过计算机的断层扫描（CT）、核磁共振成像（MRI）和血管造影作出诊断。

多发性病变由变性、血管病变、感染性疾病或肿瘤引起。关于肿瘤，常见的多发性中枢神经系统肿瘤鉴别诊断的M规则包括转移性肿瘤、恶性淋巴瘤、黑色素瘤和髓母细胞瘤[13]。

根据年龄、断层摄影密度常常足以对出血为主要成分的病变作出诊断。在CT上可以很好地观察钙化及其与颅骨之间的关系。在MRI上可以更好地对灰质、白质、水肿和黑色素进行观察。通常经过血管造影确定血管异常。

非肿瘤性病变常常由神经病学家来确诊。因而，主要的神经系统症状（如疼痛、无力或视力丧失）或者神经系统疾病（如痴呆）使鉴别诊断局限（表18.3）。

抗原/抗体生物学

绝大多数在神经系统应用的抗原、抗体已在本书的其他部分提及，胶质纤维酸性蛋白，胶质分化的一种特异性中间丝蛋白是个例外。Syn和神经微丝蛋白

神经系统的免疫组织化学 18

是检测神经元分化的主要指标。除了用于检测淀粉样血管病变的β/A4抗体外，还有少数用于神经病理诊断的新抗体。有应用前景的抗体与相关的特异性病变放在一起讨论。示意图18.1和18.2给出了神经系统病变研究最常用抗体的流程。

非肿瘤性脑部病变

反应性改变

胶质增生

胶质增生是中枢神经系统对脑和脊髓损伤的反应。虽然在早期即可有轻微的改变，但胶质增生通常在损伤2~3周后才能见到。几乎任何中枢神经系统的损伤都能导致胶质增生，因此，胶质增生不能作为特异性病变的诊断（表18.2）[14]。

抗GFAP免疫染色（图18.2）黑褐色显示出阳性反应强，核浆比例低，胶质增生中散在星形细胞。在必须要区分胶质增生和正常脑组织的情况下，应当同时做年龄和部位匹配的正常中枢神经系统的对照切片染色。胶质增生标本中GFAP阳性的细胞数量、密度和细胞突起应比正常对照多。

GFAP染色有助于区分胶质增生和胶质瘤（表18.2）。在胶质增生中GFAP阳性细胞分布均匀，细胞间距一致（图18.2）。反应性星形细胞的分布比浸润性胶质瘤边缘的星形细胞间距均匀，胶质增生的核浆比例比胶质瘤低[3]。

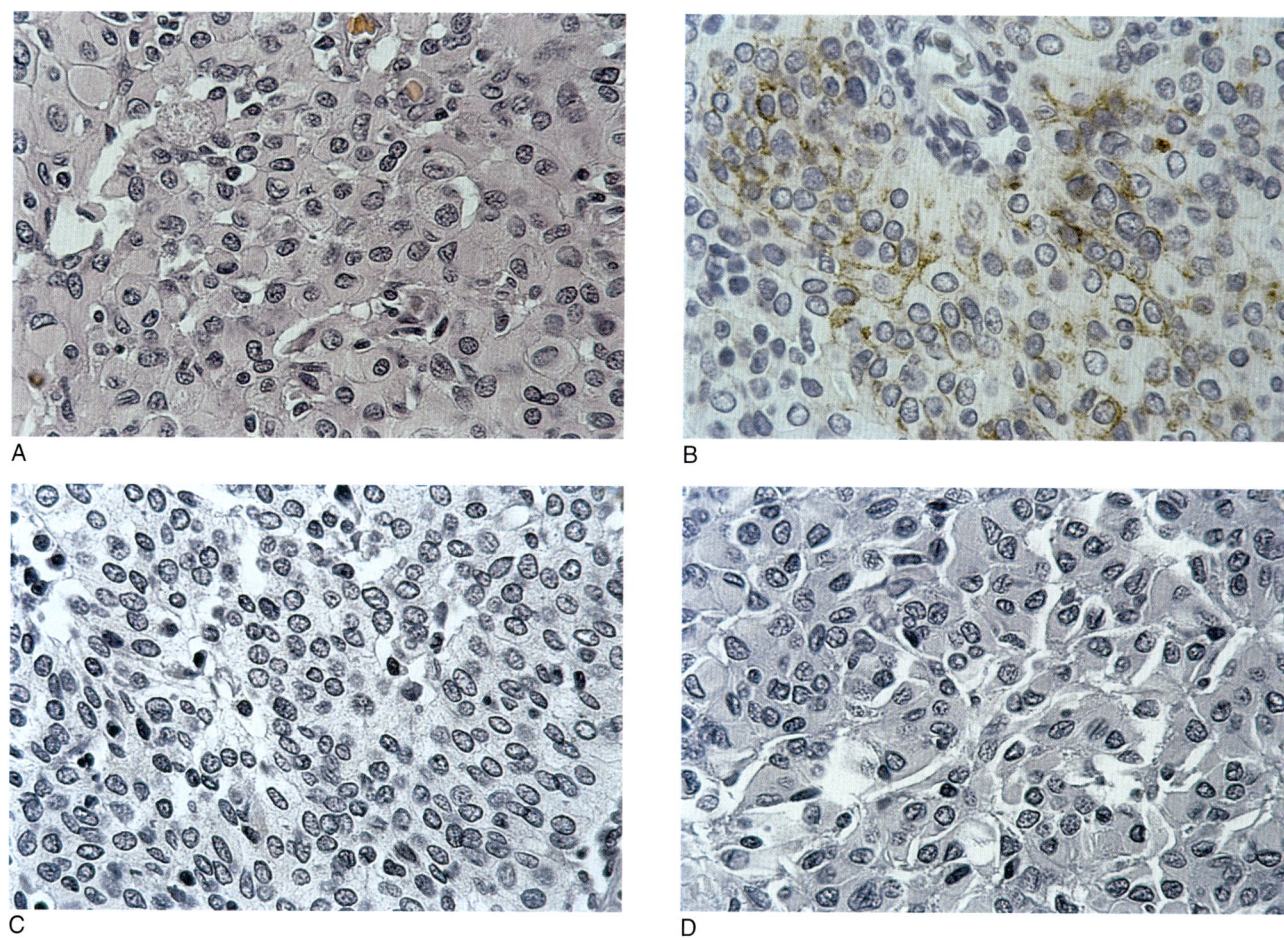

图18.1 本实例阐述了示意图（示意图18.1和18.2）、表格和正文是如何帮助从初步印象到最后诊断的。一中年妇女腰骶部大的肿块（HE）EMA局灶性阳性(B)，CAM5.2阴性(C)，CgA阴性（D）。波形蛋白阳性、GFAP和Syn阴性（图中未显示）。该肿瘤是伴有明显上皮样细胞的脑膜上皮细胞型脑膜瘤（引自 McKeever PE. New methods of brain tumor analysis. In: Mena H, ed. Dr. Kenneth M. Earle Memorial Neuropathology Review. Washington, DC: Armed Forces Institute of Pathology; Feb 24, 2000）

表18.2 中枢神经系统实质细胞内浸润细胞的鉴别诊断

诊 断	结 构	鉴别特征抗体	位 置[*]
神经胶质增生[a]	纤维性细胞，稀疏，圆/椭圆形细胞核	GFAP 位于星形胶质细胞突起	CNS
巨噬细胞	细胞和细胞核圆形或伸长；细胞内容物反映了损伤	KP-1、α-ACT	CNS、脑膜
大脑炎/脑炎	血管周围混合性炎细胞	LCA、L26、A6、κ和λIg、α-ACT、KP-1、微生物	CNS 灰质/CNS
出血	红细胞或含有含铁血黄素的巨噬细胞	纤维蛋白、KP-1	大脑深部、小脑、CNS
胶质瘤边缘[b]	纤维状细胞，互相有压迹的角形细胞核，（有丝分裂）[bc]	GFAP	CNS
淋巴瘤	血管周围缺乏黏附性的小圆细胞	LCA、L26、A6、κ和λIg	大脑深部、CNS、脑膜

[*] 先列出的为最常见或最特异性的部位
[a] 损伤的非特异性反应
[b] 冰冻切片怀疑是胶质瘤边缘时，应当要求再一次取材，活检时要靠近病变中心。有丝分裂提示为高级别胶质瘤的边缘
[c] 圆括号内是不常见的鉴别诊断特征，一旦发现对鉴别诊断非常有用
CNS，中枢神经系统；GFAP，胶质纤维酸性蛋白；α-ACT，α-抗胰凝乳蛋白酶；Ig，免疫球蛋白；LCA，白细胞共同抗原；RBC，红细胞
（改自McKeever PE, Blaivas M. The brain, spinal cord, and meninges. In: Sternberg SS, ed. Diagnostic Surgical Pathology. 2nd edn. New York: Raven Press; 1994: 409-492）

免疫组化染色反应				边缘	疾病
GFAP+	EMA−	Syn−	KP1−	弥散	少突胶质细胞瘤
					PXA
				锐利	透明细胞室管膜瘤
		Syn+			DNT
					中枢神经细胞瘤
		Syn−	KP1+		脱髓鞘
					梗死
GFAP−	EMA+		KP1−	锐利	透明细胞脑膜瘤
					肾细胞癌
	EMA−				血管母细胞瘤

[*] 未标记的方格表明肿瘤的特征或免疫组化染色反应尚未确定
DNT，胚胎期发育不良性神经上皮肿瘤；EMA，上皮细胞膜抗原；GFAP，胶质纤维酸性蛋白；PXA，多形性黄色星形细胞瘤；Syn，突触素
（改自Gokden M, Roth KA, Garroll SL, et al. Clear cell neoplasms and pseudoneoplastic lesions of the central nervous system. Semin Diagn Pathol 1997; 14:253-269）

示意图 18.1 透明细胞病变的鉴别诊断

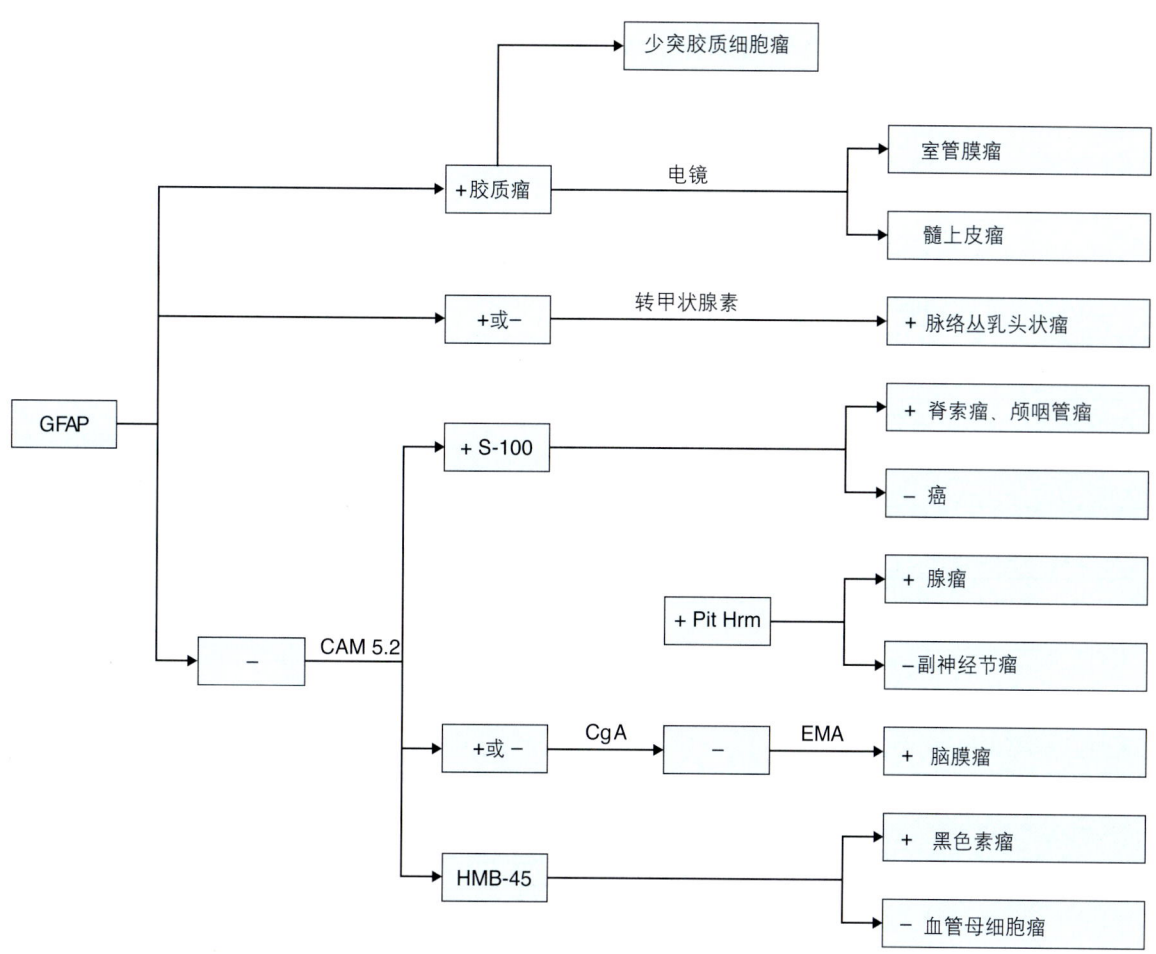

示意图 18.2　上皮样细胞肿瘤的免疫组化诊断

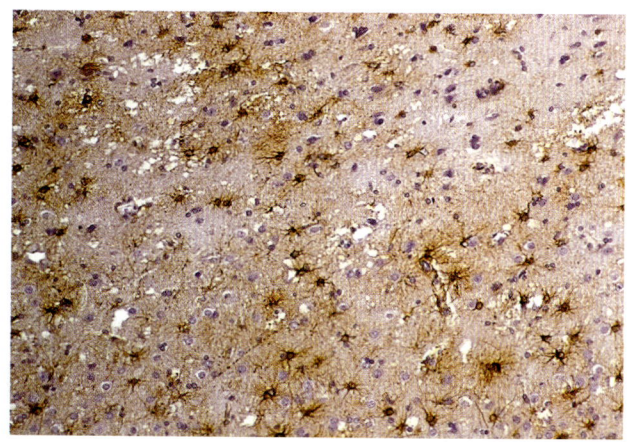

图 18.2　胶质增生的 GFAP 染色。该胶质增生来自一名克-雅病（CJD）病人的大脑皮质。神经胶质是反应性的，细胞呈星芒状，有丰富的GFAP染色棕色的胞浆，与长期的癫痫病例的少量神经胶质增生完全不同（图18.31B）。一般来讲，融合的空泡是CJD的特征而不是神经胶质增生的特征（抗GFAP和HE 染色）

巨噬细胞

任何脑组织的损伤或刺激 3 天后都可以看到吞噬的巨噬细胞（表 18.3、图 18.3A、表 18.2）。巨噬细胞富含 α-抗胰凝乳蛋白酶和溶菌酶等酶类，并且含有单核巨噬细胞的标记，可以与CD68（KP-1）和MAC387抗体相作用。所有这些特征均可用于免疫组化染色。在出血或外伤病变周围，巨噬细胞内有铁染色阳性的含铁血黄素。

脑炎仅仅意味着脑部的炎症。许多因素都能引起脑炎，从病毒感染到外科移植等[13]。

在大脑炎、脑膜炎或脑炎，巨噬细胞是多形性的细胞，某些细胞细长，其他的则含有细胞碎片（图18.3）。它们可能含有真菌或其他微生物。在中枢神经系统，巨噬细胞通过吞噬而体积增大，称为颗粒状或格子细胞。这种细胞大而圆，胞浆内充满脂滴呈泡沫状（图18.4、

表18.3 有关神经病学症状或特异性疾病的活检指南

症状/疑似疾病[*]	疑似疾病的诊断特征		
	结 构	抗 体	部 位[a]
单纯疱疹性脑炎	脑炎（表18.2），90~100 nm "目标"衣壳的 Cowdry A 嗜酸性核内包涵体	HSV	颞叶或额叶基底部，CNS，常为双侧性
弓形虫病	坏死，包含 3~5nm 的速殖体，（囊），（炎症）[b]	弓形虫属	CNS，常为多个病变
进行性多灶性白质脑病	脱髓鞘，异型胶质细胞，直径 15~25nm 或 30~40nm 的嗜酸性核内包涵体	JCV/SV40、髓鞘、NF、KP-1	大脑白质，CNS
痴呆/克-雅病	凹入胞核的胞质空泡，神经胶质增生	PrPres、GFAP	双侧大脑皮质，灰质
小血管疾病	血管炎或动脉硬化或嗜刚果红血管病变	A6、L26、CD31、淀粉样蛋白、肌动蛋白、弹性蛋白	大脑，CNS，常为多个病变
痴呆/Alzheimer 病	嗜银蛋白斑，双螺旋形丝的神经纤维缠结	NF、tau、泛肽、Alz-50	双侧大脑皮质
脱髓鞘	髓鞘脱失，神经胶质增生，网格细胞，有或无轴突保留	髓鞘、NF、KP-1	大脑白质，CNS
癫痫	低级别胶质瘤或节细胞胶质瘤，或神经胶质增生，或血管畸形	GFAP、NF、弹性蛋白	大脑皮质

[*] 表格的病变排列顺序按照正文中讨论的顺序
a 首先列出最常见或最特异的部位
b 鉴别特征旁的括号提示为少见的特征，一旦发现对鉴别诊断非常有用
CNS，中枢神经系统；GFAP，胶质纤维酸性蛋白；HSV，单纯疱疹病毒
（改自 McKeever PE, Blaivas M. The brain, spinal cord, and meninges. In: Sternberg SS, ed. Diagnostic Surgical Pathology. 2nd edn. New York: Raven Press; 1994: 409-492）

图18.3A）。胞浆稀少而体积小的巨噬细胞参与了脑炎中以血管为中心的慢性炎性浸润、形成胶质结节、围绕于正在死亡的神经元（噬神经细胞）周围，格子细胞也存在于其他炎性病变、脱髓鞘和变性疾病的过程中[3,5]。CD68 对巨噬细胞染色反应良好（图 18.3A）。

血管周围炎症

血管周围炎症由核浆比例高的小圆细胞组成，可被误诊为淋巴瘤或神经外胚层细胞团，神经外胚层细胞团在儿童脑组织中尤为常见。白细胞共同抗原（LCA，CD45/45R）、CD3ξ、CD5、CD20 和 CD79α 等标记物可以通过显示淋巴细胞的多克隆性将其与炎症相鉴别（图 18.3B、C）。

中枢神经系统的刺激可引起血管周围的炎症[16]。CD68 阳性的巨噬细胞吞噬刺激物或损伤的细胞成分，并将它们运送至血管周围间隙中[15]。脑组织中没有淋巴结，血管周围区域则是细胞与抗原反应和相互作用的地方。根据疾病的严重性和持续时间的不同，血管周围炎症是完全不同的[3]。陈旧性出血可作为反应很轻微的例子，主要特征为血管周围有含有含铁血黄素的巨噬细胞（表18.2）。外科伤口和移植导致明显的反应。病毒和过敏性脑炎可以引起强烈的反应，血管周围有大量的巨噬细胞和 CD3ξ 阳性的 T 淋巴细胞[3]。

某些疾病主要影响静脉，如静脉周围脑炎（PVE），或小动脉，如 CADASIL（伴皮质下梗死及白质脑病的常染色体显性遗传性脑动脉病）。与 PVE 不同，CADASIL 很少甚至没有炎症。累及的血管可以用抗 SMA 或肌球蛋白来鉴别，因为与大脑静脉相比，大脑动脉有梭形平滑肌细胞构成的环形厚壁血管壁。

纤维化

纤维化在脑组织中很少见。它发生于脓肿周围（图18.4）、肉芽肿、促纤维增生和肉瘤样肿瘤。纤维化在脑膜中较常见。脑膜纤维化常发生于外伤、脑膜炎、血管炎累及脑膜血管、放射性治疗和对肿瘤反应性的结缔组织增生。

胶原、纤维粘连蛋白和层粘连蛋白等纤维化的不同成分可以通过免疫组化方法检测[17]。IV型胶原对于大多数脑和脑膜组织都有作用[3]。对于常规纤维化的确定，标准的组织化学染色优于免疫组化染色（图18.4）。

神经系统的免疫组织化学 18

> **诊断要点：反应性改变**
> 1. 神经胶质增生是脑损伤常见的慢性反应。
> 2. GFAP，单一的最重要的脑免疫组化染色，清楚显示了神经胶质增生的低核浆比例、星状突起和均匀分布的反应性星形细胞。
> 3. PMN、巨噬细胞和淋巴细胞对于脑损伤的反应与全身损伤相似。脑没有淋巴结，因而它们的相互作用不很明显，而是在血管周围聚集。
> 4. 纤维化在脑组织中很少见。

感染性疾病

感染可以导致脑膜炎、大脑炎、脓肿、脑炎或脑病[18]。除了脑病外，炎症是一个显著的特征。它从急性期到慢性期的发展过程与全身性感染非常相似。感染必须与淋巴瘤相鉴别。感染常导致多克隆性炎症，以T淋巴细胞成分为主，免疫组化染色标记CD45RO、CD3ξ和CD5染色阳性（表18.1）。成熟的EMA阳性的浆细胞存在时表明为炎症。另一方面，脑组织原发性淋巴瘤体积大的恶性肿瘤细胞通常为B细胞，CD20或CD79α染色阳性。在此简要叙述每一个感染性疾病的组织病理类型并对引起感染的病原体加以讨论。

组织病理学

脑膜炎是被覆于脑和脊髓的脑脊膜的炎症。软脑膜炎累及薄层脑膜：软脑膜和蛛网膜。硬脑膜炎累及厚的硬脑膜，在非手术病例中硬脑膜炎较软脑膜炎少见。微生物通过局部鼻窦蔓延或通过血流侵犯脑脊膜。中枢神经系统的血管周隙是蛛网膜下腔的延伸，因此持续存在的脑膜炎可以通过这个周隙引起脑炎或脑脓肿。

大脑炎是脑实质的局灶性炎症（脊髓炎则位于脊髓）。大脑炎发生于脓肿形成之前，但需要早期活检才能发现（表18.2、18.10）。炎性浸润包括中性粒细胞、巨噬细胞、淋巴细胞和浆细胞，有或无实质坏死。脓毒性脑炎通常由细菌引起，多数为链球菌或葡萄球菌；少数为不常见的革兰阴性菌，如大肠杆菌、假单胞菌和流感嗜血杆菌。大脑炎也可发生于肿瘤周围、

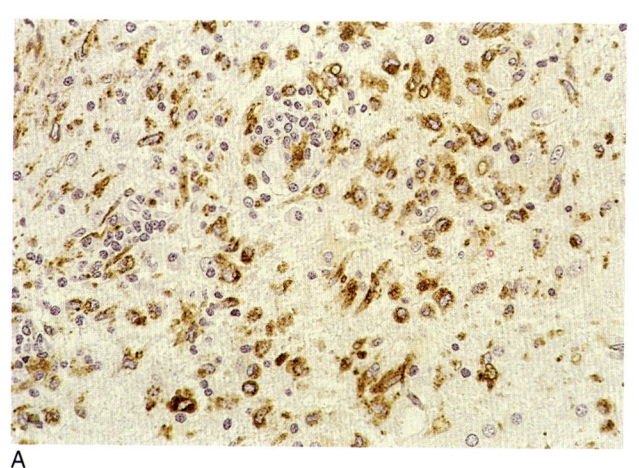

A

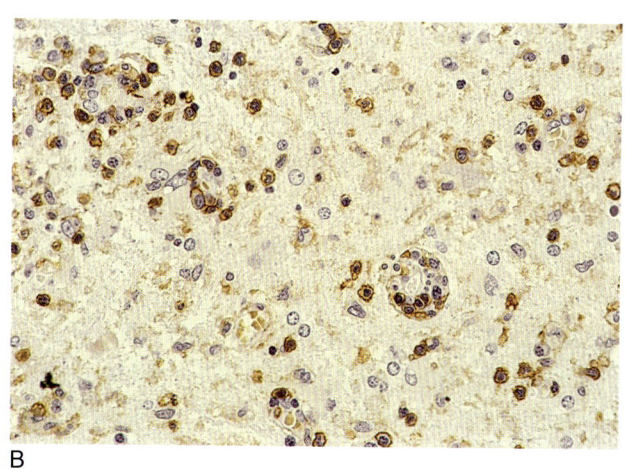

B

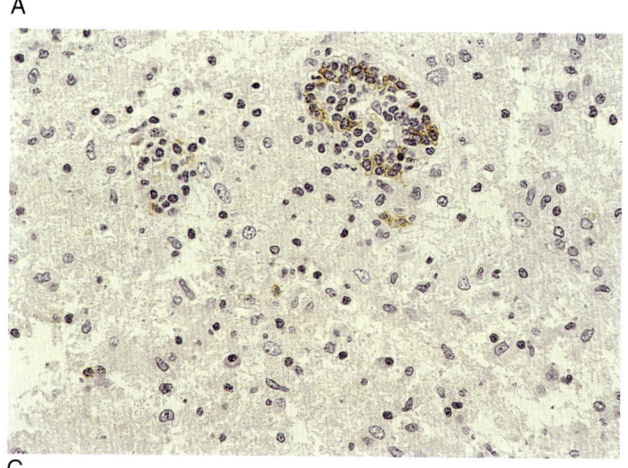

C

图18.3 重度脑炎的炎细胞包括KP-1阳性的不同形状的巨噬细胞，反映了它们直接围绕并激活的状态和吞噬胞饮产物（A）；血管周围和实质内的A6阳性的T淋巴细胞（B）；L26阳性B淋巴细胞（C）。格子细胞是大而圆的巨噬细胞，因吞噬胞饮产物而体积增大（A）

773

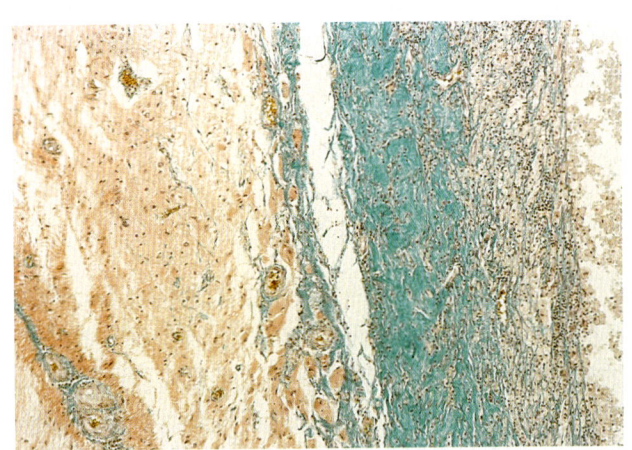

图 18.4 此标本来自脑脓肿，此炎性病变具有界限清楚的脓肿壁，Masson 三色套染显示脓肿壁的胶原呈淡绿色。胶原壁（橙色一侧）周围的脑组织包括高度反应（胖细胞型星形细胞）的星形细胞。靠近脓肿的中央（灰色一侧）是白细胞和肿胀的巨噬细胞

畸形血管破裂、梗死和外伤等病变。

肉芽肿性脑膜炎和大脑炎可见于：

1. 结核和其他分枝杆菌感染。
2. 真菌、寄生虫或螺旋体感染。
3. 特发性，如结节病、系统性红斑狼疮、Wegener 肉芽肿、淋巴样肉芽肿和组织细胞增生症 X。

某些病变是通过活检和病原体培养作出诊断，而另一些是通过与临床的联系[13, 19, 20]。

脓肿的病变包括对化脓菌的炎症反应和纤维化，病原体常常是细菌或真菌。炎症反应包括多形核白细胞、多克隆的 T 和 B 淋巴细胞、巨噬细胞和浆细胞（有或无坏死）。在疑难的病例，可以用免疫组化染色来证实炎性成分的多形性。CD45RO 和 CD20 染多克隆 T 和 B 淋巴细胞，CD68 染巨噬细胞，EMA 染浆细胞（表 18.1 和 18.10）。

脑脓肿壁包括内壁 CD31 和 CD34 阳性的血管、胶原纤维和周围 GFAP 强阳性反应性增生的神经胶质。周围的脑组织有水肿。因为在中枢神经系统中胶原很少见，胶原的存在是诊断脓肿的一个重要特征（表 18.10）。在 HE 染色切片上区分胶原与纤维性胶质增生有一定的困难。Masson 三色套染或胶原的免疫组化染色可以帮助确诊（图 18.4、表 18.1）。

脑炎是脑组织的炎症（图 18.3）。它常由病毒或立克次体引起，其造成的脑部炎症比大脑炎更弥散[7]。许多病毒性感染是自限性的，只导致脑膜炎或轻微的脑膜脑炎。在此强调的是，有些病变更为严重，需要外科处理。

脑病（常译成脑组织病变）是由炎症反应很轻或没有炎症反应的感染所致。这已在由朊蛋白引起的海绵状脑病中得以肯定，如克-雅病（CJD）[9]。脑细胞死亡导致神经胶质增生是脑病常见的特征。白质脑病（脑白质受损）损害白质。脊髓病（髓质病）一般损害脊髓。

微生物

每个脑活检标本应当以下列方式处理：如果在手术中发现炎症，应当做组织培养，包括细菌、分枝杆菌和真菌；并用特殊染色、免疫染色技术和电镜。笔者的经验认为如果病变样本相同，对于在体外生长的微生物，微生物培养优于组织化学染色、免疫组化染色或聚合酶链反应（PCR）分析。如前期采用了抗生素治疗或局灶性感染所取的标本不同则可影响相应病例的结果。

真菌和寄生虫感染在免疫缺陷的个体中很常见。常见的微生物有新型隐球菌、单核细胞增多性李斯特菌、烟曲霉菌和普通的细菌如 H 型流感杆菌、肺炎球菌、表皮葡萄球菌和假单胞菌。隐球菌脑膜炎是最常见的真菌性脑膜炎，但它的脑部炎症可以很轻微。某些微生物的慢性感染可以形成肉芽肿。可以通过培养或用特异性染色来发现这些微生物，如高碘酸-雪夫（PAS）染色和姬姆萨（GMS）染色。对于难以培养的微生物最好选择特定性反应试剂，用免疫组化方法分析[3, 13, 20]。免疫染色可以确定微生物的种属[20]。

结核可以累及中枢神经系统任何部位和脑膜。这种疾病通常引起肉芽肿性炎，有或没有干酪样坏死、脑膜炎或动脉炎。分枝杆菌的生长需要很长的时间，可通过免疫组化、PCR 分析或抗酸染色进行初步检测[19]。

梅毒的发病率正在增加，主要发生在免疫缺陷的病人。应将此放在肉芽肿性炎的鉴别诊断之列。致病微生物梅毒螺旋体难以培养，银染也可同时对脑组织染色，所产生的背景染色影响结果判断，因此免疫组化染色提供了一种新的但更为特异的检测方法[21]。

中枢神经系统最常见的寄生虫感染是神经型囊尾蚴病，主要发生在发展中国家。如果一个脑部囊肿包含一个典型的囊尾蚴（有一个特征的内陷头节），该病变无需做免疫组化即可确诊。将确诊病例的脑脊液作为原始抗体的来源来进行免疫组化分析是可行的，要使病原体破碎或变性，并仍保留其蛋白多糖[22]。血吸虫病感染脑和脊髓。可通过使用标准化高分子量 CK 免疫组化染色而诊断，因为在脑组织中几乎没有

CK，极少量的微生物即可检测到[23]。

Whipple 病极少仅有脑部疾病而无胃肠道症状[13]。致病的杆菌是 *Tropheryma whippelii*。通过光镜分析脑活检组织，链球菌B群免疫过氧化物酶染色而确诊[24]。组织学特征包括在巨噬细胞内抗淀粉酶 PAS 阳性的杆菌状小体、微小肉芽肿、血管周围 CD3ξ 和 CD20 阳性淋巴细胞，CD68 阳性的小胶质细胞。

莱姆（Lyme）病是由蜱传播、由包柔螺旋体引起的疾病。它累及中枢神经系统，可在脑脊液中检测到[25]。

非流行性脑炎中最常见原因，也是最常在活检标本中发现的是单纯疱疹病毒（HSV）（表18.3）[26]。病变过程通常并不总是局限于颞叶和额叶。最早的病变是病变区血管充血并伴有神经元缺血性改变，常规石蜡包埋组织免疫过氧化物酶染色HSV阳性。血管周围炎症变化是特征性的，以CD45RO和CD20阳性的淋巴细胞及CD68阳性的巨噬细胞为主，同时伴有不同程度的局灶性坏死和出血。核内包涵体总是有HSV，但也可由其他许多病毒如巨细胞病毒、水痘-带状疱疹、JC病毒（JCV）和类人猿病毒40（SV40）引起[7]。

HSV的Cowdry A 小体在小的脑活检标本中不易发现。需要用原位杂交（ISH）、PCR 和 IHC 等敏感特异的方法来确诊[3, 27]。电镜可以显示胞核或胞浆里的病毒颗粒，但敏感度和特异性较差。培养和连续的血清学 CSF 分析较慢，但仍是诊断包括 HSV 在内的许多病毒性 CNS 感染的最准确方法。

肠道病毒（如柯萨奇病毒、埃可病毒）和虫媒病毒感染（如Eastern equine，St.Louis，West Nile）缺乏特征性包涵体。West Nile病毒是一种虫媒病毒。蚊子和鸟可作为载体和宿主，引起人类感染[3]。通过输血和器官移植传播也有记载。有些病例是致死性的。

灶状的脑膜炎、脑炎和脊髓灰质炎可累及大脑、丘脑、基底神经节、脑干和小脑等不同部位。脑膜脑炎的证据包括 CD3ξ 和 CD68 染色显示血管周围炎症、小胶质细胞结节和噬神经细胞现象等。某些病人主要累及脊髓前角细胞[3]。

狂犬病的胞浆包涵体为圆形或椭圆形，嗜酸性，1~7μm大小[28]。免疫染色和PCR分析有助于诊断[13]。

麻疹病毒引起亚急性硬化性全脑炎和轻度脑炎。在软脑膜和血管周隙灶性淋巴细胞浸润性的炎症。在脑皮质有许多CD4阳性的细胞，GFAP片状阳性的纤维状星形细胞增多，偶尔有小胶质结节。在皮质下白质内出现弥漫性单核细胞浸润、神经胶质增生和脱髓鞘。可以在 HE 染色切片中观察到包涵体、Cowdry A，特异性的诊断需要做 IHC[29]。

获得性免疫缺陷综合征

AIDS 的中枢神经系统病变反映了神经疾病所有的病理变化。开始为大脑炎、脑膜炎、脑炎和血管病变，最后为变性代谢性病变和肿瘤。该病变已在许多综述中详细地加以总结[8, 30]。病变或由HIV直接引起或者是因免疫抑制而出现的继发性机会性感染。在发现AIDS的最初阶段CNS病变尤为常见，超过一半的病人是因神经症状而就诊并发现 CNS 异常。强有效的抗逆转录病毒治疗（HAART）已改变了疾病过程，以至于现在已很少发生 CNS 并发症[30]。

人免疫缺陷病毒的初期表现

人免疫缺陷病毒（HIV）脑炎可通过组织学分析而明确诊断。HIV脑炎的标志性改变是在脑实质和血管周围出现多核巨细胞。这些细胞与巨噬细胞和小胶质混合存在。在白质、灰质深部和皮质内形成大小不等的多个病灶。HIV p23 和 p24 抗原的免疫组化检测和 ISH 有助于诊断（图 18.5）[3]。

HIV白质脑病的特征为弥散性白质损害、髓鞘脱失、反应性星形胶质细胞增生、多核细胞和巨噬细胞浸润。IHC 或 ISH 有助于确定 HIV 与病变过程的关系。白质脑病偶尔表现为显著的髓鞘肿胀、空泡化。这在脊髓中比较常见，然而，这种多灶性的髓鞘空泡化，类似无恶性贫血的混合性系统性变性。

HIV感染的另一种表现为淋巴细胞性脑膜炎，在软脑膜和血管周围间隙内有明显的大量淋巴细胞浸润。HIV的脑血管炎和肉芽肿性血管炎可伴有脑血管壁淋巴细胞性或淋巴浆组织细胞性-多核巨细胞浸润，偶尔伴有坏死[3]。

从HAART应用以来，描述了一种新型的HIV脑炎，该病变具有严重的白质脑病和密集的血管周围巨噬细胞和淋巴细胞浸润。这可能是对重新恢复活性的免疫系统的一种反应[30]。

AIDS 的继发性感染

AIDS病人的机会性感染很常见，但也可见于其他免疫缺陷病人。弓形虫病是这些感染中最常见的。它表现为坏死性脑脊髓炎，其病变特征为散在性病灶，在病灶的坏死区周围有游离滋养体或充满寄生虫的包囊[31]。免疫过氧化物酶或免疫荧光染色可以定位不易在常规HE染色切片中发现的病原体[32]。

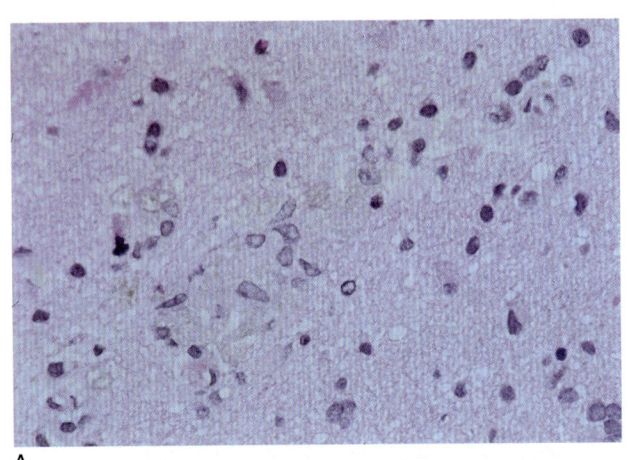
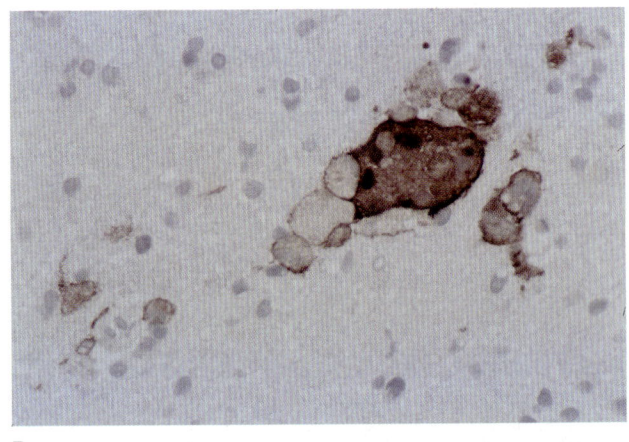

图 18.5 从巨噬细胞融合形成的多核巨细胞,胞浆的纤维状突起较周围脑组织少,锥形细胞核染色质淡染。它们在 HE 染色中难以判断(A),但在 HIV p24 抗原 IHC 染色中很显著(B)(授权自 Dr. Clayton Wiley, University of Pittsburgh, Pittsburgh, PA)

巨细胞病毒(CMV)感染经常继发于弓形虫病,病变从无炎症反应到严重坏死性脑膜脑炎和室管膜炎[33]。如果没有明显的具有核内包涵体的奇异巨细胞,免疫组化、ISH和PCR分析对于检测石蜡包埋组织中的病毒有帮助[34]。

HIV和JCV的混合感染导致重度脑炎[35]。结核和神经梅毒感染AIDS病人[36, 37]。显微镜检查显示主要在血管周围灶性淋巴细胞、浆细胞炎性浸润。AIDS病人CNS其他的感染包括阿米巴脑炎、锥虫病和类圆线虫病[13, 18]。

进行性多灶性白质脑病

进行性多灶性脑白质病(PML)是一种表现为散在的多灶性脱髓鞘疾病,轴突相对保留,通常无炎症表现。影像学观察可能类似于多发性硬化症或肿块。本病由DNA乳多空病毒引起,在免疫缺陷病人中主要由JCV引起(极少数是SV40病毒引起)(表18.3),JCV乳多空病毒通常与朊病毒无关。常见于患白血病和AIDS的病人。PML也可发生于不同类型的癌症、结核、系统性红斑狼疮、结节病或器官移植后免疫抑制的病人。

脑部活检可显示为白质进行性破坏过程,有许多吞噬脂质的巨噬细胞,胶质细胞核体积增大呈毛玻璃样,许多大的异常胶质细胞核多形性和染色质深染。在某些病例中有显著的血管周围成熟淋巴细胞浸润。尽管AIDS病人奇异型星形细胞不常见,而血管周围炎性细胞浸润很常见,有或无AIDS的病人JCV感染的病理变化是相似的[13]。

本病胶质细胞的核内充满病毒颗粒。PML应与多发性硬化、其他脱髓鞘疾病和星形细胞瘤相鉴别。星形细胞在多数含有脂质的巨噬细胞中随机分布而不是均匀分布有助于与星形细胞瘤相鉴别。其特征为奇异的星形细胞和核大、内有包涵体的异常少突胶质细胞。PML可通过电镜、ISH、免疫组化染色确诊(图18.6)或通过PCR检测JCV、SV40和BK病毒[39, 40]。

> **诊断要点:感染性疾病**
> 1. 活检发现可能为炎症时应保持无菌从OR送到微生物实验室培养。对于几乎所有体外生长的微生物而言,培养比组织染色要敏感。
> 2. 应依据临床表现和疑似的微生物选择合适的检测方法。IHC、ISH、特异染色、EM和PCR等多种血清学和组织学分析可用于检测。

海绵状脑病

海绵状脑病的特征为灰质空泡化(海绵状改变)[3]。空泡的大小不等,最大者直径可达30μm或更大(图18.7)。它们位于神经纤维网和细胞核周体。在不同的特异性疾病和不同的个体之间其神经解剖部位的分布不同。通常缺乏炎症反应。疑似为海绵状脑病的标本应当按本书在痴呆部分所述的标本处理方法处理。

海绵状脑病包括克-雅病(CJD)、众所周知的"疯牛病"、羊瘙痒病、枯疬病、Gerstmann-Sträussler-Scheinker(GSS)综合征和致死性家族性失眠症[3, 8, 41-43]。它们是由称为朊蛋白(prions)的感染性蛋白引起的。朊蛋在分析痴呆所做的脑活检标本中，一种常见的诊断就是CJD[41]。神经纤维网和神经元核周体内的空泡在CJD中是区域性的并随时间而变化（图18.2、18.7）。在疾病的晚期，海绵状改变通常减少（表18.3）。相反，GFAP阳性的神经胶质增生逐渐增加（图18.2）。抗朊蛋白（PrP）抗血清的免疫染色确定这种蛋白异构体是快速诊断CJD的有用方法[44]。通过抗蛋白酶K消化的Western blot检测朊蛋白可以确诊[9]。

1995年一位年轻的"快餐主义"者患非典型变异型CJD而神秘死亡后，1996年欧盟禁止进口英国牛肉。媒体对这些死亡病例和因饲养的牲畜中有牛海绵状脑病（BSE）的养牛人的死亡进行了大量的报道[3,45]，因而有了"疯牛病"之说。显微镜下朊蛋白免疫组化染色呈斑块状是这种非典型变异型CJD最为明显和稳定的神经病理特点[45]，当周围有海绵状改变时则更为显著。

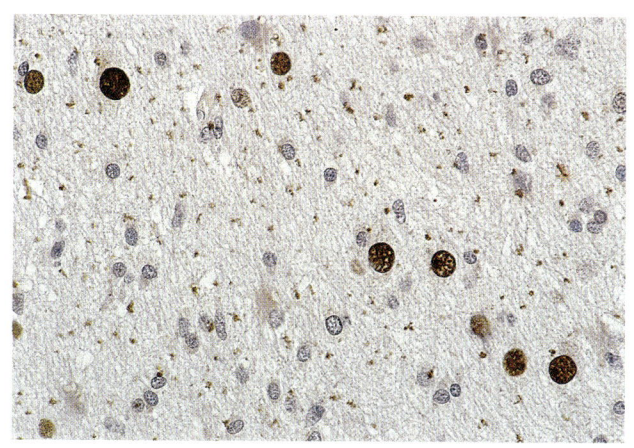

图18.6 进行性多灶性脑白质病（PML），病人系年轻女性，患系统性红斑狼疮，采用了高剂量抗炎和细胞毒性药物治疗。IHC检测JC病毒抗原，在肿胀的少突胶质细胞胞核中呈褐色染色。阴性的小圆形少突胶质细胞和伸长的星形细胞核被苏木精复染为紫蓝色（授权自 Dr. Riccardo Valdez, University of Michigan, Ann Arbor, MI）

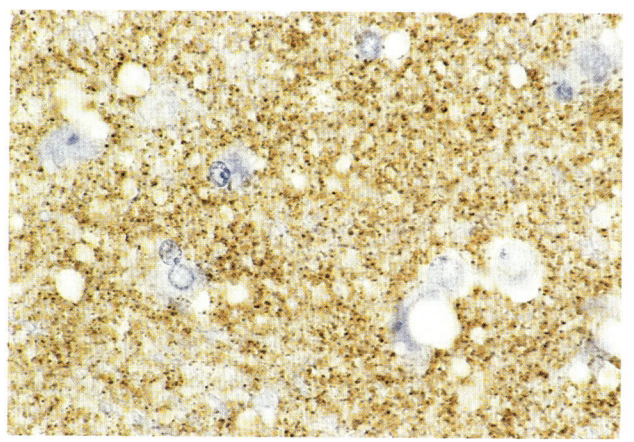

图18.7 克-雅病（CJD）。活检标本取自一老年男性额叶脑组织，患者几周来表现为进行性行为和记忆改变。在脑皮质的灰质内能看到空泡区和突触缺失。每个细小的棕色点是经Syn染色的神经纤维网中的突触。神经元胞浆内空泡使胞核有凹陷（Syn染色伴苏木精复染）

白是相应正常蛋白的转化形式。遗传性朊蛋白病如致死性家族性失眠症、GSS综合征和家族性CJD，有产生朊蛋白的基因突变。感染性朊蛋白病如疯牛病、羊瘙痒病、枯颅病和自发性CJD是由于密切接触朊蛋白而传播的。像催化剂一样，这种致病的朊蛋白通过诱导正常普遍存在的相应的蛋白质构型发生折叠成为病理性构型来传播。随着这种循环的不断重复，正常蛋白转换为病理构型蛋白的比例逐渐增加。

朊蛋白很难灭活。漂白剂、强碱和强酸（见下面痴呆部分）等能使蛋白质完全变性的试剂是有效的，而紫外线、常规甲醛固定及标准的消毒不能够消灭朊蛋白。

脑血管疾病

脑组织出血的原因有很多，经常伴有CNS其他病变。IHC的主要目的是明确出血的原因，如淀粉样变和肿瘤。淀粉样变血管病是常见的引起老年人自发性脑内出血的原因（表18.3）。在显示血管淀粉样变上β/A4蛋白抗体的免疫组化染色比刚果红染色更敏感[46]。

绝大多数引起脑出血的肿瘤是转移性的。如肾细胞癌、绒毛膜癌、黑色素瘤、白血病和胶质母细胞瘤常引起出血。胶质母细胞瘤有GFAP阳性的细胞突起，波形蛋白阳性的血管增生，在胶质瘤中MIB-1增生指数升高。癌可以表达CK。

高血压病人的出血常发生于大脑半球，尤其在基底神经节的侧面[47]。凝血障碍是脑内出血的一个重要原因，包括药物引起的凝血障碍。囊状动脉瘤偶尔破裂进入脑组织，但影像学可显示其性质。栓塞是出血性脑梗死的主要原因[48]。窦血栓形成后可发生静脉梗死，通常是先前存在的感染性或炎性疾病的并发症[3]。

非外伤性蛛网膜下腔出血通常是因为囊状动脉瘤破裂，多数位于主要动脉的分支处或Willis环。影像学上病变部位很明显。

硬膜下血肿可以发生在外伤后，也可见于老年病人、肿瘤全身播散和脑肿瘤的病人[49]。在血肿两侧形成包膜，包膜完全形成需要几个星期。5天时硬脑膜下血肿的硬膜侧包膜通常有2～5个波形蛋白阳性的纤维母细胞的厚度。最终变得与正常硬脑膜一样厚，其内有Ⅳ型胶原和纤维粘连蛋白阳性的新的胶原纤维。

小血管疾病

小血管疾病的脑活检标本需要通过整个组织块做一个切面以获得诊断材料。大量累及的血管不一定能观察到，但是通过CD31显示内皮细胞，可使血管显现出来（表18.3）；鉴于其敏感性和特异性，CD31被选择为内皮细胞的标记物[49]。与含有较多平滑肌细胞的同样直径的小动脉比较，脑的小静脉仅有很少的梭形平滑肌细胞（SMC），但是可以通过抗SMA或肌球蛋白来进行判断[50]。孤立性CNS血管炎的原因还不明确[51]。脑组织系统性血管炎可能与下列因素相关：①红斑狼疮；②药物，包括可卡因、海洛因和苯丙胺；③感染，包括带状疱疹－水痘病毒和脑膜血管梅毒；④毒素；⑤肉芽肿性疾病；⑥Wegener肉芽肿；⑦复发性多软骨炎和⑧Behçet病[7, 13, 14, 52, 53]。IHC有助于确定微生物和炎细胞的类型。

CADASIL（伴皮质下梗死及白质脑病的常染色体显性遗传性脑动脉病）影响小动脉[54]。CASADIL是Notch 3基因（染色体19）突变的一种罕见的疾病[13]。特征性血管改变可通过脑、皮肤和肌肉活检而确定。光镜下，感染的血管变粗，HE染色可观察到嗜碱性、颗粒状物质。这种物质是PAS阳性，它代替了平滑肌细胞，在SMA的IHC染色中显示得最好。EM下是黑色、颗粒状的、嗜铱酸的沉积物。可采用IHC检测Notch 3蛋白沉淀物[54]。

血管畸形

已认识5种类型的血管畸形[3, 55]：

1. 毛细血管扩张；
2. 海绵状血管瘤；
3. 动静脉畸形（AVM）；
4. 静脉畸形；
5. Sturge-Weber病（脑面部或三叉神经的血管瘤病）。

尽管AVM可以发生于CNS的任何部位，但主要发生于大脑半球（表18.4）。弹性蛋白染色可以确定中等动脉和大动脉，以及相应的异常血管。在AVM，这些染色常显示异常的血管弹性蛋白局灶性缺失或呈双层。有抗弹性蛋白的单克隆抗体，但如Movat's pentachrome等特殊染色是常用的染色方法[3]。

异常的平滑肌层可通过抗SMA显示。据报道大脑静脉缺乏大脑动脉的连续环绕的梭形平滑肌细胞层[50]，但是这些鉴别特征并没有在血管畸形的病人得到证实。IHC可用于确定和定位血管胶原、纤维粘连蛋白、肌纤维母细胞（波形蛋白和肌肉肌动蛋白）和内皮细胞（CD31）。

肿　瘤

成人和儿童常见的脑肿瘤类型不同。儿童脑肿瘤发生于后颅窝的多于前颅窝，而成人脑肿瘤与之相反。

恶性度分级

世界卫生组织（WHO）根据组织学标准建立了脑肿瘤统一的命名和分级[2]。开始为最"良性"的定为Ⅰ级，数字化的分级Ⅱ、Ⅲ和Ⅳ代表恶性度逐渐增加。在本章节中，WHO分类确定的数字分级位于该部分标题肿瘤名称之后的括号内。IHC对估计肿瘤恶性度的主要作用如下[3, 56, 57]：

1. 确定细胞的类型；
2. 利用波形蛋白、CD31、CD34、Ulex europaeus (Ulex)、Ⅷ因子内皮标记物和SM来确定增生的血管；
3. 在估计肿瘤生长潜能时，利用增生标记物，如分子免疫Borstel 1（MIB-1）作为核分裂活性的补充（图18.8）。

分级的原则为：无核分裂象，边界清楚的原发性脑肿瘤定为Ⅰ级；浸润性肿瘤倾向于是Ⅱ级或更高

表18.4 血管畸形

类型	位置	组织学
AVM	大脑半球、脑干、小脑	静脉和动脉常形成异常的弹性膜；胶质性脑组织
静脉畸形	CNS、脊髓软脑膜	静脉和胶质性或正常脑组织；无动脉
毛细血管扩张	脑桥、脑干、CNS	脑实质内薄壁扩张的毛细血管
海绵状血管瘤	CNS	异常的血管簇，常为纤维化和玻璃样变的血管，具有弹性层，血管之间无脑组织

AVM, 动静脉畸形；CNS, 中枢神经系统

(摘引自McKeever PE, Blaivas M. The brain, spinal cord, and meninges. In: Sternberg SS, ed. Diagnostic Surgical Pathology. 2nd ed. New York: Raven Press; 1994:409-492)

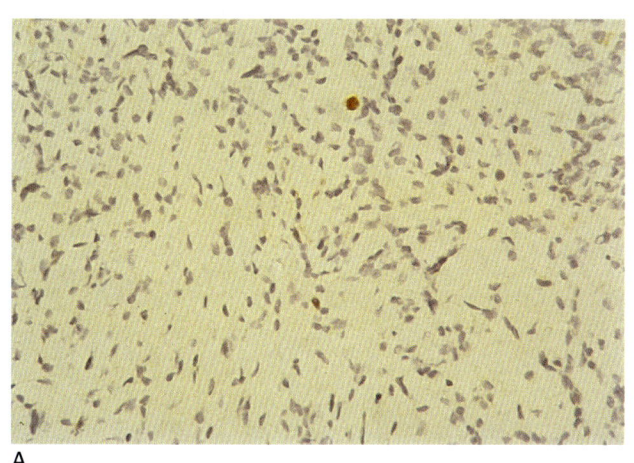 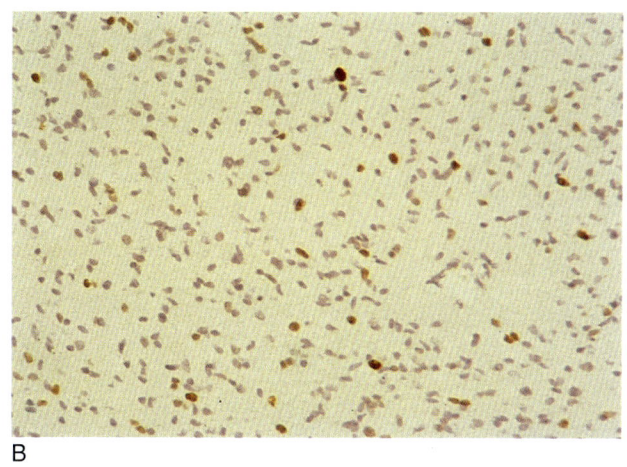

图 18.8 弥漫性纤维型星形细胞瘤，Ⅱ级。MIB-1 抗体可以区别 Ⅱ 级星形细胞瘤病人的生存期长短。(A) 取自一个存活 8 年多病人的标本，棕褐色 MIB-1 阳性细胞核很少。(B) 取自存活期不到 6 个月的一个病人标本中，有许多 MIB-1 阳性细胞核。苏木精复染使 MIB-1 阴性胞核呈紫蓝色（引自 McKeever PE, Strawderman MY, Yamini B, et al. MIB-1 proliferation index predicts survival among patients with grade Ⅱ astrocytomas. J Neuropathol Exp Neurol 1998; 57: 931-936）

级。NF 和 Syn 染色，通过对原有轴突的染色，尤其在白质中的轴突，以及灰质中原有的突触染色可以帮助分析肿瘤细胞的浸润。通过应用上述免疫组化染色，加上良好的苏木精核复染，可以非常清楚地显示浸润性的肿瘤细胞[58]。除了苏木精染色外，如果需要也可以应用伊红染色。

增生标记显示的是在细胞周期中某一个或多个增生时期出现的核抗原。可以根据它们的表达来计算标记指数（LI；也称为 PI，增生指数）[59, 60]。任何增生抗原的 LI 是指抗原标记阳性的细胞数除以肿瘤样本显微镜区域中所有细胞的数值。星形细胞瘤的组织学分级与 LI 相关[60]。

MIB-1 是检测细胞周期不同时期增生细胞的抗体。通过严格的标准化，MIB-1 LI 有助于预测病人预后[61, 62]。MIB-1 LI 可以用于鉴别 Ⅱ 级和 Ⅲ 级胶质瘤[63]。在 Ⅱ 级的星形细胞瘤的病人组中 MIB-1 标记还可用于预测患者预后，低 LI 的肿瘤患者预后好（图 18.8A）[62]。在同一实验室对一组肿瘤组织的处理过程必须严格的标准化；以便从每个病人的肿瘤的标记指数中得到最好的预后信息。因为不同实验室的染色过程和对 LI 的评判不同，从而限制了对所发表数据进行比较的价值。

PCNA 是 DNA 多聚酶的辅助蛋白[64]。笔者个人经验喜欢用 MIB-1 而不用 PCNA 来进行特异性染色和检测增殖指数 LI[60]。

凋亡是细胞的程序化死亡。凋亡指数类似前面提到的与增生相关的 LI，可以通过细胞学和细胞化学检测。细胞增生和死亡之间的平衡影响肿瘤的生长[65]。

在胶质瘤，随着肿瘤的进展其恶性度逐渐增加，最终预后较差。细胞周期素依赖性激酶 4 抑制剂（CDKN2/p16）是一种细胞周期调节蛋白，在许多人类恶性肿瘤的发生过程中，该基因由于突变、缺失或转录沉默等而失活。CDKN2/p16 免疫组化可以确诊那些低级别胶质瘤，这种胶质瘤容易进展，预后差，因而需要更积极的治疗[66]。其他不同的基因和它们的免疫活性蛋白在胶质瘤肿瘤演进中发生改变，这些已在其他部分讨论过[1, 2]。

胶质瘤

胶质瘤这一名词是描述星形细胞瘤、胶质母细胞瘤、室管膜瘤、少突胶质细胞瘤以及它们的不同的亚型及组合。胶质瘤的重要特征为实质中含有 GFAP，而缺乏胶原、网状纤维和纤维粘连蛋白，依此可以将其与非胶质肿瘤相鉴别（示意图 18.1、18.2）[67, 68]。少见的亚型如黄色星形细胞瘤，实质内可能含有网状纤维（表 18.5、18.1）。但是在少突胶质细胞瘤细胞的 GFAP 表达非常不一致，它们仅共同表达 Leu7 和 S-100 蛋白等特异性较低的胶质蛋白[3]。胶质瘤的实质无 CK 表达，但由于某些抗 CK 抗体和 GFAP 有交叉反应因而可造成误诊（图 18.9）[5]。

临床的情况使病理学家更好地解释胶质瘤。例如，伴有少突胶质细胞成分的胶质瘤，尤其伴有 1p 或 19q 染色体缺失的恶性胶质瘤对甲基苄肼-CCNU-长

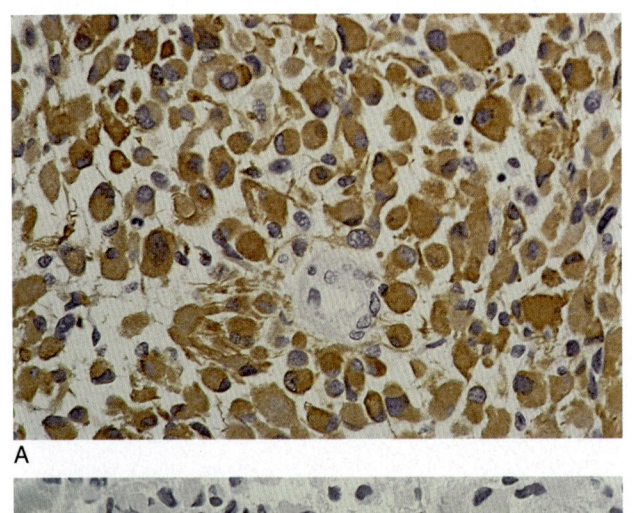
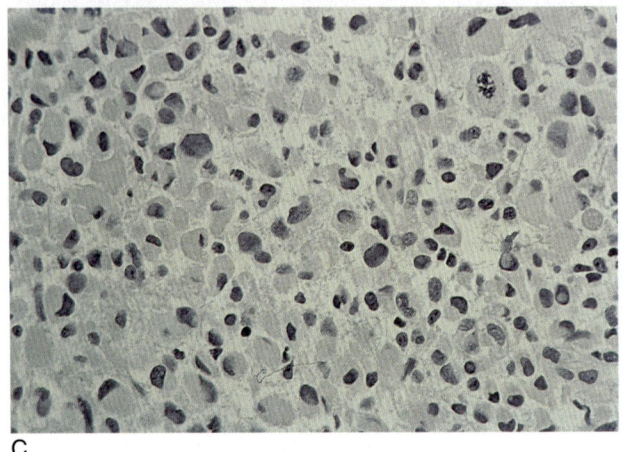
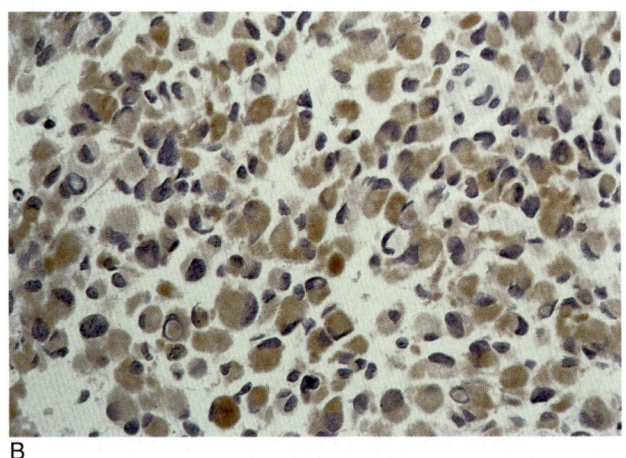

图18.9　间变型星形细胞瘤的3张切片。（A）GFAP染色显示一些纤维样细胞。（B）包括AE1/AE3 CK的单克隆抗体"鸡尾酒"染色显示AE1/AE3与GFAP有交叉反应。（C）CAM5.2单克隆抗体染色CK，显示该胶质瘤的CK阴性。这个恶性星形细胞瘤显示高级别的细胞学特征，包括核分裂活性（C），细胞核间变，细胞多形性，从胖星形细胞到几乎没有胞浆的细胞核。血管特征和间变的程度尚不足以诊断为Ⅳ级（胶质母细胞瘤），没有凝固性坏死（与图18.8相比）（苏木精复染）（引自McKeever PE. New methods of brain tumor analysis. In: Mena H, ed. Dr. Kenneth M. Earle Memorial Neuropathology Review. Washington, DC: Armed Forces Institute of Pathology; February 24, 2000）

春新碱（PCV）化疗有效[69]，对这些肿瘤的识别具有重要临床价值。另外，手术后全身性血栓形成是脑肿瘤手术的主要并发症。通过报告肿瘤（通常为恶性胶质瘤）内含有血栓形成的血管，病理学家有可能确定病人术后出现这种情况的可能性[70]。

用于星形细胞瘤和其他胶质瘤的组织学名词"低级别"不一定提示其为良性肿瘤或预后好。"良性"这个名称，是指切除胶质瘤后，肿瘤将不再复发，这种情况仅常见于 WHO Ⅰ级的星形细胞瘤、节细胞胶质瘤和室管膜瘤。此外，这些肿瘤还要位于能被完全切除的有利位置，从而使病人有治愈的可能[13]。从胶质瘤分子生物学研究而得来的资料表明Ⅰ级胶质瘤和非浸润性胶质瘤没有p53基因产物和表皮生长因子受体（EGFR）的过表达[71, 72]。相反，高级别和浸润性胶质瘤至少过表达其中的一种物质[2, 72]。

肿瘤和肿瘤边界

认识两种类型的胶质瘤标本是非常重要的（图18.10）。第一种类型是肿瘤组织本身（表18.5 ~ 18.8），细胞密度较周围脑组织高（图18.10B）。这种肿瘤病灶最适合于组织病理学分类[73, 74]。

第二种类型的标本是胶质瘤边缘浸润的脑组织，它是许多胶质瘤浸润特性的产物[3]。免疫组化染色显示脑神经解剖成分对于确定这种脑组织有很大的帮助。神经微丝蛋白可以定位白质或灰质中的轴突，这些轴突的神经解剖排列是平行的[58]。在免疫组化苏木精复染切片清楚发现在脑组织中胶质瘤细胞浸润轴突网（图18.11）。在灰质，Syn染色呈纤细的点状"地毯"状，胶质瘤细胞破坏了这个"地毯"。

如果仅能对获得的肿瘤边缘标本检测，是不可能对胶质瘤进行组织学分级和分类的，形成浸润边缘的肿瘤性胶质。另外从胶质瘤本身，CNS实质中的肿瘤胶质是难以与神经胶质增生相鉴别的（图18.12、图18.10A）。然而，通过GFAP染色显示胞浆内过量的GFAP表达和胶质增生中的胶质细胞均匀分布有助于确定神经胶质增生（图18.2）。

神经系统的免疫组织化学 18

> **诊断要点：胶质瘤**
> 1. 正确的外科取材对于弥漫性或异质性的胶质瘤的正确分类和分级是必需的。手术中病理学家和外科医师的相互交流使得取材尽可能完善。
> 2. 除了某些室管膜瘤和黄色星形细胞瘤外，大多数Ⅱ～Ⅳ级胶质瘤浸润CNS组织，使得彻底切除非常困难甚至不可能。
> 3. 增生标记物MIB-1能帮助分级和预测病人预后。

星形细胞瘤

在CNS肿瘤中，除了伸长型细胞型室管膜瘤和室管膜下瘤之外，星形细胞瘤是最呈纤维样的肿瘤，与其他胶质瘤相比更具纤维性特点（表18.5）。虽然星形细胞瘤GFAP表达的量有所不同，但几乎总是有GFAP的表达（图18.13A、图18.8A）。GFAP是区别星形细胞瘤与其他几乎所有的非胶质肿瘤唯一的和最重要的免疫组化标记[3]。神经鞘膜瘤偶尔局灶性表达GFAP，但表达量比形态相似的纤维型星形细胞瘤少。许多星形细胞瘤表达波形蛋白，当有波形蛋白表达时，可根据该特征与波形蛋白阴性的少突胶质细胞瘤相鉴别[13]。

毛细胞型星形细胞瘤（WHO Ⅰ级） 毛细胞的意思是"包含毛发样细胞"，这是毛细胞型星形细胞瘤的一个主要特征。拉长的、纤维状的、细胞浆突起组成平行束类似头发丛（图18.13A）[75]。这些毛发样突起含有大量胶质纤维，GFAP免疫过氧化物酶染色效果很好（表18.5）。

诊断毛细胞型星形细胞瘤是在星形细胞瘤中的唯一的"好消息"。这个肿瘤比其相应的弥漫型星形细胞瘤的预后好，尤其当它发生于小脑而不是第三脑室附近的其他常见部位[76,77]。Ⅱ级纤维型星形细胞瘤预后较差，因而区分毛细胞型星形细胞瘤与Ⅱ级纤维型星形细胞瘤是非常重要的。尽管毛细胞型星形细胞瘤预后好，但受下列因素影响：①能够完全外科手术切除毛细胞型星形细胞瘤依赖于肿瘤的位置，②某些毛细胞型星形细胞瘤的发生为多中心性。幕上肿瘤病人在肿瘤全切后10年生存率为100%，次全切或活检后为74%[78]。毛细胞型星形细胞瘤很少表现恶性变的特征，如细胞密度高、核分裂和坏死等。

在MRI上，毛细胞型星形细胞瘤有清楚的界限，有些肿瘤有明显的边界，但许多肿瘤与肿瘤边缘的脑组织成分相互混合。然而，弥漫性Ⅱ级星形细胞瘤比毛细胞型星形细胞瘤浸润脑组织的范围更广泛[79]。显微镜下的浸润程度可以通过连续切片来比较分析，GFAP染色来确定肿瘤边界 GFAP强阳性表达的细胞，神经微丝蛋白染色确定肿瘤边界的轴突。毛细胞型星形细胞瘤的边界很少有轴突，而Ⅱ级星形细胞瘤则有很多轴突。轴突和肿瘤细胞的混合提示为一个Ⅱ级病变。

绝大多数，但并非全部的毛细胞型星形细胞瘤发生于儿童或年轻人。它们多见于颅后窝、第三脑室旁、丘脑、下丘脑、神经垂体和视神经。大脑半球毛细胞型星形细胞瘤很少见，但是对它们的认识为保证对其进行恰当的治疗很重要[80]。

Rosenthal纤维是高度嗜酸性、玻璃样变的结构。它们呈圆形、椭圆形或串珠样伴有轻度不规则的边缘[3]。由于它们在胶质突起内形成所以出现串珠样的表现。与红细胞相比，它们是粉红色的而不是橙色的，大小和形状有很大的不同。IHC显示它们含有β-晶状体蛋白，可以用泛肽染色，重要的是Rosenthal纤维GFAP免疫染色阴性（图18.13A）。虽然Rosenthal纤维有助于毛细胞型星形细胞瘤与其他类型肿瘤的鉴别，但是由于星形细胞瘤与神经胶质增生二者均可有Rosenthal纤维，因而它们对于鉴别星形细胞瘤与神经胶质增生没有任何价值。

在毛细胞型星形细胞瘤中经常发现嗜酸性蛋白碎片（嗜酸性颗粒小体，EGB）。这些蛋白碎片通常较小，比Rosenthal纤维更加集中，通常位于细胞内，偶尔可以位于细胞外，最大直径40μm，PAS染色阳性（图18.13B）。α-B-晶状体蛋白是小热休克蛋白家族的晶状体蛋白，嗜酸性蛋白碎片和Rosenthal纤维α-B-晶状体蛋白染色阳性。据报道α-B-晶状体蛋白也可以染皮质内的Lewy小体，以及其他的星形细胞瘤、神经鞘膜、血管母细胞瘤和脊索瘤[13,81]。

观察S-100蛋白亚型提示S-100蛋白亚型可以区别毛细胞型星形细胞瘤与WHOⅡ～Ⅳ级的星形细胞瘤[82]。毛细胞型星形细胞瘤没有p53蛋白的过表达[71]。也可能没有EGFR异常[83]。这些特征有可能在将来应用于毛细胞型星形细胞瘤的诊断上。

小脑的囊性毛细胞型星形细胞瘤类似血管母细胞瘤，血管母细胞瘤可有局灶性细胞GFAP阳性表达和囊壁GFAP阳性。与血管母细胞瘤不同，毛细胞型星形细胞瘤囊腔壁的结节有高度纤维性和大量GFAP阳

表18.5 大量纤维状细胞的鉴别诊断

诊断[*]	鉴别特征结构	抗体[a]	位置[b]
纤维化	脑膜或血管周围起源的梭形细胞	Ⅳ型胶原（+）、波形蛋白（+）	脑膜，CNS
肉芽肿	类似纤维化，有"旋涡"状结构和炎症	微生物（见表18.1）	基底部脑膜，CNS
毛细胞型星形细胞瘤	细胞密度高，毛发样纤维，Rosenthal 纤维，微囊	GFAP（+）、S-100、α-B-晶状体蛋白	小脑，丘脑/下丘脑，视神经，CNS
星形细胞瘤	细胞密度高，角状核集落，相互凹入，CNS浸润	GFAP（S）、S-100	大脑，脑干，脊髓，CNS
间变型星形细胞瘤	上述特征增加，核分裂	GFAP（S）、S-100	大脑，脑干，CNS
胖细胞型星形细胞瘤	细胞密度高，细胞肿胀，胞浆红染，玻璃样变，偏位的多形性核，浸润CNS	GFAP（S）	大脑
巨细胞型星形细胞瘤	有粗纤维的巨大星形细胞，大的圆形/椭圆形细胞核	GFAP（S）	侧脑室，室管膜下
星形母细胞瘤	血管周围菊形团伴伸长的胶质细胞突起	非纤维状的GFAP（S）	大脑，CNS
多形性黄色星形细胞瘤	多形性细胞，常有空泡	GFAP（S）、Ⅳ型胶原（S）	软脑膜，大脑皮质
室管膜瘤	细胞密度高，室管膜或血管周菊形团或两个都有，圆形/椭圆形的细胞核，纤毛，基体	GFAP（S）	大脑，小脑，脊髓，CNS
伸长型细胞型室管膜瘤/室管膜下瘤	星形细胞瘤和室管膜瘤的组合，在神经纤维毯中呈簇的核圆/椭圆形的细胞	GFAP（+）	脊髓，第四脑室，室管膜下，CNS
间变型室管膜瘤	上述的特征伴有核分裂、坏死	GFAP（S）、S-100	大脑，小脑
多形性胶质母细胞瘤	凝固性坏死区，核分裂，多形性，内皮增生	GFAP（S）、S-100	大脑，CNS
胶质肉瘤	胶质母细胞瘤与纤维肉瘤的混合	GFAP（S）、纤维粘连蛋白、Ⅳ型胶原（S）、层粘连蛋白、波形蛋白（S）	大脑
节细胞肿瘤	双核和多形性神经元，诊断依靠胶质瘤和神经母细胞的成分	GFAP（S）、Syn（S）、PGP9.5、NF（S）、Ⅳ型胶原	大脑，CNS
中枢神经细胞瘤	圆形细胞和胞核，血管附近细的纤维	Syn（S）、NF（R）	透明间隔，侧脑室
松果体细胞瘤	正常松果体结构	Syn（S）、NF（R）	松果体
极性成胶质细胞瘤	纤维状细胞有规则的栅栏样排列		大脑，CNS
纤维母细胞型脑膜瘤	梭形细胞，细胞突起融合和桥粒，（厚的胶原），（旋涡结构）[c]	波形蛋白（+）、EMA（S）、S-100（R）	小脑幕镰，脑膜，脉络丛
纤维肉瘤/恶性纤维组织细胞瘤	细胞密度高，多形性梭形细胞和细胞核，核分裂，坏死	波形蛋白、胶原	脑膜，CNS
神经鞘瘤	Verocay 小体，Antoni A 和 B，薄的细胞周围基底膜	S-100（+）、Leu（7）、Ⅳ型胶原	第8对脑神经，脊神经根，PNS
神经纤维瘤	多种细胞类型伸展轴突	NF（R）、EMA、S-100（+）、Leu 7	脊神经根，PNS，脑神经

续表

诊 断*	鉴别特征结构	抗 体[a]	位 置[b]
组织细胞增生症	巨噬细胞片状排列，纤维母细胞和白细胞	α-ACT、S-100 (S)	蝶鞍旁的，CNS，全身的
黑色素瘤	间变，核分裂，坏死	HMB-45 (S)、S-100 (+)	CNS/脑膜，经常多发性转移，全身的

* 表格的病变排列顺序按照正文中讨论的顺序
a 染色结果解释：+，几乎总是弥漫强阳性；S，有时阳性；R，偶见细胞阳性
b 首先列出的是最常见或最特异的部位
c 鉴别诊断特征周围的括号提示为少见的特征，一旦发现对鉴别诊断非常有用
α-ACT，α-抗胰凝乳蛋白酶；CNS，中枢神经系统；EMA，上皮细胞膜抗原；GFAP，胶质纤维酸性蛋白；PNS，周围神经系统（改自 McKeever PE, Blaivas M. The brain, spinal cord, and meninges. In: Sternberg SS, ed. Diagnostic Surgical Pathology. 2nd ed. New York: Raven Press; 1994: 409-492）

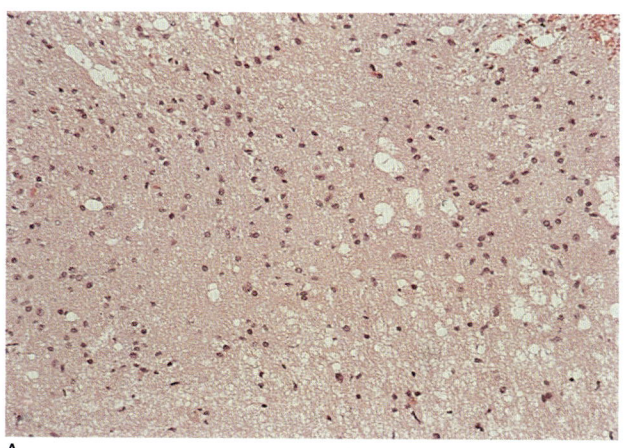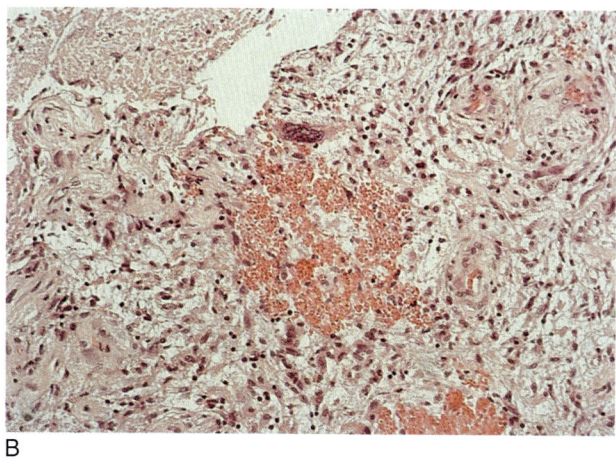

图18.10 一位老年女性左颞顶部包块立体定位活检的标本。（A）第一个标本显示了神经胶质增生、少量肿瘤性胶质、不能确定肿瘤的类型和分级；(B) 多个标本中的最后一个标本显示为胶质母细胞瘤，具有显著多形性的纤维状细胞、核分裂象、血管增生和坏死（引自 McKeever PE. New methods of brain tumor analysis. In: Mena H, ed. Dr. Kenneth M. Earle Memorial Neuropathology Review. Washington, DC: Armed Forces Institute of Pathology; February 24, 2000）

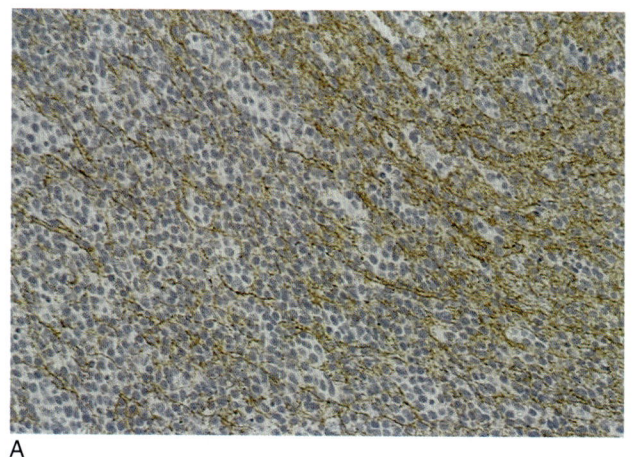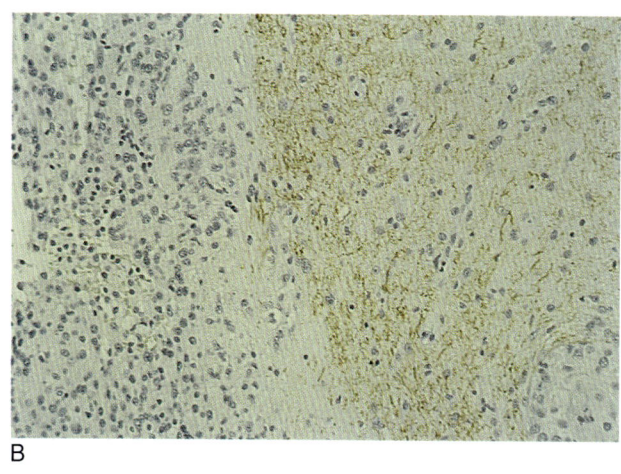

图18.11 （A）NF免疫组化染色显示脑组织中的轴突，以利于确定胶质瘤在脑组织内浸润。Ⅱ级少突星形细胞瘤中具有密集的圆形和长形的细胞核（苏木精染为紫蓝色）的细胞弥漫浸润于脑组织中长的、褐色的轴突成分中；(B) 相反，多形性黄色星形细胞瘤（PXA）不在每条褐色的轴突中间浸润，肿瘤与大脑皮质的界限清楚。在无IHC时，可以观察到PXA的其他特征，如多形性的细胞和细胞核以及脂质空泡等（图18.16）（引自McKeever PE. New methods of brain tumor analysis. In: Mena H, ed. Dr. Kenneth M. Earle Memorial Neuropathology Review. Washington, DC: Armed Forces Institute of Pathology; February 24, 2000）

表18.6　大量上皮样细胞的鉴别诊断

诊　断[*]	结　构	鉴别特征　抗体[a]	部　位[b]
格子细胞/黄色肉芽肿	密集的吞噬脂质空泡的巨噬细胞，核偏位，非黏附性细胞	α-ACT（S）、KP-1（+）、muramidase（S）	CNS
室管膜瘤/恶性室管膜瘤样细胞	室管膜瘤或恶性室管膜瘤结构加之上皮样细胞	GFAP（S）、CK（R）、EMA（R）	小脑，大脑，脊髓，CNS
黏液乳头状室管膜瘤	玻璃样变纤维血管性乳头被覆立方形/柱状上皮，不同的纤维形成	GFAP（S）	终丝区
少突胶质细胞瘤	圆形细胞和胞核有显著的核周晕，细胞巢之间为纤细的血管	Leu7（+）、S-100（+）	大脑，CNS
间变型少突胶质细胞瘤	以上特征伴核分裂和多形性	Leu7（S）、S-100（S）	大脑，CNS
脉络丛乳头状瘤	伴有脉络丛结构的大的肿块	层粘连蛋白（+）、CK（+）、转甲状腺蛋白（S）、Syn、IGF-Ⅱ	第四脑室，侧脑室，CP角，脉络丛
脉络丛乳头状癌	以上特征伴间变和核分裂，（坏死）[c]	CK（+）、CD44、Syn、转甲状腺蛋白（R）	上述部位
髓上皮瘤	柱状上皮，两面均有基底膜，乳头和小管的纤维血管性基底		大脑深部，马尾，CNS
脑膜瘤	旋涡，砂粒体，细胞突起融合和桥粒，（厚的胶原）[c]	波形蛋白（+）、EMA（S）、S-100（R）	脑镰，脑幕，脑膜，脉络丛，（颅外）[c]
脊索瘤	含空泡的细胞团或索	CK（+）、S-100（+）、EMA（+）、波形蛋白（+）	马尾，斜坡，脊柱管
颅咽管瘤	鳞状细胞，造釉上皮的	CK（+）	蝶鞍上的，蝶鞍的
癌	与CNS有明显界限，间变，核分裂，坏死	CK（+）、EMA（S）	大脑，小脑，脑膜，CNS，常见的多发的包块，全身性的
黑色素瘤	间变，核分裂，坏死	HMB-45（S）、S-100（+）	上述部位

[*] 表格的病变排列顺序按照正文中讨论的顺序
a 染色结果解释：+，几乎总是弥漫强阳性；S，有时阳性；R，罕见有细胞阳性
b 首先列出最常见或最特异的部位
c 鉴别特征旁的括号提示为少见的特征，一旦发现对鉴别诊断非常有用
α-ACT，α-抗胰凝乳蛋白酶；CNS，中枢神经系统；CP，小脑脑桥的；EMA，上皮细胞膜抗原；GFAP，胶质纤维酸性蛋白；IGF-Ⅱ，胰岛素样生长因子Ⅱ
(改自McKeever PE, Blaivas M. The brain, spinal cord, and meninges. In: Sternberg SS, ed. Diagnostic Surgical Pathology. 2nd ed. New York: Raven Press; 1994:409-492)

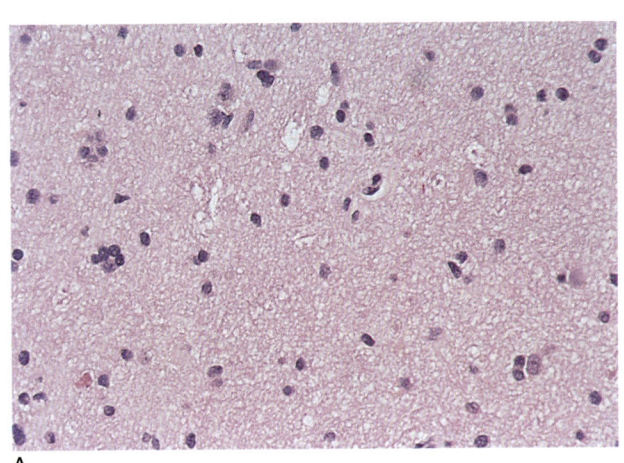
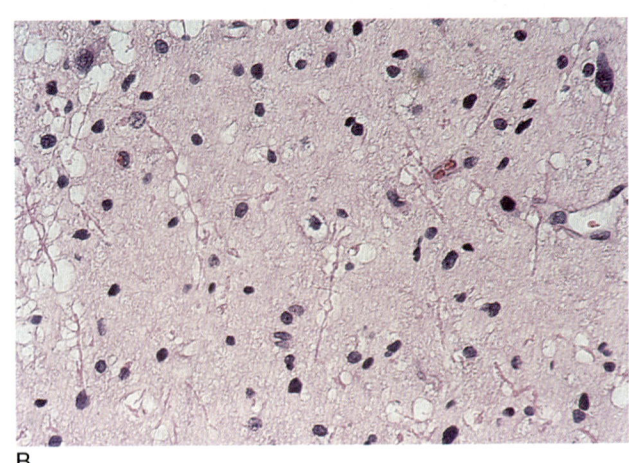

图18.12　转移癌（未示）边缘的神经胶质增生和非肿瘤性神经元周围的少突神经胶质细胞（A）与远离病灶的Ⅱ级纤维型星形细胞瘤边缘（B）相似。胞核更加多形性和染色质深染。(B)(与周围浅染的毛细血管内皮细胞核相比较)(HE)。(引自McKeever PE. New methods of brain tumor analysis. In: Mena H, ed. Dr. Kenneth M. Earle Memorial Neuropathology Review. Washington, DC: Armed Forces Institute of Pathology; February 24, 2000)

表18.7　显著不同细胞肿瘤的鉴别诊断

诊　断[*]	结　构	鉴别特征　抗体[a]	部　位[b]
少突胶质细胞瘤	星形细胞瘤（表18.5）与少突胶质细胞瘤（表18.6）的混合	GFAP（S）、Leu7（+）、S-100（+）	大脑，CNS
间变型少突胶质细胞瘤	上述特征伴核分裂和多形性	GFAP（S）、Leu7（S）、S-100（S）	大脑，CNS
胶质母细胞瘤/胶质肉瘤伴上皮样化生	胶质母细胞瘤/胶质肉瘤结构（表18.5）加之上皮区域	GFAP（S）、S-100（S）、CK（S）、EMA（S）	大脑，CNS
神经节细胞肿瘤	双核和多形性神经元加之胶质瘤（表18.5）、纤维化和炎症	GFAP（S）、Syn（S）、PGP9.5、神经微丝（R）、Ⅳ型胶原（R）	大脑，CNS
促纤维增生型髓母细胞瘤	髓母细胞瘤和纤维化区	Syn、S-100、Ⅳ型胶原、神经微丝（R）、GFAP（R）	一侧小脑，CNS，脑膜，（中轴以外）[c]
过渡型脑膜瘤	纤维性区脑膜瘤（表18.5）和合体细胞性区脑膜瘤（表18.9）	波形蛋白（+）、EMA（S）、S-100（R）	脑幕，脑镰，脑膜，脉络丛
血管母细胞瘤	在许多毛细血管间的空泡状间质细胞，血管密度高，(纤维状是冰冻切片人工产物)[c]	CD31（S）、Ⅷ因子（S）、NSE（S）	小脑，脊髓，CNS
促纤维增生型癌	癌（表18.6）和纤维化区域（表18.5），偶有炎症	CK（S）、EMA（S）	大脑，小脑，脑膜，CNS，常为多发性肿块，全身性的
黑色素瘤	纤维性区黑色素瘤和上皮样区黑色素瘤（表18.5、18.6）	HMB-45（S）、S-100（+）	大脑，小脑，脑膜，CNS，常为多发性肿块，全身性的

[*] 表格内病变的排列顺序按照正文中讨论的顺序
[a] 染色结果解释：+，几乎总是弥漫强阳性；S，有时阳性；R，罕见细胞阳性
[b] 首先列出最常见或最特异的部位
[c] 鉴别特征旁的括号提示少见的特征，一旦发现对鉴别诊断非常有用
CNS，中枢神经系统；EMA，上皮细胞膜抗原；GFAP，胶质纤维酸性蛋白；NSE，神经特异性烯醇化酶（改自McKeever PE, Blaivas M. The brain, spinal cord, and meninges. In: Sternberg SS, ed. Diagnostic Surgical Pathology. 2nd ed. New York: Raven Press; 1994: 409-492）

性的肿瘤性星形细胞，而没有含脂质的透明空泡细胞。CD31和其他内皮细胞标记显示星形细胞瘤的毛细血管比血管母细胞瘤的少。

<u>弥漫型星形细胞瘤（低级别星形细胞瘤）（WHO Ⅱ级）</u>　纤维型星形细胞瘤比原浆型星形细胞瘤常见[73]。纤维型星形细胞瘤是细胞的纤维性突起和细胞核的混合，比正常或反应性星形细胞的角度和密度更大（图18.14、图18.12B）。它们含有更多的胞质内纤维，细胞突起比原浆型星形细胞瘤的长。因而，显示纤维蛋白束的磷钨酸苏木精（PTAH）法只能使纤维型星形细胞瘤染色，两种星形细胞瘤均含有GFAP，因此均可被免疫组化染色[13]。

名词"弥漫性"恰当地描述了星形细胞瘤边缘细胞密度逐渐降低，在很宽的肿瘤边缘中，肿瘤细胞与脑实质相混合（图18.14）。NF染色清楚地显示了肿瘤细胞在白质内平行排列的轴突中浸润（见下面的毛细胞型星形细胞瘤）。弥漫性脑组织浸润也可能是明显的，形成Scherer继发性结构。

尽管"低级别"星形细胞瘤具有相对良性的组织学特征，肿瘤弥漫性生长和浸润特性是它们很少能治愈的原因。手术后存活期相当不一致，通常为3~10年。由于Ⅱ级弥漫型星形细胞瘤预后非常不同，因而要重视对每个患者预后进行更好的判断。现已明确低MIB-1 LI病人的预后好（图18.15、图18.8）[62]。p53过表达可能与肿瘤演进为胶质母细胞瘤有关[84]。

星形细胞瘤中染色体异常包括染色体13、22、X和Y的缺失及染色体7的增加[1,5]。这些改变可以通过荧光和增强的免疫组化ISH方法检测[85]。

表18.8　密集的小间变性细胞肿瘤的鉴别诊断

诊　断	结　构	鉴别特征　抗体[*]	部　位[a]
室管膜母细胞瘤	类似PNET，缎带状/索状排列细胞，真正的室管膜菊形团	波形蛋白（S）、GFAP（R）	大脑，小脑
髓母细胞瘤/松果体母细胞瘤/神经母细胞瘤/PNET	纤细纤维状，（Homer-Wright菊形团），（栅栏），"胡萝卜"样核，（神经的或胶质的病灶）[b]	Syn（S）、PGP9.5、S-100（R）、NF（R）、GFAP（R）	小脑，脑干，松果体，CNS，（中轴以外）[b]
横纹肌肉瘤/髓肌母细胞瘤	类似PNET，肌条纹	结蛋白（S）、肌特异性肌动蛋白	松果体，小脑，CNS
非典型畸胎样-横纹肌样肿瘤	类似PNET，胞浆更丰富	波形蛋白（+）、GFAP（S）、CK（S）、EMA（R）、Syn（R）、Cg（R）	小脑，脑
血管外皮细胞瘤	细胞密度高，细胞周围增厚的基质，核分裂	波形蛋白（+）	脑幕，脑镰，脑膜，（颅外）[b]
淋巴瘤	非黏附性圆形细胞，血管壁浸润	L26（+）、LCA（S）、单克隆κ和λIg	大脑深部，CNS，脑膜，可能多发
小细胞癌	黏附性细胞，（上皮样），（桥粒）[b]	CK（+）、EMA、Syn（S）	CNS，脑膜，常为多发性包块，全身性的

[*] 染色结果解释：+，几乎总是弥漫阳性；S，有时阳性；R，罕见细胞阳性
a 首先列出最常见或最特异的部位
b 鉴别特征旁的括号提示少见的特征，一旦发现对鉴别诊断非常有用
CNS，中枢神经系统；EMA，上皮细胞膜抗原；GFAP，胶质纤维酸性蛋白；Ig，免疫球蛋白；LCA，白细胞共同抗原；PNET，原始神经外胚层肿瘤
（改自McKeever PE, Blaivas M. The brain, spinal cord, and meninges.In: Sternberg SS, ed. Diagnostic Surgical Pathology. 2nd ed. New York: Raven Press; 1994: 409-492）

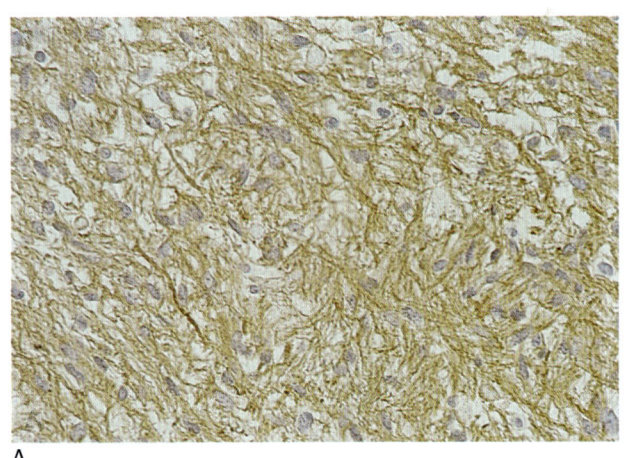
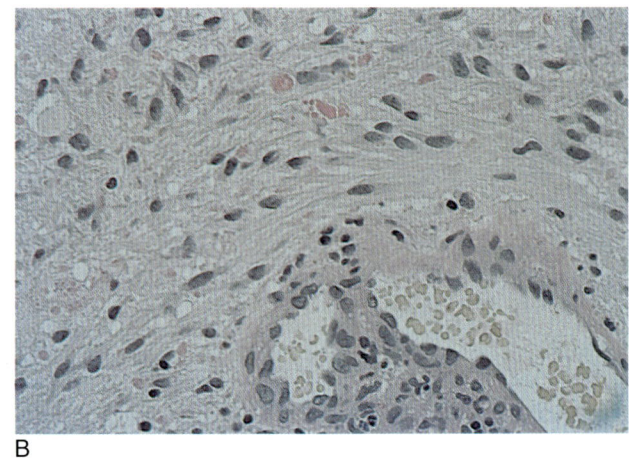

图18.13　该肿瘤位于一年轻男性的小脑中线处，患者有头痛和呕吐症状。(A) 毛细胞型星形细胞瘤特征：大量褐色的GFAP阳性的胞浆突起。浅灰色、折光的小球，某些具有褐色GFAP阳性边缘的是Rosenthal纤维。GFAP阴性的Rosenthal纤维位于星形细胞突起内。(B) 该肿瘤内浅灰色的Rosenthal纤维与粉红色、PAS染色阳性的蛋白碎片（PAS伴淀粉酶消化）相混合。与浅褐色血管内的红细胞相比，二者的直径均不一致（引自McKeever PE. New methods of brain tumor analysis. In: Mena H, ed. Dr. Kenneth M. Earle Memorial Neuropathology Review. Washington, DC: Armed Forces Institute of Pathology; February 24, 2000）

胖细胞型星形细胞瘤（WHO Ⅱ级）　胖细胞型星形细胞是含有透明的粉红色胞浆的大细胞，GFAP染色阳性（表18.5、图18.9A）。深染的和角状的胞核位于细胞边缘，形成奇异的类似反应性的星形细胞。含有20%以上的胖细胞型星形细胞的星形细胞瘤才可以诊断为胖细胞型星形细胞瘤。胖细胞型星形细胞瘤比它们相对应的非胖细胞型的星形细胞瘤更具有侵袭性。胖细胞型星形细胞瘤特别易于进展为更高级别的肿瘤。那些演进前的没有高级别特征的胖细胞型肿瘤仍考虑为Ⅱ级星形细胞瘤[2]。

胖细胞型星形细胞瘤与少突胶质细胞瘤的区别在于小胖细胞型星形细胞核更易呈角状，更具多形性，

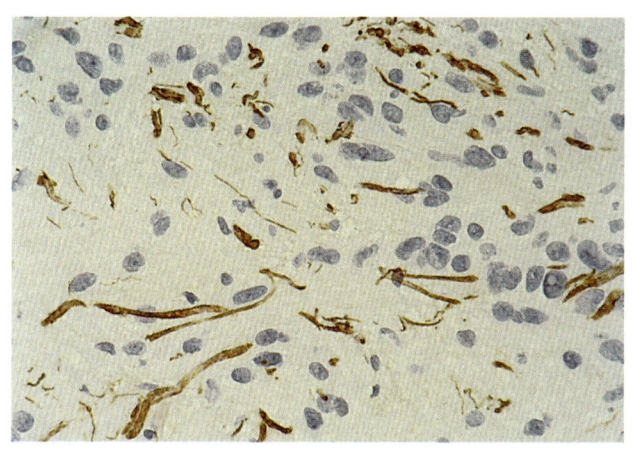

图18.14 本例为Ⅱ级弥漫型星形细胞瘤,可见多形性蓝色的细胞核与密集的、相互吻合的不规则突起。这些细胞核浸润于抗NF蛋白染色为褐色的原有的轴突之间。脑组织内的弥漫浸润可作为绝大多数Ⅱ级和更高级别的星形细胞瘤与Ⅰ级肿瘤的鉴别(免疫过氧化物酶抗NF蛋白染色,苏木精复染)[引自McKeever PE. Neurofilament(NF) and synaptophysin stains reveal diagnostic and prognostic patterns of interaction between normal and neoplastic tissues. Presented at the annual meeting of the Histochemical Society, Bethesda, MD, March 24, 2000]

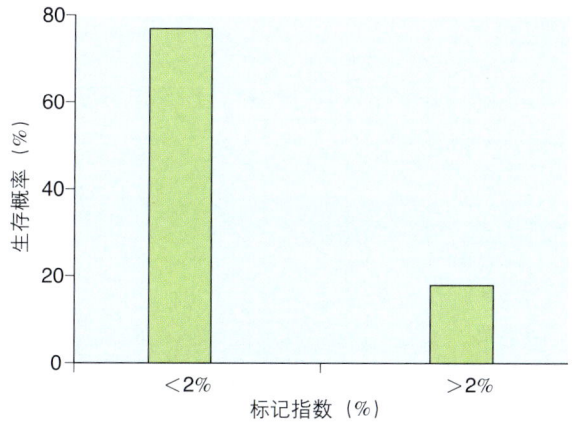

图18.15 MIB-1 标记指数 ≤ 2% 和 > 2% 的Ⅱ级星形细胞瘤病人的生存概率。柱形代表数据(引自 McKeever PE, Strawderman MY, Yamini B, et al. MIB-1 proliferation index predicts survival among patients with grade Ⅱ astrocytomas. J Neuropathol Exp Neurol 1998; 57:931-936)

GFAP阳性细胞突起更长,与节细胞胶质瘤的区别在于胖细胞型星形细胞瘤缺乏 Syn 阳性的肿瘤性神经元;与室管膜下巨细胞肿瘤区别在于胞核更小、更多角状和更易于浸润脑组织。

间变型星形细胞瘤(WHO Ⅲ级) 定义"间变性"强调了间变型星形细胞瘤是高度恶性。高级别胶质瘤的共同特征是核分裂活性高、细胞密度增加、核的多形性(图18.9)和核深染。在间变型星形细胞瘤保留 GFAP 阳性的细胞突起和间变性细胞核周围的GFAP 阳性(图 18.19A)。这一重要特征将其与陷在其他肿瘤中的反应性星形细胞区别开。在胶质瘤中它们的 MIB-1 LI 位于中间状态[60]。

星形细胞胶质瘤中同时缺乏凝固性坏死的病灶和明显的血管增生可以作为对间变型星形细胞瘤与胶质母细胞瘤的鉴别(表 18.5)[2]。间变型星形细胞瘤病人的平均存活期为2年多。在儿童患者,低MIB-1 LI 组病人的预后好[86]。

其他类型的星形细胞瘤 室管膜下巨细胞星形细胞瘤(GCA)具有特殊的病变部位和组织学特征,与结节状硬化(TS)有关[87]。在与 TS 相关的 GCA 中,可以检测到与 TS 相关的肿瘤抑制基因产物 tuberin 的丢失[88]。在TS中,巨大星形细胞构成室管膜下结节,又称为"蜡滴"(表18.5)。肿瘤从常发现"蜡滴"处的侧脑室壁内侧部位发生。肿瘤由胞核大和核仁突出的巨大"星形细胞"组成(图18.16)。虽然这些肿瘤是多形性的,但大多数核缺少锐角,巨细胞稀疏。这些细胞可能含有GFAP染色阳性程度不同的胶质微丝(图 18.16A)。

在某些 GCA 中 IHC 染色显示有部分神经元的分化(图 18.16B),这使它们作为星形细胞瘤的分类变得复杂(与节细胞胶质瘤比较)。这些巨大的星形细胞和它们特征性的粗胞浆突起形成没有方向的束状排列。认识这种组织学特点很重要,原因是:①它们的多形性与它们相对良性的生物学行为和WHO Ⅰ级不同,②许多 GCA 与 TS 相关[3]。

星形母细胞瘤罕见[2]。星形母细胞的"菊形团"与室管膜瘤血管周围的假菊形团类似,不同的是,从细胞体到血管外膜的整个距离,星形母细胞的突起仍然很粗。在靠近外膜附近的足突可能更粗。免疫组化染色与常规神经组织化学染色联合有助于对该肿瘤的确诊。虽然星形母细胞瘤局灶性表达GFAP,但不表达PTAH。这种不一致可能是由于表达的非纤维状形式的 GFAP 分子与室管膜瘤和星形细胞瘤的纤维不同,这两个肿瘤均表达 GFAP 和 PTAH。

多形性黄色星形细胞瘤是一种幕上的星形细胞瘤,经常发生于软脑膜和大脑皮质(表18.5)[89]。与大多数星形细胞瘤相比,它与脑组织的边界更清楚(图18.11B)。纤维状、多形性、玻璃样变、含有脂质的细胞以及多核细胞是诊断线索(图18.17)。在不同的肿瘤细胞内所含的脂质成分和蛋白质颗粒状变性物

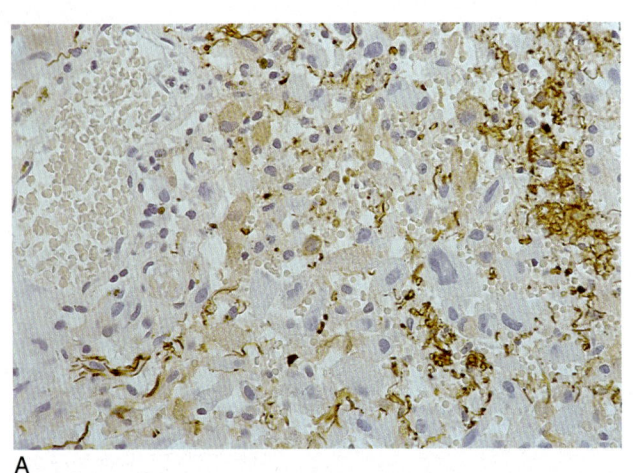
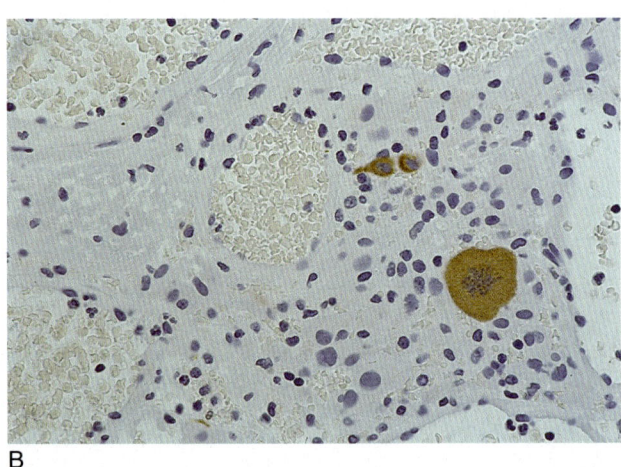

图18.16 巨细胞星形细胞瘤。（A）核体积大，核仁明显，丰富的细颗粒状胞浆，GFAP阳性程度不同的巨细胞。这些成分与粗的、黑褐色GFAP阳性的细胞突起束相混合。尽管它们的体积很大，但大多数胞核、核仁没有锐利的边缘。（B）细胞核染色质呈细颗粒状，核分裂罕见。在这个室管膜下巨细胞星形细胞瘤中有少量NF阳性的细胞和大量NF阴性的细胞。一个肿瘤细胞有核分裂，显示NF阳性反应。这种现象在该类型的肿瘤中很少见。该肿瘤发生于一位伴结节状硬化的20岁女性的透明隔（应用苏木精的免疫过氧化物酶的抗GFAP染色）（引自McKeever PE. New methods of brain tumor analysis. In: Mena H, ed. Dr. Kenneth M. Earle Memorial Neuropathology Review. Washington, DC: Armed Forces Institute of Pathology; February 24, 2000）

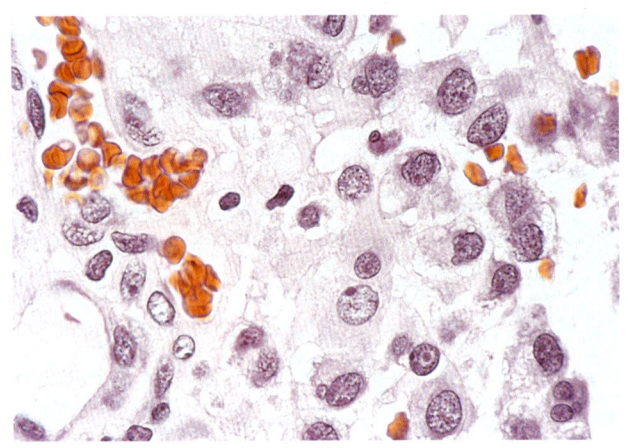

图18.17 多形性黄色星形细胞瘤。HE染色的切片，在多形性星形细胞中可以观察到圆的脂质空泡。尽管多形性的核和核仁大，但核浆比例低，染色质细颗粒状，核膜光滑

质的量不一致，可大量存在也可完全缺如。

多形性黄色星形细胞瘤（PXA）可以表现为透明细胞，此时需要用一组免疫组化试剂来明确诊断（示意图18.1）[90]。通过其GFAP强阳性而确定为星形细胞，并常常同时表达α-1-抗胰蛋白酶。稀疏的脂滴GFAP染色明显阴性，这些细胞可被网状纤维和Ⅳ型胶原阳性的基底膜所围绕，从而打破了胶质瘤细胞缺乏网硬蛋白的一般规则。某些肿瘤出现神经元成分，提示PXA可能是神经节神经胶质瘤的胶质部分[91]。Ⅱ级PXA容易与Ⅳ级胶质母细胞瘤混淆。二者的多形性均很明显。低MIB-1、缺少核分裂、EGB、轻度浸润和很少或

没有EGFR或p53的过表达可以使PXA与弥漫型星形细胞瘤尤其是胶质母细胞瘤相鉴别（图18.18）[92, 93]。

室管膜瘤

如何通过IHC显示其结构特征而作出诊断，室管膜瘤是一个最好的例子。

> **诊断要点：星形细胞瘤**
>
> 1. GFAP和良好的苏木精复染在免疫组化中是最重要的，显示由GFAP阳性围绕的肿瘤细胞核和星形细胞瘤GFAP阳性的纤维状突起。
> 2. NF染色显示肿瘤神经节的成分，更经常用于显示原来存在于脑组织内的轴突[58]，后者有助于估计肿瘤细胞的浸润。
> 3. 没有p53和EGFR过表达的非浸润性星形细胞瘤倾向于是Ⅰ级肿瘤。
> 4. MIB-1在估计肿瘤增生活性中是非常重要的，尤其是核分裂象不明显的星形细胞瘤。

室管膜瘤细胞的形态变化位于纤维状和上皮样之间，这不仅造成它与其他胶质瘤的鉴别困难，同时也造成与癌和脑膜瘤的鉴别诊断困难（表18.6、表18.5）。如果一个人能想到即使是上皮样室管膜瘤也常有GFAP染色，具有特征性的超微结构，至少少量细胞

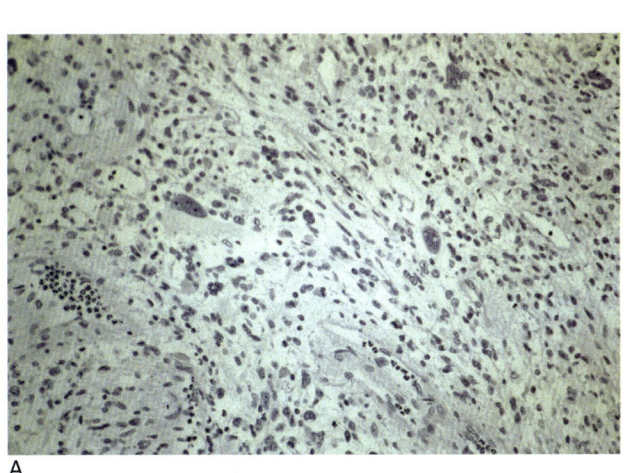
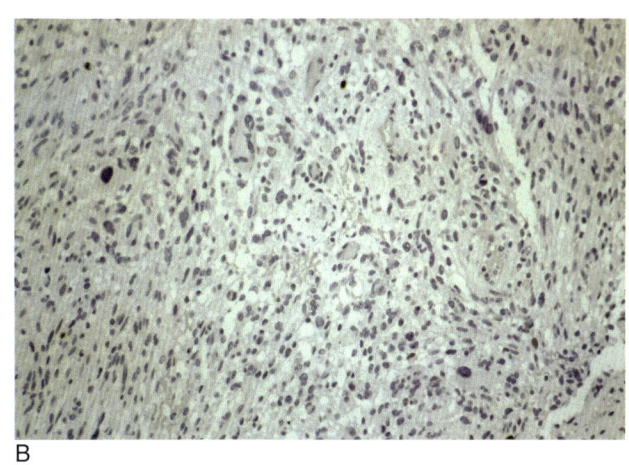

图 18.18 这个多形性黄色星形细胞瘤没有表皮生长因子受体过表达（A），很少的细胞过表达 p53（B）

有纤维状突起，则它们与癌和脑膜瘤的鉴别就会变得容易（图 18.19，示意图 18.1、18.2）。GFAP 染色清楚显示了细胞的纤维状突起，使诊断变得更容易（图 18.19A、B）。最好在血管周围寻找这些纤维状突起。

与非胶质性肿瘤相反，肿瘤实质中聚集的室管膜瘤细胞缺乏基底膜。免疫染色显示在这些肿瘤细胞中无胶原或纤维粘连蛋白[67]。低级别室管膜瘤细胞核圆形、椭圆形，染色质细、弥散。除了脑膜瘤之外，细胞核的特征使其与其他所有脑肿瘤相鉴别[3]。

当考虑为室管膜瘤时应该寻找菊形团结构（表

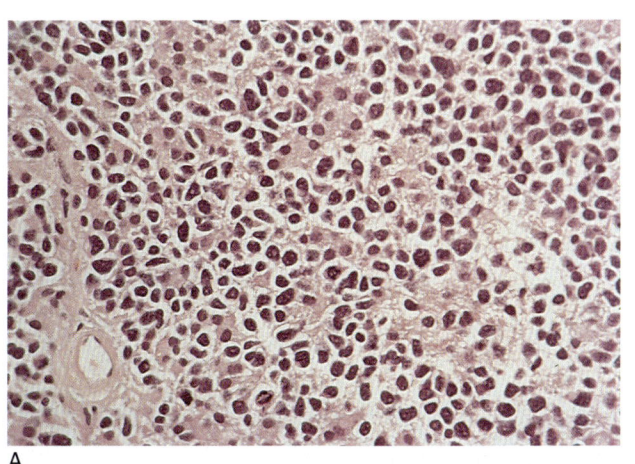
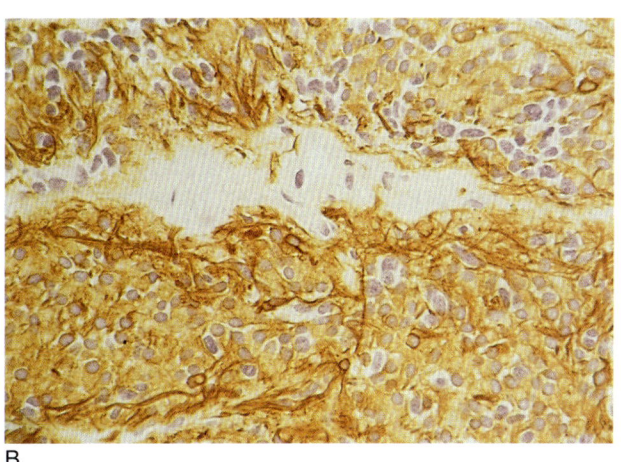
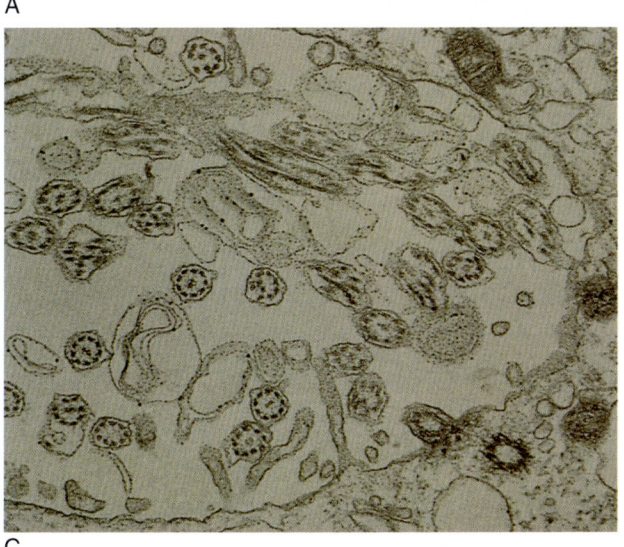

图18.19 肿瘤切片。(A)该肿瘤由上皮样细胞组成（HE）；(B)肿瘤 GFAP 阳性，在 GFAP 阴性血管的周围显示为纤细的纤维状染色；(C)电镜示室管膜瘤的纤毛和基体，该透明细胞室管膜瘤的结构特征，并非超微结构特征，与少突胶质细胞瘤类似（引自McKeever PE. New methods of brain tumor analysis. In: Mena H, ed. Dr. Kenneth M. Earle Memorial Neuropathology Review. Washington, DC: Armed Forces Institute of Pathology; February 24, 2000）

18.5、18.6）。血管周菊形团结构最有价值，几乎所有的室管膜瘤都可见到血管周菊形团。细胞围绕在中心血管的周围，纤维状区域至少有 3 个红细胞直径宽。纤维状区域 GFAP 染色阳性，因而在 GFAP 染色中很容易发现微小的纤维状区域（图 18.19B）。细胞发出的突起向血管外膜辐射时逐渐变细，从而使其有别于星形母细胞瘤的粗突起。真性室管膜菊形团是室管膜瘤的特征性结构，但有些标本缺少真性菊形团。室管膜菊形团由室管膜细胞环绕空腔排列（图 18.20）。纤毛常从室管膜内层伸入腔内。某些肿瘤有伸长形的室管膜菊形团，而有些肿瘤形成长的室管膜腔隙而没有聚集形成菊形团[3]。

与其他胶质瘤相比，许多室管膜瘤与脑组织的界限相对清楚。用 NF 免疫组化染色能够最好地显示位于白质中的肿瘤边界，NF 免疫组化染色可以显示白质中大量 NF 阳性的轴突与 NF 阴性的室管膜瘤之间的清晰界线。Syn 染色同样显示阳性反应的神经纤维网与阴性反应的肿瘤之间的边界相当清楚[58]。

对于诊断有困难的室管膜瘤电镜观察要优于 IHC（图 18.19C）。电镜可以显示纤毛、基体、细胞质内的微绒毛包涵体和伸长的细胞间连接体。

偶尔某些室管膜瘤，其高度分化的上皮细胞呈小灶状 CK、EMA 阳性反应。然而与脉络丛乳头状瘤和癌相比，室管膜瘤极少有 CAM5.2 阳性染色，因此 CAM5.2 可以用于鉴别上述肿瘤。

除了特殊病变以外，上述室管膜瘤的基本特征对本章节讨论的其他室管膜瘤变型的确诊也有帮助。

低级别室管膜瘤 其"低级别"一词经常在这组肿瘤的名字中省略，这组肿瘤简称为"室管膜瘤"。以上描述的特征和低级别室管膜瘤细胞核的特征使其与其他肿瘤相区别。室管膜瘤的核是典型的圆形或椭圆形，苏木精染色显示细胞核有明显的亮区和暗区（图 18.19A、18.20）。在菊形团周围的肿瘤实质中，细胞核的分布比低级别星形细胞瘤更均匀、密集，但不如髓母细胞瘤和原始神经外胚层肿瘤核密集（图 18.8、18.12、18.19 和 18.37）。

上皮样室管膜瘤：偶尔与脑组织有非常清楚的边界，这与非神经胶质的肿瘤边界相似（示意图 18.2）。胶质微丝的 GFAP 染色在上皮样室管膜瘤与癌、垂体腺瘤、颅咽管瘤和脑膜瘤的鉴别诊断中非常有帮助（图 18.19B、表 18.6）。GFAP 染色显示出纤维状细胞突起，由此可使室管膜瘤与其他肿瘤相鉴别[3]。

乳头状室管膜瘤：与脉络丛乳头状瘤相似。在室管膜瘤的实性区 GFAP 阳性的肿瘤细胞相互交叉生长而不是在纤维血管间质上生长，通过免疫组化染色显示其缺乏胶原和纤维粘连蛋白，可以与脉络丛乳头状瘤相鉴别[3]。组织学分级对于室管膜瘤预后的预测效果不如星形细胞瘤[13]。影像学检查显示术后有肿瘤残留者提示生存期明显缩短，因此要重视术中的正确诊断以及要将肿瘤全部切除。有大量 GFAP 表达的幕下室管膜瘤预后好[94]。

透明细胞室管膜瘤 透明细胞室管膜瘤与少突胶质细胞瘤和中枢神经细胞瘤比较相似（图 18.21A、18.19A、18.32A）。透明细胞室管膜瘤是一种上皮样室管膜瘤，具有透明的核周晕。GFAP 免疫组化染色可以显示室管膜的特征，如血管周纤维（图 18.19B）。这种透明细胞室管膜瘤需要一组抗体进行免疫组化染色，或者用电镜与其他透明细胞肿瘤进行鉴别（图 18.19C 和示意图 18.1）[90]。

伸长型细胞型室管膜瘤 伸长型细胞型室管膜瘤常见于脑内尤其是脊髓内。与室管膜瘤相似，细胞核呈圆形或椭圆形，染色质具有显著的亮区和暗区，与星形细胞瘤相似，有大量 GFAP 阳性的细胞突起，形成细胞核密集区与纤维状细胞突起区相间的结构。弥漫的、广泛的 GFAP 阳性以及缺乏Ⅳ型胶原的特征使上述结构与 Verocay 小体相鉴别。它们不像其他室管膜瘤的血管周菊形团那样局限环绕于 GFAP 阴性的血管周围。除了脊髓束 NF 阳性的轴突外，伸长型细胞型室管膜瘤与周围脑实质的分界清楚，一般可以切

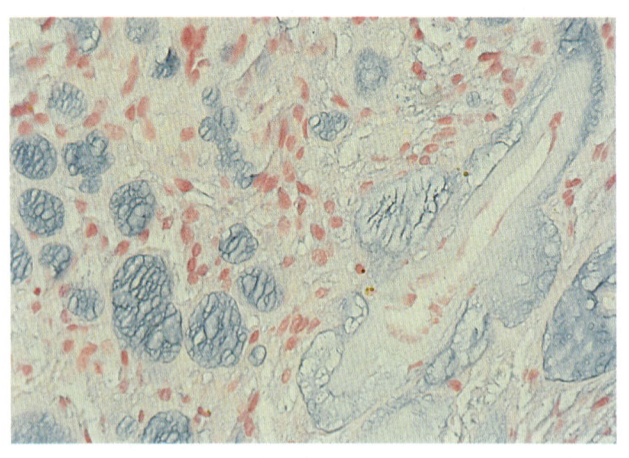

图 18.20 黏液乳头状室管膜瘤。该肿瘤来自一中年妇女的马尾，该患者有多年膝盖疼痛史。在中心部的模糊的室管膜菊形团和血管周围间隙中有上皮样细胞和淡蓝色的黏液（阿辛蓝和核固红）（引自 McKeever PE, Blaivas M. The brain, spinal cord, and meninges. In: Sternberg SS, ed. Diagnostic Surgical Pathology. 2nd ed. New York: Raven Press; 1994: 409-492）

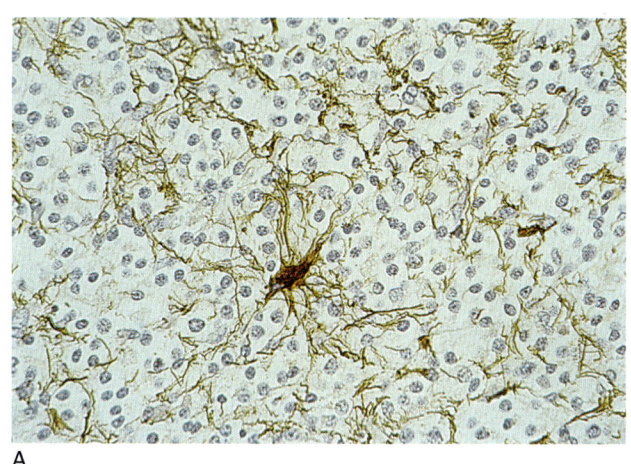
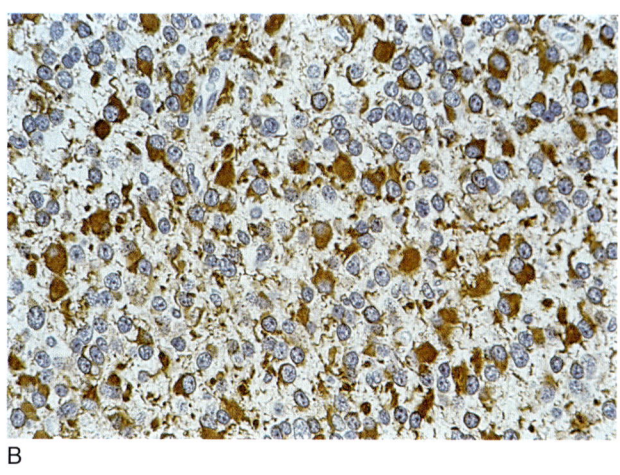
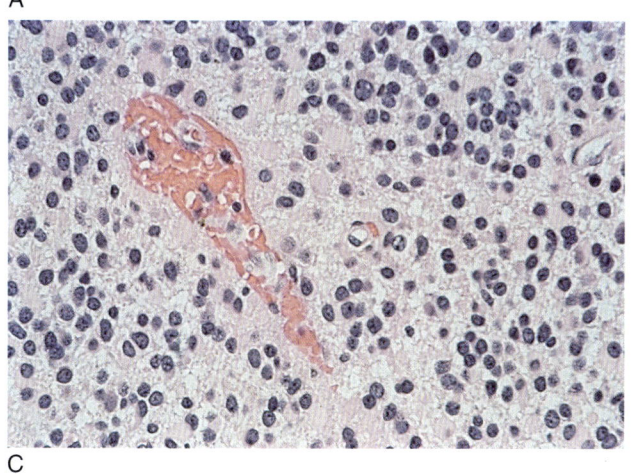

图18.21 根据目前的标准，以细胞核圆形和核周晕作为判断依据，这两个肿瘤均被认为是少突胶质细胞瘤。（A）第一个肿瘤的肿瘤细胞GFAP阴性，其交错的GFAP阳性突起来自混在肿瘤内的细胞核较小的反应性星形细胞。（B）第二个肿瘤包含大量GFAP阳性的"小胖细胞型星形细胞"，其胞质有GFAP的褐色团块和相对短的突起。（C）第二个肿瘤的HE染色切片较GFAP染色更好地显示了许多细胞的核周晕（授权自McKeever PE. Insights about brain tumors gained through immunohistochemistry and in situ hybridization of nuclear and phenotypic markers. J Histochem Cytochem 1998; 46: 585-594）

除，这也是与弥漫型星形细胞瘤很好的鉴别点。弥漫型星形细胞瘤细胞浸润于NF阳性的轴突之间[3, 58]。

室管膜下瘤（WHO Ⅰ级） 室管膜下瘤从脑室壁突入脑室腔[3]。组织学和免疫组化的特征与伸长型细胞型室管膜瘤相似（表18.5）。这种肿瘤通常为良性。

黏液乳头状室管膜瘤（WHO Ⅰ级，极少数Ⅱ级） 黏液乳头状室管膜瘤（MXPE）在HE染色切片中显示的胶质量最少。几乎总是位于终丝区、马尾、骶骨及邻近的脊椎外的软组织（图18.20、表18.6）。这种室管膜瘤产生的黏液量与其他室管膜瘤不同。其特征为在肿瘤实质和血管周围有室管膜细胞产生的黏液（图18.20）。MXPE常常呈乳头状但也可为实性。

虽然在一般性室管膜瘤讨论中有关鉴别诊断的特征可能有所帮助，但MXPE特有的形态学和生长方式提出了特别的问题。不同的MXPE可以从完全上皮样细胞到纤维状细胞而明显不同。MXPE最难以识别的类型是几乎全部为黏液样或全部为上皮样。高度黏液性变型的MXPE可以在黏液基质中出现与脊索瘤相似的细胞索，而脊索瘤也常发生于这一部位。GFAP阳性是鉴别MXPE与脊索瘤的最关键的免疫组化特征。

纤维样MXPE可能与纤维性脑膜瘤和神经鞘瘤相混淆。上皮性和乳头性变型的MXPE可能与癌或脑膜瘤相似[3]。MXPE免疫组化染色GFAP阳性可与GFAP阴性的癌和脑膜瘤相鉴别。MXPE没有环绕每个细胞的Ⅳ型胶原和纤维结合蛋白阳性的基底膜。而这正是神经鞘瘤的特征（图18.50A）。

与转移癌相反，MXPE缺乏恶性的细胞学特征。低MIB-1 LI，并且有局灶性纤维状结构[7]。副神经节瘤可能与MXPE相似，但MXPE不表达CgA而表达GFAP。

间变型室管膜瘤（恶性室管膜瘤）（WHO Ⅲ级） 间变型室管膜瘤是具有恶性特征的室管膜瘤，如明显的核分裂活性、细胞核和细胞的多形性、多核巨细胞和巨细胞、细胞密度高、坏死和血管增生等（表18.5、18.6）[3]。

间变型室管膜瘤的恶性组织病理学特征并不能准确地预测不良的预后[13]。这一问题可以最终由IHC来解决。幕下间变型室管膜瘤波形蛋白表达增加和GFAP表达降低相结合可以预示病人预后不良[94]。间变型室管膜瘤比低级别室管膜瘤更加过度表达p53或EGFR蛋白[72]。

少突胶质细胞瘤（WHO Ⅱ级）

已发现少突胶质细胞瘤，尤其是间变型少突胶质细胞瘤对于PCV的化疗有反应。这一特征引起对这两种肿瘤诊断认识的重视[2]。有染色体1p和19q缺失的肿瘤病人预后好[95,96]。除了少数的室管膜瘤外，完全性少突胶质细胞瘤与其他胶质瘤的区别在于它的上皮样形态而非纤维状形态（表18.6）。这种形态特点在含有大量密集肿瘤细胞的肿瘤中心部位最明显[3]，核周晕是甲醛固定石蜡切片中少突胶质细胞瘤的一个重要的特征（图18.21）。分化好的少突胶质细胞瘤的细胞核呈圆形，形态规则，位于细胞中央，因而类似煎蛋。肿瘤血管丰富，通常是CD31阳性纤细的毛细血管，有时血管将肿瘤实质分隔成小叶状[13]。

小胖细胞型星形细胞被认为是少突胶质细胞性的，通过其圆的细胞核和短的细胞突起而与胖细胞型星形细胞瘤的细胞相鉴别。与胖细胞型星形细胞和星形细胞瘤相比，小胖细胞型星形细胞核周围的胞浆内GFAP团块状阳性，细胞突起短（图18.21B）。

完全性少突胶质细胞瘤的上皮样形态与真正的上皮样肿瘤相似（图18.21C、表18.6）[57]。蝶鞍上的少突胶质细胞瘤可能被误诊为垂体腺瘤（示意图18.2）。少突胶质细胞瘤可能与脑膜上皮样的或透明细胞脑膜瘤，以及脑膜瘤中的脂肪化生相混淆。间变型少突胶质细胞瘤类似转移癌，尤其是肾细胞癌。肿瘤细胞GFAP阳性（图18.21B）可以将少突胶质细胞瘤与其他肿瘤相区别，但不是所有少突胶质细胞瘤都含有GFAP阳性的肿瘤细胞。如果缺乏GFAP阳性细胞，则肿瘤与脑组织的边界是诊断的关键（示意图18.1）。包括少突星形细胞瘤在内的所有类型的少突胶质细胞瘤的边界均为弥漫浸润性的（图18.11A）。在少突胶质细胞瘤中找到广泛弥散分布的反应性星形细胞也有助于鉴别诊断，在脑膜瘤中没有这种特点（图18.21A）。

与腺瘤、癌和脑膜瘤相比，即使肉眼上边界清楚的少突胶质细胞瘤也显示在肿瘤边缘的脑组织内有弥漫性肿瘤浸润。可以应用NF或Syn作为脑组织的标记[58]，在其他肿瘤，甚至是破坏大块脑组织的癌，GFAP阳性的神经胶质增生与脑组织之间有明显的边界（图18.24、18.25B）。在这些肿瘤中，继发性的结构改变只有在少突胶质细胞瘤中才能看到（见星形细胞瘤和胶质瘤的部分）。因为少突胶质细胞瘤不起源于腺垂体或硬脑膜并很少浸润这些部位，所以活检标本的确切定位对诊断是有帮助的。一组Cg和垂体激素的免疫组化染色可以确诊垂体腺瘤，但是尚没有用于石蜡切片的少突胶质细胞的特异性标记物。这种标记物的发现将是对神经病理学的一个重大贡献。

Leu7和S-100的特异性很广，限制了其在少突胶质细胞瘤免疫组化分析中的应用。然而，由于脑膜瘤是典型的Leu7阴性，浸润脑膜的少突胶质细胞瘤可以依据其与Leu7单克隆抗体的阳性反应而与合体细胞性脑膜瘤相鉴别。应当记住少突胶质细胞瘤中Syn的表达高达18%[97]，所以不要将它们与中枢神经细胞瘤（CN）和胚胎发育不良性神经上皮肿瘤（DNT）相混淆。CN和DNT二者均与脑组织有明显的边界，相反，少突胶质细胞瘤的边界是弥漫浸润性的。

MIB-1对于预测少突胶质细胞瘤病人的预后有帮助。MIB-1 LI ≤ 5%存活期长[98]。波形蛋白表达、CDKN2A、PTEN和EGFR基因的分子学改变与预后差有关[97,99]。

少突星形细胞瘤（少突胶质细胞瘤与星形细胞瘤的混合）（WHO Ⅱ级）

少突星形细胞瘤是由星形细胞瘤和少突胶质细胞瘤组成的一个混合性的胶质瘤。星形细胞瘤和少突胶质细胞瘤已在各自部分叙述过（图18.11A）。比少突星形细胞瘤少见的是在混合性胶质瘤中可以有室管膜瘤的成分[13]。

在确定单个肿瘤是含有少突胶质细胞和星形细胞的成分还是这两种成分都是肿瘤性的是困难的。为明确诊断必须每种成分都很显著。少突胶质细胞瘤细胞必须与浸润性含有脂质的巨噬细胞相鉴别。前者有肿瘤细胞的细胞核特征并缺乏KP-1等巨噬细胞的免疫组化标记（图18.3A、18.21A）。

可用苏木精染色分析星形细胞成分是否为肿瘤细胞，如果需要的话，可在调整到不遮蔽胞核的GFAP淡染后应用。对于自动染色，抗GFAP抗体可以被滴定到一个稀释度以达到能够辨别的浅棕色。对于人工染色，既可以用滴定抗体的稀释度的方法，也可以用少于常规时间的一半来进行二氨基联苯胺（DAB）底物显色。尽管胶质纤维是在胞质内，但免疫反应产物也会使胞核变得不清晰。常规的苏木精复染即可显示细胞核的微细结构，而且还没有被深褐色的免疫组化反应产物干扰，脑组织疾病的免疫组化分析必须有好的细胞核复染。不清楚的细胞边界和脑组织内的浸润需要定向复染。复染可为确定细胞类型和对肿瘤细胞的反应提供重要信息。

少突星形细胞瘤通过间变性转化为Ⅲ级肿瘤。一个常见的问题是纤维状的GFAP阳性的肿瘤性星形细胞在少突胶质细胞中过度生长。这种肿瘤可能最终演进为胶质母细胞瘤。在少突星形细胞瘤中PCV化疗的效果不如在完全少突胶质细胞瘤中肯定。

间变型少突胶质细胞瘤（恶性少突胶质细胞瘤）（WHO Ⅲ级） 少突胶质细胞瘤间变性转化的特征与间变型室管膜瘤相似（图18.22）。然而，在少突胶质细胞瘤中常有一定量的血管增生，如果仅仅是孤立性的血管增生，不能认为是恶性转化的证据（表18.6）。应用波形蛋白和CD31染色可显示血管增生。

染色体1和19的部分丢失的间变型少突胶质细胞瘤对PCV化疗有相当好的反应[2]。免疫染色增强的ISH和PCR分析两种方法均可以检测这些染色体的异常[96]。

间变型和低级别少突胶质细胞瘤可以表达神经元标记和波形蛋白（图18.23）。Syn阳性的细胞呈稀疏分散存在。

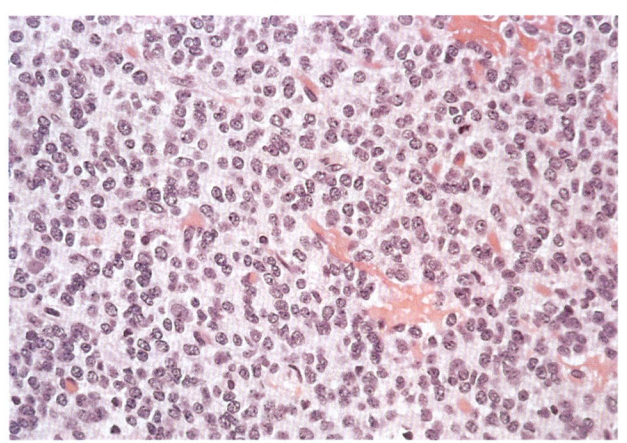

图18.22 Ⅲ级间变型少突胶质细胞瘤，比图18.21的Ⅱ级少突胶质细胞瘤细胞更密集、胞核多形性更明显。核分裂象很多（HE）（引自McKeever PE. New methods of brain tumor analysis. In: Mena H, ed. Dr. Kenneth M. Earle Memorial Neuropathology Review. Washington, DC: Armed Forces Institute of Pathology; February 24, 2000）

> **诊断要点：少突胶质细胞瘤**
> 1. 应用分子标记来检测1p和19q的缺失，缺失者提示预后好和对PCV治疗敏感。
> 2. 间变型少突胶质细胞瘤与间变型星形细胞瘤的诊断标准不同：在Ⅱ级少突胶质细胞瘤中可能偶见核分裂和一定量的血管增生。
> 3. 某些其他典型的和弥散浸润的少突胶质细胞瘤中可能有些细胞神经元标记染色阳性，尤其是Syn。

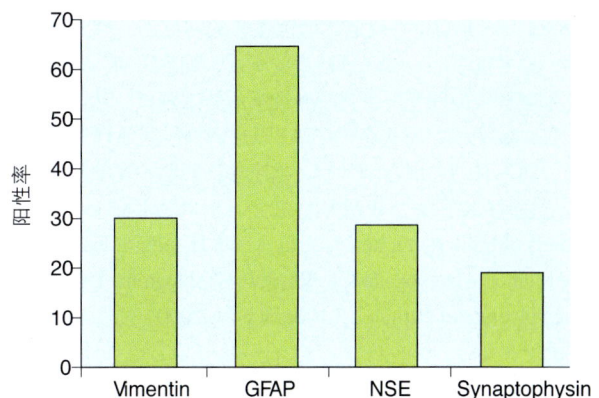

图18.23 80多例少突胶质细胞瘤（Ⅱ级和Ⅲ级）的免疫组化染色反应。直方图代表4种标记物阳性病例的比例（数据引自Dehghani F, Schachenmayr W, Laun A, et al. Prognostic implication of histopathological, immunohistochemical and clinical features of oligodendrogliomas: A study of 89 cases. Acta Neuropathol 1998; 95: 493-504）

多形性胶质母细胞瘤（胶质母细胞瘤）（WHO Ⅳ级）

大部分多形性胶质母细胞瘤由GFAP阳性的纤维状细胞突起进展而来，现认为胶质母细胞瘤是最恶性的星形细胞瘤而不是恶性胚胎性神经胶质肿瘤。它经常含有局灶性星形细胞瘤，少数含有少突胶质细胞瘤，偶尔含有室管膜瘤。一个低级别的星形细胞瘤可能随着时间进展为胶质母细胞瘤，许多这样的演进与染色体10中遗传性物质的丢失有关。这些遗传性物质的丢失可通过比较基因杂交[100]、FISH[1001]、免疫组化染色增强的ISH[102]或PCR分析观察到。染色体7 DNA的扩增也可以通过这些技术的改进而观察到[103]。

胶质母细胞瘤的诊断标准在20世纪90年代开始放松。以前，间变型星形细胞瘤的细胞学标准（核分裂活性、细胞密度高、多形性、核染色过深）必须加上血管增生、自发性坏死（图18.10B）。现在，或是血管增生或是自发性凝固性坏死加上细胞间变就足以诊断胶质母细胞瘤（与间变型星形细胞瘤相比）。

如果缺乏坏死，就必须明确血管增生（血管壁细胞的密度增加），可以通过血管内皮生长因子（VEGF）[104]、波形蛋白、Ⅳ型胶原或纤维粘连蛋白染色来显示血管。胶质母细胞瘤的其他恶性特征有奇异的细胞核、多核细胞和细胞的极度多形性（图18.10B、18.25A、18.26）。令人遗憾的是，胶质母细胞瘤这些组织学特征的异质性妨碍了来自如立体定位的针刺活检等小标本的诊断和正确分级（图18.10）[105]。

多数诊断中的困惑来自胶质母细胞瘤与恶性脑膜瘤和癌的鉴别。与癌和脑膜瘤不同，胶质母细胞瘤的纤维状肿瘤细胞突起表达GFAP（图18.24～18.26，表18.6～18.8和18.10，图18.1和18.10B）。应当注意GFAP阳性的细胞要具有间变的细胞学特征才能确定为胶质母细胞瘤，因为在癌或恶性黑色素瘤中可能有陷于其中的岛状的CNS实质并引起神经胶质增生（图18.24、18.25）。HE染色上肉瘤很容易与胶质母细胞瘤混淆，但是GFAP染色可确诊为胶质母细胞瘤（图18.26）。虽然由于胶质母细胞瘤的快速生长可以产生"假包膜"，但在这个边界之外脑组织内仍有肿瘤性胶质（图18.27）。

有两种类型的胶质母细胞瘤，一种是原发性的，一种是由低级别胶质瘤演变来的。前者经常与CDKN2A缺失、PTEN突变、表皮生长因子受体（EGFR）扩增有关。后者与p53突变有关[2, 13]。EGFR和p53的过表达可以通过免疫组化来确定（图18.28）。

胶质肉瘤（WHO Ⅳ级）　胶质肉瘤是胶质母细胞瘤和肉瘤的混合（图18.29）。胶原染色阳性、GFAP阴性的肉瘤细胞区与胶质母细胞瘤区桥接形成有大理石花纹样的结构（表18.5）。胶原的mRNA和细胞内DNA含量的不同说明了这些区域之间的不同[106, 107]。尽管胶质肉瘤看起来比胶质母细胞瘤界限更清楚，但是胶质肉瘤能够转移[74]，可以从胶质肉瘤发展为缺乏GFAP阳性细胞的纯肉瘤[108]。胶质成分和间质成分具有相似的基因改变[102, 109]。

伴有上皮样化生的胶质母细胞瘤和胶质肉瘤（WHO Ⅳ级）　偶尔，胶质肉瘤和胶质母细胞瘤内有

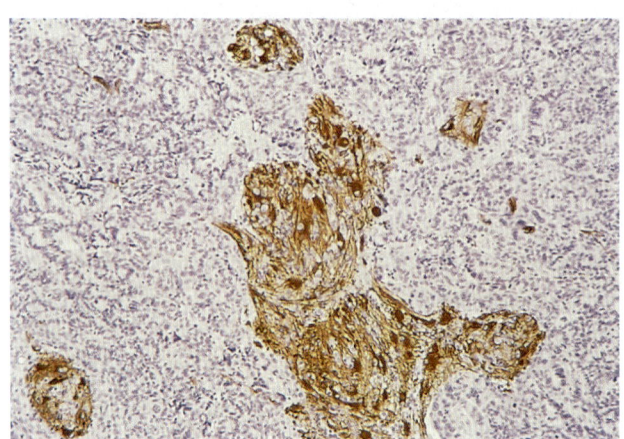

图18.24　该肿瘤是一位老年男性患者的转移癌，因为它是单发的，原发灶不明，临床诊断为胶质瘤。细胞透明、密集，间变性细胞核类似间变型少突胶质细胞瘤的细胞核。然而，在边缘它破坏脑组织，将褐色的GFAP阳性的神经胶质增生岛排除在外，而不是与之混合。其后，临床分析表明在左肺基底部有一个原发性CK阳性、GFAP阴性的癌（引自McKeever PE. New methods of brain tumor analysis. In: Mena H, ed. Dr. Kenneth M. Earle Memorial Neuropathology Review. Washington，DC: Armed Forces Institute of Pathology; February 24, 2000）

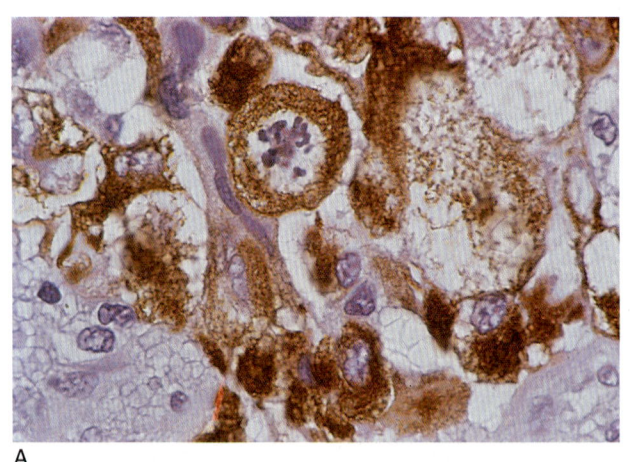

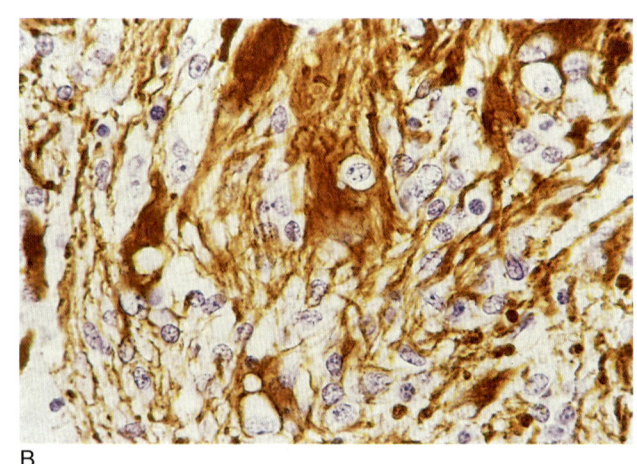

图18.25　胶质母细胞瘤与陷入的神经胶质增生对比。以标记物检测核周体（胞核周围的胞浆）的重要性在这两个不同肿瘤的GFAP染色中得以说明。（A）在胶质母细胞瘤中GFAP围绕并与肿瘤细胞核接触，有一个核分裂。（B）陷入转移癌内增生的神经胶质，GFAP只与反应性星形细胞胞核接触。癌是CK阳性（未示）。也参见图18.24（引自McKeever PE. New methods of brain tumor analysis. In: Mena H, ed. Dr. Kenneth M. Earle Memorial Neuropathology Review. Washington, DC: Armed Forces Institute of Pathology; February 24, 2000）

神经系统的免疫组织化学 18

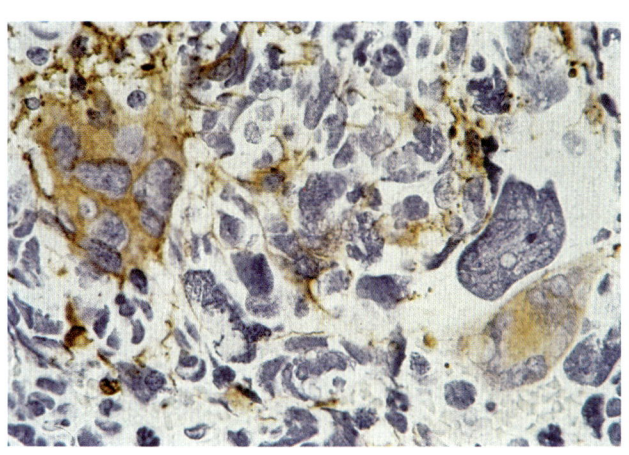

图18.26 胶质母细胞瘤的细胞和细胞核有明显的多形性，包含一个巨大的褐色的GFAP阳性的多核细胞。在认识到这些细胞GFAP阳性反应之前，巨细胞胶质母细胞瘤被称为畸异细胞性肉瘤（引自McKeever PE. New methods of brain tumor analysis. In: Mena H, ed. Dr. Kenneth M. Earle Memorial Neuropathology Review. Washington, DC: Armed Forces Institute of Pathology; February 24, 2000）

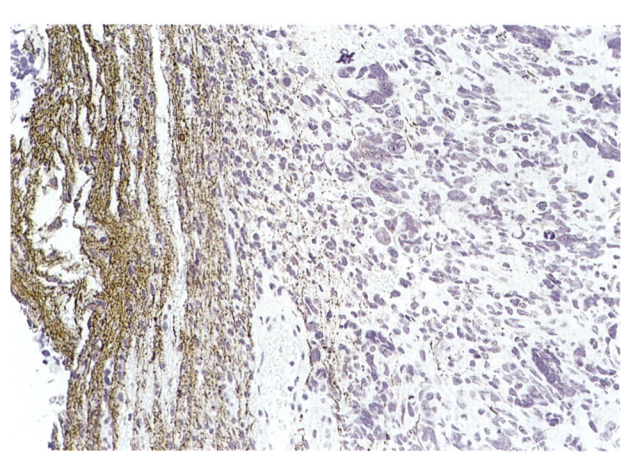

图18.27 这个巨细胞胶质母细胞瘤与NF阳性的褐色的大脑白质之间有相对清楚的边界。然而，在NF阴性的血管和大的异常核分裂附近，肿瘤细胞浸润于长的褐色的轴突之间

腺样结构或鳞状细胞分化及角化珠的上皮性病灶[3, 13]。这些区域CK和EMA免疫组化染色阳性（表18.7、图18.29D）。取材要充分，并明确这些区域是局灶性的，其他区域必须显示胶质母细胞瘤常见的纤维状特点及肿瘤细胞 GFAP 阳性，以避免将这种肿瘤与癌混淆。重要的是要记住癌细胞 GFAP 阴性。

胶质母细胞瘤可表现出其他独特的特征，极少数胶质母细胞瘤伴有颗粒细胞肿瘤。某些上皮样胶质母细胞瘤含有弥漫的胞浆内脂质[13]。

神经元肿瘤

神经元肿瘤含有异常增生的神经元。它们从最良性的节细胞瘤到间变性节细胞胶质瘤和原始神经外胚层肿瘤（以前称为节细胞神经母细胞瘤和CNS 神经母细胞瘤）（表18.5、18.7、18.8）。绝大多数低级别节细胞肿瘤比在同一部位发现的胶质瘤预后好，因此，能对它们作出正确诊断是非常重要的。

诊断和评价节细胞肿瘤分以下4个重要阶段：

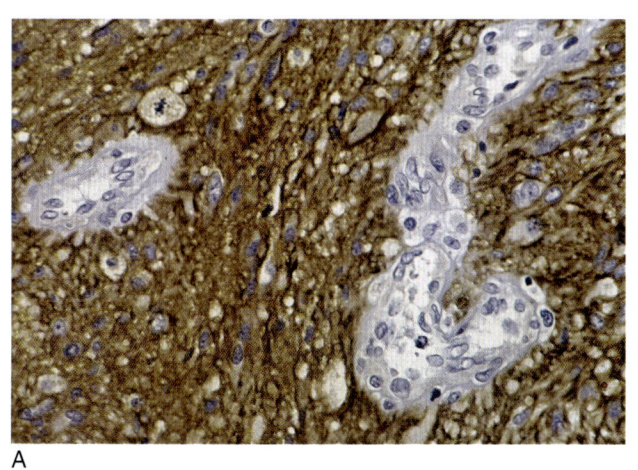

A

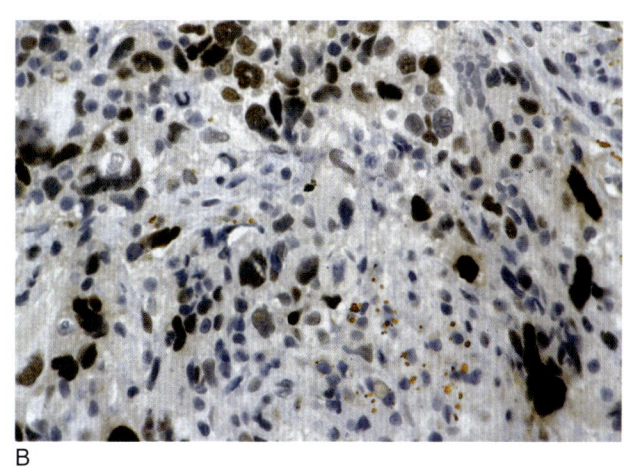

B

图18.28 胶质母细胞瘤分子标记物的表达。发生于 70 岁女性的原发性胶质母细胞瘤，伴有 2 周的头痛病史。表皮生长因子受体（EGFR）过度表达(A)，但是没有p53 的过度表达（未示）。另一个 52 岁男性的胶质母细胞瘤是从 Ⅱ 级星形细胞瘤演变而来。p53 过表达（B），但没有 EGFR 的过度表达（未示）

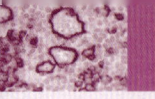

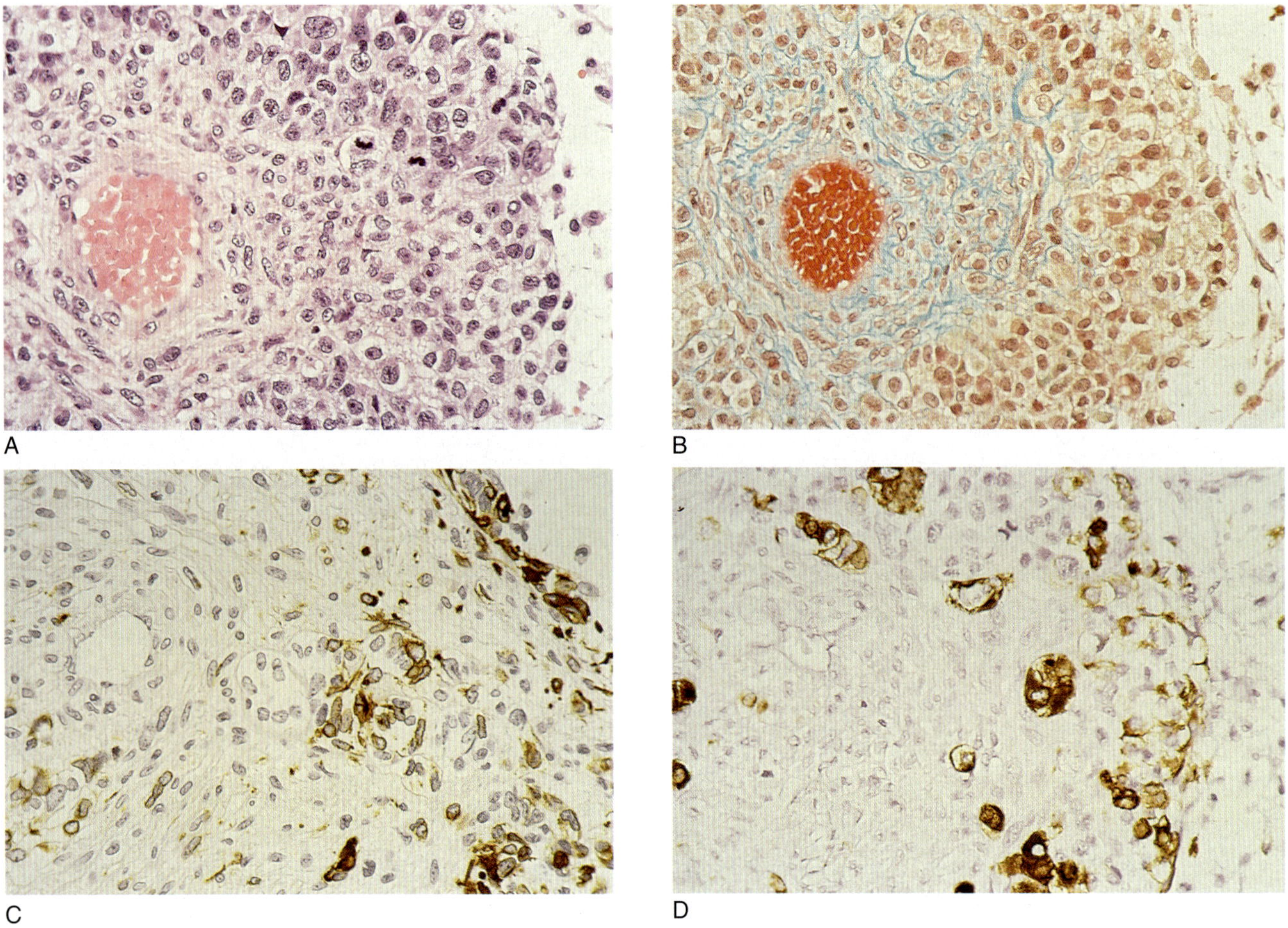

图18.29 这个胶质肉瘤显示：(A) HE染色，胶原染色阳性、GFAP阴性的肉瘤细胞区和带，以及其他GFAP阳性、胶原阴性的恶性星形细胞的区域。(B) 高倍镜显示，产生胶原的肉瘤细胞从血管伸展入肿瘤实质内（Masson三色套染）。(C) 切片附近显示大多数与胶原相关的细胞GFAP阴性，而远离血管的恶性星形细胞GFAP阳性。(D) 该胶质肉瘤另外一个区域有小灶状CAM5.2阳性的褐色上皮样化生的细胞（引自 McKeever PE. New methods of brain tumor analysis. In: Mena H, ed. Dr. Kenneth M. Earle Memorial Neuropathology Review. Washington, DC: Armed Forces Institute of Pathology; February 24, 2000）

1. 认识神经元（图 18.30）；
2. 确定神经元是肿瘤性的；
3. 确定是否存在神经胶质；
4. 对任何的肿瘤性胶质成分加以评价。

许多肿瘤细胞尤其是胶质母细胞瘤、黑色素瘤和星形细胞瘤的细胞，体积大或核仁突出而与神经元类似[110, 111]。这些细胞没有神经元的NF和Syn的标记（图 18.27、18.40D）。应用NF或Syn来确定神经元最重要的一步是确定细胞体（核周体）的标记。Syn存在于神经纤维网中，因此难以对细胞表面的染色进行分析。必须仔细选择商品化的抗NF和抗Syn的神经元免疫过氧化物酶标记物，在对未知肿瘤检测时，应该用同一批正常脑组织标本切片作为对照，最好能在同一张切片上进行（示意图 18.2）。

NSE已在综述和正文中作为一种神经元的标记予以叙述，笔者发现它还有比标记神经元肿瘤更好的用途。对于神经元肿瘤来说，NSE的缺点是神经胶质肿瘤也倾向于着色。神经胶质肿瘤常常需要与神经元肿瘤相鉴别[2, 3]。实验性的IHC染色，如Neu-N染色是通过显示它们"靶心"样的细胞核特征而不是胞浆或令人困惑的细胞表面特征来确定神经元[112, 113]。在免疫组化染色难以确定的病例，电镜可以观察到肿瘤细胞内的Nissl物质、NF、神经内分泌颗粒和突触。

在确定神经元是否为肿瘤性时，一个常见的错误是将胶质瘤细胞浸润区域内的正常神经元当作节细胞胶质瘤。如前所述，Syn或NF应当伸入到细胞体，应当利用苏木精染核的特征并根据标准确定细胞是否是肿瘤性。神经元肿瘤的证据包括Syn或NF染色阳性的细胞密度高、神经元排列紊乱、双核神经元、核

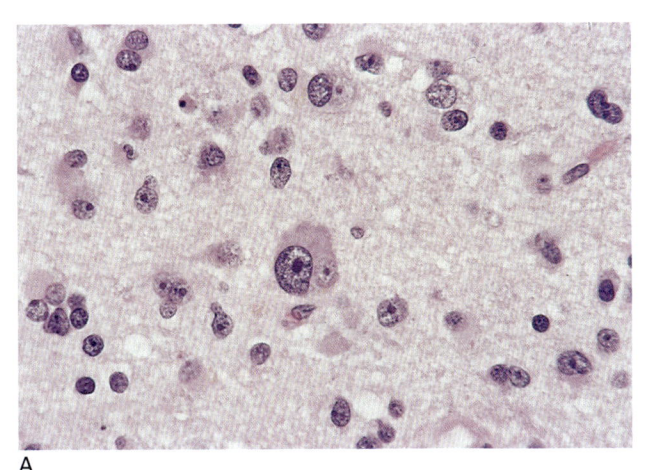
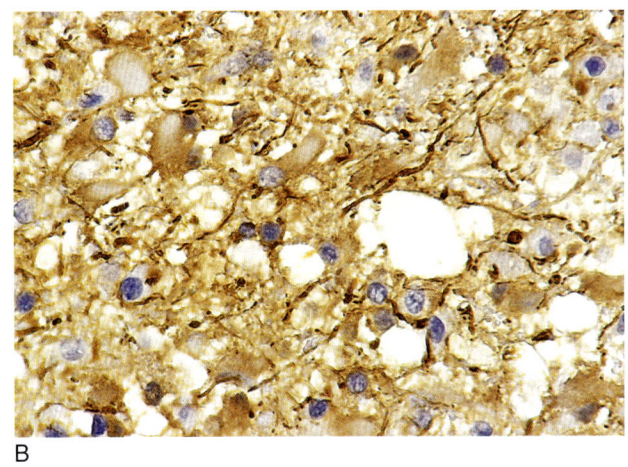

图18.30 来自一中年男性顶叶的节细胞胶质瘤，患者表现为进行性一侧协调性丧失，HE切片显示具有大的核仁和Nissl物质的双核节细胞（A）和NF染色（B）。标本B是抗NF蛋白免疫过氧化物酶并苏木精染色

异型性和多形性（图18.30B）。肿瘤性神经元可以发生变性[110]。节细胞肿瘤可能显示粗胶原带和纤维粘连蛋白阳性的纤维组织，或者显示血管周围的圆形细胞，但所有这些都不是一成不变的。

节细胞瘤（WHO Ⅰ级）、节细胞胶质瘤（WHO Ⅰ级或Ⅱ级）和间变性节细胞胶质瘤（WHO Ⅲ级或Ⅳ级）

节细胞瘤、节细胞胶质瘤和间变性节细胞胶质瘤可以发生于任何部位，在大脑尤其以颞叶最常见。

一旦确定为节细胞肿瘤，必须对胶质成分进行分析（表18.5）。用免疫过氧化物酶对切片进行GFAP淡染（或者在人工染色时应用DAB底物显色时间少于常规时间的一半，或者在自动染色中用较低的原始抗体滴定度）和充分的苏木精复染可以更好地观察神经胶质细胞的细胞核，从而易于确诊。如果浅褐色细胞为反应性的，聚集在肿瘤边缘，与在弥漫型星形细胞瘤部分叙述的肿瘤标准不一致，这个肿瘤是中枢神经细胞瘤或节细胞瘤。

节细胞瘤倾向于良性。它们常含有至少1种神经传递多肽或胺的免疫细胞化学阳性反应。其中包括生长抑素、促肾上腺皮质激素释放激素、β-内啡肽、促生长激素神经肽、血管活性肠肽、降钙素、5-羟色胺、儿茶酚胺和甲基-脑啡肽[114]。

如果GFAP阳性细胞是肿瘤性的而不是间变性的，肿瘤就是节细胞胶质瘤（图18.33B）。如果这些神经胶质成分是间变性的，这个肿瘤是一个间变性节细胞胶质瘤。节细胞肿瘤中的GFAP阳性的神经胶质成分的增生能力对于它们的组织学分级是至关重要的，可通过MIB-1或PCNA免疫组化染色分析。通常星形细胞成分对于上述增生标记呈阳性着色，但一般较弱[13]。

小脑发育不良性节细胞瘤（WHO Ⅰ级）

节细胞瘤的一个特殊变型——小脑发育不良性节细胞瘤（DGC）也称为Lhermitte-Duclos病[87]。增生的和排列紊乱的Syn阳性的颗粒细胞神经元使小脑一部分扩大为奇异的"巨叶"。这种罕见的肿瘤看起来像发育异常，但是术后易复发。不同肿瘤的生长潜能可以通过MIB-1染色检测。某些DGC是家族性的，某些与Cowden综合征或多发性错构瘤综合征相关[115]。

胚胎发育不良性神经上皮肿瘤（DNT）（WHO Ⅰ级）

胚胎发育不良性神经上皮肿瘤（DNT）可能是一种与错构瘤相似的节细胞胶质瘤。它在大脑皮质内呈多结节状，最常见于颞叶，有些病例呈囊状（图18.31A）。部分病例是偶然发现的，更多病例伴发儿童和年轻人长期的部分复杂性癫痫[116]。

DNT有一些细胞形态上近似少突胶质细胞，并有NF阳性和/或突触素阳性的神经元，漂浮在阿辛蓝阳性的酸性黏多糖中。这些细胞被称为"漂浮"神经元（图18.31B）。其他大的神经元缺少正常的空间（图18.31C）。肿瘤组织内可见数量不等的GFAP阳性的星形胶质细胞，并且这些星形胶质细胞常常围绕在肿瘤细胞周围。该肿瘤的低MIB-1表达、组织学上的成熟性表现以及伴有皮层结构不良的现象说明它是一个发育异常的疾病[13]。

少突神经胶质细胞瘤可以产生黏多糖，甚至偶尔可有正常神经元"漂浮"。胚胎发育不良性神经上皮肿

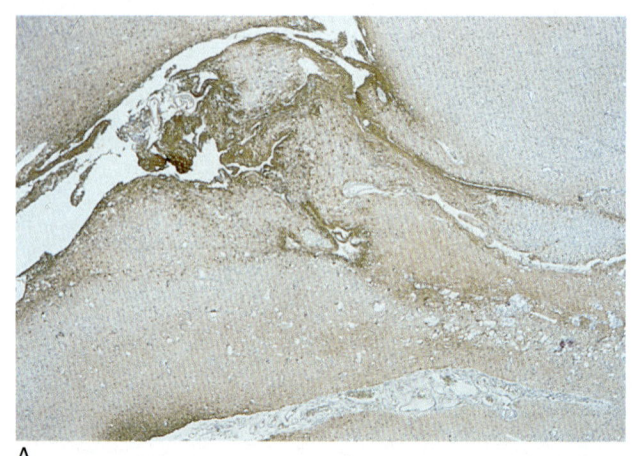
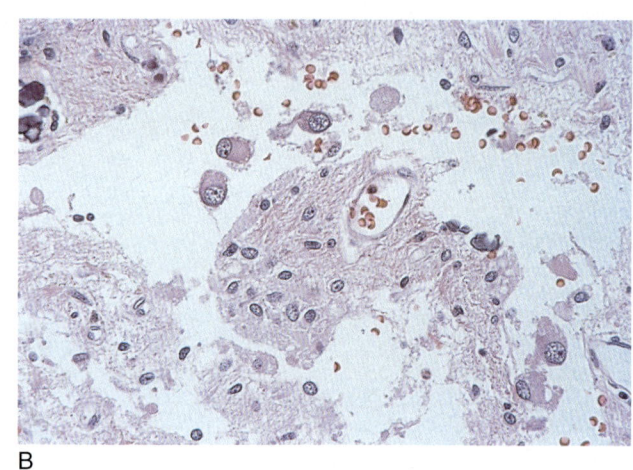
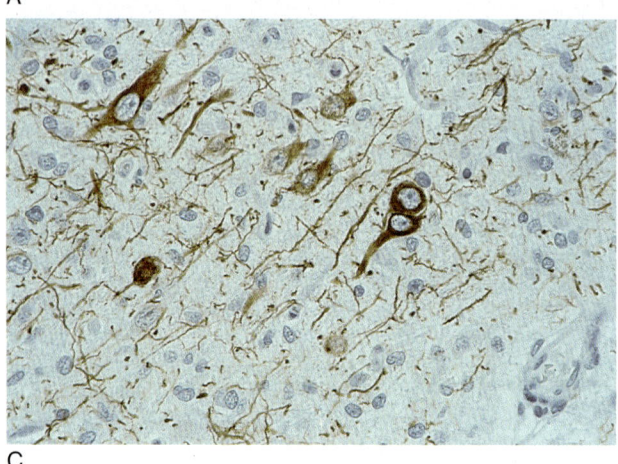

图18.31　胚胎发育不良性神经上皮肿瘤（DNT）。(A) 这是一个囊性肿瘤，塌陷的囊壁旁GFAP+的棕褐色星形胶质细胞围绕着多个皮质结节性病灶。(B) "漂浮" 在囊腔里的神经元。(C) 大的棕褐色的NF+的神经元纵横交错，相互拥挤。该病人是一位40岁男性，长期患有顽固性癫痫及右额叶多结节皮质肿瘤（引自McKeever PE. New methods of brain tumor analysis. In: Mena H, ed. Dr. Kenneth M. Earle Memorial Neuropathology Review, Washington, DC : Armed Forces Institute of Pathology; February 24, 2000）

瘤的特征性改变包括无明显肿块、皮质散在分布、低MIB-1 LI表达及缺乏脑浸润，需与少突神经胶质细胞瘤鉴别[2]。对肿瘤边缘的连续切片进行NF、MIB-1和突触素的免疫组织化学评估可显示这些特点[58]。如果神经元核抗原标记阳性的话，也可以诊断该肿瘤[117]。

婴幼儿促纤维增生性节细胞胶质瘤（WHO Ⅰ级）

婴幼儿促纤维增生性节细胞胶质瘤（DIG）往往能够达到相当大的体积，类似于纤维性胶质瘤（图18.33A）。这些肿瘤常见于3岁以内的儿童，多为囊性，常侵犯脑膜[3]。肿瘤实质细胞包括GFAP阳性的神经胶质细胞（图18.33B）、NF阳性及突触素阳性的神经元和波形蛋白阳性的纤维血管细胞。DIG低表达MIB-1，无p53的过度表达[118]。

中枢型神经细胞瘤（WHO Ⅱ级）

中枢型神经细胞瘤（CN）是最近才认识到的肿瘤。由于肿瘤结构的美观、隐匿的特性、预后的良好性及认识的不一致性（图18.32A）[3, 119]，引起了学者们的兴趣。几乎所有的CN生物学行为良好，增殖活力较低，所以以前WHO分级为Ⅰ级。该肿瘤在年轻人中是侵及透明隔最常见的肿瘤。虽然该肿瘤有轻微增多的原纤维形成，但与少突胶质瘤相似（表18.5、18.6，示意图18.1）。多年来中枢型神经细胞瘤曾被误诊为胶质瘤，应用免疫组织化学标记检查有利于该肿瘤的正确诊断（图18.32）。CN表达突触素（图18.32B）[57]，GFAP通常阴性，但可含有反应性星型胶质细胞，无EGFR扩增[120]。如果突触素染色结果不确定，建议应用电镜检查来鉴别中枢型神经细胞瘤和少突胶质细胞瘤以及室管膜瘤。

除了有些细胞内含有脂质外，少数小脑脂质神经细胞瘤与CN相似[2]。微管、100～200nm的致密核心小泡及透明空泡，可以证实这个肿瘤其实是真正的神经元肿瘤。

虽然可以进行放射治疗，但完整的手术切除通常预后良好[119]，CN极少有间变的特征。

节细胞神经母细胞瘤和神经母细胞瘤

见原始神经外胚层肿瘤章节。

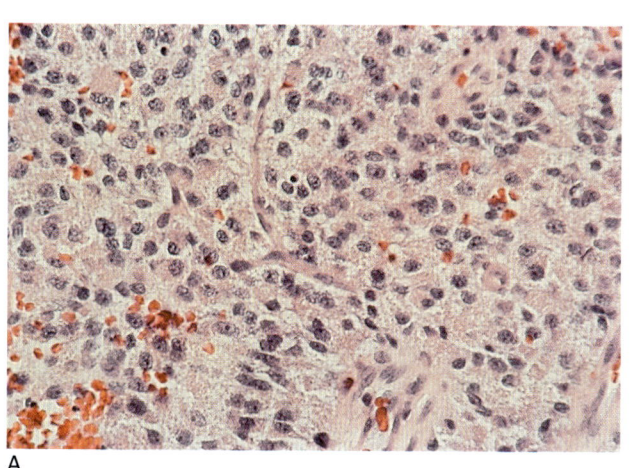
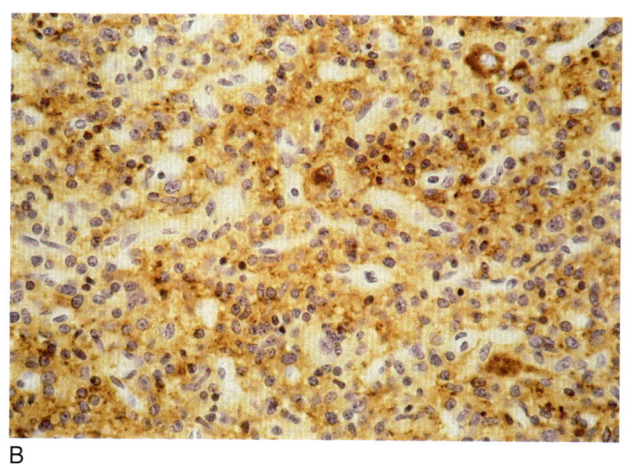

图 18.32 中枢神经细胞肿瘤。(A) 血管周围纤维性区域以及具有核周空晕圆形细胞核的圆形细胞很像室管膜瘤和少突胶质细胞瘤 (HE)。(B) 肿瘤性细胞普遍表达突触素（授权自 McKeever PE. Insights about brain tumors gained through immunohistochemistry and in situ hybridization of nuclear and phenotypic markers. J Histochem Cytochem 1998; 46: 585-594）

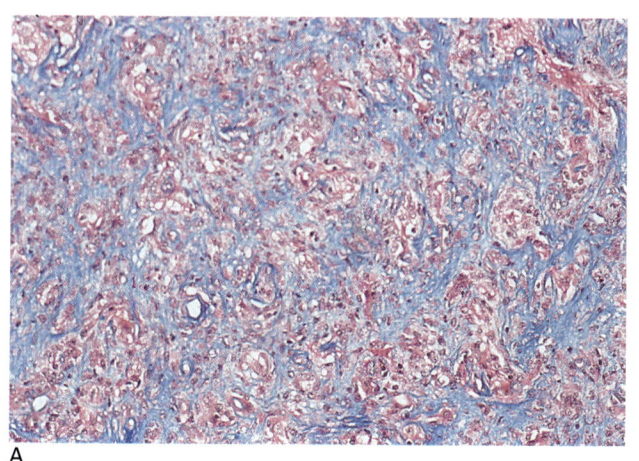
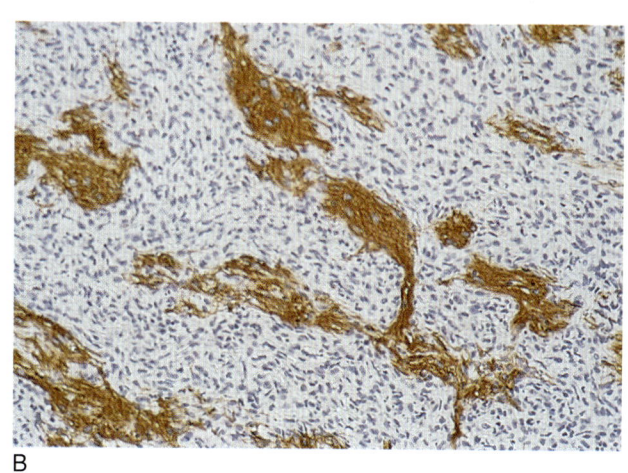

图18.33 婴幼儿促纤维增生性节细胞胶质瘤 (DIG)。(A) 这是一个男婴左大脑半球的巨大肿瘤：可见红染的异常双核神经元、神经胶质和蓝染的增生的纤维网相互交错（三色）。(B) GFAP 显示呈棕色的岛屿状星形细胞

诊断要点：神经元性肿瘤

1. 神经元性脑肿瘤与神经胶质瘤相比，病人预后较好，例如：节细胞胶质瘤与原纤维型星形胶质细胞瘤。通过近几年对恶性脑神经肿瘤如 PNET 的重新分类，使得这种趋势更加明显。
2. 关键性的神经元性肿瘤标记物：突触素和NF。阳性细胞中需要高质量的苏木精对比染色来显示肿瘤性的细胞核。
3. 许多"神经元性标记物"包括NSE对神经元性肿瘤没有特异性。在应用它们鉴别神经元性肿瘤之前，尝试新的胶质瘤标记物。
4. 低级别的神经元性肿瘤与错构瘤及发育不良相似，应用 MIB-1 和生长间期的连续 X 线照片，可以鉴别真正的肿瘤。

脉络丛上皮性肿瘤

大多数脉络丛肿瘤都出现在儿童期，可发生在脉络丛的任何部位（表 18.6），但以儿童的侧脑室和成人的第四脑室最为常见[3]。

脉络丛乳头状瘤（WHO Ⅰ级）

与乳头状室管膜瘤相比，脉络丛乳头状瘤在基底膜和纤维血管基质上有一层柱状或立方状上皮细胞。肿瘤基质内有Ⅳ型胶原及层粘连蛋白，这和室管膜瘤不同，后者有实质细胞实体分布，无胶原或层粘连蛋白（表 18.5、18.6）。某些脉络丛乳头状瘤中局灶性 GFAP 免疫组化表达阳性，表明有灶性的室管膜分化。尽管该标记物以及其他一些标记物在免疫染色反应上存在交叉反应，但脉络丛乳头状瘤表达CAM5.2 细胞角蛋白及 EMA 要强于室管膜瘤[13]。CAM5.2 常

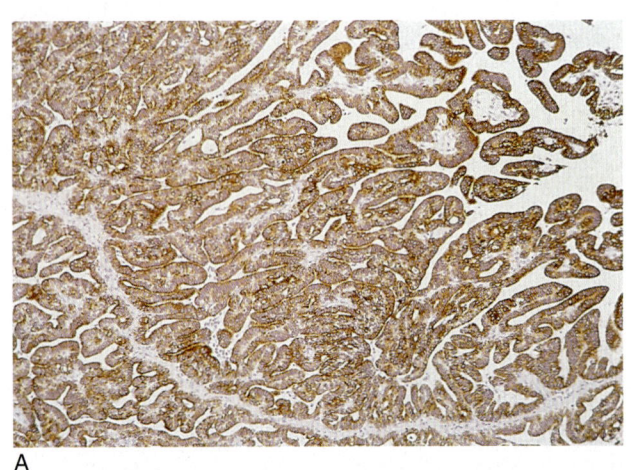
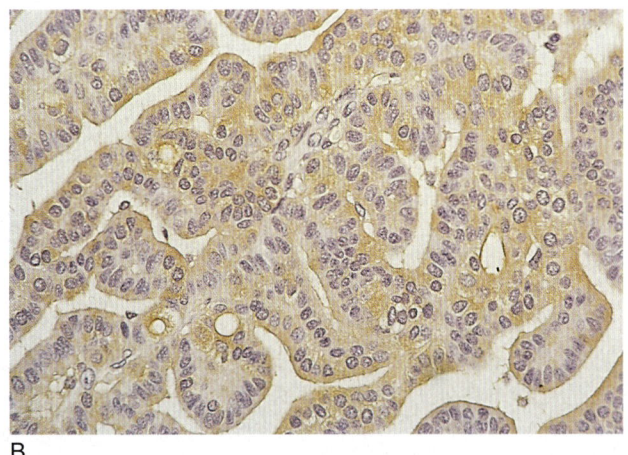

图 18.34 脉络丛乳头状瘤。儿童侧脑室的脉络丛乳头状瘤，其纤维血管基质上为分化良好的柱状上皮细胞，表达 CAM5.2 低分子量细胞角蛋白（A）和转甲状腺素(B)。细胞角蛋白阴性可确认纤维血管基质（免疫过氧化物酶，抗CAM5.2和抗前白蛋白）（引自McKeerver PE, Blaivas M. The brain, spinal cord, and meninges. In: Sternberg SS, Diagnostic Surgical Pathology. 2nd ed. New York: Raven Press; 1994, 409-492）

呈强阳性表达（图18.34A）。转甲状腺素（transthyretin）是脉络丛乳头状瘤的潜在标记物（图18.34B），但其反应谱较广泛。

新的脉络丛乳头状瘤的标记物包括胰岛素样生长因子Ⅱ（IGF-Ⅱ）和突触素。IGF-Ⅱ存在于脉络丛乳头状瘤中，但并不出现在正常的脉络丛组织中[122]。突触素在一些正常脉络丛组织、脉络丛乳头状瘤和脉络丛癌中表达，但转移性癌不表达[123]。两种标记物联合应用可能对一些肿瘤的鉴别诊断有帮助，把它们和传统的标记物结合起来会更有效。CD44 常表达在非典型性乳头状瘤和脉络丛癌中，也可能成为侵袭性脉络丛肿瘤的标记物。侵袭性肿瘤有较高的 MIB-1 标记指数，其平均值为 6%，但这些结果需要大量的病例进一步证实。

脑膜瘤和癌也需要与脉络丛乳头瘤鉴别。脉络丛乳头状瘤上皮细胞 CAM5.2 阳性，没有旋涡结构，也没有合体细胞区，可以以此来鉴别脉络丛乳头状瘤和乳头型脑膜瘤。分泌型脑膜瘤CK局灶阳性，但是其上皮细胞没有纤维血管轴心。脉络丛乳头状瘤无坏死和间变，可以以此与转移的乳头状瘤鉴别。

脉络丛癌（WHO Ⅲ～Ⅳ级）

脉络丛癌（间变性脉络丛乳头状瘤）是一种非常少见的肿瘤，很难与转移癌鉴别（表 18.6）。这类肿瘤均产生CK和转甲状腺素。脉络丛乳头状瘤和脉络丛癌之间有移行区提示为脉络丛癌。脉络丛的原发癌和转移癌十分相似，因此在诊断原发性脉络丛癌之前一定要慎重除外转移癌，隐匿的原发于肺和胃肠道的肿瘤是转移癌常见的来源。儿童罕见这些全身性的癌，此点有利于该年龄组病人的脉络丛癌诊断。一些脉络丛癌表达CD44细胞黏附分子，而大多数良性的乳头状瘤不表达。脉络丛癌平均 MIB-1 标记指数（LI）为 14%，高于乳头状瘤，但是 LI 在不同实验室间可能不同[124]。

> **诊断要点**：脉络丛肿瘤
>
> 1. 多种免疫组化标记物可用于诊断脉络丛（CP）肿瘤，但没有一个是理想的。单一标记物或者不敏感，或者缺少特异性，但免疫组化标记物的组合可确诊疑难病例。
> 2. 在许多病例中，肿瘤部位和组织学特点足够诊断脉络丛乳头状瘤。
> 3. 脉络丛癌很难与转移性癌鉴别。

松果体细胞肿瘤

这里说的松果体肿瘤是来自松果体细胞或其前体细胞的肿瘤，因为起源于松果体细胞的肿瘤是神经元性的，所以突触素免疫反应比较常见。有些松果体肿瘤还表达视网膜-S抗原（图 18.35）[125]。许多其他肿瘤如胶质瘤、脑膜瘤和生殖细胞肿瘤，也可出现在松果体区，各个有关部分将分别描述这些肿瘤。

神经系统的免疫组织化学 18

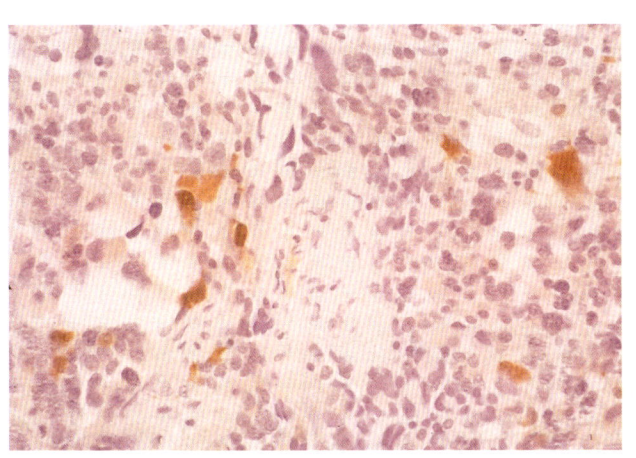

图18.35 松果体细胞瘤。瘤细胞核呈圆形，有一些表达视网膜-S 抗原（授权自 Dr. Hernando Mena, Armed Forces Institute of Pathology, Washington, DC）

松果体细胞瘤（WHO Ⅱ级）

该肿瘤和正常松果体组织相似（表18.5），瘤细胞突触素阳性，核圆形，被纤维血管间质分割成小叶，其他一些细胞围绕原纤维中心[87]，细胞发出的细纤维常围绕管腔呈放射状。NF 免疫组织化学染色可以看到这些突起的末端膨大，似棒状，电镜观察与神经元相似[3]。这些神经元的特点可以帮助鉴别松果体细胞瘤和胶质瘤。与其组织学特征容易混淆的是正常松果体，若是MIB-1表达指数高于正常松果体，标本直径大于正常松果体直径0.5cm或是侵犯松果体以外的部位就可以肯定松果体细胞瘤的诊断。

中分化的松果体细胞瘤（可能 WHO Ⅲ级）

原发性中分化松果体细胞瘤的分化低于松果体细胞瘤，高于松果体母细胞瘤。肿瘤细胞突触素阳性，中等拥挤，表现出有丝分裂活性。在靠近和松果体母细胞瘤相似的区域，肿瘤可能含有类似于松果体细胞瘤的区域。肿瘤不同区域增殖程度不一，增殖的"热点"区域要高于松果体细胞瘤区域。

松果体母细胞瘤（Ⅳ级）

松果体母细胞瘤和髓母细胞瘤相似（图 18.36、18.37），但松果体母细胞瘤起源于松果体部位（表18.8）可见纤维菊形团，比Flexner-Wintersteiner菊形团更为明显。在鉴别其神经元分化时，突触素是最有用的标记物（图 18.36A），因为 NF 的免疫反应常是阴性的（示意图 18.3）。一些肿瘤可以表达视网膜-S 抗原[125]。令人感兴趣的是，这些标记物是否在松果体母细胞瘤中比在髓母细胞瘤中更为常见。

胚胎性肿瘤（均为 WHO Ⅳ级）

髓母细胞瘤

髓母细胞瘤属于原始神经外胚层肿瘤，发生于小脑内或是第四脑室顶部（示意图 18.3、图 18.37、表18.8）。最常见于儿童，也可见于年轻人[126]，35岁以上少见[73]。常伴有 17q 等臂染色体（染色体 17 上的两个长臂组成的一个染色体），可以用免疫染色增强的ISH检测到[127]。由于它常常经脑脊液途径播散，因此治疗时要针对整个脑脊髓系统。大约有5%的髓母细胞瘤可以转移到全身其他部位，尤其是骨髓，后者可以通过突触素染色帮助诊断[13]。

由于胞核密集及核浆比例高，使得HE染色的病

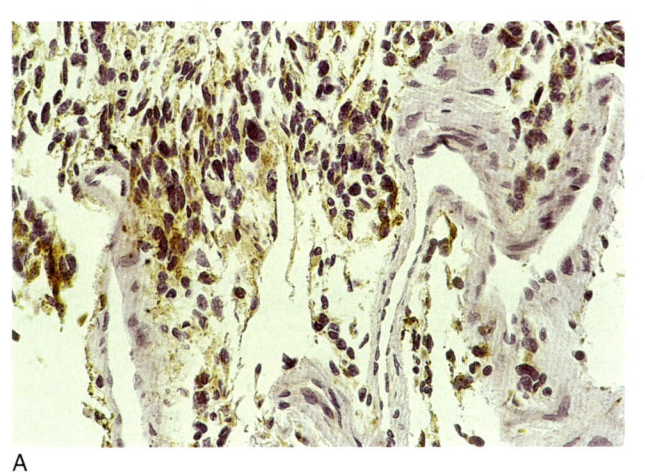

A

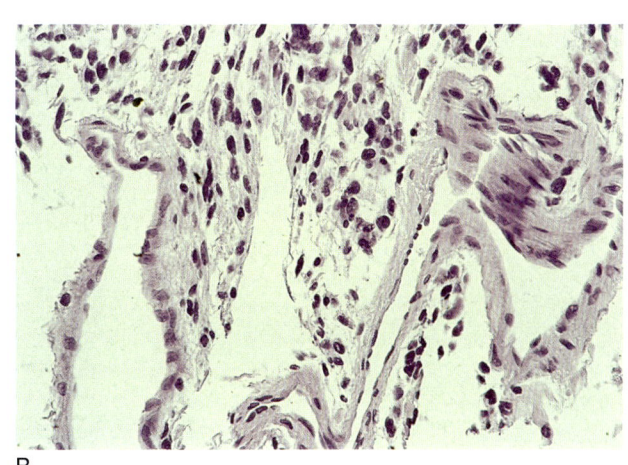

B

图18.36 在此松果体肿瘤中，恶性瘤细胞排列拥挤，呈多形性，核染色质深染，表达突触素（A）；在连续切片的松果体母细胞瘤区域不表达 GFAP（B）

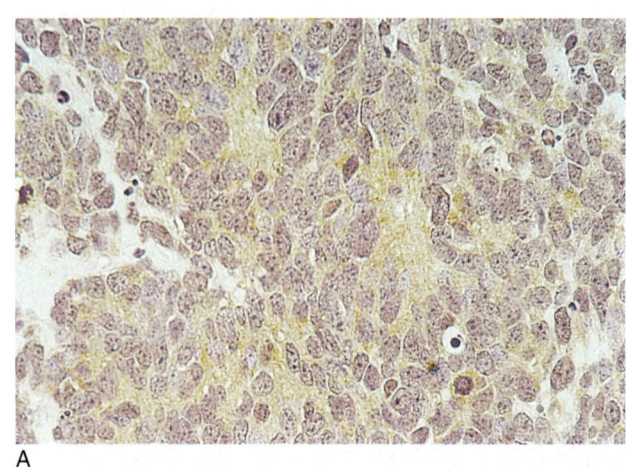
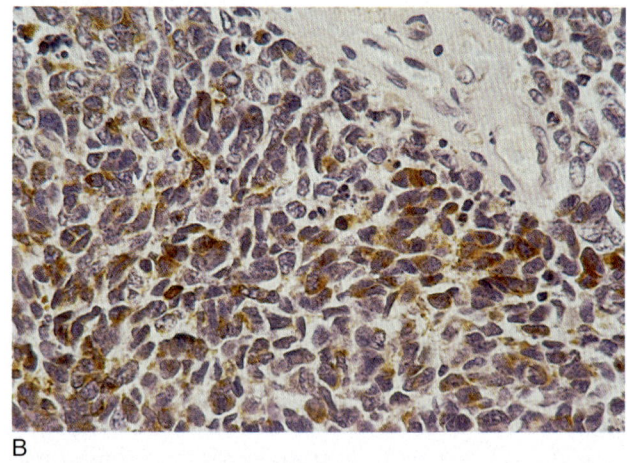

图18.37 髓母细胞瘤。（A）小学年龄女孩的颅后凹髓母细胞肿瘤，具有明显分化的Homer-Wright菊形团，NF（A）及突触素（未显示）染色均为阳性。（B）另一例为同龄男孩的颅后凹低分化的髓母细胞瘤，突触素阳性（B）而NF阴性（未显示）。突触素使稀疏的原纤维细胞突起更为显著（选自McKeever PE. New methods of brain tumor analysis. In: Mena H, ed. Dr. Kenneth M. Earle Memorial Neuropathology Review, Washington, DC: Armed Forces Institute of Pathology; February 24, 2000）

例切片肉眼看上去就显得很蓝，这些恶性瘤细胞核浆比例高于恶性胶质瘤，并且很少有EGFR扩增[128]。

髓母细胞瘤的特点是可见菊形团结构，菊形团的核心挤满了原纤维（Homer-Wright菊形团）（图18.37A）。但是，许多髓母细胞瘤的活检标本无菊形团结构，或菊形团结构模糊。没有纤维组织增生或大的恶性瘤细胞时，这种类型被称为"典型的髓母细胞瘤"。

其实，所有的髓母细胞瘤都表达突触素，这是神经元分化最可靠的标记物，在淋巴瘤和癌中不表达（图18.37B）[3]。蛋白质基因产物9.5（PGP9.5）是这些肿瘤神经元分化的另一个标记物。S-100蛋白可见于髓母细胞瘤中。笔者认为，应用PGP9.5和S-100蛋白时必须慎重，因为其他需鉴别诊断的肿瘤内也可存在S-100蛋白和PGP9.5，例如大多数胶质瘤和一些癌[3]。突触素染色和原纤维细胞突起的出现最有助于诊断（图18.37B），对于疑难病例可以检查它们的超微结构变化。

小细胞恶性瘤必须和小细胞未分化癌及淋巴瘤鉴别（表18.8）。诊断髓母细胞瘤时必须找到原纤维细胞突起，而且原纤维细胞突起必须是直接来自髓母细胞瘤的瘤细胞。突触素、S-100蛋白以及不经常表达的NF蛋白染色可以使这些突起更加明显。

髓母细胞瘤的一种不常见的变型"大细胞髓母细胞瘤"，瘤细胞有明显的核仁、核畸形及较高的有丝

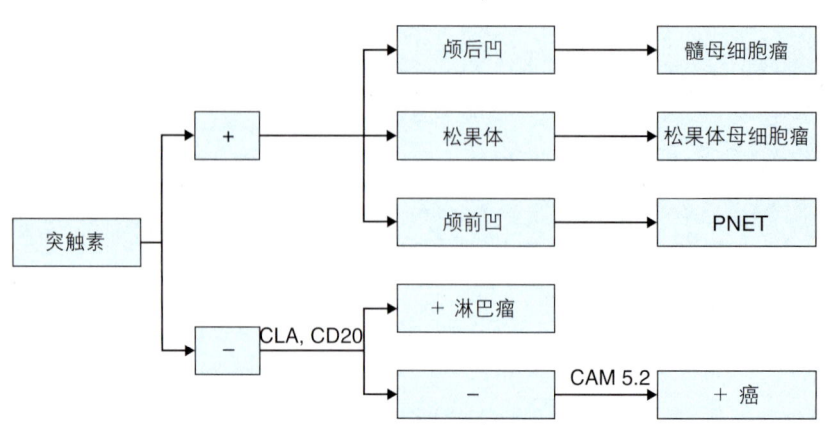

示意图18.3 具有拥挤的恶性细胞核和稀少胞浆肿瘤的免疫组化诊断

神经系统的免疫组织化学 18

分裂率和凋亡率。该变型有很强的侵袭性，因此病人的预后比较差[2]。

有资料表明 GFAP 阳性的髓母细胞瘤比 GFAP 阴性的髓母细胞瘤生存期要长，不过还需要进一步研究[129]。

促纤维增生型髓母细胞瘤

髓母细胞瘤部分区域的增殖细胞可以用网状纤维染色显示（图18.38、表18.7）。无网状纤维的灰色的岛状区域的细胞有核周空晕，多是突触素染色阳性的神经母细胞（图18.38B）[130]。促纤维增生型髓母细胞瘤近来被认为只包括那些在结节中有神经元和神经胶质分化的结节性髓母细胞瘤，且这些结节被富含细胞的结缔组织围绕，其内含有增殖活跃的能产生网状纤维的细胞[2]。现在规范治疗实施后，此组肿瘤均比典型的髓母细胞瘤预后好。

原始神经外胚层肿瘤

中枢神经原始神经外胚层肿瘤（cPNET）的特征和鉴别诊断前面已经叙述过（见髓母细胞瘤）。而大脑的神经外胚层肿瘤、小脑的髓母细胞瘤及松果体母细胞瘤在组织学上均表现为单一的神经外胚层小细胞恶性瘤，近几年的趋势是把位于大脑的肿瘤称之为神经外胚层肿瘤，位于后颅凹的称为髓母细胞瘤，位于松果体的称为松果体母细胞瘤（示意图18.3）。大脑节神经母细胞瘤和神经母细胞瘤被称为具有神经元分化的 PNET[2]。

神经元分化标记物，如突触素可以标记具有神经元分化的神经外胚层肿瘤（示意图18.3）。各种各样的其他外胚层和神经外胚层抗原的表达以及和神经管发育缺陷的关系都反映出这些肿瘤的胚胎性特征[131]。

与中枢原始神经外胚层肿瘤相比，外周原始神经

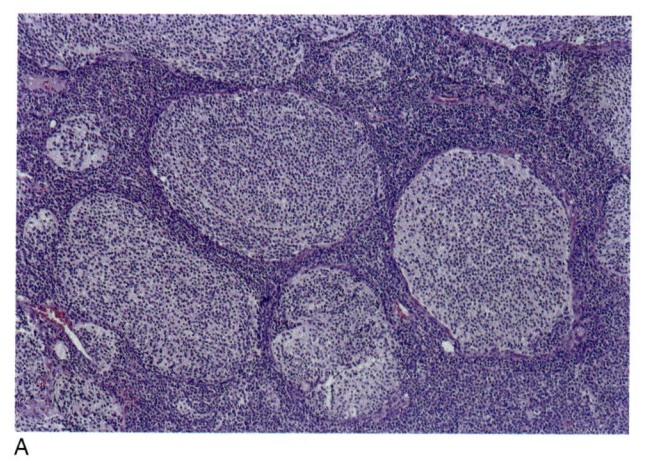
A

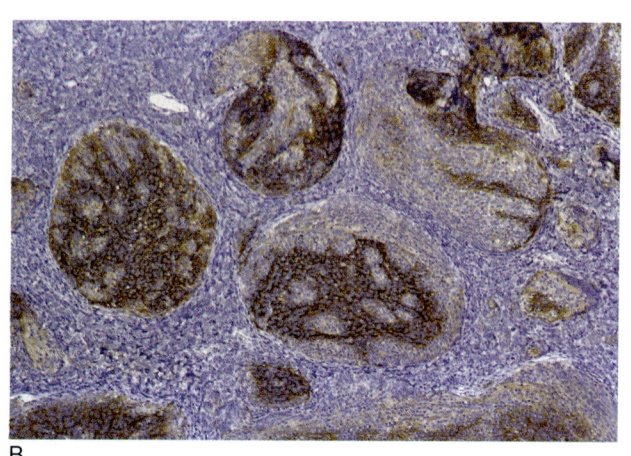
B

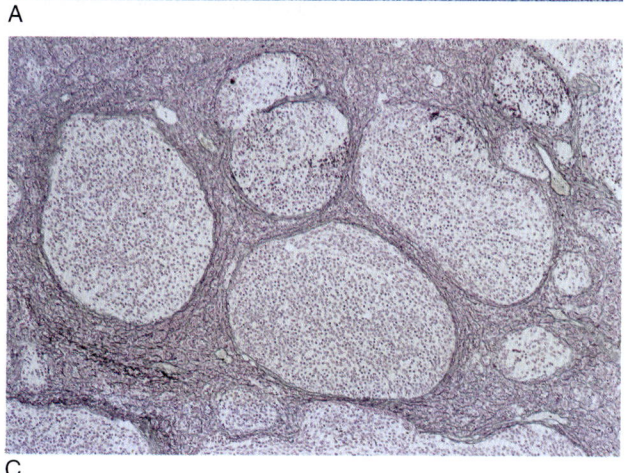
C

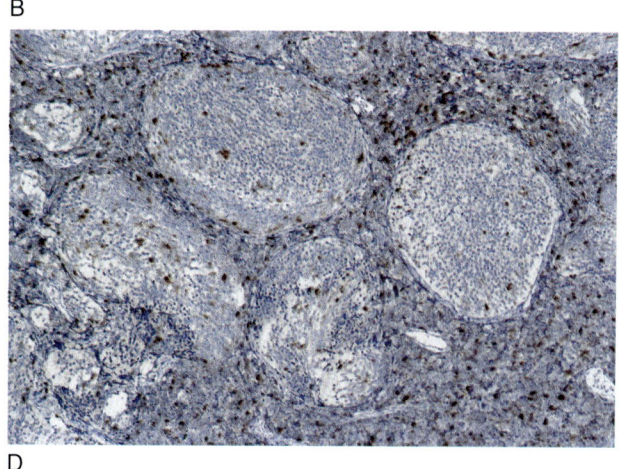
D

图18.38 促纤维增生型髓母细胞瘤在HE染色上呈灰白色岛屿状（A），内含突触素阳性细胞（B）。肿瘤同一部分的邻近区域为致密拥挤的细胞围绕灰白色岛屿形成的网状纤维阳性的条带（C），这些条带区域含有较多的 MIB-1 阳性细胞（D）

外胚层肿瘤（pPNET）和 t（11；22q24；q12）染色体易位有关，pPNET中MIC2（图18.39）和神经特异性烯醇化酶（NSE）免疫反应强阳性。pPNET的发生部位包括一些有神经嵴衍生的部位、性腺、胸壁和骨，如脊柱、颅骨及马尾[132]。pPNET是高度侵袭性肿瘤，可以局部复发或转移到特定器官[13]。

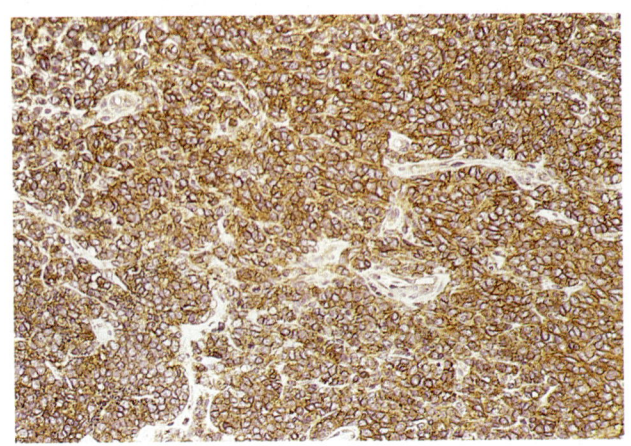

图18.39 外周原始神经外胚层肿瘤（pPNET）MIC2弥漫强阳性

髓肌母细胞瘤

这一肿瘤见于儿童颅后凹中线上，可见有平滑肌或横纹肌[73]。髓肌母细胞瘤是肌染色阳性的肌细胞和与髓母细胞瘤相似的神经外胚层小细胞的混合体。与颅内原发的横纹肌肉瘤不同，横纹肌肉瘤不包含起源于神经外胚层的细胞成分[75]。突触素和视网膜-S抗原标记物有助于检测这些神经外胚层细胞。结蛋白和MSA标记物可确定肌纤维分化（表18.8）。除肌肉外其他中胚层成分可偶然出现在髓母细胞瘤和髓肌母细胞瘤中[13]。

非典型畸胎样-横纹肌样肿瘤

该肿瘤是一个高度恶性肿瘤，主要见于婴儿和幼小的儿童，直到最近才被确认和定义（表18.8）[133]。常见于颅后凹，早期经脑脊液转移。瘤细胞具有粉红色胞浆，较髓母细胞瘤更具有上皮性特征。多种免疫组织化学标记物的表达对该肿瘤的诊断有重要意义（图18.40）。非典型畸胎样-横纹肌样肿瘤内含有多种类型的中间丝：几乎总是表达波形蛋白和EMA，且常灶状表达GFAP、CK或其他类型的中间丝，也可以表达突触素和嗜铬素。非典型畸胎样-横纹肌样肿瘤的22号染色体异常，有助于和包括髓母细胞瘤在内的PNET鉴别[133]。

少见的胚胎性肿瘤

髓上皮瘤与癌很相似，但它常见于儿童，这与癌的发病年龄不同。髓上皮瘤的假复层柱状上皮细胞拥挤，类似于衬覆于胚胎神经管的上皮。肿瘤细胞位于由Ⅳ型胶原组成的基底膜和纤维性间质上，上皮细胞基底层nestin、波形蛋白和5型微管相关蛋白免疫标记阳性，常呈局灶性分化并表达GFAP、S-100、NSE（图18.41）、NF蛋白、CK或EMA[134]。

室管膜母细胞瘤常发生在儿童的大脑（表18.8）[135]，很像PNET，有典型的菊形团，内衬有丝分裂活跃的上皮样细胞。与髓上皮瘤不同的是，室管膜母细胞瘤的菊形团镶嵌于富于细胞的恶性瘤细胞之间，没有胶原基质。室管膜母细胞瘤表达波形蛋白，其菊形团GFAP染色阴性，而室管膜细胞瘤的菊形团GFAP阳性。室管膜母细胞瘤的细胞比间变性室管膜瘤的菊形团丰富，较少见血管增生。

> **诊断要点：胚胎性肿瘤**
>
> 1. 这些多潜能肿瘤可以表达几乎所有神经外胚层标记物，但突触素多为局灶性表达。一些还可以表达其他的标记物，特别是波形蛋白。
> 2. 多见于儿童。
> 3. 细胞密度高。
> 4. 高增殖活性，MIB-1表达指数常高于20%，有丝分裂常较活跃。
> 5. 尽管被分类为Ⅳ级，但是更详细的诊断还是很有必要的，因为一些肿瘤对放疗和化疗非常敏感。

脑膜及相关肿瘤

脑膜瘤

脑膜瘤发生于脑膜部位，这是和其他原发性颅内肿瘤的一个主要鉴别点（表18.9、表18.5～18.7）。大多数的脑膜瘤附着于硬脑膜或大脑镰上，易于识别。发生于脉络丛的脑膜瘤较为少见，而发生于中枢神经系统实质内的脑膜瘤则非常罕见[136]。

脑膜瘤典型的遗传学改变是22号染色体的部分或全部缺失[1,5]，可通过染色体ISH及免疫染色进行

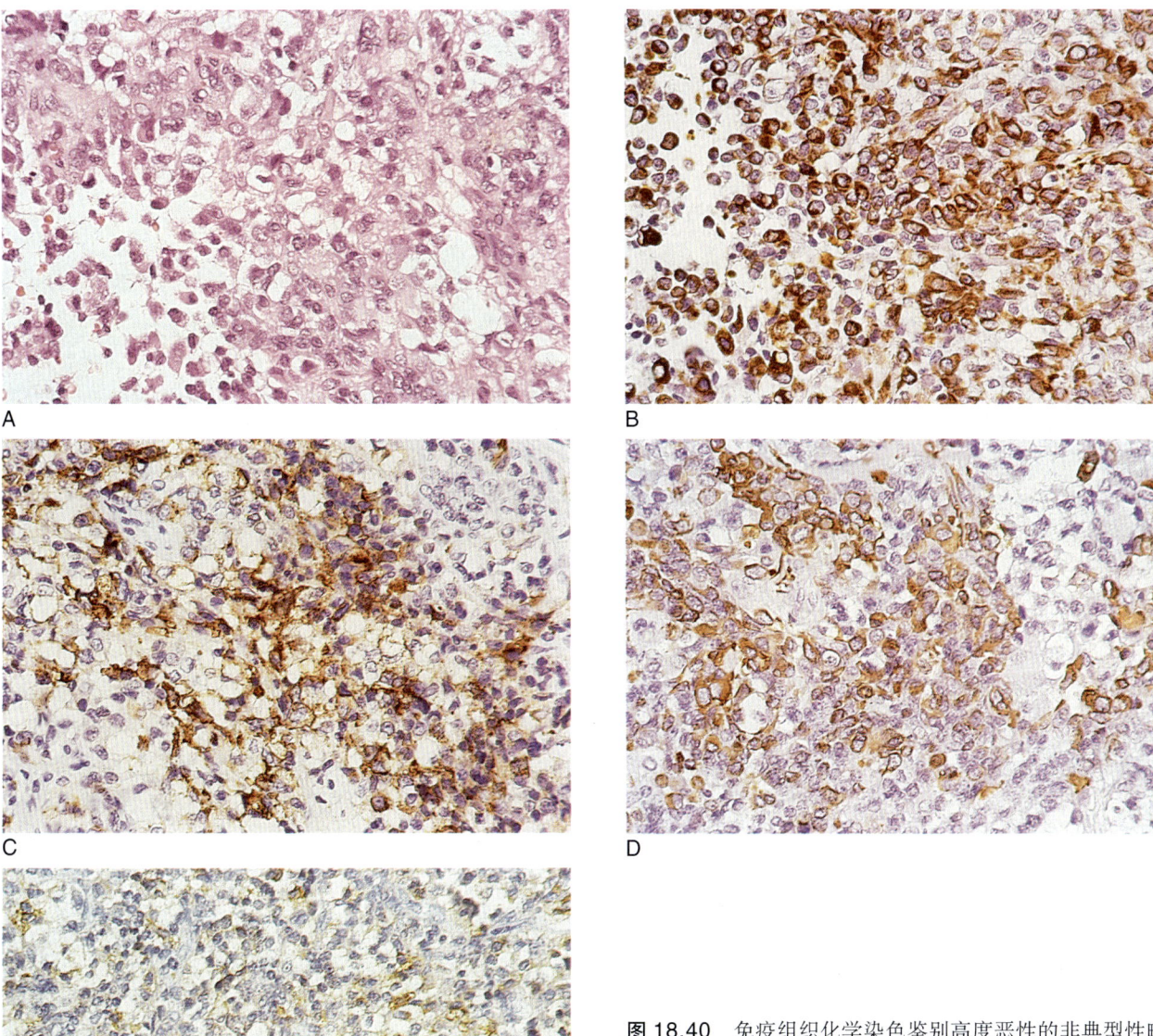

图18.40 免疫组织化学染色鉴别高度恶性的非典型性畸胎样-横纹肌样肿瘤与髓母细胞瘤。这是一个婴儿的后颅凹肿瘤（A，HE）波形蛋白阳性（B），EMA（C）和GFAP(D)局灶性阳性，突触素局灶弱阳性（E）（引自McKeever PE. New methods of brain tumor analysis. In: Mena H, ed. Dr. Kenneth M. Earle Memorial Neuropathology Review, Washington, DC : Armed Forces Institute of Pathology; February 24, 2000）

检测。

脑膜瘤的某些特点可以为其诊断提供依据。合体细胞样外观是脑膜上皮型脑膜瘤的一个特征性改变，也是其他变型脑膜瘤的局灶性特征（图18.42、表18.9）。合体细胞样外现是由桥粒紧密连接在一起的相互交错的指状细胞突起，而不是真正的合体细胞。脑膜上皮的旋涡和砂粒体是脑膜瘤的特征，砂粒体为同心圆状的钙化，HE切片上这些特征的出现减少了对免疫组化分析的需要[87]。

许多脑膜瘤表达EMA[3]，尽管常呈局灶阳性表达，一些小的标本内甚至见不到阳性表达，但是若EMA表达阳性，同时GFAP阴性，就可以同胶质瘤区别开来（图18.43、图18.1B）[137]。EMA阳性是脑膜瘤最特异的免疫组织化学标记。脑膜瘤中S-100蛋白的表达变化很大，波形蛋白在脑膜瘤中的强阳性表达使其被用于脑膜瘤的诊断，但是必须同其他标记物联合使用，因为许多其他肿瘤也表达波形蛋白。这3种标记物在脑膜瘤中的表达变化很大，但是比起低级

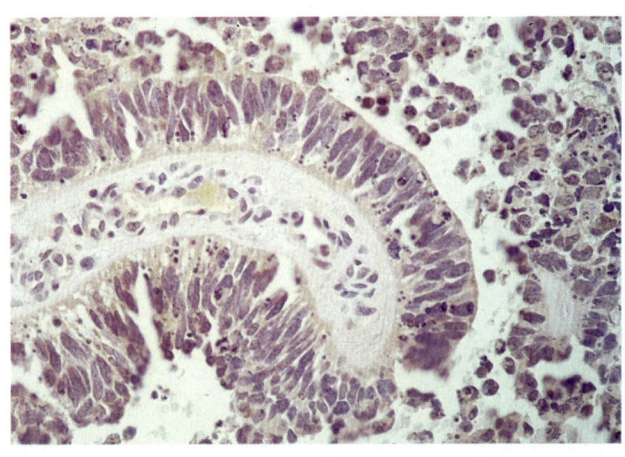

图18.41　髓上皮瘤。该乳头状肿瘤的间变细胞的神经特异性烯醇化酶弱阳性表达。瘤细胞构成假复层上皮，其表面有致密物质（引自McKeever PE. New methods of brain tumor analysis. In: Mena H, ed. Dr. Kenneth M. Earle Memorial Neuropathology Review, Washington, DC: Armed Forces Institute of Pathology; February 24, 2000）

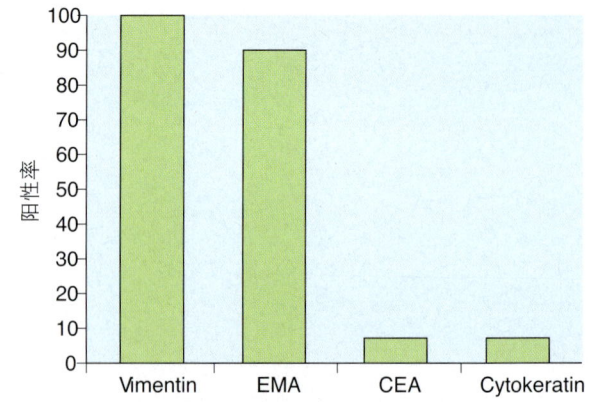

图18.43　29例脑膜瘤的广谱EMA、CEA和细胞角蛋白（AE1/AE3）免疫组化染色。除了波形蛋白，其他抗体阳性百分率均与Ng HK等报道一致（Ng HK, TseCC, Lo St. Meningomas and arachnoid cells: An immunohistochemical study of epithelial markers. Pathology 1987, 19: 253-257）

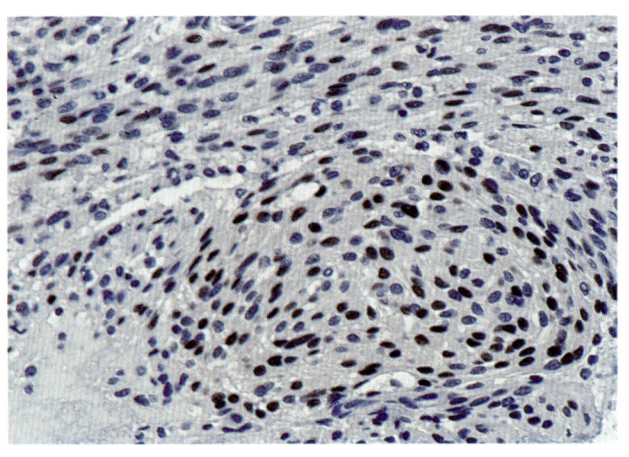

图18.42　脑膜上皮型脑膜瘤。该脑膜瘤由于位置特殊不能被完全切除。瘤细胞呈合体细胞样外观，核圆形。当病人考虑为妊娠时，则对肿瘤组织的激素受体进行了检测。图示孕激素受体阳性（核深棕色）

和毛细胞型星形细胞瘤相似[138]。HE染色显示纤维型脑膜瘤含有粗大粉染束状胶原，不同于星形细胞瘤[3]。

发生在小脑脑桥角和脊神经根周围的肿瘤，尤其是纤维型脑膜瘤跟施万细胞瘤非常相似，极易造成诊断困难。在这种情况下，可以认定为脑膜瘤的结构有以下几种，即旋涡结构、砂粒体及大量粗束的胶原。纤维型脑膜瘤可表达EMA，而施万细胞瘤不表达，前者还经常表达更多的波形蛋白和更少的S-100蛋白。

纤维型脑膜瘤可以通过免疫组织化学染色与孤立性纤维性肿瘤（SFT）鉴别[138, 139]，纤维型脑膜瘤比孤立性纤维性肿瘤较多地表达EMA、S-100、糖原，较少表达CD34（图18.44、图18.48）[138]。

脑膜上皮型脑膜瘤（合体细胞型脑膜瘤）（WHO I 级）

脑膜上皮型脑膜瘤是经典的合体细胞样脑膜瘤（图18.42），类似于正常情况下出现于脑膜和脉络丛的小巢状脑膜上皮细胞。旋涡结构和砂粒体较少见（表18.9）。一些脑膜上皮型脑膜瘤可以被它们的纤维血管基质分割成小叶结构[140]。

脑膜上皮型脑膜瘤偶尔呈现原纤维或上皮样的特点（图18.1A），与室管膜瘤相似，但是它们缺乏GFAP的表达，间质常含有很多的Ⅳ型胶原纤维、网状纤维或EMA（图18.1B）。尽管黏液乳头型室管膜瘤常有局灶性的GFAP阳性表达，但是与该肿瘤的鉴别诊断仍有困难。

脑实质内脑膜瘤可以与少突胶质细胞瘤相混淆

别的胶质瘤，脑膜瘤的实体常含有更多的网织纤维、纤维粘连蛋白和胶原。

应当对脑膜瘤尤其是那些没有被完全手术切除的脑膜瘤进行孕激素受体和雌激素受体的检测和评价，阻断激素的治疗可能对受体阳性的脑膜瘤有效。激素受体状况可能对妊娠的处理产生影响（图18.43）[1]。

纤维型脑膜瘤（纤维母细胞型脑膜瘤）（WHO I 级）

纤维型脑膜瘤由梭形细胞构成，质硬（表18.5），与施万细胞瘤、孤立性纤维性肿瘤、纤维型星形细胞瘤

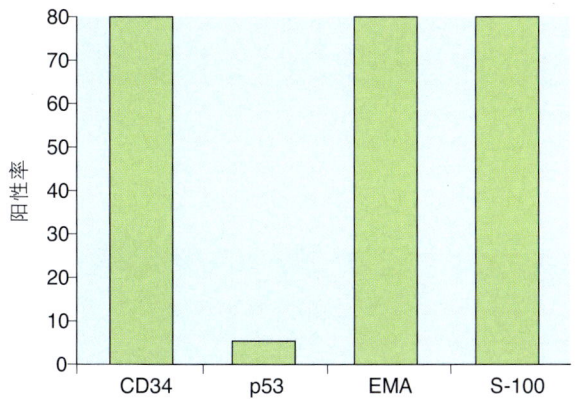

图18.44 20例纤维型脑膜瘤免疫染色柱形图，阳性百分率与PerryA等报道一致（PerryA, Scheithauer BW, Nascimento AG. The immunophenotypic spectrum of meningeal hemangiopericytoma: A comparison with fibrous meningioma and solitary fibrous tumor of meninges. Am J Surg Pathol 1997; 21: 1354-1360）

（示意图18.2）。大多数脑膜瘤EMA阳性。与胶质瘤相比，脑膜瘤与中枢神经系统实质之间的边界用GFAP、突触素、神经原纤维等CNS标记物染色分界更清。一些脑膜上皮样脑膜瘤缺乏典型的旋涡状结构和砂粒体，而其他则可以显示明显上皮样细胞边界（图18.1A）。这些肿瘤可能会与癌或腺瘤相混淆。脑实质内的脑膜瘤表达少量或不表达CAM5.2细胞角蛋白，不表达垂体肽或嗜铬素。

移行型脑膜瘤（混合型脑膜瘤）（WHO I级）

移行型脑膜瘤主要由前文所述的合体细胞成分和纤维母细胞成分组成。因其出现介于合体细胞和纤维母细胞之间的细胞成分而得名[140]。出现明显的旋涡结构、砂粒体和成堆的合体细胞使之成为最容易被识别出来的脑膜瘤之一，IHC常没有必要用于鉴别诊断（表18.7）。

砂粒体型脑膜瘤（WHO I级）

砂粒体型脑膜瘤中有大量的砂粒体[140]，好发于脊髓。在明显的、同心层状的砂粒体之间见到有合体样波形蛋白和EMA阳性的细胞，呈现良性脑膜瘤的特点。

血管瘤型脑膜瘤（WHO I级）

血管瘤型脑膜瘤是一种含有大量血管的脑膜瘤[3, 140]。其血管壁可以用CD31、CD34、Ⅷ因子、Ulex等内皮标记物和波形蛋白、肌动蛋白标记。对于这些脑膜瘤来说，CD34引起的背景染色要比其他标记物少。

其他类型的脑膜瘤

脑膜瘤其他一些类型的认定是非常重要的[3]，有助于避免将其误诊为其他需要不同治疗的实体肿瘤。脑膜瘤的变型包括脂母细胞型[141]、蛛网膜小梁型[142]、微囊型[142]、富于淋巴细胞浆细胞型[2]、成骨型[140]、软骨型[140]和分泌型（图18.45）的脑膜瘤。强的波形蛋白染色和局灶性EMA表达有助于诊断这些肿瘤[144, 145]。

细小颗粒状染色质、核分裂少见以及出现脑膜瘤的特点可将上述脑膜瘤变型与癌和肉瘤鉴别开来（表18.9）。与癌相比，脑膜瘤一般表达较多的波形蛋白和较少的CAM5.2角蛋白。

分泌型脑膜瘤是一种非常特别的肿瘤（图18.45），该肿瘤CAM5.2呈局灶阳性，紧密围绕在分泌颗粒周围。这些分泌颗粒癌胚抗原（CEA）、糖类抗

表18.9 含有"合体样"细胞的肿瘤的鉴别诊断

诊 断	结 构	抗体*	位 置[a]
脑膜瘤	旋涡结构，砂粒体，细胞间指状突起和桥粒，（厚的胶原）[b]	波形蛋白（+）、EMA（S）、S-100（R）	大脑镰，大脑幕，脑膜，脉络丛，（颅外）[b]
间变型脑膜瘤	退行性变的特点，核分裂，坏死，中枢神经系统侵犯	波形蛋白（+）、EMA（S）、S-100（R）	同上
血管外皮细胞瘤	富于细胞，血管周基质增加，核分裂	波形蛋白（+）	同上

* 染色结果：+，弥漫强阳性；S，有时阳性；R，极少的细胞阳性
a 列出最常见或最特别的部位
b 括号内的特点如果存在则对肿瘤的鉴别诊断有重要帮助
CNS，中枢神经系统；EMA，上皮细胞膜抗原
改自 McKeerver PE, Blaivas M. The brain, spinal cord, and meninges. In: Sternberg SS, Diagnostic Surgical Pathology. 2nd ed. New York: Raven Press; 1994: 409-492)

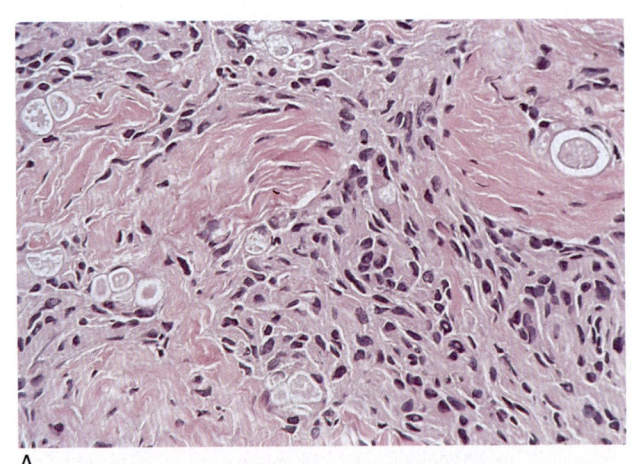

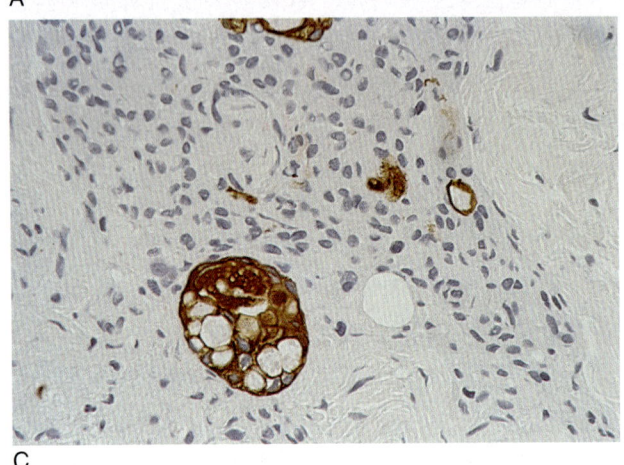

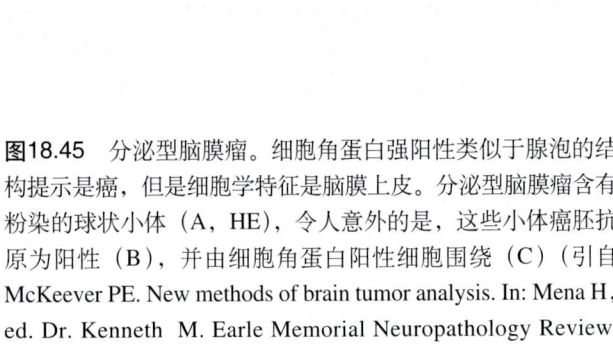

图18.45 分泌型脑膜瘤。细胞角蛋白强阳性类似于腺泡的结构提示是癌，但是细胞学特征是脑膜上皮。分泌型脑膜瘤含有粉染的球状小体（A，HE），令人意外的是，这些小体癌胚抗原为阳性（B），并由细胞角蛋白阳性细胞围绕（C）（引自 McKeever PE. New methods of brain tumor analysis. In: Mena H, ed. Dr. Kenneth M. Earle Memorial Neuropathology Review, Washington, DC: Armed Forces Institute of Pathology; February 24, 2000）

原 19-9 和 PAS 呈阳性[146]。

侵袭性或恶性脑膜瘤

脑浸润 脑组织或小血管的肿瘤浸润被认为是脑膜瘤的高危复发因素，但此时脑浸润不作为增加肿瘤级别的标准[2]。在脑膜瘤中脑浸润比硬脑膜浸润更具危险性。

脊索样型脑膜瘤（WHO Ⅱ级） 脊索样型脑膜瘤与脊索瘤相似，而且比其他大多数脑膜瘤更好发于儿童[145]。可以通过其脑膜上皮特征和不表达CK的特点作出鉴别诊断[3]。由于其有复发的趋势，因此被定为 WHO Ⅱ级。

透明细胞型脑膜瘤（颅内肿瘤 WHO Ⅱ级） 对脑膜瘤进行亚分型的理由之一就是确定那些更具侵袭性的类型。透明细胞型脑膜瘤变型就是一个范例（图 18.46），虽然看起来像良性，但有许多透明细胞型脑膜瘤在生物学行为上是侵袭性的[2]。其透明细胞与少突胶质细胞瘤和透明细胞室管膜瘤的细胞相似（示意图18.1）[90]。透明细胞和脑膜上皮特点的同时存在是其诊断的关键[3]。胞浆内见到糖原有助于证实其诊断（图18.46B、C）[90]，波形蛋白弥漫性阳性和EMA局灶性阳性有助于其脑膜上皮起源的推断（图 18.46F、表 18.9）。这一变型好发于腰脊椎和小脑脑桥角处[147]。

非典型脑膜瘤（WHO Ⅱ级） 鉴别良性脑膜瘤、非典型脑膜瘤和间变型脑膜瘤的标准已被WHO采纳（表18.10）[2]。非典型脑膜瘤的诊断标准是在10个高倍镜视野内核分裂象为 4～19 个。另一个诊断选择的标准是具备 3 个或 3 个以上的如下组织学特点：细胞丰富，具备高核浆比例的小细胞，大而突出的细胞核，无定形，片样生长，局灶性地图样坏死。非典型脑膜瘤比 Ⅰ 级脑膜瘤更具有侵袭性和容易局部复发。

该肿瘤具有介于良恶性脑膜瘤之间的组织病理学诊断特征。非典型脑膜瘤通常仍表达波形蛋白，并且至少会有局灶性轻度 EMA 的免疫活性。EMA 可能更多地在脑膜上皮瘤样的分化灶中表达。

非典型脑膜瘤倾向于侵袭和局部复发。除标准的 22 号染色体缺失之外的染色体异常和 MIB-1 的阳性细胞标记指数增加可能预示着更高的侵袭性[148]。

18 神经系统的免疫组织化学

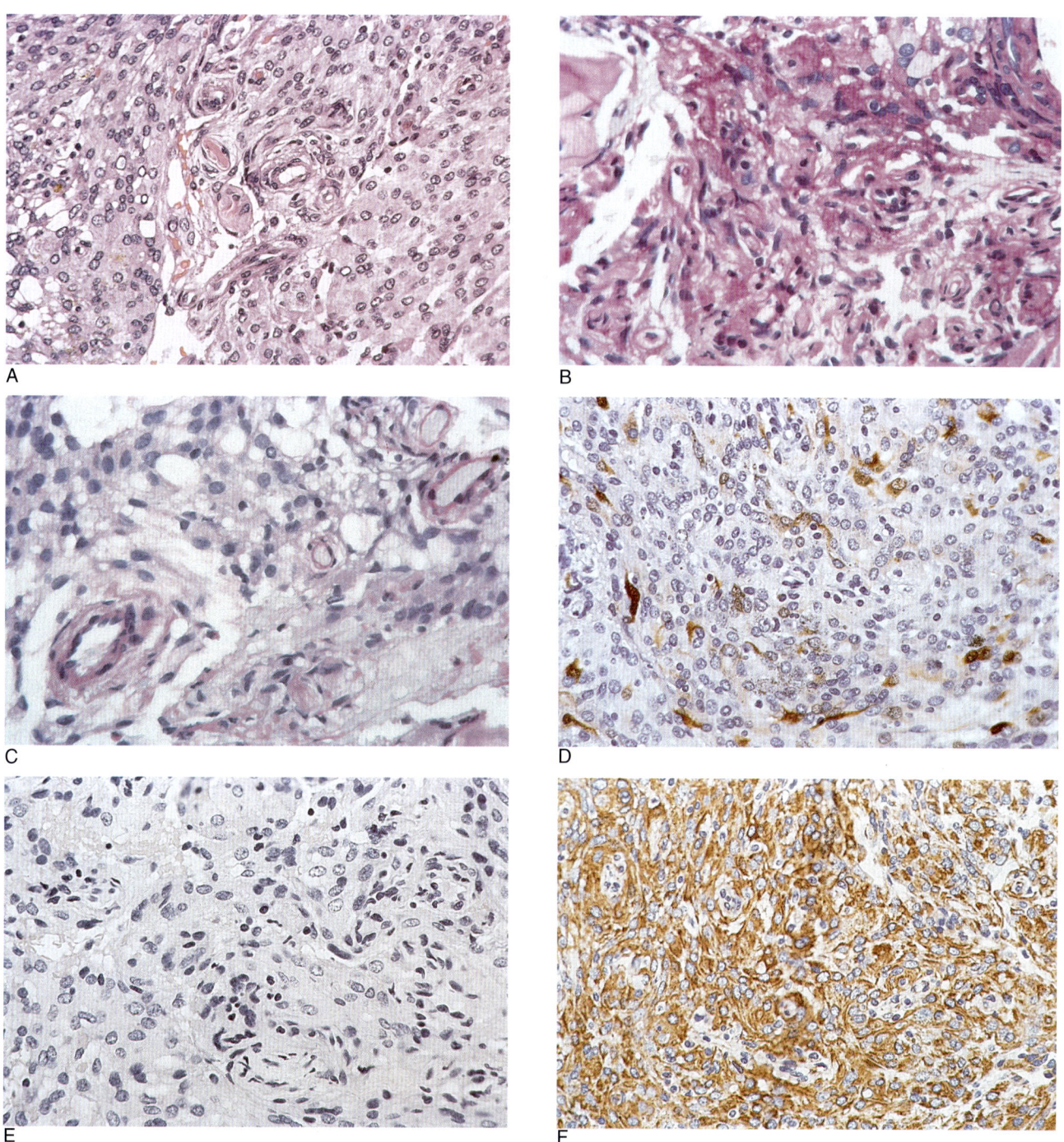

图 18.46 透明细胞型脑膜瘤。该肿瘤已经几次复发。透明细胞型脑膜瘤（HE）(A) 含有 PAS 阳性的红染的糖原 (B)，可被能够消化糖原的酶清除掉 (C)。瘤细胞散在地表达 S-100 蛋白 (D)，但 CK 表达阴性 (E)。透明细胞型脑膜瘤具有侵袭性趋势，手术切除困难。像大多数脑膜瘤一样，波形蛋白呈强阳性表达 (F)（引自 McKeever PE. New methods of brain tumor analysis. In: Mena H, ed. Dr. Kenneth M. Earle Memorial Neuropathology Review, Washington, DC: Armed Forces Institute of Pathology; February 24, 2000）

横纹肌样脑膜瘤（WHO Ⅲ 级） 横纹肌样脑膜瘤是一种高侵袭性肿瘤，肿瘤组织内几乎没有具有黏着力的细胞，细胞内可见大量的旋涡样的细丝，这些细丝波形蛋白阳性[6, 149]，把脑膜上皮细胞的细胞核推到细胞的一侧。

横纹肌样脑膜瘤难以与胖细胞型胶质瘤相鉴别。在这种情况下，波形蛋白的大量表达、EMA 阳性和缺乏 GFAP 的表达可以将二者区分开来。

乳头状脑膜瘤（WHO Ⅲ 级） 脑膜瘤中出现乳头状的结构通常会伴随高的局部复发率和转移率。乳

表18.10　脑膜瘤的WHO分级标准		
脑膜瘤（Ⅰ级）	非典型脑膜瘤（Ⅱ级）	间变型脑膜瘤（Ⅲ级）
<4个核分裂象/10HPF（0.16mm²）	核分裂活性增加：4~19/10HPF（0.16mm²）	核分裂活性增加：>19/10HPF（0.16mm²）
没有找到合适的诊断标准	OR >2： 细胞数量增加 小细胞并有高的核浆比例 明显的核仁 片状和/或无定形生长方式 局灶性地图样坏死	OR：恶性和/或间变性细胞学特点 （例如 类似于肉瘤、癌、恶性黑色素瘤）
属于高分化的亚型 （文内所述）	（透明细胞型脑膜瘤和脊索样型脑膜瘤 属于WHO Ⅱ级）	（横纹肌样脑膜瘤和乳头状脑膜瘤 属于WHO Ⅲ级）

HPF，高倍镜视野
脑侵袭并不是级别增加的标准
（改自McKeever PE, Boyer PJ. The brain, spinal cord, and meninges. In: Mills SE, Garter D, Greeson, JK， et al., eds. Sterber's Diagnostic Surgical Pathology, 4th ed. New York: Lippioncott William & Wilkins; 2004: 399-506）

头具有CD31阳性的血管轴心。脑膜瘤细胞在血管周围排列成菊形团样结构，除了表达波形蛋白和S-100蛋白外，还可以表达CK[150]。

硬脑膜是脑膜瘤发生的特征位置，在其他位置诊断乳头状脑膜瘤很困难。乳头状脑膜瘤和乳头状室管膜瘤、脉络丛乳头状瘤以及癌很相似[140]。可以通过波形蛋白与CK的高比例表达及GFAP表达的缺乏对脑膜瘤加以鉴别。

> **诊断要点：脑膜瘤**
> 1. Ⅰ级脑膜瘤大部分是"良性的"。发病部位影响手术完整切除，从而影响患者的预后。
> 2. Ⅱ级和Ⅲ级为侵袭性脑膜瘤，或是特殊的变型（如脊索样型、横纹肌样型等）；或是具有恶性特征的脑膜瘤标准变型（例如，核分裂象提示非典型或恶性脑膜瘤）。
> 3. EMA是脑膜瘤特征性的阳性标记物。
> 4. 所有的脑膜瘤都表达波形蛋白，但是很多其他肿瘤也有波形蛋白的阳性表达。

间变型脑膜瘤（恶性脑膜瘤）（WHO Ⅲ级）

间变型脑膜瘤中，每10个高倍视野有20个或更多的核分裂象，并且具有局部区域恶性肿瘤细胞的特征[2, 3, 151]。10%的恶性脑膜瘤细胞核有p53抑癌基因产物的表达。在一组20例间变型脑膜瘤中，平均MIB-1的阳性细胞标记指数为11.7%，而范围在1%至24%之间[152]。

其他脑膜肿瘤

血管外皮细胞瘤（WHO Ⅱ级或Ⅲ级）

血管外皮细胞瘤富于细胞，核分裂象多见，血管周有丰富的网织纤维，可由抗Ⅳ型胶原染色显示。80%的肿瘤会复发，23%的肿瘤发生转移[13, 153]。

与良性脑膜瘤相比，血管外皮细胞瘤更富于细胞成分，更多的核分裂象，镜下突向血管腔而不穿破内皮细胞（表18.8）。尽管有个别例外，血管外皮细胞瘤除了普遍存在的Ⅷa因子、间叶组织标记物及Leu7外，缺乏特征性肿瘤标记物[144, 154]。

血管外皮细胞瘤的免疫组化标记物与纤维型脑膜瘤的标记物相交叉，但是缺乏EMA的表达可以看做是前者的特征（图18.47、18.44）[138]。血管外皮细胞瘤在单个肿瘤细胞周围有大量网织纤维，这一点可以与恶性胶质瘤及转移癌相鉴别。并且，GEAP在胶质瘤内表达，而血管外皮细胞瘤不表达。血管外皮细胞瘤细胞核不呈多形性和梭形，可以与纤维肉瘤相鉴别。

孤立性纤维瘤

孤立性纤维瘤与纤维型脑膜瘤类似，但两者有不同的免疫组化标记物（图18.48、18.44）[3, 138, 155]。孤立性纤维瘤实质细胞表达丰富的CD34及胶原蛋白，而不表达EMA。免疫组化是鉴别孤立性纤维瘤和脑膜瘤的重要手段。根据我们的经验，孤立性纤维瘤和脑膜瘤之间的区别比血管外皮细胞瘤和脑膜瘤之间的区别更加明确。胸膜孤立性纤维瘤比脑膜孤立性纤维

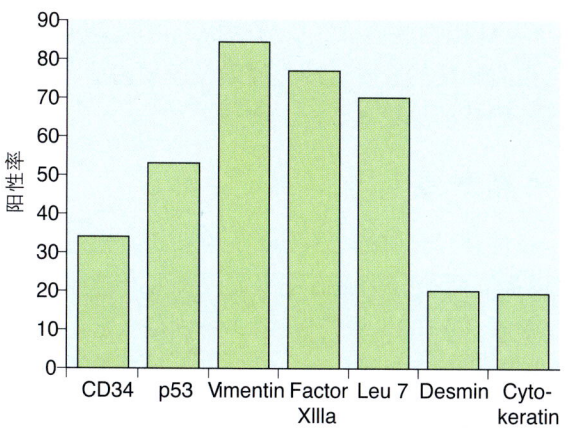

图18.47 27例脑膜血管外皮细胞瘤免疫组化染色结果。阳性百分率与Perry A 等报道一致（Perry A, Scheithauer BW, Nascimento AG. The immunophenotypic spectrum of meningeal hemangiopericytoma: A comparison with fibrous meningioma and solitary fibrous tumor of meninges. Am J Surg Pathol 1997; 21: 1354-1360）

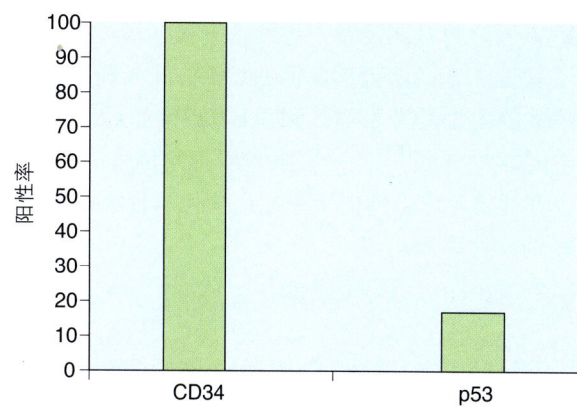

图18.48 8例孤立性纤维瘤柱形图。阳性百分率与Perry A等所报道的一致（Perry A, Scheithauer BW, Nascimento AG. The immunophenotypic spectrum of meningeal hemangiopericytoma: A comparison with fibrous meningioma and solitary fibrous tumor of meninges. Am J Surg Pathol 1997; 21: 1354-1360）

瘤更为常见。孤立性纤维瘤的恶性转化可能与8号染色体三体有关[156]。

脊索瘤和肉瘤

脊索瘤

大约40%的脊索瘤发生于颅骨斜坡，10%发生于颈椎，2%发生于胸椎，2%沿腰椎生长，45%发生于骶椎[3]。

脊索瘤的空泡细胞内含大的、特征性的空泡（图18.49、表18.6）。由于这些细胞通常呈条索状分布，细胞内空泡会偶尔出现串珠状排列，这点可以与软骨样肿瘤相鉴别，后者单个细胞包埋在软骨内[157]。脊索瘤可以表达CK（图18.49A）、EMA、5'-核苷酸酶和桥粒，而软骨肉瘤没有这些标记物的表达[157]。CK在脊索瘤中的表达是与CK阴性的软骨肉瘤相比的标准鉴别点[3]。

脊索瘤细胞内有丰富的双丝状物（图18.49），在同一个细胞中可以同时表达波形蛋白和CK。细胞内空泡富含黏液和糖原。这些结构可以与少突胶质细胞瘤的核周含水的空晕以及血管母细胞瘤的多样的小脂质空泡相鉴别（图18.21、18.49、18.54B）。

脊索瘤的恶性组织学转化比较少见，但是，临床

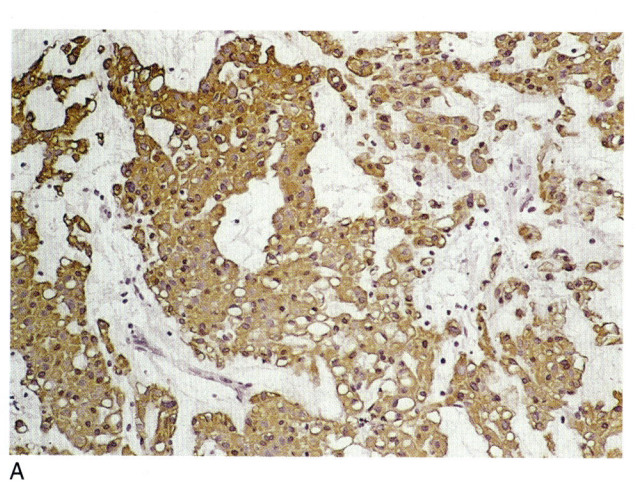

A

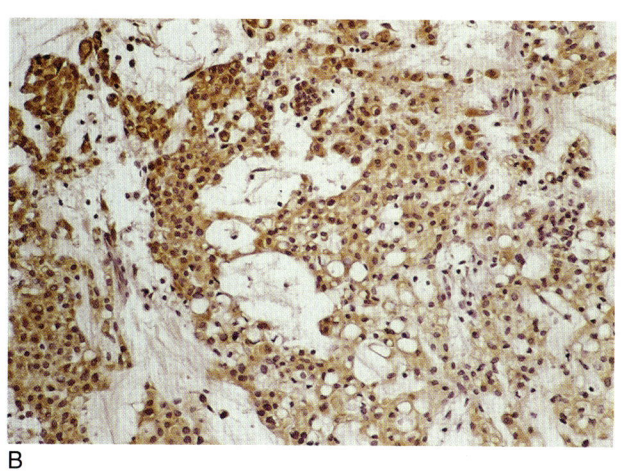

B

图18.49 脊索瘤。（A）空泡细胞索CK阳性表达是鉴别脊索瘤与CK阴性表达的软骨肉瘤最重要的免疫组化特征。（B）肿瘤波形蛋白表达也呈阳性。标本显示脊索瘤有表达一种以上中间丝的倾向

上敏感部位的局部侵袭，导致远期预后较差。

软骨样脊索瘤包括典型的 EMA、CK 和 S-100 阳性表达的典型的脊索瘤区和 S-100 阳性而 EMA 和 CK 阴性的软骨样区[157]。一些病理学家对软骨样脊索瘤的存在提出异议，他们宁愿把这些肿瘤看做脊索瘤或低级别软骨肉瘤。

肉瘤

脑肿瘤中肉瘤很少[76]。据相关资料报道，原发性颅内肉瘤的发病率在 0.08% 到 4.3% 之间，0.08% 接近现在的发病率[158]。GFAP 免疫组化分析显示以前被认为是肉瘤的肿瘤实质上是原发性脑肿瘤，特别是胶质母细胞瘤、髓母细胞瘤和原发性淋巴瘤[57]。

一些肉瘤的发病原因已经找到。令人吃惊的是，颅内放射是引发肉瘤的共同的原因[159,160]。颅内 Kaposi 肉瘤少见，大部分病例与免疫缺陷有关[161]。

脑膜间叶性软骨肉瘤少见，好发于颅内、脊膜及马尾，儿童及青少年多发[162]。脑膜间叶性软骨肉瘤除了 S-100 蛋白阳性的软骨岛外，其他特征和血管外皮细胞瘤很相似。

分化差的软骨肉瘤少见，通常好发于脑膜。这种肿瘤的重要特征是可见较少的软骨产物。在脑膜和中枢神经系统肿瘤中，将 S-100 蛋白的表达作为软骨样分化的证据，应谨慎分析判断，因为大部分的胶质瘤、脊索瘤、黑色素瘤、神经鞘瘤及小部分脑膜瘤中也有这种蛋白的表达（图 18.46D、18.50B、18.58C）[23,137]。

原发性脑横纹肌肉瘤少见[163]，突触素阴性表达可以将这种肿瘤与突触素阳性的髓肌母细胞瘤相鉴别。

GFAP 阳性肿瘤神经胶质的缺乏可以鉴别纤维肉瘤与侵袭脑膜的胶质母细胞瘤以及胶质肉瘤[3]。各种肉瘤鉴别特征见第 3 章。

神经鞘肿瘤

良性神经鞘肿瘤（WHO Ⅰ 级）如所描述的那样（表 18.5），可被分为施万细胞瘤或神经纤维瘤。恶性神经鞘瘤（WHO Ⅲ 级或 Ⅳ 级），特别是当它们失去与良性肿瘤相对应的特征时，难以进一步分类。Leu7 和 S-100 蛋白标记物可以把神经鞘瘤和其他不表达这些标记物的肿瘤区别开[13,164]。

施万细胞瘤（神经鞘瘤、神经瘤）（WHO Ⅰ 级）

周围神经旁的非侵袭性肿瘤可以提示施万细胞瘤的诊断。Verocay 小体不是在所有的施万细胞瘤中都可见到，但它们 比 Antoni A 区和 Antoni B 区更能明确施万细胞瘤的诊断。

双侧第 8 神经施万细胞瘤提示为 NF-2 型神经纤维瘤病。NF-2 型神经纤维瘤病发病部位特殊，且与脑膜增殖有关。NF-2 型神经纤维瘤病和施万细胞瘤都有第 22 号染色体的异常[1,5]。

施万细胞瘤的组织学图像和纤维型脑膜瘤、伸展细胞型室管膜细胞瘤、室管膜下瘤及星形细胞瘤很相似。施万细胞瘤实质组织内有大量Ⅳ型胶原阳性的网状纤维，可以与星形细胞瘤和室管膜瘤相鉴别（图 18.50A）。施万细胞瘤肿瘤细胞的外表面有连续的基底膜（表 18.5）。当一些施万细胞瘤呈局灶性 GFAP 阳性时，在与星形细胞瘤鉴别时要非常谨慎[3]。但是，

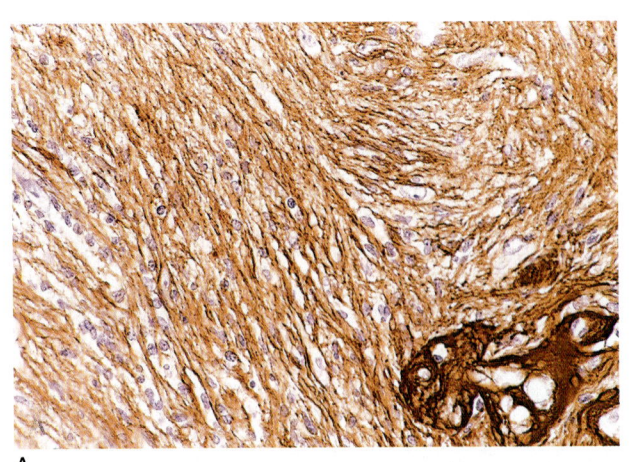
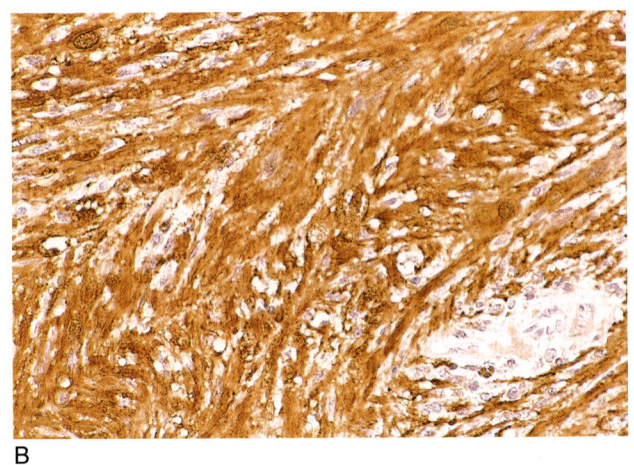

图 18.50　周围神经的施万细胞瘤，发生于臂丛神经，此例为一青年患者。（A）在致密 Antoni A 区的每个肿瘤细胞周围的基底膜可见Ⅳ型胶原阳性表达，图像右下角上的暗褐色血管有更多的胶原。（B）细胞核和细胞质示强的 S-100 表达，但是右下角的血管却没有

GFAP阴性表达支持施万细胞瘤的诊断。

当纤维型脑膜瘤缺少脑膜旋涡及砂粒体等脑膜瘤的特征时，它与施万细胞瘤的鉴别比胶质瘤与施万细胞瘤的鉴别更加困难。纤维型脑膜瘤内也有很类似施万细胞瘤中Antoni A区和Antoni B区的结构。施万细胞瘤表达Leu7和S-100蛋白，而不表达EMA，因此脑膜瘤对EMA的反应性是很有用的鉴别点。两种肿瘤都表达S-100蛋白，但是S-100蛋白在施万细胞中表达更强、更广泛（图18.50B）[3]。S-100蛋白β亚单位的单独表达被证明可以鉴别听神经施万细胞瘤与某些脑膜瘤[166]。如果施万细胞瘤存在GFAP阳性灶也可与脑膜瘤相鉴别，脑膜瘤细胞GFAP表达通常是阴性。

神经纤维瘤（WHO I级）

神经纤维瘤的诊断要点是它发生于周围神经内而不是周围神经旁（表18.5）。神经纤维瘤与施万细胞瘤的区别是神经纤维瘤NF阳性的可见神经纤维轴突穿过肿瘤而不是只局限在肿瘤周边[3]。神经纤维瘤越大，肿瘤细胞内可见轴突的机会就越少。幸运的是，现在抗NF抗体可以在杂乱的肿瘤组织中分辨出单个的轴突（图18.51）。这是因为神经纤维瘤是神经本身的膨胀，由施万细胞、纤维母细胞、胶原和黏液样物混合组成，被包裹在EMA弱阳性的神经束膜内。相反，施万细胞瘤靠近神经生长并且压迫神经，因此肿瘤内没有神经纤维丝。

丛状神经纤维瘤是多发性的肿胀的神经束，与von Recklinghausen病（NF-1）有关[1]。

恶性神经鞘瘤

见第3章。

神经内分泌肿瘤

见第9章。

生殖细胞肿瘤

在颅内，95%的原发性生殖细胞肿瘤发病部位在松果体和蝶鞍上区的中线上，特别是前者更多见。大约十分之一的肿瘤在两个区域内均可发生，四分之一肿瘤只在鞍上窝内生长。混合性生殖细胞肿瘤和淋巴瘤（gerlymphoma）仅在蝶鞍内出现[167]。生殖细胞肿瘤极少累及脊髓或周围神经[3]。

生殖细胞瘤是颅内最常见的生殖细胞肿瘤。颅内生殖细胞瘤和性腺生殖细胞瘤差别很小[168]。生殖细胞肿瘤详见第14章和16章。

造血和淋巴肿瘤

淋巴瘤（WHO III级或IV级）

原发性中枢神经系统淋巴瘤在中枢神经系统实质内生长（表18.8）。肿瘤呈弥漫性生长，边界不清。这些淋巴瘤几乎都是B细胞起源（示意图18.3、图18.52）[1, 169-171]，部分易发生在免疫抑制病人，如AIDS

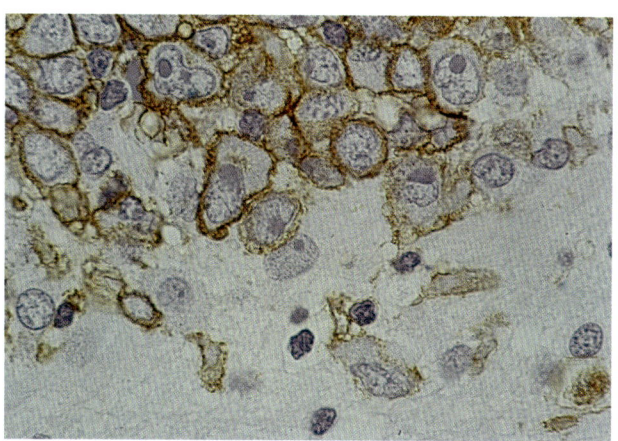

图18.52 原发性脑淋巴瘤。细胞核苏木精复染显示恶性淋巴瘤细胞内染色质凝集成块状，核仁大。免疫组化染色为L26阳性，一种B淋巴细胞标记物。T细胞及巨噬细胞标记物在恶性淋巴细胞中呈阴性反应（未显示）（引自McKeever PE.New methods of brain tumor analysis. In: Mena H, ed. Dr. Kenneth M. Earle Memorial Neuropathology Review, Washington, DC: Armed Forces Institute of Pathology; February 24, 2000）

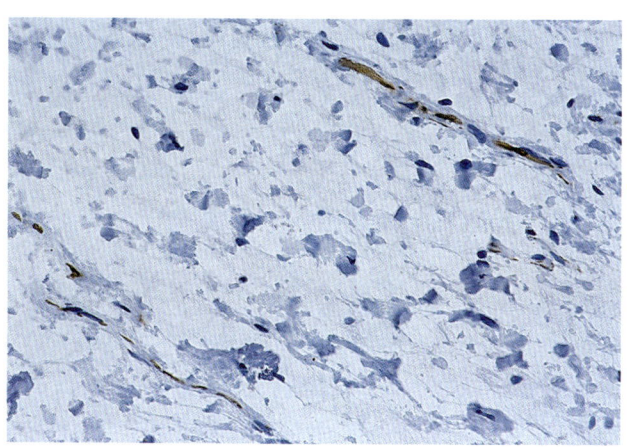

图18.51 神经纤维瘤。增生的肿瘤细胞内散在长的褐色轴突（苏木精复染抗NF染色）（授权自Andrew Flint and Victor Elner, Michigan, Ann Arbor, MI）

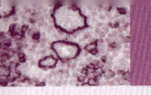

诊断免疫组织化学

患者及其他的免疫功能低下的病人[172-174]。除了极少数病例，AIDS相关的淋巴瘤预后都很差[173,175]。原发性中枢神经系统淋巴瘤中少见T细胞淋巴瘤[176]。

在石蜡切片中，B细胞标记物CD20和CD79a、T细胞标记物CD3ε和CD45RO应与LCA联合应用[13]。由于原发性中枢神经系统淋巴瘤侵犯中枢神经系统实质，对GFAP等中枢神经系统标记物的判断必须非常慎重。细胞核复染可以分辨出混杂在淋巴瘤细胞中非肿瘤性增生的神经胶质细胞核，这些细胞GFAP染色也呈阳性。B细胞（或极少数T细胞）单克隆标记物染色有助于区别淋巴瘤与中枢神经系统炎症，后者是多克隆的（图18.3B、C），也可与非淋巴肿瘤相鉴别。然而，很多淋巴瘤也有多克隆反应的淋巴细胞，这些细胞通常体积小并且有良性特征的细胞核[3]。

前面所提到的标记物适用于大部分原发性中枢神经系统淋巴瘤（示意图18.1）。有关这些和其他淋巴瘤的变型和分类详见第4章和第5章。

据估计，约5%～29%的外周淋巴瘤继发性累及中枢神经系统[3]，可累及任何部位，但常见于脑膜。

器官移植后，免疫抑制人群会出现移植后淋巴增生性疾病。组织学、免疫组织化学和基因重排可以区别淋巴或浆细胞增生（多克隆，无Ig基因重排）、非典型增生或B细胞增生及淋巴瘤（单克隆，有Ig基因重排）和免疫母细胞性弥漫性大B细胞淋巴瘤（单克隆）。大部分移植后淋巴瘤内可以发现EB病毒[170]。

淋巴瘤样肉芽肿病是与血管炎及肿瘤相似的淋巴细胞增生性疾病。淋巴瘤样肉芽肿病是EB病毒相关性疾病，因此通过原位杂交或免疫过氧化物酶对EB病毒的检测可以帮助诊断。淋巴瘤样肉芽肿病可进展为淋巴瘤。中枢神经系统的累及通常并发肺部疾病[3]。

中枢神经系统是血管内淋巴瘤的好发部位之一，血管内淋巴瘤是大B细胞淋巴瘤。肿瘤细胞可充满整个血管腔，临床表现类似血管炎。肿瘤细胞CD20染色呈阳性反应。

白血病

脑脊髓内的白血病通常是通过脑脊液细胞学检查确诊。最终的中枢神经系统实质内出血是母细胞危象的表现，白细胞的数量多于300 000/mm³，可以导致血管内白细胞淤滞。白血病很少并发脑血管炎。周围血嗜酸性粒细胞增多提示脑膜的局灶性白血病细胞聚集（绿色瘤）[13]。

组织细胞增生症

组织细胞增生症主要发生于青少年（表18.5）[3]。中枢神经系统朗格汉斯组织细胞增生症常继发于骨或全身系统疾病。非朗格汉斯型组织细胞增生症也可在中枢神经系统内发生（图18.54）[178,179]。尽管脑或脑膜的任何区域都可受累，但鞍旁区最易累及[180]。典型的病变区质硬，因为大量组织细胞、炎细胞和胶原纤维混合存在。新病变较旧病变纤维少。朗格汉斯细胞S-100蛋白染色呈阳性反应。有关文献显示CD1a在此病中有很高的敏感性，但也不是100%，故标记物的组合被推荐用于该病的诊断（表18.11）。细胞纤维内结构性GFAP缺乏可以区别组织细胞与星形细胞、室管膜细胞及室管膜下细胞。电镜下可以见到朗格汉斯组织细胞增生症中的Birbeck颗粒[8,10,13]。

组织细胞增生症不如朗格汉斯组织细胞增生症常见，可以通过免疫组化及形态学进行鉴别。中枢神经系统的Erdheim-Chester病有特征性的Touton巨细胞，该细胞CD68阳性及CD1a阴性[170]。Rosai-Dorfman病，或伴巨大淋巴结病性窦组织细胞增生症可伴或不伴全身系统疾病。它有特征性的巨噬细胞吞噬完整淋巴细胞现象。巨噬细胞CD68和S-100蛋白阳性，CD1a阴性（表18.11）。

其他颅内或脊髓内肿瘤

血管母细胞瘤（毛细血管血管母细胞瘤）（WHO I级）

毛细血管血管母细胞瘤类似于内分泌肿瘤（图18.55），肿瘤的毛细血管和间质细胞相间排列（图18.7），偶见分泌颗粒或表达红细胞生成素[181]。粉红色、空泡状间质细胞常呈NSE阳性反应，NSE在神经内分泌细胞中表达[182]。未见腺体的分化。

一些血管母细胞瘤和von Hippel-Lindau综合征有关。该综合征病人有多于一种以上的肿瘤，或有发生在特殊部位的血管母细胞瘤[183]。

因为血管母细胞瘤是非纤维性的，所以它和星形细胞瘤应该并不相似。然而，它们之间的相似性可归结为两个原因：标本处理和人工假象。小脑的血管母细胞瘤经常是囊性的，真正的肿瘤是位于囊壁中的结节。囊壁的活检标本可见明显的GFAP阳性的胶质增生。

血管母细胞瘤标本可见GFAP阳性细胞[184]。一些

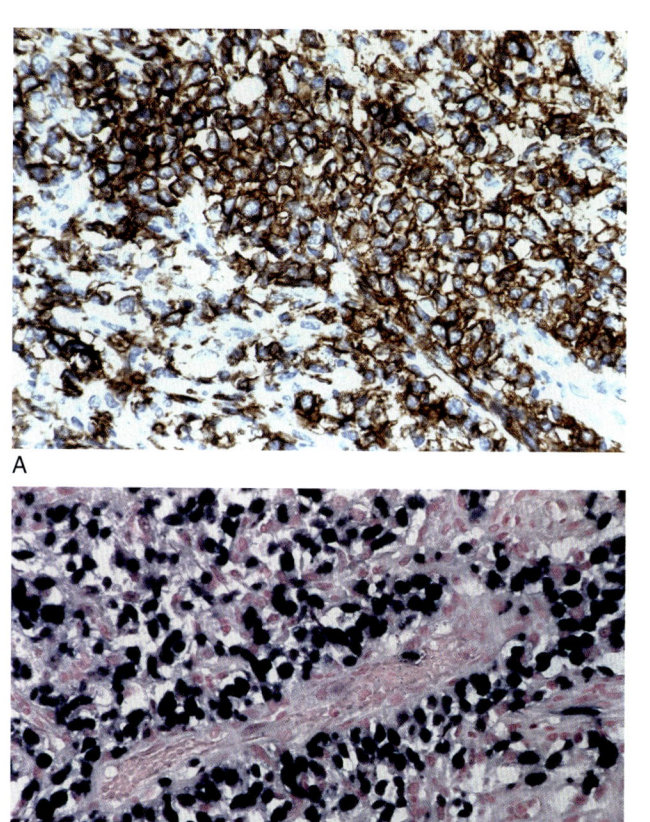

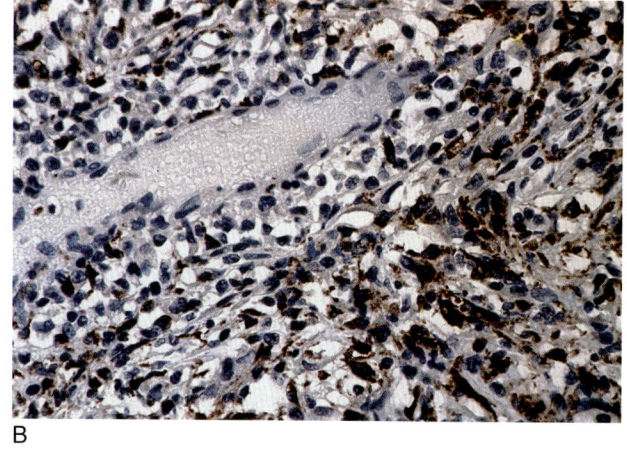

图18.53 移植后淋巴瘤。弥漫的B细胞淋巴瘤，CD20阳性（A）。混有非瘤性CD68阳性巨噬细胞（B）。苏木精染色显示CD20阳性的细胞内的恶性胞核和CD68阳性的细胞内良性的胞核。原位探针检测EB病毒阳性（C），该病例为肾移植后两年的33岁女性患者，小脑发生淋巴瘤

上皮样血管母细胞瘤和副神经节瘤[185]或肾细胞癌相似。血管母细胞瘤比副神经节瘤有更多的毛细血管，而嗜铬素A较少[186]。和肾细胞癌相比，血管母细胞瘤核染色质分布比较均一，没有坏死，核仁小，毛细血管和间质细胞紧密排列（图18.55A）。这种排列结构可见CD31、CD34、抗Ⅷ因子或抗γ-烯醇化酶（NSE）染色阳性[182]。和肾细胞癌相比，血管母细胞瘤NSE呈阳性，而EMA或CK阴性（图18.55B、C）。

颅咽管瘤（WHO Ⅰ级）

这种肿瘤常见于蝶鞍内或蝶鞍上区。颅咽管瘤的上皮细胞具有特征性。适当的颅咽管瘤标本取材应包括与颅咽管瘤囊壁相连的实性区，因为它具有特征性上皮，所以很难和其他脑肿瘤混淆，这种上皮可能是造釉细胞型、角化型或两者兼有（表18.6、18.13）[3]。四分之三的颅咽管瘤发生钙化，这是和转移癌鉴别的重要特征，脑转移癌很少钙化，也很少像颅咽管瘤那样分化。

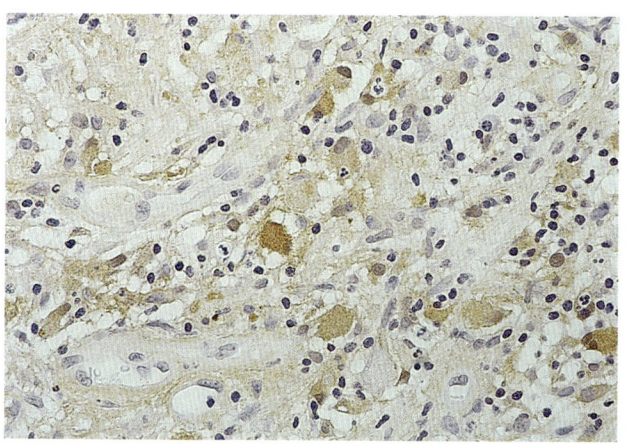

图18.54 组织细胞增生症。标本取自脑实质内肿瘤，可见S-100阳性细胞。免疫组化染色显示Rosai-Dorfman病中阴性的细胞内的白细胞

细胞是反应性的星形细胞，通常靠近肿瘤的周边部位。然而，其他的是间质细胞，最常见于血管母细胞瘤的富于细胞型和血管胶质瘤变型中，这些间质可以从邻近的反应性星形细胞中摄取GFAP或自身表达GFAP[184]。为了减少误诊，取材时应该取肿瘤实质的中间部分。

囊性颅咽管瘤标本的不适当取材可能会有一些未知来源的上皮细胞。在这些病例中，CK8和20的表达缺乏倾向于颅咽管瘤的诊断，而不是同一部位的上

表18.11 中枢神经系统的组织细胞增生症和巨噬细胞的比较

疾 病	组织学特征	CD68（KP-1）	S-100	CD1a	Birbeck 颗粒（EM）
巨噬细胞	泡沫上皮样多核巨细胞	+	−	−	−
Erdheim-Chester	Touton 巨细胞	+	S[a]	−	−
Rosai-Dorfman	吞噬淋巴细胞现象	+	+	−	−
朗格汉斯组织细胞增生症	肾形核，嗜酸性胞浆	+	+	+	+

染色结果：+，弥漫强阳性；S，有时，阳性细胞数多
a S-100 有些 Erdheim-Chester 病例阳性，但不是所有的
EM，电镜

（引自McKeer PE, Boyer PJ. The brain, spinal cord, and meninges. In : Mills SE, Carter D, Greenson, JK, et al., eds. Sternberg's Diagnostic Surgical Pathology, 4th ed. New York: Lippincott Williams & Wilkins; 2004: 399-506）

皮性囊肿[187]。颅咽管瘤与大部分的脑转移癌相比，表达更高分子量的角蛋白（图 18.56）。

仅仅当颅咽管瘤的神经胶质边缘GFAP表达阳性时，颅咽管瘤易与毛细胞型星形细胞瘤混淆。颅咽管瘤周围的高反应性纤维神经胶质增生可区分颅咽管瘤和毛细胞型星形细胞瘤，前者GFAP阳性细胞之间的间距相同，细胞较少，没有微囊。如果疑为颅咽管瘤，角蛋白免疫组化分析可以分辨出神经胶质增生中的上皮细胞[188]。

转移瘤（所有肿瘤为 WHO Ⅳ级）

癌

与中枢神经系统和脑膜相关的癌的重要特点是特殊的上皮结构（图 18.57A、表 18.6）和原发癌的转移特性。转移癌详见第7章。少数脑原发性癌发生于脉络丛，来自松果体和蝶鞍上区的生殖细胞肿瘤及囊肿[3, 189]。本节重点讨论癌（图 18.57B~D）和原

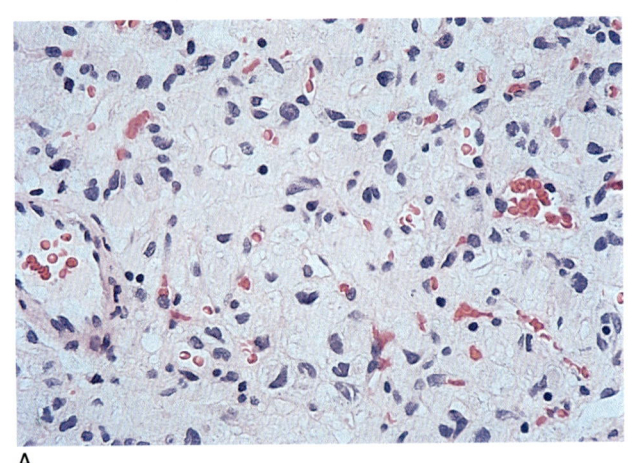
A

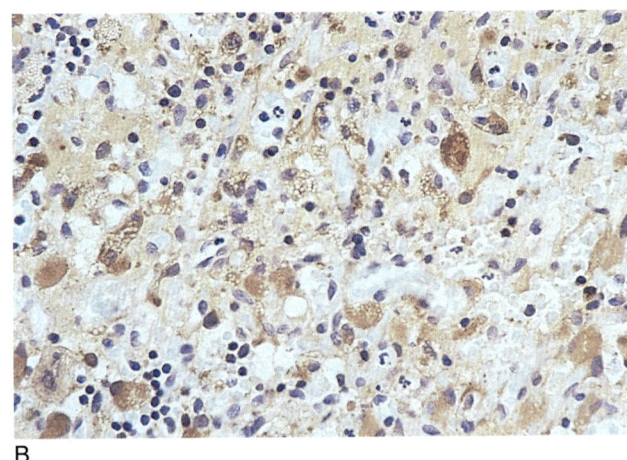
B

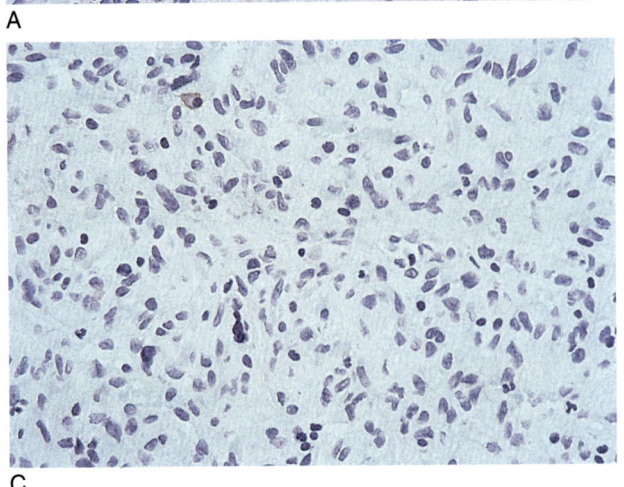
C

图 18.55 小脑血管母细胞瘤。（A）老年女性右小脑半球肿瘤，可见大量的毛细血管和空泡细胞（HE）。（B）小脑血管母细胞瘤NSE呈阳性反应。抗NSE染色的间质细胞显示出透明的、圆的脂质空泡。（C）标本EMA阴性表达。单个棕色EMA阳性浆细胞说明染色的可靠性（引自 McKeever PE.New methods of brain tumor analysis. In: Mena H, ed. Dr. Kenneth M. Earle Memorial Neuropathology Review, Washington，DC : Armed Forces Institute of Pathology; February 24, 2000. 授权自 Dr. Roger A. Hawkins, Greenville, PA）

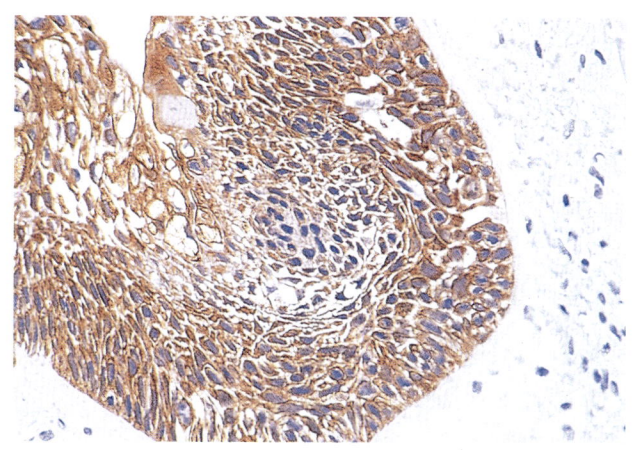

图18.56 大部分的颅咽管瘤具有特征性结构，如图示的造釉细胞型颅咽管瘤。高分子量的K903阳性可更进一步确定诊断并且可以显示收缩的上皮细胞胞浆（星状网织状）

发性颅内肿瘤（示意图18.2）的鉴别。

转移癌偶尔会伴发肿瘤性脑膜炎。尽管临床症状和炎症性脑膜炎很类似，但是脑脊液的细胞学检查可以区分它们[177,190,191]。

很多转移到中枢神经系统和脑膜的癌是腺癌，可形成腺泡并产生黏液。其他的是小细胞或未分化癌。中枢神经系统转移癌的组织学标志是上皮特征及和中枢神经系统实质之间清楚的肿瘤边界。转移癌有清楚的上皮边界及缺乏纤维性胞浆，和胶质母细胞瘤图像正好相反。中枢神经系统的实质内，除胶质母细胞瘤和间变性胶质瘤外很少有肿瘤像转移癌一样有多形性显著的核、丰富的异常核分裂象或自发性肿瘤坏死。中枢神经系统转移癌有CAM5.2细胞角蛋白强阳性表达（图18.57C），K903角蛋白阳性较少见，EMA阳性常见。这些特征和GFAP表达阴性（图18.57B）可以区分转移癌和胶质瘤[3]。在鉴别癌和胶质瘤时，要避免用AE1/AE3抗CK，它可以和GFAP交叉反应（图18.9）。其他经常犯的错误是把进展期癌的胶质增生看做GFAP阳性肿瘤（图18.24、18.25B）。

脑膜瘤通常有局灶性EMA表达，但是很多癌也是如此。除分泌性脑膜瘤的邻近分泌球形颗粒的部位外，脑膜瘤很少有CAM5.2 CK的阳性表达。这些肿瘤可以在局灶性CK染色的基础上和癌相鉴别（图18.45C）。大部分脑膜瘤和癌相比，波形蛋白表达更弥散，阳性更强，CK和波形蛋白的比例或者是零，或者至少比癌低。重要的是，除大部分恶性脑膜瘤，所有的脑膜瘤都缺乏丰富的并且常常是异常的核分裂象，而转移癌多见。

转移性肾细胞癌要与血管母细胞瘤和少突胶质细胞瘤相鉴别。这些肿瘤细胞胞浆透明，边界清晰（示意图18.1）[90]。EMA和CK阳性可以将转移性肾细胞癌和小脑血管母细胞瘤及少突胶质细胞瘤鉴别开来[3]。

小细胞癌和淋巴瘤（图18.57）、髓母细胞瘤及PNET很难鉴别（示意图18.3）。小细胞癌EMA或CK表达强阳性，髓母细胞瘤少见或局灶性表达，脑淋巴瘤表达阴性。尽管小细胞癌或髓母细胞瘤可以表达突触素、S-100蛋白或NSE，但是对于有经验的病理学家来说，这些标记物的染色是有鉴别价值的；和小细胞癌的上皮样细胞相对比，他们强调髓母细胞的纤维性基质。

对于原发于不同组织的癌，随着更精确的免疫组化标记物的出现，对于脑转移癌的原发灶的判断已经实现[192,193]。甲状腺转录因子-1（TTF-1）在一些肺癌和很多甲状腺癌中阳性表达[194]，而在大部分其他癌中阴性表达。脑部的免疫组化抗体组合应包括CAM5.2、CK7、CK20、CEA和TTF-1。在一些临床疾病，还要包括HER-2/neu、ER和PR或前列腺特异性抗原。免疫组化结果分析判断必须和组织学特征相一致。大部分脑转移的乳腺癌和肺癌都是未分化癌或腺癌，它们CAM5.2和CK7阳性，而CK20阴性。乳腺癌通常HER-2/neu或ER阳性表达。一些肺腺癌TTF-1阳性表达，TTF-1阳性可以与非肺部原发癌相鉴别。TTF-1阴性应用价值较低。结肠癌CK20和CEA典型的阳性表达，而CK7和TTF-1阴性表达。胃癌和胰腺胆管癌的诊断更具挑战性，CK7和CK20表达不一，而CEA表达一般为阳性。

事实上，所有的前列腺癌CAM5.2和PSA都是阳性表达。和中枢神经系统相比，前列腺癌更易转移到脊椎。大部分的肾细胞癌CAM5.2阳性、CK20阴性，少量有CK7阳性表达。TTF-1表达为阴性。大的透明细胞和出血倾向可以帮助对肾癌作出诊断。

黑色素细胞肿瘤

转移的黑色素瘤是神经系统最常见的黑色素细胞肿瘤（图18.58）。它的组织学特征多变（表18.5~18.7）。黑色素瘤详见第6章。黑色素瘤一般S-100蛋白强阳性表达（图18.58C）。S-100蛋白在很多中枢神经系统肿瘤中都可以表达，故特异性较差[195]。推荐用HMB-45和酪氨酸酶作为鉴别黑色素瘤和其他脑肿瘤的标记物（图18.58B）。

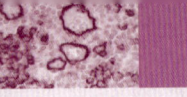

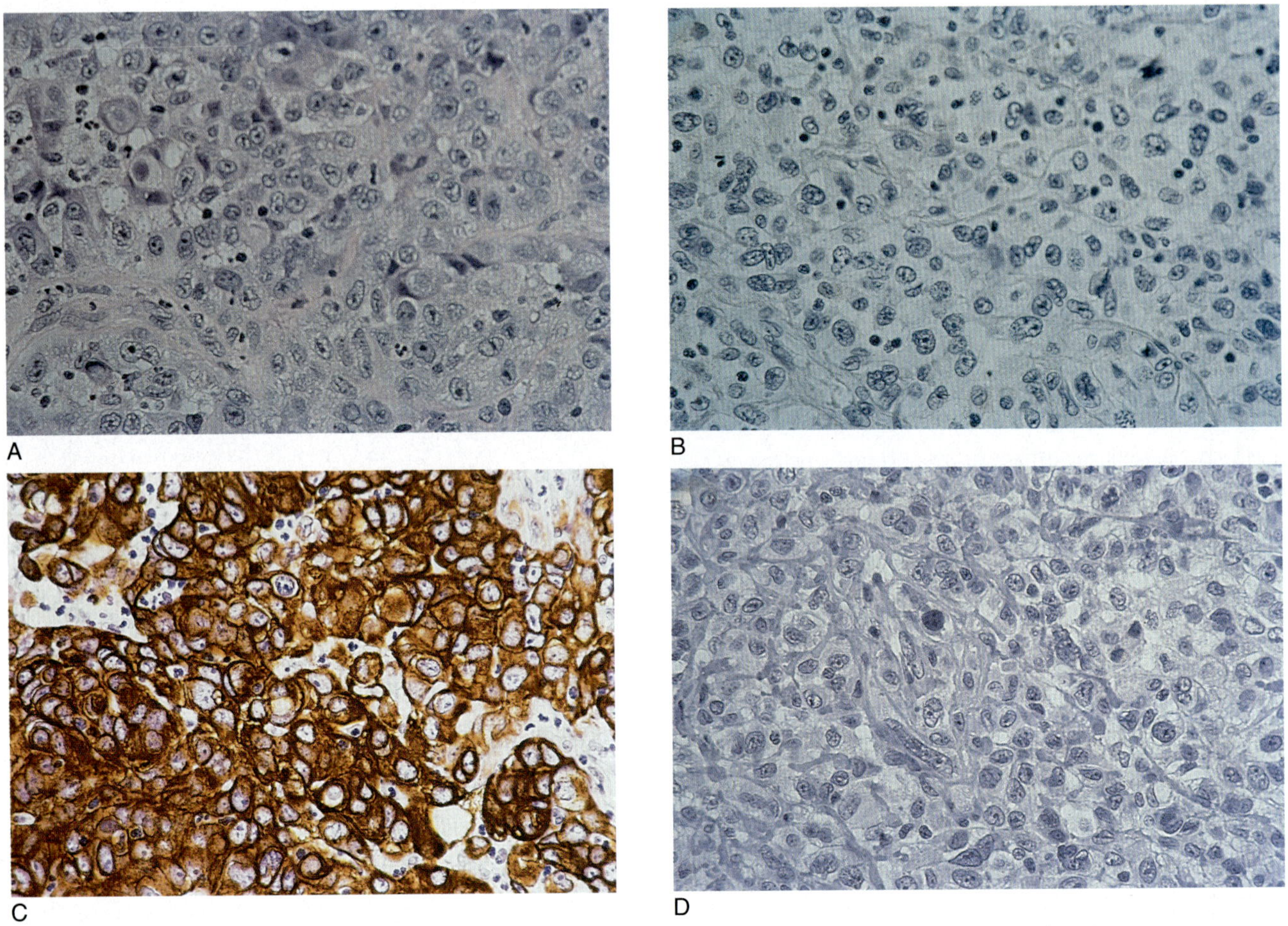

图18.57 （A）老年女性顶叶肿瘤，上皮样细胞之间边界清楚（HE），这些特殊的上皮样细胞是多形性的并且细胞核有恶性特征。示意图18.2详细分析了具有上皮样细胞的脑肿瘤的鉴别诊断方法。图A邻近的肿瘤组织切片GFAP阴性（B），细胞角蛋白CAM5.2强阳性（C），S-100蛋白阴性（D）。另外还有EMA表达阳性及嗜铬素A表达阴性（未显示）。见示意图18.2的癌的诊断步骤（引自 McKeever PE. New methods of brain tumor analysis. In: Mena H, ed. Dr. Kenneth M. Earle Memorial Neuropathology Review, Washington, DC: Armed Forces Institute of Pathology; February 24, 2000）

少数脑膜瘤、施万细胞瘤、室管膜瘤、神经母细胞瘤及PNET也含有黑色素[73]。它们可以通过各自的特征来进行鉴别。

脑脊髓的原发性黑色素瘤少见。大部分为来自脑膜的黑色素细胞。它们常原发于脑膜，通过血管周隙浸润中枢神经系统。原发性黑色素瘤恶性度较低[3]。它们可以在Meckel腔或其他部位发生。

囊　肿

囊肿和肿瘤不同，它们缺乏实性结节。这个简单的事实对区别胶质囊肿和胶质瘤、上皮囊肿和囊性颅咽管瘤非常重要。神经系统的特异性囊肿将在这里阐述[3]。其他的见它们发病部位的相关章节。

胶质囊肿、单纯性囊肿、松果体囊肿及咽鼓管壁

胶质囊肿、单纯性囊肿、松果体囊肿及咽鼓管壁这4种囊肿发生在不同的部位，病因不清楚，但是它们有一个共同的特点就是囊壁只有增生的胶质细胞（表18.12）。这些囊肿的组织学特征是神经胶质增生：GFAP强阳性的星形细胞分布均匀，它们之间夹杂有大量GFAP阳性的星形细胞纤维[196]。有时只有随着时间的推移才能证实这些囊肿与低级别的星形细胞瘤无关[3]。

神经上皮性囊肿和室管膜囊肿

神经上皮性囊肿和室管膜囊肿都有内表面的上皮样细胞，S-100和GFAP表达阳性，基底是纤维性

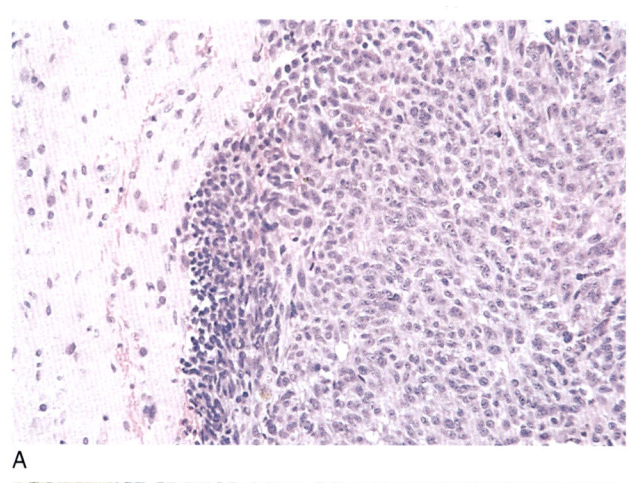
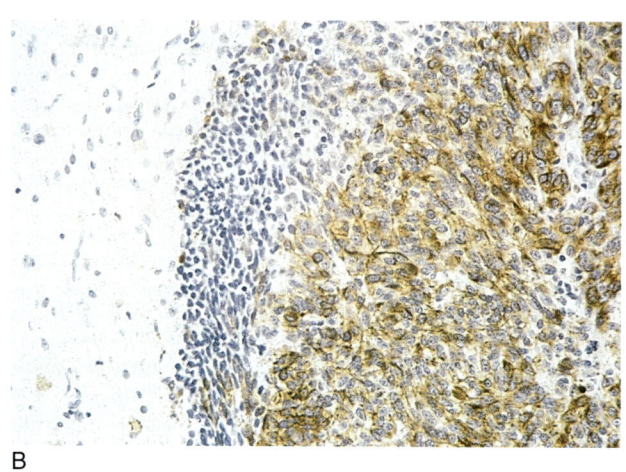
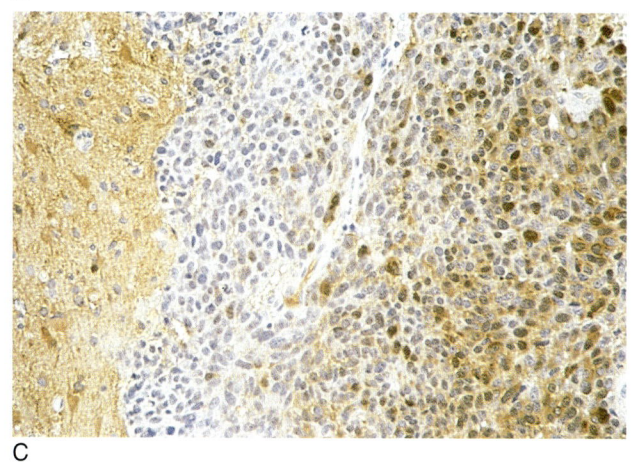

图18.58 罕见色素细胞的黑色素瘤的诊断性及辅助性的标记物。所有切片取自脑内黑色素瘤的边缘（A，HE）。（B）仅黑色素瘤HMB-45表达阳性，HMB-45是黑色素细胞的确定性标记物。（C）黑色素瘤和脑组织均S-100蛋白阳性。S-100是用于筛选的标记物，但是不能区分黑色素瘤和原发性脑肿瘤，例如胶质瘤（选自 McKeever PE. New methods of brain tumor analysis. In: Mena H, ed. Dr. Kenneth M. Earle Memorial Neuropathology Review, Washington, DC: Armed Forces Institute of Pathology; February 24, 2000）

神经胶质，这两种抗体也阳性表达[197]。这些囊肿经常在邻近脑室的部位发生（表18.13）。它们很少引起无菌性脑膜炎[13]。

胶样囊肿

发病部位是胶样囊肿的重要特征，更确切的称呼是第三脑室胶样囊肿（表18.13）。发病部位在第三脑室，通常是靠近脉络丛和室间孔，发病部位可以将胶样囊肿和其他囊肿区别开，胶样囊肿和其他囊肿表面看起来很像，但是发病部位不同。这种囊肿的上皮可以是扁平上皮、立方上皮、单纯柱状上皮或鳞状上皮，纤毛细胞和非纤毛细胞一般混杂存在[198]。运动和感觉纤毛提示嗅上皮和呼吸上皮[199]。这些细胞CK和EMA阳性表达。囊肿内容物主要是羧基黏蛋白，PAS和阿辛蓝染色阳性[200]。

皮样囊肿

皮样囊肿通常是中线囊肿，可能来自神经沟闭合时皮肤的胚胎组织包涵物（表18.13）。皮样囊肿在小脑半球之间发生，位置通常在第四脑室、脊髓的腰骶部和颅骨。这些囊肿可累及中枢神经系统、脑膜或二者兼有[73, 75]。破裂的皮样囊肿可以引起无菌性脑膜炎，这种炎症和脓肿类似。CK表达阳性的鳞状上皮细胞或伴有炎症的胆固醇结晶是诊断皮样囊肿的要点。

表皮样囊肿

表皮样囊肿更常见于大脑侧面而不是中线，但是在很多其他的地方也可发病（表18.13）。常见发病部位是小脑脑桥角、脑桥周围、鞍区附近、颞叶内、板障内及椎管内[73]。表皮样囊肿极少发生癌变[189]。

肠源性囊肿

肠源性囊肿在脑脊髓内发生。这种囊肿表面覆盖可分泌黏液的柱状上皮（表18.13）。上皮和肠上皮相似，少数情况下和支气管上皮类似。上皮表达角蛋白和EMA，有时也可有CEA和S-100蛋白的表达[201]。

表18.12　囊肿壁含有原纤维细胞时囊肿的鉴别诊断

诊　断	结　构	抗　体*	发病部位[a]
腔神经胶质增生	囊壁由增生的神经胶质组成	胶质微丝的GFAP（+）、S-100（+）	大脑，CNS
脓肿	囊壁由肉芽组织组成，纤维增生（表18.5），炎症和神经胶质增生，脓肿内容物	胶原（+）、reticulin（+）、L26（S）、A6（S）、LCA、κ和λ Ig、α-ACT、KP-1（S）、微生物	额颞叶基底部，CNS
囊性星形胶质细胞瘤	毛细胞型星形胶质细胞瘤壁	GFAP（+）、S-100（+）	小脑，CNS
血管母细胞瘤	囊壁由增生的神经胶质组成，血管母细胞瘤的囊壁结节（表18.7）	Ⅷ因子（S）、CD31（S）、NSE（S），囊壁：GFAP（+）	小脑，CNS
胶质囊肿、单纯性囊肿、松果体囊肿及咽鼓管壁	囊壁由增生的神经胶质组成，Rosenthal纤维	胶质微丝的GFAP（+）、S-100（+）、α-B-晶体蛋白	松果体，小脑，脊髓，脑干
脑膜囊肿	囊壁由硬膜、蛛网膜组成，合体细胞	胶原（S）、EMA（S）	硬脊膜外表面

* 染色结果判断：+，弥漫强阳性；S，有时阳性；R，极少阳性
a 最常见或最特异的发病位置放在首位
α-ACT，α-抗糜蛋白酶；CNS，中枢神经系统；EMA，上皮细胞膜抗原；GFAP，胶质纤维酸性蛋白；Ig，免疫球蛋白；LCA，白细胞共同抗原；NSE，神经特异性烯醇化酶
（引自McKeever PE. Blaivas M.The brain, spinal cord, and meninges. In :Sternberg SS, ed. Diagnostic Surgical Pathology, 2nd ed. New York: Raven Press; 1994: 409-492）

表18.13　囊肿壁具有内衬上皮时囊肿的鉴别诊断

诊　断	结　构	抗　体*	发病部位[a]
囊性颅咽管瘤	囊壁由造釉细胞瘤样上皮或不全角化的鳞状上皮组成，囊内容物为"油脂"	细胞角蛋白（+）	蝶鞍上区，鞍区
室管膜囊肿	通常是纤毛柱状上皮	GFAP（+）	脊髓，脑
胶样囊肿	纤维性囊壁，被覆纤毛和/或无纤毛的单层柱状上皮，囊内容物包括黏液和鬼影细胞	细胞角蛋白（+）、EMA	第三脑室
皮样囊肿	表皮样囊肿的特征加上皮肤附属器，囊内容物为皮脂、鳞屑和头发	角蛋白（+）	小脑中线，第四脑室，颅骨，硬脊膜，马尾
表皮样囊肿	纤维性囊壁衬覆角化的复层鳞状上皮，囊内容物是蜡样鳞屑	角蛋白（+）	CP角，颞叶，硬脊膜，松果体，鞍区，脑干，CNS
肠源性囊肿	被覆上皮如前，囊内容物为黏液，基底为胶原	细胞角蛋白（+）、EMA	脊髓

* 染色结果判断：+，弥漫强阳性
a 最常见或最特异的发病位置放在首位
CNS，中枢神经系统；CP，小脑脑桥；EMA，上皮细胞膜抗原；GFAP，胶质纤维酸性蛋白
（引自McKeever PE. Blaivas M. The brain, spinal cord, and meninges. In: Sternberg SS, ed. Diagnostic Surgical Pathology, 2nd ed. New York: Raven Press; 1994: 409-492）

脑膜囊肿

脑膜囊肿也称脑膜憩室，发病部位在脊髓的后面或侧面的硬膜外区，表面仅有一层和硬脊膜类似的纤维组织，无蛛网膜（表18.12）。硬膜下和蛛网膜下囊肿比硬膜外囊肿壁更薄，突入脑组织或脊髓的囊肿是蛛网膜下囊肿。普遍表达波形蛋白、孕激素受体和EMA。免疫活性表达类似于蛛网膜肉芽组织和脑膜瘤[202]。其他囊肿壁厚薄不等，很难分类。

痴　呆

痴呆是一种进行性和持续性正常认知状态的低下，其原因多种多样。病变包括变性、感染、炎症、脱髓鞘、脑血管病、肿瘤和毒性代谢疾病。本节主要讨论最常见的变性疾病。少见的病变在最近的文章

中有阐述[12]。

用来检测痴呆病因的标本应警惕临床上是否是阿尔茨海默病或克-雅病。任何用来估计痴呆病因的活检标本在证实其为其他疾病之前，应按克-雅病来处理[8]。处理过程如下，标本先用10%的福尔马林固定，然后标本的三分之一，其中必须包括大脑皮质部分，用纯甲酸或10%福尔马林加20%漂白剂做初步处理，剩下的标本在没有甲酸或漂白剂的10%福尔马林中继续固定。应避免把新鲜标本的任何部分放在没有福尔马林的漂白剂中，这样会导致组织溶解。皮质的一小部分在戊二醛中固定，以备之后的电镜观察。纯甲酸和福尔马林-漂白剂溶液可以灭活感染因子，为HE和GFAP检测克-雅病提供足够保存的组织标本。GFAP是非常稳定的具有抗氧化性的抗原。应该采用HE染色寻找灰质和神经元内的空泡，采用GFAP染色标本寻找星状细胞的胶质增生。如果这些特征都不存在，需处理未经漂白剂固定的剩下的标本，对其进行染色，以考虑其他诊断的可能（表18.3）。

所有的痴呆标本都有神经元丢失。在大多数活检标本中神经元丢失比其他的发现更难以估计。神经元的丢失需要通过神经元密度计数来估计，用形态测量学判断比肉眼观察更适合。神经元丢失引起神经胶质的增生，染色后比神经元丢失更易发现。

对照组织是从解剖标本中获得的年龄和发病部位都匹配的大脑皮质组织，它可以为估计各种各样的病变尤其是痴呆提供有价值的基线。这个对照对于估计胞浆空泡、微小的胶质增生和神经元数量尤其重要。

阿尔茨海默病

已经建立了诊断阿尔茨海默病（AD）所需的最低标准[203-205]。这些标准主要指的是在10倍和20倍镜下每个视野嗜银性斑块（老年斑）和神经原纤维缠结的数量。阿尔茨海默病的镜下判断标准主要是嗜银性斑块的数量（表18.3）。作者的方法是计算病例中斑块的数量并且和已知可信的系列样本中斑块的数量相比较[204]。AD的诊断需要结合临床资料，如果临床没有痴呆的可能性，不能通过活检标本诊断AD。

仅凭HE染色不能够完成嗜银性斑块和神经原纤维缠结的计数。推荐Bielschowsky银染法对嗜银性斑块和神经原纤维缠结进行染色（图18.59）[68]。采用荧光素荧光的蓝色光激发的硫磺素S也可以显示这两种结构[110]。神经原纤维缠结位于神经元内，由双螺旋丝组成[7,110]。这些细丝现在可以通过免疫组化的方法检测它们的蛋白结构，即tau蛋白和泛素（表18.14）[3, 206]。神经原纤维缠结Alz-50也呈强阳性表达，Alz-50是脑AD病的单克隆抗体[207]。淀粉样蛋白的抗血清可以检测在银染中的淀粉样斑块及嗜刚果红血管病[208]。

多发性脑梗死性血管性痴呆

脑缺血性损伤是老年痴呆的常见病因[13, 209]。血管性痴呆合并阿尔茨海默病也很常见。痴呆的血管性因素包括皮质下血管性痴呆、多发性梗死性痴呆、缺血性痴呆、伴皮质下梗死的脑常染色体显性动脉病和脑白质病（CADASIL）及"脑白质疏松"[3]。

路易体痴呆病

弥漫性皮质路易体痴呆病（DCLBD）是和痴呆有关的常见疾病[210]。DCLBD的统一诊断标准已经制定，并用于临床和尸检的诊断，分期系统也已经被提出来[211]。路易体痴呆病的标志性损伤是路易小体伴神经元的丢失和神经胶质增生。和脑干的帕金森病的路易小体相比较，皮质的路易小体在HE染色的切片上很难辨认。泛素和α-synuclein的免疫组化和皮质神经元内圆形褐色路易小体的存在可以帮助诊断DCLBD（表18.14）。扣带回是上述标记物的常见部位[211]。

额颞叶性痴呆症和其他痴呆症

如果通过免疫组化不能看出AD和DCLBD的组织学特征，病理学家应该考虑额颞叶性痴呆症。亚分类包括Pick病、皮质基底节变性、进行性核上性麻痹、与

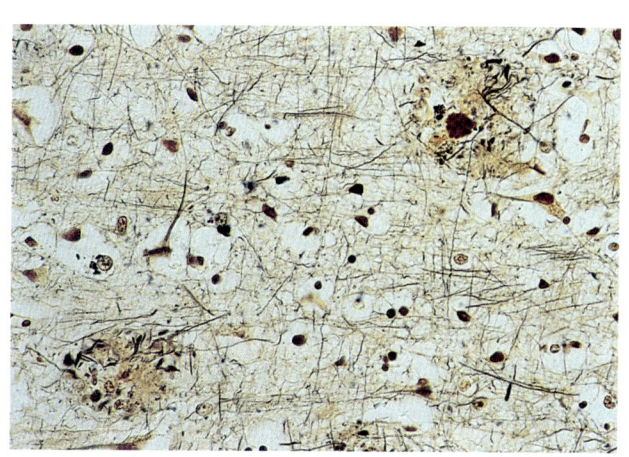

图18.59 阿尔茨海默病。切片的对角上有两个斑块，均含有黑色、扭曲的神经轴突。虽然用泛素和其他免疫组化对嗜银斑的染色对诊断很重要，但同过去一样，Bielschowsky银染色仍是诊断该病的"金标准"。本例为一中年女性病人，至少有3年的进行性痴呆病史，满足诊断阿尔茨海默病的CERAD标准[203]

17号染色体连锁的额颞叶性痴呆症合并相关性帕金森病，以及伴或不伴运动神经元疾病的额颞叶变性[212]。

额颞叶性痴呆症的病理学表现主要包括皮质浅层的空泡形成、神经元气球样变和神经胶质增生。特殊包涵体包括Pick病的银染阳性和tau（微管相关蛋白）表达阳性的Pick小体，额颞叶变性病中的泛素表达阳性的胞浆包涵体，其tau和α-synuclein表达阴性（表18.14）。

导致痴呆的另外因素有Lafora病、神经元蜡样脂褐素沉积症、肾上腺脑白质营养不良症等疾病。这些病的主要组织学特征不在本章节范围内，详细请查看其他资料[3,12,14]。

脱髓鞘疾病

除了在活检标本中发现进行性多灶性脑白质病，脱髓鞘疾病通常是在临床或尸检过程中发现的（表18.3）。

和继发于轴突脱失的髓鞘脱失相比，原发性脱髓鞘疾病仅仅累及髓鞘。原发性脱髓鞘疾病组织学特征包括髓鞘的崩解，大量的KP-1表达阳性的泡沫巨噬细胞，巨噬细胞内有髓鞘碎片和脂滴。在病变部位，NF阳性的轴突少见（图18.60）。如果病变是由病毒引起的，病变部位尤其是周边部分会查见双嗜色性包涵体。已知能引起脱髓鞘的病毒有HIV、JCV、SV40、巨细胞病毒、EB病毒和水痘-带状疱疹病毒。这些病毒可以通过免疫组化、ISH和PCR方法进行检测[39,40,213,214]。

主要的脱髓鞘疾病是多发性硬化症（MS）。MS应与其他疾病相鉴别，这些疾病的组织学表现及复发和缓解交替的临床症状都和MS相似。除了伴蛋白酶增加的大量的泡沫巨噬细胞以外，急性脱髓鞘病

变还包括血管周LCA阳性的淋巴细胞、EMA阳性和免疫球蛋白阳性的浆细胞、数量不等的GFAP阳性的神经胶质增生及少量CD34阳性的内皮细胞。巨噬细胞中Ⅱ类主要组织相容性抗原复合物（HLA-DR，Ia）表达阳性。巨噬细胞内有和吞噬作用有关的髓鞘碎片。少突胶质细胞一般仅在病变周边可见。急性斑块内可见血管壁损伤引起的血-脑屏障破裂，肌层内可见补体沉积在平滑肌细胞上以及HLA-DR阳性的巨噬细胞浸润[13]。

巨噬细胞在白质脱髓鞘的活动部位聚集，与少突胶质细胞瘤和血管母细胞瘤很相似（示意图18.1）[90,215,216]。KP-1可以用来确认巨噬细胞。少突胶质细胞瘤几乎无胞浆空泡，胞核居中，表达Leu7和S-100，这些特点可以与含脂质的巨噬细胞相鉴别。血管母细胞瘤比少突胶质细胞瘤的毛细血管有更强的Ⅷ

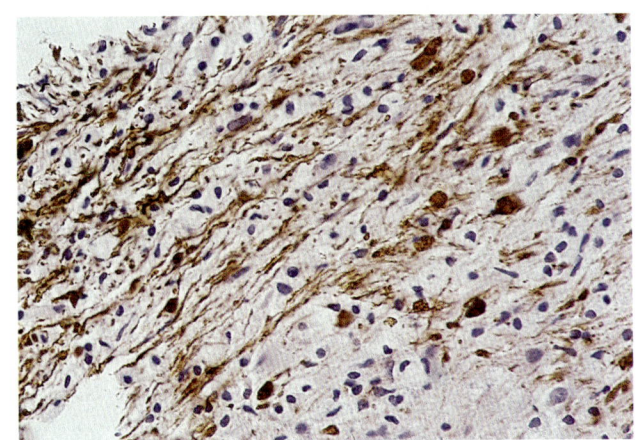

图18.60 原发性脱髓鞘病。可见棕色的NF阳性轴突存留。某些肿胀的的轴突被称为球状体。含脂质的巨噬细胞和神经胶质增生在该脑活检标本的切片中未染色，但是仍可看出它们是灰白色的

表18.14 神经变性疾病包涵体的免疫表型				
包涵体	泛素（HAR）[a]	tau（HAR）[a]	α-synuclein（甲酸）[a]	β-amyloid（甲酸）[a]
AD缠结	+	+	-	-
AD轴突斑块	+轴突	+轴突	S斑块	+斑块
路易小体	+	-	+	-
Pick小体	+	+	-[b]	-
额颞叶痴呆或运动神经元疾病	+	+	-	-
多系统萎缩	+GCIs	S GCIs	+GCIs	-

染色结果判断：+，弥漫强阳性；S，部分阳性
a 可采用抗原修复技术
b 据报道，Pick小体和轴突可用蛋白酶K抗原修复
AD，阿尔茨海默病；GCIs，胶质细胞包涵体；HAR，抗原热修复，枸橼酸盐缓冲液微波修复
（引自McKeever PE, Boyer PJ. The brain, spinal cord, and meninges. In :Mills SE, Carter D, Greenson, JK, et al., eds. Sternberg's Diagnostic Surgical Pathology, 4th ed. New York: Lippincott Williams & Wilkins; 2004: 399-506）

因子和CD31表达，Leu7（CD57）表达较弱。位于脱髓鞘部位的含脂质的巨噬细胞可以通过组织化学或电镜与肿瘤相鉴别，电镜下可见髓鞘被吞噬后形成的小的圆形球体[68]。

在周围神经中，KP-1（CD68）阳性的巨噬细胞吞噬髓鞘并在神经内膜血管周围聚集[217]。在慢性炎症性脱髓鞘性多发性神经病变（CIDP）中[218]，神经内膜周围有大量的具有CD3、CD4和CD8免疫活性的T淋巴细胞，无B淋巴细胞。在CIPD和格林-巴利综合征中都以T淋巴细胞为主（图18.61）[217]。

癫 痫

复杂部分性癫痫发作（以前称做颞叶癫痫）主要累及颞叶、额叶、顶叶或枕叶[219-223]。大约80%的复杂部分性癫痫发作位于颞叶，因此最常见的难治性癫痫的手术治疗是颞叶切除术[219]。神经元染色和GFAP染色可以对最常见的病变神经元丢失和反应性GFAP+胶质增生进行检测和神经解剖定位，对照采用年龄匹配的尸检中的颞叶组织（图18.62、18.63、表18.3）[3]。

神经元缺失可以引起神经胶质增生，两者在对缺氧敏感的海马中常见（图18.62）。大的锥体神经元非常敏感，阿蒙角（cornu ammonis）1区（CA1）的Sommer部的神经元更为敏感，而CA2区神经元敏感性稍低。神经元标记物特别是突触素经常在GFAP的对照染色中被削减。破碎的手术切除标本可能混淆上述区域（图18.62），但是CA4区明显由位于齿状回的、密集的、小的、表达突触素的神经元环绕。其他区域可以根据它们和CA4区的联系、齿状回的开放和海马回下角大神经元的增宽等表现找到（图18.62）。NF和突触素染色可以帮助辨认这些碎组织的神经解剖部位。

皮质畸形

解剖病理学家、儿科病理学家和外科病理学家通常会发现大脑结构的畸形。神经元标记物，例如Neu-N、突触素和神经丝（NF），加上HE染色、S-100和GFAP，可以用来找到皮质异常区域。它们还可以对异常细胞进行分类[3]。

微小发育不全指的是仅在显微镜下才能看到的病变：①在灰质或白质中，NF阳性的神经节细胞之间掺杂有局灶性S-100蛋白阳性的少突胶质细胞灶；②少突胶质细胞增生太小且分化很好，不能诊断少突胶质细胞瘤；并且③白质中正常情况下数量很少的神经元数量增加。皮质发育不全包括皮质结构破坏和异常增大的细胞，其中有些细胞IHC为神经元染色，有些为GFAP阳性的星形细胞，有些单个细胞为神经胶质和神经元染色均阳性[74]。结节性硬化的皮质结节是皮质的异型增生。

海马内可见锥形神经元细胞和颗粒神经元细胞丢失、大量的淀粉样小体（图18.62、18.63）、血管周巨噬细胞内含铁血黄素沉积、局灶性脑膜纤维化、钙化和大量锥体神经元的铁化[3]。在切除的颞叶新皮质中，白质和灰质的细胞结构研究可以揭示神经元细胞的发育异常，如神经元异位、神经元聚集和软脑膜下胶质增生[13]。

在将要手术切除的部位的深层和表层有时放入电极以监测和评估癫痫活动性发作。如果病人用了这种电极，手术医生应告知病理医师。这些电极可能导致伴有慢性炎症的脑软化，可见A6和L26阳性的T和B淋巴细胞、KP-1阳性的巨噬细胞，也可以导致手术标本的出血[223]。表层的电极可以导致局灶性脑膜炎。

在单个标本中可以发现各种各样临床上未预期的病理改变。对部分性癫痫发作的脑部病变进行立体定位切除时，可能发现血管畸形和神经胶质肿瘤。原发性脑肿瘤可表现为难治性癫痫，一般是低级别神经胶质瘤、神经胶质和神经元或两者兼有的混合瘤、错构瘤或胚胎发育不良性神经上皮性肿瘤（图18.13A、18.21A、18.30）[223, 224]。

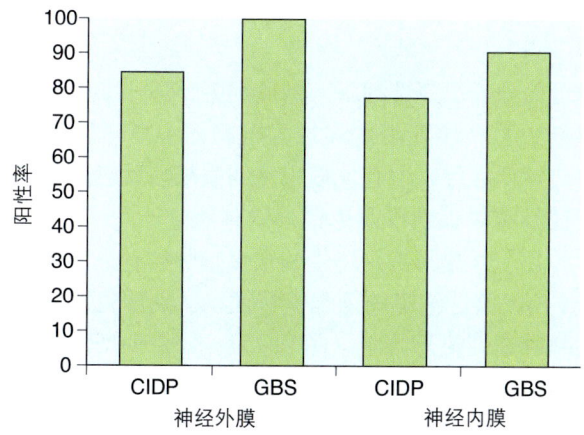

图18.61　13例慢性炎症性脱髓鞘性多发性神经病变（CIDP）和22例格林-巴利综合征中，腓肠肌神经内T淋巴细胞的定位。阳性百分数和Schmidt B等人报道的一致（Schmidt B, Toyka KV和Keifer R, et al. Inflammatory infiltrates in sural nerve biopsies in Guillain-Barré syndrome and chronic inflammatory demyelinating neuropathy. Muscle Nerve 1996;19:474-487）

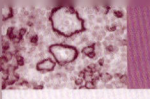

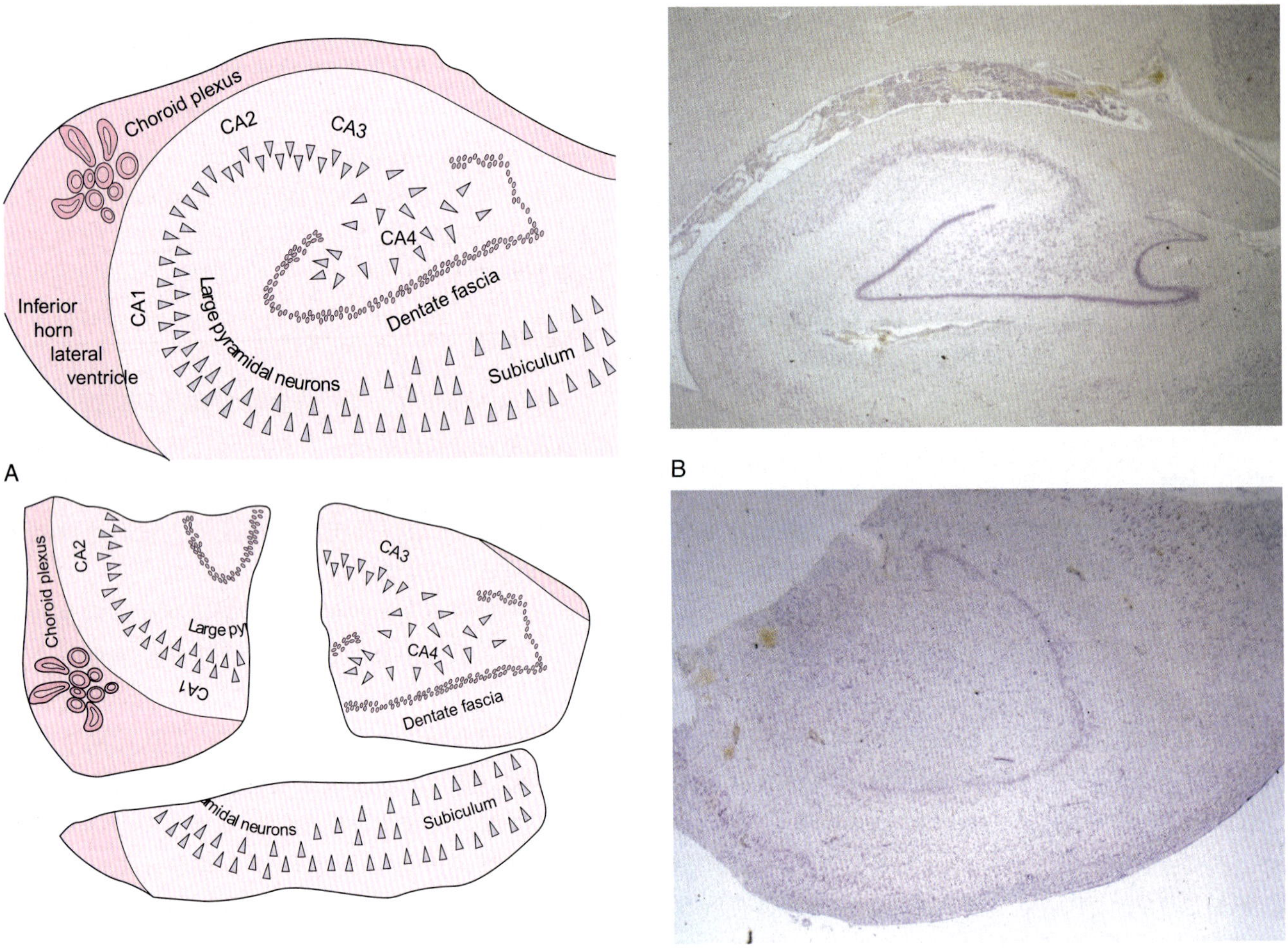

图18.62 显示海马阿蒙角（CA）的两种方式。(A) 手术切除标本或尸检标本断面的简图，可见大的锥形神经元和由密集的、小的并有圆形细胞核的神经元组成的齿状回。CA区背侧的相邻脑组织（图上方）可能呈现在尸检标本中，但不出现在手术切除标本中。侧面的颞叶组织（图左）在两种标本中都可能存在。实际尸检过程中看到的正常海马的位置和简图相似，可见Nissl染色的神经元（B）。(C) 简图示破碎的手术标本，仍可辨认出被齿状回围绕的CA4区、衬覆于脑室的室管膜细胞和齿状回连续线状分布的小的神经元之间的CA1区。实际的手术标本及比简图略大的破碎部分，可以看到神经元丢失，特别是在CA1和CA4区（D）

诊断中的陷阱

真的是阴性吗？

标本的标记物表达是否为真阴性，这个简单的问题必须要认真考虑以避免错误的判断。无论何时都要设立标记物阳性对照，像前面所描述的那样，采用已确定病变的组织块（图18.64）。阳性对照采用不同组织无效。如果对照组织没有染色，那么病变就不能用此次免疫组化染色来评价。

细胞是真阳性吗？

好的核复染对正确分析免疫组化结果很重要。复染可以分辨反应性细胞、肿瘤细胞、坏死细胞及神经解剖关系。坏死细胞表现为核固缩、核碎裂及核溶解。坏死区可以引起免疫组化的假阳性反应。这两种特征都需要识别以避免错误的判断。

反应性星形细胞增生和很多脑肿瘤有关，必须检查GFAP阳性细胞的细胞核特征以区别反应性星形细胞和肿瘤性星形细胞（图18.25）。如果免疫组化阳性反应紧邻细胞核应仔细检查，以正确确定这些细胞。这种准则普遍适用于其他标记物（图18.16B、18.52）。

肿瘤细胞有不典型或多形性细胞核，染色质分布常很特别（图18.12B）。胶质瘤的细胞核很密集。WHO Ⅲ级或更高级别的胶质瘤和其他恶性肿瘤可见较多核分裂象（图18.9A、18.9C、18.25A）。

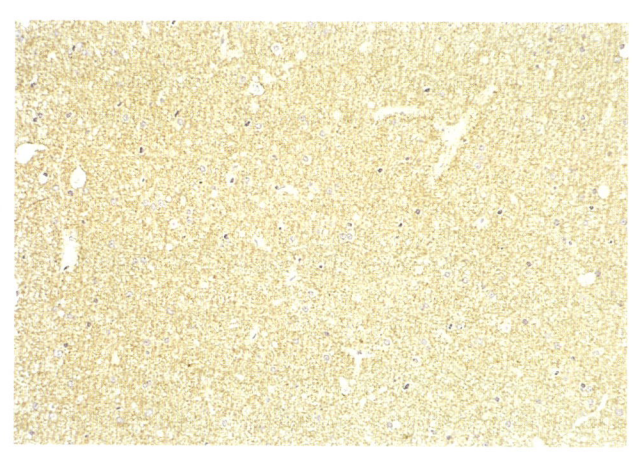

图18.63 患几十年复杂性部分性癫痫患者,图中所示为海马CA1区的锥形细胞层。在视野的一侧靠近血管的地方可见两个大的、透明的GFAP阴性神经元。其他的神经元已经死亡。尽管可见大量的棕色GFAP阳性胶质增生的纤维,但是星形细胞处于静止状态,细胞核周围几乎看不到棕色的胞浆。圆形、模糊状、淡紫色细胞核大小的小体是淀粉样小体,在此类标本中常见。神经元丢失和胶质增生在多年前已经出现

神经胶质增生和胶质瘤

脱髓鞘疾病可能和肿瘤相混淆是因为它也有大量的胶质增生[216]。细胞体积大,染色体短,在胞浆内散在分布,这些特点和胶质瘤的核分裂象很相似[215]。如果在脑实质内血管周围发现大量的KP-1阳性的含脂质的巨噬细胞,可以考虑诊断脱髓鞘疾病。诊断时应考虑髓鞘染色、轴突NF染色(示意图18.2)和下面要提到的神经胶质增生和胶质瘤的特征(图18.3A、18.12A和B、18.60)。

区分神经胶质增生和胶质瘤可能非常困难(图18.10A)[3]。弥漫性胶质瘤可以浸润脑组织并刺激胶质增生,这样使问题变得复杂起来。在胶质增生和胶质瘤中都可以发现肿胀的GFAP阳性细胞(表18.15)。区别胶质瘤细胞和胶质增生及正常脑实质的特征包括各个细胞GFAP染色各不相同、核深染(图18.12B)、核聚集、核变形(图18.14)、核分裂象和钙化。核分裂象不仅可以证实肿瘤是胶质瘤,而且可以说明恶性程度较高。在胶质瘤的边缘常见胶质细胞核大小和形状的异常。

在星形细胞瘤、室管膜瘤和星形细胞胶质瘤中,GFAP是胶质细胞的理想标记物。在胶质增生和胶质瘤中,GFAP都是在胞浆内表达,因此这些细胞的判断很容易。高的核浆比是胶质瘤的典型特征。围以较少细胞浆的核分裂(图18.25A)在胶质细胞增生中极其少见(图18.25B),反应性星形细胞核浆比较低,有大量棕褐色的星状突起,细胞间空隙很大,看上去像果园里的苹果树(图18.2)。增殖的免疫组化标记物如MIB-1可以帮助区别胶质瘤和胶质增生。

胶质瘤是膨胀性生长,与胶质增生形成对比。但是如果没有系列X射线照相,没有对肿块和边缘融合的原位观察,很难排除其他肿瘤边缘胶质增生的可能性。

颗粒性钙化在增生的神经胶质中分散存在,将胶

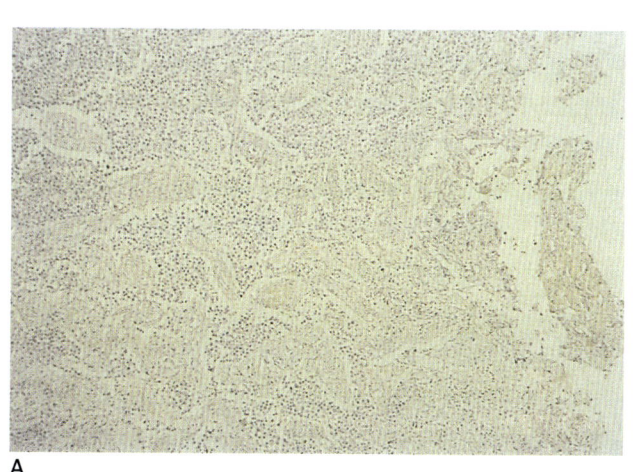
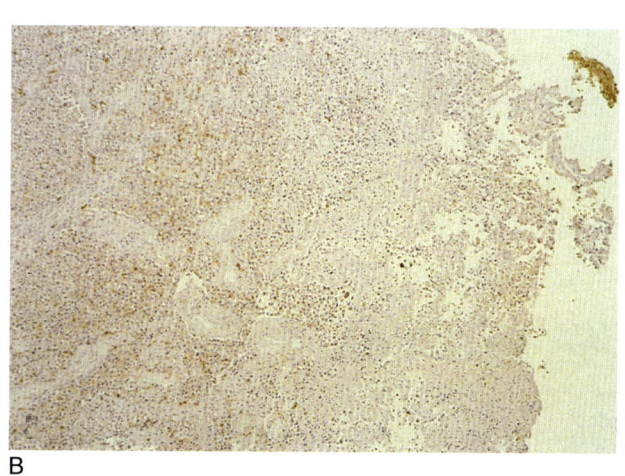

A   B

图18.64 免疫组化内对照的重要性。两个肿瘤切片边缘的小碎块组织和两张切片的角都是脑组织。脑组织总是表达S-100蛋白,因此用来作阳性内对照。两组实验都检测S-100蛋白。(A)第一组实验中肿瘤和脑组织均没有S-100的染色。(B)第二组实验脑组织和肿瘤组织都被染成棕黄色。只有第二组实验对S-100的检测是可信的,显示肿瘤组织S-100阳性。接着HMB-45染色提示转移性黑色素瘤,最终查见皮肤的原发性肿瘤(引自McKeever PE. New methods of brain tumor analysis. In: Mena H, ed. Dr. Kenneth M. Earle Memorial Neuropathology Review, Washington, DC: Armed Forces Institute of Pathology; February 24, 2000)

表18.15 肿胀的GFAP阳性细胞类型

病变	GFAP阳性细胞间的关系	GFAP的细胞内分布	细胞核特征	其他组织
反应性胶质增生	分散	低核浆比值，纤维化高，细胞突起最长	光滑，卵圆形，染色质细	NF阳性轴突正常
原浆性星形细胞瘤	黏着，凝集	部分细胞有长的突起	多形性，细长形，染色质浓染	NF阳性轴突分散
有小原浆性星形细胞的少突胶质细胞瘤	黏着，凝集	细胞突起最短，混合有阴性的少突胶质细胞	光滑，圆形，染色质浓染	NF阳性轴突分散

质瘤与胶质增生和正常的白质区分开来[150]。要注意的是，在0.5cm大的组织内不能过度诠释神经元细胞和神经纤维网间的钙化。尽管微囊、钙化和核分裂是胶质瘤的重要诊断特征，但不能在每一例肿瘤中都观察到，而且在侵犯中枢神经系统实质的胶质瘤的边缘也不常见。

另外一个区别胶质瘤边缘和神经胶质增生的重要特征是细胞密度（表18.2）。一些胶质瘤的细胞密度分部不均一（图18.11）。其他的特征是胶质瘤可能使白质和灰质之间的界限模糊。还有一些胶质瘤会产生舍雷尔（Scjerer）二级结构。这些二级结构使软脑膜下或神经元周围的肿瘤胶质集中，是软脑膜下和神经元旁神经胶质瘤病的特征性结构[171]。GFAP染色可以将二级结构和星形细胞瘤区分开。少突胶质细胞瘤的二级结构中的突触素的表达远远少于灰质的神经纤维网，并且当神经元和血管周围的细胞染色较浅时，二级结构更加明显[58]。

胶质瘤的细胞核相互密切接触甚至互相交错（图18.14、表18.15），甚至在弥散分布于胶质瘤边缘的细胞也是如此。但是胶质增生中GFAP阳性的星形细胞分布是均匀的（图18.2）。低倍镜下抗GFAP染色可以更清楚地观察到均匀的细胞间隙，高倍镜下可以看到神经胶质增生的低的核浆比。由于胶质瘤的多形性明显高于正常或胶质增生的中枢神经系统实质，多形性核和细胞核质浓染（苏木精复染最易观察）可帮助诊断胶质瘤（图18.8～18.10、18.12、18.14）[5, 87]。

浸润和非浸润细胞

非浸润性胶质瘤一般是可以手术切除的，这个特点在与浸润性胶质瘤鉴别时非常重要。但是在破碎或不完整的标本中很难判断。

在肿瘤性神经元的可能性被除外后（见神经元肿瘤部分），脑组织神经解剖对鉴别非浸润和浸润性胶质瘤来说非常有用。轴突在白质中密集平行排列，灰质中也是如此。非浸润性胶质瘤中轴突走向正常（图18.11B），但是浸润性胶质瘤中的轴突分散（图18.11A），部分发生肿胀。突触素在灰质的神经纤维中表达，呈棕色点状分布。突触素阴性的胶质瘤细胞或者突然中断，或者浸润这些纤细的点状分布[58]。

在不能分辨的脑组织中，肿瘤染色后仍然可以进行鉴别。如果胶质瘤中发现非肿瘤源性的轴突，则该肿瘤是浸润性胶质瘤（图18.14）。这个特点可以区分浸润性胶质瘤及非浸润性胶质瘤，非浸润性胶质瘤和正常脑组织有更分离的边缘。

脓肿和肿瘤

在中枢神经系统内能够产生胶原的实体性肿瘤可能与脓肿壁混淆（图18.4，表18.5、18.7、18.10、18.11）。如果组织活检过程中可疑于脓肿，无菌组织需送微生物室培养。即使组织培养结果阴性也比错过寻找有价值东西的机会好得多。若组织培养阴性，微生物染色可能会有所帮助。

肉瘤和促纤维增生性肿瘤以及具有胶原性囊壁的各类囊肿可与脓肿相似（图18.29B、18.33A、18.38）。这些肿瘤一般都没有炎症成分，而存在肿瘤性成分，可以通过这些进行鉴别。值得注意的是，如果囊肿壁破裂，并且有异物流到中枢神经系统内，例如胶样囊肿或是鳞状上皮细胞。如果HE染色不能辨别炎症反应中的这些异物，囊壁的免疫组织化学染色可以帮助诊断[188]，例如染上皮细胞的CK。这些病变局部是无菌的，不必做微生物染色（示意图18.2）。

发育不良和肿瘤

皮质发育不良和神经节细胞肿瘤鉴别比较困难。这里有一些应用IHC来鉴别发育不良和肿瘤的准则。发育不良含有不正常的组织结构，如神经元数目过多或层次增加、神经元异位，或体积异常大或小的神经元或神经胶质。它们可能很大，但不增殖。

神经性肿瘤的典型特点远不止结构的异常，还有细胞学的异常，包括双核、大核与奇异核、染色深。

以上特点在神经微丝或突触素染色以及高质量的苏木精复染中特别明显。当可疑病变与来自其他病例的同一部位的正常标本或尸检标本进行对照时，它们很容易被辨认。

肿瘤细胞增殖明显，MIB-1染色可测定肿瘤细胞的增殖潜能，其中有很多并不显示核分裂。在作者的染色中，发育不良MIB-1 LI一般低于3%，而肿瘤的则高于3%。取样和实验技术可能影响该结果。

致　谢

以下的同事提供了特别有用的帮助。Philip Boyer、Mila Blaivas、Jeanne Bell、Larry Junck 和 Ricardo Lloyd 博士提供了关键引文。感谢 Elizabeth Wawrzaszek、Dianna Banka 和 Peggy Otto 在撰写章节时给予的帮助。Mark Deming 和 Elizabeth Horn Walker精心准备了图释。Michigan大学医学中心病理学实验室的免疫病理学家和组织病理学家提供了质量上乘的切片。

本章的工作部分由美国公共医疗服务的 NIH CA68545 和 CA47558 基金资助。

参考文献

1. McKeever PE. New methods of brain tumor analysis. In: Mena H, Sandberg G, eds. Dr. Kenneth M. Earle memorial neuropathology review. Washington, DC: Armed Forces Institute of Pathology; 2004.
2. Kleihues P, Cavenee WK. World Health Organization classification of tumors: pathology and genetics of tumors of the nervous system. Lyon: IARC Press, 2000.
3. McKeever PE, Boyer P. The brain, spinal cord, and meninges. In: Mills SE, Carter D, Greenson JK, et al., eds. Sternberg's diagnostic surgical pathology. 4th edn. Philadelphia: Lippincott Williams & Wilkins; 2004:400–503.
4. Firlik KS, Martinez AJ, Lunsford LD. Use of cytological preparations for the intraoperative diagnosis of stereotactically obtained brain biopsies: a 19-year experience and survey of neuropathologists. J Neurosurg 1999; 91:454–458.
5. McKeever PE. Laboratory methods in brain tumor diagnosis. In: Nelson JS, Mena H, Parisi et al., eds. Principles and practice of neuropathology. 2nd edn. New York: Oxford University Press; 2003:272–297.
6. Kepes JJ, Moral LA, Wilkinson SB, et al. Rhabdoid transformation of tumor cells in meningiomas: A histologic indication of increased proliferative activity: Report of four cases. Am J Surg Pathol 1998; 22:231–238.
7. Graham DI, Lanto PL, eds. Greenfield's neuropathology. 7th edn. New York: Edward Arnold; 2002.
8. Garcia JH, Budka H, McKeever PE, et al, eds. Neuropathology: the diagnostic approach. Philadelphia: Mosby; 1997.
9. Castellani RJ, Parchi P, Madoff L, et al. Biopsy diagnosis of Creutzfeldt-Jakob disease by Western blot: a case report. Hum Pathol 1997; 28:623–641.
10. Mrak RE. The big eye in the 21st century: the role of electron microscopy in modern diagnostic neuropathology. J Neuropathol Exp Neurol 2002; 61:1027–1039.
11. Dickson DW, Bergeron C, Chin SS, et al. Office of Rare Diseases neuropathologic criteria for corticobasal degeneration. J Neuropathol Exp Neurol 2002; 61:935–946.
12. Dickson DW, ed. Neurodegeneration: the molecular pathology of dementia and movement disorders. Basel: ISN Neuropath Press; 2003.
13. McKeever PE. Immunohistochemistry of the nervous system. In: Dabbs D, ed. Diagnostic immunohistochemistry. Philadelphia: Churchill Livingstone; 2002:559–624.
14. Ellison D, Love S, Chimelli L, et al., eds, Neuropathology. Amsterdam: Elsevier; 2003.
15. McKeever PE, Balentine JD. Macrophage migration through the brain parenchyma to the perivascular space following particle ingestion. Am J Pathol 1978; 93:153–164.
16. Danton GH, Dietrich WD. Inflammatory mechanisms after ischemia and stroke. J Neuropathol Exp Neurol 2003; 62: 127–136.
17. McKeever PE, Fligiel SEG, Varani J, et al. Products of cells cultured from gliomas. IV: Extracellular matrix proteins of gliomas. Int J Cancer 1986; 37:867–874.
18. Thomson RB Jr, Bertram H. Laboratory diagnosis of central nervous system infections. Infec Dis Clin North Am 2001; 15:1047–1071.
19. Park Y, Kim JY, Chi KU, et al. Comparison of polymerase chain reaction with histopathologic features for diagnosis of tuberculosis in formalin-fixed, paraffin-embedded histologic specimens. Arch Pathol Lab Med 2003; 127:326–330.
20. Kaufman L, Standard PG, Jalbert M, et al. Immunohistologic identification of *Aspergillus* spp. and other hyaline fungi by using polyclonal fluorescent antibodies. J Clin Microbiol

1997; 35:2206–2209.

21. Guarner J, Greer PW, Bartlett J, et al. Congenital syphilis in a newborn: An immunopathologic study. Mod Pathol 1999; 12:82–87.

22. Shankar SK, Ravi V, Suryanarayana V, et al. Immunoreactive antigenic sites of *Cysticercus cellulosae* relevant to human neurocysticercosis – immunocytochemical localization using human CSF as source of antibody. Clin Neuropathol 1995; 14:33–36.

23. Diogo CM, Mendonca MC, Savino W, et al. Immunoreactivity of a cytokeratin-related polypeptide from adult *Schistosoma mansoni*. Int J Parasitol 1994; 24:727–732.

24. Schwartz MA, Selhorts JB, Ochs AL, et al. Oculomasticatory myorrhythmia: A unique movement disorder occurring in Whipple's disease. Ann Neurol 1986; 20:677–683.

25. Cadavid D, Barbour AG. Neuroborreliosis during relapsing fever: Review of the clinical manifestations, pathology, and treatment of infections in humans and experimental animals. Clin Infect Dis 1998; 26:151–164.

26. Cassady KA, Whitley RJ. Pathogenesis and pathophysiology of viral infections of the central nervous system. In: Scheld WM, Whitley RJ, Durack DT, eds. Infections of the central nervous system, 2nd edn. Philadelphia: Lippincott-Raven; 1997:7–22.

27. Fleming KA. Analysis of viral pathogenesis by in situ hybridization. J Pathol 1992; 166:95–96.

28. Mrak RE, Young L. Rabies encephalitis in humans: Pathology, pathogenesis and pathophysiology. J Neuropathol Exp Neurol 1994; 53:1–10.

29. McQuaid S, Cosby SL, Koffi K, et al. Distribution of measles virus in the central nervous system of HIV-seropositive children. Acta Neuropathol 1998; 96:637–642.

30. Gray F, Chretien F, Vallat-Decouvelaere AV, et al. The changing pattern of HIV neuropathology in the HAART era. J Neuropathol Exp Neurol 2003; 62:429–444.

31. Nath A, Sinai AP. Cerebral toxoplasmosis. Curr Treat Options Neurol 2003; 5:3–12.

32. Zimmer C, Daeschlein G, Patt S, et al. Strategy for diagnosis of *Toxoplasma gondii* in stereotactic brain biopsies. Stereotact Funct Neurosurg 1991; 56:66–75.

33. Rhodes RH. Histopathology of the central nervous system in the acquired immunodeficiency syndrome. Hum Pathol 1987; 18:636–643.

34. Persons DL, Moore JA, Fishback JL. Comparison of polymerase chain reaction, DNA hybridization, and histology with viral culture to detect cytomegalovirus in immunosuppressed patients. Mod Pathol 1991; 4:149–152.

35. Vazeux R, Cumont M, Girard PM, et al. Severe encephalitis resulting from coinfections with HIV and JC virus. Neurology 1990; 40:944–948.

36. Daley CL, Small PM, Schecter GF, et al. An outbreak of tuberculosis with accelerated progression among persons infected with the human immunodeficiency virus. N Engl J Med 1992; 4:231–235.

37. Feraru ER, Aronow HA, Lipton RB. Neurosyphilis in AIDS patients: Initial CSF VDRL may be negative. Neurology 1990; 40:541–543.

38. Martinez AJ, Visvesvara GS. Free-living, amphizoic and opportunistic amebas. Brain Pathol 1997; 7:583–598.

39. Prayson RA, Estes ML. Stereotactic brain biopsy for diagnosis of progressive multifocal leukoencephalopathy. South Med J 1993; 86:1381–1394.

40. Hulette CM, Downey BT, Burger PC. Progressive multifocal leukoencephalopathy: Diagnosis by in situ hybridization with a biotinylated JC virus DNA probe using an automated histomatic code-on slide stainer. Am J Surg Pathol 1991; 15: 791–797.

41. Hulette CM, Earl NL, Crain BJ. Evaluation of cerebral biopsies for the diagnosis of dementia. Arch Neurol 1992; 49:28–31.

42. Capellari S, Vital C, Parchi P, et al. Familial prion disease with a novel 144-bp insertion in the prion protein gene in a Basque family. Neurology 1997; 49:133–141.

43. Bruce ME, Will RG, Ironside JW, et al. Transmissions to mice indicate that 'new variant' CJD is caused by the BSE agent. Nature 1997; 389:498–501.

44. Kovacs GG, Head MW, Hegy I, et al. Immunohistochemistry for the prion protein: comparison of different monoclonal antibodies in human prion disease subtypes. Brain Pathol 2002; 12:1–11.

45. Ironside JW, Sutherland K, Bell JE, et al. A new variant of Creutzfeldt-Jakob disease: Neuropathological and clinical features. Cold Spring Harb Symp Quant Biol 1996; 50:523–527.

46. Vinters HV, Secor DL, Pardridge WM, et al. Immunohistochemical study of cerebral amyloid angiopathy. III: Wide-

spread Alzheimer A4 peptide in cerebral microvessel walls colocalizes with gamma trace in patients with leukoencephalopathy. Ann Neurol 1990; 28:34–42.

47. Chen ST, Chen SD, Hsu CY, et al. Progression of hypertensive intracerebral hemorrhage. Neurology 1989; 39:1509–1514.

48. Kittner SJ, Sharkness CM, Sloan MA, et al. Infarcts with a cardiac source of embolism in the NINDS stroke data bank: Neurologic examination. Neurology 1992; 42:299–302.

49. Miettinen M, Lindenmayer AE, Chaubal A. Endothelial cell markers CD31, CD34, and BNH9 antibody to H- and Yantigens – evaluation of their specificity and sensitivity in the diagnosis of vascular tumors and comparison with von Willebrand factor. Mod Pathol 1994; 7:82–90.

50. Takahashi A, Ushiki T, Abe K, et al. Cytoarchitecture of periendothelial cells in human cerebral venous vessels as compared with the scalp vein: A scanning electron microscopic study. Arch Histol Cytol 1994; 57:331–339.

51. Lanthier S, Lottie A, Michaud J, et al. Isolated angiitis of the CNS in children. Neurology 2001; 56:837–842.

52. Jennekens FG, Kater L. The central nervous system in systemic lupus erythematosus. Parts 1 and 2. Rheumatology 2002; 41:605–630.

53. McKelvie PA, Collins S, Thyagarajan D, et al. Meningoencephalomyelitis with vasculitis due to varicella zoster virus: a case report and review of the literature. Pathology 2002; 34:88–93.

54. Markus HS, Martin RJ, Simpson MA, et al. Diagnostic strategies in CADASIL. Neurology 2002; 59;1134–1138.

55. Fleetwood IG, Steinberg GK. Arteriovenous malformations. Lancet 2002; 359:863–873.

56. McKeever PE. Molecular neuropathology in brain tumor diagnosis. In: Kornblith PL, Walker MD, eds. Advances in neuro-oncology II. Armonk, New York: Futura; 1997:139–178.

57. McKeever PE. Insights about brain tumors gained through immunohistochemistry and in situ hybridization of nuclear and phenotypic markers. J Histochem Cytochem 1998; 46:585–594.

58. McKeever PE. Neurofilament (NF) and synaptophysin stains reveal diagnostic and prognostic patterns of interaction between normal and neoplastic tissues. Presented at the annual meeting of the Histochemical Society, Bethesda, MD, March 24, 2000.

59. Shi S-R, Cote RJ, Taylor CR. Antigen retrieval immunohistochemistry: Past, present, and future. J Histochem Cytochem 1997; 45:327–343.

60. McKeever PE, Ross DA, Strawderman MS, et al. A comparison of the predictive power for survival in gliomas provided by MIB-1, bromodeoxyuridine and proliferating cell nuclear antigen with histopathologic and clinical parameters. J Neuropathol Exp Neurol 1997; 7:798–805.

61. McKeever PE, Junck L, Strawderman MS, et al. Proliferation index is related to patient age in glioblastoma. Neurology 2001; 56:1216–1108.

62. McKeever PE, Strawderman MS, Yamini B, et al. MIB-1 proliferation index predicts survival among patients with grade II astrocytoma. J Neuropathol Exp Neurol 1998; 57:931–936.

63. Hsu DW, Louis DN, Efird JT, et al. Use of MIB-1 (Ki-67) immunoreactivity in differentiating grade II and grade III gliomas. J Neuropathol Exp Neurol 1997; 56:857–865.

64. Aboussekhra A, Wood RD. Detection of nucleotide excision repair incisions in human fibroblasts by immunostaining for PCNA. Exp Cell Res 1995; 221:326–332.

65. Schiffer D, Cavalla P, Migheli A, et al. Apoptosis and cell proliferation in human neuroepithelial tumors. Neurosci Lett 1995; 195:81–84.

66. Taniguchi K, Wakabayashi T, Yoshida T, et al. Immunohistochemical staining of DNA topoisomerase II alpha in human gliomas. J Neurosurg 1999; 91:477–482.

67. Chronwall BM, McKeever PE, Kornblith PL. Glial and nonglial neoplasms evaluated on frozen section by double immunofluorescence for fibronectin and glial fibrillary acidic protein. Acta Neuropathol (Berl) 1983; 59:283–287.

68. McKeever PE, Balentine JD. Histochemistry of the nervous system. In: Spicer SS, ed. Histochemistry in pathologic diagnosis. New York: Marcel-Dekker; 1987:871–957.

69. Reifenberger G, Louis DN. Oligodendroglioma: toward molecular definitions in diagnostic neuro-oncology. J Neuropathol Exp Neurol 2003; 62:111–126.

70. Rodas RA, Fenstermaker RA, McKeever PE, et al. Correlation of intraluminal thrombosis in brain tumor vessels with postoperative thrombotic complications. J Neurosurg 1998; 89:200–205.

71. Cheng Y, Pang JC, Ng HK, et al. Pilocytic astrocytomas do not show most of the genetic changes commonly seen in dif-

fuse astrocytomas. Histopathology 2000; 37:437–444.

72. Korshunov A, Golanov A, Timirgaz V. Immunohistochemical markers for intracranial ependymoma recurrence. An analysis of 88 cases. J Neurological Sciences 2000; 177:72–82.

73. Rubinstein LJ. Tumors of the central nervous system. Washington, DC: Armed Forces Institute of Pathology;1972.

74. Burger PC, Scheithauer BW, Vogel FS. Surgical pathology of the nervous system and its coverings. 4th edn. New York: Churchill Livingstone; 2002.

75. Burger PC, Scheithauer BW. Atlas of tumor pathology: tumors of the central nervous system. Washington, D.: Armed Forces Institute of Pathology; 1994.

76. McKeever PE, Blaivas M, Gebarski SS. Sellar tumors other than adenomas. In: Thapar K, Kovacs K, Scheithauer BW, et al., eds. Diagnosis and management of pituitary tumors. Totowa, NJ: Humana Press; 2001:387–447.

77. Hayostek C, Shaw EG, Scheithauer BW, et al. Astrocytomas of the cerebellum: A comparative clinicopathologic study of pilocytic and diffuse astrocytomas. Cancer 1993; 72:856–869.

78. Forsyth PA, Shaw EG, Scheithauer BW, et al. 51 cases of supratentorial pilocytic astrocytomas: a clinicopathologic, prognostic, and flow cytometric study. Cancer 1993; 72:1335–1342.

79. Coakley KJ, Huston J, Scheithauer BW, et al. Pilocytic astrocytomas: Well-demarcated magnetic resonance appearance despite frequent infiltration histologically. Mayo Clin Proc 1995; 70:747–751.

80. Clark GB, Henry JM, McKeever PE. Cerebral pilocytic astrocytoma. Cancer 1985; 56:1128–1133.

81. Hitotsumatsu T, Iwaki T, Fukui M, et al. Distinctive immunohistochemical profiles of small heat shock proteins (heat shock protein 27 and alpha B-crystallin) in human brain tumors. Cancer 1996; 77:352–361.

82. Camby I, Lefranc F, Titeca G, et al. Differential expression of S100 calcium-binding proteins characterizes distinct clinical entities in both WHO grade II and III astrocytic tumours. Neuropathol Applied Neurobiol 2000; 26:76–90.

83. Biegel JA. Genetics of pediatric central nervous system tumors. J Pediatr Hematol/Oncol 1997; 19:492–501.

84. Rao RD, James CD. Altered molecular pathways in gliomas: an overview of clinically relevant issues. Semin Oncol 2004; 31:595–604.

85. Bigner SH, Schrock E. Molecular cytogenetics of brain tumors. J Neuropathol Exp Neurol 1997; 56:1173–1181.

86. Ho DM, Wong TT, Hsu CY, et al. MIB-1 labeling index in nonpilocytic astrocytoma of childhood: A study of 101 cases. Cancer 1998; 82:2459–2466.

87. McKeever PE, Blaivas M, Nelson JS. Diagnosis of nervous system tumors by light microscopic methods. In: Garcia JH, Budka H, McKeever PE, et al, eds. Neuropathology: the diagnostic approach. Philadelphia: CV Mosby; 1997:193–218.

88. Kimura N, Watanabe M, Date F, et al. HMB-45 and tuberin in hamartomas associated with tuberous sclerosis. Mod Pathol 1997; 10:952–959.

89. Levy RA, Allen R, McKeever P. Pleomorphic xanthoastrocytoma presenting with massive intracranial hemorrhage. AJNR 1996; 17:154–156.

90. Gokden M, Roth KA, Carroll SL, et al. Clear cell neoplasms and pseudoneoplastic lesions of the central nervous system. Semin Diagn Pathol 1997; 14:253–269.

91. Powell SZ, Yachnis AT, Rorke LB, et al. Divergent differentiation in pleomorphic xanthoastrocytoma: evidence for a neuronal element and possible relationship to ganglion cell tumors. Am J Surg Pathol 1996; 20:80–85.

92. Kaulich K, Blaschke B, Numann A, et al. Genetic alterations commonly found in diffusely infiltrating cerebral gliomas are rare or absent in pleomorphic xanthoastrocytomas. J Neuropathol Exp Neurol 2002; 61:1092–1099.

93. Martinez-Diaz H, Kleinschmidt-DeMasters BK, Powell SZ, et al. Giant cell glioblastoma and pleomorphic xanthoastrocytoma show different immunohistochemical profiles for neuronal antigens and p53 but share reactivity for class III beta-tubulin. Arch Pathol Lab Med 2003; 127:1187–1191.

94. Figarella-Branger D, Gambarelli D, Dollo C, et al. Infratentorial ependymomas of childhood: Correlation between histologic features, immunohistological phenotype, silver nucleolar organizer region staining values and postoperative survival in 16 cases. Acta Neuropathol (Berl) 1991; 82:208–216.

95. Mason WP, Krol GS, DeAngelis LM. Low-grade oligodendroglioma responds to chemotherapy. Neurology 1996; 46:203–207.

96. Yong WH, Chou D, Ueki K, et al. Chromosome 19q deletions in human gliomas overlap telomeric to D19S219 and

may target a 425 kb region centromeric to D19S112. J Neuropathol Exp Neurol 1995; 54:622–626.

97. Dehghani F, Schachenmayr W, Laun A, et al. Prognostic implication of histopathological, immunohistochemical and clinical features of oligodendrogliomas: a study of 89 cases. Acta Neuropathol 1998; 95:493–504.

98. Coons SW, Johnson PC, Pearl DK. The prognostic significance of Ki-67 labeling indices for oligodendrogliomas. Neurosurgery 1997; 41:878–884.

99. Reifenberger G, Louis DN. Oligodendroglioma: toward molecular definitions in diagnostic neuro-oncology. J Neuropathol Exp Neurol 2003; 62:111–126.

100. Schröck E, Thiel G, Lozanova T, et al. Comparative hybridization of human malignant gliomas reveals multiple amplification sites and nonrandom chromosomal gains and losses. Am J Pathol 1994; 144:1203–1218.

101. McKeever PE, Dennis TR, Burgess AC, et al. Chromosomal breakpoint at 17q11.2 and insertion of DNA from three different chromosomes in a glioblastoma with exceptional glial fibrillary acidic protein expression. Cancer Genet Cytogenet 1996; 87:41–47.

102. Horiguchi H, Hirose T, Kannuki S, et al. Gliosarcoma: An immunohistochemical, ultrastructural and fluorescence in situ hybridization study. Pathol Int 1998; 48:595–602.

103. Liu L, Ichimura K, Pettersson EH, et al. Chromosome 7 rearrangements in glioblastomas: Loci adjacent to EGFR are independently amplified. J Neuropathol Exp Neurol 1998; 57:1138–1145.

104. Takekawa Y, Sawada T. Vascular endothelial growth factor and neovascularization in astrocytic tumors. Pathol Int 1998; 48:109–114.

105. Paulus W, Peiffer J. Intratumoral histologic heterogeneity of gliomas: a quantitative study. Cancer 1989; 64:442–447.

106. Davenport RD, McKeever PE. Ploidy of endothelium in high grade astrocytomas. Anal Quant Cytol Histol 1987; 9:25–29.

107. McKeever PE, Zhang K, Nelson JS, et al. Type IV collagen messenger RNA localizes within cells of abnormal vascular proliferations of glioblastoma and sarcomatous regions of gliosarcoma. J Histochem Cytochem 1993; 41:1124.

108. McKeever PE, Davenport RD, Shakui P. Patterns of antigenic expression in cultured glioma cells. Crit Rev Neurobiol 1991; 6:119–147.

109. Boerman RH, Anderl K, Herath J, et al. The glial and mesenchymal elements of gliosarcomas share similar genetic alterations. J Neuropathol Exp Neurol 1996; 55:973–981.

110. Oberc-Greenwood MA, McKeever PE, Kornblith PL, et al. A human ganglioglioma containing paired helical filaments. Hum Pathol 1984; 15:834–838.

111. Wirnsberg GH, Becker H, Ziervogel K, et al. Diagnostic immunohistochemistry of neuroblastic tumors. Am J Surg Pathol 1992; 15:49–57.

112. Laeng RH, Scheithauer BW, Altermatt HJ. Anti-neuronal nuclear autoantibodies, types 1 and 2: their utility in the study of tumors of the nervous system. Acta Neuropathol 1998; 96:329–339.

113. Goldbart A, Cheng ZJ, Brittian KR, et al. Intermittent hypoxia induces time-dependent changes in the protein kinase B signaling pathway in the hippocampal CA1 region of the rat. Neurobiology of Disease 2003; 14:440–446.

114. Felix I, Bilbao JM, Asa SL, et al. Cerebral and cerebellar gangliocytomas: a morphological study of nine cases. Acta Neuropathol 1994; 88:246–251.

115. Lindboe CF, Helseth E, Myhr G. Lhermitte-Duclos disease and giant meningioma as manifestations of Cowden's disease. Clin Neuropathol 1995; 14:327–330.

116. Daumas-Duport C, Varlet P, Bacha S, et al. Dysem-bryoplastic neuroepithelial tumors: nonspecific histological forms – a study of 40 cases. J Neurooncol 1999; 41:267–280.

117. Wolf HK, Buslei R, Blumcke I, et al. Neural antigens in oligodendrogliomas and dysembryoplastic neuroepithelial tumors. Acta Neuropathol 1997; 94:436–443.

118. Rout P, Santosh V, Mahadevan A, et al. Desmoplastic infantile ganglioglioma – clinicopathological and immunohistochemical study of four cases. Childs Nervous System 2002; 18:463–467.

119. Figarella-Branger D, Pellissier JF, Daumas-Duport C, et al. Central neurocytomas: critical evaluation of a small-cell neuronal tumor. Am J Surg Pathol 1992; 16:97–109.

120. Tong CY, Ng HK, Pang JC, et al. Central neurocytomas are genetically distinct from oligodendrogliomas and neuroblastomas. Histopathology 2000; 37:160–165.

121. Albrecht S, Rouah E, Becker LE, et al. Transthyretin immunoreactivity in choroid plexus neoplasms and brain metastases. Mod Pathol 1991; 4:610–614.

122. Kubo S, Ogino S, Fukushima T, et al. Immunocytochemical detection of insulin-like growth factor II (IGF-II) in choroid

plexus papilloma: A possible marker for differential diagnosis. Clin Neuropathol 1999; 18:74–79.

123. Kepes JJ, Collins J. Choroid plexus epithelium (normal and neoplastic) expresses synaptophysin: a potentially useful aid in differentiating carcinoma of the choroid plexus from metastatic papillary carcinomas. J Neuropathol Exp Neurol 1999; 58:398–401.

124. Varga Z, Vajtai I. Prognostic markers in the histopathological diagnosis of tumors of the choroid plexus. Orv Hetil 1998; 139:761–765.

125. Mena H, Rushing EJ, Ribas JL, et al. Tumors of pineal parenchymal cells: a correlation of histological features, including nucleolar organizer regions, with survival in 35 cases. Hum Pathol 1995; 26:20–30.

126. Roberts RO, Lynch CF, Jones MP, et al. Medulloblastoma: a population-based study of 532 cases. J Neuropathol Exp Neurol 1991; 50:134–144.

127. Gilhuis HJ, Anderi KL, Boerman RH, et al. Comparative genomic hybridization of medulloblastomas and clinical relevance: eleven new cases and a review of the literature. Neurol Clinical Neuro Neurosurg 2000; 102:203–209.

128. Tong CY, Hui AB, Yin XL, et al. Detection of oncogene amplifications in medulloblastomas by comparative genomic hybridization and array-based comparative genomic hybridization. J Neurosurg Spine 2004; 100:187–193.

129. Goldberg-Stern H, Gadoth N, Stern S, et al. The prognostic significance of glial fibrillary acidic protein staining in medulloblastoma. Cancer 1991; 68:568–573.

130. Katsetos CD, Herman MM, Frankfurter A, et al. Cerebellar desmoplastic medulloblastomas: a further immunohistochemical characterization of the reticulin-free pale islands. Arch Pathol Lab Med 1989; 113:1019–1029.

131. Freyer DR, Hutchinson RJ, McKeever PE. Primary primitive neuroectodermal tumor of the spinal cord associated with neural tube defect. Pediatr Neurosci 1989; 15:181–187.

132. Katayama Y, Kimura S, Watanabe T, et al. Peripheral-type primitive neuroectodermal tumor arising in the tentorium. J Neurosurg 1999; 90:141–144.

133. Rorke LB, Packer R, Biegel J. Central nervous system atypical teratoid/rhabdoid tumors of infancy and childhood. J Neurooncol 1995; 24:21–28.

134. Khoddami M, Becker LE. Immunohistochemistry of medulloepithelioma and neural tube. Pediatr Pathol Lab Med 1997; 17:913–925.

135. Mork SJ, Rubinstein LJ. Ependymoblastoma: A reappraisal of a rare embryonal tumor. Cancer 1985; 55:1536–1542.

136. Salvati M, Artico M, Lunardi P, et al. Intramedullary meningioma: case report and review of the literature. Surg Neurol 1992; 37:42–45.

137. Meis JM, Ordonez NG, Bruner JM. Meningiomas: An immunohistochemical study of 50 cases. Arch Pathol Lab Med 1986; 110:934–937.

138. Perry A, Scheithauer BW, Nascimento AG. The immunophenotypic spectrum of meningeal hemangiopericytoma: A comparison with fibrous meningioma and solitary fibrous tumor of meninges. Am J Surg Pathol 1997; 21:1354–1360.

139. Carneiro SS, Scheithauer BW, Nascimento AG, et al. Solitary fibrous tumor of the meninges: a lesion distinct from fibrous meningioma: a clinicopathologic and immunotochemical study. Am J Clin Pathol 1996; 106:217–224.

140. Kepes JJ. Meningiomas: biology, pathology, and differential diagnosis. Chicago: Year Book Medical; 1982.

141. Lattes R, Bigotti G. Lipoblastic meningioma: 'vacuolated meningioma.' Hum Pathol 1991; 22:164–171.

142. Ito H, Kawano N, Yada K, et al. Meningiomas differentiating to arachnoid trabecular cells: a proposal for histological subtype 'arachnoid trabecular cell meningioma.' Acta Neuropathol (Berl) 1991; 82:327–330.

143. Kulah A, Ilcayto R, Fiskeci C. Cystic meningiomas. Acta Neurochir (Wien) 1991; 111:108–113.

144. Winek RR, Scheithauer BW, Wick MR. Meningioma, meningeal hemangiopericytoma (angioblastic meningioma), peripheral hemangiopericytoma, and acoustic schwannoma: a comparative immunohistochemical study. Am J Surg Pathol 1989; 13:251–261.

145. Kobata H, Kondo A, Iwasaki K, et al. Chordoid meningioma in a child. J Neurosurg 1998; 88:319–323.

146. Probst-Cousin S, Villagran-Lillo R, Lahl R, et al. Secretory meningioma: clinical, histologic, and immunohistochemical findings in 31 cases. Cancer 1997; 79:2003–2015.

147. Alameda F, Lloreta J, Ferrer MD, et al. Clear cell meningioma of the lumbo-sacral spine with chordoid features. Ultrastruct Pathol 1999; 23:51–58.

148. Cerdá-Nicolás M, López-Ginés C, Peydró-Olaya A, et al. Histologic and cytogenetic patterns in benign, atypical, and

148. malignant meningiomas: does correlation with recurrence exist? Int J Surg Pathol 1995; 2:301–310.
149. Perry A, Scheithauer BW, Stafford SL, et al. 'Rhabdoid' meningioma: an aggressive variant. Am J Surg Pathol 1998; 22:1482–1490.
150. Kobayashi S, Haba R, Hirakawa E, et al. Cytology and immunohistochemistry of anaplastic meningiomas in squash preparations: a report of two cases. Acta Cytol 1995; 39:118–124.
151. Perry A, Scheithauer BW, Stafford SL, et al. 'Malignancy' in meningiomas: a clinicopathologic study of 116 patients, with grading implications. Cancer 1999; 85:2046–2056.
152. Prayson RA. Malignant meningioma: a clinicopathologic study of 23 patients including MIB-1 and p53 immunohistochemistry. Am J Clin Pathol 1996; 105:719–726.
153. Fletcher CD, Unni KK, Mertens F, eds. World Health Organization classification of tumors: pathology and genetics of tumors of soft tissue and bone. Lyon: IARC Press; 2002.
154. Probst-Cousin S, Rickert CH, Gullotta F. Factor XIIIa-immunoreactivity in tumors of the central nervous system. Clin Neuropathol 1998; 17:79–84.
155. Tihan T, Viglione M, Rosenblum MK, et al. Solitary fibrous tumors in the central nervous system: a clinicopathologic review of 18 cases and comparison to meningeal hemangiopericytomas. Arch Pathol Lab Med 2003; 127:432–439.
156. Miettinen MM, el-Rifai W, Sarlomo-Rikala M, et al. Tumor size-related DNA copy number changes occur in solitary fibrous tumors but not in hemangiopericytomas. Mod Pathol 1997; 10:1194–1200.
157. Persson S, Kindblom LG, Angervall L. Classical and chondroid chordoma: a light-microscopic, histochemical, ultrastructural and immunohistochemical analysis of the various cell types. Pathol Res Pract 1991; 187:828–838.
158. Paulus W, Slowik F, Jellinger K. Primary intracranial sarcomas: Histopathological features of 19 cases. Histopathology 1991; 18:395–402.
159. Powell HC, Marshall LF, Igneizi RJ. Post-irradiation pituitary sarcoma. Acta Neuropathol (Berl) 1977; 39:165–167.
160. McKeever PE, Blaivas M, Sima AAF. Neoplasms of the sellar region. In: Lloyd RV, ed. Surgical pathology of the pituitary gland. Philadelphia: Saunders; 193:141–210.
161. Ariza A, Kim JH. Kaposi's sarcoma of the dura mater. Hum Pathol 1988; 19:1461–1463.
162. Rushing EJ, Mena H, Smirniotopoulos JG. Mesenchymal chondrosarcoma of the cauda equina. Clin Neuropathol 1995; 14:150–153.
163. Matsukado Y, Yokota A, Marubayashi T. Rhabdomyosarcoma of the brain. J Neurosurg 1975; 43:215–221.
164. Scheithauer BW, Woodruff JM, Erlandson RA. Tumors of the peripheral nervous system. Washington, DC: American Registry of Pathology; 1999.
165. Geddes JF, Sutcliffe JC, King TT. Mixed cranial nerve tumors in neurofibromatosis type 2. Clin Neuropathol 1995; 14:310–313.
166. Hayashi K, Hoshida Y, Horie Y, et al. Immunohistochemical study on the distribution of alpha and beta subunits of S-100 protein in brain tumors. Acta Neuropathol (Berl) 1991; 81:657–663.
167. Valdez R, McKeever P, Finn WG, et al. Composite germ cell tumor and B-cell non-Hodgkin's lymphoma arising in the sella turcica. Hum Pathol 2002; 33:1044–1047.
168. Nakagawa Y, Perentes E, Ross GW, et al. Immunohistochemical differences between intracranial germinomas and their gonadal equivalents: an immunoperoxidase study of germ cell tumours with epithelial membrane antigen, cytokeratin, and vimentin. J Pathol 1988; 156:67–72.
169. Garvin AJ, Spicer SS, McKeever PE. The cytochemical demonstration of intracellular immunoglobulin in neoplasms of lymphoreticular tissue. Am J Pathol 1976; 82:457–478.
170. Jaffee ES, Harris NL, Stein H, et al., eds. World Health Organization classification of tumors: pathology and genetics of tumors of haematopoietic and lymphoid tissues. Lyon: IARC Press; 2001.
171. Lai R, Rosenblum MK, DeAngelis LM. Primary CNS lymphoma: a whole-brain disease? Neurology 2002; 59:1557–1562.
172. Davenport RD, O'Donnell LJ, Schnitzer B, et al. Non-Hodgkin's lymphoma of the brain following Hodgkin's disease: an immunohistochemical study. Cancer 1991; 67:440–443.
173. Morgello S. Pathogenesis and classification of primary central nervous system lymphoma: an update. Brain Pathol 1995; 5:383–393.
174. Carbone A. AIDS-related non-Hodgkin's lymphomas: from pathology and molecular pathogenesis to treatment. Hum

Pathol 2002; 33:392–404.
175. Kadan-Lottick NS, Skluzacek MC, Gurney JG. Decreasing incidence rates of primary central nervous system lymphoma. Cancer 2002; 95:193–202.
176. Ferracini R, Bergmann M, Pileri S, et al. Primary T-cell lymphoma of the central nervous system. Clin Neuropathol 1995; 14:125–129.
177. An-Foraker SH. Cytodiagnosis of malignant lesions in cerebrospinal fluid. Review and cytohistologic correlation. Acta Cytol (Baltimore) 1985; 29:286–290.
178. Deodhare SS, Ang LC, Bilbao JM. Isolated intracranial involvement in Rosai-Dorfman disease: a report of two cases and review of the literature. Arch Pathol Lab Med 1998; 122: 161–165.
179. Adle-Biassette H, Chetritt J, Bergemer-Fouquet AM, et al. Pathology of the central nervous system in Chester-Erdheim disease: report of three cases. J Neuropathol Exp Neurol 1997; 56:1207–1216.
180. McKeever P, Lloyd RV. Tumors of the pituitary region. In: Garcia JH, Budka H, McKeever PE, et al, eds. Neuropathology: the diagnostic approach. Philadelphia: CV Mosby; 1997:219–262.
181. Tachibana O, Yamashima T, Yamashita J. Immunohistochemical study of erythropoietin in cerebellar hemangioblastomas associated with secondary polycythemia. Neurosurgery 1991; 28:24–26.
182. Feldenzer JA, McKeever PE. Selective localization of gamma-enolase in stromal cells of cerebellar hemangioblastomas. Acta Neuropathol (Berl) 1987; 72:281–285.
183. Rubio A, Meyers SP, Powers JM, et al. Hemangioblastoma of the optic nerve. Hum Pathol 1994; 25:1249–1251.
184. McComb RD, Eastman PJ, Hahn FJ, et al. Cerebellar hemangioblastoma with prominent stromal astrocytosis: Diagnostic and histogenetic considerations. Clin Neuropathol 1987; 6:149–154.
185. Silverstein AM, Quint DJ, McKeever PE. Intraductal paraganglioma of the thoracic spine. Am J Neuroradiol 1990; 11:614–616.
186. Lloyd RV. Immunohistochemical localization of chromogranin in polypeptide hormone producing cells and tumors. In: Lechago J, Kameya T, eds. Endocrine pathology update. Philadelphia: Field and Wood; 1990.
187. Xin W, Rubin MA, McKeever PE. Differential expression of cytokeratins 8 and 20 distinguishes craniopharyngioma from Rathke cleft cyst. Arch Pathol Lab Med 2002; 126:1174–1178.
188. McKeever PE, Spicer SS. Pituitary histochemistry. In: Spicer SS, ed. Histochemistry in pathologic diagnosis. New York: Marcel-Dekker; 1987: 603–645.
189. Wong SW, Ducker TB, Powers JM. Fulminating parapontine epidermoid carcinoma in a four-year-old boy. Cancer 1976; 37:1525–1531.
190. Weller M, Stevens A, Sommer N, et al. Tumor cell dissemination triggers an intrathecal immune response in neoplastic meningitis. Cancer 1992; 69:1475–1480.
191. Bigner SH, Johnston WW. The cytopathology of cerebrospinal fluid. II: Metastatic cancer, meningeal carcinomatosis and primary central nervous system neoplasms. Acta Cytol (Baltimore) 1981; 25:461–479.
192. DeYoung BR, Wick MR. Immunohistologic evaluation of metastatic carcinomas of unknown origin: an algorithmic approach. Semin Diagn Pathol 2000; 17:184–193.
193. Chu P, Wu E, Weiss LM. Cytokeratin 7 and cytokeratin 20 expression in epithelial neoplasms: a survey of 435 cases. Med Pathol 2000; 13:962–972.
194. Srodon M, Westra WH. Immunohistochemical staining for thyroid transcription factor-1: a helpful aid in discerning primary site of tumor origin in patients with brain metastases. Hum Pathol 2002; 33:642–645.
195. Cochran AJ, Wen DR. S-100 protein as a marker for melanocytic and other tumors. Pathology 1985; 17:340–345.
196. Rushing EJ, Mena J, Ribas JL. Primary pineal parenchymal lesions: a review of 53 cases. J Neuropathol Exp Neurol 1991; 50:364.
197. Coca S, Martinez A, Vaquero J, et al. Immunohistochemical study of intracranial cysts. Histol Histopathol 1993; 8:651–654.
198. Ho KL, Garcia JH. Colloid cysts of the third ventricle: ultrastructural features are compatible with endodermal derivation. Acta Neuropathol 1992; 83:605–612.
199. McKeever PE, Brissie NT. Scanning electron microscopy of neoplasms removed at surgery: surface topography and comparison of meningioma, colloid cyst, ependymoma, pituitary adenoma, schwannoma and astrocytoma. J Neuropathol Exp Neurol 1977; 36:875–896.
200. McKeever PE, Hall BJ, Spicer SS. The origin of colloid cysts

of the third ventricle. J Neuropathol Exp Neurol 1978; 37: 658.
201. Bejjani GK, Wright DC, Schessel D, et al. Endodermal cysts of the posterior fossa: report of three cases and review of the literature. J Neurosurg 1998; 89:326–335.
202. Go KG, Blankenstein MA, Vroom TM, et al. Proges-terone receptors in arachnoid cysts: an immunocyto-chemical study in 2 cases. Acta Neurochirurg 1997; 139:349–354.
203. Mirra SS, Heyman A, McKeel D, et al. The Consortium to Establish a Registry for Alzheimer's Disease (CERAD). Part II: Standardization of the neuropathologic assessment of Alzheimer's disease. Neurology 1991; 41:479–486.
204. Mirra SS, Hart MN, Terry RD. Making the diagnosis of Alzheimer's disease. A primer for practicing pathologists. Arch Pathol Lab Med 1993; 117:132–144.
205. National Institute on Aging, and Reagan Institute Working Group on diagnostic criteria of the neuropathological assessment of Alzheimer's disease: consensus recommendations for the postmortem diagnosis of Alzheimer's disease. Neurobiol Aging 1997; 18:S1–S2.
206. Feany MB, Dickson DW. Neurodegenerative disorders with extensive tau pathology: a comparative study and review. Ann Neurol 1996; 40:139–148.
207. Dwork AJ, Liu D, Kaufman MA, et al. Archival, formalin-fixed tissue: its use in the study of Alzheimer's type changes. Clin Neuropathol 1998; 17:45–49.
208. Lue LF, Brachova L, Civin WH, et al. Inflammation, A beta deposition, and neurofibrillary tangle formation as correlates of Alzheimer's disease neurodegeneration. J Neuropathol Exp Neurol 1996; 55:1083–1088.
209. Jellinger KA. Vascular-ischemic dementia: an update. J Neurol Transm Suppl 2002; 62:1–23.
210. McKeith IG, Ballard CG, Perry RH, et al. Prospective validation of consensus criteria for the diagnosis of dementia with Lewy bodies. Neurology 2000; 54:1050–1058.
211. Braak H, Del Tredici K, Rub U, et al. Staging of brain pathology related to sporadic Parkinson's disease. Neurobiol Aging 2003; 24:197–211.
212. McKahann GM, Albert MS, Grossman M, et al. Clinical and pathological diagnosis of frontotemporal dementia: report of the Work Group on Frontotemporal Dementia and Pick's Disease. Arch Neurol 2001; 58:1803–1809.
213. Wanschitz J, Hainfellner JA, Simonitsch I, et al. Non-HTLV-I associated pleomorphic T-cell lymphoma of the brain mimicking post-vaccinal acute inflammatory demyelination. Neuropathol Appl Neurobiol 1997; 23:43–49.
214. Tachikawa N, Goto M, Hoshino Y, et al. Detection of *Toxoplasma gondii*, Epstein-Barr virus, and JC virus DNAs in the cerebrospinal fluid in acquired immunodeficiency syndrome patients with focal central nervous system complications. Intern Med 1999; 38:556–562.
215. Zagzag D, Miller DC, Kleinman GM, et al. Demyelinating disease versus tumor in surgical neuropathology: clues to a correct pathologic diagnosis. Am J Surg Pathol 1993; 17:537–545.
216. Reith KG, Di Chiro G, Cromwell LD, et al. Primary demyelinating disease simulating glioma of the corpus callosum. J Neurosurg 1981; 55:620–624.
217. Schmidt B, Toyka KV, Kiefer R, et al. Inflammatory infiltrates in sural nerve biopsies in Guillain-Barré syndrome and chronic inflammatory demyelinating neuropathy. Muscle Nerve 1996; 19:474–487.
218. Matsumuro K, Izumo S, Umehara F, et al. Chronic inflammatory demyelinating polyneuropathy: histological and immunopathological studies on biopsied sural nerves. J Neurol Sci 1994; 127:170–178.
219. Babb TL, Brown WJ. Pathological findings in epilepsy. In: Engel J, ed. Surgical treatment of the epilepsies. New York: Raven Press; 1987:511–540.
220. Bruton CJ. The neuropathology of temporal lobe epilepsy. In: Russel G, Marley E, Williams P, eds. Maudsley Monographs, No. 31, London: Oxford Press; 1988:1–94.
221. Prayson RA, Frater JL. Rasmussen encephalitis: a clinicopathologic and immunohistochemical study of seven patients. Am J Clin Pathol 2002; 117:776–782.
222. Frater JL, Prayson RA, Morris HH III, et al. Surgical pathologic findings of extratemporal-based intractable epilepsy: a study of 133 consecutive reactions. Arch Pathol Lab Med 2000; 124:545–549.
223. Volk EE, Prayson RA. Hamartomas in the setting of chronic epilepsy: a clinicopathologic study of 13 cases. Hum Pathol 1997; 28:227–232.
224. Smith DF, Hutton JL, Sandemann D, et al. The prognosis of primary intracerebral tumours presenting with epilepsy: the outcome of medical and surgical management. J Neurol Neurosurg Psychiatry 1991; 54:915–920.

索 引

A

A103 206
AD 缠结 823
AD 轴突斑块 823
Ad4BP 206
ALK 129, 139, 415
Arias-Stella 反应 665
α-1- 抗糜蛋白酶 422
α- 肌动蛋白 408
α- 甲基脂酰辅酶 A 消旋酶 205, 518
α- 胎球蛋白 587
α- 抑制素 206
阿尔茨海默病 821
阿根廷出血热 42
埃博拉出血热 42
埃利希病 47
癌胚抗原 196, 406, 446, 678
癌肉瘤 675

B

bcl-2 140, 418
bcl-6 124, 140
B72.3 208
BerEP4 208, 408
Bg7 124
Bg8 208

Birbeck 颗粒 419
BOB.1 125
Borst-Jadassohn（克隆）型上皮内癌 412
Bowen 病 731
Brenner 瘤 684
B 细胞慢性淋巴细胞白血病 144
B 细胞前淋巴细胞白血病 144
B 细胞特异激活蛋白 124
β- 钙黏素 668
β- 连环素 639
Ⅷ α 因子 415
Ⅷ 因子相关抗原 71, 426
巴尔通体属 44
白细胞共同抗原 680
白血病 814
伴有皮脂腺分化的浅表上皮瘤 410
伴有上皮样化生的胶质母细胞瘤和胶质肉瘤 794
杯状细胞类癌 462
鼻窦未分化癌 237
鼻咽癌 243
表皮生长因子受体 430, 570, 748
表皮样囊肿 819
表位 2
丙型肝炎病毒 40
病毒性出血热 42
波形蛋白 66, 195
玻璃样小梁状肿瘤 272
伯基特淋巴瘤/白血病 148
不标记抗体法 6

不典型乳头状瘤　725
不典型性导管上皮增生　731
部分胎块　677

C

calretinin　209，638，679
c-erbB-2　430
c-kit（CD117）　675
claudin-1　425
cyclin D1　139，415
CA125　678
CA72.4　409
CCR7　125
CD10　140，416，615，668
CD117　415，447，453
CD138　124
CD141　426
CD15　126，140，406
CD15（LeuM1）　678
CD179　415
CD19　137
CD1α　140，419
CD2　138
CD20　129，137，415
CD21　137
CD22　137
CD23　137
CD25　140
CD3　129，138，415
CD30　127，140，415
CD31　72，419
CD34　71，426
CD4　139，415
CD40　129
CD43　141，415
CD44　431
CD45　129，141，680
CD45RO　415
CD5　139，208，415
CD56　141，413
CD57　70，141，406
CD68　415

CD7　139，415
CD79a　137，415
CD8　139，415
CD99　141，406
CDX2　203，446
CG　413
CK19　187
CK20　189，413，564
CK5　193
CK7　188，409，564，678
Crimean-Congo 出血热　42
层粘连蛋白　71，692
肠病毒71　47
肠病型 T 细胞淋巴瘤　149
肠嗜铬样细胞　452
肠源性囊肿　819
成肌素　70
成人 T 细胞淋巴瘤 / 白血病　149
成熟 T 细胞肿瘤　148
痴呆　820
痴呆 / 克 - 雅病　773
川崎病　418
穿孔素　142
传染性单核细胞增多症　128
垂体腺瘤　270
雌 / 孕激素受体　210
雌激素受体　430
促结缔组织增生性毛发上皮瘤　411
促结缔组织增生性小圆细胞肿瘤　356，628
促肾上腺皮质激素　413
促纤维增生型癌　785
促纤维增生型髓母细胞瘤　785，803
促纤维增生型纤维瘤病　309
促纤维增生性小圆细胞肿瘤　82
催乳素生长激素腺瘤　270

D

desmoplakin　428
DBA.44　138
大汗腺上皮瘤　408
大汗腺腺癌　430
大细胞非霍奇金淋巴瘤　319

大细胞神经内分泌癌　666
单层上皮细胞角蛋白　187
单纯疱疹病毒　40
单纯疱疹性脑炎　773
单纯性囊肿　818
单克隆标记物染色　814
单克隆抗体　1
胆汁性糖蛋白　377
弹性蛋白染色　778
蛋白A法　8
蛋白基因产物9.5　630
导管癌　540
导管内乳头状癌　725
导管上皮增生　731
导管原位癌　731
登革出血热　42
癫痫　773
淀粉样变血管病　777
动静脉畸形　778
动脉瘤样皮肤纤维组织细胞瘤　424
多表型小圆细胞肿瘤　82
多发性内分泌肿瘤综合征　277
多发性脑梗死性血管性痴呆　821
多价系统　7
多角形/梭形细胞癌　339
多聚体标记二步法　9
多克隆抗体　2
多潜能性浆膜下细胞　367
多系统萎缩　823
多形性癌　345
多形性低度恶性腺癌　247
多形性恶性外周神经鞘瘤　91
多形性横纹肌肉瘤　91
多形性黄色星形细胞瘤　782
多形性胶质母细胞瘤　782
多形性腺瘤　246
多形性小叶癌　737
多形性脂肪肉瘤　91
多灶性进行性脑白质病　43
多组织对照切片　14

E

EB病毒潜伏膜蛋白1　142
EKH5　409
EKH6　409
EMA　666
ER/PR　668
Ewing肉瘤　81，241，314，628
E-钙黏素　570
额颞叶痴呆　823
恶性黑色素瘤　164，239
恶性横纹肌样瘤　628
恶性毛母质瘤　412
恶性神经鞘瘤　814
恶性室管膜瘤样细胞　784
恶性外周神经鞘瘤　85
恶性纤维组织细胞瘤　91，422，782

F

fascin　120，419
FLI-1　413
反应性胶质增生　827
放射性瘢痕　718
非典型畸胎瘤　629
非典型畸胎样横纹肌样肿瘤　787
非典型脑膜瘤　808
非典型纤维黄色瘤　422
非典型畸胎样-横纹肌样肿瘤　804
非连接方法　11
非特异交叉反应性物质　377
肺玻璃样变肉芽肿　349
肺的假间皮瘤样癌　381
肺间皮瘤　337
肺母细胞瘤　346
肺胎盘绒毛异位　357
分化抗原　532
分化型的VIN3　658
分泌素　267
分泌型腹泻相关血管活性肠肽　630
分叶状肿瘤　750

复层上皮角蛋白 192
复发性指纤维瘤 421
副脊索瘤 95
副神经节瘤 318
富含岩藻糖细胞膜荆豆凝集素 1 426
富于 T 细胞的 B 细胞淋巴瘤 127

G

gp100/PMel 17 相关单克隆抗体 168
GCDFP-24 409
钙调素结合蛋白 70，422
钙结合蛋白 74，167
钙结合蛋白 S100A6 522
钙黏素 532
钙周期蛋白 522
肝母细胞瘤 480
肝脾 T 细胞淋巴瘤 149
肝细胞石蜡抗原 1 447
肝硬化 479
刚果红染色 777
高碘酸 - 雪夫染色 774
格子细胞 / 黄色肉芽肿 784
弓形虫病 773
宫颈管腺癌 662
钩端螺旋体病 38
孤立性纤维瘤 77，573，810
孤立性纤维性肿瘤 309
骨钙素 72
骨化性纤维黏液瘤 77
骨连接素 73
骨桥蛋白 531
骨肉瘤 628
骨外软骨肉瘤 96
骨纤维结构不良 98
管状促结缔组织增生性假间皮瘤样腺癌 381
管状腺病 725
光化性类网状细胞增多症 417
过渡型脑膜瘤 785
过氧化物酶 - 抗过氧化物酶法 6

H

HepPar-1 197
HKN5 412
HKN6 412
HKN7 412
HMB-45 168，409
h- 钙调素结合蛋白 675
海绵状脑病 776
海绵状血管瘤 778
汉坦病毒肺综合征 46
汗腺癌 409
合并发育不良痣综合征 430
合体细胞型霍奇金淋巴瘤 319
黑色素瘤 314，409，783
黑色素瘤预后的标记物 171
黑色素细胞 - "特异性"单克隆抗体 168
横纹肌瘤 75
横纹肌肉瘤 241，311，628，727，786
横纹肌样瘤 355，629
横纹肌样脑膜瘤 809
后肾腺瘤 613
滑膜肉瘤 83，323，727
化生性癌 718
黄热病 42
黄色肉芽肿 424
混合细胞型霍奇金淋巴瘤 321
混合型小细胞肺癌 339
活动性皮肤红斑狼疮 418
霍奇金淋巴瘤 119，319

I

IKH-4 409

J

Jessner 浸润 418
Jun B 和 c-Jun 124
J 链蛋白 125
肌动蛋白 69，407，668

索 引

肌红蛋白 70
肌上皮瘤 248，726
肌上皮细胞癌 726
肌酸激酶 632
肌纤维母细胞瘤 349
姬姆萨染色 774
基底皮脂腺样上皮瘤 408
基底细胞癌 408
基底细胞样癌 450
基底细胞样鳞状细胞癌 235，309
基质蛋白酶 532
畸胎瘤 692
激素受体 745
激素原转化酶 266
极性成胶质细胞瘤 782
棘层松解性皮炎 417
脊索瘤 94，784
脊索样型脑膜瘤 808
技术问题 22
家族性腺瘤息肉 452
甲磺酸伊马替尼 453
甲硫氨酸脑啡肽 413
甲硫啡肽 283
甲胎蛋白 679
甲状旁腺癌 317
甲状旁腺激素 279
甲状腺滤泡癌 268
甲状腺球蛋白 201
甲状腺乳头状癌 268
甲状腺髓样癌 267
甲状腺转录因子-1 202，413
假间皮瘤样上皮型血管内皮瘤 381
假淋巴瘤样浸润 417
假性假淋巴瘤 419
尖锐湿疣 658
间变型脑膜瘤 807
间变型少突胶质细胞瘤 784
间变型室管膜瘤 782
间变型星形细胞瘤 781
间变性大细胞淋巴瘤 127，151，419
间变性淋巴瘤激酶-1 73
间接标记法 5
间皮瘤 320，695

间皮素 208，375，685
间叶性软骨肉瘤 82
间质水解酶-3 411
碱性磷酸酶-抗碱性磷酸酶法 8
鉴别诊断 172
浆细胞骨髓瘤 145
浆细胞瘤 145，320
浆细胞性肉芽肿 349
浆液性乳头状癌 669
浆液性肿瘤 681
降钙素 413
胶样囊肿 819
胶原蛋白 531
胶质瘤 769
胶质母细胞瘤 777
胶质囊肿 818
胶质肉瘤 782
胶质肉瘤伴上皮样化生 785
胶质纤维酸性蛋白 68，425
胶质增生 769
角蛋白 63
角蛋白 34βE12 520
节细胞神经瘤 629
节细胞神经母细胞瘤 629，798
节细胞肿瘤 782
结蛋白 66，407，668
结缔组织生长因子 638
结节性B细胞淋巴瘤大细胞型 418
结节性筋膜炎 424
结节性淋巴细胞为主型霍奇金淋巴瘤 119
结节性皮下纤维瘤 424
结节性组织细胞瘤 424
结节硬化型霍奇金淋巴瘤 123
结外NK/T细胞淋巴瘤（鼻型） 149
结外皮肤窦组织细胞增生伴巨大淋巴结病 419
结直肠锯齿状腺瘤 466
进行性多灶性白质脑病 773
浸润性导管癌 737
浸润性基底细胞癌 411
浸润性曲霉病 45
浸润性筛状癌 718
浸润性小叶癌 737
经典的鳞状细胞癌 234

经典毛发上皮瘤　411
经典型霍奇金淋巴瘤　119
荆豆凝集素　72
精确性　13
精原细胞瘤　199，307
静脉畸形　778
局灶性结节性增生　479
巨囊病囊液蛋白　207
巨细胞病毒　40
巨细胞病毒感染性淋巴结炎　128
巨细胞瘤　96
巨细胞纤维母细胞瘤　422
巨细胞血管纤维瘤　422

K

Kaposi 肉瘤　86，428
Kaposi 肉瘤相关核抗原 -1　40
Ki-1　419
Ki-67　142
KIT 蛋白　453
KP-1　419
卡波西型血管内皮瘤　78
抗 κ 和 λ 型免疫球蛋白轻链　138
抗人毛发角蛋白　412
抗生物素蛋白 - 生物素连接法　7
抗体　2
抗原　2
抗原 L1　422
抗原矩阵模型　30
抗原决定簇　2
抗原修复　2
颗粒细胞瘤　75，245，422，448，687
颗粒细胞血管肉瘤　91
颗粒细胞肿瘤　357
狂犬病　43

L

Lennert 淋巴瘤　127
Leu7　201
Leydig 细胞瘤　689

莱姆病　44
朗格汉斯细胞组织细胞增生症　419
酪氨酸酶相关抗体　170
酪氨酸信号放大系统　10
类癌　247，446
类固醇细胞瘤　689
类固醇因子 -1　206
立克次体　38
粒酶 B　142
粒细胞肉瘤　320，416
良性混合性肿瘤　409
良性淋巴细胞性血管炎　349
良性头部组织细胞增生症　419
亮氨酸脑啡肽　283
淋巴浆细胞性淋巴瘤　144
淋巴结边缘区 B 细胞淋巴瘤　146
淋巴瘤　313，666，814
淋巴瘤样丘疹病　419
淋巴瘤样肉芽肿病　148，351
淋巴母细胞白血病 / 淋巴瘤　416
淋巴母细胞淋巴瘤　308
淋巴上皮样癌　321
淋巴细胞消减型霍奇金淋巴瘤　122
淋巴细胞性间质性肺疾病 / 肺炎　349
淋巴血管平滑肌瘤病　354
淋巴组织增生　307
鳞状上皮癌　677
鳞状上皮内病变　677
鳞状上皮乳头状瘤　658
鳞状细胞癌　406，666
隆突性皮肤纤维肉瘤　421
颅咽管瘤　784，815
滤泡间淋巴结炎　129
滤泡性淋巴瘤　146
滤泡性皮肤淋巴组织增生　418
滤泡性腺瘤　272
路易小体　823
卵巢癌　410
卵巢的甲状腺肿　692
卵巢性索 - 间质肿瘤　685
卵黄囊瘤　324，684
卵黄囊肿瘤　593
卵泡膜瘤　686

螺旋腺瘤 408
落基山斑疹热 44

M

melan-A 168, 207, 419
MAC387 415
MAC-387 419
MALT 型边缘区 B 细胞淋巴瘤 350
MART-1 409
Mel-Cam 676
Merkel 细胞癌 408, 413
MOC-31 197, 209, 413
Myo-D1 70
马尔堡病 42
脉络丛癌 800
脉络丛乳头状癌 784
脉络丛乳头状瘤 784
慢性苔藓样皮炎 417
毛发癌 412
毛母质瘤 411
毛囊瘤 411
毛细胞白血病 145
毛细胞型星形细胞瘤 782
毛细血管扩张 778
毛细血管血管母细胞瘤 814
酶标记抗原法 9
酶桥接技术 6
酶消化法 1
弥漫性大 B 细胞淋巴瘤 147
弥漫性纤维型星形细胞瘤 779
免疫球蛋白 A 410
免疫球蛋白分子 2
免疫组织化学 1
免疫组织化学染色定量及标准化 25
敏感性 13
末端脱氧核苷酸转移酶（TdT） 142
末端脱氧核糖核酸转移酶 416

N

内淋巴囊肿瘤 252

内胚窦瘤 199, 317
囊内乳头状癌 718
囊泡病液体蛋白 15 409
囊性颅咽管瘤 820
囊性星形胶质细胞瘤 820
囊肿 818
脑浸润 808
脑膜瘤 804
脑膜囊肿 820
脑膜上皮型脑膜瘤 806
脑脓肿 774
尼派病毒 47
黏膜相关淋巴组织结外边缘区 B 细胞淋巴瘤 146
黏糖蛋白 A-80 538
黏液癌 541
黏液乳头状室管膜瘤 784
黏液腺癌 463
黏液性囊腺瘤 473
黏液性肿瘤 681
黏液性子宫内膜腺癌 664
黏液样软骨肉瘤 96
黏液样脂肪肉瘤 94
念珠菌属 45
尿激酶Ⅲ 684
尿路上皮癌 564
脓胸相关性淋巴瘤 352

O

Oct-2 125
OCT4 200
OKM5（CD36） 410

P

p16 657
p21 411
p53 668
p63 406, 521, 657
P504S 蛋白 518
Paget 病 210, 408, 657, 731
Paget 病样鲍温病 409

PAX-5　415，416
PGP9.5　630
Pick 小体　823
PNET　787
PNL2　170
POU5F1　200
PTEN　668
P 物质　413
胖细胞型星形细胞瘤　782
疱疹病毒　40
胚胎发育不良性神经上皮肿瘤　797
胚胎性癌　199，317，692
胚胎性横纹肌肉瘤　78
胚胎性肿瘤　801
皮肤 Merkel 细胞癌　291
皮肤 T 细胞淋巴瘤　416
皮肤恶性外周神经鞘肿瘤　425
皮肤孤立性纤维性肿瘤　422
皮肤间变性大细胞淋巴瘤　419
皮肤淋巴细胞瘤　418
皮肤淋巴腺瘤　418
皮肤隆突性纤维肉瘤　422
皮肤平滑肌瘤　424
皮肤纤维瘤　422
皮肤纤维肉瘤　421
皮肤小梁癌　413
皮肤炎性假瘤　418
皮肤原发性神经内分泌癌　413
皮下脂膜炎样 T 细胞淋巴瘤　149
皮样囊肿　819
皮脂腺瘤　410
皮脂样抗原 OV-2　410
皮质畸形　823
脾边缘区 B 细胞淋巴瘤　144
平滑肌瘤　75
平滑肌肉瘤　83，325，424，542，727
平滑肌肿瘤　670
葡萄糖转运蛋白 1　75

Q

前列腺酸性磷酸酶　517

前列腺特异性抗原　204，515
前列腺特异性膜抗原　204，517
前驱 B 淋巴母细胞白血病 / 淋巴瘤　143
前驱 T 淋巴母细胞白血病 / 淋巴瘤　148
前哨淋巴结　731
前哨淋巴结活检　171
前哨淋巴结转移　731
潜伏膜蛋白 1　123
浅表扩散性恶性黑色素瘤　409
腔神经胶质增生　820
桥粒斑蛋白　69
桥粒芯糖蛋白　69
侵袭性或恶性脑膜瘤　808
侵袭性乳腺外 Paget 病　408
侵袭性血管黏液瘤　78
球血管瘤　425
去分化脂肪肉瘤　91

R

RCC 抗体　615
人类多瘤病毒 JC 病毒　43
人类疱疹病毒 8　40
人类疱疹病毒 8 型隐匿型核抗原 -1　428
人类乳头瘤病毒　41
人绒毛膜促性腺激素　679
人胎盘催乳素　588，676
人腺体激肽释放酶 2　518
人型囊泡单胺转运体　452
绒毛蛋白　447
绒毛膜癌　200，318，677
绒毛素　203
肉瘤样癌　406，456，541，726
肉瘤样胸腺癌　324
肉芽肿性淋巴结炎　130
肉芽肿性炎　349
乳球蛋白　207
乳头瘤病毒　42
乳头脑膜瘤　809
乳头状鳞状细胞癌　236
乳腺肌纤维母细胞瘤　727
乳腺乳头状瘤　725

乳腺微浸润性癌 728
乳脂肪球相关皮脂样抗原 OV-2 410
软垂疣 430
软骨母细胞瘤 95
软骨样汗管瘤 409
软组织多形性肿瘤 90

S

S-100 蛋白 70，167，406，680
Sertoli-Leydig 细胞瘤 688
Sertoli 细胞瘤 689
Sturge-Weber 病 778
Syn 413
Sézary 综合征 150
4KB5 CD45R 415
Ⅳ型胶原纤维 71
三明治法 5
桑葚胚 346
砂粒体型脑膜瘤 807
上皮/肌上皮癌 249
上皮内鳞癌 409
上皮细胞膜抗原 69，197，406，767
上皮性/肌上皮性肿瘤 357
上皮性抗原决定簇 166
上皮样恶性外周神经鞘肿瘤 89
上皮样平滑肌肉瘤 90
上皮样肉瘤 86，429
上皮样肉瘤样血管内皮瘤 429
上皮样血管瘤 75
上皮样血管内皮瘤 77
上皮样血管肉瘤 86
上皮样滋养层细胞肿瘤 677
上皮样组织细胞瘤 424
少见的胚胎性肿瘤 804
少突胶质细胞瘤 784
少突星形细胞瘤 792
申克孢子丝菌 45
伸长型细胞型室管膜瘤/室管膜下瘤 782
神经胶质酸性蛋白 635
神经节细胞瘤 309
神经瘤 813

神经母细胞瘤 283，309，628，787，798
神经母细胞性肿瘤 628
神经内分泌癌 239，467
神经内分泌标记物 170
神经内分泌肿瘤 814
神经鞘瘤 425，782
神经鞘黏液瘤 425
神经鞘肿瘤 812
神经上皮性囊肿 818
神经生长因子受体 425
神经束膜瘤 425
神经丝 413
神经丝蛋白 67，630
神经特异性烯醇化酶 201，267，425，629
神经系统疾病 767
神经细胞黏附分子 342
神经纤维瘤 74，422，782
神经型囊尾蚴病 774
神经元肿瘤 795
肾横纹肌样瘤 611
肾母细胞瘤 611
肾上腺皮质癌 281
肾上腺外副神经节瘤 268
肾嗜酸细胞腺瘤 612
肾外横纹肌样肿瘤 91
肾细胞癌抗原 206
生长抑素 269，413
生长抑素瘤 287
生肌调节蛋白 628
生物素-抗生物素蛋白法 6
生物素-链卵白素系统 7
生殖细胞肿瘤 199，317，690，814
施万细胞瘤 309，425，813
视网膜母细胞瘤基因 569
室管膜瘤 782
室管膜母细胞瘤 787
室管膜囊肿 818
嗜铬素 200，267，406，630，657
嗜铬细胞瘤 268
鼠疫 49
双嗜色性包涵体 822
双重免疫酶标技术 20
双重染色 31

845

水痘-带状疱疹 40
松果体瘤 271
松果体母细胞瘤 271，787
松果体囊肿 818
松果体细胞瘤 782
髓过氧化物酶 415
髓肌母细胞瘤 786，804
髓母细胞瘤 787，801
髓上皮瘤 784
髓外浆细胞瘤 241
髓外髓样瘤 415
损伤后梭形细胞结节 424
梭形细胞癌 236
梭形细胞肉瘤 727
梭形细胞血管肉瘤 86
梭形细胞脂肪瘤 74

退行性非典型组织细胞增生症 419
脱髓鞘 773
脱髓鞘疾病 822
唾液腺肿瘤 357

U

Uroplakin 565
Uroplakin Ⅲ 207

V

VIP 413
VIP 生成性肿瘤 288

W

Whipple 病 44
Wilms 瘤 628
Wilms 瘤抑癌基因 208
WT-1 668
外毛根鞘癌 412
外毛根鞘瘤 411
外胚层间叶瘤 629
外皮蛋白 407
外周 T 细胞淋巴瘤（非特异性） 150
外周神经鞘瘤 309
外周神经鞘膜肿瘤和梭形细胞脂肪瘤 422
外周神经鞘肿瘤 74，425
完全性葡萄胎 677
网状细胞增生 419
微波加热法 18
微囊性腺瘤 473
微卫星不稳定型 456
微腺体增生 664
微腺型腺病 716
微血管密度 533
微转移癌 731
委内瑞拉出血热 42
未分化肉瘤 675
胃肠间质瘤 448

T

T 和 NK 细胞肿瘤 148
T 细胞前淋巴细胞白血病 149
T 细胞限制性细胞内抗原 142
胎盘部位结节 677
胎盘碱性磷酸酶 634，676
胎盘样碱性磷酸酶 587
肽类激素 201
炭疽 48
糖蛋白 A-80 539
套细胞淋巴瘤 147
特异性 13
透明细胞癌 251，478，665
透明细胞瘤/糖瘤/PEComa 353
透明细胞肉瘤 86
透明细胞软骨肉瘤 96
透明细胞肾细胞癌 614
透明细胞型脑膜瘤 808
透明质酸盐 379
突触结合蛋白 268
突触素 200，268，406，630，657
突触小泡蛋白 2 268
突触小泡相关膜蛋白 268
兔热病 48

胃泌素瘤 287
无性细胞瘤 690

X

西尼罗病毒性脑炎 47
细胞核雄激素受体蛋白 410
细胞角蛋白 186，406，655
细胞性瘢痕 424
细胞周期蛋白 D1 570
细小病毒 B19 41
先天性表浅血管外皮细胞瘤 421
先天性巨结肠病 464
先天性牙龈瘤 245
先天性自限性网状组织细胞增生症 419
纤维瘤 686
纤维瘤病 74
纤维肉瘤 83，727，782
纤维上皮性息肉 658
纤维上皮性肿瘤 750
纤维腺瘤 750
纤维组织细胞瘤 308
涎腺导管癌 250
腺病毒 41
腺管型小叶癌 742
腺肌上皮瘤 726
腺瘤样瘤 599，696
腺泡细胞癌 477
腺泡状横纹肌肉瘤 80
腺泡状软组织肉瘤 90
腺样鳞癌 406
腺样囊性癌 247，450，726
腺样囊性癌/基底细胞癌 542
小管癌 718
小汗腺癌 430
小汗腺上皮瘤 408
小淋巴细胞淋巴瘤 144
小脑发育不良性节细胞瘤 797
小无裂细胞 313
小细胞癌 666
小细胞神经内分泌癌 309
小眼基因 170

小叶原位癌 731
小叶肿瘤 737
小圆细胞横纹肌肉瘤 311
锌-α-2-糖蛋白 409
新型隐球菌 45
性腺母细胞瘤 693
胸膜的钙化纤维性假瘤 382
胸膜的原发性硬纤维瘤 382
胸膜肺母细胞瘤 383
胸膜间皮瘤样肿瘤 381
胸腺癌 314
胸腺瘤 306
雄激素受体 533
嗅神经母细胞瘤 237
血管活性肠肽 413
血管肌纤维母细胞瘤 75
血管瘤型脑膜瘤 807
血管免疫母细胞性 T 细胞淋巴瘤 150
血管母细胞瘤 785
血管内淋巴瘤 352
血管内皮生长因子 570
血管内皮细胞瘤 346，428
血管内细支气管肺泡瘤 346
血管平滑肌脂肪瘤 487
血管球瘤 425
血管球肉瘤 425
血管外皮瘤 243，308
血管外皮细胞瘤 76，787
血管周上皮样细胞肿瘤 487，675
血管周围炎症 772
血栓调节素 72，684
血小板源性生长因子-AB 链 638
血小板源性生长因子受体 α 638
血型抗原 Pr 413
蕈样霉菌病 150，417

Y

咽鼓管壁 818
严重急性呼吸性综合征 48
炎性假瘤 309，349
炎症性肌纤维母细胞瘤 309

阳性对照　14
叶状肿瘤　542
胰岛素瘤　287
胰岛素样生长因子2　638
胰多肽　413
胰腺囊实性肿瘤　477
移行细胞肿瘤　684
移行型脑膜瘤　807
移行性组织细胞瘤　424
移植后霍奇金样淋巴组织增生　127
乙肝病毒表面抗原　39
乙肝病毒核心抗原　39
异型增生　234
抑制素　588，668
阴性对照　14
印戒细胞癌　541
婴幼儿促纤维增生性节细胞胶质瘤　798
硬化性胆管炎　479
硬化性上皮样纤维肉瘤　89
硬化性腺病　540，718
硬化性血管瘤　354
硬化性纵隔炎　309
幽门螺杆菌　43，452
疣状癌　236
有小原浆性星形细胞的少突胶质细胞瘤　827
幼年性毛细血管瘤　75
原发性肺内胸腺瘤　357
原发性皮肤CD30+的T细胞淋巴组织增生性疾病　150
原发性渗出性淋巴瘤　352
原发性尤文肉瘤　413
原浆性星形细胞瘤　827
原始神经外胚层肿瘤　81，311，413，628，803
圆形细胞脂肪肉瘤　94
圆柱瘤　408
孕激素受体　430
运动神经元疾病　823

Z

杂交瘤技术　1
造血系统标记　166
造釉细胞瘤　98
增强κ轻链核因子　124
增生性毛发肿瘤　411
增殖细胞核抗原　566
栅栏样纤维组织细胞瘤　424
真皮髓样白血病　415
整合素　530，570
支气管相关淋巴样组织　347
支气管源性小细胞癌　268
脂肪酶　410
脂溢性角化病　412
直接连接-标记抗体法　5
质量控制　13
中耳腺瘤　251
中间丝　407
中间丝蛋白　62，164
中胚叶肾瘤　611
中枢型神经细胞瘤　798
肿瘤相关糖蛋白72　408
转化生长因子β-1　638
转移瘤　816
子宫浆液癌　669
子宫内膜间质肉瘤　673
子宫内膜间质肿瘤　670
子宫内膜上皮内癌　669
子宫内膜未分化癌　675
子宫内膜腺癌　662
子宫内膜样癌　669
子宫内膜增生　669
组胺脱羧酶　343
组织蛋白酶B　415
组织细胞样癌　742
组织细胞增生症　814
组织细胞增生症X　419